American
Drug Index 2015

Facts & Comparisons®

American Drug Index, Fifty-Ninth Edition.

ISBN-10: 1-57439-359-6
ISBN-13: 978-1-57439-359-0

Library of Congress Catalog Card Number 55-6286

Printed in the United States of America

The information contained in *American Drug Index* is available for licensing as source data. For more information on data licensing, please call 1-800-223-0554.

Clinical Drug Information, LLC
77 Westport Plaza, Suite 450
St. Louis, Missouri 63146-3125
Phone 314/392-0000 • 800/223-0554
Fax 317/735-5350
factsandcomparisons.com

American Drug Index

Norman F. Billups, RPh, MS, PhD
Dean and Professor Emeritus
College of Pharmacy
The University of Toledo

Shirley M. Billups, RN, LPC, MEd
Oncology Nurse
Licensed Professional Counselor

Facts & Comparisons® Publishing Group

Scot E. Walker, PharmD, MS, BCPS, BCACP	Senior Director Content Development
Joyce A. Generali, RPh, MS, FASHP	Director, Synthesized Referential Content
Paul B. Johnson, RPh **Cathy A. Meives, PharmD**	Senior Clinical Managers
Kim S. Dufner, PharmD	Clinical Manager
Christine M. Cohn, PharmD, BCPS **Patricia L. Spenard, PharmD** **Andrea L. Williams, RPh**	Senior Clinical Editors
Esta Razavi, PharmD	Clinical Editor
Arvind Subramanian, MBA	President & CEO, Clinical Solutions
Angela J. Bush **Sarah W. Gremillion**	Senior Managing Editors
Sara L. Schweain	Managing Editor
Jennifer E. Rolfes	Senior Editor
Susan H. Sunderman	Managing Editor, Quality Control
Jennifer M. Love	Senior Composition Specialist
Wendy M. Bell	Managing Technical Editor
Barbara J. Hunter	Inventory Analyst

Facts & Comparisons® Editorial Advisory Panel

Contents

[•] Denotes official name: Generic name or chemical name recognized by the *USP, NF,* or USAN.

Preface

The 59th Edition of the *American Drug Index* (*ADI*) has been prepared for the identification, explanation, and correlation of the many pharmaceuticals available to the medical, pharmaceutical, and allied health professions. The need for this index has become even more acute as the variety and number of drugs and drug products have continued to multiply. *ADI* should be useful to pharmacists, nurses, health care administrators, physicians, medical transcriptionists, dentists, sales personnel, students, and teachers in the fields that incorporate pharmaceuticals.

Special note to medical transcriptionists: Generic names are in lowercase and trade names are in upper/lowercase as appropriate to facilitate transcription. The names for officially designated products (eg, *United States Pharmacopeia* or *USP*) are preceded by a bullet (•) and should appear in lowercase in transcription.

The organization of *ADI* falls into 14 major sections:

- Monographs of Drug Products
- Standard Medical Abbreviations
- Calculations
- Common Systems of Weights and Measures
- Approximate Practical Equivalents
- International System of Units
- Normal Laboratory Values
- FDA Pregnancy Categories
- Controlled Substances Summary
- Medical Terminology Glossary
- Oral Dosage Forms That Should Not Be Crushed or Chewed
- Drug Names That Look Alike and Sound Alike
- Discontinued Drugs
- Manufacturer and Distributor Listing

MONOGRAPHS: The organization of the monograph section of *ADI* is alphabetical with extensive cross-indexing. Names listed are generic (also called nonproprietary, public name, or common name); brand (also called trademark, proprietary, or specialty); and chemical. Synonyms in general use also are included. All names used for a pharmaceutical appear in alphabetical order, with the pertinent data given under the brand name by which it is made available.

The monograph for a typical brand name product appears in upper/lowercase as appropriate, and consists of the manufacturer, generic name, composition and strength, available pharmaceutic dosage forms, package size, use, and appropriate legend designation (eg, *Rx, OTC, c-v*).

Generic names appear in lowercase in alphabetical order, followed by the pronunciation and the corresponding recognition of the drug to the *USP* (*United States Pharmacopeia*), *NF* (*National Formulary*), and USAN (*USP Dictionary of United States Adopted Names and International Drug Names*). Each of these official generic names is preceded by a bullet (•).

To minimize medication errors, The Institute for Safe Medication Practices established Tall Man lettering for look-alike pairs. Tall Man lettering was added to generic entries for the drugs involved in the name differentiation project.

Pronunciations have been included for many of the generic drugs. However, not every drug will have a corresponding pronunciation. Some of the most common pronunciations are not listed for every drug. The following list is included as a guide to very common names:

Acetate	AS-eh-tate
Besylate	BESS-ih-late
Borate	BOE-rate
Bromide	BROE-mide
Butyrate	BYOO-tih-rate
Calcium	KAL-see-uhm
Chloride	KLOR-ide
Citrate	SIH-trate
Dipotassium	die-poe-TASS-ee-uhm
Disodium	die-SO-dee-uhm
Edetate	eh-deh-TATE
Fosfatex	foss-FAH-tex
Fumarate	FEW-mah-rate
Hydrobromide	HIGH-droe-BROE-mide
Hydrochloride	HIGH-droe-KLOR-ide
Iodide	EYE-oh-dide
Lactobionate	LACK-toe-BYE-oh-nate
Maleate	MAL-ee-ate
Mesylate	MEH-sih-LATE
Monosodium	MAHN-oh-SO-dee-uhm
Nitrate	NYE-trate
Pendetide	PEN-deh-TIDE
Pentetate	PEN-teh-tate
Phosphate	FOSS-fate
Potassium	poe-TASS-ee-uhm
Propionate	PRO-pee-oh-nate
Sodium	SO-dee-uhm
Succinate	SUX-sih-nate
Sulfate	SULL-fate
Tartrate	TAR-trate
Trisodium	try-SO-dee-uhm

Because of the multiplicity of brand names used for the same therapeutic agent or the same combination of therapeutic agents, some correlation was done. Please turn to aspirin for an example of this. Here under the generic name are listed the various brand names. Following are combinations of aspirin organized in a manner to point out relationships among the many products. Reference then is made to the brand name or names having the indicated composition. Under the brand name are given manufacturer, composition, available forms, sizes, dosage, and use.

The multiplicity of generic names for the same therapeutic agent has complicated the nomenclature of these agents. Examples of multiple generic names for the same chemical substance are: (1) acetaminophen, N-acetyl-p-aminophenol; (2) guaifenesin, glyceryl guaiacolate, glyceryl guaiacol ether, guaianesin, guayanesin; and (3) pyrilamine maleate, pyranilamine maleate, pyraminyl maleate, anisopyradamine.

The cross-indexing feature of *ADI* permits the finding of drugs or drug combinations when only one major ingredient is known. For example, a combination of aluminum hydroxide gel and magnesium trisilicate is available. This combination can be found by looking under the name of either of the two ingredients, and in each case the brand names are given. A second form of cross-indexing lists drugs under various therapeutic and pharmaceutical classes (ie, antacids, antihistamines, diuretics, laxatives).

ABBREVIATIONS: The listing of standard medical abbreviations is included as an aid in interpreting medical orders. The Latin or Greek word and abbreviation are given with the meaning.

CALCULATIONS: A listing of common formulas used to calculate weight, creatinine clearance, ideal body weight, and temperature conversion between Celsius and Farenheit.

WEIGHTS AND MEASURES: Tables containing common systems of weights and measures are included to aid the practitioner in calculating dosages in the metric, apothecary, and avoirdupois systems.

CONVERSION FACTORS: A listing of approximate practical equivalents to aid in calculating and converting dosages among the metric, apothecary, and avoirdupois systems.

INTERNATIONAL SYSTEM OF UNITS: A modernized version of the metric system listed in tables for rapid reference.

NORMAL LABORATORY VALUES: Tables containing normal reference values for commonly requested laboratory tests are included as a guideline for the health care practitioner.

FDA PREGNANCY CATEGORIES: A table summarizing each of the pregnancy categories established by the FDA.

CONTROLLED SUBSTANCES: A brief summary explanation of the key points of the Controlled Substances Act of 1970.

MEDICAL TERMINOLOGY GLOSSARY: Commonly used terms are listed and defined as an aid in interpreting the use given for drug monographs included in *ADI*.

ORAL DOSAGE FORMS THAT SHOULD NOT BE CRUSHED OR CHEWED: This section alerts the health care practitioner about oral dosage forms that should not be crushed, and may serve as an aid in consulting with patients. Examples of products falling into the non-crush category are extended-release, enteric-coated, encapsulated beads, wax matrix, sublingual dosage forms, and encapsulated liquid formulations.

DRUG NAMES THAT LOOK ALIKE AND SOUND ALIKE: A listing of common drugs that look alike and sound alike. Familiarity with this list may prevent the prescriber from making a dispensing error.

DISCONTINUED DRUGS: A combined list of generic and brand products no longer available in the United States because they were withdrawn from the market or discontinued by the manufacturer.

MANUFACTURER AND DISTRIBUTOR LISTING: The name, phone number, and website of virtually every American pharmaceutical manufacturer and drug distributor are listed in alphabetical order in this section.

Direct correspondence or communication with reference to a drug or drug product listed in *ADI* to Editorial/Production, Attn: ADI, Clinical Drug Information, 77 Westport Plaza, Suite 450, St. Louis, Missouri 63146-3125, or call 1-800-223-0554.

Monographs

A

AABP. (Brookstone) 0.01% acetic acid, 5.4% antipyrine, 1.4% benzocaine, 0.01% polycosanol 410, glycerin. Soln., Otic. 15 mL w/dropper. *Rx.*
Use: Ophthalmic and otic agent, otic preparation.

A & D Tablets. (Barth's) Vitamins A 10,000 units, D 400 units. Tab. Bot. 100s, 500s. *OTC.*
Use: Vitamin supplement.

abacavir. (Various Mfr.) Abacavir sulfate 300 mg. Tab. 60s, UD 60s. *Rx.*
Use: Antiretroviral agent, nucleoside reverse transcriptase inhibitor.

•**abacavir succinate.** (ab-ah-KAV-ear SUCK-sih-nate) USAN.
Use: Antiviral.

abacavir sulfate.
Use: Antiviral; nucleoside reverse transcriptase inhibitor.
See: Ziagen.
W/Lamivudine
See: Epzicom.

abacavir sulfate/lamivudine/zidovudine. (Various Mfr.) Abacavir sulfate 300 mg/lamivudine 150 mg/zidovudine 300 mg. Tab. 60s, 100s, 500s. *Rx.*
Use: Antiretroviral agent, reverse transcriptase combination.

•**abafilcon A.** (ab-ah-FILL-kahn) USAN.
Use: Contact lens material, hydrophilic.

•**abamectin.** (abe-ah-MEK-tin) USAN.
Use: Antiparasitic.

•**abarelix.** (ab-ah-RELL-ix) USAN.
Use: Gonadotropin-releasing hormone antagonist.

•**abatacept.** (ab-a-TA-sept) USAN.
Use: Immunomodulator, immunologic agent.
See: Orencia.

Abbokinase Open-Cath. (Abbott Diagnostics) Urokinase for catheter clearance gelatin 5 mg, mannitol 15 mg, sodium chloride 1.7 mg, monobasic sodium phosphate anhydrous/mL when reconstituted, preservative free. Single-dose *Univial* 1 mL, 1.8 mL. *Rx.*
Use: Thrombolytic.

Abbott AFP-EIA. (Abbott Diagnostics) Enzyme immunoassay for the quantitative measurement of alpha-fetoprotein (AFP) in human serum and amniotic fluid. Test kits 100s.
Use: Diagnostic aid.

Abbott AFP-EIA Monoclonal. (Abbott Diagnostics) Enzyme immunoassay for the quantitative measurement of alpha-fetoprotein (AFP) in human serum and amniotic fluid.
Use: Diagnostic aid.

Abbott Anti-Delta. (Abbott Diagnostics) Radioimmunoassay for the detection of antibody to hepatitis delta antigen (HDAg) in human serum or plasma.
Use: For research only. Not for use in diagnostic procedures.

Abbott Anti-Delta EIA. (Abbott Diagnostics) Enzyme immunoassay for the detection of antibody to hepatitis delta antigen (HDAg) in human serum or plasma.
Use: For research only. Not for use in diagnostic procedures.

Abbott β-HCG 15/15. (Abbott Diagnostics) Enzyme immunoassay for the quantitative determination of human chorionic gonadotropin (hCG) in human serum.
Use: Diagnostic aid.

Abbott CA125-EIA. (Abbott Diagnostics) Enzyme immunoassay for the quantitative measurement of cancer antigen (CA) 125 in human serum.
Use: For research only. Not for use in diagnostic procedures.

Abbott CEA-EIA Monoclonal. (Abbott Diagnostics) Enzyme immunoassay for the quantitative measurement of carcinoembryonic antigen (CEA) in human serum or plasma to aid in the management of cancer patients and assessing prognosis.
Use: Diagnostic aid.

Abbott CEA-RIA. (Abbott Diagnostics) Solid phase radioimmunoassay for the quantitative measurement of carcinoembryonic antigen (CEA) in human serum or plasma to aid in the management of cancer patients and assessing prognosis.
Use: Diagnostic aid.

Abbott CMV Total AB EIA. (Abbott Diagnostics) Enzyme immunoassay for the detection of antibody to cytomegalovirus in human serum, plasma, and whole blood. Test kits 100s.
Use: Diagnostic aid.

Abbott Diagnostic Reagents. (Abbott Diagnostics) A series of diagnostic tests for cancer, cardiovascular, hepatitis, infectious disease and immunology, metabolic and digestive disease, OB/GYN, rubella, and thyroid.
Use: Diagnostic aid.

Abbott ER-EIA Monoclonal. (Abbott Diagnostics) Enzyme immunoassay for the quantitative measurement of human estrogen receptor in tissue cytosol.
Use: For research only. Not for use in diagnostic procedures.

Abbott ER-ICA Monoclonal. (Abbott Diagnostics) Immunoassay for the detection of estrogen receptor.
Use: For research only. Not for use in diagnostic procedures.

Abbott HB-EIA. (Abbott Diagnostics) Enzyme immunoassay for the detection of hepatitis Be antigen or antibody to hepatitis Be antigen.
Use: Diagnostic aid.

Abbott HBe Test. (Abbott Diagnostics) Radioimmunoassay or enzyme immunoassay for detection of hepatitis Be antigen or antibody to hepatitis Be antigen. Test kits 100s.
Use: Diagnostic aid.

Abbott HIVAB HIV-1 EIA. (Abbott Diagnostics) Enzyme immunoassay for the antibody to human immunodeficiency virus type 1 (HIV-1) in serum or plasma. Test kits 100s, 1000s.
Use: Diagnostic aid.

Abbott HIVAG-1. (Abbott Diagnostics) Enzyme immunoassay for the human immunodeficiency virus type 1 (HIV-1) antigens in serum or plasma. Test kits 100s, 1000s.
Use: Diagnostic aid.

Abbott HTLV I EIA. (Abbott Diagnostics) To detect antibody to Human T-Lymphotropic Virus Type I in serum or plasma. Test kits 100s.
Use: Diagnostic aid.

Abbott HTLV III Antigen EIA. (Abbott Diagnostics) Enzyme immunoassay for the detection of Human T-Lymphotropic Virus Type III (HIV) antigens.
Use: For research only. Not for use in diagnostic procedures.

Abbott HTLV III Confirmatory EIA. (Abbott Diagnostics) Enzyme immunoassay for confirmation of specimens found to be positive to antibody to HTL VIII. Test kits 100s.
Use: Diagnostic aid.

Abbott HTLV III EIA. (Abbott Diagnostics) Enzyme immunoassay for the detection of antibody to Human T-Lymphotropic Virus Type III (HIV) in human serum or plasma. Test kits 1s.
Use: Diagnostic aid.

Abbott IGE EIA. (Abbott Diagnostics) Enzyme immunoassay for quantitative determination of IgE in human serum and plasma. Test kits 100s.
Use: Diagnostic aid.

Abbott PAP-EIA. (Abbott Diagnostics) Enzyme immunoassay for the measurement of prostatic acid phosphatase (PAP) in serum or plasma.
Use: Diagnostic aid.

Abbott RSV-EIA. (Abbott Diagnostics) Enzyme immunoassay for the detection of respiratory syncytial virus (RSV) in nasopharyngeal washes and aspirates.
Use: Diagnostic aid.

Abbott SCC-RIA. (Abbott Diagnostics) Radioimmunoassay for the quantitative measurement of squamous cell carcinoma-associated antigen in human serum.
Use: For research only. Not for use in diagnostic procedures.

Abbott TdT EIA. (Abbott Diagnostics) Enzyme immunoassay for the quantitative measurement of terminal deoxynucleotidyl transferase (TdT), in extracts of human whole blood or isolated mononuclear cells.
Use: Diagnostic aid.

Abbott Testpak hCG-Serum. (Abbott Diagnostics) Monoclonal antibody, enzyme immunoassay for the qualitative determination of human chorionic gonadotropin (hCG) in serum. No instrumentation required.
Use: Diagnostic aid.

Abbott Testpak hCG-Urine. (Abbott Diagnostics) Monoclonal antibody, enzyme immunoassay for the qualitative determination of human chorionic gonadotropin (hCG) in urine. No instrumentation required.
Use: Diagnostic aid.

Abbott Testpack-Strep A. (Abbott Diagnostics) A rapid screening and confirmatory test for the detection of group A beta-hemolytic streptococci from throat swabs. No instrumentation required.
Use: Diagnostic aid.

Abbott Toxo-G EIA. (Abbott Diagnostics) Enzyme immunoassay for the qualitative and quantitative determination of IgG antibody to toxoplasma gondii in human serum and plasma.
Use: Diagnostic aid.

Abbott Toxo-M EIA. (Abbott Diagnostics) Enzyme immunoassay for the qualitative determination of IgM antibody to toxoplasma gondii in human serum.
Use: Diagnostic aid.

•**abciximab.** (ab-SICK-sih-mab) USAN.
Use: Monoclonal antibody; antithrombotic; antiplatelet agent, glycoprotein IIb/IIIa inhibitor.
See: ReoPro.

ABC to Z. (NBTY) Iron 18 mg, Vitamins A 5000 units, D 400 units, E 30 units, B_1 1.5 mg, B_2 1.7 mg, B_3 20 mg, B_5 10 mg, B_6 2 mg, B_{12} 6 mcg, C 60 mg, folic acid 0.4 mg, biotin 30 mcg, Ca, P, I, Mg, Cu, Mn, K, Cl, Cr, Mo, Se, Ni, Si,

Sn, V, B, vitamin K, Zn 15 mg. Tab. Bot. 100s. *OTC.*
Use: Mineral, vitamin supplement.

•**abediterol.** (A-bed-I-ter-ol) USAN.
Use: Treatment of asthma and chronic obstructive pulmonary disorder.

•**abediterol napadisylate.** (A-bed-I-ter-ol NA-pa-DIS-i-late) USAN.
Use: Treatment of asthma and chronic obstructive pulmonary disorder.

Abelcet. (Enzon) Amphotericin B 100 mg/20 mL (as lipid complex). Susp. for Inj. Single-use Vial w/5-micron filter needles 10 mL, 20 mL. *Rx.*
Use: Antifungal.

•**abetimus sodium.** (a-BE-ti-mus) USAN.
Use: Investigational immunomodulator.

•**abexinostat.** (A-bex-IN-oh-stat) USAN.
Use: Antineoplastic.

•**abexinostat hydrochloride.** (A-bex-IN-oh-stat) USAN.
Use: Antineoplastic.

Abilify. (Bristol-Myers Squibb) Aripiprazole. **Inj.:** 9.75 mg per 1.3 mL. Single-dose vials. 1.3 mL. **Oral Soln.:** 1 mg/mL. EDTA, fructose, sucrose, parabens. Orange cream flavor. 150 mL. **Tab.:** 2 mg, 5 mg, 10 mg, 15 mg, 20 mg, 30 mg. Lactose. Pkg. 30s, UD 100s (except 2 mg). *Rx.*
Use: Antipsychotic.

Abilify Discmelt. (Bristol-Myers Squibb) Aripiprazole 10 mg (phenylalanine 1.12 mg), 15 mg (phenylalanine 1.68 mg). Aspartame. Vanilla cream flavor. Orally Disintegrating Tab. Blister 30s. *Rx.*
Use: Antipsychotic.

Abilify Maintena. (Otsuka America) Aripiprazole 300 mg, 400 mg. Mannitol. Inj., lyophilized Pow. for Susp., extended release. Single-use vial w/diluent. *Rx.*
Use: Antipsychotic, quinolinone derivative.

•**abiraterone acetate.** (A-bir-A-ter-one) USAN.
Use: Antineoplastic.
See: Zytiga.

Abitrexate. (International Pharm) Methotrexate sodium 25 mg/mL. Vial 2 mL, 4 mL, 8 mL. *Rx.*
Use: Antineoplastic.

Ablavar. (Lantheus Medical Imaging) Gadofosveset trisodium 244 mg/mL (also contains fosveset 0.268 mg) (equiv. to 0.25 mmol/mL). Preservative free. Inj., Soln. Single-use vial. 10 mL, 20 mL.
Use: In vivo diagnostic aid.

•**ablukast.** (ab-LOO-kast) USAN.
Use: Antiasthmatic, leukotriene antagonist.

•**ablukast sodium.** (ab-LOO-kast) USAN.
Use: Antiasthmatic, leukotriene antagonist.
See: Ulpax.

•**abobotulinumtoxinA.** (ab-oh-BOT-ue-LYE-num-TOX-in-ay) USAN.
Use: Botulinum toxin.
See: Dysport.

abortifacients.
See: Mifepristone.
Prostaglandins.

Abraxane. (Abraxis Oncology) Paclitaxel protein bound 100 mg. Albumin (human) 900 mg. Inj., lyophilized Pow. for Susp. Single-use vial. *Rx.*
Use: Antimitotic agent.

Abreva. (GlaxoSmithKline) Docosanol 10%, benzyl alcohol, light mineral oil. Cream. Tube 2 g. *OTC.*
Use: Cold sores; fever blisters.

•**abrineurin.** (aye-bri-NOOR-in) USAN.
Previously brineurin.
Use: Amyotrophic lateral sclerosis (ALS).

absorbable cellulose cotton or gauze.
See: Oxidized Cellulose.

absorbable dusting powder.
Use: Lubricant.

absorbable gelatin film.
Use: Hemostatic, topical.
See: Gelfilm.
Gelfilm Ophthalmic.

absorbable gelatin sponge.
Use: Hemostatic.
See: Gelfoam.

absorbable surgical suture.
Use: Surgical aid.

Absorbase. (Carolina Medical Products) Petrolatum, mineral oil, ceresin wax, wool wax, alcohol. Oint. Tube 114 g, 454 g. *OTC.*
Use: Pharmaceutical aid, emollient base.

absorbent gauze.
Use: Surgical aid.

Absorbent Rub Relief Formula. (DeWitt) Green soap 11.64%, camphor 1.63%, menthol 1.63%, pine tar soap 0.87%, wintergreen oil 0.71%, sassafras oil 0.54%, benzocaine 0.48%, capsicum 0.03%, wormwood oil 0.6%, isopropyl alcohol 75%. Bot. 2 oz. *OTC.*
Use: Analgesic, topical.

Absorbine Jr. (W.F. Young) Menthol 1.27%, absinthium oil, echinacea, iodine, plant extracts of calendula, potassium iodide, thymol, wormwood. Liq., topical. 118 mL w/applicator. *OTC.*
Use: Rub and liniment.

Absorbine Jr. Arthritis Strength. (W.F. Young) Natural menthol 4%, capsaicin 0.025%, acetone, calendula plant extracts, echinacea, wormwood. Liq. *OTC.*
Use: Liniment.

Absorbine Jr. Back Patch. (W.F. Young) Menthol 5%. Aloe barbadensis, camphor, lanolin, zinc oxide. Patch. 22 × 10 cm. 4s. *OTC.*
Use: Rub and liniment.

Absorbine Jr. Extra Strength. (W.F. Young) Natural menthol 4%; plant extracts of calendula, echinacea and wormwood; acetone; chloroxylenol iodine; potassium iodide; thymol; wormwood oil. Liq. Bot. 59 mL, 118 mL. *OTC.*
Use: Liniment.

Absorbine Jr. Ultra Strength. (W.F. Young) Menthol. **Patch:** 6.5%. Alcohol, camphor, eucalyptus leaf oil, glycerin, kaolin, polysorbate 80, titanium dioxide. 6s. **Spray:** 12%. Alcohol, plant extracts of calendula, echinacea, wormwood, spearmint oil. 118 mL. *OTC.*
Use: Rub and liniment.

Absorica. (Ranbaxy) Isotretinoin 10 mg, 20 mg, 30 mg, 40 mg. Soybean oil. Cap. UD 30s. *Rx.*
Use: First-generation retinoid.

Abstral. (Galena Biopharma) Fentanyl 100 mcg, 200 mcg, 300 mcg, 400 mcg, 600 mcg, 800 mcg. Mannitol. Tab., sublingual. Blister packs. 12s (except 600 mcg, 800 mcg), 32s. *c-II.*
Use: Opioid analgesic.

Abuscreen. (Roche) An immunological and radiochemical assay for morphine and morphine glucuronide in nanogram levels. Utilizes I-125 labeled morphine requiring gamma scintillation equipment. Tests 100s.
Use: Diagnostic aid.

•**acacia syrup.** (ah-KAY-shah) *NF.*
Use: Pharmaceutic aid, suspending agent, viscosity agent.

•**acadesine.** (ack-AH-dess-een) USAN.
Use: Platelet aggregation inhibitor.

•**acamprosate calcium.** (a-kam-PROE-sate) USAN.
Use: Antialcoholic agent.
See: Campral.

acamprosate calcium. (Various Mfr.) Acamprosate calcium 333 mg. Enteric coated. May contain sulfites. Tab., delayed release. 180s, UD 100s. *Rx.*
Use: Antialchoholic agent.

Acanya. (Valeant) Benzoyl peroxide 2.5%, clindamycin phosphate 1.2%. Kit with benzoyl peroxide gel 40 g and clindamycin phosphate solution 10 g. Gel. *Rx.*
Use: Dermatologic agent, acne treatment.

•**acarbose.** (A-car-bose) USAN.
Use: Alpha-glucosidase inhibitor.
See: Precose.

acarbose. (Various Mfr.) Acarbose 25 mg, 50 mg, 100 mg. Tab. 100s, UD 100s (except 100 mg). *Rx.*
Use: Alpha-glucosidase inhibitor.

Accolate. (AstraZeneca) Zafirlukast 10 mg, 20 mg, lactose, povidone. Tab. Bot. 60s, UD 100s. *Rx.*
Use: Leukotriene receptor antagonist.

AccuHist. (Tiber) Chlorpheniramine maleate 1 mg, phenylephrine hydrochloride 2.5 mg. Glycerin, propylene glycol, saccharin, sorbitol. Alcohol free, dye free, and sugar free. Cherry flavor. Soln., Conc. 59.2 mL w/calibrated syringe. *OTC.*
Use: Upper respiratory combination, decongestant, antihistamine.

AccuNeb. (Dey) Albuterol sulfate 0.021% (0.63 mg/3 mL), 0.042% (1.25 mg/3 mL). Preservative free. Soln. for Inh. UD Vial 3 mL. *Rx.*
Use: Bronchodilator, sympathomimetic.

Accupep HPF. (Sherwood Davis & Geck) Hydrolyzed lactalbumin, maltodextrin, MCT oil, corn oil, mono- and diglycerides, vitamins A, B_1, B_2, B_3, B_5, B_6, B_{12}, C, D, E, K, Ca, Cl, Cu, Fe, I, Mg, Mn, P, Zn, biotin, and choline. Pks. 128 g. *OTC.*
Use: Nutritional supplement.

Accupril. (Pfizer) Quinapril hydrochloride 5 mg, 10 mg, 20 mg, 40 mg. Lactose. Film-coated. Tab. Bot. 90s and UD 100s (except 40 mg). *Rx.*
Use: Antihypertensive; angiotensin-converting enzyme inhibitor.

Accuretic. (Parke-Davis) Quinapril hydrochloride/hydrochlorothiazide 10 mg/12.5 mg, 20 mg/12.5 mg, 20 mg/25 mg. Lactose. Film-coated. Tab. Bot. 30s. *Rx.*
Use: Antihypertensive.

Accusens T Taste Function Kit. (Westport Pharmaceuticals, Inc.) Test for ability to distinguish among salty, sweet, sour, and bitter tastants. Kit contains 15 bottles (60 mL) tastants and 30 taste record forms.
Use: Diagnostic aid.

A-C-D Solution. Sodium citrate, citric acid, and dextrosein sterile pyrogen-free solution. (Baxter Pharmaceutical Products, Inc.). Soln. 600 mL Bot. with 70 mL, 120 mL, 300 mL Soln.; 1000 mL Bot. with 500 mL Soln. (Bayer Biologi-

cal). 500 mL Bot. with 75 mL, 120 mL Soln.; 650 mL Bot. with 80 mL, 130 mL Soln. (The Diamond Co.). 250 mL, 500 mL *Abbo-Vac. Rx.*
Use: Anticoagulant for preparation of plasma or whole blood.

A-C-D Solution Modified. (Bristol-Myers Squibb) Acid citrate dextrose anticoagulant solution modified. *Rx.*
Use: Anticoagulant, radiolabeled.

•**acebutolol hydrochloride.** (A-se-BUE-toe-lol) *USP.*
Use: Antiadrenergic/sympatholytic; beta-adrenergic blocking agent.
See: Sectral.

acebutolol hydrochloride. (Various Mfr.) Acebutolol hydrochloride 200 mg, 400 mg. Cap. Bot. 100s, 1000s. *Rx.*
Use: Antiadrenergic/sympatholytic, beta-adrenergic blocking agent.

•**acecainide hydrochloride.** (A-se-KAY-nide) USAN.
Use: Cardiovascular agent.
See: NAPA.

•**aceclidine.** (a-SEK-li-deen) USAN.
Use: Cholinergic.

•**acedapsone.** (A-se-DAP-sone) USAN.
Use: Antimalarial; antibacterial, leprostatic.

Acedoval. (Pal-Pak, Inc.) Dover's powder 15 mg, ipecac 1.5 mg, aspirin 162 mg, caffeine anhydrous 8.1 mg. Tab. Bot. 1000s, 5000s. *OTC.*
Use: Analgesic; antispasmodic; antiperistaltic.

•**aceglutamide aluminum.** (AH-see-GLUE-tah-mide ah-LOO-min-uhm) USAN.
Use: Antiulcerative.

acellular pertussis adsorbed, hepatitis B (recombinant) and inactivated poliovirus vaccine combined, diphtheria and tetanus toxoids.
Use: Active immunization, toxoid.
See: Diphtheria and Tetanus Toxoids and Acellular Pertussis Adsorbed, Hepatitis B (Recombinant) and Inactivated Poliovirus Vaccine Combined.

acellular pertussis and Haemophilus influenzae type B conjugate vaccine (DTaP-HIB), diphtheria and tetanus toxoids.
Use: Active immunization, toxoid.
See: Diphtheria and Tetanus Toxoid, Acellular Pertussis and Haemophilus Influenzae Type B Conjugate Vaccine (DTaP-HIB).

acellular pertussis vaccine, adsorbed (DTaP), diphtheria and tetanus toxoids.
Use: Active immunization, toxoid.
See: Diphtheria and Tetanus Toxoids and Acellular Pertussis Vaccine, Adsorbed (DTaP).

•**acemannan.** (ah-see-MAN-an) USAN.
Use: Antiviral; immunomodulator.

acemannan hydrogel.
Use: Mouth and throat product.
See: Oral Wound Rinse.

Aceon. (Xoma) Perindopril erbumine 4 mg, 8 mg. Lactose. Tab. 100s. *Rx.*
Use: Antihypertensive, angiotensin-converting enzyme inhibitor.

Acephen. (G & W Labs) Acetaminophen 120 mg, 325 mg, 650 mg. Glyceryl stearate (120 mg only), hydrogenated vegetable oil. Supp. 6s (120 mg only); 12s; 50s, 100s, 1000s (except 120 mg); 500s (650 mg only); UD 6s (325 mg only); UD 12s (except 650 mg); UD 50s, UD 100s (120 mg only). *OTC.*
Use: Analgesic.

•**acepromazine maleate.** (A-se-PROE-ma-zeen) *USP.*
Use: Anxiolytic.

Acerola-C. (Barth's) Vitamin C 300 mg. Wafer. Bot. 30s, 90s, 180s, 360s. *OTC.*
Use: Vitamin supplement.

Acerola-Plex. (Barth's) Vitamin C 100 mg, bioflavonoids 50 mg. Tab. Bot. 100s, 500s. *OTC.*
Use: Vitamin supplement.

Acetadote. (Cumberland) Acetylcysteine 20% (200 mg/mL). EDTA 0.5 mg/mL. Preservative-free. Inj. Single-dose vials. 30 mL. *Rx.*
Use: Antidote.

Aceta-Gesic. (Rugby) Acetaminophen 325 mg, diphenhydramine hydrochloride 12.5 mg. Mineral oil, PEG. Tab. 100s. *OTC.*
Use: Upper respiratory combination, analgesic, antihistamine.

•**acetaminophen.** (a-SEET-a-MIN-oh-fen) *USP.* APAP.
Use: Analgesic; antipyretic.
See: Acephen.
Aminofen.
Anacin Aspirin Free Extra Strength.
Apap.
Aphen.
BetaTemp Children's.
Cetafen.
Ed-Apap.
ElixSure.
FeverAll.
Genapap.

Infantaire.
Little Fevers.
Little Remedies for Fevers Children's.
Little Remedies for Fever Infant.
Mapap.
Mapap Extra Strength.
Mapap Infants'.
Masophen.
Non-Aspirin.
Nortemp.
Nortemp Infants' Drops.
Ofirmev.
Painaid ESF Extra-Strength Formula.
Pain and Fever.
Pain Relief.
Pain Reliever.
Pharbetol.
Pharbetol Extra Strength.
Q-Pap.
Quick Melts.
Silapap.
Triaminic Infants' Fever Reducer/Pain Reliever.
Tylenol.
Tylenol Meltaways Jr.
UN-Aspirin, Extra Strength.
Valorin.

W/Aluminum Hydroxide, Aspirin, Caffeine, Magnesium Hydroxide.
See: Vanquish.

W/Aspirin, Buffered.
See: Excedrin Back & Body Extra Strength.

W/Aspirin, Caffeine.
See: Anacin Advanced Headache.
Bayer Migraine.
Excedrin Extra Strength.
Excedrin Migraine.
Goody's Cool Orange.
Goody's Extra Strength.
Goody's Extra Strength Fast Pain Relief.
Goody's Migraine Relief.
Summit Extra Strength.

W/Aspirin, Caffeine, Salicylamide.
See: Levacet.
Medi-First Extra Strength Pain Relief.
Painaid.
Saleto.

W/Butalbital.
See: Bupap.
Butalbital, Acetaminophen, and Caffeine.
Butex Forte.
Dolgic.
Marten-Tab.
Orbivan CF.
Phrenilin Forte.
Sedapap.
Tencon.

W/Butalbital, Caffeine.
See: Alagesic LQ.
Americet.
Capacet.
Dolgic Plus.
Esgic.
Esgic-Plus.
Fioricet.
Margesic.
Orbivan.
Repan.
Triad.
Zebutal.

W/Butalbital, Caffeine, Codeine.
See: Fioricet with Codeine.
Phrenilin with Caffeine and Codeine.

W/Caffeine.
See: APAP-Plus.

W/Caffeine, Dihydrocodeine Bitartrate.
See: Panlor DC.
Trezix.

W/Caffeine, Isometheptene Mucate.
See: MigraTen.
Prodrin.

W/Caffeine, Magnesium Salicylate.
See: Back Pain-Off.

W/Caffeine, Magnesium Salicylate, Phenyltoloxamine Citrate.
See: Durabac Forte.

W/Caffeine, Phenyltoloxamine Citrate, Salicylamide.
See: Durabac.

W/Calcium Carbonate
See: Acid-X.

W/Chlorpheniramine Maleate.
See: Coricidin HBP Cold & Flu.

W/Chlorpheniramine Maleate, Codeine Phosphate.
See: Cotabflu.

W/Chlorpheniramine Maleate, Dextromethorphan Hydrobromide.
See: Coricidin HBP Maximum Strength Flu.
Formula 44 Custom Care Cough & Cold PM.
Triaminic Flu, Cough & Fever.
Tylenol Plus Children's Cough & Runny Nose.
Vicks Alcohol-Free NyQuil Cold & Flu Relief.
Vicks Formula 44 Custom Care Cough & Cold PM.

W/Chlorpheniramine Maleate, Dextromethorphan Hydrobromide, Phenylephrine Hydrochloride.
See: Alka-Seltzer Plus Cold & Cough.
Comtrex Maximum Strength Day & Night Cold & Cough.
Dimetapp Children's Multi-Symptom Cold & Flu.
Robitussin Cough, Cold & Flu Nighttime.

Theraflu Nighttime Severe Cold.
Tylenol Cold Head Congestion Nighttime.
Tylenol Cold Multi-Symptom Nighttime.
Tylenol Plus Children's Flu.
Tylenol Plus Children's Multi-Symptom Cold.
W/Chlorpheniramine Maleate, Phenylephrine Hydrochloride.
See: Alka-Seltzer Multi-Symptom Cold Relief.
Alka-Seltzer Plus Fast Crystal Packs.
Comtrex Maximum Strength Day & Night Flu Therapy.
Comtrex Maximum Strength Day & Night Severe Cold and Sinus.
Contac Cold + Flu.
Contac Cold + Flu Maximum Strength.
Contac Cold + Flu Night.
Dristan Cold Multi-Symptom Formula.
Dryphen Multi-Symptom Formula.
Medicidin-D.
Norel AD.
Pyrroxate Extra Strength.
Robitussin Adult Peak Cold Nighttime Nasal Relief.
Sine Off Sinus/Cold.
Tylenol Allergy Multi-Symptom.
Tylenol Allergy Multi-Symptom Convenience Pack.
Tylenol Sinus Congestion & Pain Nighttime.
W/Chlorpheniramine Maleate, Phenylephrine Hydrochloride, Phenyltoloxamine Citrate.
See: Norel SR.
Trital SR.
W/Codeine Phosphate.
See: Capital with Codeine.
Cocet.
Cocet Plus.
Vopac.
W/Dexbrompheniramine, Phenylephrine Hydrochloride.
See: Sinadrin PE.
W/Dextromethorphan Hydrobromide.
See: PediaCare Children's Cough & Sore Throat.
Triaminic Cough & Sore Throat.
Tylenol Plus Children's Cough & Sore Throat.
W/Dextromethorphan Hydrobromide, Diphenhydramine.
See: Diabetic Tussin Cold & Flu.
Diabetic Tussin Night Time Formula Cold/Flu.
W/Dextromethorphan Hydrobromide, Diphenhydramine Hydrochloride, Phenylephrine Hydrochloride.
See: Respa C & C.
W/Dextromethorphan Hydrobromide, Doxylamine Succinate.
See: Tylenol Cough & Sore Throat Nighttime.
Vicks Nature Fusion Cold & Flu Nighttime Relief.
Vicks NyQuil Cold/Flu Relief.
W/Dextromethorphan Hydrobromide, Doxylamine Succinate, Phenylephrine Hydrochloride.
See: Alka-Seltzer Plus Day & Night Cold.
Alka-Seltzer Plus Night Cold.
Alka-Seltzer Plus Severe Sinus Congestion Allergy & Cough.
Tylenol Cold Multi-Symptom Nighttime.
W/Dextromethorphan Hydrobromide, Doxylamine Succinate, Pseudoephedrine Hydrochloride.
See: All-Nite.
W/Dextromethorphan Hydrobromide, Guaifenesin, Phenylephrine Hydrochloride.
See: Mucinex Children's Cold, Cough and Sore Throat.
Mucinex Fast-Max Cold, Flu and Sore Throat.
Mucinex Fast-Max Severe Congestion and Cold.
Phenflu G.
Sine-Off Cough/Cold.
Sudafed PE Multi-Symptom Cold and Cough.
W/Dextromethorphan Hydrobromide, Guaifenesin, Pseudoephedrine Hydrochloride.
See: Duraflu.
Flutabs.
Maxiflu DM.
Maxiflu G.
Tylenol Cold Severe Congestion Daytime.
W/Dextromethorphan Hydrobromide, Phenylephrine Hydrochloride.
See: Alka-Seltzer Plus Day & Night Cold.
Alka-Seltzer Plus Day Cold.
Alka-Seltzer Plus Day Non-Drowsy Cold.
Comtrex Maximum Strength Day & Night Cold & Cough.
Mapap Cold Formula Multi-Symptom.
Theraflu Daytime Severe Cold & Cough.
Theraflu Severe Cold & Cough Daytime/Nighttime.
Theraflu Warming Relief Daytime Multi-Symptom Cold.
Tylenol Cold Head Congestion Daytime.

Tylenol Cold Multi-Symptom Daytime.
Vicks DayQuil Multi-Symptom Cold/Flu Relief.
Vicks Nature Fusion Cold & Flu Relief.
W/Dextromethorphan Hydrobromide, Pseudoephedrine Hydrochloride.
See: 666 Cold Preparation Maximum Strength.
W/Dichloralphenazone, Isometheptene Mucate.
See: Epidrin.
Midrin.
Migrazone.
Nodolor.
W/Diphenhydramine Citrate.
See: Goody's PM.
W/Diphenhydramine Hydrochloride.
See: Aceta-Gesic.
Acetaminophen PM Extra Strength.
Pain Reliever PM Extra Strength.
Percogesic Extra Strength.
Tylenol PM Extra Strength.
Tylenol Severe Allergy.
Tylenol Sore Throat Nighttime.
Unisom PM Pain.
W/Diphenhydramine Hydrochloride, Phenylephrine Hydrochloride.
See: Benadryl Allergy & Cold.
Benadryl Allergy & Sinus Headache.
Benadryl Severe Allergy & Sinus Headache Maximum Strength.
Sudafed PE Multi-Symptom Severe Cold.
Sudafed PE Nighttime Cold Maximum Strength.
Theraflu Nighttime Severe Cough & Cold.
Theraflu Severe Cold & Cough Daytime/Nighttime.
Theraflu Sugar-Free Nighttime Severe Cough & Cold.
Theraflu Warming Relief Flu & Sore Throat.
Tylenol Allergy Multi-Symptom Convenience Pack.
Tylenol Allergy Multi-Symptom Nighttime.
Tylenol Plus Children's Cold & Allergy.
W/Guaifenesin.
See: Theraflu Chest Congestion.
Tylenol Chest Congestion.
W/Guaifenesin, Phenylephrine Hydrochloride.
See: Mucinex Fast-Max Cold and Sinus.
Sine-Off Multi Symptom Relief.
Tylenol Sinus Congestion & Pain Severe Daytime.
W/Guaifenesin, Pseudoephedrine Hydrochloride.
See: Tylenol Sinus Severe Congestion.
W/Hydrocodone Bitartrate.
See: Anexsia 5/500.
Anexsia 7.5/650.
Anexsia 10/660.
Co-Gesic.
Hycet.
Hydrocodone Bitartrate and Acetaminophen.
Hydrogesic.
Liquicet.
Lorcet Plus.
Lorcet 10/650.
Lortab.
Margesic H.
Maxidone.
Norco.
Norco 5/325.
Stagesic.
T-Gesic.
Vicodin.
Xodol.
Zamicet.
Zolvit.
Zydone.
W/Magnesium Salicylate.
See: Painaid Back Relief Formula.
Painaid BRF Back Relief Formula.
W/Magnesium Salicylate, Pamabrom.
See: Pamprin Maximum Pain Relief.
W/Oxycodone.
See: Endocet.
Percocet.
Pimlev.
Xolox.
W/Pamabrom.
See: Painaid PMF Premenstrual Formula.
Women's Tylenol Multi-Symptom Menstrual Relief.
W/Pamabrom, Pyridoxine Hydrochloride.
See: Vitelle Lurline PMS.
W/Pamabrom, Pyrilamine Maleate.
See: Pamprin Multi-Symptom Maximum Strength.
Prēmsyn PMS.
W/Pheniramine Maleate, Phenylephrine Hydrochloride.
See: Theraflu Cold & Sore Throat.
Theraflu Flu & Sore Throat.
Theraflu Nighttime Severe Cold.
W/Phenylephrine Hydrochloride.
See: Alka-Seltzer Plus Sinus.
Comtrex Maximum Strength Day & Night Flu Therapy.
Comtrex Maximum Strength Day & Night Severe Cold & Sinus.
Contac Cold + Flu Day.
Dilotab II.
Excedrin Sinus Headache.
Mapap Sinus Congestion and Pain Maximum Strength.

Robitussin Adult Peak Cold Nasal Relief.
Sine-Off Non-Drowsy Maximum Strength.
Sinutab Sinus.
Sudafed PE Sinus Headache.
Tylenol Sinus Congestion & Pain Daytime.
Vicks DayQuil Sinex.
W/Phenyltoloxamine Citrate.
See: Biphenox.
Pain-gesic.
Relagesic.
Zflex.
W/Phenyltoloxamine Citrate, Salicylamide.
See: Duraxin.
Ed-Flex Plus.
W/Propoxyphene Napsalate.
See: Darvocet A500.
Darvocet-N 100.
W/Pseudoephedrine Hydrochloride.
See: Dilotab II.
Mapap Sinus Maximum Strength.
Ornex No Drowsiness.
W/Pseudoephedrine Hydrochloride, Chlorpheniramine Maleate.
See: BC Allergy, Sinus, Headache.
W/Pseudoephedrine Hydrochloride, Guaifenesin.
See: Tylenol Sinus Severe Congestion.
W/Tramadol Hydrochloride.
See: Ultracet.

acetaminophen. (Various Mfr.) Acetaminophen. **Cap.:** 500 mg. 100s. **Liq.:** 160 mg/5 mL (May contain methylparaben, saccharin, sorbitol sucrose. 118 mL, 120 mL, 473 mL, 500 mL), 166.6 mg/5 mL (237 mL). **Oral Soln.:** 160 mg/5 mL. May contain sorbitol, sucrose. 118 mL, 473 mL. **Supp.:** 120 mg, 325 mg, 650 mg. Hydrogenated vegetable oil. 12s. **Tab.:** 325 mg, 500 mg. 25s (500 mg only), 50s (325 mg only), 100s, 700s (500 mg only), 1000s, UD 100s (500 mg only). *OTC.*
Use: Analgesic.

•**acetaminophen and aspirin.** (a-SEET-a-MIN-oh-fen and AS-pihr-in) *USP.*
Use: Analgesic.

•**acetaminophen and caffeine.** (a-SEET-a-MIN-oh-fen and KAF-een) *USP.*
Use: Analgesic.

acetaminophen and codeine. (Various Mfr.) **Tab.:** Codeine phosphate 15 mg, acetaminophen 300 mg. Bot. 100s, 500s, 1000s. Codeine phosphate 30 mg, acetaminophen 300 mg. Bot. 100s, 500s, 1000s, UD 100s, RN 100s. Codeine phosphate 60 mg, acetaminophen 300 mg. Bot. 100s, 500s, 1000s. *c-iii.* **Soln.:** Codeine phosphate 12 mg, acetaminophen 120 mg/5 mL. Bot. 120 mL, 500 mL, Pt, gal, UD 5 mL, 12.5 mL, 15 mL. *c-v.*
Use: Analgesic combination, narcotic.

•**acetaminophen and codeine phosphate.** (a-SEET-a-MIN-oh-fen and KOE-deen) *USP.*
Use: Analgesic.

•**acetaminophen and diphenhydramine.** (a-SEET-a-MIN-oh-fen and die-fen-HIGH-druh-meen) *USP.*
Use: Analgesic; antihistamine.

•**acetaminophen and pseudoephedrine hydrochloride.** (a-SEET-a-MIN-oh-fen and SUE-doe-eh-FED-rin) *USP.*
Use: Analgesic; decongestant.

•**acetaminophen, aspirin, and caffeine.** (a-SEET-a-MIN-oh-fen, AS-pihr-in, and KAF-een) *USP.*
Use: Analgesic.

acetaminophen, caffeine, and dihydrocodeine bitartrate. (Boca) Acetaminophen 712.8 mg, caffeine 60 mg, dihydrocodeine bitartrate 32 mg. Tab. 30s. *c-III.*
Use: Narcotic analgesic.

acetaminophen, children's. (Geri-Care) Acetaminophen 80 mg. Aspartame, dextrose, mannitol, phenylalanine, sugar. Fruit flavor. Chew. Tab. 30s. *OTC.*
Use: Analgesic.

acetaminophen/diphenhydramine. (Various Mfr.) Acetaminophen 500 mg, diphenhydramine hydrochloride 25 mg. May contain PEG. Tab. 50s. *OTC.*
Use: Nonnarcotic analgesic combination.

•**acetaminophen, diphenhydramine hydrochloride, and pseudoephedrine hydrochloride.** (a-SEET-a-MIN-oh-fen, die-fen-HIGH-druh-meen, and SUE-doe-eh-FED-rin) *USP.*
Use: Analgesic; antihistamine, decongestant.

acetaminophen extra strength. (Akyma) Acetaminophen 500 mg. Tab. 100s, 700s, 1000s. *OTC.*
Use: Analgesic.

acetaminophenol.
See: Acetaminophen.

Acetaminophen PM Extra Strength. (Plus Pharma) Acetaminophen 500 mg, diphenhydramine hydrochloride 25 mg. Tab. 50s. *OTC.*
Use: Nonprescription sleep aid combination.

acetanilid. (Various Mfr.) Acetylaminobenzene, acetylaniline, antifebrin.
Use: Analgesic (former use).

Acetasol. (Actavis MidAtlantic) Acetic

acid 2% with propylene glycol diacetate 3%, benzethonium chloride 0.02%, sodium acetate 0.015%. Soln. Bot. 15 mL. *Rx.*
Use: Otic preparation.

Acetasol HC. (Actavis MidAtlantic) Hydrocortisone 1%, acetic acid 2%, propylene glycol diacetate 3%, sodium acetate 0.015%, benzethonium chloride 0.02%. Citric acid 0.05%. Soln. Bot. 10 mL with dropper. *Rx.*
Use: Anti-infective; corticosteroid, otic.

Aceta w/Codeine. (Century) Acetaminophen 300 mg, codeine phosphate 30 mg. Tab. Bot. 100s. *c-III.*
Use: Analgesic combination, narcotic.

•**acetazolamide.** (uh-seet-uh-ZOLE-uh-mide) *USP.*
Tall Man: acetaZOLAMIDE
Use: Carbonic anhydrase inhibitor; anticonvulsant.
See: Diamox Sequels.

acetazolamide. (Bedford Labs) Acetazolamide 500 mg. Pow. for Inj., lyophilized. Preservative-free. Vials. *Rx.*
Use: Anticonvulsant.

acetazolamide. (Various Mfr.) Acetazolamide. **Tab.:** 125 mg, 250 mg. May contain lactose. 90s (250 mg only), 100s, 500s (250 mg only), 1,000s (250 mg only). **ER Cap.:** 500 mg. 100s, UD 30s. *Rx.*
Use: Carbonic anhydrase inhibitor; anticonvulsant.

•**acetazolamide sodium, sterile.** (uh-seet-uh-ZOLE-uh-mide SO-dee-uhm) *USP.*
Tall Man: acetaZOLAMIDE
Use: Carbonic anhydrase inhibitor.

acet-dia-mer-sulfonamide. Sulfacetamide, sulfadiazine, and sulfamerazine. Susp. *Rx.*
Use: Antibacterial, sulfonamide.

•**acetic acid.** (ah-SEE-tick) *NF.*
Use: Pharmaceutic aid, acidifying agent.
See: Otic Domeboro.
W/Antipyrine, Benzocaine, Polycosanol.
See: AABP.
Auralgan.

acetic acid. (Various Mfr.) Acetic acid 0.25% (glacial acetic acid 250 mg). Preservative free. Irrigant, Soln. Single-dose, semirigid irrigation container. 250 mL, 1,000 mL.
Use: Irrigating solution.

acetic acid/antipyrine/benzocaine/polycosanol 410. (Brookstone) Acetic acid 0.01%, antipyrine 5.4%, benzocaine 1.4%, polycosanol 410 0.01%, glycerin. Soln.; Otic. 15 mL w/dropper. *Rx.*
Use: Miscellaneous otic preparation.

•**acetic acid, glacial.** (ah-SEE-tick) *USP.*
Use: Pharmaceutic aid, acidifying agent.
W/Combinations.
See: Fem ph.

acetic acid otic. (Various Mfr.) Acetic acid 2% with propylene glycol diacetate 3%, benzethonium chloride 0.02%, and sodium acetate 0.015%. Soln. Bot. 15 mL. *Rx.*
Use: Otic preparation.

acetic acid, potassium salt. Potassium Acetate.

acetic acid 2% and aluminum acetate otic. (Bausch & Lomb) Acetic acid 2% in aluminum acetate solution. Soln. 60 mL. *Rx.*
Use: Otic preparation.

•**acetohydroxamic acid.** (a-SEET-oh-HYE-drox-AM-ik) *USP.*
Use: Enzyme inhibitor, urease.
See: Lithostat.

acetomeroctol.
Use: Antiseptic, topical.

•**acetone.** (AS-e-tone) *NF.*
Use: Pharmaceutic aid, solvent.

acetone or diacetic acid test.
See: Acetest Reagent.

acetophenetidin.
Use: Analgesic; antipyretic.
See: Phenacetin.

acetorphan.
Use: Enkephalinase inhibitor.

•**acetosulfone sodium.** (ah-SET-oh-SULL-fone SO-dee-uhm) USAN.
Use: Antibacterial, leprostatic.

acetoxyphenylmercury.
See: Phenylmercuric Acetate.

acetylaniline.
See: Acetanilid.

•**acetylcholine chloride.** (ah-SEH-till-KOE-leen KLOR-ide) *USP.*
Use: Cardiovascular agent; cholinergic; miotic; vasodilator, peripheral.
See: Miochol-E.

acetylcholine-like therapeutic agents.
See: Cholinergic agents.

•**acetylcysteine.** (a-SEET-il-SIS-teen) *USP.*
Use: Antidote; mucolytic.
See: Acetadote.
Mucomyst 10.

acetylcysteine. (Various Mfr.) Acetylcysteine 10%, 20%. EDTA. Oral Soln. Vial 4 mL, 10 mL, 30 mL. *Rx.*
Use: Antidote; mucolytic.

•**acetylcysteine and isoproterenol hydrochloride inhalation solution.** (a-SEET-il-SIS-teen and eye-so-pro-TER-uh-nahl) *USP.*
Use: Mucolytic.

Acetylin.
See: Acetylsalicylic Acid.
N-acetyl-p-aminophenol. Acetaminophen.
acetylphenylisatin.
See: Oxyphenisatin Acetate.
acetylprocainamide-n.
Use: Cardiovascular agent.
See: Acecainide Hydrochloride.
NAPA.
acetylsalicylic acid.
Use: Analgesic; antipyretic; antirheumatic.
See: Aspirin.
n[1]-acetylsulfanilamide.
Use: Sulfonamide therapy.
acetyl sulfisoxazole.
See: Sulfisoxazole Acetyl.
acetyltannic acid. Tannic acid acetate.
Use: Antiperistaltic.
AC Eye. (Walgreen) Tetrahydrozoline hydrochloride 0.05%, zinc sulfate 0.25%. Ophth. Drops. Bot. 0.75 oz. *OTC.*
Use: Decongestant combination, ophthalmic.
achlorhydria therapy.
See: Glutamic Acid Hydrochloride.
Achol. (Enzyme Process) Vitamin A 4000 units, ketocholanic acids 62 mg. Tab. Bot. 100s, 250s. *OTC.*
Use: Vitamin supplement.
acid acriflavine.
See: Acriflavine Hydrochloride.
acid citrate dextrose anticoagulant solution modified.
See: A-C-D Solution Modified.
acid citrate dextrose solution.
See: A-C-D Solution.
Acid Gone. (Major Pharmaceuticals) Aluminum hydroxide 31.7 mg, magnesium carbonate 119.33 mg per 5 mL. Benzyl alcohol, edetate disodium, glycerin, saccharin, sodium alginate 13 mg, sorbitol. Liq. 355 mL. *OTC.*
Use: Antacid combination.
acidifiers.
See: Ammonium Chloride.
K-Phos M.F.
Acid Jelly. (Hope Pharm) Oxyquinoline sulfate 0.025%, ricinoleic acid 0.7%, glacial acetic acid 0.921%, glycerin 5%, propylparaben. Jelly. 85 g with applicator. *OTC.*
Use: Vaginal preparation.
acidophilus.
See: Bacid.
Lactinex.
More Dophilus.
acidophilus. (Basic Vitamins) *L. acidophilus* 7.5 mg. Maltodextrin. Preservative free, sugar free. Cap. 100s. *OTC.*
Use: Probiotic.
Acidophilus Lactobacilli. (Magno-Humphries) *L. acidophilus* 500 million cells. Cap. 100s, 250s. *OTC.*
Use: Probiotic.
Acidophilus Lactobacillin Freeze-Dried. (National Vitamin) 25 million *L. acidophilus.* Lactose. Gluten free and preservative free. Cap. 100s. *OTC.*
Use: Probiotic.
Acidophilus Pearls. (Enzymatic Therapy) 1 billion CFU blend of *L. acidophilus* and *B. longum.* Palm oil, coconut oil, glycerin, soy lecithin. Gluten free. Cap. 90s, UD 30s. *OTC.*
Use: Probiotic.
Acidophilus Probiotic. (Natrol) *L. acidophilus* 3 billion active cultures. Gluten free and preservative free. Cap. 100s, 150s. *OTC.*
Use: Probiotic.
Acidophilus Probiotic Blend High Potency. (21st Century) 175 mg blend of *L. acidophilus, L. salivarius, B. bifidum, S. thermophilus.* Preservative free and sugar free. Cap. 150s. *OTC.*
Use: Probiotic.
Acidophilus Probiotic Blend With Pectin. (Windmill) 500 million CFU blend of *L. acidophilus, L. sporogenes, L. plantarum, B. bifidum, L. casei.* Preservative free, sugar free. Tab. 100s. *OTC.*
Use: Probiotic.
Acidophilus Probiotic Extra Strength With Pectin. (Nature's Bounty) 3 billion active cultures blend of *L. acidophilus, B. lactis, L. bulgaricus, L. salivarius.* Gluten free, lactose free, preservative free, and sugar free. Cap. 100s. *OTC.*
Use: Probiotic.
acidophilus with bifidus. (Various Mfr.) *Lactobacillus acidophilus* and *Lactobacillus bifidus* 1 billion units. Wafers. 100s. *OTC.*
Use: Probiotic.
Acidophilus With Citrus Pectin Captabs. (Rugby) *L. acidophilus* 25 million, calcium 18 mg, citrus pectin 100 mg. Maltodextrin. Gluten free, preservative free, soy free, sugar fee. Tab. 100s. *OTC.*
Use: Probiotic.
acidophilus with goat milk. (Windmill) *L. acidophilus* 1 billion CFU. Lactose. Preservative free. Cap. 100s. *OTC.*
Use: Probiotic.
acidophilus with pectin. (Mason) **Cap.:** *L. acidophilus* > 100 colonies. 100s. **Wafer, Chew.:** *L. acidophilus* 10 million.

Sugar 1 g. Vanilla-banana flavor. 100s. *OTC.*
Use: Probiotic.

Acidophilus Xtra. (Rexall Sundown) 20 million CFU blend of *L. acidophilus, B. lactis, L. bulgaricus, S. thermophilus.* Dextrose. Gluten free, lactose free, preservative free. Tab. 60s. *OTC.*
Use: Probiotic.

Acid Reducer + Antacid. (Various Mfr.) Famotidine 10 mg/calcium carbonate 800 mg/magnesium hydroxide 165 mg. May contain aspartame, phenylalanine 2.2 mg. Chew. Tab. 25s. *OTC.*
Use: Histamine H_2 antagonist combination.

Acid Reducer 200. (Major) Cimetidine 200 mg. Tab. 30s. *OTC.*
Use: Histamine H_2 antagonists.

acid trypaflavine.
See: Acriflavine Hydrochloride.

Acidulated Phosphate Fluoride. (Scherer) Fluoride ion 0.31% in 0.1 molar phosphate. Soln. Bot. 64 oz. (Office Product).
Use: Dental caries agent.

Acid-X. (BDI) Acetaminophen 500 mg, calcium carbonate 250 mg. Tab. Bot. 36s. *OTC.*
Use: Antacid.

•**acifran.** (AYE-si-fran) USAN.
Use: Antihyperlipoproteinemic.

AcipHex. (Eisai) Rabeprazole sodium 20 mg. Mannitol. Enteric coated. DR Tab. 30s, 90s, UD 100s. *Rx.*
Use: Proton pump inhibitor.

AcipHex Sprinkle. (Eisai) Rabeprazole 5 mg, 10 mg. Enteric coated. Mannitol. Cap., delayed release. 30s. *Rx.*
Use: Proton pump inhibitor.

•**acitretin.** (A-si-TRE-tin) USAN.
Use: Retinoid, second generation.
See: Soriatane.
Soriatane CK.

acitretin. (Various Mfr.) Acitretin 10 mg, 17.5 mg, 25 mg. May contain maltodextrin. Cap. 30s. *Rx.*
Use: Second-generation retinoid.

•**acivicin.** (ace-ih-VIH-sin) USAN.
Use: Antineoplastic.

Aclaro PD. (JSJ Pharmaceuticals) Hydroquinone 4%. Benzyl alcohol, cetyl alcohol, EDTA, glycerin, methoxycinnamate. Emulsion. Airless pump bot. 44 mL. *Rx.*
Use: Pigment agent.

•**aclarubicin.** (ack-lah-ROO-bih-sin) USAN. *Formerly Aclacinomycin A.*
Use: Antineoplastic.

•**aclidinium bromide.** (A-kli-DIN-ee-um) USAN.
Use: Bronchodilator, anticholinergic.
See: Tudorza Pressair.

Aclophen. (Nutripharm Laboratories, Inc.) Phenylephrine hydrochloride 40 mg, chlorpheniramine maleate 8 mg, acetaminophen 500 mg, dye free. SR Tab. Bot. 100s. *Rx.*
Use: Analgesic; antihistamine; decongestant.

Aclovate. (Pharmaderm) Alclometasone dipropionate 0.05%. Cream or Oint. Tube 15 g, 45 g. *Rx.*
Use: Anti-inflammatory, topical.

A.C.N. (Person and Covey) Vitamin A 25,000 units, ascorbic acid 250 mg, niacinamide 25 mg. Tab. Bot. 100s. *OTC.*
Use: Vitamin supplement.

Acnaveen.
See: Aveenobar Medicated.

Acna-Vite. (Cenci, H.R. Labs, Inc.) Vitamins A 10,000 units, C 250 mg, hesperidin 50 mg, niacinamide 25 mg. Cap. Bot. 75s. *OTC.*
Use: Dermatologic, acne; vitamin supplement.

Acne Clear. (Altaire) Benzoyl peroxide 10%. EDTA. Gel. 45 g. *OTC.*
Use: Topical anti-infective.

Acne Medication 5. (Rugby) Benzoyl peroxide 5%. **Lot.:** Disodium edetate. 30 mL. **Gel:** Disodium edetate. 42.5 g. *OTC.*
Use: Topical anti-infective, antibiotic agent.

Acne Medication 10. (Rugby) Benzoyl peroxide 10%. Disodium edetate. Gel. 42.5 g. *OTC.*
Use: Topical anti-infective, antibiotic agent.

Acno Cleanser. (Baker Cummins Dermatologicals) Isopropyl alcohol 60%, laureth-23, tetrasodium EDTA. Bot. 240 mL. *OTC.*
Use: Dermatologic, acne.

Acnomel. (Numark) Sulfur 8%, resorcinol 2%, alcohol 11%. Cream. Tube 28 g. *OTC.*
Use: Keratolytic, acne product.

Acnotex. (C & M Pharmacal) Sulfur 8%, resorcinol 2%, isopropyl alcohol 20%, acetone. In lotion base. Bot. 60 mL. *OTC.*
Use: Dermatologic, acne.

•**acodazole hydrochloride.** (ah-KOE-dah-ZOLE) USAN.
Use: Antineoplastic.

•**acolbifene hydrochloride.** (aye-KOLE-bi-feen) USAN.
Use: Breast and uterine proliferation or cancer.

aconiazide. (Lincoln Diagnostics)
Use: Antituberculous. [Orphan Drug]

Acotus. (Whorton Pharmaceuticals, Inc.) Phenylephrine hydrochloride 5 mg, guaiacol glyceryl ether 100 mg, menthol 1 mg, alcohol by volume 10%/5 mL. Bot. 4 oz, 12 oz, gal. *OTC.*
Use: Antitussive; decongestant.

ACR. (Western Research) Ammonium chloride 7.5 g. Tab. *Handicount* 28s (36 bags of 28 tab.). *Rx.*
Use: Diuretic.

acriflavine. (Eli Lilly) Acriflavine 1.5 g. Tab. Bot. 100s.
Use: Antiseptic.

acriflavine hydrochloride. (Various Mfr.) Hydrochloride form of acriflavine. Acid acriflavine, acid trypaflavine, flavine, trypaflavine. National Aniline-Pow., Bot. 1 g, 5 g, 10 g, 25 g, 50 g. Tab. 1.5 g. Bot. 50s, 100s. *Rx.*
Use: Anti-infective.

•**acrisorcin.** (ACK-rih-sahr-sin) USAN.
Use: Antifungal.
See: Akrinol.

•**acrivastine.** (ACK-rih-VAS-teen) USAN.
Use: Antihistamine.

acrivastine and pseudoephedrine hydrochloride.
Use: Upper respiratory combination, antihistamine, decongestant.
See: Semprex-D.

•**acronine.** (ACK-row-neen) USAN.
Use: Antineoplastic.

ACT. Dactinomycin.
Use: Antineoplastic.
See: Actinomycin D.

ACT. (J & J Merck Consumer Pharm.) **Rinse:** 0.02% (from 0.05% sodium fluoride). **Mint:** Tartrazine, alcohol 8%. **Cinnamon:** Alcohol 7%. Bot. 360 mL, 480 mL. *OTC.*
Use: Dentrifice.

Actacin. (Vangard Labs, Inc.) Triprolidine hydrochloride 2.5 mg, pseudoephedrine hydrochloride 60 mg. Tab. Bot. 100s, 1000s. *Rx-OTC.*
Use: Antihistamine; decongestant.

Actacin-C. (Vangard Labs, Inc.) Codeine phosphate 10 mg, triprolidine hydrochloride 2 mg, pseudoephedrine hydrochloride 20 mg, guaifenesin 100 mg/ 5 mL. Syr. Bot. Pt, gal. *c-v.*
Use: Antihistamine; antitussive; decongestant; expectorant.

Actal Plus. (Sanofi-Synthelabo) Aluminum hydroxide, magnesium hydroxide. Tab. *OTC.*
Use: Antacid.

Actal Suspension. (Sanofi-Synthelabo) Aluminum hydroxide. Susp. *OTC.*
Use: Antacid.

Actal Tablets. (Sanofi-Synthelabo) Aluminum hydroxide. Tab. *OTC.*
Use: Antacid.

Actamin. (Buffington) Acetaminophen 325 mg. Tab. *Dispens-A-Kit* 100s, 200s, 500s. *OTC.*
Use: Analgesic.

Actamine. (H.L. Moore Drug Exchange) **Tab.:** Pseudoephedrine hydrochloride 60 mg, triprolidine hydrochloride 2.5 mg. 100s, 1000s. **Syrup:** Pseudoephedrine hydrochloride 30 mg, triprolidine hydrochloride 1.25 mg/5 mL. 120 mL, Pt, gal. *Rx-OTC.*
Use: Antihistamine; decongestant.

Actamin Extra. (Buffington) Acetaminophen 500 mg. Tab. Bot. 100s, 200s, 500s. *OTC.*
Use: Analgesic.

Actamin Super. (Buffington) Acetaminophen 500 mg, caffeine. Sugar, salt, and lactose free. Tab. *Dispens-A-Kit* 500s, *Medipak* 200s. *OTC.*
Use: Analgesic.

Actemra. (Genetech Inc) Tocilizumab. **Inj., Soln., concentrate:** 20 mg/mL. Disodium phosphate dodecahydrate, sodium dihydrogen phosphate dehydrate (as a 15 mmol/L phosphate buffer), sucrose 50 mg/mL. Preservative free. Single-use vial. 4 mL, 10 mL, 20 mL. **Inj., Soln.:** 162 mg per 0.9 mL. Polysorbate 80. Preservative free. Single-use prefilled syringe. *Rx.*
Use: Immunologic agent, immunomodulator.

ACTH. Adrenocorticotrophic hormone. Adrenocorticotropin.
Use: Corticosteroid.
See: Corticotropin.

ACTH-Actest. (Forest) Repository corticotropin 40 units or 80 units/mL. Gel. Vial 5 mL. *Rx.*
Use: Corticosteroid.

ActHIB. (Sanofi Pasteur) Purified capsular polysaccharide of *Haemophilus* b 10 mcg, tetanus toxoid 24 mcg/0.5 mL. Sucrose 8.5%. Pow. for Inj., lyophilized. Single-dose vials with 7.5 mL vials of diphtheria and tetanus toxoids and pertussis vaccine as diluents or 0.6 mL vial containing 0.4% sodium chloride diluent. *Rx.*
Use: Agent for active immunization, bacterial vaccine.

ActHIB/DTP. (Aventis Pasteur) Diphtheria and tetanus toxoids and pertussis and *Haemophilus influenzae* type b vaccines. One package consists of one

7.5 mL vial of Connaught's DTwP and 10 single-dose vials of ActHIB vaccine. *Rx.*
Use: Immunization.

Acthrel. (Ferring) Corticorelin ovine triflutate 100 mcg. Cake, lyophilized. 5 mL single-dose vial w/diluent. *Rx.*
Use: Diagnostic aid.

ActiBath. (Andrew Jergens) Colloidal oatmeal 20%. Tab. Effervescent. Pkg. 4s. *OTC.*
Use: Emollient.

Acticin. (Bertek) Permethrin 5%. Coconut oil, lanolin alcohols, light mineral oil. Cream. Tube 60 g. *Rx.*
Use: Scabicide.

Acticort 100. (Baker Cummins Dermatologicals) Hydrocortisone 1%. Lot. Bot. 60 mL. *Rx.*
Use: Corticosteroid, topical.

Actidose. (Paddock) Activated charcoal. 25 g/120 mL or 50 g/240 mL. Soln. *OTC.*
Use: Antidote.

Actidose-Aqua. (Paddock) Activated charcoal. 25 g/120 mL or 50 g/240 mL. Aqueous susp. *OTC.*
Use: Antidote.

Actidose w/Sorbitol. (Paddock) Activated charcoal. 25 g in 120 mL susp. w/sorbitol, 50 g in 240 mL susp. w/sorbitol. Liq. *OTC.*
Use: Antidote.

Actifed Cold & Allergy. (J & J) Phenylephrine hydrochloride 10 mg, chlorpheniramine maleate 4 mg. Tab. Pkg. 12s. *OTC.*
Use: Upper respiratory combination, antihistamine, decongestant.

Actifed Cold & Sinus Maximum Strength. (J & J) Pseudoephedrine hydrochloride 30 mg, chlorpheniramine maleate 2 mg, acetaminophen 500 mg. Tab. Pkg. 20s. *OTC.*
Use: Upper respiratory combination, analgesic, antihistamine, decongestant.

Actigall. (Watson) Ursodiol (Ursodeoxycholic acid) 300 mg. Cap. Bot. 100s. *Rx.*
Use: Gallstone solubilizing agent.

Actimmune. (Vidara Therapeutics) Interferon gamma-1b 100 mcg (2 million units) per 0.5 mL. Mannitol 20 mg, sodium succinate 0.36 mg, polysorbate 20 0.05 mg. Preservative free. Single-dose vials. *Rx.*
Use: Immunologic agent, immunomodulator.

actinomycin C. *Name previously used for Cactinomycin.*

actinomycin D.
Use: Antineoplastic.
See: Dactinomycin.

•**actinoquinol sodium.** (ack-TIN-oh-kwih-nole SO-dee-uhm) USAN.
Use: Ultraviolet screen.

actinospectacin. *Name previously used for Spectinomycin.*

Actiq. (Cephalon) Fentanyl citrate (as base) 200 mcg, 400 mcg, 600 mcg, 800 mcg, 1,200 mcg, 1,600 mcg. Sugar (each unit contains ≈ 2 g), berry flavor. Loz. on a stick. 30s with carton blister packs. *c-II.*
Use: Opioid analgesic.

•**actisomide.** (ackt-EYE-so-MIDE) USAN.
Use: Cardiovascular agent.

Activase. (Genentech) Alteplase recombinant 50 mg (29 million U), 100 mg (58 million U). L-arginine, phosphoric acid, polysorbate 80. Pow. for Inj., lyophilized. Vials with diluent (50 mL sterile water for injection) and vacuum (50 mg only); vials with diluent (100 mL sterile water for injection) and 1 transfer device (100 mg only). *Rx.*
Use: Thrombolytic.

activated charcoal. (W.F. Young) Activated charcoal 250 mg. Sugar. Lactose free. Tab. 125s. *OTC.*
Use: Detoxification agent, antidote.

activated charcoal liquid. (Various Mfr.) Activated charcoal 12.5 g, 25 g with propylene glycol. Liq. Bot. 60 mL (12.5 g), 120 mL (25 g). *OTC.*
Use: Antidote.

activated charcoal powder. (Various Mfr.) Activated charcoal 15 g, 30 g, 40 g, 120 g, and 140 g. Pow. *OTC.*
Use: Antidote.

activated charcoal tablets. (Cowley) Activated charcoal 5 g. Tab. Bot. 1000s. *OTC.*
Use: Antidote.

activated ergosterol.
See: Calciferol.

activated 7-dehydrocholesterol.
See: Cholecalciferol.

activated vegetable charcoal. (Mason) Activated vegetable charcoal 260 mg. Cap. 60s. *OTC.*
Use: Detoxification agent, antidote.

Active FE. (GM Pharmaceuticals) Iron 75 mg, vitamins A 2,100 units, D 400 units, E 40 units, B_1 4 mg, B_2 4 mg, B_3 20 mg, B_6 20 mg, B_{12} 30 mcg, C 160 mg, folic acid 1.25 mg, Cu, Mg, Zn. Gluten free, lactose free, sugar free. PEG. 30s. *Rx.*
Use: Multivitamin with minerals (including iron).

active immunization agents.
See: Toxoids.
Vaccines, Bacterial.
Vaccines, Viral.

Active OB. (GM Pharmaceuticals) Folic acid 1 mg, iron 20 mg, vitamins D 400 units, E 30 units, B_1 2 mg, B_2 4 mg, B_6 20 mg, B_{12} 30 mcg, C 100 mg, Cu, Zn, DHA 320 mg. Gluten free, lactose free, sugar free. Glycerin, soy lecithin, vegetable oil. Cap., softgel. 30s. *Rx.*
Use: Prenatal vitamin with minerals.

•**actodigin.** (ACK-toe-dihj-in) USAN.
Use: Cardiovascular agent.

Actonel. (Procter & Gamble) Risedronate sodium 5 mg, 30 mg, 35 mg, 150 mg. Lactose (except 150 mg). Film coated. Tab. 30s (5 mg, 30 mg only), 2000s (5 mg only), dose packs of 1s (150 mg only), dose packs of 3s (150 mg only), dose packs of 4s (35 mg only), dose pack of 12s (35 mg only). *Rx.*
Use: Bisphosphonate.

Actoplus Met. (Takeda) Pioglitazone hydrochloride and metformin hydrochloride 15 mg/500 mg, 15 mg/850 mg. Film coated. Tab. 60s, 180s. *Rx.*
Use: Antidiabetic combination.

ActoPlus Met XR. (Takeda) Pioglitazone/ER metformin hydrochloride 15 mg/1,000 mg, 30 mg/1,000 mg. Film coated. Lactose, PEG. ER Tab. 30s, 60s, 90s. *Rx.*
Use: Antidiabetic agent.

actoquinol sodium.
Use: Ultraviolet screen.

Actos. (Takeda) Pioglitazone hydrochloride 15 mg, 30 mg, 45 mg. Lactose. Tab. Bot. 30s, 90s, 500s. *Rx.*
Use: Antidiabetic, thiazolidinedione.

•**actoxumab.** (ak-TOX-ue-mab) USAN.
Use: Prevention of recurrence of *Clostridium difficile* infection.

Acucron. (Seatrace) Acetaminophen 300 mg, salicylamide 200 mg, phenyltoloxamine 20 mg. Tab. Bot. 100s, 1000s, 5000s. *OTC.*
Use: Analgesic; antihistamine.

Acu-Dyne. (Acme United Corp.) **Douche:** Povidone-iodine. Pkt. 240 mL. **Oint.:** Povidone-iodine. Jar. lb. Pkt. 1.2 g, 2.7 g (100s). **Perineal wash conc.:** Available iodine 1%. Bot. 40 mL. **Prep. Soln.:** Povidone-iodine. Bot. 240 mL, Pt, qt, gal. Pkt. 30 mL, 60 mL. **Skin Cleanser:** Povidone-iodine. Bot. 60 mL, 240 mL, Pt, qt, gal. **Soln., prep. swabs:** Available iodine 1%. Bot. 100s. **Soln., swabsticks:** Povidone-iodine. Pkt. 1 or 3 in 25s. **Whirlpool conc.:** Available iodine 1%. Bot. gal. *OTC.*
Use: Antiseptic; antimicrobial.

Acular. (Allergan) Ketorolac tromethamine 0.5%. Benzalkonium chloride 0.01%, EDTA 0.1%, octoxynol 40, sodium chloride, hydrochloric acid, and/or sodium hydroxide. Ophth. Soln. Drop. Bot. 3 mL, 5 mL, 10 mL. *Rx.*
Use: Nonsteroidal anti-inflammatory drug, ophthalmic.

Acular LS. (Allergan) Ketorolac tromethamine 0.4%. Benzalkonium chloride 0.006%, EDTA 0.015%, sodium chloride, hydrochloric acid, and/or sodium hydroxide. Ophth. Soln. Drop. Bot. 5 mL. *Rx.*
Use: Nonsteroidal anti-inflammatory drug, ophthalmic.

Acuvail. (Allergan) Ketorolac tromethamine 0.45%. Sodium chloride, hydrochloric acid, sodium hydroxide. Preservative free. Single-use vial. 0.4 mL. *Rx.*
Use: Ophthalmic and otic agent, nonsteroidal anti-inflammatory drug.

•**acyclovir.** (A-SIKE-low-vir) *USP.*
Use: Antiviral.
See: Zovirax.
W/Hydrocortisone.
See: Xerese.

acyclovir. (Various Mfr.) Acyclovir. **Tab.:** 400 mg, 800 mg. Bot. 100s, 500s, 1000s (400 mg only). **Cap.:** 200 mg. Bot. 100s. **Susp.:** 200 mg/5 mL. 473 mL. *Rx.*
Use: Antiviral.

•**acyclovir sodium.** (A-SIKE-low-vir) USAN.
Use: Antiviral.
See: Zovirax.

acyclovir sodium. (Various Mfr.) Acyclovir sodium. **Inj.:** 50 mg/mL. Ctns. of 10. **Pow. for Inj.:** 500 mg/vial, 1,000 mg/vial. Vials. 10 mL (500 mg only), 20 mL (1,000 mg only). **Oint.:** 5%. In polyethylene glycol base. Tube. 15 g. *Rx.*
Use: Antiviral.

Aczone. (Allergan) Dapsone 5%. Methylparaben. Gel, Top. 30 g. *Rx.*
Use: Topical anti-infective.

Adacel. (Aventis Pasteur) Diphtheria toxoid 2 Lf units, tetanus toxoid 5 Lf units, pertactin 3 mcg, filamentous hemagglutinin (FHA) 5 mcg, detoxified pertussis toxins 2.5 mcg, fimbriae types 2 and 3 5 mcg per 0.5 mL. Formaldehyde, phenoxyethanol. Inj. Single-dose vials. *Rx.*
Use: Immunization.

Adagen. (Enzon) Pegademase bovine 250 units/mL. Monobasic sodium phosphate 1.2 mg, dibasic sodium phosphate 5.58 mg, sodium chloride 8.5 mg,

water for inj. Preservative free. IM Soln. Single-use vial. 1.5 mL. *Rx.*
Use: Enzyme (ADA) replacement therapy.

Adalat CC. (Schering) Nifedipine 30 mg, 60 mg, 90 mg. Lactose. Film coated. ER Tab. Bot. 100s, 1000s (except 90 mg), UD 100s. *Rx.*
Use: Calcium channel blocker.

•**adalimumab.** (ah-dah-LIM-you-mab) USAN.
Use: Immunomodulator.
See: Humira.

adamantanamine hydrochloride.
See: Amantadine Hydrochloride. Symmetrel.

•**adapalene.** (ADE-ah-PALE-een) USAN.
Use: Dermatologic, acne, retinoid.
See: Differin.
W/Benzoyl Peroxide.
See: Epiduo.

adapalene. (Fougera) Adapalene 0.1%. Edetate disodium, glycerin, parabens, PEG-20, phenoxyethanol, squalane, trolamine. Cream 45 g. *Rx.*
Use: Retinoid.

adapalene. (Various Mfr.) Adapalene. **Cream:** 0.1%. Edetate disodium, glycerin, parabens, PEG-20, phenoxyethanol, squalane, trolamine. 45 g. **Gel:** 0.1%. Disodium edetate, methylparaben, propylene glycol. 45 g. *Rx.*
Use: Retinoid.

Adapettes for Sensitive Eyes. (Alcon) Povidone and other water-soluble polymers, EDTA, sorbic acid. Pkg. 15 mL. *OTC.*
Use: Contact lens care.

Adapin. (Lotus Biochemical) Doxepin hydrochloride **10 mg, 75 mg, 100 mg:** Cap. Bot. 100s, 1000s, UD 100s. **25 mg, 50 mg:** Cap. Bot. 100s, 1000s, 5000s, UD 100s. **150 mg:** Cap. Bot. 50s, 100s. *Rx.*
Use: Antidepressant.

•**adaprolol maleate.** (ad-AH-prole-ole MAL-ee-ate) USAN.
Use: Antihypertensive, β-blocker, ophthalmic.

Adapt. (Alcon) Povidone, EDTA 0.1%, thimerosal 0.004%. Bot. 15 mL. *OTC.*
Use: Contact lens care.

Adapt Wetting Solution. (Alcon) Adsorbobase with thimerosal 0.004%, EDTA 0.1%. Soln. Bot. 15 mL. *OTC.*
Use: Contact lens care.

Adasuve. (Teva) Loxapine 10 mg. Pow.; Inhal. Single-use inhaler. *Rx.*
Use: Antipsychotic.

•**adatanserin hydrochloride.** (ahd-at-AN-ser-in HIGH-droe-KLOR-ide) USAN.
Use: Antidepressant; anxiolytic.

AdatoSil 5000. (Escalon Ophthalmics, Inc.) Polydimethylsiloxane oil. Inj. Vial 10 mL, 15 mL. *Rx.*
Use: Ophthalmic.

Adavite. (Hudson Corp.) Vitamins A 5000 units, D 400 units, E 30 mg, B_1 3 mg, B_2 3.4 mg, B_3 30 mg, B_5 10 mg, B_6 3 mg, B_{12} 9 mcg, C 90 mg, folic acid 0.4 mg, biotin 35 mcg, beta-carotene 1250 units. Tab. Bot. 130s. *OTC.*
Use: Mineral, vitamin supplement.

Adavite-M. (Hudson Corp.) Iron 27 mg, Vitamins A 5000 units, D 400 units, E 30 mg, B_1 3 mg, B_2 3.4 mg, B_3 20 mg, B_5 10 mg, B_6 3 mg, B_{12} 9 mcg, C 190 mg, folic acid 0.4 mg, Ca, Cl, Cr, Cu, I, K, Mg, Mn, Mo, P, Se, Zinc 15 mg, biotin 30 mcg. Tab. Bot. 130s. *OTC.*
Use: Mineral, vitamin supplement.

Adcetris. (Seattle Genetics) Brentuximab vedotin 50 mg. Trehalose dihydrate 70 mg/mL, polysorbate 80 0.2 mg/mL. Preservative free. Inj., lyophilized Pow. for Soln. Single-use vial. *Rx.*
Use: Antineoplastic agent, antibody-drug conjugate.

Adcirca. (Eli Lilly) Tadalafil 20 mg. Film coated. Lactose. Tab. 60s. *Rx.*
Use: Impotence agent, phosphodiesterase type 5 inhibitor.

ADC with Fluoride. (Various Mfr.) Fluoride 0.5 mg, vitamins A 1500 units, D 400 units, C 35 mg, methylparaben/mL. Drops. Bot. 50 mL. *Rx.*
Use: Mineral, vitamin supplement.

Adderall. (Teva) **5 mg:** Dextroamphetamine saccharate 1.25 mg, amphetamine aspartate 1.25 mg, dextroamphetamine sulfate 1.25 mg, amphetamine sulfate 1.25 mg. **7.5 mg:** Dextroamphetamine saccharate 1.875 mg, amphetamine aspartate 1.875 mg, dextroamphetamine sulfate 1.875 mg, amphetamine sulfate 1.875 mg. **10 mg:** Dextroamphetamine sulfate 2.5 mg, dextroamphetamine saccharate 2.5 mg, amphetamine aspartate 2.5 mg, amphetamine sulfate 2.5 mg. **12.5 mg:** Dextroamphetamine saccharate 3.125 mg, amphetamine aspartate 3.125 mg, dextroamphetamine sulfate 3.125 mg, amphetamine sulfate 3.125 mg. **15 mg:** Dextroamphetamine saccharate 3.75 mg, amphetamine aspartate monohydrate 3.75 mg, dextroamphetamine sulfate 3.75 mg, amphetamine sulfate 3.75 mg. **20 mg:** Dextroamphetamine sulfate 5 mg, dextro-

amphetamine saccharide 5 mg, amphetamine aspartate 5 mg, amphetamine sulfate 5 mg. **30 mg:** Dextroamphetamine saccharate 7.5 mg, amphetamine aspartate 7.5 mg, dextroamphetamine sulfate 7.5 mg, amphetamine sulfate 7.5 mg. Lactose, sucrose. Tab. Bot. 100s. *c-II.*
Use: CNS stimulant, amphetamine.

Adderall XR. (Shire) **5 mg:** Dextroamphetamine saccharate 1.25 mg, amphetamine aspartate monohydrate 1.25 mg, dextroamphetamine sulfate 1.25 mg, amphetamine sulfate 1.25 mg. **10 mg:** Dextroamphetamine saccharate 2.5 mg, amphetamine aspartate monohydrate 2.5 mg, dextroamphetamine sulfate 2.5 mg, amphetamine sulfate 2.5 mg. **15 mg:** Dextroamphetamine saccharate 3.75 mg, amphetamine aspartate monohydrate 3.75 mg, dextroamphetamine sulfate 3.75 mg, amphetamine sulfate 3.75 mg. **20 mg:** Dextroamphetamine saccharate 5 mg, amphetamine aspartate monohydrate 5 mg, dextroamphetamine sulfate 5 mg, amphetamine sulfate 5 mg. **25 mg:** Dextroamphetamine saccharate 6.25 mg, amphetamine aspartate monohydrate 6.25 mg, dextroamphetamine sulfate 6.25 mg, amphetamine sulfate 6.25 mg. **30 mg:** Dextroamphetamine saccharate 7.5 mg, amphetamine aspartate monohydrate 7.5 mg, dextroamphetamine sulfate 7.5 mg, amphetamine sulfate 7.5 mg. Talc (except 10 mg, 20 mg, 30 mg). Sugar spheres. Cap. Bot. 100s. *c-II.*
Use: CNS stimulant, amphetamine.

Adeecon. (CMC) Vitamins A 5000 units, D 1000 units. Cap. Bot. 1000s. *OTC.*
Use: Vitamin supplement.

•**adefovir dipivoxil.** (ah-DEF-fah-vihr die-pih-vox-ill) USAN.
Use: Antiviral, treatment of HIV and HBV infections.
See: Hepsera.

adefovir dipivoxil. (Sigmapharm Laboratories) Adefovir dipivoxil 10 mg. May contain lactose. Tab. 30s. *Rx.*
Use: Anti-infective, antiviral agent.

ADEKs Pediatric. (Scandipharm, Inc.) Vitamin A 1500 units, D 400 units, E 40 units, K_1 0.1 mg, C 45 mg, B_1 0.5 mg, B_2 0.6 mg, B_3 6 mg, B_5 3 mg, B_6 0.6 mg, B_{12} 4 mcg, biotin 15 mcg, Zn 5 mg, beta-carotene 1 mg per mL. Drops. Bot. 60 mL. *OTC.*
Use: Vitamin supplement.

Adempas. (Bayer Healthcare) Riociguat 0.5 mg, 1 mg, 1.5 mg, 2 mg, 2.5 mg. Film coated. Lactose. Tab. 90s, UD 42s. *Rx.*
Use: Vasodilator, soluble guanylate cyclase stimulator.

•**adenine.** (A-de-neen) *USP.*
Use: Vitamin.

adeno-associated viral-based vector cystic fibrosis gene therapy. (Targeted Genetics)
Use: Cystic fibrosis. [Orphan Drug]

Adenocard. (Fujisawa) Adenosine 3 mg/mL, sodium chloride 9 mg/mL. Preservative free. Inj. Vial. 2 mL. Syringe. 2 mL, 5 mL. *Rx.*
Use: Antiarrhythmic.

Adenolin Forte. (Lincoln Diagnostics) Adenosine-5-monophosphate 25 mg, methionine 25 mg, niacin 10 mg/mL. Inj. Vial 15 mL. *Rx.*
Use: Anti-inflammatory.

Adenoscan. (Fujisawa Healthcare) Adenosine 3 mg/mL. Sodium chloride 9 mg/mL. Preservative free. Inj. Single-dose vial. 20 mL, 30 mL. *Rx.*
Use: Diagnostic aid.

•**adenosine.** (ah-DEN-oh-seen) *USP.*
Use: Antiarrhythmic.
See: Adenocard.
Adenoscan.

adenosine. (Medco Research)
Use: Antineoplastic. [Orphan Drug]

adenosine. (Various Mfr.) Adenosine 3 mg/mL. Sodium chloride 9 mg/mL. Preservative free. Inj. Vials. 2 mL, 4 mL. Disposable syringes. 2 mL. *Rx.*
Use: Antiarrhythmic agent.

adenosine in gelatin. (Forest) **Forte:** Adenosine-5-monophosphate 50 mg/mL. **Super:** Adenosine-5-monophosphate 100 mg/mL. *Rx.*
Use: Varicosity.

Adeno Twelve. (Forest) Adenosine-5-monophosphate 25 mg, methionine 25 mg, niacin 10 mg/mL. Gel. Inj. Vial 10 mL. *Rx.*
Use: Anti-inflammatory.

adenovirus vaccine type 4. (Wyeth) Adenovirus vaccine live type 4. At least 32,000 $TCID_{50}$. Tab. Bot. 100s. *Rx.*
Use: Immunization.

adenovirus vaccine type 7. (Wyeth) Adenovirus vaccine live type 7. At least 32,000 $TCID_{50}$. Tab. Bot. 100s. *Rx.*
Use: Immunization.

adepsine oil.
See: Petrolatum.

AdGVCFTR 10. (GenVec)
Use: Cystic fibrosis. [Orphan Drug]

•**adinazolam.** (AHD-in-AZE-oh-lam) USAN.

Use: Antidepressant; hypnotic, sedative.

•**adinazolam mesylate.** (AHD-in-AZE-oh-lam MEH-sih-LATE) USAN.
Use: Antidepressant.

Adipex-P. (Gate) **Cap.:** Phentermine hydrochloride 37.5 mg (equiv. to phentermine base 30 mg). Lactose. 100s. **Tab.:** Phentermine hydrochloride 37.5 mg (equiv. to phentermine base 30 mg). Lactose, sucrose. 30s, 100s. *c-iv.*
Use: CNS stimulant, anorexiant.

•**adiphenine hydrochloride.** (ah-DIH-feh-neen HIGH-droe-KLOR-ide) USAN.
Use: Muscle relaxant.

Adisol. (Major) Disulfiram 250 mg, 500 mg. Tab. Bot. 50s (500 mg only), 100s (250 mg only). *Rx.*
Use: Antialcoholic.

Adlerika. (Last) Magnesium sulfate 4 g/15 mL. Bot. 12 oz. *OTC.*
Use: Laxative.

Adlone. (Forest) Methylprednisolone acetate 40 mg, 80 mg. Inj. Vial 5 mL. *Rx.*
Use: Corticosteroid, topical.

Adolph's Salt Substitute. (Adolphs) Potassium chloride 2480 mg/5 g, silicon dioxide, tartaric acid. Gran. Bot. 99.2 g. *OTC.*
Use: Salt substitute.

Adolph's Seasoned Salt Substitute. (Adolphs) Potassium chloride 1360 mg/5 g, silicon dioxide, tartaric acid. Gran. Bot. 92.1 g. *OTC.*
Use: Salt substitute.

•**adomiparin.** (A-doe-mi-PAR- in) USAN.
Use: Anticoagulant.

•**adomiparin sodium.** (A-doe-mi-PAR- in) USAN.
Use: Anticoagulant.

Adonidine. (City Chemical Corp.) Bot. g. *Rx.*
Use: Cardiovascular agent.

•**adozelesin.** (ADE-oh-ZELL-eh-sin) USAN.
Use: Antineoplastic.

Adprin-B. (Pfeiffer) Aspirin 325 mg, calcium carbonate, magnesium carbonate, magnesium oxide. Tab. Bot. 130s. *OTC.*
Use: Analgesic.

ADR.
Use: Antineoplastic.
See: Doxorubicin Hydrochloride.

Adrenaclick. (Amedra Pharmaceuticals) Epinephrine 0.15 mg per 0.15 mL, 0.3 mg per 0.3 mL. Chlorobutanol, sodium bisulfite. Inj., Soln. Single-dose autoinjector. 0.15 mL (0.15 mg per 0.15 mL), 0.3 mL (0.3 mg per 0.3 mL). *Rx.*
Use: Vasopressor used in shock.

adrenalin chloride. (JHP Pharmaceuticals) Epinephrine (as hydrochloride) **Soln., intranasal:** 1:1,000 (1 mg/mL). Chlorobutanol, sodium bisulfite. 30 mL. **Inj., Soln.:** 1:1,000 (1 mg/mL) Vial. 1 mL (w/sodium bisulfite), 30 mL (w/chlorobutanol and sodium bisulfite). *Rx.*
Use: Vasopressor used in shock.

adrenalin(e).
See: Epinephrine.

adrenaline hydrochloride.
See: Epinephrine Hydrochloride.

•**adrenalone.** (ah-DREN-ah-lone) USAN.
Use: Adrenergic, ophthalmic.

adrenamine.
See: Epinephrine.

adrenergic agents.
See: Sympathomimetic agents.

adrenergic-blocking agents.
See: Sympatholytic agents.

adrenine.
See: Epinephrine.

adrenocortical steroids.
See: Corticotropin.
Corticotropin, repository injection.
Glucocorticoids.
Mineralocorticoids.

adrenocorticotrophic hormone. ACTH acts by stimulating the endogenous production of cortisone. *Rx.*
See: ACTH.
Corticotropin.

Adrenoid. (MedChem) Vitamin B_{12} 50 mcg, Cu, I, Mg, Mn, Mo, Se, Zn, ashwagandha root 100 mg, bladderwrack 25 mg, cayenne pepper 15 mg, schizandra 120 mg, L-tyrosine 150 mg. Cap. 60s. *OTC.*
Use: Multivitamin with minerals (except iron).

Adrenucleo. (Enzyme Process) Vitamin C 250 mg, d-calcium pantothenate 12.5 mg, bioflavonoids 62.5 mg. Tab. Bot. 100s, 250s. *OTC.*
Use: Vitamin supplement.

AdreView. (GE Healthcare) Iobenguane sulfate I 123 74 MBq (2 mCi) per mL at calibration (each mL contains iobenguane sulfate 0.08 mg, sodium dihydrogen phosphate dihydrate 23 mg, disodium hydrogen phosphate dihydrate 2.8 mg, benzyl alcohol 10.3 mg [1% v/v]). Preservative free. Single-use vial. 5 mL. *Rx.*
Use: Radiopharmaceutical.

Adriamycin. (Bedford Laboratories) Doxorubicin hydrochloride. **Inj., lyophilized Pow. for Soln.:** 10 mg, 20 mg,

50 mg. Single-dose vial. **Inj., Soln.:** 2 mg/mL. Single-dose vial: 5 mL, 10 mL, 25 mL. Multidose vial: 100 mL. *Rx.*
Use: Antibiotic, anthracycline.

•**adrogolide hydrochloride.** (a-DROE-goe-lide) USAN.
Use: Parkinson disease.

Adrucil. (Gensia Sicor) Fluorouracil 50 mg/mL. Inj. Vial 10 mL, 50 mL, 100 mL. *Rx.*
Use: Antineoplastic; antimetabolite.

Adsorbocarpine. (Alcon) Pilocarpine hydrochloride 1%, 2%, 4%. Bot. 15 mL. *Rx.*
Use: Miotic.

Adsorbotear. (Alcon) Hydroxyethylcellulose 0.4%, povidone 1.67%, water-soluble polymers, thimerosal 0.004%, EDTA 0.1%. Soln. Bot. dropper 15 mL. *OTC.*
Use: Artificial tears.

•**aducanumab.** (A-due-KAN-ue-mab) USAN.
Use: Treatment of Alzheimer disease.

Adult Acnomel. (Numark) Sulfur 8%. resorcinol 2%, alcohol 15%, propylene glycol. Cream. Tube. 28 g. *OTC.*
Use: Keratolytic, acne product.

Advair Diskus. (GlaxoSmithKline) Fluticasone propionate 100 mcg, salmeterol 50 mcg; fluticasone propionate 250 mcg, salmeterol 50 mcg; fluticasone propionate 500 mcg, salmeterol 50 mcg. Lactose. Pow. for Inh. Disp. device w/28 and 60 blisters. *Rx.*
Use: Respiratory inhalant combination.

Advair HFA. (GlaxoSmithKline) Fluticasone propionate/salmeterol 45 mg/21 mcg, 115 mg/21 mcg, 230 mg/21 mcg. Inh. Aerosol Spray. 12 g pressurized aluminum canister containing 120 metered inhalations. Boxes. 1s. *Rx.*
Use: Respiratory inhalant combination.

Advance. (Ross) **Ready-to-Feed Infant Formula:** (16 cal/fl oz). Can 13 fl oz. **Conc. Liq:** 32 fl oz. *OTC.*
Use: Nutritional supplement.

Advanced Care Cholesterol Test. (Johnson & Johnson)
Use: At home cholesterol test.

Advanced D5000. (Mason Vitamins) Vitamin D 5,000 units. Soybean oil. Cap., softgel. 50s. *OTC.*
Use: Fat-soluble vitamin.

Advanced Ear Health Formula. (Mason) Vitamin B_1 0.33 mg, B_2 1 mg, B_3 3.33 mg, B_5 1.66 mg, B_6 1.66 mg, B_{12} 300 mcg, Ca, bioflavonoids 300 mg, choline 111.33 mg, inositol 111.33 mg. Sugar free. Tab. 100s. *OTC.*
Use: Multivitamin with minerals.

Advanced Eye Relief. (Bausch & Lomb) Propylene glycol 0.95%, boric acid, edentate disodium, sodium borate, sodium chloride. Preservative free. Soln., Ophth. Single-use container. *OTC.*
Use: Artificial tear solution.

Advanced Eye Relief Preservative Free. (Bausch & Lomb) Propylene glycol 0.95%, boric acid, edetate disodium, sodium borate, sodium chloride. Preservative free. Soln.; Ophth. Single-use container. *OTC.*
Use: Artificial tears.

Advanced Eye Relief, Redness Instant Relief. (Bausch & Lomb) Naphazoline hydrochloride 0.012%. 0.2% of polyethylene 300, benzalkonium chloride 0.01%, boric acid, sodium borate, sodium chloride, EDTA. Soln., Ophth. 15 mL. *Rx.*
Use: Ophthalmic and otic agent, ophthalmic decongestant.

Advanced Eye Relief, Redness Maximum Relief. (Bausch & Lomb) Naphazoline hydrochloride 0.03%. Benzalkonium chloride 0.01%, boric acid, EDTA, hydroxypropyl methylcellulose 0.5%, sodium borate, sodium chloride. Soln., Ophth. 15 mL. *OTC.*
Use: Ophthalmic and otic agent, ophthalmic decongestant.

Advanced Formula Centrum Liquid. (Wyeth) Vitamins A 2500 units, E 30 units, C 60 mg, B_1 1.5 mg, B_2 1.7 mg, B_3 20 mg, B_5 10 mg, B_6 2 mg, B_{12} 6 mcg, D 400 units, iron 9 mg, biotin 300 mcg, I, Zn 3 mg, Mn, Cr, Mo, alcohol 6.7%, sucrose. Bot. 236 mL. *OTC.*
Use: Mineral, vitamin supplement.

Advanced Formula Centrum Tablets. (Wyeth) Iron 18 mg, vitamins A 5000 units, D 400 units, E 30 units, B_1 1.5 mg, B_2 1.7 mg, B_3 20 mg, B_5 10 mg, B_6 2 mg, B_{12} 6 mcg, C 60 mg, folic acid 0.4 mg, biotin 30 mcg, B, Ca, Cl, Cr, Cu, I, K, Mg, Mn, Mo, Ni, P, Se, Si, Sn, V, Zn 15 mg, vitamin K. Bot. 60s, 130s, 200s. *OTC.*
Use: Mineral, vitamin supplement.

Advanced Formula Cerovite. (Rugby) Iron 3 mg, vitamins E 10 units, B_1 0.5 mg, B_2 0.57 mg, B_3 6.7 mg, B_5 3.3 mg, B_6 0.67 mg, B_{12} 2 mcg, C 20 mg, Cr, I, Mn, Mo, Zn, biotin. BHA, citrus flavoring, EDTA, ethyl alcohol 5.7%, glycerin, lemon flavoring, polysorbate 80, potassium sorbate, propylene glycol, sodium benzoate, sucrose. Liq. 237 mL. *OTC.*
Use: Multivitamin with minerals.

Advanced Formula Zenate. (Solvay) Fe

65 mg, vitamins A 3000 units, D 400 units, E 10 units, C 70 mg, folic acid 1 mg, B_1 1.5 mg, B_2 1.6 mg, B_3 17 mg, B_6 2.2 mg, B_{12} 2.2 mcg, Ca 200 mg, I 175 mcg, Mg 100 mg, Zn 15 mg. Tab. UD 30s. *Rx.*
Use: Mineral, vitamin supplement.

Advance Pregnancy Test. (Johnson & Johnson) Can be used as early as 3 days after a missed period. Gives results in 30 min. Test kit 1s.
Use: Diagnostic aid.

Advate. (Baxter) Antihemophilic factor (recombinant) 250 units, 500 units, 1,000 units, 1,500 units, 2,000 units, 3,000 units, 4,000 units. Solvent/Detergent treated, monoclonal antibody purified. Von Willebrand factor ≤ 2 ng per AHF unit, glutathione, histidine, sodium, mannitol (except 3,000 units), polysorbate 80 (except 3,000 units). Preservative free and plasma/albumin free. Inj., lyophilized Pow. for Soln. In kits with single-use vials and diluent (5 mL of sterile water for injection). *Rx.*
Use: Antihemophilic agent.

Advera. (Ross) Protein 14.2 g, fat 5.4 g, carbohydrate 51.2 g, l-carnitine 30 mg, taurine 50 mg, vitamins A 2550 units, D 80 units, E 9 units, K 24 mcg, C 90 mg, folic acid 120 mcg, B, 0.75 mg, B_2 0.68 mg, B_6 9.5 mg, B_{12} 12 mcg, niacin 6 mg, choline 50 mg, biotin 50 mcg, B_5 3 mg, sodium 250 mg, potassium 670 mg, chloride 350 mg, Ca 260 mg, Ph 260 mg, Mg 50 mg, I 30 mcg, Mn 1.3 mg, Cu 0.5 mg, Zn 2 mg, Fe 4.5 mg, Se 14 mcg, chromium 17 mcg, Md 54 mcg/240 mL, 1.28 calories/mL, vanilla flavor. Liq. Bot. 273 mL. *OTC.*
Use: Nutritional supplement, enteral.

Advicor. (AbbVie) Niacin (extended release)/lovastatin 500 mg/20 mg, 750 mg/20 mg, 1,000 mg/20 mg, 1,000 mg/40 mg. PEG. Tab. 90s. *Rx.*
Use: Antihyperlipidemic.

Advil. (Pfizer Consumer Healthcare) Ibuprofen. **Cap.:** 200 mg. Sorbitol. 4s, 20s, 40s, 80s. **Tab.:** 200 mg. Sucrose. Tab. Bot. 8s, 24s, 50s, 72s, 100s, 165s, 250s. *OTC.*
Use: Analgesic; NSAID.

Advil Allergy Sinus. (Pfizer Consumer Healthcare) Pseudoephedrine hydrochloride 30 mg, chlorpheniramine maleate 2 mg, ibuprofen 200 mg. PEG. Tab. 20s, 40s. *OTC.*
Use: Upper respiratory combination, decongestant, antihistamine, analgesic.

Advil, Children's. (Pfizer Consumer Healthcare) Ibuprofen 100 mg/5 mL. Fruit flavor, sorbitol, sucrose, EDTA. Susp. Bot. 119 mL, 473 mL. *OTC.*
Use: Analgesic; NSAID.

Advil Children's Cold. (Pfizer Consumer Healthcare) Ibuprofen 100 mg, pseudoephedrine hydrochloride 15 mg. Edetate disodium, glycerin, polysorbate 80, sodium 3 mg, sodium benzoate, sorbitol, sucrose. Grape flavor. Susp. 120 mL. *OTC.*
Use: Upper respiratory combination, decongestant and analgesic combination.

Advil Cold & Sinus. (Pfizer Consumer Healthcare) Pseudoephedrine hydrochloride 30 mg, ibuprofen 200 mg. Parabens, sucrose. **Liqui-gels:** Liquid filled. PEG, sorbitol. 16s. **Tab.:** Bot. 20s. *OTC.*
Use: Upper respiratory combination, analgesic, decongestant.

Advil Flu & Body Ache. (Pfizer Consumer Healthcare) Pseudoephedrine hydrochloride 30 mg, ibuprofen 200 mg, parabens, sucrose. Tab. Pkg. 20s. *OTC.*
Use: Upper respiratory combination, analgesic, decongestant.

Advil Liqui-Gels. (Pfizer Consumer Healthcare) Ibuprofen 200 mg. Sorbitol. Cap. Bot. 4s, 20s, 40s, 80s. *OTC.*
Use: Analgesic; NSAID.

Advil Migraine. (Pfizer Consumer Healthcare) Ibuprofen 200 mg. Sorbitol. Cap. Bot. 20s. *OTC.*
Use: Analgesic; NSAID.

Advil Pediatric Drops. (Pfizer Consumer Healthcare) Ibuprofen 100 mg/2.5 mL. Sorbitol, sucrose, EDTA, glycerin, grape flavor. Susp. Bot. 7.5 mL. *OTC.*
Use: Analgesic; NSAID.

Advil PM. (Pfizer Consumer Healthcare) **Tab.:** Diphenhydramine citrate 38 mg, ibuprofen 200 mg. Lactose. 20s, UD 50s. **Cap.:** Diphenhydramine hydrochloride 25 mg, ibuprofen 200 mg. Sorbitol. 38s. *OTC.*
Use: Nonprescription sleep aid.

A.E.R. (Birchwood) Hamamelis water (witch hazel) 50%, glycerin 12.5%, methylparaben, benzalkonium chloride. Pads. Jar 40s. *OTC.*
Use: Dermatologic.

Aerdil. (Econo Med Pharmaceuticals) Triprolidine hydrochloride 1.25 mg, pseudoephedrine hydrochloride 30 mg/5 mL. Bot. Pt, gal. *OTC.*
Use: Antihistamine; decongestant.

Aerocell. (Health & Medical Techniques) Exfoliative cytology fixative spray. Bot. 3.5 oz.
Use: Exfoliative cytology fixative spray.

Aerofreeze. (Graham Field) Trichloro-

monofluoromethane and dichlorodifluoromethane. Spray. Cont. 240 mL. *OTC.*
Use: Anesthetic, local.

AeroHist. (Aero) Chlorpheniramine maleate 8 mg, methscopolamine nitrate 2.5 mg. ER Tab. 100s. *Rx.*
Use: Upper respiratory combination, decongestant, antihistamine, and anticholinergic combination.

AeroHist Plus. (Aero) Phenylephrine hydrochloride 20 mg, chlorpheniramine maleate 8 mg, methscopolamine nitrate 2.5 mg. ER Tab. 100s. *Rx.*
Use: Upper respiratory combination, decongestant, antihistamine, and anticholinergic combination.

AeroKid. (Aero) Phenylephrine hydrochloride 10 mg, chlorpheniramine maleate 4 mg, methscopolamine nitrate 1.25 mg per 5 mL. Sorbitol, saccharin, blue raspberry flavor. Syrup. 20 mL, 120 mL, 473 mL. *Rx.*
Use: Upper respiratory combination, decongestant, antihistamine, and anticholinergic combination.

Aeropin.
Use: Cystic fibrosis. [Orphan Drug]

Aeropure. (Health & Medical Techniques) Isopropanol 7.8%, triethylene glycol 3.9%, essential oils 3%, methyldodecyl benzyl trimethyl ammonium chloride 0.12%, methyldodecylxylene bis (trimethyl ammonium chloride) 0.03%, inert ingredients 85.15%. Bot. 0.8 oz, 4.5 oz.
Use: Antiseptic; deodorant.

Aeroseb-Dex. (Allergan) Dexamethasone 0.01%, alcohol 65.1%. Aerosol 58 g. *Rx.*
Use: Corticosteroid, topical.

Aerosil. (Health & Medical Techniques) Dimethylpolysiloxane. Bot. 4.5 oz.
Use: Lubricant; protectant.

Aerosol OT.
See: Docusate Sodium.

Aerosolv. (Health & Medical Techniques) Isopropyl alcohol, methylene chloride, silicone. Aerosol 5.5 oz.
Use: Adhesive remover.

Aerospan. (Forest) Flunisolide hemihydrate ≈ 80 mcg (flunisolide 78 mcg)/actuation. Aerosol. Canisters. 5.1 g (60 metered actuations), 8.9 g (120 metered actuations). *Rx.*
Use: Corticosteroid.

AeroTuss 12. (Aero Pharmaceuticals, Inc.) Dextromethorphan HBr 30 mg per 5 mL. Methylparaben, sodium saccharin, sucrose. Grape flavor. Susp. 237 mL. *Rx.*
Use: Nonnarcotic antitussive.

AeroZoin. (Health & Medical Techniques) Benzoin compound tincture 30%, isopropyl alcohol 44.8%. Spray Bot. 3.5 oz. *OTC.*
Use: Dermatologic, protectant.

•**afatinib.** (a-FA-ti-nib) USAN.
Use: Antineoplastic.
See: Gilotrif.

•**afatinib dimaleate.** (a-FA-ti-nib) USAN.
Use: Antineoplastic.

Afaxin. (Sanofi-Synthelabo) Vitamin A Palmitate 10,000 units, 50,000 units. Cap. Bot. *Rx-OTC.*
Use: Vitamin supplement.

Afeditab CR. (Watson) Nifedipine 30 mg, 60 mg. ER Tab. 100s. *Rx.*
Use: Calcium channel blocker.

•**afegostat.** (a-FEG-oh-stat) USAN.
Use: Gaucher disease.

•**afegostat tartrate.** (a-FEG-oh-stat) USAN.
Use: Gaucher disease.

A-Fil. (PharmaDerm) Methyl anthranilate 5%, titanium dioxide 5% in vanishing cream base. Tube 45 g. Neutral or dark. *OTC.*
Use: Sunscreen.

•**afimoxifene.** (a-fim-OX-i-feen) USAN.
Use: Antineoplastic.

Afinitor. (Novartis) Everolimus 2.5 mg, 5 mg, 7.5 mg, 10 mg. Butylated hydroxytoluene, lactose. Tab. UD 28s. *Rx.*
Use: Protein-tyrosine kinase inhibitor, mTOR inhibitor.

Afinitor Disperz. (Novartis) Everolimus 2 mg, 3 mg, 5 mg. Butylated hydroxytoluene, lactose, mannitol. Tab. for Susp. UD 28s. *Rx.*
Use: Kinase inhibitor, mTOR inhibitor.

Afko-Lube. (A.P.C.) Docusate sodium 100 mg. Cap. Bot. 100s. *OTC.*
Use: Laxative.

Afko-Lube Lax. (A.P.C.) Docusate sodium 100 mg, casanthranol 30 mg. Cap. Bot. 100s. *OTC.*
Use: Laxative.

•**aflibercept.** (A-fli-BER-sept) USAN.
Use: Selective vascular endothelial growth factor antagonist.
See: Eylea.

Afluria. (CSL Biotherapies) Hemagglutinin 15 mcg each of A/California/7/2009 NYMC X-181 (H1N1), A/Texas/50/2012 NYMC X-223 (H3N2) (an A/Victoria/361/2011-like strain), and B/Massachusetts/2/2012 NYMC BX-51B per 0.5 mL. Mercury 24.5 mcg/dose. Each dose may contain residual amounts of sodium taurodeoxycholate (≤ 10 ppm), ovalbumin (≤ 1 mcg), neomycin sulfate

(≤ 3 ng), polymyxin B (≤ 0.5 ng), and beta-propiolactone (≤ 2 ng). Inj., Susp. (purified split virus). Preservative-free, 0.5 mL prefilled single-dose syringes and 5 mL multidose vials with preservative (thimerosal). *Rx.*
Use: Viral vaccine.

•**afovirsen sodium.** (aff-oh-VEER-sen SO-dee-uhm) USAN.
Use: Antiviral.

•**afoxolaner.** (a-FOX-oh-LAN-er) USAN.
Use: Insecticide.

Afrin. (Schering-Plough) Oxymetazoline hydrochloride 0.05%. **Nose Drops:** Drop. Bot. 20 mL. **Nasal Spray:** Reg. Bot. 15 mL, 30 mL; Menthol. Bot. 15 mL. **Children's Nose Drops:** Oxymetazoline hydrochloride 0.025%. Drop. Bot. 20 mL. *OTC.*
Use: Decongestant.

Afrin All Night No Drip. (Schering-Plough) Oxymetazoline hydrochloride 0.05%. Benzalkonium chloride, benzyl alcohol, edetate disodium, flower oil, glycerin, PEG. Soln., intranasal. 15 mL. *OTC.*
Use: Nasal decongestant, imidazoline.

Afrin Extra Moisturizing. (Schering-Plough) Oxymetazoline hydrochloride 0.05%. Benzalkonium chloride, edetate disodium. Soln., Intranasal Spray. 15 mL. *OTC.*
Use: Nasal decongestant, imidazoline.

Afrin Moisturizing Saline Mist. (Schering-Plough) Sodium chloride 0.64%, benzalkonium chloride, EDTA. Soln. Bot. 30 mL. *OTC.*
Use: Decongestant.

Afrin No-Drip 12-Hour. (Schering-Plough) Oxymetazoline hydrochloride 0.05%, carboxymethylcellulose sodium, microcrystalline cellulose, benzalkonium chloride, benzyl alcohol, EDTA. Soln. Spray Bot. 15 mL. *OTC.*
Use: Nasal decongestant, imidazoline.

Afrin No-Drip 12-Hour Extra Moisturizing. (Schering-Plough) Oxymetazoline hydrochloride 0.05%, carboxymethylcellulose sodium, microcrystalline cellulose, benzalkonium chloride, benzyl alcohol, EDTA, glycerin, Soln. Spray Bot. 15 mL. *OTC.*
Use: Nasal decongestant, imidazoline.

Afrinol Repetabs. (Schering-Plough) Pseudoephedrine sulfate 120 mg. Repeat Action Tab. Box 12s, bot. 100s, dispensary pack 48s. *OTC.*
Use: Decongestant.

Afrin Severe Congestion with Menthol. (Schering-Plough) Oxymetazoline hydrochloride 0.05%, benzalkonium chloride, benzyl alcohol, camphor, EDTA, eucalyptol, menthol. Soln. Spray Bot. 15 mL. *OTC.*
Use: Nasal decongestant, imidazoline.

Afrin Sinus. (Schering-Plough) Oxymetazoline hydrochloride 0.05%, benzyl alcohol. Spray. Bot. 15 mL. *OTC.*
Use: Decongestant.

Afrin Sinus 12 Hour Relief. (Schering-Plough) Oxymetazoline hydrochloride 0.05%. Benzalkonium chloride, benzyl alcohol, camphor, EDTA, eucalyptol, menthol. Soln., Intranasal Spray. 15 mL. *OTC.*
Use: Nasal decongestant, imidazoline.

Afrin 12-Hour Original. (Schering-Plough) Oxymetazoline hydrochloride 0.05%, benzalkonium chloride, EDTA. Soln. Spray Bot. 15 mL. *OTC.*
Use: Nasal decongestant, imidazoline.

After Bite. (Tender) Ammonium hydroxide 3.5% in aqueous solution. Pen-like dispenser. *OTC.*
Use: Analgesic; antipruritic, topical.

After Burn. (Tender) Lidocaine 0.5% in aloe vera 98% solution. *OTC.*
Use: Anesthetic, local.

•**aftobetin.** (af-TOE-be-tin) USAN.
Use: Early detection of Alzheimer disease.

•**aftobetin hydrochloride.** (af-TOE-be-tin) USAN.
Use: Early detection of Alzheimer disease.

•**afuresertib.** (A-fue-re-SER-tib) USAN.
Use: Antineoplastic.

•**afuresertib hydrochloride.** (A-fue-re-SER-tib) USAN.
Use: Antineoplastic.

•**agalsidase alfa.** (aye-GAL-si-days) USAN.
Use: Fabry disease.

•**agalsidase beta.** (aye-GAL-si-days) USAN.
Use: Fabry disease.
See: Fabrazyme.

•**aganepag.** (a-GAN-e-pag) USAN.
Use: Treatment of glaucoma.

•**aganepag ethanediol.** (a-GAN-e-pag) USAN.
Use: Treatment of glaucoma.

•**aganepag isopropyl.** (a-GAN-e-pag) USAN.
Use: Treatment of glaucoma.

•**agar.** (AH-gahr) *NF.*
Use: Pharmaceutical aid, suspending agent.
W/Mineral oil.
See: Agoral.

Aggrastat. (Medicure) Tirofiban hydro-

chloride. **Inj.:** 50 mcg/mL. Preservative-free. Single-dose *IntraVia* containers 250 mL (sodium chloride 2.25 g, sodium citrate dihydrate 135 mg), 500 mL (sodium chloride 4.5 g, sodium citrate dihydrate 270 mg). **Conc. Inj.:** 250 mcg/mL. Preservative-free, sodium chloride 8 mg, sodium citrate dihydrate 2.7 mg. Vial 25 mL, 50 mL. *Rx.*
Use: Antiplatelet, glycoprotein IIb/IIIa inhibitor.

aggregation inhibitors.
Use: Antiplatelet agents.
See: Cilostazol.
Clopidogrel Bisulfate.
Prasugrel.
Ticagrelor.

Aggrenox. (Boehringer Ingelheim) Dipyridamole 200 mg extended-release, aspirin 25 mg, lactose, sucrose. Cap. Bot. 60s. *Rx.*
Use: Antiplatelet.

agomelatine.
Use: Investigational antidepressant.

Agoral. (Numark) Sennosides A and B 25 mg/15 mL, parabens. Liq. Bot. 473 mL. *OTC.*
Use: Laxative.

A/G-Pro. (Miller Pharmacal Group) Protein hydrolysate 542 mg, L-lysine 50 mg, L-methionine 12.5 mg, vitamin B_6 0.33 mg, C 16.7 mg, iron 1.66 mg, Cu, I, K, Mg, Mn, Zn. Tab. Bot. 180s. *OTC.*
Use: Nutritional supplement, amino acid.

Agriflu. (Novartis Vaccines) Hemagglutinin 15 mcg each of A/California/7/2009, NYMC X-181 (H1N1); A/Victoria/361/2011, IVR-165 (H3N2); and B/Hubei-Wujiagang/158/2009, NYMC BX-39 (a B/Wisconsin/1/2010-like virus) per 0.5 mL. Each 0.5 mL dose may contain residual amounts of egg proteins (< 0.4 mcg), formaldehyde (≤ 10 mcg), polysorbate 80 (≤ 50 mcg), and cetyltrimethylammonium bromide (≤ 12 mcg). Each dose may also contain residual amounts of neomycin (≤ 0.02 mcg by calculation), and kanamycin (≤ 0.03 mcg by calculation). Preservative free. Inj., Susp. (purified split virus). 0.5 mL prefilled, single-dose syringe (the tip caps of the prefilled syringes may contain natural latex rubber; the rubber plungers do not contain latex). *Rx.*
Use: Viral vaccine.

Agrylin. (Shire) Anagrelide hydrochloride 0.5 mg. Lactose. Cap. 100s. *Rx.*
Use: Thrombocythemia; polycythemia vera; essential thrombocythemia; thrombocytosis in chronic myelogenous leukemia. [Orphan Drug]

agurin.
See: Theobromine Sodium Acetate.

Ah-Chew. (Dexo Pharma) Phenylephrine tannate equiv. to phenylephrine hydrochloride 10 mg, chlorpheniramine tannate equiv. to chlorpheniramine maleate 2 mg, methscopolamine nitrate 1.5 mg per 5 mL. Parabens, sucralose. Susp. 20 mL, 118 mL. *Rx.*
Use: Upper respiratory combination, anticholinergic, antihistamine, decongestant combination.

Ah-Chew Ultra. (Dexo Pharma) Phenylephrine hydrochloride 10 mg (as phenylephrine tannate), chlorpheniramine maleate 2 mg (as chlorpheniramine tannate), methscopolamine nitrate 1.5 mg. Saccharin, sugar. Chew. Tab. 100s. *Rx.*
Use: Upper respiratory combination, decongestant, antihistamine, and anticholinergic combination.

AHF.
See: Antihemophilic Factor.

Ahist. (Magna Pharmaceuticals) Chlorcyclizine hydrochloride 25 mg. Tab. UD 30s. *OTC.*
Use: Antihistamine, nonselective piperazine.

A-Hydrocort. (Hospira) Hydrocortisone sodium succinate 100 mg/2 mL or 250 mg/2 mL, 500 mg/4 mL; 1000 mg/8 mL. *Rx.*
Use: Corticosteroid.

AIDS vaccine. (Various Mfr.) Phase I to III AIDS, HIV prophylaxis and treatment. Investigational.
Use: Immunization.

Airacof. (Centurion Labs) Codeine phosphate 7.5 mg, diphenhydramine hydrochloride 12.5 mg, phenylephrine hydrochloride 7.5 mg per 5 mL. Propylene glycol, saccharin, sodium benzoate, sorbitol. Alcohol free, dye free, and sugar free. Strawberry flavor. Liq. 473 mL. *c-v.*
Use: Upper respiratory combination, antitussive combination.

air and surface disinfectant. (Health & Medical Techniques) Aerosol 16 oz.
Use: Antiseptic; deodorant.

•**air, medical.** *USP.*
Use: Gas, medicinal.

AK-Beta. (Akorn) Levobunolol hydrochloride 0.25%, 0.5%, polyvinyl alcohol 1.4%, benzalkonium chloride 0.004%, sodium metabisulfite, EDTA, dibasic sodium phosphate, monobasic potassium phosphate, NaCl, hydrochloric acid, sodium hydroxide. Ophth. Soln. Bot.

2 mL, 5 mL, 10 mL, 15 mL. *Rx.*
Use: Antiglaucoma.

AK-Con. (Akorn) Naphazoline hydrochloride 0.1%. Benzalkonium chloride 0.01%, EDTA. Ophth. Soln. Bot. 15 mL. *Rx.*
Use: Ophthalmic decongestant; mydriatic, vasoconstrictor.

AK-Dilate. (Akorn) Phenylephrine hydrochloride 2.5%, 10%. Benzalkonium chloride 0.01%, sodium phosphate mono- and dibasic. Bot. 2 mL (2.5% only), 5 mL (10% only), 15 mL (2.5% only). *Rx.*
Use: Mydriatic, vasoconstrictor; ophthalmic decongestant.

AKEDamins. (Macoven Pharmaceuticals) Vitamins A 9,000 units, C 60 mg, D 400 units, E 150 units, K 150 mcg, B_1 1.2 mg, B_2 1.3 mg, B_3 10 mg, B_5 10 mg, B_6 1.5 mg, B_{12} 12 mcg, folic acid 200 mcg. Biotin 50 mcg, Zn. Dextrose, fructose, sorbitol, xylitol. Gluten free. Orange flavor. Chew. Tab. 60s. *OTC.*
Use: Multivitamin with minerals.

AK-Fluor. (Akorn) Fluorescein sodium 10%. Amp. 5 mL, Vial 5 mL.
Use: Diagnostic aid, ophthalmic.

Akineton Lactate. (Knoll) Biperiden lactate 5 mg in aqueous 1.4% sodium lactate soln/mL. Amp. 1 mL. Box 10s. *Rx.*
Use: Antiparkinsonian.

AK-NaCl. (Akorn) **Oint.:** Sodium chloride hypertonic 5%. Tube 3.5 g. **Soln.:** Sodium chloride hypertonic 5%. Bot. 15 mL. *OTC.*
Use: Ophthalmic.

Akne Drying Lotion. (Alto) Zinc oxide 12%, urea 10%, sulfur 6%, salicylic acid 2%, benzalkonium chloride 0.2%, isopropyl alcohol 70%, in a base containing menthol, silicon dioxide, iron oxide, perfume. Bot. ¾ oz, 2.25 oz. *OTC.*
Use: Dermatologic, acne.

Akne-Mycin. (Valeant) Erythromycin 2%. Cetostearyl alcohol, petrolatum, mineral oil. Oint. Tubes. 25 g. *Rx.*
Use: Topical anti-infective, antibiotic.

AK-Neo-Dex. (Akorn) Dexamethasone sodium phosphate 0.1%, neomycin sulfate 0.35%. Ophth. Soln. Bot. 5 mL. *Rx.*
Use: Anti-infective; corticosteroid, ophthalmic.

Akne Scrub. (Alto) Povidone-iodine with polyethylene granules. Bot. ¾ oz. *OTC.*
Use: Dermatologic, acne.

AK-Pentolate. (Akorn) Cyclopentolate hydrochloride 1%, benzalkonium chloride 0.01%, EDTA. Soln. Bot. 2 mL, 15 mL. *Rx.*
Use: Cycloplegic, mydriatic.

AK-Poly-Bac. (Akorn) Polymyxin B sulfate 10,000 units, bacitracin zinc 500 units/g, white petrolatum, mineral oil. Oint. Tube 3.5 g. *Rx.*
Use: Anti-infective, ophthalmic.

AK-Ramycin. (Akorn) Doxycycline hyclate 100 mg. Cap. Bot. 50s, 100s, 200s, 250s, 500s, UD 100s. *Rx.*
Use: Anti-infective, tetracycline.

AK-Ratabs. (Akorn) Doxycycline hyclate 100 mg. Tab. Bot. 50s. *Rx.*
Use: Anti-infective, tetracycline.

Akrinol. (Schering-Plough) Acrisorcin.
Use: Antifungal.

AK-Sulf. (Akorn) **Soln.:** Sodium sulfacetamide 10%. Dropper Bot. 2 mL, 5 mL, 15 mL. **Oint.:** Sodium sulfacetamide 10%. Tube 3.5 g. *Rx.*
Use: Anti-infective, ophthalmic.

AK-Taine. (Akorn) Proparacaine hydrochloride 0.5%, glycerin, chlorobutanol, benzalkonium chloride. Dropper bot. 2 mL, 15 mL. *Rx.*
Use: Anesthetic, ophthalmic.

AK-Tate. (Akorn) Prednisolone acetate 1%, benzalkonium chloride, EDTA, polysorbate 80, polyvinyl alcohol, hydroxyethyl cellulose. Susp. Dropper bot. 5 mL, 10 mL, 15 mL. *Rx.*
Use: Corticosteroid, ophthalmic.

Akten. (Akorn) Lidocaine hydrochloride 3.5%. Preservative free. Gel, Ophth. Single-use dropper bottle. 5 mL. *Rx.*
Use: Ophthalmic local anesthetic.

Ala-Bath. (Del-Ray) Bath oil. Bot. 8 oz. *OTC.*
Use: Emollient.

Ala-Cort. (Del-Ray) Hydrocortisone 1%. **Cream:** Tube 1 oz, 3 oz. **Lot.:** Bot. 4 oz. *Rx.*
Use: Corticosteroid, topical.

Ala-Derm. (Del-Ray) Lot. Bot. 8 oz, 12 oz.
Use: Emollient.

•**aladorian.** (AL-a-DOR-i-an) USAN.
Use: Cardiovascular agent.

•**aladorian sodium.** (AL-a-DOR-i-an) USAN.
Use: Cardiovascular agent.

Aladrine. (Scherer) Ephedrine sulfate 8.1 mg, secobarbital sodium 16.2 mg. Tab. Bot. 100s. *c-II.*
Use: Decongestant; hypnotic, sedative.

•**alagebrium chloride.** (al-A-je-BREE-um) USAN.
Use: Cardiovascular complications.

Alagesic LQ. (Poly Pharmaceuticals) Acetaminophen 325 mg, butalbital 50 mg, caffeine 40 mg per 15 mL. Alcohol 7.368%, glucose, parabens, saccharin, sorbitol, sucrose. Tropical fruit

punch flavor. Soln. 473 mL. *Rx.*
Use: Nonnarcotic analgesic combination, nonnarcotic analgesic with barbiturate.

Alahist DHC. (Poly Pharmaceuticals) Dihydrocodeine bitartrate 3 mg, phenylephrine hydrochloride 7.5 mg per 5 mL. Saccharin, sorbitol. Mango flavor. Liq. 473 mL. *c-v.*
Use: Upper respiratory combination, analgesic, decongestant.

Alahist DM. (Poly Pharmaceuticals) Brompheniramine maleate 4 mg, dextromethorphan HBr 15 mg, phenylephrine hydrochloride 7.5 mg per 5 mL. Saccharin, sorbitol. Alcohol free, dye free, sugar free. Strawberry flavor. Liq. 473 mL. *Rx.*
Use: Upper respiratory combination; antitussive, antihistamine, decongestant.

Alahist IR. (Poly Pharmaceuticals) Dexbrompheniramine maleate 2 mg. Tab. 60s. *Rx.*
Use: Antihistamine, nonselective alkylamine.

Ala-Hist PE. (Poly Pharmaceuticals) Dexchlorpheniramine maleate 2 mg, phenylephrine hydrochloride 10 mg. Tab. 60s. *OTC.*
Use: Upper respiratory combination, decongestant and antihistamine.

Alamag. (Ivax) Aluminum hydroxide 225 mg, magnesium hydroxide 200 mg, sorbitol, sucrose, parabens. Susp. Bot. 355 mL. *OTC.*
Use: Antacid.

Alamag Plus. (Ivax) Magnesium hydroxide 200 mg, aluminum hydroxide 225 mg, simethicone 25 mg/5 mL. Susp. Bot. 355 mL. *OTC.*
Use: Antacid.

•**alamecin.** (al-ah-MEE-sin) USAN.
Use: Anti-infective.

•**alanine.** (AL-ah-NEEN) *USP.*
Use: Amino acid.

•**alaproclate.** (AL-ah-PRO-klate) USAN.
Use: Antidepressant.

Ala-Quin 0.5%. (Del-Ray) Hydrocortisone, iodochlorhydroxyquinoline cream. Tube 1 oz. *Rx-OTC.*
Use: Corticosteroid, topical.

Ala-Scalp HP 2%. (Del-Ray) Hydrocortisone Lot. Bot. 1 oz. *Rx.*
Use: Corticosteroid, topical.

Ala-Seb. (Del-Ray) Salicylic acid 2%, sulfur 2%. Shampoo. 355 mL. *OTC.*
Use: Antiseborrheic.

Ala-Seb T. (Del-Ray) Shampoo **118 mL:** Sulfur 2%, salicylic acid 2%, coal tar 1%, PEG-20. **4 oz:** Coal tar, colloidal sulfur, salicylic acid. **12 oz:** Coal tar, colloidal sulfur, salicylic acid. *OTC.*
Use: Antiseborrheic combination.

Alasulf. (Major) Sulfanilamide 15%, aminacrine hydrochloride 0.2%, allantoin 2%. Vaginal Cream. Tube w/applicator 120 g. *Rx.*
Use: Anti-infective, vaginal.

Alatone. (Major) Spironolactone 25 mg. Tab. Bot. 100s, 250s, 500s, 1000s, UD 100s. *Rx.*
Use: Antihypertensive.

Alavert. (Wyeth) Loratadine 10 mg. Lactose. Orally Disintegrating Tab. 6s, 12s, 15s, 30s, 48s. *OTC.*
Use: Antihistamine, peripherally selective piperidine.

Alavert Allergy & Sinus D-12 Hour. (Wyeth) Pseudoephedrine sulfate 120 mg, loratadine 5 mg. Lactose. ER Tab. 12s, 24s. *OTC.*
Use: Upper respiratory combination, decongestant, antihistamine.

Alavert Children's. (Wyeth) Loratadine 5 mg/5 mL. Sucrose. Syrup. 118 mL. *OTC.*
Use: Antihistamine, peripherally selective piperidine.

Alaway. (Bausch & Lomb) Ketotifen fumarate 0.025%. Benzalkonium chloride 0.01%, glycerin, sodium hydroxide, and/or hydrochloric acid. Soln., Ophth. 10 mL. *OTC.*
Use: Ophthalmic decongestant.

Alaway Children's. (Bausch & Lomb) Ketotifen fumarate 0.025%. Benzalkonium chloride 0.01%, glycerin, sodium hydroxide, and/or hydrochloric acid. Soln., Ophth. 5 mL. *OTC.*
Use: Ophthalmic antihistamine.

Alaxin. (Delta Pharmaceutical Group) Oxyethlene oxypropylene polymer 240 mg. Cap. Bot. 100s. *OTC.*
Use: Laxative.

alazanine triclofenate.
Use: Anthelmintic.

Alazide. (Major) Spironolactone w/hydrochlorothiazide. Tab. Bot. 250s, 1000s. *Rx.*
Use: Antihypertensive, diuretic.

Alazine. (Major) Hydralazine 10 mg, 25 mg, 50 mg. Cap. Bot. 100s, 1000s. *Rx.*
Use: Antihypertensive.

•**albaconazole.** (Al-ba-KON-a-zole) USAN.
Use: Antifungal agent.

Albafort. (Baroli) Ferrous fumarate 110 mg, B_{12} 15 mcg, intrinsic factor (as concentrate or from stomach preparations) 240 mg, vitamin C 100 mg, folic

acid 0.8 mg. Cap. 100s. *Rx.*
Use: Trace element, iron.

Albatussin. (Baroli) Carbetapentane citrate 25 mg, guaifenesin 400 mg, phenylephrine hydrochloride 10 mg. Cap. 100s. *Rx.*
Use: Upper respiratory combination, antitussive and expectorant combination.

Albatussin SR. (Lambda Pharmacal) Dextromethorphan HBr 40 mg, potassium guaiacolsulfonate 600 mg, phenylephrine hydrochloride 20 mg, pyrilamine maleate 25 mg. ER Cap. 100s. *Rx.*
Use: Antitussive and expectorant combination.

•**albendazole.** (AL-BEND-ah-zole) *USP.*
Use: Anthelmintic.
See: Albenza.

Albenza. (Amedra Pharmaceuticals) Albendazole 200 mg. Lactose, saccharin. Tab. 112s. *Rx.*
Use: Anthelmintic; hydatid disease. [Orphan Drug]

•**albiglutide.** (al-bi-GLOO-tide) USAN.
Use: Treatment of type 2 diabetes.
See: Tanzeum.

•**albinterferon alfa-2b.** (AL-bin-ter-FEER-on) USAN.
Use: Treatment of chronic hepatitis C.

Albolene. (DSE Healthcare) Mineral oil, petrolatum. Fragrance free. Soap. 340 g. *OTC.*
Use: Emollient.

Albuconn 25%. (Cryosan) Normal serum albumin (human) 12.5 g in 50 mL solution for IV administration. Vial 50 mL. *Rx.*
Use: Treatment of plasma or blood volume deficit, acute hypoproteinemia, oncotic deficit.

•**albumin, aggregated.** (al-BYOO-min AGG-reh-GAY-tuhd) USAN.
Use: Diagnostic aid, lung-imaging.
See: Technescan MAA.

•**albumin, aggregated iodinated I 131 injection.** (al-BYOO-min AGG-reh-GAY-tuhd) *USP.*
Use: Radiopharmaceutical.

•**albumin, aggregated iodinated I 131 serum.** (al-BYOO-min AGG-reh-GAY-tuhd) USAN. Blood serum aggregates of albumin labeled with iodine-131.
Use: Radiopharmaceutical.
See: Albumotope I-131.

Albuminar-5. (ZLB Behring) Albumin (human) 5%. Soln. with administration set. Bot. 50 mL, 1000 mL. *Rx.*
Use: Plasma protein fraction.

Albuminar-25. (ZLB Behring) Albumin (human) 25%. Soln. Vials. 20 mL with administration set. *Rx.*
Use: Plasma protein fraction.

•**albumin, chromated Cr 51 serum.** (al-BYOO-min) USAN. Blood serum albumin labeled with chromium-51.
Use: Radiopharmaceutical.

•**albumin human.** (al-BYOO-MIN) *USP.*
Formerly Albumin, Normal Human Serum.
Use: Plasma protein fraction; blood volume supporter.
See: Albuminar-5 and Albuminar-25.
Albutein 5%.
Albutein 25%.
Buminate.
Kedbumin.
Optison.
Plasbumin-5.
Plasbumin-25.
W/Combinations.
See: Monarc-M.

albumin human, 5%. (Baxter Healthcare) Normal serum albumin 5%. Inj. Vial 250 mL. *Rx.*
Use: Plasma protein fraction.

albumin human, 25%. (Baxter Healthcare) Normal serum albumin 25%. Inj. Vial 10 mL, 50 mL. *Rx.*
Use: Plasma protein fraction.

•**albumin, iodinated I 131 injection.** (al-BYOO-min) *USP.* Albumin labeled with iodine-131. Inj.
Use: Diagnostic aid, blood volume determination, intrathecal imaging; radiopharmaceutical.

•**albumin, iodinated I 131 serum.** (al-BYOO-min) *USP.*
Use: Diagnostic aid, blood volume determination, intrathecal imaging; radioactive agent.

•**albumin, iodinated I 125 injection.** (al-BYOO-min) *USP.* Albumin labeled with iodine-125.
Use: Diagnostic aid, blood volume determination; radiopharmaceutical.

•**albumin, iodinated I 125 serum.** (al-BYOO-min) *USP.*
Use: Diagnostic aid, blood volume determination; radiopharmaceutical.

albumin, normal serum 5%. (Baxter Healthcare) Albumin human 5%. Inj. Vial 120 mL. *Rx.*
Use: Plasma protein fraction.

albumin, normal serum 25%. (Baxter Healthcare) Albumin human 25%. Inj. Vial 10 mL, 50 mL. *Rx.*
Use: Plasma protein fraction.

albumin-saline diluent. (Bayer Consumer Care) Dilute allergenic extracts

and venom products for patient testing and treating. Pre-measured vials 1.8 mL, 4 mL, 4.5 mL, 9 mL, 30 mL. Vial 2 mL, 5 mL, 10 mL, 30 mL.
Use: Pharmaceutical necessity, diluent.

Albumotope I-131. (Bristol-Myers Squibb) Albumin, iodinated I-131 serum (50 uCi).
Use: Diagnostic aid.

Albustix Reagent Strips. (Siemens Medical) Firm paper reagent strips impregnated with tetrabromophenol blue, citrate buffer and a protein-adsorbing agent. Bot. 50s, 100s.
Use: Diagnostic aid.

Albutein 5%. (Grifols Biologicals) Normal serum albumin 5%. Inj. Vial w/IV set 250 mL, 500 mL. *Rx.*
Use: Plasma protein fraction.

Albutein 25%. (Grifols Biologicals) Normal serum albumin 25%. Inj. Vial w/IV set 50 mL. *Rx.*
Use: Plasma protein fraction.

•**albuterol.** (al-BYOO-ter-ahl) *USP.*
Use: Bronchodilator, sympathomimetic.
See: Proventil.
Ventolin.
W/Ipratropium Bromide.
See: Combivent Respimat.

albuterol. (Nephron) Albuterol sulfate 0.042% (1.25 mg/3 mL). Preservative free. Soln. for Inh. 3 mL UD vials. *Rx.*
Use: Bronchodilator.

albuterol. (Various Mfr.) Albuterol 90 mcg per actuation. Aer. Can. 6.8 g (≥ 80 inhalations), 17 g (≥ 200 inhalations). *Rx.*
Use: Bronchodilator, sympathomimetic.

albuterol. (Watson) Albuterol sulfate 0.021%. Preservative free. Soln., Inh. 3 mL UD vials. *Rx.*
Use: Bronchodilator, sympathomimetic.

•**albuterol sulfate.** (al-BYOO-teh-rahl SULL-fate) *USP.*
Use: Bronchodilator, sympathomimetic.
See: AccuNeb.
ProAir HFA.
Proventil HFA.
Ventolin HFA.
VoSpire ER.
W/Ipratropium Bromide.
See: Combivent.
DuoNeb.

albuterol sulfate. (Mylan) Albuterol 4 mg, 8 mg. Polydextrose. Film coated. ER Tab. 100s, 500s. *Rx.*
Use: Bronchodilator.

albuterol sulfate. (Various Mfr.) Albuterol sulfate. **Tab.:** 2 mg, 4 mg. May contain lactose. Bot. 100s, 500s, 600s. **Syrup:** 2 mg/5 mL. May contain sorbitol. Bot. 473 mL. **Inh. Soln.:** 0.083% (2.5 mg/3 mL), 0.5% (5 mg/mL). UD 3 mL (0.083% only). Vials. 0.5 mL (0.5% only), 20 mL with dropper (0.5% only) *Rx.*
Use: Bronchodilator, sympathomimetic.

albuterol sulfate and ipratropium bromide. (al-BYOO-ter-ahl SULL-fate and IH-pruh-TROE-pee-uhm BROE-mide)
Use: Chronic obstructive pulmonary disease (COPD).

•**albutoin.** (al-BYOO-toe-in) USAN.
Use: Anticonvulsant.

•**alcaftadine.** (al-KAF-ta deen) USAN.
Use: Antihistamine.
See: Lastacaft.

Alcaine. (Alcon) Proparacaine hydrochloride 0.5%. Glycerin, benzalkonium chloride 0.01%. Soln. Bot. 15 mL *Drop-Tainers. Rx.*
Use: Anesthetic, ophthalmic.

Alcare. (GlaxoSmithKline) Ethyl alcohol 62%. Foam Bot. 210 mL, 300 mL, 600 mL. *OTC.*
Use: Antiseptic.

Alclear Eye. (Walgreen) Sterile isotonic fluid. Lot. Bot. 8 oz. *OTC.*
Use: Anti-irritant, ophthalmic.

•**alclofenac.** (al-KLOE-feh-nak) USAN.
Use: Analgesic; anti-inflammatory.
See: Mervan.

•**alclometasone dipropionate.** (al-kloe-MEH-tah-zone die-PRO-pee-oh-nate) *USP.*
Use: Anti-inflammatory, topical.
See: Aclovate.

alclometasone dipropionate. (Taro) Alclometasone dipropionate 0.05%. Hexylene glycol, propylene glycol stearate, petrolatum. Oint. 15 g, 45 g, 60 g. *Rx.*
Use: Anti-inflammatory agent.

alclometasone dipropionate. (Various Mfr.) Alclometasone dipropionate 0.05%. Cream. 15 g, 45 g, 60 g. *Rx.*
Use: Anti-inflammatory agent.

•**alcloxa.** (al-KLOX-ah) USAN.
Use: Astringent; keratolytic.

Alco-Gel. (Tweezerman) Ethyl alcohol 60%. Gel. Tube 60 g, 480 g. *OTC.*
Use: Dermatologic, cleanser.

•**alcohol.** (AL-koe-hol) *USP.* Ethanol, ethyl alcohol.
Use: Anti-infective, topical; pharmaceutic aid, solvent.
See: Anbesol.
Anbesol Maximum Strength.

alcohol, dehydrated.
Use: Solvent, vehicle.

•**alcohol, diluted.** (AL-koe-hol) *NF.*
Use: Pharmaceutic aid, solvent.

•**alcohol, rubbing.** (AL-koe-hol) *USP.*
Use: Rubefacient.
See: Lavacol.

Alcojet. (Alconox) Biodegradable machine washing detergent and wetting agent. Ctn. 9 × 4 lb, 25 lb, 50 lb, 100 lb, 300 lb. *OTC.*
Use: Detergent, wetting agent.

Alcolec. (American Lecithin) Lecithin w/choline base, cephalin, lipositol. Cap. 100s. Gran. 8 oz, lb. *OTC.*
Use: Nutritional supplement.

Alcon Enzymatic Cleaning Tablets for Extended Wear. (Alcon) Pancreatin. Tab. Pkg. 12s. *OTC.*
Use: Contact lens care.

Alcon Opti-Pure Sterile Saline Solution. (Alcon) Sterile unpreserved saline solution. Aerosol 8 oz. *OTC.*
Use: Contact lens care.

Alconox. (Alconox) Biodegradable detergent and wetting agent. Box 4 lb, Container 25 lb, 50 lb, 100 lb, 300 lb. *OTC.*
Use: Contact lens care, detergent; wetting agent.

Alcortin A. (Primus Pharmaceuticals) Hydrocortisone acetate 2%. Aloe polysaccharide 1%, benzyl alcohol, glycerin, iodoquinol 1%, amino methylpropanol, propylene glycol, SD alcohol. Gel. Individual pack. 2 g. *Rx.*
Use: Anti-inflammatory agent, topical corticosteroid.

Alcotabs. (Alconox) Tab. Box 6s, 100s.
Use: Cleanser.

•**alcuronium chloride.** (al-cure-OH-nee-uhm KLOR-ide) USAN. Diallyldinortoxiferin dichloride.
Use: Muscle relaxant.

Aldactazide. (Pfizer US) Spironolactone and hydrochlorothiazide. **25 mg/25 mg:** Bot. 100s, 500s, 1000s, 2500s, UD 100s. **50 mg/50 mg:** Bot. 100s, UD 32s, UD 100s. Tab. *Rx.*
Use: Antihypertensive, diuretic.

Aldactone. (Searle) Spironolactone 25 mg, 50 mg, 100 mg. PEG. Film coated. Tab. 100s, 500s (25 mg only). *Rx.*
Use: Diuretic.

Aldara. (Valeant) Imiquimod 5%. Cetyl alcohol, stearyl alcohol, white petrolatum, benzyl alcohol, parabens. Cream. Boxes. 12s. Single-use packets. *Rx.*
Use: Topical immunomodulator.

•**aldesleukin.** (al-dess-LOO-kin) USAN. Recombinant form of interleukin-2.
Use: Biological response modifier.
See: Proleukin.

Aldex-CT. (Zyber) Diphenhydramine hydrochloride 12.5 mg, phenylephrine hydrochloride 5 mg. Mannitol, saccharin. Strawberry flavor. Chew. Tab. 100s. *Rx.*
Use: Upper respiratory combination; antihistamine, decongestant.

Aldex GS. (Pernix) Guaifenesin 190 mg, pseudoephedrine hydrochloride 30 mg. Tab. 100s. *OTC.*
Use: Upper respiratory combination, decongestant and expectorant combination.

Aldex GS DM. (Pernix) Dextromethorphan hydrobromide 15 mg, guaifenesin 190 mg, pseudoephedrine hydrochloride 30 mg. Tab. 100s. *Rx.*
Use: Upper respiratory combination, antitussive and expectorant combination.

•**aldioxa.** (al-DIE-ox-ah) USAN. Aluminum dihydroxy allantoinate.
Use: Astringent; keratolytic.

Aldomet Ester Hydrochloride. (Merck & Co.) Methyldopate hydrochloride 250 mg/5 mL, citric acid anhydrous 25 mg, sodium bisulfite 16 mg, disodium edetate 2.5 mg, monothioglycerol 10 mg, sodium hydroxide to adjust pH, methylparaben 0.15%, propylparaben 0.02% w/water for inj. q.s. to 5 mL. Inj. Vial 5 mL. *Rx.*
Use: Antihypertensive.

Aldomet Oral Suspension. (Merck & Co.) Methyldopa 250 mg/5 mL, alcohol 1%, benzoic acid 0.1%, sodium bisulfite 0.2%. Oral Susp. Bot. 473 mL. *Rx.*
Use: Antihypertensive.

Aldomet Tablets. (Merck & Co.) Methyldopa. **125 mg Tab.:** Bot. 100s. **250 mg Tab.:** Bot. 100s, 1000s, UD 100s, unit-of-use 100s. **500 mg Tab.:** Bot. 100s, 500s, UD 100s, unit-of-use 60s, 100s. *Rx.*
Use: Antihypertensive.

Aldosterone RIA Diagnostic Kit. (Abbott Diagnostics) Test kits 50s.
Use: Diagnostic aid.

•**aldoxorubicin.** (al-DOX-oh-ROO-bi-sin) USAN.
Use: Antineoplastic.

•**aldoxorubicin hydrochloride.** (al-DOX-oh-ROO-bi-sin) USAN.
Use: Antineoplastic.

Aldurazyme. (BioMarin) Laronidase 2.9 mg/5 mL, albumin (human) 0.1% after dilution, NaCl 43.9 mg, sodium phosphate monobasic monohydrate 63.5 mg, sodium phosphate dibasic heptahydrate 10.7 mg, preservative free. Inj. Single-use vials. 5 mL. *Rx.*
Use: Treatment of mucopolysaccharidosis.

ALEC. (Forum Products, Inc.) Dipalmitoyl phosphatidylcholine/phosphatidylglycerol.
Use: Neonatal respiratory distress syndrome. [Orphan Drug]

•**alectinib.** (al-EK-ti-nib) USAN.
Use: Antineoplastic.

•**alefacept.** (ah-LEE-fah-sept) USAN.
Use: Immunologic agent, immunosuppressive.
See: Amevive.

•**aleglitazar.** (AL-e-GLI-ta-zar) USAN.
Use: Antidiabetic agent.

•**alemcinal.** (al-EM-si-nal) USAN.
Use: Gastrointestinal prokinetic.

•**alemtuzumab.** (al-em-TUE-zue-mab) USAN.
Use: Monoclonal antibody.

•**alendronate sodium.** (al-LEN-droe-nate) *USP.*
Use: Bisphosphonate.
See: Fosamax.
W/Cholecalciferol.
See: Fosamax Plus D.

alendronate sodium. (Various Mfr.) Alendronate sodium. **Tab.:** 5 mg, 10 mg, 35 mg, 40 mg, 70 mg. 30s; 100s (5 mg and 10 mg only); UD 1s, UD 4s, UD 12s (35 mg and 70 mg only); UD 20s (10 mg, 35 mg, and 70 mg only). **Soln.:** 70 mg. May contain parabens, saccharin. UD 75 mL. *Rx.*
Use: Bisphosphonate.

Alenic Alka. (Rugby) **Liq.:** Aluminum hydroxide 31.7 mg, magnesium carbonate 137.3 mg, sodium alginate, EDTA, sodium 13 mg. Bot. 355 mL. **Chew. Tab.:** Aluminum hydroxide 80 mg, magnesium trisilicate 20 mg, sodium bicarbonate, calcium stearate, sugar. Bot. 100s. *OTC.*
Use: Antacid.

•**alentemol hydrobromide.** (al-EN-teh-mole HIGH-droe-BROE-mide) USAN.
Use: Antipsychotic; dopamine agonist.

•**aleplasinin.** (al-e-PLAS-in-in) USAN.
Use: Alzheimer disease.

Alersule. (Edwards) Chlorpheniramine maleate 8 mg, phenylephrine hydrochloride 20 mg. Cap. Bot. 100s. *Rx-OTC.*
Use: Antihistamine; decongestant.

Alert-Pep. (Health for Life Brands) Caffeine 200 mg. Cap. Bot. 16s. *OTC.*
Use: CNS stimulant.

•**aletamine hydrochloride.** (al-ETT-ah-meen HIGH-droe-KLOR-ide) USAN.
Use: Antidepressant.

Aleve. (Bayer) Naproxen 200 mg (naproxen sodium 220 mg). Tab. Bot. 24s, 50s, 100s, 150s. Cap. Bot. 24s, 50s, 100s, 150s, 200s. Gelcap. Bot. 20s, 40s, 80s. *OTC.*
Use: Nonsteroidal anti-inflammatory agent.

Aleve-D Sinus & Cold. (Bayer) Pseudoephedrine hydrochloride 120 mg, naproxen sodium 220 mg (naproxen 200 mg). Sodium 20 mg, lactose. ER Tab. Pkg. 10s, 20s, 24s, 30s. *OTC.*
Use: Upper respiratory combination, analgesic, decongestant.

Aleve PM. (Bayer) Diphenhydramine hydrochloride 25 mg, naproxen sodium 220 mg. PEG. Tab. 20s, 40s, 80s. *OTC.*
Use: Nonprescription sleep aid.

•**alexidine.** (ah-LEX-ih-DEEN) USAN.
Use: Anti-infective.

alfa interferon-2a.
See: Roferon A.

alfa interferon-2b.
See: Intron A.

•**alfentanil hydrochloride.** (al-FEN-tuh-NILL HIGH-droe-KLOR-ide) USAN.
Use: Opioid analgesic.

alfentanil hydrochloride. (Abbott) Alfentanil hydrochloride (as base) 500 mcg/mL. Preservative free. Inj. Amps. 2 mL, 5 mL, 10 mL. *c-II.*
Use: Opioid analgesic.

•**alferminogene tadenovec.** (AL-fer-MIN-oh-jeen ta-DEN-oh-vek) USAN.
Use: Gene therapy.

•**alfimeprase.** (AL-fi-me-prace) USAN.
Use: Thrombolytic.

•**alfuzosin hydrochloride.** (al-FEW-zoe-sin HIGH-droe-KLOR-ide) USAN.
Use: Antihypertensive, alpha-blocker.
See: Uroxatral.

alfuzosin hydrochloride. (Various Mfr.) Alfuzosin hydrochloride 10 mg. May contain lactose. ER Tab. 30s, 100s, 500s, 1,000s, 8,000s, UD 90s, UD 100s. *Rx.*
Use: Antiadrenergic agent, peripherally acting; alpha-1 adrenergic blocker.

Algel. (Faraday) Magnesium trisilicate 0.5 g, aluminum hydroxide 0.25 g. Tab. Bot. 100s. Susp. Bot. gal. *OTC.*
Use: Antacid.

•**algeldrate.** (AL-jell-drate) USAN.
Use: Antacid.

Algemin. (Thurston) Macrocystis pyrifera alga. Pow. Jar 8 oz. Tab. Bot. 300s. *OTC.*
Use: Dietary aid.

Algenic Alka. (Rugby) Aluminum hydroxide 31.7 mg/mL, magnesium carbonate 137 mg/mL, sodium alginate, sorbitol. Liq. Bot. 355 mL. *OTC.*
Use: Antacid.

Algenic Alka Improved. (Rugby) Aluminum hydroxide 240 mg, magnesium hydroxide 100 mg/Chew. Tab. Bot. 100s, 500s. *OTC.*
Use: Antacid.

•**algenpantucel-L.** (AL-jen-pan-TOO-sel-el) USAN.
Use: Antineoplastic.

•**algestone acetonide.** (al-JESS-tone ah-SEE-toe-nide) USAN.
Use: Anti-inflammatory.

•**algestone acetophenide.** (al-JESS-tone ah-SEE-toe-FEN-ide) USAN.
Use: Hormone, progestin.

Algex. (Health for Life Brands) Menthol, camphor, methylsalicylate, eucalyptus. Liniment. Bot. 4 oz. *OTC.*
Use: Analgesic, topical.

algin.
See: Sodium Alginate.

Algin-All. (Barth's) Sodium alginate from kelp. Tab. Bot. 100s, 500s.

•**alginic acid.** (al-JIN-ik) *NF.*
Use: Pharmaceutic aid, tablet binder, emulsifying agent.
W/Combinations.
See: Pretts Diet-Aid.

•**alglucerase.** (al-GLUE-ser-ACE) USAN.
Formerly Macrophage-targeted β-*glucocerebrosidase.*
Use: Enzyme replacement, type 1 Gaucher disease; enzyme replacement, types 2 and 3 Gaucher disease. [Orphan Drug]

•**alglucosidase alfa.** (al-gloo-KOSE-i-dase) USAN.
Use: Enzyme replacement therapy.
See: Lumizyme.
Myozyme.

•**alicaforsen sodium.** (a-li-KA-for-sen) USAN.
Use: Anti-inflammatory.

alidine dihydrochloride or phosphate.
See: Anileridine.

•**aliflurane.** (al-IH-flew-rane) USAN.
Use: Anesthetic, inhalation.

Align Daily Probiotic Supplement. (Procter & Gamble) *Bifidobacterium infantis* 35624 1 billion CFU. Sugar. Gluten free and lactose free. Cap. 28s. *OTC.*
Use: Oral nutritional supplement, probiotic.

Alikal. (Sanofi-Synthelabo) Sodium bicarbonate, tartaric acid powder. *OTC.*
Use: Antacid.

Alimentum. (Ross) Casein hydrolysate, sucrose, tapioca starch, MCT (fractionated coconut oil), safflower oil, soy oil. Qt. Ready-to-use. *OTC.*
Use: Nutritional supplement-enteral.

Alimta. (Lilly) Pemetrexed 100 mg (mannitol 106 mg), 500 mg (mannitol 500 mg). Inj., Lyophilized, Pow. for Soln. Single-use vials. *Rx.*
Use: Antimetabolite.

Alinia. (Romark Laboratories) Nitazoxanide. **Pow. for Oral Susp.:** 100 mg/5 mL (after reconstitution). Sugar, sucrose 1.48 mg/5 mL, strawberry flavor. Bot. 60 mL. **Tab.:** 500 mg. Polyvinyl alcohol, sucrose, talc. Film coated. 60s, UD 6s. *Rx.*
Use: Antiprotozoal.

•**alipamide.** (al-IH-pam-ide) USAN.
Use: Antihypertensive; diuretic.

•**alirocumab.** (Al-i-ROK-ue-mab) USAN.
Use: Antihyperlipidemic agent.

•**alisertib.** (A-li-SER-tib) USAN.
Use: Antineoplastic.

•**alisertib sodium.** (A-li-SER-tib) USAN.
Use: Antineoplastic.

•**aliskiren.** (a-LIS-kir-EN) USAN.
Use: Renin angiotensin system antagonist; direct renin inhibitor.
See: Tekturna.
W/Amlodipine Besylate.
See: Tekamlo.
W/Amlodipine Besylate, Hydrochlorothiazide.
See: Amturnide.
W/Hydrochlorothiazide.
See: Tekturna HCT.

•**aliskiren fumarate.** (a-LIS-kir-EN) USAN.
Use: Cardiovascular agent.

alisobumal.
See: Butalbital.

•**alisporivir.** (AL-is-POR-i-vir) USAN.
Use: Antiviral.

•**alitame.** (AL-ih-TAME) USAN.
Use: Sweetener.

•**alitretinoin.** (a-li-TRET-i-noyn) USAN.
Use: Retinoid, second generation.
See: Panretin.

Alive! Men's Energy. (Nature's Way Products) Vitamins A 3,500 units, D 800 units, E 45 units, B_1 4.5 mg, B_2 5.1 mg, B_3 40 mg, B_5 15 mg, B_6 6 mg, B_{12} 18 mcg, C 90 mg, K 60 mcg, folic acid 0.4 mg, B, Ca, Cl, Cr, Cu, I, K, Mg, Mn, Mo, Na, Se, Zn, biotin 40 mcg, *Garden Veggies Blend* 50 mg, lutein 100 mcg, lycopene 600 mcg, *Orchard Fruits Blend* 50 mg, resveratrol 700 mcg, saw palmetto 50 mg. Maltodextrin, polydextrose. Preservative free. Tab. 50s. *OTC.*
Use: Multivitamin with minerals (except iron).

Alive! Once Daily Women's 50+ Ultra Potency. (Nature's Way Products) Vi-

tamins A 7,500 units, D 1,000 units, E 100 units, B_1 25 mg, B_2 25 mg, B_3 50 mg, B_5 40 mg, B_6 40 mg, B_{12} 225 mcg, C 120 mg, K 100 mcg, folic acid 0.8 mg, B, Ca, Cr, Cu, I, Mg, Mn, Mo, Se, Zn, biotin 325 mcg, *Cardiovascular Blend* with *Resveratrol* 20 mg, choline 10 mg, *Citrus Bioflavonoid Complex* 20 mg, *CranRx* 20 mg, *Digestive Enzyme Blend* 20 mg, *Flax Lignan Blend* 20 mg, *Garden Veggies Blend* 30 mg, *Green Food/Spirulina Blend* 20 mg, inositol 10 mg, lutein 1 mg, *Mind & Body Energy Blend* 30 mg, *Orchard Fruits Blend* 30 mg, *Organic Mushroom Defense Blend* 20 mg, rutin 5 mg. Glycerin. Preservative free. Tab. 60s. *OTC.*
Use: Multivitamin with minerals.

Alive! Women's 50+. (Nature's Way Products) Vitamins A 3,500 units, D 1,000 units, E 30 units, B_1 4.5 mg, B_2 5.1 mg, B_3 20 mg, B_5 15 mg, B_6 6 mg, B_{12} 100 mcg, C 90 mg, K 60 mcg, folic acid 0.4 mg, B, Ca, Cr, Cu, I, Mg, Mn, Mo, Na, Se, Zn, biotin 300 mcg, *Garden Veggies Blend* 50 mg, lutein 300 mcg, *Orchard Fruits Blend* 50 mg, resveratrol 900 mcg. Maltodextrin, polydextrose. Preservative free. Tab. 50s. *OTC.*
Use: Multivitamin with minerals (except iron).

alkalinizers, minerals and electrolytes.
See: Bicitra.
Oracit.
Polycitra.

alkalinizers, systemic.
See: Citrate and Citric Acid.

alkalinizers, urinary tract products.
See: Bicitra.
Citrolith.
Polycitra.
Potassium Citrate.
Sodium Bicarbonate.
Urocit-K.

Alkalol. (Alkalol) Thymol, eucalyptol, menthol, camphor, benzoin, potassium alum, potassium chlorate, sodium bicarbonate, sodium chloride, sweet birch oil, spearmint oil, pine and cassia oil, alcohol 0.05%. Bot. Pt. Nasal douche cup pkg. 1s. *OTC.*
Use: Eyes, nose, throat, and all inflamed mucous membranes.

Alka-Med Liquid. (Halsey Drug) Aluminum hydroxide 200 mg, magnesium hydroxide 200 mg/5 mL. Bot. 8 oz. *OTC.*
Use: Antacid.

Alka-Med Tablets. (Halsey Drug) Magnesium hydroxide, aluminum hydroxide. Bot. 60s. *OTC.*
Use: Antacid.

Alka-Mints. (Bayer Consumer Care) Calcium carbonate 850 mg (elemental calcium 340 mg). Sorbitol, sugar, sodium < 5 mg. Assorted flavors and spearmint. Chew. Tab. 75s. *OTC.*
Use: Mineral supplement; antacid.

Alka-Seltzer Gold. (Bayer Consumer Care) Citric acid 1,000 mg, potassium bicarbonate 344 mg, sodium bicarbonate 1,050 mg. Mannitol, sodium 309 mg. Effervescent Tab. 36s. *OTC.*
Use: Antacid combination

Alka-Seltzer Heartburn Relief. (Bayer Consumer Care) Citric acid 1,000 mg, sodium bicarbonate 1,940 mg. Acesulfame K, aspartame, phenylalanine 5.6 mg, mannitol. Lemon-lime flavor. Tab. 36s. *OTC.*
Use: Antacid combination.

Alka-Seltzer Lemon Lime. (Bayer Consumer Care) Citric acid 1,000 mg, aspirin 325 mg, sodium bicarbonate 1,700 mg. Aspartame, phenylalanine 9 mg, sodium 504 mg. Lemon-lime flavor. Tab. 24s. *OTC.*
Use: Antacid combination.

Alka-Seltzer Multi-Symptom Cold Relief. (Bayer Consumer Care) Acetaminophen 250 mg, chlorpheniramine maleate 2 mg, phenylephrine hydrochloride 5 mg. Maltodextrin. Sodium 503 mg per tablet. Effervescent Tab. 20s. *OTC.*
Use: Upper respiratory combination; decongestant, antihistamine, and analgesic combination.

Alka-Seltzer Original. (Bayer Consumer Care) Aspirin 325 mg, citric acid 1,000 mg, sodium bicarbonate 1,916 mg. Sodium 567 mg. Effervescent Tab. 24s. *OTC.*
Use: Antacid combination.

Alka Seltzer Plus Cold. (Bayer Consumer Care) Aspirin 325 mg, chlorpheniramine maleate 2 mg, phenylephrine bitartrate 7.8 mg. Acesulfame K, aspartame, mannitol, phenylalanine 8.4 mg (original flavor) or 10 mg (cherry burst and orange zest flavors), sodium 474 mg (original flavor) and 476 mg (cherry burst and orange zest flavors). Effervescent Tab. 20s, 36s, 72s. *OTC.*
Use: Upper respiratory combination; decongestant, antihistamine, and analgesic combination.

Alka-Seltzer Plus Cold & Cough. (Bayer Consumer Care) **Effervescent Tab.:** Aspirin 325 mg, chlorpheniramine maleate 2 mg, dextromethorphan hydrobromide

10 mg, phenylephrine bitartrate 7.8 mg. Acesulfame, aspartame, mannitol, phenylalanine 9 mg, sodium 415. Citrus flavor. 20s. **Liq.:** Acetaminophen 162.5 mg, chlorpheniramine maleate 1 mg, dextromethorphan hydrobromide 5 mg, phenylephrine hydrochloride 2.5 mg per 5 mL. Edetate disodium, PEG 400, sorbitol, sucralose. Alcohol free. 180 mL. **Liqui-Gels:** Dextromethorphan HBr 10 mg, chlorpheniramine maleate 2 mg, phenylephrine hydrochloride 5 mg, acetaminophen 325 mg, Liquid filled. Sorbitol. 12s. *OTC.*
Use: Upper respiratory combination, antitussive combination.

Alka-Seltzer Plus Day & Night Cold. (Bayer Consumer Care) **Effervescent Tab.: Day:** Aspirin 325 mg, dextromethorphan hydrobromide 10 mg, phenylephrine bitartrate 7.8 mg. Acesulfame K, aspartame, mannitol, phenylalanine 9 mg, sodium 416 mg. 10s. **Night:** Aspirin 500 mg, dextromethorphan hydrobromide 10 mg, doxylamine succinate 6.25 mg, phenylephrine bitartrate 7.8 mg. Acesulfame K, aspartame, phenylalanine 5.6 mg, sodium 474 mg, sorbitol. 10s. **Liq. Gels: Day:** Acetaminophen 325 mg, dextromethorphan hydrobromide 10 mg, phenylephrine hydrochloride 5 mg. Mannitol, PEG 400, sorbitol. 10s. **Night:** Acetaminophen 325 mg, dextromethorphan hydrobromide 10 mg, doxylamine succinate 6.25 mg, phenylephrine hydrochloride 5 mg. Mannitol, PEG 400, sorbitol. 10s. *OTC.*
Use: Upper respiratory combination, antitussive combination.

Alka-Seltzer Plus Day Non-Drowsy Cold. (Bayer Consumer Care) **Cap. Liquid filled:** Acetaminophen 325 mg, dextromethorphan HBr 10 mg, phenylephrine hydrochloride 5 mg. Mannitol, PEG 400/600, sorbitol. 12s, 20s. **Liq.:** Acetaminophen 162.5 mg, dextromethorphan hydrobromide 5 mg, phenylephrine hydrochloride 2.5 mg/5 mL. Edetate disodium, PEG 400, sorbitol, sucralose. Alcohol free. 180 mL. *OTC.*
Use: Upper respiratory combination, antitussive combination.

Alka-Seltzer Plus Fast Crystal Packs. (Bayer Consumer Care) Acetaminophen 650 mg, chlorpheniramine maleate 4 mg, phenylephrine hydrochloride 10 mg. Acesulfame K, aspartame, phenylalanine 6 mg, sucralose, sucrose. Taste free. Pow. 10s. *OTC.*
Use: Upper respiratory combination; decongestant, antihistamine, and analgesic combination.

Alka-Seltzer Plus Mucus & Congestion. (Bayer Consumer Care) **Effervescent Tab:** Dextromethorphan HBr 10 mg, guaifenesin 200 mg. Acesulfame K, aspartame, mannitol, phenylalanine 6.7 mg, sodium 296 mg, sucralose. Lemon-lime flavor. 20s. **Cap., liquid filled:** Dextromethorphan hydrobromide 10 mg, guaifenesin 200 mg. Mannitol, PEG 400, PEG 600, sorbitan, sorbitol. 20s. *OTC.*
Use: Upper respiratory combination, expectorant.

Alka-Seltzer Plus Night Cold. (Bayer Consumer Care) **Effervescent Tab.:** Aspirin 500 mg, dextromethorphan HBr 10 mg, doxylamine succinate 6.25 mg, phenylephrine bitartrate 7.8 mg. Acesulfame K, aspartame, phenylalanine 5.6 mg, saccharin, sodium 474 mg, sorbitol. 20s. **Liq.:** Acetaminophen 162.5 mg, dextromethorphan hydrobromide 5 mg, doxylamine succinate 3.125 mg, phenylephrine hydrochloride 2.5 mg per 5 mL. Edetate disodium, PEG 400, sodium 3 mg, sorbitol, sucralose. Alcohol free. 180 mL. **Liquid-Gels:** Dextromethorphan HBr 10 mg, doxylamine succinate 6.25 mg, phenylephrine hydrochloride 5 mg, acetaminophen 325 mg. Sorbitol. 12s. *OTC.*
Use: Upper respiratory combination, antitussive combination.

Alka-Seltzer Plus Severe Sinus Congestion Allergy & Cough. (Bayer Consumer Care) Acetaminophen 325 mg, dextromethorphan hydrobromide 10 mg, doxylamine succinate 6.25 mg, phenylephrine hydrochloride 5 mg. Glycerin, mannitol, PEG, sorbitol. Cap., liquid filled. 40s. *OTC.*
Use: Upper respiratory combination, antitussive combination.

Alka-Seltzer Plus Sinus. (Bayer Consumer Care) Phenylephrine hydrochloride 5 mg, acetaminophen 250 mg. Acesulfame K, phenylalanine 4.2 mg, saccharin, sodium 477 mg, sorbitol. Effervescent Tab. 20s. *OTC.*
Use: Upper respiratory combination, decongestant and analgesic combination.

Alka-Seltzer Plus Sparkling Original Cold Formula. (Bayer Consumer Care) Aspirin 325 mg, chlorpheniramine maleate 2 mg, phenylephrine bitartrate 5 mg. Acesulfame K, aspartame, mannitol, phenylalanine 8.4 mg, sodium 474 mg, sorbitol. Effervescent Tab. 20s.

OTC.
Use: Upper respiratory combination, antihistamine and decongestant.

Alka-Seltzer PM. (Bayer Consumer Care) Aspirin 325 mg, diphenhydramine citrate 38 mg. Phenylalanine 4 mg, acesulfame K, aspartame, mannitol. Effervescent Tab. 24s. *OTC.*
Use: Upper respiratory combination, analgesic, antihistamine.

Alka-Seltzer Wake-Up Call. (Bayer Consumer Care) Aspirin 500 mg, caffeine 65 mg. Phenylalanine 9 mg, acesulfame K, aspartame, mannitol. Effervescent Tab. 16s. *OTC.*
Use: Analgesic.

Alkavite. (Vitality) Vitamins A 5000 units, C 250 mg, D 400 units, E 30 units, B_1 100 mg, B_6 3 mg, B_{12} 12 mcg, folic acid 1 mg, B_2 3 mg, niacin 20 mg, biotin 0.03 mg, Ca 68.5 mg, Fe 60 mg, Mg, Zn 4 mg, Se. ER Tab. UD 100s *OTC.*
Use: Vitamin supplement.

Alkeran. (APO Pharma USA) Melphalan. **Inj., Lyophilized, Pow. for Reconstitution:** 50 mg (as melphalan hydrochloride). Single-use vials (with povidone 20 mg) with 10 mL of sterile diluent (water for injection with sodium citrate 0.2 g, propylene glycol 6 mL, ethanol 0.52 mL). **Tab.:** 2 mg. Film-coated. Amber Glass Bot. 50s. *Rx.*
Use: Alkylating agent, nitrogen mustard.

alkylamines, nonselective.
Use: Antihistamine
See: Brompheniramine Maleate.
Chlorpheniramine Maleate.
Chlorpheniramine Tannate.
Dexbrompheniramine Maleate.
Dexchlorpheniramine Maleate.
Triprolidine Hydrochloride.

alkylating agents.
See: Alkyl Sulfonates.
Estrogen/Nitrogen Mustard.
Ethylenimines/Methylmelamines.
Nitrogen Mustards.
Nitrosoureas.
Triazenes.

alkylbenzyldimethylammonium chloride. Benzalkonium Chloride.

•**alkyl (C12-15) benzoate.** (al-kil-BEN-zoe-ate) *NF.*
Use: Pharmaceutical aid, oleaginous vehicle emollient.

alkyl sulfonates.
Use: Alkylating agents.
See: Busulfan.

•**allantoin.** (al-AN-toe-in) USAN.
Use: Vulnerary, topical.
See: Cutemol Emollient.
W/Camphor, Menthol.
See: Nose Better.
W/Combinations.
See: Anbesol Cold Sore Therapy.
Nil Vaginal Cream.
Par.
Tegrin.

Allay. (LuChem Pharmaceuticals, Inc.) Acetaminophen 650 mg, hydrocodone bitartrate 7.5 mg. Cap. Bot. 100s. *c-III.*
Use: Analgesic combination; narcotic.

Allbee C-800. (Wyeth) Vitamins E 45 units, C 800 mg, B_1 15 mg, B_2 17 mg, B_3 100 mg, B_5 25 mg, B_{12} 12 mcg. Tab. Bot. 60s. *OTC.*
Use: Vitamin supplement.

Allbee C-800 Plus Iron. (Wyeth) Vitamins E 45 units, C 800 mg, B_1 15 mg, B_2 17 mg, niacin 100 mg, B_6 25 mg, B_{12} 12 mcg, pantothenic acid 25 mg, iron 27 mg, folic acid 0.4 mg. Tab. Bot. 60s. *OTC.*
Use: Mineral, vitamin supplement.

Allbee-T. (Wyeth) Vitamins B_1 15.5 mg, B_2 10 mg, B_6 8.2 mg, B_5 23 mg, B_3 100 mg, C 500 mg, B_{12} 5 mcg. Tab. Bot. 100s, 500s. *OTC.*
Use: Vitamin supplement.

Allbee w/C. (Wyeth) Vitamins B_1 15 mg, B_6 5 mg, B_2 10.2 mg, B_3 50 mg, B_5 10 mg, C 300 mg. Cap. Bot. 30s. *OTC.*
Use: Vitamin supplement.

Allbex. (Health for Life Brands) Vitamins B_1 5 mg, B_2 2 mg, B_6 0.25 mg, calcium pantothenate 3 mg, niacinamide 20 mg, ferrous sulfate 194.4 mg, inositol 10 mg, choline 10 mg, B_{12} (concentrate) 3 mcg. Cap. Bot. 100s, 1000s. *OTC.*
Use: Mineral, vitamin supplement.

All Day Allergy. (Major) Cetirizine hydrochloride 10 mg. Tab. 14s. *OTC.*
Use: Antihistamine; piperazine, peripherally selective.

All Day Allergy Children's. (Major) Cetirizine hydrochloride 10 mg. Acesulfame K, benzyl alcohol, lactose, maltodextrin, propylene glycol. Tutti frutti flavor. Chew. Tab. 24s. *OTC.*
Use: Antihistamine, peripherally selective piperazine.

All-Day-C. (Barth's) Vitamin C 200 mg. or 500 mg. Cap (200 mg). Tab (500 mg). with rose hip extract. Bot. 30s, 90s, 180s, 360s. *OTC.*
Use: Vitamin supplement.

All-Day Iron Yeast. (Barth's) Iron 20 mg, Vitamins B_1 2 mg, B_2 4 mg, niacin 0.57 mg. Cap. Bot. 30s, 90s, 180s. *OTC.*
Use: Mineral, vitamin supplement.

All Day Relief. (Rugby) Naproxen so-

dium. **Tab.:** 220 mg. 50s, 100s. **Caplets:** 220 mg. 50s, 100s. *OTC.*
Use: Nonsteroidal anti-inflammatory agent.

All-Day-Vites. (Barth's) Vitamins A 10,000 units, D 400 units, B_1 3 mg, B_2 6 mg, niacin 1 mg, C 120 mg, B_{12} 10 mcg, E 30 units. Cap. Bot. 30s, 90s, 180s, 360s. *OTC.*
Use: Vitamin supplement.

Allegra Allergy. (Chattem) Fexofenadine hydrochloride 60 mg, 180 mg. PEG. Tab. 12s (60 mg), 70s (180 mg). *OTC.*
Use: Antihistamine, peripherally selective piperidine.

Allegra Children's Allergy. (Chattem) Fexofenadine hydrochloride. **Tab.:** 30 mg. PEG. 6s. **Tab., orally disintegrating:** 30 mg. Aspartame, mannitol, phenylalanine 5.3 mg, sodium 5 mg. 12s. **Susp.:** 30 mg per 5 mL. Edetate disodium, parabens, propylene glycol, sodium 18 mg, sucrose, xylitol. Alcohol free and dye free. Berry flavor. 120 mL. *OTC.*
Use: Antihistamine, peripherally selective piperidine.

Allegra-D 12 Hour Allergy & Congestion. (Chattem) Fexofenadine hydrochloride 60 mg (immediate release), pseudoephedrine hydrochloride 120 mg (extended release). Film coated. ER Tab. 100s. *OTC.*
Use: Upper respiratory combination, antihistamine, decongestant.

Allegra-D 24 Hour Allergy & Congestion. (Chattem) Pseudoephedrine hydrochloride 240 mg, fexofenadine hydrochloride 180 mg. PEG, isopropyl and methyl alcohols. Film-coated. ER Tab. 100s. *OTC.*
Use: Decongestant and antihistamine, upper respiratory combination.

Allegron. Nortriptyline.
Use: Antidepressant.

Allent. (B.F. Ascher) Pseudoephedrine hydrochloride 120 mg, brompheniramine maleate 12 mg. SR Cap. Bot. 100s. *Rx.*
Use: Antihistamine; decongestant.

AllePak Dose Pack. (Everton Pharmaceuticals) **Day:** Pseudoephedrine hydrochloride 120 mg, methscopolamine nitrate 2.5 mg. Tab. 10s. **Night:** Chlorpheniramine maleate 8 mg, methscopolamine nitrate 2.5 mg. Tab. 10s. *Rx.*
Use: Decongestant, antihistamine, and anticholinergic combination.

Allerben. (Forest) Diphenhydramine 10 mg/mL. Inj. Vial 30 mL. *Rx.*
Use: Antihistamine.

Aller-Chlor. (Rugby) Chlorpheniramine maleate. **Tab.:** 4 mg. Bot. 24s, 100s, 1000s. **Syr.:** 2 mg/5 mL, alcohol 5%, parabens, sugar. Bot. 118 mL. *OTC.*
Use: Antihistamine, nonselective alkylamine.

Allercon. (Parmed Pharmaceuticals, Inc.) Pseudoephedrine hydrochloride 60 mg, triprolidine hydrochloride 2.5 mg. Tab. Bot. 24s, 100s, 1000s. *OTC.*
Use: Antihistamine; decongestant.

Allerest. (Insight) **Headache Strength Tab.:** Acetaminophen 325 mg, pseudoephedrine hydrochloride 30 mg, chlorpheniramine maleate 2 mg. Tab. Pkg. 24s. **Nasal Spray:** Oxymetazoline hydrochloride 0.05%. Bot. 0.5 oz. *OTC.*
Use: Analgesic (Headache Strength Tab. only); antihistamine; decongestant.

Allerest Allergy & Sinus Relief Maximum Strength. (Insight) Pseudoephedrine hydrochloride 30 mg, acetaminophen 325 mg. Tab. 24s. *OTC.*
Use: Decongestant and analgesic.

Allergan Hydrocare Cleaning & Disinfecting Solution. (Allergan) Tris (2-hydroxyethyl) tallow ammonium chloride 0.013%, thimerosal 0.002%, bis (2-hydroxyethyl) tallow ammonium chloride, sodium bicarbonate, dibasic, monobasic and anhydrous sodium phosphate, hydrochloric acid, propylene glycol, polysorbate 80, special soluble polyhema. Bot. 4 oz, 8 oz, 12 oz. *OTC.*
Use: Contact lens care.

Allergan Hydrocare Preserved Saline Solution. (Allergan) Sodium chloride, sodium hexametaphosphate, sodium hydroxide, boric acid, sodium borate, EDTA 0.01%, thimerosal 0.001%. Bot. 8 oz, 12 oz. *OTC.*
Use: Contact lens care.

allergenic extracts. Allergenic extracts of pollens, foods, inhalants, epidermals, fungi, insects, miscellaneous antigens.
Use: Diagnostic aid, allergens.
See: Grass Pollen Allergen Extract.
Short Ragweed Pollen Allergen Extract.

allergenic extracts, alum-precipitated.
See: Allpyral.
Center-Al.

Allergen Patch Test Kit. (Healthpoint Medical) Box of tubes of semi-solid pastes or solutions. Allergens are either suspended in 4.5 g petrolatum, USP, or dissolved in 5.5 g water. Kit includes 20 reclosable syringes for topical use only (not for injection), each exuding sufficient allergen to test 150 patients, housed in a plastic case with two drawers. Allergens include benzocaine, mercaptobenzothiazole, colophony, p-phenylenediamine, imidazolidinyl urea (Germall115), cinnamon aldyhyde, lanolin alcohol (woolwax alcohols), carba-rubber mix, neomycin sulfate, thiuram rubber mix, formaldehyde, ethylenediamine dihydrochloride, epoxyresin, quaternium 15, p-tert-butylphenol formalde hyderesin, mercapto rubber mix, black rubber p-phenylenediamine mix, potassium dichromate, balsam of Peru and nickel sulfate.

allergen test patches.
Use: Diagnostic aid; allergic dermatitis.
See: T.R.U.E. Test.

Allergex. (Bayer Consumer Care) Silicones, polyethylene and triethylene glycol, antioxidants, mineral oil concentrate. Bot. Pt. Aerosol pt.
Use: Antiallergic.

Allergy. (Major) Chlorpheniramine maleate 4 mg, lactose. Tab. Bot. 24s, 100s. *OTC.*
Use: Antihistamine, nonselective alkylamine.

Allergy-D. (Major) Cetirizine hydrochloride 5 mg, pseudoephedrine hydrochloride 120 mg. Lactose. ER Tab. 12s. *OTC.*
Use: Upper respiratory combination, decongestant and antihistamine.

Allergy DN. (Breckenridge) **Day:** Pseudoephedrine hydrochloride 120 mg, methscopolamine nitrate 2.5 mg. **Night:** Chlorpheniramine maleate 8 mg, methscopolamine nitrate 2.5 mg. Tab. 20s (10 day, 10 night). *Rx.*
Use: Upper respiratory combination, decongestant, antihistamine, and anticholinergic combination.

allergy preparations.
See: Antihistamines.

Allergy Relief. (Zee Medical) Chlorpheniramine maleate 4 mg. Tab. 12s. *OTC.*
Use: Antihistamine.

Allergy Relief & Nasal Decongestant. Loratadine 10 mg, pseudoephedrine sulfate 240 mg. Lactose, PEG. ER Tab. 10s. *OTC.*
Use: Upper respiratory combination, decongestant and antihistamine.

Allergy Tablets. (Major) Chlorpheniramine 4 mg. Tab. Bot. 24s and 100s. *OTC.*
Use: Antihistamine.

Allergy-Time. (Time-Cap Labs) Chlorpheniramine maleate 4 mg. Lactose. Tab. 1,000s. *OTC.*
Use: Antihistamine, nonselective alkylamine.

AllerMax. (Pfeiffer) Diphenhydramine hydrochloride 12.5 mg/5 mL, alcohol 0.5%, glucose, saccharin, sorbitol, sucrose, menthol, raspberry flavor. Liq. Bot. 118 mL. *OTC.*
Use: Antihistamine, nonselective ethanolamine, nonnarcotic antitussive.

AllerMax Allergy & Cough Formula. (Pfeiffer) Diphenhydramine hydrochloride 6.25 mg/5 mL, alcohol 0.5%, raspberry flavor, menthol, sucrose, glucose, saccharin, sorbitol. Bot. 118 mL. *OTC.*
Use: Antihistamine.

AllerMax Caplets, Maximum Strength. (Pfeiffer) Diphenhydramine hydrochloride 50 mg, lactose. Tab. Bot. 24s. *OTC.*
Use: Antihistamine, nonselective ethanolamine.

Allersone. (Roberts) Hydrocortisone 0.5%, diperodon hydrochloride 0.5%, zinc oxide 5%, sodium lauryl sulfate, propylene glycol, cetyl alcohol, petrolatum, methyl- and propylparabens. Oint. Tube 15 g. *Rx-OTC.*
Use: Corticosteroid, topical.

Allersule Forte. (Edwards) Phenylephrine hydrochloride 20 mg, chlorpheniramine maleate 8 mg, methscopolamine nitrate 2.5 mg. Cap. Bot. 100s. *Rx-OTC.*
Use: Anticholinergic; antihistamine; decongestant.

AlleRx DF Dose Pack. (Cornerstone) **Day:** Chlorpheniramine maleate 4 mg, methscopolamine nitrate 2.5 mg. Lactose. **Night:** Chlorpheniramine maleate 8 mg, methscopolamine nitrate 2.5 mg. Lactose.Tab. 20s (10 day, 10 night), 60s (30 day, 30 night). *Rx.*
Use: Upper respiratory combination; decongestant, antihistamine, and anticholinergic combination.

Allfen C. (MCR American) Carbetapentane citrate 5 mg, guaifenesin 1000 mg. ER Tab. 100s. *Rx.*
Use: Antitussives with expectorant.

Allfen CDX. (MCR) Codeine phosphate 20 mg, guaifenesin 200 mg. Parabens, sorbitol, sucralose. Liq. 473 mL. *c-III.*
Use: Upper respiratory combination, antitussive with expectorant.

Alli. (GlaxoSmithKline) Orlistat 60 mg. Cap. 60s, 90s, 120s. *OTC.*
Use: Lipase inhibitor.

All-Nite. (Major) Dextromethorphan HBr 5 mg, doxylamine succinate 2.1 mg, acetaminophen 166.7 mg per 5 mL. Alcohol 10%, saccharin. Liq. Bot.

177 mL. *OTC.*
Use: Upper respiratory combination, antitussive combination.

All-Nite Children's Cold/Cough Relief. (Major) Pseudoephedrine hydrochloride 10 mg, chlorpheniramine maleate 0.67 mg, dextromethorphan HBr 5 mg per 5 mL. Alcohol free. Sucrose. Cherry flavor. Liq. 118 mL. *OTC.*
Use: Antihistamine; antitussive; decongestant.

•**allobarbital.** (AL-low-BAR-bih-tal) USAN. *Formerly Diallybarbituric acid.*
Use: Hypnotic; sedative.

•**allopurinol.** (AL-oh-PURE-ee-nahl) *USP.*
Use: Antigout; xanthine oxidase inhibitor; antimetabolite.
See: Aloprim.
Zyloprim.

allopurinol. (Various Mfr.) Allopurinol 100 mg, 300 mg. Tab. Bot. 100s, 500s, 1000s, UD 100s. *Rx.*
Use: Antimetabolite.

allopurinol sodium. (Bedford Labs) Allopurinol sodium 500 mg. Preservative free. Pow. for Inj., lyophilized. Vials with rubber stopper. 30 mL. *Rx.*
Use: Antimetabolite.

Allpyral. (Bayer Consumer Care) Allergenic extracts, alum-precipitated. For subcutaneous inj. pollens, molds, epithelia, house dust, other inhalants, stinging insects.
Use: Diagnostic aid, allergens.

Allres DS. (Allegis) Chlorpheniramine maleate 4 mg (as 8 mg chlorpheniramine tannate), dextromethorphan hydrobromide 30 mg (as 60 mg dextromethorphan tannate), pseudoephedrine hydrochloride 30 mg (as 60 mg pseudoephedrine tannate) per 5 mL. Acesulfame K, aspartame, methylparaben, phenylalanine 25.25 mg, sucralose. Grape bubble gum flavor. Susp. 473 mL. *Rx.*
Use: Upper respiratory combination, antitussive combination.

allylamine antifungal.
Use: Antifungal agent.
See: Terbinafine Hydrochloride.

allylbarbituric acid. Allylisobutylbarbituric acid, butalbital.
Use: Sedative.
W/A.P.C.
See: Anti-Ten.
Fiorinal.
W/Acetaminophen.
See: Panitol.

allyl-isobutylbarbituric acid.
See: Allylbarbituric Acid.

•**allyl isothiocyanate.** (AL-il EYE-soe-THYE-oh-SYE-a-nate) *USP.*
Use: Counterirritant in neuralgia.

Almacone. (Rugby) **Chew Tab.:** Aluminum hydroxide 200 mg, magnesium hydroxide 200 mg, simethicone 20 mg. Bot. 100s, 1000s. **Liq.:** Aluminum hydroxide 200 mg, magnesium hydroxide 200 mg, simethicone 20 mg, sodium 0.75 mg/5 mL. Bot. 360 mL, gal. *OTC.*
Use: Antacid.

Almacone II Double Strength Liquid. (Rugby) Aluminum hydroxide 400 mg, magnesium hydroxide 400 mg, simethicone 40 mg/5 mL. Bot. 360 mL, gal. *OTC.*
Use: Antacid.

•**almadrate sulfate.** (AL-ma-drate SULL-fate) USAN. Aluminum magnesium hydroxide-oxide-sulfate-hydrate.
Use: Antacid.

•**almagate.** (AL-mah-gate) USAN.
Use: Antacid.

almagucin. Gastric mucin, dried aluminum hydroxide gel, magnesium trisilicate. *OTC.*
Use: Antacid.

Almebex Plus B_{12}. (Dayton) Vitamins B_1 1 mg, B_2 2 mg, B_3 5 mg, B_6 0.4 mg, B_{12} 5 mcg, choline 33 mg/5 mL. Bot. 473 mL (with B_{12} in separate container). *OTC.*
Use: Vitamin supplement.

•**almond oil.** *NF.*
Use: Pharmaceutic aid, emollient, oleaginous vehicle, perfume.

•**almotriptan.** (al-moe-TRIP-tan) USAN.
Use: Antimigraine.

•**almotriptan malate.** (al-moe-TRIP-tan MAL-ee-ate) USAN.
Use: Antimigraine agent, serotonin 5-HT_1 receptor agonist.
See: Axert.

•**alniditan dihydrochloride.** (al-nih-DIH-tan die-HIGH-droe-KLOR-ide) USAN.
Use: Antimigraine.

Alnyte. (Mayer Lab) Scopolamine aminoxide HBr 0.2 mg, salicylamide 250 mg. Tab. Pkg. 16s. *Rx.*
Use: Analgesic; anticholinergic.

Alocass Laxative. (Western Research) Aloin 0.25 g, cascara sagrada 0.5 g, rhubarb 0.5 g, ginger 1⁄32 g, powdered extract of belladonna g. Tab. Bot. 1000s. Pak 28s. *OTC.*
Use: Laxative.

Alocril. (Allergan) Nedocromil sodium 2% (20 mg/mL), benzalkonium chloride 0.01%, NaCl 0.5%, EDTA 0.05%. Ophth.

Soln. Bot. 5 mL w/dropper tip. *Rx.*
Use: Ophthalmic agent, mast cell stabilizer.

Alodox Convenience Kit. (OcuSoft) Doxycycline hyclate 20 mg. Film coated. Lactose, polydextrose. Tab. 60s. *Rx.*
Use: Tetracycline.

•**aloe.** (AL-oh) *USP.*
Use: See Compound Benzoin Tincture.

Aloe Grande Creme. (Gordon Laboratories) Aloe, vitamins E 1500 units, A 100,000 units/oz in cream base. Jar 2.5 oz. *OTC.*
Use: Emollient.

Aloe Vesta. (ConvaTec) **Cloth:** Aloe barbadensis leaf juice, dimethicone, parabens, urea. 24s. **Lot.:** Dimethicone 3%. Alcohols, aloe, glycerin, petrolatum. 60 mL. **Oint:** Miconazole nitrate 2%. Aloe, mineral oil, white petrolatum. 56 g, 141 g. **Spray:** Petrolatum 36%, mineral oil, aloe extract. 60 g. *OTC.*
Use: Emollient.

Aloe Vesta Perineal. (ConvaTec) Solution of sodium C14-16 olefin sulfonate, propylene glycol, aloe vera gel, hydrolyzed collagen. Bot. 118 mL, 236 mL, gal. *OTC.*
Use: Perianal hygiene.

•**alofilcon A.** (AL-oh-FILL-kahn) USAN.
Use: Contact lens material, hydrophilic.

•**alogliptin benzoate.** (AL-oh-GLIP-tin BEN-zoe-ate) USAN.
Use: Antidiabetic.
See: Nesina.
W/Pioglitazone Hydrochloride.
See: Oseni.

aloin. (J.T. Baker) A mixture of crystalline pentosides from various aloes. Bot. oz. *OTC.*
Use: Laxative.

Alomide. (Alcon) Lodoxamide tromethamine 0.1%. Soln. *Drop-tainers* 10 mL. *Rx.*
Use: Antiallergic, ophthalmic.

•**alonimid.** (ah-LAHN-ih-mid) USAN.
Use: Hypnotic; sedative.

Alophen. (Numark) Bisacodyl 5 mg. Sugar. Tab., delayed release. 100s. *OTC.*
Use: Laxative.

Aloprim. (Nabi) Allopurinol 500 mg. Preservative free. Pow. for Inj., lyophilized. Vial 30 mL with rubber stoppers. *Rx.*
Use: Antimetabolite.

Aloquin. (Primus Pharma) Aloe polysaccharides 1%, iodoquinol 1.25%, benzyl alcohol, PEG-20, SDA alcohol 40 B. Gel. 60 g. *Rx.*
Use: Miscellaneous topical combination.

Alora. (Actavis) Estradiol 0.77 mg (0.025 mg/day), 1.5 mg (0.05 mg/day), 2.3 mg (0.075 mg/day), 3.1 mg (0.1 mg/day). Transdermal System. Calendar packs 8 systems. *Rx.*
Use: Estrogen, sex hormone.

•**alosetron hydrochloride.** (al-OH-seh-trahn HIGH-droe-KLOR-ide) USAN.
Use: Antiemetic.
See: Lotronex.

Alotone. (Major) Triamcinolone 4 mg. Tab. Bot. 100s. *Rx.*
Use: Corticosteroid.

•**alovudine.** (al-OHV-you-deen) USAN.
Use: Antiviral.

Aloxi. (Eisai Inc.) Palonosetron hydrochloride 0.05 mg/mL. Disodium edetate. Inj., Soln. Single-use vials. 1.5 mL (mannitol 83 mg), 5 mL (mannitol 207.5 mg). *Rx.*
Use: 5-HT_3 receptor antagonist, antiemetic/antivertigo agent.

•**alpertine.** (al-PURR-teen) USAN.
Use: Antipsychotic.

l-alpha-acetyl-methadol (LAAM). (Bio Development Corp.) *Rx.*
Use: Treatment of heroin addicts. [Orphan Drug]

•**alpha amylase.** (AL-fah AM-ih-lace) USAN. A concentrated form of alpha amylase produced by a strain of nonpathogenic bacteria.
Use: Digestive aid; anti-inflammatory.
See: Kutrase Capsules.
Ku-Zyme Capsules.

alpha-amylase w-100. W/Proteinase W-300, cellase W-100, lipase, estrone, testosterone, vitamins, minerals. *Rx.*
Use: Digestive aid.

alpha/beta-adrenergic blocking agent.
See: Carvedilol.
Labetalol Hydrochloride.

alpha-chymotrypsin.
See: Chymotrypsin.

Alphaderm. (Teva) Hydrocortisone 1%. Cream. Tube 30 g, 100 g. *Rx-OTC.*
Use: Corticosteroid, topical.

alpha-d-galactosidase.
Use: Antiflatulent.

Alpha-E. (Barth's) d-Alpha tocopherol. **50 units or 100 units:** Cap. Bot. 100s, 500s, 1000s. **200 units:** Cap. Bot. 100s, 250s. **400 units:** Cap. Bot. 100s, 250s, 500s. *OTC.*
Use: Vitamin supplement.

alpha-estradiol. Known as beta-estradiol.
See: Estradiol.

Alpha Fast. (Eastwood) Bath oil. Bot. 16 oz. *OTC.*
Use: Emollient.

alpha-fetoprotein with Tc-99m.
Use: Diagnostic aid.

•**alphafilcon A.** (al-fah-FILL-kahn) USAN.
Use: Contact lens material, hydrophilic.

alpha-galactosidase.
See: Aspergillus niger enzyme.

alpha-galactosidase A.
Use: Fabry disease. [Orphan Drug]

alpha-galactoside A.
Use: Treatment of Fabry disease. [Orphan Drug]

Alphagan P. (Allergan) Brimonidine tartrate 0.1%, 0.15%, *Purite* 0.005%, boric acid, potassium chloride, sodium borate, sodium chloride. Hydrochloric acid and/or sodium hydroxide to adjust pH. Soln. Bot. 5 mL, 10 mL, 15 mL. *Rx.*
Use: Agent for glaucoma.

alpha-glucosidase inhibitor.
Use: Antidiabetic agent.
See: Acarbose.
Miglitol.

alpha-glucosidase, recombinant human acid. (Pharmain BV)
Use: Glycogen storage disease type II. [Orphan Drug]

alpha-hypophamine.
See: Oxytocin.

alpha interferon-2b.
See: Intron A.

•**alpha lipoic acid.** *NF.*
Use: Antioxidant.

Alpha-Keri. (Novartis Consumer) **Shower & Bath:** Mineral oil, lanolin oil, PEG-4-dilaurate, benzophenone-3, D&C green #6, fragrance. Bot. 4 oz, 8 oz, 16 oz. **Cleansing Bar:** Bar containing sodium tallowate, sodium cocoate, water, mineral oil, fragrance, PEG-75, glycerin, titanium dioxide, lanolin oil, sodium chloride, BHT, EDTA, D&C green #5, D&C yellow #10. 120 g. *OTC.*
Use: Emollient.

alpha-methyldopa. *Name previously used for Methyldopa.*

AlphaNine. (Grifols) Purified heat-treated/solvent preparation of coagulation Factor IX from human plasma. With ≥ 50 units Factor IX per mg protein, < 5 units each Factor II (prothrombin) and Factor VII (proconvertin) per 100 IU Factor IX and < 20 units Factor X (Stuart-Power Factor) per 100 IU Factor IX. In single-dose vials with diluent, double-ended needle, and microaggregated filter. Pow. for Inj. *Rx.*
Use: Antihemophilic.

AlphaNine SD. (Grifols) Factor IX (human) 500 units, 1,000 units, 1,500 units. Actual factor IX activity in units is stated on the label of each vial. Inj., lyophilized Pow. for Soln. Single-dose vial (contains not more than 0.04 units of heparin, 0.2 mg of dextrose, 1 mcg of polysorbate 80, and 0.1 mcg tri-n-butyl phosphate per unit of factor IX) w/diluent and a *Mix2Vial* filter transfer set. *Rx.*
Use: Antihemophilic agent.

alpha-1-adrenergic blockers.
Use: Antihypertensives.
See: Alfuzosin.
Silodosin.
Tamsulosin Hydrochloride.

alpha-1 antitrypsin. Alpha-1 trypsin inhibitor; human alpha-1 protease inhibitor.
Use: Glycoprotein.

alpha-1-proteinase inhibitor.
Use: Treatment of alpha-1-antitrypsin deficiency.
See: Aralast NP.
Glassia.
Prolastin-C.
Zemaira.

alphasone acetophenide. Name previously used for Algestone acetonide.

alpha-tocopherol.
See: Vitamin E.

alpha-2 adrenergic agonist.
Use: Glaucoma agent.
See: Brimonidine tartrate.

Alpha Vee-12. (Schlicksup) Hydroxocobalamin 1000 mcg/mL. Vial 10 mL. *Rx.*
Use: Vitamin supplement.

Alphosyl. (Schwarz Pharma) Allantoin 1.7%, special crude coal tar extracts 5%. **Lot.:** Bot. 8 fl oz. **Cream:** 2 oz. *OTC.*
Use: Antipruritic.

•**alpidem.** (AL-PIH-dem) USAN.
Use: Antianxiety; anxiolytic.

•**alprazolam.** (al-PRAY-zoe-lam) *USP.*
Tall Man: ALPRAZolam
Use: Hypnotic; sedative; antianxiety agent.
See: Niravam.
Xanax.
Xanax XR.

alprazolam. (Par Pharmaceuticals) Alprazolam 0.25 mg, 0.5 mg, 1 mg, 2 mg. Aspartame, mannitol, peppermint and vanilla flavoring, phenylalanine, sorbitol, xylitol. Tab. UD 100s. *c-IV.*
Use: Antianxiety agent, benzodiazepine.

alprazolam. (Various Mfr.) Alprazolam. **ER Tab.:** 0.5 mg, 1 mg, 2 mg, 3 mg. May contain lactose. 60s, 500s. **Tab.:** 0.25 mg, 0.5 mg, 1 mg, 2 mg. Bot. 100s, 500s, 1000s (except 2 mg), UD 100s

(except 2 mg). *c-iv.*
Use: Management of anxiety disorders.

alprazolam intensol. (Roxane) Alprazolam 1 mg/mL. Flavorless. Oral Soln. 30 mL with calibrated dropper. *c-iv.*
Use: Antianxiety agent.

•**alprenolol hydrochloride.** (al-PREH-no-lole HIGH-droe-KLOR-ide) USAN.
Use: Antiadrenergic; β-receptor.

•**alprenoxime hydrochloride.** (al-PREN-ox-eem) USAN.
Use: Antiglaucoma agent.

Alprolix. (Biogen Idec) Coagulation factor IX (recombinant) Fc fusion protein 500 units, 1,000 units, 2,000 units, 3,000 units. Mannitol, sucrose. Preservative free. Inj., lyophilized Pow. for Soln. Single-use vial w/diluent. *Rx.*
Use: Antihemophilic agent.

•**alprostadil.** (al-PRAHST-uh-dill) *USP. Formerly Prostaglandin* E_1, *PGE*$_1$.
Use: Vasodilator; anti-impotence agent; arterial patency agent.
See: Caverject.
Edex.
Muse.
Prostin VR Pediatric.

alprostadil. (Teva Parenteral Medicines) Alprostadil 500 mcg/mL (in dehydrated alcohol 1 mL). Inj., Soln.; concentrate. Single-dose vial. 1 mL. *Rx.*
Use: Agent for patent ductus arteriosus.

•**alrestatin sodium.** (AHL-reh-STAT-in SO-dee-uhm) USAN.
Use: Enzyme inhibitor, aldose reductase.

Alrex. (Bausch & Lomb) Loteprednol etabonate 0.2%. Benzalkonium chloride 0.01%, EDTA, glycerin, povidone. Ophth. Susp. Bot. 5 mL, 10 mL. *Rx.*
Use: Corticosteroid, ophthalmic.

AL-721. (Matrix) Phase I/II AIDS, ARC, HIV positive.
Use: Antiviral.

Alsorb Gel. (Standex) Magnesium and aluminum hydroxide. Colloidal Susp. *OTC.*
Use: Antacid.

Alsorb Gel, C.T. (Standex) Calcium carbonate 2 g, glycine 3 g, magnesium trisilicate 3 g. Tab. *OTC.*
Use: Antacid.

Alsuma. (US Worldmeds) Sumatriptan succinate 6 mg per 0.5 mL. Sodium chloride 3.5 mg. Inj., Soln. Pack containing 6 mg single-dose prefilled auto-injectors. *Rx.*
Use: Agent for migraine, serotonin 5-HT_1 receptor agonist (triptan).

Altabax. (GlaxoSmithKline) Retapamulin 1%. White petrolatum. Top. Oint. Tubes. 15 g, 30 g. *Rx.*
Use: Topical anti-infective.

Altacaine. (Altaire) Tetracaine hydrochloride 0.5%. Chlorobutanol, boric acid, potassium chloride, hydrochloric acid or sodium hydroxide. Soln. 15 mL, 30 mL. *Rx.*
Use: Ophthalmic local anesthetic.

Altace. (Monarch) Ramipril 1.25 mg, 2.5 mg, 5 mg, 10 mg. Cap. Bot. 100s, 500s (except 1.25 mg), 1000s (except 1.25 mg), UD 100s (except 10 mg), bulk pack 5000s (2.5 mg, 5 mg only). *Rx.*
Use: Antihypertensive; renin angiotensin system antagonist.

Altafed. (Altaire Pharmaceuticals) Pseudoephedrine hydrochloride 30 mg, triprolidine hydrochloride 1.25 mg per 5 mL. Methylparaben, sorbitol. Syrup. 118 mL. *OTC.*
Use: Upper respiratory combination, decongestant and antihistamine.

Altafluor. (Altaire) Benoxinate hydrochloride 0.4%, fluorescein sodium 0.25%. Soln.; Ophth. 5 mL w/dropper (w/povidone, boric acid, chlorobutanol 1%). *Rx.*
Use: Ophthalmic local anesthetic.

Altafrin. (Altaire) Phenylephrine hydrochloride 2.5%, 10%. Ophth. Soln. 5 mL (benzalkonium chloride, sodium phosphate mono- and dibasic), 15 mL (benzalkonium chloride, boric acid, sodium phosphate mono- and dibasic) (except 10%). *OTC.*
Use: Ophthalmic decongestant.

•**altanserin tartrate.** (AL-TAN-ser-in TAR-trate) USAN.
Use: Serotonin antagonist.

Altarussin. (Altaire) Guaifenesin 100 mg/5 mL. Alcohol-free. Corn syrup, menthol, saccharin. Syrup. 118 mL. *OTC.*
Use: Expectorant.

Altarussin-PE. (Altaire) Pseudoephedrine hydrochloride 30 mg, guaifenesin 100 mg per 5 mL. Alcohol free. Corn syrup, saccharin. Liq. 118 mL. *OTC.*
Use: Upper respiratory combination, decongestant and expectorant combination.

Altaryl Children's Allergy. (Altaire) Diphenhydramine (as hydrochloride) 12.5 mg per 5 mL. Alcohol free. Sodium 9 mg, glycerin, saccharin, sugar. Cherry flavor. Liq. 118 mL. *OTC.*
Use: Antihistamine.

Altavera. (Sandoz) Ethinyl estradiol 30 mcg, levonorgestrel 0.15 mg. Film coated. Lactose, PEG. Tab. Blister card 28s (w/7 white round inert tablets). *Rx.*
Use: Oral contraceptive.

Altazine. (Altaire) Tetrahydrozoline hydrochloride 0.05%. Soln., Ophth. 15 mL, 30 mL. *OTC.*
Use: Ophthalmic decongestant.

•**alteplase, recombinant.** (AL-teh-PLACE) USAN.
Use: Plasminogen activator.
See: Activase.
Cathflo Activase.

AlternaGEL. (J & J Merck Consumer Pharm.) Aluminum hydroxide 600 mg/5 mL. Liq. Bot. 150 mL, 360 mL. *OTC.*
Use: Antacid.

•**althiazide.** (al-THIGH-azz-ide) USAN.
Use: Antihypertensive; diuretic.

•**altinicline maleate.** (AL-ti-ni-kleen) USAN.
Use: Antiparkinsonian agent.

Altoprev. (Sciele) Lovastatin 20 mg, 40 mg, 60 mg. Sugar, lactose. ER Tab. 30s. *Rx.*
Use: Antihyperlipidemic.

Altracin. (Alra) Bacitracin.
Use: Antibiotic. [Orphan Drug]

•**altretamine.** (ahl-TRETT-uh-meen) USAN.
Use: Antineoplastic.
See: Hexalen.

al12. (JSJ Pharmaceuticals) Ammonium lactate. **Aer. Foam:** 12%. *Butyrospermum parkii*, cetyl alcohol, *Helianthus annuus* seed oil. 113.4 g. **Lot:** 12%. Cetyl alcohol, glycerin, mineral oil, PEG-40, PEG-100, parabens. 423 mL. *OTC.*
Use: Emollient.

Al-U-Creme. (MacAllister) Aluminum hydroxide equivalent to 4% aluminum oxide. Susp. Bot. Pt, gal. *OTC.*
Use: Antacid.

Aludrox. (Wyeth) Aluminum hydroxide gel 307 mg, magnesium hydroxide 103 mg/5 mL. Susp. Bot. 355 mL. *OTC.*
Use: Antacid.

alukalin. Activated kaolin.
Use: Antidiarrheal.

Alulex. (Lexington) Magnesium trisilicate 3.25 g, aluminum hydroxide gel 3.5 g, phenobarbital ⅛ g, homatropine methylbromide g. Tab. Bot. 100s. *Rx.*
Use: Agent for peptic ulcer.

alum. Sulfuric acid, aluminum ammonium salt (2:1:1), dodecahydrate. Sulfuric acid, aluminum potassium salt (2:1:1), dodecahydrate.
Use: Astringent.

•**alum, ammonium.** (AL-um) *USP.*
Use: Astringent.

Alumate-HC. (Dermco) Hydrocortisone 0.125%, 0.25%, 0.5%, 1%. Cream. Pkg. 0.5 oz, 1 oz, 4 oz. *OTC.*
Use: Corticosteroid, topical.

Alumate Mixture. (Schlicksup) Aluminum hydroxide gel, milk of magnesia/5 mL. Bot. 12 oz, gal. *OTC.*
Use: Antacid.

alumina and magnesia.
Use: Antacid.

alumina and magnesium carbonate.
Use: Antacid.

alumina and magnesium trisilicate.
Use: Antacid.

alumina hydrated. W/Activated attapulgite, pectin. *OTC.*
Use: Antidiarrheal.

alumina, magnesia, and calcium carbonate.
Use: Antacid.

alumina, magnesia, and calcium chloride.
Use: Antacid.

alumina, magnesia, and simethicone. (Roxane) Aluminum hydroxide 213 mg, magnesium hydroxide 200 mg, simethicone 20 mg, parabens, sorbitol/5 mL. Susp. Bot. UD 15, 30 mL. *OTC.*
Use: Antacid.

alumina, magnesia, calcium carbonate, and simethicone.
Use: Antacid.

alumina, magnesium carbonate, and magnesium oxide.
Use: Antacid.

•**aluminum acetate topical solution.** (ah-LOO-min-uhm) *USP.*
Use: Astringent.
See: Buro-Sol Antiseptic.
Domeboro Otic.

aluminum aminoacetate, dihydroxy.
See: Dihydroxyaluminum Aminoacetate.

aluminum chlorhydroxide.
See: Aluminum Chlorohydrate.

•**aluminum chloride.** (ah-LOO-min-uhm KLOR-ide) *USP.* Aluminum chloride hexahydrate.
Use: Astringent; drying agent.
See: Drysol.
Xerac AC.

aluminum chloride (hexahydrate). (Glades) Aluminum chloride hexahydrate 20% in SD alcohol 40-2 88.5%. Soln. Bot. 37.5 mL, *Dab-O-Matic* applicator bottle 35 mL, 60 mL. *Rx.*
Use: Drying agent.

•**aluminum chlorohydrate.** (ah-LOO-min-uhm) *USP. Formerly Aluminum chlorhydroxide, aluminum hydroxychloride.*
Use: Anhidrotic.
See: Ostiderm Roll-On.

•**aluminum chlorohydrex.** (ah-LOO-min-uhm) USAN. *Formerly Aluminum chlorhydroxide alcohol soluble complex, alu-*

minum chlorohydrol propylene glycol complex.
Use: Astringent.

•**aluminum chlorohydrex polyethylene glycol.** (ah-LOO-min-uhm) *USP.*
Use: Anhidrotic.

•**aluminum chlorohydrex propylene glycol.** (ah-LOO-min-uhm) *USP.*
Use: Anhidrotic.

•**aluminum dichlorohydrate.** (ah-LOO-min-uhm) *USP.*
Use: Anhidrotic.

•**aluminum dichlorohydrex polyethylene glycol.** (ah-LOO-min-uhm) *USP.*
Use: Anhidrotic.

•**aluminum dichlorohydrex propylene glycol.** (ah-LOO-min-uhm) *USP.*
Use: Anhidrotic.

aluminum dihydroxyaminoacetate. (ah-LOO-min-uhm)
See: Dihydroxyaluminum Aminoacetate.

aluminum glycinate, basic.
See: Dihydroxyaluminum Aminoacetate.

aluminum hydroxide.
Use: Antacid.
W/Aspirin, Magnesium Hydroxide.
See: Arthritis Pain Formula.
W/Aspirin, Magnesium Hydroxide, Calcium Carbonate.
See: Ascriptin Maximum Strength.
W/Magnesium Carbonate.
See: Acid Gone.
Gaviscon Extra Strength Antacid.
W/Magnesium Hydroxide.
See: Delcid.
Maagel.
W/Magnesium Hydroxide, Simethicone.
See: Di-Gel.
Gas Ban DS.
Maalox Advanced Maximum Strength.
Maalox Advanced Regular Strength.
Maalox Regular Strength.
Mi-Acid Maximum Strength.
Mintox.
Trial AG.

•**aluminum hydroxide gel.** (ah-LOO-min-uhm) *USP.*
Use: Antacid.
See: AlternaGEL.
Al-U-Creme.
Amphojel.
W/Aminoacetic acid, magnesium trisilicate.
See: Maracid-2.
W/Calcium carbonate, magnesium carbonate, magnesium trisilicate.
See: Marblen.
W/Magnesium hydroxide.
See: Alsorb Gel.
Aludrox.
W/Magnesium hydroxide, aspirin.
See: Ascriptin.
Calciphen.
W/Magnesium hydroxide, simethicone.
See: Di-Gel.
Maalox Maximum Strength Multi-Symptom.
W/Magnesium trisilicilate.
See: Gacid.
Gaviscon.
Maracid 2.
W/Phenindamine tartrate, phenylephrine hydrochloride, aspirin, caffeine, magnesium carbonate.
See: Dristan.

aluminum hydroxide gel. (Various Mfr.) Aluminum hydroxide 320 mg/5 mL. Susp. Bot. 360 mL, 480 mL, UD 15 and 30 mL. *OTC.*
Use: Antacid.

aluminum hydroxide gel, concentrated. (Roxane) Susp. **450 mg/5 mL:** Bot. 500 mL, UD 30 mL; **675 mg/5 mL:** Bot. 180 mL, 500 mL, UD 20 mL and 30 mL. *OTC.*
Use: Antacid.

aluminum hydroxide gel, concentrated. (Various Mfr.) Aluminum hydroxide 600 mg/5 mL. Liq. Bot. 30 mL, 180 mL, 480 mL. *OTC.*
Use: Antacid.

aluminum hydroxide gel, dried.
Use: Antacid.
W/Combinations.
See: Aludrox.
Alurex.
Banacid.
Delcid.
Eulcin.
Gaviscon.
Mylanta Maximum Strength.
Mylanta Regular Strength.
Presalin.

aluminum hydroxide glycine.
See: Dihydroxyaluminum aminoacetate.

aluminum hydroxide magnesium carbonate.
Use: Antacid.
See: Di-Gel.

•**aluminum monostearate.** (ah-LOO-min-uhm) *NF.*
Use: Pharmaceutic necessity for preparation of penicillin G procaine w/aluminum stearate suspension.
See: Penicillin G procaine w/aluminum stearate suspension, sterile.

aluminum paste. (Paddock) Metallic aluminum 10%. Oint. Jar lb. *OTC.*
Use: Dermatologic, protectant.

•**aluminum phosphate gel.** (ah-LOO-min-uhm FOSS-fate) *USP.*
Use: Antacid.

•**aluminum sesquichlorohydrate.** (ah-LOO-min-uhm sess-kwih-KLOR-oh-HIGH-drate) *USP.*
Use: Anhidrotic.

•**aluminum sesquichlorohydrex polyethylene glycol.** (ah-LOO-min-uhm sess-kwih-KLOR-oh-HIGH-drex poli-eth-uh-leen gli-cawl) *USP.*
Use: Anhidrotic.

•**aluminum sesquichlorohydrex propylene glycol.** (ah-LOO-min-uhm sess-kwih-KLOR-oh-HIGH-drex) *USP.*
Use: Anhidrotic.

aluminum sodium carbonate hydroxide.
See: Dihydroxyaluminum sodium carbonate.

•**aluminum subacetate.** (ah-LOO-min-uhm sub-AS-e-tate) *USP.*
Use: Astringent.

•**aluminum sulfate.** (ah-LOO-min-uhm SULL-fate) *USP.*
Use: Pharmaceutic necessity for preparation of aluminum subacetate solution.
See: Aluminum subacetate topical solution.
Ostiderm.

•**aluminum zirconium octachlorohydrate.** (ah-LOO-min-uhm zihr-KOE-nee-uhm) *USP.*
Use: Anhidrotic.

•**aluminum zirconium octachlorohydrex gly.** (ah-LOO-min-uhm zihr-KOE-nee-uhm) *USP.*
Use: Anhidrotic.

•**aluminum zirconium pentachlorohydrate.** (ah-LOO-min-uhm zihr-KOE-nee-uhm) *USP.*
Use: Anhidrotic.

•**aluminum zirconium pentachlorohydrex gly.** (ah-LOO-min-uhm zihr-KOE-nee-uhm) *USP.*
Use: Anhidrotic.

•**aluminum zirconium tetrachlorohydrate.** (ah-LOO-min-uhm zihr-KOE-nee-uhm teh-trah-KLOR-oh-HIGH-drate) *USP.*
Use: Anhidrotic.

•**aluminum zirconium tetrachlorohydrex gly.** (ah-LOO-min-uhm zihr-KOE-nee-uhm teh-trah-KLOR-oh-HIGH-drex Gly) *USP.*
Use: Anhidrotic.

•**aluminum zirconium trichlorohydrate.** (ah-LOO-min-uhm zihr-KOE-nee-uhm try-KLOR-oh-HIGH-drate) *USP.*
Use: Anhidrotic.

•**aluminum zirconium trichlorohydrex gly.** (ah-LOO-min-uhm zihr-KOE-nee-uhm try-KLOR-oh-HIGH-drex Gly) *USP.*
Use: Anhidrotic.

•**alum, potassium.** (AL-um) *USP.*
Use: Astringent.

alum-precipitated allergenic extracts.
See: Allpyral.
Center-Al.

Alurex. (Rexall Group) Magnesium-aluminum hydroxide. **Susp.:** 150 mg, 200 mg/5 mL. Bot. 12 oz. **Tab:** 300 mg, 400 mg. Box 50s. *OTC.*
Use: Antacid.

Aluvea. (Merz Pharmaceutical) Urea 39%. Glycerin, wax. Cream. 227 g. *Rx.*
Use: Emollient.

•**alvameline maleate.** (al-va-MEL-een) USAN.
Use: Partial M_1 agonist, M_2/M_3 antagonist.

Alvedil. (Luly-Thomas) Theophylline 4 g, pseudoephedrine hydrochloride 50 mg, butabarbital 15 mg. Cap. Bot. 100s. *Rx.*
Use: Bronchodilator; decongestant; hypnotic; sedative.

•**alverine citrate.** (AL-ver-een SIH-trate) USAN.
Use: Anticholinergic.

Alvesco. (Sepracor) Ciclesonide 80 mcg/actuation, 160 mcg/actuation. Soln.; Inhal. 6.1 g canister (60 actuations) w/actuator. *Rx.*
Use: Respiratory inhalant product, corticosteroid.

•**alvespimycin hydrochloride.** (al-VES-pi-MYE-sin) USAN.
Use: Antineoplastic.

•**alvimopan.** (al-VI-moe-pan) USAN.
Use: Gastrointestinal agent.
See: Entereg.

•**alvircept sudotox.** (AL-vihr-sept SOOD-ah-tox) USAN.
Use: Antiviral.

•**alvocidib.** (al-VOE-si-dib) USAN.
Use: Antineoplastic.

•**alvocidib hydrochloride.** (al-VOE-si-dib) USAN.
Use: Antineoplastic.

Alyacen 1/35. (Glenmark Generics) Ethinyl estradiol 35 mcg, norethindrone 1 mg. Lactose. Tab. 28s (w/7 inert tablets). *Rx.*
Use: Oral monophasic contraceptive.

Alyacen 7/7/7. (Glenmark Generics) **Phase 1:** Norethindrone 0.5 mg, ethinyl estradiol 35 mcg (7 white to off-white tablets). **Phase 2:** Norethindrone 0.75 mg, ethinyl estradiol 35 mcg (7 lt.

peach tablets). **Phase 3:** Norethindrone 1 mg, ethinyl estradiol 35 mcg (7 peach tablets). Tab. 28s (w/7 inert tablets). *Rx.*
Use: Oral triphasic contraceptive.

Alzapam. (Major) Lorazepam 0.5 mg, 1 mg, 2 mg. Tab. Bot. 100s, 500s. *c-IV.*
Use: Antianxiety.

ALZ-NAC. (Macoven) Vitamin B_{12} 2,000 mcg (as methylcobalamin), L-methylfolate calcium 6 mg, N-acetylcysteine 600 mg. PEG, saccharin. Tab. 90s. *Rx.*
Use: Multivitamin.

Ama. (Wampole) Antimitochondrial antibodies test by IFA. Test 48s.
Use: Diagnostic aid.

amacetam sulfate.
See: Pramiracetam sulfate.

•**amadinone acetate.** (aim-AD-ih-nohn AS-e-tate) USAN.
Use: Hormone, progestin.

•**amantadine hydrochloride.** (uh-MAN-tuh-deen) *USP.*
Use: Antiviral.
See: Symmetrel.

amantadine hydrochloride. (Upsher-Smith) Amantadine hydrochloride 100 mg. Tab. 100s, 500s. *Rx.*
Use: Antiparkinson agent; antiviral agent.

amantadine hydrochloride. (Various Mfr.) **Cap.:** 100 mg. Bot. 100s, 500s, UD 100s. **Syrup:** 50 mg/5 mL. May contain sorbitol and parabens. Bot. 480 mL. *Rx.*
Use: Antiviral; treatment of Parkinson disease.

A-Mantle. (PharmaDerm) Beeswax, cetearyl alcohol, glycerin, methylparaben, mineral oil, petrolatum. Cream. 30 g, 120 g, 454 g. *OTC.*
Use: Ointment, lotion base.

amaranth.
Use: Color (Not for internal use).

Amaryl. (Aventis) Glimepiride 1 mg, 2 mg, 4 mg. Lactose. Tab. Bot. 100s, UD 100s (4 mg only). *Rx.*
Use: Antidiabetic.

Amatine. (Roberts) Midodrine hydrochloride.
Use: Orthostatic hypotension. [Orphan Drug]

•**amatuximab.** (A-ma-TUX-i-mab) USAN.
Use: Antineoplastic.

Ambenyl Cough. (Forest) Codeine phosphate 10 mg, bromodiphenhydramine hydrochloride 12.5 mg/5 mL, alcohol 5%. Syr. Bot. 4 oz, Pt, gal. *c-V.*
Use: Antihistamine; antitussive.

Amberlite. (Rohm and Haas) I.R.P.-64. Polacrilin.

AMBI 80/780/40. (AMBI) Dextromethorphan HBr 40 mg, guaifenesin 780 mg, pseudoephedrine hydrochloride 80 mg. Dye free. ER Tab. 100s. *Rx.*
Use: Antitussive and expectorant combination.

AMBI 80/700/40. (AMBI) Dextromethorphan HBr 40 mg, guaifenesin 700 mg, pseudoephedrine hydrochloride 80 mg. Dye free. ER Tab. 100s. *Rx.*
Use: Antitussive and expectorant combination.

Ambien. (Sanofi Aventis) Zolpidem tartrate 5 mg, 10 mg. Lactose, PEG. Film coated. Tab. 100s, 500s (10 mg only). *c-IV.*
Use: Hypnotic/sedative, nonbarbiturate, imidazopyridine.

Ambien CR. (Sanofi Aventis) Zolpidem tartrate 12.5 mg. Lactose. ER Tab. 100s, 500s (12.5 mg only), UD 30s. *c-IV.*
Use: Nonbarbiturate sedative and hypnotic, imidazopyridine.

Ambifed CD. (MCR/American Pharmaceutical) Codeine phosphate 10 mg, guaifenesin 400 mg, pseudoephedrine hydrochloride 30 mg. Tab. 100s. *c-III.*
Use: Upper respiratory combination, antitussive and expectorant combination.

Ambifed CDX. (MCR/American Pharmaceutical) Codeine phosphate 20 mg, guaifenesin 400 mg, pseudoephedrine hydrochloride 30 mg. Tab. 100s. *c-III.*
Use: Upper respiratory combination, antitussive and expectorant combination.

Ambifed-G DM. (MCR American) **Tab:** Dextromethorphan hydrobromide 20 mg, guaifenesin 400 mg, pseudoephedrine hydrochloride 20 mg. 100s. **ER Tab:** Dextromethorphan hydrobromide 30 mg, guaifenesin 1,000 mg, pseudoephedrine hydrochloride 60 mg. 100s. *Rx.*
Use: Upper respiratory combination, antitussive and expectorant combination.

AMBI 40PSE/400GFN/20DM. (AMBI) Dextromethorphan HBr 20 mg, guaifenesin 400 mg, pseudoephedrine hydrochloride 40 mg. Cap. 100s. *Rx.*
Use: Upper respiratory combination; antitussive, expectorant, decongestant.

AMBI 60/580/30. (Ambi) Dextromethorphan HBr 30 mg, guaifenesin 580 mg, pseudoephedrine hydrochloride 60 mg. Dye free. ER Tab. 100s. *Rx.*
Use: Antitussive and expectorant combination, upper respiratory combination.

AMBI 60PSE/4CPM. (AMBI) Pseudoephedrine hydrochloride 60 mg, chlorpheniramine maleate 4 mg. Tab. 100s. *OTC.*
Use: Upper respiratory combination, decongestant and antihistamine.

AMBI 60PSE/4CPM/20DM. (AMBI) Pseudoephedrine hydrochloride 60 mg, chlorpheniramine maleate 4 mg, dextromethorphan hydrobromide 20 mg. Tab. 100s. *Rx.*
Use: Upper respiratory combination, decongestant and antihistamine.

AMBI 60PSE/400GFN/20DM. (AMBI) Dextromethorphan HBr 20 mg, guaifenesin 400 mg, pseudoephedrine hydrochloride 60 mg. Cap. 100s. *Rx.*
Use: Upper respiratory combination, antitussive, expectorant, decongestant.

AmBisome. (Astellas) Amphotericin B 50 mg (as liposomal), sucrose. Pow. for Inj. Single-dose Vial w/5-micron filter. *Rx.*
Use: Antifungal.

AMBI 10PEH/4CPM. (AMBI) Phenylephrine hydrochloride 10 mg, chlorpheniramine maleate 4 mg. Tab. 100s. *OTC.*
Use: Upper respiratory combination, decongestant and antihistamine.

AMBI 10PEH/4CPM/20DM. (AMBI) Phenylephrine hydrochloride 10 mg, chlorpheniramine maleate 4 mg, dextromethorphan hydrobromide 20 mg. Tab. 100s. *Rx.*
Use: Upper respiratory combination, antitussive combination.

AMBI 10PEH/400GFN/20DM. (AMBI) Dextromethorphan HBr 20 mg, guaifenesin 400 mg, phenylephrine hydrochloride 10 mg. Cap. 100s. *Rx.*
Use: Upper respiratory combination, antitussive, expectorant, decongestant.

AMBI 20DM/4CPM. (AMBI) Dextromethorphan hydrobromide 20 mg, chlorpheniramine maleate 4 mg. Tab. 100s. *Rx.*
Use: Upper respiratory combination, decongestant and antihistamine.

•**ambomycin.** (AM-boe-MY-sin) USAN. Isolated from filtrates of *Streptomyces ambofaciens.*
Use: Antineoplastic.

ambrisentan. (am-brih-SEN-tan)
Use: Vasodilator, endothelin receptor antagonist.
See: Letairis.

•**ambruticin.** (am-brew-TIE-sin) USAN.
Use: Antifungal.

ambucaine. Ambutoxate hydrochloride.

•**ambuphylline.** (AM-byoo-fill-in) USAN.
Formerly Bufylline.
Use: Diuretic; muscle relaxant.

•**ambuside.** (AM-buh-SIDE) USAN.
Use: Diuretic.

ambutonium bromide.
Use: Antispasmodic.

AMC. (Schlicksup) Ammonium chloride 7.5 g. Tab. Bot. 1000s. *Rx.*
Use: Diuretic; expectorant.

Amcill. (Parke-Davis) Ampicillin trihydrate. **Cap.:** 250 mg, 500 mg. Bot. 100s, 500s, UD 100s. **Oral Susp.:** 125 mg, 250 mg/5 mL. Bot. 100 mL, 200 mL.
Use: Anti-infective, penicillin.

•**amcinafal.** (am-SIN-ah-fal) USAN.
Use: Anti-inflammatory.

•**amcinafide.** (am-SIN-ah-fide) USAN.
Use: Anti-inflammatory.

•**amcinonide.** (am-SIN-oh-nide) *USP.*
Use: Corticosteroid, topical.

amcinonide. (Taro) **Cream:** Amcinonide 0.1%. 15 g, 30 g, 60 g. **Oint.:** 0.1%. Benzyl alcohol 2.2%, glycerin, white petrolatum. 15 g, 30 g, 60 g. *Rx.*
Use: Corticosteroid, topical.

•**amdinocillin.** (am-DEE-no-SILL-in) USAN.
Use: Anti-infective.

•**amdinocillin pivoxil.** (am-DEE-no-SILL-in pihv-OX-ill) USAN.
Use: Anti-infective.

•**amdoxovir.** (am-DOX-oh-veer) USAN.
Use: Antiviral; reverse transcriptase inhibitor.

Amdry-D. (Prasco Laboratories) Pseudoephedrine hydrochloride 120 mg, methscopolamine nitrate 2.5 mg. ER Tab. 60s. *Rx.*
Use: Upper respiratory combination, decongestant and anticholinergic combination.

ameban.
See: Carbarsone.

amebicides.
See: Carbarsone.
Chiniofon.
Chloroquine Hydrochloride.
Chloroquine Phosphate.
Emetine Hydrochloride.
Iodoquinol.
Metronidazole.

Amechol.
Use: Diagnostic aid.
See: Methacholine Chloride.

•**amedalin hydrochloride.** (ah-MEH-dah-lin) USAN.
Use: Antidepressant.

•**ameltolide.** (AH-mell-TOE-lide) USAN.
Use: Anticonvulsant.

Amerge. (GlaxoSmithKline) Naratriptan hydrochloride 1 mg, 2.5 mg, lactose. Tab. Blister pack 9s. *Rx.*
Use: Antimigraine; serotonin 5-HT_1 receptor agonist.

Americaine. (Insight Pharmaceuticals) Benzocaine 20%. Polyethylene glycol 300, isobutene, normal butane, propane. Spray. 57 g. *OTC.*
Use: Topical anesthetic.

Americaine Hemorrhoidal. (Insight Pharmaceuticals) Benzocaine 20%. Benzethonium chloride, polyethylene glycol 300, polyethylene glycol 3350. Oint. 28 g. *OTC.*
Use: Anorectal preparation.

Americet. (MCR American) Acetaminophen 325 mg, caffeine 40 mg, butalbital 50 mg. Tab. 100s. *Rx.*
Use: Nonnarcotic analgesic combination with barbiturates.

Amerifed. (Ambi) Pseudoephedrine hydrochloride 80 mg, chlorpheniramine maleate 4 mg per 5 mL. Parabens, aspartame, phenylalanine, alcohol free, sugar free, raspberry flavor. Liq. 30 mL, 473 mL. *Rx.*
Use: Decongestant and antihistamine.

Amerigel. (Amerx Health Care Corp.) **Lot.:** Glycerin, lemon oil, parabens, oak extract (Oakin). Bot. 228 g. **Oint.:** Meadowsweet extract, oakbark extract, polyethylene glycol 400, polyethylene glycol 3350, zinc acetate. Tube. 28.3 g. *OTC.*
Use: Diaper rash product.

Amerituss AD. (Ambi) Dextromethorphan HBr 15 mg, chlorpheniramine maleate 3 mg, phenylephrine hydrochloride 10 mg per 5 mL. Phenylalanine, aspartame, alcohol free, sugar free. Liq. 473 mL. *Rx.*
Use: Upper respiratory combination.

AmeriWash. (AmeriDerm Laboratories) Triclosan. Eucalyptus oil, glycerin, parabens, tetrasodium EDTA, triethanolamine. Soap. 473 mL. *OTC.*
Use: Topical anti-infective, antiseptic and germicide.

Ames Dextro System Lancets. (Bayer Consumer Care) Sterile disposable lancet. Box 100s.
Use: Diagnostic aid.

•**amesergide.** (am-eh-SIR-jide) USAN.
Use: Serotonin antagonist.

•**ametantrone acetate.** (am-ETT-an-TRONE) USAN.
Use: Antineoplastic.

A-Methapred. (Hospira) Methylprednisolone sodium succinate 40 mg/vial, 125 mg/vial. Inj. Pow. for Soln. *Univial.* 1 mL (40 mg only) with sodium phosphate anhydrous (monobasic 1.6 mg, dibasic 17.5 mg), lactose 25 mg, benzyl alcohol 9 mg; 2 mL with sodium phosphate anhydrous (monobasic 1.6 mg, dibasic 17.4 mg), benzyl alcohol ≈ 18 mg. *Rx.*
Use: Adrenocortical steroid, glucocorticoid.

Amethia. (Watson) **Phase 1:** Ethinyl estradiol 30 mcg, levonorgestrel 0.15 mg. Lactose. Tab. 84s. **Phase 2:** Ethinyl estradiol 10 mcg. Lactose. Tab. 7s. *Rx.*
Use: Biphasic oral contraceptive.

Amethia Lo. (Watson) **Phase 1:** Ethinyl estradiol 20 mcg, levonorgestrel 0.1 mg. Lactose. Tab. 84s. **Phase 2:** Ethinyl estradiol 10 mcg. Lactose. Tab. 7s. *Rx.*
Use: Biphasic oral contraceptive.

amethocaine hydrochloride.
Use: Anesthetic, local.
See: Tetracaine hydrochloride.

amethopterin.
Use: Antineoplastic.
See: Methotrexate.

Amethyst. (Watson) Ethinyl estradiol 20 mcg, levonorgestrel 0.09 mg. Lactose. Tab. 28s. *Rx.*
Use: Monophasic oral contraceptive.

Amevive. (Astellas) Alefacept 15 mg. Sucrose 12.5 mg, preservative free. Pow. for Inj., lyophilized. Dose pack. 1s, 4s (in single-use vials with 10 mL single-use diluent [sterile water for injection]). *Rx.*
Use: Immunologic agent, immunosuppressive.

•**amfenac sodium.** (AM-fen-ack SO-dee-uhm) USAN.
Use: Anti-inflammatory.

•**amfilcon A.** (AM-FILL-kahn A) USAN.
Use: Contact lens material, hydrophilic.

•**amflutizole.** (am-FLEW-tih-zole) USAN.
Use: Treatment of gout.

amfodyne.
See: Imidecyl iodine.

•**amfonelic acid.** (am-fah-NEH-lick) USAN.
Use: Central nervous system stimulant.

Amgenal Cough. (Ivax) Bromodiphenhydramine hydrochloride 12.5 mg, codeine phosphate 10 mg/5 mL, alcohol 5%. Syr. Bot. 120 mL, pt, gal. *c-v.*
Use: Antihistamine; antitussive.

AMG 531.
Use: Investigational thrombopoiesis-stimulating peptibody.

amibiarson.
See: Carbarsone.

Amicar. (Xanodyne) **Tab.:** Aminocaproic acid 500 mg, 1,000 mg. Bot. 100s. **Soln.:** Aminocaproic acid 250 mg/mL, parabens, EDTA, sorbitol, saccharin, raspberry flavor. Bot. 473 mL. *Rx.*
Use: Hemostatic, systemic.

•**amicycline.** (AM-ee-SIGH-kleen) USAN.
Use: Anti-infective.

Amidate. (Hospira) Etomidate 2 mg/mL, propylene glycol 35%. Single-dose Amp 20 mg/10 mL, 40 mg/20 mL; *Abboject* syringe 40 mg/20 mL. *Rx.*
Use: Anesthetic, general.

amide local anesthetics.
See: Articaine Hydrochloride.
Bupivacaine Hydrochloride.
Bupivacaine Hydrochloride with Epinephrine 1:200,000.
Bupivacaine Spinal.
Carbocaine.
Carbocaine with Neo-Cobefrin.
Chirocaine.
Citanest Forte.
Citanest Plain.
Dibucaine.
Lidocaine and Epinephrine.
Lidocaine Hydrochloride.
Lidocaine Hydrochloride and Epinephrine.
Marcaine.
Mepivacaine Hydrochloride.
Mepivacaine Hydrochloride and Levonordefrin.
Naropin.
Octocaine.
Polocaine.
Polocaine MPF.
Polocaine with Levonordefrin.
Prilocaine Hydrochloride.
Ropivacaine Hydrochloride.
Sensorcaine.
Sensorcaine MPF.
Sensorcaine-MPF Spinal.
Septocaine.
Xylocaine.
Xylocaine MPF.

•**amidephrine mesylate.** (AM-ee-DEH-frin MEH-sih-LATE) USAN.
Use: Adrenergic.

amidofebrin.
See: Aminopyrine.

amidone hydrochloride.
Use: Analgesic; narcotic.
See: Methadone hydrochloride.

amidopyrazoline.
See: Aminopyrine.

amidotrizoate, sodium.
See: Diatrizoate sodium.

•**amifloxacin.** (am-ih-FLOX-ah-SIN) USAN.
Use: Anti-infective.

•**amifloxacin mesylate.** (am-ih-FLOX-ah-SIN MEH-sih-LATE) USAN.
Use: Anti-infective.

•**amifostine.** (am-ih-FOSS-teen) USAN.
Formerly Ethiofos.
Use: Cytoprotective agent.
See: Ethyol.

amifostine. (Caraco Pharmaceutical) Amifostine 500 mg (as amifostine trihydrate). Inj. Pow. for Soln. Single-use vials. 10 mL. *Rx.*
Use: Cytoprotective agent.

Amigen. (Baxter PPI) Protein hydrolysate. **5%, 10%:** Bot. 500 mL, 1000 mL. **5% w/dextrose 5%:** Bot. 500 mL, 1000 mL. **5% w/dextrose 5%, alcohol 5%:** Bot. 1000 mL. **5% w/fructose 10%:** Bot. 1000 mL. **5% w/fructose 12.5%, alcohol 2.4%:** Bot. 1000 mL. *Rx.*
Use: Nutritional supplement.

•**amikacin.** (am-ih-KAE-sin) *USP.*
Use: Anti-infective.
See: Amikin.

amikacin. (Bedford) Amikacin sulfate 250 mg, sodium metabisulfite 0.66%, sodium citrate dihydrate 2.5%/mL. Inj. Vial 2 mL, 4 mL. *Rx.*
Use: Anti-infective.

amikacin. (Various Mfr.) Amikacin 50 mg (as sulfate) per mL, sodium metabisulfite 0.13%, sodium citrate dihydrate 0.5%. Inj. Vial 2, 4 mL. 10s. *Rx.*
Use: Anti-infective.

•**amikacin sulfate.** (am-ih-KAE-sin) *USP.*
Use: Anti-infective.

amikacin sulfate. (Various Mfr.) Amikacin sulfate 50 mg/mL. Inj. Vial 2 mL, 4 mL (10s). *Rx.*
Use: Anti-infective.

•**amiloride hydrochloride.** (uh-MILL-oh-ride) *USP.*
Tall Man: aMILoride
Use: Diuretic.
See: Midamor.

amiloride hydrochloride. (AvKARE) Amiloride hydrochloride 5 mg. Lactose. Tab. 90s. *Rx.*
Use: Potassium-sparing diuretic.

amiloride hydrochloride and hydrochlorothiazide.
Use: Antihypertensive; diuretic.
See: Moduretic.

•**amiloxate.** (A-mil-Ox-ate) *USP. Formerly isoamyl methoxycinnamate.*
Use: Sunscreen.

•**aminacrine hydrochloride.** (ah-MEE-nah-kreen) USAN.
Use: Anti-infective, topical.

aminarsone.
See: Carbarsone.

Amina-21. (Miller Pharmacal Group) Free-form amino acids 556 mg. Cap. Bot. 100s, 300s. *OTC.*
Use: Dermatologic, wound therapy.

Aminicotin.
Use: Vitamin supplement.
See: Nicotinamide.

aminoacetic acid.
Use: Myasthenia gravis; irrigant.
See: Glycine.
W/Magnesium trisilicate, aluminum hydroxide.
See: Maracid-2.
W/Phenylephrine hydrochloride, chlorpheniramine maleate, acetaminophen, caffeine.
See: Codimal.

amino acid and protein.
See: Aminoacetic Acid.
Glutamic Acid.
Lysine.
Phenylalanine.
Thyroxine.

amino acid combinations.
See: A/G-Pro.
Amina-21.
Body Fortress Natural Amino.
Dequasine.
EMF.
Jets.
NeuRecover-DA.
NeuRecover-SA.
NeuroSlim.
PDP Liquid Protein.
PowerMate.
PowerSleep.

amino acid derivatives.
See: Carnitor.
L-Carnitine.
Levocarnitine.

amino acids.
Use: Amino acid supplement.
See: Aminosyn.

aminoacridine. (ah-MEE-no-ACK-rih-deen)
See: Aminacrine hydrochloride.

9-aminoacridine hydrochloride. Aminacrine hydrochloride.
Use: Anti-infective, vaginal.
See: Vagisec Plus.
W/Polyoxyethylene nonyl phenol, sodium edetate, docusate sodium.
See: Vagisec Plus.
W/Sulfanilamide, allantoin.
See: Nil Vaginal Cream.

p-aminobenzene-sulfonylacetylimide.
See: Sulfacetamide.

•**aminobenzoate potassium.** (ah-MEE-no-BEN-zoe-ate) *USP.*
Use: Analgesic, water-soluble vitamin.
See: Potaba.
W/Potassium salicylate.
See: Pabalate-SF.

aminobenzoate potassium. (Hope Pharm) Aminobenzoate potassium 500 mg. Cap. 250s. *Rx.*
Use: Water-soluble vitamin.

•**aminobenzoate sodium.** (ah-MEE-no-BEN-zoe-ate) *USP.*
Use: Analgesic.
See: PABA Sodium.
W/Phenobarbital, colchicine salicylate, vitamin B_1, aspirin.
See: Doloral.
W/Salicylamide, sodium salicylate, ascorbic acid, butabarbital sodium.
See: Bisalate.

•**aminobenzoic acid.** (a-MEE-noe-ben-ZOE-ik) *USP. Formerly Para-aminobenzoic acid.*
Use: Ultraviolet screen.

•**aminocaproic acid.** (uh-mee-no-kuh-PRO-ik) *USP.*
Use: Hemostatic.
See: Amicar.

aminocaproic acid. (Orphan Medical)
Use: Topical treatment of traumatic hyphema of the eye.

aminocaproic acid. (Various Mfr.) Aminocaproic acid 250 mg/mL. Inj. Vial 20 mL. *Rx.*
Use: Antifibrinolytic; hemostatic, systemic.

aminocaproic acid. (VersaPharm) Aminocaproic acid. **Oral Soln.:** 250 mg/mL, saccharin, sorbitol, parabens, raspberry flavor. Bot. 237 mL, 473 mL. **Tab.:** 500 mg. 100s. *Rx.*
Use: Hemostatic.

aminocardol.
Use: Bronchodilator.
See: Aminophylline.

Amino-Cerv. (Cooper Surgical) Urea 8.34%, sodium propionate 0.5%, methionine 0.83%, cystine 0.35%, inositol 0.83%, benzalkonium chloride, water miscible base. Tube with applicator 82.5 g. *Rx.*
Use: Vaginal agent.

2-aminoethanethiol.
Use: Urinary tract agent.

amino-ethyl-propanol.
See: Aminoisobutanol.
W/Bromotheophyllin.
See: Pamabrom.

Aminofen. (Dover Pharmaceuticals) Acetaminophen 325 mg. Tab. 500s. *OTC.*
Use: Analgesic.

Aminofen Max Extra Strength. (Dover Pharmaceuticals) Acetaminophen 500 mg. Tab. 500s. *OTC.*
Use: Analgesic.

aminoform.
Use: Anti-infective, urinary.
See: Methenamine.

Aminogen. (Christina) Vitamin B complex, folic acid. Amp. 2 mL Box 12s, 24s, 100s. Vial 10 mL. *Rx.*
Use: Vitamin supplement.

•**aminoglutethimide.** (ah-MEE-no-glue-TETH-ih-mide) *USP.*
Use: Treatment of Cushing syndrome; adrenocortical suppressant; antineoplastic.

aminoglycosides, parenteral.
See: Gentamicin.
Kanamycin Sulfate.
Streptomycin Sulfate.
Tobramycin.

aminohippurate sodium. (Merck & Co.) Aminohippurate sodium 0.2 g/10 mL. Amp 10 mL, 50 mL.
Use: IV diagnostic aid for renal plasma flow and function determination.

•**aminohippurate sodium injection.** (ah-MEE-no-HIP-your-ate) *USP.*
Use: Diagnostic aid, renal function determination.

•**aminohippuric acid.** (ah-MEE-no-hip-YOUR-ik) *USP.*
Use: Component of aminohippurate sodium (Inj.); diagnostic aid, renal function determination.

aminoisobutanol.
See: Butaphyllamine.
Pamabrom for combinations.

aminoisometradine.
See: Methionine.

•**aminolevulinic acid hydrochloride.** (ah-MEE-no-lev-you-LIN-ik AS-id HIGH-droe-KLOR-ide) USAN.
Use: Antineoplastic.
See: Levulan Kerastick.

Amino-Min-D. (Tyson) Ca 250 mg, D 100 units, Fe 7.5 mg, Zn 5.6 mg, Mg, I, Mn, Cu, K, Cr, Se, betaine hydrochloride, glutamic acid hydrochloride. Cap. Bot. 100s. *OTC.*
Use: Mineral, vitamin supplement.

Aminonat. Protein hydrolysates (oral).

aminonitrozole.
Use: Antitrichomonal.

Amino-Opti-C. (Tyson) Vitamin C 1000 mg, lemon bioflavonoids 250 mg. Rutin, hesperidin, rose hips powder, dicalcium phosphate, hydrogenated soybean oil. SR Tab. Bot. 100s. *OTC.*
Use: Water-soluble vitamin.

aminopenicillins.
Use: Anti-infective.
See: Amoxicillin.
Amoxicillin and Clavulanate Potassium.
Ampicillin.
Ampicillin Sodium and Sulbactam Sodium.

•**aminopentamide sulfate.** (a-MEE-noe-PEN-ta-mide) *USP.*
Use: Anticholinergic.

•**aminophylline.** (am-in-AHF-ih-lin) *USP.*
Formerly Theophylline ethylenediamine.
Use: Muscle relaxant.
W/Combinations.
See: Mudrane.
Mudrane GG-2.

aminophylline. (Various Mfr.) Aminophylline. **Inj.:** 25 mg (equivalent to theophylline 19.75 mg) per mL. Amps, vials. 10 mL, 20 mL. **Tab.:** 100 mg (equivalent to theophylline 79 mg), 200 mg (equivalent to theophylline 158 mg). 100s, UD 100s. *Rx.*
Use: Bronchodilator.

Aminoprel. (Taylor Pharmaceuticals) L-lysine 60 mg, dl-methionine 15 mg, hydrolyzed protein 750 mg, iron 2 mg, Cu, I, K, Mg, Mn, Zn. Cap. Bot. 180s.
Use: Nutritional supplement.

aminopromazine. (I.N.N.) Proquamezine.

4-aminopyridine.
Use: Relief of symptoms of multiple sclerosis. [Orphan Drug]

aminopyrine.
Use: Antipyretic; analgesic.
See: Dipyrone.

8-aminoquinoline derivatives.
Use: Antimalarial.
See: Primaquine Phosphate.

4-aminoquinoline compounds.
Use: Antimalarial.
See: Aralen.
Chloroquine Phosphate.

•**aminorex.** (am-EE-no-rex) USAN.
Use: Anorexic.

aminosalicylate calcium. (Dumas-Wilson) Aminosalicylate calcium 7.5 g. Bot. 1000s.
Use: Tuberculosis therapy.

aminosalicylate potassium. Monopotassium 4-aminosalicylate.
Use: Antibacterial; tuberculostatic.

•**aminosalicylate sodium.** (uh-MEE-no-suh-LIS-ih-LATE) *USP.*
Use: Anti-infective; tuberculostatic.

•**aminosalicylic acid.** (ah-MEE-no-sal-ih-SILL-ik) *USP.*
Use: Antituberculosis agent.
See: Paser.

5-aminosalicylic acid.
See: Mesalamine.

4-aminosalicylic acid.
Use: Treatment of ulcerative colitis in patients intolerant to sulfasalazine. [Orphan Drug]

p-aminosalicylic acid salts.
See: Aminosalicylate Calcium.
Aminosalicylate Potassium.
Aminosalicylate Sodium.

aminosidine.
Use: Mycobacterium avium complex; tuberculosis; visceral leishmaniasism (KALA-AZAR). [Orphan Drug]
See: Gabbromicina.

Aminosyn. (Hospira) Crystalline amino acid solution. **3.5%:** 1,000 mL. **5%:** 500 mL, 1,000 mL. **7%:** 500 mL. **8.5%:** 500 mL, 1,000 mL. **10%:** 500 mL, 1,000 mL. **W/Electrolytes: 7%:** 500 mL. **8.5%:** 500 mL. *Rx.*
Use: Nutritional supplement, parenteral.

Aminosyn-HBC 7%. (Hospira) Crystalline amino acid infusion for high metabolic stress. 500 mL, 1,000 mL. *Rx.*
Use: Nutritional supplement, parenteral.

Aminosyn II. (Hospira) Crystalline amino acid. Inj. **3.5%:** 1,000 mL. **5%:** 500 mL, 1,000 mL. **7%:** 500 mL. **8.5%:** 500 mL, 1,000 mL. **10%:** 500 mL, 1,000 mL. **15%:** 2,000 mL. **W/Dextrose: 3.5% in 5% dextrose:** 1,000 mL. **4.25% in 10% dextrose:** 1,000 mL. **4.25% in 20% dextrose:** 500 mL. **4.25% in 25% dextrose:** 500 mL. **W/Electrolytes: 8.5%:** 1,000 mL. *Rx.*
Use: Nutritional supplement, parenteral.

Aminosyn II M. (Hospira) Crystalline amino acid w/electrolytes in dextrose. Inj. **3.5% in 5% dextrose:** 500 mL. **4.25% in 10% dextrose:** 500 mL. *Rx.*
Use: Nutritional supplement, parenteral.

Aminosyn M 3.5%. (Hospira) Crystalline amino acid infusion with electrolytes. 1,000 mL. *Rx.*
Use: Nutritional supplement, parenteral.

Aminosyn-PF. (Hospira) Crystalline amino acid infusions for pediatric use. **7%:** 500 mL. **10%:** 1,000 mL. *Rx.*
Use: Nutritional supplement, parenteral.

Aminosyn-RF. (Hospira) Crystalline amino acid infusion for renal failure patients. 5.2%. Inj. 500 mL. *Rx.*
Use: Nutritional supplement, parenteral.

Amino-Thiol. (Marcen) Sulfur 10 mg, casein 50 mg, sodium citrate 5 mg, phenol 5 mg, benzyl alcohol 5 mg/mL. Vial 10 mL, 30 mL. *Rx.*
Use: Treatment of arthritis; neuritis.

aminotrate phosphate. Trolnitratephosphate.
See: Triethanolamine.

Aminoxin. (Tyson & Assoc.) Pyridoxal-5′-phosphate 20 mg. EC Tab. Bot. 100s. *OTC.*
Use: Water-soluble vitamin.

aminoxytropine tropate hydrochloride. Atropine-N-oxide hydrochloride.

Amio-Aqueous. (Academic Pharmaceuticals) Amiodarone.
Use: Antiarrhythmic. [Orphan Drug]

•**amiodarone hydrochloride.** (A-MEE-oh-duh-rone) USAN.
Use: Cardiovascular agent; antiarrhythmic; ventricular.
See: Amio-Aqueous.
Cordarone.
Nexterone.
Pacerone.

amiodarone hydrochloride. (Various Mfr.) Amiodarone hydrochloride. **Inj.:** 50 mg/mL, may contain benzyl alcohol. 3 mL vials and amps. **Tab.:** 100 mg, 200 mg, 400 mg. May contain lactose. 30s (except 200 mg); 60s, 100s, 250s, 500s, 1,000s (200 mg only); UD 100s (except 100s). *Rx.*
Use: Antiarrhythmic.

Amipaque. (Sanofi-Synthelabo) Metrizamide 18.75%/20 mL Vial.
Use: Radiopaque agent.

•**amiprilose hydrochloride.** (ah-MIH-prih-LOHS) USAN.
Use: Anti-infective; antifungal; anti-inflammatory; antineoplastic; antiviral; immunomodulator.

•**amiquinsin hydrochloride.** (AM-ih-KWIN-sin) USAN. Under study.
Use: Antihypertensive.

•**amitifadine.** (AM-i-TIF-a-deen) USAN.
Use: Antidepressant.

•**amitifadine hydrochloride.** (AM-i-TIF-a-deen) USAN.
Use: Antidepressant.

Amitin. (Thurston) Vitamin C 200 mg, lemon bioflavonoid 100 mg, niacinamide 60 mg, methionine 100 mg. Tab. Bot. 100s, 500s. *Rx.*
Use: Vitamin supplement.

Amitiza. (Sucampo Pharmaceuticals) Lubiprostone 8 mcg, 24 mcg. Sorbitol. Cap. 60s. *Rx.*
Use: Treatment of chronic constipation.

•**amitraz.** (AM-ih-trazz) *USP.*
Use: Scabicide.

•**amitriptyline hydrochloride.** (am-ee-TRIP-tih-leen) *USP.*

Use: Antidepressant.
See: Endep.
W/Chlordiazepoxide.
See: Limbitrol.
W/Perphenazine.
See: Etrafon.

amitriptyline hydrochloride. (Various Mfr.) Amitriptyline hydrochloride 10 mg, 25 mg, 50 mg, 75 mg, 100 mg, 150 mg. Tab. Bot. 100s, 500s (75 mg and 100 mg only), 1000s, UD 100s, blister pack 25s (25 mg and 50 mg only), 100s (except 150 mg), 600s (10 mg, 25 mg, 50 mg only). *Rx.*
Use: Antidepressant.

AmLactin Foot Cream Therapy. (Upsher-Smith) Ammonium lactate, emulsifying wax, glycerin, light mineral oil, parabens, potassium lactate, white petrolatum. Cream. 85 g. *OTC.*
Use: Emollient.

AmLactin Ultra. (Upsher-Smith) Ammonium lactate, glycerin, mineral oil, petrolatum, propylene glycol, parabens, wax. Cream. 140 g. *OTC.*
Use: Emollient.

AmLactin XL. (Upsher-Smith) Ammonium lactate, potassium lactate, sodium lactate, light mineral oil, white petrolatum, glycerin, xanthan gum, parabens. Lot. 160 g. *OTC.*
Use: Emollient.

•**amlexanox.** (am-LEX-an-ox) USAN.
Use: Mouth and throat product.

•**amlintide.** (AM-lin-tide) USAN.
Use: Treatment of type I diabetes mellitus; antidiabetic.

•**amlodipine.** (am-LOW-dih-PEEN)
Tall Man: amLODIPine
Use: Calcium channel blocker.
See: Norvasc.
W/Benazepril Hydrochloride.
See: Lotrel.
W/Hydrochlorothiazide/Valsartan.
See: Exforge HCT.

•**amlodipine besylate.** (am-LOW-dih-PEEN) USAN.
Tall Man: amLODIPine
Use: Antianginal; antihypertensive.
See: Norvasc.
W/Aliskiren.
See: Tekamlo.
W/Aliskiren Hemifumarate, Hydrochlorothiazide.
See: Amturnide.
W/Atorvastatin Calcium.
See: Caduet.
W/Olmesartan Medoxomil.
See: Azor.
W/Valsartan.
See: Exforge.

amlodipine besylate. (Various Mfr.) Amlodipine besylate 2.5 mg, 5 mg, 10 mg. Tab. 90s, 100s, 300s, 500s, 1000s (except 2.5 mg), 2500s (5 mg only), UD 100s, UD 300s (5 mg only). *Rx.*
Use: Calcium channel blocking agent.

amlodipine besylate and benazepril hydrochloride. (Various Mfr.) Amlodipine/benazepril hydrochloride 2.5 mg/10 mg, 5 mg/10 mg, 5 mg/20 mg, 5 mg/40 mg, 10 mg/20 mg, 10 mg/40 mg. May contain lactose. Cap. 100s, 500s (5 mg/40 mg, 10 mg/40 mg). *Rx.*
Use: Antihypertensive combination.

amlodipine besylate/atorvastatin calcium. (Various Mfr.) Amlodipine/atorvastatin 2.5 mg/10 mg, 2.5 mg/20 mg, 2.5 mg/40 mg, 5 mg/10 mg, 5 mg/20 mg, 5 mg/40 mg, 5 mg/80 mg, 10 mg/10 mg, 10 mg/20 mg, 10 mg/40 mg, 10 mg/80 mg. May contain calcium carbonate. Tab. 30s, 90s, 500s. *Rx.*
Use: Antihyperlipidemic combination product.

•**amlodipine maleate.** (am-LOW-dih-PEEN) USAN.
Tall Man: amLODIPine
Use: Antianginal; antihypertensive.

Ammens Medicated. (Bristol-Myers Squibb) Boric acid 4.55%, zinc oxide 9.10%, talc, starch. Pow. Can 6.25 oz, 11 oz. *OTC.*
Use: Dermatologic; protectant.

ammoidin. Methoxsalen.
Use: Psoralen.

•**ammonia N 13 injection.** (ah-MOE-nee-ah N13) *USP.*
Use: Diagnostic aid, cardiac imaging, liver imaging; radiopharmaceutical.

•**ammonia solution, strong.** (ah-MOE-nee-ah) *NF.*
Use: Pharmaceutic aid, solvent; source of ammonia.

•**ammonia spirit, aromatic.** (ah-MOE-nee-ah) *USP.*
Use: Respiratory.

•**ammonio methacrylate copolymer.** (ah-MOE-nee-oh meth-ah-KRILL-ate koe-PAHL-ih-mer) *NF.*
Use: Pharmaceutic aid, coating agent.

ammonium benzoate.
Use: Antiseptic, urinary.

ammonium biphosphate, sodium biphosphate, and sodium acid pyrophosphate.
Use: Genitourinary.

•**ammonium carbonate.** (ah-MOE-nee-uhm) *NF.*
Use: Pharmaceutic aid, source of ammonia.

•**ammonium chloride.** (ah-MOE-nee-uhm) *USP.*
Use: Acidifier; diuretic.

ammonium chloride. (Hospira) Ammonium chloride 26.75% (5 mEq/mL). To be diluted before infusion. Inj. Vials. 20 mL (100 mEq) with EDTA 2 mg. *Rx.*
Use: Intravenous nutritional therapy.

•**ammonium lactate.** (ah-MOE-nee-uhm LACK-tate) USAN.
Use: Antipruritic, topical.
See: al12.
AmLactin Foot Cream Therapy.
Geri-Hydrolac 12.
Lac-Hydrin.
LAC-Lotion.

ammonium lactate. (Glades) Ammonium lactate (equiv. to 12% lactic acid), cetyl alcohol, glycerin, glyceryl stearate, light mineral oil, parabens. Lot. 225 g, 400 g. *Rx.*
Use: Emollient.

ammonium mandelate. Ammonium salt of mandelic acid 8 g/fl oz. Syr. Bot. Pt, gal.
Use: Urinary antiseptic, oral.

•**ammonium molybdate.** (ah-MOE-nee-uhm) *USP.*

ammonium nitrate.
See: Reditemp-C.

•**ammonium phosphate.** (ah-MOE-nee-uhm) *NF.* Phosphoric acid diammonium salt. Diammonium phosphate.
Use: Pharmaceutic aid.

•**ammonium sulfate.** (ah-MOE-nee-uhm) USAN.
Use: Pharmaceutic aid.

ammonium tetrathiomolybdate.
Use: Treatment of Wilson disease. [Orphan Drug]

ammonium valerate.
Use: Sedative.

Ammonul. (Ucyclyd Pharma) Sodium benzoate 100 mg and sodium phenylacetate 100 mg per mL. Inj. Single-use vials. 50 mL. *Rx.*
Use: Hyperammonemia.

ammophyllin.
Use: Bronchodilator.
See: Aminophylline.

Amnesteem. (Mylan) Isotretinoin 10 mg, 20 mg, 40 mg. Cap. 30s, 100s (except 10 mg), UD 30s (10 mg only), UD 100s (10 mg only). *Rx.*
Use: Retinoid, first generation.

•**amobarbital sodium.** (am-oh-BAR-bih-tahl) *USP.*
Use: Hypnotic; sedative.

amobarbital sodium. (Various Mfr.) **Cap. 1 g:** Bot. 100s, 500s. **3 g:** Bot. 100s, 500s, 1000s. (Various Mfr.) **Tab. 30 mg:** Bot. 100s. **50 mg:** Bot. 100s. **100 mg:** Bot. 100s. (Eli Lilly and Co.) Vial 250 mg, 500 mg. (Eli Lilly and Co.)
Use: Sedative; hypnotic.
W/Ephedrine hydrochloride, theophylline, chlorpheniramine maleate.
See: Amytal Sodium.
W/Secobarbital sodium.
See: Dusotal.
Tuinal.

Amoclan. (West-ward) Amoxicillin/clavulanic acid (as potassium salt) 200 mg/28.5 mg (potassium 0.143 mEq per 5 mL), 400 mg/57 mg (potassium 0.286 mEq per 5 mL) (after reconstitution) per 5 mL. Phenylalanine 7 mg/5 mL, aspartame. Golden syrup and orange flavor. Pow. for Oral Susp. 50 mL, 75 mL, 100 mL. *Rx.*
Use: Penicillin, aminopenicillin.

•**amodiaquine.** (am-oh-DIE-ah-kwin) *USP.*
Use: Antiprotozoal.

•**amodiaquine hydrochloride.** (am-oh-DIE-ah-kwin) *USP.*
Use: Antimalarial.

Amodopa. (Major) Methyldopa 125 mg, 250 mg, 500 mg. Bot. 100s, 500s, (500 mg only), 1000s (250 mg only), UD 100s. *Rx.*
Use: Antihypertensive.

Amol. Mono-n-amyl-hydroquinone ether.
See: B-F-I.

Amoline. (Major) Aminophylline 100 mg, 200 mg. Tab. Bot. 100s, 1000s, UD 100s. *Rx-OTC.*
Use: Bronchodilator.

•**amonafide.** (a-MOE-na-fide) USAN.
Use: Antineoplastic.

•**amonafide L-malate.** (a-MOE-na-fide) USAN.
Use: Antineoplastic.

amopyroquin hydrochloride.
See: Propoquin.

•**amorolfine.** (am-OH-role-feen) USAN.
Use: Antimycotic.

Amosan. (Oral-B) Sodium perborate, saccharin. Single-dose packet box. 1.76 g. 20s, 40s. *OTC.*
Use: Mouth and throat preparation.

•**amotosalen hydrochloride.** (a-moe-TOE-sa-len) USAN.
Use: Photochemical treatment for plasma.

Amotriphene. *Rx.*
Use: Coronary vasodilator.

•**amoxapine.** (am-OX-uh-peen) *USP.*
Use: Antidepressant.

amoxapine. (Various Mfr.) Amoxapine 25 mg, 50 mg, 100 mg, 150 mg. Tab. Bot. 30s, 100s, 500s (50 mg only), 1000s, blister pack 100s (25 mg and 50 mg only). *Rx.*
Use: Antidepressant.

•**amoxicillin.** (a-MOX-ih-sil-in) *USP.*
Use: Penicillin, aminopenicillin.
See: Amoxil.
DisperMox.
Moxatag.
Trimox.

amoxicillin. (Ranbaxy) Amoxicillin. **Chew. Tab.:** 200 mg, 400 mg. Bot. 20s, 100s (400 mg only). **Pow. for Oral Susp.:** 200 mg/5 mL, 400 mg/5 mL when reconstituted. Fruit flavor. 50 mL, 75 mL, 100 mL. *Rx.*
Use: Penicillin, aminopenicillin.

amoxicillin. (Various Mfr.) Amoxicillin. **Cap.:** 250 mg, 500 mg. 50s (500 mg only), 100s, 500s, 1000s (250 mg only). **Chew. Tab.:** 125 mg, 250 mg. 100s; 250s, 500s (250 mg only). **Pow. for Susp., Oral:** 125 mg/5 mL, 250 mg/5 mL when reconstituted. 80 mL, 100 mL, 150 mL. **Tab.:** 500 mg, 875 mg. 20s, 100s, 500s (875 mg only). *Rx.*
Use: Penicillin, aminopenicillin.

•**amoxicillin and clavulanate potassium.** (a-MOX-ih-sil-in and CLAV-you-lon-ate poe-TASS-ee-uhm) *USP.*
Use: Aminopenicillin, penicillin.
See: Amoclan.
Augmentin.
Augmentin XR.

amoxicillin, clavulanate potassium. (Geneva) **Chew. Tab.:** Amoxicillin trihydrate 200 mg/clavulanic acid 28.5 mg, amoxicillin trihydrate 400 mg/clavulanic acid 57 mg. Bot. UD 20s. **Pow. for Oral Susp.:** Amoxicillin trihydrate 200 mg/clavulanic acid 28.5 mg, amoxicillin trihydrate 400 mg/clavulanic acid 57 mg. Vial. 100 mL. *Rx.*
Use: Anti-infective, penicillin.

amoxicillin/clavulanate potassium. (Lek) Amoxicillin/clavulanic acid (as the potassium salt) 250 mg/125 mg. Tab. 30s. *Rx.*
Use: Penicillin, aminopenicillin.

amoxicillin/clavulanate potassium. (Sandoz) Amoxicillin 1,000 mg, clavulanic acid 62.5 mg. Film coated. PEG, potassium 0.31 mEq, sodium 1.25 mEq. ER Tab. 28s (7-day XR pack) and 40s (10-day XR pack). *Rx.*
Use: Penicillin, aminopenicillin.

amoxicillin/clavulanate potassium. (Various Mfr.) **Chew. Tab.:** Amoxicillin/clavulanic acid (as the potassium salt) 125 mg/31.25 mg, 200 mg/28.5 mg, 250 mg/62.5 mg, 400 mg/57 mg. May contain aspartame, mannitol, phenylalanine, saccharin. 20s, UD 20s (200 mg/28.5 mg, 400 mg/57 mg); 30s (125 mg/31.25 mg, 250 mg/62.5 mg). **Pow. for Oral Susp.:** Amoxicillin/clavulanic acid (as the potassium salt) 125 mg/31.25 mg, 200 mg/28.5 mg, 250 mg/62.5 mg, 400 mg/57 mg, 600 mg/42.9 mg per 5 mL after reconstitution. May contain aspartame, mannitol, phenylalanine, saccharin. 50 mL (200 mg/28.5 mg, 400 mg/57 mg), 75 mL, 100 mL, 150 mL (125 mg/31.25 mg, 250 mg/62.5 mg), 200 mL. **Tab.:** Amoxicillin/clavulanic acid (as the potassium salt) 500 mg/125 mg, 875 mg/125 mg. Bot. 20s, 100s, UD 100s. *Rx.*
Use: Anti-infective, penicillin.

amoxicillin intramammary infusion.
Use: Anti-infective; penicillin.

•**amoxicillin sodium.** (a-MOX-ih-sil-in) USAN.
Use: Antibiotic.

amoxicillin trihydrate. (Various Mfr.) Amoxicillin trihydrate. **Chew. Tab.:** 125 mg, 250 mg. Bot. 100s, 250s (250 mg only), 500s (250 mg only). **Tab.:** 500 mg, 875 mg. Bot. 20s, 100s, 500s (875 mg only). **Cap.:** 250 mg, 500 mg. Bot. 50s (500 mg only), 100s, 500s, 1000s (250 mg only). **Pow. for Oral Susp.:** 125 mg/5 mL, 250 mg/mL when reconstituted. Bot. 80 mL, 100 mL, 150 mL. *Rx.*
Use: Anti-infective; penicillin.

Amoxil. (Dr. Reddy's) Amoxicillin. **Cap.:** 500 mg. 500s. **Pow. for Oral Susp.:** 125 mg/5 mL when reconstituted. Sucrose. Strawberry flavor. 80 mL, 150 mL. **Tab.:** 875 mg. Film coated. 20s, 100s, 500s. *Rx.*
Use: Aminopenicillin, penicillin.

AMP. Adenosine Phosphate, USAN.
Use: Nutrient.

d-AMP. (Oxypure) Ampicillin trihydrate 500 mg. Cap. Bot. 100s. *Rx.*
Use: Anti-infective; penicillin.

Amperil. (Armenpharm Ltd.) Ampicillin trihydrate 250 mg or 500 mg. Cap. Bot. 100s, 500s. *Rx.*
Use: Anti-infective; penicillin.

Amphadase. (Amphastar) Hyaluronidase (bovine source) 150 units/mL. Contains no more than 0.1 mg thimerosal. Soln. for Inj. Vials. 2 mL. *Rx.*
Use: Physical adjunct.

•**amphecloral.** (AM-feh-klahr-ahl) USAN.
Use: Sympathomimetic; anorexic.

amphenidone.
Use: CNS stimulant.
amphetamine aspartate.
W/Amphetamine Sulfate, Dextroamphetamine Saccharate, Dextroamphetamine Sulfate.
See: Adderall.
Adderall XR.
MAS-ER.
amphetamine/dextroamphetaime. (Various Mfr.) Amphetamine/dextroamphetamine. **Tab.:** 5 mg, 7.5 mg, 10 mg, 12.5 mg, 15 mg, 20 mg, 30 mg (1.25 mg [5 mg], 1.875 mg [7.5 mg], 2.5 mg [10 mg], 3.125 mg [12.5 mg], 3.75 mg [15 mg], 5 mg [20 mg], and 7.5 mg [30 mg] each of dextroamphetamine sulfate, dextroamphetamine saccharate, amphetamine aspartate, and amphetamine sulfate). 100s. **ER Cap.:** 5 mg, 10 mg, 15 mg, 20 mg, 25 mg, 30 mg (1.25 [5 mg], 2.5 mg [10 mg], 3.75 mg [15 mg], 5 mg [20 mg], 6.25 mg [25 mg], and 7.5 mg [30 mg] each of dextroamphetamine saccharate, amphetamine aspartate, dextroamphetamine sulfate, and amphetamine sulfate). 100s. *c-II.*
Use: CNS stimulant, amphetamine.
amphetamine hydrochloride. (Various Mfr.) Amphetamine hydrochloride 20 mg/mL, 1 mL. Amp. *Rx.*
Use: Vasoconstrictor; CNS stimulant.
amphetamine, levo.
Use: CNS stimulant.
amphetamine phosphate.
Use: CNS stimulant.
amphetamine phosphate, dextro. (Various Mfr.) Dextroamphetamine phosphate. Tab.
Use: CNS stimulant.
amphetamine phosphate, dibasic. (Various Mfr.) Racemic amphetamine phosphate 5 mg, 10 mg. Cap. or Tab. Bot. *Rx.*
Use: CNS stimulant.
amphetamines.
See: Amphetamine Sulfate.
Dextroamphetamine Sulfate.
Lisdexamfetamine Dimesylate.
Methamphetamine Hydrochloride.
•**amphetamine sulfate.** (am-FET-a-meen) *USP.*
Use: CNS stimulant.
W/Amphetamine Aspartate, Dextroamphetamine Saccharate, Dextroamphetamine Sulfate.
See: Adderall.
Adderall XR.
MAS-ER.
amphetamine sulfate. (Various Mfr.) Amphetamine sulfate 5 mg, 10 mg. Cap. Tab. Bot. Inj. 20 mg/mL. Vial.
Use: CNS stimulant.
amphetamine sulfate, dextro.
Use: CNS stimulant.
See: Dextroamphetamine Sulfate.
amphetamine with dextroamphetamine as resin complexes.
Use: Appetite depressant.
Amphocaps. (Halsey Drug) Ampicillin 250 mg, 500 mg. Cap. Bot. 100s. *Rx.*
Use: Anti-infective; penicillin.
Amphojel. (Wyeth) Aluminum hydroxide gel. 300 mg, 600 mg. Tab. Bot. 100s. *OTC.*
Use: Antacid.
•**amphomycin.** (AM-foe-MY-sin) USAN. An antibiotic produced by *Streptomyces canus.*
Use: Anti-infective.
Amphotec. (Sequus) Amphotericin B (as cholesteryl) 50 mg, 100 mg. Pow. for Inj. Single-use Vial 20 mL (50 mg), 50 mL (100 mg). *Rx.*
Use: Antifungal.
•**amphotericin B.** (am-foe-TER-ih-sin B) *USP.*
Use: Antifungal.
See: Abelcet.
Amphotec.
amphotericin B. (Pharma-Tek) Amphotericin B 50 mg as desoxycholate. Pow. for Inj. Vial. *Rx.*
Use: Antifungal.
amphotericin B desoxycholate.
Use: Antifungal.
amphotericin B, lipid-based.
Use: Antifungal.
See: Abelcet.
AmBisome.
Amphotec.
amphotericin B lipid complex.
Use: Invasive fungal infections. [Orphan Drug]
See: Abelcet.
•**ampicillin.** (am-pih-SILL-in) *USP.*
Use: Anti-infective.
See: Principen With Probenecid.
•**ampicillin sodium.** (am-pih-SILL-in) *USP.*
Use: Anti-infective.
See: Omnipen-N.
ampicillin sodium. (Various Mfr.) Ampicillin sodium 125 mg, 250 mg, 500 mg, 1 g, 2 g, 10 g. Sodium 2.9 mEq/g. Pow. for Inj. Vials. *Rx.*
Use: Anti-infective.
•**ampicillin sodium and sulbactam sodium.** (am-pih-SILL-in and sull-BAK-tam) *USP.*
Use: Aminopenicillin, penicillin.
See: Unasyn.

ampicillin/sulbactam. (ESI Lederle) Ampicillin sodium 1 g/sulbactam sodium 0.5 g, ampicillin sodium 2 g/sulbactam sodium 1 g. Inj. Pow. for Soln. Vials. *Rx.*
Use: Aminopenicillin, penicillin.

ampicillin/sulbactam. (Various Mfr.) Ampicillin sodium 10 g/sulbactam sodium 5 g. Inj., Pow. for Soln. Bulk package. *Rx.*
Use: Penicillin, aminopenicillin.

ampicillin trihydrate. (Various Mfr.) Ampicillin (as trihydrate) 250 mg, 500 mg. Cap. Bot. 100s, 500s. *Rx.*
Use: Anti-infective; penicillin.

Amplicor. (Roche) Kits 10s, 96s, 100s. *Rx.*
Use: Diagnostic aid, chlamydia.

Amplicor HIV-1 Monitor. (Roche) Reagent kit for plasma HIV-1 tests. Kit. 24 tests.
Use: Diagnostic aid.

Ampligen. (HEM Research) Poly I: Poly C12U. Phase II/III HIV.
Use: Immunomodulator.

•**amprenavir.** (am-PREN-a-vir) USAN.
Use: Antiviral.

Ampyra. (Acorda) Dalfampridine 10 mg. Film coated. ER Tab. 60s. *Rx.*
Use: Potassium channel blocker.

•**ampyzine sulfate.** (AM-pih-zeen) USAN.
Use: Central nervous system stimulant.

•**amquinate.** (am-KWIN-ate) USAN.
Use: Antimalarial.

•**amrinone.** (AM-rih-nohn) *USP.*
Use: Cardiovascular agent.
See: Inocor Lactate.

Amrix. (Teva Pharmaceuticals) Cyclobenzaprine hydrochloride 15 mg, 30 mg. Sugar spheres. ER Cap. 60s. *Rx.*
Use: Skeletal muscle relaxant.

•**amsacrine.** (AM-sah-KREEN) USAN.
Use: Investigational antineoplastic. [Orphan Drug]

Amturnide. (Novartis) Aliskiren hemifumarate/amlodipine besylate/hydrochlorothiazide 150 mg/5 mg/12.5 mg, 300 mg/5 mg/12.5 mg, 300 mg/5 mg/25 mg, 300 mg/10 mg/12.5 mg, 300 mg/10 mg/25 mg. Film coated. PEG. Tab. 30s. *Rx.*
Use: Antihypertensive combination.

•**amuvatinib.** (AM-ue-VA-ti-nib) USAN.
Use: Antineoplastic.

•**amuvatinib hydrochloride.** (AM-ue-VA-ti-nib) USAN.
Use: Antineoplastic.

Amvisc. (Bausch & Lomb) Sodium hyaluronate 12 mg/mL. Inj. Disp. syringe 0.5 mL, 0.8 mL. *Rx.*
Use: Viscoelastic.

Amvisc Plus. (Bausch & Lomb) Sodium hyaluronate 16 mg/mL. Inj. Disp. syringe 0.5 mL, 0.8 mL. *Rx.*
Use: Viscoelastic.

Am-Wax. (AmLab) Urea, benzocaine, propylene glycol, glycerin. Bot. 10 mL. *OTC.*
Use: Otic.

amyl. Phenyl phenol, phenyl mercuric nitrate.
See: Lubraseptic.

amylase.
W/Lipase, Protease.
See: Bio-Zyme.
Creon.
Palcaps 10.
Pancreatin Quadruple Strength.
Pancreaze.
Pancrelipase.
Pertzye.
Tri-Pase 8.
Tri-Pase 16.
Tyler Panplex 2-Phase.
Tyler Similase Jr.
Ultresa.
Viokace.
Zenpep.

•**amylene hydrate.** (AM-ih-leen HIGH-drate) *NF.*
Use: Pharmaceutic aid, solvent.

amylin analog.
Use: Antidiabetic agent.
See: Pramlintide Acetate.

•**amyl nitrite.** (A-mill NYE-trite) *USP.*
Use: Vasodilator.
W/Sodium nitrite, sodium thiosulfate.
See: Cyanide Antidote Pkg.

amyl nitrite. (Various Mfr.) Amyl nitrite 0.3 mL. Inh. Covered glass capsules. 12s. *Rx.*
Use: Vasodilator.

amylolytic enzyme.
W/Calcium carbonate, glycine, proteolytic and cellulolytic enzymes.
See: Converspaz.
W/Proteolytic, cellulolytic, lipolytic enzymes.
See: Arco-Lase.
W/Proteolytic, cellulolytic, lipolytic enzymes, iron, ox bile.
See: Ku-Zyme.

Amytal Sodium. (Marathon) Amobarbital sodium 500 mg. Pow. for Inj. Vial. *c-II.*
Use: Hypnotic; sedative.

Ana. (Wampole) Antinuclear antibodies test by IFA. Test 54s.
Use: Diagnostic aid.

anabolic agents. These agents stimulate constructive processes leading to reten-

tion of nitrogen and increasing the body protein.
See: Anadrol-50.
Anavar.

anabolic steroids.
Use: Sex hormone.
See: Nandrolone Decanoate.
Oxandrolone.
Oxymetholone.

Anacaine. (Gordon Laboratories) Benzocaine 10%. Jar oz, lb. *OTC.*
Use: Anesthetic, local.

Anacin. (Insight Pharmaceutical) Aspirin 400 mg, caffeine 32 mg. Tab. Bot. 30s, 50s, 100s, 200s, 300s. Cap. Bot. 100s. *OTC.*
Use: Analgesic.

Anacin Advanced Headache. (Insight Pharmaceutical) Acetaminophen 250 mg, aspirin 250 mg, caffeine 65 mg. Tab. 75s. *OTC.*
Use: Nonnarcotic analgesic.

Anacin Aspirin Free. (Insight Pharmaceutical) Acetaminophen 500 mg. Film coated. Parabens. Tab. 100s. *OTC.*
Use: Analgesic.

Anacin Maximum Strength. (Insight Pharmaceutical) Aspirin 500 mg, caffeine 32 mg. Tab. Bot. 20s, 40s, 75s. *OTC.*
Use: Analgesic.

Anadrol-50. (Alaven) Oxymetholone 50 mg. Lactose. Tab. Bot. 100s. *c-III.*
Use: Anabolic steroid.

anafebrina.
See: Aminopyrine.

Anafranil. (Mallinckrodt) Clomipramine hydrochloride 25 mg, 50 mg, 75 mg. Parabens. Cap. 30s. *Rx.*
Use: Antidepressant.

•**anagestone acetate.** (AN-ah-JEST-ohn) USAN.
Use: Hormone, progestin.

•**anagrelide hydrochloride.** (AN-AGG-reh-lide) USAN.
Use: Antiplatelet agent.
See: Agrylin.

anagrelide hydrochloride. (Mallinckrodt) Anagrelide hydrochloride 0.5 mg, 1 mg. Lactose. Cap. 100s. *Rx.*
Use: Antiplatelet agent.

Ana-Guard. (Bayer Consumer Care) Epinephrine 1:1000. Syr. 1 mL. *Rx.*
Use: Bronchodilator; sympathomimetic.

Ana Hep-2. (Wampole) Antinuclear antibodies test by IFA. Tests 60s.
Use: Diagnostic aid.

•**anakinra.** (an-ah-KIN-rah) USAN.
Use: Immunologic agent, immunomodulator.
See: Kineret.

Ana-Kit. (Bayer Consumer Care) Syringe, epinephrine 1:1000 in 1 mL; four (each 2 mg) chlorpheniramine maleate; two sterilized swabs, tourniquet, instructions/kit. *Rx.*
Use: Anaphylactic therapy.

analeptics. Usually a term applied to agents with stimulant action, particularly on the central nervous system.
See: Armodafinil.
Caffeine.
Doxapram Hydrochloride.
Modafinil.

Analgesia. (Rugby) Trolamine sulfate 10%. Cream. Tube 85 g. *OTC.*
Use: Liniment.

analgesic and antihistamine combinations.
Use: Upper respiratory combination.
See: Acetaminophen, Chlorpheniramine Maleate.
Acetaminophen, Diphenhydramine Maleate.
Acetaminophen, Phenyltoloxamine Citrate.

analgesic and decongestant combinations.
Use: Upper respiratory combination.
See: Acetaminophen, Phenylephrine Hydrochloride.
Acetaminophen, Pseudoephedrine Hydrochloride.
Ibuprofen, Pseudoephedrine Hydrochloride.
Naproxen, Pseudoephedrine Hydrochloride.

analgesic, antihistamine, and antitussive combinations.
Use: Upper respiratory combination.

analgesic, antihistamine, and decongestant combinations.
Use: Upper respiratory combination.

analgesic, antihistamine, antitussive, and decongestant combinations.
Use: Upper respiratory combination.

analgesic, antitussive, and decongestant combinations.
Use: Upper respiratory combination.

analgesic, antitussive, decongestant, expectorant combinations.
Use: Upper respiratory combination.

Analgesic Balm. (Various Mfr.) Menthol w/methylsalicylate in a suitable base. *OTC.*
Use: Counterirritant.

Analgesic Balm-GRX. (Geritrex) Methyl salicylate 14%, menthol 6%. Balm. 28 g. *OTC.*
Use: Rub and liniment.

Analgesic Creme Rub. (Major) Trolamine salicylate 10%. Aloe vera, cetyl al-

cohol, glycerin, mineral oil, parabens, triethanolamine. Cream. 85 g. *OTC.*
Use: Rub and liniment.

Analgesic Liquid. (Weeks & Leo) Triethanolamine salicylate 20% in an alcohol base. Liq. Bot. 4 oz. *OTC.*
Use: Analgesic, topical.

Analgesic Lotion. (Weeks & Leo) Methyl nicotinate 1%, methyl salicylate 10%, camphor 0.1%, menthol 0.1%. Lot. Bot. 4 oz. *OTC.*
Use: Analgesic, topical.

analgesics, central.
See: Clonidine Hydrochloride.

analgesics, miscellaneous.
See: Ziconotide.

analgesics, opioid.
See: Opioid analgesics.

analgesics, topical.
See: Camphor.
Diphenhydramine Hydrochloride.

Analpram-E. (Sebela) Hydrocortisone acetate 2.5%, pramoxine hydrochloride 1%. Cetostearyl alcohol, mineral oil, propylparaben, white petrolatum. Cream. Kit with 4 g single-use tubes of cream and 18 Prax wipes. 30s. *Rx.*
Use: Anti-inflammatory agent; corticosteroid, topical.

Analpram-HC. (Sebela) **Cream:** Hydrocortisone acetate 1%, 2%, pramoxine hydrochloride 1%. Tube 30 g. **Lot.:** Hydrocortisone acetate 2.5%, pramoxine hydrochloride 1%. Hydrophilic. Alcohol, glycerin. 60 mL. *Rx.*
Use: Anesthetic; corticosteroid, local.

Analval. (Pal-Pak, Inc.) Aspirin 227 mg, acetaminophen 162 mg, caffeine 32 mg. Tab. Bot. 1000s. *OTC.*
Use: Analgesic combination.

Anamine. (Merz) Pseudoephedrine hydrochloride 30 mg, chlorpheniramine maleate 2 mg/5 mL. Syr. Bot. 473 mL. *Rx.*
Use: Antihistamine; decongestant.

Anamine HD. (Merz) Phenylephrine hydrochloride 5 mg, chlorpheniramine maleate 2 mg, hydrocodone bitartrate 1.67 mg. Syr. Bot. *c-III.*
Use: Antihistamine; antitussive; decongestant.

Anamine TD. (Merz) Chlorpheniramine maleate 8 mg, pseudoephedrine hydrochloride 120 mg. TD Cap. Bot. 100s. *Rx.*
Use: Antihistamine; decongestant.

•**anamorelin hydrochloride.** (AN-a-moe-REL-in) USAN.
Use: Treatment of cancer anorexia and cancer cachexia.

ananain, comosain.
Use: Burn therapy. [Orphan Drug]
See: Vianain.

Anaprox. (Roche) Naproxen 250 mg (naproxen sodium 275 mg). Tab. Bot. 100s. *Rx.*
Use: Nonsteroidal anti-inflammatory agent.

Anaprox DS. (Roche) Naproxen 500 mg (naproxen sodium 550 mg). Film coated. Tab. Bot. 100s, 500s. *Rx.*
Use: Nonsteroidal anti-inflammatory agent.

anarel. Guanadrel sulfate.

•**anaritide acetate.** (an-NAR-ih-TIDE) USAN.
Use: Antihypertensive; diuretic.

Anascorp. (Accredo Health Group) *Centruroides* (scorpion) immune $f(ab')_2$ (equine) ≤ 120 mg total protein per vial (each vial will neutralize at least 150 LD_{50} of *Centruroides* scorpion venom). Glycine, sodium chloride, sucrose. Inj., lyophilized Pow. for Soln. Single-use vial. *Rx.*
Use: Antitoxin/antivenin.

Anaspaz. (B.F. Ascher & Company Inc) Hyoscyamine sulfate 0.125 mg. Lactose, mannitol, sorbitol. Tab., disintegrating. 100s. *Rx.*
Use: Gastrointestinal anticholinergic/antispasmodic, belladonna alkaloid.

•**anastrozole.** (an-AS-troe-zole) *USP.*
Use: Antineoplastic; hormone.
See: Arimidex.

anastrozole. (Various Mfr.) Anastrozole 1 mg. May contain lactose, PEG, polydextrose. Tab. 30s, 90s, 500s. *Rx.*
Use: Hormone, aromatase inhibitor.

Anatrast. (Mallinckrodt) Barium sulfate 100%. Simethicone, sorbitol, parabens. Paste. Tube 500 g, enema tip assemblies. *Rx.*
Use: Radiopaque agent, GI contrast agent.

Anatuss LA. (Merz) Guaifenesin 400 mg, pseudoephedrine hydrochloride 120 mg. Tab. Bot. 100s. *Rx.*
Use: Decongestant; expectorant.

Anavar. (Pharmacia) Oxandrolone 2.5 mg. Tab. Bot. 100s. *Rx.*
Use: Anabolic steroid.

anayodin.
See: Chiniofon.

•**anazolene sodium.** (an-AZZ-oh-leen) USAN. Sodium anoxynaphthonate.
Use: Diagnostic aid, blood volume, cardiac output determination.

Anbesol. (Pfizer) Benzocaine 6.3%. Phenol 0.5%, alcohol 70%. Sugar free. Gel. Tube 7.5 g. *OTC.*
Use: Anesthetic combination, topical.

Anbesol Baby. (Pfizer) Benzocaine 7.5%.

Benzoic acid, edetate disodium, glycerin, parabens, PEG, saccharin. Alcohol free. Grape flavor. Gel; dental. 7.1 g. *OTC.*
Use: Topical local anesthetic, ester local anesthetic.

Anbesol Cold Sore Therapy. (Pfizer) Benzocaine 20%. Allantoin 1%, camphor 3%, petrolatum 64.9%, aloe, benzyl alcohol, parabens, menthol, vitamin E. Oint. 7.1 g. *OTC.*
Use: Topical local anesthetic, ester local anesthetic.

Anbesol Maximum Strength. (Pfizer) **Gel:** Benzocaine 20%. Benzyl alcohol, glycerin, methylparaben, PEG, propylene glycol, saccharin. 9 g. **Liq.; dental:** Benzocaine 20%. Benzyl alcohol, methylparaben, PEG, saccharin. 9 mL. *OTC.*
Use: Anesthetic, local.

Anbesol Regular Strength. (Pfizer) Benzocaine 10%. Benzyl alcohol, glycerin, methylparaben, PEG, propylene glycol, saccharin. Cool mint flavor. Gel; dental. 9 g. *OTC.*
Use: Topical local anesthetic, ester local anesthetic.

•**ancestim.** (an-SESS-tim) USAN.
Use: Investigational for treatment of anemia; hematopoietic adjuvant, stem cell factor.

Ancid. (Sheryl) Calcium aluminum carbonate, di-amino acetate complex. Tab. Bot. 100s. Susp. Bot. Pt. *OTC.*
Use: Antacid.

Ancobon. (ICN) Flucytosine 250 mg, 500 mg, lactose, parabens, talc. Cap. Bot. 100s. *Rx.*
Use: Anti-infective; antifungal.

•**ancriviroc.** (AN-kri-VIR-ok) USAN.
Use: Antiviral.

•**ancrod.** (AN-krahd) USAN. An active principle obtained from the venom of the Malayan pit viper Agkistrodon rhodostoma.
Use: Anticoagulant.

Andesterone. (Lincoln Diagnostics) Estrone 2 mg, testosterone 6 mg/mL. Susp. Vial 15 mL. **Forte:** Estrone 1 mg, testosterone 20 mg/mL. Inj. Vial 15 mL. *Rx.*
Use: Androgen, estrogen combination.

Andrest 90-4. (Seatrace) Testosterone enanthate 90 mg, estradiol valerate 4 mg/mL. Vial 10 mL. *Rx.*
Use: Androgen, estrogen combination.

Androderm. (Watson Pharma) Testosterone. Patch; transdermal. **2 mg/day:** 9.7 mg (total content); 32 cm^2 contact surface area. Alcohol. 60s. **4 mg/day:** 19.5 mg (total content); 39 cm^2 contact surface area. Alcohol. 30s. *c-III.*
Use: Sex hormone, androgen.

Andro-Estro 90-4. (Rugby) Estradiol valerate 4 mg, testosterone enanthate 90 mg/mL with chlorobutanol in sesame oil. Inj. Vial. 10 mL. *Rx.*
Use: Androgen, estrogen combination.

AndroGel. (AbbVie) Testosterone. Gel. **1% (50 mg):** Ethanol 67%. UD 30s (in 2.5 g [testosterone 25 mg] or 5 g [testosterone 50 mg]), 75 g metered multiple-dose pumps (60 metered 1.25 g [testosterone 12.5 mg] doses). **1.62% (20.25 mg):** Ethyl alcohol. UD 30s (in 1.25 g [testosterone 20.25 mg] or 2.5 g [testosterone 40.5 mg]), 75 g metered multiple-dose pumps (60 metered 1.25 g [testosterone 20.25 mg] doses). *c-III.*
Use: Sex hormone, androgen.

AndroGel-DHT. (Unimed Pharm) Dihydrotestosterone.
Use: AIDS. [Orphan Drug]

androgen hormone inhibitors.
See: Dutasteride.
Finasteride.

androgens. Substances that possess masculinizing activities.
Use: Sex hormone.
See: Fluoxymesterone.
Methyltestosterone.
Testosterone.
Testosterone, Buccal.
Testosterone Cypionate.
Testosterone Enanthate.
Testosterone Heptanoate.
Testosterone Phenylacetate.
Testosterone Undecanoate.

androgens and estrogens.
Use: Sex hormone.
See: Covaryx.
Covaryx H.S.
Estratest.
Estratest H.S.

Androlin. (Lincoln Diagnostics) Testosterone 100 mg/mL. Vial 10 mL. *c-III.*
Use: Androgen.

Andronaq-50. (Schwarz Pharma) Testosterone 50 mg/mL, sodium carboxymethylcellulose, methylcellulose, povidone, DSS, thimerosal. Inj. Vial. 10 mL. *c-III.*
Use: Androgen.

Andronaq LA. (Schwarz Pharma) Testosterone cypionate 100 mg, benzyl alcohol 0.9% in cottonseed oil. Vial 10 mL. Bot. 12s. *c-III.*
Use: Androgen.

Andronate 100. (Taylor Pharmaceuticals) Testosterone cypionate 100 mg/mL with benzyl alcohol in cottonseed oil. Vial

10 mL. *c-III.*
Use: Androgen.

Andronate 200. (Taylor Pharmaceuticals) Testosterone cypionate 200 mg/mL with benzyl alcohol, benzyl benzoate in cottonseed oil. Vial 10 mL. *c-III.*
Use: Androgen.

Andro 100. (Forest) Testosterone 100 mg/mL. Vial 10 mL. *c-III.*
Use: Androgen.

androstanazole.
See: Stanozold.

androstenopyrazole. Anabolic steroid; pending release.

Androtest P.
See: Testosterone propionate.

Androvite. (Optimox) Iron 3 mg, vitamins A 4167 units, D 67 units, E 67 units, B_1 8.3 mg, B_2 8.3 mg, B_3 8.3 mg, B_5 16.7 mg, B_6 16.7 mg, B_{12} 20.8 mcg, C 167 mg, folic acid 0.06 mg, PABA, inositol, biotin, betaine, B, Cr, Cu, I, Mg, Mn, Se, Zn 8.3 mg, pancreatin, hesperidin, rutin. Tab. Bot. 180s. *OTC.*
Use: Mineral, vitamin supplement.

Androxy. (Upsher-Smith) Fluoxymesterone 10 mg. Lactose. Tab. 100s. *c-III.*
Use: Sex hormone.

Andylate. (Vita Elixir) Sodium salicylate 10 g. Tab. *OTC.*
Use: Analgesic.

Andylate Forte. (Vita Elixir) Acetaminophen 3 g, salicylamide 3 g, caffeine 0.25 g. Tab. *OTC.*
Use: Analgesic combination.

Andylate Rub. (Vita Elixir) Methylnicotinate, methyl salicylate, camphor, dipropylene glycol salicylate, oil of cassia, oleo resin of capsicum, oleo resin of ginger. *OTC.*
Use: Analgesic, topical.

•**anecortave acetate.** (an-eh-CORE-tave AS-eh-tate) USAN.
Use: Angiostatic steroid.

AneCream. (Focus Health Group) Lidocaine hydrochloride 4%. Benzyl alcohol, cholesterol, polysorbate 80, propylene glycol, trolamine. Cream. 15 g, 30 g; 5 g kits w/*Tegaderm* patches 5s and 10s. *Rx.*
Use: Topical local anesthetic, amide local anesthetic.

AneCream5. (Focus Health Group) Lidocaine 5%. Benzyl alcohol, cholesterol, polysorbate 80, propylene glycol, trolamine. Cream; rectal. 30 g. *OTC.*
Use: Topical local anesthetic, amide local anesthetic.

Anectine. (GlaxoSmithKline) Succinylcholine chloride. **Soln.:** 20 mg/mL. Multidose Vial 10 mL. **Sterile Pow.:** 500 mg, 1000 mg. Flo-Pak Box 12s. *Rx.*
Use: Muscle relaxant.

Anefrin Nasal Spray, Long Acting. (Walgreen) Oxymetazoline hydrochloride 0.05%. Bot. 0.5 oz. *OTC.*
Use: Decongestant.

Anergan 50. (Forest) Promethazine hydrochloride 50 mg/mL, EDTA, phenol. Vial 10 mL. *Rx.*
Use: Antihistamine.

anertan.
See: Testosterone propionate.

Anestacon. (PolyMedica) Lidocaine hydrochloride 2%. Hydroxypropylmethyl cellulose 1%, benzalkonium chloride 0.01%. Jelly. Disposable units. 15 mL, 240 mL. *Rx.*
Use: Topical local anesthetic, amide local anesthetic.

Anesthesin. (Ethyl-p-aminobenzoate).
Use: Anesthetic, local.
See: Benzocaine.

anesthetics, combination local.
See: Duocaine.

anesthetics, general.
See: Barbiturates.
Diprivan.
Droperidol.
Inapsine.
Propofol.
Sevoflurane.
Ultane.
Volatile Liquids.

anesthetics, injectable local.
See: Amide Local Anesthetics.
Anesthetics, Combination Local.
Bupivacaine Hydrochloride.
Chloroprocaine Hydrochloride.
Ester Local Anesthetics.
Lidocaine Hydrochloride.
Mepivacaine Hydrochloride.
Prilocaine Hydrochloride.
Procaine Hydrochloride.
Ropivacaine Hydrochloride.
Tetracaine Hydrochloride.

anesthetics, ophthalmic local.
See: Proparacaine Hydrochloride.
Tetracaine Hydrochloride.

anesthetics, topical local.
See: Amide Local Anesthetics.
Benzethonium Chloride w/Lidocaine Hydrochloride.
Benzocaine.
Ester Local Anesthetics.
Pramoxine Hydrochloride.

anethaine.
See: Tetracaine Hydrochloride.

•**anethole.** (AN-eh-thole) *NF.*
Use: Pharmaceutic aid, flavor.

aneurine hydrochloride.
See: Thiamine hydrochloride.
Anexsia 5/500. (Mallinckrodt) Hydrocodone bitartrate 5 mg, acetaminophen 500 mg. Tab. Bot. 100s. *c-III.*
Use: Analgesic combination; narcotic.
Anexsia 7.5/650. (Mallinckrodt) Hydrocodone bitartrate 7.5 mg, acetaminophen 650 mg. Tab. Bot. 100s. *c-III.*
Use: Analgesic combination, narcotic.
Anexsia 10/660. (Mallinckrodt) Hydrocodone bitartrate 10 mg, acetaminophen 660 mg. Tab. Bot. 100s, 1000s. *c-III.*
Use: Analgesic combination, narcotic.
Angeliq. (Bayer) Drospirenone/estradiol 0.25 mg/0.5 mg, 0.5 mg/1 mg. Film coated. Lactose. Tab. Blister packs 28s. *Rx.*
Use: Sex hormone, estrogen and progestin combined.
Angel Sweet. (Garrett) Vitamins A and D_2. Cream. Tube 90 g. *OTC.*
Use: Dermatologic, protectant.
Angen. (Davis & Sly) Estrone 2 mg, testosterone 25 mg/mL. Aqueous Susp. Vial 10 mL. *Rx.*
Use: Androgen, estrogen combination.
Angerin. (Kingsbay) Nitroglycerin 1 mg. Cap. Bot. 60s. *Rx.*
Use: Coronary vasodilator.
Angex. (Janssen) Lidoflazine. *Rx.*
Use: Coronary vasodilator.
Angio-Conray. (Mallinckrodt) Iothalamate sodium 80% (48% iodine), EDTA. Inj. Vial 50 mL.
Use: Radiopaque agent.
Angiomax. (Medicines Company) Bivalirudin 250 mg. Inj., lyophilized. Single-use vial. *Rx.*
Use: Anticoagulant.
•**angiotensin amide.** (an-JEE-oh-TEN-sin AH-mid) USAN.
Use: Vasoconstrictor.
angiotensin-converting enzyme inhibitors.
Use: Antihypertensive; congestive heart failure.
See: Benazepril Hydrochloride.
Captopril.
Enalapril Maleate.
Fosinopril Sodium.
Lisinopril.
Moexipril Hydrochloride.
Perindopril Erbumine.
Quinapril Hydrochloride.
Ramipril.
Trandolapril.
angiotensin II receptor antagonists.
See: Azilsartan Medoxomil.
Candesartan Cilexetil.
Eprosartan Mesylate.
Irbesartan.
Losartan Potassium.
Telmisartan.
Valsartan.
Angiovist 370. (Berlex) Diatrizoate meglumine 66%, diatrizoate sodium 10%, (iodine 37%). Vial 50 mL, 100 mL, 150 mL, or 200 mL. Box 10s.
Use: Radiopaque agent.
Angiovist 282. (Berlex) Diatrizoate meglumine 60% (iodine 28%). Vial 50 mL, 100 mL, 150 mL. Box 10s.
Use: Radiopaque agent.
Angiovist 292. (Berlex) Diatrizoate meglumine 52%, diatrizoate sodium 8% (iodine 29.2%). Vial 30 mL, 50 mL, 100 mL. Box 10s.
Use: Radiopaque agent.
anhydrohydroxyprogesterone.
Ethisterone.
•**anidoxime.** (AN-ih-DOX-eem) USAN.
Use: Analgesic.
•**anidulafungin.** (AN-ih-doo-la-FUN-jin) USAN.
Use: Antifungal.
See: Eraxis.
•**anifrolumab.** (AN-i-FROL-ue-mab) USAN.
Use: Monoclonal antibody.
A-Nil. (Vangard Labs, Inc.) Codeine phosphate 10 mg, bromodiphenhydramine hydrochloride 3.75 mg, diphenhydramine hydrochloride 8.75 mg, ammonium chloride 80 mg, potassium guaiacolsulfonate 80 mg, menthol 0.5 mg/5 mL, alcohol 5%. Bot. Pt. gal. *c-v.*
Use: Antitussive; expectorant.
•**anileridine.** (an-ih-LURR-ih-deen) *USP.*
Use: Analgesic, narcotic.
•**anileridine hydrochloride.** (an-ih-LURR-ih-deen) *USP.*
Use: Analgesic, narcotic.
•**anilopam hydrochloride.** (AN-ih-low-pam) USAN.
Use: Analgesic.
Animal Shapes. (Major) Vitamin A 2500 units, D 400 units, E 15 units, C 60 mg, B_1 1.05 mg, B_2 1.2 mg, B_3 13.5 mg, B_6 1.05 mg, B_{12} 4.5 mcg, folic acid 0.3 mg. Chew. Tab. Bot. 100s, 250s. *OTC.*
Use: Vitamin supplement.
Animal Shapes + Iron. (Major) Vitamin A 2500 units, D 400 units, E 15 units, C 60 mg, B_1 1.05 mg, B_2 1.2 mg, B_3 13.5 mg, B_6 1.05 mg, B_{12} 4.5 mcg, folic acid 0.3 mg, iron 15 mg. Chew. Tab. Bot. 100s, 250s. *OTC.*
Use: Mineral, vitamin supplement.
Animi-3. (PBM Pharm) Omega-3 acids

500 mg (eicosapentaenoic acid [EPA] 35 mg and docosahexaenoic acid [DHA] 350 mg), vitamin B_6 12.5 mg, B_{12} 500 mcg, folic acid 1 mg. Sunflower oil. Cap. 60s. *Rx.*
Use: Dietary supplement.

Animi-3 With Vitamin D. (PBM Pharm) Omega-3 500 mg (DHA 350 mg, EPA 35 mg), vitamins D 1,000 units, B_6 12.5 mg, B_{12} 500 mcg, folic acid 1 mg, phytosterols 200 mg. Lecithin. Cap. 60s. *Rx.*
Use: Multivitamin and mineral with omega-3 polyunsaturated fatty acids.

•**aniracetam.** (AN-ih-RA-se-tam) USAN.
Use: Mental performance enhancer.

•**anirolac.** (ah-NIH-role-ACK) USAN.
Use: Analgesic; anti-inflammatory.

•**anise oil.** (AN-is) *NF.*
Use: Flavoring.

anisopyradamine.
See: Pyrilamine maleate.

•**anisotropine methylbromide.** (ah-NIH-so-TROE-peen meth-ill-BROE-mide) USAN.
Use: Anticholinergic.

•**anitrazafen.** (AN-ih-TRAY-zaff-en) USAN.
Use: Anti-inflammatory, topical.

•**anivamersen.** (AN-i-va-MER-sen) USAN.
Use: Reversal of pegnivacogin anticoagulation.

•**anivamersen sodium.** (AN-i-va-MER-sen) USAN.
Use: Reversal of pegnivacogin anticoagulation.

anodynon.
See: Ethyl Chloride.

Anodynos. (Buffington) Aspirin 420.6 mg, salicylamide 34.4 mg, caffeine 34.4 mg. Sugar, lactose, and salt free. Tab. Dis-pens-A-Kit 500s, Bot. 100s, 500s, Medipak 200s. *OTC.*
Use: Analgesic combination.

Anodynos-DHC. (Buffington) Hydrocodone bitartrate 5 mg, acetaminophen 500 mg. Tab. Bot. 100s. *c-III.*
Use: Analgesic combination; narcotic.

anorectal preparations.
See: Hydrocortisone.
Nitroglycerin.

Anorex. (Oxypure) Phendimetrazine 35 mg. Tab. Bot. 100s. *c-III.*
Use: Anorexiant.

anorexiants.
Use: Appetite suppressants.
See: Benzphetamine Hydrochloride.
Diethylpropion Hydrochloride.
Phendimetrazine Tartrate.
Phentermine Hydrochloride.
Serotonin 2C Receptor Agonists.
Sibutramine Hydrochloride.

Anoro Ellipta. (GlaxoSmithKline) Umeclidinium 62.5 mcg/vilanterol 25 mcg per actuation (equiv. to umeclidinium bromide 74.2 mcg/vilanterol trifenatate 40 mcg). Lactose. Pow.; Inhal. Disposable inhaler (30 inhalations). *Rx.*
Use: Respiratory inhalant combination.

Anovlar. Norethindrone plus ethinyl estradiol. *Rx.*
Use: Contraceptive.

•**anoxomer.** (an-OX-ah-MER) USAN.
Use: Pharmaceutic aid, antioxidant; food additive.

anoxynaphthonate sodium. Anazolene sodium.

Anspor. (GlaxoSmithKline) Cephradine (a semisynthetic cephalosporin). **Cap.:** 250 mg, 500 mg. Bot. 20s (500 mg only), 100s, UD 100s. **Oral Susp.:** 125 mg, 250 mg/5 mL. Bot. 100 mL.
Use: Anti-infective; cephalosporin.

Answer. (Carter-Wallace) Reagent in-home pregnancy test kit for urine testing. Test kit box 1s.
Use: Diagnostic aid.

Answer One-Step Pregnancy Test. (Carter-Wallace) Pregnancy test kit for urine testing. Stick. Test kit box 1s. *OTC.*
Use: Diagnostic aid.

Answer Plus. (Carter-Wallace) Reagent in-home pregnancy test kit for urine testing. Test kit box 1s.
Use: Diagnostic aid.

Answer Plus 2. (Carter-Wallace) Reagent in-home pregnancy test kit for urine testing. Test kit box 2s.
Use: Diagnostic aid.

Answer Quick & Simple. (Carter-Wallace) Reagent in-home kit for urine testing. Test kit box 1s.
Use: Diagnostic aid.

Answer 2. (Carter-Wallace) Reagent in-home pregnancy test kit for urine testing. Test kit box 2s.
Use: Diagnostic aid.

Antabuse. (Barr/Duramed) Disulfiram 250 mg, 500 mg. Lactose. Tab. 50s (500 mg only), 100s, 500s (500 mg only). *Rx.*
Use: Antialcoholic.

Antacid. (Walgreen) Calcium carbonate 500 mg. Tab. Bot. 75s. *OTC.*
Use: Antacid.

Antacid Extra Strength. (Various Mfr.) Calcium carbonate 750 mg. Tab. Bot. 96s. *OTC.*
Use: Antacid.

Antacid M. (Walgreen) Aluminum oxide 225 mg, magnesium hydroxide 200 mg/5 mL. Liq. Bot. 12 oz, 26 oz. *OTC.*
Use: Antacid.

Antacid No. 6. (Jones Pharma) Calcium carbonate 0.42 g, glycine 0.18 g. Tab. Bot. 100s. *OTC.*
Use: Antacid.
Antacid #2. (Global Source) Calcium carbonate 5.5 g, magnesium carbonate 2.5 g. Tab. Bot. 100s. *OTC.*
Use: Antacid.
Antacid Relief. (Walgreen) Dihydroxyaluminum sodium carbonate 334 mg. Tab. Bot. 75s. *OTC.*
Use: Antacid.
antacids. Drugs that neutralize excess gastric acid.
See: Alka-Seltzer.
Aluminum Hydroxide.
Aluminum Hydroxide Gel.
Aluminum Hydroxide Gel Dried.
Aluminum Hydroxide Magnesium Carbonate.
Aluminum Phosphate Gel.
Calcium Carbonate.
Calcium Carbonate, Precipitated.
Ceo-Two.
Chooz.
Citrocarbonate.
Di-Gel.
Dicarbosil.
Dihydroxyaluminum Aminoacetate.
Dihydroxyaluminum Sodium Carbonate.
Magaldrate.
Magnesium Carbonate.
Magnesium Hydroxide.
Magnesium Oxide.
Magnesium Trisilicate.
Rolaids.
Romach Antacid.
Simethicone.
Sodium Bicarbonate.
Tums.
Antacid Suspension. (Geneva) Aluminum hydroxide 225 mg, magnesium hydroxide 200 mg/5 mL. Bot. 360 mL. *OTC.*
Use: Antacid.
Antacid Tablets. (Goldline) Calcium carbonate 500 mg (elemental calcium 200 mg). Sucrose, sodium up to 2 mg. Assorted flavors. Chew. Tab. Bot. 150s. *OTC.*
Use: Mineral supplement; antacid.
Anta-Gel. (Halsey Drug) Aluminum hydroxide 200 mg, magnesium hydroxide 200 mg, simethicone 20 mg/5 mL. Bot. 12 oz. *OTC.*
Use: Antacid; antiflatulent.
antagonists of curariform drugs.
See: Neostigmine Methylsulfate.
Tensilon.
Antara. (Lupin Pharmaceuticals) Fenofibrate (micronized) 30 mg, 43 mg, 90 mg, 130 mg. Sugar spheres. Cap. 30s, 90s (90 mg only), 100s (except 30 mg). *Rx.*
Use: Antihyperlipidemic agent, fibric acid derivatives.
antazoline hydrochloride. Antastan.
•**antazoline phosphate.** (an-TAZ-oh-leen) *USP.*
Use: Antihistamine.
anterior pituitary.
See: Pituitary, anterior.
Anthelios 40. (La Roche-Posay) Avobenzone 2%, *Mexoryl SX* 3%, octocrylene 10%, titanium dioxide 5%. PABA free. Cream. 50 g. *OTC.*
Use: Sunscreen.
Anthelios SX. (La Roch-Posay) Avobenzone 2%, ecamsule 2%, octocrylene 10%. EDTA, glycerin, parabens, stearyl alcohol. SPF 15. Cream. 100 g. *OTC.*
Use: Sunscreen.
anthelmintics.
Use: A remedy for worms.
See: Biltricide.
Carbon Tetrachloride.
Gentian Violet.
Ivermectin.
Mintezol.
Piperazine.
Praziquantel.
Stromectol.
Tetrachloroethylene.
Vermox.
•**anthelmycin.** (AN-thell-MY-sin) USAN.
Use: Anthelmintic.
Anthelvet. Tetramisole hydrochloride.
anthracenedione.
See: Mitoxantrone Hydrochloride.
Novantrone.
anthracyclines.
See: Daunorubicin Citrate Liposomal.
Daunorubicin Hydrochloride.
Doxorubicin Hydrochloride.
Doxorubicin Hydrochloride, Liposomal.
Epirubicin Hydrochloride.
Idarubicin Hydrochloride.
•**anthralin.** (AN-thrah-lin) *USP.*
Use: Antipsoriatic.
See: Dritho-Scalp.
Zithranol.
Zithranol-RR.
anthralin. (Rising Pharmaceuticals) Anthralin 1%. Cream. 50 g. *Rx.*
Use: Antipsoriatic agent.
•**anthramycin.** (an-THRAH-MY-sin) USAN.
Use: Antineoplastic.
anthraquinone of cascara.
See: Cascara Sagrada.

anthrax vaccine. (Michigan Biological Products Institute) Vial 5 mL. *Rx.*
Use: Immunization.
•**anthrax vaccine, adsorbed.** (AN-thrax VAX-een) *USP.*
Use: Immunization.
See: BioThrax.
anti-a blood grouping serum.
Use: Diagnostic aid, blood in vitro.
Antiacid. (Hillcrest North) Aluminum hydroxide, magnesium trisilicate, calcium carbonate. Tab. Bot. 100s. *OTC.*
Use: Antacid.
antiadrenergic agents, centrally acting.
See: Clonidine Hydrochloride.
Guanfacine Hydrochloride.
antiadrenergic agents, peripherally acting.
Use: Antiadrenergic/sympatholytic.
See: Alfuzosin Hydrochloride.
Alpha-1 Adrenergic Blockers.
Doxazosin Mesylate.
Prazosin Hydrochloride.
Reserpine.
Tamsulosin Hydrochloride.
Terazosin Hydrochloride.
antiadrenergics/sympatholytics.
See: Alpha/Beta-Adrenergic Blocking Agents.
Antiadrenergic Agents, Centrally Acting.
Antiadrenergic Agents, Peripherally Acting.
Beta-Adrenergic Blocking Agents.
antialcoholic agents.
See: Acamprosate Calcium.
Disulfiram.
antiandrogens.
See: Abiraterone Acetate.
Bicalutamide.
Eulexin.
Flutamide.
Nilandron.
Nilutamide.
antianginal agents, miscellaneous.
See: Ranolazine.
antianxiety agents.
See: Alprazolam.
Benzodiazepines.
Buspirone Hydrochloride.
Chlordiazepoxide Hydrochloride.
Clonazepam.
Clorazepate Dipotassium.
Diazepam.
Doxepin Hydrochloride.
Hydroxyzine.
Lorazepam.
Meprobamate.
Oxazepam.
antiarrhythmic agents.
See: Adenosine.
Amiodarone Hydrochloride.
Bretylium Tosylate.
Disopyramide.
Dofetilide.
Dronedarone.
Flecainide Acetate.
Ibutilide Fumarate.
Lidocaine Hydrochloride.
Procainamide Hydrochloride.
Propafenone Hydrochloride.
Quinidine.
antiasthmatic combinations.
See: Cromolyn Sodium.
Ephedrine Hydrochloride.
Ephedrine Sulfate.
Isoephedrine Hydrochloride.
Isoetharine.
Isoetharine Hydrochloride.
Isoetharine Mesylate.
Isoproterenol Hydrochloride.
Isoproterenol Sulfate.
Methoxyphenamine Hydrochloride.
Phenylephrine Hydrochloride.
Pseudoephedrine Hydrochloride.
Racephedrine Hydrochloride.
Xanthine Combinations.
antiasthmatic inhalants.
See: AsthmaNefrin.
antibason.
See: Methylthiouracil.
anti-b blood grouping serum.
Use: Diagnostic aid, blood in vitro.
AntibiOtic. (Parnell) **Otic Susp.:** Polymyxin B sulfate 10,000 units, neomycin (as sulfate) 3.5 mg, hydrocortisone 10 mg/mL, thimerosal 0.01%. Bot. 10 mL w/dropper. **Otic Soln.:** Polymyxin B sulfate 10,000 units, neomycin sulfate 5 mg, hydrocortisone 1%. Propylene glycol, glycerin, potassium metabisulfite. Bot. 10 mL. *Rx.*
Use: Anti-infective; anti-inflammatory.
antibiotic and steroid combinations.
See: Ciprofloxacin/Dexamethasone.
Ciprofloxacin/Hydrocortisone.
Dexamethasone Phosphate/Neomycin Sulfate.
Dexamethasone/Tobramycin.
Hydrocortisone Acetate/Chloramphenicol/Polymyxin B.
Hydrocortisone/Neomycin Sulfate.
Hydrocortisone/Neomycin Sulfate/Bacitracin Zinc/Polymyxin B Sulfate.
Loteprednol Etabonate/Tobramycin.
Neomycin and Polymyxin B Sulfates and Dexamethasone.
Neomycin/Polymyxin B Sulfates/Hydrocortisone.
Prednisolone Acetate/Gentamicin Sulfate.
Prednisolone Acetate/Neomycin Sulfate/Polymyxin B Sulfate.

antibiotic combinations.
See: AK-Poly-Bac.
AK-Spore.
Bacitracin Zinc and Polymyxin B Sulfate.
Betadine Plus First Aid Antibiotics and Pain Reliever.
Betadine First Aid Antibiotics Plus Moisturizer.
Double Antibiotic.
Lanabiotic.
Neomycin and Polymyxin B Sulfates and Bacitracin Zinc.
Neomycin and Polymyxin B Sulfates and Gramicidin.
Neosporin.
Neosporin Original.
Neosporin Plus Pain Relief.
Polysporin.
Polytrim.
Terramycin w/Polymyxin B Sulfate.
Tri-Biozene.
Triple Antibiotic.

Antibiotic Ear. (Various Mfr.) **Soln.:** Hydrocortisone 1%, neomycin sulfate 5 mg, polymyxin B 10,000 units. 10 mL. **Susp.:** Hydrocortisone 1%, neomycin sulfate 5 mg, polymyxin B 10,000 units. 10 mL with dropper. *Rx.*
Use: Steroid and antibiotic combination.

antibiotics/anti-infectives.
See: Amebicides, General.
Amikacin Sulfate.
Amoxicillin.
Amoxicillin and Clavulanate Potassium.
Ampicillin.
Anthelmintics.
Anthracyclines.
Antifungal Agents.
Antimalarial Agents.
Antiprotozoal Agents.
Antituberculosis Agents.
Antiviral Agents.
Azithromycin.
Aztreonam.
Bacampicillin Hydrochloride.
Bacitracin.
Benzoyl Peroxide.
Betadine First Aid Antibiotics Plus Moisturizer.
Betadine Plus First Aid Antibiotics and Pain Reliever.
Bicillin C-R.
Blenoxane.
Bleomycin Sulfate.
Capecitabine.
Cefaclor.
Cefadroxil.
Cefazolin Sodium.
Cefditoren Pivoxil.
Cefixime.
Cefmetazole Sodium.
Cefoperazone Sodium.
Cefotaxime Sodium.
Cefotetan Disodium.
Cefoxitin Sodium.
Cefpodoxime Proxetil.
Cefprozil.
Ceftazidime.
Ceftizoxime Sodium.
Ceftriaxone Sodium.
Cefuroxime.
Cephalexin.
Cephalothin Sodium.
Cephradine.
Chloramphenicol.
Ciprofloxacin.
Clarithromycin.
Clindamycin.
Clindamycin Phosphate.
Clioquinol.
Clofazimine.
Cloxacillin Sodium.
Colistimethate Sodium.
Cruex.
Dactinomycin.
Dapsone.
Daunorubicin Hydrochloride.
Demeclocycline.
Desenex.
Dicloxacillin.
Doxycycline.
Enoxacin.
Erythromycin.
Fungicides.
Furazolidone.
Gentamicin Sulfate.
Kanamycin Sulfate.
Lanabiotic.
Levofloxacin.
Lincomycin.
Lomefloxacin Hydrochloride.
Loprox.
Loracarbef.
Lotrimin AF.
Methenamine.
Methicillin Sodium.
Methylene Blue.
Metronidazole.
Minocycline.
Mitomycin.
Mupirocin.
Nafcillin Sodium.
Nalidixic Acid.
Neomycin Sulfate.
Neosporin Original.
Netilmicin Sulfate.
Nitrofurantoin.
Norfloxacin.
Ocuflox.
Ofloxacin.

Oxacillin Sodium.
Oxytetracycline.
Penicillin G Benzathine.
Penicillin G Potassium.
Penicillin G Procaine.
Penicillin G Procaine Combinations.
Penicillin G Sodium.
Penicillin V Potassium.
Penlac Nail Lacquer.
Pentamidine Isethionate.
Phenoxymethyl Penicillin.
Piperacillin Sodium.
Piperacillin Sodium w/Comb.
Polymyxin B Sulfate.
Polysporin.
Pyrimidine Analogs.
Quixin.
Retapamulin.
Rubex.
Sodium Sulfacetamide.
Spectazole.
Spectinomycin.
Spectracef.
Sulfadiazine.
Sulfamethoxazole.
Sulfasalazine.
Sulfisoxazole.
Sulfonamides.
Tetracycline Hydrochloride.
Ticarcillin Disodium.
Tobramycin.
Tobramycin Sulfate.
Tri-Biozene.
Triple Antibiotic.
Trimethoprim.
Vancomycin Hydrochloride.
Xeloda.

antibiotics, ophthalmic.
See: Azithromycin.
Bacitracin.
Chloramphenicol.
Ciprofloxacin Hydrochloride.
Erythromycin.
Gatifloxacin.
Gentamicin Sulfate.
Moxifloxacin Hydrochloride.
Ofloxacin.
Polymyxin B.
Sulfacetamide Sodium.
Tobramycin.

antibiotics, otic.
See: Ciprofloxacin Hydrochloride.

antibodies, monoclonal.
See: Alemtuzumab.
Campath.
Herceptin.
Rituxan.
Rituximab.
Trastuzumab.

antibody-drug conjugates.
See: Brentuximab Vedotin.

anti-CD45 monoclonal antibodies.
Use: Prevention of graft rejection in organ transplants. [Orphan Drug]

anticholinergic agents.
Use: Antiemetic/antivertigo agents; antiparkinson agents; bronchodilators.
See: Antispasmodics.
Belladonna Alkaloids.
Benztropine Mesylate.
Biperiden.
Buclizine Hydrochloride.
Cyclizine.
Darifenacin Hydrobromide.
Dimenhydrinate.
Diphenhydramine.
Fesoterodine Fumarate.
Flavoxate Hydrochloride.
Glycopyrrolate.
Ipratropium Bromide.
Ipratropium Bromide/Albuterol Sulfate.
Meclizine Hydrochloride.
Mepenzolate Bromide.
Methscopolamine Bromide.
Nabilone.
Oxybutynin Chloride.
Propantheline Bromide.
Scopolamine.
Solifenacin Succinate.
Tiotropium Bromide.
Tolterodine Tartrate.
Trihexyphenidyl Hydrochloride.
Trimethobenzamide Hydrochloride.
Trospium Chloride.

anticholinergic and antitussive combinations.
Use: Upper respiratory combination.

anticholinergic and decongestant combinations.
Use: Upper respiratory combination.

anticholinergic, antihistamine, and decongestant combinations.
Use: Upper respiratory combination.

anticholinergics, urinary.
See: Oxybutynin Chloride.
Tolterodine Tartrate.

anticholinesterase muscle stimulants.
See: Neostigmine Methylsulfate.

•**anticoagulant citrate dextrose solution.** (an-tee-koe-ag-ue-lant) *USP.*
Use: Anticoagulant for storage of whole blood.
See: A-C-D.

•**anticoagulant citrate phosphate dextrose adenine solution.** *USP.*
Use: Anticoagulant for storage of whole blood.

•**anticoagulant citrate phosphate dextrose solution.** *USP.*
Use: Anticoagulant for storage of whole blood.

•**anticoagulant heparin solution.** *USP.*
Use: Anticoagulant for storage of whole blood.

anticoagulants.
See: Antithrombin Agents.
Direct Factor Xa Inhibitors.
Heparin.
Low Molecular Weight Heparins.
Selective Factor Xa Inhibitor.
Thrombin Inhibitors.
Warfarin.

•**anticoagulant sodium citrate solution.** *USP.*
Use: Anticoagulant for plasma and blood fractionation.

anticonvulsants.
See: Acetazolamide.
Benzodiazepines.
Carbamazepine.
Clonazepam.
Clorazepate Dipotassium.
Diazepam.
Divalproex Sodium.
Eslicarbazepine Acetate.
Felbamate.
Gabapentin.
Hydantoins.
Lacosamide.
Lamotrigine.
Levetiracetam.
Lorazepam.
Magnesium Sulfate.
Mephobarbital.
Methsuximide.
Oxcarbazepine.
Perampanel.
Phenobarbital.
Phenytoin.
Phenytoin Sodium.
Potassium Channel Openers.
Pregabalin.
Primidone.
Rufinamide.
Succinimides.
Sulfonamides.
Tiagabine Hydrochloride.
Topiramate.
Valproate.
Valproic Acid.
Vigabatrin.
Zonisamide.

anticytomegalovirus monoclonal antibodies.
Use: Treatment of cytomegalovirus.

antidepressants.
See: Bupropion Hydrochloride.
Monoamine Oxidase Inhibitors.
Nefazodone Hydrochloride.
Selective Serotonin Reuptake Inhibitors.
Serotonin and Norepinephrine Reuptake Inhibitors.
Tetracyclic Compounds.
Trazodone Hydrochloride.
Tricyclic Antidepressants.
Vortioxetine.

antidiabetic combinations.
See: Glipizide/Metformin Hydrochloride.
Glyburide/Metformin Hydrochloride.
Pioglitazone Hydrochloride/Glimepiride.
Pioglitazone Hydrochloride/Metformin Hydrochloride.
Rosiglitazone Maleate/Glimepiride.
Rosiglitazone Maleate/Metformin Hydrochloride.
Sitagliptin/Metformin Hydrochloride.

antidiabetics.
See: Alpha-Glucosidase Inhibitors.
Amylin Analog.
Antidiabetic Combination Products.
Biguanides.
Dipeptidyl Peptidase-4 Inhibitor.
Glucagon-Like Peptide 1 Receptor Agonists.
Incretin Mimetic Agents.
Insulin.
Meglitinides.
Sodium-Glucose Cotransporter 2 Inhibitors.
Sulfonylureas.
Thiazolidinediones.

antidiarrheals.
See: Attapulgite, Activated.
Bismuth Subsalicylate.
Cantil.
Diasorb.
Furoxone.
Imodium.
Imodium A-D.
Kaodene Non-Narcotic.
Kaolin.
Kaolin Colloidal.
Kaopectate.
Kao-Spen.
Kapectolin.
K-C.
Lactinex.
Lactobacillus acidophilus and *bulgaricus* mixed culture.
Lactobacillus acidophilus, viable culture.
Logen.
Lomanate.
Lomotil.
Lonox.
Loperamide Hydrochloride.
Milk of Bismuth.
Motofen.
Pepto-Bismol.
Pink Bismuth.

antidiuretics.
See: Pitressin.
Pituitary Posterior Injection.

antidopaminergics.
Use: Antiemetic/antivertigo agents.
See: Chlorpromazine.
Metoclopramide.
Nabilone.
Perphenazine.
Prochlorperazine.
Promethazine.
Thiethylperazine Maleate.

antidotes.
See: Acetylcysteine.
Atropine/Pralidoxime Chloride.
Charcoal, Activated.
Digoxin Immune Fab (Ovine).
Flumazenil.
Fomepizole.
Glucarpidase.
Hydroxocobalamin.
Ipecac.
Methylene Blue.
Methylnaltrexone Bromide.
Nalmefene Hydrochloride.
Naloxone Hydrochloride.
Naltrexone Hydrochloride.
Physostigmine Salicylate.
Pralidoxime Chloride.
Sodium Nitrite.
Sodium Thiosulfate.

antiemetic/antivertigo agents.
See: Anticholinergic Agents.
Antidopaminergics.
Antiemetic/Antivertigo Agents, Miscellaneous.
Doxylamine Succinate/Pyridoxine Hydrochloride.
5-HT_3 Receptor Antagonists.

antiemetic/antivertigo agents, miscellaneous.
See: Aprepitant.
Dronabinol.
Fosaprepitant.
Nabilone.
Phosphorated Carbohydrate Solution.

antiepilepsirine.
Use: Treatment for drug-resistant generalized tonic-clonic epilepsy. [Orphan Drug]

antiepileptic agents.
See: Anticonvulsants.

antiestrogens.
Use: Hormone for cancer therapy.
See: Fulvestrant.
Tamoxifen Citrate.
Toremifene Citrate.

antifebrin.
See: Acetanilid.

antiflatulents.
See: Di-Gel.
Simethicone.

Antifoam A Compound. (Hoechst)
Use: Antiflatulent.
See: Simethicone.

antifolic acid.
See: Methotrexate.

Antiformin. Sodium hypochlorite in sodium hydroxide 7.5%, available chlorine 5.2%; may be colored with meta cresol purple.
Use: Antiseptic; antimicrobial.

antifungal agents.
See: Allylamine Antifungals.
Amphotericin B Desoxycholate.
Amphotericin B, Lipid-based.
Anidulafungin.
Butenafine Hydrochloride.
Caspofungin Acetate.
Ciclopirox.
Clioquinol.
Clotrimazole.
Echinocandins.
Econazole Nitrate.
Fluconazole.
Flucytosine.
Fungicides.
Gentian Violet.
Griseofulvin.
Imidazole Antifungals.
Itraconazole.
Ketoconazole.
Luliconazole.
Micafungin Sodium.
Miconazole Nitrate.
Naftifine Hydrochloride.
Nystatin.
Polyene Antifungals.
Posaconazole.
Sertaconazole Nitrate.
Sulconazol Nitrate.
Terbinafine Hydrochloride.
Tolnaftate.
Triazole Antifungals.
Undecylenic Acid.
Voriconazole.

antiglaucoma agents.
See: AK-Beta.
Betagan Liquifilm.
Betaxolol Hydrochloride.
Betimol.
Betoptic.
Betoptic S.
Bimatoprost.
Carteolol Hydrochloride.
Levobetaxolol Hydrochloride.
Levobunolol Hydrochloride.
Lumigan.
Metipranolol Hydrochloride.
OptiPranolol.
Timolol.
Timolol Maleate.
Timoptic.
Timoptic-XE.
Travatan.
Travoprost.

antihemophilic agents.
See: Antihemophilic Factor (Factor VIII; AHF).
Anti-Inhibitor Coagulant Complex.
Coagulation Factor IX (Recombinant).
Coagulation Factor VIIa, Recombinant.
Coagulation Factor XII A-Subunit (Recombinant).
Factor IX Concentrates.
Factor IX (Recombinant).
Factor XIII Concentrate.

•**antihemophilic factor.** (AN-tee-HEE-moe-FIL-ik) *USP.* Factor VIII; AHF.
Use: Antihemophilic.
See: Advate.
Helixate FS.
Hemofil M.
Koate-DVI.
Kogenate FS.
Monoclate-P.
Novoeight.
Recombinate.
ReFacto.
Xyntha.

antihemophilic factor combinations.
See: Antihemophilic Factor/von Willebrand Factor Complex (Factor VIII/VWF; AHF/VWF).

antihemophilic factor, human.
Use: Treatment of von Willebrand disease. [Orphan Drug]

antihemophilic factor (recombinant).
Use: Prophylaxis/treatment of bleeding in hemophilia A. [Orphan Drug]
See: Kogenate FS.

antihemophilic factor/von Willebrand factor complex (factor VIII/VWF; AHF/VWF).
Use: Antihemophilic.
See: Humate-P.

antiheparin.
See: Protamine Sulfate.

antiherpes virus agents.
Use: Antiviral.
See: Acyclovir.
Famciclovir.
Valacyclovir Hydrochloride.

antihistamine, analgesic, and decongestant combinations.
Use: Upper respiratory combination.

antihistamine and analgesic combinations.
Use: Upper respiratory combination.
See: Analgesic and antihistamine combinations.

antihistamine and antitussive combinations.
Use: Upper respiratory combination.

antihistamine and decongestant combinations.
Use: Upper respiratory combination.

antihistamine, anticholinergic, and decongestant combinations.
Use: Upper respiratory combination.

antihistamine, antitussive, analgesic, and decongestant combinations.
Use: Upper respiratory combination.

antihistamine, antitussive, and analgesic combinations.
Use: Upper respiratory combination.

antihistamine, antitussive, and decongestant combinations.
Use: Upper respiratory combination.

antihistamine, antitussive, decongestant, expectorant combinations.
Use: Upper respiratory combination.

Antihistamine Cream. (Towne) Methapyrilene hydrochloride 10 mg, pyrilamine maleate 5 mg, allantoin 2 mg, diperodon hydrochloride 2.5 mg, benzocaine 10 mg, menthol 2 mg/g. Cream. Jar 2 oz. *OTC.*
Use: Antihistamine, topical.

antihistamine, decongestant, and expectorant combinations.
Use: Upper respiratory combination.
See: Acetaminophen, Dextromethorphan Hydrobromide, Guaifenesin, Phenylephrine Hydrochloride.
Chlorpheniramine Maleate, Guaifenesin, Phenylephrine Hydrochloride.
Guaifenesin, Phenylephrine Tannate, Pyrilamine Tannate.

antihistamines.
See: Alkylamines, Nonselective.
Ethanolamines, Nonselective.
Phenothiazines, Nonselective.
Phthalazinones, Peripherally Selective.
Piperazines, Nonselective.
Piperazines, Peripherally Selective.
Piperidines, Nonselective.
Piperidines, Peripherally Selective.

antihistamines, inhalant.
See: Azelastine.
Olopatadine.

Antihist-1. (Various Mfr.) Clemastine fumarate 1.34 mg. Tab. Pkg. 16s. *OTC.*
Use: Antihistamine.

antihyperlipidemic agents.
See: Bile Acid Sequestrants.
Ezetimibe.
Fibric Acid Derivatives.
HMG-CoA Reductase Inhibitors.
Icosapent Ethyl.
Lomitapide.
Niacin.

antihyperlipidemic combinations.
See: Amlodipine Besylate/Atorvastatin Calcium.
Atorvastatin/Ezetimibe.
Ezetimibe/Simvastatin.

Guanoxyfen Sulfate.
Harbolin.
H.H.R.
Hiwolfia.
Hydralazine.
Hydralazine Hydrochloride.
Hydralazine Polistirex.
Hydrochloroserpine.
Hydroflumethiazide.
Hydropine.
Hydropine H.P.
Hydroxyisoindolin.
Indacrinone.
Indapamide.
Indolapril Hydrochloride.
Indoramin.
Indoramin Hydrochloride.
Indorenate Hydrochloride.
Ingadine.
Inhibace.
Inversine.
Irbesartan.
Ismelin.
Labetalol Hydrochloride.
Leniquinsin.
Levcromakalim.
Lofexidine Hydrochloride.
Losartan Potassium.
Losulazine Hydrochloride.
Mebutamate.
Mecamylamine Hydrochloride.
Medroxalol.
Medroxalol Hydrochloride.
Methalthiazide.
Methyclodine.
Methylclothiazide.
Methyldopa.
Metipranolol.
Metipranolol Hydrochloride.
Metolazone.
Metoprolol Fumarate.
Metoprolol Succinate.
Metyrosine.
Moexipril Hydrochloride.
Muzolimine.
Nadolol.
Natrico.
Nebivolol.
Nitrendipine.
Nitroprusside Sodium.
Pargyline Hydrochloride.
Pelanserin Hydrochloride.
Pentolinium Tartrate.
Perindopril Erbumine.
Pheniprazine Hydrochloride.
Phenoxybenzamine Hydrochloride.
Phentolamine Hydrochloride.
Prazosin Hydrochloride.
Prizidilol Hydrochloride.
Quinapril Hydrochloride.
Quinazosin Hydrochloride.
Quinelorane Hydrochloride.
Quinuclium Bromide.
Raunescine.
Rauwolfia Serpentina.
Rauwolscine.
Rawfola.
Saprisartan Potassium.
Saralasin Acetate.
Sodium Nitroprusside.
Sulfinalol Hydrochloride.
Teludipine Hydrochloride.
Temocapril Hydrochloride.
Terazosin Hydrochloride.
Tiamenidine Hydrochloride.
Timolol Maleate.
Tipentosin Hydrochloride.
Trimazosin Hydrochloride.
Trimethamide.
Trimoxamine Hydrochloride.
Univasc.
Valsartan.
Zankiren Hydrochloride.
Zofenoprilat Arginine.

anti-infectives.
See: Aminoglycosides, Parenteral.
Antibiotics/Anti-infectives.
Antifungal Agents.
Antiprotozoal Agents.
Antituberculosis Agents.
Antiviral Agents.
Carbapenems.
Cephalosporins and Related Antibiotics.
Fluoroquinolones.
Lincosamides.
Lipoglycopeptides.
Macrolides.
Methenamines.
Metronidazole.
Monobactams.
Nitrofurans.
Sulfonamides.
Tetracyclines.

anti-infectives, miscellaneous.
See: Clindamycin Phosphate.
Metronidazole.
Vancomycin.

anti-infectives, topical.
See: Amphotericin B.
Antibiotic Agents.
Antifungal Agents.
Antiseptics and Germicides.
Antivirals.
Boric Acid.
Burn Preparations.
Chloroxine.
Dapsone.

anti-inflammatory agents.
See: Corticosteroids, Topical.
Nonsteroidal Anti-Inflammatory Drugs, Topical.

anti-inhibitor coagulant complex.
Use: Antihemophilic agent.
See: Feiba NF.
Anti-Itch. (Taro) Diphenhydramine 2%, zinc acetate 0.1%. Cetyl alcohol, parabens. Cream. 28.4 g. *OTC.*
Use: Topical antihistamine.
Antilerge. (Merz) Chlorpheniramine maleate 8 mg, phenylephrine hydrochloride 12 mg. Tab. Bot. 30s. *OTC.*
Use: Antihistamine; decongestant.
antileukemia.
See: Antineoplastic agents.
antimalarial agents.
See: Atovaquone and Proguanil Hydrochloride.
Cinchona Alkaloid.
Folic Acid Antagonists.
4-Aminoquinolone Compounds.
Mefloquine Hydrochloride.
Pyrimethamine.
Sulfadoxine and Pyrimethamine.
antimetabolites.
See: Allopurinol.
Capecitabine.
Cladribine.
Clofarabine.
Cytarabine.
Floxuridine.
Fludarabine Phosphate.
Fluorouracil.
Folic Acid Antagonists.
Gemcitabine Hydrochloride.
Mercaptopurine.
Methotrexate.
Pemetrexed.
Pentostatin.
Purine Analogs and Related Agents.
Pyrimidine Analogs.
Rasburicase.
Thioguanine.
antimigraine agents.
See: Almotriptan Maleate.
Amerge.
Axert.
Frova.
Frovatriptan Succinate.
Imitrex.
Maxalt.
Maxalt-MLT.
Midrin.
Naratriptan Hydrochloride.
Rizatriptan Benzoate.
Serotonin 5-HT_1 Receptor Agonists.
Sumatriptan Succinate.
Zolmitriptan.
Zomig.
Zomig ZMT.
antimitotic agents.
See: Epothilones.
Halichondrin B Analogs.
Paclitaxel.
Taxoids.
Vinca Alkaloids.
Vincristine Sulfate.
Vinorelbine Tartrate.
•**antimony potassium tartrate.** (AN-ti-MOE-nee) *USP.*
Use: Antischistosomal; leishmaniasis; expectorant; emetic.
W/Guaifenesin, codeine phosphate.
See: Cheracol.
W/Guaifenesin, dextromethorphan HBr.
See: Cheracol D.
antimony preparations.
See: Antimony Potassium Tartrate.
Antimony Sodium Thioglycollate.
Tartar Emetic.
•**antimony sodium tartrate.** *USP.*
Use: Antischistosomal.
antimony sodium thioglycollate. (Various Mfr.). *Rx.*
Use: Schistosomiasis; leishmaniasis; filariasis.
•**antimony trisulfide colloid.** (AN-ti-MOE-nee trye-SUL-fide KOL-oid) USAN.
Use: Pharmaceutic aid.
anti-my9-blocked ricin.
Use: Leukemia treatment. [Orphan Drug]
antinauseants.
See: Antiemetic/antivertigo agents
antineoplastic agents.
See: Adriamycin.
Allopurinol Sodium.
Aloprim.
Amifostine.
Amsacrine.
Antimetabolites.
Antineoplastic Antibiotics.
Arsenic Trioxide.
Azacitidine.
Blenoxane.
Brentuximab Vedotin.
Cosmegen.
Decitabine.
DNA Demethylation Agents.
Elspar.
Emcyt.
Enzymes.
Epipodophyllotoxins.
Estinyl.
Ethyol.
FUDR.
Gefitinib.
Herceptin.
Hexalen.
Hormones.
Hydrea.
Idamycin PFS.
Imidazotetrazine Derivatives.
Kadcyla.

Kinase Inhibitors.
Leukeran.
Lysodren.
Matulane.
Medroxyprogesterone Acetate.
Megace.
Mercaptopurine.
Methotrexate.
Methotrexate Sodium.
Mitotane.
Monoclonal Antibodies.
Mustargen.
Myleran.
Oncovin.
Oxaliplatin.
Platinum Coordination Complex.
Protein Synthesis Inhibitors.
Purinethol.
Tamoxifen Citrate.
Temodar.
Temozolomide.
Teniposide.
Thioguanine.
Thiotepa.
Trastuzumab.
Trisenox.
Vismodegib.

antineoplastic antibiotics.
See: Dactinomycin.

antineoplastics, miscellaneous.
See: Mitotane.
Porfimer Sodium.
Sipuleucel-T.
Talc Powder, Sterile.

antiobesity agents.
See: Adderall.
Adipex-P.
Amphetamines.
Anorex.
Bontril.
Dextroamphetamine.
Didrex.
Diethylpropion Hydrochloride.
Ionamin.
Levo-Amphetamine.
Mazanor.
Phendimetrazine Tartrate.
Phentermine Hydrochloride.
Prelu-2.
Tenuate.
Tenuate Dospan.
Tepanil.
Trimstat.
Xenical.

Antiox. (Merz) Vitamin C 120 mg, vitamin E 100 units, beta-carotene 25 mg. Cap. Bot. 60s. *OTC.*
Use: Vitamin supplement.

Antioxidant Formula. (Rugby) Vitamins 5,000 units, E 200 units, C 250 mg, Cu, Mn, Se, Zn. Corn oil, glycerin, soy lecithin, soybean oil. Gluten free, preservative free, sugar free. Cap., softgel. 50s. *OTC.*
Use: Multivitamin with minerals (except iron).

Anti-Pak Compound. (Lowitt) Phenylephrine hydrochloride 5 mg, salicylamide 0.23 g, acetophenetidin 0.15 g, caffeine 0.03 g, ascorbic acid 50 mg, hesperidin complex 50 mg, chlorprophenpyridamine maleate 2 mg. Tab. Bot. 30s, 100s. *OTC.*
Use: Analgesic; antihistamine; decongestant combination.

antiparasympathomimetics.
See: Parasympatholytic agents.

antiparkinson agents.
See: Amantadine Hydrochloride.
Anticholinergic Agents.
Bromocriptine Mesylate.
Carbidopa.
Carbidopa and Levodopa.
Dopaminergics.
Entacapone.
Pergolide Mesylate.
Rasagiline.
Selegiline Hydrochloride.
Tolcapone.

antipellagra vitamin.
See: Nicotinic acid.

antipernicious anemia principle.
See: Vitamin B_{12}.

Antiphlogistine. (Denver Chemical Inc.) Medicated poultice. Jar 5 oz, lb. Tube 8 oz. Can 5 lb. *OTC.*
Use: Counterirritant.

antiplatelet agents.
See: Aggregation Inhibitors.
Anagrelide Hydrochloride.
Dipyridamole.
Glycoprotein IIb/IIIa Inhibitors.

antiprotozoal agents.
See: Atovaquone.
Diiodohydroxyquinoline.
Emetine Hydrochloride.
Furazolidone.
Levofuraltadone.
Miltefosine.
Nitazoxanide.
Quinoxyl.
Sodium Suramin.
Tinidazole.

antipsoriatic agents.
See: Anthralin.
Calcipotriene.
Calcipotriene and Betamethasone Dipropionate.
Methotrexate.
Selenium Sulfide.

antipsychotics.
See: Benzisoxazole Derivatives.

Benzoisothiazol Derivatives.
Dibenzapine Derivatives.
Dihydroindolone Derivatives.
Lithium.
Phenothiazine Derivatives.
Phenylbutylpiperadine Derivatives.
Quinolinone Derivatives.
Thioxanthene Derivatives.

•**antipyrine.** (an-tee-PYE-reen) *USP.*
Use: Analgesic; antipyretic.
W/Acetic Acid, Benzocaine, Polycosanol.
See: AABP.
W/Benzocaine.
See: Aurax.
W/Benzocaine, Chlorobutanol.
See: G.B.A.
W/Benzocaine, Phenylephrine Hydrochloride.
See: Ear-Gesic.
W/Benzocaine, u-Polycosanol 410.
See: Treagan.
W/Carbamide, Benzocaine, Cetyldimethylbenzylammonium Hydrochloride.
See: Auralgesic.

antipyrine and benzocaine.
Use: Anesthetic, local.
See: Auro Ear Drops.

antipyrine and benzocaine otic. (URL) Benzocaine 1.4%, antipyrine 5.4%, glycerin. Soln. 15 mL with dropper. *Rx.*
Use: Otic preparation.

antipyrine, benzocaine, and phenylephrine hydrochloride.
Use: Anesthetic, local; decongestant eardrop.

antiretroviral agents.
See: Cellular Chemokine Receptor Antagonist.
Fusion Inhibitors.
Integrase Inhibitors.
Non-Nucleoside Reverse Transcriptase Inhibitors.
Nucleoside Analog Reverse Transcriptase Inhibitor Combination.
Nucleoside Reverse Transcriptase Inhibitors.
Nucleotide Analog Reverse Transcriptase Inhibitors.
Protease Inhibitor Combination.
Protease Inhibitors.

antirheumatic agents.
See: Arava.
Azulfidine.
Azulfidine EN-tabs.
Hydroxychloroquine Sulfate.
Leflunomide.
Sulfasalazine.

antirickettsial agents.
See: Chloromycetin.

antiscorbutic vitamin.
See: Ascorbic Acid.

antiseptic, dyes.
See: Acriflavine.
Bismuth Violet.
Crystal Violet.
Fuchsin, Basic.
Gentian Violet.
Methyl Violet.
Pyridium.

antiseptic, mercurials.
See: Merthiolate.
Phenylmercuric Acetate.
Phenylmercuric Borate.
Phenylmercuric Nitrate.
Phenylmercuric Picrate.
Thimerosal.

antiseptic, n-chloro compounds.
See: Chloramine-T.
Chlorazene.
Dichloramine T.
Halazone.

antiseptic, phenols.
See: Anthralin.
Creosote.
Hexachlorophene.
Hexylresorcinol.
Methylparaben.
Parachlorometaxylenol.
Phenol.
o-Phenylphenol.
Propylparaben.
Pyrogallol.
Resorcinol.
Resorcinol Monoacetate.
Thymol.
Trinitrophenol.

antiseptics.
See: Furacin.
Iodine Products, Anti-infective.
Phenol.

antiseptics and germicides.
See: Benzalkonium Chloride.
Benzethonium Chloride w/Menthol.
Chlorhexidine Gluconate.
Iodine.
Triclosan.

antiseptic, surface-active agents.
See: Bactine.
Bactine Pain Relieving Cleansing.
Benzalkonium Chloride.
Benzethonium Chloride.
Ceepryn.
Diaparene.
Methylbenzethonium Chloride.
Zephiran.

Antiseptic Wound & Skin Cleanser. (MPM Medical) Benzethonium chloride 0.1%, EDTA, glycerin, methylparaben. Liq. 120 mL. *OTC.*
Use: Topical anti-infective.

antisickling agents.
See: Droxia.

Hydroxyurea.

Antispasmodic. (Teva) Phenobarbital 16.2 mg, hyoscyamine sulfate 0.1037 mg, atropine sulfate 0.0194 mg, scopolamine HBr 0.0065 mg. Cap. Bot. 1000s. *Rx.*
Use: Anticholinergic; antispasmodic; hypnotic; sedative.

Antispasmodic. (Various Mfr.) Atropine sulfate 0.0194 mg, scopolamine HBr 0.0065 mg, hyoscyamine HBr or sulfate 0.1037 mg, phenobarbital 16.2 mg/mL. Alcohol 23%, sugar, sorbitol. Elix. Bot. 120 mL, Pt, gal. *Rx.*
Use: GI anticholinergic combination.

antispasmodic agents. Parasympatholytic agents.
See: Anticholinergic Agents.
Belladonna Alkaloids.
Dicyclomine Hydrochloride.
Spasmolytic Agents.

antistreptolysin-O.
Use: Titration procedure.

anti-tac, humanized. (Roche)
Use: Prevention of acute renal allograft rejection. [Orphan Drug]

Anti-Ten. (Century) Allylisobutylbarbituric acid ¾ g, aspirin 3 g, phenacetin 2 g, caffeine g. Tab. Bot. 100s, 1000s. *Rx.*
Use: Analgesic; sedative; stimulant.

antithrombin.
Use: Anticoagulant.
See: ATryn.

antithrombin agents.
Use: Anticoagulant.
See: Antithrombin.
Antithrombin III (Human).

•**antithrombin III human.** *USP.*
Use: Thromboembolic.
See: Thrombate III.

antithrombin III (human) concentrate IV.
Use: Prophylaxis/treatment of thromboembolic episodes in AT-III deficiency. [Orphan Drug]

antithymocyte globulin (equine).
Use: Immune globulin.
See: Atgam.

antithymocyte globulin (rabbit).
Use: Immunosuppressant.
See: Thymoglobulin.

antithyroid agents.
See: Iothiouracil Sodium.
Methimazole.
Methylthiouracil.
Propylthiouracil.
Sodium Iodide I 131.
Tapazole.

antitoxins.
See: Antivenin (Crotalidae) Polyvalent (Equine Origin).
Antivenin (Lactrodectus mactans) (Black Widow Spider Antivenin) (Equine Origin).
Botulism Antitoxin.
Botulism Antitoxin Heptavalent.
Centruroides (Scorpion) Immune $F(ab')_2$ (Equine).
Crotalidae Polyvalent Immune Fab (Ovine Origin).
Tetanus Immune Globulin.

antitrypsin, alpha-1.
See: Alpha-1 Antitrypsin.

antituberculosis agents.
See: Aminosalicylic Acid.
Bedaquiline.
Capreomycin.
Cycloserine.
Ethambutol Hydrochloride.
Ethionamide.
Isoniazid.
Pyrazinamide.
Rifabutin.
Rifampin.
Rifapentine.

Anti-Tuss DM. (Century) Guaifenesin 100 mg, dextromethorphan HBr 15 mg/5 mL. Syr. Bot. 120 mL, 3.8 L. *OTC.*
Use: Antitussive; expectorant.

antitussive, analgesic, antihistamine, and decongestant combinations.
Use: Upper respiratory combination.

antitussive, analgesic, decongestant, expectorant combinations.
Use: Upper respiratory combination.

antitussive and anticholinergic combinations.
Use: Upper respiratory combination.

antitussive and antihistamine combinations.
Use: Upper respiratory combination.

antitussive and decongestant combinations.
Use: Upper respiratory combination.

antitussive and expectorant combinations.
Use: Upper respiratory combination.

antitussive, antihistamine, and decongestant combinations.
Use: Upper respiratory combination.

antitussive, antihistamine, decongestant, expectorant combinations.
Use: Upper respiratory combination.

antitussive combinations.
Use: Upper respiratory combination.

Antitussive Cough Syrup. (Weeks & Leo) Chlorpheniramine 2 mg, phenylephrine hydrochloride 5 mg, dextromethorphan 15 mg, ammonium chloride 50 mg/5 mL. Syr. Bot. *OTC.*
Use: Antihistamine; antitussive; decongestant; expectorant.

Antitussive Cough Syrup with Codeine. (Weeks & Leo) Chlorpheniramine maleate 2 mg, phenylephrine hydrochloride 5 mg, codeine phosphate 10 mg, ammonium chloride 50 mg/5 mL. Syr. Bot. 4 oz. *c-v.*
Use: Antihistamine; antitussive; decongestant; expectorant.

antitussive, decongestant, and expectorant combinations.
Use: Upper respiratory combination.

antitussive hydrocodone bitartrate and homatropine methylbromide. (Actavis) Hydrocodone bitartrate 5 mg, homatropine HBr 1.5 mg. Lactose. Tab. 100s, 500s. *c-III.*
Use: Upper respiratory combination, antitussive combination.

antitussives, narcotic.
See: Narcotic antitussive.

antivenin Centruroides sculpturatus. (Arizona State University) Available in Arizona only. 5 mL vials. *Rx.*
Use: Antivenin.

•**antivenin (Crotalidae) polyvalent.** (AN-tee-VEN-in kro-TAL-i-dee POL-ee-VAY-lent) *USP.*
Use: Immunization.

antivenin, Crotalidae polyvalent immune fab (ovine).
Use: Bites of North American crotalid snakes. [Orphan Drug]
See: CroFab.

•**antivenin (Latrodectus mactans).** (AN-tee-VEN-in LAT-roe-DEK-tus MAK-tans) *USP. Formerly Widow spider species antivenin (Latrodectus mactans).*
Use: Immunization.

antivenin (Latrodectus mactans). (Merck) Black widow spider antivenin (equine origin) ≥ 6000 antivenin units/vial. Thimerosal 1:10,000. Pow. for Inj. Single-use Vial with 1 vial diluent (Sterile Water for Injection 2.5 mL) and normal horse serum 1 mL (1:10 dilution) for sensitivity testing. *Rx.*
Use: Treatment of black widow spider bites.

•**antivenin (Micrurus fulvius).** (AN-tee-VEN-in mye-KROO-rus FUL-vi-us) *USP.*
Use: Immunization.

antivenin (Micrurus fulvius). North American coral snake antivenin (equine origin), phenol 0.25%, thimerosal 0.005%, phenylmercuric nitrate 1:100,000. Pow. for Inj., lyophilized. Single-use Vial with 1 vial diluent (Water for Injection 10 mL). *Rx.*
Use: Bites of North American coral snake and Texas coral snake.

antivenins.
See: Antivenin (Crotalidae) Polyvalent.
Antivenin (Latrodectus mactans).
Antivenin (Micrurus fulvius).
Crotalidae Polyvalent Immune Fab (Ovine origin).

antivenom (Crotalidae) purified (avian). (Ophidian Pharmaceuticals, Inc.)
Use: Bites of snakes of the Crotalidae family. [Orphan Drug]

Antivert. (Pfizer US) Meclizine hydrochloride 12.5 mg. Tab. Bot. 100s, 1000s, UD 100s. *Rx.*
Use: Antiemetic/antivertigo agent.

Antivert/50. (Pfizer US) Meclizine hydrochloride 50 mg, Tab. Bot. 100s. *Rx.*
Use: Antiemetic/antivertigo agent.

Antivert/25. (Pfizer US) Meclizine hydrochloride 25 mg. Tab. Bot. 100s, 1000s, UD 100s. *Rx.*
Use: Antiemetic/antivertigo agent.

antiviral agents.
See: Abacavir Sulfate.
Acyclovir.
Adefovir Dipivoxil.
Amantadine Hydrochloride.
Antiherpes Virus Agents.
Boceprevir.
Cidofovir.
Entecavir.
Famciclovir.
Foscarnet Sodium.
Ganciclovir.
Nevirapine.
Oseltamivir Phosphate.
Ribavirin.
Rimantadine Hydrochloride.
Simeprevir.
Sofosbuvir.
Valacyclovir Hydrochloride.
Valganciclovir Hydrochloride.
Zanamivir.

antiviral agents, ophthalmic.
See: Ganciclovir.

antiviral antibodies.
See: Cytomegalovirus Immune Globulin (Human).
Hepatitis B Immune Globulin.
Immune Globulin IV.
Rabies Immune Globulin.
Vaccinia Immune Globulin.
Varicella-Zoster Immune Globulin.

antixerophthalmic vitamin.
See: Vitamin A.

Antizol. (Paladin Labs) Fomepizole 1 g/mL. Preservative free. Inj. Conc. Vial 1.5 mL. *Rx.*
Use: Antidote.

Antril. (Amgen) Interleukin-1 receptor antagonist (human recombinant).
Use: Arthritis; organ rejection. [Orphan Drug]

Antrizine. (Major) Meclizine hydrochloride 12.5 mg. Tab. Bot. 100s, 500s, 1000s. *Rx.*
Use: Antiemetic/antivertigo agent.

Antrocol. (ECR) Atropine sulfate 0.195 mg, phenobarbital 16 mg per 5 mL. Alcohol 20%. Sugar free. Elix. Bot. Pt. *Rx.*
Use: GI anticholinergic combination.

Antrypol. Suramin. *Rx.*
Use: CDC anti-infective agent.

Anucaine. (Calvin) Procaine 50 mg, butyl-p-aminobenzoate 200 mg, benzyl alcohol 265 mg in sweet almond oil/ 5 mL. Amp. 5 mL. Box 6s, 24s, 100s. *OTC.*
Use: Anorectal preparation.

Anucort-HC. (G & W) Hydrocortisone acetate 25 mg in a hydrogenated vegetable oil base. Supp. Box 12s, 24s, 100s. *Rx.*
Use: Anorectal preparation.

Anuject. (Roberts) Procaine. Soln. Vial 5 mL, 10 mL. *Rx.*
Use: Anorectal preparation.

Anu-Med. (Major) Phenylephrine hydrochloride 0.25%, hard fat 88.7%. Corn starch, parabens. Supp. 12. *OTC.*
Use: Anorectal preparation.

Anumed HC. (Major) Hydrocortisone acetate 10 mg. Supp. Box 12s. *Rx.*
Use: Anorectal preparation.

Anuprep HC. (Great Southern) Hydrocortisone acetate 25 mg. Supp. Box 12s.
Use: Anorectal preparation.

Anuprep Hemorrhoidal. (Great Southern) Bismuth subgallate 2.25%, bismuth resorcin compound 1.75%, benzyl benzoate 1.2%, peruvian balsam 1.8%, and zinc oxide 11% in a hydrogenated vegetable oil base. Supp. Box 12s, 24s. *Rx.*
Use: Anorectal preparation.

Anusol-HC. (Salix) Hydrocortisone 2.5%. Cream. Tube 30 g. *Rx.*
Use: Corticosteroid, topical.

Anzemet. (Aventis) Dolasetron mesylate. **Tab.:** 50 mg, 100 mg. Lactose. Film coated. 5s, blister pack 5s, UD 10s. **Inj.:** 20 mg/mL. Mannitol 38.2 mg/mL. Single-use amp. 0.625 mL. 0.625 mL fill in 2 mL *Carpu-ject.* Single-use vial. 5 mL. Multi-dose vial. 25 mL. *Rx.*
Use: Antiemetic; antivertigo.

A1cNow. (Metrika) Reagent kit for blood tests. Box 1s, 2s with lancet(s), monitor, dilution kit. *Rx.*
Use: In vitro diagnostic aid.

AOSEPT. (Ciba Vision) **AODISC Neutralizer:** Platinum-coated tablet. Tab. good for 100 uses or 3 months of daily use. **Disinfecting Soln.:** Hydrogen peroxide 3%, sodium chloride 0.85%, phosphonic acid, phosphate buffer. Soln. Bot. 120 mL, 240 mL, 360 mL. *OTC.*
Use: Contact lens disinfection system.

•**apadenoson.** (a-pa-DEN-oh-son) USAN.
Use: Imaging agent.

•**apafant.** (APP-ah-fant) USAN.
Use: Platelet activating factor antagonist; antiasthmatic.

•**apalcillin sodium.** (APE-al-SIH-lin) USAN.
Use: Anti-infective.

APAP.
See: Acetaminophen.

Apap. (Cypress) Acetaminophen 325 mg, 500 mg. Film coated. Tab. 150s (325 mg only), UD 100s (500 mg only). *OTC.*
Use: Analgesic.

Apap 500. (Cypress) Acetaminophen 500 mg/5 mL. Alcohol and sugar free. Liq. 237 mL. *OTC.*
Use: Analgesic.

Apap Infant's. (Various Mfr.) Acetaminophen 100 mg/mL. May contain butylparaben, saccharin. Oral Soln., Conc. 15 mL. *OTC.*
Use: Analgesic.

•**apatorsen.** (A-pa-TOR-sen) USAN.
Use: Antineoplastic.

•**apatorsen sodium.** (A-pa-TOR-sen) USAN.
Use: Antineoplastic.

•**apaxifylline.** (A-pock-SIH-fih-leen) USAN.
Use: Selective adenosine A_1 antagonist.

•**apaziquone.** (a-PA-zi-kwone) USAN.
Use: Antineoplastic.

•**apazone.** (APP-ah-zone) USAN.
Use: Anti-inflammatory.

Apcogesic. (Apco) Sodium salicylate 5 g, colchicine 1/320 g, calcium carbonate 65 mg, dried aluminum hydroxide gel 130 mg, phenobarbital ⅛ g. Tab. Bot. 100s. *Rx.*
Use: Antigout; hypnotic; sedative.

Apcoretic. (A.P.C) Caffeine anhydrous 100 mg, ammonium chloride 325 mg. Tab. Bot. 90s. *Rx.*
Use: Diuretic.

Ap Creme. (T.E. Williams Pharmaceuticals) Hydrocortisone 0.5%, iodochlorhydroxyquin 3%. Tube. *Rx-OTC.*
Use: Antifungal; corticosteroid, topical.

A.P.C. with gelsemium combinations.
See: Valacet.

ApexiCon E. (Sandoz) Diflorasone diacetate 0.05%. Stearyl alcohol, cetyl alco-

hol. Cream. 30 g, 60g. *Rx.*
Use: Anti-inflammatory.

APF.
Use: Analgesic.
See: Arthritis Pain Formula.

Aphco Hemorrhoidal Combination. (A.P.C) Combination package of Aphco Hemorrhoidal ointment 1.5 oz tube, Aphco Hemorrhoidal supp. Box 12s, 1000s. *OTC.*
Use: Anorectal preparation.

Aphen. (MedChem) Acetaminophen 325 mg. Tab. 150s. *OTC.*
Use: CNS agent.

Aphrodyne. (Star) Yohimbine hydrochloride 5.4 mg. Tab. Bot. 100s, 1000s. *Rx.*
Use: Anti-impotence agent, alpha-adrenergic blocker.

Apicillin.
See: Ampicillin.

Apidra. (Sanofi Aventis) Insulin glulisine 100 units/mL. Inj. Vials. 10 mL. Cartridge system for use with *OptiClik.* 3 mL. *Rx.*
Use: Antidiabetic agent, insulin.

•**apitolisib.** (a-PIT-oh-LIS-ib) USAN.
Use: Antineoplastic.

•**apixaban.** (a-PIX-a-ban) USAN.
Use: Anticoagulant.
See: Eliquis.

•**aplaviroc hydrochloride.** (AP-la-VIR-ok) USAN.
Use: Antiretroviral agent.

Aplenzin. (Sanofi-Aventis) Bupropion hydrobromide 174 mg, 348 mg, 522 mg. Polyethylene glycol. ER Tab. 30s. *Rx.*
Use: Antidepressant.

APL 400-020 V-Beta DNA vaccine. (Apollon)
Use: Treatment of cutaneous T-cell lymphoma. [Orphan Drug]

•**aplindore fumarate.** (AP-lin-dor) USAN.
Use: Antischizophrenic.

Aplisol. (JHP Pharmaceuticals) Tuberculin purified protein derivative 5 units/0.1 mL, polysorbate 80, potassium and sodium phosphates, phenol 0.35%. Vial 1 mL (10 tests), 5 mL (50 tests). *Rx.*
Use: Diagnostic aid.

Aplitest. (Parke-Davis) Purified tuberculin protein derivative buffered with potassium and sodium phosphates, phenol 0.5%/single-use, multipuncture unit. 25s. *Rx.*
Use: Diagnostic aid.

A + D Ointment. (Schering-Plough) Fish liver oil, cholecalciferol. Oint. Tube 1.5 oz, 4 oz. Jar lb. *OTC.*
Use: Emollient.

A + D Zinc Oxide Cream. (Schering-Plough) Dimethicone 1%, zinc oxide 10%. Aloe, benzyl alcohol, coconut oil, cod liver oil, light mineral oil. Cream. 113 g. *OTC.*
Use: Emollient.

Apokyn. (US WorldMeds) Apomorphine hydrochloride 10 mg/mL. Sodium metabisulfite. Inj. Glass Amps. 2 mL. Cartridges. 3 mL. *Rx.*
Use: Antiparkinson agent, dopaminergic.

•**apolizumab.** (ap-ol-IZ-yoo-mab) USAN.
Use: Anti-cancer agent.

•**apomorphine hydrochloride.** (ah-poh-MORE-feen) *USP.*
Use: Treatment of Parkinson disease.
See: Apokyn.

aporphine-10, 11-diol hydrochloride.
See: Apomorphine hydrochloride.

appetite depressants.
See: Anorexiants

APPG.
See: Aqueous Procaine Penicillin G.

•**apraclonidine hydrochloride.** (app-rah-KLOE-nih-deen) *USP.*
Use: Adrenergic, α_2-agonist.
See: Iopidine.

•**apramycin.** (APP-rah-MY-sin) USAN.
Use: Anti-infective.

Aprazone. (Major) Sulfinpyrazone 100 mg. Tab. Bot. 100s. *Rx.*
Use: Antigout agent.

apremilast.
Use: Immunomodulator.
See: Otezla.

•**aprepitant.** (ap-REH-pih-tant) USAN.
Use: Antiemetic/antivertigo agent, miscellaneous.
See: Emend.

Apresodex. (Rugby) Hydrochlorothiazide 15 mg, hydralazine hydrochloride 25 mg. Tab. Bot. 100s, 1000s. *Rx.*
Use: Antihypertensive.

Apresoline. (Novartis) Hydralazine hydrochloride. **Amp.:** 20 mg w/propylene glycol, methyl and propyl parabens/mL. Pkg. 5s. **Tab.:** 10 mg Bot. 100s, 1200s; 25 mg or 50 mg Bot. 100s, 1000s; 100 mg Bot. 100s. Consumer pack 100s. *Rx.*
Use: Antihypertensive.

Apresoline-Esidrix. (Novartis) Hydralazine hydrochloride 25 mg, hydrochlorothiazide 15 mg. Tab. Bot. 100s. *Rx.*
Use: Antihypertensive.

Apri. (Barr) Desogestrel 0.15 mg, ethinyl estradiol 30 mcg. Lactose. Tab. Blister cards 28s with 7 inert tabs. *Rx.*
Use: Sex hormone, contraceptive hormone.

•**apricoxib.** (AP-ri-KOX-ib) USAN.
Use: Anti-inflammatory agent.

•**aprindine.** (APE-rin-deen) USAN.
Use: Cardiovascular agent.

•**aprindine hydrochloride.** (APE-rin-deen) USAN.
Use: Cardiovascular agent.

•**aprinocarsen sodium.** (ap-ri-NOE-kar-sen) USAN.
Use: Protein kinase inhibitor.

Apriso. (Salix) Mesalamine 375 mg. Aspartame, phenylalanine. Enteric coated granules. ER Cap. 4s, 120s. *Rx.*
Use: Gastrointestinal agent.

Aprobee w/C. (Health for Life Brands) Vitamins B_1 15 mg, B_2 10 mg, B_6 5 mg, niacinamide 50 mg, calcium pantothenate 10 mg, C 250 mg. Cap. Bot. 100s, 1000s. Tab. Bot. 50s, 100s, 1000s. *OTC.*
Use: Mineral, vitamin supplement.

Aprodine. (Major) Pseudoephedrine hydrochloride 60 mg, triprolidine hydrochloride 2.5 mg. Lactose, PEG. Tab. 24s. *OTC.*
Use: Upper respiratory combination, antihistamine and decongestant.

Aprodine w/Codeine. (Major) Pseudoephedrine hydrochloride 30 mg, triprolidine hydrochloride 1.25 mg, codeine phosphate 10 mg. Syr. Bot. Pt, gal. *c-v.*
Use: Antihistamine; decongestant.

•**aprotinin.** (app-row-TIE-nin) USAN.
Use: Enzyme inhibitor, proteinase.
See: Trasylol.

Aprozide 50/50. (Major) Hydrochlorothiazide 50 mg, hydralazine 50 mg. Cap. Bot. 100s, 250s. *Rx.*
Use: Antihypertensive.

Aprozide 25/25. (Major) Hydralazine 25 mg, hydrochlorothiazide 25 mg. Cap. Bot. 100s, 250s. *Rx.*
Use: Antihypertensive.

A.P.S. Aspirin, phenacetin, and salicylamide.

APSAC. Thrombolytic enzyme.

•**aptazapine maleate.** (app-TAZZ-ah-PEEN MAL-ee-ate) USAN.
Use: Antidepressant.

•**aptiganel hydrochloride.** (app-tih-GAN-ehl) USAN.
Use: Stroke and traumatic brain injury treatment (NMDA ion channel blocker).

Aptiom. (Sunovion) Eslicarbazepine acetate 200 mg, 400 mg, 600 mg, 800 mg. Tab. 30s (except 600 mg), 60s (600 mg only), 90s (600 mg, 800 mg). *Rx.*
Use: Anticonvulsant.

Aptivus. (Boehringer Ingelheim) Tipranavir. **Cap.:** 250 mg. Dehydrated alcohol 7% w/w, polyoxyl 35 castor oil. 120s. **Soln.:** 100 mg/mL. Buttermint-toffee flavor. Unit-of-use w/syringe. 95 mL. *Rx.*
Use: Antiretroviral, protease inhibitor.

Apyron.
See: Magnesium acetylsalicylate.

AQ-4B. (Western Research) Trichlormethiazide 4 mg. Tab. Bot. 1000s. *Rx.*
Use: Diuretic.

Aqua-Ban, Maximum Strength.
See: Maximum Strength Aqua-Ban.

Aquabase. (Pal-Pak, Inc.) Cetyl alcohol, propylene glycol, sodium lauryl sulfate, white wax, purified water. Jar lb. *OTC.*
Use: Pharmaceutic aid; ointment base.

Aquacare. (Numark) Urea 10%. **Cream:** Benzyl alcohol, glycerin, lanolin alcohol, lanolin oil, mineral oil, petrolatum. 75 g. **Lot.:** Mineral oil, parabens, petrolatum. 240 mL. *OTC.*
Use: Emollient.

Aquacillin G. (Armenpharm Ltd.) Penicillin G. *Rx.*
Use: Anti-infective, penicillin.

Aquacycline. (Armenpharm Ltd.) Tetracycline hydrochloride. *Rx.*
Use: Anti-infective, tetracycline.

Aquaderm. (Baker Norton) Octyl methoxycinnamate 7.5%, oxybenzone 6%. SPF 15. Cream. Tube. 105 g. *OTC.*
Use: Sunscreen.

Aquaderm. (C & M Pharmacal) Purified water, glycerin 25%, salicylic acid 0.1%, octoxynol-9 0.03%, FD&C Red #40 0.0001%. Bot. 2 oz. *OTC.*
Use: Emollient.

Aqua-E. (Yasoo) Vitamin E 30 units/mL. PEG 1000. Gluten free and sugar free. Liq. 120 mL, 237 mL. *OTC.*
Use: Fat-soluble vitamin.

Aquaflex Ultrasound Gel Pad. (Parker) Clear, solid, flexible, moist, standoff gel pad for use where transducer movement is impeded by bony or irregular body surfaces. 2 cm × 9 cm.
Use: Ultrasound aid.

Aquafuren. (Armenpharm Ltd.) Nitrofurantoin. *Rx.*
Use: Anti-infective, urinary.

Aquagen. (ALK) Allergenic extracts. Vials.

Aqua Glycolic Face. (Merz) Cetyl ricinoleate, C12-15 alkyl benzoate, glycolic acid, hyaluronic acid, ceresin, ammonium glycolate, glyceryl stearate, PEG-100 stearate, sorbitan stearate, sorbitol, propylene glycol, diazolidinyl urea, parabens, magnesium aluminum silicate, dimethicone, xanthan gum, trisodium EDTA. Cream. 50 mL. *OTC.*
Use: Emollient.

Aqua Glycolic Hand & Body. (Merz) Glycolic acid, ammonium glycolate, cetyl alcohol, glyceryl stearate, PEG-100 stearate, C12-15 alkyl benzoate, mineral oil, stearyl alcohol, magnesium aluminum silicate, xanthan gum, parabens, disodium EDTA. Lot. 117 mL. *OTC.*
Use: Emollient.

Aquakay.
See: Menadione.

Aqua Lacten. (Allergan) Demineralized water, urea, petrolatum, propylene glycol monostearate, sorbitan monostearate, lactic acid. Lot. Bot. 8 oz. *OTC.*
Use: Emollient.

Aqua Mist. (Faraday) Nasal spray. Squeeze Bot. 20 mL.

Aquamycin. (Armenpharm Ltd.) Erythromycin. *Rx.*
Use: Anti-infective, erythromycin.

Aquanil. (Sigma-Tau) Mersalyl 100 mg, theophylline (hydrate) 50 mg, methylparaben 0.18%, propylparaben 0.02%. Vial 10 mL. *OTC.*
Use: Bronchodilator; diuretic.

Aquanil Cleanser. (Person & Covey) Glycerin, cetyl, stearyl, and benzyl alcohol, sodium laureth sulfate, xanthan gum. Lipid free. Lot. Bot. 240 mL, 480 mL. *OTC.*
Use: Dermatologic, cleanser.

Aquanil HC. (Person & Covey) Hydrocortisone 1%. Alcohols, benzyl alcohol, glycerin. Fragrance free. Lot. 118 mL. *OTC.*
Use: Anti-inflammatory agent, topical corticosteroid.

Aquanine. (Armenpharm Ltd.) Quinine hydrochloride. *Rx.*
Use: Antimalarial.

Aquaoxy. (Armenpharm Ltd.) Oxytetracycline hydrochloride. *Rx.*
Use: Anti-infective, tetracycline.

Aquaphenicol. (Armenpharm Ltd.) Chloramphenicol. *Rx.*
Use: Anti-infective.

Aquaphilic Ointment. (Medco Lab) Hydrated hydrophilic oint. Jar 16 oz. *OTC.*
Use: Emollient; ointment base.

Aquaphilic Ointment with Carbamide 10% and 20%. (Medco Lab) Stearyl alcohol, white petrolatum, sorbitol, propylene glycol, sodium lauryl sulfate, lactic acid, methylparaben, propylparaben.
Use: Prescription compounding; emollient.

Aquaphor. (BSN Medical) Cholesterolized anhydrous petrolatum ointment base. Tube 1.75 oz, 3.25 oz, 16 oz, Jar 5 lb, Bar 3 oz. *OTC.*
Use: Pharmaceutic aid; ointment base.
See: Eucerin (Duke).

Aquaphor Antibiotic. (Beiersdorf) Polymyxin B sulfate 10,000 units, bacitracin zinc 500 units/g in a cholesterolized ointment base. Oint. Tube 15 g. *OTC.*
Use: Anti-infective, topical.

Aquaphor Healing Ointment. (Beiersdorf) Petrolatum, mineral oil, lanolin, alcohol, panthenol, glycerin. Oint. Tubes. 10 g, 50 g. Jars. 99 g, 396 g. *OTC.*
Use: Emollient.

Aquapool Concentrate. (Parker) Color additive for hydrotherapy to control foaming. Bot. Pt, gal.

Aquasol A. (Hospira) Vitamin A palmitate 50,000 IU/mL. Chlorobutanol 0.5%, polysorbate 80, butylated hydroxyanisole, butylated hydroxytoluene. Inj. Vial 2 mL. *Rx.*
Use: Vitamin supplement.

Aquasol E. (Hospira) Vitamin E (as dl-alpha tocopheryl acetate) 15 units per 0.3 mL. Drops. 12 mL, 30 mL. *OTC.*
Use: Fat soluble vitamin.

Aquasonic 100. (Parker) Water-soluble, viscous, contact medium gel for ultrasonic transmission. Bot. 250 mL, 1 L, 5 L.
Use: Ultrasound aid.

Aquasonic 100 Sterile. (Parker) Water-soluble, sterile gel for ultrasonic transmission. Overwrapped Foil Pouches 15 g, 50 g.
Use: Ultrasound aid.

Aquasulf. (Armenpharm Ltd.) Triple sulfa tablet. *Rx.*
Use: Anti-infective.

Aquatab C. (Deston Therapeutics) Carbetapentane citrate 30 mg, guaifenesin 400 mg, phenylephrine hydrochloride 10 mg. Tab. 100s. *Rx.*
Use: Upper respiratory combination, antitussive and expectorant combination.

Aquatab D. (Adams) Guaifenesin 1200 mg, pseudoephedrine hydrochloride 75 mg. ER Tab. Bot. 100s. *Rx.*
Use: Upper respiratory combination, expectorant, decongestant.

Aquatab D Dose Pack. (Adams) Pseudoephedrine hydrochloride 60 mg, guaifenesin 600 mg. SR Tab. Bot. 56s. *Rx.*
Use: Upper respiratory combination, decongestant, expectorant.

Aquatab DM. (Adams) **Syrup:** Guaifenesin 200 mg, dextromethorphan HBr 10 mg per 5 mL. Acesulfame K, aspartame, menthol, methylparaben, phenylalanine. 473 mL. **Tab.:** Guaifenesin

1200 mg, dextromethorphan HBr 60 mg. Bot. 100s. *Rx.*
Use: Upper respiratory combination, expectorant, antitussive.

Aquavite. (Armenpharm Ltd.) Soluble multivitamin.
Use: Vitamin supplement.

Aquavit-E. (Cypress) Dl-alpha tocopheryl acetate 15 IU/0.3 mL. Drops. Bot. 30 mL. *OTC.*
Use: Vitamin supplement.

Aquazide. (Western Research) Trichlormethiazide 4 mg. Tab. Bot. 100s. *Rx.*
Use: Antihypertensive; diuretic.

Aquazide H. (Western Research) Hydrochlorothiazide 50 mg. Tab. Bot. 1000s. *Rx.*
Use: Diuretic.

Aquazol. (Armenpharm Ltd.) Sulfisoxazole.
Use: Anti-infective.

Aqueous Allergens. (Bayer Consumer Care)
Use: Antiallergic.

aquinone.
See: Menadione.

Aquol Bath Oil. (Lamond) Vegetable oil, olive oil. Bot. 4 oz, 6 oz, 16 oz, qt, gal. *OTC.*
Use: Antipruritic; emollient.

Aquoral. (Mission Pharmacal) Aspartame, oxidized glycerol triesters, phenylalanine, silicon dioxide. Spray, Soln. 40 mL spray pump (400 sprays per pump). *Rx.*
Use: Saliva substitute.

ARA-C.
See: Cytarabine.

Aralast NP. (Baxter Healthcare) Alpha-1 proteinase inhibitor (human) 500 mg, 1,000 mg. Preservative free. Inj., lyophilized Cake for Soln. Single-dose vial (diluent is sterile water for inj.) w/25 mL of diluent (500 mg) or 50 mL of diluent (1,000 mg) and needleless transfer device. *Rx.*
Use: Respiratory enzyme.

Aralen Phosphate. (Sanofi-Synthelabo) Chloroquine phosphate 500 mg (equiv. to 300 mg base). Film coated. Tab. 25s. *Rx.*
Use: Amebicide; antimalarial.

Aralis. (Sanofi-Synthelabo) Glycobiarsol, chloroquine phosphate. Tab. *Rx.*
Use: Amebicide.

Aranelle. (Barr) **Phase 1:** Norethindrone 0.5 mg, ethinyl estradiol 35 mcg. 7 tabs. **Phase 2:** Norethindrone 1 mg, ethinyl estradiol 35 mcg. 9 tabs. **Phase 3:** Norethindrone 0.5 mg, ethinyl estradiol 35 mcg. Lactose. 5 tabs. Tab. 28s with 7 inert tabs. *Rx.*
Use: Contraceptive hormone, sex hormone.

Aranesp. (Amgen) Darbepoetin alfa 25 mcg/0.42 mL, 25 mcg/mL, 40 mcg/0.4 mL, 40 mcg/mL, 60 mcg/0.3 mL, 60 mcg/mL, 100 mcg/0.5 mL, 100 mcg/mL, 150 mcg/0.3 mL, 150 mcg/0.75 mL, 200 mcg/0.4 mL, 200 mcg/mL, 300 mcg/0.6 mL, 300 mcg/mL, 500 mcg/mL. Preservative-free. In polysorbate or albumin solutions. The polysorbate solution contains polysorbate 80 0.05 mg, sodium phosphate monobasic monohydrate 2.12 mg, sodium phosphate dibasic anhydrous 0.66 mg, sodium chloride 8.18 mg, and water for injection. The albumin solution contains human albumin 2.5 mg, sodium phosphate monobasic monohydrate 2.23 mg, sodium phosphate dibasic anhydrous 0.53 mg, sodium chloride 8.18 mg, and water for injection. Soln. for Inj. Single-dose prefilled *SingleJect* syringe, single-dose prefilled *SureClick* autoinjectors (25 mcg/0.42 mL, 40 mcg/0.4 mL, 60 mcg/0.3 mL, 100 mcg/0.5 mL, 150 mcg/0.3 mL, 200 mcg/0.4 mL, 300 mcg/0.6 mL, 500 mcg/mL only). Single-dose vial 1 mL (25 mcg/mL, 40 mcg/mL, 60 mcg/mL, 100 mcg/mL, 150 mcg/0.75 mL, 200 mcg/mL, 300 mcg/mL, 500 mcg/mL only). *Rx.*
Use: Hematopoietic agent, recombinant human erythropoietin.

•**aranotin.** (AR-ah-NO-tin) USAN.
Use: Antiviral.

Arava. (Hoechst) Leflunomide 10 mg, 20 mg. Film coated. Lactose, PEG. Tab. 30s. *Rx.*
Use: Antirheumatic.

•**arbaclofen.** (ar-BAK-loe-fen) USAN.
Use: CNS agent.

•**arbaprostil.** (ahr-bah-PRAHST-ill) USAN.
Use: Antisecretory, gastric.

Arbinoxa. (Hawthorn Pharmaceuticals) Carbinoxamine maleate. **Tab.:** 4 mg. Lactose. 100s. **Soln.:** 4 mg per 5 mL. Glycerin, parabens, propylene glycol, sorbitol. Bubble gum flavor. 473 mL. *Rx.*
Use: Antihistamine, nonselective ethanolamine.

Arbolic. (Burgin-Arden) Methandriol dipropionate 50 mg/mL. Vial 10 mL. *Rx.*
Use: Anabolic steroid.

Arbutal. (Arcum) Butalbital 0.75 g, phenacetin 2 g, aspirin 3 g, caffeine g. Tab. Bot. 100s, 1000s. *Rx.*
Use: Analgesic; hypnotic; sedative.

•**arbutamine hydrochloride.** (ahr-BYOO-tah-meen) USAN.
Use: Cardiovascular agent.

ARC. (Xttrium Laboratories) Petrolatum 28.5%, zinc oxide 9.14%. Beeswax, lanolin, mineral oil, parabens. Oint. 113 g. *OTC.*
Use: Miscellaneous protectant.

Arcalyst. (Regeneron) Rilonacept 220 mg. Preservative free. PEG 3350, sucrose. Inj., Lyophilized, Pow. for Soln. Single-use vials. 20 mL. *Rx.*
Use: Immunomodulator, immunologic agents.

Arcapta Neohaler. (Novartis) Indacaterol 75 mcg (equiv. to indacaterol maleate 97 mcg). Lactose. Cap., Pow. for Inhal. UD 30s w/*Neohaler* inhaler. *Rx.*
Use: Bronchodilator, sympathomimetic.

Arcet. (Econo Med Pharmaceuticals) Butalbital 50 mg, acetaminophen 325 mg, caffeine 40 mg. Tab. Bot. 100s. *Rx.*
Use: Analgesic; hypnotic; sedative.

•**arcitumomab.** (ahr-sigh-TOO-moe-mab) USAN.
Use: Monoclonal antibody.
See: CEA-Scan.

•**arclofenin.** (AHR-kloe-FEN-in) USAN.
Use: Diagnostic aid for hepatic function determination.

Arcoban. (Arcum) Meprobamate 400 mg. Tab. Bot. 50s, 1000s. *Rx.*
Use: Anxiolytic.

Arcobee w/C. (NBTY) Vitamins B_1 15 mg, B_2 10.2 mg, B_3 50 mg, B_5 10 mg, B_6 5 mg, C 300 mg, tartrazine. Cap. Box 100s. *OTC.*
Use: Vitamin supplement.

Arco-Lase. (Arco) Trizyme 38 mg (amylase 30 mg, protease 6 mg, cellulase 2 mg), lipase 25 mg. Tab. Bot. 50s. *Rx.*
Use: Digestive aid.

Arcosterone. (Arcum) Methyltestosterone. **Oral:** 10 mg, 25 mg. Tab. Bot. 100s, 1000s. **Sublingual Tab.:** 10 mg. Bot. 100s, 1000s. *Rx.*
Use: Androgen.

Arco-Thyroid. (Arco) Thyroid 1.5 g. Tab. Bot. 1000s. *Rx.*
Use: Hormone, thyroid.

Arcotrate. (Arcum) Pentaerythritol tetranitrate 10 mg. Tab. **No. 2:** Pentaerythritol tetranitrate 20 mg. **No. 3:** Pentaerythritol tetranitrate 20 mg, phenobarbital ⅛ g. Bot. 100s, 1000s. *Rx.*
Use: Antianginal.

Arcoval Improved. (Arcum) Vitamin A palmitate 10,000 units, D 400 units, thiamine mononitrate 15 mg, B_2 10 mg, nicotinamide 150 mg, B_6 5 mg, calcium pantothenate 10 mg, B_{12} 5 mcg, C 150 mg, E 5 units. Cap. Bot. 100s, 1000s. *OTC.*
Use: Mineral, vitamin supplement.

Arcum V-M. (Arcum) Vitamin A palmitate 5000 units, D 400 units, B_1 2.5 mg, B_2 2.5 mg, B_6 0.5 mg, B_{12} 2 mcg, C 50 mg, niacinamide 20 mg, calcium pantothenate 5 mg, iron 18 mg. Cap. Bot. 100s, 1000s. *OTC.*
Use: Mineral, vitamin supplement.

A-R-D. (Birchwood) Anatomically shaped dressing. Dispenser 24s.
Use: Antipruritic; counterirritant, rectal.

Ardeben. (Burgin-Arden) Diphenhydramine hydrochloride 10 mg, chlorobutanol 0.5%. Inj. Vial 30 mL. *Rx.*
Use: Antihistamine.

Ardecaine 1%. (Burgin-Arden) Lidocaine hydrochloride 1%. Inj. Vial 30 mL. *Rx.*
Use: Anesthetic, local.

Ardecaine 1% w/Epinephrine. (Burgin-Arden) Lidocaine hydrochloride 1%, epinephrine. Inj. Vial 30 mL. *Rx.*
Use: Anesthetic, local.

Ardecaine 2%. (Burgin-Arden) Lidocaine hydrochloride 2%. Inj. Vial 30 mL. *Rx.*
Use: Anesthetic, local.

Ardecaine 2% w/Epinephrine. (Burgin-Arden) Lidocaine hydrochloride 2%, epinephrine. Inj. Vial 30 mL. *Rx.*
Use: Anesthetic, topical.

Ardefem 40. (Burgin-Arden) Estradiol valerate 40 mg/mL. Vial 10 mL. *Rx.*
Use: Estrogen.

Ardefem 10. (Burgin-Arden) Estradiol valerate 10 mg/mL. Vial 10 mL. *Rx.*
Use: Estrogen.

Ardefem 20. (Burgin-Arden) Estradiol valerate 20 mg/mL. Vial 10 mL. *Rx.*
Use: Estrogen.

•**ardenermin.** (ar-den-ER-min) USAN.
Use: Tumor necrosis factor.

•**ardeparin sodium.** (ahr-dee-PA-rin) USAN.
Use: Anticoagulant.

Ardepred Soluble. (Burgin-Arden) Prednisolone 20 mg, niacinamide 25 mg, disodium edetate 0.5 mg, sodium bisulfite 1 mg, phenol 5 mg/mL. Vial 10 mL. *Rx.*
Use: Corticosteroid combination.

Ardevila. (Sanofi-Synthelabo) Inositol hexanicotinate. Tab. *Rx.*
Use: Vasodilator.

Ardiol 90/4. (Burgin-Arden) Testosterone enanthate 90 mg, estradiol valerate 4 mg/mL. Vial 10 mL. *Rx.*
Use: Androgen, estrogen combination.

Arestin. (Cord Logistics) Minocycline hydrochloride (as base) 1 mg. ER Dental Pow. Microspheres. UD 12s. *Rx.*
Use: Anti-infective, tetracycline.

•**arformoterol tartrate.** (ar-for-MOE-ter-ole) USAN.
Use: Bronchodilator; sympathomimetic.
See: Brovana.

•**argatroban.** (ahr-GAT-troe-ban) USAN.
Use: Anticoagulant.

argatroban. (West-Ward) Argatroban 100 mg/mL. Dehydrated alcohol, propylene glycol. Inj., Soln., Conc. Single-use vials. 2.5 mL. *Rx.*
Use: Anticoagulant, direct thrombin inhibitor.

argatroban in sodium chloride. (Eagle Pharmaceuticals) Argatroban 1 mg/mL. Inj., Soln. Single-use vial. 50 mL. *Rx.*
Use: Anticoagulant, direct thrombin inhibitor.

Arginaid Extra. (Novartis Nutrition) Protein (whey protein isolate, L-arginine, L-cysteine) 25.3 g, carbohydrate (sugar, hydrolyzed corn starch) 219.4 g/L, vitamins A, B_1, B_2, B_3, B_5, B_6, B_{12}, C, D, E, K, biotin, folic acid, Cu, Fe, I, Mn, P, Zn, Na < 295 mg, K < 93 mg/L, 1.05 cal/mL, orange and wild berry flavors. Liq. *Tetra Brik Paks. OTC.*
Use: Enteral nutritional therapy.

•**arginine.** (AHR-jih-neen) *USP.*
Use: Ammonia detoxicant; diagnostic aid, pituitary function determination.

arginine butyrate. (AHR-jih-neen)
Use: Sickle cell disease; beta-thalassemia. [Orphan Drug]

•**arginine glutamate.** (AHR-jih-neen GLUE-tah-mate) USAN.
Use: Ammonia detoxicant.

•**arginine hydrochloride.** (AHR-jih-neen) *USP.*
Use: Ammonia detoxicant.

arginine hydrochloride. (AHR-jih-neen)
Use: Diagnostic aid.
See: R-Gene 10.

8-arginine-vasopressin.
See: Vasopressin.

•**argipressin tannate.** (AHR-JIH-press-in TAN-ate) USAN.
Use: Antidiuretic.

argyn.
See: Mild Silver Protein.

•**arhalofenate.** (AR-hal-oh-FEN-ate) USAN.
Use: Agent for gout.

Aricept. (Eisai/Pfizer) Donepezil hydrochloride 5 mg, 10 mg, 23 mg. Film coated. Lactose. Tab. 30s, 90s, UD blister pack 100s (except 23 mg). *Rx.*
Use: Treatment of mild to moderate dementia associated with Alzheimer disease.

Aricept ODT. (Eisai/Pfizer) Donepezil hydrochloride 5 mg, 10 mg. Mannitol. Orally Disintegrating Tab. UD blister pack 30s. *Rx.*
Use: Treatment of mild to moderate dementia associated with Alzheimer disease.

Aridex-D Pediatric. (Gentex) Phenylephrine hydrochloride 2 mg, carbinoxamine maleate 1 mg per 1 mL. Sugar and alcohol free. Sorbitol, sucralose. Bubble gum flavor. Drops. 30 mL. *Rx.*
Use: Pediatric decongestant and antihistamine.

Aridex Pediatric. (Gentex) Phenylephrine hydrochloride 2 mg, carbinoxamine maleate 1 mg, carbetapentane citrate 4 mg per mL. Sorbitol. Sugar free. Bubble gum flavor. Drops. Bot. 30 mL. *Rx.*
Use: Pediatric antitussive combination.

•**arildone.** (AR-ill-dohn) USAN.
Use: Antiviral.

Arimidex. (AstraZeneca) Anastrozole 1 mg, lactose. Tab. Bot. 30s. *Rx.*
Use: Hormone; aromatase inhibitor.

•**aripiprazole.** (AR-i-PIP-ra-zole) USAN.
Tall Man: ARIPiprazole
Use: Antipsychotic; antischizophrenic.
See: Abilify.
Abilify Maintena.

•**aripiprazole cavoxil.** (AR-i-PIP-ra-zole ka-VOX-il) USAN.
Use: CNS agent.

•**aripiprazole lauroxil.** (AR-i-PIP-ra-zole lawr-OX-il) USAN.
Use: CNS agent.

Aris Phenobarbital Reagent Strips. (Bayer Consumer Care) Box 25s.
Use: Diagnostic aid.

Aris Phenytoin Reagent Strips. (Bayer Consumer Care) Box 25s.
Use: Diagnostic aid.

Aristocort Acetonide, Sodium Phosphate Salt. (Fujisawa Healthcare)
Use: Corticosteroid, topical.

Aristo-Pak. (Wyeth) Triamcinolone 4 mg. Tab. 16s. *Rx.*
Use: Corticosteroid.

Aristospan Intra-articular. (Sandoz) Triamcinolone hexacetonide 20 mg/mL suspension. Polysorbate 80, sorbitol, benzyl alcohol. Inj. Vials. 1 mL, 5 mL. *Rx.*
Use: Adrenocortical steroid, glucocorticoid.

Aristospan Intralesional. (Sandoz) Triamcinolone hexacetonide 5 mg/mL suspension. Polysorbate 80, sorbitol, benzyl alcohol. Inj. Vials. 5 mL. *Rx.*
Use: Adrenocortical steroid, glucocorticoid.

Arixtra. (GlaxoSmithKline) Fondaparinux sodium 2.5 mg per 0.5 mL, 5 mg per 0.4 mL, 7.5 mg per 0.6 mL, 10 mg per 0.8 mL. Preservative free. Inj. Single-dose prefilled syringes with 27-gauge needle. 10s. *Rx.*
Use: Anticoagulant, selective factor Xa inhibitor.

Arlacel C. (AstraZeneca) Sorbitan sesquioleate. Mixture of oleate esters of sorbitol and its anhydrides.
Use: Surface active agent.

Arlacel 83. (AstraZeneca) Sorbitan sesquioleate.
Use: Surface active agent.

Arlacel 165. (AstraZeneca) Glyceryl monostearate, PEG-100 stearate nonionic self-emulsifying.
Use: Surface active agent.

Arlamol E. (AstraZeneca) Polyoxypropylene (15), stearyl ether, BHT 0.1%.
Use: Emollient.

Arlatone 507. (AstraZeneca) Padimate O. *OTC.*
Use: Sunscreen.

Arm-a-Med Metaproterenol Sulfate. (Centeon) Metaproterenol sulfate 0.4%, 0.6%, sodium chloride, EDTA. Soln. for nebulization. Vial UD 2.5 mL for use with IPPB device. *Rx.*
Use: Bronchodilator.

Arm-a-Vial. (Centeon) Sterile water, sodium chloride 0.45%, 0.9%. Box 100s. Plastic vial 3 mL, 5 mL.
Use: Electrolyte supplement.

•**armodafinil.** (ar-moe-DAF-in-il) USAN.
Use: Analeptic.
See: Nuvigil.

Armour Thyroid. (Forest) Thyroid desiccated 15 mg (1/4 gr), 30 mg (1/2 gr), 60 mg (1 gr), 90 mg (1 1/2 gr), 120 mg (2 gr), 180 mg (3 gr), 240 mg (4 gr), 300 mg (5 gr), dextrose. Tab. Bot. 100s, 1000s (except 15 mg, 90 mg, 240 mg, 300 mg), 5000s (30 mg, 60 mg only), 50,000s (60 mg, 120 mg only), UD 100s (30 mg, 60 mg, 120 mg only). *Rx.*
Use: Thyroid hormone.

Arnica Tincture. (Eli Lilly) Arnica 20% in alcohol 66%. Bot. 120 mL, 480 mL. *OTC.*
Use: Analgesic, topical.

•**arofylline.** (ah-ROE-fih-lin) USAN.
Use: Bronchodilator; asthma prophylactic.

Aromasin. (Pharmacia) Exemestane 25 mg, mannitol, methylparaben, polyvinyl alcohol. Tab. Bot. 30s. *Rx.*
Use: Hormone, breast cancer.

aromatase inhibitors.
See: Anastrozole.
Arimidex.
Aromasin.
Exemestane.
Femara.
Letrozole.

Aromatic Ammonia Vaporole. (GlaxoSmithKline) Inhalant. Vial 5 min. Box 10s, 12s, 100s. *Rx.*
Use: Respiratory.

Aromatic Cascara Fluid Extract. (Various Mfr.) Cascara sagrada. 19% alcohol. Liq. 473 mL. *OTC.*
Use: Irritant or stimulant laxative.

•**aromatic elixir.** (AR-oh-MAT-ik ee-LIX-ir) *NF.*
Use: Pharmaceutic aid, vehicle, flavored, sweetened.

aromatic elixir. (Eli Lilly) Alcohol 22%. Bot. 16 fl. oz.
Use: Pharmaceutic aid, flavoring.

AR-121. (Argus) Phase I/II HIV. *Rx.*
Use: Antiviral.

•**arprinocid.** (ahr-PRIN-oh-sid) USAN.
Use: Coccidiostat.

Arranon. (GlaxoSmithKline) Nelarabine 250 mg (5 mg/mL). Sodium chloride 4.5 mg/mL. Inj. Vials. 50 mL. *Rx.*
Use: DNA demethylation agent; antineoplastic.

arseclor.
See: Dichlorophenarsine hydrochloride.

arsenic compounds.
Use: Rarely employed in modern medicine; there are no longer any official compounds.
See: Arsphenamine.
Carbarsone.
Dichlorophenarsine Hydrochloride.
Ferric Cacodylate.
Glycobiarsol.

•**arsenic trioxide.** (AR-se-nik) USAN.
Use: Antineoplastic.
See: Trisenox.

arsenobenzene.
See: Arsphenamine.

arsenphenolamine.
See: Arsphenamine.

Arsobal. Melarsoprol (Mel B).
Use: CDC anti-infective agent.

arsphenamine. Arsenobenzene, arsenobenzol, arsenophenolamine, Ehrlich 606, salvarsan.
Use: Formerly used as antisyphilitic.

arsthinol. Cyclic.
Use: Antiprotozoal.

Artarau. (Archer-Taylor) Rauwolfia serpentina 50 mg, 100 mg. Tab. Bot. 100s, 1000s. *Rx.*
Use: Antihypertensive.

Arta-Vi-C. (Archer-Taylor) Multivitamins with Vitamin C 100 mg. Tab. Bot. 100s.

OTC.
Use: Vitamin supplement.

Artazyme. (Archer-Taylor) Bot. 13 mL.
Use: Autolyzed proteolytic enzyme.

•**arteflene.** (AHR-teh-fleen) USAN.
Use: Antimalarial.

•**artegraft.** (AHR-teh-graft) USAN. Arterial graft composed of a section of bovine carotid artery that has been subjected to enzymatic digestion with ficin and tanned with dialdehyde starch.
Use: Prosthetic aid, arterial.

•**artemether.** (ar-TEM-ee-ther) USAN.
Use: Antimalarial.

artemether/lumefantrine.
See: Coartem.

arterenol.
See: Norepinephrine bitartrate.

•**artesunate.** (ar-TES-oo-nate) USAN.
Use: Investigational antimalarial agent.

Arthralgen. (Wyeth) Salicylamide 250 mg, acetaminophen 250 mg. Tab. Bot. 30s, 100s, 500s. *OTC.*
Use: Analgesic combination.

ArthriCare Daytime Formula. (Del) Menthol 1.25%, methyl nicotinate 0.25%, capsaicin 0.025%, with aloe vera gel, carbomer 940, DMDM hydantoin, glyceryl stearate SE, myristyl propionate, propylparaben, triethanolamine. Cream. Jar 90 g. *OTC.*
Use: Analgesic, topical.

Arthritic Pain. (Walgreen) Triethanolamine salicylate 10%. Lot. Bot. 6 oz. *OTC.*
Use: Analgesic, topical.

Arthritis Bayer Timed Release Aspirin. (Bayer Consumer Care) Aspirin 650 mg. TR Tab. Bot. 30s, 72s, 125s. *OTC.*
Use: Analgesic.

Arthritis Hot Creme. (Thompson Medical) Methyl salicylate 15%, menthol 10%, glyceryl stearate, carbomer 934, lanolin, PEG-100 stearate, propylene glycol, trolamine, parabens. Cream. Jar 90 g. *OTC.*
Use: Liniment.

Arthritis Pain Formula. (Whitehall-Robins) Aspirin 500 mg, aluminum hydroxide 27 mg, magnesium hydroxide 100 mg. Tab. Bot. 40s, 100s, 175s. *OTC.*
Use: Salicylate, buffered aspirin.

Arthritis Pain Formula, Aspirin Free. (Whitehall-Robins) Acetaminophen 500 mg. Tab. Bot. 30s, 75s. *OTC.*
Use: Analgesic.

Arthrotec. (Searle) Diclofenac sodium 50 mg/misoprostol 200 mcg, diclofenac sodium 75 mg/misoprostol 200 mcg. Lactose. Film coated. Tab. Bot. 60s, 90s (50 mg only), UD 100s. *Rx.*
Use: Analgesic.

Arthrotrin. (Whiteworth Towne) Enteric-coated aspirin 325 mg. Tab. Bot. 100s.
Use: Analgesic.

•**articaine.** (AR-ti-kane) USAN.
Use: Anesthetic, injectable local amide.

Articulose L.A. (Seatrace) Triamcinolone diacetate 40 mg/mL. Vial 5 mL. *Rx.*
Use: Corticosteroid.

artificial tanning agent.
See: Sudden Tan.

artificial tear insert.
See: Lacrisert.

artificial tears. (Rugby) White petrolatum, anhydrous liquid lanolin, mineral oil. Ophth. Oint. Tube 3.5 g. *OTC.*
Use: Lubricant, ophthalmic.

artificial tears. (Various Mfr.) Benzalkonium chloride 0.01%. May also contain EDTA, NaCl, polyvinyl alcohol, hydroxypropyl methylcellulose Soln. Bot. 15 mL, 30 mL. *OTC.*
Use: Lubricant, ophthalmic.

artificial tear solutions.
Use: Lubricant, ophthalmic.
See: Advanced Eye Relief.
Advanced Eye Relief Preservative Free.
Artificial Tears.
Artificial Tears Plus.
Blink Tears.
Blink Tears Preservative Free.
Celluvisc.
Comfort Tears.
Moisture Eyes Preservative Free.
Murine Tears for Dry Eyes.
Natural Balance Tears.
Optive.
OptiZen.
Puralube Tears.
Refresh Optive Advanced.
Refresh Plus.
Soothe Hydration.
Soothe Preservative Free.
Systane.
Systane Balance.
Systane Ultra.
Tears Naturale Forte.
TheraTears.
Visine for Contacts.
Visine Pure Tears.
Visine Tears.
Visine Tears Preservative Free.

Artificial Tears Plus. (Various Mfr.) Polyvinyl alcohol 1.4%, povidone 0.6%, chlorobutanol 0.5%, NaCl. Soln. Bot. 15 mL. *OTC.*
Use: Lubricant, ophthalmic.

•**artilide fumarate.** (AHR-tih-lide) USAN.
Use: Cardiovascular agent.

Artiss. (Baxter) Fibrin sealant (human). **Pow. for Soln. Top.:** Total protein 96 to 125 mg/mL, fibrinogen 67 to 106 mg/mL, fibrinolysis inhibitor (synthetic) 2,250 to 3,750 kallikrein-inhibiting units/mL, thrombin (human) 2.5 to 6.5 units/mL, calcium chloride 36 to 44 mcmol/mL (when reconstituted). Single-use vials with or without *Duploject* system. 2 mL, 4 mL, 10 mL. *Artiss Kit* contains the following substances in 4 separate vials: sealer protein concentrate (human), fibrinolysis inhibitor solution (synthetic), thrombin (human), and calcium chloride solution. **Soln. Top.:** Total protein 96 to 125 mg/mL, fibrinogen 67 to 106 mg/mL, thrombin (human) 2.5 to 6.5 units/mL. Single-use prefillled (frozen) syringe with *Duo Set.* 2 mL, 4 mL, 10 mL. *Rx.*
Use: Fibrin agent.

Artra Beauty Bar. (Schering-Plough) Triclocarban 1% in soap base. Cake 3.6 oz. *OTC.*
Use: Dermatologic; cleanser.

Artra Skin Tone Cream. (Schering-Plough) Hydroquinone 2%. Oint. Tube 1 oz (normal only), 2 oz, 4 oz.
Use: Dermatologic.

arylalkylamines.
Use: Nasal decongestant.
See: Adrenalin Chloride.
Afrin Children's.
AH-Chew D.
Cenafed.
Decofed.
Dimetapp Decongestant Pediatric.
Dimetapp, Maximum Strength, Non-Drowsy.
Dimetapp, Maximum Strength 12-Hour, Non-Drowsy.
Drixoral 12 Hour Non-Drowsy Formula.
Efidac 24.
Ephedrine Sulfate.
Epinephrine Hydrochloride.
4-Way Fast Acting.
Genaphed.
Kid Kare.
Little Colds for Infants and Children.
Little Noses Gentle Formula, Infants & Children.
Medi-First Sinus Decongestant.
Nasal Decongestant, Children's Non-Drowsy.
Nasal Decongestant Oral.
Neo-Synephrine 4-Hour Extra Strength.
Neo-Synephrine 4-Hour Mild Formula.
Neo-Synephrine 4-Hour Regular Strength.
PediaCare Decongestant, Infants'.
Phenylephrine Hydrochloride.
Pretz-D.
Pseudoephedrine Hydrochloride.
Pseudoephedrine Sulfate.
Rhinall.
Silfedrine, Children's.
Simply Stuffy.
Sinustop.
Sudafed, Children's Non-Drowsy.
Sudafed Non-Drowsy, Maximum Strength.
Sudafed Non-Drowsy 12 Hour Long-Acting.
Sudafed Non-Drowsy 24 Hour Long-Acting.
Triaminic Allergy Congestion.
Vicks Sinex.

Arzol Silver Nitrate Applicators. (Arzol) Silver nitrate 75% and potassium nitrate 25%. Applicator. 100s. *Rx.*
Use: Topical anti-infective.

•**arzoxifene hydrochloride.** (ar-ZOX-i-feen) USAN.
Use: Uterine fibroids; endometriosis; dysfunctional uterine bleeding; breast cancer.

5-ASA. Mesalamine.
See: Asacol.
Rowasa.

ASA. (Wampole) Anti-skin antibodies test by IFA. Test 48s.
Use: Diagnostic aid.

A.S.A. (Eli Lilly) Aspirin. Acetylsalicylic acid. **Enseal:** 5 g, 10 g. Bot. 100s, 1000s. **Supp.:** 5 g, 10 g. Pkg. 6s, 144s. *OTC.*
Use: Analgesic.

Asacol HD. (Warner Chilcott) Mesalamine 800 mg. Lactose, PEG. Tab., delayed release. 180s. *Rx.*
Use: Gastrointestinal agent.

asafetida, emulsion of. Milk of Asafetida.

Asaped. (Sanofi-Synthelabo) Acetylsalicylic acid. Tab. *OTC.*
Use: Analgesic.

Asawin. (Sanofi-Synthelabo) Acetylsalicylic acid. Tab. *OTC.*
Use: Analgesic.

A.S.B. (Femco) Calcium carbonate, magnesium carbonate, bismuth subcarbonate, sodium bicarbonate, kaolin. Pow. Can 3 oz. Tab. Bot. 50s. *OTC.*
Use: Antacid.

Asclera. (Merz Aesthetics) Polidocanol 0.5%, 1%. Ethanol 5%. Preservative free. Inj., Soln. Single-use ampule. 2 mL. *Rx.*
Use: Sclerosing agent.

Asclerol. (Spanner) Liver injection crude (2 mcg/mL) 50%, Vitamins B_1 20 mg, B_2 3 mg, B_6 1 mg, B_{12} 30 mcg, niacinamide 100 mg, panthenol 2.8 mg, choline chloride 20 mg, inositol 10 mg/mL. Multiple dose vial 10 mL. *Rx.*
Use: Vitamin supplement.

ASC Lotionized. (Geritrex) Triclosan 0.3%. Aloe vera gel, sweet almond oil, parabens, tartrazine. Liq. 8 oz. *OTC.*
Use: Topical anti-infective.

Ascocid. (Key) Vitamin C (as calcium ascorbate). **Gran.:** 4,000 mg per tsp. 8 oz. **Pow.:** 5,000 mg per tsp. 227 g. *OTC.*
Use: Water-soluble vitamin.

Ascomp with Codeine. (Breckenridge) Codeine phosphate 30 mg, aspirin 325 mg, caffeine 40 mg, butalbital 50 mg. Cap. Bot. 100s, 500s. *c-III.*
Use: Narcotic analgesic combination.

ascorbate sodium. Antiscorbutic vitamin.

•**ascorbic acid.** (AS-kore-bik AS-id) *USP.*
Use: Water-soluble vitamin, antiscorbutic; acidifier, urinary.
See: Ascocid.
Ascorbineed.
Ascor L 500.
Cenolate.
C-500.
C-Gel.
Complex C.
C-250.
Dull-C.
Hall's Defense.
Neo-Vadrin.
N'Ice.
Pure C 500.
Sunkist Vitamin C.
Vita-C.

ascorbic acid. (Freeda) Ascorbic acid 1000 mg. TR Tab. 100s, 250s, 500s. *OTC.*
Use: Water-soluble vitamin.

ascorbic acid. (Humco) Ascorbic acid 60 mg/¼ tsp. Pow. 454 g. *OTC.*
Use: Water-soluble vitamin.

ascorbic acid. (Various Mfr.) Ascorbic acid. **Tab.:** 250 mg, 500 mg, 1,000 mg, 1,500 mg. 100s, 250s (500 mg, 1,000 mg only), 1,000s (500 mg only), UD 100s (250 mg, 500 mg only). **Chew. Tab.:** 500 mg. 100s. **TR Tab.:** 500 mg. 100s, 250s, 500s. **Inj.:** 500 mg/mL. Vials. 50 mL. **Liq.:** 500 mg/5 mL. 120 mL, 480 mL. *OTC.*
Use: Water-soluble vitamin.

ascorbic acid and sodium ascorbate.
Use: Water-soluble vitamin.
See: Chewable Vitamin C.
Chew C.
Fruit C 500.
Fruit C 100.
Fruit C 200.
Sunkist Vitamin C.
Vicks Vitamin C.

ascorbic acid injection.
Use: Vitamin supplement.

ascorbic acid salts.
See: Calcium Ascorbate.
Sodium Ascorbate.

Ascorbineed. (Hanlon) Vitamin C 500 mg. T-Cap. Bot. 100s. *OTC.*
Use: Vitamin supplement.

Ascorbin/11. (Taylor Pharmaceuticals) Lemon bioflavonoids 110 mg, Vitamin C 1 g, rosehips powder 50 mg, rutin 25 mg. SR Tab. Bot. 100s. *OTC.*
Use: Vitamin supplement.

Ascorbocin. (Paddock) Vitamin C 500 mg, niacin 500 mg, B_1 50 mg, B_6 50 mg, d-α-tocopheryl, polyethylene glycol 1000 succinate 50 units, lactose/ 3 g. Pow. Bot. lb. *OTC.*
Use: Vitamin supplement.

•**ascorbyl palmitate.** (ah-SCORE-bill PAL-mih-tate) *NF.*
Use: Preservative; pharmaceutic aid, antioxidant.

Ascor L 500. (McGuff) Ascorbic acid 500 mg/mL. EDTA 0.025%, preservative free. Inj. 50 mL. *Rx.*
Use: Water-soluble vitamin.

Ascorvite S.R. (Eon Labs) Vitamin C 500 mg. SR Cap. *OTC.*
Use: Vitamin supplement.

Ascriptin. (Novartis) Aspirin 325 mg, magnesium hydroxide 50 mg, aluminum hydroxide 50 mg. Tab. Bot. 50s, 100s, 225s, 500s. *OTC.*
Use: Analgesic; antacid.

Ascriptin Maximum Strength. (Novartis) Aspirin 500 mg, calcium carbonate 237 mg, magnesium hydroxide 33 mg, aluminum hydroxide 33 mg. Tab. 85s. *OTC.*
Use: Salicylate, buffered aspirin.

asenapine. (a-SEN-a-peen)
Use: Antipsychotic agent.
See: Saphris.

•**asenapine maleate.** (a-SEN-a-peen) USAN.
Use: Serotonin antagonist.

aseptichrome.
See: Merbromin.

•**asfotase alfa.** (AS-oh-FOS-tase) USAN.
Use: Treatment of hypophosphatasia.

Aslum. (Drug Products) Carbolic acid 1%, aluminum acetate, ichthammol, zinc oxide, aromatic oils in a petrolatum-stearin base. Tube. Jar.
Use: Astringent.

Asma. (Wampole) Anti-smooth muscle antibody test by IFA. Test 48.
Use: Diagnostic aid.

AsmalPred Plus. (Tiber Labs) Prednisolone 15 mg per 5 mL (equiv. to prednisolone sodium phosphate 20.2 mg). Alcohol 1.8%, glycerin, sodium benzoate, sorbitol, sucrose. Grape flavor. Soln. 237 mL. *Rx.*
Use: Adrenocortical steroid, glucocorticoid.

Asmanex Twisthaler. (Schering) Mometasone furoate 110 mcg (delivers mometasone fuorate 100 mcg)/actuation, 220 mcg (delivers mometasone furoate 200 mcg)/actuation. Lactose. Pow. for Inh. Inhalation device. 7 units (110 mcg only), 14 units (220 mcg only), 30 units, 60 units (220 mcg only), 120 units (220 mcg only). *Rx.*
Use: Corticosteroid, respiratory inhalant.

Asma-Tuss. (Halsey Drug) Phenobarbital 4 mg, theophylline 15 mg, ephedrine sulfate 12 mg, guaifenesin 50 mg/5 mL. Bot. 4 oz. *Rx.*
Use: Bronchodilator.

Asolectin. (Associated Concentrates) Chemical lecithin 25%, chemical cephalin 22%, inositol phosphatides 16%, soybean oil 2.5%, other miscellaneous sterols and lipids 34.5%. *OTC.*
Use: Diet supplement.

•**asoprisnil.** (as-oh-PRIS-nil) USAN.
Use: Endometriosis.

•**asparaginase.** (as-PAR-uh-jin-aze) USAN.
Use: Antineoplastic.
See: Erwinaze.

•**asparaginase** ***Erwinia chrysanthemi.*** (as-PAR-uh-jin-aze) USAN.
Use: Antineoplastic.

•**aspartame.** (as-PAR-tame) *NF.*
Use: Sweetener.

•**aspartic acid.** (as-PAR-tik) *USP.* Aspartic acid; aminosuccinic acid.
Use: Management of fatigue; amino acid.

•**aspartocin.** (AS-par-TOE-sin) USAN.
Use: Anti-infective.

Aspercreme. (Chattem) Triethanolamine salicylate 10% in cream base. *OTC.*
Use: Analgesic, topical.

Aspercreme Max Roll-On. (Chattem) Menthol 16%, capsaicin, glycerin, propylene glycol, SD alcohol, triethanolamine. Liq. 73 mL. *OTC.*
Use: Rub and liniment.

Aspercreme with Aloe. (Chattem) Trolamine salicylate 10%. Aloe vera, cetyl alcohol, glycerin, mineral oil, parabens. Cream. 85 g. *OTC.*
Use: Rub and liniment.

aspergillus niger enzyme. Alpha-galactosidase. *OTC.*
See: Beano.

aspergillus oryzae enzyme. Diastase.

asperkinase. Proteolytic enzyme mixture derived from aspergillus oryzae.

•**asperlin.** (AS-per-lin) USAN.
Use: Anti-infective; antineoplastic.

Aspermin. (Buffington) Aspirin 325 mg. Sugar, caffeine, lactose, and salt free. Tab. *Dispens-A-Kit* 500s. *OTC.*
Use: Analgesic.

Aspermin Extra. (Buffington) Aspirin 500 mg. Sugar, caffeine, lactose, and salt free. Tab. *Dispens-A-Kit* 500s. *OTC.*
Use: Analgesic.

•**aspirin.** (AS-pihr-in) *USP.*
Use: Analgesic; antipyretic; antirheumatic. Prophylactic to reduce risk of death or non-fatal MI in patients with a previous infarction or unstable angina pectoris.
See: A.S.A.
Aspirin Low Dose.
Aspir Low.
Bayer Buffered Aspirin.
Bayer Children's Chewable Aspirin.
Bayer, 8-Hour Timed-Release.
Bayer Extra Strength Advanced Aspirin.
Bayer Extra Strength Back & Body Pain.
Bayer Low Adult Strength.
Bayer Women's Aspirin Plus Calcium.
Easprin.
Ecotrin Low Strength.
Ecotrin Regular Strength.
Genprin.
Genuine Bayer Aspirin.
Halfprin 81.
Heartline.
Maximum Bayer Aspirin.
Miniprin Low Dose.
Norwich Extra Strength.
Norwich Regular Strength.
St. Joseph Adult Chewable Aspirin.
St. Joseph Aspirin for Adults.
ZORprin.

W/Acetaminophen, Aluminum Hydroxide, Caffeine, Magnesium Hydroxide.
See: Vanquish.

W/Acetaminophen, Caffeine.
See: Anacin Advanced Headache.
Bayer Migraine.
Excedrin Extra Strength.
Excedrin Migraine.
Goody's Cool Orange.
Goody's Extra Strength.
Goody's Extra Strength Fast Pain Relief.

Goody's Migraine Relief.
W/Acetaminophen, Caffeine, Phenyltoloxamine Citrate, Salicylamide.
See: Levacet.
W/Acetaminophen, Caffeine, Salicylamide.
See: Medi-First Extra Strength Pain Relief.
Saleto.
W/Aluminum Hydroxide, Magnesium Hydroxide.
See: Ascriptin.
W/Caffeine.
See: Alka-Seltzer Wake-Up Call.
Anacin.
Anacin Maximum Strength.
Bayer Quick Release Crystals.
BC Fast Pain Relief.
BC Fast Pain Relief Arthritis.
P-A-C Analgesic.
Painaid ESF Extra-Strength Formula.
W/Caffeine, Orphenadrine Citrate.
See: Orphenadrine Compound.
Orphenadrine Compound-DS.
W/Caffeine, Salicylamide.
See: BC Powder Arthritis Strength.
Painaid.
Stanback Headache Powders.
W/Chlorpheniramine Maleate, Dextromethorphan Hydrobromide, Phenylephrine Bitartrate.
See: Alka-Seltzer Plus Cold & Cough.
W/Chlorpheniramine Maleate, Phenylephrine Bitartrate.
See: Alka-Seltzer Plus Cold.
Alka-Seltzer Plus Sparkling Cold Formula.
W/Citric Acid, Sodium Bicarbonate.
See: Alka-Seltzer Lemon Lime.
Alka-Seltzer Original.
W/Dextromethorphan Hydrobromide, Doxylamine Succinate, Phenylephrine Bitartrate.
See: Alka-Seltzer Plus Day & Night Cold.
Alks-Seltzer Plus Night Cold.
W/Dextromethorphan Hydrobromide, Phenylephrine Bitartrate.
See: Alka-Seltzer Plus Day & Night Cold.
W/Diphenhydramine Citrate.
See: Alka-Seltzer PM.
W/Magnesium Salicylate, Phenyltoloxamine.
See: Mobigesic.

aspirin, alumina, and magnesia.
Use: Analgesic; antacid.

aspirin, alumina, and magnesium oxide.
Use: Analgesic; antacid.

aspirin and barbiturate combinations.
Use: Analgesic; sedative; hypnotic.
See: BAC.
Butalbital.
Fiorinal.

aspirin and codeine phosphate. (Vintage Pharmaceuticals) Codeine phosphate 15 mg/aspirin 325 mg. Tab. 100s, 500s, 1,000s. *c-III.*
Use: Analgesic, narcotic.

aspirin and dipyridamole.
Use: Antiplatelet.
See: Aggrenox.

aspirin and narcotic combinations.
See: Alor 5/500.
Ascomp with Codeine.
Butalbital, Aspirin, and Caffeine.
Butalbital Compound.

aspirin and oxycodone. (Various Mfr.) Oxycodone hydrochloride 4.5 mg, oxycodone terephthalate 0.38 mg, aspirin 325 mg. Tab. Bot. 100s, 500s, 1000s, UD 25s. *c-II.*
Use: Analgesic combination, narcotic.

aspirin, buffered.
Use: Salicylate.
See: Arthritis Pain Formula.
Ascriptin Maximum Strength.
Bufferin.
Bufferin Extra Strength.
Extra Strength Bayer Plus.
W/Acetaminophen.
See: Excedrin Back & Body Extra Strength.

Aspirin-Free Bayer Select Allergy Sinus. (Bayer Consumer Care) Pseudoephedrine hydrochloride 30 mg, chlorpheniramine maleate 2 mg, acetaminophen 500 mg. Cap. Pkg. 16s. *OTC.*
Use: Analgesic; antihistamine; decongestant.

Aspirin-Free Bayer Select Headache. (Bayer Consumer Care) Acetaminophen 500 mg, caffeine 65 mg. Cap. Bot. 50s. *OTC.*
Use: Analgesic combination.

Aspirin-Free Bayer Select Head & Chest Cold. (Bayer Consumer Care) Pseudoephedrine hydrochloride 30 mg, dextromethorphan HBr 10 mg, guaifenesin 100 mg, acetaminophen 325 mg. Capl. Bot. 16s. *OTC.*
Use: Analgesic; decongestant; expectorant.

Aspirin Free Excedrin. (Bristol-Myers Squibb) Acetaminophen 500 mg, caffeine 65 mg. Tab., Capl. Bot. 20s, 40s, 80s. *OTC.*
Use: Analgesic combination.

Aspirin Low Dose. (Time-Cap Labs) Aspirin 81 mg. Orange flavor. Chew. Tab. 36s. *OTC.*
Use: Salicylate.

Aspirin Plus. (Walgreen) Aspirin 400 mg,

caffeine 32 mg. Tab. Bot. 100s. *OTC.*
Use: Analgesic combination.

aspirin salts.
See: Calcium Acetylsalicylate.

Aspirin Uniserts. (Upsher-Smith) Aspirin 125 mg, 300 mg, 650 mg. Supp. Ctn. 12s, 50s. *OTC.*
Use: Analgesic.

aspirin w/codeine no. 4. (Various Mfr.) Codeine phosphate 60 mg, aspirin 325 mg Tab. Bot. 100s, 500s, 1000s. *c-III.*
Use: Analgesic combination, narcotic.

aspirin w/codeine no. 3. (Various Mfr.) Codeine phosphate 30 mg, aspirin 325 mg. Tab. Bot. 100s, 1000s. *c-III.*
Use: Analgesic combination, narcotic.

Aspir Low. (Major) Aspirin 81 mg. Enteric coated. PEG, polydextrose. Tab. 1,000s. *OTC.*
Use: CNS agent, salicylate.

Aspirtab. (Dover Pharmaceuticals) Aspirin 325 mg. Sugar, lactose, and salt free. Tab. UD Box 500s. *OTC.*
Use: Analgesic.

Aspirtab Max. (Dover Pharmaceuticals) Aspirin 500 mg. Sugar, lactose, and salt free. Tab. UD Box 500s. *OTC.*
Use: Analgesic.

Astagraf XL. (Astellas) Tacrolimus 0.5 mg, 1 mg, 5 mg. Lactose. ER Cap. 30s. *Rx.*
Use: Immunosuppressive.

Astaril. (Sanofi-Synthelabo) Theophylline anhydrous, ephedrine sulphate. Tab. *Rx.*
Use: Bronchodilator.

Astelin. (Medpointe) Azelastine 137 mcg/spray. Benzalkonium chloride, EDTA. Nasal Spray. Bot. 17 mg (100 metered sprays) per bottle. 2s. *Rx.*
Use: Antihistamine, peripherally selective phthalazinone.

•**astemizole.** (a-STEM-i-zole) *USP.*
Use: Antihistamine; antiallergic.

Astepro. (MEDA Pharmaceuticals) Azelastine 0.15% (205.5 mcg/spray). Equiv. to azelastine base 187.6 mcg. Benzalkonium chloride, edetate disodium. 30 mL (200 metered sprays), 17 mL (106 metered sprays). *Rx.*
Use: Respiratory inhalant, intranasal antihistamine.

asterol.
Use: Antifungal.

Asthmalixir. (Reese) Theophylline 45 mg, ephedrine sulfate 36 mg, guaifenesin 150 mg, phenobarbital 12 mg/15 mL, alcohol 19%. Bot. *Rx.*
Use: Bronchodilator; expectorant; hypnotic; sedative.

Asthmanefrin. (Nephron Pharmaceuticals) Epinephrine 1% (equiv. to racepinephrine hydrochloride 2.25%). Edetate disodium. Preservative free. Soln. Inhal. Single-use vial. 0.5 mL. *OTC.*
Use: Vasopressor used in shock.

Asthmanefrin Refill. (Nephron Pharmaceuticals) Racepinephrine 2.25%. Edetate disodium. Soln., Inhal. Single-use vial. 30s. *OTC.*
Use: Vasopressor used in shock.

Asthmanefrin Starter Kit. (Nephron Pharmaceuticals) Racepinephrine 2.25%. Edetate disodium. Soln., Inhal. 10 single-use vials w/*EZ Breathe Atomizer* inhalation device. *OTC.*
Use: Vasopressor used in shock.

•**astifilcon A.** (AS-ti-FIL-kon) USAN.
Use: Contact lens material, hydrophilic.

•**astodrimer.** (as-TOE-dri-mer) USAN.
Use: Anti-infective.

•**astodrimer sodium.** (as-TOE-dri-mer) USAN.
Use: Anti-infective.

Astramorph PF. (APP Pharmaceutical) Morphine sulfate 0.5 mg/mL, 1 mg/mL. Inj. Amp. 2 mL, 10 mL. Single-use vial 10 mL. *c-II.*
Use: Analgesic, narcotic agonist.

astringents.
See: Aluminum Acetate.

AstrinGyn. (Cooper Surgical) Ferric subsulfate 259 mg/g. Benzalkonium chloride, povidone, glycerin. Soln., Top. Single-use bottle. 8 g. *Rx.*
Use: Topical hemostatic.

Astroglide. (Biofilm) Purified water, glycerin, propylene glycol, parabens. Vaginal gel. Bot 66.5 mL. Travel pks. 5 mL. *OTC.*
Use: Lubricant.

•**astromicin sulfate.** (AS-troe-MYE-sin) USAN.
Use: Anti-infective.

Astro-Vites. (Faraday) Vitamins A 3500 units, D 400 units, C 60 mg, B_1 0.8 mg, B_2 1.3 mg, niacinamide 14 mg, B_6 1 mg, B_{12} 2.5 mcg, folic acid 0.05 mg, pantothenic acid 5 mg, iron 12 mg. Tab. Bot. 100s, 250s. *OTC.*
Use: Mineral, vitamin supplement.

AST/SGOT Reagent Strips. (Bayer Consumer Care) Seralyzer reagent strip. A quantitative strip test for aspartate transaminase/serum glutamic oxaloacetic transaminase in serum or plasma. Bot. Strip 25s.
Use: Diagnostic aid.

•**astuprotimut-R.** (AS-tu-PROE-ti-mut) USAN.
Use: Immunologic.

•**asunaprevir.** (A-soo-NA-pre-vir) USAN.
Use: Treatment of hepatitis C.

Asupirin. (Suppositoria Laboratories, Inc.) Aspirin 60 mg, 120 mg, 200 mg, 300 mg, 600 mg, 1.2 g. Supp. Box 12s, 100s, 1000s. *OTC.*
Use: Analgesic.

Atabee TD. (Defco) Vitamins C 500 mg, B_1 15 mg, B_2 10 mg, B_6 2 mg, nicotinamide 50 mg, calcium pantothenate 10 mg. Cap. Bot. 30s, 1000s. *OTC.*
Use: Vitamin supplement.

Atabex EC Prenatal. (Advanced Medical Enterprises) Folic acid 0.8 mcg, Ca 100 mg, Fe 18 mg, vitamins D 400 units, B_6 10 mg, B_{12} 6 mcg, C 60 mg. Stevia leaf extract, sugar. Gluten free, preservative free. Chew. Tab. 30s. *Rx.*
Use: Prenatal vitamin with minerals.

Atacand. (AstraZeneca) Candesartan cilexetil 4 mg, 8 mg, 16 mg, 32 mg. Lactose. Tab. Bot. Unit-of-use 30s, 90s (16 mg, 32 mg only); UD 100s (only 16 mg, 32 mg). *Rx.*
Use: Antihypertensive.

Atacand HCT. (AstraZeneca) Candesartan cilexetil/hydrochlorothiazide 16 mg/12.5 mg, 32 mg/12.5 mg, 32 mg/25 mg. Lactose. Tab. UD 100s (16 mg/12.5 mg and 32 mg/12.5 mg only), unit-of-use 90s. *Rx.*
Use: Antihypertensive.

•**atagabalin.** (A-ta-GAB-a-lin) USAN.
Use: CNS agent.

•**ataluren.** (AT-a-LUR-en) USAN.
Use: Genetic mutation disorders.

•**atazanavir sulfate.** (AT-ah-zah-NAH-veer) USAN.
Use: Antiretroviral, protease inhibitor.
See: Reyataz.

Atelvia. (Warner Chilcott) Risedronate sodium 35 mg. Edetate disodium, polysorbate 80. Tab., delayed release. Dose pack 4s. *Rx.*
Use: Bisphosphonate.

•**atenolol.** (ah-TEN-oh-lahl) *USP.*
Use: Beta-adrenergic blocker.
See: Tenormin.
W/Chlorthalidone.
See: Tenoretic.

atenolol. (Various Mfr.) Atenolol. 25 mg, 50 mg, 100 mg. Tab. 30s, 60s, 90s, 100s, 500s (100 mg only), 1,000s. *Rx.*
Use: Antiadrenergic/sympatholytic; beta-adrenergic blocking agent.

atenolol/chlorthalidone. (Various Mfr.) Atenolol/chlorthalidone 50 mg/25 mg, 100 mg/25 mg. Tab. Bot. 50s, 100s, 250s, 500s, 1000s. *Rx.*
Use: Antihypertensive.

•**atevirdine mesylate.** (at-TEH-vihr-DEEN) USAN.
Use: Antiviral.

Atgam. (Pharmacia) Lymphocyte immune globulin, antithymocyte globulin horse gamma globulin 50 mg/mL. Glycine 0.3 M. Inj. Amps. 5 mL. *Rx.*
Use: Immunosuppressant.

Athlete's Foot. (Walgreen) Zinc undecylenate 20%, undecylenic acid 5%. Oint. Tube 1.5 oz. *OTC.*
Use: Antifungal, topical.

•**atilmotin.** (A-til-MOE-tin) USAN.
Use: Gastrointestinal agent.

•**atipamezole.** (AT-ih-pam-EH-zole) USAN.
Use: Antagonist, α_2-receptor.

•**atiprimod dihydrochloride.** (at-TIH-prih-mahd) USAN.
Use: Antiarthritic, immunomodulator, suppressor cell inducing agent; anti-inflammatory; antirheumatic, disease-modifying.

•**atiprimod dimaleate.** (at-TIH-prih-mahd) USAN.
Use: Antiarthritic; anti-inflammatory; immunomodulator; antirheumatic, disease-modifying.

•**atiprosin maleate.** (ah-TIH-pro-SIN) USAN.
Use: Antihypertensive.

Ativan. (West-Ward) Lorazepam. **Tab.:** 0.5 mg, 1 mg, 2 mg. Lactose. 100s, 1,000s (1 mg only). **Inj.:** 2 mg/mL, 4 mg/mL. Inj. Single and 10 mL multidose vials (PEG 400, propylene glycol, benzyl alcohol 2%), boxes of 10 *Tubex. c-iv.*
Use: Anxiolytic.

•**atlafilcon A.** (at-LAH-FILL-kahn A) USAN.
Use: Contact lens material, hydrophilic.

ATnativ. (Bayer) Antithrombin III (human), lyophilized powder/500 units. Inj. Bot. 50 mL w/10 L sterile water. *Rx.*
Use: Thromboembolic. [Orphan Drug]

•**atolide.** (ATE-oh-lide) USAN. Under study.
Use: Anticonvulsant.

•**atomoxetine hydrochloride.** (AT-oh-mox-ah-teen) USAN.
Use: Psychotherapeutic agent.
See: Strattera.

atomoxetine hydrochloride. (Actavis Elizabeth) Atomoxetine 10 mg, 18 mg, 25 mg, 40 mg, 60 mg, 80 mg, 100 mg. Cap. 30s, 90s, 500s (100 mg only), 1,000s (except 100 mg). *Rx.*
Use: Psychotherapeutic agent.

atomoxetine hydrochloride. (Mylan) Atomoxetine hydrochloride 10 mg,

18 mg, 25 mg, 40 mg, 60 mg, 80 mg, 100 mg. Cap. 30s, 500s. *Rx.*
Use: Miscellaneous psychotherapeutic agent.

•**atopaxar.** (A-toe-PAX-ar) USAN.
Use: Cardiovascular agent.

•**atopaxar hydrobromide.** (A-toe-PAX-ar) USAN.
Use: Cardiovascular agent.

Atopiclair. (Medicis) Ethylhexyl palmitate, pentylene glycol, shea butter, caprylol glycine, glyceryl, PEG-100, arachidyl glucoside, behenyl alcohol, arachidyl alcohol, bisabolol, tocopheryl acetate (anti-oxidant), glycyrrhetinic acid, carbomer, ethylhexylglycerin, piroctone olamine, sodium hydroxide, allantoin, DMDM hydantoin, vitis vinifer, disodium EDTA, ascorbyl tetraisopalmitate, sodium hyaluronate, propyl gallate, parabens, telmesteine, butylene glycol. Cream. 100 g. *Rx.*
Use: Emollient, miscellaneous.

atorvastatin.
Use: HMG-CoA reductase inhibitor.
W/Ezetimibe.
See: Liptruzet.

•**atorvastatin calcium.** (a-TORE-va-sta-tin) USAN.
Use: HMG-CoA reductase inhibitor; antihyperlipidemic agent.
See: Lipitor.
W/Amlodipine Besylate.
See: Caduet.

atorvastatin calcium. (Various Mfr.) Atorvastatin 10 mg, 20 mg, 40 mg, 80 mg. May contain lactose, PEG. Tab. 90s, 500s, 1,000s, UD 30s (80 mg only), UD 100s (except 80 mg). *Rx.*
Use: Antihyperlipidemic agent, HMG-CoA reductase inhibitor (statin).

•**atosiban.** (at-OH-sih-ban) USAN.
Use: Antagonist; oxytocin.

•**atovaquone.** (uh-TOE-vuh-KWONE) *USP.*
Use: Antipneumocystic.
See: Mepron.

atovaquone. (Various Mfr.) Atovaquone 750 mg per 5 mL. May contain benzyl alcohol, saccharin. Susp. 210 mL. *Rx.*
Use: Anti-infective agent, antiprotozoal.

atovaquone and proguanil hydrochloride.
Use: Antimalarial.
See: Malarone.
Malarone Pediatric.

atovaquone/proguanil hydrochloride. (Various Mfr.) Atovaquone 250 mg/proguanil hydrochloride 100 mg. Tab. 60s, 90s, 100s, 1,000s, UD 12s, UD 24s. *Rx.*
Use: Antimalarial preparation.

Atozine. (Major) Hydroxyzine hydrochloride. 10 mg, 25 mg, 50 mg. Tab. Bot. 100s, 250s, 500s (50 mg only), 1000s (except 50 mg), UD 100s. *Rx.*
Use: Anxiolytic.

Atpeg. (AstraZeneca) Polyethylene glycol available as 300, 400, 600, or 4000.
Use: Humectant; surfactant.

Atrac-Tain. (Coloplast) Urea. **Cream:** 10%. Alpha hydroxy acid 4%. Preservative free. 57 g, 142 g. **Lot.:** 5%. 118 mL, 237 mL. *OTC.*
Use: Emollient.

•**atracurium besylate.** (AT-rah-CUE-ree-uhm BESS-ih-late) *USP.*
Use: Neuromuscular blocker; muscle relaxant.
See: Tracrium.

atracurium besylate. (Bedford Labs) Atracurium besylate 10 mg/mL. Inj. Single-dose vials. 5 mL. Multidose vials (benzyl alcohol 0.9%). 10 mL. *Rx.*
Use: Muscle relaxant.

Atralin. (Coria) Tretinoin 0.05%. Benzyl alcohol, parabens. Gel. 45 g. *Rx.*
Use: First-generation retinoid.

atrasentan.
Use: Investigational selective endothelin-A receptor antagonist.

•**atreleuton.** (at-reh-LOO-tuhn) USAN.
Use: Antiasthmatic.

Atripla. (Bristol-Myers Squibb/Gilead Sciences) Efavirenz 600 mg, emtricitabine 200 mg, tenofovir disoproxil fumarate 300 mg (equiv. to tenofovir disproxil 245 mg). Film coated. Tab. 30s. *Rx.*
Use: Antiretroviral agent, non-nucleoside reverse transcriptase inhibitor.

Atrocap. (Freeport) Atropine sulfate 0.06 mg, hyoscyamine sulfate 0.3 mg, hyoscine hydrobromide 0.02 mg, phenobarbital 50 mg. TR Cap. Bot. 1000s. *Rx.*
Use: Anticholinergic; antispasmodic; hypnotic; sedative.

Atrocholin. (GlaxoSmithKline) Dehydrocholic acid 130 mg. Tab. Bot. 100s. *OTC.*
Use: Laxative.

Atrofed. (Genetco, Inc.) Pseudoephedrine hydrochloride 60 mg, triprolidine hydrochloride 2.5 mg. Tab. Bot. 24s, 100s, 1000s. *OTC.*
Use: Antihistamine; decongestant.

Atrohist LA. (Medeva) Pseudoephedrine hydrochloride 120 mg, brompheniramine maleate 4 mg, phenyltoloxamine citrate 50 mg. SR Tab with atropine sulfate 0.0242 mg available for immediate

release. Bot. 100s. *Rx.*
Use: Antihistamine; decongestant.

Atrohist Pediatric Capsules. (Medeva) Chlorpheniramine maleate 4 mg, pseudoephedrine hydrochloride 60 mg. SR Cap. Bot. 100s. *Rx.*
Use: Antihistamine; decongestant.

Atrohist Pediatric Suspension. (Medeva) Phenylephrine tannate 5 mg, chlorpheniramine tannate 2 mg, pyrilamine tannate 12.5 mg. Susp. Bot. 473 mL. Unit-of-use 118 mL. *Rx.*
Use: Antihistamine; decongestant.

Atrohist Sprinkle. (Medeva) Pseudoephedrine hydrochloride 120 mg, brompheniramine maleate 2 mg, phenyltoloxamine citrate 25 mg. SR Cap. Bot. 100s. *Rx.*
Use: Antihistamine; decongestant.

AtroPen. (Meridian Medical Technologies) Atropine sulfate 0.5 mg, 1 mg, 2 mg. Glycerin, phenol. Inj. Auto-injectors prefilled. *Rx.*
Use: Gastrointestinal anticholinergic/antispasmodic.

•**atropine.** (AT-troe-peen) *USP.*
Use: Anticholinergic.

Atropine Care. (Akorn) Atropine sulfate 1%. Benzalkonium chloride 0.01%, hypromellose 0.5%, edetate disodium. Soln.; Ophth. 2 mL, 5 mL, 15 mL. *Rx.*
Use: Ophthalmic and otic agent, cycloplegic mydriatic.

atropine-hyoscine-hyoscyamine combinations. (Also see Belladonna Products).
See: Barbella.
Barbeloid.
Belbutal No. 2 Kaptabs.
Brobella-P.B.
Spabelin.
Spasmolin.
Urogesic.

atropine-n-oxide hydrochloride.
See: Atropine Oxide Hydrochloride.

•**atropine oxide hydrochloride.** (AT-row-peen OX-ide) USAN.
Use: Anticholinergic.

atropine/pralidoxime chloride.
Use: Detoxification agent, antidote.
See: DuoDote.

•**atropine sulfate.** (AT-row-peen) *USP.*
Use: Anticholinergic/antispasmodic, ophthalmic.
See: AtroPen.
Atropine Care.
Atropine Sulfate S.O.P.
Bellahist-D LA.
W/Benzoic Acid, Hyoscyamine Sulfate, Methenamine, Methylene Blue, Phenyl Salicylate.
See: Uritact DS.
W/Chlorpheniramine Maleate, Hyoscyamine Sulfate, Phenylephrine Hydrochloride, Scopolamine Hydrobromide.
See: Bellahist-D LA.
W/Chlorpheniramine Maleate, Hyoscyamine Sulfate, Pseudoephedrine Hydrochloride, Scopolamine Hydrobromide.
See: Respa A.R.
Stahist.
W/Hyoscyamine Hydrobromide or Sulfate, Phenobarbital, Scopolamine Hydrobromide.
See: Antispasmodic.
Belladonna Alkaloids with Phenobarbital.
Donnatal.
Donnatal Extentabs.
PB-Hyos.
Quadrapax.
Se-Donna PB Hyos.
W/Phenobarbital.
See: Antrocol.
Barbeloid.
Brobella-P.B.
Donnatal.
Palbar No. 2.
Spabelin.

atropine sulfate. (Hospira) Atropine sulfate 0.05 mg/mL, 0.1 mg/mL. *Abboject* syringes. 5 mL, 10 mL (0.1 mg/mL only). *Rx.*
Use: Anticholinergic/antispasmodic.

atropine sulfate. (Various Mfr.). Atropine sulfate 0.3 mg/mL. Vial 1 mL, 30 mL; 0.4 mg/mL. Amp. 1 mL, vial 20 mL, 30 mL; 0.5 mg/mL. Vials. 1 mL, 30 mL. Syringes. 5 mL; 0.8 mg/mL. Amp. 0.5 mL, 1 mL. Syringes. 0.5 mL; 1 mg/mL. Amp., vial 1 mL, syringe 10 mL Inj. *Rx.*
Use: Gastrointestinal anticholinergic/antispasmodic, belladonna alkaloid.

atropine sulfate. (Various Mfr.) Atropine sulfate. **Oint:** 1%. 3.5 g, UD 1 g. **Soln.:** 1%. 2 mL, 5 mL, 15 mL, UD 1 mL. *Rx.*
Use: Ophthalmic and otic agent, cycloplegic mydriatic.

atropine sulfate and edrophonium chloride. Anticholinesterase muscle stimulant.
See: Enlon-Plus.

atropine sulfate S.O.P. (Allergan) Atropine sulfate 0.5%, 1%. Oint. Tube 3.5 g. *Rx.*
Use: Cycloplegic; mydriatic.

Atrosed. (Freeport) Atropine sulfate 0.0195 mg, hyoscine HBr 0.0065 mg, hyoscyamine sulfate 0.104 mg, phenobarbital 0.25 g. Tab. Bot. 1000s, 5000s. *Rx.*
Use: Anticholinergic; antispasmodic; hypnotic; sedative.

Atrosept. (Geneva) Methenamine 40.8 mg, phenyl salicylate 18.1 mg, atropine sulfate 0.03 mg, hyoscyamine 0.03 mg, benzoic acid 4.5 mg, methylene blue 5.4 mg. Tab. Bot. 100s, 1000s. *Rx.*
Use: Anti-infective, urinary.

Atrovent. (Boehringer Ingelheim) Ipratropium bromide 0.03% (21 mcg/spray). Nasal Spray. Bot. with spray pump. 30 mL (345 sprays); 0.06% (42 mcg/spray). Bot. with spray pump. 15 mL (165 sprays). *Rx.*
Use: Bronchodilator.

Atrovent HFA. (Boehringer Ingelheim) Ipratropium bromide 17 mcg per actuation. Aerosol. 12.9 g metered-dose inhaler with mouthpiece (200 inhalations). *Rx.*
Use: Bronchodilator.

ATryn. (GTC Biotherapeutics) Antithrombin 1,750 units (recombinant). Sodium chloride 79 mg, sodium citrate 26 mg. Preservative free. Inj., lyophilized Pow. for Soln. Single-dose vial. *Rx.*
Use: Anticoagulant, antithrombin agent.

A/T/S. (Medicis) Erythromycin. **Gel:** 2%. Alcohol 92%. Tubes. 30 g. **Top. Soln.:** 2%. Alcohol 66%. Bot. 60 mL. *Rx.*
Use: Topical anti-infective, antibiotic.

AT-Solution. (Sanofi-Synthelabo) Dihydrotachysterol solution.
Use: Antihypocalcemic.

Attain. (Sherwood Davis & Geck) Sodium caseinate, calcium caseinate, maltodextrin, corn oil, soy lecithin. Liq. Can 250 mL and 1000 mL closed system. *OTC.*
Use: Nutritional supplement.

•**attapulgite, activated.** (at-ah-PULL-gyte) *USP.*
Use: Antidiarrheal; pharmaceutic aid, suspending agent.
W/Pectin, hydrated alumina.
See: Sebasorb.

A.T. 10.
See: Dihydrotachysterol.

Atuss-12 DM. (Atley) Pseudoephedrine hydrochloride (as polistirex) 30 mg, chlorpheniramine maleate (as polistirex) 6 mg, dextromethorphan HBr (as polistirex) 30 mg/5 mL. Corn syrup, parabens. ER Susp. 20 mL, 473 mL. *Rx.*
Use: Pediatric antitussive combination.

Atuss-12 DX. (Atley) Dextromethorphan polistirex (equiv. to dextromethorphan HBr 30 mg), guaifenesin 200 mg/5 mL. Parabens, honey. Honey-lemon flavor. ER Susp. 20 mL, 473 mL. *Rx.*
Use: Antitussive, expectorant.

Aubagio. (Genzyme) Teriflunomide 7 mg, 14 mg. Film coated. Lactose. Tab. UD 5s, UD 28s. *Rx.*
Use: Immunomodulator.

augmented betamethasone dipropionate.
Use: Corticosteroid, topical.
See: Diprolene.

Augmentin. (Dr. Reddy's) **Tab.:** Amoxicillin/clavulanic potassium 500 mg/125 mg, 875 mg/125 mg. PEG, potassium 0.63 mEq. Film coated (500 mg/125 mg only). 20s, UD 100s. **Pow. for Oral Susp.:** Amoxicillin/clavulanic acid (as potassium salt) 125 mg/31.25 mg per 5 mL, 250 mg/62.5 mg per 5 mL. Mannitol, saccharin. Banana flavor (125 mg/31.25 mg), orange flavor (250 mg/62.5 mg). 75 mL, 100 mL, 150 mL. *Rx.*
Use: Aminopenicillin, penicillin.

Augmentin XR. (Dr. Reddy's) Amoxicillin 1000 mg, clavulanic acid 62.5 mg. Potassium 0.32 mEq, sodium 1.27 mEq, PEG. Film coated. ER Tab. Pkg. 28s (7-day XR pack), 40s (10-day XR pack). *Rx.*
Use: Aminopenicillin, penicillin.

Auralgesic. (Wesley) Carbamide 10%, antipyrine 5%, benzocaine 2.5%, cetyldimethylbenzylammonium hydrochloride 0.2%. Bot. 0.5 oz. *Rx.*
Use: Otic.

•**auranofin.** (or-RAIN-oh-fin) USAN.
Use: Antirheumatic.
See: Ridaura.

Aurax. (Acella Pharmaceuticals) Antipyrine 5.5%, benzocaine 1.4%. Glycerin, oxyquinoline sulfate. Soln.; Otic. 14 mL dropper tip bottle. *Rx.*
Use: Miscellaneous otic preparation.

Aureoquin Diamate. *Name previously used for Quinetolate.*

Aurinol Ear Drops. (Various Mfr.) Chloroxylenol and acetic acid, w/benzalkonium chloride and glycerin. Soln. Bot. 15 mL. *Rx.*
Use: Otic.

Aurocein. (Christina) Gold naphthyl sulfhydryl derivative 5%, 12.5%. Inj. Amp. 10 mL. *Rx.*
Use: Antirheumatic.

Aurodex. (Major) Antipyrine 5.4%, benzocaine 1.4%, glycerin, oxyquinoline sulfate. Soln.; Otic. 10 mL and 15 mL w/dropper. *Rx.*
Use: Otic preparation.

Auro-Dri. (Commerce) Boric acid 2.75% in isopropyl alcohol. Soln. 30 mL with dropper. *OTC.*
Use: Otic preparation.

Auro Ear Drops. (Commerce) Carba-

mide peroxide 6.5% in an anhydrous glycerine base. Soln. 15 mL. *OTC.*
Use: Otic.

Aurolate. (Taylor Pharmaceuticals) Gold sodium thiomalate 50 mg, benzyl alcohol 0.5%/mL. Inj. Vial 2 mL, 10 mL. *Rx.*
Use: Antirheumatic.

Aurolin.
See: Gold sodium thiosulfate.

Auropin.
See: Gold sodium thiosulfate.

Aurosan.
See: Gold sodium thiosulfate.

•**aurothioglucose.** (or-oh-THIGH-oh-GLUE-kose) *USP.*
Use: Antirheumatic.

aurothiomalate, sodium.
See: Gold Sodium Thiomalate.

Aurstat Skin and Wound HydroGel. (Onset Dermatologies) Sodium magnesium fluorosilicate 3%, sodium phosphate 0.4%, sodium chloride 0.066%, hypochlorous acid 0.008%, sodium hypochlorite 0.002%. Gel. 225 mL kit w/100 mg of *Hylatopic Plus* cream. *Rx.*
Use: Miscellaneous topical combination.

Ausab. (Abbott Diagnostics) Radioimmunoassay or enzyme immunoassay for detection of antibody to hepatitis B surface antigen. Test kit 100s.
Use: Diagnostic aid.

Ausab EIA. (Abbott Diagnostics) Enzyme immunoassay for the detection of antibody to hepatitis B surface antigen.
Use: Diagnostic aid.

Auscell. (Abbott Diagnostics) Reverse passive hemagglutination test for hepatitis B surface antigen. Test kit 110s, 450s, 1800s.
Use: Diagnostic aid.

Ausria II-125. (Abbott Diagnostics) Radioimmunoassay for detection of hepatitis B surface antigen. Test kit 100s, 500s, 600s, 700s, 800s, 900s, 1000s.
Use: Diagnostic aid.

Auszyme II. (Abbott Diagnostics) Enzyme immunoassay for detection of hepatitis B surface antigen (HBsAg) in human serum or plasma. Test kit 100s, 500s.
Use: Diagnostic aid.

Auszyme Monoclonal. (Abbott Diagnostics) Qualitative third generation enzyme immunoassay for the detection of hepatitis B surface antigen (HBsAg) in human serum or plasma.
Use: Diagnostic aid.

Autoantibody Screen. (Wampole) Autoantibody screening system. To screen serum for the presence of a variety of autoantibodies. Test 48s.
Use: Diagnostic aid.

Autolet Kit. (Bayer Consumer Care) Automatic bloodletting spring-loaded device to obtain capillary blood samples from fingertips, ear lobes, or heels.
Use: Diagnostic aid.

autolymphocyte therapy; ALT. (Cellcor, Inc.)
Use: Treatment of renal cancer. [Orphan Drug]

Autrinic. Intrinsic factor concentrate. *Rx.*
Use: To increase absorption of vitamin B_{12}.

Auxotab Enteric 1 & 2. (Colab) Rapid identification of enteric bacteria and *Pseudomonas.* Test contains capillary units with selective biochemical reagents.
Use: Diagnostic aid.

•**avagacestat.** (A-va-GAY-se-stat) USAN.
Use: CNS agent.

Avage. (Allergan) Tazarotene 0.1%, benzyl alcohol 1%, EDTA, medium chain triglycerides, mineral oil. Cream. 15 g, 30 g. *Rx.*
Use: Retinoid.

Avail. (Menley & James Labs, Inc.) Iron 18 mg, vitamin A 5000 units, D 400 units, E 30 mg, B_1 2.25 mg, B_2 2.55 mg, B_3 20 mg, B_6 3 mg, B_{12} 9 mcg, C 90 mg, folic acid 0.4 mg, Ca, Cr, I, Mg, Se, Zn 22.5 mg. Tab. Bot. 60s. *OTC.*
Use: Mineral, vitamin supplement.

Avalgesic. (Various Mfr.) Methyl salicylate, menthol, camphor, methylnicotinate, dipropylene glycol salicylate, oil of cassia, oleoresins capsicum, ginger. Bot. 120 mL, Pt, gal. *OTC.*
Use: Analgesic, topical.

Avalide. (Sanofi-Aventis U.S.) Irbesartan/hydrochlorothiazide 150 mg/12.5 mg, 300 mg/12.5 mg, 300 mg/25 mg (film coated). Lactose. Tab. Bot. 30s, 90s; 500s, blister pack 100s (except 300 mg/25 mg). *Rx.*
Use: Antihypertensive.

A-Van. (Stewart-Jackson Pharmacal) Dimenhydrinate 50 mg. Cap. Bot. 100s.
Use: Antivertigo.

•**avanafil.** (av-AN-a-fil) USAN.
Use: Erectile dysfunction.
See: Stendra.

Avandamet. (GlaxoSmithKline) Rosiglitazone maleate/metformin hydrochloride 2 mg/500 mg, 4 mg/500 mg, 2 mg/1000 mg, 4 mg/1000 mg. Lactose, polyethylene glycol 400. Film coated. Tab. Bot. 60s. *Rx.*
Use: Antidiabetic combination.

Avandaryl. (GlaxoSmithKline) Rosiglitazone (as rosiglitazone maleate) and

glimepiride 4 mg/1 mg, 4 mg/2 mg, 4 mg/4 mg, 8 mg/2 mg, 8 mg/4 mg. Lactose, PEG. Tab. 30s. *Rx.*
Use: Antidiabetic combination.

Avandia. (GlaxoSmithKline) Rosiglitazone maleate 2 mg, 4 mg, 8 mg. Lactose, PEG 3000. Film coated. Tab. Bot. 30s (except 2 mg), 60s (2 mg only), 90s (except 2 mg). *Rx.*
Use: Antidiabetic, thiazolidinedione.

Avapro. (Bristol-Myers Squibb Sanofi-Synthelabo Partnership) Irbesartan 75 mg, 150 mg, 300 mg. Lactose. Tab. Bot. 30s, 90s, 500s (except 75 mg), UD 100s (150 mg only). *Rx.*
Use: Renin angiotensin system antagonist, angiotensin II receptor antagonist.

Avar. (Mission) Sulfur/sodium sulfacetamide. **Cleanser:** 5%/10%. Cetyl alcohol, stearyl alcohol. 226.8 g. **Pads:** 5%/9.5%. Alcohols, benzyl alcohol, glyceryl stearate, PEG, propylene glycol. 30s, 60s. *Rx.*
Use: Keratolytic agent.

Avar-e Emollient. (Kylemore) Sulfur 5%, sodium sulfacetamide 10%, glycerin, EDTA, benzyl alcohol, cetyl alcohol. Cream. 45 g. *Rx.*
Use: Acne product.

Avar-e LS. (Mission) Sodium sulfacetamide 10%, sulfur 2%. Benzyl alcohol, cetyl alcohol, disodium EDTA, glycerin, glyceryl, PEG 100, phenoxyethanol, polawax, zinc oxide. Cream. 45 g. *Rx.*
Use: Acne product combination.

Avar LS. (Mission) Sodium sulfacetamide 10%, sulfur 2%. Alcohols, benzyl alcohol, glyceryl stearate, PEG, propylene glycol. Pads; topical. 30s, 60s. *Rx.*
Use: Acne product combination.

Avar LS Cleanser. (Kylemore) Sodium sulfacetamide 10%, sulfur 2%. Benzyl alcohol, cetyl alcohol, phenoxyethanol, propylene glycol, stearyl alcohol. Soap. 226.8 g. *Rx.*
Use: Acne production combination.

•**avarofloxacin.** (a-VAR-oh-FLOX-a-sin) USAN.
Use: Anti-infective, fluoroquinolone.

•**avarofloxacin hydrochloride.** (a-VAR-oh-FLOX-a-sin) USAN.
Use: Anti-infective, fluoroquinolone.

•**avasimibe.** (a-VA-si-mibe) USAN.
Use: Antiatherosclerotic; hypolipidemic (acylCoA: Cholesterol acyltransferase [ACAT] inhibitor).

Avastin. (Genentech) Bevacizumab 25 mg/mL. Preservative-free. Inj., Soln., Conc. Single-use vials. 4 mL (with α, α-trehalose dihydrate 240 mg, sodium phosphate [monobasic] 23.3 mg, sodium phosphate [dibasic] 4.8 mg), 16 mL (with α, α-trehalose dihydrate 960 mg, sodium phosphate [monobasic] 92.8 mg, sodium phosphate [dibasic] 19.2 mg). *Rx.*
Use: Monoclonal antibody.

•**avatrombopag.** (A-va-TROM-boe-pag) USAN.
Use: Treatment of thrombocytopenia.

•**avatrombopag maleate.** (A-va-TROM-boe-pag) USAN.
Use: Treatment of thrombocytopenia.

Aveed. (Endo) Testosterone undecanoate 250 mg/mL. Castor oil. Inj., Soln. Single-use vial. 3 mL. *c-III.*
Use: Sex hormone, androgen.

Aveeno Active Naturals Hydrocortisone. (J & J Consumer) Hydrocortisone 1%. Aloe, benzyl alcohol, cetearyl alcohol, glycerin, methylparaben, oat kernel oil. Cream. 28 g. *OTC.*
Use: Emollient.

Aveeno Anti-Itch. (J & J Consumer) Calamine 3%, pramoxine hydrochloride 1%. Camphor, cetyl alcohol, petrolatum. Cream. 28 g. *OTC.*
Use: Poison ivy treatment.

Aveeno Baby. (J & J Consumer) Dimethicone 1.2%. Benzyl alcohol, cetyl alcohol, glycerin, petrolatum. Lot. 227 mL. *OTC.*
Use: Emollient.

Aveeno Bath. (J & J Consumer) Colloidal oatmeal. Box 1 lb, 4 lb. *OTC.*
Use: Emollient.

Aveeno Cleansing Bar. (Rydelle) **Combination Skin:** Soap free. Colloidal oatmeal 51%, sodium cocoyl isethionate, glycerin, lactic acid, sodium lactate, petrolatum, magnesium aluminum silicate, potassium sorbate, titanium dioxide, PEG 14M. Bar 90 g. **Dry Skin:** Soap free. Colloidal oatmeal 51%, sodium cocoyl isethionate, vegetable oil and shortening, glycerin, PEG-75, lauramide DEA, lactic acid, sodium lactate, sorbic acid, titanium dioxide. Bar 90 g. *OTC.*
Use: Dermatologic; cleanser.

Aveeno Colloidal Oatmeal. (Rydelle) Colloidal oatmeal. Box 1 lb, 4 lb. *OTC.*
Use: Emollient.

Aveeno Daily Moisturizing. (J & J Consumer) Dimethicone 1.25%, benzyl alcohol, cetyl alcohol, glycerin, petrolatum. Lot. 354 mL. *OTC.*
Use: Emollient.

Aveeno Dry. (Rydelle) Dry skin formula,

soap free, emollient colloidal oatmeal, vegetable oils, lanolin derivative, and glycerin 29% in mild surfactant base. Cleansing bar 90 g. *OTC.*
Use: Dermatologic; cleanser.

Aveeno Lotion. (J & J Consumer) Colloidal oatmeal 1%, glycerin, petrolatum, dimethicone, phenylcarbinol. Lot. Bot. 354 mL. *OTC.*
Use: Emollient.

Aveeno Moisturizing Cream. (J & J Consumer) Colloidal oatmeal, glycerin, petrolatum, dimethicone, phenylcarbinol. Cream. Tube 120 g. *OTC.*
Use: Emollient.

Aveeno Oilated. (Rydelle) Aveeno colloidal oatmeal impregnated with 35% liquid petrolatum, refined olive oil. Box 8 oz, 2 lb. *OTC.*
Use: Emollient.

Aveeno Shave. (J & J Consumer) Oatmeal flour. Gel. Can 210 g. *OTC.*
Use: Emollient.

Aveeno Shower & Bath. (J & J Consumer) Colloidal oatmeal, 5% mineral oil, glyceryl stearate, PEG 100 stearate, laureth-4, benzyl alcohol, silica benzaldehyde. Oil. Bot. 240 mL. *OTC.*
Use: Emollient.

Avelox. (Merck Sharp & Dohme) Moxifloxacin hydrochloride 400 mg, lactose. Tab. Bot. 30s, UD 50s, *ABC* Packs of 5. *Rx.*
Use: Anti-infective; fluoroquinolone.

Avelox I.V. (Merck Sharp & Dohme) Moxifloxacin hydrochloride 400 mg per 250 mL. Sodium chloride 0.8%. Preservative free. Premix Inj. Flexible bag (latex free) 250 mL. *Rx.*
Use: Anti-infective, fluoroquinolone.

Aviane. (Barr) Ethinyl estradiol 20 mcg, levonorgestrel 0.1 mg. Lactose. Tab. Pkg. 28s with 7 inert tabs. *Rx.*
Use: Sex hormone, contraceptive hormone.

•**avibactam.** (A-vi-BAK-tam) USAN.
Use: Beta-lactamase inhibitor.

•**avibactam sodium.** (A-vi-BAK-tam) USAN.
Use: Beta-lactamase inhibitor.

Avidoxy. (Avidas) Doxycycline monohydrate 100 mg. Film coated. Lactose, PEG. Tab. 50s and *Avidoxy DK Kit* w/*Defence Solare Sun Protection* 56.7 g and *Defence Acne Wash* 118 mL. *Rx.*
Use: Anti-infective, tetracycline.

•**avilamycin.** (ah-VILL-ah-MY-sin) USAN.
Use: Anti-infective.

Avinar. Uredepa.
Use: Antineoplastic.

Avinza. (King Pharmaceuticals) Morphine sulfate 30 mg, 45 mg, 60 mg, 75 mg, 90 mg, 120 mg (for use only in opioid-tolerant patients). Sugar starch spheres, fumaric acid. ER Pellets Cap. 100s. *c-II.*
Tall Man: AVINza
Use: Opioid analgesic.

Avita. (Mylan) Tretinoin. **Cream:** 0.025%, stearyl alcohol. Tube 20 g, 45 g. **Gel:** 0.025%, ethanol 83%. Tube. 20 g, 45 g. *Rx.*
Use: Dermatologic, retinoid.

•**avitriptan fumarate.** (av-ih-TRIP-tan FEW-mah-rate) USAN.
Use: Antimigraine.

•**avobenzone.** (AV-ah-BENZ-ohn) USAN.
Use: Sunscreen.
W/Combinations.
See: PreSun Ultra.
TI-Screen Sports.
W/Ecamsule, Octocrylene.
See: Anthelios SX.
UV Protective.
W/Ecamsule, Octocrylene, Titanium Dioxide.
See: Capital Soleil 20.
W/Homosalate, Octisalate, Octocrylene, Oxybenzone.
See: Neutrogena Ultra Sheer Dry-Touch Sunblock.
W/Mexoryl SX, Octocrylene, Titanium Dioxide.
See: Anthelios 40.

Avodart. (GlaxoSmithKline) Dutasteride 0.5 mg. Cap. 30s, 90s. *Rx.*
Use: Sex hormone, androgen hormone inhibitor.

Avonex. (Biogen Idec) Interferon beta-1A **Inj., lyophilized Pow. for Inj.:** 33 mcg (30 mcg/vial when reconstituted). Albumin (human) 16.5 mg, sodium. Preservative free. Administration dose packs (single-use vial w/diluent [sterile water for injection], alcohol wipes, gauze pad, syringe, *MicroPin* vial access pin, needle, and bandage). 4s. **Inj., Soln.:** 30 mcg/0.5 mL. Albumin free. Administration dose packs (0.5 mL single-use prefilled syringe or autoinjector, needle, reclosable accessory pouch, alcohol wipes, gauze pads, and bandages). 4s. *Rx.*
Use: Immunologic agent, immunomodulator.

Avonique. (Armenpharm Ltd.) Vitamins A 4000 units, D 400 units, B_1 1 mg, B_2 1.2 mg, B_6 2 mg, B_{12} 2 mcg, calcium pantothenate 5 mg, B_3 10 mg, C 30 mg, calcium 100 mg, phosphorus 76 mg, iron 10 mg, manganese 1 mg, magne-

sium 1 mg, zinc 1 mg. *OTC.*
Use: Mineral, vitamin supplement.

•**avoparcin.** (AVE-oh-PAR-sin) USAN.
Use: Anti-infective.

Avosil. (Avocet) BHT 0.2%, parabens 0.3%, PEG, sodium salicylate 2%. Oint. 56.7 g. *OTC.*
Use: Dermatological agent.

•**avridine.** (AV-rih-deen) USAN.
Use: Antiviral.

Awake. (Walgreens) Caffeine 100 mg. Tab. Bot. 36s. *OTC.*
Use: CNS stimulant.

axerophthol.
See: Vitamin A.

Axert. (Janssen) Almotriptan malate 6.25 mg, 12.5 mg. Mannitol. Tab. UD 6s (6.25 mg), 12s (12.5 mg). *Rx.*
Use: Antimigraine agent, serotonin 5-HT_1 receptor agonist.

Axid. (Braintree) Nizatidine 15 mg/mL. Parabens, saccharin, sucrose. Bubble gum flavor. Oral Soln. 480 mL. *Rx.*
Use: Histamine H_2 antagonist.

Axid AR. (Wyeth Consumer) Nizatidine 75 mg. Tab. Bot. 12s, 30s. *OTC.*
Use: Histamine H_2 antagonist.

Axid Pulvules. (GlaxoSmithKline) Nizatidine 150 mg. Cap. 60s. *Rx.*
Use: Histamine H_2 antagonist.

Axiron. (Lilly) Testosterone 30 mg per 1.5 mL. Ethanol, isopropyl alcohol. Soln. 110 mL metered-dose pump w/applicator (each metered-dose pump delivers 60 metered 30 mg doses). *C-III.*
Use: Sex hormone, androgen.

•**axitinib.** (AX-i-TI-nib) USAN.
Use: Antineoplastic.
See: Inlyta.

•**axitirome.** (ax-i-TYE-rome) USAN.
Use: Hypolipidemic.

•**axomadol.** (ax-OH-ma-dole) USAN.
Use: Analgesic.

Axona. (Accera) Caprylidene 40 g (20 g medium-chain triglycerides). Acesulfame potassium, sucralose. Vanilla flavor. 40 g packets. 30s (also contains potassium caseinate [milk-derived protein]), maltodextrin, whey protein [milk-derived], sugar, sunflower oil, dimagnesium phosphate, tricalcium phosphate, dipotassium phosphate, soy lecithin, distilled monoglyceride, sodium ascorbate [vitamin C], silicon dioxide, natural vanilla bean extract, vitamin E acetate, vitamin A palmitate, zinc sulfate, pyridoxine hydrochloride [vitamin B_6], folic acid, and chromium chloride). *Rx.*
Use: Nutritional supplement.

Axsain. (Rodlen Labs) Capsaicin 0.25% in an emollient base, lidocaine, alcohols, white petrolatum. Cream. 60 g. *OTC.*
Use: Counterirritant.

Aygestin. (Duramed) Norethindrone acetate 5 mg. Lactose. Tab. Bot. 50s, blister pack 10s. *Rx.*
Use: Sex hormone, progestin.

Ayr Saline. (B.F. Ascher) Sodium chloride 0.65%, benzalkonium chloride, EDTA. Soln. **Drops:** Bot. 5 mL. **Gel:** Aloe vera gel, glycerin, parabens. Tube. 14 g. **Mist:** Bot. 50 mL. *OTC.*
Use: Dermatologic; moisturizer.

•**azabon.** (AZE-ah-bahn) USAN.
Use: CNS stimulant.

•**azacitidine.** (AZE-ah-SIGH-tih-deen) USAN. *Formerly Ladakamycin.*
Tall Man: azaCITIDine
Use: DNA demethylation agent.
See: Vidaza.

azacitidine. (Various Mfr.) Azacitidine 100 mg. May contain mannitol. Inj., lyophilized Pow. Single-use vial. *Rx.*
Use: Antineoplastic.

•**azaclorzine hydrochloride.** (AZE-ah-KLOR-zeen) USAN. *Formerly Nonachlazine.*
Use: Coronary vasodilator.

•**azaconazole.** (AZE-ah-CONE-ah-zole) USAN. *Formerly Azoconazole.*
Use: Antifungal.

AZA-CR. NCI Investigational agent.
See: Azacitidine.

Azactam. (Bristol-Myers Squibb) Aztreonam 1 g, 2 g (≈ 780 mg L-arginine/g of aztreonam). Inj., lyophilized cake for Soln. Single-dose vial and single-dose infusion bottle. 100 mL. *Rx.*
Use: Anti-infective.

•**azalanstat dihydrochloride.** (aze-ah-LAN-stat) USAN.
Use: Hypolipidemic.

Azaline. (Major) Sulfasalazine 500 mg. Tab. Bot. 100s, 500s, 1000s.
Use: Anti-inflammatory.

•**azaloxan fumarate.** (aze-ah-LOX-ahn) USAN.
Use: Antidepressant.

•**azanator maleate.** (AZE-an-nay-tore) USAN.
Use: Bronchodilator.

•**azanidazole.** (AZE-ah-NIH-dah-zole) USAN.
Use: Antiprotozoal.

•**azaperone.** (AZE-app-eh-RONE) *USP.*
Use: Antipsychotic.

•**azaribine.** (aze-ah-RYE-bean) USAN.
Use: Dermatologic.

•**azarole.** (AZE-ah-role) USAN.
Use: Immunoregulator.
Azasan. (Various Mfr.) Azathioprine 25 mg, 50 mg, 75 mg, 100 mg. Lactose. Tab. 100s. *Rx.*
Use: Immunosuppressant.
•**azaserine.** (AZE-ah-SER-een) USAN.
Use: Antifungal.
AzaSite. (Inspire) Azithromycin 1%. EDTA, benzalkonium chloride 0.003%, sodium chloride, sodium citrate, poloxamer 407, polycarbophil. Ophth. Soln. 2.5 mL. *Rx.*
Use: Ophthalmic antibiotic.
•**azatadine maleate.** (aze-AT-ad-EEN) *USP.*
Use: Antihistamine.
See: Optimine.
W/Combinations.
See: Rynatan.
•**azathioprine.** (AZE-uh-THIGH-oh-preen) *USP.*
Tall Man: azaTHIOprine
Use: Immunosuppressant.
See: Azasan.
Imuran.
azathioprine. (aaiPharma) Azathioprine 50 mg. Tab. 100s. *Rx.*
Use: Immunosuppressant.
•**azathioprine sodium for injection.** (AZE-uh-THIGH-oh-preen) *USP.*
Use: Immunosuppressant.
5-aza-2′-deoxycytidine.
Use: Treatment of acute leukemia. [Orphan Drug]
5-AZC.
See: Azacitidine.
•**azelaic acid.** (aze-eh-LAY-ik) USAN.
Use: Dermatologic; acne.
See: Azelex.
Finacea.
Finevin.
•**azelastine hydrochloride.** (AY-ze-LAS-teen) USAN.
Use: Antiallergic, antiasthmatic, antihistamine, peripherally selective phthalazinone.
See: Astelin.
Astepro.
Optivar.
W/Fluticasone Propionate.
See: Dymista.
azelastine hydrochloride. (Sun Pharmaceutical) Azelastine hydrochloride 0.1% (137 mcg/spray; equiv. to azelastine base 125 mcg). Benzalkonium chloride, edetate disodium. Spray, Soln., intranasal. 30 mg (1 mg/mL) (200 metered sprays) per bottle. *Rx.*
Use: Respiratory inhalant, intranasal antihistamine.
azelastine hydrochloride. (Various Mfr.) Azelastine hydrochloride 0.05% (equiv. to azelastine 0.457 mg). Benzalkonium chloride 0.25 mg, disodium edetate dihydrate, hydroxypropylmethylcellulose, sodium hydroxide. Soln., Ophth. 6 mL w/dropper. *Rx.*
Use: Ophthalmic antihistamine.
Azelex. (Allergan) Azelaic acid 20%, glycerin, cetearyl alcohol, benzoic acid. Cream. Tube 30 g, 50 g. *Rx.*
Use: Dermatologic, acne.
•**azepindole.** (AZE-eh-PIN-dole) USAN.
Use: Antidepressant.
•**azetepa.** (AZE-eh-teh-pah) USAN.
Use: Antineoplastic.
•**azficel-T.** (az-FYE-sel) USAN.
Use: Treatment of nasolabial fold wrinkles.
azidothymidine.
See: Zidovudine.
•**3-azido-2, 3 dideoxyuridine.** USAN.
Use: Antiviral, HIV.
Azidouridine. (Berlex) Phase I HIV-positive symptomatic, ARC, AIDS. *Rx.*
Use: Antiviral.
Azilect. (Teva) Rasagiline (as base) 0.5 mg, 1 mg. Mannitol. Tab. 30s. *Rx.*
Use: Antiparkinson agent.
•**azilsartan medoxomil.** (AY-zil-SAR-tan me-DOX-oh-mil) USAN.
Use: Angiotensin II receptor antagonist.
See: Edarbi.
W/Chlorthalidone.
See: Edarbyclor.
•**azimilide dihydrochloride.** (azz-IM-ih-lide die-HIGH-droe-KLOR-ide) USAN.
Use: Cardiovascular agent.
•**azipramine hydrochloride.** (aze-IPP-RAH-meen) USAN.
Use: Antidepressant.
•**azithromycin.** (UHZ-ith-row-MY-sin) *USP.*
Use: Anti-infective, macrolide; ophthalmic antibiotic.
See: AzaSite.
Zithromax.
ZMax.
azithromycin. (Greenstone) Azithromycin (as azithromycin dihydrate) 100 mg/5 mL and 200 mg/5 mL when reconstituted, 1 g/packet. Sucrose. Cherry/banana/creme de vanilla flavors (100 mg/5 mL and 200 mg/5 mL), cherry/banana flavor (1 g/packet). Pow. for Susp. 15 mL, 22.5 mL (200 mg/mL), 30 mL (200 mg/mL). Single-dose packet. 3s, 10s (1 g/packet). *Rx.*
Use: Macrolide.
azithromycin. (Various Mfr.) Azithromycin. **Tab.:** 250 mg, 500 mg, 600 mg.

May contain lactose. 1s (250 mg); 3s, 6s (250 mg and 500 mg); 30s; UD 9s (500 mg); UD 18s (250 mg); UD 50s (250 mg and 500 mg); UD 100s (250 mg). **Inj., lyophilized Pow. for Soln.:** 500 mg, 2.5 g. May contain sodium. Vial (500 mg), pharmacy bulk package (2.5 g). *Rx.*
Use: Macrolide.

•**azlocillin.** (AZZ-low-SILL-in) USAN.
Use: Anti-infective.

Azma-Aid. (Purepac) Theophylline 118 mg, ephedrine 24 mg, phenobarbital 8 mg. Tab. Bot. 100s, 250s, 1000s. *Rx.*
Use: Bronchodilator.

azoconazole.
See: Azaconazole.

Azodyne Hydrochloride.
See: Pyridium.

Azolen Tincture. (Stratus) Miconazole nitrate 2%. Benzyl alcohol, isopropyl alcohol. Soln. 29.57 mL. *OTC.*
Use: Topical anti-infective, antifungal agent.

•**azolimine.** (aze-OLE-ih-meen) USAN.
Use: Diuretic.

AZO Negacide. (Sanofi-Synthelabo) Nalidixic acid, phenazopyridine hydrochloride. Tab. *Rx.*
Use: Anti-infective, urinary.

AZO-100. (Scruggs) Phenylazodiaminopyridine hydrochloride 100 mg. Tab. Bot. 100s, 1000s. *OTC.*
Use: Analgesic, urinary.

Azopt. (Alcon) Brinzolamide 1%. Benzalkonium chloride 0.01%, mannitol, carbomer 974P tyloxapol, sodium chloride, hydrochloric acid and/or sodium hydroxide, and EDTA. Ophth. Susp. *Drop-Tainers* 2.5 mL, 5 mL, 10 mL, 15 mL. *Rx.*
Use: Glaucoma treatment.

Azor. (Daiichi Sankyo) Amlodipine besylate/olmesartan medoxomil 5 mg/20 mg, 5 mg/40 mg, 10 mg/20 mg, 10 mg/40 mg. Tab. 30s, 90s, 1000s, blister 100s. *Rx.*
Use: Antihypertensive combination.

•**azosemide.** (AZE-oh-SEH-mide) USAN.
Use: Diuretic.

AZO Standard. (Amerifit Brands) Phenazopyridine hydrochloride 95 mg. Tab. Bot. 30s. *OTC.*
Use: Interstitial cystitis agent.

AZO Standard Maximum Strength. (Amerifit Brands) Phenazopyridine hydrochloride 97.5 mg. PEG. Tab. 12s *OTC.*
Use: Interstitial cystitis agent.

Azostix Reagent Strips. (Bayer Consumer Care) Bromthymol blue, urease, buffers. Colorimetric test for blood urea nitrogen level. Bot 25 strips.
Use: Diagnostic aid.

•**azotomycin.** (aze-OH-toe-MY-sin) USAN. Antibiotic isolated from broth filtrates of *Streptomyces ambofaciens.*
Use: Antineoplastic.

Azovan Blue.
See: Evans Blue Dye (City Chemical; Harvey).

AZO Wintomylon. (Sanofi-Synthelabo) Nalidixic acid, phenazopyridine hydrochloride. *Rx.*
Use: Anti-infective, urinary.

AZT.
See: Zidovudine.

AZT-P-ddi. (Baker Norton) Phase I AIDS. Investigational.
Use: Antiviral.

•**aztreonam.** (AZZ-TREE-oh-nam) *USP.*
Use: Antimicrobial.
See: Azactam.

aztreonam. (APP Pharmaceutical) Aztreonam 500 mg, 1 g, 2 g. L-arginine (≈ 780 mg per gram aztreonam). Inj., lyophilized cake for Soln. Single-dose vial. *Rx.*
Use: Anti-infective agent, monobactam.

Azulfidine. (Pfizer) Sulfasalazine 500 mg. Tab. Bot. 100s, 300s, UD 100s. *Rx.*
Use: Anti-inflammatory, antirheumatic.

Azulfidine EN-tabs. (Pfizer) Sulfasalazine 500 mg. Enteric coated. DR Tab. Bot. 100s, 300s. *Rx.*
Use: Anti-inflammatory, antirheumatic.

•**azumolene sodium.** (AH-ZUH-moe-leen) USAN.
Use: Muscle relaxant.

Azurette. (Watson) **Phase 1:** Desogestrel 0.15 mg, ethinyl estradiol 20 mcg. **Phase 2:** Ethinyl estradiol 10 mcg. Lactose. Tab. Blister pack 21s w/2 inert green tablets. *Rx.*
Use: Oral monophasic contraceptive.

B

B_1. Thiamine hydrochloride.
B_2. Riboflavin.
B_3. Niacin, nicotinamide.
B_5. Calcium pantothenate.
B_6. Pyridoxine hydrochloride.
B_6 50. (Western Research) Vitamin B_6 50 mg. Tab. Bot. 1000s. *OTC.*
Use: Vitamin supplement.
B_{12}. Cyanocobalamin. *OTC.*
Babee Teething. (SmithKline Beecham Consumer) Benzocaine 2.5%. Camphor, cetalkonium chloride 0.02%, eucalyptol, menthol. Dye free, sugar free. Lot.; dental. 15 mL. *OTC.*
Use: Anesthetic, local.
Baby Anbesol. (Whitehall-Robins) Benzocaine 7.5%, saccharin. Gel. Tube 7.2 g. *OTC.*
Use: Mouth and throat preparation.
BabyBIG. (California Dept. of Health Sciences) Botulism immune globulin IV (human) 100 ± 20 mg (50 mg/mL when reconstituted). Sucrose 5%, albumin (human) 1%. Solvent/detergent-treated. Preservative free. Pow. for Inj., lyophilized. Single-dose vial with 2 mL vial of diluent. *Rx.*
Use: Infant botulism, immune globulin.
Baby Ddrops. (J.R. Carlson Labs) Vitamin D_3 (cholecalciferol) 400 units per 0.03 mL. Gluten free, preservative free, and sugar free. Drops. 11 mL. *OTC.*
Use: Fat-soluble vitamin.
Baby Gas-X Infant. (Novartis Consumer Health) Simethicone 20 mg/0.3 mL. Mannitol. Alcohol free. Drops. 30 mL. *OTC.*
Use: Antiflatulent.
Baby Orajel. (Del) Benzocaine. **Gel:** 7.5%. Saccharin, sorbitol, alcohol free. Tube 9.45 g. **Liq.:** 7.5%. Parabens, saccharin, sorbitol. Berry flavor. 13.3 mL. *OTC.*
Use: Mouth and throat preparation.
Baby Orajel Nighttime Formula. (Del) Benzocaine 10%, saccharin, sorbitol, alcohol free. Gel. Tube 6 g. *OTC.*
Use: Mouth and throat preparation.
Baby Orajel Teeth & Gum Cleanser. (Del) Poloxamer 407 2%, simethicone 0.12%, parabens, saccharin, sorbitol. Gel. Tube 14.2 g. *OTC.*
Use: Mouth and throat preparation.
Baby Vitamin. (Ivax) Vitamins A 1500 units, D 400 units, E 5 units, B_1 0.5 mg, B_2 0.6 mg, B_3 8 mg, B_6 0.4 mg, B_{12} 2 mcg, C 35 mg/mL. Drop. Bot. 50 mL. *OTC.*
Use: Vitamin supplement.
Baby Vitamin Drops with Iron. (Ivax) Iron 10 mg, vitamins A 1500 units, D 400 units, E 5 units, B_1 0.5 mg, B_2 0.6 mg, B_3 8 mg, B_6 0.4 mg, C 35 mg/mL. Bot. 50 mL. *OTC.*
Use: Mineral, vitamin supplement.
BAC. Benzalkonium Chloride.
•**bacampicillin hydrochloride.** (BACK-am-PIH-sill-in) *USP.*
Use: Anti-infective.
See: Spectrobid.
Bacco-Resist. (Vita Elixir) Lobeline sulfate 1/64 g.
Use: Smoking deterrent.
Bacid. (Insight Pharmaceuticals) *L. acidophilus* 800 million cultures, *L. bulgaricus* 100 million, *B. bifidum* 50 million, *S. thermophilus* 50 million. Preservative free. Tab. 100s. *OTC.*
Use: Probiotic.
Bacillus Calmette-Guérin.
See: BCG vaccine.
Bacillus coagulans.
Use: Probiotic.
See: Probiotic With Prebiotic.
Sustenex.
•**bacitracin.** (bass-ih-TRAY-sin) *USP.*
Use: Anti-infective.
See: Altracin.
W/Neomycin, Polymyxin B Sulfate.
See: Mycitracin.
Neosporin Original.
Neo-Thrycex.
Tigo.
W/Neomycin Sulfate.
See: Bacitracin-Neomycin.
W/Polymyxin B sulfate
See: Polysporin.
W/Polymyxin B Sulfate and Neomycin Sulfate.
See: Trimixin.
bacitracin. (Various Mfr.) An antibiotic produced by a strain of *Bacillus subtilis.* Diagnostic Tabs., Oint., Ophth. Oint. 500 units/g. Tube 3.5 g, 3.75 g. Soluble Tab., Systemic Use, Vial, Topical Use, Vial, Troche. Vaginal Tab.
Use: Anti-infective. [Orphan Drug]
bacitracin. (Various Mfr.) Bacitracin 500 units/g. Oint. 3.5 g, 3.75 g. *Rx.*
Use: Anti-infective, ophthalmic.
bacitracin-neomycin ointment. (Various Mfr.) Neomycin sulfate equivalent to 3.5 mg base, bacitracin 500 units/g. Topical Oint. Tube 0.5 oz, 1 oz, Ophth. Oint. 1/8 oz. *OTC.*
Use: Anti-infective, topical.
bacitracin/neomycin/polymyxin B ointment. (Various Mfr.) Polymyxin B sulfate 10,000 units/g, neomycin sulfate 3.5 mg/g, bacitracin zinc 400 units/g.

Tube 3.5 g. *Rx.*
Use: Anti-infective, ophthalmic.

•**bacitracin zinc.** (bass-ih-TRAY-sin) *USP. Rx.*
Use: Anti-infective.
W/Hydrocortisone Acetate, Neomycin Sulfate, Polymyxin B.
See: Coracin.
W/Neomycin Sulfate, Polymyxin B Sulfate.
See: Bacitracin Zinc and Polymyxin B Sulfate.
Mycitracin.
Neomycin and Polymyxin B sulfates and Bacitracin Zinc.
Neosporin Maximum Strength.
Neosporin Original.
Neotal.
Neo-Thrycex.
Ocutricin.
Tigo.
Trimixin.
Triple Antibiotic.
W/Hydrocortisone Acetate, Neomycin Sulfate, Polymyxin B Sulfate.
See: Coracin.
W/Polymyxin B sulfate.
See: AK-Poly-Bac.
Double Antibiotic.
Polysporin.
W/Polymyxin B Sulfate, Lidocaine, Neomycin.
See: Lanabiotic.
W/Polymyxin B Sulfate, Neomycin, Pramoxine Hydrochloride.
See: Neosporin Plus Pain Relief.
Tri-Biozene.
W/Pramoxine Hydrochloride.
See: Bacitraycin Plus.

bacitracin zinc. (Pharmacia) Bacitracin zinc 10,000 units, 50,000 units. Sterile pow. Vial. *Rx.*
Use: Anti-infective.

bacitracin zinc and polymyxin B sulfate. (Roerig) Polymyxin B sulfate 10,000 units, bacitracin zinc 500 units/g, white petrolatum, mineral oil. Ophth. Oint. Tube 3.5 g. *Rx.*
Use: Antibiotic.

bacitracin zinc/neomycin sulfate/polymyxin B sulfate/hydrocortisone. (Various Mfr.) Hydrocortisone 1%, neomycin sulfate 0.35%, bacitracin zinc 400 units, polymyxin B sulfate 10,000 units. Tube 3.5 g. *Rx.*
Use: Anti-infective; corticosteroid ophthalmic.

bacitracin zinc ointment. (Alpharma) Bacitracin zinc is an anhydrous ointment base. Polymyxin B sulfate 10,000 units, bacitracin zinc 500 units. Oint. Tube 3.5 g. *OTC.*
Use: Anti-infective, topical.

Bacitraycin Plus. (First Aid Research) Bacitracin zinc 500 units/g, pramoxine hydrochloride 10 mg/g. Aloe vera, lt. mineral oil, petrolatum. Oint. 28 g. *OTC.*
Use: Topical anti-infective, antibiotic.

Bacit White. (Whiteworth Towne) Bacitracin. Oint. Tube 0.5 oz, 1 oz. *OTC.*
Use: Anti-infective, topical.

Backache Maximum Strength Relief. (Bristol-Myers Squibb) Magnesium salicylate anhydrous (as tetrahydrate) 467 mg. Cap. Bot. 24s, 50s. *OTC.*
Use: Analgesic.

Back Pain-Off. (Medique Products) Acetaminophen 250 mg, caffeine 50 mg, magnesium salicylate 290 mg. Film coated. Maltodextrin, PEG. Tab. UD 2s (100s, 200s, and 500s). *OTC.*
Use: Nonnarcotic analgesic combination.

•**baclofen.** (BACK-low-fen) *USP. Rx.*
Use: Muscle relaxant.
See: Gablofen.
Lioresal.

baclofen. (Various Mfr.) Baclofen 10 mg, 20 mg. Tab. 30s, 100s, 250s, 500s, 1,000s. *Rx.*
Use: Muscle relaxant.

baclofen. *Rx.*
Use: Treatment of muscle spasticity; dystonia. [Orphan Drug]

l-baclofen. *Rx.*
Use: Trigeminal neuralgia. [Orphan Drug]

Bacmin. (Marnel) Iron 27 mg, Vitamin A 5000 units, E 30 units, C 500 mg, B_1 20 mg, B_2 20 mg, B_3 100 mg, B_5 25 mg, B_6 25 mg, B_{12} 50 mcg, biotin 0.15 mg, folic acid 0.8 mg, Cr, Cu, Mg, Mn, Zn 22.5 mg. Tab. Bot. 100s. *Rx.*
Use: Mineral, vitamin supplement.

Bac-Neo-Poly. (Burgin-Arden) Bacitracin 400 units, neomycin sulfate 5 mg, polymyxin B sulfate 5000 units/g. Oint. Tube 5 oz. *OTC.*
Use: Anti-infective, topical.

Bactal Soap. (Whittaker General) Triclosan 0.5%, anhydrous soap 10%. Liq. Bot. 240 mL, ½ gal. *OTC.*
Use: Antiseptic; cleaner.

•**bacteriostatic water for injection.** *USP.*
Use: Pharmaceutic aid, diluting and dissolving drugs for injection.

bacteriostatic water for injection. (Abbott) 30 mL. Multiple-dose fliptop vial (plastic).
Use: Pharmaceutic aid, diluting and dissolving drugs for injection.

bacteriuria tests. In vitro diagnostic aids.

See: Microstix-3.
Uricult.

Bacti-Cleanse. (Pedinol Pharmacal) Benzalkonium chloride, mineral oil, isopropyl palmitate, cetyl alcohol, glycerine, glyceryl stearate, PEG-100 stearate, dimethicone, diazolidinyl urea, parabens, DMDM hydantoin, EDTA. Liq. Bot. 453.6 g. *OTC.*
Use: Dermatologic cleanser.

Bacticort. (Rugby) Hydrocortisone 1%, neomycin sulfate equivalent to 0.35% neomycin base, polymyxin B sulfate 10,000 units/mL, benzalkonium Cl, cetyl alcohol, glyceryl monostearate, mineral oil, polyoxyl 40 stearate, propylene glycol. Ophth. Soln. Bot. 7.5 mL. *Rx.*
Use: Anti-infective; corticosteroid, ophthalmic.

Bactigen Group A Streptococcus. (Wampole) Latex agglutination slide test for the qualitative detection of group A streptococcal antigen directly from throat swabs. Test kit 60s.
Use: Diagnostic aid.

Bactigen Group A Streptococcus with Gast Trak Slides. (Wampole) Latex agglutination slide test for qualitative detection of group A streptococcal antigen directly from throat swabs. Test 24s. Kit 48s.
Use: Diagnostic aid.

Bactigen H. Influenzae. (Wampole) Rapid latex agglutination slide test for the qualitative detection of *Haemophilus influenzae* type b antigen in cerebrospinal fluid, serum, and urine. Test kit 15s, 30s.
Use: Diagnostic aid.

Bactigen Meningitis Panel. (Wampole) Rapid latex agglutination slide test for the qualitative detection of *Haemophilus influenzae* type b, *Neisseria meningitidis* A/B/C/Y/W135, and *Streptococcus pneumoniae* antigens in cerebrospinal fluid, serum, and urine. Test kit 18s.
Use: Diagnostic aid.

Bactigen Salmonella-Shigella. (Wampole) Latex agglutination slide test for the qualitative detection of *Salmonella* or *Shigella* from cultures. Test kit 96s.
Use: Diagnostic aid.

Bactine Antiseptic Anesthetic. (Bayer Consumer Care) Benzalkonium Cl 0.13%, lidocaine 2.5%, EDTA, alcohol 3.17%. **Spray:** 60 mL, 120 mL, 480 mL. **Aerosol:** 90 g. *OTC.*
Use: Topical local anesthetic.

Bactine First Aid Antibiotic. (Bayer Consumer Care) Polymyxin B sulfate 5000 units, bacitracin 500 units, neomycin sulfate 5 mg/g in mineral oil, white petrolatum. Oint. Tube 15 g. *OTC.*
Use: Anti-infective, topical.

Bactine Hydrocortisone Skin Cream. (Bayer Consumer Care) Hydrocortisone 0.5%. Tube 0.5 oz. *OTC.*
Use: Corticosteroid, topical.

Bactine Maximum Strength. (Bayer Consumer Care) Hydrocortisone 1%, glycerin, mineral oil, methylparaben, white petrolatum. Cream. Tube 30 g. *OTC.*
Use: Corticosteroid, topical.

Bactine Pain Relieving Cleansing. (Bayer Consumer Care) Lidocaine 2.5%, benzalkonium chloride 0.13%. EDTA. Spray. 150 mL. *OTC.*
Use: Topical local anesthetic.

Bactocill. (GlaxoSmithKline) Oxacillin sodium 500 mg, 1 g, 2 g, 4 g, 10 g. Pow. for Inj. Vial (except 10 g); piggyback and *ADD-Vantage* vial (only 1 g and 2 g); Bulk vial (10 g only). *Rx.*
Use: Anti-infective; penicillin.

Bacto Shield Foam. (Steris) Chlorhexidine gluconate 4%, isopropyl alcohol 4%. Foam. Aerosol. 180 mL. *OTC.*
Use: Dermatologic, cleanser.

Bacto Shield Solution. (Steris) Chlorhexidine gluconate 4%, isopropyl alcohol 4%. Soln. Bot. 960 mL. *OTC.*
Use: Dermatologic, cleanser.

Bacto Shield 2. (Steris) Chlorhexidine gluconate 2%, isopropyl alcohol 4%. Soln. Bot. 960 mL. *OTC.*
Use: Preoperative skin preparation, cleanser.

Bactrim. (Roche) Sulfamethoxazole 400 mg, trimethoprim 80 mg. Tab. 100s, 500s. *Rx.*
Use: Anti-infective.

Bactrim DS. (Roche) Trimethoprim 160 mg, sulfamethoxazole 800 mg. Tab. 100s, 500s. *Rx.*
Use: Anti-infective.

Bactrim Suspension. (Roche) Sulfamethoxazole 200 mg, trimethoprim 40 mg/5 mL. Susp. Bot. 16 oz. *Rx.*
Use: Anti-infective.

Bactroban. (GlaxoSmithKline) Mupirocin. **Oint.:** 2% (20 mg/g). Polyethylene glycol base. Tube 22 g. **Cream:** Mupirocin 2% (as calcium 2.15%). Oil/water base, benzyl alcohol, cetyl alcohol, stearyl alcohol. Tubes. 15 g, 30 g. *Rx.*
Use: Topical local anesthetic antibiotic.

Bactroban Nasal. (GlaxoSmithKline) Mupirocin 2% (as calcium 2.15%). Glycerin esters. Oint. 1 g. *Rx.*
Use: Anti-infective used in adult patients and health care workers during institutional outbreaks.

Bacturcult. (Wampole) A urinary bacteria culture medium diagnostic urine culture system for urine collection, bacteriuria screening, and presumptive bacterial identification. Test kit 10s, 100s.
Use: Diagnostic aid.

•**bafetinib.** (ba-FE-ti-nib) USAN. Antineoplastic.

B.A. Gradual. (Federal) Theophylline 260 mg, pseudoephedrine hydrochloride 50 mg, butabarbital 15 mg. Gradual. Bot. 50s, 1000s. *Rx.*
Use: Bronchodilator; decongestant; hypnotic; sedative.

Bain de Soleil All Day For Kids SPF 30. (Procter & Gamble) Ethylhexyl p-methoxycinnamate, 2-ethylhexyl 2-cyano-3, 3-diphenyl acrylate, oxybenzone, titanium dioxide, stearyl alcohol, tocopheryl acetate, EDTA. PABA free. Waterproof. Lot. Bot. 120 mL. *OTC.*
Use: Sunscreen.

Bain de Soleil All Day Waterproof Sunblock. (Procter & Gamble) SPF 15, 30. Ethylhexyl p-methoxycinnamate, 2-ethylhexyl 2-cyano-3, 3-diphenyl acrylate, oxybenzone, titanium dioxide, stearyl alcohol, vitamin E, EDTA. Lot. Bot. 120 mL. *OTC.*
Use: Sunscreen.

Bain de Soleil All Day Waterproof Sunfilter. (Procter & Gamble) SPF 4, 8. 2-ethylhexyl 2-cyano-3, 3-diphenyl acrylate, ethylhexyl p-methoxycinnamate, titanium dioxide, stearyl alcohol, vitamin E, EDTA. Lot. Bot. 120 mL. *OTC.*
Use: Sunscreen.

Bain de Soleil Body Silkening Creme. (Procter & Gamble) Padimate O, ethylhexyl p-methoxycinnamate, oxybenzone, benzyl alcohol. Waterproof. Cream. Bot. 94 g. *OTC.*
Use: Sunscreen.

Bain de Soleil Body Silkening Spray. (Procter & Gamble) Padimate O, oxybenzone, ethylhexyl p-methoxycinnamate. Waterproof. Lot. Bot. 240 mL. *OTC.*
Use: Sunscreen.

Bain de Soleil Body Silkening Stick. (Procter & Gamble) Padimate O, ethylhexyl p-methoxycinnamate, oxybenzone, dioxybenzone. Stick 53 g. *OTC.*
Use: Sunscreen.

Bain de Soleil Face Creme. (Procter & Gamble) Padimate O, ethylhexyl p-methoxycinnamate, oxybenzone. Waterproof. Cream. Bot. 60 g. *OTC.*
Use: Sunscreen.

Bain de Soleil Kids Sport. (Procter & Gamble) SPF 25. Ethylhexyl p-methoxycinnamate, 2-ethylhexyl 2-cyano-3, 3-diphenyl acrylate, titanium dioxide, PVP/eicosene copolymer, dimethicone, cyclomethicone, triethanolamine, glyceryl tribehenate, tocopheryl acetate, carbomer, EDTA, DMDM hydantoin. PABA free. Waterproof, all day protection. Lot. Bot. 120 mL. *OTC.*
Use: Sunscreen.

Bain de Soleil Lip Protecteur. (Procter & Gamble) Ethylhexyl p-methoxycinnamate, oxybenzone, 2-ethylhexyl salicylate, oleyl alcohol, petrolatum. PABA free. Lip balm 3 g. *OTC.*
Use: Sunscreen.

Bain de Soleil Megatan. (Procter & Gamble) Ethylhexyl p-methoxycinnamate, 2-ethylhexyl salicylate, lanolin, cocoa butter, palm oil, aloe, DMDM hydantoin, xanthan gum, shea butter, EDTA. Lot. Bot. 120 mL. *OTC.*
Use: Sunscreen.

Bain de Soleil Orange Gelee SPF 4. (Procter & Gamble) Ethylhexyl p-methoxycinnamate, 2-ethylhexyl salicylate. PABA free. Gel. Tube 93.75 g. *OTC.*
Use: Sunscreen.

Bain de Soleil SPF 8+ Color. (Procter & Gamble) Octyl methoxycinnamate, octocrylene, mineral oil, cetyl alcohol, EDTA. Lot. Bot. 118 mL. *OTC.*
Use: Sunscreen.

Bain de Soleil SPF 15+ Color. (Procter & Gamble) Octyl methoxycinnamate, octocrylene, oxybenzone, mineral oil, cetyl alcohol, EDTA. Lot. Bot. 118 mL. *OTC.*
Use: Sunscreen.

Bain de Soleil SPF 30+ Color. (Procter & Gamble) Octocrylene, octyl methoxycinnamate, oxybenzone, mineral oil, cetyl alcohol, EDTA. Lot. Bot. 118 mL. *OTC.*
Use: Sunscreen.

Bain de Soleil Sport. (Procter & Gamble) SPF 15. 2-ethylhexyl 2-cyano-3, 3-diphenyl acrylate, ethylhexyl p-methoxycinnamate, titanium dioxide, dimethicone, cyclomethicone, panthenol, tocopheryl acetate, carbomer, EDTA, DMDM hydantoin. PABA free. Waterproof, sweatproof, all day protection. Lot. Bot. 180 mL. *OTC.*
Use: Sunscreen.

Bain de Soleil Tropical Deluxe SPF 4. (Procter & Gamble) Ethylhexyl p-methoxycinnamate, 2-ethylhexyl salicylate, cetyl alcohol, EDTA. PABA free. Waterproof. Lot. Bot. 240 mL. *OTC.*
Use: Sunscreen.

Bain de Soleil Under Eye. (Procter & Gamble) Ethylhexyl p-methoxycinna-

mate, oxybenzone, 2-ethylhexyl salicylate. Stick 1.5 g. *OTC.*
Use: Sunscreen.

Bakers Best. (Scherer) Water, alcohol 38%, propylene glycol, extract of capsicum, glycerin, boric acid, Tween 80, diethylphthalate, rose oil, pyrilamine maleate, glacial acetic acid, Uvinul MS 40, hexetidine, benzalkonium Cl 50%, sodium hydroxide 76%. Bot. 8 oz. *OTC.*
Use: Antipruritic; antiseborrheic, topical.

•**balafilcon A.** (ba-lah-FILL-kahn A) USAN.
Use: Contact lens material, hydrophilic.

Balamine DM. (Ballay) Chlorpheniramine maleate 2 mg, dextromethorphan hydrobromide 10 mg, phenylephrine hydrochloride 5 mg. Glycerin, sodium benzoate, sorbitol, strawberry flavoring. Alcohol free, dye free, sugar free. Syrup. 473 mL. *OTC.*
Use: Upper respiratory combination, antitussive combination.

Balanced B_{100}. (Fibertone) Vitamins B_1 100 mg, B_2 100 mg, B_3 100 mg, B_5 100 mg, B_6 100 mg, B_{12} 100 mcg, folic acid 0.1 mg, PABA 100 mg, inositol 100 mg, d-biotin 100 mcg. SR Tab. Bot. 50s. *OTC.*
Use: Mineral, vitamin supplement.

Balanced Salt Solution. (Various Mfr.) Sodium Cl 0.64%, potassium Cl 0.075%, calcium Cl 0.048%, magnesium Cl 0.03%, sodium acetate 0.39%, sodium citrate 0.17%, sodium hydroxide or hydrochloric acid. Soln. *Drop-Tainer* 18 mL, 500 mL.
Use: Irrigant, ophthalmic.

•**balapiravir.** (BAL-a-PIR-a-vir) USAN.
Use: Anti-infective.

•**balapiravir hydrochloride.** (BAL-a-PIR-a-vir) USAN.
Use: Anti-infective.

Baldex Ophthalmic. (Bausch & Lomb) Dexamethasone phosphate. **Oint.:** 0.05%. Tube 3.75 g. **Soln.:** 0.01%. Dropper Bot. 5 mL. *Rx.*
Use: Corticosteroid, ophthalmic.

BAL in Oil. (Akorn) 2, 3-dimercaptopropanol 100 mg, benzylbenzoate 210 mg, peanut oil 680 mg/mL. Amp. 3 mL. Box 10s. *Rx.*
Use: Antidote.

Balmex. (Block Drug) Zinc oxide. **Cream:** 11.3%. Mineral oil, parabens, soybean oil. 118 g. **Oint.:** 11.3%, aloe vera gel, parabens, mineral oil. Tubes. 30 g, 60 g, 120 g, 454 g. *OTC.*
Use: Emollient.

Balmex Baby Powder. (Block Drug) Specially purified balsam Peru, zinc oxide, starch, calcium carbonate. Shaker top can. 4 oz. *OTC.*
Use: Adsorbent, emollient.

Balmex Diaper Rash Cream Stick. (Chattem) Zinc oxide 11.3%, soybean oil, parabens, mineral oil, evening primrose seed extract, olive leaf extract, propylene glycol, beeswax, benzoic acid, dimethicone. Cream. 56 g. *OTC.*
Use: Diaper rash product.

Balneol. (Alaven) Glyceryl, lanolin oil, mineral oil, methylparaben, PEG-4, PEG-40, PG-100, propylene glycol. Lot. 88 mL. *OTC.*
Use: Anorectal preparation, perianal hygiene product.

Balneol For Her. (Alaven) Glyceryl, lanolin oil, mineral oil, methylparaben, PEG-4, PEG-40, PEG-100, propylene glycol. Lot. 89 mL. *OTC.*
Use: Anorectal preparation, perianal hygiene product.

Balneol For Her Convenience Packets. (Alaven) Glyceryl, hydrocortisone 0.25%, lanolin oil, methylparaben, mineral oil, PEG-4, PEG-40, PEG-100, propylene glycol. Lot. 20s. *OTC.*
Use: Anorectal preparation, perianal hygiene product.

Balneol Hygienic Cleansing. (Alaven) Mineral oil, lanolin oil, methylparaben. Bot. 120 mL. *Formerly Balneol Perianal Cleansing. OTC.*
Use: Anorectal preparation.

Balnetar. (Westwood Squibb) Coal tar 2.5% in mineral oil, lanolin oil. Liq. 221 mL. *OTC.*
Use: Dermatologic.

•**balsalazide disodium.** (bahl-SAL-ah-zide) USAN.
Use: Anti-inflammatory, gastrointestinal agent.
See: Colazal.

balsalazide disodium. (Various Mfr.) Balsalazide disodium 750 mg. Sodium ≈ 79 to 86 mg. Cap. 30s, 280, 350s, 500s, UD 100s. *Rx.*
Use: Anti-inflammatory, gastrointestinal agent.

balsam Peru.
W/Combinations.
See: Vasolex.
Xenaderm-T.

Balsan. Specially purified balsam Peru.
See: Balmex Baby Powder.

•**balugrastim.** (BAL-ue-GRA-stim) USAN.
Use: Hematopoietic agent, colony-stimulating factor.

Balziva. (Barr Laboratories) Ethinyl estradiol 35 mcg, norethindrone 0.4 mg. Lactose. Tab. 28s with 7 inert tablets. *Rx.*
Use: Contraceptive hormone, sex hormone.

•**bambermycins.** (BAM-ber-MY-sinz) USAN.
Use: Anti-infective.

•**bamethan sulfate.** (BAM-eth-an) USAN.
Use: Vasodilator.

•**bamifylline hydrochloride.** (BAM-ih-FILL-in) USAN.
Use: Bronchodilator.

•**bamnidazole.** (bam-NIH-DAH-zole) USAN.
Use: Antiprotozoal, trichomonas.

Banacid. (Buffington) Magnesium trisilicate 220 mg. Tab. Bot. 100s, 200s, 500s. *OTC.*
Use: Antacid.

Banadyne-3. (Norstar Consumer) Lidocaine 4%, menthol 1%, alcohol 45%. Soln. Bot. 7.5 mL. *OTC.*
Use: Mouth and throat preparation.

B & A. (Eastern Research) Sodium bicarbonate, potassium, aluminum, borax. Hygienic pow. Jar 8 oz, 5 lb. *Rx.*
Use: Vaginal agent.

•**bandage, adhesive.** *USP.*
Use: Surgical aid.

•**bandage, gauze.** *USP.*
Use: Surgical aid.

B and O Supprettes No. 15A & No. 16A. (Amerifit) Opium 30 mg, 60 mg, belladonna extract 16.2 mg. Supp. Jar 12s. *c-II.*
Use: Analgesic; antispasmodic; narcotic.

Banflex. (Forest Pharm) Orphenadrine citrate 30 mg/mL. Inj. Vial 10 mL. *Rx.*
Use: Muscle relaxant.

Bangesic. (H.L. Moore Drug Exchange) Menthol, camphor, methyl salicylate, eucalyptus oil in nongreasy base. Bot. 2 oz, gal. *OTC.*
Use: Analgesic, topical.

Banocide.
See: Diethylcarbamazine citrate.

Banophen. (Major) Diphenhydramine hydrochloride. **Tab.:** 25 mg. Bot. 24s, 100s. **Cap.:** 25 mg. Bot. 24s, 100s. *OTC.*
Use: Antihistamine, nonselective ethanolamine.

Banophen Allergy. (Major) Diphenhydramine hydrochloride 12.5 mg/5 mL. Glycerin, saccharin, sodium 5 mg, sodium benzoate, sorbitol. Alcohol free. Cherry flavor. Liq. 118 mL. *OTC.*
Use: Antihistamine, nonselective ethanolamine.

Banophen Children's Allergy. (Major) Diphenhydramine hydrochloride 12.5 mg per 5 mL. Corn syrup, glycerin, sodium 15 mg, sodium benzoate, sorbitol. Alcohol free. Cherry flavor. Liq. 118 mL. *OTC.*
Use: Antihistamine, nonselective ethanolamine.

Banophen Decongestant. (Major) Diphenhydramine 25 mg, pseudoephedrine 60 mg. Cap. 24s. *OTC.*
Use: Antihistamine; decongestant.

Bansmoke. (Thompson Medical) Benzocaine 6 mg, corn syr., dextrose, lecithin, sucrose. Gum. Pack 24s. *OTC.*
Use: Smoking deterrent.

Banzel. (Eisai) Rufinamide. **Tab.:** 200 mg, 400 mg. Film coated. Lactose, PEG. 30s (200 mg), 120s (400 mg). **Susp.:** 40 mg/mL. Parabens, potassium sorbate, propylene glycol. Orange flavor. 460 mL. *Rx.*
Use: Anticonvulsant.

•**bapineuzumab.** (BAP-ee-NUE-zoo-mab) USAN.
Use: Alzheimer disease.

Baraclude. (Bristol-Myers Squibb Company) Entecavir. **Oral Soln.:** 0.05 mg/mL. Parabens. Orange flavor. 210 mL. **Tab.:** 0.5 mg, 1 mg. Lactose. Film-coated. 30s. *Rx.*
Use: Antiviral agent.

Barbased. (Major) **Tab.:** Butabarbital 0.25 g, 0.5 g. Tab. Bot. 1000s. **Elix.:** Butabarbital 30 mg/5 mL, alcohol 7%. Bot. 480 mL. *Rx.*
Use: Hypnotic; sedative.

Barbatose No. 2. (Pal-Pak, Inc.) Barbital 64.8 mg, hyoscyamus sulfate, passiflora, valerian. Tab. Bot. 1000s. *Rx.*
Use: Sedative.

Barbella Elixir. (Forest) Phenobarbital 0.25 g, hyoscyamine sulfate 0.1037 mg, atropine sulfate 0.0194 mg, scopolamine HBr 0.0065 mg, alcohol 24%/5 mL. Elix. Bot. 4 oz, gal. *Rx.*
Use: Anticholinergic; antispasmodic; hypnotic; sedative.

Barbella Tablets. (Forest) Phenobarbital 16.2 mg, atropine sulfate 0.0194 mg, hyoscyamine sulfate 0.1037 mg, hyoscine HBr 0.0065 mg. Tab. Bot. 100s, 1000s, 5000s. *Rx.*
Use: Anticholinergic; antispasmodic; hypnotic; sedative.

Barbeloid. (Pal-Pak, Inc.) Phenobarbital 16.2 mg, hyoscyamine sulfate 0.1037 mg, atropine sulfate 0.0194 mg, scopolamine HBr 0.0065 mg. Tab. Bot. 100s, 1000s. *Rx.*
Use: Anticholinergic; antispasmodic; hypnotic; sedative.

Barbenyl.
See: Phenobarbital.

Barbiphenyl.
See: Phenobarbital.

barbital. Barbitone, Deba, Dormonal, Hypnogene, Malonal, Sedeval, Uronal, Veronal, Vesperal, diethylbarbituric acid, diethylmalonylurea.
Use: Hypnotic; sedative.

barbital sodium. Barbitone sodium, diethylbarbiturate monosodium, diethylmalonylurea sodium, Embinal, Medinal, Veronal sodium.
Use: Hypnotic; sedative.

barbitone.
See: Barbital.

barbitone sodium.
See: Barbital Sodium.

barbiturate-aspirin combinations.
See: Aspirin-barbiturate combinations.

barbiturates.
See: Methohexital Sodium.

barbiturates, intermediate duration.
See: Butabarbital.

barbiturates, long duration.
See: Barbital.
Mebaral.
Mephobarbital.
Phenobarbital.
Phenobarbital Sodium.

barbiturates, short duration.
See: Amobarbital.
Amobarbital Sodium.
Butalbital.
Pentobarbital Salts.
Secobarbital.

barbiturates, ultrashort duration.
See: Pentothal Sodium.
Thiopental Sodium.

•**bardoxolone.** (bar-DOX-oh-lone) USAN.
Use: Anti-inflammatory.

•**bardoxolone methyl.** (bar-DOX-oh-lone) USAN.
Use: Anti-inflammatory.

•**baricitinib.** (BAR-i-SYE-ti-nib) USAN.
Use: Immunomodulator.

Baricon. (Mallinckrodt) Barium sulfate 98%. Simethicone, sorbitol, sucrose, lemon-vanilla flavor. Pow. for Susp. UD 340 g. *Rx.*
Use: Radiopaque agent, GI contrast agent.

Baridium. (Pfeiffer) Phenazopyridine hydrochloride 100 mg. Tab. Bot. 32s. *OTC.*
Use: Interstitial cystitis agent.

Bari-Stress M. (Alpharma) Vitamins B_1 10 mg, B_2 10 mg, niacinamide 100 mg, C 300 mg, B_6 2 mg, B_{12} 4 mcg, folic acid 1.5 mg, calcium pantothenate 20 mg. **Cap.:** Bot. 30s, 100s, 1000s. **Tab.:** Bot. 100s, 1000s. *Rx.*
Use: Mineral, vitamin supplement.

•**barium hydroxide lime.** (BA-ree-uhm) *USP.*
Use: Carbon dioxide absorbent.

•**barium sulfate.** (BA-ree-uhm) *USP.* Paste; For suspension; Suspension; Tablets.
Use: Radiopaque agent, miscellaneous GI contrast agent.
See: Anatrast.
Baricon.
Barobag.
Baro-cat.
Barosperse.
Bar-test.
Bear-E-Yum CT.
Bear-E-Yum GI.
Cheetah.
Digibar 190.
Enecat CT.
Enhancer.
Entero VU.
Entrobar.
Epi-C.
E-Z-HD.
E-Z-Paque.
E-Z-Paque Liquid.
E-Z-Paste.
Flo-Coat.
HD 85.
HD 200 Plus.
Imager ac.
Intropaste.
Liqui-Coat HD.
Liquid Barosperse.
Liquid Polibar.
Liquid Polibar Plus.
Medebar Plus.
MedeScan.
Prepcat.
Readi-Cat.
Readi-Cat 2.
Tomocat.
Tonopaque.
Varibar Honey.
Varibar Nectar.
Varibar Pudding.
Varibar Thin Honey.
Varibar Thin Liquid.

barium sulfate preparation.
See: Fleet.

Barlevite. (Barth's) Vitamins B_6 0.6 mg, B_{12} 3 mcg, pantothenic acid 0.6 mg, D 3 units, l-lysine 20 mg/0.6 mL. 100-day supply. *OTC.*
Use: Vitamin, mineral supplement.

•**barmastine.** (BAR-mast-een) USAN.
Use: Antihistamine.

BarnesHind Cleaning and Soaking Solution. (PBH Wesley Jessen) Cleaning and buffering agents, benzalkonium chloride 0.01%, disodium edetate 0.2%.

Soln. Bot. 1.2 oz, 4 oz. *OTC.*
Use: Contact lens care.

BarnesHind Wetting & Soaking Solution. (PBH Wesley Jessen) Polyvinyl alcohol, povidone, hydroxyethyl cellulose, octylphenoxy (oxyethylene) ethanol, benzalkonium chloride, edetate disodium. Soln. Bot. 4 oz. *OTC.*
Use: Contact lens care.

BarnesHind Wetting Solution. (PBH Wesley Jessen) Polyvinyl alcohol, edetate disodium 0.02%, benzalkonium chloride 0.004%. Soln. Bot. 35 mL, 60 mL. *OTC.*
Use: Contact lens care.

Barobag. (Mallinckrodt) Barium sulfate 95%. Simethicone. Vanilla flavor. Pow. for Susp. Enema kit. 340 g, 454 g. UD bot. 225 g, 900 g. Bulk. 25 lb. *Rx.*
Use: Radiopaque agent, GI contrast agent.

Baro-Cat. (Mallinckrodt) Barium sulfate 1.5%. Simethicone, sorbitol, pineapple-banana flavor. Susp. Bot. 300 mL, 900 mL, 1900 mL. *Rx.*
Use: Radiopaque agent, GI contrast agent.

Baroset. (Lafayette) Air contrast stomach. Unit-of-use kit. Case 12s.
Use: Radiopaque agent.

barosmin.
See: Diosmin.

Barosperse. (Mallinckrodt) Barium sulfate 95%. Simethicone, sorbitol, cherry flavor. Pow. for Susp. UD Bot. 180 g, 1200 g. Container. 25 lb. *Rx.*
Use: Radiopaque agent, GI contrast agent.

Bar-test. (Glenwood) Barium sulfate 650 mg. Tab. 100s. *Rx.*
Use: Radiopaque agent, GI contrast agent.

Basa. (Freeport) Acetylsalicylic acid 324 mg. Tab. Bot. 1000s. *OTC.*
Use: Analgesic.

basic aluminum carbonate.
See: Basaljel.

basic aluminum glycinate.
See: Dihydroxyaluminum aminoacetate.

basic bismuth carbonate.
See: Bismuth subcarbonate.

basic bismuth gallate.
See: Bismuth subgallate.

basic bismuth nitrate.
See: Bismuth subnitrate.

basic bismuth salicylate.
See: Bismuth subsalicylate.

basic fuchsin.
See: Carbol-Fuchsin.

•**basifungin.** (bass-ih-FUN-jin) USAN.
Use: Antifungal.

•**basiliximab.** (bass-ih-LICK-sih-mab) USAN.
Use: Immunosuppressant.
See: Simulect.

Basis, Glycerin Soap. (Beiersdorf) Tallow, coconut oil, glycerin. Sensitive and normal to dry. Bar 90 g, 150 g. *OTC.*
Use: Dermatologic, cleanser.

Basis, Superfatted Soap. (Beiersdorf) Sodium tallowate, sodium cocoate, petrolatum, glycerin, zinc oxide, sodium Cl, titanium dioxide, lanolin, alcohol, beeswax, BHT, EDTA. Bar 99 g, 225 g. *OTC.*
Use: Dermatologic, cleanser.

•**batabulin sodium.** (bat-a-BUE-lin) USAN.
Use: Antineoplastic agent.

•**batanopride hydrochloride.** (bah-TAN-oh-pride) USAN.
Use: Antiemetic.

•**batefenterol.** (BA-te-FEN-ter-ol) USAN.
Use: Bronchodilator, sympathomimetic.

•**batefenterol succinate.** (BA-te-FEN-ter-ol) USAN.
Use: Bronchodilator, sympathomimetic.

•**batelapine maleate.** (bat-EH-lap-EEN) USAN.
Use: Antipsychotic.

•**batimastat.** (bat-IM-ah-stat) USAN.
Use: Antineoplastic.

•**bavisant.** (BAV-i-sant) USAN.
Use: CNS agent.

•**bavisant dihydrochloride.** (BAV- i-sant) USAN.
Use: CNS agent.

•**bavituximab.** (bav-i-TUX-i-mab) USAN.
Use: Antineoplastic.

Baycadron. (Wockhardt) Dexamethasone 0.5 mg per 5 mL. Alcohol 5.1%, benzoic acid 0.1%, sugar. Raspberry flavor. Elix. 237 mL.
Use: Corticosteroid.

Bayer Aspirin, Genuine. (Bayer Consumer Care) Aspirin 325 mg. Tab. Bot. 50s, 100s, 200s, 300s. Pkg. 12s, 24s. *OTC.*
Use: Analgesic.

Bayer Aspirin, Maximum. (Bayer Consumer Care) Aspirin 500 mg. Tab. Bot. 30s, 60s, 100s. *OTC.*
Use: Analgesic.

Bayer Buffered Aspirin. (Bayer Consumer Care) Buffered aspirin 325 mg. Tab. Bot. 100s. *OTC.*
Use: Analgesic.

Bayer Children's Chewable Aspirin. (Bayer Consumer Care) Aspirin 1.25 g (81 mg). Chew. Tab. Bot. 30s. *OTC.*
Use: Analgesic.

Bayer 8-Hour Timed-Release Aspirin. (Bayer Consumer Care) Aspirin 10 g (650 mg). TR Tab. Bot. 30s, 72s, 125s. *OTC.*
Use: Analgesic.

Bayer Enteric Coated Caplets, Regular Strength. (Bayer Consumer Care) Aspirin 325 mg. EC Tab. Bot. 50s, 100s. *OTC.*
Use: Analgesic.

Bayer Enteric 500 Aspirin, Extra Strength. (Bayer Consumer Care) Aspirin 500 mg. EC Tab. Bot. 60s. *OTC.*
Use: Analgesic.

Bayer Extra Strength Advanced Aspirin. (Bayer Consumer Care) Aspirin 500 mg. Sodium 72 mg. Tab. 20s, 40s, 80s. *OTC.*
Use: Salicylate.

Bayer Extra Strength Back & Body Pain. (Bayer Consumer Care) Aspirin 500 mg, caffeine 32.5 mg. Tab. 50s, 100s. *OTC.*
Use: Analgesic; CNS stimulant.

Bayer Low Adult Strength. (Bayer Consumer Care) Aspirin 81 mg, lactose. DR Tab. Bot. 120s. *OTC.*
Use: Analgesic.

Bayer Migraine. (Bayer Consumer Care) Acetaminophen 250 mg, aspirin 250 mg, caffeine 65 mg. Saccharin. Tab. 50s, 200s. *OTC.*
Use: Nonnarcotic analgesic combination.

Bayer Muscle & Joint Cream. (Bayer Consumer Care) Menthol 10%, camphor 4%, methyl salicylate 30%. EDTA, glyceryl, lanolin, stearyl alcohol. Cream 56 g, 114 g. *OTC.*
Use: Rub and liniment.

Bayer PM Extra Strength Aspirin Plus Sleep Aid. (Bayer Consumer Care) Aspirin 500 mg, diphenhydramine hydrochloride 25 mg. Cap. 24s. *OTC.*
Use: Analgesic.

Bayer Quick Release Crystals. (Bayer Consumer Care) Aspirin 850 mg, caffeine 65 mg. Acesulfame K, aspartame, phenylalanine 6 mg per packet, sucralose. Crystals. 20s. *OTC.*
Use: Nonnarcotic analgesic combination.

Bayer Select Chest Cold. (Bayer Consumer Care) Dextromethorphan HBr 15 mg, acetaminophen 500 mg. Cap. Pkg. 16s. *OTC.*
Use: Analgesic; antitussive.

Bayer Select Maximum Strength Backache. (Bayer Consumer Care) Magnesium salicylate tetrahydrate 580 mg. Cap. Bot. 24s, 50s. *OTC.*
Use: Analgesic.

Bayer Select Maximum Strength Night Time Pain Relief. (Bayer Consumer Care) Acetaminophen 500 mg, diphenhydramine hydrochloride. Tab. Bot. 24s, 50s. *OTC.*
Use: Antihistamine.

Bayer Select Maximum Strength Sinus Pain Relief. (Bayer Consumer Care) Acetaminophen 500 mg, pseudoephedrine hydrochloride 30 mg. Tab. Bot. 50s. *OTC.*
Use: Analgesic; decongestant.

Bayer Women's Aspirin Plus Calcium. (Bayer Consumer Care) Aspirin 81 mg, calcium 300 mg, lactose, mineral oil, polydextrose. Tab. 60s, 90s. *OTC.*
Use: Analgesic; mineral supplement.

Baylocaine 4%. (Bay Labs) Lidocaine 4% w/methylparaben. Soln. Bot. 50 mL, 100 mL.
Use: Anesthetic, local.

Baylocaine 2% Viscous. (Bay Labs) Lidocaine 2% w/sodium carboxymethylcellulose. Soln. Bot. 100 mL. *OTC.*
Use: Local anesthetic, topical.

BayRho-D. (Bayer) Rh_o(D) immune globulin (human). Prefilled single-dose syringe. Single-dose syringe. Single-dose vial. *Rx.*
Use: Immunization.

BayRho-D Full Dose Pharmaceutical. (Bayer) Rh_o(D) immune globulin 15% to 18% protein. Glycine 0.21 to 0.32 M, solvent/detergent treated, preservative free. Soln. for Inj. Individual and multiple-pack single-dose syringes w/attached needles and vials. *Rx.*
Use: Immune globulin.

Baza Antifungal. (Coloplast) Miconazole nitrate 2%. Alcohol, cod liver oil, glyceryl, lanolin oil, PEG, petrolatum, propylene glycol, urea, zinc oxide. Cream. 57 g. *OTC.*
Use: Topical anti-infective, antifungal.

•**bazedoxifene acetate.** (bay-ze-DOX-i-feen) USAN.
Use: Osteoporosis; estrogen receptor modulator.
W/Conjugated Estrogens.
See: Duavee.

BCAD 2. (Mead Johnson Nutritionals) Protein 24 g (L-glutamine, potassium aspartate, L-lysine hydrochloride, L-tyrosine, L-proline, L-alanine, L-arginine, L-phenylalanine, L-threonine, L-serine, glycine, L-histidine, L-methionine, L-tryptophan, L-cystine, L-carnitine, taurine), carbohydrate 57 g (corn syr. solids, sugar, modified corn starch), fat 8.5 g (soy oil)/100 g, vitamins, A, B_1, B_2, B_3, B_5, B_6, B_{12}, C, D, E, K, biotin, cho-

line, folic acid, inositol, Ca, chloride, Cr, Cu, Fe, I, Mg, Mn, Mo, P, Se, Zn, Na 610 mg, K 1220 mg/g, 410 cal/100 g. Pow. Can 1 lb. *OTC.*
Use: Enteral nutritional therapy.

BC Allergy, Sinus, Headache. (GlaxoSmithKline Consumer Healthcare) Pseudoephedrine hydrochloride 60 mg, chlorpheniramine maleate 4 mg, acetaminophen 650 mg. Pow. 6s, 12s. *OTC.*
Use: Decongestant, antihistamine, and analgesic combination, upper respiratory combination.

BC Arthritis Strength. (Block Drug) Aspirin 742 mg, salicylamide 222 mg, caffeine 36 mg. Pow. Bot. 6s, 24s, 50s. *OTC.*
Use: Analgesic combination.

BC Fast Pain Relief. (GlaxoSmithKline Consumer Healthcare) Aspirin 845 mg, caffeine 65 mg. Lactose, potassium 55 mg per packet. Pow. 2s, 6s, 24s. *OTC.*
Use: Analgesic combination.

BC Fast Pain Relief Arthritis. (GlaxoSmithKline Consumer Health Care) Aspirin 1,000 mg, caffeine 65 mg. Potassium 65 mg per packet, lactose. Pow. 2s, 6s, 50s. *OTC.*
Use: Nonnarcotic analgesic combination.

BCG, live.
Use: Biological response modifier.
See: TheraCys.
Tice BCG.

•**BCG vaccine.** *USP.*
Use: Active immunization, bacterial vaccine.
See: BCG vaccine.
TheraCys.

BCG vaccine. (Organon) Tice strain (1 to 8×10^8 CFU equiv. to ≈ 50 mg). Preservative free. Pow. for Inj., lyophilized. Vials. *Rx.*
Use: Active immunization, bacterial vaccine.

BCNU.
Use: Antineoplastic.
See: BiCNU.

BCO. (Western Research) Vitamins B_1 10 mg, B_2 2 mg, B_6 1.5 mg, B_{12} 25 mcg, niacinamide 50 mg. Tab. Bot. 1000s. *OTC.*
Use: Vitamin supplement.

B-Com. (Century) Vitamins B_1 3 mg, B_2 3 mg, B_6 0.5 mg, niacinamide 20 mg, calcium pantothenate 5 mg, B_{12} 1 mcg, desiccated liver (undefatted) 60 mg, debittered brewer's dried yeast 60 mg. Cap. Bot. 100s, 1000s. *OTC.*
Use: Mineral, vitamin supplement.

B•Compleet•50. (J.R. Carlson) Vitamins B_1 50 mg, B_2 50 mg, B_3 100 mg, B_5 200 mg, B_6 50 mg, B_{12} 50 mcg, biotin 50 mg, choline 50 mg, folic acid 0.4 mg, inositol 50 mg, PABA 50 mg. Maltodextrin. Gluten free, preservative free, soy free, and sugar free. Tab. 250s. *OTC.*
Use: Multivitamin.

B•Compleet•100. (J.R. Carlson) Vitamins B_1 100 mg, B_2 100 mg, B_3 100 mg, B_5 100 mg, B_6 100 mg, B_{12} 100 mcg, biotin 100 mg, choline 100 mg, folic acid 0.4 mg, inositol 100 mg, PABA 100 mg. Gluten free, preservative free, soy free, and sugar free. Tab. 100s. *OTC.*
Use: Multivitamin.

B-Complex and B_{12}. (NBTY) Vitamins B_1 7 mg, B_2 14 mg, B_3 4.5 mg, B_{12} 25 mcg, protease 10 mg. Tab. Bot. 90s. *OTC.*
Use: Vitamin supplement.

B-Complex Capsules. (Arcum) Vitamins B_1 1.5 mg, B_2 2 mg, niacinamide 10 mg, B_6 0.1 mg, calcium pantothenate 1 mg, desiccated liver 70 mg, dried yeast 100 mg. Cap. Bot. 100s, 1000s. *OTC.*
Use: Mineral, vitamin supplement.

B-Complex Capsules J.F. (Bryant) Vitamins B_1 1 mg, B_2 0.3 mg, nicotinic acid 0.3 mg, B_6 0.25 mg, desiccated liver 0.15 g, yeast powder, dried 0.15 g. Cap. Bot. 100s, 1000s. *OTC.*
Use: Mineral, vitamin supplement.

B-Complex Elixir. (Nion Corp.) B_1 2.3 mg, B_2 1 mg, B_3 6.7 mg, B_6 0.3 mg, alcohol 10%. Elix. Bot. 240 mL, 480 mL. *OTC.*
Use: Mineral, vitamin supplement.

B-Complex-50. (Nion Corp.) Vitamins B_1 50 mg, B_2 50 mg, B_3 50 mg, B_5 50 mg, B_6 50 mg, B_{12} 50 mcg, FA 0.4 mg, biotin 50 mcg, PABA 50 mg, choline bitartrate 50 mg, inositol 50 mg. SR Tab. Bot. 100s. *OTC.*
Use: Mineral, vitamin supplement.

B-Complex "50". (Vitaline) Vitamins B_1 50 mg, B_2 50 mg, B_3 50 mg, B_4 50 mg, B_5 50 mg, B_6 50 mg, B_{12} 50 mcg, FA 0.1 mg, PABA 30 mg, inositol 50 mg, biotin 50 mcg, choline bitartrate 50 mg. Reg. or TR Tab. Bot. 90s, 1000s. *OTC.*
Use: Vitamin supplement.

B-Complex 100. (Rabin-Winters) Vitamins B_1 100 mg, B_2 2 mg, B_6 2 mg, niacinamide 125 mg, panthenol 10 mg/mL. Inj. Vial 30 mL. *Rx.*
Use: Vitamin supplement.

B-Complex-150. (Nion Corp.) Vitamins B_1 150 mg, B_2 150 mg, B_3 150 mg, B_5 150 mg, B_6 150 mg, B_{12} 1 mcg, FA 0.4 mg, biotin 150 mcg, PABA 100 mg,

choline bitartrate 150 mg, inositol 150 mg. SR Tab. Bot. 30s. *OTC.*
Use: Mineral, vitamin supplement.

B-Complex 100/100. (Sandia) Vitamins B_1 100 mg, B_2 2 mg, B_6 2 mg, niacinamide 100 mg/mL. Inj. Vial 30 mL. *Rx.*
Use: Vitamin supplement.

B-Complex + C. (NBTY) Vitamins C 200 mg, B_1 10 mg, B_2 10 mg, B_3 50 mg, B_5 10 mg, B_6 5 mg. Tab. Bot. 100s. *OTC.*
Use: Vitamin supplement.

B Complex + C. (Various Mfr.) Vitamins B_1 15 mg, B_2 10 mg, B_3 100 mg, B_5 20 mg, B_6 5 mg, B_{12} 10 mcg, C 500 mg. Tab. Bot. 100s. *OTC.*
Use: Vitamin supplement.

B-Complex 25-25. (Forest) Niacinamide 100 mg, vitamins B_1 25 mg, B_2 1 mg, B_6 2 mg, pantothenic acid 2 mg/mL. Inj. Vial 30 mL. *Rx.*
Use: Vitamin supplement.

B-Complex/Vitamin C Caplets. (Geneva) Vitamins B_1 15 mg, B_2 10.2 mg, B_3 50 mg, B_5 10 mg, B_6 5 mg, C 300 mg. Cap. Bot. 100s. *OTC.*
Use: Vitamin supplement.

B-Complex with B-12. (Ivax) B_1 1.5 mg, B_2 1.7 mg, B_3 20 mg, B_5 10 mg, B_6 2 mg, B_{12} 6 mcg, FA 0.4 mg. Tab. Bot. 100s. *OTC.*
Use: Mineral, vitamin supplement.

B Complex with B_{12} Capsules. (Bryant) Vitamins B_1 2 mg, B_2 2 mg, B_6 0.5 mg, niacinamide 10 mg, B_{12} 2 mcg, biotin 10 mcg, calcium pantothenate 1.5 mg, choline dihydrogen citrate 40 mg, inositol 30 mg, desiccated liver 1 g, brewer's yeast 3 g. Cap. Bot. 100s, 1000s. *OTC.*
Use: Mineral, vitamin supplement.

B Complex with C and B-12. (Ivax) Vitamins B_1 50 mg, B_2 5 mg, B_3 125 mg, B_5 6 mg, B_6 5 mg, B_{12} 1000 mcg, C 50 mg. Inj. Vial 10 mL. *Rx.*
Use: Vitamin supplement.

B-Complex with Vitamin C and B_{12}-10,000. (Fujisawa Healthcare) Vitamins B_1 20 mg, B_2 3 mg, B_3 75 mg, B_5 5 mg, B_6 5 mg, B_{12} 1000 mcg, C 100 mg. Covial. 10 mL multiple dose. *Rx.*
Use: Vitamin supplement.

BC-1000. (Solvay) Vitamins B_1 50 mg, B_2 5 mg, B_{12} 1000 mcg, B_6 5 mg, d-panthenol 6 mg, niacinamide 125 mg, ascorbic acid 50 mg, benzyl alcohol 1%/mL. Vial 10 mL. *OTC.*
Use: Vitamin supplement.

BC Powder, Arthritis Strength. (GlaxoSmithKline Consumer Healthcare) Aspirin 742 mg, salicylamide 222 mg, caffeine 38 mg. Lactose. Pow. Pkg. 50s. *OTC.*
Use: Analgesic combination.

BC Tablets. (Block Drug) Aspirin 325 mg, salicylamide 95 mg, caffeine 16 mg. Tab. Pkg 4s. Bot. 50s, 100s. *OTC.*
Use: Analgesic combination.

B-C w/Folic Acid. (Geneva) Vitamins B_1 15 mg, B_2 15 mg, B_3 100 mg, B_5 18 mg, B_6 4 mg, B_{12} 5 mcg, C 500 mg, folic acid 0.5 mg. Tab. Bot. 100s. *Rx.*
Use: Mineral, vitamin supplement.

B-C w/Folic Acid Plus. (Geneva) Fe 27 mg, vitamins A 5000 units, E 30 units, B_1 20 mg, B_2 20 mg, B_3 100 mg, B_5 25 mg, B_6 25 mg, B_{12} 50 mcg, C 500 mg, FA 0.8 mg, biotin 0.15 mg, Cr, Cu, Mg, Mn, Zn 22.5 mg. Tab. Bot. 100s. *Rx.*
Use: Mineral, vitamin supplement.

B-Day. (Barth's) Vitamins B_1 7 mg, B_2 14 mg, niacin 4.67 mg, B_{12} 5 mcg. Tab. Bot. 100s, 500s. *OTC.*
Use: Vitamin supplement.

B-D Glucose. (Becton Dickinson & Co.) Glucose 5 g. Chew. Tab. Bot. 36s. *OTC.*
Use: Hyperglycemic.

B Dozen. (Standex) Vitamin B_{12} 25 mcg Tab. Bot. 1000s. *OTC.*
Use: Vitamin supplement.

B-Dram w/C Computabs. (Dram) Vitamins B_1 5 mg, B_2 10 mg, B_6 5 mg, nicotinamide 50 mg, calcium pantothenate 20 mg. Tab. Bot. 100s. *OTC.*
Use: Mineral, vitamin supplement.

Beano. (Prestige) Alpha-D-galactosidase derived from *Aspergillus niger*, a fungal source in carrier of water and glycerol. Liq. Bot. 75 serving size at 5 drops per dose. Tab. Pkg. 12s. Bot. 30s, 100s. *OTC.*
Use: Antiflatulent.

Bear-E-Yum CT. (Mallinckrodt) Barium sulfate 1.5%. Simethicone, sorbitol. Susp. Bot. 200 mL, 1900 mL. *Rx.*
Use: Radiopaque agent, GI contrast agent.

Bear-E-Yum GI. (Mallinckrodt) Barium sulfate 60%. Simethicone. Susp. Bot. 200 mL. *Rx.*
Use: Radiopaque agent, GI contrast agent.

Bebatab No. 2. (Freeport) Belladonna ⅙ g, phenobarbital 0.25 g. Tab. Bot. 1000s. *Rx.*
Use: Anticholinergic; antispasmodic; hypnotic; sedative.

Bebulin VH. (Baxter) Factor IX, II, X, and low amounts of VII (human). Vapor-treated. Actual number of units shown on each bottle. Heparin, dry natural rub-

ber latex. Inj., Pow. for Soln. Single-dose vials with sterile water for injection. *Rx.*
Use: Antihemophilic agent.

•**becanthone hydrochloride.** (BEE-kan-thone) USAN.
Use: Antischistosomal.

•**becaplermin.** (beh-kah-PLER-min) USAN.
Use: Chronic dermal ulcers treatment.
See: Regranex.

•**becatecarin.** (BE-Ka-TEK-ar-in) USAN.
Use: Antineoplastic.

Beceevite. (Halsey Drug) Vitamins C 300 mg, B_1 15 mg, B_2 10 mg, niacin 50 mg, B_6 5 mg, pantothenic acid 10 mg. Cap. Bot. 100s. *OTC.*
Use: Vitamin supplement.

•**beclomethasone dipropionate.** (BEK-low-METH-uh-zone die-PRO-peo-uh-NATE) *USP.*
Use: Corticosteroid; intranasal steroid.
See: Beconase AQ.
QNASL.
QVAR.
Vanceril.
Vanceril Double Strength.

beclomycin dipropionate.
Use: Corticosteroid.

Beclovent. Beclomethasone dipropionate. *Rx.*
Use: Respiratory inhalant, corticosteroid.

•**becocalcidiol.** (BE-koe-KAL-si-DYE-ol) USAN.
Use: Psoriasis.

Becomp-C. (Cenci, H.R. Labs, Inc.) Vitamins C 250 mg, B_1 25 mg, B_2 10 mg, nicotinamide 50 mg, B_6 2 mg, calcium pantothenate 10 mg, hesperidin complex 50 mg. Cap. Bot. 100s, 500s. *OTC.*
Use: Mineral, vitamin supplement.

Beconase AQ. (GlaxoSmithKline) Beclomethasone dipropionate 0.042% (42 mcg/actuation), dextrose, polysorbate 80, benzalkonium chloride, 0.25% w/w phenylethyl alcohol. Spray. Bot. 25 g (180 metered doses per bottle) with metering pump and nasal adaptor. *Rx.*
Use: Corticosteroid; intranasal steroid.

Becotin-T. (Eli Lilly) Vitamins B_1 15 mg, B_2 10 mg, B_6 5 mg, niacinamide 100 mg, pantothenic acid 20 mg, B_{12} 4 mcg, C 300 mg. Tab. Bot. 100s, 1000s, Blister pkg. 10 × 10s. *OTC.*
Use: Vitamin supplement.

•**bectumomab.** (beck-TYOO-moe-mab) USAN.
Use: Monoclonal antibody, diagnosis of non-Hodgkin lymphoma and detection of AIDS-related lymphoma.

•**bedaquiline.** (bed-AK-wi-leen) USAN.
Use: Treatment of tuberculosis.
See: Sirturo.

•**bedaquiline fumarate.** (bed-AK-wi-leen) USAN.
Use: Treatment of tuberculosis.

•**bederocin.** (be-DER-oh-sin) USAN.
Use: Antibacterial agent.

Bedoce. (Lincoln Diagnostics) Crystalline anhydrous vitamin B_{12} 1000 mcg/mL. Vial 10 mL. *Rx.*
Use: Vitamin supplement.

Bedoce-Gel. (Lincoln Diagnostics) Vitamin B_{12} 1000 mcg/mL in 17% gelatin soln. Vial 10 mL. *Rx.*
Use: Vitamin supplement.

•**bedoradrine sulfate.** (bed-OR-a-dreen) USAN.
Use: Tocolytic agent.

Bedside Care. (Sween) Bot. 8 oz, gal.
Use: Dermatologic.

beechwood creosote.
See: Creosote.

Bee-Forte w/C. (Rugby) Vitamins B_1 25 mg, B_2 12.5 mg, B_3 50 mg, B_5 10 mg, B_6 3 mg, B_{12} 2.5 mcg, C 250 mg. Cap. Bot. 100s. *OTC.*
Use: Vitamin supplement.

beef peptones. (Sandia) Water-soluble peptones derived from beef 20 mg/2 mL. Inj. Vial 30 mL. *Rx.*
Use: Nutritional supplement, parenteral.

Beelith. (Beach) Pyridoxine hydrochloride 20 mg, magnesium oxide 600 mg. Tab. Bot. 100s. *OTC.*
Use: Mineral, vitamin supplement.

Beepen-VK. (GlaxoSmithKline) Penicillin V. **Tab.:** 250 mg, Bot. 1000s; 500 mg, Bot. 500s. **Pow. for Oral Soln.:** 125 mg/5 mL; 250 mg/5 mL. Bot. 100 mL, 200 mL. *Rx.*
Use: Anti-infective; penicillin.

Bee-Thi. (Burgin-Arden) Cyanocobalamin 1000 mcg, thiamine hydrochloride 100 mg in isotonic soln. of sodium chloride/mL. Vial 10 mL, 20 mL. *Rx.*
Use: Vitamin supplement.

Bee-Twelve 1000. (Burgin-Arden) Cyanocobalamin 1000 mcg/mL. Vial 10 mL, 30 mL. *Rx.*
Use: Vitamin supplement.

Bee-Zee. (Rugby) Vitamins E 45 mg, B_1 15 mg, B_2 10.2 mg, B_3 100 mg, B_5 25 mg, B_6 10 mg, B_{12} 6 mcg, C 600 mg, zinc 5.2 mg. Tab. Bot. 60s. *OTC.*
Use: Mineral, vitamin supplement.

•**befetupitant.** (BEF-et-UE-pi-tant) USAN.
Use: CNS agent.

Behepan.
See: Cyanocobalamin.

•**belagenpumatucel-L.** (BEL-a-JEN-pum-a-too-sel) USAN.
Use: Antineoplastic.

•**belatacept.** (bel-a-TA-sept) USAN.
Use: Immunosuppressive agent.
See: Nulojix.

Belatol. (Cenci, H.R. Labs) **No. 1:** Belladonna leaf extract 1/8 g, phenobarbital 0.25 g. Tab. Bot. 100s, 1000s. **No. 2:** Belladonna leaf extract, phenobarbital 0.5 g. Tab. Bot. 100s, 1000s. *Rx.*
Use: Anticholinergic; antispasmodic; hypnotic; sedative.

Belatol Elixir. (Cenci, H.R. Labs, Inc.) Phenobarbital 20 mg, belladonna 6.75 mg/5 mL w/alcohol 45%. Bot. Pt, gal. *Rx.*
Use: Anticholinergic; antispasmodic; hypnotic; sedative.

Belbutal No. 2 Kaptabs. (Churchill) Phenobarbital 32.4 mg, hyoscyamine sulfate 0.1092 mg, atropine sulfate 0.0215 mg, hyoscine HBr 0.0065 mg. Tab. Bot. 100s. *Rx.*
Use: Anticholinergic; antispasmodic; hypnotic; sedative.

Beldin. (Halsey Drug) Diphenhydramine hydrochloride 12.5 mg/5 mL w/alcohol 5%. Bot. Gal. *OTC.*
Use: Antihistamine.

Belexal. (Pal-Pak, Inc.) Vitamins B_1 1.5 mg, B_2 2 mg, B_6 0.167 mg, calcium pantothenate 1 mg, niacinamide 10 mg, brewer's yeast. Tab. Bot. 1000s, 5000s. *OTC.*
Use: Mineral, vitamin supplement.

Belexon Fortified Improved. (A.P.C.) Liver fraction No. 2, 3 g, yeast extract 3 g, vitamins B_1 5 mg, B_2 6 mg, niacinamide 10 mg, calcium pantothenate 2 mg, cyanocobalamin 1 mcg, iron 10 mg. Cap. Bot. 100s. *OTC.*
Use: Mineral, vitamin supplement.

Belfer. (Forest) Vitamins B_1 2 mg, B_2 2 mg, B_{12} 10 mcg, B_6 2 mg, C 50 mg, iron 17 mg. Tab. Bot. 100s. *OTC.*
Use: Mineral, vitamin supplement.

•**belfosdil.** (bell-FOSE-dill) USAN.
Use: Antihypertensive; calcium channel blocker.

Belganyl.
See: Suramin.

•**belimumab.** (bel-LIM-oo-mab) USAN.
Use: Monoclonal antibody.
See: Benlysta.

•**belladonna.** (bell-a-DON-a) *USP.*
Use: Gastrointestinal anticholinergic/antispasmodic.

belladonna alkaloids.
Use: Anticholinergic; antispasmodic.
See: Hyoscyamine Sulfate.
W/Chlorpheniramine Maleate, Pseudoephedrine Hydrochloride.
See: Respa A.R.
W/Combinations.
See: Atropine Sulfate.
Belladonna.
L-Hyoscyamine Sulfate.

belladonna alkaloids with phenobarbital. (Various Mfr.) Atropine sulfate 0.0194 mg, scopolamine HBr 0.0065 mg, hyoscyamine HBr or sulfate 0.1037 mg, phenobarbital 16.2 mg. Tab. Bot. 50s, 100s, 1000s, UD 100s. *Rx.*
Use: GI anticholinergic combination.

belladonna and phenobarbital combinations.
Use: Anticholinergic; antispasmodic; hypnotic; sedative.
See: Bebatab No. 2.
Belatol.
Chardonna-2.
Spabelin No. 2.

•**belladonna extract.** (bell-a-DON-a) *USP.*
Use: Antispasmodic.
W/Butabarbital Sodium.
See: Butibel.

belladonna extract. (Eli Lilly) Belladonna extract 15 mg (0.187 mg belladonna). Tab. *Rx.*
Use: Antispasmodic.

belladonna extract combinations.
Use: Anticholinergic; antispasmodic.
See: B & O Supprettes.

•**belladonna leaf.** (bell-a-DON-a) *USP.*
Use: Antispasmodic.

belladonna leaf, phenobarbital, and benzocaine.
Use: Anticholinergic.

•**belladonna tincture.** (bell-a-DON-a) *USP.*
Use: Antispasmodic.

Bellahist-D LA. (Cypress) Phenylephrine hydrochloride 20 mg, chlorpheniramine maleate 8 mg, hyoscyamine sulfate 0.19 mg, atropine sulfate 0.04 mg, scopolamine HBr 0.01 mg. Alcohol and dye free. ER Tab. 100s. *Rx.*
Use: Upper respiratory combination, decongestant, antihistamine, anticholinergic combination.

Bellaneed. (Hanlon) Belladonna, phenobarbital 16 mg. Cap. Bot. 100s. *Rx.*
Use: Anticholinergic; antispasmodic; hypnotic; sedative.

Bell/ans. (C.S. Dent & Co.) Sodium bicarbonate 520 mg (sodium content 144 mg). Tab. Bot. 30s, 60s. *OTC.*
Use: Antacid.

Bellastal. (Wharton) Atropine sulfate

0.0194 mg, scopolamine HBr 0.0065 mg, hyoscyamine HBr or SO_4 0.1037 mg, phenobarbital 16.2 mg. Cap. Bot. 1000s. *Rx.*
Use: Anticholinergic; antispasmodic.

•**belnacasan.** (bel-NA-ka-san) USAN.
Use: Antiepileptic.

•**belotecan hydrochloride.** (BEL-oh-TEE-kan) USAN.
Use: Antineoplastic.

•**beloxamide.** (bell-OX-ah-mid) USAN.
Use: Antihyperlipoproteinemic.

•**beloxepin.** (beh-LOX-eh-pin) USAN.
Use: Antidepressant.

Belviq. (Eisai) Lorcaserin 10 mg (equiv. to lorcaserin hydrochloride 10.4 mg). Film coated. PEG. Tab. 100s, UD 10s. *c-iv.*
Use: Anorexiant, serotonin 2C receptor agonist.

•**bemarinone hydrochloride.** (BEH-mah-rih-NOHN) USAN.
Use: Cardiovascular agent, positive inotropic, vasodilator.

•**bemesetron.** (beh-meh-SET-rone) USAN.
Use: Antiemetic.

Beminal 500. (Whitehall-Robins) Vitamins B_1 25 mg, B_2 12.5 mg, B_3 100 mg, B_6 10 mg, B_5 20 mg, C 500 mg, B_{12} 5 mcg. Tab. Bot. 100s. *OTC.*
Use: Vitamin supplement.

•**bemitradine.** (beh-MIH-trah-DEEN) USAN.
Use: Antihypertensive; diuretic.

•**bemoradan.** (beh-MOE-rah-DAN) USAN.
Use: Cardiovascular agent.

•**bemotrizinol.** (be-MOE-trye-zi-nol) USAN.
Use: Sunscreen.

Benacen. (Cenci, H.R. Labs, Inc.) Probenecid 0.5 g. Tab. Bot. 100s, 1000s. *Rx.*
Use: Antigout.

Benacol. (Cenci, H.R. Labs, Inc.) Dicyclomine hydrochloride 20 mg. Tab. Bot. 100s, 1000s. *Rx.*
Use: Anticholinergic; antispasmodic.

benactyzine hydrochloride. 2-Diethylaminoethyl benzilate hydrochloride.
Use: Anxiolytic.

benactyzine/meprobamate. Psychotherapeutic combination.

Benadryl Allergy Dye-Free. (McNeil) Diphenhydramine hydrochloride 25 mg. Glycerin, polyethylene glycol, sorbitol. Dye free. Cap., liquid filled. 24s. *OTC.*
Use: Antihistamine, nonselective ethanolamine.

Benadryl Allergy KapGels. (McNeil) Diphenhydramine hydrochloride 25 mg. Butylparaben, calcium 35 mg, methylparaben, polyethylene glycol, polysorbate 80, propylparaben. Gel coated. Tab. 24s, 48s. *OTC.*
Use: Antihistamine.

Benadryl Allergy Plus Sinus Headache. (McNeil) Acetaminophen 325 mg, diphenhydramine hydrochloride 12.5 mg, phenylephrine hydrochloride 5 mg. PEG. Tab. 24s, 48s. *OTC.*
Use: Upper respiratory combination; decongestant, antihistamine, and analgesic combination.

Benadryl Allergy ULTRATAB. (McNeil) Diphenhydramine hydrochloride 25 mg. Tab. 24s, 48s, 100s. *OTC.*
Use: Antihistamine, nonselective ethanolamine.

Benadryl Anti-Itch Gel for Kids. (McNeil) Camphor 0.45%. Benzyl alcohol, EDTA, menthol, SD alcohol 40-B, trolamine. Gel. 85 g. *OTC.*
Use: Topical analgesic.

Benadryl Children's Allergy. (McNeil) Diphenhydramine hydrochloride 12.5 mg/5 mL. Glycerin, glycyrrhizinate, sodium benzoate, sucrose. Cherry flavor. Liq. 118 mL, 236 mL. *OTC.*
Use: Antihistamine, nonselective ethanolamine.

Benadryl Children's Dye-Free Allergy. (McNeil) Diphenhydramine hydrochloride 12.5 mg/5 mL. Glycerin, saccharin sodium, sodium benzoate, sorbitol. Alcohol free. Bubblegum flavor. Liq. 118 mL. *OTC.*
Use: Antihistamine, nonselective ethanolamine.

Benadryl-D Allergy & Sinus, Children's. (McNeil) Diphenhydramine hydrochloride 12.5 mg, phenylephrine hydrochloride 5 mg. Edetate disodium, glycerin, sodium benzoate, sorbitol, sucralose. Alcohol free, sugar free. Grape flavor. Liq. 118 mL. *OTC.*
Use: Upper respiratory combination, decongestant and antihistamine.

Benadryl Extra Strength. (McNeil) Diphenhydramine hydrochloride 2%, zinc acetate 0.1%. Alcohol, glycerin, povidone, tromethamine. Spray. 59 mL. *OTC.*
Use: Topical analgesic.

Benadryl Extra Strength Itch Relief Stick. (McNeil) Diphenhydramine hydrochloride 2%, zinc acetate 0.1%. Alcohol, glycerin, povidone, tromethamine. Stick. 14 mL. *OTC.*
Use: Topical analgesic.

Benadryl Extra Strength Itch Stopping Cream. (McNeil) Diphenhydramine

hydrochloride 2%, zinc acetate 0.1%. Cetyl alcohol, urea, methylparaben, polyethylene glycol monostearate, propylene glycol, propylparaben. Cream. 14.2 g. *OTC.*
Use: Topical analgesic.

Benadryl Itch Stopping Extra Strength. (McNeil) Diphenhydramine hydrochloride 2%. SD alcohol, camphor, urea, glycerin, methylparaben, propylene glycol, propylparaben. Gel. 118 mL. *OTC.*
Use: Topical analgesic.

Benadryl Original Strength Itch Stopping. (McNeil) Diphenhydramine hydrochloride 1%, zinc acetate 0.1%. Cetyl alcohol, urea, methylparaben, polyethylene glycol monostearate, propylene glycol, propylparaben. Cream. 14.2 g. *OTC.*
Use: Topical analgesic.

Benadryl ReadyMist Itch Stopping Spray. (McNeil) Diphenhydramine hydrochloride 2%, zinc acetate 0.1%. Alcohol, glycerin, povidone, tromethamine. Spray. 7.7 mL. *OTC.*
Use: Topical analgesic.

Benadryl Severe Allergy & Sinus Headache, Maximum Strength. (McNeil) Phenylephrine hydrochloride 5 mg, diphenhydramine hydrochloride 25 mg, acetaminophen 325 mg. PEG. Tab. 20s. *OTC.*
Use: Upper respiratory combination, decongestant, antihistamine, and analgesic combination.

Benahist 50. (Keene Pharmaceuticals) Diphenhydramine 50 mg/mL. Vial 10 mL. *Rx.*
Use: Antihistamine.

Benahist 10. (Keene Pharmaceuticals) Diphenhydramine 10 mg/mL. Vial 30 mL. *Rx.*
Use: Antihistamine.

benanserin hydrochloride.
Use: Serotonin antagonist.

Benaphen Caps. (Major) Diphenhydramine 25 mg, 50 mg. Cap. Bot. 100s, 1000s. *OTC.*
Use: Antihistamine.

•**benapryzine hydrochloride.** (BEN-ah-PRY-zeen) USAN.
Use: Anticholinergic.

Benase. (Ferndale) Proteolytic enzymes extracted from Carica papaya 20,000 units enzyme activity. Tab. Bot. 1000s. *Rx.*
Use: Reduction of edema, relief of episiotomy.

•**benazeprilat.** (BEN-AZE-eh-prill-at) USAN.
Use: Angiotensin-converting enzyme inhibitor.

•**benazepril hydrochloride.** (BEN-AZE-eh-prill) USAN.
Use: Angiotensin-converting enzyme inhibitor, renin angiotensin system antagonist.
See: Lotensin.
W/Combinations.
See: Lotensin HCT.
Lotrel.

benazepril hydrochloride. (Various Mfr.) Benazepril hydrochloride 5 mg, 10 mg, 20 mg, 40 mg. May contain lactose, maltodextrin. Tab. 30s, 100s, 500s, 1,000s. *Rx.*
Use: Angiotensin-converting enzyme inhibitor, renin angiotensin system antagonist.

benazepril hydrochloride/hydrochlorothiazide. (Sandoz) Hydrochlorothiazide/benazepril hydrochloride 6.25 mg/5 mg, 12.5 mg/10 mg, 12.5 mg/20 mg, 25 mg/20 mg. Lactose. Tab. 100s. *Rx.*
Use: Antihypertensive.

•**bendacalol mesylate.** (ben-DACK-ah-LOLE) USAN.
Use: Antihypertensive.

•**bendamustine hydrochloride.** (BEN-da-MUS-teen) USAN.
Use: Mechlorethamine derivative, ethylenimine/methylmelamine; alkylating agent.
See: Treanda.

•**bendazac.** (BEN-dah-ZAK) USAN.
Use: Anti-inflammatory.

•**bendroflumethiazide.** (ben-droe-floo-meth-EYE-a-zide) *USP.*
Use: Antihypertensive; diuretic.
W/Combinations.
See: Corzide.

bendroflumethiazide and rauwolfia.
See: Rauwolfia/Bendroflumethiazide.

Benefiber. (Novartis) Fiber. **Chew. Tab.:** 1 g. Acesulfame K, aspartame, dextrates, phenylalanine, sorbitol, sucralose, wheat dextrin. Gluten free and sugar free. Assorted fruit and orange crème flavors. 100s. **Pow.:** 1.5 g per teaspoon. Wheat dextrin. Gluten free and sugar free. 70 g, 133 g, 217 g, 315 g, 437.5 g, 665 g. *OTC.*
Use: Laxative, bulk-producing laxative.

Benefiber Drink Mix. (Novartis) Fiber 3 g per packet. Acesulfame K, aspartame, maltodextrin, phenylalanine, potassium citrate, wheat dextrin. Sugar free. Cherry pomegranate, citrus punch, kiwi strawberry, and raspberry tea flavors. Pow. 8s, 16s. *OTC.*
Use: Laxative, bulk-producing laxative.

Benefiber for Children. (Novartis) Fiber

1.5 g per teaspoon. Wheat dextrin. Gluten free and sugar free. Pow. 153 g. *OTC.*
Use: Laxative, bulk-producing laxative.

Benefiber Plus Calcium. (Novartis) Fiber. **Chew. Tab.:** 1 g. Acesulfame K, aspartame, calcium 100 mg, dextrates, maltodextrin, phenylalanine, sorbitol, sucralose, wheat dextrin. Gluten free and sugar free. Berry flavor. Chew. 90s. **Pow.:** 3 g per tablespoon. Calcium 300 mg, wheat dextrin. Gluten free and sugar free. 423.8 g. *OTC.*
Use: Laxative, bulk-producing laxative.

Benefiber Plus Heart Health. (Novartis) Fiber. **Tab.:** 1 g. Folic acid 44.7 mcg, vitamin B_6 0.23 mg, B_{12} 0.67 mcg, wheat dextrin. Gluten free and sugar free. 60s. **Pow.:** 1.5 g per teaspoon. Folic acid 67 mg, vitamin B_6 0.35 mg, B_{12} 1 mcg, wheat dextrin. Gluten free and sugar free. 181.4 g. *OTC.*
Use: Laxative, bulk-producing laxative.

Benefiber Sticks. (Novartis) Fiber 3 g per packet. Acesulfame K, aspartame, maltodextrin, phenylalanine (all except unflavored), tartrazine (citrus punch flavor), wheat dextrin. Sugar free. Unflavored, cherry pomegranate, citrus punch, kiwi strawberry, and raspberry tea flavors. Pow. 8s, 16s, 28s. *OTC.*
Use: Laxative, bulk-producing laxative.

Benefiber Ultra. (Novartis) Fiber 1 g. Wheat dextrin. Sugar free and gluten free. Tab. 72s, 114s. *OTC.*
Use: Laxative, bulk-producing laxative.

BeneFIX. (Wyeth) Factor IX (recombinant) 250 units, 500 units, 1,000 units, 2,000 units, 3,000 units. Actual number of units shown on each bottle. Glycine, L-histidine, polysorbate 80, sucrose. Preservative free. Inj., lyophilized Pow. for Soln. Kit (contains sodium chloride 0.234%, L-histidine 8 mM, sucrose 0.8%, glycine 208 mM, 0.004% polysorbate 80 when reconstituted) w/single-dose vial (kits include 5 mL of sterile water for injection, double-ended needle for reconstitution, vented filter spike for withdrawal, winged infusion set, and alcohol swabs). *Rx.*
Use: Antihemophilic agent.

Benemid. (Merck & Co.) Probenecid 0.5 g. Tab. Bot. 100s, 1000s, UD 100s. *Rx.*
Use: Antigout.

Benepro Tabs. (Major) Probenecid 500 mg. Tab. Bot. 100s, 1000s. *Rx.*
Use: Antigout.

bengal gelatin.
See: Agar.

Bengay Children's Vaporizing Rub. (Pfizer) Camphor, menthol, w/oils of turpentine, eucalyptus, cedar leaf, nutmeg, thyme in stainless white base. Jar 1.125 oz. *OTC.*
Use: Analgesic, topical.

Bengay Extra Strength. (Pfizer) Methyl salicylate 30%, menthol 8%. Balm. Jar 3.75 oz. *OTC.*
Use: Analgesic, topical.

Bengay Extra Strength Sports. (Pfizer) Methyl salicylate 28%, menthol 10%. Balm. Tube 1.25 oz, 3 oz. *OTC.*
Use: Analgesic, topical.

Bengay Gel. (Pfizer) Methyl salicylate 15%, menthol 7%, alcohol 40%. Gel. Tube 1.25 oz, 3 oz. *OTC.*
Use: Analgesic, topical.

Bengay Greaseless. (Pfizer) Methyl salicylate 18.3%, menthol 16%. Oint. Tube 1.25 oz, 3 oz, 5 oz. *OTC.*
Use: Analgesic, topical.

Bengay Lotion. (Pfizer) Methyl salicylate 15%, menthol 7% in lotion base. Lot. Bot. 2 oz, 4 oz. *OTC.*
Use: Analgesic, topical.

Bengay Ointment. (Pfizer) Methyl salicylate 15%, menthol 10% in ointment base. Oint. Tube 1.25 oz, 3 oz, 5 oz. *OTC.*
Use: Analgesic, topical.

Bengay Original. (Pfizer) Methyl salicylate 18.3%, menthol 16%. Oint. Tube. 37.5 g, 90 g, 150 g. *OTC.*
Use: Analgesic, topical.

Bengay Patch. (Pfizer) Menthol 1.4%. Glycerin. Patch, regular and large size. 1s. *OTC.*
Use: Liniment.

Bengay Sports Gel. (Pfizer) Methyl salicylate, menthol, alcohol 40%. Gel. Tube 1.25 oz, 3 oz. *OTC.*
Use: Analgesic, topical.

Benicar. (Sankyo Pharm) Olmesartan medoxomil 5 mg, 20 mg, 40 mg. Lactose. Film-coated. Tab. Bot. 30s, 90s (except 5 mg), blister card 100s (except 5 mg). *Rx.*
Use: Antihypertensive.

Benicar HCT. (Sankyo Pharma) Hydrochlorothiazide/olmesartan medoxomil. 12.5 mg/20 mg, 12.5 mg/40 mg, 25 mg/40 mg. Lactose. Film-coated. Tab. 30s, 90s, 1000s, blister card 10s. *Rx.*
Use: Antihypertensive.

Benlysta. (GlaxoSmithKline) Belimumab 120 mg, 400 mg. Polysorbate 80, sucrose 80 mg/mL. Latex free, preservative free. Inj., lyophilized Pow. for Soln. Single-use vial. 20 mL. *Rx.*
Use: Monoclonal antibody.

•**benorterone.** (bee-NAHR-ter-ohn) USAN.
Use: Antiandrogen.
•**benoxaprofen.** (ben-OX-ah-PRO-fen) USAN.
Use: Anti-inflammatory; analgesic.
•**benoxinate hydrochloride.** (ben-OX-ih-nate) *USP.*
Use: Anesthetic, topical.
W/Fluorescein Sodium.
See: Altafluor.
Fluress.
Flurox.
W/Fluorexon Disodium.
See: FluraSafe.
•**benperidol.** (BEN-peh-rih-dahl) USAN.
Use: Antipsychotic.
•**benralizumab.** (BEN-ra-LIZ-oo-mab) USAN.
Use: Respiratory agent.
•**bensalan.** (BEN-sal-an) USAN.
Use: Disinfectant.
Bensal HP. (7 Oaks) Benzoic acid 6%, salicylic acid 3%, extract of oak bark. Oint. Tube 15 g, 30 g. Jar 30 g, 60 g. *Rx.*
Use: Anti-infective, topical.
•**benserazide.** (ben-SER-ah-zide) USAN.
Use: Inhibitor, decarboxylase; antiparkinson.
Benson's Bottom Paint. (Benson's Bottom Paint) Cetyl alcohol, emulsifying wax, glycerin, paraffin, petrolatum, stearyl alcohol, triethanolamine, zinc oxide. Oint. 56.7 g. *OTC.*
Use: Diaper rash product.
•**bentazepam.** (BEN-tay-zeh-pam) USAN.
Use: Hypnotic; sedative.
Bentical. (Lamond) Bentonite, zinc oxide, zinc carbonate, titanium dioxide. Bot. 4 oz, 6 oz, 8 oz, 16 oz, 32 oz, 0.5 gal, gal.
Use: Emollient.
•**bentiromide.** (ben-TEER-oh-mide) USAN.
Use: Diagnostic aid, pancreas function determination.
•**bentonite.** (BEN-tun-ite) *NF.*
Use: Pharmaceutic aid, suspending agent.
bentonite magma.
Use: Pharmaceutic aid, suspending agent.
bentonite, purified.
Use: Pharmaceutic aid.
•**bentoquatam.** (BEN-toe-KWAH-tam) USAN.
Use: Barrier for prevention of allergic contact dermatitis.
See: Ivy Block.
Bentyl. (Axcan Scandipharm) Dicyclomine hydrochloride. **Cap.:** 10 mg. Bot. 100s, 500s, UD 100s. **Tab.:** 20 mg. Bot. 100s, 500s, 1000s, UD 100s. **Syr.:** 10 mg/5 mL. Saccharin. Bot. Pt. **Inj.:** 10 mg/mL. Amps. 2 mL. Vials. 10 mL. *Rx.*
Use: GI anticholinergic/antispasmodic.
•**benurestat.** (BEN-YOU-reh-stat) USAN.
Use: Enzyme inhibitor, urease.
Benylin Expectorant. (Warner Lambert) Dextromethorphan HBr 5 mg, guaifenesin 100 mg per 5 mL. Saccharin, sorbitol, raspberry flavor, alcohol free, sugar free. Bot. Liq. 118 mL. *OTC.*
Use: Upper respiratory combination, antitussive, expectorant.
Benza. (Century) Benzalkonium chloride. **Soln.:** 1:750. 60 mL, 120 mL. **Disinfectant concentrate:** 17%. 120 mL, gal. **Tincture:** 1:750. Gal. **Tissue:** 1:750. Chlorothymol, isopropyl alcohol, alcohol (20%). Individual single-use packet. *OTC.*
Use: Topical anti-infective, antiseptic and germicide.
Benzac AC 5 & 10. (Galderma) **Gel:** Benzoyl peroxide 5%, 10%. Glycerine and EDTA in water base. Tube 60 g, 90 g. **Liq.:** Benzoyl peroxide 5%, 10%. Glycerin. 240 mL. *Rx.*
Use: Antiacne.
Benzac 5 & 10. (Galderma) Benzoyl peroxide 5%, 10%, alcohol 12%. Tube 60 g, 90 g. *Rx.*
Use: Antiacne.
BenzaClin. (Valeant) Clindamycin 1%, benzoyl peroxide 5%. Gel. 25 g, 50 g. Pump. 35 g, 50 g. *BenzaClin Care Kit* w/50 g pump and 20 topical ampules of viscontour serum. *Rx.*
Use: Anti-infective, antibiotic, topical.
Benzac W Wash 5 & 10. (Galderma) Benzoyl peroxide 5%, 10%, Bot. 120 mL (5% only), 240 mL. *Rx.*
Use: Antiacne.
Benzagel Wash. (Dermik) Benzoyl peroxide 10%, alcohol 14%. Gel. 60 g. *Rx.*
Use: Dermatologic, acne.
•**benzalkonium chloride.** (benz-al-KOE-nee-uhm) USAN.
Use: Surface antiseptic; pharmaceutical aid, preservative.
See: Bacti-Cleanse.
Eye-Stream.
Germicin.
Otrivin.
Remedy.
Ultra Tears.
Zephiran.
W/Benzocaine, Butamben, Tetracaine Hydrochloride.
See: Cetacaine.

W/Chloroxylenol, Hydrocortisone, Pramoxine Hydrochloride.
See: Cortic-ND.
Mediotic-HC.
W/Lidocaine.
See: Bactine Pain Relieving Cleansing.
W/Lidocaine Hydrochloride.
See: Bactine Antiseptic Anesthetic.
Medi-First With Lidocaine.
Medi-Quik.
W/Combinations.
See: Bite Rx.
Cortane-B Lotion.
Dacriose.
Garamycin.
Ionax Foam.
Isopto Plain & Tears.
Mycomist.
Oxyzal Wet Dressing.
SalineX.
Tearisol.

Benzamycin. (Valeant) Benzoyl peroxide 5%, erythromycin 3%, alcohol 20%. Gel. 8 g, 23 g, 46 g. *Rx.*
Use: Anti-infective, topical.

Benzamycin Pak. (Valeant) Benzoyl peroxide 5%, erythromycin 3%, SD alcohol 40B. Gel. 0.8 g pouches. 60s. *Rx.*
Use: Anti-infectives, topical.

•**benzbromarone.** (BENZ-brome-ah-rone) USAN.
Use: Uricosuric.

Benzedrex. (B.F. Ascher) Propylhexedrine 250 mg, menthol, lavender oil. Inhaler. *OTC.*
Use: Nasal decongestant.

BenzEFoam. (Onset Therapeutics) Benzoyl peroxide 5.3%. Cetearyl alcohol, disodium EDTA, glycerin, parabens. Foam. 60 g. *Rx.*
Use: Anti-infective, topical; antibiotic agent.

•**benzethonium chloride.** (benz-eth-OH-nee-uhm) *USP.* Topical solution; Tincture.
Use: Anti-infective, topical; pharmaceutic aid, preservative.
See: Antiseptic Wound & Skin Cleanser.
Dermoplast Antibacterial.
W/Benzocaine.
See: Ivy-Rid.
W/Diphenhydramine Hydrochloride, Zinc Acetate.
See: Calagel Maximum Strength.
W/Lidocaine Hydrochloride.
See: StaphAseptic.
W/Menthol.
See: Gold Bond Antiseptic First Aid Quick Spray.

•**benzetimide hydrochloride.** (benz-ETT-ih-mide) USAN.
Use: Anticholinergic.

•**benzilonium bromide.** (BEN-zill-oh-nih-uhm) USAN.
Use: Anticholinergic.

•**benzindopyrine hydrochloride.** (BENZ-in-doe-pie-reen) USAN.
Use: Antipsychotic.

Benziq. (Graceway Pharmaceuticals) Benzoyl peroxide 5.25%. Benzyl alcohol, disodium EDTA, glycerin. Gel. 50 g. *Rx.*
Use: Anti-infective, topical; antibiotic agent.

Benziq LS. (Graceway Pharmaceuticals) Benzoyl peroxide 2.75%. Benzyl alcohol, disodium EDTA, glycerin. Gel. 50 g. *Rx.*
Use: Anti-infective, topical; antibiotic agent.

Benziq Wash. (Graceway Pharmaceuticals) Benzoyl peroxide 5.25%. Benzyl alcohol, cetyl alcohol, disodium EDTA, glycerin, PEG-100. Soap. 175 g. *Rx.*
Use: Anti-infective, topical; antibiotic agent.

benzisoxazole derivatives.
Use: Antipsychotic.
See: Iloperidone.
Paliperidone.
Risperidone.
Ziprasidone.

benzoate and phenylacetate.
Use: Treatment of hyperammonemia. [Orphan Drug]

Benzo-C. (Freeport) Benzocaine 5 mg, cetalkonium Cl 5 mg, ascorbic acid 50 mg. Troche. Bot. 1000s, cello-packed boxes 1000s. *OTC.*
Use: Anesthetic, local.

•**benzocaine.** (BEN-zoe-kane) *USP.* Ethyl-p-aminobenzoate. Anesthesin, orthesin, parathesin.
Use: Anesthetic, topical.
See: Americaine.
Americaine Hemorrhoidal.
Anbesol.
Anbesol Baby.
Anbesol Cold Sore Therapy.
Anbesol Maximum Strength.
Anbesol Regular Strength.
Bansmoke.
Benz-O-Sthetic.
Boil-Ease.
Cēpacol Sore Throat Lozenges.
Dent-O-Kain/20.
Dermoplast.
Dermoplast Antibacterial.
Detane.
Foille Medicated First Aid.
Hurricaine.

Hurricaine ONE.
Kank-A Mouth Pain.
Kank-A Soothing Beads.
Lanacane.
Maximum Strength Anbesol.
Orabase.
Orajel.
Orajel Baby.
Orajel Baby Nighttime.
Orajel Brace-Aid.
Orajel D.
Orajel Maximum Strength.
Orajel Mouth-Aid.
Orajel P.M. Nighttime Formula Toothache Pain Relief.
Orajel Regular Strength.
Oral Pain Relief Maximum Strength.
OraMagic Plus.
SensoGARD.
Solarcaine.
Solarcaine Medicated First Aid.
Tanac.
Tanac Roll-On.
Toothache Gel.
Toothache Relief 3 in 1.
Trocaine.

W/Acetic Acid, Antipyrine, Polycosanol.
See: AABP.

W/Antipyrine.
See: Aurax.

W/Antipyrine, Phenylephrine Hydrochloride.
See: Ear-Gesic.

W/Antipyrine, u-Polycosanol 410.
See: Treagan.

W/Benzalkonium Chloride, Butamben, Tetracaine Hydrochloride.
See: Cetacaine.

W/Benzethonium Chloride.
See: Ivy-Rid.

W/Camphor, Menthol.
See: Chiggerex.

W/Cetylpyridinium Chloride, Menthol.
See: Orasep.

W/Chloroxylenol, Hydrocortisone Acetate.
See: TriOxin.

W/Dextromethorphan Hydrobromide.
See: Cēpacol Sore Throat Plus Cough Relief.
Chloraseptic Total Sore Throat + Cough.
Cough-X.
Tetra-Formula.

W/Dextromethorphan Hydrobromide, Glycerin.
See: Cēpacol Dual Relief Sore Throat + Cough.

W/Glycerin.
See: Cēpacol Dual Relief Sore Throat & Coating Spray.

W/Menthol.
See: Cēpacol Maximum Numbing Sore Throat.
Cēpacol Sore Throat Pain Relief Maximum Numbing.
Sting-Kill.

W/Menthol, Methyl Salicylate.
See: Dendracin Neurodendtraxin.

W/Pectin.
See: Cēpacol Sore Throat & Coating Relief Maximum Numbing.

W/Phenol.
See: Anbesol.

W/Resorcinol.
See: Unguentine Maximum Strength.
Vagisil.
Vagisil Maximum Strength.

W/Sulfur.
See: Chigg Away.

W/Combinations.
See: Anacaine.
Auralgesic.
Benzo-C.
Benzodent.
Bicozene.
Boil-Ease Salve.
Chloraseptic Children's.
Chloraseptic Kids Sore Throat.
Chloraseptic Sore Throat.
Chloraseptic Sore Throat Relief.
Culminal.
Dent's Extra Strength Toothache Gum.
Dent's Lotion-Jel.
Dent's Maximum Strength Toothache Drops.
Dent's Toothache Gum.
Denture Orajel.
Dent-Zel-Ite.
Dermoplast.
Dermoplast Antibacterial.
Foille.
Foille Medicated First Aid.
Foille Plus.
Hurricaine.
Jiffy.
Lanacane.
Orabase B.
Orabase Baby.
Orabase Lip.
Orabase with Benzocaine.
Orajel Mouth-Aid.
Rectal Medicone.
Rectal Medicone Unguent.
Solarcaine.
Spec-T Sore Throat Anesthetic.
Tanac Liquid.
Tanac Stick.
Toothache.
Zilactin-B Medicated.

benzocaine. (Various Mfr.) Benzocaine 5%. Cream. 480 g. *OTC.*

Use: Topical local anesthetic, ester local anesthetic.

benzochlorophene sodium. Sodium salt of ortho-benzyl-para-chlorophenol.

•**benzoctamine hydrochloride.** (benz-OCK-tah-meen) USAN.
Use: Hypnotic; muscle relaxant; sedative.

Benzodent. (Procter & Gamble) Benzocaine 20%. 30 g. *OTC.*
Use: Anesthetic, local.

•**benzodepa.** (BEN-zoe-DEH-pah) USAN.
Use: Antineoplastic.

benzodiazepines.
Use: Antianxiety agents; anticonvulsants; sedative/hypnotics, nonbarbiturates.
See: Alprazolam.
Clobazam.
Clonazepam.
Clorazepate Dipotassium.
Chlordiazepoxide Hydrochloride.
Diazepam.
Estazolam.
Flurazepam Hydrochloride.
Lorazepam.
Oxazepam.
Quazepam.
Temazepam.
Triazolam.

•**benzoic acid.** (ben-ZOE-ik) *USP.*
Use: Pharmaceutic aid, antifungal.
W/Atropine Sulfate, Hyoscyamine Sulfate, Methenamine, Methylene Blue, Phenyl Salicylate.
See: Uritact DS.
W/Boric Acid, Zinc Oxide, Zinc Stearate.
See: Whitfield's.
W/Hyoscyamine Sulfate, Methenamine, Methylene Blue, Phenyl Salicylate.
See: Hyophen.

benzoic acid. (Various Mfr.) Benzoic acid. Pkg. 0.25 lb, 1 lb. *OTC.*
Use: Antifungal; fungistatic.

benzoic acid, 2-hydroxy. Salicylic acid.

benzoic and salicylic acids.
Use: Antifungal, topical.
See: Whitfield's.

•**benzoin.** (BEN-zoyn) *USP.*
Use: Protectant, topical; expectorant.
See: Sprayzoin.
W/Podophyllum resin.
See: Podoben.

benzoin. (Morton International) Benzoin, tolu balsam, styrax, alcohol w/propellant. Aerosol. Can 7 oz. *OTC.*
Use: Skin protectant.

benzoisothiazol derivatives.
See: Lurasidone Hydrochloride.

benzol. Usually refers to benzene.

Benzo-Menth. (Pal-Pak, Inc.) Benzocaine 2.2 mg. Tab. Bot. 1000s. *OTC.*
Use: Anesthetic, topical.

•**benzonatate.** (ben-ZOE-nah-tate) *USP.*
Use: Nonnarcotic antitussive.
See: Tessalon.
Tessalon Perles.
Zonatuss.

benzonatate softgels. (Various Mfr.) Benzonatate 100 mg, 200 mg. Cap. Bot. 100s, 500s. *Rx.*
Use: Nonnarcotic antitussive.

benzoquinonium chloride.
Use: Muscle relaxant.

Benz-O-Sthetic. (Geritrex) Benzocaine 20%. Benzyl alcohol, PEG. Gel; dental. 29 g. *OTC.*
Use: Local anesthetic, topical.

benzosulfimide.
See: Saccharin.

benzosulphinide sodium. *Name previously used for Saccharin sodium.*

•**benzoxiquine.** (benz-OX-ee-kwine) USAN.
Use: Disinfectant.

•**benzoylpas calcium.** (benz-oe-ILL-pass) USAN.
Use: Anti-infective, tuberculostatic.

•**benzoyl peroxide.** (BEN-zoyl per-OX-ide) *USP.*
Use: Keratolytic.
See: Acne Clear.
Acne Medication 5.
Acne Medication 10.
Benzac AC Wash.
Benzac W Wash.
BenzEFoam.
Benziq.
Benziq LS.
Benziq Wash.
BP 5.25%.
BP Foam.
BP 4.25%.
BP Gel.
BP 7% Wash.
Brevoxyl Cleansing.
Brevoxyl-8 Acne Wash Kit.
Brevoxyl-4 Acne Wash Kit.
Clearasil Maximum Strength Acne Treatment.
Clinac BPO.
Delos.
Desquam-E.
Desquam-X.
Desquam-X Wash.
Effaclar Duo.
Inova Easy Pad.
Lavoclen-8.
Lavoclen-4.
NeoBenz Micro SD.

NeoBenz Micro Wash.
Neutrogena Clear Pore.
OC8.
On-the-Spot-Acne Treatment.
Oxy Oil-Free Maximum Strength Acne Wash.
Pacnex HP.
Pacnex LP.
PanOxyl.
PanOxyl AQ.
RE Benzoyl Peroxide.
Riax.
SE BPO.
SE BPO 7%.
Soluclenz Rx.
Theroxide.
Triaz.
ZoDerm.
W/Adapalene.
See: Epiduo.
W/Chlorhydroxyquinoline, Hydrocortisone.
See: Vanoxide-HC.
W/Clindamycin.
See: Acanya.
Duac.
Duac CS.
W/Hydrocortisone.
See: Vanoxide-HC.
W/Polyoxyethylene Lauryl Ether.
See: Benzac 5 & 10.
Desquam-X 5.
Desquam-X 10.
W/Salicylic Acid, Tocopherol.
See: Inova 8/2 Acne Control Therapy.
Inova 4/1 Acne Control Therapy.
W/Sulfur.
See: NuOx.

benzoyl peroxide. (Fougera) Benzoyl peroxide 4.5%, 6.5%, 8.5%. Cetyl alcohol, disodium EDTA, glycerin, glyceryl stearate, PEG-100, urea 10%. Cleanser. 400 mL. *Rx.*
Use: Anti-infective, topical; antibiotic agent.

benzoyl peroxide. (Kylemore Pharmaceuticals) Benzoyl peroxide 4%. Alcohol, propylene glycol. Lot. 297 g. *Rx.*
Use: Topical anti-infective, antibiotic.

benzoyl peroxide. (River's Edge) Benzoyl peroxide. **5.75%:** Cetyl alcohol, disodium EDTA, glycerin, urea 10%. **7%:** Alcohols, aloe, glycerin, green tea extract, PEG, propylene glycol, triethanolamine.Soap. 473 mL (5.75%), 180 g (7%). *Rx.*
Use: Anti-infective, topical; antibiotic agent.

benzoyl peroxide. (Various Mfr.) Benzoyl peroxide. **Mask:** 5%. In 30 mL. **Lot.:** 5%, 10%. Bot. 30 mL. **Gel:** 2.5%, 4%, 5%, 8%, 10%. Tube 42.5 g (4%, 8%), 60 g (2.5%, 5%, 10%), 90 g (except 2.5%). *Rx.*
Use: Anti-infective, topical; antibiotic agent.

benzoyl peroxide wash. (Various Mfr.) Benzoyl peroxide 2.5%, 5%, 10%. Liq. Bot. 118 mL (5% only) 148 mL (except 2.5%), 237 mL. *Rx.*
Use: Keratolytic.

n′-benzoylsulfanilamide.
See: Sulfabenzamide.

benzphetamine hydrochloride. (benz-FEET-a-meen)
Use: CNS stimulant, anorexiant.
See: Didrex.
Regimex.

benzphetamine hydrochloride. (Various Mfr.) Benzphetamine hydrochloride 50 mg. May contain lactose, polydextrose, sorbitol. Tab. 30s, 90s, 100s, 500s. *Rx.*
Use: CNS stimulant, anorexiant.

•**benzquinamide.** (benz-KWIN-ah-mid) USAN.
Use: Antiemetic.

•**benztropine mesylate.** (BENZ-troe-peen) *USP.*
Use: Parasympatholytic, antiparkinsonian.

benztropine mesylate. (West-Ward) Benztropine mesylate 1 mg/mL. Inj., Soln. Amp. 2 mL. *Rx.*
Use: Antiparkinson agent, anticholinergic.

benztropine mesylate. (Various Mfr.) Benztropine mesylate 0.5 mg, 1 mg, 2 mg. Tab. 100s, 1000s (except 0.5 mg), UD 100s. *Rx.*
Use: Antiparkinson agent, anticholinergic.

benztropine methanesulfonate.
See: Benztropine mesylate.

•**benzydamine hydrochloride.** (ben-ZIH-dah-meen) USAN.
Use: Analgesic; anti-inflammatory; antipyretic.

benzydroflumethiazide.
See: Bendroflumethiazide.

•**benzyl alcohol.** (BEN-zil) *NF.* Phenylcarbinol.
Use: Anesthetic; antiseptic, topical; pharmaceutic aid, antimicrobial.
See: Topic.
Ulesfia.
Zilactin-L.

•**benzyl benzoate.** (BEN-zil) *USP.*
Use: Pharmaceutical necessity for Dimercaprol Inj.

benzyl benzoate saponated. (Various Mfr.) Triethanolamine 20 g, oleic acid 80 g, benzyl benzoate q.s. 1000 mL.
Use: Scabicide, pediculicides.

benzyl carbinol.
See: Phenylethyl alcohol.

benzylpenicillin, benzylpenicilloic, benzylpenilloic acid. (Kremers Urban)
Use: Assessment of penicillin sensitivity. [Orphan Drug]
See: Pre-Pen/MDM.

benzyl penicillin-C-14. (Nuclear-Chicago) Carbon-14 labelled penicillin. Vacuum-sealed glass vial 50 microcuries, 0.5 millicuries.
Use: Radiopharmaceutical.

benzyl penicillin G, potassium.
See: Penicillin G potassium.

benzyl penicillin G, sodium.
See: Penicillin G sodium.

•**benzylpenicilloyl polylysine concentrate.** (BEN-zil-PEN-i-SIL-oh-il POL-ee-LYE-seen) *USP.*
Use: In vivo diagnostic aid.
See: Pre-Pen.

Bepanthen.
See: Panthenol.

Bephedin. Benzyl ephedrine.

bephenium hydroxynaphthoate.
Use: Anthelmintic, hookworms.

•**bepotastine.** (BEP-oh-TAS-teen) USAN.
Use: Mast cell stabilizer.

•**bepotastine besilate.** (BEP-oh-TAS-teen) USAN.
Use: Mast cell stabilizer.
See: Bepreve.

Bepreve. (ISTA Pharmaceuticals) Bepotastine besilate 1.5% (equiv. to bepotastine 10.7 mg base). Benzalkonium chloride 0.005%, monobasic sodium phosphate dihydrate, sodium chloride, sodium hydroxide. Soln., Ophth. Bot. 10 mL. *Rx.*
Use: Ophthalmic and otic agent, mast cell stabilizer.

•**beractant.** (ber-ACT-ant) USAN.
Use: Lung surfactant; respiratory distress syndrome. Respiratory failure; pulmonary hypertension; pneumonia; sepsis. [Orphan Drug]
See: Survanta.

•**beraprost.** (BEH-reh-prahst) USAN.
Use: Platelet aggregation inhibitor, improves ischemic syndromes.

•**beraprost sodium.** (BEH-reh-prahst) USAN.
Use: Platelet aggregation inhibitor, improves ischemic action.

berberine sulfate. (BUR-bur-een)
Use: Antimicrobial.

•**berefrine.** (BEH-reh-FREEN) USAN. *Formerly Burefrine.*
Use: Mydriatic.

Ber-Ex. (Dolcin) Calcium succinate 2.8 g, acetyl salicylic acid 3.7 g. Tab. Bot. 100s, 500s. *OTC.*
Use: Antiarthritic; antirheumatic.

Berinert. (CSL Behring) C1 inhibitor (human) 500 units. Preservative free. Total protein 50 to 80 mg, glycine 85 to 115 mg, sodium chloride 70 to 100 mg, sodium citrate 25 to 35 mg per vial. Kit includes one 10 mL single-use vial of diluent (sterile water), one *Mix2Vial* filter transfer set, and an alcohol swab. Inj., lyophilized Pow. for Soln. Single-use kit. *Rx.*
Use: Protein C1 inhibitor.

Berinert P. (Aventis Behring) C1-Esterase-inhibitor, human, pasteurized.
Use: Hereditary angioedema. [Orphan Drug]

Berocca Plus. (Roche) Vitamins A 5000 units, E 30 units, C 500 mg, B_1 20 mg, B_2 20 mg, B_3. Tab. Bot. 100s. *Rx.*
Use: Iron, vitamin supplement.

Berri-Freez. (Geritrex) Menthol 3.5%, camphor, glycerin, isopropyl alcohol, parabens, triethanolamine. Gel. 473 g. *OTC.*
Use: Rub and liniment.

•**berythromycin.** (beh-RITH-row-MY-sin) USAN.
Use: Antiamebic; anti-infective.

Beserol. (Sanofi-Synthelabo) Acetaminophen, chlormezanone. Tab. *Rx.*
Use: Analgesic; tranquilizer; muscle relaxant.

•**besifloxacin hydrochloride.** (BE-si-FLOX-a-sin) USAN.
Use: Ophthalmic and otic agent, antibiotic.
See: Besivance.

•**besipirdine hydrochloride.** (beh-SIH-pihr-deen) USAN.
Use: Cognition enhancer; Alzheimer disease.

Besivance. (Bausch & Lomb) Besifloxacin 0.6%. Besifloxacin hydrochloride 6.63 mg equiv. to 6 mg base. Benzalkonium chloride 0.01%, edetate disodium dihydrate. Susp.; Ophth. Bot. 5 mL. *Rx.*
Use: Ophthalmic and otic agent, antibiotic.

•**besonprodil.** (be-son-PROE-dil) USAN.
Use: Parkinson disease.

Besta. (Roberts) Vitamins B_1 20 mg, B_2 15 mg, niacinamide 100 mg, calcium pantothenate 20 mg, E 50 units, magnesium sulfate 70 mg, zinc 18.4 mg, B_{12} 4 mcg, B_6 25 mg, C 300 mg. Cap. Bot. 100s. *OTC.*
Use: Vitamin, mineral supplement.

Best C. (Roberts) Ascorbic acid 500 mg. TR Cap. Bot. 100s. *OTC.*
Use: Vitamin supplement.

Bestrone. (Bluco) Estrone in aqueous susp. 2 mg/mL, 5 mg/mL. Inj. Vial 10 mL. *Rx.*
Use: Hormone, estrogen.

beta-adrenergic blockers, ophthalmic.
See: AKBeta.
Betagan Liquifilm.
Betaxolol Hydrochloride.
Betimol.
Betoptic.
Betoptic S.
Levobunolol Hydrochloride.
Metipranolol Hydrochloride.
OptiPranolol.
Timolol.
Timolol Maleate.
Timoptic.
Timoptic in Ocudose.
Timoptic-XE.

beta-adrenergic blocking agents.
See: Acebutolol Hydrochloride.
Atenolol.
Betaxolol Hydrochloride.
Bisoprolol Fumarate.
Carteolol Hydrochloride.
Esmolol Hydrochloride.
Metoprolol.
Nadolol.
Nebivolol.
Penbutolol Sulfate.
Pindolol.
Propranolol Hydrochloride.
Sotalol Hydrochloride.
Timolol Maleate.

beta alethine.
Use: Antineoplastic. [Orphan Drug]
See: Betathine.

•**beta carotene.** (BAY-tah CARE-oh-teen) *USP.*
Use: Ultraviolet screen.
See: Lumitene.

beta carotene. (Various Mfr.) Beta carotene 15 mg (vitamin A 25,000 units). Softgel cap. Bot. 60s, 100s. *OTC.*
Use: Vitamin supplement.

•**beta cyclodextrin.** (BAY-tah sigh-kloe-DEX-trin) *NF.*
See: Betadex.

•**betadex.** (BAY-tah-dex) USAN. *Formerly beta cyclodextrin.*
Use: Pharmaceutical aid.

Betadine. (Purdue) Povidone-iodine.
Available as: Aerosol Spray, Bot. 3 oz. Antiseptic Gz. Pads 3" × 9". Box 12s. Antiseptic Lubricating Gel, Tube 5 g. Disposable Medicated Douche, concentrated packette w/cannula and 6 oz water. Douche, Bot. 1 oz, 4 oz, 8 oz. Douche Packette, 0.5 oz (6 per carton). *Helafoam* Solution Canister 250 g. Mouthwash/Gargle, Bot. 6 oz. Oint. Tube 1 oz. Jar 1 lb, 5 lb. Oint., Packette. Perineal Wash Conc. Kit, Bot. 8 oz w/dispenser. Skin Cleanser, Bot. 1 oz, 4 oz. Skin Cleanser Foam, Canister 6 oz. Solution, 0.5 oz, 8 oz, 16 oz, 32 oz, gal. Solution Packette, oz. Solution Swab Aid, 100s. Solution Swabsticks, 1s Box 200s; 3s Box 50s. Surgical Scrub, Bot. Pt w/dispenser, qt, gal, packette 0.5 oz. Surgi-prep Sponge-Brush 36s. Vaginal Suppositories, Box 7s w/vaginal applicator. Viscous Formula Antiseptic Gauze Pads: 3" × 9", 5" × 9". Box 12s. Whirlpool Concentrate, Bot. Gal. *OTC.*
Use: Antiseptic.

Betadine Cream. (Purdue) Povidone-iodine 5% mineral oil, polyoxyethylene stearate, polysorbate, sorbitan monostearate, white petrolatum. Cream. Tube 14 g. *OTC.*
Use: Antimicrobial; antiseptic.

Betadine 5% Sterile Ophthalmic Prep Solution. (Alcon) Povidone-iodine 5%. Soln. Bot. 50 mL. *Rx.*
Use: Antiseptic, ophthalmic.

Betadine Medicated Disposable Douche. (Purdue) Povidone-iodine 10%. Soln (0.3% when diluted). Vial 5.4 mL with 180 mL bot. Sanitized water. 1 and 2 packs. *OTC.*
Use: Vaginal agent.

Betadine Medicated Douche. (Purdue) Povidone-iodine 10% (0.3% when diluted). Soln. In 15 mL (6s) packettes and 240 mL. *OTC.*
Use: Vaginal agent.

Betadine Medicated Premixed Disposable Douche. (Purdue) Povidone-iodine 10%. Soln. (0.3% when diluted). Bot. 180 mL. 1s, 2s. *OTC.*
Use: Vaginal agent.

Betadine Medicated Suppositories. (Purdue) Povidone-iodine 10%. Supp. In 7s w/applicator. *OTC.*
Use: Vaginal agent.

Betadine PrepStick. (Purdue) Povidone-iodine 10%. Soln. Prep Swab. Box 150s, 600s. *OTC.*
Use: Anti-infective, topical.

Betadine PrepStick Plus. (Purdue) Povidone-iodine 10%, alcohol. Soln. Prep Swab. Box 150s, 600s. *OTC.*
Use: Anti-infective, topical.

Betadine Shampoo. (Purdue) Povidone-iodine 7.5%. Shampoo. Bot. 118 mL. *OTC.*
Use: Antiseborrheic.

beta-estradiol.
See: Estradiol.

beta eucaine hydrochloride. *Name previously used for Eucaine hydrochloride.*

Betagan Liquifilm. (Allergan) Levobunolol hydrochloride 0.5%. Liquifilm. Bot. 2 mL (0.5%), 5 mL, 10 mL, 15 mL (0.5%) w/B.I.D. C Cap and Q.D. C Cap (0.5%). *Rx.*
Use: Antiglaucoma, beta-adrenergic blocker.

Betagen. (Enzyme Process) Vitamins B_1 1 mg, B_2 1.2 mg, niacin 15 mg, B_6 18 mg, pantothenic acid 18 mg, choline 1.8 g, betaine 96 mg. 6 Tab. Bot. 100s, 250s. *OTC.*
Use: Mineral, vitamin supplement.

Betagen Surgical Scrub. (Ivax) Povidone-iodine. Bot. Pt, gal. *OTC.*
Use: Antiseptic.

•**betahistine hydrochloride.** (BEE-tah-HISS-teen) USAN.
Use: Vasodilator, Meniere disease; diamine oxidase inhibitor, increase microcirculation.

beta-hypophamine.
See: Vasopressin.

betaine. (Orphan Medical)
Use: Treatment of homocystinuria. [Orphan Drug]
See: Cystadane.

•**betaine hydrochloride.** (BEE-tane) *USP.* Acidol hydrochloride, lycine hydrochloride.
Use: Replenisher adjunct, electrolytes.
W/Ferrous fumarate, docusate sodium, desiccated liver, vitamins, minerals.
See: Hemaferrin.

Betalin S. (Eli Lilly) Thiamine hydrochloride 50 mg, 100 mg. Tab. Bot. 100s. *OTC.*
Use: Vitamin supplement.

•**betamethasone.** (BAY-tuh-METH-uh-zone) *USP.*
Use: Adrenocortical steroid, glucocorticoid.
See: Celestone.

•**betamethasone acetate.** (BAY-tuh-METH-uh-zone) *USP.*
Use: Corticosteroid, topical.

•**betamethasone dipropionate.** (BAY-tuh-METH-uh-zone) *USP.*
Use: Corticosteroid, topical.
See: Diprolene.
Diprosone.
Psorion.
W/Calcipotriene.
See: Taclonex.
Taclonex Scalp.
W/Clotrimazole.
See: Clotrimazole and Betamethasone Dipropionate.

betamethasone dipropionate, augmented. (Various Mfr.) Betamethasone (augmented). **Cream:** 0.05%, propylene glycol, sorbitol solution, white petrolatum. 15 g, 50 g. **Gel:** 0.05%, propylene glycol. 15 g, 50 g. *Rx.*
Use: Anti-inflammatory.

betamethasone dipropionate (augmented). (Fougera) Betamethasone dipropionate 0.05%. Hydroxypropylcellulose, isopropyl alcohol 30%, propylene glycol. Lot. 30 mL, 60 mL. *Rx.*
Use: Anti-inflammatory agent, topical corticosteroid.

betamethasone sodium phosphate and betamethasone acetate.
Use: Adrenocortical steroid, glucocorticoid.
See: Celestone Soluspan.

betamethasone sodium phosphate and betamethasone acetate. (American Regent) Betamethasone acetate 3 mg/betamethasone sodium phosphate 3 mg per mL. May contain benzalkonium chloride and edetate disodium. Inj., Susp. Multiple-dose vial. 5 mL. *Rx.*
Use: Adrenocortical steroid, glucocorticoid.

•**betamethasone valerate.** (BAY-tuh-METH-uh-zone) *USP.*
Use: Corticosteroid, topical.
See: Beta-Val.
Luxiq.
Valisone.
Valnac.

betamethasone valerate. (Perrigo) Betamethasone valerate 0.12%. May contain alcohols, propylene glycol. Foam; topical. 50 g, 100 g. *Rx.*
Use: Anti-inflammatory agent, topical corticosteroid.

•**betamicin sulfate.** (bay-tah-MY-sin) USAN.
Use: Anti-infective.

betanaphthol. 2-Naphthol.
Use: Parasiticide.

Betapace. (Bayer) Sotalol hydrochloride 80 mg, 120 mg, 160 mg, 240 mg, lactose. Tab. Bot. 100s, UD 100s. *Rx.*
Use: Antiadrenergic/sympatholytic, beta-adrenergic blocker.

Betapace AF. (Bayer) Sotalol hydrochloride 80 mg, 120 mg, 160 mg, lactose. Tab. UD 60s, 100s. *Rx.*
Use: Antiadrenergic/sympatholytic, beta-adrenergic blocker.

Betapen-VK. (Bristol-Myers Squibb) Penicillin V potassium. **Oral Soln.:** 125 mg/mL, 250 mg/5 mL Bot. 100 mL, 200 mL (250 mg/5mL only). **Tab.:** 250 mg, 500 mg. Tab. Bot. 100s, 1000s (250 mg

only). *Rx.*
Use: Anti-infective, penicillin.
beta-phenyl-ethyl-hydrazine. Phenelzine dihydrogen sulfate.
See: Nardil.
beta-pyridyl-carbinol. Nicotinyl alcohol. Alcohol corresponding to nicotinic acid.
BetaRx. (VivoRx, Inc.) Encapsulated porcine islet preparation.
Use: Type I diabetic patients already on immunosuppression. [Orphan Drug]
Betasept. (Purdue) Chlorhexidine gluconate 4%, isopropyl 4%, alcohol. Liq. Bot. 946 mL. *OTC.*
Use: Dermatologic.
Betaseron. (Bayer) Interferon beta-1b 0.3 mg. Albumin (human) 15 mg, mannitol 15 mg per vial. Preservative free. Inj., lyophilized Pow. for Soln. Single-use vial (capacity 3 mL) w/1.2 mL prefilled syringe of diluent (sodium chloride 0.54%), alcohol prep pads, and vial adaptor with attached needle for each drug vial. Blister units. 14s. *Rx.*
Use: Immunologic agent, immunomodulator.
BetaTemp Children's. (Beta Dermaceuticals) Acetaminophen 160 mg per 5 mL. Butylparaben, corn syrup, glycerin, *Magnasweet*, propylene glycol, sodium benzoate, sorbitol. Cotton candy flavor. Susp. 118 mL. *OTC.*
Use: CNS agent.
Betathine. (Dovetail Technologies, Inc.) Beta alethine.
Use: Antineoplastic. [Orphan Drug]
Beta-2. (Nephron) Isoetharine hydrochloride 1% with glycerin, sodium bisulfite, parabens. Liq. Bot. 10 mL, 30 mL. *Rx.*
Use: Respiratory product.
Beta-Val. (Teva) Betamethasone valerate equivalent to 0.1% betamethasone base in cream base. Cream. Tube 15 g, 45 g. *Rx.*
Use: Corticosteroid, topical.
Beta XMA. (Beta Dermaceuticals) Aloe, C14-22 alcohols, castor oil, cetyl alcohol, *butyrospermum parkii*, dimethicone, emu oil, methylparaben, PEG-40, PEG-100, triethanolamine. Cream. 118 g. *OTC.*
Use: Emollient.
betaxolol. (KVK-Tech) Betaxolol hydrochloride 10 mg, 20 mg. Lactose, PEG. Film coated. Tab. 100s. *Rx.*
Use: Antiadrenergic/sympatholytic, beta-adrenergic blocking agent.
•**betaxolol hydrochloride.** (BAY-TAX-oh-lahl) *USP.*
Use: Antiadrenergic/sympatholytic, beta-adrenergic blocking agent.
See: Betoptic S.
Kerlone.
betaxolol hydrochloride. (Various Mfr.) Betaxolol hydrochloride 5.6 mg (equiv. to 5 mg base)/mL (0.5%). Ophth. Soln. Bot. 2.5 mL, 5 mL, 10 mL, 15 mL. *Rx.*
Use: Antiglaucoma, beta-adrenergic blocker.
•**bethanechol chloride.** (beth-AN-ih-kole) *USP.*
Use: Cholinergic.
See: Myotonachol.
Urabeth.
Urecholine.
bethanechol chloride. (Various Mfr.) Bethanechol chloride 5 mg, 10 mg, 25 mg, 50 mg. Tab. Bot. 100s, 250s (10 mg, 25 mg only), 500s (50 mg only), 1000s, UD 100s. *Rx.*
Use: Urinary cholinergic.
•**bethanidine sulfate.** (beth-AN-ih-deen) USAN.
Use: Antihypertensive.
Bethaprim. (Major) Trimethoprim 40 mg, sulfamethoxazole 200 mg/5 mL, alcohol 0.26%, saccharin, sorbitol. Susp. *Rx.*
Use: Anti-infective.
Bethaprim DS Tabs. (Major) Trimethoprim 160 mg, sulfamethoxazole 800 mg. Tab. Bot. 100s, 500s, UD 100s. *Rx.*
Use: Anti-infective.
Bethaprim SS Tabs. (Major) Trimethoprim 80 mg, sulfamethoxazole 400 mg. Tab. Bot. 100s, 500s. *Rx.*
Use: Anti-infective.
Bethkis. (Cornerstone) Tobramycin 300 mg per 4 mL. Preservative free. Soln.; Inhal. Single-use amp. 4 mL (w/sodium chloride, sodium hydroxide, sulfuric acid). *Rx.*
Use: Anti-infective, parenteral aminoglycoside.
•**betiatide.** (BEH-tie-ah-tide) USAN.
Use: Pharmaceutic aid.
Betimol. (Akorn) Timolol maleate (as hemihydrate) 0.25%, 0.5%, benzalkonium Cl 0.01%, monosodium and disodium phosphate dihydrate. Soln. Bot. 2.5 mL, 5 mL, 10 mL, 15 mL. *Rx.*
Use: Antiglaucoma, beta-adrenergic blocker.
Betoptic S. (Alcon) Betaxolol hydrochloride 2.8 mg (equiv. to 2.5 mg base) per mL (0.25%), benzalkonium chloride 0.01%, mannitol, polysulfonic acid, hydrochloric acid or sodium hydroxide, EDTA. Susp. *Drop-Tainer* dispenser 2.5 mL, 5 mL, 10 mL, 15 mL. *Rx.*
Use: Antiglaucoma, beta-adrenergic blocker.

•**bevacizumab.** (beh-vuh-SIZ-uh-mab) USAN.
Use: Antiangiogenic; monoclonal antibody.
See: Avastin.

•**bevantolol hydrochloride.** (beh-VAN-toe-LOLE) USAN.
Use: Antianginal; antihypertensive; cardiac depressant, antiarrhythmic.

•**bevenopran.** (be-VEN-oh-pran) USAN.
Use: Treatment of chronic opioid-induced constipation.

•**bevirimat dimeglumine.** (be-VIR-i-mat) USAN.
Use: Antiretroviral.

•**bexarotene.** (bex-AIR-oh-teen) USAN.
Use: Antineoplastic; antidiabetic; rexinoid.
See: Targretin.

•**bexlosteride.** (bex-LOW-ster-ide) USAN.
Use: Prostate cancer.

Bexomal-C. (Roberts) Vitamins B_1 6 mg, B_2 7 mg, B_3 80 mg, B_5 10 mg, B_6 5 mg, B_{12} 6 mcg, C 250 mg. Tab. Bot. 50s. *OTC.*
Use: Vitamin supplement.

Beyaz. (Bayer Healthcare) **Drospirenone/ethinyl estradiol Tab.:** 3 mg/0.02 mg. Film coated. Lactose, PEG. 24s. **Levomefolate calcium Tab.:** 0.451 mg. Film coated. Lactose, PEG. 4s. *Rx.*
Use: Oral contraceptive, oral monophasic contraceptive.

•**bezafibrate.** (BEH-zah-FIE-brate) USAN.
Use: Antihyperlipoproteinemic.

•**bezlotoxumab.** (BEZ-loe-TOX-ue-mab) USAN.
Use: Prevention of recurrence of *Clostridium difficile* infection.

Bezon. (Whittier) Vitamins B_1 5 mg, B_2 3 mg, niacinamide 20 mg, pantothenic acid 3 mg, B_6 0.5 mg, C 50 mg, B_{12} 1 mcg. Cap. Bot. 30s, 100s. *OTC.*
Use: Vitamin supplement.

Bezon Forte. (Whittier) Vitamins B_1 25 mg, B_2 12.5 mg, niacinamide 50 mg, pantothenic acid 10 mg, B_6 5 mg, C 250 mg. Cap. Bot. 30s, 100s. *OTC.*
Use: Vitamin supplement.

B-F-I. (Numark Labs) Bismuth-formic-iodide, zinc phenolsulfonate, bismuth subgallate, amol, potassium alum, boric acid, menthol, eucalyptol, thymol, and inert diluents. Pow. Can. 0.25 oz, 1.25 oz, 8 oz. *OTC.*
Use: Antiseptic, topical.

B-50. (NBTY) Vitamins B_1 50 mg, B_2 50 mg, B_3 50 mg, B_5 50 mg, B_6 50 mg, B_{12} 50 mcg, folic acid 0.1 mg, d-biotin 50 mcg, PABA, choline bitartrate, inositol. Tab. Bot. 50s, 100s. *OTC.*
Use: Mineral, vitamin supplement.

B-50 Time Release. (NBTY) Vitamins B_1 50 mg, B_2 50 mg, B_3 50 mg, B_5 50 mg, B_6 50 mg, B_{12} 50 mcg, folic acid 0.1 mg, d-biotin 50 mcg, PABA 50 mg, choline bitartrate 50 mg, inositol 50 mg, lecithin. Tab. Bot. 100s. *OTC.*
Use: Mineral, vitamin supplement.

B.G.O. (Calotabs) Iodoform, salicylic acid, sulfur, zinc oxide, phenol (liquefied) 1%, calamine, menthol, petrolatum, lanolin, mineral oil, undecylenic acid 1%. Jar ⅞ oz, Tube 1 oz. *OTC.*
Use: Antifungal, topical; antiseptic.

Biafine. (OrthoNeutrogene) Avocado oil, liquid paraffin, parabens, paraffin wax, propylene glycol, triethanolamine. Emuls.; topical. Tube. 45 g, 90 g. *Rx.*
Use: Flexible hydroactive dressings and granules.

•**bialamicol hydrochloride.** (bye-AH-lam-IH-KAHL) USAN.
Use: Antiamebic.

•**biapenem.** (bye-ah-PEN-en) USAN.
Use: Anti-infective.

biaphasic insulin. A suspension of insulin crystals in a solution of insulin buffered at pH 7. Insulin Novo Rapitard. Inj.

Biaxin. (AbbVie) **Gran. for Oral Susp.:** Clarithromycin 250 mg/5 mL. Castor oil, maltodextrin, sucrose, fruit punch flavor. 50 mL, 100 mL. **Tab.:** Clarithromycin 250 mg, 500 mg. Film-coated. 60s, *ABBO-PAC* UD 100s (500 mg only). *Rx.*
Use: Anti-infective, macrolide.

Biaxin XL. (AbbVie) Clarithromycin 500 mg. Lactose. Film-coated. ER Tab. Bot. 60s, *BIAXIN XL PAC* blister pack 4 × 14s. *Rx.*
Use: Anti-infective, macrolide.

•**bibapcitide.** (bib-APP-sih-tide) USAN.
Use: Radionuclide carrier; detection and localization of deep vein thrombosis.

•**bicalutamide.** (bye-kah-LOO-tah-mide) USAN.
Use: Antineoplastic; antiandrogen.
See: Casodex.

bicalutamide. (Various Mfr.) Bicalutamide 50 mg. May contain lactose, PEG. Tab. 30s, 100s, 500s, 1,000s, UD 30s. *Rx.*
Use: Hormone, antiandrogen.

Bicarsim. (Kramer-Novis) Simethicone 80 mg. Sugar. Tab. 60s. *OTC.*
Use: Antiflatulent.

Bicarsim Forte. (Kramer-Novis) Simethicone 125 mg. Sugar. Tab. 60s. *OTC.*
Use: Antiflatulent.

•**bicifadine hydrochloride.** (bye-SIGH-fah-deen) USAN.
Use: Analgesic.

Bicillin C-R. (Monarch) **600,000 units/dose:** Penicillin G benzathine 300,000 units, penicillin G procaine 300,000 units. *Tubex* 1 mL. **1,200,000 units/dose:** Penicillin G benzathine 600,000, penicillin G procaine 600,000. *Tubex* 2 mL. Inj. *Rx.*
Use: Anti-infective.

Bicillin C-R 900/300. (Monarch) 1,200,000 units/dose (penicillin G benzathine 900,000, penicillin G procaine 300,000), parabens, lecithin, povidone. *Tubex* 2 mL. *Rx.*
Use: Anti-infective.

Bicillin L-A. (Monarch) Penicillin G benzathine 600,000 units/dose, 1,200,000 units/dose, 2,400,000 units/dose, povidone, parabens. Inj. *Tubex* 1 mL (600,000 only), 2 mL (1,200,000 only); Prefilled syringes 4 mL (2,400,000 only). *Rx.*
Use: Anti-infective.

•**biciromab.** (bye-SIH-rah-mab) USAN.
Use: Monoclonal antibody, antifibrin.

•**biclodil hydrochloride.** (BYE-kloe-DILL) USAN.
Use: Antihypertensive, vasodilator.

Biclora. (Hawthorn) Chlophedianol hydrochloride/chlorcyclizine hydrochloride. **Tab.:** 25 mg/25 mg. 60s. **Liq.:** 12.5 mg/12.5 mg. Glycerin, propylene glycol, sorbitol, sucralose. Alcohol free and dye free. Cherry flavor. 240 mL. *OTC.*
Use: Upper respiratory combination, antitussive combination.

Biclora-D. (Hawthorn) Chlophedianol hydrochloride/chlorcyclizine hydrochloride/pseudoephedrine hydrochloride. **Tab.:** 25 mg/25 mg/60 mg. 60s. **Liq.:** 12.5 mg/12.5 mg/30 mg. Glycerin, propylene glycol, sorbitol, sucralose. Alcohol free and dye free. Grape flavor. 240 mL. *OTC.*
Use: Upper respiratory combination, antitussive combination.

BiCNU. (Heritage Pharmaceuticals) Carmustine (BCNU) 100 mg, sterile diluent 3 mL. Pow. for Inj., lyophilized. Preservative free. Single-dose vial. *Rx.*
Use: Antineoplastic, alkylating agent.

Bicycline. (Knight) Tetracycline hydrochloride 250 mg. Cap. Bot. 100s. *Rx.*
Use: Anti-infective.

Bidex-400. (SJ Pharmaceuticals) Guaifenesin 400 mg. Maltodextrin. Tab. 100s. *OTC.*
Use: Respiratory agent, expectorant.

BiDil. (Arbor Pharmaceuticals) Isosorbide dinitrate 20 mg, hydralazine hydrochloride 37.5 mg. Lactose. Film-coated. Tab. 180s. *Rx.*
Use: Vasodilator.

•**bidisomide.** (bye-DIH-so-mide) USAN.
Use: Cardiovascular agent, antiarrhythmic.

•**bifeprunox.** (bye-fee-PRUE-nox) USAN.
Use: Antipsychotic agent.

•**bifeprunox mesylate.** (bye-fee-PRUE-nox) USAN.
Use: Antipsychotic agent.

BiferaRx. (Meda Pharmaceuticals) Fe 28 mg (as polysaccharide iron complex 22 mg and heme iron polypeptide [bovine source] 6 mg), B_{12} 25 mcg, folate 1 mg. Film coated. PEG. Tab. 90s. *Rx.*
Use: Multivitamin with iron.

Bifidobacterium infantis 35624.
See: Align Daily Probiotic Supplement.

•**bifonazole.** (BYE-FONE-ah-zole) USAN.
Use: Antifungal.

biguanides.
Use: Antidiabetic agent.
See: Metformin Hydrochloride.

bile acid sequestrants.
See: Cholestyramine.
Colesevelam Hydrochloride.
Colestipol Hydrochloride.

bile acids, oxidized. Note also dehydrocholic acid.
W/Atropine methyl nitrate, ox and hog bile extract, phenobarbital.
See: G.B.S.

bile extract.
W/Combinations
See: Biloric.
Enzobile Improved.

bile extract, ox. (Eli Lilly) Purified ox gall. Enseal 5 g, Bot. 100s, 500s, 1000s. (C.D. Smith) Tab. 5 g, Bot. 1000s. (Stoddard) Tab. 3 g, Bot. 100s, 500s, 1000s.
Use: Digestive enzymes.

bilein. Bile salts obtained from ox bile.

bile-like products. Bile products.
See: Bile salts.
Dehydrocholic acid.

bile salts. (Eli Lilly) Sodium glycocholate and taurocholate.

bile salts and belladonna. (Various Mfr.) Belladonna, nux vomica compound bile salts 60 mg, belladonna leaf extract 5 mg, nux vomica extract 2 mg, phenolphthalein 30 mg, sodium salicylate 15 mg, aloin 15 mg. Tab. Bot. 1000s. *Rx.*
Use: Laxative; antispasmodic.

Bili-Labstix SG Reagent Strips. (Bayer Consumer Care) Urinalysis reagent strip test for specific gravity, pH, pro-

tein, glucose, ketone, bilirubin, and blood. Bot. 100s.
Use: Diagnostic aid.

Bilirubin Reagent Strips. (Bayer Consumer Care) Seralyzer reagent strip. Quantitative strip test for total bilirubin serum or plasma. Bot. 25s.
Use: Diagnostic aid.

bilirubin test.
See: Ictotest.

Bilivist. (Berlex) Ipodate sodium 500 mg. Cap. Bot. 120s. *Rx.*
Use: Radiopaque agent.

Biloric. (Arcum) Pepsin 9 mg, ox bile 160 mg. Cap. Bot. 100s, 1000s. *OTC.*
Use: Antispasmodic.

Bilstan. (Standex) Bile salts 0.5 g, cascara sagrada powder extract 0.5 g, phenolphthalein 0.5 g, aloin ⅛ g, podophyllin g. Tab. Bot. 100s. *OTC.*
Use: Laxative.

Biltricide. (Schering) Praziquantel 600 mg. Tab. Bot. 6s. *Rx.*
Use: Anthelmintic.

•**bimatoprost.** (bi-MA-toe-prost) USAN.
Use: Antiglaucoma; prostaglandin agonist.
See: Latisse.
Lumigan.

•**bimosiamose disodium.** (bye-moh-SYE-a-mose) USAN.
Use: Anti-inflammatory agent.

•**bindarit.** (BIN-dah-rit) USAN.
Use: Antirheumatic.

•**binetrakin.** (bih-NEH-trah-kin) USAN.
Use: Gastrointestinal carcinoma; rheumatoid arthritis; dendritic cell activation; immunomodulatory.

•**biniramycin.** (bih-NEER-ah-MY-sin) USAN.
Use: Anti-infective.

•**binodenoson.** (bi-NOE-den-oh-son) USAN.
Use: Vasodilator.

•**binospirone mesylate.** (bih-NO-spy-rone) USAN.
Use: Anxiolytic.

Bintron. (Madland) Liver fraction 4.6 g, ferrous sulfate 5 g, vitamins B_1 3 mg, B_2 0.5 mg, B_6 0.15 mg, C 20 mg, calcium pantothenate 0.3 mg, niacinamide 10 mg. Tab. Bot. 100s, 1000s. *OTC.*
Use: Mineral, vitamin supplement.

BioBeads. (Natrol) 2.5 billion live cultures blend of *L. acidophilus, L. rhamnosus, B. bifidum, B. longum.* Coconut and palm kernel oil, glycerin. Gluten free and preservative free. Tab. 30s. *OTC.*
Use: Probiotic.

Biobrane. (Sanofi-Synthelabo) Temporary skin substitute available in various sizes. *OTC.*
Use: Dermatologic.

Biobron SF. (Advanced Generic) Dextromethorphan hydrobromide 15 mg, guaifenesin 350 mg, phenylephrine hydrochloride 10 mg per 5 mL. Parabens, propylene glycol, saccharin. Alcohol free and sugar free. Cherry flavor. Liq. 473 mL. *OTC.*
Use: Upper respiratory combination, antitussive and expectorant combination.

Biocal 500. (Bayer Consumer Care) Calcium 500 mg. Tab. Bot. 75s. *OTC.*
Use: Mineral supplement.

Biocal 250. (Bayer Consumer Care) Calcium 250 mg. Chew. Tab. Bot. 75s. *OTC.*
Use: Calcium supplement.

Biocult-GC. (Orion) Swab test for gonorrhea. For endocervical, urethral, rectal, and pharyngeal cultures. Box 1 test per kit.
Use: Diagnostic aid.

bioflavonoid compounds.
See: Amino-Opti-C.
Bioflex.
C Factors "1000" Plus.
Ester-C Plus 500 mg Vitamin C.
Ester-C Plus Multi-Mineral.
Ester-C Plus 1000 mg Vitamin C.
Flavons.
Flavons-500.
Pan C-500.
Peridin-C.
Quercetin.
Span C.
Tri-Super Flavons 1000.

Bioflex. (Advanced Generic) Vitamin C 500 mg, citrus bioflavonoids 50 mg, hawthorn berry extract 25 mg, horse chestnut extract 25 mg, hesperidin complex 25 mg, rutin 40 mg, witch hazel extract 25 mg. Tab. 60s. *OTC.*
Use: Water-soluble vitamin.

Biofreeze. (Performance Health Products) Menthol. **Gel:** 4%. Alcohol, aloe, camphor, glycerin, triethanolamine. 118 mL. **Liq. Roll-on:** 4%. Alcohol, aloe, camphor, glycerin, triethanolamine. 89 mL. **Spray:** 10%. Chamomile, *Echinacea*, ethanol, juniper berry, white tea. 118 mL. *OTC.*
Use: Rub and liniment.

BioGaia. (Nutraceutics) 100 million *Lactobacillus reuteri* Protectis. Hydrogenated palm oil, xylitol. Preservative free and sugar free. Lemon-lime flavor. Chew. Tab. 30s. *OTC.*
Use: Oral nutritional supplement, probiotic product.

BioGaia Probiotic Drops. (Nutraceutics) *L. reuteri protectis* 100 million CFU per 5 drops. Medium chain triglyceride oil, sunflower oil. Preservative free, sugar free. Soln. 5 mL. *OTC.*
Use: Probiotic.

BioGaia Probiotic Straws. (Nutraceutics) *L. reuteri protectis* 100 million CFU. Rapeseed oil. Preservative free and sugar free. Oil; oral. Straws. 30s. *OTC.*
Use: Probiotic.

BioGaia ProTectis Baby. (Everidis) *L. reuteri protectis* 100 million CFU per 5 drops. MTC oil, sunflower oil. Soln. 5 mL. *OTC.*
Use: Probiotic.

Biogastrone.
See: Carbenoxolone.

Biogil. (Advanced Generic) Dextromethorphan hydrobromide 15 mg, guaifenesin 300 mg, phenylephrine hydrochloride 10 mg. Parabens, sorbitol. Alcohol free and sugar free. Grape flavor. Liq. 473 mL. *Rx.*
Use: Upper respiratory combination, antitussive and expectorant combination.

BioGlo. (Hub Pharmaceuticals) Fluorescein sodium 1 mg. Strip. 100s. *OTC.*
Use: Diagnostic aid, ophthalmic.

BioGtuss. (Advanced Generics) Dextromethorphan hydrobromide 15 mg, guaifenesin 300 mg, phenylephrine hydrochloride 10 mg. Aspartame, glycerin, parabens, phenylalanine 17 mg per 5 mL, propylene glycol. Alcohol free and sugar free. Grape flavor. Liq. 473 mL. *Rx.*
Use: Upper respiratory combination, antitussive and expectorant combination.

Biohist-LA. (IVAX) Chlorpheniramine maleate 12 mg, pseudoephedrine hydrochloride 120 mg. SR Tab. Bot. 100s. *Rx.*
Use: Upper respiratory combination, antihistamine, decongestant.

•**biological indicator for dry-heat sterilization, paper strip.** *USP.*
Use: Biological indicator, sterilization.

•**biological indicator for ethylene oxide sterilization, paper strip.** *USP.*
Use: Biological indicator, sterilization.

•**biological indicator for steam sterilization, paper strip.** *USP.*
Use: Biological indicator, sterilization.

•**biological indicator for steam sterilization, self-contained.** *USP.*
Use: Biological indicator, sterilization.

biological response modifiers.
See: Aldesleukin.
BCG, Live.
Denileukin Diftitox.
Ontak.
TheraCys.
TICE BCG.

Bionate 50-2. (Seatrace) Testosterone cypionate 50 mg, estradiol cypionate 2 mg/mL. Vial 10 mL. *Rx.*
Use: Androgen; estrogen combination.

Bionect. (Innocutis) Hyaluronic acid. **Cream:** 0.2%. As sodium salt. Parabens, PEG. 25 g. **Gel:** 0.2%. As sodium salt. Parabens. 30 g. **Spray:** 0.2%. As sodium salt. Parabens. 20 mL. *Rx.*
Use: Physical adjunct.

Bionel. (Advanced Generic) Dextromethorphan hydrobromide 15 mg, guaifenesin 200 mg, pseudoephedrine hydrochloride 30 mg per 5 mL. Aspartame, glycerin, parabens, phenylalanine 19 mg per 5 mL. Alcohol free, dye free, and sugar free. Liq. 473 mL. *OTC.*
Use: Upper respiratory combination, antitussive and expectorant combination.

Bionel Pediatric. (Advanced Generic) Dextromethorphan hydrobromide 5 mg, guaifenesin 50 mg, pseudoephedrine hydrochloride 15 mg per 5 mL. Aspartame, parabens, phenylalanine 14 mg. Alcohol free. Liq. 473 mL. *Rx.*
Use: Upper respiratory combination antitussive and expectorant combination.

Bion Tears. (Alcon) Dextran 70 0.1%, hydroxypropyl methylcellulose 2910 0.3%, NaCl, KCl, sodium bicarbonate. Preservative free. Soln. In single-use 0.45 mL containers (28s). *OTC.*
Use: Artificial tears.

Biopatch. (Johnson & Johnson) Chlorhexidine gluconate 52.5 mg (¾-inch [1.9 cm]; 1.5 mm center hole with radial slit), 86.8 mg (1-inch [2.5 cm]; 7 mm center hole with radial slit), 92 mg (1-inch [2.5 cm]; 4 mm center hole with radial slit). Disk, foam. 10s. *OTC.*
Use: Topical anti-infective, antiseptic and germicide.

Bioral.
See: Carbenoxolone.

Bio-Rescue. (Biomedical Frontiers) Dextran and deferoxamine.
Use: Acute iron poisoning. [Orphan Drug]

Bios I.
See: Inositol.

Biospec DMX. (Deliz Pharmaceutical) Dextromethorphan hydrobromide 15 mg, guaifenesin 25 mg. Glucose,

saccharin. Alcohol free. Cherry flavor. Liq. 473 mL. *OTC.*
Use: Upper respiratory combination, antitussive with expectorant.

Biosynject. (Chembiomed, Inc.) Trisaccharides A and B.
Use: Hemolytic disease of the newborn. [Orphan Drug]

Bio-Tab. (International Ethical Labs) Doxycycline hyclate 100 mg. Tab. Bot. 50s, 100s, 500s. *Rx.*
Use: Anti-infective, tetracycline.

Biotect Plus. (Advanced Generic) Vitamins A 1,666.67 units, D 133.33 units, E 33.33 units, B_1 16.67 mg, B_2 16.67 mg, B_3 16.67 mg, B_5 16.67 mg, B_6 16.67 mg, B_{12} 16.67 mcg, C 166.67 mg, Fe 3.33 mg, folate 0.33 mg, Cr, Cu, Mg, Mn, Mo, Se, Zn, biotin, choline, inositol, lysine. Acesulfame K, glycerin, methylparaben, polysorbate 80, xylitol. Alcohol free, dye free, and sugar free. Strawberry flavor. Liq. 473 mL. *OTC.*
Use: Multivitamin with minerals.

Biotel U.T.I. (Biotel Corp.) In vitro diagnostic home test to detect urinary tract infections by screening for nitrate in urine. Test kit 12s.
Use: Diagnostic aid.

Biotène Dry Mouth. (GlaxoSmithKline) Sodium monofluorophosphate. Glucose, glycerin, lactoferrin, lactoperoxidase, sodium benzoate, sorbitol, xylitol. Fresh mint flavor. Paste; dental. 127.6 g. *OTC.*
Use: Mouth and throat product, preparation for sensitive teeth.

Biotène with Calcium. (Laclede) Propylene glycol, xylitol, poloxamer 407, hydroxyethylcellulose, sodium benzoate, peppermint, benzoic acid, zinc gluconate, aloe vera, calcium lactate, lactoferrin, lysozyme, lactoperoxidase, potassium thiocyanate, glucose oxidase. Alcohol free. Mouthwash. 474 mL. *OTC.*
Use: Mouth and throat products.

Bio-Therm Pain Relieving Lotion. (Weeks & Leo) Capsaicin 0.002%, menthol 10%, methyl salicylate 20%. Aloe, cetearyl alcohol, glycerin, methylisothiazolinone, trolamine, vitamin E. Lot. 113.4 g. *OTC.*
Use: Rub and liniment.

Biothesin. (Pal-Pak, Inc.) Phosphorated carbohydrate solution ceriumoxalate 120 mg, bismuth subnitrate 120 mg, benzocaine 15 mg, aromatics. Tab. 1000s. *OTC.*
Use: Antiemetic; antivertigo.

BioThrax. (Emergent BioDefense Operations Lansing) Anthrax vaccine. *Bacillus anthracis* 83 kDa. Aluminum 1.2 mg/mL, benzethonium chloride 25 mcg/mL, formaldehyde 100 mcg/mL. Inj., Susp. Multidose vial. 5 mL. *Rx.*
Use: Active immunization agent, bacterial vaccine.

Bio-Throid. (Bio-Tech) Thyroid desiccated 7.5 mg (1/8 g), 15 mg (1/4 g), 30 mg (1/2 g), 60 mg (1 g), 90 mg (1 1/2 g), 120 mg (2 g), 150 mg (2 1/2 g), 180 mg (3 g), 240 mg (4 g). Cap. Bot. 100s, 1,000s. *Rx.*
Use: Hormone, thyroid.

Bio T Pres. (Advanced Generic) Dextromethorphan hydrobromide 10 mg, guaifenesin 200 mg, phenylephrine hydrochloride 5 mg. Aspartame, glycerin, parabens, phenylalanine 17 mg per 5 mL, propylene glycol. Alcohol free and sugar free. Cherry flavor. Liq. 473 mL. *Rx.*
Use: Upper respiratory combination, antitussive and expectorant combination.

Bio T Pres Pediatric. (Advanced Generics) Dextromethorphan hydrobromide 5 mg, guaifenesin 75 mg, phenylephrine hydrochloride 2.5 mg. Aspartame, glycerin, parabens, phenylalanine 5 mg per 5 mL, propylene glycol. Alcohol free, dye free, and sugar free. Orange flavor. Liq. 473 mL. *Rx.*
Use: Upper respiratory combination, antitussive and expectorant combination.

Biotrue Multi-Purpose. (Bausch & Lomb) Polyaminopropyl biguanide 0.00013%, polyquaternium 0.0001%, boric acid, edetate disodium, hyaluronan, poloxamine, sodium borate, sodium chloride, sulfobetaine. Soln., Ophth. 60 mL, 118 mL, 296 mL, 473 mL. *OTC.*
Use: Contact lens product, soft.

Biotuss. (GIL) Dextromethorphan HBr 15 mg, guaifenesin 300 mg, phenylephrine hydrochloride 10 mg per 5 mL. Phenylalanine 3.75 mg/5 mL. Alcohol and sugar free. Grape flavor. Liq. 473 mL. *Rx.*
Use: Upper respiratory combination, antitussive and expectorant combination.

Bio-Tussi. (Advanced Generic) Dextromethorphan hydrobromide 10 mg, guaifenesin 200 mg, phenylephrine hydrochloride 5 mg per 5 mL. Aspartame, glycerin, parabens, phenylalanine 19 mg per 5 mL, propylene glycol. Alcohol free and sugar free. Cherry flavor. Liq. 473 mL. *OTC.*

Use: Upper respiratory combination, antitussive and expectorant combination.

Bio-Tussi Pediatric. (Advanced Generic) Dextromethorphan hydrobromide 5 mg, guaifenesin 75 mg, phenylephrine hydrochloride 2.5 mg. Aspartame, glycerin, parabens, phenylalanine 14 mg per 5 mL, propylene glycol. Alcohol free, dye free, and sugar free. Orange flavor. Liq. 473 mL. *OTC.*
Use: Upper respiratory combination, antitussive and expectorant combination.

Bio-Tytra. (Health for Life Brands) Neomycin sulfate 2.5 mg, gramicidin 0.25 mg, benzocaine 10 mg. Troche. Box 10s. *Rx.*
Use: Anti-infective.

Bio-Zyme. (Integrative Therapeutics) Amylase 40,625 units, lipase 3,250 units, protease 40,625 units. Soy. Tab. 100s. *OTC.*
Use: Digestive enzyme.

•**bipenamol hydrochloride.** (bye-PEN-ah-MAHL) USAN.
Use: Antidepressant.

•**biperiden.** (by-PURR-ih-den) *USP.*
Use: Anticholinergic; antiparkinson.

•**biperiden hydrochloride.** (by-PURR-ih-den) *USP.*
Use: Anticholinergic; antiparkinson.
See: Akineton.

•**biperiden lactate, injection.** (by-PURR-ih-den) *USP.*
Use: Anticholinergic; antiparkinsonian.

•**biphenamine hydrochloride.** (bye-FEN-ah-meen) USAN.
Use: Anesthetic, local; anti-infective; antimicrobial.

Biphenox. (MedChem) Acetaminophen 325 mg, phenyltoloxamine citrate 30 mg. Lactose. Tab. 100s. *OTC.*
Use: Nonnarcotic analgesic combination.

Bipole-S. (Spanner) Testosterone 25 mg, estrone 2 mg/mL. Inj. Vial. 10 mL. *Rx.*
Use: Androgen, estrogen combination.

•**biricodar dicitrate.** (BYE-rih-koe-dahr die-SIH-trate) USAN.
Use: Chemotherapy agent, multidrug resistance inhibitor.

•**birinapant.** (bir-IN-a-pant) USAN.
Use: Antineoplastic.

Bisac-Evac. (G & W) Bisacodyl. **EC Tab.:** 5 mg. Bot. 25s. **Supp.:** 10 mg. Pkg. 8s, 12s, 50s, 100s, 500s, 1000s. *OTC.*
Use: Laxative.

•**bisacodyl.** (BISS-uh-koe-dill) *USP.*
Use: Laxative, irritant or stimulant laxative.
See: Alophen.
Bisac-Evac.
Bisacodyl Uniserts.
Bisa-Lax.
Correctol.
Dacodyl.
Deficol.
Delco-Lax.
Dulcagen.
Dulcolax.
Dulcolax Bowel Prep Kit.
Ex-Lax Ultra.
Feen-a-mint.
Fleet Laxative.
Modane.
Women's Gentle Laxative.

bisacodyl. (Various Mfr.) Bisacodyl. **Enteric-coated Tab.:** 5 mg. Bot. 25s, 50s, 100s, 1000s, UD 100s. **Supp.:** 10 mg. Pkg. 12s, 16s, 100s. *OTC.*
Use: Laxative.

•**bisacodyl tannex.** (BISS-uh-koe-dill) USAN.
Use: Laxative.

Bisacodyl Uniserts. (Upsher-Smith) Bisacodyl 10 mg. Supp. Pack. 12s. *OTC.*
Use: Laxative.

Bisalate. (Allison) Sodium salicylate 5 g, salicylamide 2.5 g, sodium paraminobenzoate 5 g, ascorbic acid 50 mg, butabarbital sodium ⅛ g. Tab. Bot. 100s, 1000s. *Rx.*
Use: Antirheumatic.

Bisa-Lax. (Bergen Brunswig) **Supp.:** Bisacodyl 10 mg. Hydrogenated vegetable oil. 50s. **Tab., delayed release:** Bisacodyl 5 mg. 25s, 50s. *OTC.*
Use: Laxative.

•**bisantrene hydrochloride.** (BISS-an-TREEN) USAN.
Use: Antineoplastic.

bisatin.
See: Oxyphenisatin.

•**bisdisulizole disodium.** (bis-dye-SU-li-zole) USAN.
Use: Dermatologic agent; sunscreen.

bishydroxycoumarin.
See: Dicumarol.

Bismapec. (Pal-Pak, Inc.) Bismuth hydroxide 137.7 mg, colloidal kaolin 648 mg, citrus pectin 129.6 mg. Tab. Bot. 1000s. *OTC.*
Use: Antidiarrheal.

Bismatrol. (Major) Bismuth subsalicylate. **Chew. Tab.:** 262 mg. Sodium 0.1 mg, saccharin, mannitol. 30s. **Liq.:** 262 mg per 15 mL. Benzoic acid, saccharin. 236 mL. *OTC.*
Use: Antidiarrheal.

Bismatrol Maximum Strength. (Major) Bismuth subsalicylate 525 mg per 15 mL. Saccharin, sodium 6 mg. Liq. 237 mL. *OTC.*
Use: Antidiarrheal.

bismuth. (Contract Pharmacal Corporation) Bismuth subsalicylate 262 mg. Cherry flavoring, mannitol, saccharin, sorbitol, wintergreen oil flavoring. Sugar free. Chew. Tab. 30s. *OTC.*
Use: Antidiarrheal.

•**bismuth aluminate.** (BISS-muth) USAN. Aluminum bismuth oxide.

•**bismuth carbonate.** (BISS-muth) USAN.
Use: Protectant, topical.

•**bismuth citrate.** (BISS-muth) *USP.*
Use: Antacid.

bismuth glycolylarsanilate.
Use: Antiamebic.
See: Glycobiarsol.

bismuth hydroxide.
See: Bismuth, Milk of.

bismuth, insoluble products.
See: Bismuth subgallate.
Bismuth subsalicylate.
Bismuth tribromophenate.

bismuth magma. *Name previously used for Milk of Bismuth.*

•**bismuth, milk of.** (BISS-muth) *USP. Formerly Bismuth Magma.*
Use: Astringent; antacid.

bismuth oxycarbonate.
See: Bismuth subcarbonate.

bismuth potassium tartrate. Basic bismuth potassium bismuthotartrate. (Brewer) 25 mg/mL. Amp. 2 mL. (Miller Pharmacal Group) 0.016 g/mL. Amp. 2 mL. Box 12s, 100s; Bot. 30 mL, 60 mL. (Raymer) 2.5%. Amp. 2 mL. Box 12s, 100s. *Rx.*
Use: Agent for syphilis.

bismuth resorcin compound.
W/Bismuth subgallate, balsam Peru, benzocaine, zinc oxide, boric acid.
See: Bonate.

bismuth sodium tartrate.
Use: Syphilis.

bismuth subbenzoate.
Use: Dusting powder for wounds.

•**bismuth subcarbonate.** (BISS-muth sub-KAR-bo-nate) *USP.*
Use: Protectant, topical.

bismuth subcarbonate.
Use: Gastroenteritis; diarrhea.
W/Hydrocortisone acetate, belladonna extract, ephedrine sulfate, zinc oxide, boric acid, balsam Peru, cocoa butter.
See: K-C.

bismuth subcitrate potassium.
W/Metronidazole, Tetracycline Hydrochloride.
See: Pylera.

•**bismuth subgallate.** (BISS-muth sub-GAL-ate) *USP.*
Use: Topically for skin conditions; orally as an antidiarrheal.
See: Devrom.
W/Balsam Peru, Bismuth Resorcin Compound, Zinc Oxide.
See: Versal.
W/Opium Powder, Pectin, Kaolin, Zinc Phenolsulfonate.
See: Paregoric.
Pectin.

•**bismuth subnitrate.** (BISS-muth sub-NYE-trate) *USP.*
Use: Pharmaceutic necessity; gastroenteritis; amebic dysentery; locally for wounds.

•**bismuth subsalicylate.** (BISS-muth sub-sa-LIS-i-late) *USP.* Basic bismuth salicylate. Agent for syphilis. Used in combination with metronidazole and tetracycline hydrochloride to treat active duodenal ulcer associated with *Helicobacter pylori* infection.
Use: Antidiarrheal; antacid; antiulcerative.
See: Bismatrol.
Bismatrol Maximum Strength.
Kaopectate.
Kaopectate Children's.
Kaopectate Extra Strength.
Kao-Tin.
Maalox Total Relief.
Peptic Relief.
Pepto-Bismol InstaCool.
W/Calcium Carbonate.
See: Pepto-Bismol.
W/Pectin, Salol, Kaolin, Zinc Sulfocarbolate, Aluminum Hydroxide.
See: Pepto-Bismol.

bismuth tannate. (Various Mfr.) Tan bismuth. *OTC.*
Use: Astringent and protective in GI disorders.

bismuth tribromophenate.
Use: Intestinal antiseptic.

bismuth, water-soluble products.
See: Bismuth potassium tartrate.

•**bisnafide dimesylate.** (BISS-nah-fide die-MEH-sih-late) USAN.
Use: Antineoplastic.

•**bisobrin lactate.** (BISS-oh-brin LACK-tate) USAN.
Use: Fibrinolytic.

•**bisoctrizole.** (bis-OK-trye-zole) USAN.
Use: Sunscreen.

•**bisoprolol.** (bih-SO-pro-lahl) *USP.*
Use: Antiadrenergic/sympatholytic, beta-adrenergic blocking agent.

•**bisoprolol fumarate.** (bih-SO-pro-lahl) *USP.*
Use: Antiadrenergic/sympatholytic, beta-adrenergic blocking agent.
See: Zebeta.
W/Combinations.
See: Ziac.

bisoprolol fumarate. (Eon) Bisoprolol fumarate 5 mg, 10 mg. Tab. Bot. 30s, 100s. *Rx.*
Use: Antiadrenergic/sympatholytic, beta-adrenergic blocking agent.

bisoprolol fumarate and hydrochlorothiazide. (Various Mfr.) Bisoprolol fumarate/hydrochlorothiazide 2.5 mg/6.25 mg, 5 mg/6.25 mg, 10 mg/6.25 mg. Tab. Bot. 30s (10 mg/6.25 mg only), 100s, 500s, 1000s. *Rx.*
Use: Antihypertensive, diuretic.

•**bisoxatin acetate.** (biss-OX-at-in) USAN.
Use: Laxative.

bisphosphonates.
Use: Antihypercalcemic; bone resorption inhibitor.
See: Alendronate Sodium.
Alendronate Sodium/Vitamin D_3.
Etidronate Disodium.
Ibandronate Sodium.
Pamidronate Disodium.
Risedronate/Calcium Carbonate.
Risedronate Sodium.
Tiludronate Disodium.
Zoledronic Acid.

•**bispyrithione magsulfex.** (BISS-PIHR-ih-thigh-ohn mag-sull-fex) USAN.
Use: Antidandruff; anti-infective; antimicrobial.

bis-tropamide. Tropicamide.
See: Mydriacyl.

Bite & Itch Lotion. (Weeks & Leo) Pramoxine hydrochloride 1%, pyrilamine maleate 2%, pheniramine maleate 0.2%, chlorpheniramine maleate 0.2%. Bot. 4 oz. *OTC.*
Use: Dermatologic, topical.

Bite Rx. (International Lab. Tech.) Aluminum acetate 0.5%, benzalkonium chloride. Soln. Bot. 120 mL. *OTC.*
Use: Astringent.

bithionol. (bye-THYE-oh-nole)
Use: Anti-infective.

•**bithionolate, sodium.** (bye-THIGH-oh-noe-late) USAN.
Use: Topical anti-infective.

Bitin. CDC anti-infective agent.
See: Bithionol.

•**bitolterol mesylate.** (by-TOLE-tor-ole) USAN.
Use: Bronchodilator, sympathomimetic.

•**bitopertin.** (BYE-toe-PER-tin) USAN.
Use: CNS agent.

Bitrate. (Arco) Phenobarbital 15 mg, pentaerythritol tetranitrate 20 mg. Tab. Bot. 100s. *Rx.*
Use: Antianginal; hypnotic; sedative.

•**bivalirudin.** (bye-VAL-ih-ruh-din) USAN.
Use: Anticoagulant; antithrombotic.
See: Angiomax.

Bivigam. (Biotest Pharmaceuticals) Immune globulin (human) 10% (100 mg/mL). Glycine 0.2 to 0.29 M, polysorbate 80 0.15% to 0.25%. Preservative free. Inj., Soln. Single-use vial. 50 mL, 100 mL. *Rx.*
Use: Immune globulin.

•**bixalomer.** (bix-AL-oh-mer) USAN.
Use: Hyperphosphatemia.

•**bizelesin.** (bye-ZELL-eh-sin) USAN.
Use: Antineoplastic.

Black and White Bleaching Cream. (Schering-Plough) Hydroquinone 2%. Cream. Tube 0.75 oz, 1.5 oz. *Rx.*
Use: Dermatologic.

Black and White Ointment. (Schering-Plough) Resorcinol 3%. Oint. Tube 0.62 oz, 2.25 oz.
Use: Antiseptic; dermatologic, topical.

Black Draught. (Lee Pharmaceuticals) Sennosides. **Chew. Tab.:** 10 mg. Sugar. Bot. 30s. **Tab.:** 6 mg, sucrose. Bot. 30s. **Gran.:** 20 mg/5 mL, tartrazine, sucrose. Bot. 22.5 g. *OTC.*
Use: Laxative.

black widow spider, antivenin.
See: Antivenin (Latrodectus mactans).

Bladder 2.2. (Theralogix) Vitamins A 9,000 units, D 1,000 units, E 100 units, B_1 0.75 mg, B_2 0.85 mg, B_3 10 mg, B_5 5 mg, B_6 50 mg, B_{12} 3 mcg, C 500 mg, folate 200 mcg, B, Ca, Cr, Cu, I, Mg, Mn, Mo, P, Se, Zn. Biotin 15 mcg, chloride 23 mg, lycopene 5 mg, potassium 25 mg. Tab. 180s. *OTC.*
Use: Nutritional supplement.

Blairex Hard Contact Lens Cleaner. (Blairex) Anionic detergent. Liq. Bot. 60 mL. *OTC.*
Use: Contact lens care.

Blairex Sterile Saline Solution. (Blairex) Sodium Cl, boric acid, sodium borate. Soln. Bot. Aerosol. 90 mL, 240 mL, 360 mL. *OTC.*
Use: Contact lens care.

Blairex System. (Blairex) Sodium Cl 135 mg. Tab. 200s, 365s w/15 mL bot. *OTC.*
Use: Contact lens care.

Blairex System II. (Blairex) Sodium Cl 250 mg. Tab. 90s, 180s w/27.7 mL bot. *OTC.*
Use: Contact lens care.

Blaud Strubel. (Strubel) Ferrous sulfate 5 g. Cap. Bot. 100s. *OTC.*
Use: Mineral supplement.

Blefcon. (Madland) Sodium sulfacetamide 30%. Oint. Tube 1/8 oz. *Rx.*
Use: Anti-infective, ophthalmic.

bleomycin. (Various Mfr.) Bleomycin 15 units, 30 units. Pow. for Inj. Vial. *Rx.*
Use: Antineoplastic; antibiotic.

bleomycin sulfate. (Various Mfr.) Bleomycin sulfate 15 units, 30 units. Pow. for Inj. Vial. *Rx.*
Use: Antineoplastic.

•**bleomycin sulfate, sterile.** (BLEE-oh-MY-sin) *USP.* Antibiotic obtained from cultures of *Streptomyces verticillus.*
Use: Antineoplastic; antibiotic.

Blephamide. (Allergan) Sulfacetamide sodium 10%, prednisolone acetate 0.2%. EDTA, polyvinyl alcohol 1.4%, polysorbate 80, sodium thiosulfate, benzalkonium chloride. Susp. 2.5 mL, 5 mL, 10 mL. *Rx.*
Use: Anti-inflammatory; anti-infective, ophthalmic.

Blephamide Ophthalmic Ointment. (Allergan) Prednisolone acetate 0.2%, sulfacetamide sodium 10%. Phenylmercuric acetate 0.0008%, mineral oil, white petrolatum, lanolin alcohol. Ophth. Oint. Tube 3.5 g. *Rx.*
Use: Anti-inflammatory; anti-infective, ophthalmic.

Bleph-10. (Allergan) Sulfacetamide sodium 10%. Polyvinyl alcohol 1.4%, benzalkonium chloride 0.005%, polysorbate 80, sodium thiosulfate, EDTA. Soln. 2.5 mL, 5 mL, 15 mL. *Rx.*
Use: Ophthalmic and otic agent, antibiotic.

•**blinatumomab.** (BLIN-a-toom-oh-mab) USAN.
Use: Antineoplastic agent.

Blink Gel Tears Lubricating Eye Drops. (Abbott Medical Optics) 0.25% PEG 400, boric acid, potassium chloride, sodium borate, sodium chlorite, sodium hyaluronate. Gel; Ophth. 10 mL. *OTC.*
Use: Ocular lubricant.

Blink Tears. (Abbott Medical Optics) Polyethylene glycol 400 0.25%. Soln.; Ophth. 15 mL. *OTC.*
Use: Artificial tears.

Blink Tears Preservative Free. (Abbott Medical Optics) Polyethylene glycol 400 0.25%. Preservative free. Soln.; Ophth. Single-use container. 0.4 mL (25s). *OTC.*
Use: Artificial tears.

Blis. (Del) Boric acid 47.5%, salicylic acid 17%. Bot. 7 oz. *OTC.*
Use: Antifungal, topical.

•**blisibimod.** (blye-SIB-i-mod) USAN.
Use: Immunomodulator.

BlisterGard. (Medtech) Alcohol 6.7%, pyroxylin solution, oil of cloves, B-hydroxyquinolone. Liq. Bot. 30 mL. *OTC.*
Use: Dermatologic, protectant.

Blistex. (Blairex) Camphor 0.5%, phenol 0.5%, allantoin 1%, lanolin, mineral oil. Tube 4.2 g, 10.5 g. *OTC.*
Use: Lip protectant.

Blistex Five Star Lip Protection. (Blistex) Homosalate 9.6%, octinoxate 7.5%, octisalate 5%, oxybenzone 5%, petrolatum 30.1%, calendula officinalis flower extract, safflower oil, candelilla wax, glycerin, sunflower seed oil, coconut oil, jojoba esters, lanolin, microcrystalline wax, saccharin, cocoa seed butter, titanium dioxide, tocopheryl acetate, wheat germ oil. SPF 30. Lip balm. 4.25 g. *OTC.*
Use: Sunscreen.

Blistex Lip Balm. (Blairex) SPF 10. Camphor 0.5%, phenol 0.5%, allantoin 1%, dimethicone 2%, pamidate 0.25%, oxybenzone, parabens, petrolatum. Tube 4.5 g. *OTC.*
Use: Lip protectant.

Blistex Ultra Protection. (Blairex) Octyl methoxycinnamate, oxybenzone, octylsalicylate, menthylanthranilate, homosalate, dimethicone. Tube 4.2 g. *OTC.*
Use: Lip protectant.

Blistik. (Blairex) Padimate O 6.6%, oxybenzone 2.5%, dimethicone 2%. Lip-balm stick 4.5 g. *OTC.*
Use: Lip protectant.

Blis-To-Sol. (Oakhurst) **Liq.:** Tolnaftate 1%. 30 mL. **Pow.:** Zinc undecylenate 12%. 60 g. **Soln.:** Tolnaftate 1%. 30 mL, 55.5 mL. *OTC.*
Use: Antifungal, topical.

BLM.
See: Bleomycin Sulfate.

Blocadren. (Merck & Co.) Timolol maleate 5 mg, 20 mg. Tab. Bot. 100s. *Rx.*
Use: Antiadrenergic/sympatholytic, beta-adrenergic blocker.

Block Out by Sea & Ski. (Carter-Wallace) Padimate O, octyl methoxycinnamate, oxybenzone. Cream. Tube 120 g. *OTC.*
Use: Sunscreen.

Block Out Clear by Sea & Ski. (Carter-Wallace) Padimate O, octyl methoxy-

cinnamate, octyl salicylate, SD alcohol 40. Lot. Bot. 120 mL. *OTC.*
Use: Sunscreen.

blood, anticoagulants.
See: Anticoagulants.

•**blood cells, red.** *USP. Formerly Blood cells, human red.*
Use: Blood replenisher.

blood coagulation.
See: Hemostatics.

blood glucose concentrator.
See: Glucagon.

blood glucose test.
See: Chemstrip bG.
First Choice.
Glucostix.

•**blood grouping serum, anti-A.** *USP.*
Use: Diagnostic aid, blood, in vitro.

•**blood grouping serum, anti-B.** *USP.*
Use: Diagnostic aid, blood, in vitro.

•**blood grouping serums anti-D, anti-C, anti-E, anti-c, anti-e.** *USP. Formerly Anti-Rh typing serums.*
Use: Diagnostic aid, blood, in vitro.

blood group specific substances A, B and AB. *Formerly Blood Grouping specific substances A and B.*
Use: Blood neutralizer.

Blood Sugar Balance. (Mason) Magnesium 200 mg (magnesium content expressed in mg elemental magnesium), biotin 600 mcg, bitter melon 200 mg, chromium 48 mcg, ginkgo 120 mg, gymnema 300 mg, iron oxide, lipoic acid 150 mg, mineral oil, quercetin 50 mg, vanadium 40 mcg, zinc 30 mg. PEG. Gluten free, lactose free, preservative free, and sugar free. Tab. 60s. *OTC.*
Use: Nutritional supplement, multimineral.

•**blood, whole.** *USP. Formerly Blood, whole human.*
Use: Blood replenisher.

•**blosozumab.** (bloe-SOZ-ue-mab) USAN.
Use: Treatment of osteoporosis.

Bloxiverz. (Éclat Pharmaceuticals) Neostigmine methylsulfate 0.5 mg/mL, 1 mg/mL. Phenol 4.5 mg/mL. Inj., Soln. Multiple-dose vial. 10 mL. *Rx.*
Use: Cholinergic muscle stimulant, anticholinesterase muscle stimulant.

Bludex. (Burlington) Methenamine 40.8 mg, methylene blue 5.4 mg, phenylsalicylate 18.1 mg, atropine sulfate 0.03 mg, hyoscyamine 0.03 mg, benzoic acid 4.5 mg. Tab. Bot. 100s, 1000s. *Rx.*
Use: Antiseptic; antispasmodic, urinary.

Blue. (Various Mfr.) Pyrethrins 0.3%, piperonyl butoxide 3%, petroleum distillate 1.2%. Gel. Bot. 30 g, 480 g. *OTC.*
Use: Pediculicide.

Blue-Emu Maximum Strength. (NFI Consumer Products) Menthol 2.5%. Aloe vera gel, balm mint extract, boswella extract, citrus extract, emu oil, eucalyptus oil, ginger extract, isopropyl alcohol, nettle leaf extract, peppermint extract, rosemary oil, urea. Spray. 59.15 mL. *OTC.*
Use: Topical analgesic.

Blue Gel Muscular Pain Reliever. (Rugby) Menthol in a specially formulated base. Gel. Tube 240 g. *OTC.*
Use: Liniments.

Blue Ice. (Geritrex) Menthol 2%, isopropyl alcohol. Gel. 227 g. *OTC.*
Use: Rub and liniment.

Blue Star. (McCue Labs.) Salicylic acid, benzoic acid, methyl salicylate, camphor, lanolin, petrolatum. Oint. Jar 2 oz. *OTC.*
Use: Dermatologic, counterirritant.

Blu-12 100. (Bluco) Cyanocobalamin 100 mcg/mL. Vial 30 mL. *Rx.*
Use: Vitamin supplement.

Blu-12 1000. (Bluco) Cyanocobalamin 1000 mcg/mL. Vial 30 mL. *Rx.*
Use: Vitamin supplement.

B-Major. (Barth's) Vitamins B_1 7 mg, B_2 14 mg, niacin 2.35 mg, B_{12} 7.5 mcg, B_6 0.15 mg, pantothenic acid 0.37 mg, choline 85 mg, inositol 6 mg, biotin, folic acid, aminobenzoic acid. Cap. Bot. 1s, 3s, 6s, 12s. *Rx-OTC.*
Use: Mineral, vitamin supplement.

B-N. (Eric, Kirk & Gary) Bacitracin 500 units, neomycin sulfate 5 mg. Oint. Tube 0.5 oz. *OTC.*
Use: Anti-infective, topical.

b-naphthyl salicylate. Betol, naphthosalol, salinaphthol.
Use: gastrointestinal and genitourinary, antiseptic.

B-Nexa. (Upsher-Smith) Folic acid 1.22 mg, calcium 124.23 mg, vitamin B_6 42 mg, ginger root powder extract 100 mg. Film coated. Maltodextrin. Tab. 60s. *Rx.*
Use: Prenatal vitamin with minerals.

•**boceprevir.** (boe-SE-pre-vir) USAN.
Use: Treatment of hepatitis C infection.
See: Victrelis.

•**bococizumab.** (BOE-koe-SIZ-ue-mab) USAN.
Use: Treatment of dyslipidemia.

Bodi Kleen. (Geritrex) Triethanolamine lauryl sulfate, 2-phenoxy-ethanol, hexylene glycol, aloe vera gel. Spray. 8 oz. *OTC.*
Use: Anorectal preparation.

Body Fortress Natural Amino. (Nature's Bounty) Protein 1.67 g, lactalbumin hydrolysate 1500 mg, yeast and preservative free. Tab. Bot. 150s. *OTC.*
Use: Amino acid.

Boil-Ease. (Del) Benzocaine 20% with camphor, lanolin, eucalyptus oil, menthol, petrolatum, phenol. Oint. 30 g. *OTC.*
Use: Topical local anesthetic, ester local anesthetic.

BoilnSoak. (Alcon) Sodium Cl 0.7%, boric acid, sodium borate, thimerosal 0.001%, disodium edetate 0.1%. Bot. 8 oz, 12 oz. *OTC.*
Use: Contact lens care.

•**bolandiol dipropionate.** (bole-AN-die-ole die-PRO-pee-oh-nate) USAN.
Use: Anabolic.

•**bolasterone.** (BOLE-ah-STEE-rone) USAN.
Use: Anabolic.

Bolax. (Boyd) Docusate sodium 240 mg, phenolphthalein 30 mg, dihydrocholic acid ¾ g. Cap. Bot. 100s. *OTC.*
Use: Laxative.

•**boldenone undecylenate.** (BOLE-deen-ohn uhn-deh-sih-LEN-ate) USAN. Parenabol. Under study.
Use: Anabolic.

•**bolenol.** (BOLE-ee-nahl) USAN.
Use: Anabolic.

•**bolmantalate.** (BOLE-MAN-tah-late) USAN.
Use: Anabolic.

Bonacal Plus. (Kenwood) Vitamins A 5000 units, D 400 units, C 100 mg, B_1 3 mg, B_2 3 mg, B_6 10 mg, B_{12} 4 mcg, niacinamide 20 mg, d-calcium pantothenate 3.3 mg, iron 42 mg, calcium 350 mg, manganese 0.33 mg, zinc 0.1 mg, magnesium 1.67 mg, potassium 1.67 mg. Tab. Bot. 100s. *OTC.*
Use: Mineral, vitamin supplement.

Bonamil Infant Formula with Iron. (Wyeth) Protein 2.3 g (from nonfat milk, taurine), fat 5.4 g (from soybean and coconut oils, soy lecithin), carbohydrate 10.7 g (from lactose), linoleic acid 1300 mg, vitamin A 300 units, D 60 units, E 2.85 units, K 8 mcg, $B_1$100 mcg, B_2 150 mcg, B_6 63 mcg, B_{12} 0.2 mcg, B_3 750 mcg, folic acid 7.5 mcg, B_5 315 mcg, biotin 2.2 mcg, vitamin C 8.3 mg, choline 15 mg, Ca 69 mg, P 54 mg, Mg 6 mg, Fe 1.8 mg, Zn 0.75 mg, Mn 15 mcg, Cu 70 mcg, I 5 mcg, Na 27 mg, K 93 mg, Cl 63 mg/100 cal (5.3 cal/g). Conc., Liq. Bot. 453 g. Conc. 384 mL. Ready-to-feed liq. 946 mL. *OTC.*
Use: Nutritional supplement, enteral.

Bonate. (Suppositoria Laboratories, Inc.) Bismuth subgallate, balsam Peru, benzocaine, zinc oxide. Supp. Box 12s, 100s, 1000s. *OTC.*
Use: Anorectal preparation.

Bonefos. (Leiras) Disodium clodronate tetrahydrate.
Use: Bone resorption inhibitor. [Orphan Drug]

B 100. (Fibertone) Vitamins B_1 100 mg, B_2 100 mg, B_3 100 mg, B_5 100 mg, B_6 100 mg, B_{12} 100 mcg, FA 0.4 mg, biotin 50 mcg, PABA 100 mg, choline bitartrate 100 mg, inositol 100 mg. SR Tab. Bot. 100s. *OTC.*
Use: Vitamin supplement.

B-100. (NBTY) Vitamins B_1 100 mg, B_2 100 mg, B_3 100 mg, B_5 100 mg, B_6 100 mg, B_{12} 100 mcg, folic acid 0.1 mg, d-biotin 100 mcg, PABA 100 mg, choline bitartrate, inositol, lecithin. Tab. Bot. 50s, 100s. *OTC.*
Use: Mineral, vitamin supplement.

B150. (NBTY) Vitamins B_1 150 mg, B_2 150 mg, B_3 150 mg, B_5 150 mg, B_6 150 mg, B_{12} 150 mcg, folic acid 0.1 mg, d-biotin 150 mcg, PABA 150 mg, choline bitartrate 150 mg, inositol 150 mg, lecithin. Tab. Bot. 100s. *OTC.*
Use: Mineral, vitamin supplement.

B125. (NBTY) Vitamins B_1 125 mg, B_2 125 mg, B_3 125 mg, B_5 125 mg, B_6 125 mg, B_{12} 125 mcg, folic acid 0.1 mg, d-biotin 125 mcg, PABA 125 mg, choline bitartrate 125 mg, inositol 125 mg, lecithin. Tab. Bot. 100s. *OTC.*
Use: Mineral, vitamin supplement.

Bone Meal w/Vitamin D. (Nature's Bounty) Calcium 220 mg, vitamin D 100 units, phosphorus 100 mg, iron 0.45 mg, copper 3.25 mg, zinc 20 mcg, manganese 2.75 mcg, magnesium 0.925 mg. Tab. Bot. 100s, 250s. *OTC.*
Use: Mineral, vitamin supplement.

Bonine. (Insight) Meclizine hydrochloride 25 mg. Lactose, saccharin. Raspberry flavor. Chew. Tab. 8s. *OTC.*
Use: Antiemetic/antivertigo agent, anticholinergic.

Bonine for Kids. (Insight) Cycliziine hydrochloride 25 mg. Mannitol, sorbitol, sucralose. Berry flavor. Chew. Tab. 8s. *OTC.*
Use: Antiemetic/antivertigo agent, antidopaminergic.

Boniva. (Roche) Ibandronate sodium (as base). **Inj.:** 1 mg/mL. Single-use prefilled syringe. 5 mL. **Tab.:** 150 mg. Lactose. Film coated. UD 1s. *Rx.*
Use: Bisphosphonate.

Bontril PDM. (Valeant) Phendimetrazine tartrate 35 mg, sugar, isopropyl alcohol, lactose. Tab. Bot. 100s, 1000s. *c-III.*
Use: CNS stimulant, anorexiant.

Bontril Slow Release. (Valeant) Phendimetrazine tartrate 105 mg. SR Cap. Bot. 100s. *c-III.*
Use: CNS stimulant, anorexiant.

Boost. (Nestle Nutrition) Protein 41.7 g (milk protein), carbohydrate 171 g (corn syr., sugar), fat 16.7 g (soy lecithin, vegetable oil), Na 542.1 mg, K 1,668 mg, vitamin A, B_1, B_2, B_3, B_5, B_6, B_{12}, C, D, E, K, Ca, Cl, Cr, Cu, Fe, I, Mg, Mo, Mn, P, Se, Zn, biotin, choline, folic acid. Lactose free. Butter pecan, chocolate, strawberry, and vanilla flavors. Liq. 240 mL. *OTC.*
Use: Defined formula diet, supplemental nutritional formula.

Boost Glucose Control. (Nestle Nutrition) Protein 66.72 g (Ca caseinate, Na caseinate, L-arginine, milk protein), carbohydrate 66.72 g (fructose, maltodextrin, sucralose, tapioca dextrin), fat 29.9 g (soy lecithin, vegetable oil), Na 750.6 mg, K 271.05 mg, vitamin A, B_1, B_2, B_3, B_5, B_6, B_{12}, C, D, E, K, Ca, Cl, Cr, Cu, Fe, I, Mg, Mo, Mn, P, Se, Zn, biotin, choline, folic acid. Lactose free. Chocolate, strawberry, and vanilla flavors. Liq. 240 mL. *OTC.*
Use: Defined formula diet, supplemental nutritional formula.

Boost High Protein. (Nestle Nutrition) Protein 70.5 g (Ca caseinate, Na caseinate, milk protein), carbohydrate 137.61 g (corn syr., sugar), fat 25.02 g (soy lecithin, vegetable oil, Na 708.9 mg, K 1,584.6 mg, vitamin A, B_1, B_2, B_3, B_5, B_6, B_{12}, C, D, E, K, Ca, Cl, Cr, Cu, Fe, I, Mg, Mo, Mn, P, Se, Zn, biotin, choline, folic acid. Lactose free. Chocolate, strawberry, and vanilla flavors. Liq. 240 mL. *OTC.*
Use: Defined formula diet, supplemental nutritional formula.

Boost Kid Essentials. (Nestle Nutrition) Protein 28.68 g (L-carnitine, Ca caseinate, Na caseinate, taurine, whey protein), carbohydrate 135.25 g (fructose, maltodextrin, sugar), fat 36.89 g (medium chain triglycerides, soybean oil, soy lecithin, sunflower oil) Na 737.7 mg, K 1,106.6 mg, vitamin A, B_1, B_2, B_3, B_5, B_6, B_{12}, C, D, E, K, Ca, Cl, Cr, Cu, Fe, I, Mg, Mn, Mo, P, Se, Zn, biotin, choline, folic acid, inositol. Lactose free. Chocolate, strawberry, and vanilla flavors. Liq. 244 mL w/probiotic straw. *OTC.*
Use: Defined formula diet, supplemental nutritional formula.

Boost Kid Essentials 1.5. (Nestle Nutrition) Protein 42.19 g (Ca caseinate, L-carnitine, M-inositol, Na caseinate, taurine, whey protein) carbohydrate 164.56 g (maltodextrin, sugar), fat 75.11 g (medium chain triglycerides, soybean oil, soy lecithin, sunflower oil), Na 691.98 mg, K 1,303.8 mg, vitamin A, B_1, B2, B_3, B_5, B_6, B_{12}, C, D, E, K, Ca, Cl, Cr, Cu, Fe, I, Mg, Mn, Mo, P, Se, Zn, biotin, choline, folic acid. Lactose free. Vanilla flavor. Liq. 237 mL. *OTC.*
Use: Defined formula diet, supplemental nutritional formula.

Boost Kid Essentials 1.5 with Fiber. (Nestle Nutrition) Protein 42.19 g (Ca caseinate, L-carnitine, M-inositol, Na caseinate, taurine, whey protein), carbohydrate 164.56 g (maltodextrin, sugar), fat 75.11 g (medium chain triglycerides, soybean oil, soy lecithin, sunflower oil), Na 691.98 mg, K 1,303.8 mg, vitamin A, B_1, B_2, B_3, B_5, B_6, B_{12}, C, D, E, K, Ca, Cl, Cr, Cu, Fe, I, Mg, Mn, Mo, P, Se, Zn, biotin, choline, folic acid. Lactose free. Vanilla flavor. Liq. 237 mL. *OTC.*
Use: Defined formula diet, supplemental nutritional formula.

Boost Nutritional Pudding. (Nestle Nutrition) Protein 7 g, fat 9 g, carbohydrate 32 g, sodium 120 mg, potassium 320 mg, calories 240/serving, vitamins A, C, D, E, K, B_6, B_{12}, B_1, B_2, B_3, B_5, Ca, Fe, folic acid, biotin, P, I, Mg, Zn, Se, Cu, Mn, Cr, Mo, sugar. Pudding Cont. 142 g. *OTC.*
Use: Nutritional supplement.

Boost Plus. (Nestle Nutrition) Protein 58.38 g (Ca caseinate, Na caseinate, milk protein), carbohydrate 187.65 g (corn syr., sugar), fat 58.38 g (soy lecithin, vegetable oil), Na 708.9 mg, K 1,584.6 mg, vitamins A, B_1, B_2, B_3, B_5, B_6, B_{12}, C, D, E, K, Ca, Cl, Cr, Cu, Fe, I, Mg, Mo, Mn, P, Se, Zn, biotin, choline, folic acid. Lactose free. Chocolate, strawberry, and vanilla flavors. Liq. 240 mL. *OTC.*
Use: Defined formula diet, supplemental nutritional formula.

Boostrix. (GlaxoSmithKline) Diphtheria toxoid 2.5 Lf units, tetanus toxoid 5 Lf units, pertactin 2.5 mcg, FHA (filamentous hemagglutinin) 8 mcg, inactivated pertussis toxins 8 mcg per 0.5 mL. Sodium chloride, formaldehyde. Inj. Single-dose vials, disposable prefilled *Tip-Lok* syringes. *Rx.*
Use: Agent for active immunization.

Boost VHC. (Nestle Nutrition) Protein 22 g (calcium-protein caseinate, soy lecithin, soy protein, taurine), carbohydrate 46 g (corn syrup, sugar), fat 30 g (canola oil, corn oil), Na 280 mg, K 420 mg, 2.25 Kcal/mL. Vitamins A, C, D, E, K, B_1, B_2, B_3, B_5, B_6, B_{12}, folic acid, choline 115 mg, I, Zn, Ca, Cu, Cr, Fe, P, Mg, Se, Mn, Mo, Cl, biotin. Lactose free and gluten free. Vanilla flavor. Liq. 237 mL. *OTC.*
Use: Supplemental nutritional formula.

Bopen-VK. (Boyd) Potassium phenoxymethyl penicillin 400,000 units. Tab. Bot. 100s.
Use: Anti-infective, penicillin.

borax. Sodium borate.

•**boric acid.** (BOR-ik) *NF.*
Use: Antiseptic, pharmaceutic necessity; topical anti-infective.
W/Combinations.
See: Saratoga.

2-bornanone. Camphor.

•**bornelone.** (BORE-neh-LONE) USAN.
Use: Ultraviolet screen.

•**bornyl acetate.** (BOR-nil) USAN.
Use: Flavoring agent.

•**borocaptate sodium B 10.** (bore-oh-CAP-tate) USAN.
Use: Antineoplastic; radiopharmaceutical.

Borocell. (Neutron Technology) Sodium monomercaptoundecahdrocloso-dodecaborate.
Use: Boron neutron capture therapy (BNCT) in glioblastoma multiforme.

boroglycerin. (Emerson) Glycerol borate. Bot. Pt.
Use: Agent for dermatitis.

boroglycerin glycerite. Boric acid 31 parts, glycerin 96 parts.
Use: Agent for dermatitis.

borotannic complex. Boric acid 31 mg, tannic acid 50 mg.
Use: Dermatologic agent.

•**bortezomib.** (bore-TEZZ-oh-mib) USAN.
Use: Antineoplastic.
See: Velcade.

•**bosentan.** (boe-SEN-tan) USAN.
Use: Vasodilator, endothelin receptor antagonist.
See: Tracleer.

Boston Advance Cleaner. (Polymer Technology) Concentrated homogenous surfactant with friction-enhancing agents. Soln. Bot. 30 mL. *OTC.*
Use: Contact lens care.

Boston Advance Comfort Formula. (Polymer Technology) Buffered, slightly hypertonic. Polyaminopropyl biguanide 0.00015%, EDTA 0.05%, cationic cellulose derivative polymer. Soln. Bot. 120 mL. *OTC.*
Use: Contact lens care.

Boston Advance Conditioning Solution. (Polymer Technology) Sterile, buffered, slightly hypertonic. Polyaminopropyl biguanide 0.0015%, EDTA 0.05%. Soln. Bot. 120 mL or with cleaner in a convenience pack. *OTC.*
Use: Contact lens care.

Boston Advance Rewetting Drops. (Polymer Technology) Buffered, slightly hypertonic. Polyaminopropyl biguanide 0.0015%, EDTA 0.05%. Drops. Bot. 10 mL. *OTC.*
Use: Contact lens care.

Boston Cleaner. (Bausch & Lomb) Concentrated homogeneous surfactant with friction-enhancing agents, sodium Cl. Soln. Bot. 30 mL. *OTC.*
Use: Contact lens care.

Boston Conditioning Solution. (Polymer Technology) Sterile, buffered, slightly hypertonic, low viscosity. EDTA 0.05%, chlorhexidine gluconate 0.006%. Soln. Bot. 120 mL. *OTC.*
Use: Contact lens care.

Boston Reconditioning Drops. (Polymer Technology) Hydrophilic polyelectrolyte, polyvinyl alcohol, hydroxyethylcellulose, chlorhexidine gluconate, EDTA. Soln. Bot. 120 mL. *OTC.*
Use: Contact lens care.

Boston Rewetting Drops. (Polymer Technology) Buffered, slightly hypertonic. Chlorhexidine gluconate 0.006%, EDTA 0.05%, cationic cellulose derivative polymer. Soln. Bot. 10 mL. *OTC.*
Use: Contact lens care.

Boston Simplicity Multi-Action. (Polymer Technology) PEO sorbitan monolaurate, silicone glycol copolymer, cellulosic viscosifier, derivatized PEG, chlorhexidine gluconate, polyaminopropyl biguanide, EDTA. 0.05%. Soln. Bot. 60 mL, 90 mL, 120 mL. *OTC.*
Use: Contact lens product.

Bosulif. (Pfizer) Bosutinib 100 mg, 500 mg. Film coated. PEG. Tab. 120s (100 mg), 30s (500 mg). *Rx.*
Use: Kinase inhibitor, tyrosine kinase inhibitor.

•**bosutinib.** (boe-SUE-ti-nib) USAN.
Use: Antineoplastic.
See: Bosulif.

Botox. (Allergan) OnabotulinumtoxinA 100 units (one unit corresponds to the calculated median lethal intraperitoneal dose [LD_{50}] in mice). Human albumin 0.5 mg, sodium chloride 0.9 mg. Preservative free. Pow. for Inj. (vacuum

dried). Single-use vial. *Rx.*
Use: Ophthalmic; treatment of cervical dystonia; axillary hyperhidrosis, strabismus and blepharospasm.

Botox Cosmetic. (Allergan) OnabotulinumtoxinA 100 units (one unit corresponds to the calculated median lethal intraperitoneal dose [LD_{50}] in mice). Human albumin 0.5 mg, sodium chloride 0.9 mg. Preservative free. Pow. for Inj. (vacuum dried). Single-use vial. *Rx.*
Use: Treatment of glabellar lines.

botulinum toxins.
See: AbobotulinumtoxinA.
Botulinum toxin type A.
Botulinum toxin type B.
Botulinum toxin type F.
IncobotulinumtoxinA.
Myobloc.
OnabotulinumtoxinA.

botulinum toxin type A.
Use: Ophthalmic; treatment of cervical dystonia, glabellar lines; axillary hyperhidrosis, strabismus and blepharospasm.
See: Botox.
Botox Cosmetic.

botulinum toxin type B.
Use: Cervical dystonia.
See: Myobloc.

botulinum toxin type F. (Porton Product Limited)
Use: Cervical dystonia; essential blepharospasm. [Orphan Drug]

•**botulism antitoxin.** (BOT-yoo-lism) *USP.*
Use: Prophylaxis and treatment of the toxins of *Clostridium botulinum*, types A or B; passive immunizing agent.

botulism antitoxin heptavalent. (Cangene Corporation) Botulism antitoxin heptavalent, equine (serotype A antitoxin ≥ 4,500 units, serotype B antitoxin 3,300 units, serotype C antitoxin 3,000 units, serotype D antitoxin 600 units, serotype E antitoxin 5,100 units, serotype F antitoxin 3,000 units, serotype G antitoxin 600 units. Polysorbate 80. Preservative free. Inj., Soln. Single-use vial. 10 mL, 22 mL. *Rx.*
Use: Antitoxin/antivenin.

botulism immune globulin.
Use: Infant botulism.
See: BabyBIG.

Boudreaux's All Natural Butt Paste. (Fleet Pharmaceuticals) Zinc oxide 16%, aloe, beeswax, castor oil, Peruvian balsam oil, wax. Oint. 56.7 g. *OTC.*
Use: Diaper rash product.

Boudreaux's Butt Paste. (Fleet Pharmaceuticals) Zinc oxide 16%, castor oil, mineral oil, Peruvian balsam, paraffin, petrolatum. Oint. Single foil pack. 28.3 g, 56.7 g, 85 g, 113.4 g, 453.6 g. *OTC.*
Use: Diaper rash product.

Boudreaux's Maximum Strength Butt Paste. (Fleet Pharmaceuticals) Zinc oxide 40%, castor oil, mineral oil, Peruvian balsam, paraffin, petrolatum. Oint. 56.7 g, 113.4 g. *OTC.*
Use: Diaper rash product.

Bounty Bears. (NBTY) Vitamins A 2500 units, D 400 units, E 15 units, C 60 mg, B_1 1.05 mg, B_2 1.2 mg, B_3 13.5 mg, B_6 1.05 mg, B_{12} 4.5 mcg, folic acid 0.3 mg. Tab. Bot. 100s. *OTC.*
Use: Mineral, vitamin supplement.

Bounty Bears Plus Iron. (NBTY) Vitamins A 2500 units, D 400 units, E 15 units, C 60 mg, B_1 1.05 mg, B_2 1.2 mg, B_3 13.5 mg, B_6 1.05 mg, B_{12} 4.5 mcg, folic acid 0.3 mg, iron 15 mg. Tab. Bot. 100s. *OTC.*
Use: Mineral, vitamin supplement.

bourbonal.
See: Ethyl Vanillin.

bovine colostrum.
Use: AIDS-related diarrhea. [Orphan Drug]

bovine immunoglobulin concentrate, Cryptosporidium parvum.
Use: Anti-infective. [Orphan Drug]

bovine whey protein concentrate.
Use: Treatment of cryptosporidiosis. [Orphan Drug]
See: Immuno-C.

bowel evacuants.
Use: Laxative.
See: CoLyte.
Fleet Prep Kit 1.
Fleet Prep Kit 3.
Fleet Prep Kit 2.
GoLYTELY.
MiraLax.
NuLYTELY.
OCL.
Polyethylene Glycol.
Polyethylene Glycol and Electrolytes.
Tridrate Bowel Cleansing System.
X-Prep Bowel Evacuant Kit-1.

Bowman's Poison Antidote Kit. (Jones Pharma) Syr. of ipecac 1 oz, 1 bottle; activated charcoal liquid 2 oz, 3 bottles. *OTC.*
Use: Antidote.

Bowsteral. (Jones Pharma) Isopropanol 60%. Bot. Pt, gal.
Use: Disinfectant.

•**boxidine.** (BOX-ih-deen) USAN.
Use: Adrenal steroid blocker; antihyperlipoproteinemic.

Boylex. (Health for Life Brands) Diperodon, hexachlorophene, rosin cerate,

ichthammol, carbolic acid, thymol, camphor, juniper tar. Tube oz. *OTC.*
Use: Drawing salve.

B-Pap. (Wren) Acetaminophen 120 mg, sodium butabarbital 15 mg/5 mL. Bot. Pt, gal. *Rx.*
Use: Analgesic; sedative.

b-pas.
See: Calcium Benzoyl PAS.

BP Cleansing Wash. (Brookstone) Sodium sulfacetamide 10%, sulfur 4%. Cetyl alcohol, disodium EDTA, glyceryl stearate, parabens, PEG 100 stearate, stearyl alcohol, urea 10%. Soap. 473 mL. *Rx.*
Use: Acne product, combination.

BP 8 Cough. (Macoven Pharmaceuticals) Dextromethorphan hydrobromide 15 mg, guaifenesin 175 mg, pseudoephedrine hydrochloride 30 mg per 5 mL. Parabens, saccharin, sorbitol. Alcohol free. Grape flavor. Susp. 473 mL. *Rx.*
Use: Upper respiratory combination, antitussive and expectorant combination.

BP-50. (Brookstone) Urea 50%. Cetyl alcohol, disodium EDTA, glycerin, lactic acid, PEG-6, titanium dioxide, vitamin E. Emulsion. 284 g. *Rx.*
Use: Emollient.

BP 5.25%. (River's Edge Pharmaceuticals) Benzoyl peroxide 5.25%. Alcohols, aloe, glycerin, PEG, propylene glycol, triethanolamine. Soap. 175 g. *Rx.*
Use: Topical anti-infective, antibiotic agent.

BP Foam. (Cintex) Benzoyl peroxide 9.8%. Parabens, wax. Foam. 100 g. *Rx.*
Use: Topical anti-infective, antibiotic agent.

BP 4.25%. (River's Edge Pharmaceuticals) Benzoyl peroxide 4.25%. Alcohols, aloe, glycerin, green tea extract, PEG, propylene glycol, triethanolamine. Soap. 473 mL. *Rx.*
Use: Topical anti-infective, antibiotic agent.

BP Gel. (Cintex) Benzoyl peroxide 10%. Aloe, benzyl alcohol, disodium EDTA, glycerin, panthenol, PEG, sodium hyaluronate, triethanolamine. Gel. 60 g. *OTC.*
Use: Topical anti-infective, antibiotic.

B-Plex. (Ivax) Vitamins B_1 15 mg, B_2 15 mg, B_3 100 mg, B_5 18 mg, B_6 4 mg, B_{12} 5 mcg, C 500 mg, folic acid 0.5 mg. Tab. Bot. 100s. *Rx.*
Use: Mineral, vitamin supplement.

BPM-DM-PHEN. (Cintex) Brompheniramine maleate 2 mg, dextromethorphan hydrobromide 10 mg, phenylephrine hydrochloride 5 mg. Benzoic acid, disodium EDTA, propylene glycol, saccharin, sorbitol. Syrup. 473 mL. *OTC.*
Use: Upper respiratory combination, antitussive combination.

BPM Pseudo 6/45 mg. (Boca Pharmacal) Pseudoephedrine hydrochloride 45 mg, brompheniramine maleate 6 mg. ER Tab. 30s, 100s. *Rx.*
Use: Decongestant and antihistamine, upper respiratory combination.

BP 7% Wash. (River's Edge) Benzoyl peroxide 7%. Aloe barbadensis, benzyl alcohol, camellia oleifera leaf (green tea) extract, cetyl alcohol, glycerin, PEG-100. Soap. 473 mL. *Rx.*
Use: Anti-infective, topical; antibiotic agent.

Brace. (GlaxoSmithKline) Denture adhesive. Tube 1.4 oz, 2.4 oz.

Bradosol Bromide. (Novartis) Domiphen bromide.
Use: Antiseptic.

bradykinin inhibitors.
See: Icatibant Acetate.

BRAF inhibitors.
See: Dabrafenib.
Vemurafenib.

Brainstrong Prenatal Multivitamin Plus DHA. (iHealth) Folic acid 0.8 mg, calcium 300 mg, iron 33 mg, vitamins A 6,000 units, D 800 units, E 30 units, B_1 1.7 mg, B_2 2 mg, B_3 20 mg, B_5 12 mg, B_6 2.5 mg, B_{12} 12 mcg, C 60 mg, Cr, Cu, I, Mg, P, Zn, biotin 330 mcg. **Tab.:** 30s. **Cap., softgel:** DHA 350 mg. 30s. *OTC.*
Use: Prenatal vitamin with minerals.

branched chain amino acids.
Use: Nutritional supplement; amyotrophic lateral sclerosis agent. [Orphan Drug]

Brasivol Fine, Medium, and Rough. (GlaxoSmithKline) Aluminum oxide scrub particles in a surfactant cleansing base. **Fine:** Jar 153 g. **Medium:** Jar 180 g. **Rough:** Jar 195 g. *OTC.*
Use: Scrub cleanser.

•**brasofensine maleate.** (brah-so-FEN-seen) USAN.
Use: Antiparkinsonian.

Bravelle. (Ferring) Urofollitropin 75 units FSH activity. Contains up to 2% luteinizing hormone activity. Pow. for Inj., lyophilized. Vials with NaCl 2 mL as diluent and lactose monohydrate 23 mg. *Rx.*
Use: Ovulation stimulant.

Breatheasy. (Pascal Co. Inc.) Racemic epinephrine hydrochloride 2.2%. Soln. inhaled by use of nebulizer. Bot. 0.25 oz,

0.5 oz, 1 oz. *OTC.*
Use: Bronchodilator.

Breathe Free. (Thompson Medical) Sodium chloride 0.65%, benzalkonium chloride. Soln. Spray Bot. 45 mL. *OTC.*
Use: Nasal decongestant.

Breathe Right Menthol Nasal Strips. (GlaxoSmithKline) Menthol. Strip. Pkg. 10s, 28s. *OTC.*
Use: Upper respiratory combination, topical.

Breathe Right Nasal Strips. (GlaxoSmithKline) Strip. Pkg. 2s, 10s, 26s, 44s. *OTC.*
Use: Upper respiratory product, topical.

•**brecanavir.** (bre-KAN-a-vir) USAN.
Use: Antiretroviral.

Breezee Mist Foot Powder. (Pedinol Pharmacal) Isobutane, talc, aluminum chlorhydrate, cyclomethicone, isopropyl myristate, propylene carbonate, stearalkonium hectorite, undecylenic acid, menthol. Pow. Aerosol can. 113 g. *OTC.*
Use: Antifungal, topical.

•**bremelanotide.** (BRE-mel-AN-oh-tide) USAN.
Use: Melanocortin agent.

•**brentuximab vedotin.** (bren-TUK-see-mab ve-DOE-tin) USAN.
Use: Antineoplastic.
See: Adcetris.

Breo Ellipta. (GlaxoSmithKline) Fluticasone furoate 100 mcg/vilanterol 25 mcg per actuation. Lactose. Pow.; Inhal. Blister 28s and 60s and plastic inhaler device. *Rx.*
Use: Respiratory inhalant combination.

•**brequinar sodium.** (BREh-kwih-NAHR) USAN.
Use: Antineoplastic.

•**bretazenil.** (bret-AZZ-eh-nill) USAN.
Use: Anxiolytic.

Brethancer. (Novartis)
Use: Inhaler, complete unit to be used with *Brethaire.*

•**bretylium tosylate.** (bre-TILL-ee-uhm TAH-sill-ate) *USP.*
Use: Hypotensive; antiadrenergic; cardiovascular agent, antiarrhythmic.

Brevibloc. (Baxter) Esmolol hydrochloride 10 mg/mL, 250 mg/mL. Inj. **10 mg/mL:** Vial 10 mL. **250 mg/mL:** Amp 10 mL, propylene glycol 25%, alcohol 25%. *Rx.*
Use: Antiadrenergic/sympatholytic, beta-adrenergic blocker.

Brevicon. (Watson) Norethindrone 0.5 mg, ethinyl estradiol 35 mcg. Lactose. Tab. *Wallette* 28s with 7 inert tabs. *Rx.*
Use: Sex hormone, contraceptive.

Brevital Sodium. (JHP Pharm) Methohexital sodium 200 mg, 500 mg, 2.5 g. Sodium carbonate. Inj., lyophilized Pow. for Soln. 20 mL single-use vial (200 mg only); 50 mL multiple-dose vial (500 mg and 2.5 g only). *c-IV.*
Use: General anesthetic, barbiturate.

Brevoxyl-8. (GlaxoSmithKline) Benzoyl peroxide 8%. Cetyl alcohol, stearyl alcohol. Gel. Tube 42.5 g, 90 g. *Rx.*
Use: Anti-infective; antibiotic, topical.

Brevoxyl-8 Acne Wash Kit. (GlaxoSmithKline) Benzoyl peroxide 8%. Castor oil, glycerin, mineral oil, parabens. Cream. 170 g. Kit w/SFC lotion (106.6 mL). *Formerly Brevoxyl Creamy Wash. Rx.*
Use: Anti-infective; antibiotic, topical.

Brevoxyl-8 Cleansing. (GlaxoSmithKline) Benzoyl peroxide 8%. Cetyl alcohol. Lot. Bot. 297 g. *Rx.*
Use: Anti-infective, antibiotic, topical.

Brevoxyl-4. (GlaxoSmithKline) Benzoyl peroxide 4%. Cetyl alcohol, stearyl alcohol. Gel. Tube 42.5 g, 90 g. *Rx.*
Use: Antiacne.

Brevoxyl-4 Acne Wash Kit. (GlaxoSmithKline) Benzoyl peroxide 4%. Glycerin, castor oil, parabens, mineral oil. Cream. 170 g. Kit w/SFC lotion (106.6 mL). *Formerly Brevoxyl Creamy Wash. Rx.*
Use: Anti-infective; antibiotic, topical.

Brevoxyl-4 Cleansing. (GlaxoSmithKline) Benzoyl peroxide 4%. Cetyl alcohol. Lot. Bot. 297 g. *Rx.*
Use: Anti-infective, antibiotic, topical.

brewer's yeast. (NBTY) Vitamins B_1 0.06 mg, B_2 0.02 mg, B_3 0.2 mg. Tab. Bot. 250s. *OTC.*
Use: Vitamin supplement.

Brexin EX. (Savage) **Liq.:** Pseudoephedrine hydrochloride 30 mg, guaifenesin 200 mg/5 mL. **Tab.:** Pseudoephedrine hydrochloride 60 mg, guaifenesin 400 mg. Bot. 100s. *OTC.*
Use: Decongestant, expectorant.

•**brexpiprazole.** (brex-PIP-ra-zole) USAN.
Use: CNS agent.

•**briakinumab.** (BRYE-a-kin-ue-mab) USAN.
Use: Immunomodulator.

Briellyn. (Glenmark) Ethinyl estradiol 35 mcg, norethindrone 0.4 mg. Lactose. Tab. 28s (w/7 inert tablets). *Rx.*
Use: Monophasic oral contraceptive.

•**brifentanil hydrochloride.** (brih-FEN-tah-NILL) USAN.
Use: Analgesic; narcotic.

Brigen-G. (Grafton) Chlordiazepoxide 5 mg, 10 mg, 25 mg. Tab. Bot. 500s. *c-IV.*
Use: Anxiolytic.

Brij 96 and 97. (ICI) Polyoxyl 10 oleyl ether available as 96 and 97.
Use: Surface active agent.

Brij-721. (ICI) Polyoxyethylene 21 stearyl ether (100% active).
Use: Surface active agent.

•**brilacidin.** (BRIL-a-SYE-din) USAN.
Use: Antibiotic.

•**brilacidin tetrahydrochloride.** (BRIL-a-SYE-din) USAN.
Use: Antibiotic.

Brilinta. (AstraZeneca) Ticagrelor 90 mg. Film coated. Mannitol, PEG. Tab. 60s, 180s, UD 100s. *Rx.*
Use: Antiplatelet agent, aggregation inhibitor.

•**brimonidine tartrate.** (brih-MOE-nih-DEEN) USAN.
Use: Agent for glaucoma.
See: Alphagan P.
Mirvaso.
W/Brinzolamide.
See: Simbrinza.

brimonidine tartrate. (Falcon) Brimonidine tartrate 0.15%. Soln.; Ophth. 5 mL, 10 mL, 15 mL bottle (with 0.001% *Polyquad*, boric acid, potassium chloride, sodium borate, sodium chloride, hydrochloric acid and/or sodium hydroxide adjusted to pH. *Rx.*
Use: Agent for glaucoma.

brimonidine tartrate. (Various Mfr.) Brimonidine tartrate 0.2%. Soln. 5 mL, 10 mL, 15 mL. *Rx.*
Use: Agent for glaucoma.

brimonidine tartrate/timolol maleate.
Use: Agent for glaucoma.
See: Combigan.

•**brincidofovir.** (BRIN-sye-DOF-oh-vir) USAN.
Use: Antiviral.

brineurin.
See: Abrineurin.

•**brinolase.** (BRIN-oh-laze) USAN. Fibrinolytic enzyme produced by *Aspergillus oryzae.*
Use: Fibrinolytic.

Brintellix. (Takeda Pharmaceuticals) Vortioxetine 5 mg (equiv. to vortioxetine hydrobromide 6.355 mg), 10 mg (equiv. to vortioxetine hydrobromide 12.71 mg), 15 mg (equiv. to vortioxetine hydrobromide 19.065 mg), 20 mg (equiv. to vortioxetine hydrobromide 25.42 mg). Film coated. Mannitol. Tab. 30s, 90s, 500s. *Rx.*
Use: Antidepressant.

•**brinzolamide.** (brin-ZOE-lah-mide) *USP.*
Use: Antiglaucoma agent.
See: Azopt.
W/Brimonidine Tartrate.
See: Simbrinza.

Brioschi. (Brioschi-USA) Sodium bicarbonate 500 mg per capful or packet. Corn syrup, sugar, tartaric acid. Sodium 500 mg/dose. Lemon flavor. Gran. 120.5 g, 241 g, UD packets. *OTC.*
Use: Systemic alkalinizer.

Brisdelle. (Noven Therapeutics) Paroxetine 7.5 mg (equiv. to paroxetine mesylate 9.69 mg). Cap. UD 30s. *Rx.*
Use: Antidepressant, selective serotonin reuptake inhibitor.

Bristoject. (Bristol-Myers Squibb) Prefilled disposable syringes w/needle.
Available with: Aminophylline: 250 mg/10 mL. Atropine sulfate: 5 mg/5 mL or 1 mg/mL. 10s. Calcium Cl: 10%. 10 mL. 10s. Dexamethasone: 20 mg/5 mL. Dextrose: 50%. 50 mL. 10s. Diphenhydramine: 50 mg/5 mL. Dopamine hydrochloride: 200 mg/5 mL, 400 mg/10 mL. Ephedrine: 50 mg/10 mL. Epinephrine: 1:10,000. 10 mL. 10s. Lidocaine hydrochloride: 1%: 5 mL, 10 mL; 2%: 5 mL; 4%: 25 mL, 50 mL; 20%: 5 mL, 10 mL. Magnesium sulfate: 5 g/10 mL, 10s. Metaraminol: 1%. 10 mL. Sodium bicarbonate: 75%: 50 mL; 84%: 50 mL. 10s.
Use: Medical device.

British anti-Lewisite. Dimercaprol.
See: BAL.

•**brivanib.** (bri-VAN-ib) USAN.
Use: Antineoplastic.

•**brivaracetam.** (BRIV-a-RA-se-tam) USAN.
Use: Anticonvulsant.

Brobella-P.B. (Brothers) Atropine sulfate 0.0195 mg, hyoscine HBr 0.0065 mg, hyoscyamine sulfate 0.1040 mg, phenobarbital 0.25 g. Tab. Bot. 100s, 1000s. *Rx.*
Use: Anticholinergic; antispasmodic; hypnotic; sedative.

•**brocresine.** (broe-KREE-seen) USAN.
Use: Histidine decarboxylase inhibitor.

•**brocrinat.** (BROE-krih-NAT) USAN.
Use: Diuretic.

Brocycline. (Brothers) Tetracycline hydrochloride 250 mg. Cap. Bot. 100s, 1000s. *Rx.*
Use: Anti-infective, tetracycline.

•**brodalumab.** (broe-DAL-ue-mab) USAN.
Use: Immunomodulator.

Brofed. (Marnel) Pseudoephedrine hydrochloride 30 mg, brompheniramine maleate 4 mg/5 mL, parabens, saccharin, sorbitol, sucrose, corn syr., menthol, mint flavor. Liq. Bot. 473 mL. *Rx.*

Use: Upper respiratory combination, antihistamine, decongestant.

•**brofoxine.** (BROE-fox-een) USAN.
Use: Antipsychotic.

Brohist D. (Allegis Pharmaceuticals) Brompheniramine maleate 4 mg, phenylephrine hydrochloride 10 mg. Tab. 60s. *OTC.*
Use: Upper respiratory combination, decongestant and antihistamine.

•**bromadoline maleate.** (BROE-mah-DOE-leen) USAN.
Use: Analgesic.

bromaleate.
See: Pamabrom.

Bromanate. (Alpharma) Brompheniramine maleate 1 mg/5 mL, pseudoephedrine hydrochloride 15 mg, alcohol free, grape flavor. Elix. Bot. 118 mL, 237 mL, 473 mL, gal. *OTC.*
Use: Upper respiratory combination, antihistamine, decongestant.

Bromanate DM Cold & Cough. (Alpharma) Pseudoephedrine hydrochloride 15 mg, brompheniramine maleate 1 mg, dextromethorphan HBr 5 mg per 5 mL. Alcohol free, grape flavor. Elixir. Bot. 118 mL. *OTC.*
Use: Upper respiratory combination, decongestant, antihistamine, antitussive.

Bromanyl. (Various Mfr.) Bromodiphenhydramine hydrochloride 12.5 mg, codeine phosphate 10 mg, alcohol 5%. Syr. Bot. Pt, gal. *c-v.*
Use: Antihistamine; antitussive.

Bromarest DX. (Warner Chilcott) Pseudoephedrine hydrochloride 30 mg, brompheniramine maleate 2 mg, dextromethorphan HBr 10 mg, alcohol 0.95%. Butterscotch flavor. Syr. Bot. 480 mL. *Rx.*
Use: Antihistamine; antitussive; decongestant.

Bromatap. (Ivax) Brompheniramine maleate 2 mg, phenylephrine hydrochloride 12.5 mg, alcohol 2.3%/5 mL. Liq. Bot. 4 oz, 8 oz, pt, gal. *OTC.*
Use: Antihistamine; decongestant.

bromauric acid. Hydrogen tetrabromoaurate.

•**bromazepam.** (broe-MAY-zeh-pam) USAN.
Use: Anxiolytic.

Brombay. (Rosemont) Brompheniramine maleate 2 mg/5 mL, alcohol 3%. Elix. Bot. 4 oz, pt, gal. *OTC.*
Use: Antihistamine.

•**bromchlorenone.** (brome-KLOR-ee-nohn) USAN.
Use: Anti-infective, topical.

•**bromelains.** (BROE-meh-lanes) USAN.
Use: Anti-inflammatory.
See: Dayto-Anase.

Brometane DX Cough. (Hi-Tech) Pseudoephedrine hydrochloride 30 mg, brompheniramine maleate 2 mg, dextromethorphan HBr 10 mg per 5 mL. Alcohol, saccharin, sorbitol. Sugar free. Syr. Bot. 473 mL. *Rx.*
Use: Upper respiratory combination, antitussive combination.

Bromfed DM. (Wockhardt) Brompheniramine maleate 2 mg, dextromethorphan hydrobromide 10 mg, pseudoephedrine hydrochloride 30 mg. Alcohol 0.95%, methylparaben, sugar. Butterscotch flavor. Syr. 118 mL, 473 mL. *Rx.*
Use: Upper respiratory combination, antitussive combination.

•**bromfenac.** (BROME-fen-ak) USAN.
Use: Nonsteroidal anti-inflammatory agent, ophthalmic.
See: Prolensa.
Xibrom.

bromfenac sodium. (Mylan) Bromfenac sodium 0.09%. Benzalkonium chloride 0.05 mg/mL, disodium edetate 0.2 mg/mL, povidone 20 mg/mL, sodium sulfite 2 mg/mL, boric acid, sodium borate, sodium hydroxide. Soln., Ophth. 2.5 mL, 5 mL w/dropper bottles. *Rx.*
Use: Ophthalmic nonsteroidal anti-inflammatory drug.

bromhexine. (Boehringer Ingelheim)
Use: Mild/moderate keratoconjunctivitis sicca. [Orphan Drug]

•**bromhexine hydrochloride.** (brome-HEX-een) USAN.
Use: Expectorant; mucolytic.

Bromhist-DM. (Cypress) Brompheniramine maleate 1 mg, dextromethorphan HBr 4 mg, pseudoephedrine hydrochloride 15 mg per mL. Alcohol, sugar, and dye free. Maltitol, saccharin, sorbitol. Grape flavor. Drops. 30 mL. *Rx.*
Use: Upper respiratory combination, antitussive combination.

Bromhist-DM Pediatric. (Cypress) Pseudoephedrine hydrochloride 30 mg, brompheniramine maleate 2 mg, dextromethorphan hydrobromide 5 mg, guaifenesin 50 mg per 5 mL. Alcohol free, dye free. Saccharin, sorbitol. Grape flavor. Syr. 473 mL. *Rx.*
Use: Upper respiratory combination, antitussive and expectorant combination.

Bromhist PDX. (Cypress) Phenylephrine hydrochloride 5 mg, dextromethorphan hydrobromide 5 mg, guaifenesin 50 mg, brompheniramine maleate 2 mg/5 mL. Alcohol free. Parabens, sugar. Grape

flavor. Syr. 473 mL. *Rx.*
Use: Upper respiratory combination, antitussive combination, antitussive and expectorant.

bromides.
See: Peacock's Bromides.

bromide salts.
See: Ferrous Bromide.
Strontium Bromide.

Bromi-Lotion. (Gordon Laboratories) Aluminum hydroxychloride 20%, emollient base. Lot. Bot. 1.5 oz, 4 oz. *OTC.*
Use: Antiperspirant.

•**bromindione.** (BROME-in-die-ohn) USAN.
Use: Anticoagulant.

Bromi-Talc. (Gordon Laboratories) Potassium alum, bentonite, talc. Shaker can 3.5 oz, 1 lb, 5 lb. *OTC.*
Use: Bromidrosis; hyperhidrosis.

•**bromocriptine.** (BROE-moe-KRIP-teen) USAN.
Use: Enzyme inhibitor, prolactin.

•**bromocriptine mesylate.** (BROE-moe-KRIP-teen) *USP.*
Use: Enzyme inhibitor, prolactin.
See: Cycloset.
Parlodel.

bromocriptine mesylate. (Mylan) Bromocriptine mesylate. **Cap.:** 5 mg. 30s, 100s. **Tab.:** 2.5 mg. May contain lactose, EDTA. 30s, 100s. *Rx.*
Use: Enzyme inhibitor, prolactin; antiparkinson agent.

bromodiethylacetylurea.
See: Carbromal.

•**bromodiphenhydramine hydrochloride.** (BROE-moe-die-fen-HIGH-drah-meen) *USP.*
Use: Antihistamine.

•**bromodiphenhydramine hydrochloride/codeine phosphate.** (BROE-moe-die-fen-HIGH-drah-meen) *USP.* Antitussive combination.

bromodiphenhydramine hydrochloride/codeine phosphate. (Rosemont) Bromodiphenhydramine hydrochloride 12.5 mg, codeine phosphate 10 mg. Syr. Bot. 480 mL. *c-v.*
Use: Antitussive combination.

bromoform. Tribromomethane.

bromoisovaleryl urea. Alpha, bromoisovaleryl urea.

Bromophin.
See: Apomorphine Hydrochloride.

bromotheophyllinate aminoisobutanol.
See: Pamabrom.

bromotheophyllinate pyranisamine.
See: Pyrabrom.

bromotheophyllinate pyrilamine.
See: Pyrabrom.

8-bromotheophylline.
See: Pamabrom.

Bromotuss w/Codeine. (Rugby) Bromodiphenhydramine hydrochloride 12.5 mg, codeine phosphate 10 mg, alcohol 5%. Syr. Bot. 120 mL, pt, gal. *c-v.*
Use: Antihistamine; antitussive.

•**bromoxanide.** (broe-MOX-ah-nide) USAN.
Use: Anthelmintic.

Brom/PE/DM. (Brighton Pharmaceuticals) Brompheniramine maleate 2 mg, dextromethorphan hydrobromide 10 mg, phenylephrine hydrochloride 5 mg per 5 mL. Glycerin, prosweet, saccharin, sodium benzoate, sorbitol. Strawberry flavor. Syr. 473 mL. *Rx.*
Use: Upper respiratory combination, antitussive combination.

•**bromperidol.** (brome-PURR-ih-dahl) USAN.
Use: Antipsychotic.

•**bromperidol decanoate.** (brome-PURR-ih-dole deh-KAN-oh-ate) USAN.
Use: Antipsychotic.

Bromphen DX. (Rugby) Pseudoephedrine hydrochloride 30 mg, brompheniramine maleate 2 mg, dextromethorphan HBr 10 mg, alcohol 0.95%. Syr. Bot. 480 mL. *Rx.*
Use: Antihistamine; antitussive; decongestant.

brompheniramine.
Use: Antihistamine, nonselective alkylamine.
See: Lodrane D.

Brompheniramine Cough. (Geneva) Pseudoephedrine hydrochloride 30 mg, brompheniramine maleate 2 mg, dextromethorphan HBr 10 mg, alcohol 0.95%. Syr. Bot. 480 mL. *Rx.*
Use: Antihistamine; antitussive; decongestant.

brompheniramine/hydrocodone/PSE. (Varsity) Hydrocodone bitartrate 2.5 mg, brompheniramine maleate 3 mg, pseudoephedrine hydrochloride 30 mg per 5 mL. Alcohol and sugar free. Saccharin, sorbitol. Bubble gum flavor. Liq. 473 mL. *c-III.*
Use: Upper respiratory combination, antitussive combination.

•**brompheniramine maleate.** (brome-fen-AIR-uh-meen) *USP.*
Use: Antihistamine.
See: J-Tan PD.
Lodrane 12 Hour.

W/Carbetapentane Citrate, Phenylephrine Hydrochloride
See: Vazotan.
V-Cof.
W/Chlophedianol Hydrochloride, Pseudoephedrine Hydrochloride.
See: Dicel CD.
W/Codeine Phosphate, Phenylephrine Hydrochloride.
See: M-End PE.
Poly-Tussin AC.
W/Codeine Phosphate, Pseudoephedrine Hydrochloride.
See: CPB WC.
Mar-Cof BP.
M-END WC.
Mesehist WC.
W/Dextromethorphan Hydrobromide, Guaifenesin, Phenylephrine Hydrochloride.
See: Bromhist-PDX.
W/Dextromethorphan Hydrobromide, Guaifenesin, Pseudoephedrine Hydrochloride.
See: Bromhist DM Pediatric.
Histacol DM Pediatric.
Pediahist DM.
W/Dextromethorphan Hydrobromide, Phenylephrine Hydrochloride.
See: Alahist DM.
BPM-DM-PHEN.
BROM/PE/DM.
Brōvex PEB DM.
Children's Dimaphen DM.
Dimetapp Children's Cold & Cough.
LoHist-DM.
LoHist PEB DM.
TGQ 7.5PEH/4BRM/15DM.
TL-Hist DM.
W/Dextromethorphan Hydrobromide, Pseudoephedrine Hydrochloride.
See: Brometane-DX Cough.
Bromhist-DM.
Bromhist PDX.
Bromphenex DM.
Brotapp DM.
BrōveX PSE DM.
Dimaphen DM Cough, Cold & Allergy.
DM/PSE/BPM.
Myphetane DX Cough.
Neo DM.
Pediahist DM.
Prohist DM.
Q-Tapp DM Cold and Cough.
TGQ 50PSE/3BRM/30DM.
W/Dihydrocodeine Bitartrate, Phenylephrine Hydrochloride.
See: Poly-Tussin DHC.
W/Dihydrocodeine Bitartrate, Pseudoephedrine Hydrochloride.
See: J-COF DHC.
W/Phenylephrine Hydrochloride.
See: Brohist D.
Brōvex PEB.
Cenhist.
Dimetapp Children's Cold & Allergy.
Entre-B.
LoHist PEB.
Ru-Hist D.
Rynex PE.
Vazobid-PD.
W/Pseudoephedrine Hydrochloride.
See: BPM Pseudo 6/45 mg.
Brotapp.
Brōvex PSB.
BrōveX PSE.
J-Tan D PD.
Lodrane D.
Lodrane LD.
LoHist PSB.
Rynex PSE.
SymPak II.

brompheniramine maleate. (River's Edge) Brompheniramine maleate 1 mg. Saccharin. Alcohol free, dye free, and sugar free. Strawberry-banana flavor. Drops. 30 mL. *Rx.*
Use: Antihistamine; alkylamine, nonselective.

brompheniramine maleate/pseudoephedrine hydrochloride. (River's Edge Pharmaceuticals) Brompheniramine maleate 1 mg, pseudoephedrine hydrochloride 7.5 mg per mL. Saccharin, sorbitol. Alcohol free, dye free, and sugar free. Cotton candy flavor. Soln., Conc. 30 mL w/dropper. *Rx.*
Use: Upper respiratory combination, decongestant and antihistamine.

brompheniramine/pseudoephedrine DM. (Macoven) Brompheniramine 4 mg, dextromethorphan hydrobromide 20 mg, pseudoephedrine hydrochloride 20 mg. Parabens, potassium citrate, propylene glycol, sorbitol, sucralose. Alcohol free, dye free, gluten free, and sugar free. Cotton candy flavor. Liq. 473 mL. *OTC.*
Use: Upper respiratory combination, antitussive combination.

brompheniramine tannate.
See: J-Tan.
P-Tex.
W/Carbetapentane Tannate, Phenylephrine Tannate.
See: Vazotan Tannate.
W/Dextromethorphan Tannate, Phenylephrine Tannate.
See: Neo DM.
W/Phenylephrine Tannate.
See: Brōvex ADT.
Relhist.

W/Pseudoephedrine Tannate.
See: B-Vex PD
Lodrane D.

brompheniramine tannate. (Ani Pharmaceuticals, Inc.) Brompheniramine tannate. **Chew. Tab.:** 12 mg. Sugar. Banana flavor. 60s. **Oral Susp.:** 12 mg per 5 mL. Methylparaben, sucrose, tartrazine. Banana flavor. 118 mL. *Rx.*
Use: Antihistamine.

brompheniramine tannate. (Various Mfr.) Brompheniramine tannate 12 mg. Chew. Tab. 60s. *Rx.*
Use: Antihistamine.

Brompton's cocktail. Heroin or morphine 10 mg, cocaine 10 mg, alcohol, chloroform water, syr. *c-II.*
Use: Analgesic, narcotic.

bronchodilators.
See: Anticholinergics.
Sympathomimetics.
Xanthine Derivatives.

Broncholate. (Sanofi-Aventis) Ephedrine hydrochloride 12.5 mg, guaifenesin 200 mg. **Cap.:** 100s, 1,000s. **Softgels:** 100s. *Rx.*
Use: Bronchodilator; expectorant.

Broncomar. (Marlop Pharmaceuticals) Guaifenesin 50 mg, pseudoephedrine hydrochloride 10 mg, theophylline 50 mg. Alcohol, parabens, saccharin, sucrose. Grape flavor. Elix. 473 mL. *Rx.*
Use: Antiasthmatic combination, xanthine combination.

Broncotron-D. (Seyer Pharmatec) Dextromethorphan HBr 20 mg, guaifenesin 200 mg, phenylephrine hydrochloride 5 mg per 5 mL. Phenylalanine, aspartame, sorbitol. Cherry flavor. Susp. 30 mL, 473 mL. *Rx.*
Use: Antitussive and expectorant combination, upper respiratory combination.

Brondecon. (Parke-Davis) **Tab.:** Oxtriphylline 200 mg, guaifenesin 100 mg. Bot. 100s. **Elix.:** Oxtriphylline 100 mg, guaifenesin 50 mg/5 mL w/alcohol 20%. Bot. 8 oz, 16 oz. *Rx.*
Use: Bronchodilator; expectorant.

Bronitin. (Whitehall-Robins) Theophylline hydrous 120 mg, guaifenesin 100 mg, ephedrine hydrochloride 24.3 mg, pyrilamine maleate 16.6 mg. Tab. Bot. 24s, 60s. *OTC.*
Use: Bronchodilator.

Bronitin Mist. (Whitehall-Robins) Epinephrine bitartrate in inhalation aerosol. Each spray releases 0.3 mg epinephrine bitartrate equivalent to 0.16 mg epinephrine base. Bot. 15 mL or 15 mL refills. *OTC.*
Use: Bronchodilator.

Bronkaid Dual Action. (Bayer Consumer Care) Ephedrine sulfate 25 mg, guaifenesin 400 mg. Tab. Bot. 24s. *OTC.*
Use: Bronchodilator; upper respiratory combination, decongestant, expectorant.

Bronkometer. (Sanofi-Synthelabo) Isoetharine mesylate 0.61%, saccharin, menthol, alcohol 30%. Metered dose of 340 mcg isoetharine in fluorohydrocarbon propellant. Bot. w/nebulizer 10 mL, 15 mL. Refill 10 mL, 15 mL. *Rx.*
Use: Bronchodilator.

Bronkosol. (Sanofi-Synthelabo) Isoetharine hydrochloride 1% w/glycerin, sodium bisulfite, parabens for oral inhalation. Bot. 10 mL, 30 mL. *Rx.*
Use: Bronchodilator.

Bronkotuss. (Hyrex) Chlorpheniramine maleate 4 mg, guaifenesin 100 mg, ephedrine sulfate 8.216 mg, hydriodic acid syr. 1.67 mg/5 mL w/alcohol 5%. Bot. Pt, gal. *Rx.*
Use: Antihistamine; decongestant; expectorant.

Brontex Liquid. (Procter & Gamble) Codeine phosphate 2.5 mg, guaifenesin 75 mg/5 mL, methylparaben, saccharin, sucrose. Liq. Bot. 473 mL. *c-v.*
Use: Antitussive expectorant; narcotic.

Brontuss DX. (Portal) Dextromethorphan hydrobromide 20 mg, guaifenesin 200 mg, phenylephrine hydrochloride 10 mg. Cherry flavoring, maltitol, propylene glycol, saccharin, sorbitol. Alcohol free, dye free, gluten free, and sugar free. Liq. 118 mL. *OTC.*
Use: Upper respiratory combination, antitussive and expectorant combination.

•**broperamole.** (BROE-PURR-ah-mole) USAN.
Use: Anti-inflammatory.

•**bropirimine.** (broe-PIE-rih-MEEN) USAN.
Use: Antineoplastic; antiviral.

Broserpine. (Brothers) Reserpine 0.25 mg. Tab. Bot. 250s, 100s.
Use: Antihypertensive.

Brotapp. (Silarx) Brompheniramine maleate 1 mg, pseudoephedrine hydrochloride 15 mg. Grape flavoring, propylene glycol, saccharin, sodium benzoate, sorbitol. Alcohol free and sugar free. Liq. 118 mL, 237 mL, 437 mL. *OTC.*
Use: Upper respiratory combination, decongestant and antihistamine.

Brotapp DM. (Silarx) Brompheniramine maleate 1 mg, dextromethorphan hydrobromide 5 mg, pseudoephedrine hydrochloride 15 mg. Saccharin, sorbi-

tol. Alcohol free and sugar free. Grape flavor. Liq. 118 mL, 237 mL. *OTC.*
Use: Upper respiratory combination, antitussive combination.

•**brotizolam.** (broe-TIE-zoe-LAM) USAN.
Use: Hypnotic; sedative.

Bro-T's. (Brothers) Bromisovalum 0.12 g, carbromal 0.2 g. Tab. Bot. 100s, 1000s. *Rx.*
Use: Sedative; anxiolytic.

Bro-Tuss. (Brothers) Dextromethorphan HBr 15 mg, chlorpheniramine maleate 2 mg, phenylephrine hydrochloride 5 mg, ammonium Cl 100 mg, sodium citrate 150 mg, vitamin C 30 mg/10 mL. Bot. 4 oz, pt, gal. *OTC.*
Use: Antihistamine; antitussive; decongestant; expectorant.

Bro-Tuss A.C. (Brothers) Acetaminophen 120 mg, codeine phosphate 10 mg, phenylephrine hydrochloride 5 mg, chlorpheniramine maleate 2 mg, menthol 1 mg, alcohol 10%/5 mL. Bot. Pt, gal. *c-v.*
Use: Analgesic; antihistamine; antitussive; decongestant.

Brovana. (Sunovion) Arformoterol (as base) 7.5 mcg/mL. Soln. for Inh. Unit-dose vials. 2 mL. *Rx.*
Use: Bronchodilator, sympathomimetic.

BrōveX ADT. (MCR American) Brompheniramine tannate 12 mg, phenylephrine tannate 10 mg per 5 mL. Aspartame, parabens, phenylalanine 7 mg per 5 mL. Bubble gum flavor. Susp. 473 mL. *Rx.*
Use: Upper respiratory combination, decongestant and antihistamine.

BrōveX-D. (MCR American) Phenylephrine tannate 20 mg, brompheniramine tannate 12 mg per 5 mL. Aspartame, parabens. Bubble gum flavor. Susp. 473 mL. *Rx.*
Use: Decongestant and antihistamine.

BrōveX PEB. (Pernix Therapeutics) Brompheniramine maleate 4 mg, phenylephrine hydrochloride 10 mg. Parabens, potassium citrate, potassium sorbate, propylene glycol, sorbitol, sucralose. Alcohol free, dye free, gluten free, and sugar free. Bubble gum flavor. Liq. 473 mL. *OTC.*
Use: Upper respiratory combination, decongestant and antihistamine.

BrōveX PEB DM. (Pernix Therapeutics) Brompheniramine maleate 4 mg, dextromethorphan hydrobromide 20 mg, phenylephrine hydrochloride 10 mg per 5 mL. Parabens, potassium citrate, potassium sorbate, propylene glycol, sorbitol, sucralose. Alcohol free, dye free, gluten free, and sugar free. Bubble gum flavor. Liq. 473 mL. *OTC.*
Use: Upper respiratory combination, antitussive combination.

BrōveX PSB. (Pernix Therapeutics) Brompheniramine maleate 4 mg, pseudoephedrine hydrochloride 20 mg per 5 mL. Parabens, potassium citrate, potassium sorbate, propylene glycol, sorbitol, sucralose. Alcohol free, dye free, gluten free, and sugar free. Cotton candy flavor. Liq. 473 mL. *OTC.*
Use: Upper respiratory combination, decongestant and antihistamine.

BrōveX PSE. (Pernix Therapeutics) Brompheniramine maleate 4 mg, pseudoephedrine hydrochloride 40 mg. Tab. 100s. *OTC.*
Use: Upper respiratory combination, decongestant and antihistamine.

BrōveX PSE DM. (Pernix Therapeutics) Brompheniramine maleate 4 mg, dextromethorphan hydrobromide 20 mg, pseudoephedrine hydrochloride 40 mg. Tab. 100s. *OTC.*
Use: Upper respiratory combination, antitussive combination.

Bryrel. (Sanofi-Synthelabo) Piperazine citrate anhydrous 110 mg/mL. Syr. Bot. oz. *Rx.*
Use: Anthelmintic.

B-Scorbic. (Pharmics) Vitamins C 300 mg, B_1 25 mg, B_2 10 mg, calcium pantothenate 10 mg, niacinamide 50 mg, lemon flavored complex 200 mg. Tab. Bot. 100s, 1000s. *OTC.*
Use: Mineral, vitamin supplement.

BSS. (Alcon) Sodium Cl 0.64%, potassium Cl 0.075%, magnesium Cl 0.03%, calcium Cl 0.048%, sodium acetate 0.39%, sodium citrate 0.17%, sodium hydroxide or hydrochloric acid. Bot. 15 mL, 30 mL, 250 mL, 500 mL. *Rx.*
Use: Irrigant, ophthalmic.

BSS Plus. (Alcon) **Part I:** Sodium Cl 7.44 mg, potassium Cl 0.395 mg, dibasic sodium phosphate 0.433 mg, sodium bicarbonate 2.19 mg, hydrochloric acid, or sodium hydroxide/mL. Soln. Bot. 240 mL. **Part II:** Calcium chloride dihydrate 3.85 mg, magnesium chloride hexahydrate 5 mg, dextrose 24 mg, glutathione disulfide 4.5 mg/mL. Soln. Bot. 10 mL. *Rx.*
Use: Irrigant, ophthalmic.

BTA Rapid Urine Test. (Bard) Reagent kit for detection of bladder tumor associated analytes in urine to aid in management of bladder cancer. Kits of 15 and 30 tests.
Use: Diagnostic aid.

B-12. (Mason Natural) Vitamin B_{12} (cyanocobalamin) 1,500 mcg. Gluten free, preservative free, and sugar free. ER Tab. 60s. *OTC.*
Use: Water-soluble vitamin.

B-12. (21st Century) Vitamin B_{12} 1,000 mcg, Ca 100 mg. Gluten free and preservative free. ER Tab. 110s. *OTC.*
Use: Water-soluble vitamin.

B-12 Dots. (Twinlab) Cyanocobalamin (B_{12}) 500 mcg. Cherry flavoring, sorbitol. Preservative free. Tab., disintegrating. 100s. *OTC.*
Use: Water-soluble vitamin.

B-12-SL. (J.R. Carlson) Cyanocobalamin 1,000 mcg. Mannitol, sorbitol, lemon flavoring. Gluten free, preservative free. Tab., sublingual. 90s, 180s. *OTC.*
Use: Water-soluble vitamin.

B_2-400. (Bio-Tech) Riboflavin 400 mg. Preservative free and dye free. Cap. 100s. *OTC.*
Use: Water-soluble vitamin.

•**bucainide maleate.** (byoo-CANE-ide) USAN.
Use: Cardiovascular agent, antiarrhythmic.

buchu.
See: Diosmin.

•**bucindolol hydrochloride.** (BYOO-SIN-doe-lole) USAN.
Use: Investigative; antihypertensive.

Buckley's Chest Congestion. (Novartis) Guaifenesin 100 mg/5 mL. Alcohol and sugar free. Acesulfame potassium, menthol, parabens. Liq. 118 mL. *OTC.*
Use: Expectorant.

Buckley's Cough Mixture. (Novartis) Dextromethorphan HBr 12.5 mg/5 mL. Alcohol and sugar free. Menthol, parabens, pine needle oil. Liq. 118 mL. *OTC.*
Use: Nonnarcotic antitussive.

•**buclizine hydrochloride.** (BYOO-klih-zeen) USAN.
Use: Antiemetic; antinauseant.

•**bucromarone.** (byoo-KROE-mah-rone) USAN.
Use: Cardiovascular agent, antiarrhythmic.

•**bucrylate.** (BYOO-krih-late) USAN.
Use: Surgical aid, tissue adhesive.

•**budesonide.** (BYOO-DESS-oh-nide) USAN.
Use: Anti-inflammatory; adrenocortical steroid, glucocorticoid; corticosteroid, intranasal steroid.
See: Entocort EC.
Pulmicort Flexhaler.
Pulmicort Respules.
Rhinocort Aqua.
Uceris.
W/Formoterol.
See: Symbicort.

budesonide. (Mylan) Budesonide (micronized) 3 mg. Enteric coated. Lactose. Cap. 100s, 500s. *Rx.*
Use: Adrenocortical steroid, glucocorticoid.

budesonide. (Teva) Budesonide 0.25 mg per 2 mL, 0.5 mg per 2 mL. Disodium edetate. Susp., Inhal. Single-dose vial. 30s. *Rx.*
Use: Respiratory inhalant product, corticosteroid.

•**budiodarone.** (BUE-di-OH-da-rone) USAN.
Use: Antiarrhythmic.

•**budiodarone tartrate.** (BUE-di-OH-da-rone) USAN.
Use: Antiarrhythmic.

Buf Acne Cleansing Bar. (3M) Salicylic acid 1%, sulfur 1%. Bar. 3.5 oz. *OTC.*
Use: Antiacne.

Buf-Bar. (3M) Sulphur 3% and titanium dioxide. Bar 105 g. *OTC.*
Use: Antiacne.

Buf Body Scrub. (3M) Round cleansing sponge on plastic handles. *OTC.*
Use: Cleansing sponge.

Buff-A. (Merz) Aspirin acid 5 g buffered w/magnesium hydroxide, aluminum hydroxide dried gel. Tab. Bot. 100s, 1000s. *OTC.*
Use: Analgesic; antacid.

Buffaprin. (Buffington) Aspirin 325 mg buffered with magnesium oxide. Sugar, caffeine, lactose, salt free. Tab. *Dispense-A-Kit* 500s. *OTC.*
Use: Analgesic.

Buffasal. (Dover Pharmaceuticals) Aspirin 325 mg, magnesium oxide. Sugar, lactose, salt free. Tab. UD Box 500s. *OTC.*
Use: Analgesic.

Buffasal Max. (Dover Pharmaceuticals) Aspirin 500 mg, magnesium oxide. Sugar, lactose, salt free. Tab. *OTC.*
Use: Analgesic.

Buffered Aspirin. (Various Mfr.) Aspirin 325 mg with buffers. Tab. Bot. 100s, 500s, 1000s, UD 100s and 200s. *OTC.*
Use: Analgesic.

buffered intrathecal electrolyte/dextrose injection.
Use: Diluent. [Orphan Drug]
See: Elliot's B.

Bufferin. (Novartis) Aspirin 325 mg with calcium carbonate 158 mg, magnesium oxide 63 mg, magnesium carbonate 34 mg. Coated. Tab. 12s, 36s, 60s, 100s, 200s, UD 150s. *OTC.*
Use: Salicylate, aspirin, buffered.

Bufferin Extra Strength. (Novartis) Aspirin 500 mg with calcium carbonate, magnesium carbonate, and magnesium oxide. Tab. 130s. *OTC.*
Use: Salicylate, aspirin, buffered.

Buffex. (Roberts) Aspirin 325 mg w/ dihydroxyaluminum aminoacetate. Tab. Bot. 1000s, *Sanipack* 1000s. *OTC.*
Use: Analgesic.

Buf Foot Care Kit. (3M) Cleansing system for the feet. *OTC.*
Use: Foot preparation.

Buf Foot Care Lotion. (3M) Moisturizing lotion for feet. *OTC.*
Use: Foot preparation.

Buf Foot Care Soap. (3M) Bar 3.5 oz. *OTC.*
Use: Foot preparation.

•**bufilcon A.** (BYOO-fill-kahn A) USAN.
Use: Contact lens material, hydrophilic.

Buf Kit for Acne. (3M) Cleansing sponge, cleansing bar 3.5 oz w/booklet, holding tray. *OTC.*
Use: Antiacne.

Buf Lotion. (3M) Moisturizing lotion. *OTC.*
Use: Emollient.

•**buformin.** (BYOO-FORE-min) USAN.
Use: Antidiabetic.

Bufosal. (Table Rock) Sodium salicylate 15 g/dram w/calcium carbonate, sodium bicarbonate as granulated effervescent powder. Bot. 4 oz. *OTC.*
Use: Analgesic; antacid.

Buf-Ped Non-Medicated Cleansing Sponge. (3M) Abrasive cleansing sponge. *OTC.*
Use: Cleansing skin or feet.

Buf-Puf Bodymate. (3M) Oval two-sided cleansing sponge. Abrasive/gentle. *OTC.*
Use: Cleansing all areas of the body.

Buf-Puf Medicated. (3M) Water-activated. Salicylic acid 0.5% (reg. strength), alcohols, benzoate, EDTA, triethanolamine, and vitamin E acetate. Salicylic acid 2% (max. strength). Pads. Jar 30s. *OTC.*
Use: Antiacne.

Buf-Puf Non-Medicated Cleansing Sponge. (3M) Abrasive cleansing sponge. *OTC.*
Use: Skin cleansing.

Buf-Sul. (Sheryl) Sulfacetamide 167 mg, sulfadiazine 167 mg, sulfamerazine 167 mg. Tab. Bot. 100s. Susp. Bot. Pt. *Rx.*
Use: Anti-infective, sulfonamide.

Buf-Tabs. (Halsey Drug) Aspirin 5 g. Tab. w/aluminum hydroxide, glycine magnesium carbonate. Bot. 100s. *OTC.*
Use: Analgesic; antacid.

Bugs Bunny Chewable Vitamins and Minerals. (Bayer Consumer Care) Vitamins A 5000 units, D 400 units, E 30 units, C 60 mg, folic acid 0.4 mg, B_1 1.5 mg, B_2 1.7 mg, niacin 20 mg, B_6 2 mg, B_{12} 6 mcg, biotin 40 mcg, pantothenic acid 10 mg, iron 18 mg, calcium 100 mg, phosphorus 100 mg, iodine 150 mcg, magnesium 20 mg, copper 2 mg, zinc 15 mg. Chew. Tab. Bot. 60s. *OTC.*
Use: Mineral, vitamin supplement.

Bugs Bunny Complete. (Bayer Consumer Care) Ca 100 mg, iron 18 mg, vitamins A 5000 units, D 400 units, E 30 mg, B_1 1.5 mg, B_2 1.7 mg, B_3 20 mg, B_5 10 mg, B_6 2 mg, C 60 mg, folic acid 0.4 mg, biotin 40 mcg, Cu, I, Mg, P, aspartame, phenylalanine, Zn 15 mg. Tab. Bot. 60s. *OTC.*
Use: Mineral, vitamin supplement.

Bugs Bunny Plus Iron. (Bayer Consumer Care) Vitamins A 2500 units, E 15 units, C 60 mg, folic acid 0.3 mg, B_1 1.05 mg, B_2 1.2 mg, niacin 13.5 mg, B_6 1.05 mg, B_{12} 4.5 mcg, D 400 units, iron 15 mg. Chew. Tab. Bot. 60s. *OTC.*
Use: Mineral, vitamin supplement.

Bugs Bunny With Extra C. (Bayer Consumer Care) Vitamins A 2500 units, D 400 units, E 15 units, C 250 mg, folic acid 0.3 mg, B_1 1.05 mg, B_2 1.2 mg, niacin 13.5 mg, B_6 1.05 mg, B_{12} 4.5 mcg. Tab. Bot. 60s. *OTC.*
Use: Mineral, vitamin supplement.

Bulk Forming Fiber Laxative. (Goldline Consumer) Calcium polycarbophil 625 mg (equiv. to polycarbophil 500 mg). Tab. Bot. 60s. *OTC.*
Use: Laxative.

bulkogen. A mucin extracted from the seeds of Cyanopsis tetragonaloba.

bulk-producing laxatives.
See: Bulk Forming Fiber Laxative.
Citrucel.
Citrucel Sugar Free.
Equalactin.
Fiber.
Fiberall Orange Flavor.
Fiberall Tropical Fruit Flavor.
FiberCon.
Fiber-Lax.
FiberNorm.
Genfiber.
Genfiber, Orange Flavor.
Hydrocil Instant.
Konsyl.
Konsyl-D.
Konsyl Easy Mix Formula.
Konsyl Fiber.

Konsyl-Orange.
Maltsupex.
Metamucil.
Metamucil Orange Flavor, Original Texture.
Metamucil Orange Flavor, Smooth Texture.
Metamucil Original Texture.
Metamucil, Sugar Free, Orange Flavor, Smooth Texture.
Metamucil, Sugar Free, Smooth Texture.
Modane.
Natural Fiber Laxative.
Perdiem Fiber Therapy.
Polycarbophil.
Psyllium.
Reguloid.
Reguloid, Orange.
Reguloid, Sugar Free Orange.
Reguloid, Sugar Free Regular.
Serutan.
Syllact.
Unifiber.

BullFrog. (Chattem) Benzophenone-3, octyl methoxycinnamate, isostearyl alcohol, aloe, hydrogenated vegetable oil, vitamin E. Waterproof. Stick 16.5 g. *OTC*.
Use: Sunscreen.

BullFrog Extra Moisturizing. (Chattem) Benzophenone-3, octocrylene, octyl methoxycinnamate, vitamin E, aloe. SPF 18. Gel. Tube 90 g. *OTC*.
Use: Sunscreen.

BullFrog for Kids. (Chattem) SPF 18. Octocrylene, octyl methoxycinnamate, octyl salicylate, vitamin E, aloe, alcohols, benzoate. Gel. Tube 60 g. *OTC*.
Use: Sunscreen.

BullFrog Marathon Mist With UV Extender. (Chattem) Avobenzone 3%, homosalate 15%, octisalate 5%, octocrylene 10%, oxybenzone 6%. Aloe, glycerin, propylene glycol, SD alcohol. SPF 50. Spray. 177 mL. *OTC*.
Use: Sunscreen.

BullFrog Quik Gel With UV Extender. (Chattem) Avobenzone 3%, homosalate 15%, octisalate 5%, octocrylene 10%, oxybenzone 6%. Aloe, glycerin, propylene glycol, SD alcohol. SPF 50. Gel. 147 mL. *OTC*.
Use: Sunscreen.

BullFrog Sport. (Chattem) SPF 18. Benzophenone-3, octocrylene, octyl methoxycinnamate, octyl salicylate, titanium dioxide, diazolidinyl urea, EDTA, parabens, vitamin E, aloe. Lot. Bot. 120 mL. *OTC*.
Use: Sunscreen.

BullFrog Sunblock. (Chattem) SPF 18, 36. Benzophenone-3, octocrylene, octyl methoxycinnamate, aloe, vitamin E, isostearyl alcohol. PABA free. Waterproof. Gel. Tube 120 g. *OTC*.
Use: Sunscreen.

•**bumetanide.** (BYOO-MET-uh-hide) *USP.*
Use: Loop diuretic.

bumetanide. (Teva) Bumetanide 0.5 mg, 1 mg, 2 mg. Lactose. Tab. 100s, 1000s (except 0.5 mg). *Rx*.
Use: Loop diuretic.

bumetanide. (Various Mfr.) Bumetanide. **Tab:** 0.5 mg, 1 mg, 2 mg. Bot. 100s. **Inj.:** 0.25 mg/mL. Amp. 2 mL. Vial 2 mL, 4 mL, 10 mL; 4 mL fill in 5 mL. *Rx*.
Use: Loop diuretic.

•**bumetrizole.** (BYOO-meh-TRY-zole) USAN.
Use: Ultraviolet screen.

Buminate. (Baxter PPI) Normal serum albumin (human). **25%:** Soln. in 20 mL w/o administration set; 50 mL and 100 mL w/administration set. **5%:** Soln. in 250 mL, 500 mL w/administration set. *Rx*.
Use: Albumin replacement.

•**bunamidine hydrochloride.** (BYOO-NAM-ih-deen) USAN.
Use: Anthelmintic.

bunamiodyl sodium.
Use: Diagnostic aid, radiopaque medium.

•**bunaprolast.** (BYOO-nah-PROLE-ast) USAN.
Use: Antiasthmatic.

•**bunolol hydrochloride.** (BYOO-no-lole) USAN.
Use: Antiadrenergic, β-receptor.

Bun Reagent Strips. (Bayer Consumer Care) *Seralyzer* reagent strips. A quantitative strip test for BUN in serum or plasma. Bot. 25s.
Use: Diagnostic aid.

Bupap. (ECR) Butalbital 50 mg, acetaminophen 650 mg. Tab. Bot. 100s. *Rx*.
Use: Analgesic.

•**buparlisib.** (BUE-par-LIS-ib) USAN.
Use: Antineoplastic.

•**buparlisib hydrochloride.** (BUE-par-LIS-ib) USAN.
Use: Antineoplastic.

Buphenyl. (Medicis) Sodium phenylbutyrate. **Tab.:** 500 mg. 250s, 500s. **Pow.:** 3 g per 5 mL. 500 mL bottle w/measurer. *Rx*.
Use: Antihyperammonemic.

•**bupicomide.** (byoo-PIH-koe-mide) USAN.
Use: Antihypertensive.

•**bupivacaine.** (bue-PIV-a-kane) USAN.
Use: Anesthetic, local.

bupivacaine and epinephrine.
Use: Anesthetic, local.
See: Marcaine w/Epinephrine.

•**bupivacaine hydrochloride.** (byoo-PIH-vah-cane) *USP.*
Use: Anesthetic, local.
See: Bupivacaine Hydrochloride.
Bupivacaine Hydrochloride with Epinephrine 1:200,000.
Bupivacaine Spinal.
Marcaine.
Marcaine Spinal.
Marcaine w/Epinephrine.
Sensorcaine.
Sensorcaine MPF.
Sensorcaine MPF Spinal.

bupivacaine hydrochloride. (Abbott) Bupivacaine hydrochloride 0.25%, 0.5%, 0.75%. Inj. Amp. 20 mL, 30 mL, 50 mL (0.25% only). Vial 10 mL, 30 mL. Multidose vial 50 mL (except 0.75%) with methylparaben 1 mg/mL. *Abboject* 30 mL (0.5% only), 50 mL (0.25% only). *Rx.*
Use: Anesthetic, local.

bupivacaine hydrochloride with epinephrine 1:200,000. (Hospira) Bupivacaine hydrochloride 0.25%, 0.5%, 0.75% with epinephrine 1:200,000. Inj. Amp. 30 mL (except 0.25%), 50 mL (0.25% only). Vial 10 mL, 30 mL (except 0.75%). Fliptop multidose vial 50 mL (except 0.75%). *Rx.*
Use: Anesthetic, local.

bupivacaine in dextrose.
Use: Anesthetic, local.

bupivacaine liposome.
Use: Local anesthetic.
See: Exparel.

Bupivacaine Spinal. (Abbott) Bupivacaine hydrochloride 0.75% in dextrose 8.25%. Preservative free. Inj. Amp. 2 mL. *Rx.*
Use: Anesthetic, local.

Buprenex. (Reckitt & Benckiser) Buprenorphine hydrochloride 0.3 mg/mL w/50 mg anhydrous dextrose. Inj. Amp. 1 mL. *c-III.*
Use: Analgesic; narcotic.

buprenorphine. (Roxane Labs) Buprenorphine hydrochloride 2 mg, 8 mg. Lactose, mannitol. Tab., sublingual. 30s. *c-III.*
Use: Opioid agonist-antagonist analgesic.

•**buprenorphine hydrochloride.** (BYOO-preh-NAHR-feen) *USP.*
Use: Analgesic.
See: Buprenex.
Butrans.
W/Naloxone Hydrochloride.
See: Suboxone.
Zubsolv.

buprenorphine hydrochloride. (Hospira) Buprenorphine hydrochloride 0.3 mg/mL with anhydrous dextrose 50 mg. Inj. *Carpu-ject* 1 mL. *c-III.*
Use: Analgesic.

buprenorphine hydrochloride/naloxone hydrochloride dehydrate. (Various Mfr.) Buprenorphine/naloxone 2 mg/0.5 mg, 8 mg/2 mg. May contain acesulfame potassium, lactose, mannitol. Tab.; sublingual. 30s, 90s. *c-III.*
Use: Opioid agonist-antagonist analgesic.

Buproban. (Teva) Bupropion hydrochloride 150 mg. Film coated. Polydextrose. ER Tab. 60s, 100s. *Rx.*
Use: Antidepressant.

•**bupropion hydrobromide.** (bue-PRO-pee-ahn) USAN.
Use: CNS agent.

•**bupropion hydrochloride.** (byoo-PRO-pee-ahn) USAN.
Tall Man: buPROPion.
Use: Antidepressant; smoking deterrent.
See: Aplenzin.
Buproban.
Forfivo XL.
Wellbutrin.
Wellbutrin SR.
Wellbutrin XL.
Zyban.

bupropion hydrochloride. (Reckitt & Colman)
Use: Treatment of opiate addiction. [Orphan Drug]

bupropion hydrochloride. (Various Mfr.) **ER Tab. (24 hour):** 150 mg, 300 mg. 30s, 60s, 90s, 500s. **ER Tab (12 hour):** 100 mg, 150 mg, 200 mg. 60s, 100s, 180s (200 mg only), 250s (150 mg only), 500s, 1,000s (200 mg only). **Tab.:** Bupropion hydrochloride 75 mg, 100 mg. 30s, 100s, 500s, 1,000s. *Rx.*
Use: Antidepressant.

•**buramate.** (BYOO-rah-mate) USAN.
Use: Anticonvulsant; antipsychotic; anxiolytic.

Burdeo. (Hill Dermaceuticals) Aluminum subacetate 100 mg, boric acid 300 mg/oz. Bot. 3 oz. Roll-on 8 oz. *OTC.*
Use: Deodorant.

Burn-a-Lay. (Ken-Gate) Chlorobutanol 0.75%, oxyquinoline benzoate 0.025%, zinc oxide 2%, thymol 0.5%. Cream. Tube oz. *OTC.*
Use: Burn therapy.

Burnate. (Burlington) Vitamins A

4000 units, D_2 400 units, thiamine hydrochloride 3 mg, riboflavin 2 mg, niacinamide 10 mg, pyridine hydrochloride 2 mg, cyanocobalamin 5 mcg, calcium pantothenate 0.5 mg, folic acid 0.4 mg, ascorbic acid 50 mg, ferrous fumarate 300 mg, calcium 200 mg, iodine 0.15 mg, copper 1 mg, magnesium 5 mg, zinc 1.5 mg. Tab. Bot. 100s. *OTC.*
Use: Mineral, vitamin supplement.

Burn-O-Jel. (S.S.S. Company) Lidocaine hydrochloride 0.5%. Aloe vera gel, EDTA, glycerin, ethyl alcohol. Gel. 58 g. *OTC.*
Use: Topical local anesthetic, amide local anesthetic.

burn preparations.
Use: Topical anti-infective.
See: Mafenide.
Nitrofurazone.
Silver Sulfadiazine.

Burn-Quel. Halperin aerosol dispenser 1 oz, 2 oz.
Use: Burn therapy.

burn therapy.
See: Burn-A-Lay.
Burn-Quel.
Foille.
Nupercainal.
Silvadene.
Solarcaine.
Sulfamylon.
Unguentine.

Buro-Sol Antiseptic. (Doak Dermatologics) Contents make a diluted Burow's Solution. Aluminum acetate topical soln. plus benzethonium Cl. Pow. Pkg. (2.36 g) 12s, 100s. Bot. Pow. 4 oz, 1 lb, 5 lb. *OTC.*
Use: Astringent.

Burow's Otic. (Rugby) Acetic acid 2% in aluminum acetate solution. Soln. 60 mL. *Rx.*
Use: Otic preparation.

Bursul. (Burlington) Sulfamethizole 500 mg. Tab. Bot. 100s. *Rx.*
Use: Anti-infective; sulfonamide.

Bur-Zin. (Lamond) Aluminum acetate solution 2%, zinc oxide 10%. Bot. 4 oz, 8 oz, pt, qt, gal. Also w/o lanolin. *OTC.*
Use: Antipruritic, counterirritant.

•**buserelin acetate.** (BYOO-seh-REH-lin ASS-eh-tate) USAN.
Use: Gonad-stimulating principle.

•**buspirone hydrochloride.** (byoo-SPY-rone) *USP.*
Tall Man: busPIRone.
Use: Anxiolytic.

buspirone hydrochloride. (Mylan) Buspirone hydrochloride 30 mg. Tab. Bot. 60s, 100s, 180s. *Rx.*
Use: Anxiolytic.

buspirone hydrochloride. (Par) Buspirone hydrochloride 7.5 mg. May contain lactose. Tab. 100s, 500s. *Rx.*
Use: Anxiolytic.

buspirone hydrochloride. (Various Mfr.) Buspirone hydrochloride 5 mg, 10 mg, 15 mg. May contain lactose. Tab. Bot. 100s, 500s. *Rx.*
Use: Anxiolytic.

•**busulfan.** (bue-SUL-fan) *USP.*
Use: Alkylating agent.
See: Busulfex.
Myleran.

Busulfex. (Ben Venue Labs) Busulfan 6 mg/mL. Inj. Single-use ampules 10 mL w/syringe filters. *Rx.*
Use: Alkylating agent.

•**butabarbital.** (byoo-tah-BAR-bih-tahl) *USP.*
Use: Hypnotic; sedative.
See: Butisol.
Da-Sed.
Expansatol.
W/Hyoscyamine Hydrobromide, Phenazopyridine Hydrochloride.
See: Phenazopyridine Plus.
W/Combinations
See: Dapco.
Monosyl.
Petn.
Quibron Plus.
Sedapap.

•**butabarbital sodium.** (byoo-tah-BAR-bih-tahl) *USP.*
Use: Hypnotic; sedative.
See: Butalan.
Butisol Sodium.
Quiebar.
Renbu.
W/Belladonna Extract.
See: Butibel.
W/Combinations.
See: Bisalate.
Eulcin.
Indogesic.
Monosyl.
Phrenilin.
Quiebel.

butacaine.
Use: Anesthetic, local.

•**butacetin.** (byoot-ASS-ih-tin) USAN.
Use: Analgesic; antidepressant.

•**butaclamol hydrochloride.** (byoo-tah-KLAM-ole) USAN.
Use: Antipsychotic.

Butagen Caps. (Ivax) Phenylbutazone 100 mg. Cap. Bot. 100s, 500s. *Rx.*
Use: Antirheumatic; hypnotic; sedative.

Butalan. (Lannett) Sodium butabarbital 0.2 g/30 mL. Elix. Bot. Pt, gal.
Use: Hypnotic; sedative.

•**butalbital.** (BYOO-TAL-bih-tuhl) *USP.*

Formerly Allybarbituric acid.
Use: Hypnotic; sedative.
W/Acetaminophen.
See: Bupap.
Butex Forte.
Dolgic.
Marten-Tab.
Orbivan CF.
Phrenilin Forte.
Promacet.
Sedapap.
Tencon.
W/Acetaminophen, Caffeine.
See: Alagesic LQ.
Americet.
Arbutal.
Arcet.
Capacet.
Dolgic LQ.
Dolgic Plus.
Esgic.
Esgic-Plus.
Fioricet.
Margesic.
Medigesic Plus.
Orbivan.
Repan.
Triad.
Zebutal.
W/Acetaminophen, Caffeine, Codeine Phosphate.
See: Phrenilin w/Caffeine and Codeine.
W/Aspirin, Caffeine.
See: Butalbital Compound.
Fiorinal.
Medigesic Plus.
W/Aspirin, Caffeine, Codeine Phosphate.
See: Ascomp with Codeine.
Butalbital, Aspirin, Caffeine with Codeine Phosphate.
Fiorinal with Codeine.
Floricet with Codeine.
W/Aspirin, Caffeine, Phenacetin.
See: Arbutal.
W/Hyoscyamine Hydrobromide, Phenazopyridine Hydrochloride.
See: PhenazoForte Plus.

butalbital, acetaminophen, and caffeine. (Various Mfr.) **Cap.:** Acetaminophen 300 mg, butalbital 50 mg, caffeine 40 mg. 100s, 500s. **Tab.:** Acetaminophen 325 mg, 500 mg, caffeine 40 mg, butalbital 50 mg. 30s, 50s, 100s, 500s, 1000s, UD 100s. *Rx.*
Use: Nonnarcotic analgesic with barbiturates.

butalbital, acetaminophen, caffeine, and codeine phosphate. (Breckenridge) Codeine phosphate 30 mg, acetaminophen 325 mg, caffeine 40 mg, butalbital 50 mg. Cap. 100s, 500s. *c-III.*
Use: Narcotic analgesic.

butalbital and aspirin.
Use: Analgesic; sedative.

butalbital, aspirin, and caffeine. (Various Mfr.) **Tab.:** Aspirin 325 mg, caffeine 40 mg, butalbital 50 mg. Bot. 30s, 50s, 100s, 500s, 1000s, UD 100s. **Cap.:** Aspirin 325 mg, caffeine 40 mg, butalbital 50 mg. Bot. 100s, 1000s. *c-III.*
Use: Analgesic combination.

butalbital, aspirin, caffeine with codeine phosphate. (Watson) Aspirin 325 mg, butalbital 50 mg, caffeine 40 mg, codeine phosphate 30 mg. Cap. 100s, 500s. *c-III.*
Use: Opioid analgesic combination.

butalbital compound. (Various Mfr.) Aspirin 325 mg, caffeine 40 mg, butalbital 50 mg. Tab., Cap. Bot. 100s, 1000s (Tab. only). *c-III.*
Use: Analgesic.

butalgin.
See: Methadone hydrochloride.

•**butamben.** (BYOO-tam-ben) *USP. Formerly Butyl aminobenzoate.*
Use: Anesthetic, local.
W/Benzocaine, Tetracaine Hydrochloride, Bezalkonium Chloride.
See: Cetacaine.

•**butamirate citrate.** (byoo-tah-MY-rate SIH-trate) USAN.
Use: Antitussive.

•**butane.** (BUE-tane) *NF.*
Use: Aerosol propellant.

•**butaperazine.** (BYOO-tah-PURR-ah-zeen) USAN.
Use: Antipsychotic.

•**butaperazine maleate.** (BYOO-tah-PURR-ah-zeen) USAN.
Use: Antipsychotic.

butaphyllamine. Ambuphylline. Theophylline aminoisobutanol. Theophylline with 2-amino-2-methyl-1-propanol.

Butapro. (Health for Life Brands) Butabarbital sodium 0.2 g/30 mL. Elix. Bot. Pt, gal. *c-v.*
Use: Hypnotic; sedative.

•**butaprost.** (BYOO-tah-PRAHST) USAN.
Use: Bronchodilator.

Butazone. (Major) Phenylbutazone 100 mg. Cap. Tab. Bot. 100s (Cap. only), 500s. *Rx.*
Use: Antirheumatic.

•**butedronate tetrasodium.** (BYOO-teh-DROE-nate TET-rah-SO-dee-uhm) USAN.
Use: Diagnostic aid, bone imaging.

butelline.
See: Butacaine Sulfate.

•**butenafine hydrochloride.** (byoo-TEN-ah-feen) USAN.
Use: Topical anti-infective, antifungal.
See: Lotrimin Ultra.
Mentax.

butenafine hydrochloride. (Penederm)
Use: Treatment of interdigital tinea pedis, athlete's foot.

•**buterizine.** (byoo-TER-ih-ZEEN) USAN.
Use: Vasodilator, peripheral.

butethanol.
See: Tetracaine.

Butex Forte. (Athlon) Acetaminophen 650 mg, butalbital 50 mg, benzyl alcohol, EDTA, parabens. Cap. Bot. 100s. *Rx.*
Use: Analgesic.

•**buthiazide.** (byoo-THIGH-azz-IDE) USAN.
Use: Antihypertensive; diuretic.

Butibel. (Wallace) Butabarbital sodium 15 mg, belladonna extract 15 mg. **Tab.:** Bot. 100s. **Elix.:** Per 5 mL. Alcohol 7%, sucrose, saccharin. Orange flavor. Bot. Pt. *Rx.*
Use: GI anticholinergic combination.

•**butikacin.** (BYOO-tih-KAY-sin) USAN.
Use: Anti-infective.

•**butilfenin.** (BYOO-till-FEN-in) USAN.
Use: Diagnostic aid, hepatic function determination.

•**butirosin sulfate.** (byoo-TIHR-oh-sin) USAN. A mixture of the sulfates of the A and B forms of an antibiotic produced by *Bacillus circularis.*
Use: Anti-infective.

Butisol Sodium. (Medpointe) Butabarbital sodium. **Elix.:** 30 mg/5 mL. Pt, gal. **Tab.:** 30 mg, 50 mg. 100s. *c-III.*
Use: Hypnotic; sedative.

•**butixirate.** (BYOO-TIX-ih-rate) USAN.
Use: Analgesic; antirheumatic.

•**butoconazole nitrate.** (BYOO-toe-KOE-nuh-zole) *USP.*
Use: Antifungal.

butolan. Benzylphenyl carbamate.

•**butonate.** (BYOO-tahn-ate) USAN.
Use: Anthelmintic.

•**butopamine.** (BYOO-TOE-pah-meen) USAN.
Use: Cardiovascular agent.

•**butoprozine hydrochloride.** (byoo-TOE-pro-ZEEN) USAN.
Use: Cardiovascular agent, antiarrhythmic; antianginal.

butopyronoxyl. (Indalone) Butylmesityl oxide.
Use: Insect repellant.

•**butorphanol.** (BYOO-TAR-fan-ahl) USAN.
Use: Analgesic; antitussive.

•**butorphanol tartrate.** (BYOO-TAR-fan-ahl) *USP.*
Use: Analgesic; antitussive.

butorphanol tartrate. (Various Mfr.) Butorphanol tartrate. **Inj.:** 1 mg/mL, 2 mg/mL. Vials 1 mL (1 mg/mL only), 2 mL. **Nasal Spray:** 10 mg/mL. Vials 2.5 mL. *c-IV.*
Use: Analgesic; antitussive.

•**butoxamine hydrochloride.** (byoo-TOX-ah-meen) USAN.
Use: Antidiabetic; antihyperlipoproteinemic.

Butrans. (Purdue) Buprenorphine 5 mcg/h, 10 mcg/h, 15 mcg/h, 20 mcg/h. Patch. Carton of 4 individually packaged systems and a pouch containing 4 patch-disposal units. *c-III.*
Use: Opioid agonist-antagonist analgesic.

•**butriptyline hydrochloride.** (BYOO-TRIP-till-een) USAN.
Use: Antidepressant.

•**butyl alcohol.** (BUE-til AL-ka-hol) *NF.* Butyl alcohol is n-butyl alcohol.
Use: Pharmaceutic aid, solvent.

butyl aminobenzoate. n-butyl p-aminobenzoate. Scuroforme.
Use: Anesthetic, local.
W/Benzocaine, Tetracaine Hydrochloride.
See: Cetacaine.
W/Benzyl Alcohol, Phenylmercuric Borate, Benzocaine.
See: Dermathyn.
W/Procaine, Benzyl Alcohol, in Sweet Almond Oil.
See: Anucaine.

•**butylated hydroxyanisole.** (BUE-ti-LAY-ted hye-drox-ee-AN-i-sole) *NF.*
Use: Pharmaceutic aid, antioxidant.

•**butylated hydroxytoluene.** (BUE-ti-LAY-ted hye-drox-ee-TOL-yoo-een) *NF.*
Use: Pharmaceutic aid, antioxidant.

•**butylparaben.** (byo-till-PAR-ah-ben) *NF.*
Use: Pharmaceutic aid, antifungal.

butylphenylsalicylamide.
See: Butylphenamide.

butyrophenone. Class of antipsychotic agents. *Rx.*
See: Haloperidol.

butyrylcholinesterase. (Pharmavene)
Use: Treat cocaine overdose; postsurgical apnea. [Orphan Drug]

B-Vex PD. (Midlothian Laboratories) Brompheniramine tannate 6 mg, pseudoephedrine tannate 30 mg per 5 mL. Aspartame, methylparaben, phenylalanine 5 mg per 5 mL, prosweet, saccharin, sorbitol. Cotton candy flavor.

Susp. 473 mL. *Rx.*
Use: Upper respiratory combination, decongestant and antihistamine.

B vitamins with vitamin C, oral.
See: Dialyvite Multi-Vitamins for Dialysis Patients.
Dialyvite with Zinc.

B vitamins with vitamin C, parenteral.
See: Neurodep.
Vicam.

B-Vite Injection. (Bluco) Vitamins B_1 50 mg, B_2 5 mg, B_6 5 mg, niacinamide 125 mg, B_{12} 1000 mcg, dexpanthenol 6 mg, C 50 mg/10 mL. Mono vial w/benzyl alcohol 1% in water for injection. *Rx.*
Use: Vitamin supplement.

Bydureon. (AstraZeneca) Exenatide 2 mg. Inj., Pow. for Susp. (extended release). Single-dose trays (1 vial of exenatide, 1 vial connector, 1 prefilled diluent syringe, 2 needles). *Rx.*
Use: Antidiabetic agent, glucagon-like peptide 1 receptor agonist.

Bydureon Pen. (AstraZeneca) Exenatide 2 mg. Inj., Pow. for Susp. (extended release). Single-dose pen. *Rx.*
Use: Antidiabetic agent, glucagon-like peptide 1 receptor agonist.

Byetta. (Amylin Pharmaceuticals, Inc.) Exenatide 250 mcg/mL. Metacresol. Inj. Soln. Prefilled pens. 1.2 mL (provides 5 mcg/dose), 2.4 mL (provides 10 mcg/dose). *Rx.*
Use: Antidiabetic agent; incretin mimetic agent.

Bystolic. (Forest Laboratories) Nebivolol (as nebivolol hydrochloride) 2.5 mg, 5 mg, 10 mg, 20 mg. Lactose. Tab. 30s, 100s, UD 100s (except 2.5 mg). *Rx.*
Use: Antiadrenergic/sympatholytic, beta-adrenergic blocking agent.

C

•**cabazitaxel.** (ka-BAZ-i-TAX-el) USAN.
Use: Taxoid.
See: Jevtana.

•**cabergoline.** (cab-ERR-go-leen) USAN.
Use: Antidyskinetic; antihyperprolactinemic; antiparkinsonian; dopamine agonist; hyperprolactinemic disorders treatment.

cabergoline. (Various Mfr.) Cabergoline 5 mg. May contain lactose. Tab. 8s. *Rx.*
Use: Agent for gout.

•**cabozantinib.** (KA-boe-ZAN-ti-nib) USAN.
Use: Antineoplastic.
See: Cometriq.

•**cabozantinib s-malate.** (KA-boe-ZAN-ti-nib) USAN.
Use: Antineoplastic.

•**cabufocon A.** (cab-YOU-FOE-kahn A) USAN.
Use: Contact lens material, hydrophobic.

•**cabufocon B.** (cab-YOU-FOE-kahn B) USAN.
Use: Contact lens material.

Cachexon. (Telluride) L-Glutathione.
Use: AIDS-associated cachexia. [Orphan Drug]

cacodylic acid. Dimethylarsinic acid.

•**cactinomycin.** (KACK-tih-no-MY-sin) USAN. Antibiotic produced by *Streptomyces chrysomallus. Formerly Actinomycin C.*
Use: Antineoplastic.

cade oil.
See: Juniper Tar.

•**cadexomer iodine.** (kad-EX-oh-mer) USAN.
Use: Antiseptic; antiulcerative.

Caduet. (Pfizer) Amlodipine besylate/atorvastatin calcium (as base) 2.5 mg/10 mg, 2.5 mg/20 mg, 2.5 mg/40 mg, 5 mg/10 mg, 5 mg/20 mg, 5 mg/40 mg, 5 mg/80 mg, 10 mg/10 mg, 10 mg/20 mg, 10 mg/40 mg, 10 mg/80 mg. Calcium carbonate. Film-coated. Tab. 30s. *Rx.*
Use: Antihyperlipidemic.

Cafatine-PB. (Major) Ergotamine tartrate 2 mg, caffeine 100 mg, belladonna alkaloids 0.25 mg, pentobarbital 60 mg. Supp. Box foil 10s. *Rx.*
Use: Antimigraine.

Cafcit. (Bedford) Caffeine citrate. **Oral Soln.:** 20 mg/mL. **Inj.:** 20 mg/mL (caffeine citrate 2 mg equivalent to caffeine base 1 mg). Preservative free. Vial 3 mL. *Rx.*
Use: CNS stimulant.

Cafenol. (Sanofi-Synthelabo) Aspirin, caffeine. *OTC.*
Use: Analgesic combination.

Cafergot P-B Suppositories. (Novartis) Ergotamine tartrate 2 mg, caffeine 100 mg, bellafoline 0.25 mg, pentobarbital 60 mg. Supp. Box 12s. *Rx.*
Use: Antimigraine.

Cafergot P-B Tablets. (Novartis) Ergotamine tartrate 1 mg, caffeine 100 mg, bellafoline 0.125 mg, pentobarbital sodium 30 mg. Tab. *SigPak* dispensing pkg. of 90s, 250s. *c-IV.*
Use: Antimigraine.

Cafergot Tablets. (Novartis) Ergotamine tartrate 1 mg, caffeine 100 mg. Sugar coated. Parabens, sugar. Tab. 100s. *SigPak* dispensing pkg. of 90s. *Rx.*
Use: Antimigraine.

Caffedrine. (Various Mfr.) Caffeine 200 mg. Tab. Pkg. 16s. *OTC.*
Use: CNS stimulant.

•**caffeine.** (ka-FEEN) *USP.*
Use: CNS stimulant; apnea of prematurity.
See: Cafcit.
Caffedrine.
Enerjets.
Fastlene.
.44 Magnum.
Keep Alert.
Keep Going.
Lucidex.
Maximum Strength NoDoz.
Overtime.
Stay Alert.
Stay Awake.
357 HR Magnum.
20-20.
Valentine.
Vivarin.

W/Acetaminophen.
See: APAP-Plus.
Excedrin Tension Headache.

W/Acetaminophen, Aluminum Hydroxide, Aspirin, Magnesium Hydroxide.
See: Vanquish.

W/Acetaminophen, Aspirin.
See: Anacin Advanced Headache.
Bayer Migraine.
Excedrin Extra Strength.
Excedrin Migraine.
Goody's Cool Orange.
Goody's Extra Strength.
Goody's Extra Strength Fast Pain Relief.
Goody's Migraine Relief.
Painaid ESF Extra-Strength Formula.

W/Acetaminophen, Aspirin, Salicylamide.
See: Medi-First Extra Strength Pain Relief.

Painaid.
Saleto.
W/Acetaminophen, Butalbital.
See: Alagesic LQ.
Americet.
Butalbital, Acetaminophen, and Caffeine.
Capacet.
Dolgic Plus.
Esgic.
Esgic-Plus.
Margesic.
Orbivan.
Triad.
Zebutal.
W/Acetaminophen, Butalbital, Codeine Phosphate.
See: Butalbital, Acetaminophen, Caffeine, and Codeine Phosphate.
Phrenilin w/Caffeine and Codeine.
W/Acetaminophen, Dihydrocodeine Bitartrate.
See: Panlor DC.
Trezix.
W/Acetaminophen, Isometheptene Mucate.
See: Prodrin.
W/Acetaminophen, Magnesium Salicylate.
See: Back Pain-Off.
W/Acetaminophen, Magnesium Salicylate, Phenyltoloxamine Citrate.
See: Durabac Forte.
W/Acetaminophen, Phenyltoloxamine, Salicylamide.
See: Durabac.
Levacet.
W/Acetaminophen, Pyrilamine Maleate.
See: Midol Menstrual Complete.
W/Aspirin.
See: Alka-Seltzer Wake-Up Call.
Anacin.
Anacin Maximum Strength.
Bayer Quick Release Crystals.
BC Fast Pain Relief.
BC Fast Pain Relief Arthritis.
Summit Extra Strength.
W/Aspirin, Butalbital.
See: Butalbital, Aspirin, and Caffeine.
Butalbital Compound.
Fiorinal.
W/Aspirin, Butalbital, Codeine Phosphate.
See: Butalbital, Aspirin, Caffeine w/Codeine Phosphate.
W/Aspirin, Orphenadrine Citrate.
See: Orphenadrine Compound.
Orphenadrine Compound-DS.
W/Aspirin, Salicylamide.
See: BC Powder Arthritis Strength.
Stanback Headache Powders.
W/Butalbital, Codeine Phosphate.
See: Fiorinal with Codeine.
W/Isometheptene Mucate, Acetaminophen.
See: MigraTen.

caffeine and sodium benzoate. (Bedford, American Regent) Caffeine and sodium benzoate 250 mg/mL (caffeine 121 mg, sodium benxoate 129 mg). Inj. Single-use vial. 2 mL. *Rx.*
Use: CNS stimulant.

•**caffeine citrate.** (ka-FEEN) *USP.*
Use: CNS stimulant.
W/Phenylephrine Hydrochloride, Pheniramine Maleate, Sodium Salicylate.
See: Scot-Tussin Original Multi-Action Cold and Allergy Formula.
W/Sodium Citrate, Phenylephrine Hydrochloride, Pheniramine Maleate, Sodium Salicylate, Codeine Phosphate.
See: Tussirex.
Tussirex Sugar Free.

caffeine citrate. (Paddock) Caffeine citrate. **Inj.:** 20 mg/mL. Preservative free. Vials. 3 mL. **Oral Soln.:** 20 mg/mL. Preservative free. Vials. 3 mL. *Rx.*
Use: Analeptic, central nervous system stimulant.

caffeine citrated.
Use: CNS stimulant.

caffeine sodio-benzoate.
See: Caffeine Sodium Benzoate.

caffeine sodium salicylate. (Various Mfr.) Caffeine sodium salicylate. Bot. 1 oz; Pkg. 0.25 lb, 1 lb. *OTC.*
Use: CNS stimulant.

Cagol. (Harvey) Guaiacol 0.1 g, eucalyptol 0.08 g, iodoform 0.2 g, camphor 0.05 g/2 mL in olive oil. Vial 30 mL. *Rx.*
Use: Expectorant.

Calaclear. (Humco) Pramoxine hydrochloride 1%, zinc acetate 0.1%. Alcohol, camphor, glycerin, parabens, polysorbate 80, propylene glycol, urea. Lot. 177 mL. *OTC.*
Use: Poison ivy product.

Caladryl. (Pfizer) Calamine 8%, pramoxine hydrochloride 1%, alcohol, camphor, diazolidinyl urea, parabens. Lot. Bot. 177 mL. *OTC.*
Use: Antipruritic, topical; poison ivy treatment.

Caladryl Clear. (Pfizer) Pramoxine hydrochloride 1%, zinc acetate 0.1%, alcohol, camphor, diazolidinyl urea, parabens. Lot. Bot. 177 mL. *OTC.*
Use: Antipruritic, topical; poison ivy treatment.

Calafol. (Alaven) Vitamin B_6 25 mg, vitamin B_{12} 425 mg, FA 1.6 mg, Ca 400 mg, D_3 400 units. Tab. 90s. *Rx.*
Use: Nutritional product.

Calaformula. (Eric, Kirk & Gary) Ferrous gluconate 130 mg, calcium lactate

130 mg, vitamins A 1000 units, D 400 units, B_1 2 mg, B_2 2 mg, niacinamide 5 mg, ascorbic acid 20 mg, folic acid 0.13 mg, Mg 0.25 mg, Cu 0.25 mg, Zn 0.25 mg, Mn 0.25 mg, K 0.075 mg. Cap. Bot. 50s, 100s, 500s, 1000s, 5000s. *OTC.*
Use: Mineral, vitamin supplement.

Calaformula F. (Eric, Kirk & Gary) Calaformula plus fluorine 0.333 mg. Tab. Bot. 100s. *Rx.*
Use: Mineral, vitamin supplement; dental caries agent.

Calagel Maximum Strength. (Tec Labs) Benzethonium chloride 0.15%, diphenhydramine hydrochloride 2%, zinc acetate 0.215%. Disodium edetate, menthol. Gel. 177.44 mL. *OTC.*
Use: Antihistamine preparation, topical.

Calagesic. (Humco) Calamine 8%, pramoxine hydrochloride 1%. Alcohol, camphor, glycerin, parabens, polysorbate 80, propylene glycol, urea. Lot. 177 mL. *OTC.*
Use: Poison ivy product.

Calahist. (Walgreen) Diphenhydramine hydrochloride 1%, calamine 8.1%, camphor 0.1%. Lot. Bot. 6 oz. *OTC.*
Use: Antipruritic, topical.

•**calamine.** (kal-a-MINE) *USP.*
Use: Protectant, topical.
W/Diphenhydramine Hydrochloride.
See: Ivarest Maximum Strength.
W/Pramoxine Hydrochloride.
See: Aveeno Anti-Itch.
Caladryl.
Calagesic.

calamine. (Various Mfr.) Calamine 6.97%, zinc oxide 6.97%, glycerin. Lot. Bot. 118 mL, 240 mL, 480 mL. *OTC.*
Use: Antiseptic; astringent; poison ivy treatment.

calamine, phenolated. (Humco) Calamine, zinc oxide, glycerin, liquefied phenol 1%. Lot. Bot. 177 mL. *OTC.*
Use: Antiseptic; astringent; poison ivy treatment.

Calamycin. (Pfeiffer) Pyrilamine maleate, zinc oxide 10%, calamine 10%, benzocaine, chloroxylenol, zirconium oxide, isopropyl alcohol 10%. Lot. Bot. 120 mL. *OTC.*
Use: Antipruritic, topical.

Calan. (Pfizer) Verapamil hydrochloride 80 mg, 120 mg. Film coated. Lactose, polyethylene glycol. Tab. 100s. *Rx.*
Use: Calcium channel blocking agent.

Calan SR. (Pfizer) Verapamil hydrochloride 120 mg, 180 mg, 240 mg. Film-coated. ER Tab. Bot. 100s, 500s (240 mg only), UD 100s. *Rx.*
Use: Calcium channel blocker.

•**calaspargase pegol.** (kal-AS-par-jase PEG-ol) USAN.
Use: Antineoplastic.

Cal-Bid. (Roberts) Elemental calcium 250 mg, ascorbic acid 100 mg, vitamin D 125 units. Tab. Bot. 100s. *OTC.*
Use: Mineral, vitamin supplement.

Cal-Carb Forte. (Vitaline) Calcium carbonate. **Cap.:** 1250 mg (elemental calcium 500 mg). Bot. 100s. **Chew Tab.:** 1250 mg (elemental calcium 500 mg). Mint flavor. Bot. 100s. *OTC.*
Use: Mineral supplement.

Cal-C-Caps. (Key) Elemental calcium (as calcium citrate) 180 mg. Cap. 100s. *OTC.*
Use: Mineral supplement.

Cal-Cee. (Key) Calcium citrate 1150 mg (elemental calcium 250 mg). Tab. 100s. *OTC.*
Use: Mineral supplement.

Calcet. (Mission) Calcium 150 mg, vitamin D_3 100 units. Tab. Bot. 100s. *OTC.*
Use: Mineral, vitamin supplement.

Calcet Plus. (Mission Pharmacal) Elemental calcium 152.8 mg, elemental iron 18 mg, vitamins A 5000 units, D 400 units, E 30 mg, B_1 2.25 mg, B_2 2.55 mg, B_3 30 mg, B_5 15 mg, B_6 3 mg, B_{12} 9 mcg, C 500 mg, folic acid 0.8 mg, zinc 15 mg, sugar. Tab. Bot 60s. *OTC.*
Use: Mineral, vitamin supplement.

Calcibind. (Mission) Inorganic phosphate content 31% to 36%, sodium content ≈ 11%. Pow. 300 g bulk pack. *Rx.*
Use: Antiurolithic.

CalciCaps. (Nion Corp.) Calcium (dibasic calcium phosphate, calcium gluconate, calcium carbonate) 125 mg, vitamin D 67 units, phosphorus 60 mg. Tab. Bot. 100s, 500s. *OTC.*
Use: Mineral, vitamin supplement.

CalciCaps M-Z. (Nion Corp.) Ca 400 mg, Mg 133 mg, Zn 5 mg, vitamin A 1667 mg, D 133 units, Se. Tab. Bot. 90s. *OTC.*
Use: Mineral, vitamin supplement.

CalciCaps, Super. (Nion Corp.) Calcium 400 mg, phosphorus 41.7 mg, vitamin D 100 units. Tab. Bot. 90s. *OTC.*
Use: Mineral, vitamin supplement.

CalciCaps with Iron. (Nion Corp.) Calcium 125 mg, phosphorus 60 mg, vitamin D 67 units, ferrous gluconate 7 mg, tartrazine. Tab. Bot. 100s, 500s. *OTC.*
Use: Mineral, vitamin supplement.

Calci-Chew. (Rugby) Calcium carbonate 1250 mg (elemental calcium 500 mg). Sugar. Cherry and assorted flavors.

Chew. Tab. Bot. 100s. *OTC.*
Use: Mineral supplement.
Calcidrine. (Abbott) Codeine 8.4 mg, calcium iodide anhydrous 152 mg, alcohol 6%/5 mL. Syr. Bot. 120 mL, 480 mL. *c-v.*
Use: Antitussive; expectorant.
Calciferol. (Schwarz Pharma) Ergocalciferol (vitamin D_2) 8000 units/mL in propylene glycol. Liq. 60 mL. *OTC.*
Use: Refractory rickets; familial hypophosphatemia; hypoparathyroidism.
Calcijex. (Abbott) Calcitriol 1 mcg/mL, polysorbate 20 4 mg, sodium chloride 1.5 mg, sodium ascorbate 10 mg, dibasic sodium phosphate 7.6 mg, anhydrous, EDTA. Inj. Amp. 1 mL. *Rx.*
Use: Antihypocalcemic; antihypoparathyroid; vitamin.
Calci-Mix. (Watson) Calcium carbonate 1250 mg (elemental calcium 500 mg). Cap. Bot. 100s. *OTC.*
Use: Mineral supplement.
Calcionate. (Various Mfr.) Calcium glubionate 1.8 g/5 mL. Syr. Bot. 473 mL. *OTC.*
Use: Mineral supplement.
•**calcipotriene.** (kal-sih-POE-try-een) USAN.
Use: Antipsoriatic.
See: Calcitrene.
Dovonex.
Sorilux.
W/Betamethasone Dipropionate.
See: Taclonex.
Taclonex Scalp.
calcipotriene. (Taro Pharmaceuticals) Calcipotriene 0.005%. Alpha tocopherol, edetate disodium, mineral oil, petrolatum, propylene glycol. Oint. 60 g. *Rx.*
Use: Antipsoriatic agent.
calcipotriene. (Various Mfr.) Calcipotriene 0.005%. **Soln.:** May contain menthol, propylene glycol. 60 mL. **Cream:** May contain alcohol, edetate disodium, glycerin, mineral oil, urea, white petrolatum. 60 g, 120 g. *Rx.*
Use: Antipsoriatic.
Calciquid. (Breckenridge) Calcium glubionate 1.8 g/5 mL. Syr. Bot. 473 mL. *OTC.*
Use: Mineral supplement.
•**calcitonin.** (kal-sih-TOE-nin) USAN.
Use: Treatment of Paget disease, calcium regulator.
See: Calcimar.
Cibacalcin.
Miacalcin.
Osteocalcin.
calcitonin-human for injection. Hormone from thyroid gland.
Use: Plasma hypocalcemic hormone; symptomatic Paget disease of bone. [Orphan Drug]
See: Cibacalcin.
calcitonin-salmon.
Use: Antihypercalcemic.
See: Fortical.
Miacalcin.
calcitonin-salmon. (Various Mfr.) Calcitonin-salmon 200 units per 0.09 mL spray. Soln., Intranasal. Glass bottle. 3.7 mL. *Rx.*
Use: Endocrine and metabolic agent.
Cal-Citrate. (Bio-Tech) Elemental calcium. **Tab.:** 250 mg. Bot. 250s. **Cap.:** 225 mg. 100s, 250s. *OTC.*
Use: Mineral supplement.
Calcitrene. (Taro Pharmaceuticals) Calcipotriene 0.005%. Edetate disodium, mineral oil, petrolatum propylene glycol. Oint. 60 g. *Rx.*
Use: Antipsoriatic agent.
•**calcitriol.** (KAL-sih-TRY-ole) USAN.
Use: Antihypocalcemic, calcium regulator; vitamin.
See: Calcijex.
Rocaltrol.
Vectical.
calcitriol. (Roxane) Calcitriol 1 mcg/mL. Oral Soln. 15 mL with single-use graduated oral dispensers. *Rx.*
Use: Antihypocalcemic, calcium regulator; vitamin.
calcitriol. (Teva) Calcitriol 0.25 mcg, 0.5 mcg. Mannitol, sorbitol. Cap. 100s. *Rx.*
Use: Vitamin.
calcitriol injection. (aaiPharma) Calcitriol 1 mcg/mL, 2 mcg/mL, sodium chloride, EDTA. Inj. 1 mL vial. *Rx.*
Use: Antihypocalcemic, calcium regulator; vitamin.
calcium.
Use: Mineral.
See: Calcium Acetate.
Calcium Ascorbate.
Calcium Carbonate.
Calcium Citrate.
Calcium Gluconate.
Calcium Lactate.
Tricalcium Phosphate.
W/Chloride, Magnesium.
See: Slow Magnesium Chloride With Calcium.
W/Selenium.
See: Vitaline Selenium.
W/Vitamin D.
See: Calcium 1000 + D.
Oyster Shell Calcium 500 mg + D.
Oyster Shell Calcium With Vitamin D.
Vitamin D_3 400 IU.

•**calcium acetate.** (KAL-see-um) *USP.*
Use: Pharmaceutic aid, buffering agent; hyperphosphatemia; mineral.
See: Calphron.
Eliphos.
PhosLo.

calcium acetate. (Paddock Laboratories) Calcium acetate 667 mg (elemental calcium 169 mg). PEG. Tab. 200s. *Rx.*
Use: Mineral.

calcium acetylsalicylate. Kalmopyrin, kalsetal, soluble aspirin, tylcalsin.
Use: Analgesic.

calcium aluminum carbonate.
W/DI-Amino Acetate Complex.
See: Ancid.

•**calcium aminosalicylate.** (KAL-see-um) *NF.* Aminosalicylate calcium.

calcium amphomycin.
See: Amphomycin.

calcium and magnesium carbonates.
Use: Mineral; antacid.

•**calcium and vitamin D with minerals.** (KAL-see-um) *USP.*
Use: Mineral, vitamin supplement.

Calcium Antacid Extra Strength. (Various Mfr.) Calcium carbonate 750 mg (elemental calcium 300 mg). Chew. Tab. Bot. 96s. *OTC.*
Use: Mineral supplement; antacid.

•**calcium ascorbate.** (KAL-see-uhm a-skor-bate) *USP.*
Use: Water-soluble vitamin.
See: Ascocid.

calcium ascorbate. (Freeda) **Tab.:** Calcium ascorbate 500 mg. Calcium 75 mg. Sugar free. Buffered. Bot. 100s, 250s, 500s. **Pow.:** Calcium ascorbate 814 mg per ¼ tsp. Calcium 100 mg per ¼ tsp. Sugar free. Buffered. Bot. 120 g, 1 lb. *OTC.*
Use: Water-soluble vitamin.

calcium benzoyl-p-aminosalicylate.
See: Benzoylpas Calcium.

calcium benzoylpas.
See: Benzoylpas Calcium.

calcium bis-dioctyl sulfosuccinate.
See: Dioctyl Calcium Sulfosuccinate.

calcium carbimide. Calcium cyanamide. Sulfosuccinate.

•**calcium carbonate.** (KAL-see-um KAR-bo-nate) *USP. Formerly calcium carbonate, precipitated.*
Use: Antacid; mineral; hyperphosphatemia.
See: Alka-Mints.
Antacid Tablets.
Cal-Carb Forte.
Calci-Chew.
Calci-Mix.
Calcium Antacid Extra Strength.
Calcium 600.
Cal•Gest.
Chooz.
Dicarbosil.
Equilet.
Maalox Children's.
Maalox Regular Strength.
Nephro-Calci.
Os-Cal 500.
Oysco 500.
Oyst-Cal 500.
Oyster Shell Calcium.
Pepto Children's.
Rolaids Extra Strength Softchews.
Surpass.
Surpass Extra Strength.
Titralac.
Trial Antacid.
Tums Calcium for Life Bone Health.
Tums Calcium for Life PMS.
Tums E-X.
Tums Freshers.
Tums Kids.
Tums Quik Pak.
Tums Smooth Dissolve.
Tums Smoothies.
Tums Ultra.

W/Acetaminophen.
See: Acid-X.

W/Aspirin, Magnesium Hydroxide, Aluminum Hydroxide.
See: Ascriptin Maximum Strength.

W/Aspirin, Magnesium Oxide, Magnesium Carbonate.
See: Bufferin.
Bufferin Extra Strength.
Extra Strength Bayer Plus.

W/Famotidine, Magnesium Hydroxide.
See: Acid Reducer + Antacid.
Dual Action Complete.
Pepcid Complete Dual Action.
Tums Dual Action.

W/Magnesium Carbonate.
See: MagneBind 400 Rx.
MagneBind 300.
MagneBind 200.
Marblen.

W/Magnesium Hydroxide.
See: Rolaids.
Rolaids Calcium Rich.
Rolaids Extra Strength.

W/Magnesium Hydroxide, Simethicone.
See: Rolaids Multi-Symptom.

W/Sodium Fluoride.
See: Florical.

W/Simethicone.
See: Gas Ban.
Gas-X With Maalox Extra Strength.
Maalox Advanced Maximum Strength.
Maalox Junior.

Rolaids Extra Strength Plus Gas Relief.
Titralac Plus.
Tums Plus.
W/Vitamin D_3
See: Citrus Calcium With Vitamin D.
D-1000 Extra Strength.
Liquid Calcium With D_3 Maximum Strength.
Super Calcium 600 + D_3 400.

calcium carbonate. (Various Mfr.) Calcium carbonate. **Tab.:** 500 mg (elemental calcium 200 mg). 100, 120s, UD 100s. 600 mg (elemental calcium 240 mg). 60s, 72s, 150s, UD 100s. 648 to 650 mg (elemental calcium 260 mg). 100s, 250s, 500s, 1,000s. 1,250 mg (elemental calcium 500 mg). 100s. 1,500 mg (elemental calcium 600 mg). 60s, 150s. **Chew. Tab.:** 1,250 mg (elemental calcium 500 mg). 60s. **Oral Susp.:** 1,250 mg per 5 mL (elemental calcium 500 mg per 5 mL). 500 mL, UD 5 mL. **Pow.:** 454 g. *OTC.*
Use: Mineral supplement; antacid.

calcium carbonate. (Various Mfr.) Precipitated chalk; carbonic acid, calcium salt (1:1).
Use: Antacid; calcium supplement.

calcium carbonate, aromatic. (Eli Lilly) Calcium carbonate 10 g. Tab. Bot. 100s, 1000s. *OTC.*
Use: Antacid.

Calcium Carbonate 600 mg + Vitamin D. (Major) Ca 600 mg, D 125 units. Tab. Bot. 60s. *OTC.*
Use: Mineral, vitamin supplement.

calcium carbonate, sodium chloride, and potassium chloride.
Use: Salt replacement.
See: Sustain.

calcium caseinate.
Use: Mineral supplement.

calcium channel blockers.
Use: Angina pectoris; vasospastic and unstable angina.
See: Amlodipine.
Clevidipine Butyrate.
Diltiazem Hydrochloride.
Felodipine.
Isradipine.
Nicardipine Hydrochloride.
Nifedipine.
Nimodipine.
Nisoldipine.
Verapamil Hydrochloride.

Calcium Chel 330. (Novartis)
Use: Antidote, heavy metals.
See: Calcium Trisodium Pentetate.

•**calcium chloride.** (KAL-see-um) *USP.*
Use: Electrolyte, calcium replenisher.
W/Dibasic Sodium Phosphate, Monobasic Sodium Phosphate, Sodium Chloride.
See: Cephosol.
W/Dibasic Sodium Phosphate, Monobasic Sodium Phosphate, Silicon Dioxide, Sodium Chloride, Sodium Bicarbonate.
See: NeutraSal.
W/Fibrinogen, Fibrinolysis Inhibitor, Protein, Thrombin.
See: Tisseel.

calcium chloride. (Pharmacia) Calcium chloride. 1 g. Inj. Amp. 10 mL, 25s. (Torigian) 1 g. Inj. Amp. 10 mL 12s, 25s, 100s. (Trent) 10%. Inj. Amp. 10 mL. (Bayer Consumer Care) 13.6 mEq/ 10 mL Inj. Vial.
Use: Antihypocalcemic.

•**calcium chloride Ca 45.** (KAL-see-um) USAN.
Use: Radiopharmaceutical.

•**calcium chloride Ca 47.** (KAL-see-um) USAN.
Use: Radiopharmaceutical.

•**calcium citrate.** (KAL-see-um) *USP.*
Use: Mineral supplement.
See: Cal-C-Caps.
Cal-Cee.
Cal-Citrate.
Citracal.
Citrus Calcium.

calcium citrate. (Various Mfr.) **Tab.:** Elemental calcium 250 mg. Bot. 100s, 120s, 250s, 500s, 1000s. Calcium citrate 950 mg. Bot. 100s. **Pow. for Susp.:** Elemental calcium 760 mg/5 mL. Pow. Bot. 454 g. *OTC.*
Use: Mineral supplement.

calcium cyclamate. Calcium cyclohexanesulfamate.

calcium cyclobarbital.
Use: Central depressant.

calcium cyclohexanesulfamate.
See: Calcium Cyclamate.

•**calcium dioctyl sulfosuccinate.** (KAL-see-uhm die-OC-tuhl sul-foe-SUCK-sih-nate) *USP.* Docusate calcium.
See: Surfak.

•**calcium disodium edathamil.** (KAL-see-uhm die-SO-dee-uhm eh-DA-tha-mill) *USP.*

•**calcium disodium edetate.** (KAL-see-uhm die-SO-dee-uhm ed-deh-TATE) *USP.* Edetate calcium disodium.
Use: Antidote for acute and chronic lead poisoning, lead encephalopathy.
See: Calcium Disodium Versenate.

calcium disodium versenate. (Graceway) Calcium disodium edetate 200 mg/mL. Inj. Amp 5 mL. *Rx.*

Use: IV or IM for lead poisoning and lead encephalopathy.

•**calcium dl-pantothenate.** (KAL-see-uhm dl pan-toe-THEH-nate) *USP.* Calcium Pantothenate, Racemic.

calcium edetate sodium.
See: Calcium Disodium Edetate.

calcium EDTA.
See: Calcium Disodium Edetate.

Calcium 500. (Rugby) Vitamin D 100 units (as cholecalciferol), calcium 500 units (as calcium carbonate). Malted milk powder, nonfat dried milk, sugar. Vanilla flavor. Chew. Tab. 60s. *OTC.*
Use: Nutritional combination product.

Calcium 500+D. (21st Century) Vitamin D 800 units (as cholecalciferol), calcium 1,000 mg (as oyster shell). Preservative free. Tab. 200s. *OTC.*
Use: Nutritional combination product.

Calcium-Folic Acid Plus D. (Brookstone) Vitamin D_3 300 units, B_6 10 mg, B_{12} 125 mcg, folate 100 mcg B, Ca, Mg. fructose. Chocolate flavor. Wafers, chewable. 60s. *Rx.*
Use: Multivitamin with minerals.

calcium 4-benzamidosalicylate. Calcium aminacyl B-PAS. Benzoylpas calcium.

•**calcium glubionate.** (KAL-see-uhm glue-BYE-oh-nate) *USP.*
Use: Calcium replenisher.
See: Calcionate.
Calciquid.

calcium glucoheptonate. (Various Mfr.) Cal. D-glucoheptonate O. *OTC.*
Use: Nutritional supplement.

•**calcium gluconate.** (KAL-see-uhm glue-KAHN-nate) *USP.*
Use: Mineral supplement.
See: Cal-G.

calcium gluconate. (Bio-Tech) Calcium gluconate 500 mg. Cap. 100s. *OTC.*
Use: Mineral supplement.

calcium gluconate. (Freeda) Calcium gluconate. **Tab.:** ≈555.6 mg (equiv. to elemental calcium 50 mg). Gluten free, sugar free. 100s, 500s. **Pow.:** 1,040 mg per 15 mL (equiv. to elemental calcium 346.7 mg/15 mL). Gluten free, sugar free. 448 g. *OTC.*
Use: Mineral supplement.

calcium gluconate. (Various Mfr.) Calcium gluconate. **Tab.:** 648 to 650 mg (equiv. to elemental calcium 58.5 to 60 mg), 972 to 975 mg (equiv. to elemental calcium 87.75 to 90 mg). 100s, 1,000s (648 to 650 mg only); UD 100s, UD 1,000s (972 to 975 mg only). **Chew. Tab.:** 650 mg. Sugar free. 30s, 60s, 90s, 100s, 120s. **Inj. Soln.:** 10% (equiv. to elemental calcium 0.465 mEq/mL [9.3 mg]). Preservative free. 10 mL and 50 mL single-dose vials and 100 mL and 200 mL pharmacy bulk vials. *Rx-OTC.*
Use: Mineral supplement.

calcium gluconate gel 2.5%. (LTR Pharmaceuticals, Inc.)
Use: Topical treatment of hydrogen fluoride burns. [Orphan Drug]
See: H-F.

calcium glycerophosphate. Neurosin.
W/Phosphorus.
See: Prelief.

•**calcium hydroxide.** (KAL-see-uhm) *USP.*
Use: Astringent; pharmaceutic necessity for calamine lotion.

calcium hydroxide. (Eli Lilly) Calcium hydroxide. Pow. Bot. 4 oz.
Use: Lime water.

calcium hydroxylapatite.
Use: Physical adjunct.
See: Radiesse.

calcium hypophosphite.
Use: Mineral supplement.

calcium iodide.
W/Codeine Phosphate.
See: Calcidrine.

calcium iodized.
See: Cal-Lime-1.

calcium iodobehenate. Calioben.

•**calcium ipodate.** (KAL-see-uhm ip-OH-date) *USP.* Ipodate calcium.
See: Oragrafin Calcium.

calcium kinate gluconate. Kinate is hexahydrotetrahydroxybenzoate. Calcium quinate.

•**calcium lactate.** (KAL-see-um LAK-tate) *USP.*
Use: Mineral supplement.
See: Cal-Lac.
W/Calcium Glycerophosphate.
See: Calphosan.
W/Niacinamide, Folic Acid, Ferrous Gluconate, Vitamins.
See: Pergrava No. 2.

calcium lactate. (Various Mfr.) Calcium lactate 648 to 650 mg (elemental calcium 84.5 mg). Tab. Bot. 100s, 1000s. Elemental calcium 100 mg. Tab. Bot. 100s, 250s. *OTC.*
Use: Mineral supplement.

•**calcium lactobionate.** (KAL-see-um) *USP.*
Use: Mineral supplement.

calcium lactophosphate. Lactic acid hydrogen phosphate calcium salt.

calcium leucovorin.
Use: For overdosage of folic acid an-

tagonists; megaloblastic anemias.
See: Leucovorin Calcium.

•**calcium levulinate.** (KAL-see-uhm LEV-you-lih-nate) *USP.*
Use: Calcium replenisher.

calcium/magnesium. (Nature's Bounty) Calcium 500 mg, magnesium 250 mg. Gluten free, lactose free, and preservative free. Tab. 100s. *OTC.*
Use: Nutritional supplement, multimineral.

calcium/magnesium. (Windmill) Ca 1,000 mg (calcium content expressed in mg elemental calcium), Mg 500 mg (magnesium content expressed in mg elemental magnesium). Preservative free and sugar free. Tab. 60s. *OTC.*
Use: Nutritional supplement, multimineral.

Calcium Magnesium Chelated. (NBTY) Ca 500 mg, Mg 250 mg. Tab. Bot. 50s, 100s. *OTC.*
Use: Mineral supplement.

Calcium Magnesium Zinc. (NBTY) Ca 333 mg, Mg 133 mg, Zn 8.3 mg. Tab. Bot. 100. *OTC.*
Use: Mineral supplement.

calcium microcrystalline hydroxyapatite. (Pure Encapsulations) Calcium microcrystalline hydroxyapatite 150 mg, 300 mg. Bovine, vitamin C. Cap. 90s, 180s. *OTC.*
Use: Mineral.

calcium novobiocin. Calcium salt of an antibacterial substance produced by *Streptomyces niveus.*
Use: Anti-infective.

Calcium 1000 + D. (21st Century) Calcium 1,000 mg, vitamin D (as cholecalciferol) 800 mg. Polydextrose, PEG. Tab. 90s. *OTC.*
Use: Nutritional supplement.

•**calcium oxytetracycline.** (KAL-see-uhm ox-EE-tet-rah-SYE-kleen) *NF.* Oxytetracycline calcium.

•**calcium pantothenate.** (KAL-see-uhm pan-toe-THEH-nate) *USP.*
Use: Pantothenic acid (B_5) deficiency; coenzyme A precursor; vitamin, enzyme cofactor.
W/Combinations.
See: Arcum-VM.
Maintenance Vitamin Formula.
Mulvidren-F.
Probec-T.
Uplex.
Vicon-C.
Vicon Forte.
W/Zinc Sulfate, Niacinamide, Magnesium Sulfate, Manganese Sulfate, Vitamin Complex.
See: Vicon Plus.

calcium pantothenate. (Various Mfr.) Calcium pantothenate 100 mg (equiv. to 92 mg pantothenic acid), 218 mg (equiv. to 200 mg pantothenic acid), 545 mg (equiv. to 500 mg pantothenic acid). Tab. Bot. 100s, 250s. *OTC.*
Use: Pantothenic acid deficiency, water-soluble vitamin.

•**calcium pantothenate, racemic.** (KAL-see-uhm pan-toe-THEH-nate, ray-SEE-mik) *USP.*
Use: Vitamin B, enzyme cofactor.

•**calcium phosphate, dibasic.** (KAL-see-um) *USP.*
Use: Calcium replenisher; pharmaceutic aid, tablet base.

calcium phosphate, monocalcium.
See: Dicalcium Phosphate.

•**calcium phosphate, tribasic.** (KAL-see-um) *NF.* Tricalcium phosphate.
Use: Mineral supplement.
See: Posture.

•**calcium polycarbophil.** (KAL-see-uhm PAHL-ee-CAR-boe-fill) *USP.*
Use: Laxative.
See: Equalactin.
Fibercon.
FiberNorm.
Konsyl Fiber.

calcium polysulfide.
Use: Wet dressing, soak.

calcium quinate.
See: Calcium Kinate Gluconate.

calcium receptor agonists.
See: Cinacalcet Hydrochloride.

•**calcium saccharate.** (KAL-see-uhm SACK-uh-rate) *USP.*
Use: Pharmaceutic aid, sweetener, stabilizer.

calcium saccharin. Saccharin calcium.
Use: Pharmaceutic aid, sweetener.

•**calcium silicate.** (KAL-see-uhm SILL-eh-cate) *NF.*
Use: Pharmaceutic aid, tablet excipient.

Calcium 600. (Various Mfr.) Calcium carbonate 1500 mg (elemental calcium 600 mg). Tab. Bot. 60s, 100s. *OTC.*
Use: Mineral supplement.

Calcium 600-D. (Rugby) Vitamin D 400 units (as cholecalciferol), calcium 600 mg (as calcium carbonate). Maltodextrin, propylene glycol, sodium 5 mg. Tab. 60s. *OTC.*
Use: Nutritional combination product.

Calcium 600 + D. (NBTY) Calcium 600 mg, vitamin D 125 units. Film-coated. Tab. Bot. 60s. *OTC.*
Use: Mineral, vitamin supplement.

Calcium 600/Vitamin D. (Schein) Ca 600 mg, D 125 units. Tab. Bot. 60s.

OTC.
Use: Mineral, vitamin supplement.

•**calcium stearate.** (KAL-see-uhm STEE-uh-rate) *NF.*
Use: Pharmaceutic aid, tablet and capsule lubricant.

calcium succinate.
W/Aspirin.
See: Ber-Ex.
Dolcin.

•**calcium sulfate.** (KAL-see-um) *NF.*
Use: Pharmaceutic aid, tablet and capsule diluent.

calcium thiosulfate.
Use: Wet dressing, soak.

calcium trisodium pentetate.
Use: Antidote, heavy metals.
See: Calcium Chel 330.

•**calcium undecylenate.** (KAL-see-uhm un-DES-eye-lie-nate) *USP.*
Use: Antifungal.
See: Caldesene.
Cruex Squeeze Powder.

calcium with vitamin D. (Rexall Sundown) Vitamin D 400 units (as cholecalciferol), calcium 1,000 mg (as oyster shell). Sodium 10 mg. Gluten free, preservative free. Tab. 250s. *OTC.*
Use: Nutritional combination product.

Caldesene. (Insight) Calcium undecylenate 10%. Pow. 60 g, 120 g. *OTC.*
Use: Antifungal agent.

Caldesene. (Insight) Cod liver oil (vitamins A and D), zinc oxide 15%, lanolin oil, petrolatum 54%, parabens, talc. Oint. 37.5 g. *OTC.*
Use: Emollient.

Caldesene. (Insight) Talc 81%, zinc oxide 15%. Pow., Top. 142 g. *OTC.*
Use: Diaper rash product, topical.

•**caldiamide sodium.** (KAL-DIE-ah-MIDE) USAN.
Use: Pharmaceutic aid.

Cal-D-Mint. (Enzyme Process) Ca 800 mg, Mg 150 mg, Fe 18 mg, iodine 0.1 mg, Cu 2 mg, vitamin D 200 units. Tab. Bot. 100s, 250s. *OTC.*
Use: Mineral, vitamin supplement.

Caldolor. (Cumberland Pharmaceuticals) Ibuprofen 100 mg/mL. Arginine 78 mg/mL. Inj., Soln. Single-dose vial. 4 mL, 8 mL. *Rx.*
Use: Nonsteroidal anti-inflammatory agent.

Cal-D-Phos. (Archer-Taylor) Dicalcium phosphate 4.5 g, calcium gluconate 3 g, vitamin D. Tab. Bot. 1000s. *OTC.*
Use: Mineral, vitamin supplement.

calfactant.
Use: Lung surfactant.
See: Infasurf.

Cal-G. (Key) Calcium gluconate 700 mg (as elemental calcium 50 mg). Cap. 100s, 250s. *OTC.*
Use: Mineral supplement.

Cal•Gest. (Rugby) Calcium carbonate 500 mg (elemental calcium 200 mg). Dextrose. Assorted flavors. Chew. Tab. 150s. *OTC.*
Use: Mineral supplement.

Calicylic. (Gordon Laboratories) Salicylic acid 10%, mineral oil, cetyl alcohol, propylene glycol, white wax, sodium lauryl sulfate, oleic acid, methyl- and propylparabens, triethanolamine. Cream. Tube. 60 g. *OTC.*
Use: Keratolytic.

Cal-Im. (Standex) Calcium glycerophosphate 1%, calcium levulinate 1.5%. Vial 30 mL. *Rx.*
Use: Mineral supplement.

Calinate-FA. (Solvay) Ca 250 mg, vitamins A 4000 units, D 400 units, B_1 3 mg, B_2 3 mg, B_6 5 mg, B_{12} 1 mcg, folic acid 1 mg, C 50 mg, B_3 (niacinamide) 20 mg, B_5 (d-panthenol) 1 mg, Fe 60 mg, I 0.02 mg, Mn 0.2 mg, Mg 0.2 mg, Zn 0.1 mg, Cu 0.15 mg. Tab. Bot. 100s. *Rx.*
Use: Mineral, vitamin supplement.

calioben.
See: Calcium Iodobehenate.

Calivite. (Apco) Calcium carbonate 885 mg, ferrous sulfate 199 mg, vitamins A 3600 units, D 400 units, C 75 mg, B_1 1.5 mg, B_2 1.95 mg, B_6 0.75 mg, nicotinic acid 15 mg, B_{12} activity 0.025 mcg, choline 1500 mcg, inositol 2500 mcg, pantothenic acid 75 mcg, folic acid 25 mcg, p-aminobenzoic acid 12 mcg, K 10 mg, Mg 1 mg, Zn 0.075 mg, Mn 0.02 mg, Cu 0.01 mg, cobalt 0.02 mcg. Tab. Bot. 100s. *OTC.*
Use: Mineral, vitamin supplement.

Cal-Lac. (Bio-Tech) Calcium lactate 500 mg (elemental calcium 96 mg). Cap. Bot. 100s. *OTC.*
Use: Mineral supplement.

Callergy Clear. (Major) Pramoxine hydrochloride 1%, zinc acetate 0.1%. Alcohol, camphor, glycerin, lavender oil, parabens, propylene glycol, rosemary oil, urea. Lot. 177 mL. *OTC.*
Use: Poison ivy treatment.

Cal-Lime-1. (Scrip) Calcium iodized 1 g. Tab. Bot. 1000s.

Calmasyn. (Links Medical Products) Menthol 0.45%, zinc oxide 20%, aloe, calamine, chamomile oil, cod liver oil, disodium EDTA, glycerin, lanolin, mineral oil, parabens, petrolatum, tocoph-

erol. Oint. 113 g. *OTC.*
Use: Skin protectant.

Calmol 4. (Mentholatum Co.) Cocoa butter 80%, zinc oxide 10%, parabens. Supp. Box 12s, 24s. *OTC.*
Use: Anorectal preparation.

Calmoseptine. Menthol 0.44%, zinc oxide 20.625%. Glycerin, lanolin. Top. Oint. 71 g, 113 g. *OTC.*
Use: Protectant.

Calmosin. (Spanner) Calcium gluconate, strontium bromide. Amp. 10 mL. 100s.

Cal-Nor. (Vortech Pharmaceuticals) Calcium glycerophosphate 100 mg, calcium levulinate 150 mg/10 mL. Inj. Vial 100 mL. *Rx.*
Use: Mineral supplement.

Calocarb. (Pal-Pak, Inc.) Calcium carbonate 648 mg, cinnamon flavor. Tab. Bot. 1000s. *OTC.*
Use: Antacid.

calomel. Mercurous chloride.
Use: Cathartic.

CaloMist. (Fleming) Cyanocobalamin 25 mcg/0.1 mL. Benzyl alcohol, benzalkonium chloride. Spray, Intranasal. 18 mL (60 sprays). *Rx.*
Use: Water-soluble vitamin.

Calotabs. (Calotabs) Docusate sodium 100 mg, casanthranol 30 mg. Tab. Box 10s. *OTC.*
Use: Laxative.

caloxidine (iodized calcium).
See: Calcium Iodized.

Calphosan. (Glenwood) Calcium glycerophosphate 50 mg, calcium lactate 50 mg/10 mL sodium chloride solution. Contains calcium 0.08 mEq/mL. Inj. Amp. 10 mL, Vial 60 mL. *Rx.*
Use: Mineral supplement.

Calphron. (Nephro-Tech) Calcium acetate 667 mg (elemental calcium 169 mg). Tab. 200s. *Rx.*
Use: Mineral supplement.

Calsan. (Burgin-Arden) Calcium glycerophosphate 10 mg, calcium levulinate 15 mg, chlorobutanol 0.5% mL. Inj. Vial 100 mL. *Rx.*
Use: Calcium supplement.

Cal Sup Instant 1000. (3M) Elemental calcium 1000 mg, vitamins D 400 units, C 60 mg. Pow. Packet 12s. *OTC.*
Use: Mineral, vitamin supplement.

Cal Sup 600 Plus. (3M) Elemental calcium 600 mg, vitamins D 200 units, C 30 mg. Tab. Bot. 60s. *OTC.*
Use: Mineral, vitamin supplement.

•**calteridol calcium.** (KAL-TER-ih-dahl KAL-see-uhm) USAN.
Use: Pharmaceutic aid.

Caltrate Plus. (Wyeth) Vitamin D 200 units, Ca 600 mg, Zn 7.5 mg, Mg, Cu, Mn, B. Sugar free. Tab. Bot. 60s. *OTC.*
Use: Mineral, vitamin supplement.

Caltrate 600 + D. (Wyeth) Vitamin D 200 units, Ca 600 mg. Sugar free. Tab. Bot. 60s. *OTC.*
Use: Mineral, vitamin supplement.

Caltrate 600 + Iron. (Wyeth) Calcium carbonate 600 mg, iron 18 mg, vitamin D 125 units. Tab. Bot. 60s. *OTC.*
Use: Mineral, vitamin supplement.

Caltro. (Geneva) Elemental calcium 250 mg, vitamin D 125 units. Tab. Bot. 100s, 1000s. *OTC.*
Use: Mineral, vitamin supplement.

•**calusterone.** (kal-YOO-ster-ohn) USAN.
Use: Antineoplastic.

Cam-Ap-Es. (Camall) Hydrochlorothiazide 15 mg, reserpine 0.1 mg, hydralazine hydrochloride 25 mg. Tab. Bot. 100s. *Rx.*
Use: Antihypertensive.

•**cambendazole.** (kam-BEND-ah-zole) USAN.
Use: Anthelmintic.

Cambia. (Depomed) Diclofenac 50 mg. Aspartame, mannitol, saccharin. Pow. for Soln. Boxes of 9 individual packets. *Rx.*
Use: CNS agent, nonsteroidal anti-inflammatory agent.

Camellia. (O'Leary) Moisturizer for face, hands and body. For normal to oily skin. Lot. Bot. 4 oz. *OTC.*
Use: Emollient.

Cameo. (Medco Lab) Mineral oil, isopropyl myristate, lanolin oil, PEG-8-Dioleate. Oil. Plastic Bot. 8 oz, 16 oz, 32 oz. *OTC.*
Use: Emollient.

•**camicinal.** (kam-I-si-nal) USAN.
Use: Gastrointestinal agent.

•**camiglibose.** (kah-mih-GLIE-bose) USAN.
Use: Antidiabetic, glucohydrolase inhibitor.

Camila. (Barr) Norethindrone 0.35 mg. Lactose. Tab. 28s. *Rx.*
Use: Sex hormone, contraceptive hormone.

•**camobucol.** (kam-oh-BUE-kol) USAN.
Use: Anti-inflammatory.

Camouflage Crayon. (O'Leary) Coverup for minor skin discolorations, under eye concealer, lipstick fixer. Available in 6 shades. Crayon 0.05 oz. *OTC.*
Use: Skin coverup.

Campho-Phenique. (Bayer) Camphor 10.8%, phenol 4.7%. **Liq.:** Bot. 22.5 mL, 45 mL, 120 mL. **Gel:** Tube. 6.9 g, 15 g.

OTC.
Use: Analgesic; antiseptic, local.

Campho-Phenique Cold Sore Treatment and Scab Relief. (Bayer Consumer) Pramoxine hydrochloride 1%. Petrolatum 30%, alcohols, EDTA, glycerin, parabens, ureas. Mint flavor. Cream. 6.5 g. *OTC.*
Use: Local anesthetics, topical.

•**camphor.** (KAM-fore) *USP.*
Use: Topical antipruritic; anti-infective; pharmaceutic necessity for camphorated phenol; paregoric and flexible collodion; antitussive; expectorant, local counterirritant; nasal decongestant.
See: Benadryl Anti-Itch Gel for Kids.
W/Allantoin, Menthol.
See: Nose Better.
W/Benzocaine, Menthol.
See: Chiggerex.
W/Menthol.
See: Mentholatum.
TheraPatch Vapor Patch for Kids Cough Suppressant.
Tiger Balm.
Tom's of Maine Natural Cough & Cold Rub Cough Suppressant.
W/Menthol, Eucalyptus Oil.
See: Vicks VapoRub.
W/Menthol, Methyl Salicylate.
See: Bayer Muscle and Joint.

camphorated, parachlorophenol.
Use: Anti-infective, dental.

camphoric acid ester. Ester of p-Tolylmethylcarbinal as Diethanolamine Salt.

Campral. (Forest) Acamprosate calcium 333 mg. DR Tab. 180s, 1,080s, Dose pak 180s. *Rx.*
Use: Antialcoholic agent.

Camptosar. (Pfizer) Irinotecan hydrochloride 20 mg/mL, sorbitol 45 mg. Inj. Vial. 2 mL, 5 mL. *Rx.*
Use: Antineoplastic, DNA topoisomerase inhibitor.

Camrese. (Teva) **Phase 1:** Ethinyl estradiol 30 mcg, levonorgestrel 0.15 mg. Film coated. Lactose. Tab. 84s. **Phase 2:** Ethinyl estradiol 10 mcg. Film coated. Lactose, PEG. Tab. 7s. *Rx.*
Use: Biphasic oral contraceptive.

Camrese Lo. (Teva) **Phase 1:** Ethinyl estradiol 20 mcg, levonorgestrel 0.1 mg. Film coated. Lactose. Tab. 84s. **Phase 2:** Ethinyl estradiol 10 mcg. Film coated. Lactose, PEG. Tab. 7s. *Rx.*
Use: Biphasic oral contraceptive.

•**canagliflozin.** (KAN-a-gli-FLOE-zin) USAN.
Use: Antidiabetic.
See: Invokana.

•**canakinumab.** (KAN-a-KIN-ue-mab) USAN.
Use: Immunomodulator.
See: Ilaris.

Canasa. (Aptalis Pharma) Mesalamine 1000 mg (in base of hard fat). Supp. 30s. *Rx.*
Use: Anti-inflammatory.

Cancidas. (Merck) Caspofungin acetate 50 mg, 70 mg. Pow. for Inj., lyophilized. Single-use Vial. *Rx.*
Use: Antifungal, echinocandins.

C & E Capsules. (NBTY) Vitamins C 500 mg, E 400 mg. Cap. Bot. 50s, 100s. *OTC.*
Use: Vitamin supplement.

•**candesartan.** (kan-deh-SAHR-tan) USAN.
Use: Antagonist, angiotensin II receptor; antihypertensive.

•**candesartan cilexetil.** (kan-deh-SAHR-tan sigh-LEX-eh-till) USAN.
Use: Antagonist, angiotensin II receptor; antihypertensive.
See: Atacand.
W/Hydrochlorothiazide.
See: Atacand HCT.

candesartan cilexetil/hydrochlorothiazide. (Mylan Pharmaceuticals) Candesartan cilexetil/hydrochlorothiazide 16 mg/12.5 mg, 32 mg/12.5 mg, 32 mg/25 mg. Lactose. Tab. 90s, 500s. *Rx.*
Use: Antihypertensive combination.

C & E Softgels. (NBTY) Vitamins E 400 mg, C 500 mg. Cap. Bot. 50s.
Use: Vitamin supplement.

•**candicidin.** (KAN-dih-SIDE-in) *USP.* An antifungal antibiotic derived from *Strepomyces griseus.*
Use: Antifungal.

candida albicans skin test antigen.
Use: Diagnostic aid.
See: Candin.

candida test. (SmithKline Diagnostics) Culture test for *Candida.* Box 4s.
Use: Diagnostic aid.

Candin. (ALK) *Candida albicans* skin test antigen prepared from the culture filtrate and cells of 2 strains of *Candida albicans.* Vial 1 mL. *Rx.*
Use: Evaluation of cell-mediated immunity; diagnostic aid.

•**candoxatril.** (kan-DOXE-at-trill) USAN.
Use: Antihypertensive.

•**candoxatrilat.** (kan-DOXE-at-trill-at) USAN.
Use: Antihypertensive.

Candycon. (Allison) Chlorprophenpyridamine maleate 2 mg, phenylephrine

hydrochloride 5 mg. Tab. Bot. 50s. *OTC.*
Use: Antihistamine; decongestant.

•**canertinib dihydrochloride.** (can-ER-tin-ib) USAN.
Use: Epithelial tumors.

•**canfosfamide hydrochloride.** (kan-FOS-fa-mide) USAN.
Use: Antineoplastic.

•**cangrelor.** (KAN-grel-or) USAN.
Use: Antiplatelet.

•**cangrelor tetrasodium.** (KAN-grel-or) USAN.
Use: Antiplatelet.

Cankaid Liquid. (Dickinson) Carbamide peroxide 10% in anhydrous glycerol, EDTA. Soln. 22.5 mL. *OTC.*
Use: Mouth and throat product.

cannabinoids.
Use: Antiemetic; antivertigo agent.
See: Dronabinol.

cannabis.
Use: Antiemetic; antivertigo.
See: Dronabinol.

•**canrenoate potassium.** (kan-REN-oh-ate) USAN.
Use: Aldosterone antagonist.

•**canrenone.** (kan-REN-ohn) USAN.
Use: Aldosterone antagonist.

cantharidin.
Use: Keratolytic.

Cantil. (Hoechst Marion Roussel) Mepenzolate bromide 25 mg. Tab. Bot. 100s. *Rx.*
Use: Anticholinergic; antispasmodic.

•**cantuzumab mertansine.** (can-TUE-zue-mab mer-TAN-seen) USAN.
Use: Colorectal and pancreatic cancer.

•**cantuzumab ravtansine.** (kan-TOOZ-ue-mab rav-TAN-seen) USAN.
Use: Antineoplastic.

Ca-Orotate. (Miller Pharmacal Group) Calcium (as calcium orotate) 50 mg. Tab. Bot. 100s. *OTC.*
Use: Mineral supplement.

C-A-P. (Eastman Kodak) Cellulose acetate phthalate.

Capacet. (Magna Pharmaceuticals) Acetaminophen 325 mg, butalbital 50 mg, caffeine 40 mg. Cap. 100s. *Rx.*
Use: Nonnarcotic analgesic combination, nonnarcotic analgesic with barbiturate.

Capastat Sulfate. (Akorn) Capreomycin 1 g/10 mL. Vial 10 mL. *Rx.*
Use: Antituberculosis agent.

•**capecitabine.** (cap-eh-SITE-ah-bean) USAN.
Use: Antineoplastic, antimetabolite.
See: Xeloda.

capecitabine. (Various Mfr.) Capecitabine 150 mg, 500 mg. May contain lactose. Tab. 60s (150 mg only), 120s (500 mg only). *Rx.*
Use: Antineoplastic, antimetabolite, pyrimidine analog.

Capex. (Galderma) Fluocinolone acetonide 0.01%, dibasic calcium phosphate dihydrate 5.48 mg. Shampoo. In 12 mg capsule with shampoo base to be mixed by pharmacist before dispensing. *Formerly Fs Shampoo (Hill) Rx.*
Use: Anti-inflammatory; corticosteroid, topical.

Caphosol. (EUSA Pharma) Dibasic sodium phosphate 3.2 g, monobasic sodium phosphate 0.9 g, calcium chloride 5.2 g, sodium chloride 56.9 g. Vanilla flavor. Soln. Dose box. 30s, 120s (1 dose = two 15 mL amps mixed together). *Rx.*
Use: Mouth and throat product, saliva substitute.

•**capimorelin tartrate.** (CAP-eh-mohr-lyn) USAN.
Use: Prevention of frailty; congestive heart failure; catabolic illness.

Capital Soleil 20. (Vichy) Avobenzone 2%, ecamsule 2%, octocrylene 10%, titanium dioxide 2%. SFP 20. Cream. 100 g. *OTC.*
Use: Sunscreen.

Capital with Codeine. (Carnrick) **Susp.:** Acetaminophen 120 mg, codeine phosphate 12 mg/5 mL. Bot. 473 mL. *c-v.* **Tab.:** Codeine phosphate 30 mg, acetaminophen 325 mg. Bot. 100s. *c-III.*
Use: Analgesic combination, narcotic.

•**caplacizumab.** (KAP-la-SIZ-ue-mab) USAN.
Use: Treatment of thrombotic thrombocytopenic purpura, thrombosis.

Capmist DM. (Capital) Dextromethorphan hydrobromide 30 mg, guaifenesin 400 mg, pseudoephedrine hydrochloride 30 mg. Maltodextrin. Tab. 30s. *OTC.*
Use: Upper respiratory combination, antitussive and expectorant combination.

Capnitro. (Freeport) Nitroglycerin 6.5 mg. TR Cap. Bot. 100s. *Rx.*
Use: Antianginal agent.

•**capobenate sodium.** (CAP-oh-BEN-ate) USAN.
Use: Cardiovascular agent, antiarrhythmic.

•**capobenic acid.** (CAP-oh-BEN-ik) USAN.
Use: Cardiovascular agent, antiarrhythmic.

•**capravirine.** (cap-ruh-VYE-reen) USAN.
Use: Antiviral.

Caprelsa. (AstraZeneca) Vandetanib 100 mg, 300 mg. Film coated. Tab. 30s. *Rx.*
Use: Tyrosine kinase inhibitor.

•**capreomycin.** (CAP-ree-oh-MY-sin) *USP.* An antibiotic derived from *Streptomyces capreolus.* Caprocin.
Use: Antituberculosis agent.
See: Capastat Sulfate.

•**capromab pendetide.** (KAP-row-mab PEN-deh-TIDE) USAN.
Use: Monoclonal antibody; in vivo diagnostic aid.
See: ProstaScint.

•**capromorelin tartrate.** (kap-roe-moor-lyn) USAN.
Use: Prevention of frailty; congestive heart failure; carabolic illness.

Capron DM. (Capital Pharmaceutical) Dextromethorphan hydrobromide 7.5 mg, pyrilamine maleate 7.5 mg. *Magnasweet*, parabens, potassium sorbate, propylene glycol, sorbitol, sucralose. Candy apple flavor. Liq. 473 mL. *OTC.*
Use: Upper respiratory combination, antitussive combination.

caprylate, salts.
See: Caprylate Sodium.

caprylate sodium. (Ingram) Caprylate sodium 33%. Inj. Amp. 1 mL. Pkg. 12s, 25s, 100s.
Use: Antifungal.

caprylidene.
Use: Nutritional supplement.
See: Axona.

•**capsaicin.** (kap-SAY-uh-sin) *USP.*
Use: Analgesic, topical; antineuralgic; specific pain syndromes, topical.
See: Axsain.
Capsin.
Capzasin-P.
Icy Hot PM.
No Pain-HP.
Pain Doctor.
Qutenza.
Rid-a-Pain-HP.
Zostrix.
Zostrix Diabetic Foot Pain.
Zostrix Diabetic Joint & Arthritis Pain Relief.
Zostrix Maximum Strength.
W/Lidocaine, Menthol, Methyl Salicylate.
See: Terocin.
W/Menthol.
See: Capzasin Quick Relief.
Zostrix Hot and Cold Therapy.
W/Menthol, Methyl Salicylate.
See: Bio-Therm Pain Relieving Lotion.
Medi-Derm.
Medrox.
New Terocin.
Ultracin.
Xoten-C Pain Relief.
Ziks.

capsaicin. (Various Mfr.) Capsaicin 0.025%, 0.075%. Cream. Tube. 45 g (0.025% only), 60 g. *OTC.*
Use: Analgesic, topical; antineuralgic; specific pain syndromes, topical.

•**capsicum.** (KAP-see-kum) *USP.*
Use: Carminative; counterirritant, external; stomachic.

•**capsicum oleoresin.** (KAP-see-kum OH-lee-oh-RES-in) *USP.*
Use: Carminative; counterirritant, external; stomachic.

Capsin. (Fleming & Co.) Capsaicin 0.025%, 0.075%, benzyl alcohol, propylene glycol, denatured alcohol. Lot. Bot. 59 mL. *OTC.*
Use: Analgesic, topical.

capsules, empty gelatin. (Eli Lilly) Lilly markets clear empty gelatin capsules in sizes 000, 00, 0, 1, 2, 3, 4, 5.

•**captamine hydrochloride.** (KAP-tam-een) USAN.
Use: Depigmentor.

•**captopril.** (KAP-toe-prill) *USP.*
Use: Angiotensin-converting enzyme inhibitor, renin angiotensin system antagonist.

captopril. (Various Mfr.) Captopril 12.5 mg, 25 mg, 50 mg, 100 mg. Tab. Bot. 100s, 500s, 1000s, 5000s (except 100 mg), UD 100s, blister 600s. *Rx.*
Use: Angiotensin-converting enzyme inhibitor, renin angiotensin system antagonist.

captopril and hydrochlorothiazide. (Teva) Hydrochlorothiazide/captopril 15 mg/25 mg, 15 mg/50 mg, 25 mg/25 mg, 25 mg/50 mg. Tab. Bot. 100s, 1000s. *Rx.*
Use: Antihypertensive; diuretic.

•**capuride.** (CAP-you-ride) USAN.
Use: Hypnotic; sedative.

Capzasin. (Chattem) Capsaicin 0.025%, menthol 10%. Aloe barbadensis leaf juice, glycerin, parabens, SD alcohol 15%. Gel. 42.5 g. *OTC.*
Use: Counterirritant.

Capzasin•HP. (Chattem) Capsaicin 0.1%. Alcohols, petrolatum. Cream. 42.5 g. *OTC.*
Use: Counterirritant.

Capzasin•P. (Chattem) Capsaicin 0.035%. Alcohols, petrolatum. Cream. Tube 42.5 g. *OTC.*
Use: Analgesic, topical.

Carac. (Valeant) Fluorouracil 0.5%. Glycerin, parabens. Cream. Tubes. 30 g. *Rx.*
Use: Pyrimidine antagonist, topical.

•**caracemide.** (car-ASS-eh-MIDE) USAN.
Use: Antineoplastic.

Carafate. (Axcan Scandipharm) **Tab.:** Sucralfate 1 g. Bot. 100s, 120s, 500s. **Susp.:** Sucralfate 1 g/10 mL, sorbitol, methylparaben. Bot. 415 mL. *Rx.*
Use: Antiulcerative.

•**caramel.** (KAR-uh-mel) *NF.*
Use: Pharmaceutic aid, color.

caramiphen hydrochloride.
Use: Proposed antiparkinson.

•**caraway.** (KAR-uh-way) *NF.*
Use: Flavoring.

•**caraway oil.** (KAR-uh-way) *NF.*
Use: Flavoring.

•**carbachol.** (KAR-bah-kole) *USP.*
Use: Parasympathomimetic; cholinergic, ophthalmic.
See: Miostat Intraocular.
W/Methylcellulose.
See: Isopto Carbachol.

carbacrylamine resins.
Use: Cation-exchange resin.

•**carbadox.** (KAR-bah-dox) USAN.
Use: Anti-infective.

Carbaglu. (Accredo Health Group Inc) Carglumic acid 200 mg. Tab., dispersible. 5s, 60s. *Rx.*
Use: Endocrine and metabolic agent.

•**carbamazepine.** (KAR-bam-AZE-uh-peen) *USP.*
Tall Man: carBAMazepine
Use: Analgesic; anticonvulsant.
See: Carbatrol.
Epitol.
Equetro.
Tegretol.
Tegretol-XR.

carbamazepine. (Nostrum Labs) Carbamazepine 300 mg. PEG. ER Cap. 120s. *Rx.*
Use: Anticonvulsant.

carbamazepine. (Taro) Carbamazepine. **Chew. Tab.:** 200 mg. Sorbitol. Cherry flavor. 100s, 400s. **ER Tab.:** 100 mg, 200 mg, 400 mg. Lactose. 30s, 100s, 1,000s. *Rx.*
Use: Anticonvulsant.

carbamazepine. (Various Mfr.) Carbamazepine. **Chew. Tab.:** 100 mg. May contain lactose, sorbitol, sucrose. 100s, 500s, UD 100s. **Tab.:** 200 mg. May contain lactose. 100s, 500s, 1,000s, UD 25s, UD 100s, UD 750s. **ER Tab.:** 100 mg, 200 mg, 400 mg. May contain lactose. 30s (100 mg only), 100s, UD 30s (except 100 mg). **ER Cap.:** 100 mg, 200 mg, 300 mg. May contain lactose, PEG. 120s. **Susp.:** 100 mg/5 mL. May contain sorbitol, sucrose. 450 mL, UD 10 mL. *Rx.*
Use: Anticonvulsant.

carbamide.
Use: Emollient.
See: Urea.

carbamide compounds.
See: Acetylcarbromal.
Carbromal.

•**carbamide peroxide.** (CAR-bah-mide purr-ox-ide) *USP.* Urea compound w/hydrogen peroxide (1:1).
Use: Anti-inflammatory; mouth and throat product.
See: Cankaid Liquid.
Gly-Oxide.
Orajel Perioseptic.

carbamide peroxide 6.5% in glycerin.
Use: Otic.
See: Murine Ear Drops.
Murine Ear Wax Removal System.

carbamylcholine chloride.
See: Carbachol.

carbamylmethylcholine chloride.
See: Urecholine.

•**carbantel lauryl sulfate.** (CAR-ban-tell LAH-ruhl) USAN.
Use: Anthelmintic.

carbapenems.
Use: Anti-infective.
See: Doripenem.
Ertapenem.
Imipenem-Cilastatin.
Meropenem.

carbarsone. (Various Mfr.) N-carbamoylarsanilic acid. Amabevan, ameban, amibiarson, arsambide, fenarsone, leucarsone, aminarsone, amebarsone. p-Ureidobenzenearsonic acid. Caps.
Use: Acute and chronic amebiasis and trichomoniasis.

•**carbaspirin calcium.** (kar-ba-SPEER-in) USAN.
Use: Analgesic.

Carbatab-12. (GM) Carbetapentane citrate 60 mg, guaifenesin 600 mg, phenylephrine hydrochloride 15 mg. ER Tab. 100s. *Rx.*
Use: Antitussive and expectorant combination, upper respiratory combination.

Carbatrol. (Shire) Carbamazepine 100 mg, 200 mg, 300 mg. Lactose. ER Cap. 120s. *Rx.*
Use: Anticonvulsant.

Carbatuss. (GM Pharmaceuticals) Carbetapentane citrate 20 mg, guaifenesin 100 mg, phenylephrine hydrochlo-

ride 10 mg per 5 mL. Alcohol free. Spearmint flavor. Liq. 15 and 473 mL. *Rx.*
Use: Upper respiratory combination; antitussive, expectorant, decongestant.

Carbatuss CL. (GM Pharmaceuticals) Carbetapentane citrate 20 mg, potassium guaiacolsulfonate 100 mg, phenylephrine hydrochloride 10 mg per 5 mL. Sugar free. Saccharin, sorbitol, menthol. Liq. 15 mL, 473 mL. *Rx.*
Use: Antitussive and expectorant combination.

Carbaxefed RF. (Morton Grove) Pseudoephedrine hydrochloride 15 mg, carbinoxamine maleate 1 mg per 1 mL. Sugar and alcohol free. Saccharin, sorbitol. Cherry flavor. Oral Drops. 30 mL bottle with dropper. *Rx.*
Use: Pediatric decongestant and antihistamine.

•**carbazeran.** (KAR-BAY-zeh-ran) USAN.
Use: Cardiovascular agent.

•**carbenicillin disodium, sterile.** (KAR-ben-ih-SILL-in die-SO-dee-uhm, STEER-ill) *USP.*
Use: Anti-infective.
See: Geopen.

•**carbenicillin indanyl sodium.** (car-BEN-ih-SILL-in IN-duh-nil) *USP.*
Use: Extended-spectrum penicillin.

•**carbenicillin phenyl sodium.** (CAR-ben-ih-SILL-in FEN-ill) USAN.
Use: Anti-infective.

•**carbenicillin potassium.** (CAR-ben-ih-SILL-in) USAN.
Use: Anti-infective.

•**carbenoxolone sodium.** (CAR-ben-ox-ah-lone) USAN.
Use: Corticosteroid, topical.

carbetapentane citrate.
Use: Antitussive.
W/Brompheniramine Maleate, Phenylephrine Hydrochloride.
See: V-Cof.
W/Brompheniramine Tannate, Carbetapentane Tannate, Phenylephrine Tannate.
See: Vazotan.
W/Dexchlorpheniramine Maleate, Phenylephrine Hydrochloride.
See: Corzall-PE.
W/Guaifenesin.
See: XPect-AT.
W/Guaifenesin, Phenylephrine Hydrochloride.
See: Albatussin.
Carbatab-12.
Extendryl GCP.
Gentex 30.
Levall.
Phencarb GG.
Zinx GCP.
W/Guaifenesin, Pseudoephedrine Hydrochloride.
See: Exall-D.

carbetapentane tannate.
Use: Nonnarcotic antitussive.
W/Brompheniramine Tannate, Phenylephrine Tannate.
See: Vazotan Tannate.
W/Chlorpheniramine Tannate.
See: Tannic-12 S.
Tussi-12.
W/Chlorpheniramine Tannate, Phenylephrine Tannate.
See: D-Tann CT.
Dytan CS.
W/Guaifenesin, Phenylephrine Hydrochloride.
See: Carbatuss.
W/Phenylephrine Tannate, Pyrilamine Tannate.
See: Tussi-12D S.

Carbetaplex. (Breckenridge Pharmaceutical) Carbetapentane citrate 20 mg, guaifenesin 100 mg, phenylephrine hydrochloride 15 mg per 5 mL. Sugar, alcohol, and dye free. Saccharin. Strawberry flavor. Liq. 480 mL. *Rx.*
Use: Antitussive and expectorant combination.

•**carbetimer.** (kar-BEH-tih-MER) USAN.
Use: Antineoplastic.

•**carbidopa.** (KAR-bih-doe-puh) *USP.*
Use: Decarboxylase inhibitor.
See: Lodosyn.
W/Levodopa.
See: Carbidopa and Levodopa.
Parcopa.
Sinemet CR.
Sinemet-10/100.
Sinemet-25/100.
Sinemet-25/250.
W/Levodopa and Entacapone.
See: Stalevo 50.
Stalevo 100.
Stalevo 150.
Stalevo 125.
Stalevo 75.
Stalevo 200.

carbidopa and levodopa. (Various Mfr.) **ER Tab.:** Carbidopa 25 mg, levodopa 100 mg. 100s, 500s. **Tab.:** Carbidopa 10 mg, levodopa 100 mg; carbidopa 25 mg, levodopa 100 mg; carbidopa 25 mg, levodopa 250 mg; carbidopa 50 mg, levodopa 200 mg. Bot. 100s, 500s, 1000s. **Orally disintegrating Tab.:** Carbidopa 10 mg, levodopa 100 mg; carbidopa 25 mg, levodopa

100 mg; carbidopa 25 mg, levodopa 250 mg. May contain aspartame, mannitol, phenylalanine, sorbitol. 100s, 500s. *Rx.*
Use: Antiparkinson agent.

carbidopa/levodopa/entacapone. (Caraco Pharmaceutical Laboratories) Carbidopa/levodopa/entacapone 12.5 mg/50 mg/200 mg, 18.75 mg/75 mg/200 mg, 25 mg/100 mg/200 mg, 31.25 mg/125 mg/200 mg, 37.5 mg/150 mg/200 mg, 50 mg/200 mg/200 mg. Film coated. Mannitol, sucrose. Tab. 100s. *Rx.*
Use: Antiparkinson agent.

•**carbinoxamine maleate.** (KAR-bin-OX-a-meen) *USP.*
Use: Antihistamine.
See: Arbinoxa.
Histex CT.
Histex I/E.
Histex Pd.
Karbinal ER.
Palgic.
Pediatex.
Pediatex 12.

carbinoxamine maleate. (Boca) Carbinoxamine maleate. **Tab.:** 4 mg. Lactose 100s. **Soln.:** 4 mg per 5 mL. Parabens, sorbitol. Bubble gum flavor. 118 mL, 473 mL. *Rx.*
Use: Antihistamine.

carbinoxamine maleate and carbinoxamine tannate. (Brighton) Carbinoxamine maleate 2 mg, carbinoxamine tannate 6 mg/5 mL. Alcohol, dye, and sugar free. Saccharin, sorbitol, parabens. Bubble-gum flavor. Oral Susp. 118 mL, 473 mL. *Rx.*
Use: Antihistamine.

carbinoxamine maleate, pseudoephedrine hydrochloride, dextromethorphan HBr. (Cypress) **Syrup:** Carbinoxamine maleate 4 mg, pseudoephedrine hydrochloride 60 mg, dextromethorphan HBr 15 mg/5 mL. Bot. 120 mL, pt, gal. **Drops:** Carbinoxamine maleate 2 mg, pseudoephedrine hydrochloride 25 mg, dextromethorphan HBr 4 mg/mL. Bot. 30 mL w/dropper. *Rx.*
Use: Antihistamine; decongestant; antitussive.

carbinoxamine oral drops. (Morton Grove) Carbinoxamine maleate 2 mg, pseudoephedrine hydrochloride 25 mg/mL, sorbitol, parabens, alcohol free, raspberry, fruit flavors. Bot. 30 mL w/calibrated dropper. *Rx.*
Use: Upper respiratory combination, antihistamine, decongestant.

carbinoxamine syrup. (Morton Grove) Carbinoxamine maleate 4 mg, pseudoephedrine hydrochloride 60 mg/5 mL, sorbitol, parabens, alcohol free, raspberry, fruit flavors. Bot. 118 mL, 237 mL, 473 mL. *Rx.*
Use: Upper respiratory combination, antihistamine, decongestant.

carbinoxamine tannate.
Use: Antihistamine.
W/Combinations.
See: Pediatex 12 D.
W/Dextromethorphan Tannate, Pseudoephedrine Tannate.
See: Carb PSE 12 DM.

•**carbiphene hydrochloride.** (KAR-bih-FEEN) USAN.
Use: Analgesic.

Carbiset. (Nutripharm Laboratories, Inc.) Pseudoephedrine 60 mg, carbinoxamine maleate 4 mg. Tab. Bot. 100s, 500s. *Rx.*
Use: Antihistamine; decongestant.

Carbiset-TR. (Nutripharm Laboratories, Inc.) Pseudoephedrine hydrochloride 120 mg, carbinoxamine maleate 8 mg. Tab. Bot. 100s. *Rx.*
Use: Antihistamine; decongestant.

Carbocaine. (Hospira) Mepivacaine hydrochloride. **1%:** Methylparaben. Inj. Multidose vial 50 mL. **1.5%:** Inj. Single-dose vial 30 mL. **2%:** Inj. Single-dose vial 20 mL. Multidose vial 50 mL, methylparaben. **3%:** Acetone sodium bisulfite. Inj. Dental Cartridge 1.8 mL. *Rx.*
Use: Anesthetic, local amide, injectable.

Carbocaine with Neo-Cobefrin. (Eastman-Kodak) Mepivacaine hydrochloride 2% with levonordefrin 1:20,000, acetone sodium bisulfite. Inj. Dental cartridge 1.8 mL. *Rx.*
Use: Anesthetic, local amide, injectable.

•**carbocloral.** (KAR-boe-KLOR-uhl) USAN.
Use: Hypnotic; sedative.
See: Chloralurethane.

•**carbocysteine.** (kar-boe-SIS-teen) USAN.
Use: Mucolytic.

Carbodec DM. (Rugby) **Syr.:** Pseudoephedrine hydrochloride 60 mg, carbinoxamine maleate 4 mg, dextromethorphan HBr 15 mg, alcohol < 0.6%/5 mL. Bot. 30 mL, 120 mL, pt, gal. **Drops:** (Pediatric Pharmaceuticals) Pseudoephedrine hydrochloride 25 mg, carbinoxamine maleate 2 mg, dextromethorphan HBr 4 mg, alcohol 0.6%/mL. Bot. 30 mL. *Rx.*
Use: Antihistamine, antitussive, decongestant.

Carbodec Syrup. (Rugby) Pseudoephedrine hydrochloride 60 mg, carbinoxamine maleate 4 mg/5 mL. Syr. Bot. 473 mL. *Rx.*
Use: Antihistamine, decongestant.

Carbodec Tablets. (Rugby) Pseudoephedrine hydrochloride 60 mg, carbinoxamine maleate 4 mg. Tab. Bot. 100s. *Rx.*
Use: Antihistamine, decongestant.

Carbodec TR. (Rugby) Pseudoephedrine hydrochloride 120 mg, carbinoxamine maleate 8 mg. Tab. Bot. 100s. *Rx.*
Use: Antihistamine, decongestant.

Carbodex DM. (Tri-Med) **Drops:** Carbinoxamine maleate 2 mg, pseudoephedrine hydrochloride 15 mg, dextromethorphan HBr 4 mg per 1 mL. Bot. 30 mL. **Syrup:** Dextromethorphan HBr 15 mg, brompheniramine maleate 4 mg, pseudoephedrine hydrochloride 45 mg per 5 mL. Menthol, sorbitol. Bot. 473 mL. *Rx.*
Use: Upper respiratory combination, antihistamine, antitussive, decongestant.

Carbofed DM. (Hi-Tech) **Drops:** Pseudoephedrine hydrochloride 15 mg, carbinoxamine maleate 1 mg, dextromethorphan HBr 4 mg per 1 mL. Alcohol and sugar free. Bot. 30 mL w/dropper. *Rx.*
Use: Upper respiratory combination, antitussive combination.

Carb-O-Lac HP. (Geritrex) Ammonium lactate 10%, urea 20%, lactic acid, petrolatum, propylene glycol, stearyl alcohol. Cream. 277 g. *OTC.*
Use: Emollient.

carbol-fuchsin paint. Original fuchsin formula known as Castellani's Paint. Basic Fuchsin 0.3%, phenol 4.5%, resorcinol 10%, acetone 5%, alcohol 10%. Paint. Bot. 30 mL, 120 mL, 480 mL.
Use: Antifungal, topical.
See: Castellani's Paint.

•**carbol-fuchsin, topical solution.** (KAR-buhl-FOOK-sin) *USP.*
Use: Antifungal.

•**carbomer.** (KAR-boe-mer) *NF.* A polymer of acrylic acid, crosslinked with a polyfunctional agent.
Use: Pharmaceutic aid, emulsifying, suspending agent.

•**carbomer copolymer.** (KAR-boe-mer) *NF.*
Use: Pharmaceutic aid.

•**carbomer interpolymer.** (KAR-boe-mer) *NF.*
Use: Pharmaceutic aid; emulsifying, suspending agent.

•**carbomer 940.** (KAR-boe-mer 940) *NF.*
Use: Pharmaceutic aid, emulsifying, suspending agent.

•**carbomer 941.** (KAR-boe-mer 941) *NF.*
Use: Pharmaceutic aid, emulsifying, suspending agent.

•**carbomer 910.** (KAR-boe-mer 910) *NF.*
Use: Pharmaceutic aid, emulsifying, suspending agent.

•**carbomer 934.** (KAR-boe-mer 934) *NF.*
Use: Pharmaceutic aid, emulsifying, suspending agent.

•**carbomer 934p.** (KAR-boe-mer 934) *NF.*
Formerly carpolene.
Use: Pharmaceutic aid, emulsifying, suspending, viscosity, thickening agent.

•**carbomer 1342.** (KAR-boe-mer 1342) *NF.*
Use: Pharmaceutic aid, emulsifying, suspending agent.

carbomycin. An antibiotic from *Streptomyces halstedii.*
Use: Anti-infective.

•**carbon dioxide.** (KAR-bahn dye-OX-ide) *USP.*
Use: Inhalation, respiratory.

•**carbonic acid, dilithium salt.** (KAR-bahn-ik acid, dye-LITH-ee-uhm) *USP.* Lithium Carbonate.

•**carbonic acid, disodium salt.** (KAR-bahn-ik) *USP.* Sodium Carbonate.

•**carbonic acid, monosodium salt.** (KAR-bahn-ik) *USP.* Sodium Bicarbonate.

carbonic anhydrase inhibitors.
See: Acetazolamide.
Brinzolamide.
Dorzolamide Hydrochloride.
Methazolamide.

Carbonis Detergens, Liquor.
See: Coal Tar Topical Solution.

•**carbon monoxide C 11.** (KAR-bahn moe-NOX-ide C11) *USP.*
Use: Diagnostic aid, blood volume determination; radiopharmaceutical.

•**carbon tetrachloride.** (KAR-bahn teh-truh-KLOR-ide) *NF.* Benzinoform.
Use: Pharmaceutic aid, solvent.

carbonyl diamide.
See: Chap Cream.

carbonyl iron.
Use: Trace element.
See: Feosol.
Ferralet 90.
Icar.
Ircon.
Iron Chews.
Wee Care.

Carb-O-Philic/10. (Geritrex) DMDM hydantoin, lactic acid, lemon oil, petrola-

tum, propylene glycol, urea. Cream. 454 g. *OTC.*
Use: Emollient.

Carb-O-Philic/20. (Geritrex) DMDM hydantoin, lactic acid, lemon oil, petrolatum, propylene glycol, urea. Cream. 454 g. *OTC.*
Use: Emollient.

•**carboplatin.** (kar-boe-PLATT-in) *USP.*
Tall Man: CARBOplatin
Use: Antineoplastic.
See: Paraplatin.

carboplatin. (Mayne) Carboplatin 10 mg/mL. Inj. Single-use vials. 5 mL, 15 mL, 45 mL. *Rx.*
Use: Antineoplastic.

carboplatin. (Various Mfr.) Carboplatin 50 mg, 150 mg, 450 mg. Mannitol. Pow. for Inj., lyophilized. Single-dose vials. *Rx.*
Use: Antineoplastic.

•**carboprost.** (KAR-boe-prahst) USAN.
Use: Oxytocic.

•**carboprost methyl.** (KAR-boe-prahst METH-ill) USAN.
Use: Oxytocic.

•**carboprost tromethamine.** (KAR-boe-prahst troe-METH-ah-meen) *USP.*
Use: Oxytocic.

carbose D.
See: Carboxymethylcellulose Sodium.

carbowax. Polyethylene glycol 300, 400, 1540, 4000.

carboxymethylcellulose.
Use: Ocular lubricant.
See: Refresh Tears.

•**carboxymethylcellulose calcium.** (kar-BOX-ee-meth-ill-SELL-you-lohs) *NF.*
Use: Pharmaceutic aid, tablet disintegrant.

carboxymethylcellulose salt of dextroamphetamine. Carboxyphen.

•**carboxymethylcellulose sodium.** (kar-BOX-ee-meth-ill-SELL-you-lohs) *USP.*
Use: Pharmaceutic aid, suspending agent, tablet excipient, viscosity-increasing agent; cathartic.
W/Combinations.
See: Clear Eyes for Dry Eyes.
Ex-Caloric Wafers.
Foxalin.
Refresh.
W/Glycerin.
See: Optive.

•**carboxymethylcellulose sodium 12.** (car-BOX-ee-meth-ill-SELL-you-lohs) *NF.*
Use: Pharmaceutic aid, suspending, viscosity-increasing agent; mucolytic agent.

Carb PSE 12 DM. (River's Edge) Dextromethorphan tannate 27.5 mg, carbinoxamine tannate 3.2 mg, pseudoephedrine tannate 45.2 mg per 5 mL. Methylparaben, saccharin, sorbitol. Candy apple flavor. Susp. Bot. 473 mL. *Rx.*
Use: Antitussive combination, upper respiratory combination.

Carbromal. (Various Mfr.) Bromodiethylacetylurea, bromadel, nyctal, planadalin, uradal. *Rx.*
Use: Sedative; hypnotic.
W/Bromisovalum (Bromural).
See: Bro-T's.

carbutamide.
Use: Hypoglycemic.

•**carbuterol hydrochloride.** (kar-BYOO-ter-ole) USAN.
Use: Bronchodilator.

•**cardamon.** (KAR-duh-mohn) *NF.* Oil, seed, Cpd. Tincture.
Use: Flavoring.

Cardec. (Macoven Pharmaceuticals) Chlorpheniramine maleate 1 mg, phenylephrine hydrochloride 3.5 mg. Glycerin, parabens, potassium citrate, potassium sorbate, propylene glycol, sucralose. Alcohol free, gluten free, and sugar free. Grape flavor. Drops. 30 mL w/dropper. *OTC.*
Use: Upper respiratory combination, decongestant and antihistamine.

Cardec DM. (Macoven Pharmaceuticals) Chlorpheniramine maleate 1 mg, dextromethorphan hydrobromide 3 mg, phenylephrine hydrochloride 3.5 mg. Glycerin, maltitol, propylene glycol, sodium benzoate, sorbitol, sucralose. Alcohol free, gluten free, and sugar free. Grape flavor. Drops. 30 mL. *OTC.*
Use: Upper respiratory combination, antitussive combination.

Cardene I.V. (Cornerstone Therapeutics) Nicardipine hydrochloride. **Inj., Soln.:** 0.1 mg/mL, 0.2 mg/mL. 200 mL premixed, single-use *Galaxy* container in either dextrose 4.8% or sodium chloride 0.86% (0.1 mg/mL), 200 mL premixed single-use *Galaxy* container in either dextrose 5% or sodium chloride 0.83% (0.2 mg/mL). **Inj., Soln., concentrate:** 2.5 mg/mL. 10 mL ampule. *Rx.*
Use: Calcium channel blocker.

Cardene SR. (Roche) Nicardipine hydrochloride 30 mg, 45 mg, 60 mg. Lactose. ER Cap. Bot. 60s, 200s (except 60 mg). *Rx.*
Use: Calcium channel blocker.

Cardenz. (Miller Pharmacal Group) Vitamins C 25 mg, E 5 mg, inositol 30 mg, p-aminobenzoic acid 9 mg, A 2000 units,

B_6 1.5 mg, B_{12} 1 mcg, D 100 units, niacinamide 20 mg, Mg 23 mg, I 0.05 mg, K 8 mg. Tab. Bot. 100s. *OTC.*
Use: Mineral, vitamin supplement.

cardiac glycosides.
Use: Inotropic agent.
See: Digoxin.

Cardilate. (GlaxoSmithKline) Erythrityl tetranitrate 10 mg. Tab. Bot. 100s.
Use: Antianginal.

Cardio-Green Disposable Unit. (Becton Dickinson & Co.) Cardio-Green 10 mg. Vial. Amp. Aqueous solvent and calibrated syringe.
Use: Diagnostic aid.

Cardi-Omega 3. (Thompson Medical) EPA 180 mg, DHA 120 mg, cholesterol 5 mg, < 2% RDA of vitamins A, B_1, B_2, B_3, C, D, Fe, Ca. Cap. Bot. 60s. *OTC.*
Use: Mineral, vitamin supplement.

Cardio Omega Benefits With Vitamin D-3. (Physician Recommended Nutriceuticals) Omega-3 667 mg (DHA 280 mg, EPA 280 mg, other omega-3s 107 mg), vitamin D 250 units. Soy. Dairy free, gluten free. Cap., softgel. 120s. *OTC.*
Use: Multivitamin and mineral with omega-3 polyunsaturated fatty acids.

cardioplegic solution.
Use: During open heart surgery.
See: Plegisol.

Cardiopress. (MedChem) Vitamins B_3 2.5 mg, B_6 5 mg, B_{12} 100 mcg, C 60 mg, folate 0.1 mg, buchu leaves, garlic, green tea, hawthorn berry, hibiscus flower powder, juniper berry, olive leaf, uva ursi. Cap. 60s. *OTC.*
Use: Multivitamin.

Cardiotek Rx. (Stewart-Jackson) Vitamin B_6 50 mg, B_{12} 500 mcg, FA 2 mg. With L-arginine hydrochloride. Coated. Tab. 30s. *Rx.*
Use: Nutritional product.

Cardio Tone. (MDR Fitness Corp) Vitamins A 1,700 units, E 100 units, B_1 1 mg, B_2 1 mg, B_6 3 mg, B_{12} 3 mcg, C 100 mg, folic acid 0.1 mg, Cr, Mg, Se, alpha lipoic acid 50 mg, L-carnitine 100 mg, coenzyme Q10 50 mg, grape seed extract 25 mg, green tea leaf extract 25 mg, hawthorn berries 2.5 mg, lutein 500 mcg, lycopene 2,000 mcg, quercetin 2.5 mg, zeaxanthin 25 mcg. PEG, peppermint oil. Gluten free, sugar free. Tab. 120s. *OTC.*
Use: Multivitamin with minerals (except iron).

Cardiotrol-CK. (Roche) Lyophilized human serum containing 3 CK isoenzymes from human tissue source. 10 × 2 mL.
Use: Diagnostic aid, quality control.

Cardiotrol-LD. (Roche) Lyophilized human serum containing all LD isoenzymes from human tissue source. 10 × 1 mL.
Use: Diagnostic aid, quality control.

Cardizem. (Valeant) Diltiazem hydrochloride 30 mg, 60 mg, 90 mg, 120 mg. Lactose, methylparaben. Tab. 100s, 500s (30 mg, 60 mg only), UD 100s. *Rx.*
Use: Calcium channel blocker.

Cardizem CD. (Valeant) Diltiazem hydrochloride 120 mg, 180 mg, 240 mg, 300 mg, 360 mg. Sucrose. ER Cap. Bot. 30s (except 360 mg), 90s, UD 100s (except 360 mg). *Rx.*
Use: Calcium channel blocker.

Cardizem LA. (AbbVie) Diltiazem hydrochloride 120 mg, 180 mg, 240 mg, 300 mg, 360 mg, 420 mg. Sucrose. ER Tab. Bot. 7s, 30s, 90s, 1000s. *Rx.*
Use: Calcium channel blocker.

Cardoxin. (Vita Elixir) Digoxin 0.25 mg. Tab. *Rx.*
Use: Cardiovascular agent.

Cardura. (Pfizer) Doxazosin mesylate (as base) 1 mg, 2 mg, 4 mg, 8 mg. Lactose. Tab. Bot. 100s, UD 100s. *Rx.*
Use: Antihypertensive.

Cardura XL. (Pfizer) Doxazosin mesylate (as base) 4 mg, 8 mg. ER Tab. 30s. *Rx.*
Use: Antiadrenergic agent, peripherally acting.

Ca-Rezz. (FNC Medical Corporation) Triclosan. **Soap: 0.2%:** Alcohol, aloe vera, parabens, polysorbate 80, propylene glycol, urea. 237 mL. **0.25%:** Alcohol, aloe vera, parabens, polysorbate 80, propylene glycol. 361 mL. **0.3%:** Disodium EDTA, parabens, propylene glycol, urea. 355 mL. **Cream:** 0.3%. Alcohol, aloe vera, glyceryl, mineral oil, parabens, PEG, propylene glycol, safflower oil, triethanolamine, urea, vitamins A, D, and E. 275 g. *OTC.*
Use: Topical anti-infective, antiseptic and germicide.

•**carfentanil citrate.** (kar-FEN-tah-NILL SIH-trate) USAN.
Use: Analgesic; narcotic.

•**carfilzomib.** (car-FIL-zoe-mib) USAN.
Use: Antineoplastic, proteasome inhibitor.
See: Kyprolis.

Cargentos.
See: Silver protein, mild.

•**carglumic acid.** (kar-GLOO-mik) USAN.
Use: Treatment of hyperammonemia due to N-acetylglutamate synthase deficiency.

Carimune NF. (ZLB Bioplasma) Immune

globulin IV 3 g, 6 g, 12 g. Preservative-free. With 1.67 g sucrose/g protein. Pow. for Inj., lyophilized. Vials. 3 g, 6 g, 12 g. *Rx.*
Use: Immune globulin.

•**cariporide mesylate.** (kar-ee-POR-ide) USAN.
Use: Cardiovascular agent.

•**cariprazine.** (kar-IP-ra-zeen) USAN.
Use: CNS agent.

•**cariprazine hydrochloride.** (kar-IP-ra-zeen) USAN.
Use: CNS agent.

•**carisoprodol.** (car-eye-so-PRO-dole) *USP.*
Use: Muscle relaxant.
See: Soma.

carisoprodol. (Various Mfr.) Carisoprodol 350 mg. Tab. 30s, 60s, 100, 500s, 1000s, UD 100s. *c-IV.*
Use: Muscle relaxant.

carisoprodol. (Wallace) Carisoprodol 250 mg. Potassium sorbate. Tab. 100s. *c-IV.*
Use: Skeletal muscle relaxant, centrally acting.

carisoprodol and aspirin. (Various Mfr.) Carisoprodol 200 mg, aspirin 325 mg. Tab. 15s, 30s, 40s, 100s, 500s, 1000s. *c-IV.*
Use: Analgesic; muscle relaxant.

carisoprodol, aspirin, and codeine phosphate. (Amide) Carisoprodol 200 mg, aspirin 325 mg, codeine phosphate 16 mg. Tab. 100s, 500s. *c-III.*
Use: Skeletal muscle relaxant.

Cari-Tab. (Jones Pharma) Fluoride 0.5 mg, vitamins A 2000 units, D 200 units, C 75 mg. Softab. Bot. 100s. *Rx.*
Use: Vitamin supplement; dental caries agent.

•**carlumab.** (KAR-lue-mab) USAN.
Use: Immunomodulator.

•**carmantadine.** (kar-MAN-tah-deen) USAN.
Use: Antiparkinsonian.

•**carmegliptin.** (kar-mee-GLIP-tin) USAN.
Use: Antidiabetic.

•**carmegliptin dihydrochloride.** (kar-mee-GLIP-tin) USAN.
Use: Antidiabetic.

Carmol HC Cream 1%. (Pharmaderm) Micronized hydrocortisone acetate 1%, urea 10% in water-washable base. Tube 1 oz, Jar 4 oz. *Rx.*
Use: Corticosteroid, topical.

•**carmustine.** (KAR-muss-teen) USAN. BCNU.
Use: Antineoplastic, alkylating agent.
See: BiCNU.
Gliadel.

Carnation Follow-Up. (Carnation) Protein (from nonfat milk) 18 g, carbohydrate (from lactose and corn syrup) 89.2 g, fat 27.7 g, vitamins A, D, E, K, C, B_1, B_2, B_3, B_6, B_{12}, B_5, biotin, choline, Ca, P, Cl, Mg, I, Mn, Cu, Zn, Fe 13 mg, inositol, cholesterol 11.4 mg, taurine, Na 264 mg, K 913 mg. Pow. 360 g. Conc. 390 mL. *OTC.*
Use: Nutritional supplement.

Carnation Good-Start. (Carnation) Protein 16 g, carbohydrate 74.4 g, fat 34.5 g, vitamins A, D, E, K, B_1, B_2, B_3, B_5, B_6, B_{12}, C, biotin, choline, inositol, cholesterol 68 mg, taurine, Ca, P, Mg, Fe 10 mg, Zn, Mn, Cu, I, Cl, Na 162 mg, K 663 mg. Pow 360 g. Conc. 390 mL. *OTC.*
Use: Nutritional supplement.

Carnation Instant Breakfast. (Carnation) Nonfat instant breakfast containing 280 K calories w/15 g protein and 8 oz whole milk. Pkt. 35 g, Ctn. 6s. Six flavors. *OTC.*
Use: Nutritional supplement.

•**carnidazole.** (kar-NIH-dah-zole) USAN. Methylnitroimidazole.
Use: Antiparasitic; antiprotozoal.

Carnitor. (Sigma-Tau) Levocarnitine. **Soln.:** 100 mg/mL, sucrose, parabens, cherry flavor. Bot. 118 mL. **Tab.:** 330 mg. Bot. 90s. **Inj.:** 200 mg/mL, preservative-free. Single-dose vial, amp. *Rx.*
Use: Amino acid derivative.

•**caroxazone.** (kar-OX-ah-zone) USAN.
Use: Antidepressant.

•**carphenazine maleate.** (kar-FEN-azz-een) USAN.
Use: Antipsychotic.

•**carprofen.** (car-PRO-fen) USAN.
Use: Investigational analgesic, NSAID.

•**carrageenan.** (ka-rah-GEE-nan) *NF.*
Use: Pharmaceutic aid, suspending, viscosity-increasing agent.

Carrasyn. (Carrington) Phase I AIDS, ARC. *Rx.*
Use: Antiviral, immunomodulator.

•**carsatrin succinate.** (car-SAT-rin) USAN.
Use: Cardiovascular agent.

•**cartazolate.** (kar-TAZZ-oh-late) USAN.
Use: Antidepressant.

•**carteolol hydrochloride.** (KAR-tee-oh-lahl) *USP.*
Use: Antiadrenergic/sympatholytic, beta-adrenergic blocking agent; antiglaucoma.

carteolol hydrochloride. (Various Mfr.) Carteolol hydrochloride 1%. Soln. Bot. 5 mL, 10 mL, 15 mL. *Rx.*
Use: Antiglaucoma; beta-adrenergic blocker.

Carter's Little Pills. (Carter-Wallace) Bisacodyl 5 mg. Bot. 30s, 85s. *OTC.*
Use: Laxative.

Cartia XT. (Watson Pharma) Diltiazem hydrochloride 120 mg, 180 mg, 240 mg, 300 mg. Sucrose. ER Cap. Box 30s, 90s, 500s, 1000s. *Rx.*
Use: Calcium channel blocker.

•**carubicin hydrochloride.** (kah-ROO-bih-sin) USAN. *Formerly carminomycin hydrochloride.*
Use: Antineoplastic.

•**carumonam sodium.** (kah-roo-MOE-nam) USAN.
Use: Anti-infective.

•**carvedilol.** (CAR-veh-DILL-ole) USAN.
Use: Antianginal; antihypertensive; antiadrenergic/sympatholytic.
See: Coreg.

carvedilol. (Various Mfr.) Carvedilol 3.125 mg, 6.25 mg, 12.5 mg, 25 mg. May contain lactose, mannitol, sucrose. Tab. 28s, 30s, 100s, 500s, 1000s, UD 100s, blister 100s. *Rx.*
Use: Antiadrenergic/sympathomimetic, alpha/beta-adrenergic blocking agent.

carvedilol phosphate.
Use: Antiadrenergic/sympatholytic.
See: Coreg CR.

Car-Vit. (Mericon Industries) Ascorbic acid 60 mg, vitamins A acetate 4000 units, D-2 400 units, ferrous fumarate 90 mg (elemental iron 30 mg), oyster shell 600 mg (calcium 230 mg). Cap. Bot. 90s, 1000s. *OTC.*
Use: Mineral, vitamin supplement.

•**carvotroline hydrochloride.** (car-VAH-trah-leen) USAN.
Use: Antipsychotic.

•**carzelesin.** (car-ZELL-eh-sin) USAN.
Use: Antineoplastic, site-selective DNA binding.

carzenide.
Use: Carbonic anhydrase inhibitor.

casa-dicole. (Halsey Drug) Docusate sodium 100 mg, casanthrol 30 mg. Cap. Bot. 100s. *OTC.*
Use: Laxative.

•**casanthranol.** (kass-AN-thrah-nole) *USP.* A purified mixture of the anthranol glycosides derived from cascara sagrada.
Use: Laxative.
W/Docusate Sodium.
See: Calotabs.
Dio-Soft.
Docusate with Casanthranol.
Easy-Lax Plus.
Laxative & Stool Softener.

cascara fluid extract, aromatic.
Use: Laxative.
See: Aromatic Cascara Fluid Extract.

cascara glycosides.
Use: Laxative.

•**cascara sagrada.** (kass-KA-rah sah-GRAH-dah) *USP.*
Use: Cathartic.
See: Aromatic Cascara Fluid Extract.
Bilstan.
Nature's Remedy.

cascarin.
See: Casanthranol.

Casodex. (AstraZeneca) Bicalutamide 50 mg, lactose. Tab. Bot. 30s, 100s, UD 30s. *Rx.*
Use: Antineoplastic; hormone, antimutagenic.

•**casopitant mesylate.** (KAS-oh-pi-tant) USAN.
Use: CNS agent.

•**caspofungin acetate.** (KASS-poe-FUN-jin) USAN.
Use: Antifungal.
See: Cancidas.

CAST. (Biomerica) Reagent test for immunoglobulin E in serum. Tube Kit 25s.
Use: Diagnostic aid.

Castellani Paint Modified. (Pedinol Pharmacal) Basic fuchsin, phenol resorcinol, acetone, alcohol. Bot. 30 mL, 120 mL, 480 mL. Also available as colorless solution without basic fuchsin. Bot. 30 mL, 120 mL, 480 mL. *Rx.*
Use: Antifungal, topical.

Castellani's Paint. (Penta) Carbolfuchsin solution. Fuchsin 0.3%, phenol 4.5%, resorcinol 10%, acetone 1.5%, alcohol 13%. Bot. 1 oz, 4 oz, pt. *Rx.*
Use: Antifungal, topical.

•**castor oil.** (KASS-ter) *USP.*
Use: Laxative; pharmaceutic aid, plasticizer.
See: Emulsoil.
W/Combinations.
See: Xenaderm.

castor oil. (Various Mfr.) Castor oil. Liq. Bot. 60 mL, 120 mL, 480 mL. *OTC.*
Use: Laxative; pharmaceutic aid, plasticizer.

castor oil, hydrogenated.
Use: Laxative.

Cataflam. (Novartis) Diclofenac 50 mg (as potassium). Sucrose. Tab. Bot. 100s, UD 100s. *Rx.*
Use: Analgesic, NSAID.

Catapres. (Boehringer Ingelheim) Clonidine hydrochloride 0.1 mg, 0.2 mg, 0.3 mg. Lactose. Tab. 100s. *Rx.*
Use: Antiadrenergic/sympatholytic; antiadrenergic agent, centrally acting.

Catapres-TTS-1. (Boehringer Ingelheim) Clonidine hydrochloride 0.1 mg/24 h (surface area, 3.5 cm^2) (total clonidine content, 2.5 mg). Mineral oil. Transdermal patch. 12s. *Rx.*
Use: Antiadrenergic/sympatholytic; antiadrenergic agent, centrally acting.

Catapres-TTS-3. (Boehringer Ingelheim) Clonidine hydrochloride 0.3 mg/24 h (surface area, 10.5 cm^2) (total clonidine content, 7.5 mg). Mineral oil. Transdermal patch. 4s. *Rx.*
Use: Antiadrenergic/sympatholytic; antiadrenergic agent, centrally acting.

Catapres-TTS-2. (Boehringer Ingelheim) Clonidine hydrochloride 0.2 mg/24 h (surface area, 7 cm^2) (total clonidine content, 5 mg). Mineral oil. Transdermal patch. 12s. *Rx.*
Use: Antiadrenergic/sympatholytic; antiadrenergic agent, centrally acting.

Catatrol. (AstraZeneca) Viloxazine.
Use: Antidepressant.

catechins.
Use: Treatment of external genital and perianal warts.
See: Kunecatechins.

Cathflo Activase. (Genentech) Alteplase 2 mg, L-arginine, phosphoric acid, polysorbate 80. Pow. for Inj., lyophilized. Vials. *Rx.*
Use: Thrombolytic.

cathomycin calcium. Calcium novobiocin.
Use: Anti-infective.

cathomycin sodium. Novobiocin sodium.
Use: Anti-infective.

cationic resins.
See: Sodium-Removing Resins.

•**catramilast.** (ka-TRA-mil-ast) USAN.
Use: Dermatologic.

Cavan-EC SOD DHA Tablets and Softgel Capsules. (Seton) Folic acid 1 mg, calcium 230 mg, iron 30 mg, vitamins A 3,000 units, D 410 units, E 30 units, B_1 1.8 mg, B_2 4 mg, B_3 20 mg, B_6 28 mg, B_{12} 12 mcg, C 130 mg, Cu, Mg, Zn. **Tab.:** 30s. **Cap., softgels:** Omega-3 fatty acids ≥ 440 mg (including DHA ≥ 295 mg, other omega-3 fatty acids ≥ 145 mg) in fish oil ≥ 628 mg. Enteric coated. Soy. 30s. *Rx.*
Use: Prenatal vitamin with minerals.

Caverject. (Pharmacia & Upjohn) Alprostadil. **Inj., aqueous:** 10 mcg/mL, 20 mcg/mL, 40 mcg/2 mL Amps. 1 mL and kit with 2 mL *Luer-lock* syringe, 2½-inch needles (one 27-gauge and one 30-gauge) alcohol swab. **Pow. for Inj., lyophilized:** 5 mcg/mL, 10 mcg/mL, 20 mcg/mL, 40 mcg/mL, benzyl alcohol 8.4 mg, lactose. Vials, vials with diluent syringes (except 40 mcg/mL). *Rx.*
Use: Anti-impotence agent.

Caverject Impulse. (Pharmacia & Upjohn) Alprostadil 10 mcg/0.5 mL, 20 mcg/0.5 mL, benzyl alcohol 4.45 mg, lactose. Blister tray containing 1 dual chamber syringe system, 1 needle, 2 alcohol swabs. *Rx.*
Use: Anti-impotence agent.

Cav-X Fluoride Treatment. (Palisades Pharmaceuticals) Stannous fluoride 0.4%. Gel. Bot. 121.9 g. *Rx.*
Use: Dental caries agent.

Cayston. (Gilead Sciences) Aztreonam 75 mg. Lysine 46.7 mg. Preservative free and arginine free. Pow. for Soln., lyophilized; Inhal. Single-dose vial. 2 mL w/1 mL ampule of sodium chloride 0.17% diluent. *Rx.*
Use: Anti-infective agent, monobactam.

Caziant. (Watson) **Phase 1:** Desogestrel 0.1 mg, ethinyl estradiol 25 mcg. **Phase 2:** Desogestrel 0.125 mg, ethinyl estradiol 25 mcg. **Phase 3:** Desogestrel 0.15 mg, ethinyl estradiol 25 mcg. Lactose. 28-day blister card w/7 green inert tablets. Tab. *Rx.*
Use: Oral contraceptive, oral triphasic contraceptive.

C-Bio. (Barth's) Vitamin C 150 mg, citrus bioflavonoid complex 100 mg, rutin 50 mg. Tab. Bot. 100s, 500s, 1000s. *OTC.*
Use: Vitamin supplement.

C-B Time. (Arco) Vitamins C 300 mg, B_1 15 mg, B_2 10 mg, B_3 100 mg, B_5 20 mg, B_6 5 mg, B_{12} 5 mcg. Liq. Bot. 120 mL. *OTC.*
Use: Vitamin supplement.

CC-Galactosidase. Alpha-galactosidase A.
Use: Fabry disease. [Orphan Drug]

CCNU. Lomustine.
Use: Antineoplastic.
See: CeeNU.

C-Crystals. (NBTY) Vitamin C 5000 mg/tsp. Crystals. Bot. 180 g. *OTC.*
Use: Vitamin supplement.

CDDP.
Use: Antineoplastic.
See: Cisplatin.

C.D.P. (Ivax) Chlordiazepoxide hydrochloride 5 mg, 10 mg, 25 mg. Cap. Bot. 100s, 500s, 1000s. *c-IV.*
Use: Anxiolytic.

Cea. (Abbott Diagnostics) Radioimmunoassay or enzyme immunoassay for quantitative measurement of carcinoembryonic antigen in human serum or plasma. Test Kit 100s.
Use: Diagnostic aid.

Cea-Roche. (Roche) Radioimmunoassay capable of detecting and measuring plasma levels of CEA in the nanogram range. Sensitivity-0.5 ng/mL of CEA.
Use: Diagnostic aid.

Cea-Roche Test Kit. (Roche) Carcinoembryonic antigen, a glycoprotein which is a constituent of the glycocalyx of embryonic entodermal epithelium. Test Kit.
Use: Diagnostic aid.

CEA-Scan. (Immunomedics; Mallinckrodt-Baker) Arcitumomab 1.25 mg. Reconstitute with Tc 99m sodium pertechnetate in NaCl for Inj. Inj. Single-dose Vial. *Rx.*
Use: For detection of recurrent or metastatic colorectal carcinoma of the liver, extrahepatic abdomen and pelvis; radioimmunoscintigraphy.

Ceb Nuggets. (Scot-Tussin) Vitamins B_1 15 mg, B_2 15 mg, B_6 5 mg, B_{12} 5 mcg, C 600 mg, niacinamide 100 mg, E 40 units, calcium pantothenate 20 mg, folic acid 0.1 mg. Nugget. Bot. 60s. *OTC.*
Use: Mineral, vitamin supplement.

Cebo-Caps. (Forest) Placebo capsules. *OTC.*

•**cebranopadal.** (SEB-ran-OH-pa-dol) USAN.
Use: Analgesic.

Cedax. (Pernix Therapeutics) **Cap.:** Ceftibuten 400 mg. Parabens. Bot. 20s. **Pow. for Oral Susp.:** Ceftibuten 90 mg/5 mL, 180 mg/5 mL. Polysorbate 80, sodium benzoate, sucrose. Cherry flavor. 30 mL (180 mg/5 mL only); 60 mL; 90 mL, 120 mL (90 mg/5 mL only). *Rx.*
Use: Anti-infective, cephalosporin.

•**cedefingol.** (seh-deh-FIN-gole) USAN.
Use: Antineoplastic, adjunct; antipsoriatic.

•**cedelizumab.** (sed-eh-LIE-zoo-mab) USAN.
Use: Monoclonal antibody; immunosuppressant.

Ceebevim. (NBTY) Vitamins B_1 15 mg, B_2 10.2 mg, B_3 50 mg, B_5 10 mg, B_6 5 mg, C 300 mg. Cap. Bot. 100s, 300s. *OTC.*
Use: Vitamin supplement.

CeeNU. (Bristol Labs Oncology) Lomustine (CCNU) 10 mg, 40 mg, 100 mg, mannitol. Cap. 20s, dose pk. of 2 cap. each of all 3 strengths. *Rx.*
Use: Antineoplastic, alkylating agent.

Ceepa. (Geneva) Theophylline 130 mg, ephedrine hydrochloride 24 mg, phenobarbital 8 mg. Tab. Bot. 100s, 1000s. *Rx.*
Use: Bronchodilator; decongestant; hypnotic; sedative.

Ceepryn. Cetylpyridinium chloride. *OTC.*
Use: Antiseptic.
See: Cēpacol.

Cee with Bee. (Wesley) Vitamins B_1 15 mg, B_2 10.2 mg, B_3 50 mg, B_5 10 mg, B_6 5 mg, C 300 mg, tartrazine. Bot. 100s, 1000s. *OTC.*
Use: Vitamin supplement.

•**cefaclor.** (SEFF-uh-klor) *USP.*
Use: Anti-infective, cephalosporin.

cefaclor. (Various Mfr.) Cefaclor. **Cap.:** 250 mg, 500 mg. Bot. 15s (500 mg), 30s (250 mg), 100s, 500s, 1000s (250 mg). **Pow. for Oral Susp.:** 125 mg/5 mL, 187 mg/5 mL, 250 mg/5 mL, 375 mg/5 mL. Bot. 50 mL (187 mg/5 mL, 375 mg/5 mL only), 75 mL (125 mg/5 mL, 250 mg/5 mL only), 100 mL (187mg/5 mL, 375 mg/5 mL only), 150 mL (125 mg/5 mL, 250 mg/5 mL only). *Rx.*
Use: Anti-infective.

cefaclor. (Zenith Goldline) Cefaclor 375 mg, 500 mg. ER Tab. Bot. 100s. *Rx.*
Use: Anti-infective.

•**cefadroxil.** (SEFF-uh-DROX-ill) *USP.*
Use: Anti-infective, cephalosporin.

cefadroxil. (Various Mfr.) Cefadroxil. **Cap.:** 500 mg. 20s, 50s, 100s. **Tab.:** 1 g. 50s. **Pow. for Susp.:** 250 mg per 5 mL (may contain sodium benzoate, sucrose), 500 mg per 5 mL (may contain sodium benzoate, sucrose, sulfur dioxide). 75 mL (500 mg per 5 mL only), 100 mL. *Rx.*
Use: Anti-infective, cephalosporin.

•**cefamandole.** (SEFF-ah-MAN-dole) USAN.

•**cefamandole sodium for injection.** (SEFF-ah-MAN-dole) *USP.*
Use: Anti-infective, cephalosporin.

Cefanex. (Apothecon) Cephalexin monohydrate 250 mg, 500 mg. Cap. Bot. 100s. *Rx.*
Use: Anti-infective, cephalosporin.

•**cefaparole.** (SEFF-ah-pah-ROLE) USAN.
Use: Anti-infective.

•**cefatrizine.** (SEFF-ah-TRY-zeen) USAN.
Use: Anti-infective, cephalosporin.

•**cefazaflur sodium.** (seff-AZE-ah-flure) USAN.
Use: Anti-infective, cephalosporin.

•**cefazolin sodium.** (seff-AH-zoe-lin) USAN.
Tall Man: ceFAZolin
Use: Anti-infective; cephalosporin.

cefazolin sodium. (Apothecon) Cefazolin sodium 500 mg, 1 g, 5 g, 10 g, 20 g. Sodium 2.1 mEq/g. Pow. for Inj. Vials, piggyback vials (except 10 g, 20 g); phar-

macy bulk packages (10 g, 20 g only). *Rx.*
Use: Anti-infective.

cefazolin sodium and dextrose. (B. Braun Medical) Cefazolin 1 g (contains sodium 48 mg/g), 2 g (contains sodium 48 mg/g). Inj., lyophilized Pow. for Soln. *Duplex* drug delivery system. *Rx.*
Use: Anti-infective agent, cephalosporin and related antibiotic.

•**cefbuperazone.** (SEFF-byoo-PURR-ah-zone) USAN.
Use: Anti-infective, cephalosporin.

•**cefdinir.** (SEFF-dih-ner) USAN.
Use: Anti-infective, cephalosporin.

cefdinir. (Various Mfr.) Cefdinir. **Cap.:** 300 mg. 60s, 100s, UD 10s, UD 50s. **Susp.:** 125 mg/5 mL, 250 mg/5 mL. May contain sucrose. Strawberry or cherry flavor. 60 mL, 100 mL. *Rx.*
Use: Anti-infective, cephalosporin.

•**cefditoren pivoxil.** (SEFF-dih-TOR-en pih-VOX-ill) USAN.
Use: Anti-infective.
See: Spectracef.

cefditoren pivoxil. (Aristos) Cefditoren (as cefditoren pivoxil) 200 mg, 400 mg. May contain mannitol, sodium cassinate. Tab. Blister pack. 20s, 28s (400 mg only). *Rx.*
Use: Anti-infective agent, cephalosporin and related antibiotic.

•**cefepime.** (SEFF-eh-pim) USAN.
Use: Anti-infective.

cefepime. (Baxter) Cefepime. Inj., Soln. **1 g:** Dextrose 1.03 g. 50 mL single-dose *Galaxy* containers. **2 g:** Dextrose 2.06 g. 100 mL single-dose *Galaxy* containers. *Rx.*
Use: Anti-infective agent, cephalosporin and related antibiotic.

•**cefepime hydrochloride.** (SEFF-eh-pim) USAN.
Use: Anti-infective.
See: Maxipime.

cefepime hydrochloride. (Apotex USA) Cefepime hydrochloride 500 mg, 1 g, 2 g. Inj., Pow. for Soln. Vials. 1s, 10s. *Rx.*
Use: Anti-infective.

•**cefetecol.** (seff-EH-teh-kahl) USAN.
Use: Antibacterial, cephalosporin.

Cefinal II. (Alto) Salicylamide 150 mg, acetaminophen 250 mg, doxylamine succinate 25 mg. Tab. Bot. 100s. *OTC.*
Use: Analgesic combination.

•**cefixime.** (sef-IX-eem) *USP.*
Use: Anti-infective, cephalosporin.
See: Suprax.

•**cefmenoxime hydrochloride, sterile.** (SEFF-men-ox-eem) *USP.*
Use: Anti-infective, cephalosporin.

•**cefmetazole.** (seff-MET-ah-zole) *USP.*
Use: Anti-infective, cephalosporin.

•**cefmetazole for injection.** (seff-MET-ah-zole) *USP.*
Use: Anti-infective, cephalosporin.

•**cefmetazole sodium.** (seff-MET-ah-zole) *USP.*
Use: Anti-infective, cephalosporin.

•**cefonicid monosodium.** (seh-FAHN-ih-SID MAHN-oh-SO-dee-uhm) USAN.
Use: Anti-infective, cephalosporin.

•**cefoperazone sodium.** (SEFF-oh-PUR-uh-zone) *USP.*
Use: Anti-infective, cephalosporin.

•**ceforanide for injection.** (seh-FAR-ah-NIDE) *USP.*
Use: Anti-infective, cephalosporin.

cefotaxime. (Cura) Cefotaxime 1 g, 2 g. Sodium 2.2 mEq/g. Inj. Infusion bottles. Packages of 25. *Rx.*
Use: Antibiotic.

cefotaxime. (Various Mfr.) Cefotaxime 500 mg, 1 g, 2 g, 10 g. Sodium 2.2 mEq/g. Pow. for Inj. Vials. Packages of 10 (500 mg only), packages of 25 (1 g, 2 g only), bottles (10 g only). *Rx.*
Use: Antibiotic.

•**cefotaxime sodium.** (seff-oh-TAX-eem) *USP.*
Use: Anti-infective, cephalosporin.
See: Claforan.

•**cefotetan.** (SEFF-oh-tee-tan) *USP.*
Tall Man: cefoTEtan
Use: Anti-infective, cephalosporin.

•**cefotetan disodium.** (SEFF-oh-tee-tan die-SO-dee-uhm) *USP.*
Use: Anti-infective.

cefotetan disodium. (Abraxis) Cefotetan 1 g, 2 g, 10 g. Sodium 3.5 mEq/mL. Inj., Pow. for Soln. 10 mL (1 g only), 20 mL (2 g and 10 g only). *Rx.*
Use: Anti-infective, cephalosporin.

•**cefotiam hydrochloride sterile.** (SEFF-oh-TIE-am) *USP.*
Use: Anti-infective, cephalosporin.

•**cefovecin sodium.** (sef-OH-vee-sin) USAN.
Use: Antibacterial (veterinary).

•**cefoxitin.** (seff-OX-ih-tin) USAN.
Tall Man: cefOXitan
Use: Anti-infective, cephalosporin.

cefoxitin. (American Pharmaceutical Partners) Cefoxitin (as sodium) 1 g, 2 g, 10 g. Pow. for Inj. Vials and infusion

bottles (1 g, 2 g); pharmacy bulk packages (10 g). *Rx.*
Use: Anti-infective, cephalosporin.

cefoxitin and dextrose. (B. Braun McGaw) Cefoxitin sodium 1 g, 2 g. Dextrose 50 mL. Preservative free. Inj., Pow. for Soln. Single-use *Duplex* drug delivery system container. *Rx.*
Use: Anti-infective agent, cephalosporin and related antibiotic.

•**cefoxitin sodium.** (seff-OX-ih-tin) *USP.*
Tall Man: cefOXitan
Use: Anti-infective, cephalosporin.

•**cefpimizole.** (seff-PIH-mih-zole) USAN.
Use: Anti-infective, cephalosporin.

•**cefpimizole sodium.** (seff-PIH-mih-zole) USAN.
Use: Anti-infective, cephalosporin.

•**cefpiramide.** (SEFF-PIHR-am-ide) USAN.
Use: Anti-infective, cephalosporin.

•**cefpiramide sodium.** (SEFF-PIHR-am-ide) USAN.
Use: Anti-infective, cephalosporin.

•**cefpirome sulfate.** (SEFF-pihr-ome) USAN.
Use: Anti-infective, cephalosporin.

•**cefpodoxime proxetil.** (SEFF-pode-OX-eem PROX-uh-til) *USP.*
Use: Anti-infective, cephalosporin.
See: Vantin.

cefpodoxime proxetil. (Aurobindo) Cefpodoxime proxetil. **Tab.:** 100 mg, 200 mg. Lactose. Film-coated. 20s. **Susp.:** 50 mg/5 mL, 100 mg/5 mL. Lactose, sucrose. 50 mL, 75 mL, 100 mL. *Rx.*
Use: Cephalosporin.

•**cefprozil.** (SEFF-pro-zill) *USP.*
Use: Anti-infective, cephalosporin.

cefprozil. (Various Mfr.) **Pow. for Oral Susp.:** Cefprozil (as anhydrous when reconstituted) 125 mg per 5 mL, 250 mg per 5 mL. May contain aspartame, sucrose, phenylalanine. 50 mL, 75 mL, 100 mL. **Tab.:** Cefprozil (as anhydrous) 250 mg, 500 mg. 50s (500 mg only), 100s. *Rx.*
Use: Anti-infective.

•**cefroxadine.** (SEFF-ROX-ah-deen) USAN.
Use: Anti-infective, cephalosporin.

•**cefsulodin sodium.** (SEFF-SULL-oh-din) USAN.
Use: Anti-infective, cephalosporin.

•**ceftaroline fosamil.** (sef-TAR-oh-leen FOS-a-mil) USAN.
Use: Anti-infective, cephalosporin.
See: Teflaro.

•**ceftazidime.** (seff-TAZE-ih-deem) *USP.*
Tall Man: cefTAZidime
Use: Anti-infective, cephalosporin.
See: Fortaz.
Tazicef.

ceftazidime and dextrose. (B. Braun) Ceftazidime 1 g, 2 g. Inj., Pow. for Soln. 50 mL single-use *Duplex* container (with dextrose 5%). *Rx.*
Use: Anti-infective, cephalosporin and related antibiotic.

•**ceftibuten.** (seff-TIE-byoo-ten) USAN.
Use: Anti-infective.
See: Cedax.

Ceftin. (GlaxoWellcome) Cefuroxime (as axetil). **Tab.:** 125 mg, 250 mg, 500 mg. Film-coated. Bot. 10s (250 mg only), 20s, 60s (except 125 mg), UD 50s (500 mg only), 100s (except 500 mg). **Susp.:** 125 mg/5 mL, 250 mg/5 mL. Sucrose. Tutti-frutti flavor. Bot. 50 mL, 100 mL. *Rx.*
Use: Anti-infective, cephalosporin.

•**ceftizoxime sodium.** (SEFF-tih-ZOX-eem) *USP.*
Use: Anti-infective, cephalosporin.

•**ceftobiprole.** (sef-TOE-bye-prole) USAN.
Use: Antibiotic.

•**ceftobiprole medocaril.** (sef-TOE-bye-prole me-DOK-a-ril) USAN.
Use: Antibiotic.

•**ceftolozane.** (sef-TOL-oh-zane) USAN.
Use: Antibiotic.

•**ceftolozane sulfate.** (sef-TOL-oh-zane) USAN.
Use: Antibiotic.

•**ceftriaxone sodium.** (SEFF-TRY-AXE-own) *USP.*
Tall Man: cefTRIAXone
Use: Anti-infective, cephalosporin.
See: Rocephin.

ceftriaxone sodium. (Various Mfr.) Ceftriaxone sodium (as base). **Inj.:** 1 g, 2 g. May contain dextrose. Sodium 3.6 mEq/g. 50 mL *ADD-Vantage* vials. **Pow. for Inj.:** 250 mg, 500 mg, 1 g, 2 g, 10 g. Sodium 3.6 mEq per g. Vials (except 10 g), bulk containers (10 g only). *Rx.*
Use: Anti-infective.

•**cefuroxime.** (SEFF-yur-OX-eem) USAN.
Use: Anti-infective, cephalosporin.

•**cefuroxime axetil.** (SEFF-your-OX-eem ACK-seh-TILL) *USP.*
Use: Anti-infective, cephalosporin.
See: Ceftin.

cefuroxime axetil. (Ranbaxy) Cefuroxime (as axetil). **Oral Susp.:** 125 mg/5 mL, 250 mg/5 mL when reconstituted. Aspartame, mannitol, phenylalanine 4.5 mg/5 mL, sucrose. Fruit flavor.

50 mL, 100 mL. **Tab.:** 125 mg, 250 mg, 500 mg. 20s (250 mg, 500 mg), 60s, 100s. *Rx.*
Use: Anti-infective, cephalosporin.

•**cefuroxime pivoxetil.** (SEFF-your-OX-eem pih-VOX-eh-till) USAN.
Use: Anti-infective, cephalosporin.

•**cefuroxime sodium.** (SEFF-your-OX-eem) *USP.*
Use: Anti-infective, cephalosporin.
See: Zinacef.

cefuroxime sodium. (Various Mfr.) Cefuroxime sodium 750 mg, 1.5 g, 7.5 g. Sodium 2.4 mEq/g. Pow. for Inj. Vials. 10 mL (750 mg only), 20 mL (1.5 g only), 100 mL piggyback vials (750 mg, 1.5 g only), pharmacy bulk package (7.5 g only). *Rx.*
Use: Anti-infective, cephalosporin.

Celebrex. (Searle) Celecoxib 50 mg, 100 mg, 200 mg, 400 mg. Lactose. Cap. Bot. 60s (50 mg, 400 mg only); 100s, 500s (except 50 mg, 400 mg); UD 100s (except 50 mg). *Rx.*
Tall Man: CeleBREX
Use: Nonsteroidal anti-inflammatory agent.

•**celecoxib.** (cell-ih-COX-ib) USAN.
Use: Nonsteroidal anti-inflammatory agent.
See: Celebrex.

Celestone. (Schering) Betamethasone 0.6 mg/5 mL. Alcohol, sorbitol, sugar. Soln. Bot. 118 mL. *Rx.*
Use: Adrenocortical steroid, glucocorticoid.

Celestone Soluspan. (Schering) Betamethasone sodium phosphate 3 mg, betamethasone acetate 3 mg/mL, EDTA, benzalkonium chloride. Multidose vials. 5 mL. *Rx.*
Use: Adrenocortical steroid, glucocorticoid.

Celexa. (Forest) Citalopram hydrobromide 10 mg, 20 mg, 40 mg. Lactose, polyethylene glycol. Tab. 100s. *Rx.*
Tall Man: CeleXA
Use: Antidepressant, SSRI.

•**celgosivir hydrochloride.** (sell-GO-sih-vihr) USAN.
Use: Antiviral; inhibitor, alpha-glucoside.

•**celiprolol hydrochloride.** (SEE-lih-PRO-lahl) USAN.
Use: Investigational beta-adrenergic blocking agent.

Cellaburate. (Eastman Kodak) Cellulose acetate butyrate.
Use: Pharmaceutic aid, plastic-filming agent.

cellacefate.
Use: Pharmaceutic aid, tablet coating agent.
See: Cellulose Acetate Phthalate.

CellCept. (Genentech USA) Mycophenolate mofetil. **Cap.:** 250 mg. Bot. 100s, 120s, 500s. **Pow. for Soln., Inj., lyophilized:** 500 mg (as mycophenolate mofetil hydroxide). Preservative free. Vials. 20 mL. **Pow. for Oral Susp.:** 200 mg/mL (when reconstituted). Aspartame, methylparaben, sorbitol, phenylalanine 0.56 mg/mL, mixed fruit flavor. Bot. 225 mL. **Tab.:** 500 mg. Alcohols, PEG. Film-coated. Bot. 100s, 500s. *Rx.*
Use: Immunosuppressant.

Cellepacbin. (Arthrins) Vitamins A 1200 units, B_1 1.5 mg, B_2 1.5 mg, B_6 0.75 mg, niacinamide 7.5 mg, panthenol 3 mg, C 20 mg, B_{12} 2 mcg, E 1 units. Cap. Bot. 180s. *OTC.*
Use: Vitamin supplement.

Cellothyl. (Numark) Methylcellulose 0.5 g. Tab. Bot. 100s, 1000s. *OTC.*
Use: Laxative.

cellular chemokine receptor (CCR5) antagonist.
Use: Antiretroviral agent.
See: Maraviroc.

•**cellulase.** (SELL-you-lace) USAN. A concentrate of cellulose-splitting enzymes derived from *Aspergillus niger* and other sources.
Use: Enzyme, digestive adjunct.

cellulolytic enzyme.
See: Cellulase.

cellulose.
W/Combinations.
See: Zeasorb.

•**cellulose acetate.** (SELL-you-lohs) *NF.*
Use: Pharmaceutic aid, coating agent; polymer membrane, insoluble.

•**cellulose acetate phthalate.** (SELL-you-lohs ASS-eh-tate THAL-ate) *NF.*
Use: Pharmaceutic aid, tablet coating agent.
See: Cellacefate.

•**cellulose, carboxymethyl, sodium salt.** (SELL-you-lohs kar-BOX-ee-meth-ill) *USP.* Carboxymethylcellulose sodium.

•**cellulose, hydroxypropyl methyl ether.** (SELL-you-lohs, hi-DROX-ee-pro-pill meth-ill E-thur) *USP.* Hydroxypropyl methylcellulose.

cellulose methyl ether.
See: Methylcellulose.

•**cellulose microcrystalline.** (SELL-you-lohs my-KROE-cris-tahl-een) *NF.*
Use: Pharmaceutic aid, tablet and capsule diluent.

cellulose, nitrate. Pyroxylin.

•**cellulose, oxidized.** (SELL-you-lohs, OX-ih-dized) *USP.*
Use: Hemostatic.

•**cellulose, oxidized regenerated.** (SELL-you-lohs, OX-ih-dized) *USP.*
Use: Hemostatic.

cellulose, powdered.
Use: Tablet and capsule diluent.

•**cellulose sodium phosphate.** (SELL-you-lohs) *USP.*
Use: Antiurolithic.
See: Calcibind.

cellulosic acid.
See: Oxidized Cellulose.

Celluvisc. (Allergan) Carboxymethylcellulose 1%, NaCl, KCl, sodium lactate. Ophth. Soln. Single-use containers 0.3 mL (UD 30s). *OTC.*
Use: Artificial tears.

Celontin. (Pfizer US) Methsuximide 300 mg. Cap. 100s. *Rx.*
Use: Anticonvulsant.

Cena-K. (Century) Potassium and chloride 20 mEq/15 mL (10% KCl), saccharin. Bot. Pt, gal. *Rx.*
Use: Electrolyte supplement.

Cenalax. (Century) Bisacodyl. **Tab.:** 5 mg. Bot. 100s, 1000s. **Supp.:** 10 mg. Pkg. 12s, 1000s. *OTC.*
Use: Laxative.

•**cenderitide.** (sen-DER-i-tide) USAN.
Use: Cardiovascular agent.

Cenestin. (Barr/Duramed) Synthetic conjugated estrogens, A, 0.3 mg, 0.45 mg, 0.625 mg, 0.9 mg, 1.25 mg. Lactose. Film-coated. Tab. Bot. 30s, 100s, 1000s. *Rx.*
Use: Estrogen, sex hormone.

CenFol. (Centurion Labs) Folate 2.3 mg, B_6 24.5 mg, B_{12} 2,000 mcg. Lactose free. Tab. 90s. *Rx.*
Use: Multivitamin.

Cenhist. (Centurion Labs) Brompheniramine maleate 6 mg, phenylephrine hydrochloride 15 mg, Saccharin, sucralose, xylitol. Orange flavor. Chew. Tab. 60s. *OTC.*
Use: Upper respiratory combination, decongestant and antihistamine.

•**cenicriviroc.** (SEN-i-kri-VIR-ok) USAN.
Use: Treatment of HIV infection and arthritis.

•**cenicriviroc mesylate.** (SEN-i-kri-VIR-ok) USAN.
Use: Treatment of HIV infection and arthritis.

•**cenplacel-L.** (SEN-pla-sel-el) USAN.
Use: Immunomodulator.

•**censavudine.** (sen-SAV-ue-deen) USAN.
Use: Antiretroviral agent.

Centany. (Medimetriks Pharmaceuticals) Mupirocin 2%. Alcohol, carylic/capric/myristic/stearic triglyceride, castor oil, propylene glycol. Oint. 30 g; kits w/gauze pads and latex-free cloth tape strips. *Rx.*
Use: Topical anti-infective, antibiotic.

Centeon Thyroid. (Aventis) Desiccated animal thyroid glands (active thyroid hormones) T-4 thyroxine, T-3 thyronine 0.25 g, 0.5 g, 1 g, 1.5 g, 2 g, 3 g, 4 g, 5 g. Tab. Bot. 100s, 1000s. Handy Hundreds, Carton Strip 100s. *Rx.*
Use: Hormone, thyroid.

Center-Al. (Center) Allergenic extracts, alum precipitated 10,000 PNU/mL, 20,000 PNU/mL. Vial 10 mL, 30 mL. *Rx.*
Use: Antiallergic.

Centoxin. (Centocor) Nebacumab.
Use: Antibacterial. [Orphan Drug]

Centrafree. (NBTY) Iron 27 mg, vitamins A 5000 units, D 400 units, E 30 units, B_1 2.25 mg, B_2 2.6 mg, B_3 20 mg, B_5 10 mg, B_6 3 mg, B_{12} 9 mcg, C 90 mg, folic acid 0.4 mg, biotin 45 mcg, Ca, Cl, Cr, Cu, I, K, Mg, Mn, Mo, P, Se, Zn. Tab. Bot. 100s. *OTC.*
Use: Mineral, vitamin supplement.

central nervous system depressants.
See: Sedative/Hypnotic Agents.

central nervous system stimulants.
See: Amphetamines.
Analeptics.
Anorexiants.
Dexmethylphenidate Hydrochloride.
Methylphenidate Hydrochloride.

Centrovite Advanced Formula. (Rugby) Fe 18 mg, A 5000 units, D 400 units, E 30 units, B_1 1.5 mg, B_2 1.7 mg, B_3 20 mg, B_5 10 mg, B_6 2 mg, B_{12} 6 mcg, C 60 mg, Fa 0.4 mg, biotin 30 mcg, Ca, Cl, Cr, Cu, I, vitamin K, Mg, Mn, Mo, Ni, P, Se, Si, Sn, V, Zn, K. Tab. Bot. 100s. *OTC.*
Use: Mineral, vitamin supplement.

Centrovite Jr. (Rugby) Iron 18 mg, vitamins A 5000 units, D 400 units, E 15 units, B_1 1.5 mg, B_2 1.7 mg, B_3 20 mg, B_5 10 mg, B_6 2 mg, B_{12} 6 mcg, C 60 mg, folic acid 0.4 mg, biotin 45 mcg, Cr, Cu, I, Mg, Mn, Mo, Zn. Chew. Tab. Bot. 60s. *OTC.*
Use: Mineral, vitamin supplement.

Centrum. (Wyeth) Vitamins A 5000 units, E 30 units, C 90 mg, folic acid 400 mcg, B_1 2.25 mg, B_2 2.6 mg, B_6 3 mg, niacinamide 20 mg, B_{12} 9 mcg, D 400 units, biotin 45 mcg, pantothenic acid 10 mg, Ca 162 mg, P 125 mg, I 150 mcg, Fe

27 mg, Mg 100 mg, K 30 mg, Mn 5 mg, chromium 25 mcg, Se 25 mcg, Mo 25 mcg, Zn 15 mg, Cu 2 mg, vitamin K 25 mcg, Cl 27.2 mg. Tab. *OTC.*
Use: Mineral, vitamin supplement.

Centrum, Advanced Formula. (Wyeth) Vitamins A 2500 units, E 30 units, C 60 mg, B_1 1.5 mg, B_2 1.7 mg, B_3 20 mg, B_5 10 mg, B_6 2 mg, B_{12} 6 mcg, D_2 400 units, Fe 9 mg, biotin 300 mcg per 15 mL. With I, Zn, Mn, Cr, Mo, alcohol. 6.6%. Liq. Bot. 236 mL. *OTC.*
Use: Mineral, vitamin supplement.

Centrum Jr. (Wyeth) Vitamins A 5000 units, D 400 units, E 30 units, C 60 mg, folic acid 400 mcg, B_1 1.5 mg, B_6 2 mg, B_{12} 6 mcg, riboflavin 1.7 mg, niacinamide 20 mg, Fe 18 mg, Mg 25 mg, Cu 2 mg, Zn 10 mg, biotin 45 mcg, panthothenic acid 10 mg, Mo 20 mcg, chromium 20 mcg, I 150 mcg, Mn 1 mg. Chew. Tab. Bot. 60s. *OTC.*
Use: Mineral, vitamin supplement.

Centrum Performance. (Wyeth) Ca 100 mg, Fe 18 mg, A 5000 units, D 400 units, E 60 units, B_1 4.5 mg, B_2 5.1 mg, B_3 40 mg, B_5 10 mg, B_6 6 mg, B_{12} 18 mcg, C 120 mg, folic acid 400 mcg, K 25 mcg, biotin 40 mcg, chloride 72 mcg, Ginkgo biloba leaf 60 mg, ginseng root 50 mg, B, Cr, Cu, I, K, Mg, Mn, Mo, Ni, P, Se, Si, Sn, V, Zn 15 mg, glucose, lactose, maltodextrin, sucrose. Tab. Bot. 120s. *OTC.*
Use: Mineral, vitamin supplement.

Centrum Silver. (Wyeth) Vitamin A 3500 units, D 400 units, E 45 units, B_1 1.5 mg, B_2 1.7 mg, B_3 20 mg, B_5 10 mg, B_6 3 mg, B_{12} 25 mcg, C 60 mg, folic acid 400 mcg, Zn 15 mg, vitamin K 10 mcg, biotin 30 mcg, chloride, lutein 250 mcg, B, Ca, Cr, Cu, I, K, Mg, Mn, Mo, Ni, P, Se, Si, V, sucrose, glucose. Tab. Bot. 220s. *OTC.*
Use: Mineral, vitamin supplement.

Centrum Silver Gel-Tabs. (Wyeth) Vitamins A 6000 units, D 400 units, E 45 units, B_1 1.5 mg, B_2 1.7 mg, B_3 20 mg, B_5 10 mg, B_6 3 mg, B_{12} 25 mcg, C 60 mg, K 10 mcg, biotin 30 mcg, folic acid 200 mcg, Fe 9 mg. With Ca 200 mg, Cu, I, Mg, P, Zn, Cl, Cr, Mn, Mo, Ni, K, Se, Si, V. Tab. Bot. 60s. *OTC.*
Use: Mineral, vitamin supplement.

Centrum Silver Ultra Women's. (Pfizer Consumer Healthcare) Vitamins A (43% as beta-carotene) 3,500 units, B_1 1.1 mg, B_2 1.1 mg, B_3 14 mg, B_5 5 mg, B_6 5 mg, B_{12} 50 mcg, C 100 mg, D 800 units, E 35 units, K, folic acid 400 mcg, biotin 30 mcg, Ca, Fe 8 mg, P, I, Mg, Zn, Se, Cu, Mn, Cr, Mo, Cl, potassium, Ni, Si, V, boron, lutein 300 mcg. Gelatin, hydrogenated palm oil, MCTs, PEG, polyvinyl alcohol, sucrose, maltodextrin, sunflower oil, soy. Tab. 100s. *OTC.*
Use: Nutritional supplement.

centruroides (scorpion) immune F(ab′)$_2$ (equine).
Use: Antitoxin/antivenin.
See: Anascorp.

Centurion A-Z. (Mission Pharmacal) Fe 27 mg, A 5000 units, D 400 units, E 30 units, B_1 2.25 mg, B_2 2.6 mg, B_3 20 mg, B_5 10 mg, B_6 3 mg, B_{12} 9 mcg, C 90 mg, FA 0.4 mg, biotin 0.45 mg, Ca, Cl, Cr, Cu, I, K, Mg, Mn, Mo, P, Se, Zn, vitamin K. Tab. Bot. 130s. *OTC.*
Use: Mineral, vitamin supplement.

Ceo-Two. (Beutlich) Potassium bitartrate, sodium bicarbonate in polyethylene glycol base. Supp. Box 10s. *OTC.*
Use: Laxative.

Cēpacol. (Combe) Cetylpyridinium chloride 0.05%, alcohol denatured 14%, disodium EDTA, glycerin, polysorbate 80, saccharin. Mouthwash. 24 oz, 32 oz. *OTC.*
Use: Mouth and throat product.

Cēpacol Dual Relief Sore Throat + Coating Spray. (Combe) Benzocaine 5%, glycerin 33%. Acesulfame K, PEG, SD alcohol 38B. Sugar free. Cherry flavor. Spray 22.2 mL. *OTC.*
Use: Topical anesthetic.

Cēpacol Dual Relief Sore Throat + Cough. (Combe) Benzocaine 5%, dextromethorphan hydrobromide 5 mg, glycerin 30%. SD alcohol 38B, sucralose. Sugar free. Cherry flavor. Spray, Soln. 20.2 mL. *OTC.*
Use: Nonnarcotic antitussive.

Cēpacol Fizzlers. (Combe) Benzocaine 6 mg. Corn syrup, mannitol, sodium bicarbonate, sucralose. Grape flavor. Tab., orally disintegrating. 12s. *OTC.*
Use: Mouth and throat product.

Cēpacol Maximum Numbing Sore Throat. (Combe) **Cherry flavor:** Benzocaine 15 mg, menthol 3.6 mg. Glucose, acesulfame K, propylene glycol, sucrose. Loz. 18s. **Citrus flavor:** Benzocaine 15 mg, menthol 2.1 mg. Maltitol, sucrose. Loz. 18s. **Honey-lemon flavor:** Benzocaine 15 mg, menthol 2.6 mg. Maltitol, sucrose. Loz. 18s. *OTC.*
Use: Mouth and throat product.

Cēpacol Menthol Regular Strength. (Combe) Menthol 3 mg. Glucose, peppermint oil, propylene glycol, sucrose.

Loz. Blister 648s. *OTC.*
Use: Mouth and throat product.

Cēpacol Sore Throat From Post Nasal Drip. (Combe) Menthol 5.4 mg. Glucose, sucrose. Cherry flavor. 18s. *OTC.*
Use: Mouth and throat product.

Cēpacol Sore Throat Pain Relief Maximum Numbing. (Combe) Benzocaine 15 mg, menthol 4 mg. Acesulfame K, maltitol. Sugar free. Cherry flavor. Loz. 16s. *OTC.*
Use: Mouth and throat product.

Cēpacol Sore Throat + Coating Relief Maximum Numbing. (Combe) Benzocaine 15 mg, pectin 5 mg. Acesulfame K. Sugar free. Lemon lime flavor. Loz. 18s. *OTC.*
Use: Mouth and throat product.

Cēpacol Sore Throat Plus Cough Relief. (Combe) Benzocaine 7.5 mg, dextromethorphan HBr 5 mg. Glucose, sucrose. Mixed berry flavor. Loz. 18s. *OTC.*
Use: Nonnarcotic antitussive.

Cēpastat Cherry Lozenges. (GlaxoSmithKline) Phenol 14.5 mg, menthol, sorbitol, saccharin. Sugar free. Loz. Box 18s. *OTC.*
Use: Anesthetic.

Cēpastat Extra Strength. (GlaxoSmithKline) Phenol 29 mg, menthol, sorbitol, eucalyptus oil. Sugar free. Loz. Pkg. 18s. *OTC.*
Use: Anesthetic.

•**cephacetrile sodium.** (SEFF-ah-seh-TRILE) USAN.
Use: Anti-infective, cephalosporin.

•**cephalexin.** (SEFF-ah-LEX-in) *USP.*
Use: Anti-infective, cephalosporin.
See: Keflex.

cephalexin. (Various Mfr.) Cephalexin. **Cap.:** 250 mg, 333 mg, 500 mg, 750 mg. 20s, 40s (250 mg and 500 mg only), 50s (750 mg only), 100s (333 mg, 500 mg, and 750 mg only), 500s, 1,000s, UD 100s (250 mg, 333 mg, and 500 mg only). **Tab.:** 250 mg, 500 mg. Bot. 20s, 100s, 500s. **Pow. for Oral Susp.:** 125 mg/5 mL, 250 mg/5 mL. Bot. 100 mL, 200 mL. *Rx.*
Use: Anti-infective, cephalosporin.

cephalin.
W/Lecithin with Choline Base, Lipositol.
See: Alcolec.

•**cephaloglycin.** (SEFF-ah-low-GLIE-sin) USAN.
Use: Anti-infective.

•**cephaloridine.** (SEFF-ah-lor-ih-deen) USAN.
Use: Anti-infective, cephalosporin.

cephalosporins and related antibiotics.
Use: Antibiotics.
See: Cefaclor.
Cefadroxil.
Cefazolin Sodium.
Cefdinir.
Cefditoren Pivoxil.
Cefepime Hydrochloride.
Cefixime.
Cefmetazole Sodium.
Cefoperazone Sodium.
Cefotaxime Sodium.
Cefotetan Disodium.
Cefoxitin Sodium.
Cefpodoxime Proxetil.
Cefprozil.
Ceftaroline Fosamil.
Ceftazidime.
Ceftibuten.
Ceftizoxime Sodium.
Ceftriaxone Sodium.
Cefuroxime Axetil.
Cephalexin.
Cephradine.

•**cephalothin sodium.** (seff-AY-low-thin) *USP.*
Use: Anti-infective, cephalosporin.

•**cephapirin benzathine.** (SEFF-uh-PIE-rin BEN-zuh-theen) *USP.*

•**cephapirin sodium.** (SEFF-uh-PIE-rin) *USP.*
Use: Anti-infective.

cephazolin sodium.
See: Cefazolin Sodium.

•**cephradine.** (SEFF-ruh-deen) *USP.*
Use: Anti-infective, cephalosporin.

Cephulac. (Hoechst) Lactulose 10 g/15 mL (< galactose 1.6 g, lactose 1.2 g, other sugars 1.2 g). Soln. Bot. 473 mL, 1.9 L, UD 30 mL. *Rx.*
Use: Laxative.

Ceprotin. (Baxter) Protein C concentrate (human) 500 units, 1,000 units. Inj. Lyophilized Pow. for Soln. Single-dose vials. Each vial contains human albumin 8 mg/mL, trisodium citrate dihydrate 4.4 mg/mL, sodium chloride 8.8 mg/mL when reconstituted. *Rx.*
Use: Thrombolytic agent, human protein C.

ceramide trihexosidase/alpha-galactosidase A. (Genzyme)
Use: Fabry disease. [Orphan Drug]

CeraORS 75. (Cera Products) Sodium 2.9 g, potassium 1.5 g, citrate 2.9 g per liter. Gluten free. Pow. for Soln. Packet. *OTC.*
Use: Electrolyte mixture.

Cerapon. (Purdue) Triethanolamine polypeptide oleate condensate.

CeraSport. (Cera Products) Sodium 115 mg, potassium 40 mg per 10.5 g. Gluten free. Citrus flavor. Pow. for Soln. Packet. *OTC.*
Use: Electrolyte mixture.

CeraSport EX1. (Cera Products) Sodium 200 mg, potassium 100 mg per 6 g. Gluten free. Orange flavor. Pow. for Soln. Pouch. *OTC.*
Use: Electrolyte mixture.

CeraVe. (Coria Labs) Caprylic/capric triglyceride, cetyl alcohol, cetearyl alcohol, dimethicone, disodium EDTA, glycerin, parabens, petrolatum. Cream. 453 g. *OTC.*
Use: Emollient.

CeraVe AM. (Coria Labs) Homosalate 12%, octinoxate 7.5%, octocrylene 2%, zinc oxide 3.5%, cetearyl alcohol, dimethicone, disodium EDTA, glycerin, hyaluronic acid, parabens. SPF 30. Lot. 89 mL. *OTC.*
Use: Sunscreen.

CeraVe Moisturizing. (Valeant Pharmaceuticals) Alcohols, caprylic/capric triglyceride, dimethicone, disodium EDTA, glycerin, hyaluronic acid, parabens. Lot. 354 mL. *OTC.*
Use: Emollient.

CeraVe PM. (Coria Labs) Caprylic/capril triglyceride, ceramide, cetearyl alcohol, cholesterol, dimethicone, disodium EDTA, glycerin, glyceryl, hyaluronic acid, methosulfate, niacinamide, parabens. Lot., controlled-release. 89 mL. *OTC.*
Use: Emollient.

CeraVe SA Renewing. (Valeant Pharmaceuticals) Alcohols, cholecalciferol in corn oil, disodium EDTA, glycerin, glyceryl, hyaluronic acid, mineral oil, parabens, salicylic acid, trolamine, PEG, dimethicone. Lot. 237 mL. *OTC.*
Use: Emollient.

Cerebyx. (Pfizer) Fosphenytoin sodium 75 mg/mL (equivalent to phenytoin sodium 50 mg/mL). Inj., Soln.; concentrate. Vial. 2 mL. *Rx.*
Use: Anticonvulsant, hydantoin.

Cerefolin. (Pamlab) Vitamin B_2 5 mg, vitamin B_6 50 mg, vitamin B_{12} 1 mg. L-methylfolate 5.635 mg. Tab. 90s. *Rx.*
Use: Multivitamin.

CerefolinNAC. (Pamlab) Vitamin B_{12} 2,000 mcg, folate 6 mg, N-acetyl-L-cysteine 600 mg, algae-S powder 90.314 mg. PEG. Gluten free, lactose free. Tab. 90s. *Rx.*
Use: Multivitamin.

cerelose.
See: Glucose.

Ceretex. (Enzyme Process) Iron 15 mg, vitamins B_{12} 10 mcg, B_1 2 mg, B_6 1 mg, niacinamide 1 mg, pantothenic acid 0.15 mg, B_2 2 mg, iodine 15 mg/2 mL. Bot. 60 mL, 240 mL. *OTC.*
Use: Mineral, vitamin supplement.

Cerezyme. (Genzyme) Imiglucerase 212 units (equiv. to a withdrawal dose of 200 units) (mannitol 170 mg, sodium citrate 70 mg [trisodium citrate 52 mg, disodium hydrogen citrate 18 mg] per vial), 424 units (equiv. to a withdrawal dose of 400 units) (mannitol 340 mg, sodium citrate 140 mg [trisodium citrate 104 mg, disodium hydrogen citrate 36 mg] per vial). Preservative free. Pow. for Inj., lyophilized. Vials. *Rx.*
Use: Treatment for Gaucher disease.

Cerisa. (Stratus Pharmaceuticals) Sodium sulfacetamide 10%, sulfur 1%. Cetyl alcohol, disodium EDTA, glyceryl stearate, lactic acid, parabens, PEG-100, stearyl alcohol, white petrolatum. Wash. 170.1 g. *Rx.*
Use: Acne product combination.

•**ceritinib.** (se-RI-ti-nib) USAN.
Use: Tyrosine kinase inhibitor.
See: Zykadia.

•**cerlapirdine.** (ser-LA-pir-deen) USAN.
Use: CNS agent.

•**cerlapirdine hydrochloride.** (ser-LA-pir-deen) USAN.
Use: CNS agent.

Cernevit-12. (Baxter Healthcare) Vitamin A 3500 units, D_3 200 units, E (as dl-alpha tocopheryl) 11.2 units, C 125 mg, B_3 46 mg, B_5 17.25 mg, B_6 4.53 mg, B_2 4.14 mg, B_1 3.51 mg, folic acid 414 mcg, d-biotin 60 mcg, B_{12} 5.5 mcg. Pow. for Inj., lyophilized. Single-dose vial 5 mL. *Rx.*
Use: Vitamin supplement.

•**ceronapril.** (seh-ROE-nap-rill) USAN.
Use: Antihypertensive.

Cerovite. (Rugby) Iron 18 mg, vitamins A 5000 units, D 400 units, E 30 units, B_1 1.5 mg, B_2 1.7 mg, B_3 20 mg, B_5 10 mg, B_6 2 mg, B_{12} 6 mcg, C 60 mg, folic acid 0.4 mg, Ca, Cl, Cr, Cu, I, Mg, Mn, Mo, Ni, P, Se, Si, SN, V, biotin 30 mcg, vitamin K, Zn 15 mg. Tab. Bot. 130s. *OTC.*
Use: Mineral, vitamin supplement.

Cerovite Advanced Formula. (Rugby) Iron (as ferrous fumarate) 18 mg, A 3500 units, D 400 units, E 30 units, B_1 1.5 mg, B_2 1.7 mg, B_3 20 mg, B_5 10 mg, B_6 2 mg, B_{12} 6 mcg, C 60 mg, folic acid 0.4 mg, biotin 30 mcg, B, Ca, P, I, Mg, Cu, Mn, K, Cl, Cr, Mo, Se, Ni, Si, Sn, V,

vitamin K, Zn 15 mg, vitamin K_1, lutein, lycopene. Tab. Bot. 130s. *OTC.*
Use: Iron with vitamin supplement.

Cerovite Jr. (Rugby) Iron 18 mg, vitamins A 3,500 units, D 400 units, E 30 units, B_1 1.5 mg, B_2 1.7 mg, B_3 20 mg, B_5 10 mg, B_6 2 mg, B_{12} 6 mcg, C 60 mg, Ca 108 mg, folic acid 0.4 mg, Cu, I, K 10 mcg, Mg, Zn, Mn, Mo, P, biotin 45 mcg, Cr. Aspartame, maltodextrin, mannitol, phenylalanine 4.5 mg, various flavorings. Chew. Tab. 60s. *OTC.*
Use: Mineral, vitamin supplement.

Cerovite Senior. (Rugby) Vitamins A 6000 units, D 400 units, E 45 units, B_1 1.5 mg, B_2 1.7 mg, B_3 20 mg, B_5 10 mg, B_6 3 mg, B_{12} 25 mcg, C 60 mg, iron 9 mg, folic acid 0.2 mg, Ca 200 mg, Zn 15 mg, biotin 30 mcg, Cu, I, Mg, P, Cl, Cr, Mn, Mo, Ni, Se, Si, V, vitamin K. Tab. Bot. 60s. *OTC.*
Use: Mineral, vitamin supplement.

Certagen Liquid. (Ivax) Vitamins A 2500 units, B_1 1.5 mg, B_2 1.7 mg, B_3 20 mg, B_5 10 mg, B_6 2 mg, B_{12} 6 mcg, C 60 mg, D_3 400 units, E 30 units, biotin 300 mcg, iron 9 mg, Zn 3 mg, Cr, I, Mn, Mo/15 mL. Alcohol 6.6%. Liq. Bot. 237 mL. *OTC.*
Use: Mineral, vitamin supplement.

Certagen Tablets. (Ivax) Iron 18 mg, A 5000 units, D 400 units, E 30 units, B_1 1.5 mg, B_2 1.7 mg, B_3 20 mg, B_5 10 mg, B_6 2 mg, B_{12} 6 mcg, C 60 mg, folic acid 0.4 mg, biotin 30 mcg, Ca, P, I, Mg, Cu, Mn, K, Cl, Cr, Mo, Se, Ni, Si, Sn, V, vitamin K, Zn 15 mg. Tab. Bot. 130s, 1000s. *OTC.*
Use: Mineral, vitamin supplement.

CertaVite Senior with Antioxidant Nutrients. (Major) Vitamins A 2,500 units, D 500 units, E 50 units, B_1 1.5 mg, B_2 1.7 mg, B_3 20 mg, B_5 10 mg, B_6 3 mg, B_{12} 25 mcg, C 60 mg, K 30 mcg, folic acid 0.4 mg, B, Ca, Cl, Cr, Cu, I, K, Mg, Mn, Mo, Ni, P, Se, Si, V, Zn, biotin 30 mcg, lutein 250 mcg, lycopene 300 mcg. Gluten free, lactose free, preservative free, sugar free. Tab. 60s. *OTC.*
Use: Multivitamin with minerals (except iron).

CertaVite With Antioxidants. (Major) Iron 3 mg, vitamins E 10 units, B_1 0.5 mg, B_2 0.57 mg, B_3 6.67 mg, B_5 3.33 mg, B_6 0.67 mg, B_{12} 2 mcg, C 20 mg, Cr, I, Mn, Mo, Zn, biotin per 5 mL. BHA, citrus flavoring, EDTA, ethyl alcohol 5.7%, glycerin, lemon flavoring, polysorbate 80, potassium sorbate, propylene glycol, sodium benzoate, sucrose. Liq. 236 mL. *OTC.*
Use: Multivitamin with minerals.

•**certolizumab pegol.** (SER-toe-LIZ-oo-mab PEG-ol)
Use: Immunologic agent, immunomodulator.
See: Cimzia.

Certuss-D. (Capellon) Chlophedianol hydrochloride 25 mg, guaifenesin 400 mg, pseudoephedrine hydrochloride 60 mg. Tab. 90s. *OTC.*
Use: Upper respiratory combination, antitussive and expectorant combination.

Cerubidine. (Bedford) Daunorubicin hydrochloride 21.4 mg (equivalent to daunorubicin 20 mg), mannitol 100 mg. Pow. for Inj., lyophilized. Single-dose vial. *Rx.*
Use: Antibiotic, anthracycline.

•**ceruletide.** (seh-ROO-leh-tide) USAN.
Use: Stimulant, gastric secretory.

•**ceruletide diethylamine.** (seh-ROO-leh-tide die-ETH-ill-ah-meen) USAN.
Use: Stimulant, gastric secretory.

Cervarix. (GlaxoSmithKline) Human papillomavirus (types 16, 18) bivalent vaccine, recombinant ≈ 20 mcg of HPV 16 L1 protein, 20 mcg of HPV 18 L1 protein per 0.5 mL (each 0.5 mL dose contains approximately 50 mcg of 3-O-desacyl-4′-monophosphoryl lipid A [MPL], aluminum hydroxide 0.5 mg, sodium chloride 4.4 mg, sodium dihydrogen phosphate dihydrate 0.624 mg). Preservative free. Inj., Susp. Single-dose vial and prefilled *TIP-LOK* syringes (tip cap and rubber plunger of the needleless prefilled syringes contain dry natural latex rubber). *Rx.*
Use: Agent for active immunization, viral vaccine.

cervical ripening agents.
See: Dinoprostone.

Cervidil. (Forest) Dinoprostone 10 mg. Insert. 1s. *Rx.*
Use: Cervical ripening.

Ces. (ICN) Conjugated estrogens 0.625 mg, 1.25 mg, 2.5 mg. Tab. *Rx.*
Use: Estrogen.

Cesamet. (Meda) Nabilone 1 mg. Corn starch. Cap. 20s. *c-II.*
Use: Antiemetic/antivertigo agent.

Cesia. (Prasco) **Phase 1:** Desogestrel 0.1 mg, ethinyl estradiol 25 mcg. 7 tabs. **Phase 2:** Desogestrel 0.125 mg, ethinyl estradiol 25 mcg. 7 tabs. **Phase 3:** Desogestrel 0.15 mg, ethinyl estradiol 25 mcg. 7 tabs. Lactose, talc. Tab. 28s

with 7 inert tabs. *Rx.*
Use: Contraceptive hormone, sex hormone.

•**cesium chloride Cs 131.** (SEE-zee-uhm KLOR-ide) USAN.
Use: Radiopharmaceutical agent.

Ceta. (C & M Pharmacal) Soap-free. Propylene glycol, hydroxyethylcellulose, cetyl and cetearyl alcohols, sodium lauryl sulfate, parabens. Liq. Bot. 240 mL. *OTC.*
Use: Dermatologic cleanser.

•**cetaben sodium.** (SEE-tah-ben) USAN.
Use: Antihyperlipoproteinemic.

Cetacaine. (Cetylite) Benzocaine 14%, tetracaine hydrochloride 2%, butamben 2%, benzalkonium chloride 0.5%, cetyl dimethyl ethyl ammonium bromide 0.005% in a bland water-soluble base. **Aerosol:** 56 g. **Liq.:** 56 mL. **Oint.:** 37 g. **Gel:** 29 g. *Rx.*
Use: Topical local anesthetic.

Cetacort. (Galderma) Hydrocortisone 0.25%, 0.5%, 1% w/cetyl alcohol, propylene glycol, stearyl alcohol, sodium lauryl sulfate, butylparaben, methylparaben, propylparaben, purified water. Bot. 120 mL (0.25% only), 60 mL (0.5%, 1% only). *Rx.*
Use: Corticosteroid, topical.

Cetafen. (Hart Health & Safety) Acetaminophen 325 mg. Sugar free. Film-coated. Tab. UD 100s, UD 250s. *OTC.*
Use: Analgesic.

Cetafen Extra. (Hart Health & Safety) Acetaminophen 500 mg. Sugar free. Film-coated. Tab. UD 100s. *OTC.*
Use: Analgesic.

Cetaklenz. (Geritrex) Cetyl alcohol, propylene glycol, sodium lauryl sulfate, stearyl alcohol, DMDM hydantoin, parabens. Fragrance free. Cleanser. 120 mL. *OTC.*
Use: Cleanser.

•**cetalkonium chloride.** (SEET-al-KOE-nee-uhm) USAN.
Use: Anti-infective, topical.

•**cetamolol hydrochloride.** (SEET-AM-oh-lahl) USAN.
Use: Anti-adrenergic, beta-receptor.

Cetaphil. (Galderma) **Cream, Lot.:** Cetyl alcohol, stearyl alcohol, propylene glycol (cream only), sodium lauryl sulfate, methylparaben, propylparaben, butylparaben. Bot. 480 g (cream), 120 mL, 240 mL, 480 mL (lotion). **Antibacterial Bar:** Triclosan, petrolatum. Soap-free. 127 g. **Bar:** Petrolatum. Soap-free. 127 g. **Cleanser:** Cetyl alcohol, stearyl alcohol, parabens. Bot. 236 mL. *OTC.*
Use: Dermatologic cleanser.

Cetaphil Daily Advance. (Galderma) Benzyl alcohol, butyrospermum parkii, cetearyl alcohol, glycerin, macadamia seed oil, stearyl alcohol. Lot. 226 g. *OTC.*
Use: Emollient.

Cetazol. (Professional Pharmacal) Acetazolamide 250 mg. Tab. Bot. 100s. *Rx.*
Use: Anticonvulsant; diuretic.

•**cethromycin.** (ceth-roe-MYE-sin) USAN.
Use: Antibacterial.

•**cetiedil citrate.** (see-TIE-eh-DILL SIH-trate) USAN.
Use: Vasodilator, peripheral.

•**cetilistat.** (ce-tye-LI-stat) USAN.
Use: Treatment of obesity.

cetirizine. (Apotex) Cetirizine hydrochloride 5 mg. Lactose. Tab. 100s. *OTC.*
Use: Antihistamine, peripherally selective piperazine.

cetirizine. (Various Mfr.) Cetirizine hydrochloride 10 mg. May contain lactose, polydextrose. Tab. 100s, 300s. *OTC.*
Use: Antihistamine, peripherally selective piperazine.

•**cetirizine hydrochloride.** (seh-TIH-rih-zeen) USAN.
Use: Antihistamine, peripherally selective piperazine.
See: All Day Allergy.
All Day Allergy Children's.
Zyrtec Allergy.
Zyrtec Children's Allergy.
Zyrtec Children's Hives Relief.
Zyrtec Hives Relief.
W/Pseudoephedrine Hydrochloride.
See: All Day Allergy-D.
Zyrtec-D.
Zyrtec-D 12 Hour.

cetirizine hydrochloride. (Various Mfr.) Cetirizine hydrochloride 1 mg/mL. May contain parabens, saccharin, sucrose. Syr. 118 mL, 473 mL. *OTC.*
Use: Antihistamine, peripherally selective piperazine.

•**cetocycline hydrochloride.** (SEE-toe-SIGH-kleen) USAN. *Formerly cetotetrine hydrochloride.*
Use: Anti-infective.

•**cetophenicol.** (see-toe-FEN-ih-kole) USAN.
Use: Antibacterial.

•**cetostearyl alcohol.** (SEE-toe-STEER-il) *NF.*
Use: Pharmaceutic aid, emulsifying agent.

Cetraxal. (WraSer Pharmaceuticals) Ciprofloxacin 0.2%. Preservative free. Soln., Otic. Single-use container. 14s.

Rx.
Use: Otic preparation, otic antibiotic.

•**cetraxate hydrochloride.** (seh-TRAX-ate) USAN.
Use: Antiulcerative; gastrointestinal.

cetrorelix acetate.
Use: Sex hormone; gonadotropin-releasing hormone antagonist.
See: Cetrotide.

Cetrotide. (Serono) Cetrorelix acetate 0.25 mg, 3 mg. Inj. Trays containing 1 vial of 0.26 to 0.27 mg or 3.12 to 3.24 mg cetorelix acetate, 1 mL or 3 mL syr. of Sterile Water for Inj., 20-gauge needle, 27-gauge needle, alcohol swabs. 1s, 7s (0.25 mg only). *Rx.*
Use: Sex hormone; gonadotropin-releasing hormone antagonist.

•**cetuximab.** (seh-TUCKS-ih-mab) USAN.
Use: Monoclonal antibody.
See: Erbitux.

•**cetyl alcohol.** (SEE-till) *NF.*
Use: Pharmaceutic aid, emulsifying and stiffening agent.

Cetylcide Solution. (Cetylite Industries) Cetyldimethylethyl ammonium bromide 6.5%, benzalkonium chloride 6.5%, isopropyl alcohol 13%. Inert ingredients 74%, including sodium nitrite. Bot. 16 oz, 32 oz.
Use: Disinfectant.

•**cetyl esters wax.** (SEE-till ess-ters) *NF. Formerly synthetic spermacet.*
Use: Pharmaceutic aid, stiffening agent.

•**cetylpyridinium chloride.** (SEE-till-pihr-ih-DIH-nee-uhm) *USP.*
Use: Anti-infective, topical; pharmaceutic aid, preservative.
See: Cēpacol.
W/Benzocaine, Menthol.
See: Orasep.

cetyltrimethyl ammonium bromide. (Bioline Labs) Cetrimide B.P., Cetavlon, CTAB.
Use: Antiseptic.

•**cevimeline hydrochloride.** (seh-vih-MEH-leen) USAN.
Use: Treatment of Alzheimer disease, adjunct; dry mouth.
See: Evoxac.

cevimeline hydrochloride. (Various Mfr.) Cevimeline hydrochloride 30 mg. May contain lactose. Cap. 100s, 500s, 1,000s. *Rx.*
Use: Mouth and throat product.

cevitamic acid.
See: Ascorbic Acid.

cevitan.
See: Ascorbic Acid.

Cewin. (Sanofi-Synthelabo) Ascorbic acid. *OTC.*
Use: Vitamin supplement.

Ceylon gelatin.
See: Agar.

Cezin. (Forest) Vitamins B_1 20 mg, B_2 10 mg, B_3 100 mg, B_5 20 mg, B_6 5 mg, C 300 mg, magnesium sulfate 70 mg, zinc sulfate 80 mg. Cap. Bot. 100s. *OTC.*
Use: Vitamin supplement.

Cezin-S. (Forest) Vitamins A 10,000 units, D 50 units, E 50 units, B_1 10 mg, B_2 5 mg, B_3 50 mg, B_5 10 mg, B_6 2 mg, C 200 mg, folic acid 0.5 mg, Zn 18 mg, Mg, Mn. Cap. Bot. 100s. *Rx.*
Use: Vitamin supplement.

C Factors "1000" Plus. (Solgar) Vitamin C 1000 mg, rose hips 25 mg, citrus bioflavonoids complex 250 mg, rutin 50 mg, hesperidin 25 mg. Sodium free, sugar free. Tab. Bot. 50s. *OTC.*
Use: Water-soluble vitamin.

C-500. (Nature's Bounty) Ascorbic acid 500 mg. **Tab.:** Gluten free, lactose free, preservative free, and sugar free. 100s, 250s, 500s. **Cap., timed release:** Sucrose. Gluten free, lactose free, and preservative free. 100s. *OTC.*
Use: Water-soluble vitamin.

C.G. (Sigma-Tau) Chorionic gonadotropin (lyophilized) 10,000 units, mannitol 100 mg, supplied with diluent. Univial 10 mL. *Rx.*
Use: Hormone, chorionic gonadotropin.

CG Disposable Unit.
See: Cardio Green.

C-Gel. (JR Carlson) Ascorbic acid 1,000 mg. Cap., softgels. 60s, 100s, 250s. *OTC.*
Use: Water-soluble vitamin.

CG Ria. (Abbott Diagnostics) Radioimmunoassay for the quantitative measurement of total circulating serum cholylglycine.
Use: Diagnostic aid.

CGU WC. (Elge) Codeine phosphate 6.3 mg, guaifenesin 100 mg per 5 mL. Alcohol and sugar free. PEG, saccharin, sorbitol. Liq. 473 mL. *c-v.*
Use: Upper respiratory combination, antitussive with expectorant.

Chantel Vitamin E. (National Vitamin) dl-alpha tocopheryl acetate, ergocalciferol, cetyl alcohol, panthenol, parabens, safflower oil, urea, vegetable oil. Cream. 454 g. *OTC.*
Use: Emollient.

Chantix. (Pfizer) Varenicline tartrate 0.5 mg (as base), 1 mg (as base). Film-coated. Tab. First-month packs (1 card of eleven 0.5-mg Tab. and 3 cards of

fourteen 1-mg Tab.), Continuing-therapy packs (4 cards of fourteen 1-mg Tab.), Bot. 56s. *Rx.*
Use: Smoking cessation.

Chap Cream. (Ar-Ex) Carbonyl diamide. Cream. Tube 1.5 oz, 3.25 oz. Jar 4 oz, 9 oz, 18 oz. *OTC.*
Use: Emollient.

Chapoline Cream Lotion. (Wade) Glycerin, boric acid, chlorobutanol 0.5%, alcohol 10%. Lot. Bot. 4 oz, pt, gal. *OTC.*
Use: Emollient.

Chapstick Medicated Lip Balm. (Wyeth) **Jar:** Petrolatum 60%, camphor 1%, menthol 0.6%, phenol 0.5%, microcrystalline wax, mineral oil, cocoa butter, lanolin, paraffin wax, parabens 7 g. **Squeezable tube:** Petrolatum 67%, camphor 1%, menthol 0.6%, phenol 0.5%, microcrystalline wax, mineral oil, cocoa butter, lanolin, parabens 10 g. **Stick:** Petrolatum 41%, camphor 1%, menthol 0.6%, phenol 0.5%, paraffin wax, mineral oil, cocoa butter, 2-octyl dodecanol, arachydil propionate, polyphenyl methylsiloxane 556, white wax, oleyl alcohol, isopropyl lanolate, carnuba wax, isopropyl myristate, lanolin, cetyl alcohol, parabens. 4.2 g. *OTC.*
Use: Mouth and throat preparation.

Chapstick Sunblock 15. (Wyeth) Padimate O 0.7%, oxybenzone 3%. Stick 4.25 g. *OTC.*
Use: Lip protectant.

Chapstick Sunblock 15 Petroleum Jelly Plus. (Wyeth) White petrolatum 89%, padimate O 7%, oxybenzone 3%, aloe, lanolin. Stick 10 g. *OTC.*
Use: Lip protectant.

charcoal. (Various Mfr.) Cap., Tab. *OTC.*
Use: Antiflatulent.

•**charcoal, activated.** (CHAR-kole) *USP.*
Use: Antidote, general purpose; pharmaceutic aid, adsorbent.
See: Actidose-Aqua.
Charcocaps.
Kerr Insta-Char.

Charcoal Plus. (Kramer) Activated charcoal 250 mg, sugar. EC Tab. Bot. 120s. *OTC.*
Use: Antiflatulent.

CharcoCaps. (W.F. Young) Activated charcoal 260 mg. Cap. Bot. 36s. *OTC.*
Use: Antiflatulent.

Charo Scatter-Paks. (Requa, Inc.) Activated charcoal 5 g. Packet.
Use: Odor absorbent.

Chateal. (Alfaxys) Ethinyl estradiol 30 mcg, levonorgestrel 0.15 mg. Lactose. Tab. 28s (w/7 inert tablets [lactose]). *Rx.*
Use: Monophasic oral contraceptive.

Chaz Scalp Treatment Dandruff Shampoo. (Revlon) Zinc pyrithione 1% in liquid shampoo. *OTC.*
Use: Antiseborrheic.

Chealamide. (Vortech Pharmaceuticals) Disodium edetate 150 mg/mL. Inj. Vial. 20 mL. *Rx.*
Use: Chelating agent.

Checkmate. (Oral-B) Acidulated phosphate fluoride 1.23%. Bot. 2 oz, 16 oz. *Rx.*
Use: Dental caries agent.

Cheetah. (Mallinckrodt) Barium sulfate 2.2%. Simethicone, sorbitol, saccharin, sodium benzoate. Susp. Bot. 250 mL, 450 mL, 900 mL, 1900 mL. *Rx.*
Use: Radiopaque agent, GI contrast agent.

Chek-Stix Urinalysis Control Strips. (Bayer Consumer Care) Bot. 25s.
Use: Diagnostic aid.

chelafrin.
See: Epinephrine.

Chelated Calcium Magnesium. (NBTY) Ca^{++} 500 mg, Mg 250 mg. Tab. Protein coated. Bot. 50s. *OTC.*
Use: Mineral supplement.

Chelated Calcium Magnesium Zinc. (NBTY) Ca^{++} 333 mg, Mg 133 mg, Zn 8.3 mg. Tab. Bot. 100s. *OTC.*
Use: Mineral supplement.

Chelated Manganese. (Freeda) Manganese 20 mg, 50 mg. Tab. 100s, 250s, 500s. *OTC.*
Use: Mineral supplement.

chelating agents.
See: Deferasirox.
Deferoxamine Mesylate.
Diferiprone.
Dimercaprol.
Edetate Calcium Disodium.
Pentetate Calcium Trisodium.
Pentetate Zinc Trisodium.
Prussian Blue Oral.
Succimer.
Trientine Hydrochloride.

Chelen.
See: Ethyl Chloride.

Chemet. (Recordati Rare Diseases) Succimer 100 mg. Cap. Bot. 100s. *Rx.*
Use: Chelating agent.

Chemipen. Potassium phenethicillin.
Use: Anti-infective, penicillin.

Chemovag. (Forest) Sulfisoxazole 0.5 g. Supp. Bot. 12s w/applicators. *Rx.*
Use: Anti-infective, sulfonamide.

Chemozine. (Tennessee Pharmaceutic) Sulfadiazine, 0.167 g, sulfamerazine 0.167 g, sulfamethazine 0.167 g. Tab.

Bot. 100s, 1000s. Susp. Bot. Pt, gal. *Rx.*
Use: Anti-infective, sulfonamide.

Chemstrip K. (Boehringer Mannheim) Reagent papers for ketones in urine. Paper Bot. 25s, 100s.
Use: Diagnostic aid.

Chemstrip Micral. (Boehringer Mannheim) In vitro reagent strips to detect albumin in urine. Strip Pkg. 5s, 30s.
Use: Diagnostic aid.

Chemstrip Mineral. (Boehringer Mannheim) In vitro reagent strips used to detect albumin in urine. Strip Pkg. 5s, 30s.
Use: In vitro diagnostic aid.

Chemstrip 9. (Boehringer Mannheim) Broad range test for glucose, protein, pH, blood, ketones, bilirubin, urobilinogen, nitrite, leukocytes in urine. Strip Bot. 100s.
Use: Diagnostic aid.

Chemstrip 7. (Boehringer Mannheim) Broad range test for glucose, protein, pH, blood, ketones, bilirubin, leukocytes. Strip Bot. 100s.
Use: Diagnostic aid.

Chemstrip 10 SG. (Boehringer Mannheim) Broad range test for glucose, protein, pH, blood, ketones, bilirubin, urobilinogen, nitrite, leukocytes in urine. Strip Bot. 100s.
Use: Diagnostic aid.

Chemstrip 2 GP. (Boehringer Mannheim) Broad range test for glucose and protein. Strip Bot. 100s.
Use: Diagnostic aid.

Chemstrip 2 LN. (Boehringer Mannheim) Broad range test for nitrite and leukocytes. Strip Bot. 100s.
Use: Diagnostic aid.

Chemstrip uGK. (Boehringer Mannheim) Broad range test for glucose and ketones. Strip Bot. 50s, 100s.
Use: Diagnostic aid.

Chenatal. (Miller Pharmacal Group) Calcium 580 mg, Mg 200 mg, vitamins C 100 mg, folic acid 0.4 mg, A 5000 units, D 400 units, B_1 3 mg, B_2 3 mg, B_6 5 mg, B_{12} 9 mcg, niacinamide 30 mg, pantothenic acid 5 mg, tocopherols (mixed) 10 mg, Fe 20 mg, Cu 1 mg, Mn 2 mg, K 10 mg, Zn 25 mg, I 0.1 mg. 2 Tabs. Bot. 100s. *OTC.*
Use: Mineral, vitamin supplement.

Chenix. (Solvay) Chenodil.
Use: Anticholelithogenic. [Orphan Drug]

Chenodal. (Manchester Pharmaceuticals) Chenodiol 250 mg. Film coated. Tab. 100s. *Rx.*
Use: Gallstone solubilizing agent.

chenodeoxycholic acid.
Use: Urolithic.
See: Chenodiol.

•**chenodiol.** (KEEN-oh-DIE-ahl) USAN.
Formerly chenic acid.
Use: Anticholelithogenic.
See: Chenodal.

Cheracol. (Lee Pharmaceuticals) Codeine phosphate 10 mg, guaifenesin 100 mg/5 mL, alcohol 4.75%. Bot. 2 oz, 4 oz, pt. *c-v.*
Use: Antitussive; expectorant.

Cheracol Cough. (Lee Pharmaceuticals) Codeine phosphate 10 mg, guaifenesin 100 mg per 5 mL. Alcohol 4.75%, fructose, sucrose. Syr. Bot. 60 mL, 120 mL, 480 mL. *c-v.*
Use: Upper respiratory combination, antitussive, expectorant.

Cheracol D Cough Formula. (Lee Pharmaceuticals) Dextromethorphan HBr 10 mg, guaifenesin 100 mg per 5 mL. Alcohol 4.75%, fructose, sucrose. Syrup. Bot. 118 mL, 180 mL. *OTC.*
Use: Upper respiratory combination, antitussive with expectorant.

Cheracol Plus. (Lee Pharmaceuticals) Dextromethorphan HBr 10 mg, guaifenesin 100 mg per 5 mL. Alcohol 4.75%, fructose, sucrose. Liq. Bot. 118 mL. *OTC.*
Use: Upper respiratory combination, antitussive with expectorant.

Cheracol Sore Throat. (Lee Pharmaceuticals) Phenol 1.4%, saccharin, sorbitol, alcohol 12.5%. Spray Bot. 180 mL. *OTC.*
Use: Mouth and throat product.

Cheratussin AC Expectorant Cough Suppressant. (Qualitest Pharmaceuticals) Codeine phosphate 10 mg, guaifenesin 100 mg per 5 mL. Sugar free. Alcohol 3.5%, saccharin, sorbitol. Syrup. 118 mL, 236 mL, 473 mL, 3785 mL. *c-v.*
Use: Antitussive with expectorant, upper respiratory combination.

Cheratussin DAC. (Qualitest) Codeine phosphate 10 mg, guaifenesin 100 mg, pseudoephedrine hydrochloride 30 mg per 5mL. Alcohol 2.1%. Menthol, saccharin, sorbitol. Sugar free. Soln. 473 mL. *c-v.*
Use: Upper respiratory combination; analgesic, expectorant, decongestant.

Chero-Trisulfa-V. (Vita Elixir) Sulfadiazine 0.166 g, sulfacetamide 0.166 g, sulfamerazine 0.166 g, sodium citrate 0.5 g/5 mL. Susp. Bot. Pt.
Use: Anti-infective, sulfonamide.

•**cherry juice.** *NF.*
Use: Flavoring.

•**cherry syrup.** *NF.*
Use: Pharmaceutic aid, vehicle.

Chest Throat. (Lane) Eucalyptol, anise, horehound, tolu balsam, benzoin tincture, sugar, corn syrup. Loz. Pkg. 30s. *OTC.*
Use: Antiseptic.

Chewable Multivitamins w/Fluoride. (H.L. Moore Drug Exchange) Fluoride 1 mg, vitamins A 2500 units, D 400 units, E 15 units, B_1 1.05 mg, B_2 1.2 mg, B_3 13.5 mg, B_6 1.05 mg, B_{12} 4.5 mcg, C 60 mg, folic acid 0.3 mg, sucrose. Tab. Bot. 100s. *Rx.*
Use: Mineral, vitamin supplement; dental caries agent.

Chewable Vitamin C. (Various Mfr.) Vitamin C (as sodium ascorbate and ascorbic acid) 250 mg, 500 mg. Chew. Tab. Bot. 100s. *OTC.*
Use: Water-soluble vitamin.

Chew-C. (Key Company) Vitamin C (as ascorbic acid and sodium ascorbate) 500 mg. Sugar. Orange flavor. Chew. Tab. 100s. *OTC.*
Use: Water-soluble vitamin.

Chew-Vims. (Barth's) Vitamins A 5000 units, D 400 units, B_1 3 mg, B_2 6 mg, niacin 1.71 mg, C 100 mg, B_{12} 5 mcg, E 5 units. Tab. Bot. 30s, 90s, 180s, 360s. *OTC.*
Use: Water-soluble vitamin.

Chew-Vi-Tab. (Halsey Drug) Vitamins A 2500 units, D 400 units, E 15 units, C 60 mg, folic acid 0.3 mg, B_1 1.05 mg, B_2 1.2 mg, niacin 13.5 mg, B_6 1.05 mg, B_{12} 4.5 mcg. Tab. Bot. 100s. *OTC.*
Use: Vitamin supplement.

Chew-Vi-Tab with Iron. (Halsey Drug) Vitamins A 5000 units, C 60 mg, E 15 units, folic acid 0.4 mg, B_1 1.5 mg, B_2 1.7 mg, niacin 20 mg, B_6 2 mg, B_{12} 6 mcg, D 400 units, iron 18 mg. Tab. Bot. 100s. *OTC.*
Use: Mineral, vitamin supplement.

chicken pox vaccine.
See: Varivax.

Chigg Away. (Pierson Labs) Benzocaine 5%, sulfur 10%. Cetyl alcohol, glycerin, glyceryl, isopropyl alcohol, parabens, petrolatum, triethanolamine. Lot. 118 mL. *OTC.*
Use: Local anesthetic, topical combination.

Chiggerex. (Scherer) Benzocaine with camphor, menthol. Oint. 50 g. *OTC.*
Use: Topical local anesthetic.

Children's Advil. (Wyeth) Ibuprofen 100 mg/5 mL. Sorbitol, sucrose, EDTA, fruit flavor. Susp. Bot. 119 mL, 473 mL. *OTC.*
Use: Analgesic, NSAID.

Children's Advil. (Wyeth) Ibuprofen 50 mg. Aspartame, phenylalanine 2.1 mg, fruit and grape flavor. Chew. Tab. Bot. 24s, 50s. *OTC.*
Use: Analgesic, NSAID.

Children's Advil Cold. (Wyeth) Pseudoephedrine hydrochloride 15 mg, ibuprofen 100 mg per 5 mL. Sorbitol, sucrose. Alcohol free. Grape flavor. Susp. 120 mL. *OTC.*
Use: Decongestant and analgesic.

Children's Dimaphen DM. (Major) Brompheniramine maleate 1 mg, dextromethorphan hydrobromide 5 mg, phenylephrine hydrochloride 2.5 mg. Sodium 3 mg, sorbitol, sucralose. Alcohol free. Grape flavor. Elix. 118 mL. *OTC.*
Use: Upper respiratory combination, antitussive combination.

Children's Elixir DM Cough & Cold. (AmerisourceBergen) Pseudoephedrine hydrochloride 15 mg, brompheniramine maleate 1 mg, dextromethorphan HBr 5 mg per 5 mL. Saccharin, sorbitol, grape flavor, alcohol free. Elixir. Bot. 118 mL. *OTC.*
Use: Upper respiratory combination, decongestant, antihistamine, antitussive.

Children's Formula Cough. (Pharmakon) Guaifenesin 50 mg, dextromethorphan HBr 5 mg/5 mL, sucrose, corn syrup. Alcohol free. Grape flavor. Syr. Bot. 118 mL, 236 mL. *OTC.*
Use: Expectorant; antitussive.

Children's Ibuprofen Cold. (Major) Pseudoephedrine hydrochloride 15 mg, ibuprofen 100 mg/5 mL. Alcohol-free. Corn syrup. Berry flavor. Susp. 120 mL. *OTC.*
Use: Decongestant, analgesic.

Children's Kaopectate. (Pharmacia) Attapulgite 600 mg/5 mL. Liq. Bot. 180 mL. *OTC.*
Use: Antidiarrheal.

Children's Loratadine. (Taro) Loratadine 5 mg per 5 mL. Fruit flavor. Syrup. 120 mL. *OTC.*
Use: Antihistamine, peripherally selective piperidine.

Children's Motrin. (McNeil Consumer) Ibuprofen. **Chew. Tab.:** 50 mg. Aspartame, phenylalanine 3 mg, orange flavor. Bot. 24s. **Susp.:** 100 mg/5 mL. Sucrose. Grape and bubble gum flavors. Bot. 60 mL, 120 mL. *OTC.*
Use: Analgesic, NSAID.

Children's Motrin Cold. (McNeil Consumer) Ibuprofen 100 mg, pseudo-

ephedrine hydrochloride 15 mg/5 mL. Dye free. Acesulfame K, sucralose, sucrose. Berry, grape, or tropical punch flavors. Susp. 118 mL. *OTC.*
Use: Analgesic and decongestant, upper respiratory combination.

Children's NasalCrom. (Pharmacia) Cromolyn sodium 40 mg/mL (cromolyn sodium 5.2 mg/spray), benzalkonium chloride 0.01%, EDTA 0.01%. Spray. Bot. 13 mL, 26 mL. *OTC.*
Use: Analgesic; prophylactic.

Children's No Aspirin Elixir. (Walgreen) Acetaminophen 80 mg/2.5 mL. Nonalcoholic. Elix. Bot. 4 oz. *OTC.*
Use: Analgesic.

Children's No-Aspirin Tablets. (Walgreen) Acetaminophen 80 mg. Tab. Bot. 30s. *OTC.*
Use: Analgesic.

Children's Probiotic Pearls. (Integrative Therapeutics) 500 million CFU blend of *L. acidophilus, L. casei, L. reuteri, L. rhamnosus, B. longum.* Vegetable glycerin, vegetable oil. Preservative free, sugar free. Cap. 30s. *OTC.*
Use: Probiotic.

Children's Probiotic with Acidophilus. (Windmill) 75 million CFU blend of *L. sporogenes, B. bifidum, L. acidophilus, B. longum, L. casei, L. rhamnosus.* Sucralose. Preservative free and sugar free. Raspberry flavor. Chew. Tab. 100s. *OTC.*
Use: Probiotic.

Children's Silfedrine. (Silarx) Pseudoephedrine hydrochloride 30 mg/5 mL. Liq. Bot. 118 mL. *OTC.*
Use: Decongestant, nasal.

Children's Sunkist Multivitamins Complete. (Novartis) Iron 18 mg, vitamin A 5000 units, D_3 400 units, E 30 units, B_1 1.5 mg, B_2 1.7 mg, B_3 20 mg, B_5 10 mg, B_6 2 mg, B_{12} 6 mcg, C 60 mg, folic acid 0.4 mg, Ca, Cu, I, K, Mg, Mn, P, Zn 10 mg, biotin 40 mcg, vitamin K, sorbitol, aspartame, phenylalanine, tartrazine. Chew. Tab. Bot. 60s. *OTC.*
Use: Mineral, vitamin supplement.

Children's Sunkist Multivitamins + Extra C. (Novartis) Vitamin A 2500 units, E 15 units, D_3 400 units, B_1 1.05 mg, B_2 1.2 mg, B_3 13.5 mg, B_6 1.05 mg, B_{12} 4.5 mcg, C 250 mg, folic acid 0.3 mg, vitamin K_1 5 mcg, sorbitol, aspartame, phenylalanine, tartrazine. Chew. Tab. Bot. 60s. *OTC.*
Use: Mineral, vitamin supplement.

Children's Ty-Tabs. (Major) Acetaminophen 80 mg. Tab. Bot. 100s, 1000s. *OTC.*
Use: Analgesic.

Chinese gelatin.
See: Agar.

Chinese isinglass.
Use: Amebicide.

chiniofon.
Use: Amebicide.

Chinositol. (Vernon) 8-Hydroxyquinoline sulfate 7.5 g. Tab. Vial 6s. Trit. Tab. (600 mg) Bot. 50s. Vial 110s. Pow. 1 oz.
Use: Antiseptic.

ChiRhoStim. (ChiRhoClin) Secretin 16 mcg, 40 mcg. Mannitol 20 mg (16 mcg), 50 mg (40 mcg), L-cysteine 1.5 mg (16 mcg), 3.75 mg (40 mcg). Inj. lyophilized Pow. for Soln. Vial. *Rx.*
Use: Diagnostic aid, gastrointestinal function test.

chlamydia trachomatis test.
Use: Diagnostic aid.
See: MicroTrak.

Chlamydiazyme. (Abbott Diagnostics) Enzyme immunoassay for detection of *Chlamydia trachomatis* from urethral or urogenital swabs. Test Kit 100s.
Use: Diagnostic aid.

•**chlophedianol hydrochloride.** (KLOE-fee-DIE-ah-nole) USAN.
Use: Antitussive.
W/Brompheniramine Maleate, Pseudoephedrine Hydrochloride.
See: Dicel CD.
W/Chlorcyclizine Hydrochloride.
See: Biclora.
W/Chlorcyclizine Hydrochloride, Pseudoephedrine Hydrochloride.
See: Biclora-D.
W/Chlorpheniramine Maleate, Pseudoephedrine Hydrochloride.
See: DryMax AF.
W/Dexbrompheniramine Maleate, Pseudoephedrine Hydrochloride.
See: Chlo Tuss.
W/Guaifenesin.
See: Chlo Tuss Ex.
W/Guaifenesin, Phenylephrine Hydrochloride.
See: Vanacof GPE.
W/Guaifenesin, Pseudoephedrine Hydrochloride.
See: Certuss-D.
Vanacof Dx.
W/Phenylephrine Hydrochloride, Thonzylamine Hydrochloride.
See: Vanacof APE.
W/Pseudoephedrine Hydrochloride.
See: Clofera.
W/Pyrilamine Maleate.
See: Vanacof-8.
W/Triprolidine Hydrochloride.
See: ProHist CF.

Chloracol 0.5%. (Horizon) Chlorampheni-

col 5 mg/mL with chlorobutanol, hydroxypropyl methylcellulose. Dropper bot. 7.5 mL. *Rx.*
Use: Anti-infective, ophthalmic.

Chlorafed. (Roberts) Chlorpheniramine maleate 2 mg, pseudoephedrine hydrochloride 30 mg/5 mL, alcohol, dye, sugar, and corn free. Liq. Bot. 120 mL, 480 mL. *OTC.*
Use: Antihistamine; decongestant.

Chlorafed H.S. Timecelles. (Roberts) Chlorpheniramine maleate 4 mg, pseudoephedrine hydrochloride 60 mg. SR Cap. Bot. 100s. *Rx.*
Use: Antihistamine; decongestant.

Chlorafed Timecelles. (Roberts) Chlorpheniramine maleate 8 mg, pseudoephedrine hydrochloride 120 mg. SA Timecelles. Bot. 100s. *Rx.*
Use: Antihistamine; decongestant.

Chlorahist. (Evron) Chlorpheniramine maleate. **Tab:** 4 mg. Bot. 100s, 1000s. **Cap:** 8 mg, 12 mg. Bot. 250s, 1000s. **Syr:** 2 mg/4 mL. Bot. qt. *Rx-OTC.*
Use: Antihistamine.

•**chloral betaine.** (KLOR-uhl BEE-tah-een) USAN.
Use: Hypnotic; sedative.

•**chloral hydrate.** (KLOR-uhl HIGH-drate) *USP.*
Use: Hypnotic/sedative, nonbarbiturate.
See: Somnote.

chloral hydrate. (Various Mfr.) Chloral hydrate 500 mg. Cap. 100s, 500s, 1,000s, UD 100s. *c-IV.*
Use: Hypnotic/sedative, nonbarbiturate.

chloral hydrate betaine (1:1) compound. Chloral Betaine.

chloralpyrine dichloralpyrine.
See: Dichloralantipyrine.

chloralurethane. *Name used for Carbochloral.*

•**chlorambucil.** (klor-AM-byoo-sill) *USP.*
Use: Antineoplastic; alkylating agent; nitrogen mustard.
See: Leukeran.

Chloramine-T. Sodium paratoluenesulfan chloramide, chloramine, chlorozone. **Eli Lilly:** Tab. (0.3 g), Bot. 100s, 1000s. **Robinson:** Pow., 1 oz.
Use: Antiseptic; deodorant.
See: Chlorazene.

•**chloramphenicol.** (KLOR-am-FEN-ih-kole) *USP.*
Use: Anti-infective; antirickettsial; treatment of superficial ocular infections involving the conjunctiva or cornea caused by susceptible organisms.
W/Hydrocortisone Acetate.
See: Chloromycetin/Hydrocortisone.

•**chloramphenicol palmitate.** (KLOR-am-FEN-ih-kahl pal-mih-tate) *USP.*
Use: Anti-infective; antirickettsial.

•**chloramphenicol pantothenate complex.** (KLOR-am-FEN-ih-kahl PAN-toe-THEH-nate) USAN.
Use: Anti-infective; antirickettsial.

•**chloramphenicol sodium succinate.** (KLOR-am-FEN-ih-kahl) *USP.*
Use: Anti-infective; antirickettsial.
See: Mychel-S.

chloramphenicol sodium succinate. (Various Mfr.) Chloramphenicol sodium succinate 100 mg/mL. Inj. Vial. 1 g in 15 mL.
Use: Anti-infective; antirickettsial.

ChloraPrep One-Step. (CareFusion) Chlorhexidine gluconate 2% w/70% isopropyl alcohol. Soln.; topical. 3 mL. *OTC.*
Use: Topical anti-infective, antiseptic and germicide.

Chlorascrub. (PDI) Chlorhexidine gluconate 3.15% with isopropyl alcohol 70%. Swab; top. 1 mL. *OTC.*
Use: Topical anti-infective, antiseptic and germicide.

Chlorascrub Maxi Swabstick. (PDI) Chlorhexidine gluconate 3.15% with isopropyl alcohol 70%. Swab; top. 5.1 mL. *OTC.*
Use: Topical anti-infective, antiseptic and germicide.

Chlorascrub Swabstick. (PDI) Chlorhexidine gluconate 3.15% with isopropyl alcohol 70%. Swab; top. 1.6 mL. *OTC.*
Use: Topical anti-infective, antiseptic and germicide.

Chloraseptic Children's. (Prestige) Benzocaine 5 mg. Loz. Pkg. 18s. *OTC.*
Use: Anesthetic, local.

Chloraseptic Kids' Sore Throat. (Prestige) Benzocaine 2 mg, menthol 2 mg. Glycerin, sucralose. Strips. 20s. *OTC.*
Use: Mouth and throat products.

Chloraseptic Kids' Sore Throat. (Prestige) Phenol 0.5%. Sugar and alcohol free. Saccharin. Grape flavor. Spray. Bot. 177 mL. *OTC.*
Use: Mouth and throat product.

Chloraseptic Liquid. (Prestige) Total phenol 1.4% as phenol and sodium phenolate, saccharin. Menthol and cherry flavors. Liq. Bot. 180 mL, 360 mL (mouthwash/gargle); 45 mL, 240 mL, 360 mL (throat spray). *OTC.*
Use: Anesthetic; antiseptic, local.

Chloraseptic Lozenge. (Prestige) Total phenol 32.5 mg as phenol and sodium phenolate. Menthol and cherry flavors. Pkg. 18s, 36s. *OTC.*
Use: Anesthetic; antiseptic.

Chloraseptic Sore Throat. (Prestige) Acetaminophen 166.6 mg per 5 mL. Corn syrup, menthol, saccharin, sorbitol. Cherry flavor. Liq. 283 mL. *OTC.*
Use: Analgesic.
Chloraseptic Sore Throat. (Prestige) **Loz.:** Benzocaine 6 mg, menthol 10 mg. Pkg. 18s. **Spray:** Phenol 1.4%. Saccharin. Alcohol free. Cherry, mint, menthol, and citrus flavors. 177 mL. *OTC.*
Use: Mouth and throat product.
Chloraseptic Sore Throat Relief. (Prestige) Benzocaine 3 mg, menthol 3 mg. Acesulfame, sucralose. Cherry and citrus flavors. Strips. 40s. *OTC.*
Use: Mouth and throat products.
Chloraseptic Total Sore Throat + Cough. (Medtech) Benzocaine 6 mg, dextromethorphan hydrobromide 5 mg. Corn syrup, glycerin, menthol 10 mg, soy, sucrose. Wild cherry flavor. Loz. 15s. *OTC.*
Use: Nonnarcotic antitussive.
Chloraseptic Warming Sore Throat. (Prestige) Phenol 1.4%. Glycerin, saccharin, sucralose, tartrazine. Alcohol free and sugar free. Honey lemon flavor. Throat spray. 177 mL. *OTC.*
Use: Mouth and throat product.
Chlorazene. (Badger) Chloramine-T, sodium p-toluene-sulfonchloramide. **Pow.:** UD Pkg. 20 g, 38 g, 50 g, 88 g, 200 g, 240 g, 320 g, Bot. 1 lb, 5 lb. **Aromatic Pow. (5%):** Bot. 1 lb, 5 lb. **Tab. (0.3 g):** Bot. 20s, 100s, 1000s, 5000s. *OTC.*
Use: Antiseptic; deodorant.
chlorazepate dipotassium.
See: Clorazepate Dipotassium.
chlorazepate monopotassium.
See: Clorazepate Monopotassium.
Chlorazine. (Major) Prochlorperazine 5 mg, 10 mg. Tab. Bot. 100s.
Use: Antiemetic; antipsychotic; antivertigo.
chlorbutanol.
See: Chlorobutanol.
chlorbutol.
See: Chlorobutanol.
•**chlorcyclizine hydrochloride.** (klor-SIK-lih-zeen) *NF.*
Use: Antihistamine.
See: Ahist.
W/Chlophedianol Hydrochloride.
See: Biclora.
W/Chlophedianol Hydrochloride, Pseudoephedrine Hydrochloride.
See: Biclora-D.
W/Codeine Phosphate.
See: Poly-Tussin.
W/Codeine Phosphate, Phenylephrine Hydrochloride.
See: Nasotuss.
W/Codeine Phasphate, Pseudoephedrine Hydrochloride.
See: Poly-Tussin D.
W/Phenylephrine Hydrochloride.
See: Dallergy.
W/Pseudoephedrine Hydrochloride.
See: NasOpen.
Stahist AD.
•**chlordantoin.** (KLOR-dan-toe-in) USAN.
Use: Antifungal.
Chlordex GP. (Cypress) Dextromethorphan HBr 7.5 mg, guaifenesin 100 mg, phenylephrine hydrochloride 10 mg, chlorpheniramine maleate 2 mg per 5 mL. Alcohol and sugar free. Saccharin, sorbitol. Grape flavor. Syrup. 473 mL. *Rx.*
Use: Upper respiratory combination, antitussive and expectorant combination.
•**chlordiazepoxide.** (klor-DIE-aze-ee-POX-side) *USP.*
Tall Man: chlordiazePOXIDE
Use: Anxiolytic.
See: Brigen-G.
W/Amitriptyline.
See: Limbitrol.
Limbitrol DS.
•**chlordiazepoxide hydrochloride.** (klor-DIE-aze-ee-POX-ide) *USP.*
Tall Man: chlordiazePOXIDE
Use: Hypnotic; sedative; anxiolytic.
W/Clidinium Bromide.
See: Librax.
RE Chlordiazepoxide/Clidinium.
chlordiazepoxide hydrochloride. (Various Mfr.) Chlordiazepoxide hydrochloride 5 mg, 10 mg, 25 mg. Cap. 20s, 100s, 500s, 1000s, UD 100s. *c-iv.*
Use: Anxiolytic.
chlordiazepoxide with clidinium bromide. (Various Mfr.) Clidinium 2.5 mg, chlordiazepoxide hydrochloride 5 mg. Cap. Bot. 100s, 500s, 1000s, UD 100s. *Rx.*
Use: Gastrointestinal anticholinergic combination.
Chlordrine S.R. (Rugby) Pseudoephedrine hydrochloride 120 mg, chlorpheniramine maleate 8 mg. SR Cap. Bot. 100s. *Rx.*
Use: Antihistamine; decongestant.
Chloren 8 T.D. (Wren) Chlorpheniramine maleate 8 mg. Tab. Bot. 100s, 1000s. *OTC.*
Use: Antihistamine.
Chloren 12 T.D. (Wren) Chlorpheniramine

maleate 12 mg. Tab. Bot. 100s, 1000s. *Rx-OTC.*
Use: Antihistamine.

Chloresium Tooth Paste. (Rystan) Chlorophyllin copper complex. Tube 3.25 oz. *OTC.*
Use: Deodorant, oral.

chlorethyl.
See: Ethyl Chloride.

chlorguanide hydrochloride.
See: Chloroguanide Hydrochloride.

•**chlorhexidine gluconate.** (klor-HEX-ih-deen GLUE-koe-nate) USAN.
Use: Antimicrobial.
See: Bacto Shield.
Bacto Shield 2.
Biopatch.
Chloraprep One-Step.
Chlorascrub.
Chlorascrub Maxi Swabstick.
Chlorascrub Swabstick.
Hibistat.
Peridex.
PerioChip.
PerioGard.
Surgilube.

chlorhexidine gluconate. (Various Mfr.) Chlorhexidine gluconate. **Oral rinse:** 0.12%. 473 mL. **Cloth:** 2%. Aloe vera, glycerin. Alednol free. 6s. *Rx.*
Use: Mouth and throat product.

chlorhexidine gluconate mouthrinse.
Use: Amelioration of oral mucositis associated with cytoreductive therapy for conditioning patients for bone marrow transplantation. [Orphan Drug]
See: Peridex.
PerioGard.

•**chlorhexidine hydrochloride.** (klor-HEX-ih-deen) USAN.
Use: Anti-infective, topical.

•**chlorhexidine phosphanilate.** (klor-HEX-ih-deen FOSS-fah-nih-LATE) USAN.
Use: Anti-infective.

chlorinated and iodized peanut oil. Chloriodized oil.

•**chlorindanol.** (klor-IN-dah-nahl) USAN.
Use: Antiseptic, spermaticide.

chlorine compound, antiseptic. Antiseptic, chlorine.

chloriodized oil. Chlorinated and iodized peanut oil.

•**chlormadinone acetate.** (klor-MAD-ih-nohn) USAN.
Use: Hormone, progestin.

Chlor Mal w/Sal + APAP S.C. (Global Source) Chlorpheniramine maleate 2 mg, acetaminophen 150 mg, salicylamide 175 mg. Tab. Bot. 1000s. *OTC.*
Use: Analgesic; antihistamine.

chlormerodrin. Mercloran. *Rx.*
Use: Diuretic.

•**chlormerodrin Hg 197.** (klor-MER-oh-drin) USAN.
Use: Diagnostic aid, renal function determination; radiopharmaceutical.

•**chlormerodrin Hg 203.** (klor-MER-oh-drin) USAN.
Use: Diagnostic aid, renal function determination; radiopharmaceutical.

chlormezanone. Chlormethazanone.
Use: Anxiolytic.

Chlor-Niramine Allergy Tabs. (Whiteworth Towne) Chlorpheniramine maleate 4 mg. Tab. Bot. 24s, 100s. *OTC.*
Use: Antihistamine.

chloroacetic acids.
See: Monochloroacetic Acid.

•**chlorobutanol.** (Klor-oh-BYOO-tah-nole) *NF.*
Use: Anesthetic; antiseptic; hypnotic; pharmaceutic aid, antimicrobial.

W/Combinations.
See: Ardeben.
Depo-Testadiol.
Efedron NaSal.
Lacril.
Lacri-Lube.
Minirin.
Pred-G.

•**chlorocresol.** (KLOR-oh-KREE-sole) *NF.*
Use: Antiseptic; disinfectant.

chloroethane.
Use: Anticholinergic; antispasmodic; topical anesthetic.
See: Gebauer's Ethyl Chloride.

Chlorofair. (Bausch & Lomb) **Soln.:** Chloramphenicol 5 mg/mL. Bot. 7.5 mL. **Oint.:** Chloramphenicol 10 mg/g in white petrolatum base with mineral oil, polysorbate 60. Tube 3.5 g. *Rx.*
Use: Anti-infective, ophthalmic.

chloroguanide hydrochloride. (Various Mfr.) Proguanil hydrochloride. *Rx.*
Use: Antimalarial.

Chlorohist-LA. (Roberts) Xylometazoline hydrochloride 0.1%. Soln. Spray 15 mL. *OTC.*
Use: Decongestant.

Chloromag. (Merit) Magnesium chloride hexahydrate 200 mg/mL (1.97 mEq/mL). Benzyl alcohol 1%, sodium chloride 9 mg. Inj., Soln. Multiple-dose vials. 50 mL. *Rx.*
Use: Intravenous nutritional therapy, mineral.

chloromethapyrilene citrate.
See: Chlorothen Citrate.

Chloromycetin/Hydrocortisone. (Parke-Davis) Hydrocortisone acetate 0.5% (2.5% as powder), chloramphenicol 0.25% (1.25% as powder). Pow. Bot. with dropper 5 mL. *Rx.*
Use: Anti-infective, ophthalmic.

chlorophenothane.
Use: Pediculicide.

chlorophyll. (Freeda) Chlorophyll 20 mg, sugar free. Tab. Bot. 100s, 250s, 500s. *OTC.*
Use: Deodorant, oral.

chlorophyll derivatives, systemic.
See: Chlorophyll.
Derifil.

chlorophyllin.
Use: Deodorant; healing agent.

•**chlorophyllin copper complex.** (KLOR-oh-FILL-in KAHP-uhr) USAN.
Use: Deodorant.
See: Chloresium.
Derifil.
Nullo.
PALS.

•**chlorophyllin copper complex sodium.** (KLOR-oh-FILL-in KAHP-uhr) *USP.*
Use: Deodorant.

•**chloroprocaine hydrochloride.** (klor-oh-PRO-cane) *USP.*
Use: Anesthetic, local ester, injectable.
See: Nesacaine.
Nesacaine-MPF.

chloroprocaine hydrochloride. (Bedford) Chloroprocaine hydrochloride 2% (20 mg/mL), 3% (30 mg/mL). Preservative-free. Inj. Single-dose vials. 20 mL. *Rx.*
Use: Anesthetic, local ester, injectable.

•**chloroquine.** (KLOR-oh-kwin) *USP.*
Use: Antiamebic; antimalarial.

•**chloroquine phosphate.** (KLOR-oh-kwin) *USP.*
Use: Antiamebic; antimalarial; lupus erythematosus agent.
See: Aralen Phosphate.

chloroquine phosphate. (Ranbaxy) Chloroquine phosphate (equiv. to 300 mg base). Film coated. PEG. Tab. 10s, 25s, 500s. *Rx.*
Use: Antimalarial preparation, 4-aminoquinoline compound.

chloroquine phosphate. (Various Mfr.) Chloroquine phosphate 250 mg (equiv. to 150 mg base), 500 mg (equiv. to 300 mg base). May contain lactose (500 mg only). Tab. Bot. 20s, 22s (250 mg only); 25s (500 mg only); 30s (250 mg only); 100s; 500s (500 mg only); 1000s, UD 100s (250 mg only). *Rx.*
Use: Amebicide.

chlorothen.
Use: Antihistamine.

chlorothen citrate. (Whittier) Chlorothen citrate. Tab. Bot. 100s.
Use: Antihistamine.
W/Pyrilamine, Thenylpyramine.
See: Derma-Pax.

chlorothenylpyramine. Chlorothen.

•**chlorothiazide.** (KLOR-oh-THIGH-uh-zide) *USP.*
Use: Diuretic.
See: Diuril.
W/Methyldopa.
See: Aldoclor.

chlorothiazide. (Various Mfr.) Chlorothiazide 250 mg, 500 mg. Tab. 100s. *Rx.*
Use: Diuretic.

•**chlorothiazide sodium for injection.** (KLOR-oh-THIGH-uh-zide) *USP.*
Use: Antihypertensive; diuretic.

chlorothymol.
Use: Anti-infective.

•**chlorotrianisene.** (klor-oh-try-AN-ih-seen) *USP.*
Use: Estrogen.

•**chloroxine.** (KLOR-ox-een) USAN.
Use: Topical anti-infective.

•**chloroxylenol.** (KLOR-oh-ZIE-len-ole) *USP.*
Use: Antibacterial.
W/Benzalkonium Chloride, Hydrocortisone, Pramoxine Hydrochloride.
See: Cortic-ND.
Mediotic-HC.
W/Benzocaine, Hydrocortisone Acetate.
See: TriOxin.
W/Hydrocortisone, Pramoxine.
See: Oto-End 10.
Otomar-HC.
Pramoxine-HC.
Zoto-HC.
W/Methyl Salicylate, Menthol, Camphor, Thymol, Eucalyptus Oil, Isopropyl Alcohol.
See: Gordobalm.
W/Pramoxine Hydrochloride, Zinc Acetate Dihydrate.
See: ZinOtic ES.

chlorozone.
See: Chloramine-T.

Chlorpazine. (Major) Prochlorperazine maleate 5 mg, 10 mg, 25 mg. Tab. Bot. 100s, UD 100s (5 mg, 10 mg only). *Rx.*
Use: Antipsychotic.

Chlorphed. (Roberts) Brompheniramine maleate 10 mg/mL. Inj. Vial 10 mL. *Rx.*
Use: Antihistamine.

Chlorphed-LA. (Roberts) Oxymetazoline 0.05%. Soln. Spray 15 mL. *OTC.*
Use: Decongestant.

Chlorphedrine SR. (Ivax) Chlorpheniramine maleate 8 mg, pseudoephedrine hydrochloride 120 mg. Cap. Bot. 100s. *Rx.*
Use: Antihistamine; decongestant.

•**chlorphenesin carbamate.** (KLOR-fen-ee-sin CAR-bah-mate) USAN.
Use: Muscle relaxant.

chlorpheniramine. (KVK Tech) Chlorpheniramine maleate 12 mg. Calcium 28 mg, lactose, propyl parahydroxybenzoate, sodium benzoate, sucrose, sugar. ER Tab. 24s, 60s. *OTC.*
Use: Antihistamine; alkylamine, nonselective.

chlorpheniramine/codeine. (Breckenridge) Chlorpheniramine maleate 2 mg, codeine phosphate 10 mg per 5 mL. Glycerin, parabens, saccharin, sorbitol. Alcohol free, dye free, and sugar free. Grape flavor. Liq. 473 mL. *c-v.*
Use: Upper respiratory combination, antitussive combination.

•**chlorpheniramine maleate.** (klor-fen-IHR-ah-meen) *USP.*
Use: Antihistamine, nonselective alkylamine.
See: Aller-Chlor.
Allergy.
Allergy Relief.
Allergy-Time.
Chlor-Trimeton Allergy 4 Hour.
Ed ChlorPed.
Ed ChlorPed Jr.
Ed-Chlortan.
Pediox-S.
Pharbechlor.

W/Acetaminophen.
See: Coricidin HBP Cold & Flu.

W/Acetaminophen, Codeine Phosphate.
See: Cotabflu.

W/Acetaminophen, Dextromethorphan Hydrobromide.
See: Coricidin HBP Maximum Strength Flu.
Formula 44 Custom Care Cough & Cold PM.
Theraflu Nighttime Severe Cold.
Triaminic Flu, Cough & Fever.
Tylenol Plus Children's Cough & Runny Nose.
Vicks Alcohol-Free NyQuil Cold & Flu Relief.
Vicks Formula 44 Custom Care Cough & Cold PM.

W/Acetaminophen, Dextromethorphan Hydrobromide, Phenylephrine Hydrochloride.
See: Alka-Seltzer Plus Cold & Cough.
Comtrex Maximum Strength Day & Night Cold & Cough.
Dimetapp Children's Multi-Symptom Cold & Flu.
Robitussin Cough, Cold & Flu Nighttime.
Theraflu Nighttime Severe Cold.
Tylenol Cold Head Congestion Nighttime.
Tylenol Cold Multi-Symptom Nighttime.
Tylenol Plus Children's Flu.
Tylenol Plus Children's Multi-Symptom Cold.

W/Acetaminophen, Phenylephrine Hydrochloride.
See: Alka-Seltzer Multi-Symptom Cold Relief.
Alka-Seltzer Plus Fast Crystal Packs.
Comtrex Maximum Strength Day & Night Flu Therapy.
Comtrex Maximum Strength Day & Night Severe Cold & Sinus.
Contac Cold + Flu.
Contac Cold + Flu Maximum Strength.
Contac Cold + Flu Night.
Dristan Cold Multi-Symptom Formula.
Dryphen Multi-Symptom Formula.
Medicidin-D.
Norel AD.
Onset Forte Micro-Coated.
Pyrroxate Extra Strength.
Robitussin Adult Peak Cold Nighttime Nasal Relief.
Sine Off Sinus/Cold.
Tylenol Allergy Multi-Symptom.
Tylenol Allergy Multi-Symptom Convenience Pack.
Tylenol Plus Children's Cold.
Tylenol Sinus Congestion & Pain Nighttime.

W/Acetaminophen, Phenylephrine Hydrochloride, Phenyltoloxamine Citrate.
See: Trital SR.

W/Acetaminophen, Pseudoephedrine Hydrochloride.
See: BC Allergy, Sinus, Headache.

W/Aspirin, Phenylephrine Bitartrate.
See: Alka-Seltzer Plus Cold.
Alka-Seltzer Plus Sparkling Original Cold Formula.

W/Belladonna Alkaloids, Pseudoephedrine Hydrochloride.
See: Respa A.R.

W/Chlophedianol Hydrochloride, Pseudoephedrine Hydrochloride.
See: DryMax AF.

W/Codeine Phosphate.
See: Cotab A.
Cotab AX.
EndaCof-C.
Lexuss 210.

TL-Hist CM.
Zodryl AC 40.
Zodryl AC 30.
Zodryl AC 35.
Zodryl AC 25.
W/Codeine Phosphate, Pseudoephedrine Hydrochloride.
See: Phenylhistine DH.
W/Dextromethorphan Hydrobromide.
See: AMBI 20 DM/4CPM.
Coricidin HBP Cough & Cold.
Dimetapp Children's Long Acting Cough Plus Cold.
Robitussin Children's Cough & Cold Long-Acting.
Robitussin Pediatric Cough & Cold Long Acting.
Scot-Tussin DM.
Triaminic Cough & Runny Nose.
Tricodene Sugar Free.
Vicks Children's NyQuil Cold & Cough Relief.
W/Dextromethorphan Hydrobromide, Guaifenesin, Phenylephrine Hydrochloride.
See: Chlordex GP.
DM/CPM/PE/GG.
Donatussin.
W/Dextromethorphan Hydrobromide, Phenylephrine Hydrochloride.
See: AMBI 10PEH/4CPM/20DM.
Amerituss AD.
Balamine DM.
Cardec DM.
Corfen-DM.
CP DEC-DM.
DM/PE/CPM.
Donatussin DM.
Ed-A-Hist DM.
Father John's Medicine Plus.
Maxichlor PEH DM.
Nasohist DM.
Neo DM.
PE-Hist DM.
Relahist-DM.
Rondec-DM.
Rondex-DM.
Sonahist DM.
TGQ 15DM/5PEH/2CPM.
Trigofen DM.
Virdec DM.
Z-Dex 120.
ZoDen DM.
W/Dextromethorphan Hydrobromide, Pseudoephedrine Hydrochloride.
See: Allres DS.
AMBI 60PSE/4CPM/20DM.
Atuss DS.
CPM/PSE DM.
Dicel DM.
Esocor P.
KidKare Children's Cough/Cold.
Mesehist DM.
Neutrahist PDX.
Pedia Relief Cough-Cold.
Pediatric Cough & Cold.
Pediatric Cough & Cold Medicine.
Rescon DM.
Triaminic-D Children's.
W/Guaifenesin, Hydrocodone Bitartrate, Pseudoephedrine Hydrochloride.
See: ZTuss Expectorant.
W/Hydrocodone Bitartrate
See: Hydro-PC.
TussiCaps Full Strength.
TussiCaps Half Strength.
Vituz.
W/Hydrocodone Bitartrate, Phenylephrine Hydrochloride.
See: Neo HC.
Notuss-Forte.
Relacon-HC.
W/Hydrocodone Bitartrate, Pseudoephedrine Hydrochloride.
See: Notuss-Forte.
W/Methscopolamine Nitrate.
See: AeroHist.
AllePak Dose Pack.
Allergy ND.
AlleRx DF Dose Pack.
NoHist EXT.
RelCof CPM.
W/Methscopolamine Nitrate, Phenylephrine Hydrochloride.
See: AeroHist Plus.
AeroKid.
CPM 8/PE 20/MSC 1.25.
Dehistine.
Denaze.
DriHist SR.
Drysec.
Duradryl.
Duravent.
Duravent-DA.
Extendryl.
NoHist-Plus.
OMNIhist II LA.
PCM.
PE-CPM-MSN 8-2-0.75.
PE HCL-CPM-MSN 10-2-0.75.
Phenylephrine CM.
QV Allergy.
Ralix.
RelCof PE.
Relcof PSE.
Rescon-MX.
ScopoHist.
ScopoHist-PE.
SymPak.
SymPak PDX.
Triall.
Zinx PCM.

W/Methscopolamine Nitrate, Pseudoephedrine Hydrochloride.
See: CPM 8/PSE 90/MSC 2.5.
DryMax.
Histatab.
Relcof PSE.
ScopoHist.
Time-Hist QD.
W/Phenylephrine Hydrochloride.
See: AccuHist.
Actifed Cold & Allergy.
AMBI 10PEH/4CPM.
Cardec.
Dallergy.
Ed A-Hist.
Ed ChlorPed D.
Extendryl PEM.
LoHist.
Nasohist.
NoHist LQ.
Rescon-Jr.
Virdec.
W/Phenylephrine Hydrochloride, Pyrilamine Maleate.
See: Polyhist PD.
Pyrichlor PE.
W/Pseudoephedrine Hydrochloride.
See: AMBI 60PSE/4CPM.
Colfed-A.
Deconamine.
Duratuss DA.
LoHist-D.
Neutrahist.
Sudafed Sinus & Allergy.
SudaHist.
SudoGest Sinus & Allergy Maximum Strength.
Zinx Chlor-D.

d-chlorpheniramine maleate.
See: Polaramine Expectorant.

chlorpheniramine maleate. (KVK Tech) Chlorpheniramine maleate 12 mg. Calcium 28 mg, lactose, propyl parahydroxybenzoate, sodium benzoate, sucrose, sugar. ER Tab. 24s, 60s. *OTC.*
Use: Antihistamine, nonselective alkylamine.

chlorpheniramine maleate. (Various Mfr.) Chlorpheniramine maleate 4 mg. Tab. 24s, 100s, 1,000s. *Rx.*
Use: Antihistamine, nonselective alkylamine.

chlorpheniramine maleate/phenylephrine hydrochloride. (Silarx) **Liq.:** Phenylephrine hydrochloride 3.5 mg, chlorpheniramine maleate 1 mg per 5 mL. Alcohol and sugar free. Saccharin, sorbitol. Raspberry flavor. 30 mL with dropper. **Syrup:** Phenylephrine hydrochloride 12.5 mg, chlorpheniramine maleate 4 mg per 5 mL. Alcohol and sugar free. Saccharin, sorbitol. Raspberry flavor. 118 mL, 473 mL. *Rx.*
Use: Upper respiratory combination, decongestant and antihistamine.

•**chlorpheniramine maleate with pseudoephedrine hydrochloride.** (klor-fen-IHR-ah-meen MAL-ee-ate with SOO-do-ee-fed-rin) *USP.*
Use: Antihistamine, decongestant.

•**chlorpheniramine polistirex.** (klor-fen-IHR-ah-meen pahl-ee-STIE-rex) USAN.
Use: Antihistamine.
W/Combinations.
See: Atuss-12 DM.
Codeprex.
W/Hydrocodone Polistirex.
See: Tussionex PennKinetic.

chlorpheniramine polistirex/hydrocodone polistirex. (Various Mfr.) Chlorpheniramine maleate (as chlorpheniramine polistirex) 8 mg, hydrocodone bitartrate (as hydrocodone polistirex) 10 mg. May contain corn syrup, parabens, polysorbate 80, propylene glycol, sucrose. ER Susp. 473 mL. *c-III.*
Use: Upper respiratory combination, antitussive combination.

chlorpheniramine tannate.
See: Ed-Chlor-Tan.
Pediatan.
TanaHist PD.
W/Carbetapentane Tannate.
See: Tannic-12 S.
Tussi-12.
W/Methscopolamine Nitrate.
See: Dexodryl.
W/Methscopolamine Nitrate, Phenylephrine Tannate.
See: AH-Chew.
AH-Chew Ultra Tannate.
Redur-PCM.
W/Phenylephrine Tannate.
See: Phenyl Chlor-Tan Pediatric.
Ry-Tann.
TanaHist-D Pediatric.
Tannate Pediatric.

chlorpheniramine tannate and pseudoephedrine tannate. (Various Mfr.) Pseudoephedrine tannate 75 mg, chlorpheniramine tannate 4.5 mg/5 mL, strawberry/banana flavor, alcohol free. Susp. Bot. 118 mL, 473 mL. *Rx.*
Use: Upper respiratory combination, decongestant, antihistamine.

•**chlorphentermine hydrochloride.** (klor-FEN-ter-meen) USAN.
Use: Anorexic.

chlorphthalidone.
See: Chlorthalidone.

•**chlorpromazine.** (klor-PRO-muh-zeen) *USP.*
Tall Man: chlorproMAZINE
Use: Antiemetic; antipsychotic.

•**chlorpromazine hydrochloride.** (klor-PRO-muh-zeen) *USP.*
Tall Man: chlorproMAZINE
Use: Antiemetic; antipsychotic.
See: Promachlor.

chlorpromazine hydrochloride injection. (Various Mfr.) Chlorpromazine hydrochloride 25 mg/mL. sodium metabisulfite, sodium sulfite. Amp. 1 mL, 2 mL. *Rx.*
Use: Antipsychotic.

chlorpromazine hydrochloride tablets. (Various Mfr.) Chlorpromazine hydrochloride 10 mg, 25 mg, 50 mg, 100 mg, 200 mg. Tab. Bot. 100s, 1000s, UD 100s. *Rx.*
Use: Antipsychotic.

•**chlorpropamide.** (klor-PRO-puh-mide) *USP.*
Tall Man: chlorproPAMIDE
Use: Antidiabetic.

chlorpropamide. (Various Mfr.) Chlorpropamide 100 mg, 250 mg. Tab. Bot. 100s, 250s (250 mg only), 500s, 1000s, UD 100s, UD 600s. *Rx.*
Use: Antidiabetic.

chlorprophenpyridamine maleate.
See: Chlorpheniramine maleate.

Chlor-Pro 10. (Schein) Chlorpheniramine maleate 10 mg/mL, benzyl alcohol. Inj. Vial 30 mL. *Rx.*
Use: Antihistamine.

chlorquinol. Mixture of the chlorinated products of 8-hydroxyquinoline containing about 65% of 5,7-dichloro-8-hydroxyquinoline.

chlortetracycline and sulfamethazine bisulfates.
Use: Anti-infective.

•**chlortetracycline bisulfate.** (klor-the-trah-SIGH-kleen) *USP.*
Use: Anti-infective; antiprotozoal.

•**chlorthalidone.** (klor-THAL-ih-dohn) *USP.*
Use: Diuretic.
See: Thalitone.
W/Atenolol.
See: Tenoretic.
W/Azilsartan Medoxomil.
See: Edarbyclor.
W/Clonidine Hydrochloride.
See: Clorpres.

chlorthalidone. (Various Mfr.) Chlorthalidone 25 mg, 50 mg, 100 mg. Tab. Bot. 100s, 250s (50 mg only), 500s (100 mg only). *Rx.*
Use: Diuretic.

Chlor-Trimeton Allergy. (Schering-Plough) Chlorpheniramine maleate 4 mg, lactose. Tab. Box. 24s. *OTC.*
Use: Antihistamine.

Chlor-Trimeton Allergy•D 4 Hour. (Schering-Plough) Pseudoephedrine sulfate 60 mg, chlorpheniramine maleate 4 mg, lactose. Tab. Box. 24s. *OTC.*
Use: Upper respiratory combination, decongestant, antihistamine.

Chlor-Trimeton Allergy•D 12 Hour. (Schering-Plough) Pseudoephedrine sulfate 120 mg, chlorpheniramine maleate 8 mg, butylparaben, sugar, lactose. Tab. Bot. 24s. *OTC.*
Use: Upper respiratory combination, decongestant, antihistamine.

Chlor-Trimeton Allergy 4 Hour. (Schering-Plough) Chlorpheniramine maleate 4 mg. Lactose. Tab. 24s. *OTC.*
Use: Antihistamine; alkylamine, nonselective.

Chlor-Trimeton 4 Hour Relief. (Schering-Plough) Chlorpheniramine maleate 4 mg, pseudoephedrine sulfate 60 mg. Tab. Box 24s, 48s. *OTC.*
Use: Antihistamine; decongestant.

Chlor-Trimeton 12 Hour Allergy. (Schering-Plough) Chlorpheniramine maleate 8 mg, pseudoephedrine sulfate 120 mg. SR Tab. Box 24s, 48s. UD 96s. *OTC.*
Use: Antihistamine; decongestant.

Chlor-Trimeton 12 Hour Relief. (Schering-Plough) Chlorpheniramine 8 mg, pseudoephedrine sulfate 120 mg. Tab. Box 12s. Bot. 36s. *OTC.*
Use: Antihistamine; decongestant.

•**chlorzoxazone.** (klor-ZOX-uh-zone) *USP.*
Use: Muscle relaxant.
See: Lorzone.
Paraflex.
Parafon Forte DSC.
Remular-S.

chlorzoxazone. (Various Mfr.) Chlorzoxane 250 mg, 500 mg. Tab. Bot. 100s, 500s (500 mg only), 1000s.
Use: Muscle relaxant.

chlorzoxazone and acetaminophen.
Use: Analgesic; muscle relaxant.

Chlo Tuss. (R.A. McNeil) Chlophedianol hydrochloride 12.5 mg, dexbrompheniramine maleate 1 mg, pseudoephedrine hydrochloride 30 mg. Glycerin, propylene glycol, saccharin, sorbitol. Alcohol free, dye free, gluten free, sugar free. Tutti frutti flavor. Liq. 473 mL. *OTC.*
Use: Upper respiratory combination, antitussive combination.

Chlo Tuss EX. (R.A. McNeil) Chlophedianol hydrochloride 12.5 mg, guaifene-

sin 100 mg. Glycerin, propylene glycol, saccharin, sorbitol, sucralose. Alcohol free, dye free, gluten free, and sugar free. Berry vanilla flavor. Liq. 473 mL. *OTC.*
Use: Upper respiratory combination, antitussive with expectorant.

•**chocolate.** (CHOK-a-lat) *NF.*
Use: Flavoring.

Choice DM. (Bristol-Myers Squibb) Protein 38.1 g, carbohydrate 101.5 g, fat 42.3 g, Na 846 mg, K 1818.9 mg per liter, 0.93 Cal/mL; vitamins A, D, E, K, C, B_1, B_2, B_3, B_5, B_6, B_{12}, FA, biotin, Ca, P, I, Mg, Zn, Mn, Cl, K, Na, Se, Cr, Mo, sucrose. Vanilla and chocolate flavors. Liq. 237 mL ready-to-use cans. *OTC.*
Use: Enteral nutrition therapy.

Choice DM AIC Home Blood Test. (Bristol-Myers Squibb) Kit for blood samples. 1 single-use test kit. *OTC.*
Use: In vitro diagnostic aid.

Choice DM Daily Moisturizing. (Bristol-Myers Squibb) Petrolatum, glycerin, dimethicone, steareth-2, alcohols, laureth-23, magnesium aluminum silicate, carbomer, potassium sorbate, sodium hydroxide, aloe. Fragrance free. Lot. 226.8 mL. *OTC.*
Use: Emollient.

Choice DM Gentle Care. (Bristol-Myers Squibb) Sorbitol, poloxamer 407, sodium, saccharin, cetylpyridinium chloride, citric acid. Alcohol and sugar free. Fresh mint flavor. Mouthwash. 500 mL. *OTC.*
Use: Mouth and throat product.

Choice DM Sugar Free Shakes. (Bristol-Myers Squibb) **Mocha cappuccino flavor:** Protein 30.7 g, carbohydrate 33.8 g, fat 7.7 g, Na 460.5 mg. K 1043.8 mg per liter, 0.38 Cal/mL; vitamins A, D, E, K, B_1, B_2, B_3, B_5, B_6, B_{12}, Ca, Fe, FA, biotin, P, I, Mg, Zn, Se, Cu, Cr, Mo. Liq. 325 mL. **Chocolate fudge flavor:** Protein 30.7 g, carbohydrate 36.8 g, fat 6.1 g, Na 460.5 mg. K 1043.8 mg per liter, 0.38 Cal/mL; vitamins A, D, E, K, B_1, B_2, B_3, B_5, B_6, B_{12}, Ca, Fe, FA, biotin, P, I, Mg, Zn, Se, Cu, Cr, Mo. Liq. 325 mL. **French vanilla flavor:** Protein 30.7 g, carbohydrate 24.6 g, fat 6.1 g, Na 399.1 mg. K 337.7 mg per liter, 0.31 Cal/mL; vitamins A, D, E, K, B_1, B_2, B_3, B_5, B_6, B_{12}, Ca, Fe, FA, biotin, P, I, Mg, Zn, Se, Cu, Cr, Mo. Liq. 325 mL. **Strawberries'n cream flavor:** Protein 30.7 g, carbohydrate 21.5 g, fat 7.7 g, Na 399.1 mg. K 337.7 mg per liter, 0.31 Cal/mL; vitamins A, D, E, K, B_1, B_2, B_3, B_5, B_6, B_{12}, Ca, Fe, FA, biotin, P, I, Mg, Zn, Se, Cu, Cr, Mo. Liq. 325 mL. *Rx.*
Use: Enteral nutrition therapy.

Choice 10. (Whiteworth Towne) Potassium chloride 10%. Soln., unflavored. Bot. Gal. *Rx.*
Use: Electrolyte supplement.

Choice 20. (Whiteworth Towne) Potassium chloride 20%. Soln., unflavored. Bot. Gal. *Rx.*
Use: Electrolyte supplement.

cholacrylamine resin. Anion exchange resin consisting of a water-soluble polymer having a molecular weight equivalent between 350 and 360 in which aliphatic quaternary amine groups are attached to an acrylic backbone by ester linkages.

cholalic acid. Cholic acid.

Cholan-DH. (Medeva) Dehydrocholic acid 250 mg. Tab. Bot. 100s.
Use: Laxative.

cholanic acid. Dehydrodesoxycholic acid.

Cholebrine. (Mallinckrodt) Iocetamic acid (62% iodine) 750 mg. Tab. Bot. 100s, 150s.
Use: Radiopaque agent.

•**cholecalciferol.** (kole-eh-kal-SIH-fer-ole) *USP. Formerly 7-Dehydrocholesterol, activated.*
Use: Vitamin D_3 (antirachitic).
See: A and D Ointment.
Advanced D5000.
Baby Ddrops.
Ddrops.
Delta-D.
D-5000 Super Strength.
D400.
D1000.
D_3 Dots.
D_3-50.
D_3 Healthy Kids.
D-Vita.
Enfamil D•Vi•Sol.
High Potency D-1000.
Maximum D3.
Maximum Strength D-2000.
Replesta Children's.
Super Strength D-2000 IU.
Ultra Strength D2000.
Ultra Strength Vitamin D_3.
Vitamin D_3.
W/Alendronate Sodium.
See: Fosamax Plus D.

choleretic. Bile salts.
See: Bile Preps and Forms.
Dehydrocholic Acid.
Tocamphyl.

cholesterin.
See: Cholesterol.

•**cholesterol.** (koe-LESS-ter-all) *NF.*
Use: Pharmaceutic aid, emulsifying agent.

cholesterol reagent strips. (Bayer Consumer Care) A quantitative strip test for cholesterol in serum. Seralyzer reagent strips. Bot. 25s.
Use: Diagnostic aid.

cholestyramine. (Various Mfr.) Anhydrous cholestyramine resin 4 g/9 g powder. May contain sucrose, sorbitol. Pow. for Oral Susp. 9 g Packet. 42s, 60s. Cans. 378 g. *Rx.*
Use: Antihyperlipidemic; bile acid sequestrant.

cholestyramine light. (Various Mfr.) Anhydrous cholestyramine resin 4 g/5.7 g powder. May contain aspartame. Pow. for Oral Susp. 5 g and 5.7 g Packets. 60s. Cans. 210 g, 231 g, 239 g. *Rx.*
Use: Antihyperlipidemic; bile acid sequestrant.

•**cholestyramine resin.** (koe-less-TEER-uh-meen) *USP.*
Use: Antihyperlipidemic; ion-exchange resin, bile acid sequestrants.
See: Cholestyramine Light.
Prevalite.
Questran.
Questran Light.

Choletec. (Bracco) Mebrofenin 45 mg (when sodium pertechnetate Tc-99m injection is added to the vial, the diagnostic agent technetium Tc-99m mebrofenin is formed containing up to 3,700 MBq [100 millicuries] of Tc-99m). Parabens. Also contains stannous fluoride dihydrate (minimum) and total tin 1.03 mg maximum (as stannous fluoride dihydrate). Inj., Lyophilized Pow. for Soln. Kits of 10 multidose vials. *Rx.*
Use: Radiopaque agent.

Cholidase. (Freeda) Choline 450 mg, inositol 150 mg, vitamins B_6 2.5 mg, B_{12} 5 mcg, E 7.5 mg. Tab. Bot. 100s, 250s, 500s. *OTC.*
Use: Lipid, vitamin supplement.

choline. (Various Mfr.) Choline 650 mg. Tab. 90s, 100s. *OTC.*
Use: Lipotropic.

•**choline bitartrate.** (koe-leen bye-TAR-trait) *USP.*

•**choline chloride.** (koe-leen) *USP.* (Various Mfr.).
Use: Liver supplement. [Orphan Drug]

choline chloride, carbamate. Carbachol.

choline chloride succinate.
See: Succinylcholine Chloride.

choline dihydrogen citrate. 2-Hydroxyethyl trimethylammonium citrate US vitamin 0.5 g. Bot. 100s, 500s.
Use: Lipotropic.

choline magnesium trisalicylate. (Sidmak) Choline magnesium trisalicylate 500 mg, 750 mg, 1000 mg. Tab. Bot. 100s, 500s. *Rx.*
Use: Analgesic.

cholinergic agents.
Use: Parasympathomimetic agents.
See: Mecholyl Ointment.
Mestinon.
Mytelase.
Pilocarpine.
Tensilon.
Urecholine.
Urinary Cholinergics.

cholinergic blocking agents.
See: Parasympatholytic Agents.

cholinergic muscle stimulants.
See: Anticholinesterase Muscle Stimulant.

•**choline salicylate.** (koe-leen suh-lih-sih-late) USAN.
Use: Analgesic.

cholinesterase inhibitors. Agents that inhibit the enzyme cholinesterase and enhance the effects of endogenous acetylcholine.
Use: Glaucoma therapy; Alzheimer disease; muscle stimulant.
See: Donepezil Hydrochloride.
Eserine Salicylate.
Eserine Sulfate.
Galantamine Hydrobromide.
Neostigmine Methylsulfate.
Rivastigmine Tartrate.
Tacrine Hydrochloride.

choline theophyllinate.
See: Oxtriphylline.

Chol Meth in B. (Esco) Choline bitartrate 235 mg, inositol 112 mg, methionine 70 mg, betaine anhydrous 50 mg, vitamins B_{12} 6 mcg, B_1 6 mg, B_6 3 mg, niacin 10 mg. Cap. Bot. 500s, 1000s. *OTC.*
Use: Vitamin supplement.

Chografin Meglumine. (Bracco Diagnostics) Iodipamide meglumine 520 mg, iodine 257 mg/mL. EDTA. Inj. Vials. 20 mL. *Rx.*
Use: Radiopaque agent; parenteral agent.

cholylglycine.
See: CG RIA.

chondodendron tomentosum.
See: Curare.

•**chondroitin sulfate and sodium hyaluronate.** (kon-DRO-ih-tin SULL-fate and SO-dee-uhm HIGH-ah-loo-rohn-ate) *USP.* Surgical aid in anterior segment procedures including cataract extraction and intraocular lens implanta-

tion. *Rx.*
See: DisCoVisc.
Viscoat.

•**chondroitin sulfate sodium.** (kon-DRO-ih-tin SULL-fate SO-dee-uhm) *NF.*
Use: Dietary supplement.

chondrus. Irish Moss.
See: Kondremul.

Chooz. (Schering-Plough) Calcium carbonate 500 mg (elemental calcium 200 mg). Sucrose, glucose. Mint flavor. Gum Tab. Pkg. 16s. *OTC.*
Use: Mineral supplement; antacid.

•**choriogonadotropin alfa.** (kore-ee-oh-goe-NAD-oh-troe-pin) USAN.
Use: Sex hormone, ovulation stimulant.
See: Ovidrel.

chorionic gonadotropin.
Use: Ovulation stimulant.
See: Pregnyl.

chorionic gonadotropin. (Various Mfr.) Chorionic gonadotropin 10,000 units per vial with 10 mL diluent (1,000 units per mL). May contain mannitol. Inj., lyophilized Pow. for Soln. Multidose vial. 10 mL. *Rx.*
Use: Ovulation stimulant.

Chromagen FA. (Ther-Rx) Fe (as elemental iron) 70 mg, vitamins B_{12} 10 mcg, C 150 mg, folic acid 1 mg. Parabens. Cap. UD 100s. *Rx.*
Use: Mineral, vitamin supplement.

Chromagen Forte. (Ther-Rx) Elemental iron (from ferrous asparto glycinate and ferrous fumarate) 151 mg, succinic acid 50 mg, vitamin C (as calcium ascorbate and calcium threonate) 60.8 mg, folic acid 1 mg, B_{12} 10 mcg. Lactose. Film-coated. Tab. 90s. *Rx.*
Use: Mineral, vitamin supplement.

Chromagen OB. (Savage) Ca 200 mg, Cu, folic acid 1 mg, Fe 28 mg, Mn, B_2 1.8 mg, B_1 1.6 mg, B_6 20 mg, C 60 mg, D 400 units, Zn 25 mg, E 30 units, niacinamide 5 mg, B_{12} 12 mcg, docusate calcium 25 mg. Cap. Bot. 100s. *Rx.*
Use: Vitamin supplement.

chromargyre.
See: Merbromin.

chromated. Solution (Cr^{51}).
See: Chromitope Sodium.

Chromelin Complexion Blender. (Summers) Dihydroxyacetone 5%, isopropyl alcohol, propylene glycol. Susp. 30 mL. *OTC.*
Use: Hyperpigmenting.

chromic acid, disodium salt. Sodium Chromate Cr^{51}.

•**chromic chloride.** (kroe-MIK) *USP.*
Use: Supplement, trace mineral.

chromic chloride. (American Regent) Chromium 4 mcg/mL (as chromic chloride 20.5 mcg/mL). Preservative free. Inj., Soln. Single-use vial. 10 mL. *Rx.*
Use: Trace metal.

chromic chloride. (Hospira) Chromium 4 mcg/mL (as chromic chloride 20.5 mcg/mL). Preservative free. Inj., Soln. Vial. 10 mL. *Rx.*
Use: Trace metal.

•**chromic chloride Cr 51.** (kroe-MIK) USAN.
Use: Radiopharmaceutical.

•**chromic phosphate Cr 51.** (kroe-MIK) USAN.
Use: Radiopharmaceutical.

•**chromic phosphate P 32 suspension.** (kroe-MIK) *USP.*
Use: Radiopharmaceutical.

Chromitope Sodium. (Bristol-Myers Squibb) Chromate Cr^{51}, sodium for Inj. 0.25 mCi.
Use: Radiopharmaceutical.

chromium. A trace metal used in IV nutritional therapy that helps maintain normal glucose metabolism and peripheral nerve function.
See: Chromic Chloride.

•**chromium Cr 51 edetate.** (KRO-me-um) *USP.*
Use: Radiopharmaceutical.

chromium picolinate. (Rugby) Chromium picolinate 200 mcg. Soybean oil, soy lecithin oil, tartrazine. Gluten free, preservative free, sugar free. Cap., softgel. 60s. *OTC.*
Use: Nutritional supplement.

•**chromonar hydrochloride.** (kroe-moe-NAHR) USAN.
Use: Coronary vasodilator.

Chur-Hist. (Churchill) Chlorpheniramine 4 mg. Kaptab. Bot. 100s.
Use: Antihistamine.

•**chymotrypsin.** (kye-moe-TRIP-sin) *USP.*
Use: Proteolytic enzyme.

Cialis. (Lilly) Tadalafil 2.5 mg, 5 mg, 10 mg, 20 mg. Lactose. Film-coated. 30s (except 2.5 mg), blisters of 2 × 15 (2.5 mg, 5 mg). *Rx.*
Use: Erectile dysfunction.

Cibacalcin. (Novartis) Calcitonin-human for injection.
Use: Paget disease. [Orphan Drug]

CI basic violet 3. Gentian Violet.

Ciba Vision Cleaner. (Ciba Vision) Cocoamphocarboxyglycinate, sodium lauryl sulfate, sorbic acid 0.1%, hexylene glycol, EDTA 0.2%. Soln. 5 mL, 15 mL. *OTC.*
Use: Contact lens care.

Ciba Vision Saline. (Ciba Vision) Buffered, isotonic with NaCl, boric acid. Soln. Bot. 90 mL, 240 mL, 360 mL. *OTC.*
Use: Contact lens care, rinsing, storage.

cibenzoline.
See: Cifenline Succinate.

•**ciclafrine hydrochloride.** (SIK-lah-freen) USAN.
Use: Antihypotensive.

•**ciclazindol.** (sigh-CLAY-zin-dole) USAN.
Use: Antidepressant.

•**ciclesonide.** (sye-KLES-oh-nide) USAN.
Use: Respiratory inhalant, intranasal steroid.
See: Alvesco.
Omnaris.
Zetonna.

•**cicletanine.** (sik-LET-ah-neen) USAN.
Use: Antihypertensive.

Ciclodan. (Medimetriks Pharmaceuticals) Ciclopirox olamine. **Soln.; topical:** 8%. Isopropyl alcohol. 6.6 mL w/brush. **Cream:** 0.77%. Alcohols, benzyl alcohol 1%, lactic acid, lt. mineral oil. 90 g and in kits w/*Rehyla Wash* in 454 g (alcohols, betaine, chamomile flower extract, cholesterol, edetate disodium, glycerin, phenoxyethanol, propylene glycol, salicylic acid, sodium hyaluronate). *Rx.*
Use: Topical anti-infective, antifungal agent.

•**ciclopirox.** (sigh-kloe-PEER-ox) USAN.
Use: Antifungal agent, topical anti-infective.
See: Ciclodan.
CNL8 Nail Kit.
Loprox.
Pedipirox Nail Lacquer.
Penlac Nail Lacquer.

ciclopirox. (Fougera) Ciclopirox 0.77%. Isopropyl alcohol. Gel. 30 g, 45 g. *Rx.*
Use: Antifungal agent, topical anti-infective.

ciclopirox. (Paddock) Ciclopirox 1%. Shampoo, Susp. 120 mL. *Rx.*
Use: Topical anti-infective, antifungal agent.

ciclopirox. (Perrigo) Ciclopirox 0.77%. Benzyl alcohol, cetyl alcohol, myristyl alcohol, stearyl alcohol, lactic acid, mineral oil. Lot. 30 mL, 60 mL. *Rx.*
Use: Antifungal agent, topical anti-infective.

ciclopirox. (Various Mfr.) Ciclopirox 0.77%. Top. Susp. 30 mL, 60 mL. *Rx.*
Use: Antifungal agent, topical anti-infective.

ciclopirox nail lacquer. (Various Mfr.) Ciclopirox 8%. May contain isopropyl alcohol. Top. Soln. 3.3 mL, 6.6 mL with brushes. *Rx.*
Use: Topical anti-infective, antifungal agent.

•**ciclopirox olamine.** (sigh-kloe-PEER-ox OLE-ah-meen) *USP.*
Use: Antifungal.

•**cicloprofen.** (SIK-low-pro-fen) USAN.
Use: Anti-inflammatory.

•**cicloprolol hydrochloride.** (SIGH-kloe-PRO-lahl) USAN.
Use: Antiadrenergic, beta-receptor.

Cidex Plus. (Johnson & Johnson) Glutaraldehyde 3.2%. Soln. Gal.
Use: Disinfectant, sterilizing.

Cidex-7. (Johnson & Johnson) Glutaraldehyde 2% and vial of activator with aqueous potassium salt as buffer and sodium nitrite as a corrosive inhibitor. Soln. Bot. Qt., gal., 5 gal.
Use: Disinfectant, sterilizing.

C.I. direct blue 53 tetrasodium salt. Evans Blue. *Rx.*

•**cidofovir.** (sigh-DAH-fah-vihr) USAN.
Use: Antiviral.
See: Vistide.

cidofovir. (Heritage) Cidofovir 75 mg/mL. Preservative free. Inj., Soln. Single-use vial. 5 mL. *Rx.*
Use: Anti-infective, antiviral agent.

•**cidoxepin hydrochloride.** (sih-DOX-eh-PIN) USAN.
Use: Antidepressant.

•**cifenline.** (sigh-FEN-leen) USAN. *Formerly cibenzoline.*
Use: Cardiovascular, antiarrhythmic.

•**cifenline succinate.** (sigh-FEN-leen) USAN.
Use: Cardiovascular agent, antiarrhythmic.

•**ciglitazone.** (sigh-GLIE-tah-ZONE) USAN.
Use: Antidiabetic.

cignolin.
See: Anthralin.

•**ciladopa hydrochloride.** (SIGH-lah-doe-pah) USAN.
Use: Antiparkinsonian, dopaminergic.

•**cilansetron.** (sil-an-SE-tron) USAN.
Use: Gastrointestinal agent; irritable bowel syndrome.

•**cilansetron hydrochloride.** (sil-an-SE-tron) USAN.
Use: Gastrointestinal agent; irritable bowel syndrome.

cilastatin-imipenem. A formulation of imipenem, a thienamycin antibiotic, and

cilastatin sodium, the inhibitor of the renal dipeptidase, dehydropeptidase-1.
Use: Anti-infective.
See: Primaxin I.V.

•**cilastatin sodium.** (SIGH-lah-STAT-in) *USP.*
Use: Enzyme inhibitor.
W/Imipenem.
See: Primaxin.

•**cilazapril.** (sile-AZE-ah-PRILL) USAN.
Use: Investigational antihypertensive.

•**cilengitide.** (sye-LEN-gi-tide) USAN.
Use: Angiogenesis inhibitor.

•**cilexetil.** (sigh-LEX-eh-till) USAN.
Use: Anti-infective.

Cilfomide. (Sanofi-Synthelabo) Inositol hexanicotinate. Tab. *Rx.*
Use: Hypolipidimic, peripheral vasodilator.

Cillium. (Whiteworth Towne) Psyllium seed husk 4.94 g, 14 calories/rounded tsp. Pow. Bot. 420 g, 630 g. *OTC.*
Use: Laxative.

•**cilmostim.** (SILL-moe-stim) USAN. *Formerly rhM-CSF, M-CSF, CSF-1.*
Use: Hematopoietic, macrophage colony-stimulating factor.

•**cilobamine mesylate.** (SIGH-low-BAM-een) USAN. *Formerly clobamine mesylate.*
Use: Antidepressant.

•**cilofungin.** (SIGH-low-FUN-jin) USAN.
Use: Antifungal.

•**cilomilast.** (sill-OH-mih-last) USAN.
Use: Investigational drug for asthma; COPD; arthritis; atopic dermatitis; multiple sclerosis.

•**cilostazol.** (sill-OH-stah-zole) USAN.
Use: Antithrombotic; platelet inhibitor; vasodilator.
See: Pletal.

cilostazol. (Various Mfr.) Cilostazol 50 mg, 100 mg. Tab. 60s, 500s (100 mg only). *Rx.*
Use: Antiplatelet agent.

Ciloxan. (Alcon) Ciprofloxacin. **Oint.:** 3.33 mg (equivalent to 3 mg base)/g. Mineral oil, white petrolatum. Tube. 3.5 g. **Soln.:** 3.5 mg/mL (equiv. to 3 mg base). Benzalkonium chloride 0.006%, mannitol 4.6%, EDTA 0.05%. *Drop-Tainers* 2.5 mL, 5 mL. *Rx.*
Use: Anti-infective.

•**ciluprevir.** (sigh-loo-PRAH-veer) USAN.
Use: Hepatitis C.

•**cimaglermin alfa.** (SYE-ma-GLER-min) USAN.
Use: Treatment of congestive heart failure.

•**cimaterol.** (sigh-MAH-teh-role) USAN.
Use: Repartitioning agent.

•**cimetidine.** (sigh-MET-ih-deen) *USP.*
Use: Histamine H_2 antagonist.
See: Acid Reducer 200.
Tagamet.
Tagamet HB 200.

cimetidine. (Various Mfr.) Cimetidine. **Soln.; oral:** 300 mg (as hydrochloride)/5 mL. May contain alcohol, parabens, saccharin, sorbitol. Bot. 240 mL, 480 mL, UD 5 mL. **Tab.:** 200 mg, 300 mg, 400 mg, 800 mg. Tab. Bot. 30s (800 mg only); 60s (400 mg only); 100s; 250s (800 mg only); 500s, 1,000s (except 800 mg). *Rx.*
Use: Histamine H_2 receptor antagonist.

cimetidine. (Various Mfr.) Cimetidine 200 mg. Tab. Bot. 30s, 50s. *OTC.*
Use: Histamine H_2 receptor antagonist.

•**cimetidine hydrochloride.** (sigh-MET-ih-deen) USAN.
Use: Histamine H_2 receptor antagonist.

Cimzia. (UCB) Certolizumab pegol. **Inj., lyophilized Pow. for Soln:** 200 mg. Preservative free. Single-use vials. **Inj., Soln:** 200 mg. Preservative free. Single-use prefilled syringe. 1 mL. *Rx.*
Use: Immunologic agent, immunomodulator.

•**cinacalcet hydrochloride.** (sin-a-KAL-set) USAN.
Use: Hyperparathyroidism agent.
See: Sensipar.

Cinacort Span. (Foy Laboratories) Triamcinolone acetonide 40 mg/mL. Vial 5 mL. *Rx.*
Use: Corticosteroid.

•**cinalukast.** (sin-ah-LOO-kast) USAN.
Use: Antiasthmatic; leukotriene antagonist.

•**cinanserin hydrochloride.** (sin-AN-ser-in) USAN.
Use: Serotonin inhibitor.

cinchona alkaloid.
Use: Antimalarial.
See: Quinine Sulfate.

cinchona bark. (Various Mfr.).
Use: Antimalarial, tonic.
W/Anhydrous Quinine, Cinchonidine, Cinchonine, Quinidine, Quinine.
See: Totaquine.

cinchonine salts. (Various Mfr.).
Use: Quinine dihydrochloride.

cinchophen.
Use: Analgesic.

•**cindunistat.** (sin-DOO-ni-stat) USAN.
Use: Disease-modifying osteoarthritis drug.

•**cindunistat hydrochloride maleate.** (sin-DOO-ni-stat) USAN.
Use: Disease-modifying osteoarthritis drug.

•**cinepazet maleate.** (SIN-eh-PAZZ-ett) USAN.
Use: Antianginal.
•**cinflumide.** (SIN-flew-mide) USAN.
Use: Muscle relaxant.
•**cingestol.** (sin-JESS-tole) USAN.
Use: Hormone, progestin.
•**cinnamedrine.** (sin-am-ED-reen) USAN.
Use: Muscle relaxant.
cinnamic aldehyde. *Name previously used for Cinnamaldehyde.*
cinnamon.
Use: Flavoring.
cinnamon oil. (Various Mfr.).
Use: Pharmaceutic aid.
•**cinnarizine.** (sin-NAHR-ih-zeen) USAN.
Use: Antihistamine.
cinnopentazone. INN for Cintazone.
Cinobac. (Oclassen) Cinoxacin 250 mg. Cap. Bot. 40s. *Rx.*
Use: Anti-infective, urinary.
•**cinoxate.** (sin-OX-ate) USAN.
Use: Ultraviolet screen.
•**cinperene.** (SIN-peh-reen) USAN.
Use: Antipsychotic.
Cin-Quin. (Solvay) Quinidine sulfate. (Contains 83% anhydrous quinidine alkaloid.) **Tab.:** 100 mg, 200 mg, 300 mg. Bot. 100s, 1000s, UD 100s. **Cap.:** 200 mg. Bot. 100s. 300 mg. Bot. 100s, 1000s, UD 100s. *Rx.*
Use: Antiarrhythmic.
•**cinromide.** (SIN-row-mide) USAN.
Use: Anticonvulsant.
Cinryze. (Lev Pharmaceuticals) C1 inhibitor (human) 500 units. Sodium chloride 4.1 mg/mL, sucrose 21 mg/mL, trisodium citrate 2.6 mg/mL, L-valine 2 mg/mL, L-alanine 1.2 mg/mL, L-threonine 4.5 mg/mL when reconstituted w/5 mL of sterile water for inj. Preservative free. Inj., lyophilized Pow. for Soln. Single-use vial. *Rx.*
Use: Hematological agent, protein C1 inhibitor.
•**cintazone.** (SIN-tah-zone) USAN.
Use: Anti-inflammatory.
•**cintriamide.** (sin-TRY-ah-mid) USAN.
Use: Antipsychotic.
•**cioteronel.** (SIGH-oh-TEH-row-nell) USAN.
Use: Dermatologic, acne; androgenic alopecia and keloid, antimutagenic.
•**cipamfylline.** (sigh-PAM-fih-lin) USAN.
Use: Antiviral.
Cipralan. (Roche) Cifenline succinate. *Formerly cibenzoline. Rx.*
Use: Antiarrhythmic.
•**cipralisant maleate.** (ci-PRAL-is-ant) USAN.
Use: Histamine H_3 antagonist; ADHD.
•**ciprefadol succinate.** (sih-PREH-fah-dahl) USAN.
Use: Analgesic.
Cipro. (Bayer) Ciprofloxacin. **Tab.:** As ciprofloxacin hydrochloride 250 mg, 500 mg. Film coated. PEG. 100s. **Microcapsules for Oral Susp.:** 250 mg/5 mL (5%), 500 mg/5 mL (10%) when reconstituted. Sucrose, strawberry flavor. 100 mL with diluent. *Rx.*
Use: Anti-infective, fluoroquinolone.
•**ciprocinonide.** (sih-PRO-SIN-oh-nide) USAN.
Use: Adrenocortical steroid.
Ciprodex. (Alcon) Ciprofloxacin 0.3%, dexamethasone 0.1%. Benzalkonium chloride, boric acid, EDTA. Susp. 5 mL, 7.5 mL. *Drop-Tainer. Rx.*
Use: Steroid and antibiotic combination.
•**ciprofibrate.** (sip-ROW-FIE-brate) USAN.
Use: Antihyperlipoproteinemic.
•**ciprofloxacin.** (sip-ROW-FLOX-ah-sin) *USP.*
Use: Anti-infective, fluoroquinolone.
See: Cetraxal.
Ciloxan.
Cipro.
Cipro I.V.
W/Dexamethasone.
See: Ciprodex.
W/Hydrocortisone.
See: Cipro HC Otic.
ciprofloxacin. (Barr) Ciprofloxacin 250 mg/5 mL (5%), 500 mg/5mL (10%) (when reconstituted). Sucrose, strawberry flavor. Pow. for Oral Susp. Bot. of microcapsules, diluent, and a teaspoon. *Rx.*
Use: Anti-infective, fluoroquinolone.
ciprofloxacin. (Xspire Pharma) Ciprofloxacin hydrochloride 0.2%. Glycerin. Preservative free. Soln.; Otic. 14 single-use containers. *Rx.*
Use: Otic antibiotic.
ciprofloxacin. (Various Mfr.) Ciprofloxacin. **Tab.:** As ciprofloxacin hydrochloride. 100 mg, 250 mg, 500 mg, 750 mg. 10s, 20s, 60s, 100s, 500s, 650s, 4,500s, UD 100s (500 mg); 50s, 100s (750 mg); 100s, 500s, UD 100s (250 mg); UD 6s (100 mg). **ER Tab.:** A bilayer tablet containing both ciprofloxacin base and ciprofloxacin hydrochloride. 500 mg, 1,000 mg. 50s. **Inj., Soln., Conc.:** 10 mg/mL (1%). May contain lactic acid. Vial. 20 mL, 40 mL. *Rx.*
Use: Fluoroquinolone.

•**ciprofloxacin hydrochloride.** (sip-ROW-FLOX-ah-sin) *USP.*
Use: Anti-infective, ophthalmic.
See: Ciloxan.

ciprofloxacin in dextrose 5%. (Various Mfr.) Ciprofloxacin 2 mg/mL. Inj., Soln. Single-dose premix flexible container. 100 mL, 200 mL. *Rx.*
Use: Fluoroquinolone.

Cipro HC Otic. (Alcon) Ciprofloxacin 0.2%, hydrocortisone 1%/mL. Benzyl alcohol. Susp. Bot. 10 mL. *Rx.*
Use: Steroid and antibiotic combination.

Cipro I.V. (Schering-Plough) Ciprofloxacin 2 mg/mL (0.2%). Lactic acid. Latex free. Inj. Premix flexible containers w/dextrose 5%. 100 mL, 200 mL. *Rx.*
Use: Anti-infective, fluoroquinolone.

•**ciprostene calcium.** (sigh-PRAHS-teen) USAN.
Use: Platelet aggregation inhibitor.

Cipro XR. (Schering-Plough) Ciprofloxacin 500 mg, 1,000 mg (as a bilayer tablet containing both ciprofloxacin base and ciprofloxacin hydrochloride). Film coated. Polyethylene glycol. ER Tab. 50s; UD 30s (1,000 mg only). *Rx.*
Use: Anti-infective, fluoroquinolone.

•**ciramadol.** (sihr-AM-ah-dole) USAN.
Use: Analgesic.

•**ciramadol hydrochloride.** (sihr-AM-ah-dole) USAN.
Use: Analgesic.

Circavite-T. (Circle) Iron 12 mg, vitamins A 10,000 units, D 400 units, E 15 mg, B_1 10.3 mg, B_2 10 mg, B_3 100 mg, B_5 18.4 mg, B_6 4.1 mg, B_{12} 5 mcg, C 200 mg, Cu, I, Mg, Mn, Zn 1.5 mg. Bot. 100s. *OTC.*
Use: Mineral, vitamin supplement.

•**cirolemycin.** (sih-ROW-leh-MY-sin) USAN.
Use: Anti-infective; antineoplastic.

•**cisapride.** (SIS-uh-PRIDE) USAN.
Note: Withdrawn from US market. Available from the manufacturer on a limited-access protocol.
Use: Gastrointestinal; stimulant, peristaltic.

•**cisatracurium besylate.** (sis-ah-trah-CURE-ee-uhm BESS-ih-late) USAN.
Use: Nondepolarizing neuromuscular blocking agent; muscle relaxant.
See: Nimbex.

cisatracurium besylate. (Sandoz) Cisatracurium besylate 2 mg/mL, 10 mg/mL. Inj., Soln. 5 mL single-use vial (benzenesulfonic acid), 10 mL multiple-use vial (contains benzyl alcohol 0.9%). *Rx.*
Use: Muscle relaxant—adjunct to anesthesia, nondepolarizing neuromuscular blocker.

•**cisconazole.** (SIS-KOE-nah-zahl) USAN.
Use: Antifungal.

•**cisplatin.** (SIS-plat-in) *USP. Formerly cis-Platinum II.*
Tall Man: CISplatin
Use: Antineoplastic.

cisplatin. (Various Mfr.) Cisplatin 1 mg/mL. Inj. Multidose vial 50 mL, 100 mL, 200 mL. *Rx.*
Use: Antineoplastic.

cis-retinoic acid. (13-cis-Retinoic Acid).
Use: Antiacne.
See: Accutane.
Isotretinoin.

9-cis retinoic acid. (Allergan)
Use: Promyelocytic leukemia treatment; prevention of retinal detachment caused by proliferative vitreoretinopathy. [Orphan Drug]

•**citalopram hydrobromide.** (sih-TAHL-oh-pram) USAN.
Use: Antidepressant.
See: Celexa.

citalopram hydrobromide. (Various Mfr.) Citalopram hydrobromide. **Tab.:** 10 mg, 20 mg, 40 mg. May contain lactose. 30s, 60s, 100s, 500s, 1,000s, 5,000s (except 10 mg), UD 100s (except 10 mg). **Soln.:** 2 mg/mL. May contain parabens, propylene glycol, sorbitol. 240 mL. *Rx.*
Use: Antidepressant.

Citanest Forte. (Dentsply Pharm) Prilocaine hydrochloride 4% with epinephrine 1:200,000, sodium metabisulfite. Inj. Dental cartridge 1.8 mL. *Rx.*
Use: Anesthetic, local amide, injectable.

Citanest Plain. (Dentsply Pharm) Prilocaine hydrochloride 4%. Inj. Dental Cartridge. 1.8 mL. *Rx.*
Use: Anesthetic, local amide, injectable.

•**citenamide.** (sigh-TEN-ah-MIDE) USAN.
Use: Anticonvulsant.

Cithal. (Table Rock) Watermelon seed extract 2 g, theobromine 4 g, phenobarbital 0.25 g. Cap. Bot. 100s, 500s. *Rx.*
Use: Antihypertensive.

•**citicoline sodium.** (SIGH-tih-koe-leen) USAN.
Use: Poststroke and posthead trauma treatment.

Citracal. (Mission) Elemental calcium 200 mg. Tab. Bot. 100s. *OTC.*
Use: Calcium supplement.

Citracal 1500 + D. (Mission) Calcium citrate 1500 mg, vitamin D 200 units. Tab. Bot. 60s. *OTC.*
Use: Mineral, vitamin supplement.

Citracal + D_3 Maximum. (Bayer) Calcium 315 mg, vitamin D 200 units. PEG, propylene glycol. Coated. Tab. 240s. *OTC.*
Use: Nutritional supplement.

Citracal Plus with Magnesium. (Mission) Ca 250 mg, vitamin D 125 units, B_6 5 mg, B, Cu, Mg, Mn, Zn. Tab. Bot. 150s. *OTC.*
Use: Mineral, vitamin supplement.

Citracal Prenatal 90 + DHA. (Mission) **Cap.:** Docosahexaenoic acid 250 mg. 6 blister packs of 5s. **Tab.:** Calcium 200 mg, iron 90 mg, vitamin A 2700 units, D_3 400 units, E 30 units, thiamin 30 mg, riboflavin 3.4 mg, niacinamide 20 mg, B_6 20 mg, B_{12} 12 mcg, C 120 mg, folic acid 1 mg, iodine 150 mcg, zinc 25 mg, copper 2 mg, docusate sodium 50 mg. 6 blister packs of 5s. *Rx.*
Use: Prenatal vitamin.

Citracal Prenatal + DHA. (Mission) **Cap.:** Docosahexaenoic acid 250 mg. 6 blister packs of 5s. **Tab.:** Calcium 125 mg, iron 27 mg, vitamin A 2700 units, D_3 400 units, E 30 units, thiamin 3 mg, riboflavin 3.4 mg, niacinamide 20 mg, B_6 20 mg, C 120 mg, folic acid 1 mg, iodine 150 mcg, zinc 25 mg, copper 2 mg, docusate sodium 50 mg. 6 blister packs of 5s. *Rx.*
Use: Prenatal vitamin.

Citra Forte. (Boyle and Co. Pharm.) Hydrocodone bitartrate 5 mg, ascorbic acid 30 mg, pheniramine maleate 2.5 mg, pyrilamine maleate 3.33 mg, potassium citrate 150 mg/5 mL. Bot. Pt, gal. *c-III.*
Use: Antihistamine; antitussive; vitamin supplement.

CitraNatal B-Calm. (Mission Pharmacal) Folic acid 1 mg, Ca 120 mg, Fe 20 mg, vitamins D_3 400 units, B_6 25 mg, C 120 mg. Gluten free. Tab. UD 30s w/blister card 6s of 5 prenatal tablets (coated) and 10 vitamin B_6 tablets (25 mg each). *Rx.*
Use: Prenatal vitamin with minerals.

Citranox. (Alconox)
Use: Liquid acid detergent for manual and ultrasonic washers.

Citra pH. (ValMed, Inc.) Sodium citrate dihydrate 450 mg/30 mL. Soln. 30 mL. *OTC.*
Use: Antacid.

Citrasan B. (Sandia) Lemon bioflavonoid complex 300 mg, vitamins C 300 mg, B_1 30 mg, B_2 10 mg, B_6 5 mg, B_{12} 4 mcg, calcium pantothenate 10 mg, niacinamide 50 mg. Tab. Bot. 100s, 1000s. *OTC.*
Use: Mineral, vitamin supplement.

Citrasan K. (Sandia) Vitamins C 125 mg, K 0.66 mg, lemon bioflavonoid complex 125 mg/5 mL. Liq. Bot. Pt, gal. *OTC.*
Use: Vitamin supplement.

Citrasan K-250. (Sandia) Vitamins C 250 mg, K 1 mg, lemon bioflavonoid 250 mg. Tab. Bot. 100s, 1000s. *OTC.*
Use: Vitamin supplement.

citrate acid.
Use: Systemic alkalinizer.

citrate and citric acid.
Use: Alkalinizer.
See: Oracit.
Taron-Crystals.

citrated normal human plasma.
See: Plasma, Normal Human.

Citresco-K. (Esco) Vitamins C 100 mg, K 0.7 mg, citrus bioflavonoid complex 100 mg. Cap. Bot. 100s, 500s, 1000s. *OTC.*
Use: Vitamin supplement.

•**citric acid.** (SI-trik) *USP.*
Use: Component of anticoagulant solutions and drug products.
W/Aspirin, Sodium Bicarbonate.
See: Alka-Seltzer Lemon Lime.
Alka-Seltzer Original.
W/Magnesium Oxide, Sodium Picosulfate.
See: Prepopik.
W/Potassium Bicarbonate, Sodium Bicarbonate.
See: Alka-Seltzer Gold.
W/Sodium Bicarbonate.
See: Alka-Seltzer Heartburn Relief.
W/Simethicone, Sodium Bicarbonate.
See: E-Z Gas II.

citric acid, glucono-delta-lactone and magnesium carbonate.
Use: Renal and bladder calculi of the apatite or struvite variety. [Orphan Drug]

citric acid, magnesium oxide, and sodium carbonate irrigation.
Use: Irrigant, ophthalmic.

citric acid monohydrate.
W/Potassium Citrate Monohydrate.
See: Taron-Crystals.

citrin.
See: Vitamin P.

Citrin Capsules. (Table Rock) Watermelon seed extract 4 g. Bot. 100s, 500s. *Rx.*
Use: Antihypertensive.

Citrocarbonate. (Lee) Sodium bicarbonate 0.78 g, sodium citrate anhydrous 1.82 g/3.9 g. Bot. 4 oz, 8 oz. *OTC.*
Use: Antacid.

Citrocarbonate Effervescent Granules. (Lee) Sodium bicarbonate 780 mg, so-

dium citrate anhydrous 1820 mg, sodium 700.6 mg/5 mg. Bot. 150 g. *OTC*.
Use: Analgesic; antacid.

Citro Cee, Super. (Marlyn Nutraceuticals) Bioflavonoids 500 mg, rutin 50 mg, vitamin C 500 mg, rose hips powder 500 mg. Tab. Bot. 50s, 100s. *OTC*.
Use: Vitamin supplement.

Citrolith. (Beach) Potassium citrate 50 mg, sodium citrate 950 mg. Tab. Bot. 100s, 500s. *Rx*.
Use: Alkalinizer, urinary.

Citroma. (Century) Magnesium citrate. Oral Soln. Bot. 10 oz. *OTC*.
Use: Laxative.

Citroma Low Sodium. (National Magnesia) Magnesium citrate, lemon or cherry flavor in sugar-free vehicle. Oral soln. Bot. 10 oz. *OTC*.
Use: Laxative.

Citrotein. (Novartis) Sucrose, pasteurized egg white solids, amino acids, maltodextrin, citric acid, natural and artificial flavors, mono- and diglycerides, partially hydrogenated soybean oil, 0.66 cal/mL, protein 40.7 g, carbohydrate 120.7 g, fat 1.55 g, Na 698 mg, K 698 mg/L. Tartrazine (orange flavor only). Orange, grape, and punch flavors. Pow. 1.57 oz. Pkt., Can 14.16 oz. *OTC*.
Use: Nutritional supplement, enteral.

•**citrovorum factor.** (sih-troe-VOHR-uhm) *USP.*
See: Leucovorin calcium.

Citrucel. (GlaxoSmithKline) Methylcellulose. **Pow.:** 2 g/heaping tbsp., sucrose, orange flavor. Can. 480 g, 846 g. **Tab.:** 500 mg. Maltodextrin. 164s. *OTC*.
Use: Laxative

Citrucel Fiber Shake. (GlaxoSmithKline) Methylcellulose 2 g per scoop. Aspartame, phenylalanine 49 mg, maltodextrin, soy lecithin, sunflower oil. Calcium 40 mg, potassium 150 mg, sodium 20 mg. Gluten free. Chocolate flavor. Pow. 413 g. *OTC*.
Use: Laxative.

Citrucel Sugar Free. (GlaxoSmithKline) Methylcellulose 2 g, aspartame, phenylalanine 52 mg/levelled scoop. Pow. Can. 245 g, 480 g. *OTC*.
Use: Laxative.

citrus bioflavonoid compound.
See: Bioflavonoid Compounds. Vitamin P.

Citrus Calcium. (Rugby) Calcium citrate 200 mg. Lactose free. Coated Tab. 100s. *OTC*.
Use: Mineral supplement.

Citrus Calcium + D. (Rugby) Vitamin D (as cholecalciferol) 200 units, calcium (as calcium citrate) 315 mg. Lactose free. PEG. Tab. 60s. *OTC*.
Use: Nutritional combination product.

Citrus Calcium with Vitamin D. (Rugby) Vitamin D_3 250 units, calcium carbonate 200 mg. Tab. 100s. *OTC*.
Use: Nutritional supplement.

Citrus Calcium with Vitamin D. (Rugby) Vitamin D_3 250 units, calcium citrate 200 mg. Propylene glycol. Tab. 100s. *OTC*.
Use: Nutritional supplement.

•**cixutumumab.** (SIKS-ue-TUE-mue-mab) USAN.
Use: Antineoplastic.

CKA Canker Aid. (Pannett Prod.) Benzocaine, aluminum hydrate, magnesium trisilicate, sodium acid carbonate. Pow. *OTC*.
Use: Cancer; cold sores.

CK (CPK) Reagent Strips. (Bayer Consumer Care) Seralyzer reagent strips for creatinine phosphokinase in serum or plasma. Bot. 25s.
Use: Diagnostic aid.

•**cladribine.** (KLAD-rih-BEAN) USAN.
Use: Antineoplastic.

cladribine. (Bedford) Cladribine 1 mg/mL, sodium chloride 9 mg/mL. Soln. for Inj. Single-use Vial 20 mL w/10 mL fill. *Rx*.
Use: Antineoplastic.

Claforan. (Hospira) Cefotaxime sodium. **Pow. for Inj. (sodium 2.2 mEq/g):** 500 mg. Vial Pkg. 10s. 1 g, 2 g. Vial. Pkg. 10s, 25s, 50s. Infusion bot. 10s, *ADD-Vantage* system Vial 25s, 50s. 10 g. Bot. **Inj. (sodium 2.2 mEq/g):** 1 g, 2 g. Premixed, frozen. 50 mL Pkg. 12s. *Rx*.
Use: Anti-infective, cephalosporin.

•**clamoxyquin hydrochloride.** (KLAM-OX-ee-kwin) USAN.
Use: Amebicide.

Claravis. (Teva) Isotretinoin 10 mg, 20 mg, 30 mg, 40 mg. EDTA. Cap. Blister packs. 30s, 100s (except 30 mg). *Rx*.
Use: Retinoid, first generation.

Clarifoam EF. (Onset) Sodium sulfacetamide 10%, sulfur 5%. Cetyl alcohol, parabens. Aer. Foam. 60 g. *Rx*.
Use: Dermatological agent, acne combination product.

Clarinex. (Schering) Desloratadine. **Syrup:** 2.5 mg/5 mL. Sugar, EDTA. Bubble gum flavor. 480 mL. **Tab.:** 5 mg. Lactose. Film-coated. Bot. 100s, 500s, unit-of-use 30s, UD hospital pack 100s. *Rx*.
Use: Antihistamine, peripherally selective piperidine.

Clarinex-D 12 Hour. (Schering) Pseudoephedrine sulfate 120 mg, desloratadine 2.5 mg. EDTA. ER Tab. 100s. *Rx.*
Use: Decongestant and antihistamine.

Clarinex-D 24 Hour. (Schering) Pseudoephedrine sulfate 240 mg, desloratadine 5 mg. EDTA. ER Tab. 100s. *Rx.*
Use: Decongestant and antihistamine, upper respiratory combination.

Clarinex RediTabs. (Schering) Desloratadine 2.5 mg (phenylalanine 1.4 mg), 5 mg (phenylalanine 2.9 mg). Mannitol, aspartame, tutti frutti flavor. Rapidly disintegrating Tab. Blister packs. 30s. *Rx.*
Use: Antihistamine, peripherally selective piperidine.

Claris. (Stratus) Sodium sulfacetamide 10%, sulfur 1%. Cetyl alcohol, disodium EDTA, glyceryl stearate, parabens, PEG-100, stearyl alcohol, urea. Soap. 473 mL. *Rx.*
Use: Acne product, combination.

•**clarithromycin.** (kluh-RITH-row-MY-sin) *USP.*
Use: Anti-infective.
See: Biaxin.
Biaxin XL.

clarithromycin. (Dava) Clarithromycin 125 mg/5 mL, 250 mg/5 mL (after reconstitution). Maltodextrin, sucrose. Fruit punch flavor. Gran. for Susp., Oral. 50 mL, 100 mL. *Rx.*
Use: Macrolide, anti-infective.

clarithromycin. (Teva) Clarithromycin. **ER Tab.:** 500 mg. Lactose. Film-coated. 60s. **Tab.:** 250 mg, 500 mg. Film-coated. Tab. 60s. *Rx.*
Use: Macrolide, anti-infective.

Claritin. (Schering-Plough) Loratadine 5 mg/5 mL. Sugar, sucrose, EDTA. Fruit flavor. Syrup. Bot. 120 mL. *OTC.*
Use: Antihistamine, peripherally selective piperidine.

Claritin Allergy, Children's. (Schering-Plough) **Chew. Tab.:** Loratadine 5 mg. Phenylalanine 1.4 mg, aspartame, mannitol. Grape flavor. 5s, 10s. **Syrup:** Loratadine 5 mg/5 mL. Maltitol, sorbitol, sucralose. Grape flavor. 60 mL, 120 mL. *OTC.*
Use: Antihistamine, peripherally selective piperidine.

Claritin-D. (Schering-Plough) Loratadine 5 mg, pseudoephedrine sulfate 120 mg. Tab, SR Tab. Bot. 30s (except Tab.), 100s, unit-of-use 10s, 30s (except SR Tab.), UD 100s. *OTC.*
Use: Antihistamine, decongestant.

Claritin-D 12-Hour. (Schering-Plough) Pseudoephedrine sulfate 120 mg, loratadine 5 mg. Lactose. ER Tab. Bot. 10s, 20s, 30s. *OTC.*
Use: Upper respiratory combination, decongestant, antihistamine.

Claritin-D 24-Hour. (Schering-Plough) Loratadine 10 mg, pseudoephedrine sulfate 240 mg. PEG, sugar. ER Tab. Bot. 15s. *OTC.*
Use: Upper respiratory combination, antihistamine, decongestant.

Claritin Eye. (Schering-Plough) Ketotifen fumarate 0.025%. Glycerol, sodium hydroxide and/or hydrochloric acid, benzalkonium chloride 0.01%. Soln., Ophth. 5 mL. *OTC.*
Use: Ophthalmic and otic agent, ophthalmic antihistamine.

Claritin Hives Relief. (Schering-Plough) Loratadine 10 mg. Lactose. Tab. 10s. *OTC.*
Use: Antihistamine, peripherally selective piperidine.

Claritin Non-Drowsy Liqui-Gels. (Schering-Plough) Loratadine 10 mg. Sorbitol. Cap., Liquid filled. 70s. *OTC.*
Use: Antihistamine; piperidine, peripherally selective.

Claritin Reditabs. (Schering-Plough) Loratadine 5 mg, 10 mg. Mannitol, mint flavor. Orally Disintegrating Tab. 4s (10 mg only), 10s, 20s (10 mg only), 30s, 40s (5 mg only). *OTC.*
Use: Antihistamine, peripherally selective piperidine.

Claritin 24-Hour Allergy. (Schering-Plough) Loratadine 10 mg. Lactose. Tab. 1s, 2s, 5s, 10s, 20s, 30s, 40s. *OTC.*
Use: Antihistamine, peripherally selective piperidine.

Classic Prenatal. (Rugby) Folic acid 800 mcg, calcium 200 mg, Fe 28 mg, vitamins A 8,000 units, D 400 units, E 30 units, B_1 1.7 mg, B_2 2 mg, B_3 20 mg, B_6 4 mg, B_{12} 8 mcg, C 60 mg, I, Mg. BHT, maltodextrin, PEG, sodium benzoate. Coated. Gluten free and sugar free. Tab. 100s. *OTC.*
Use: Prenatal vitamin with minerals.

•**clavulanate potassium.** (CLAV-you-lah-nate) *USP.*
Use: Inhibitor, β-lactamase.

clavulanate potassium/amoxicillin.
Use: Penicillin, aminopenicillin.
See: Amoclan.
Augmentin.
Augmentin XR.

clavulanate/ticarcillin.
Use: Extended-spectrum penicillin.
See: Timentin.

clavulanic acid/amoxicillin.
Use: Penicillin, aminopenicillin.
See: Amoclan.

Augmentin.
Augmentin XR.

clavulanic acid/ticarcillin.
Use: Extended-spectrum penicillin.
See: Timentin.

•**clazakizumab.** (KLAZ-a-KIZ-ue-mab) USAN.
Use: Immunomodulator.

•**clazolam.** (CLAY-zoe-lam) USAN.
Use: Anxiolytic.

•**clazolimine.** (clay-ZOLE-ih-meen) USAN.
Use: Diuretic.

Clean and Clear Foaming Facial Cleanser. (Johnson & Johnson) Triclosan 0.25%. BHT, glycerin, parabens, triethanolamine. Oil free. Soap. 240 mL. *OTC.*
Use: Topical anti-infective, antiseptic and germicide.

Clearasil Adult Care Cream. (Procter & Gamble) Sulfur, resorcinol, alcohol 10%, parabens. Cream. Tube. 17 g. *OTC.*
Use: Dermatologic, acne.

Clearasil Adult Care Medicated Blemish Stick. (Procter & Gamble) Sulfur 8%, resorcinol 1%, bentonite 4%, laureth-4, titanium dioxide. Stick ⅛ oz. *OTC.*
Use: Dermatologic, acne.

Clearasil Antibacterial Soap. (Procter & Gamble) Triclosan 0.75%. Bar 92 g. *OTC.*
Use: Dermatologic, acne.

Clearasil Clearstick for Sensitive Skin, Maximum Strength. (Procter & Gamble) Salicylic acid 2%, alcohol 39%, aloe vera gel, menthol, EDTA. Liq. 35 mL. *OTC.*
Use: Dermatologic, acne.

Clearasil Clearstick, Maximum Strength. (Procter & Gamble) Salicylic acid 2%, alcohol 39%, menthol, EDTA. Liq. 35 mL. *OTC.*
Use: Dermatologic, acne.

Clearasil Clearstick, Regular Strength. (Procter & Gamble) Salicylic acid 1.25%, alcohol 39%, aloe vera gel, menthol, EDTA. Liq. 35 mL. *OTC.*
Use: Dermatologic, acne.

Clearasil Daily Face Wash. (Procter & Gamble) Triclosan 0.3%, glycerin, aloe vera gel, EDTA. Liq. Bot. 135 mL. *OTC.*
Use: Dermatologic, acne.

Clearasil Double Clear. (Procter & Gamble) **Pads, maximum strength:** Salicylic acid 2%, alcohol 40%, witch hazel distillate, menthol. Jar 32s. **Pads, regular strength:** Salicylic acid 1.25%, alcohol 40%, witch hazel distillate, menthol. Jar 32s. *OTC.*
Use: Dermatologic, acne.

Clearasil Double Textured Pads. (Procter & Gamble) **Pads, regular strength:** Salicylic acid 2%, alcohol 40%, glycerin, aloe vera gel, EDTA. Pkg. 32s, 40s. **Pads, maximum strength:** Salicylic acid 2%, alcohol 40%, menthol, aloe vera gel, EDTA. Pkg. 32s, 40s. *OTC.*
Use: Dermatologic, acne.

Clearasil Maximum Strength Acne Treatment. (Procter & Gamble) Benzoyl peroxide 10%, parabens in vanishing base. Cream. Tube 18 g. *OTC.*
Use: Dermatologic, acne.

Clearasil Medicated Deep Cleanser. (Procter & Gamble) Salicylic acid 0.5%, alcohol 42%, menthol, EDTA, aloe vera gel, hydrogenated castor oil. Liq. Bot. 229 mL. *OTC.*
Use: Dermatologic, acne.

Clearasil 10%. (Procter & Gamble) Benzoyl peroxide 10%. Bot. oz. *OTC.*
Use: Dermatologic, acne.

Clear-Atadine Children's. (Major) Loratadine 5 mg/5 mL. Alcohol free. Sucrose. Fruit flavor. Syrup. 120 mL. *OTC.*
Use: Antihistamine, peripherally selective piperidine.

Clear-Atadine D. (Major) Pseudoephedrine sulfate 240 mg, loratadine 10 mg. Lactose, PEG. ER Tab. 10s, 15s. *OTC.*
Use: Decongestant and antihistamine, upper respiratory combination.

Clear Away. (Schering-Plough) Salicylic acid 40%. Disc Pck. 18s. *OTC.*
Use: Dermatologic, acne.

Clear Away Plantar. (Schering-Plough) Salicylic acid 40%. Disc (for feet) Pck. 24s. *OTC.*
Use: Dermatologic, acne.

Clearblue Easy Ovulation Test. (Iverness) For urine test. Kit. Contains 7 test sticks. *OTC.*
Use: Ovulation test.

Clearblue Easy Pregnancy Test. (Iverness) Dip stick for pregnancy test. Kit 2s. *OTC.*
Use: Diagnostic aid.

Clearex Acne. (Health for Life Brands) Allantoin, sulfur, resorcinol, d-panthenol, isopropanol. Cream. Tube 1.5 oz. *OTC.*
Use: Dermatologic, acne.

Clear Eyes ACR Seasonal Relief. (Medtech) Naphazoline hydrochloride 0.012%. Benzalkonium chloride, EDTA, zinc sulfate 0.25%, glycerin 0.2%, boric acid, sodium citrate, sodium chloride. Ophth. Soln. Bot. 15 mL. *OTC.*
Use: Mydriatic, vasoconstrictor; ophthalmic decongestant.

Clear Eyes Contact Lens Relief. (Medtech) Sorbic acid 0.25%, EDTA 0.1%, sodium chloride, hypromellose, glycerin. Drops. 15 mL. *OTC.*
Use: Artificial tears.

Clear Eyes Eye Drops. (Ross) Naphazoline hydrochloride 0.012%. Bot. 15 mL, 30 mL. *OTC.*
Use: Mydriatic, vasoconstrictor.

Clear Eyes for Dry Eyes. (Medtech) Carboxymethylcellulose sodium 1%, glycerin 0.25%. Boric acid, EDTA. Soln. 15 mL. *OTC.*
Use: Artificial tears.

Clear Eyes for Redness Relief. (Medtech) Naphazoline hydrochloride 0.012%. Glycerin 0.2%, benzalkonium chloride, boric acid, EDTA, sodium borate. Ophth. Soln. 6 mL, 15 mL, 30 mL. *OTC.*
Use: Ophthalmic decongestant.

Clear Eyes Tears Plus Redness Relief. (Medtech) Naphazoline hydrochloride 0.012%. Hypromellose 0.8%, glycerin 0.25%, benzalkonium chloride, EDTA, boric acid, calcium chloride, magnesium chloride, potassium chloride, sodium borate, sodium chloride. Ophth. Soln. 15 mL. *OTC.*
Use: Ophthalmic decongestant.

Clearly CalaGel. (Tec) Diphenhydramine hydrochloride, zinc acetate, menthol, EDTA. Gel. Tube. 180 g. *OTC.*
Use: Antipruritic, topical.

•**clebopride.** (KLEH-boe-PRIDE) USAN.
Use: Antiemetic.

•**clemastine.** (KLEM-ass-teen) USAN.
Use: Antihistamine.

•**clemastine fumarate.** (KLEM-ass-teen) *USP.*
Use: Antihistamine, nonselective ethanolamine.
See: Antihist-D.
Dayhist-1.
Tavist.
Tavist Allergy.
W/Combinations.
See: Tavist Allergy/Sinus/Headache.

clemastine fumarate. (Various Mfr.) Clemastine fumarate. 0.67 mg/5 mL, may contain alcohol. Syr. Bot. 118 mL, 120 mL. *Rx.*
Use: Antihistamine, nonselective ethanolamine.

clemastine fumarate. (Various Mfr.) Clemastine fumarate 1.34 mg, 2.68 mg. Tab. Bot. 100s. *OTC.*
Use: Antihistamine, nonselective ethanolamine.

Clenia. (Upsher-Smith) Sodium sulfacetamide 10%, sulfur 5%. Butylated hydroxytoluene, disodium EDTA, glyceryl, parabens, propylene glycol. Soap. 170 g, 340 g. *Rx.*
Use: Keratolytic.

Clens. (Alcon) Cleansing agent with benzalkonium chloride 0.02%, EDTA 0.1%. Soln. Bot. 60 mL. *OTC.*
Use: Contact lens care.

•**clentiazem maleate.** (klen-TIE-ah-zem) USAN.
Use: Antianginal; antihypertensive; antagonist, calcium channel.

Cleocin. (Pfizer) Clindamycin phosphate 2%. Benzyl alcohol, cetostearyl alcohol, mineral oil. Vag. Cream. Tube. 40 g with 7 disposable applicators. *Rx.*
Use: Vaginal preparation; anti-infective.

Cleocin HCl. (Pfizer) Clindamycin hydrochloride 75 mg, 150 mg, 300 mg, tartrazine, lactose. Cap. 100s (75 mg); 100s, UD 100s (150 mg, 300 mg). *Rx.*
Use: Anti-infective.

Cleocin Pediatric. (Pfizer) Clindamycin palmitate 75 mg/5 mL. Ethylparaben, sucrose. Gran. for Oral Soln. 100 mL. *Rx.*
Use: Anti-infective.

Cleocin Phosphate. (Pfizer) Clindamycin phosphate 150 mg/mL. Benzyl alcohol, disodium edetate. Vial 2 mL, 4 mL, 6 mL; *ADD-Vantage* Vial 4 mL, 6 mL. *Rx.*
Use: Anti-infective.

Cleocin Phosphate IV. (Pfizer) Clindamycin phosphate 300 mg, 600 mg, 900 mg. Disodium edetate. Inj. *Galaxy* container w/dextrose 5%. *Rx.*
Use: Anti-infective agent, lincosamide.

Cleocin T. (Pfizer) Clindamycin phosphate. **Gel:** 1%. Methylparaben. 30 g, 60 g. **Lotion:** 1%. Cetostearyl alcohol 2.5%, glycerin, isostearyl alcohol 2.5%, methylparaben 0.3%. 60 mL. **Top. Susp.:** 1%. Isopropyl alcohol 50%. 30 mL, 60 mL, single-use pledget applicators. *Rx.*
Use: Anti-infective.

Cleocin Vaginal Ovules. (Pfizer) Clindamycin phosphate 100 mg (as base). Vag. Supp. Cartons of 3s with applicator. *Rx.*
Use: Anti-infective, vaginal.

Clerz Drops for Hard Lenses. (Alcon) Hypertonic solution with hydroxyethylcellulose, sorbic acid, poloxamer 407, EDTA 0.1%, thimerosal 0.001%. Soln. Bot. 25 mL. *OTC.*
Use: Contact lens care.

Clerz Drops for Soft Lenses. (Alcon) Hypertonic solution with hydroxyethylcellu-

lose, sodium borate, poloxamer 407, sorbic acid, thimerosal 0.001%, EDTA 0.1%. Soln. Bot. 25 mL. *OTC.*
Use: Contact lens care.

Clerz Plus. (Alcon) Buffered, isotonic, citrate buffer, NaCl, EDTA 0.05%, polyquaternium-1 0.001%, PEG-11. Drops. Bot. 5 mL, 8 mL, 10 mL. *OTC.*
Use: Contact lens product.

Clerz 2 for Hard Lenses. (Alcon) Isotonic solution with hydroxyethylcellulose, poloxamer 407, sodium chloride, potassium chloride, sodium borate, boric acid, sorbic acid, EDTA. Soln. Bot. 5 mL, 15 mL, 30 mL. *OTC.*
Use: Contact lens care.

•**clevidipine.** (klev-ID-i-peen) USAN.
Use: Cardiovascular agent.

•**clevidipine butyrate.** (klev-ID-i-peen) USAN.
Use: Cardiovascular agent, calcium channel blocking agent.
See: Cleviprex.

Cleviprex. (The Medicines Company) Clevidipine butyrate 0.5 mg/mL. Glycerin 22.5 mg/mL, purified egg yolk phospholipids 12 mg/mL, soybean oil 200 mg/mL. Inj., Emulsion. Single-use vial. 50 mL, 100 mL. *Rx.*
Use: Cardiovascular agent, calcium channel blocking agent.

•**clevudine.** (cleh-VOO-deen) USAN.
Use: Antiviral.

clidinium bromide.
Use: Anticholinergic.
W/Chlordiazepoxide Hydrochloride.
See: Librax.
See: RE Chlordiazepoxide/Clidinium.

Climara. (Bayer Healthcare) Estradiol 2 mg (0.025 mg/day), 2.85 mg (0.0375 mg/day), 3.8 mg (0.05 mg/day), 4.55 mg (0.06 mg/day), 5.7 mg (0.075 mg/day), 7.6 mg (0.1 mg/day). Transdermal System. Box 4s. *Rx.*
Use: Estrogen, sex hormone.

ClimaraPro. (Bayer Healthcare) Estradiol 0.045 mg/levonorgestrel 0.015 mg/day. Transdermal Patch (22 cm^2). 4s. *Rx.*
Use: Sex hormone, estrogen and progestin combined.

Clinac BPO. (Ferndale) Benzoyl peroxide 7%, EDTA. Gel. Tube. 45 g, 90 g. *Rx.*
Use: Anti-infective, topical.

•**clinafloxacin hydrochloride.** (klin-ah-FLOX-ah-sin) USAN.
Use: Anti-infective.

Clindacin ETZ. (Medimetriks Pharmaceuticals) Clindamycin 1%. Isopropyl alcohol 50%, propylene glycol. Pledget; topical. 60s. *Rx.*
Use: Anti-infective, antibiotic agent.

Clindacin P. (Medimetriks Pharmaceuticals) Clindamycin 1%. Isopropyl alcohol 50%, propylene glycol. Pledget; topical. 69s. *Rx.*
Use: Topical anti-infective, antibiotic agent.

Clindagel. (Onset Dermatologics) Clindamycin phosphate 1%, methylparaben. Gel. Tube. 7.5 g, 42 g, 77 g. *Rx.*
Use: Anti-infective, topical.

ClindaMax. (PharmaDerm) Clindamycin phosphate 2%. Benzyl alcohol, cetostearyl alcohol, mineral oil. Cream. 40 g tube with 7 disposable applicators. *Rx.*
Use: Anti-infective, topical.

•**clindamycin.** (KLIN-dah-MY-sin) USAN.
Use: Anti-infective; dermatologic, acne. Oral as antibiotic. Vaginal as anti-infective. AIDS-associated pneumonia. [Orphan Drug]
See: BenzaClin.
Clindacin ETZ.
Evoclin.
W/Benzoyl Peroxide.
See: Duac CS.

•**clindamycin hydrochloride.** (KLIN-dah-MY-sin) *USP.*
Use: Anti-infective.
See: Cleocin HCl.

clindamycin hydrochloride. (Lannett Company) Clindamycin hydrochloride 75 mg. Lactose. Cap. 100s, 200s. *Rx.*
Use: Anti-infective, lincosamide.

clindamycin hydrochloride. (Various Mfr.) Clindamycin hydrochloride 150 mg, 300 mg. May contain lactose. Cap. 16s (300 mg only), 100s, UD 25s (150 mg only), UD 50s (300 mg only). *Rx.*
Use: Lincosamide.

clindamycin in 5% dextrose. (Sandoz) Clindamycin phosphate 300 mg, 600 mg, 900 mg. Disodium edetate. Inj., Soln. Single-dose container. 50 mL. *Rx.*
Use: Anti-infective agent, lincosamide.

clindamycin 1%/benzoyl peroxide 5%. (Mylan) Benzoyl peroxide 5%, clindamycin 1%. Gel. 50 g. *Rx.*
Use: Acne product combination.

•**clindamycin palmitate.** (KLIN-dah-MY-sin PAL-mih-tate) *USP.*
Use: Anti-infective.
See: Cleocin Pediatric.

clindamycin palmitate hydrochloride. (Paddock) Clindamycin palmitate hydrochloride 75 mg per 5 mL. May contain cherry flavoring, dextrin, ethylparaben, sucrose. Granules for Soln. 100 mL. *Rx.*
Use: Anti-infective agent, lincosamide.

•**clindamycin phosphate.** (KLIN-dah-MY-sin) *USP.*
Use: Anti-infective.
See: Cleocin.
Cleocin Phosphate.
Cleocin T.
Cleocin Vaginal Ovules.
Clindacin P.
Clindagel.
ClindaMax.
Clindesse.
PledgaClin.
W/Benzoyl Peroxide.
See: Duac.
W/Tretinoin.
See: Ziana.

clindamycin phosphate. (Greenstone) Clindamycin phosphate 2%. Cream. Tube. 40 g with 7 disposable applicators. *Rx.*
Use: Anti-infective.

clindamycin phosphate. (VersaPharm) Clindamycin phosphate 1%. Isopropyl alcohol 50%, propylene glycol. Pledget, topical. 60s. *Rx.*
Use: Topical anti-infective, antibiotic.

clindamycin phosphate. (Various Mfr.) Clindamycin phosphate. **Inj.:** 150 mg/mL. May contain benzyl alcohol, disodium edetate. Vial. 2 mL, 4 mL, 6 mL. *ADD-Vantage* vial. 2 mL, 4 mL, 6 mL. **Top. Susp.:** 1%. Bot. 30 mL, 60 mL. **Gel:** 1%. Tube 30 g, 60 g. **Lot.:** 1%. Bot. 60 mL. *Rx.*
Use: Lincosamide; dermatologic, acne.

Clindesse. (Ther-Rx) Clindamycin phosphate 2%. EDTA, mineral oil, parabens. Cream. Carton of 1 single-dose, prefilled, disposable applicator. *Rx.*
Use: Vaginal preparation.

Clinical Nutrients 50-Plus Men. (Integrative Therapeutics) Vitamins A 1,250 units, D 200 units, E 16.75 units, B_1 15 mg, B_2 15 mg, B_3 30 mg, B_5 25 mg, B_6 6.25 mg, B_{12} 200 mcg, C 75 mg, K 30 mcg, folic acid 0.2 mg, B, Ca, Cr, Cu, I, K, Mg, Mn, Mo, Na, Se, V, Zn, *Antioxidant blend* 28 mg, betaine 6.25 mg, bilberry 2.5 mg, biotin 150 mcg, choline 68.75 mg, cinnamon 50 mg, *Digestive blend* 18.5 mg, ginseng root extract 3.75 mg, inositol 7.5 mg, lutein 0.375 mg, lycopene 0.5 mg, saw palmetto 20 mg, *Vegetable blend* 10 mg, zeaxanthin 18.75 mcg. Glycerin, maltodextrin, soy lecithin, soybean oil. Gluten free, preservative free. Tab. 120s. *OTC.*
Use: Multivitamin with minerals (except iron).

Clinical Nutrients Prenatal Formula. (Integrative Therapeutics) Folic acid 0.2 mg, Ca 250 mg, Fe 7.5 mg, vitamins A 2,500 units, D 50 units, E 50 units, C 75 mg, B_1 15 mg, B_2 15 mg, B_3 11.25 mg, B_5 25 mg, B_6 25 mg, B_{12} 200 mcg. B, Cr, Cu, I, K, Mg, Mn, Mo, Na, P, Se, Si, V, Zn. Vitamin K 125 mcg, biotin 150 mcg, choline bitartrate 22.5 mg, inositol 22.5 mg, mixed bioflavonoids 50% 22.5 mg, dandelion root extract 15 mg. Soy, soybean oil. Gluten free, preservative free. Tab. 120s. *OTC.*
Use: Prenatal vitamin with minerals.

clinocaine hydrochloride.
See: Procaine Hydrochloride.

Clinolipid. (Baxter Healthcare) Lipids 0.2 g/mL. Egg phospholipids 1.2 g, glycerin 2.25 g, olive oil 16 g, sodium oleate 0.03 g, soybean oil 4 g per 100 mL. Inj., Emuls. 1,000 mL. *Rx.*
Use: Intravenous nutritional therapy.

Clinoril. (Merck) Sulindac 200 mg. Tab. 100s. *Rx.*
Use: Analgesic; NSAID.

Clinoxide. (Geneva) Clidinium bromide 2.5 mg, chlordiazepoxide hydrochloride, 5 mg. Cap. Bot. 100s, 500s. *c-IV.*
Use: Gastrointestinal; anticholinergic.

•**clioquinol.** (KLYE-oh-KWIN-ole) *USP.*
Formerly Iodochlorhydroxyquin.
Use: Antiamebic; anti-infective, topical.
W/Hydrocortisone.
See: Dermasorb AF.
Hysone.
W/Hydrocortisone, Pramoxine Hydrochloride.
See: 1 + 1-F Creme.

•**clioxanide.** (klie-OX-ah-nide) USAN.
Use: Anthelmintic.

Clipoxide. (Schein) Clidinium bromide 2.5 mg, chlordiazepoxide hydrochloride 5 mg. Cap. Bot. 100s, 500s. *c-V.*
Use: Anticholinergic; antispasmodic.

•**cliprofen.** (klih-PRO-fen) USAN.
Use: Anti-inflammatory.

clobamine mesylate. *Name previously used for cilobamine mesylate.*
Use: Antidepressant.

•**clobazam.** (KLOE-bazz-am) USAN.
Use: Investigational anxiolytic.
See: Onfi.

•**clobetasol propionate.** (kloe-BEE-tah-sahl PRO-ee-oh-nate) *USP.*
Use: Anti-inflammatory.
See: Clobex.
Cormax.
Olux.
Olux-E.
Temovate.

clobetasol propionate. (Actavis Mid Atlantic) Clobetasol propionate 0.05%.

Mineral oil, propylene glycol. Lot. 30 mL, 59 mL, 118 mL. *Rx.*
Use: Topical corticosteroid.

clobetasol propionate. (Glades Pharmaceutical) Clobetasol propionate 0.05%. Cetyl alcohol, ethanol 60%, stearyl alcohol. Top. Foam. 50 g, 100 g. *Rx.*
Use: Anti-inflammatory agent, topical corticosteroid.

clobetasol propionate. (Taro) Clobetasol propionate 0.05%. Soln. 25 mL, 50 mL. *Rx.*
Use: Anti-inflammatory agent.

clobetasol propionate. (Various Mfr.) Clobetasone propionate 0.05%. **Gel:** Tube. 15 g, 30 g, 60 g. **Cream:** Tube. 15 g, 30 g, 45 g. **Ointment:** White petrolatum. Tube. 15 g, 30 g, 45 g. **Shampoo:** May contain alcohol. 118 mL. *Rx.*
Use: Anti-inflammatory; corticosteroid, topical.

•**clobetasone butyrate.** (kloe-BEE-tih-sone BYOO-tah-rate) USAN.
Use: Corticosteroid; anti-inflammatory.

Clobex. (Galderma) Clobetasol propionate 0.05%. **Lot.:** Mineral oil. 15 mL, 30 mL, 59 mL, 118 mL. **Shampoo:** Alcohol. 118 mL. **Spray:** 0.05%. Alcohol. 60 mL. *Rx.*
Use: Anti-inflammatory; corticosteroid, topical.

•**clocortolone acetate.** (kloe-CORE-toe-lone) USAN.
Use: Corticosteroid, topical.

•**clocortolone pivalate.** (kloe-CORE-toe-lone PIH-vah-late) *USP.*
Use: Corticosteroid, topical.

clocortolone pivalate. (Various Mfr.) Clocortolone pivalate 0.1%. May contain edetate disodium, mineral oil, parabens, stearyl alcohol, white petrolatum. Cream. 45 g and 90 g tube; 30 g and 75 g pump bottle. *Rx.*
Use: Anti-inflammatory agent, topical corticosteroid.

Clocream. (Pharmacia) Vitamins A and D in vanishing base. Tube oz. *OTC.*
Use: Emollient.

•**clodanolene.** (Kloe-DAN-oh-leen) USAN.
Use: Muscle relaxant.

•**clodazon hydrochloride.** (KLOE-dah-zone) USAN.
Use: Antidepressant.

Cloderm. (Valeant) Clocortolone pivalate 0.1%. Cream. Tube 15 g, 45 g. *Rx.*
Use: Corticosteroid, topical.

•**clodronate disodium.** (kloe-DRAHN-ate) USAN.
Use: Bone calcium regulator.

•**clodronic acid.** (kloe-DRAHN-ik) USAN.
Use: Calcium regulator.

•**clofarabine.** (kloe-FAR-a-bine) USAN.
Use: Antimetabolite.
See: Clolar.

•**clofazimine.** (kloe-FAZZ-ih-meen) *USP.*
Use: Investigational tuberculostatic, leprostatic. [Orphan Drug]

Clofera. (Centrix) Chlophedianol hydrochloride 12.5 mg, pseudoephedrine hydrochloride 30 mg. Saccharin, sorbitol. Alcohol free, dye free, gluten free, and sugar free. Grape flavor. Liq. 473 mL. *OTC.*
Use: Upper respiratory combination, antitussive combination.

•**clofilium phosphate.** (KLOE-FILL-ee-uhm) USAN.
Use: Cardiovascular agent, antiarrhythmic.

•**cloflucarban.** (KLOE-flew-CAR-ban) USAN.
Use: Antiseptic; disinfectant.

•**clogestone acetate.** (kloe-JESS-tone) USAN. Under study.
Use: Hormone, progestin.

Clolar. (Genzyme Corporation) Clofarabine 1 mg/mL. Preservative free. Soln. for Inj. Vials. 20 mL. *Rx.*
Use: Antimetabolite.

•**clomacran phosphate.** (KLOE-mah-KRAN) USAN. Under study.
Use: Antipsychotic.

•**clomegestone acetate.** (KLOE-meh-JESS-tone) USAN. Under study.
Use: Hormone, progestin.

•**clometherone.** (kloe-METH-ehr-OHN) USAN.
Use: Antiestrogen.

Clomid. (Aventis Pasteur) Clomiphene citrate 50 mg. Tab. Bot. 30s. *Rx.*
Use: Sex hormone, ovulation stimulant.

•**clominorex.** (kloe-MEE-no-rex) USAN.
Use: Anorexic.

•**clomiphene citrate.** (KLOE-mih-feen SIH-trate) *USP.*
Tall Man: clomiPHENE
Use: Antiestrogen; sex hormone, ovulation stimulant.
See: Clomid.
Milophene.
Serophene.

clomiphene citrate. (Various Mfr.) Clomiphene citrate 50 mg. Tab. Bot. 10s, 30s. *Rx.*
Use: Sex hormone, ovulation stimulant.

•**clomipramine hydrochloride.** (kloe-MIH-pruh-meen) USAN.
Tall Man: clomiPRAMINE
Use: Antidepressant.
See: Anafranil.

clomipramine hydrochloride. (Various Mfr.) Clomipramine hydrochloride 25 mg, 50 mg, 75 mg. Cap. 30s, 90s, 100s. *Rx.*
Use: Antidepressant.

•**clonazepam.** (kloe-NAY-ze-pam) *USP.*
Tall Man: clonazePAM
Use: Anticonvulsant; antianxiety agent.
See: Klonopin.

clonazepam. (Barr) Clonazepam 0.125 mg, 0.25 mg, 0.5 mg, 1 mg, 2 mg. May contain phenylalanine, aspartame, mannitol, sorbitol, xylitol. Strawberry flavor. Orally Disintegrating Tab. Blister pack. 60s. *c-IV.*
Use: Antianxiety agent; anticonvulsant.

clonazepam. (Various Mfr.) Clonazepam 0.5 mg, 1 mg, 2 mg. May contain lactose, PEG. Tab. 15s (except 2 mg), 30s, 45s (except 2 mg), 60s, 90s, 100s, 120s (1 mg only), 500s, 1,000s, UD 100s, UD 300s (except 2 mg). *c-IV.*
Use: Anticonvulsant; antianxiety agent.

•**clonidine.** (KLOE-nih-DEEN) USAN.
Tall Man: cloNIDine
Use: Antihypertensive.
See: Catapres.

clonidine. (Par Pharmaceutical) Clonidine hydrochloride 0.1 mg/24 h (surface area, 10.8 cm^2) (total clonidine content, 3.67 mg); 0.2 mg/24 h (surface area, 21.6 cm^2) (total clonidine content, 7.34 mg); 0.3 mg/24 h (surface area, 32.4 cm^2) (total clonidine content, 11.02 mg). Transdermal patch. 4s. *Rx.*
Use: Antiadrenergic/sympatholytic; antiadrenergic agent, centrally acting.

clonidine. (Various Mfr.) Clonidine hydrochloride. **Tab.:** 0.1 mg, 0.2 mg, 0.3 mg. May contain lactose. 30s, 100s, 500s, 1,000s, UD 25s (except 0.3 mg), UD 100s, UD 300s (0.2 mg only). **ER Tab.:** 0.1 mg (equiv. to clonidine base 0.087 mg), 0.2 mg (equiv. to clonidine base 0.174 mg). 60s, 180s, 500s. *Rx.*
Use: Antiadrenergic/sympatholytic; antiadrenergic agent, centrally acting.

•**clonidine hydrochloride.** (KLOE-nih-DEEN) *USP.*
Tall Man: cloNIDine
Use: Antihypertensive. Epidural use for pain in cancer patients.
See: Catapres.
Duraclon.
Jenloga.
Kapvay.
W/Chlorthalidone
See: Clorpres.

clonidine hydrochloride. (American Regent) Clonidine hydrochloride. **Inj., Soln.:** 100 mcg/mL. Preservative free. Single-dose vial. 10 mL. **Inj., Soln., concentrate:** 500 mcg/mL. Preservative free. Vial. 10 mL. *Rx.*
Use: Central analgesic.

•**clonitrate.** (KLOE-nye-trate) USAN.
Use: Coronary vasodilator.

•**clonixeril.** (kloe-NIX-ehr-ill) USAN.
Use: Analgesic.

•**clonixin.** (kloe-NIX-in) USAN.
Use: Analgesic.

•**clopamide.** (kloe-PAM-id) USAN.
Use: Antihypertensive; diuretic.

•**clopenthixol.** (KLOE-pen-THIX-ole) USAN.
Use: Antipsychotic.

•**cloperidone hydrochloride.** (KLOE-per-ih-dohn) USAN.
Use: Hypnotic; sedative.

clophenoxate hydrochloride.
Use: Cerebral stimulant.

•**clopidogrel bisulfate.** (kloe-PIH-doe-grell bye-SULL-fate) *USP.*
Use: Platelet inhibitor.
See: Plavix.

clopidogrel bisulfate. (Apotex) Clopidogrel bisulfate (as base) 75 mg. Lactose. Film-coated. Tab. 30s, 90s, 1000s, UD 100s. *Rx.*
Use: Antiplatelet agent; aggregation inhibitor.

clopidogrel bisulfate. (Various Mfr.) Clopidogrel 75 mg (equiv. to clopidogrel bisulfate 97.875 mg), 300 mg (equiv. to clopidogrel bisulfate 391.5 mg). May be film coated. May contain lactose, mannitol (75 mg), polydextrose, PEG. Tab. 30s, 90s, 500s (75 mg and 300 mg); 1,000s, 3,100s, UD 100s (75 mg only). *Rx.*
Use: Antiplatelet agent, aggregation inhibitor.

•**clopimozide.** (KLOE-PIM-oh-zide) USAN.
Use: Antipsychotic.

•**clopipazan mesylate.** (KLOE-pip-ah-ZAN) USAN.
Use: Antipsychotic.

•**clopirac.** (KLOE-pih-rack) USAN.
Use: Anti-inflammatory.

•**cloprednol.** (kloe-PRED-nahl) USAN.
Use: Corticosteroid, topical.

•**cloprostenol sodium.** (kloe-PROSTE-een-ole) USAN.
Use: Prostaglandin.

•**clorazepate dipotassium.** (klor-AZE-eh-PATE DIE-poe-TASS-ee-uhm) *USP.*
Use: Anxiolytic; anticonvulsant.
See: Tranxene.

clorazepate dipotassium. (Various Mfr.) Clorazepate dipotassium 3.75 mg, 7.5 mg, 15 mg. Tab. Bot. 20s (7.5 mg only), 100s, 500s, 1000s, UD 100s, UD 500s (7.5 mg only). *c-iv.*
Use: Anxiolytic; anticonvulsant.

•**clorazepate monopotassium.** (clor-AZE-eh-PATE MAHN-oh-poe-TASS-ee-uhm) USAN.
Use: Anxiolytic.

•**clorethate.** (klahr-ETH-ate) USAN.
Use: Hypnotic; sedative.

•**clorexolone.** (KLOR-ex-oh-LONE) USAN.
Use: Diuretic.

Clorfed Capsules. (Stewart-Jackson Pharmacal) Chlorpheniramine 8 mg, pseudoephedrine 120 mg. Bot. 100s. *Rx-OTC.*
Use: Antihistamine; decongestant.

Clorfed Expectorant. (Stewart-Jackson Pharmacal) Pseudoephedrine 30 mg, guaifenesin 100 mg, codeine 10 mg/5 mL. Bot. Pt. *c-v.*
Use: Antitussive; decongestant; expectorant.

Clorfed II. (Stewart-Jackson Pharmacal) Chlorpheniramine 4 mg, pseudoephedrine 60 mg. Tab. Bot. 100s. *OTC.*
Use: Antihistamine; decongestant.

•**cloroperone hydrochloride.** (KLOR-oh-PURR-ohn) USAN.
Use: Antipsychotic.

•**clorophene.** (KLOR-oh-feen) USAN.
Use: Disinfectant.

Clorpactin WCS-90. (Guardian Laboratories) Sodium oxychlorosene 2 g. Bot. 5s.
Use: Antiseptic.

•**clorprenaline hydrochloride.** (klor-PREN-ah-leen) USAN.
Use: Bronchodilator.

Clorpres. (Mylan) Clonidine hydrochloride/chlorthalidone. 0.1 mg/15 mg, 0.2 mg/15 mg, 0.3 mg/15 mg. Tab. 100s. *Rx.*
Use: Antihypertensive.

•**clorsulon.** (KLOR-sull-ahn) *USP.*
Use: Antiparasitic; fasciolicide.

•**clortermine hydrochloride.** (klor-TER-meen) USAN.
Use: Anorexic.

•**closantel.** (KLOSE-an-tell) USAN.
Use: Anthelmintic.

•**closiramine aceturate.** (kloe-SIH-rah-meen ah-SEE-tur-ate) USAN.
Use: Antihistamine.

clostridial collagenase.
Use: Dupuytren disease. [Orphan Drug]

•**clothiapine.** (KLOE-THIGH-ah-peen) USAN.
Use: Antipsychotic.

•**clothixamide maleate.** (kloe-THIX-ah-mid) USAN.
Use: Antipsychotic.

•**cloticasone propionate.** (kloe-TIK-ah-SONE PRO-pee-oh-nate) USAN.
Use: Anti-inflammatory.

•**clotrimazole.** (kloe-TRIM-uh-zole) *USP.*
Use: Antifungal.
See: Cruex.
Desenex.
Fungi Cure Intensive.
Gyne-Lotrimin 3.
Gyne-Lotrimin 3 Combination Pack.
Lotrimin AF.
Mycelex.
Mycelex-7.
Mycelex-7 Combination Pack.
3 Day Vaginal.

clotrimazole. (Alra) Clotrimazole 1%, benzyl alcohol. Vaginal cream. In 45 g with 7 disposable applicators. *OTC.*
Use: Antifungal, vaginal.

clotrimazole. (Roxane) Clotrimazole 10 mg. Troches. 70s, 140s, 500s, UD 70s. *Rx.*
Use: Mouth and throat product.

clotrimazole. (Various Mfr.) Clotrimazole. **Cream:** 1%. Vanishing base, benzyl alcohol 1%, cetostearyl alcohol. Tubes. 15 g, 30 g, 45 g, 2 × 45 g. **Top. Soln.:** 1%, PEG 400. Bot. 30 mL. *Rx-OTC.*
Use: Antifungal, topical anti-infective.

clotrimazole. (Various Mfr.) Clotrimazole. **Vaginal Insert.:** 200 mg. Box 3s with applicator. **Vaginal Cream:** 2%. Tube 21 g with 3 disp. applicators. 1%. Tube 15 g, 30 g. 45 g with applicators. *Rx-OTC.*
Use: Antifungal, *Candida* infections.

clotrimazole and betamethasone dipropionate. (Fougera) Clotrimazole 1%, betamethasone dipropionate 0.05%, mineral oil, white petrolatum, cetearyl alcohol, benzyl alcohol. Cream. 15 g. 45 g. *Rx.*
Use: Antifungal; anti-inflammatory.

clotrimazole and betamethasone dipropionate. (Various Mfr.) Betamethasone (as dipropionate) 0.05%, clotrimazole 1%. Lot. 30 mL. *Rx.*
Use: Anti-inflammatory agent.

clotrimazole combination pack. (Various Mfr.) Clotrimazole. **Vag. Supp.:** 200 mg. 3s w/applicator. **Top. Cream:** 1%. Tube. Pack. *OTC.*
Use: Antifungal.

•**clove oil.** (klove) *NF.*
Use: Pharmaceutic aid, flavor.
Cloverine. (Medtech) White salve. Tin Oz. *OTC.*
Use: Dermatologic, counterirritant.
•**clover, red.** (KLOE-ver) *NF.*
Use: Dietary supplement.
Clovocain. (Vita Elixir) Benzocaine, oil of cloves. *OTC.*
Use: Anesthetic, local.
•**cloxacillin benzathine.** (KLOX-ah-SILL-in BENZ-ah-theen) *USP.*
Use: Anti-infective.
•**cloxacillin sodium.** (KLOX-ah-SILL-in) *USP.*
Use: Anti-infective, penicillin.
See: Cloxapen.
cloxacillin sodium. (Various Mfr.) Cloxacillin sodium. **Cap.:** 250 mg, 500 mg. Bot. 100s, UD 100s (250 mg only). **Pow. for Oral Soln.:** 125 mg/5 mL when reconstituted. Bot. 100 mL, 200 mL. *Rx.*
Use: Anti-infective, penicillin.
Cloxapen. (GlaxoSmithKline) Cloxacillin sodium 250 mg, 500 mg. Cap. Bot. 30s (500 mg only), 100s, UD 100s (500 mg only). *Rx.*
Use: Anti-infective, penicillin.
•**cloxyquin.** (KLOX-ee-kwin) USAN.
Use: Anti-infective.
•**clozapine.** (KLOE-zuh-PEEN) *USP.*
Tall Man: cloZAPine
Use: Antipsychotic.
See: Clozaril.
Fazalco.
Versacloz.
clozapine. (Teva) Clozapine. **Tab.:** 200 mg. 100s, 500s, UD 100s **Tab., disintegrating:** 12.5 mg, 25 mg, 100 mg. Aspartame; mannitol; phenylalanine 0.87 mg (12.5 mg), 1.74 mg (25 mg), or 6.96 mg (100 mg). 100s, UD 48s (except 12.5 mg). *Rx.*
Use: Antipsychotic agent, dibenzapine derivative.
clozapine. (Various Mfr.) Clozapine 25 mg, 50 mg, 100 mg. Tab. 100s, 500s, UD 100s. *Rx.*
Use: Antipsychotic.
Clozaril. (Novartis) Clozapine 25 mg, 100 mg. Lactose, talc. Tab. 100s, 500s, UD 100s. *Rx.*
Use: Antipsychotic.
C-Max. (Bio-Technology General) Vitamin C 1000 mg, Mg 40 mg, Zn 5 mg, K 10 mg, Mn 1 mg, pectin 10 mg. Gradual release Tab. Bot. 100s. *OTC.*
Use: Mineral, vitamin supplement.
C.M.C. Cellulose Gum.
See: Carboxymethylcellulose Sodium.
CMV. (Wampole) Cytomegalovirus antibody test system for the qualitative and semi-quantitative detection of CMV antibody in human serum. Test 100s.
Use: Diagnostic aid.
CMV-IGIV.
Use: Immunization.
See: Cytogam.
Cytomegalovirus Immune Globulin Intravenous.
CNL8 Nail Kit. (JSJ Pharmaceuticals) Ciclopirox 8%. Isopropyl alcohol. Top. Soln. Kit w/nail lacquer, remover swabs, emery board, 28 topical vitamin E 5% capsules. 5 mL. 3s. *Rx.*
Use: Anti-infective, topical; antifungal agent.
CNS stimulants.
See: Amphetamines.
Analeptics.
Central Nervous System Stimulants.
Dexmethylphenidate Hydrochloride.
Methylphenidate Hydrochloride.
Coadvil. (Whitehall-Robins) Ibuprofen 200 mg, pseudoephedrine hydrochloride 30 mg. Tab. Bot. 100s. *OTC.*
Use: Analgesic; decongestant.
CoaguChek PT. (Roche) In vitro. PT/INR. Test strips. 48s. *OTC.*
Use: Diagnostic aid.
coagulants.
See: Heparin Antagonists.
coagulation factor IX.
Use: Antihemophilic. [Orphan Drug]
See: Factor IX Complex, Vapor Heated Bebulin VH Immuno.
Mononine.
coagulation factor IX (human).
Use: Antihemophilic. [Orphan Drug]
See: AlphaNine.
coagulation factor IX (recombinant).
Use: Antihemophilic. [Orphan Drug]
See: Alprolix.
BeneFix.
coagulation factor VIIa, recombinant.
Use: Antihemophilic agent.
See: NovoSeven RT.
coagulation factor XII A-subunit (recombinant).
Use: Antihemophilic agent.
See: Tretten.
•**coal tar.** (kole tar) *USP.*
Use: Topical antieczematic; antipsoriatic.
See: Balnetar.
Creamy Tar.
Ionil T.
L.C.D. Compound.
MG217 Medicated Tar.
PC-Tar.
Polytar Soap.

PsoriGel.
PsoriNail.
Psovent.
Tera-Gel.
Zetar.
W/Allantoin.
See: Alphosyl.
W/Salicylic Acid.
See: Ionil T.
coal tar, distillate.
Use: Dermatologic, topical.
See: Doak Tar.
Doak Tar Oil Forte.
Lavatar.
W/Hydrocortisone, Zinc Oxide.
See: Tarpaste.
coal tar extract.
Use: Dermatologic, topical.
W/Salicylic Acid.
See: Neutrogena T/Sal.
coal tar paste.
Use: Dermatologic, topical.
W/Zinc Paste.
See: Tarpaste.
coal tar topical solution. Liquor Carbonis Detergens. L.C.D.
Use: Antieczematic, topical.
Co-Apap. (Various Mfr.) Pseudoephedrine hydrochloride 30 mg, chlorpheniramine maleate 2 mg, dextromethorphan HBr 15 mg, acetaminophen 325 mg. Tab. Bot. 24s, 50s, 1000s. *OTC.*
Use: Analgesic; antihistamine; antitussive; decongestant.
Coartem. (Novartis) Artemether 20 mg/lumefantrine 120 mg. Tab. 24s. *Rx.*
Use: Anti-infective agent, antimalarial preparation.
Coats Aloe Vera Liniment. (Coats Aloe) Methyl salicylate 10%, alcohol, aloe, coconut oil, disodium EDTA, eucalyptus oil, menthol, apricot oil, petrolatum, phenoxyethanol. Liq., Top. 237 mL. *OTC.*
Use: Liquid rub and liniment.
•**cobalamine concentrate.** (koe-BALL-uh-meen kahn-SEN-trate) *USP.*
Use: Hematopoietic vitamin.
See: Vitamin B_{12}.
cobalt gluconate.
W/Ferrous Gluconate, Vitamin B_{12} Activity, Desiccated Stomach Substance, Folic Acid.
See: Chromagen.
cobalt-labeled vitamin B_{12}.
See: Rubratope-57.
•**cobaltous chloride Co 57.** (koe-BALL-tuss) USAN.
Use: Radiopharmaceutical.
See: Cobatope-57
•**cobaltous chloride Co 60.** (koe-BALL-tuss) USAN.
Use: Radiopharmaceutical.
cobalt standards for vitamin B_{12}.
See: Cobatope-57.
Cobatope-57. (Bristol-Myers Squibb) Cobaltous Chloride Co 57.
•**cobicistat.** (koe-BIS-i-stat) USAN.
Use: Treatment of HIV infection.
W/Elvitegravir, Emtricitabine, Tenofovir Disoproxil Fumarate.
See: Stribild.
Co-Bile. (Western Research) Hog bile 64.8 mg, pancreas substance 64.8 mg, papain-pepsin complex 97.2 mg, diatase malt 16.2 mg, papain 48.6 mg, pepsin 48.6 mg. Tab. Bot. 1000s. *Rx-OTC.*
Use: Digestive enzyme.
•**cobimetinib.** (KOE-bi-ME-ti-nib) USAN.
Use: Antineoplastic.
•**cobimetinib fumarate.** (KOE-bi-ME-ti-nib) USAN.
Use: Antineoplastic.
•**cocaine.** (koe-CANE) *USP.*
Use: Topical local anesthetic, ester local anesthetic.
•**cocaine hydrochloride.** (koe-KANE) *USP.*
Use: Anesthetic, local.
cocaine hydrochloride. (Roxane) **Top. Soln.:** Cocaine hydrochloride 4%, 10%. Bot. Multidose 10 mL. UD 4 mL. **Pow.:** (Mallinckrodt). Cocaine hydrochloride 5 g, 25 g. *c-II.*
Use: Topical local anesthetic, ester local anesthetic.
cocaine viscous. (Roxane) Cocaine viscous 4%, 10%. Soln. Top. Bot. Multidose 10 mL. UD 4 mL. *c-II.*
Use: Topical local anesthetic, ester local anesthetic.
•**coccidioidin.** (cox-id-ee-OY-din) *USP.*
Use: Diagnostic aid, dermal reactive indicator.
cocculin.
See: Picrotoxin.
Cocet. (Poly Pharmaceuticals) Acetaminophen 650 mg, codeine phosphate 30 mg. Tab. 100s, 500s. c-iii.
Use: Opioid analgesic combination.
Cocet Plus. (Poly Pharmaceuticals) Codeine phosphate 60 mg, acetaminophen 650 mg. Tab. 100s, 500s. *c-III.*
Use: Opioid analgesic combination.
Cocilan. (Health for Life Brands) Euphorbia, wild lettuce, cocillana, squill, senega, cascarin (bitterless). Syr. Bot. Gal. Available w/codeine. Bot. Gal.
cocoa.
Use: Pharmaceutic aid, flavored vehicle.

•**cocoa butter.** (koe-koe) *NF.*
Use: Pharmaceutic aid, suppository base.

Coconut Oil Beauty Cream. (Mason Natural) Caprylic/capric triglyceride, alcohols, urea, glycerin, glyceryl, parabens, PEG, propylene glycol, disodium EDTA, coconut oil, shea butter, dimethicone, triethanolamine, vitamin E. Cream. 57 g. *OTC.*
Use: Emollient.

Codanol. (A.P.C.) Vitamins A, D, hexachlorophene, zinc oxide. Oint. Tube 1.5 oz, 4 oz. Jar lb. *OTC.*
Use: Dermatologic, counterirritant.

Codap. (Solvay) Codeine phosphate 32 mg, acetaminophen 325 mg. Tab. Bot. 250s. *c-III.*
Use: Analgesic combination.

Codehist DH. (Geneva) Pseudoephedrine 30 mg, chlorpheniramine maleate 2 mg, codeine phosphate 10 mg/5 mL, alcohol 5.7%. Elix. Bot. 120 mL, 480 mL. *c-V.*
Use: Antihistamine; antitussive; decongestant.

•**codeine.** (KOE-deen) *USP.*
Use: Opioid analgesic.
See: Codeine Phosphate.
Codeine Sulfate.

codeine methylbromide. Eucodin.
Use: Antitussive.

•**codeine phosphate.** (KOE-deen) *USP.*
Use: Analgesic; antitussive, narcotic.
W/Acetaminophen.
See: Acetaminophen and Codeine Phosphate.
Capital w/Codeine.
Cocet.
Cocet Plus.
Vopac.
W/Acetaminophen, Caffeine, Butalbital.
See: Fioricet with Codeine.
Phrenilin w/Caffeine and Codeine.
W/Acetaminophen, Chlorpheniramine Maleate.
See: Cotabflu.
W/Aspirin.
See: Aspirin and Codeine Phosphate.
W/Aspirin, Butalbital, Caffeine.
See: Ascomp with Codeine.
Butalbital, Aspirin, Caffeine w/Codeine Phosphate.
Fiorinal with Codeine.
W/Brompheniramine Maleate, Phenylephrine Hydrochloride.
See: M-End PE.
Poly-Tussin AC.
W/Brompheniramine Maleate, Pseudoephedrine Hydrochloride.
See: CPB WC.
Mar-Cof BP.
M-END WC.
Mesehist WC.
W/Chlorcyclizine Hydrochloride.
See: Poly-Tussin.
W/Chlorcyclizine Hydrochloride, Phenylephrine Hydrochloride.
See: Nasotuss.
W/Chlorcyclizine Hydrochloride, Pseudoephedrine Hydrochloride.
See: Poly-Tussin D.
W/Chlorpheniramine Maleate.
See: Cotab A.
Cotab AX.
EndaCof-C.
Lexuss 210.
TL-Hist CM.
Zodryl AC 80.
Zodryl AC 50.
Zodryl AC 40.
Zodryl AC 60.
Zodryl AC 30.
Zodryl AC 35.
Zodryl AC 25.
W/Chlorpheniramine Maleate, Pseudoephedrine Hydrochloride.
See: Phenylhistine DH.
W/Dexbrompheniramine Maleate, Pseudoephedrine Hydrochloride.
See: M-End Max D.
W/Diphenhydramine Hydrochloride, Phenylephrine Hydrochloride.
See: Airacof.
W/Guaifenesin.
See: Allfen CDX.
Brontex.
CGU WC.
Cheratussin AC Expectorant Cough Suppressant.
Iophen C-NR.
Mar-Cof-CG.
M-Clear.
M-Clear WC.
Tussi-Organidin-S NR.
Virtussin A/C.
W/Guaifenesin, Phenylephrine Hydrochloride.
See: Giltuss Ped-C.
W/Guaifenesin, Pseudoephedrine Hydrochloride.
See: Ambifed CD.
Ambifed CDX.
Guiatuss DAC.
Lortuss EX.
Tusnel C.
Zodryl DEC 80.
Zodryl DEC 50.
Zodryl DEC 40.
Zodryl DEC 60.
Zodryl DEC 30.
Zodryl DEC 35.

Zodryl DEC 25.
Z-Tuss E.
W/Phenylephrine Hydrochloride.
See: Cheratussin DAC.
W/Phenylephrine Hydrochloride, Promethazine Hydrochloride.
See: Promethazine VC w/Codeine.
W/Phenylephrine Hydrochloride, Pyrilamine Maleate.
See: Pro-Red AC.
W/Pseudoephedrine Hydrochloride.
See: EndaCof-DC.
W/Pseudoephedrine Hydrochloride, Triprolidine Hydrochloride.
See: Poly Hist NC.

codeine phosphate and aspirin.
See: Aspirin and Codeine Phosphate.

codeine phosphate and guaifenesin. (Ethex) Codeine phosphate 10 mg, guaifenesin 300 mg. Sugar, PEG. Tab. Bot. 100s. *c-III.*
Use: Upper respiratory combination, antitussive combination.

•**codeine polistirex.** (KOE-deen pahl-ee-STIE-rex) USAN.
Use: Antitussive.
W/Combinations.
See: Codeprex.

codeine resin complex combinations.
See: Omni-Tuss.

•**codeine sulfate.** (KOE-deen) *USP.*
Use: Analgesic; antitussive, narcotic.
See: Golacol.

codeine sulfate. (Roxane) Codeine 30 mg per 5 mL. Disodium edetate, glycerin, sodium benzoate, sorbitol, sucralose. Soln. 500 mL. *c-II.*
Use: Opioid analgesic.

codeine sulfate. (Various Mfr.) Codeine sulfate 15 mg, 30 mg, 60 mg. Tab. Bot. 100s (except 15 mg), UD 100s (except 60 mg). *c-II.*
Use: Opioid analgesic.

codelcortone.
See: Prednisolone.

Codeprex. (Celltech Pharmaceuticals) Codeine polistirex 20 mg, chlorpheniramine polistirex 4 mg per 5 mL. EDTA, parabens, sucrose, vegetable oil. Cherry-cream flavor. ER Susp. 473 mL. *c-III.*
Use: Antitussive combination.

Codimal. (Schwarz Pharma) Chlorpheniramine maleate 2 mg, pseudoephedrine hydrochloride 30 mg, acetaminophen 325 mg. Cap.Tab. Bot. 24s, 100s, 1000s. *OTC.*
Use: Antihistamine, decongestant, analgesic.

Codimal-L.A. (Schwarz Pharma) Chlorpheniramine maleate 8 mg, pseudoephedrine hydrochloride 120 mg. SR Cap. Bot. 100s, 1000s. *Rx.*
Use: Antihistamine, decongestant.

Codimal-L.A. Half Capsules. (Schwarz Pharma) Pseudoephedrine hydrochloride 60 mg, chlorpheniramine maleate 4 mg, sucrose. Cap. Bot. 100s. *Rx.*
Use: Antihistamine; decongestant.

cod liver oil. Emulsion.
Use: Vitamin A and D therapy.
See: Cod Liver Oil Concentrate.
W/Zinc Oxide.
See: Caldesene.
Desitin.

cod liver oil concentrate. (Schering-Plough) Concentrate of cod liver oil with vitamins A and D added. **Cap.:** Bot. 40s, 100s. **Tab.:** Bot. 100s, 240s. Also w/vitamin C. Bot. 100s. *OTC.*
Use: Vitamin supplement.

codorphone hydrochloride. *Name previously used for Conorphone hydrochloride.*
Use: Analgesic.
See: Conorphone Hydrochloride.

•**codoxime.** (CODE-ox-eem) USAN.
Use: Antitussive.

Codoxy. (Halsey Drug) Oxycodone hydrochloride 4.5 mg, oxycodone terephthalate 0.38 mg, aspirin 325 mg. Tab. Bot. 100s. *c-II.*
Use: Analgesic combination.

Coease. (Advance Medical) Sodium hyaluronate 12 mg/mL, NaCl 9 mg/mL. Inj. Disp. syringe. 0.5 mL, 0.8 mL. *Rx.*
Use: Ophthalmic surgical adjunct.

Cogentin. (Akorn) Benztropine mesylate 1 mg/mL. Amp. 2 mL. *Rx.*
Use: Antiparkinsonian.

coenzyme Q10.
Use: Enzyme.
See: Co Q10, Vitamin E & Fish Oil.

Co-Gesic. (Schwarz Pharma) Hydrocodone bitartrate 5 mg, acetaminophen 500 mg. Tab. Bot. 100s, 500s. *c-III.*
Use: Analgesic combination.

Co-Hep-Tral. (Davis & Sly) Folic acid 10 mg, vitamin B_{12} 100 mcg, liver injection q.s./mL. Vial 10 mL. *Rx.*
Use: Mineral, vitamin supplement.

Co-Hist. (Roberts) Pseudoephedrine hydrochloride 30 mg, chlorpheniramine 2 mg, acetaminophen 325 mg. Tab. Bot. 500s, 1000s. *OTC.*
Use: Analgesic; antihistamine; decongestant.

Colabid. (Major) Probenecid 500 mg, colchicine 0.5 mg. Tab. Bot. 100s, 1000s. *Rx.*
Use: Antigout.

Colace. (Purdue) Docusate sodium.

Cap.: 50 mg, 100 mg. Bot. 30s, 60s, 250s (100 mg only), 1000s (100 mg only), UD 100s. **Syrup:** 60 mg/15 mL with alcohol less than 1%, menthol, parabens, sucrose. Bot. 237 mL, 473 mL. **Liq.:** 150 mg/15 mL, parabens. Bot. 30 mL, 480 mL. *OTC.*
Use: Laxative.

Colace Infant/Child. (Purdue) Glycerin. Supp.; rectal. 12s, 24s. *OTC.*
Use: Laxative.

Colagyn. (Smith & Nephew) Zinc sulfocarbolate, potassium, oxyquinoline sulfate, lactic acid, boric acid. Jelly. Tube w/applicator and refill 6 oz. Douche Pow. 3 oz, 7 oz, 14 oz. *OTC.*

Colana. (Hance) Euphorbia pilulifera tincture 8 mL, wild lettuce syrup 8 mL, cocillana tincture 2.5 mL, squill compound syrup 1.5 mL, cascara 0.25 g, menthol 4.8 mg/fl oz. Bot. 4 fl oz, gal. Also w/Dionin 15 mg/fl oz. Syr. Bot. gal.

Colazal. (Salix) Balsalazide disodium 750 mg (equiv. to mesalamine 267 mg). Sodium ≈ 86 mg. Cap. Bot. 280s, 500s. *Rx.*
Use: Treatment of ulcerative colitis.

•**colchicine.** (KOHL-chih-seen) *USP.*
Use: Gout suppressant. Treat multiple sclerosis; familial Mediterranean fever; Behçet syndrome [Orphan Drug].
See: Colcrys.

W/Sodium Salicylate, Calcium Carbonate, Dried Aluminum Hydroxide Gel, Phenobarbital.
See: Apcogesic.

colchicine. (Various Mfr.) Colchicine 0.6 mg (1/100 g). Tab. Bot. 30s, 60s, 100s, 100s. *Rx.*
Use: Gout suppressant. Treat multiple sclerosis; familial Mediterranean fever; Behçet syndrome [Orphan Drug].

colchicine salicylate.
W/Phenobarbital, Sodium Para-Aminobenzoate, Vitamin B_1, Aspirin.
See: Doloral.

Colcrys. (Takeda Pharmaceuticals America) Colchicine 0.6 mg. Film coated. Lactose, polydextrose. Tab. 30s, 60s, 100s, 250s, 500s, 1,000s. *Rx.*
Use: Agent for gout.

Cold & Cough Tussin. (Amerisource Bergen) Dextromethorphan HBr 10 mg, guaifenesin 200 mg, pseudoephedrine hydrochloride 30 mg. Sorbitol. Softgels. Pkg. 12s. *OTC.*
Use: Upper respiratory combination, antitussive, expectorant, decongestant.

Cold & Hot Pain Relief Therapy Patch. (Major Pharmaceuticals) Menthol 5%. Aloe vera, disodium EDTA, methylparaben. Patch. 8 × 12 cm. 5s. *OTC.*
Use: Rub and liniment.

•**cold cream.** *USP.*
Use: Emollient; water in oil emulsion ointment base.

Coldec D. (Breckenridge) Pseudoephedrine hydrochloride 80 mg, carbinoxamine maleate 8 mg. Tab. Bot. 100s. *Rx.*
Use: Upper respiratory combination, decongestant, antihistamine.

Coldec DM. (Silarx) Dextromethorphan HBr 15 mg, brompheniramine maleate 4 mg, pseudoephedrine hydrochloride 60 mg per 5 mL. Saccharin, sorbitol, grape flavor, alcohol free, sugar free. Syrup. Bot. 480 mL. *Rx.*
Use: Upper respiratory combination, antitussive, antihistamine, decongestant.

Cold-Eeze. (Prophase Labs) Zinc gluconate 13.3 g. Corn syrup, sucrose. Preservative free. Cherry, citrus, honey lemon, menthol, and tropical flavors. Loz. 6s, 18s. *OTC.*
Use: Trace element.

Cold-Gest Cold. (Major) Chlorpheniramine maleate 8 mg, pseudoephedrine hydrochloride 75 mg. Cap. Pkg. 10s, 20s. *OTC.*
Use: Antihistamine, decongestant.

Coldran. (Halsey Drug) Phenylephrine hydrochloride 5 mg, chlorpheniramine maleate 2 mg, salicylamide 1.5 g, acetaminophen 0.5 g, caffeine. Tab. Bot. 30s. *OTC.*
Use: Decongestant, analgesic, antihistamine.

Coldrine. (Roberts) Acetaminophen 325 mg, pseudoephedrine hydrochloride 30 mg, sodium metabisulfite. Tab. Bot. 1000s, 500s (packets), 4-dose boxes. *OTC.*
Use: Analgesic, decongestant.

Cold Sore. (Purepac) Camphor, benzoin, aluminum chloride. Lot. Bot. 0.5 oz. *OTC.*
Use: Cold sores, fever blisters.

Cold Symptoms Relief. (Major) Pseudoephedrine hydrochloride 30 mg, chlorpheniramine maleate 2 mg, dextromethorphan HBr 10 mg, acetaminophen 325 mg. Tab. Bot. 50s. *OTC.*
Use: Decongestant, antihistamine, antitussive, analgesic.

Cold Symptoms Relief Maximum Strength. (Major) Dextromethorphan HBr 15 mg, chlorpheniramine maleate 2 mg, pseudoephedrine hydrochloride 30 mg, acetaminophen 500 mg. Tab. Pkg. 24s. *OTC.*
Use: Upper respiratory combination, antitussive, antihistamine, decongestant, analgesic.

Cold Tablets. (Walgreen) Phenylephrine hydrochloride 5 mg, chlorpheniramine maleate 2 mg, acetaminophen 325 mg. Tab. Bot. 50s. *OTC.*
Use: Decongestant, analgesic, antihistamine.

Cold Tablets Multiple Symptom. (Walgreen) Acetaminophen 500 mg, pseudoephedrine hydrochloride 30 mg, chlorpheniramine maleate 2 mg, dextromethorphan HBr 10 mg. Tab. Bot. 50s. *OTC.*
Use: Analgesic, decongestant, antihistamine, antitussive.

•**coleneuramide.** (COL-e-NURE-a-mide) USAN.
Use: Diabetic neuropathy.

•**colesevelam hydrochloride.** (koe-leh-SEH-veh-lam) USAN.
Use: Antihyperlipidemic; bile acid sequestrant.
See: Welchol.

Colestid. (Pharmacia) Colestipol hydrochloride 5 g/7.5 g granules. Gran. for Oral Susp. **Unflavored Gran.:** Bot. 300 g, 500 g. Packets. 5 g (30s, 90s). **Flavored Gran.:** Aspartame, mannitol, orange flavor. Bot. 450 g (60 doses). Packets. 7.5 g (60s). **Tab.:** 1 g. Bot. 120s, 500s. *Rx.*
Use: Antihyperlipidemic; bile acid sequestrant.

•**colestilan chloride.** (koe-LES-ti-lan) USAN.
Use: Hyperphosphatemia/hypercholesterolemia.

•**colestipol hydrochloride.** (koe-LESS-tih-pole) *USP.*
Use: Antihyperlipidemic.
See: Colestid.

colestipol hydrochloride. (Global) Colestipol hydrochloride 5 mg. Gran. for Oral Susp. Packets. 5 g (30s and 90s). Bot. 500 g. *Rx.*
Use: Antihyperlipidemic agent, bile acid sequestrant.

colestipol hydrochloride. (Various Mfr.) Colestipol hydrochloride 1 g. Tab. 120s, 500s. *Rx.*
Use: Antihyperlipidemic agent, bile acid sequestrant.

•**colestolone.** (koe-LESS-toe-LONE) USAN.
Use: Hypolipidemic.

Col-Evac. (Forest) Potassium bitartrate, bicarbonate of soda and a blended base of polyethylene glycols. Supp. Box. 2s, 12s.
Use: Laxative.

•**colforsin.** (kole-FAR-sin) USAN.
Use: Antiglaucoma agent.

colfosceril palmitate, cetyl alcohol, tyloxapol.
Use: Hyaline membrane disease; adult respiratory distress syndrome. [Orphan Drug]

Colgate Dry Mouth Relief. (Colgate Oral Pharmaceuticals) Sodium fluoride 2.1 mg per 10 mL. Glycerin, propylene glycol, saccharin, sorbitol, sodium benzoate. Alcohol free. Liq., rinse; dental. 473 mL. *OTC.*
Use: Mouth and throat product.

colimycin sodium methanesulfonate. (Parke-Davis)
See: Colistimethate Sodium.

colimycin sulfate.
See: Coly-Mycin.

•**colistimethate sodium.** (koe-LISS-tih-METH-ate) *USP.*
Use: Anti-infective.
See: Coly-Mycin M Parenteral.

colistimethate sodium. (Paddock) Colistin base as colistimethate sodium or pentasodium colistimethanesulfonate 150 mg. Lyophilized Cake for Inj. Vials. *Rx.*
Use: Anti-infective.

colistin and neomycin sulfates and hydrocortisone acetate.
Use: Anti-infective; anti-inflammatory.

colistin base.
W/Neomycin Base, Hydrocortisone Acetate, Thonzonium Bromide, Polysorbate 80, Acetic Acid, Sodium Acetate.
See: Coly-Mycin S Otic Drops.

colistin methanesulfonate.
See: Colistimethate Sodium.

colistin sulfate.
W/Hydrocortisone Acetate, Neomycin Sulfate, Thonzonium Bromide.
See: Coly-Mycin S Otic.
Cortisporin-TC Otic.

Co-Liver. (Standex) Folic acid 1 mg, vitamin B_{12} 100 mcg, liver 10 mcg/mL. Inj. Vial 10 mL. *Rx.*
Use: Mineral, vitamin supplement.

Colladerm. (C & M Pharmacal) Glycerin, soluble collagen, hydrolysed elastin, allantoin, ethylhydroxycellulose, sorbic, octoxynol-9. Bot. 2.3 oz. *OTC.*
Use: Emollient.

collagenase.
Use: Enzyme preparation.
See: Collagenase Santyl.

collagenase ABC. (Advance Biofactures) Collagenase 250 units/g in white petrolatum. Oint. Tube. 25 g, 50 g. *OTC.*
Use: Enzyme, topical.

•**collagenase clostridium histolyticum.** (kol-AJ-e-nase klos-TRID-ee-um HIS-toe-LIT-ik-um) USAN.

Use: Enzyme; Dupuytren contracture.
See: Xiaflex.

collagenase (lyophilized) for injection.
Use: Peyronie disease. [Orphan Drug]

Collagenase Santyl. (Ross) Collagenase enzyme 250 units/g, white petrolatum. Oint. Tube. 15 g, 30 g. *Rx.*
Use: Enzyme preparation.

collagen implant. (Lacrimedics) Collagen 0.2 mm, 0.3 mm, 0.4 mm, 0.5 mm, 0.6 mm. Box 12s. *Rx.*
Use: Collagen implant, ophthalmic.
See: Zyderm I.
Zyderm II.

•**collodion.** (koe-LOE-dee-on) *USP.*
Use: Topical protectant.

colloidal aluminum hydroxide.
See: Aluminum Hydroxide Gel.

colloidal oatmeal.
Use: Emollient.
See: Actibath.
Aveeno.

colloidal sulfur.
Use: Antiseborrheic.
W/Combinations.
See: MG217 Medicated Tar-Free.

Colloral. (AutoImmune) Purified type II collagen.
Use: Juvenile rheumatoid arthritis. [Orphan Drug]

Collyrium for Fresh Eyes Wash. (Wyeth-Ayerst) Boric acid, sodium borate, benzalkonium chloride. Soln. Bot. 120 mL. *OTC.*
Use: Irrigant, ophthalmic.

ColoCARE. (Helena Laboratories) In-home fecal test. Kit. 3s.
Use: Diagnostic aid.

Colocort. (Paddock Laboratories) Hydrocortisone 100 mg/60 mL. Methylparaben. Rectal Susp. Single-dose bot. with lubricated rectal applicator tips. 60 mL. *Rx.*
Use: Anorectal preparation.

Coloctyl. (Eon Labs) Docusate sodium 100 mg. Cap. Bot. 100s, 1000s, UD 1000s. *OTC.*
Use: Laxative.

Cologel. (Eli Lilly) Methylcellulose 450 mg/5 mL, alcohol 5%, saccharin. Bot. 16 fl oz. *OTC.*
Use: Laxative.

colony-stimulating factor.
Use: Hematopoietic agent.
See: Filgrastim.
Pegfilgrastim.
Sargramostim.

color allergy screening test.
See: CAST.

ColoScreen. (Helena Laboratories) Occult blood screening test. Kit 12s, 25s, 50s. 3 tests per kit.
Use: Diagnostic aid.

ColoScreen/VPI. (Helena Laboratories) Occult blood screening test. Box 100s, 1000s.
Use: Diagnostic aid.

Coltab Children's. (Roberts) Phenylephrine hydrochloride 2.5 mg, chlorpheniramine maleate 1 mg. Chew. Tab. Bot. 30s. *OTC.*
Use: Antihistamine; decongestant.

•**colterol mesylate.** (KOLE-ter-ole) USAN.
Use: Bronchodilator.

Columbia Antiseptic Powder. (F.C. Sturtevant) Zinc oxide, talc, carbolic acid, boric acid. Pow. 30 g, 420 g. *OTC.*
Use: Topical combination.

Coly-Mycin M Parenteral. (JHP Pharmaceuticals) Colistimethate sodium equivalent to 150 mg colistin base. Inj. Vial. *Rx.*
Use: Anti-infective.

Coly-Mycin S Otic. (JHP Pharmaceuticals) Hydrocortisone acetate 1%, neomycin sulfate 4.71 mg, colistin sulfate 3 mg, thonzonium bromide 0.5 mg/mL. Polysorbate 80, acetic acid, sodium acetate, thimerosal. Susp. Dropper bot. 5 mL, 10 mL. *Rx.*
Use: Steroid and antibiotic combination.

Colyte. (Meda) Polyethylene glycol-electrolyte 3350. **Gal:** PEG 3350 227.1 g, sodium sulfate 21.5 g, sodium bicarbonate 6.36 g, sodium chloride 5.53 g, potassium chloride 2.82 g. **4 L:** PEG 3350 240 g, sodium sulfate 22.72 g, sodium bicarbonate 6.72 g, sodium chloride 5.84 g, potassium chloride 2.98 g. Soln. Bot. 1 gal, 4 L. *Rx.*
Use: Bowel evacuant.

Combichole. (Trout) Dehydrocholic acid 2 g, desoxycholic acid 1 g. Tab. Bot. 100s, 1000s. *Rx.*
Use: Hydrocholeretic.

Combigan. (Allergan) Brimonidine tartrate 0.2%, timolol 0.5% (as timolol maleate 6.8 mg/mL). Benzalkonium chloride 0.005%. Soln., Ophth. 5 mL, 10 mL, 15 mL. *Rx.*
Use: Agent for glaucoma.

CombiPatch. (Novartis) **Transdermal Patch 9 cm^2:** Estradiol 0.05 mg/norethindrone acetate 0.14 mg per day. **Transdermal Patch 16 cm^2:** Estradiol 0.05 mg/norethindrone acetate 0.25 mg per day. Box. 8s. *Rx.*
Use: Sex hormone, estrogen and progestin combination.

Combistix. (Bayer Consumer Care) Urine test for glucose, protein and pH. In 100s.
Use: Diagnostic aid.

Combistix Reagent Strips. (Siemans Medical) Protein test area: tetrabrom-

phenol blue, citrate buffer, protein-absorbing agent; glucose test area: glucose oxidase, orthotolidin and a catalyst; pH test area methyl red and bromthymol blue. Strip Box 100s. *Rx.*
Use: Diagnostic aid.

Combivent. (Boehringer Ingelheim) Ipratropium bromide 18 mcg, albuterol sulfate 103 mcg/actuation (equivalent to albuterol base 90 mcg). Aer. Metered dose inhaler 14.7 g (200 inhalations) w/mouthpiece. *Rx.*
Use: Bronchodilator, anticholinergic.

Combivent Respimat. (Boehringer Ingelheim) Ipratropium bromide 20 mcg, albuterol sulfate 120 mcg (equiv. to albuterol base 100 mcg). Spray; Inhal. 4 g cartridge w/inhaler (120 actuations). *Rx.*
Use: Bronchodilator, anticholinergic.

Combivir. (GlaxoSmithKline) Lamivudine 150 mg, zidovudine 300 mg. Tab. Bot. 60s, UD 120s. *Rx.*
Use: Antiviral, nucleoside analog reverse transcriptase inhibitor combination.

Cometriq. (Exelixis) Cabozantinib maleate 20 mg, 80 mg. Cap. Cartons. 60s (20 mg). The 140 mg daily dose carton contains four 140 mg daily dose blister cards (each blister card containing seven 80 mg and twenty-one 20 mg capsules). The 100 mg daily dose carton contains four 100 mg daily dose blister cards (each blister card containing seven 80 mg and seven 20 mg capsules). The 60 mg daily dose carton contains four 60 mg daily dose blister cards (each blister card containing twenty-one 20 mg capsules). *Rx.*
Use: Kinase inhibitor, tyrosine kinase inhibitor.

•**comfilcon A.** (kom-FIL-kon) USAN.
Use: Contact lens material, hydrophilic.

ComfortCare GP Wetting & Soaking. (PBH Wesley Jessen) Buffered, isotonic. Chlorhexidine gluconate 0.005%, EDTA 0.02%, octylphenoxy (oxyethylene) ethanol, povidone, polyvinyl alcohol, propylene glycol, hydroxyethylcellulose, NaCl. Soln. Bot. 120 mL, 240 mL. *OTC.*
Use: Contact lens care.

Comfort Drops. (PBH Wesley Jessen) Isotonic solution containing naphazoline 0.03%, benzalkonium chloride 0.005%, edetate disodium 0.02%. Bot. 15 mL. *OTC.*
Use: Contact lens care.

Comfort Gel Liquid. (Walgreen) Aluminum hydroxide compressed gel 200 mg, magnesium hydroxide 200 mg, simethicone 20 mg/5 mL. Gel. Bot. 12 oz. *OTC.*
Use: Antacid; antiflatulent.

Comfort Gel Tablets. (Walgreen) Magnesium hydroxide 85 mg, simethicone 25 mg, aluminum hydroxide-magnesium carbonate co-dried gel 282 mg. Tab. Bot. 100s. *OTC.*
Use: Antacid; antiflatulent.

Comfort Tears. (Allergan) Hydroxyethylcellulose, benzalkonium chloride 0.005%, edetate disodium 0.02%. Soln. Bot. 15 mL. *OTC.*
Use: Artificial tear solution.

Comhist. (Roberts) Phenylephrine hydrochloride 10 mg, chlorpheniramine maleate 2 mg, phenyltoloxamine citrate 25 mg. Tab. Bot. 100s. *Rx.*
Use: Antihistamine; decongestant.

Comhist L.A. (Roberts) Phenylephrine hydrochloride 20 mg, chlorpheniramine maleate 4 mg, phenyltoloxamine citrate 50 mg. Cap. Bot. 100s. *Rx.*
Use: Antihistamine; decongestant.

Compal. (Solvay) Dihydrocodeine 16 mg, acetaminophen 356.4 mg, caffeine 30 mg. Cap. Bot. 100s. *c-III.*
Use: Analgesic combination.

Companion Multi for Men. (Theralogix) Vitamins A 3,500 units, C 100 mg, E 30 units, B_1 5 mg, B_2 5 mg, B_3 20 mg, B_5 10 mg, B_6 5 mg, B_{12} 30 mcg, folic acid 400 mcg, Ca, I, Mg, Zn, Se, Mn, Cu, Cr, Mo, B, V, choline 100 mg, biotin 30 mcg. Tab. 180s. *OTC.*
Use: Multivitamin with minerals.

Compat Nutrition Enteral Delivery System. (Novartis) Top fill feeding containers 600 mL, 1400 mL. Gravity delivery set. Pump delivery set. Compat enteral feeding pump.
Use: Nutritional supplement.

Compete. (Mission Pharmacal) Iron 27 mg, vitamins A 5000 units, D 400 units, E 45 units, B_1 2 mg, B_2 2.6 mg, B_3 30 mg, B_6 20.6 mg, B_{12} 9 mcg, C 90 mg, folic acid 0.4 mg, Zn 22.5 mg. Tab. Bot. 100s. *OTC.*
Use: Mineral, vitamin supplement.

Compleat. (Nestle Nutrition) Protein 48 g (Na caseinate), carbohydrate 128 g (corn syrup, maltodextrin), fat 40 g (canola oil, chicken puree), sodium 1,000 mg, potassium 1,720 mg. Vitamin A, B_1, B_2, B_3, B_5, B_6, B_{12}, C, D, E, K, Ca, Cl, Cr, Cu, Fe, I, Mg, Mo, Mn, P, Se, Zn, biotin, choline, folic acid. Chocolate and vanilla flavors. Liq. 1,000 mL, 1,500 mL. *OTC.*
Use: Milk-based formula.

Compleat B Meat Base Formula. (Novartis) Beef, nonfat milk, hydrolyzed cereal solids, maltodextrin, pureed fruits and vegetables, corn oil, mono- and diglycerides. Bot. 250 mL, Can 250 mL. *OTC.*
Use: Nutritional supplement, eternal.

Compleat Modified Formula Meat Base. (Novartis) Hydrolyzed cereal solids, calcium caseinate, pureed fruits and vegetables, corn oil, beef puree, mono- and diglycerides. Can 250 mL. *OTC.*
Use: Enteral nutritional supplement.

Compleat Regular Formula. (Novartis) Deionized water, beef puree, hydrolyzed cereal solids, green bean puree, pea puree, nonfat milk, corn oil, maltodextrin, peach puree, orange juice, mono- and diglycerides, carrageenan, vitamins, minerals. Bot. 250 mL, Can 250 mL. *OTC.*
Use: Nutritional supplement, eternal.

Complera. (Gilead Sciences) Emtricitabine 200 mg/rilpivirine 25 mg/tenofovir disoproxil fumarate 300 mg (equiv. to rilpivirine hydrochloride 27.5 mg and tenofovir disoproxil 245 mg). Film coated. Lactose. Tab. 30s. *Rx.*
Use: Antiretroviral agent, nonnucleoside reverse transcriptase inhibitor.

Complete Prenatal Multivitamin. (VitaMed MD) Folic acid 0.975 mg, Ca 150 mg, Fe 30 mg, vitamins D 600 units, E 30 units, B_1 3 mg, B_2 3.4 mg, B_3 20 mg, B_5 10 mg, B_6 25 mg, B_{12} 12 mcg, C 60 mg, Cu, Mn, Mo, Se, Zn, biotin 300 mcg. PEG, orange flavoring. Tab. 30s. *OTC.*
Use: Prenatal vitamin with minerals.

Complete Prenatal Multivitamin/Prenatal DHA Combo Pack. (VitaMed MD) **Tab.:** Vitamin C 60 mg, D_2 600 units, E 30 units, B_1 3 mg, B_2 3.4 mg, B_3 20 mg, B_5 10 mg, B_6 25 mg, B_{12} 12 mcg, Ca 150 mg, Fe 30 mg, folic acid 975 mcg, biotin 300 mcg, Zn, Se, Cu, Mn, Mo. PEG. 30s. **Cap., softgels:** DHA 300 mg. Sunflower oil. 30s (in vegan and regular). *Rx.*
Use: Prenatal vitamin.

Complete Vitamins. (Mission Pharmacal) Vitamins A 5000 units, D 400 units, E 45 units, C 90 mg, B_1 2.25 mg, folic acid 0.4 mg, B_2 2.6 mg, B_3 30 mg, B_6 25 mg, B_{12} 9 mcg, ferrous gluconate 233 mg, zinc 22.5 mg. Tab. Bot. 100s, 1000s. *OTC.*
Use: Mineral, vitamin supplement.

Completone Elixir Fort. (Sanofi-Synthelabo) Ferrous gluconate.
Use: Mineral supplement.

Complex C. (National Vitamin Company) Ascorbic acid 500 mg, 1,000 mg. Polydextrose. Gluten free, preservative free, and sugar free. Tab., timed release. 100s (500 mg), 60s (1,000 mg). *OTC.*
Use: Water-soluble vitamin.

Complex 15 Cream. (Baker Cummins Dermatologicals) Jar 4 oz. *OTC.*
Use: Emollient.

Complex 15 Lotion. (Baker Cummins Dermatologicals) Bot. 8 oz. *OTC.*
Use: Emollient.

Complex Zinc Carbonates.
Use: Mineral supplement.

Comply Liquid. (Sherwood Davis & Geck) sodium caseinate, calcium caseinate, hydrolyzed cornstarch, sucrose, corn oil, soy lecithin, vitamins A, B_1, B_2, B_3, B_5, B_6, B_{12}, C, D, E, K, folic acid, biotin, choline, Ca, Cl, Cu, Fe, I, Mg, Mn, P, Zn. Can 250 mL, Bot. 200 mL. *OTC.*
Use: Nutritional supplement, enteral.

compound cb3025.
See: Alkeran.

compound E.
See: Cortisone Acetate.

compound F.
See: Hydrocortisone.

compound 42.
See: Warfarin.

compound Q.
Use: Antiviral.

compound S.
Use: Antiviral.
See: Retrovir.
Zidovudine.

Compound 347. (Piramal Critical Care) Enflurane. Liq. for Inh. 250 mL. *Rx.*
Use: General anesthetic.

Compound W. (Medtech) Salicylic acid 17% w/w in flexible collodion vehicle w/ether 63.5%. Bot. 0.31 oz. *OTC.*
Use: Keratolytic.

Compound W for Kids. (Medtech) Salicylic acid 40% in a plaster vehicle, lanolin, rubber. Pad. Box. 12s. *OTC.*
Use: Keratolytic.

Compound W Freeze Off. (Medtech) Dimethyl ether, propane, isobutane. Spray. 80 mL with 12 applicators. *OTC.*
Use: Removal of warts.

Compound W One Step Invisible. (Medtech Products) Salicylic acid 40%. Lanolin, rosin ester, rubber. Strips; topical. 14s. *OTC.*
Use: Keratolytic agent.

Compound W One Step Wart Remover for Kids. (Medtech) Salicylic acid 40% in a plaster vehicle, lanolin, rubber. Pad. Box 12s. *OTC.*
Use: Keratolytic.

Compoz. (Medtech) **Tab.:** Diphenhydramine hydrochloride 50 mg. Pkg. 12s, 24s. **Cap.:** Diphenhydramine hydrochloride 25 mg. Pkg. 16s. *OTC.*
Use: Antihistamine, nonselective ethanolamine.

Compro. (Paddock) Prochlorperazine 25 mg. Supp. Box 12s. *Rx.*
Use: Antiemetic; antipsychotic.

Comtan. (Novartis) Entacapone 200 mg. Film coated. Mannitol, sucrose. Tab. 100s. *Rx.*
Use: Antiparkinsonian.

Comtrex Maximum Strength Day & Night Cold & Cough. (Novartis Consumer) **Day:** Dextromethorphan HBr 10 mg, phenylephrine hydrochloride 5 mg, acetaminophen 325 mg. **Night:** Dextromethorphan HBr 10 mg, chlorpheniramine maleate 2 mg, phenylephrine hydrochloride 6 mg, acetaminophen 325 mg. Tab. 20s (10 day, 10 night). *OTC.*
Use: Upper respiratory combination, antitussive combination.

Comtrex Maximum Strength Day & Night Flu Therapy. (Novartis Consumer) **Day:** Phenylephrine hydrochloride 5 mg, acetaminophen 325 mg. PEG. **Night:** Phenylephrine hydrochloride 5 mg, chlorpheniramine maleate 2 mg, acetaminophen 325 mg. PEG. Tab. 20s (10 day, 10 night). *OTC.*
Use: Upper respiratory combination, decongestant, antihistamine, analgesic.

Comtrex Maximum Strength Day & Night Severe Cold & Sinus. (Novartis Consumer) **Day:** Phenylephrine hydrochloride 5 mg, acetaminophen 325 mg. PEG. **Night:** Phenylephrine hydrochloride 5 mg, chlorpheniramine maleate 2 mg, acetaminophen 325 mg. PEG. Tab. 20s (10 day, 10 night). *OTC.*
Use: Upper respiratory combination, decongestant, antihistamine, and analgesic combination.

Comtrex Maximum Strength Nighttime Cold & Cough. (Novartis Consumer) Dextromethorphan 5 mg, chlorpheniramine maleate 0.67 mg, pseudoephedrine hydrochloride 10 mg, acetaminophen 166.7 mg per 5 mL. Alcohol 10%, saccharin, sucrose. Liq. 240 mL. *OTC.*
Use: Antitussive combination, upper respiratory combination.

Comtrex Multi-Symptom Deep Chest Cold. (Novartis Consumer) Guaifenesin 200 mg, acetaminophen 325 mg. PEG, polyvinyl alcohol. Cap. 24s. *OTC.*
Use: Expectorant with analgesic combination, upper respiratory combination.

Comvax. (Merck) *Haemophilus* b PRP 7.5 mcg, *Neisseria meningitidis* OMPC 125 mcg, hepatitis B surface antigen 5 mcg, aluminum hydroxide ≈ 225 mcg, sodium borate decahydrate 35 mcg/0.5 mL, sodium chloride 0.9%. Inj. Single-dose vials. 0.5 mL *Rx.*
Use: Agent for active immunization, bacterial vaccine.

Concentraid. (Ferring) Desmopressin acetate 0.1 mg/mL (0.1 mg equals 400 units arginine vasopressin). Soln. Disposable intranasal pipettes containing 20 mcg/2 mL. *Rx.*
Use: Hormone.

Concentrated Cleaner. (Bausch & Lomb) Anionic sulfate surfactant with friction-enhancing agents and sodium chlorine. Soln. Bot. 30 mL. *OTC.*
Use: Contact lens care.

Concentrated Milk of Magnesia. (Roxane) Magnesium hydroxide 2,400 mg per 10 mL. Benzyl alcohol, lemon oil, sorbitol, sugar. Lemon flavor. Susp., Conc. 400 mL. *OTC.*
Use: Antacid; Laxative.

Concentrated Milk of Magnesia-Cascara. (Roxane) Milk of magnesia-cascara 15 mL equivalent to milk of magnesia 30 mL and aromatic cascara fluid extract 5 mL, alcohol 7%. *OTC.*
Use: Laxative.

Concentrated Multiple Trace Element. (American Regent) Zinc (as sulfate) 5 mg, copper (as sulfate) 1 mg, manganese (as sulfate) 0.5 mg, chromium (as chloride) 10 mcg. Vial. 10 mL. *Rx.*
Use: Trace element supplement.

concentrated oleovitamin A and D.
See: Oleovitamin A & D.

Concentrated Phillips' Milk of Magnesia. (Roxane) Magnesium hydroxide 800 mg/5 mL, sorbitol, and sugar. Strawberry and orange vanilla creme flavors. Liq. 8 fl. oz. *OTC.*
Use: Antacid; laxative.

Concentrin. (Parke-Davis) Dextromethorphan HBr 15 mg, pseudoephedrine hydrochloride 30 mg, guaifenesin 100 mg. Cap. Bot. 12s. *OTC.*
Use: Antitussive; decongestant; expectorant.

Concerta. (McNeil) Methylphenidate hydrochloride 18 mg, 27 mg, 36 mg, 54 mg, lactose. ER Tab. Bot. 100s. *c-II.*
Use: Central nervous system stimulant.

•**condoliase.** (kon-DOE-li-ase) USAN.
Use: Treatment of lumbar disc herniation.

Condol Suspension. (Sanofi-Synthelabo) Dipyrone, chlormezanone. *Rx.*
Use: Analgesic; muscle relaxant.

Condol Tablets. (Sanofi-Synthelabo) Dipyrone, chlormezanone. *Rx.*
Use: Analgesic; muscle relaxant.

Condylox. (Watson) Podofilox 0.5%, alcohol 95%. Soln. Bot. 3.5 mL. *Rx.*
Use: Keratolytic.

C1-esterase-inhibitor, human, pasteurized.
Use: Prevention, treatment of angioedema.
See: Berinert P.

C1-esterase-inhibitor, human, pasteurized. (Alpha Therapeutic)
Use: Prevention, treatment of angioedema. [Orphan Drug]

C1-inhibitor. (Osterreichisches Baxter Healthcare)
Use: Treatment of angioedema. [Orphan Drug]

C1-inhibitor (human).
See: Berinert.
Cinryze.

C1-inhibitor (human) vapor heated. (Immuno Therapeutics)
Use: Treatment of angioedema. [Orphan Drug]

Conest. (Grafton) Conjugated estrogens 0.625 mg, 1.25 mg, 2.5 mg. Tab. Bot. 100s, 1000s. *Rx.*
Use: Estrogen.

Confident. (Block Drug) Carboxymethylcellulose gum, ethylene oxide polymer, petrolatum/mineral oil base. Tube 0.7 oz, 1.4 oz, 2.4 oz. *OTC.*
Use: Denture adhesive.

Congess. (Fleming & Co.) **Sr.:** Guaifenesin 250 mg, pseudoephedrine hydrochloride 120 mg. SR Cap. **Jr.:** Guaifenesin 125 mg, pseudoephedrine hydrochloride 60 mg. TR Cap. Bot. 100s, 1000s. *Rx-OTC.*
Use: Decongestant; expectorant.

Congestac. (B.F. Ascher) Pseudoephedrine hydrochloride 60 mg, guaifenesin 400 mg. Tab. Bot. 12s, 24s. *OTC.*
Use: Upper respiratory combination, decongestant, expectorant.

Congesta DM. (TriMarc Labs) Dextromethorphan hydrobromide 20 mg, guaifenesin 400 mg. Maltodextrin. Tab. 90s. *OTC.*
Use: Upper respiratory combination, antitussive with expectorant.

Congestaid. (Zee Medical) Pseudoephedrine hydrochloride 30 mg. Tab. 24s. *OTC.*
Use: Decongestant.

congo red. Injection.
Use: Hemostatic in hemorrhagic disorders.

•**conivaptan hydrochloride.** (kahn-ih-VAP-tahn) USAN.
Use: Hyponatremia; vasopressin receptor antagonist.
See: Vaprisol Premixed in Dextrose 5%.

conjugated estrogens.
Use: Estrogen.
See: Estrogens, Conjugated.

•**conorphone hydrochloride.** (KOE-nahr-fone) USAN. *Formerly Codorphone.*
Use: Analgesic.

Conray. (Mallinckrodt) Iothalamate meglumine 600 mg, iodine 282 mg/mL. EDTA. Inj. Vials. 30 mL, 50 mL, 100 mL. Bot. 100 mL, 150 mL, 200 mL. Prefilled power injector syringes. 50 mL, 125 mL. *Rx.*
Use: Radiopaque agent.

Conray 43. (Mallinckrodt) Iothalamate meglumine 430 mg, iodine 202 mg/mL. EDTA. Inj. Vials. 50 mL, 100 mL. Bot. 150 mL, 200 mL, 250 mL. Prefilled syringes. 50 mL. *Rx.*
Use: Radiopaque agent.

Conray 30. (Mallinckrodt) Iothalamate meglumine 300 mg, iodine 141 mg/mL. EDTA. Inj. Vials. 50 mL. Bot. 150 mL, 300 mL. *Rx.*
Use: Radiopaque agent.

Consin Compound Salve. (Wisconsin Pharmacal Co.) Carbolic acid ointment. Jar 2 oz, lb. *OTC.*
Use: Minor skin irritations.

Constonate 60. Docusate sodium 100 mg, 250 mg. Cap. Bot. 100s, 1000s. *OTC.*
Use: Laxative.

Constulose. (Alra) Lactulose 10 g/15 mL (< galactose 1.6 g, lactose 1.2 g, other sugars). Soln. Bot. 237 mL, 946 mL. *Rx.*
Use: Analgesic; laxative.

Contac Cold + Flu. (GlaxoSmithKline) Phenylephrine hydrochloride 5 mg, chlorpheniramine maleate 7 mg, acetaminophen 500 mg. Tab. 24s, 36s. *OTC.*
Use: Upper respiratory combination, decongestant, antihistamine, and analgesic combination.

Contac Cold + Flu Day & Night. (Meda Pharmaceuticals) **Day:** Phenylephrine hydrochloride 5 mg, acetaminophen 500 mg. **Night:** Phenylephrine hydrochloride 5 mg, chlorpheniramine maleate 2 mg, acetaminophen 500 mg. Tab. 28s (16 day and 12 night). *OTC.*
Use: Upper respiratory combination, decongestant, antihistamine, and analgesic combination.

Contac Cold + Flu Maximum Strength. (Meda Pharmaceuticals) Acetamino-

phen 500 mg, chlorpheniramine maleate 2 mg, phenylephrine hydrochloride 5 mg. PEG. Caplets. 24s, 36s. *OTC.*
Use: Upper respiratory combination; decongestant, antihistamine, and analgesic combination.

Contac Cold + Flu Non-Drowsy Maximum Strength. (Meda Pharmaceuticals) Acetaminophen 500 mg, phenylephrine hydrochloride 5 mg. PEG, potassium sorbate. Tab. 8s, 24s. *OTC.*
Use: Upper respiratory combination, decongestant and analgesic combination.

Contac Cough & Chest Cold. (GlaxoSmithKline) Pseudoephedrine hydrochloride 15 mg, dextromethorphan HBr 5 mg, guaifenesin 50 mg, acetaminophen 125 mg/5 mL, alcohol 10%, saccharin, sorbitol. Liq. Bot. 4 fl. oz. *OTC.*
Use: Analgesic; antitussive; decongestant; expectorant.

Contac Cough and Sore Throat Formula. (GlaxoSmithKline) Dextromethorphan HBr 5 mg, acetaminophen 125 mg/5 mL, alcohol 10%. Bot. 120 mL. *OTC.*
Use: Analgesic; antitussive.

Contac Day & Night Allergy/Sinus Relief. (GlaxoSmithKline) **Day:** Pseudoephedrine hydrochloride 60 mg, acetaminophen 650 mg. Capl. **Night:** Pseudoephedrine hydrochloride 60 mg, diphenhydramine hydrochloride 50 mg, acetaminophen 650 mg. Tab. Pkg. 20 (15 day; 5 night). *OTC.*
Use: Upper respiratory combination, decongestant, antihistamine, analgesic.

Contac Day & Night Cold & Flu. (GlaxoSmithKline) **Day:** Pseudoephedrine hydrochloride 60 mg, dextromethorphan HBr 30 mg, acetaminophen 650 mg. **Night:** Pseudoephedrine hydrochloride 60 mg, diphenhydramine hydrochloride 50 mg, acetaminophen 650 mg. Tab. Pkg. 20s (15 day, 5 night). *OTC.*
Use: Upper respiratory combination, decongestant, antihistamine, antitussive, analgesic.

Contac Nighttime Cold. (GlaxoSmithKline) Acetaminophen 167 mg, dextromethorphan HBr 5 mg, pseudoephedrine hydrochloride 10 mg, doxylamine succinate 1.25 mg/5 mL, alcohol 25%. Bot. 177 mL. *OTC.*
Use: Analgesic, decongestant, antitussive, antihistamine.

Contac Non-Drowsy Formula Sinus. (GlaxoSmithKline) Pseudoephedrine hydrochloride 30 mg, acetaminophen 500 mg. Capl. Tab. Pkg. 24s. *OTC.*
Use: Decongestant, analgesic.

Contac Severe Cold & Flu Maximum Strength. (GlaxoSmithKline) Dextromethorphan HBr 15 mg, chlorpheniramine maleate 2 mg, pseudoephedrine hydrochloride 30 mg, acetaminophen 500 mg. Tab. Bot. 30s. *OTC.*
Use: Upper respiratory combination, antitussive, antihistamine, decongestant, analgesic.

Contac Severe Cold & Flu Nighttime. (GlaxoSmithKline) Pseudoephedrine hydrochloride 10 mg, chlorpheniramine maleate 0.67 mg, dextromethorphan HBr 5 mg, acetaminophen 167 mg, alcohol 18.5%, saccharin, sorbitol, glucose. Liq. Bot. 180 mL. *OTC.*
Use: Antihistamine; antitussive; decongestant.

contact lens products, disinfectant. *OTC.*
See: Allergan Hydrocare Cleaning and Disinfecting.
Aosept.
Biotrue Multi-Purpose.
Disinfecting Solution.
Flex-Care.
Hydrocare.
Lensept.
Lens Plus Oxysept.
Opti-Free.
Opti-One.
Oxysept.
ReNu MultiPurpose.
Ultra-Care.

contact lens products, enzymatic cleaners. *OTC.*
See: Ultrazyme Enzymatic Cleaner.

contact lens products, rewetting solutions. *OTC.*
See: Adapettes for Sensitive Eyes.
Clerz.
Clerz 2.
Comfort Tears.
Lens Fresh.
Lens-Wet.
Opti-Free.
Opti-One.
Sensitive Eyes Drops.
Sterile Lens Lubricant.

contact lens products, soft. *OTC.*
Use: Contact lens care, rinsing, storage.
See: Allergan Hydrocare Preserved Saline.
Biotrue Multi-Purpose.
Blairex Sterile Saline Solution.
BoilnSoak.
Ciba Vision Saline.
Hypoclear.
Lens Plus Preservative Free.

Lensrins.
Opti-Soft.
ReNu Saline.
Saline Solution.
Sensitive Eyes Plus.
Sensitive Eyes Saline.
Sterile Saline.
Unisol.
Unisol 4.

contact lens products, surfactant cleaning solutions. *OTC.*
See: Ciba Vision Cleaner.
Daily Cleaner.
LC-65 Daily Contact Lens Cleaner.
Lens Clear.
MiraFlow Extra Strength.
Pliagel.
Preflex Daily Cleaning Especially for Sensitive Eyes.
Sensitive Eyes Saline/Cleaning Solution.
Sof/Pro-Clean.

contraceptive hormones.
Use: Sex hormone.
See: Biphasic Oral Contraceptives.
Contraceptives, Emergency.
Etonogestrel.
Etonogestrel/Ethinyl Estradiol.
Levonorgestrel.
Levonorgestrel/Ethinyl Estradiol.
Levonorgestrel-Releasing Intrauterine System.
Medroxyprogesterone.
Medroxyprogesterone Acetate/Estradiol Cypionate.
Monophasic Oral Contraceptives.
Norelgestromin/Ethinyl Estradiol.
Norethindrone.
Norgestrel.
Oral Contraceptives.
Progestin-Only Products.
Triphasic Oral Contraceptives.
Ulipristal Acetate.

contraceptives, biphasic oral.
See: Amethia.
Amethia Lo.
Camrese.
Camrese Lo.
Daysee.
Jenest-28.
Lo Loestrin Fe.
Lo Minastrin Fe.
LoSeasonique.
Mircette.
Necon 10/11.
Ortho-Novum 10/11.
Viorele.

contraceptives, emergency.
See: Levonorgestrel.
Next Choice One Dose.
Plan B.
Plan B One.

contraceptives, 4-phasic oral.
See: Natazia.
Quartette.

contraceptives, intrauterine system.
See: Mirena.

contraceptives, miscellaneous.
See: Depo-Provera.
Oral Contraceptives.

contraceptives, monophasic oral.
Use: Sex hormone, contraceptive hormone.
See: Alesse.
Apri.
Aviane.
Azurette.
Balziva.
Beyaz.
Brevicon.
Briellyn.
Chateal.
Cryselle.
Cyclafem.
Dasetta 1/35.
Desogen.
Elinest.
Emoquette.
Estarylla.
Falmina.
Femcon Fe.
Generess Fe.
Gildagia.
Gildess Fe 1.5/30.
Gildess 1.5/30.
Introvale.
Jolessa.
Junel Fe 1/20.
Junel Fe 1.5/30.
June 21 Day 1/20.
Junel 21 Day 1.5/30.
Kariva.
Kelnor 1/35.
Kurvelo.
Larin 1/20.
Lessina.
Levlen.
Levlite.
Levora.
Loestrin Fe 1/20.
Loestrin Fe 1.5/30.
Loestrin 24 Fe.
Loestrin 21 1/20.
Loestrin 21 1.5/30.
Lo/Ovral.
Low-Ogestrel.
Lutera.
Lybrel.
Microgestin Fe 1/20.
Microgestin Fe 1.5/30.
Microgestin 1/20.
Minastrin 24 Fe.

Mircette.
Modicon.
MonoNessa.
Necon 1/50.
Necon 1/35.
Necon 0.5/35.
Nordette-28.
Norethindrone Acetate/Ethinyl Estradiol and Ferrous Fumarate.
Norinyl 1 + 50.
Norinyl 1 + 35.
Nortrel 1/35.
Nortrel 0.5/35.
Ogestrel 0.5/50.
Orsythia.
Ortho-Cept.
Ortho-Cyclen.
Ortho-Novum 1/50.
Ortho-Novum 1/35.
Ovcon-50.
Ovcon-35.
Ovral.
Philith.
Pirmella 1/35.
Portia.
Quasense.
Reclipsen.
Safyral.
Seasonale.
Solia.
Sprintec.
Sronyx.
Vestura.
Wera.
Yasmin.
YAZ.
Zenchent.
Zenchent FE.
Zeosa.
Zovia 1/50E.
Zovia 1/35E.

contraceptives, oral.
See: Oral Contraceptives.

contraceptives, triphasic oral.
See: Caziant.
Cyclafem 7/7/7.
Dasetta 7/7/7.
Estrostep Fe.
Levonest.
Ortho-Novum 7/7/7.
Ortho Tri-Cyclen.
Pirmella 7/7/7.
Tri-Estarylla.
Tri-Legest Fe.
Tri-Levlen.
Tri-Linyah.
TriNessa.
Tri-Norinyl.
Tri-Sprintec.
Trivora.

contraceptives, vaginal jellies and creams.
See: Colagyn.
Ortho-Gynol.

Contrin. (Geneva) Iron (from ferrous fumarate) 110 mg, B_{12} 15 mcg, IFC (intrinsic factor as concentrate or from stomach preparations) 240 mg, C 75 mg, folic acid 0.5 mg. Cap. Bot. 100s. *Rx.*
Use: Mineral, vitamin supplement.

ControlRx. (Omnii Oral) Neutral sodium fluoride 1.1%, *Microdent* (emulsion of dimethicone and poloxamer 407) 2%. Sorbitol, saccharin. Berry and vanilla mint flavors. Paste. 56 g. *Rx.*
Use: Prevention of dental caries.

Converspaz. (B.F. Ascher) Cellulase 5 mg, protease 10 mg, amylase 30 mg, lipase 13 mg, l-hyoscamine sulfate 0.0625 mg. Cap. Bot. 100s. *Rx.*
Use: Decongestant; expectorant.

ConZip. (Vertical) Tramadol hydrochloride 100 mg (total dose of 100 mg in a combination of 25 mg immediate-release and 75 mg ER tramadol), 200 mg (total dose of 200 mg in a combination of 50 mg immediate-release and 150 mg ER tramadol), 300 mg (total dose of 300 mg in a combination of 50 mg immediate-release and 250 mg ER tramadol). Lactose, sucrose. ER Cap. 30s. *Rx.*
Use: Opioid analgesic.

Cool-Mint Listerine. (Warner Lambert) Thymol, eucalyptol, methyl salicylate, menthol, alcohol 21.6%. Liq. Bot. 90 mL, 180 mL, 360 mL, 540 mL, 720 mL, 960 mL. *OTC.*
Use: Mouthwash.

CooperVision Balanced Salt. (Ciba Vision) Sterile intraocular irrigation soln. Bot. 15 mL, 500 mL.
Use: Irrigant, ophthalmic.

Copavin Pulvules. (Eli Lilly) Codeine sulfate 15 mg, papaverine hydrochloride 15 mg. Cap. Bot. 100s. *c-v.*
Use: Antitussive.

Copaxone. (Teva) Glatiramer acetate 20 mg/mL, 40 mg/mL. Mannitol 40 mg. Preservative free. Inj. Single-use premixed prefilled syringes. *Rx.*
Use: Multiple sclerosis agent; immunosuppressant.

COPE. (Mentholatum Co.) Aspirin 421 mg, magnesium hydroxide 50 mg, aluminum hydroxide 25 mg, caffeine 32 mg. Tab. Bot. 36s, 60s. *OTC.*
Use: Analgesic; antacid.

Copegus. (Genentech) Ribavirin 200 mg. Film-coated. Tab. 168s. *Rx.*
Use: Antiviral agent.

copper. (Freeda) Copper 2 mg (as copper gluconate). Tab. 100s. *OTC.*
Use: Trace element.

copper. (Hospira) Copper 0.4 mg/mL (as 1.07 mg of cupric chloride). Inj. Vial. 10 mL. *Rx.*
Use: Trace metal.

Copper Caps. (Twinlab) Copper 2 mg (as copper gluconate). Cap. 100s. *OTC.*
Use: Trace element.

•**copper gluconate.** (KAHP-er GLUE-kohn-ate) *USP.*
Use: Supplement, trace mineral.
See: Copper Caps.
Coppermin.

copperhead bite therapy.
See: Antivenin, (Crotalidae) Polyvalent.

Copperin. (Vernon) Iron ammonium citrate, copper (6 g). "A" adult dose, "B" children dose. Bot. 30s, 100s, 500s.
Use: Mineral supplement.

Coppermin. (Key Co) Copper 5 mg. Tab. 100s. *OTC.*
Use: Trace element.

copper sebicate.
Use: Trace element.
See: Cu-5.

Coppertone. (Schering-Plough) A series of sun-care products marketed under the Coppertone name including Waterproof Lotions SPF 4, 6, 8, 15, and 25. Bot. 4 fl oz, 8 fl oz. Oil SPF 2: Bot. 4 fl oz, 8 fl oz; Lite Formula Oil SPF 2: Bot. 4 fl oz; Lite Lotion SPF 4: Bot. 4 fl oz; Dark Tanning Body Mousse SPF 4: Tube 4 oz; Suntanning Gel SPF 4: Tube 3 oz; Noskote SPF 8: Tube 0.44 oz, Jar 1 oz; Noskote SPF-15, Jar 1 oz. Contain one or more of the following ingredients: Padimate O, oxybenzone, homosalate, ethylhexyl p-methocinnamate. *OTC.*
Use: Sunscreen.

Coppertone Bug and Sun Adult Formula. (Schering-Plough) Ethylhexyl p-methoxycinnamate, oxybenzone, 2-ethylhexyl salicylate, homosalate. SPF 15. Waterproof. PABA-free. Aloe vera. Lot. Bot. 237 mL. *OTC.*
Use: Sunscreen; insect repellant.

Coppertone Bug and Sun Kid's Formula. (Schering-Plough) Octocrylene, ethylhexyl p-methoxycinnamate, oxybenzone. SPF 30. Waterproof. PABA-free. Hypoallergenic. Aloe vera. Lot. Bot. 237 mL. *OTC.*
Use: Sunscreen; insect repellant.

Coppertone Dark Tanning. (Schering-Plough) Padimate O in spray base (SPF 2). Spray. Bot. 8 fl oz. *OTC.*
Use: Sunscreen.

Coppertone Face. (Schering-Plough) A series of sunscreen lotions with SPF 2, 4, 6 and 15 in a nongreasy base with padimate O, oxybenzone (SPF 15 only). *OTC.*
Use: Sunscreen.

Coppertone Kids Sunblock. (Schering-Plough) **SPF 15:** Ethylhexyl p-methoxycinnamate, oxybenzone, 2-ethylhexyl salicylate, homosalate. Lot. Bot. 120 mL, 240 mL. **SPF 30:** Octocrylene, ethylhexyl p-methoxycinnamate, oxybenzone, 2-ethylhexyl salicylate. Lot. Bot. 120 mL, 240 mL. *OTC.*
Use: Sunscreen.

Coppertone Lipkote. (Schering-Plough) Ethylhexyl p-methoxycinnamate, oxybenzone. SPF 15. Stick 4.5 g. *OTC.*
Use: Sunscreen.

Coppertone Moisturizing Sunblock. (Schering-Plough) **SPF 45:** Ethylhexyl p-methoxycinnamate, 2-ethylhexyl salicylate, octocrylene, oxybenzone. Lot. Bot. 120 mL, 300 mL. **SPF 25, 30:** Ethylhexyl p-methoxycinnamate, oxybenzone, 2-ethylhexyl salicylate, homosalate. Lot. Bot. SPF 30: 120 mL, 240 mL; SPF 25: 120 mL. **SPF 15:** Ethylhexyl p-methoxycinnamate, oxybenzone. Lot. Bot. 120 mL, 240 mL, 300 mL. *OTC.*
Use: Sunscreen.

Coppertone Moisturizing Sunscreen. (Schering-Plough) Ethylhexyl p-methoxycinnamate, oxybenzone, benzyl alcohol, vitamin E, aloe. PABA free. SPF 6, 8. Waterproof. Lot. Bot. 120 mL, 240 mL. *OTC.*
Use: Sunscreen.

Coppertone Moisturizing Suntan. (Schering-Plough) **SPF 2:** Homosalate, vitamin E, aloe. PABA free. Waterproof. Oil. Bot. 120 mL. **SPF 4:** Ethylhexyl p-methoxycinnamate, oxybenzone, benzyl alcohol, vitamin E, aloe. PABA free. Waterproof. Lot. Bot. 120 mL, 240 mL. *OTC.*
Use: Sunscreen.

Coppertone Noskote. (Schering-Plough) Homosalate 8%, oxybenzone 3%. (SPF 8) Oint. Jar 13.2 g, 30 g. *OTC.*
Use: Sunscreen.

Coppertone SPF-25 Sunblock Lotion. (Schering-Plough) Ethylhexyl p-methoxycinnamate, oxybenzone, padimate O in lotion base (SPF 25). Bot. 120 mL. *OTC.*
Use: Sunscreen.

Coppertone Sport. (Schering-Plough) Ethylhexyl p-methoxycinnamate, oxybenzone. SPF 4, 8, 15, 30. Lot. Bot.

120 mL. *OTC.*
Use: Sunscreen.

Coppertone Tan Magnifier Suntan. (Schering-Plough) **SPF 2:** Triethanolamine salicylate. Oil Bot. 120 mL. **SPF 4 Lotion:** Ethylhexyl p-methoxycinnamate. Bot. 120 mL. **Gel:** 2-phenylbenzimidazole-5-sulfonic acid. Tube 120 g. *OTC.*
Use: Sunscreen.

Coppertone Water Babies. (Schering-Plough) SPF 30, SPF 45. Ethylhexyl p-methoxycinnamate, 2-ethylhexyl salicylate, oxybenzone, homosalate, alcohol, aloe, parabens. PABA free. Waterproof. Lot. Bot. 118 mL. *OTC.*
Use: Sunscreen.

copper trace metal additive. (I.M.S., Ltd.) Copper 1 mg. Inj. Vial 10 mL. *Rx.*
Use: Copper supplement.

•**copper undecylenate.** (KAHP-er un-deh-sil-EN-ate) USAN.
Use: Copper supplement.

Co-Pyronil 2. (Eli Lilly) Chlorpheniramine maleate 4 mg, pseudoephedrine hydrochloride 60 mg. Pulvule. Bot. 100s. *OTC.*
Use: Antihistamine, decongestant.

Co Q10, Vitamin E & Fish Oil. (Mason) Coenzyme Q10 25 mg, DHA 60 mg, EPA 90 mg, vitamin E 200 units, marine lipid concentrate 500 mg. Glycerin, soybean oil. Preservative free. Cap., softgels. 60s. *OTC.*
Use: Enzyme.

Corab. (Abbott Diagnostics) Radioimmunoassay for detection of antibody to hepatitis B core antigen. Test kit 100s.
Use: Diagnostic aid.

Corab-M. (Abbott Diagnostics) Radioimmunoassay for the qualitative determination of specific Ig antibody to hepatitis B virus core antigen (Anti-HBc Ig) in human serum or plasma and may be used as an aid in the diagnosis of acute or recent hepatitis B infection.
Use: Diagnostic aid.

Corace. (Forest) Cortisone acetate 50 mg/mL. Inj. Vial 10 mL. *Rx.*
Use: Corticosteroid, topical.

Coracin. (Roberts) Hydrocortisone acetate 1%, neomycin sulfate 0.5%, bacitracin zinc 400 units, polymyxin B sulfate 10,000 units/g in white petrolatum and mineral oil base. Oint. Tube 3.5 g. *Rx.*
Use: Anti-infective; corticosteroid, ophthalmic.

Coral. (Young Dental) Fluoride ion 1.23%, 0.1 molar phosphate. Jar 250 g, Coral II: 180 disposable cup units/carton. *Rx.*
Use: Fluoride, dental.

Coral Calcium Plus Vitamin D & Magnesium. (Mason) Ca, Mg, vitamin D_3 200 units. Gluten free, preservative free, and soy free. Cap. 60s. *OTC.*
Use: Nutritional supplement.

Coral/Plus. (Young Dental) Free fluoride ion 2.2%, recrystallized kaolinite. Tube 250 g. *Rx.*

coral snake antivenin. (NABI)
See: Antivenin (*Micrurus fulvius*).

Cordarone. (Wyeth-Ayerst) Amiodarone hydrochloride. **Tab.:** 200 mg. Lactose. Bot. 60s, UD 100s. **Inj.:** 50 mg/mL. Benzyl alcohol 20.2 mg/mL. Amp. 3 mL. *Rx.*
Use: Antiarrhythmic.

Cordran. (Aqua Pharmaceuticals) Flurandrenolide 0.05%, 0.025%. White petrolatum. Tube 15 g (0.05% only), 30 g, 60 g. *Rx.*
Use: Corticosteroid, topical.

Cordran Lotion. (Aqua Pharmaceuticals) Flurandrenolide 0.05%, cetyl alcohol, benzyl alcohol, stearic acid, glyceryl monostearate, polyoxyl 40 stearate, glycerin, mineral oil, menthol, purified water. Squeeze bot. 15 mL, 60 mL. *Rx.*
Use: Corticosteroid, topical.

Cordran SP. (Aqua Pharmaceuticals) Flurandrenolide 0.05%, 0.025% in emulsified base w/cetyl alcohol, mineral oil. Tube 15 g (0.05% only), 30 g, 60 g. *Rx.*
Use: Corticosteroid, topical.

Cordran Tape. (Watson) Flurandrenolide 4 mcg/sq. cm. Roll 7.5 cm × 60 cm, 7.5 cm × 200 cm. *Rx.*
Use: Corticosteroid, topical.

Cordrol. (Vita Elixir) Prednisolone 5 mg, 10 mg, 20 mg. Tab. Bot. 100s. *Rx.*
Use: Corticosteroid.

Coreg. (GlaxoSmithKline) Carvedilol 3.125 mg, 6.25 mg, 12.5 mg, 25 mg. Lactose, sucrose. Tab. Bot. 100s. *Rx.*
Use: Antihypertensive.

Coreg CR. (GlaxoSmithKline) Carvedilol (as phosphate) 10 mg, 20 mg, 40 mg, 80 mg. ER Cap. (contains immediate- and controlled-release microparticles). 30s, 90s. *Rx.*
Use: Antiadrenergic/sympatholytic.

Corfen-DM. (Cypress) Chlorpheniramine maleate 4 mg, dextromethorphan hydrobromide 15 mg, phenylephrine hydrochloride 10 mg. Saccharin, sorbitol. Alcohol free, dye free, and sugar free. Grape flavor. Liq. 473 mL. *Rx.*
Use: Upper respiratory combination, antitussive combination.

Corgard. (Pfizer) Nadolol 20 mg, 120 mg, 160 mg. Tab. Bot. 100s, 1000s (except 20 mg, 160 mg), *Unimatic* 100s (except 120 mg, 160 mg). *Rx.*
Use: Antiadrenergic/sympatholytic, beta-adrenergic blocker.

•**coriander oil.** (kor-ee-ANN-der oil) *NF.*
Use: Pharmaceutic aid, flavor.

Coricidin HBP Chest Congestion & Cough. (Schering-Plough) Dextromethorphan HBr 10 mg, guaifenesin 200 mg. Softgel Cap. 20s. *OTC.*
Use: Upper respiratory combination, antitussive with expectorant.

Coricidin HBP Cold & Flu. (Schering-Plough) Chlorpheniramine maleate 2 mg, acetaminophen 325 mg. Tab. Bot. 12s. *OTC.*
Use: Upper respiratory combination, antihistamine, analgesic.

Coricidin HBP Cough & Cold. (Schering-Plough) Dextromethorphan HBr 30 mg, chlorpheniramine maleate 4 mg. Sugar. Tab. Pkg. 16s. *OTC.*
Use: Upper respiratory combination, antitussive combination.

Coricidin HBP Maximum Strength Flu. (Schering-Plough) Dextromethorphan HBr 15 mg, chlorpheniramine maleate 2 mg, acetaminophen 500 mg. Lactose. Tab. Pkg. 20s. *OTC.*
Use: Upper respiratory combination, antitussive combination.

Corifact. (CSL Behring) Factor XIII concentrate (human) 1,000 to 1,600 units (the actual units of potency of factor XIII are stated on each vial label and carton). Preservative free. Inj., lyophilized Pow. for Soln. Kit w/single-dose vial (each vial contains human albumin 120 to 200 mg, total protein 120 to 320 mg, and glucose 80 to 120 mg) and diluent. *Rx.*
Use: Antihemophilic agent.

Corlopam. (Hospira) Fenoldopam mesylate 10 mg/mL. Sodium metabisulfite 1 mg. Inj. Concentrate. Single-dose Amp. 1 mL, 2 mL. *Rx.*
Use: Antihypertensive.

Cormax. (ECR Pharmaceuticals) Clobetasol propionate. **Oint.:** 0.05%. White petrolatum, sorbitan sesquioleate. Tube. 15 g, 45 g. **Soln.:** 0.05%. Alcohol 40%. 25 mL, 50 mL. *Rx.*
Use: Corticosteroid, topical.

•**cormethasone acetate.** (core-METH-ah-sone) USAN.
Use: Anti-inflammatory, topical.

Corn Huskers. (Warner Lambert) Glycerin 6.7%, SD alcohol, algin, TEA-oleoyl sarcosinate, guar gum, methylparaben, calcium sulfate, calcium chloride, TEA-fumarate, TEA-borate. Bot. 4 oz, 7 oz. *OTC.*
Use: Emollient.

•**corn oil.** (korn) *NF.*
Use: Pharmaceutic aid, solvent, oleaginous vehicle.

Corotrope. (Sanofi-Synthelabo) Milrinone for IV use. *Rx.*
Use: Cardiovascular agent.

corpus luteum, extract (water soluble).
See: Progesterone.

Corque. (Geneva) Hydrocortisone 1%, iodochlorhydroxyquin 3%. Cream. Tube 20 g. *Rx.*
Use: Corticosteroid, topical.

Correctol. (Schering-Plough) Bisacodyl 5 mg, talc, lactose, sugar. EC Tab. Bot. 30s, 60s, 90s. *OTC.*
Use: Laxative.

Cortan. (Halsey Drug) Prednisone 5 mg. Tab. Bot. 1000s. *Rx.*
Use: Corticosteroid.

Cortane-B. (Blansett) Hydrocortisone 1%, pramoxine hydrochloride 1%, chloroxylenol 0.1%, benzalkonium chloride. Lot. 60 mL. *Rx.*
Use: Corticosteroid, topical.

Cortane-B Aqueous. (Blansett) Hydrocortisone 1%, pramoxine hydrochloride 1%, chloroxylenol 0.1%. Drops. 10 mL. *Rx.*
Use: Otic preparation.

Cortane-B Otic. (Blansett) Hydrocortisone 1%, pramoxine hydrochloride 1%, chloroxylenol 0.1%. Drops. 10 mL. *Rx.*
Use: Otic preparation.

Cort-Dome. (Bayer Consumer Care) Hydrocortisone alcohol. **Cream:** 0.25%: 1 oz, 4 oz; 0.5%, 1%: 1 oz. **Lot.:** 0.25%, 0.5%: 4 oz; 1%: 1 oz. *Rx.*
Use: Corticosteroid, topical.

Cort-Dome High Potency. (Bayer Consumer Care) Hydrocortisone acetate 25 mg in a monoglyceride base. *Rx.*
Use: Corticosteroid, topical.

Cortef. (Pfizer) Hydrocortisone. Tab. **5 mg:** Bot. 50s. **10 mg, 20 mg:** Bot. 100s. *Rx.*
Use: Corticosteroid.

cortenil.
See: Desoxycorticosterone Acetate.

cortical hormone products.
See: Aristocort.
Betamethasone.
Betamethasone Sodium Phosphate.
Betamethasone Sodium Phosphate and Betamethasone Acetate.
Budesonide.
Celestone.
Celestone Phosphate.
Celestone Soluspan.
Corticotropin.
Cortisone Acetate.
Decadron.
Desoxycorticosterone Acetate.
Dexamethasone.
Entocort EC.

Fludrocortisone Acetate.
Hydrocortisone.
Hydrocortone Acetate.
Hydrocortone Phosphate.
Medrol.
Methylprednisolone.
Prednisolone.
Prednisone.
Triamcinolone.

Cortic-ND. (Everett) Hydrocortisone 1%, pramoxine hydrochloride 1%, chloroxylenol 0.1%, benzalkonium chloride. Drops. 15 mL. *Rx.*
Use: Otic preparation.

Corticool. (Tec Laboratories) Hydrocortisone 1%. Alcohol, castor oil, menthol, propylene glycol. Gel. 45 g. *OTC.*
Use: Anti-inflammatory agent, topical corticosteroid.

•**corticorelin acetate.** (core-tih-kah-REH-lin) USAN.
Use: Hormone

•**corticorelin ovine triflutate.** (core-tih-kah-REH-lin OH-vine TRY-flew-TATE) USAN.
Use: Hormone, corticotropin-releasing; diagnostic aid, adrenocortical insufficiency; Cushing syndrome. [Orphan Drug]
See: Acthrel.

corticosteroid/mydriatic combination, ophthalmic. Prednisolone acetate 0.25%, atropine sulfate 1%. *Rx.*
Use: Treatment of anterior uveitis.

corticosteroids.
Use: Respiratory inhalant; ophthalmic conditions.
See: Beclomethasone Dipropionate.
Budesonide.
Ciclesonide.
Dexamethasone.
Difluprednate.
Flunisolide.
Fluocinolone Acetonide.
Fluorometholone.
Fluticasone Propionate.
Loteprednol Etabonate.
Mometasone Furoate.
Prednisolone.
Rimexolone.
Triamcinolone Acetonide.

corticosteroids, otic.
See: Fluocinolone Acetonide.

corticosteroids, topical.
See: Betamethasone Valerate.
Clobetasol Propionate.
Clocortolone Pivalate.
Desonide.
Fluocinolone Acetonide.
Fluticasone Propionate.
Halobetasol Propionate.
Hydrocortisone.
Hydrocortisone Acetate.
Mometasone furoate.
Prednicarbate.
Triamcinolone Acetonide.

•**corticotropin.** (core-tih-koe-TROE-pin) *USP.*
Use: Adrenocortical steroids.
See: Corticotropin Injection, Repository.
Cosyntropin.

•**corticotropin, repository, injection.** (core-tih-koe-TROE-pin) *USP.*
Use: Hormone, adrenocorticotrophic; corticosteroid, topical; diagnostic aid, adrenocortical insufficiency.
See: H.P. Acthar Gel.

Cortifoam. (Schwarz Pharma) Hydrocortisone acetate 10% in an aerosol foam w/propylene glycol, emulsifying wax, steareth 10, cetyl alcohol, methylparaben, propylparaben, trolamine, inert propellants. Container 20 g w/rectal applicator for 14 applicatorsful. *Rx.*
Use: Corticosteroid, topical.

cortisol.
Note: Cortisol was the official published name for hydrocortisone in *USP 24.* The name was changed back to Hydrocortisone, *USP.* in Supplement 1 to the *USP 24.*
See: Hydrocortisone.

cortisol cyclopentylpropionate.
See: Cortef Fluid.

cortisone.
Use: Adrenocortical steroid, glucocorticoid.
See: Cortisone Acetate.

•**cortisone acetate.** (CORE-tih-sone) *USP.*
Use: Corticosteroid, topical.
See: Cortistan.
Cortone Acetate.

cortisone acetate. (Various Mfr.) Cortisone acetate 25 mg. Tab. 8s, 100s, 500s, 1,000s, UD 100s. *Rx.*
Use: Adrenocortical steroid, glucocorticoid.

Cortisporin. (Monarch) Polymyxin B sulfate 10,000 units/g, neomycin sulfate 3.5 mg as base, hydrocortisone acetate 0.5%. Methylparaben 0.25%, white, liquid petrolatum. Cream. Tube 7.5 g. *Rx.*
Use: Anti-infective; corticosteroid, topical.

Cortisporin-TC. (Monarch) Neomycin sulfate 3.3 mg, hydrocortisone 1%, colistin sulfate 3 mg, thonzonium bromide 0.5 mg. Susp. Bot. 10 mL w/dropper. *Rx.*
Use: Steroid and antibiotic combination, otic.

Cortistan. (Standex) Cortisone 25 mg/ 10 mL. *Rx.*
Use: Corticosteroid.

•**cortivazol.** (core-TIH-vah-zole) USAN.
Use: Corticosteroid, topical.

Cortizone•5. (Pfizer Consumer Healthcare) Hydrocortisone 0.5%. White petrolatum. Oint. Tube 30 g. *OTC.*
Use: Corticosteroid, topical.

Cortizone•10 Anti-Itch. (Chattem) Hydrocortisone 1%. **Cream:** Aloe, beeswax, cetearyl alcohol, glycerin, mineral oil, parabens, petrolatum. Tube. 14 g, 28 g, 57 g. **Oint.:** Petrolatum. Tube. 28 g, 57 g. *OTC.*
Use: Anti-inflammatory agent, topical corticosteroid.

Cortizone•10 Children's Cooling Cream. (Chattem) Hydrocortisone 1%. Aloe, beeswax, glycerin, mineral oil, parabens, petrolatum. Cream. Tube. 27 g. *OTC.*
Use: Anti-inflammatory agent, topical corticosteroid.

Cortizone•10 Cooling Relief Anti-Itch. (Chattem) Hydrocortisone 1%. Aloe, disodium EDTA, glycerin, parabens, SD alcohol 40. Gel. Tube. 28 g. *OTC.*
Use: Anti-inflammatory agent, topical corticosteroid.

Cortizone•10 Easy Relief Applicatory Anti-Itch. (Chattem) Hydrocortisone 1%. Alcohol, aloe, disodium EDTA, glycerin, menthyl lactate, PEG. Liq. 36 mL. *OTC.*
Use: Anti-inflammatory agent, topical corticosteroid.

Cotizone•10 Hydratensive Anti-Itch. (Chattem) Hydrocortisone 1%. **Eczema Natural Oatmeal Formula:** Alcohol, aloe, caprylic/capric triglyceride, cetyl alcohol, dipropylene glycol, disodium EDTA, glycerin, glyceryl stearate, parabens, petrolatum, retinyl palmitate, shea butter extract. Lot. 113 g. **Healing Natural Aloe Formula:** Aloe, caprylic/ capric triglyceride, cetyl alcohol, dipropylene glycol, disodium EDTA, glycerin, glyceryl stearate, glycerin, petrolatum, parabens, retinyl palmitate, shea butter extract. Lot. 113 g. *OTC.*
Use: Anti-inflammatory agent, topical corticosteroid.

Cortizone•10 Intensive Healing Eczema. (Chattem) Hydrocortisone 1%. Aloe, cetyl alcohol, dimethicone, dipropylene glycol, disodium EDTA, glycerin, glyceryl stearate, parabens, petrolatum. Lot. Tube. 3.5 oz. *OTC.*
Use: Anti-inflammatory agent, topical corticosteroid.

Cortizone•10 Intensive Healing Formula Anti-Itch. (Chattem) Hydrocortisone 1%. Alcohols, benzyl alcohol, EDTA, glycerin, glyceryl stearate, parabens, petrolatum, propylene glycol, diazolidinyl urea. Cream. Tube. 28 g, 57 g. *OTC.*
Use: Anti-inflammatory agent, topical corticosteroid.

Cortizone•10 Plus Ultra Moisturizing. (Chattem) Hydrocortisone 1%. Alcohols, aloe, beeswax, cetearyl alcohol, cetyl alcohol, glycerin, mineral oil, parabens, petrolatum, propylene glycol, retinyl palmitate. Cream. 28 g, 57 g. *OTC.*
Use: Anti-inflammatory agent, topical corticosteroid.

Cortizone•10 Poison Ivy Relief Pads. (Chattem) Hydrocortisone 1%. Aloe, dimethicone, disodium EDTA, glycerin, menthyl lactate, parabens, SD alcohol 40. Pads. 10s (self-contained *Snapplicators*). *OTC.*
Use: Anti-inflammatory agent, topical corticosteroid.

Cortizone•10 Quick Shot. (Chattem) Hydrocortisone 1%. Alcohol, aloe, disodium EDTA, glycerin, menthyl lactate, PEG. Spray. 44 mL. *OTC.*
Use: Anti-inflammatory agent, topical corticosteroid.

•**cortodoxone.** (CORE-toe-dox-OHN) USAN.
Use: Anti-inflammatory.

Cortone Acetate. (Merck & Co.) Cortisone acetate 50 mg/mL, sodium chloride, sodium carboxymethylcellulose, benzyl alcohol. Susp. Inj. Vial 10 mL. *Rx.*
Use: Corticosteroid.

Cortrosyn. (Amphastar) Cosyntropin 0.25 mg, mannitol 10 mg, Pow. for Inj., lyophilized. Vials with diluent. *Rx.*
Use: Corticosteroid.

Corubeen. (Spanner) Vitamin B_{12} crystalline 1000 mcg/mL. Vial 10 mL. *Rx.*
Use: Vitamin supplement.

Corvert. (Pharmacia) Ibutilide fumarate 0.1 mg/mL. Soln. Vial. 10 mL. *Rx.*
Use: Antiarrhythmic.

Corvita. (Trigen) Iron 13 mg, vitamins A 750 units, D 315 units, E 125 units, B_1 25 mg, B_2 3.4 mg, B_3 35 mg, B_5 5 mg, B_6 35 mg, B_{12} 70 mcg, C 375 mg, folic acid 1.25 mg, Cr, Cu, Mg, Se, Zn, alpha lipoic acid, biotin, lutein, lycopene. Tartrazine. Gluten free, lactose free, sugar free. Tab. 100s. *Rx.*
Use: Multivitamin with minerals (including iron).

Corvite FE. (Vertical Pharmaceuticals)

Fe 150 mg, vitamins B_6 10 mg, B_{12} 15 mcg, C 160 mg, folate 1 mg, Ca 5 mg, Mg 15 mg, Zn 25 mg. PEG, povidone, vegetable oil. Tab. UD 30s. *Rx.*
Use: Multivitamin with iron.

Corvite Free. (Vertical Pharmaceuticals) Vitamin D_3 400 units, E 125 units, C 500 mg, B_1 25 mg, B_2 3.4 mg, B_3 35 mg, B_5 5 mg, B_6 35 mg, B_{12} 70 mcg, folic acid 1.25 mcg, biotin 75 mcg, alpha-lipoic acid 10 mg, coenzyme Q_{10} 35 mg, lutein 400 mcg, lycopene 125 mcg. Dye free, gluten free, lactose free, sugar free. Tab. 100s. *Rx.*
Use: Multivitamin with minerals.

Corvite 150. (Vertical Pharmaceuticals) Fe 150 mg, vitamins B_6 10 mg, B_{12} 15 mcg, C 120 mg, folate 1.25 mg, Zn 25 mg. Gluten free, lactose free, sugar free. Tab. UD 100s. *Rx.*
Use: Multivitamin with iron.

CoryZa-D. (Larken) Dexchlorpheniramine maleate 3.5 mg, methscopolamine nitrate 1 mg, pseudoephedrine hydrochloride 45 mg. Lactose. ER Tab. 100s. *Rx.*
Use: Upper respiratory combination; decongestant, antihistamine, and anticholinergic combination.

Corzall-PE. (Hawthorn) Carbetapentane citrate 20 mg, dexchlorpheniramine maleate 1 mg, phenylephrine hydrochloride 10 mg. Glycerin, propylene glycol, saccharin, sorbitol. Alcohol free, dye free, and sugar free. Cherry flavor. Liq. 473 mL. *Rx.*
Use: Upper respiratory combination, antitussive combination.

Corzide. (King Pharma) Nadolol/bendroflumethiazide 40 mg/5 mg, 80 mg/5 mg. Lactose. Tab. Bot. 100s. *Rx.*
Use: Antihypertensive.

Corzyme. (Abbott Diagnostics) Enzyme immunoassay for detection of antibody to hepatitis B core antigen in serum or plasma. Test kit 100s.
Use: Diagnostic aid.

Corzyme-M. (Abbott Diagnostics) Enzyme immunoassay for the detection of Ig antibody to hepatitis B core antigen (Anti-HBc Ig). In human serum or plasma. Test kit 100s.
Use: Diagnostic aid.

•**cositecan.** (COS-eye-TEE-kan) USAN.
Use: Antineoplastic agent.

Cosmegen. (Recordati Rare Diseases) Actinomycin D (dactinomycin) 500 mcg. Mannitol 20 mg. Pow. for Inj., lyophilized. Vials. *Rx.*
Use: Antineoplastic; antibiotic.

Cosmoline.
See: Petrolatum.

Cosopt. (Merck) Dorzolamide 2%, timolol 0.5%. Benzalkonium chloride 0.0075%, mannitol. Soln. *Ocumeters.* 5 mL, 10 mL. *Rx.*
Use: Antiglaucoma agent.

Cosopt PF. (Merck) Dorzolamide hydrochloride 2%, timolol 0.5%. Preservative free. Soln., Ophth. Single-use container. 0.2 mL. *Rx.*
Use: Agent for glaucoma.

Cosulid. (Novartis) Sulfachloropyridazine.

•**cosyntropin.** (koe-sin-TROE-pin) USAN.
Use: Hormone, adrenocorticotrophic.
See: Cortrosyn.

cosyntropin. (Sandoz) Cosyntropin 0.25 mg/mL. Mannitol 10 mg, sodium chloride 6.4 mg. Preservative free. Inj., Soln. Vial. 1 mL. *Rx.*
Use: Adrenocortical steroid, corticotropin (ACTH).

Cotab A. (MCR American) Chlorpheniramine maleate 4 mg, codeine phosphate 10 mg. Cap. 100s. *c-III.*
Use: Upper respiratory combination, antitussive, antihistamine.

Cotab AX. (MCR American) Chlorpheniramine maleate 4 mg, codeine phosphate 20 mg. Tab. 100s. *c-III.*
Use: Upper respiratory combination, antitussive combination.

Cotabflu. (MCR American) Acetaminophen 500 mg, chlorpheniramine maleate 4 mg, codeine phosphate 20 mg. Tab. 100s. *c-III.*
Use: Upper respiratory combination, antitussive combination.

Cotaphylline. (Major) Oxtriphylline 100 mg, 200 mg. Tab. Bot. 100s, 500s. *Rx.*
Use: Bronchodilator.

cotarnine chloride. Cotarnine hydrochloride.
Use: Astringent.

cotarnine hydrochloride.
See: Cotarnine Chloride.

•**cotinine fumarate.** (koe-TIH-neen) USAN.
Use: Antidepressant; psychomotor stimulant.

Cotolate. (Major) Benztropine 1 mg, 2 mg. Tab. Bot. 100s, 1000s. *Rx.*
Use: Antiparkinsonian.

•**cotton, purified.** (KAHT-uhn) *USP.*
Use: Surgical aid.

•**cottonseed oil.** (KAHT-uhn-seed) *NF.*
Use: Pharmaceutic aid; solvent, oleaginous vehicle.

Co-Tuss V. (Rugby) Hydrocodone bitartrate 5 mg, guaifenesin 100 mg. Liq. Bot. 480 mL. *c-III.*
Use: Antitussive; expectorant.

CO_2-releasing suppositories.
See: Ceo-Two.

Cotylenol Children's Chewable Cold Tablet. (McNeil Consumer) Acetaminophen 80 mg, chlorpheniramine maleate 0.5 mg, pseudoephedrine hydrochloride 7.5 mg. Chew. Tab. Bot. 24s. *OTC.*
Use: Analgesic; antihistamine; decongestant.

Cotylenol Children's Liquid Cold Formula. (McNeil Consumer) Acetaminophen 160 mg, chlorpheniramine maleate 1 mg, pseudoephedrine hydrochloride 15 mg, sorbitol/5 mL. Bot. 4 oz. *OTC.*
Use: Analgesic; antihistamine; decongestant.

Cotylenol Cold Formula. (McNeil Consumer) Chlorpheniramine maleate 2 mg, dextromethorphan HBr 15 mg, pseudoephedrine hydrochloride 30 mg, acetaminophen 325 mg. **Tab.:** Box 24s, Bot. 50s, 100s. **Capl.:** Bot. 24s, 50s. *OTC.*
Use: Analgesic; antihistamine; antitussive; decongestant.

Cotylenol Liquid Cold Formula. (McNeil Consumer) Acetaminophen 650 mg, chlorpheniramine maleate 4 mg, pseudoephedrine hydrochloride 60 mg, dextromethorphan hydrochloride 30 mg/30 mL, alcohol 7.5%, sorbitol. Bot. 5 oz. *OTC.*
Use: Analgesic; antihistamine; antitussive; decongestant.

Cough Formula Comtrex. (Bristol-Myers Squibb) Pseudoephedrine hydrochloride 15 mg, dextromethorphan HBr 7.5 mg/5 mL, guaifenesin, saccharin, sucrose. Liq. Bot. 120 mL, 240 mL. *OTC.*
Use: Antitussive; expectorant.

Cough Syrup. (Ivax) Phenylephrine hydrochloride 5 mg, dextromethorphan HBr 10 mg, guaifenesin 100 mg, alcohol free. Bot. 120 mL. *OTC.*
Use: Antitussive; decongestant; expectorant.

Coumadin. (Bristol-Myers Squibb) Warfarin sodium. **Tab.:** 1 mg, 2 mg, 2.5 mg, 3 mg, 4 mg, 5 mg, 6 mg, 7.5 mg, 10 mg. Dye-free (10 mg only). Lactose. Bot. 100s, 1000s (except 7.5 mg, 10 mg), UD 100s. **Pow. for Soln., Inj., lyophilized:** Warfarin sodium 5 mg (2 mg/mL when reconstituted). Mannitol, preservative-free. Single-use vials. 5 mg. *Rx.*
Use: Anticoagulant.

coumarin.
Use: Anticoagulant; treat renal cell carcinoma. [Orphan Drug]

coumarin and indandione derivatives.
Use: Anticoagulant.
See: Coumadin.
Warfarin Sodium.

•**coumermycin.** (KOO-mer-MY-sin) USAN.
Use: Anti-infective.

•**coumermycin sodium.** (KOO-mer-MY-sin) USAN.
Use: Anti-infective.

counterirritants.
See: Capsaicin.

Counterpain Rub. (Bristol-Myers Squibb) Methylsalicylate, eugenol, menthol. Oint. Tube 1 oz. *OTC.*
Use: Analgesic, topical.

Covaryx. (Centrix) Esterified estrogens 1.25 mg, methyltestosterone 2.5 mg. Lactose, tartrazine. Film-coated. Tab. 100s. *Rx.*
Use: Estrogen and androgen combination, sex hormone.

Covaryx H.S. (Centrix) Esterified estrogens 0.625 mg, methyltestosterone 1.25 mg. Lactose, tartrazine. Film-coated. Tab. 100s. *Rx.*
Use: Estrogen and androgen combination, sex hormone.

Covera-HS. (Pfizer) Verapamil hydrochloride 180 mg, 240 mg. Film-coated. ER Tab. Bot. 100s, UD 100s. *Rx.*
Use: Calcium channel blocker.

Covermark. (O'Leary) Neutral cream, hypoallergenic, opaque, greaseless. Jar 1 oz, 3 oz, available in 11 shades. *OTC.*
Use: Conceals birthmarks and skin discolorations.

Covermark Stick. (O'Leary) For normal to oily skin, available in 7 shades. *OTC.*
Use: Conceals birthmarks and skin discolorations.

Co-Xan. (Schwarz Pharma) Theophylline anhydrous 150 mg, ephedrine hydrochloride 25 mg, guaifenesin 100 mg, codeine phosphate 15 mg, alcohol 10%/15 mL. Syr. Bot. Pt. *Rx.*
Use: Antitussive; bronchodilator; decongestant; expectorant.

Cozaar. (Merck) Losartan potassium 25 mg (potassium 2.12 mg), 50 mg (potassium 4.24 mg), 100 mg (potassium 8.48 mg). Lactose. Film-coated. Tab. Bot. 1000s, unit-of-use 30s (except 25 mg), 90s, 100s, UD 100s. *Rx.*
Use: Renin angiotensin system antagonist, angiotensin II receptor antagonist.

CPB WC. (Elge) Brompheniramine maleate 1.3 mg, codeine phosphate 6.3 mg, pseudoephedrine hydrochloride 10 mg per 5 mL. Saccharin, sorbitol. Cherry flavor. Liq. 473 mL. *c-v.*

Use: Upper respiratory combination, antitussive combination.

CP DEC-DM. (Hi-Tech) **Syrup:** Dextromethorphan HBr 15 mg, chlorpheniramine maleate 4 mg, phenylephrine hydrochloride 12.5 mg per 5 mL. Alcohol and sugar free. Saccharin, sorbitol. Grape flavor. 118 mL, 473 mL. *Rx.*
Use: Upper respiratory combination, antitussive combination.

C.P.-DM. (Hi-Tech) Pseudoephedrine hydrochloride 15 mg, carbinoxamine maleate 1 mg, dextromethorphan HBr 4 mg per 1 mL. Saccharin, sorbitol, grape flavor. Drops. Bot. 30 mL w/dropper. *Rx.*
Use: Upper respiratory combination, decongestant, antihistamine, antitussive.

C-Phed Tannate. (Morton Grove) Pseudoephedrine tannate 75 mg, chlorpheniramine tannate 4.5 mg/5 mL, strawberry/banana flavor. Susp. Bot. 118 mL. *Rx.*
Use: Upper respiratory combination, decongestant, antihistamine.

Cplex. (Arcum) Vitamins B_1 10 mg, B_2 10 mg, B_6 5 mg, B_{12} 10 mcg, niacinamide 100 mg, calcium pantothenate 25 mg, C 150 mg, liver 50 mg, dried yeast 50 mg. Cap. Bot. 100s, 1000s. *OTC.*
Use: Mineral, vitamin supplement.

C.P.M. (Ivax) Chlorpheniramine 4 mg. Tab. Bot. 1000s. *OTC.*
Use: Antihistamine.

CPM 8/PE 20/MSC 1.25. (Cypress) Phenylephrine hydrochloride 20 mg, chlorpheniramine maleate 8 mg, methscopolamine nitrate 1.25 mg. Lactose. ER Tab. 100s. *Rx.*
Use: Decongestant, antihistamine, and anticholinergic, upper respiratory combination.

CPM 8/PSE 90/MSC 2.5. (Cypress) Pseudoephedrine hydrochloride 90 mg, chlorpheniramine maleate 8 mg, methscopolamine nitrate 2.5 mg. Dye free. ER Tab. Bot. 100s. *Rx.*
Use: Upper respiratory combination, decongestant, antihistamine, anticholinergic.

CPM/PSE DM. (Trigen Laboratories) Chlorpheniramine maleate 0.8 mg, dextromethorphan hydrobromide 3 mg, pseudoephedrine hydrochloride 9 mg per 5 mL. Glycerin, parabens, potassium sorbate, propylene glycol, sorbitol, sucralose. Grape flavor. Drops. 30 mL. *Rx.*
Use: Upper respiratory combination, antitussive combination.

CP-TANNIC. (Cypress) Pseudoephedrine tannate 75 mg, chlorpheniramine tannate 4.5 mg/5 mL, strawberry/banana flavor. Susp. Bot. 473 mL. *Rx.*
Use: Upper respiratory combination, decongestant, antihistamine.

Crantex ER. (Breckenridge) Phenylephrine hydrochloride 10 mg, guaifenesin 300 mg. Sugar. ER Cap. 100s. *Rx.*
Use: Decongestant and expectorant.

Cream Camellia. (O'Leary) Jar 2 oz. *OTC.*
Use: Emollient.

•**creatinine.** (kree-OT-ih-nihn) *NF.*
Use: Bulking agent for freeze drying.

creatinine reagent strips. (Bayer Consumer Care) Seralyzer reagent strips. A quantitative strip test for creatinine in serum or plasma. Bot. 25s.
Use: Diagnostic aid.

Cremagol. (Cremagol) Emulsion of liquid petrolatum, agar agar, acacia, glycerin. Bot. 14 oz. W/cascara 11 g/oz, Bot. 14 oz. W/phenolphthalein 2 g/oz, Bot. 14 oz. *OTC.*
Use: Laxative.

•**crenezumab.** (kree-NEZ-ue-mab) USAN.
Use: CNS agent.

•**crenolanib.** (kree-NOE-la-nib) USAN.
Use: Antineoplastic.

•**crenolanib besylate.** (kree-NOE-la-nib) USAN.
Use: Antineoplastic.

Creomulsion Adult Formula. (Summit) Dextromethorphan HBr 20 mg/15 mL. Alcohol free. Sucrose. Syrup. 118 mL. *OTC.*
Use: Nonnarcotic antitussive.

Creomulsion for Children. (Creomulsion) Dextromethorphan HBr 5 mg/5 mL. Alcohol free. Sucrose. Cherry flavor. Syrup. 118 mL. *OTC.*
Use: Nonnarcotic antitussive.

Creon Delayed Release. (AbbVie) Lipase/protease/amylase 3,000 units/9,500 units/15,000 units; 6,000 units/19,000 units/30,000 units; 12,000 units/38,000 units/60,000 units; 24,000 units/76,000 units/120,000 units; 36,000 units/114,000 units/180,000 units. Enteric-coated spheres. Cap., delayed release. 100s, 250s. *Rx.*
Use: Digestive enzyme.

creosote. Wood creosote, creosote, beechwood creosote.

Creo-Terpin. (Lee) Dextromethorphan HBr 10 mg/15 mL (3.33 mg/5 mL). Tartrazine, alcohol 25%, saccharin, corn syrup. Liq. Bot. 120 mL. *OTC.*
Use: Nonnarcotic antitussive.

Crescormon. (Pharmacia) Somatotropin 4 units. Vial. IM administration. *Rx.*
Note: Crescormon will be available only for patients who qualify for treatment. Apply to Kabi Group Inc. for approval.
Use: Hormone, growth.

•**cresol.** (KREE-sole) *NF.*
Use: Antiseptic; disinfectant.

cresol preparations.
Use: Antiseptic; disinfectant.
See: Saponated Cresol.

Crestor. (AstraZeneca) Rosuvastatin calcium (as base) 5 mg, 10 mg, 20 mg, 40 mg. Lactose. 30s (40 mg only), 90s (except 40 mg), UD 100s (except 5 mg). *Rx.*
Use: HMG-CoA reductase inhibitors, antihyperlipidemic agent.

m-cresyl-acetate.
See: Cresylate.

Cresylate. (Recsei) M-cresyl-acetate 25%, isopropanol 25%, chlorobutanol 1%, benzyl alcohol 1%, castor oil 5%, propylene glycol. Bot. 15 mL with dropper, pt. *Rx.*
Use: Otic preparation.

cresylic acid. Same as Cresol.

•**crilvastatin.** (krill-vah-STAT-in) USAN.
Use: Antihyperlipidemic.

Crinone. (Watson Labs) Progesterone 4% (45 mg), 8% (90 mg). Glycerin, mineral oil, palm oil. Vaginal Gel. Single-use, prefilled, disposable applicator. 6s (4%), 15s (8%). *Rx.*
Use: Assisted reproductive technology treatment.

•**crisnatol mesylate.** (KRISS-nah-tole) USAN.
Use: Antineoplastic.

Critic-Aid Clear AF. (Coloplast) Miconazole nitrate 2%. Petrolatum. Oint. 57 g. *OTC.*
Use: Topical anti-infective, antifungal.

Criticare HN. (Bristol-Myers Squibb) High nitrogen elemental diet. Protein 14%, fat 4.3%, carbohydrate 81.5%. Bot. 8 oz. *OTC.*
Use: Nutritional supplement, enteral.

Crixivan. (Merck) Indinavir sulfate 200 mg, 333 mg, 400 mg (corresponding to 125 mg, 250 mg, 416.3 mg, 500 mg indinavir sulfate, respectively). Lactose. Cap. Unit-of-use 18s, 90s, 120s (400 mg only); 135s (333 mg only); 180s (400 mg only); 360s (200 mg only); unit dose 42s (400 mg only). *Rx.*
Use: Antiretroviral agent, protease inhibitor.

•**crizotinib.** (kriz-OH-ti-nib) USAN.
Use: Antineoplastic.
See: Xalkori.

CroFab. (Altana) Crotalidae polyvalent immune Fab (ovine origin). Total protein 1 g, thimerosal (mercury 0.11 mg)/vial. Single-use Vial. Diluent not included. *Rx.*
Use: Antivenin.

•**crofelemer.** (kroe-FEL-e-mer) USAN.
Use: Antidiarrheal.
See: Fulyzaq.

Croferrin. (Forest) Iron peptonate 50 mg, liver injection 2.5 mcg, vitamin B_{12} 12.5 mcg, lidocaine hydrochloride 1%, phenol 0.5%, sodium citrate 0.125%, sodium bisulfite 0.009%/mL. Vial 10 mL, 30 mL. *Rx.*
Use: Mineral, vitamin supplement.

•**crofilcon A.** (kroe-FILL-kahn A) USAN.
Use: Contact lens material, hydrophilic.

•**crolibulin.** (KROE-li-BUE-lin) USAN.
Use: Antineoplastic.

Cro-Man-Zin. (Freeda) Cr 200 mcg, Mn 5 mg, Zn 25 mg, kosher, sugar free. Tab. Bot. 100s, 250s. *OTC.*
Use: Electrolyte, mineral supplement.

•**cromitrile sodium.** (KROE-mih-TRILE) USAN.
Use: Antiasthmatic.

•**cromolyn sodium.** (KROE-moe-lin) *USP.*
Use: Antiasthmatic; prophylactic; mastocytosis. [Orphan Drug]
See: Children's NasalCrom.
Gastrocrom.
Intal.
NasalCrom.

cromolyn sodium. (Major Pharmaceuticals) Cromolyn sodium 40 mg/mL (5.2 mg/spray). Soln., Nasal. 26 mL. *OTC.*
Use: Respiratory inhalant, mast cell stabilizer.

cromolyn sodium. (Various Mfr.) Cromolyn sodium. **Inhalation:** 20 mg per 2 mL. Vial or Amps. 60 mL, 120 mL. **Soln. for Nebulization:** 20 mg. Vial. 2 mL. **Soln., Conc.:** 100 mg per 5 mL. Preservative free. Amp. 5 mL. *Rx.*
Use: Antiasthmatic; prophylactic.

cromolyn sodium. (Various Mfr.) Cromolyn sodium 4%. Soln. 10 mL, 15 mL. *Rx.*
Use: Ophthalmic mast cell stabilizer.

Cronetal.
See: Disulfiram.

•**croscarmellose sodium.** (KRAHS-CAR-mell-ose) *NF. Formerly Cross-linked Carboxymethylcellulose Sodium and Modified Cellulose Gum.*
Use: Pharmaceutic aid, tablet disintegrant.

•**crospovidone.** (krahs-PAV-ih-dohn) *NF.*
Use: Pharmaceutic aid, tablet excipient.

Cross Aspirin. (Cross) Aspirin 325 mg. Sugar, salt and lactose free. Tab. Bot. 100s, 1000s. *OTC.*
Use: Analgesic.

CroTAb. (CroFab)

Crotalidae antivenin polyvalent. (Wyeth) 1 vial of lyophilized serum, 1 vial of bacteriostatic water 10 mL, USP, 1 vial normal horse serum. Inj. Vial Combination Pkg. *Rx.*
Use: Antivenin.

Crotalidae polyvalent immune Fab (ovine origin).
Use: Antivenin.
See: CroFab.

•**crotaline antivenin, polyvalent.** (kroe-TAHL-een an-tee-VEH-nen pahl-ee-VAY-lent) *USP.* Antivenin Crotalidae Polyvalent, North and South American antisnakebite serum. *Rx.*
Use: Immunizing agent.

•**crotamiton.** (kroe-TAM-ih-tuhn) *USP.*
Use: Scabicide.
See: Eurax.

CRPA Latex Test. (Laboratory Diagnostics) Rapid latex agglutination test for the qualitative determination of C-reactive protein. CRPA, 1 mL CRP Positest Control, 0.5 mL CRPA Latex Test Kit.
Use: Diagnostic aid.

Cruex. (Novartis Consumer Health) **Aer., Pow:** Miconazole nitrate 2%. Aloe, SD alcohol 10%. 85 g. **Cream:** Clotrimazole 1%. Benzyl alcohol 1%, cetostearyl alcohol. Tube. 15 g. *OTC.*
Use: Anti-infective, topical; antifungal agent.

Cruex Spray Powder. (Novartis Consumer Health) Undecylenic acid 2% and zinc undecylenate 20%. Pow. Aerosol can 1.8 oz, 3.5 oz, 5.5 oz. *OTC.*
Use: Antifungal, topical.

Cruex Squeeze Powder. (Novartis Consumer Health) Calcium undecylenate 10%. Pow. Plastic squeeze bot. 1.5 oz. *OTC.*
Use: Antifungal, topical.

cryptosporidium hyperimmune bovine colostrum IgG concentrate. (Immucell)
Use: Treat diarrhea in AIDS patients. [Orphan Drug]

Cryselle. (Barr) Norgestrel 0.3 mg, ethinyl estradiol 30 mcg. Packs. 21s. 28s with 7 inert tabs. *Rx.*
Use: Sex hormone, contraceptive hormone.

crystalline trypsin. Highly purified preparation of enzyme as derived from mammalian pancreas glands.

crystal violet.
See: Methylrosaniline Chloride.

Crysti-Liver. (Roberts) Liver injection (equivalent to B_{12} 10 mcg), crystalline B_{12} 100 mcg, folic acid 0.4 mg. Inj. Vial 10 mL. *Rx.*
Use: Mineral, vitamin supplement.

Crystodigin. (Eli Lilly) Digitoxin 0.05 mg, 0.1 mg. Tab. Bot. 100s. *Rx.*
Use: Cardiovascular agent.

CTab.
See: Cetyl Trimethyl Ammonium Bromide.

C-Tussin. (Century) Codeine phosphate 10 mg, pseudoephedrine hydrochloride 30 mg, guaifenesin 100 mg/5 mL, alcohol 7.5%. Bot. 120 mL, gal. *c-IV.*
Use: Antitussive; decongestant; expectorant.

C-250. (Nature's Bounty) Ascorbic acid 250 mg. Gluten free, lactose free, preservative free, and sugar free. Tab. 100s. *OTC.*
Use: Water-soluble vitamin.

Cubicin. (Cubist) Daptomycin 500 mg. Preservative free. Pow. for Inj., lyophilized Cake. Single-use vials. 10 mL. *Rx.*
Use: Anti-infective.

Cu-5. (BioTech) Copper 5 mg (as copper sebicate). Dye free, preservative free, and sugar free. Cap. 100s. *OTC.*
Use: Trace element.

Culminal. (Culminal) Benzocaine 3% in water-miscible cream base. Tube 1 oz. *OTC.*
Use: Anesthetic, local.

Culturelle Dairy Free. (Amerifit) *L. rhamnosus* 10 billion cells. Insulin 245 mg. Gluten free. Cap. 30s. *OTC.*
Use: Probiotic.

Culturelle Digestive Health. (Amerifit) *L. rhamnosus* 10 billion cells. Insulin 245 mg. Gluten free. Cap. 30s. *OTC.*
Use: Probiotic.

Culturelle Kids. (Amerifit) *Lactobacillus GG.* **Chew. Tab.:** 2.5 billion cells. Xylitol. Gluten free, sugar free. Berry flavor. 30s. **Pow.:** 1.5 billion cells. Inulin, mannitol. Gluten free. Packets. 30s. *OTC.*
Use: Probiotic.

Culturelle Natural Health and Wellness. (Amerifit) *L. rhamnosus* 10 billion cells. Gluten free. Cap. 30s. *OTC.*
Use: Probiotic.

Culturelle Probiotic for Kids. (Amerifit) *L. rhamnosus GG* 1 billion cells. Mannitol. Gluten free, lactose free, and preservative free. Pow. Packet. 30s. *OTC.*
Use: Probiotic.

Culturette 10 Minute Group A Step ID. (Hoechst) Latex slide agglutination test

for group A streptococcal antigen on throat swabs. Kit 55 determinations.
Use: Diagnostic aid.

•**cupric acetate Cu 64.** (koo-PRIK) USAN.
Use: Radioactive agent.

•**cupric chloride.** (koo-PRIK) *USP.*
Use: Supplement, trace mineral.

•**cupric sulfate.** (koo-PRIK) *USP.*
Use: Antidote to phosphorus.

cupric sulfate. (American Regent) Copper 0.4 mg/mL (as 1.57 mg of sulfate). Inj. Vial 10 mL. *Rx.*
Use: Trace metal.

Cuprid. (Merck & Co.) Trientine hydrochloride 250 mg. Cap. Bot. 100s. *Rx.*
Use: Chelating agent.

Cuprimine. (Aton Pharma) Penicillamine 250 mg. Cap. 100s. *Rx.*
Use: Chelating agent.

•**cuprimyxin.** (KUH-prih-mix-in) USAN.
Use: Antifungal.

Cupri-Pak. (SoloPak Pharmaceuticals, Inc.) Copper. **0.4 mg/mL:** Vial 10 mL, 30 mL. **2 mg/mL:** Vial 5 mL. *Rx.*
Use: Nutritional supplement, parenteral.

curare.
Use: Muscle relaxant.

curare antagonist.
See: Neostigine Methylsulfate.
Tensilon.

Curel. (Bausch & Lomb) Glycerin, petrolatum, dimethicone, parabens. Lot. 180, 300, 390 mL. Cream. Tube. 90 g. *Rx-OTC.*
Use: Emollient.

Curity Sponge Sticks. (Kendall) Iodine 1%. Latex free. Stick, topical. 2s. *OTC.*
Use: Topical anti-infective, antiseptic and germicide.

Curity Wet Skin Scrub Pack. (Kendall) Iodine 0.75% to 1%. Latex free. Soln. Kit w/2 large winged rib sponges, 2 sponge sticks, wrap, gloves, applicators, and towels. *OTC.*
Use: Topical anti-infective, antiseptic and germicide.

Curosurf. (Cornerstone Biopharma) Poractant alfa (porcine origin). Phospholipids 80 mg/mL (including phosphatidylcholine 54 mg, of which 30.5 mg is dipalmitoyl phosphatidylcholine and 1 mg of protein, including 0.3 mg of SP-B), preservative free. Intratracheal Susp. Single-use vials. 1.5 mL, 3 mL. *Rx.*
Use: Lung surfactant; respiratory distress syndrome.

curral.
See: Diallyl Barbituric Acid.

Cutar Emulsion. (Summers) LCD 7.5% (coal tar 1.5%) in mineral oil, lanolin alcohols extract, parabens. Liq. 177 mL, 1 gal. *OTC.*
Use: Dermatologic.

Cutemol Emollient. (Summers) Allantoin 0.2%, liquid petrolatum, acetylated lanolin, lanolin alcohols extract, isopropyl myristate, water. Cream. Jar 2 oz. *OTC.*
Use: Emollient.

Cutivate. (Pharmaderm) Fluticasone propionate. **Cream:** 0.05%. Jar 15 g, 30 g, 60 g. **Lot.:** 0.05%. Cetostearyl alcohol, parabens. 60 mL. **Oint.:** 0.005%. Jar 15 g, 30 g, 60 g. *Rx.*
Use: Corticosteroid, topical.

Cutter Insect Repellent. (Bayer Consumer Care) N,N-Diethyl-meta-toluamide 28.5%, other isomers 1.5%. Vial 1 oz; Foam, Can 2 oz; Spray 7 oz, Aerosol can 14 oz; Assortment Pack; First Aid Kits, Trial Pack, 6s; Marine Pack 3s; Camp Pack 4s; Pocket Pack, Travel Pack. *OTC.*
Use: Insect repellent.

Cuvposa. (Merz Pharmaceuticals) Glycopyrrolate 1 mg per 5 mL. Glycerin, parabens, propylene glycol, saccharin, sorbitol. Cherry flavor. Soln. 473 mL. *Rx.*
Use: Gastrointestinal anticholinergic/antispasmodic, quaternary anticholinergic.

C vitamin.
See: Ascorbic Acid.

CY 1899. (Cytel Corp.)
Use: Antiviral, hepatitis B. [Orphan Drug]

CY 1503. (Cytel Corp.)
Use: Antithromboembolic. [Orphan Drug]

Cyanide Antidote Package. (Various Mfr.) 2 amp. (300 mg/10 mL) sodium nitrite; 2 vials (12.5 g/50 mL), sodium thiosulfate; 12 amps amyl nitrite inhalant 5 minim/0.3 mL, disposable syringes, stomach tube, tourniquet, and instructions. *Rx.*
Use: Antidote, cyanide poisoning.

Cyanocob. (Paddock) Vitamin B_{12} 1000 mcg/mL. Bot. 1000 mL, Vial 10 mL. *Rx.*
Use: Vitamin supplement.

•**cyanocobalamin.** (sigh-an-oh-koe-BAL-uh-min) *USP. Formerly Vitamin B_{12}.*
Use: Water-soluble vitamin, hematopoietic.
See: B-12.
B-12 Dots.
B-12-SL.
CaloMist.
Nascobal.
Rapid B-12 Energy.
Twelve Resin-K.
Vitamin B_{12}.

W/Combinations.
See: Folgard.
FOLTX.

•**cyanocobalamin Co 58.** (sigh-an-oh-koe-BAL-uh-min) *USP.*
Use: Diagnostic aid, pernicious anemia; radioactive agent.

•**cyanocobalamin Co 57.** (sigh-an-oh-koe-BAL-uh-min) *USP.*
Use: Diagnostic aid, pernicious anemia; radioactive agent.

•**cyanocobalamin Co 60.** (sigh-an-oh-koe-BAL-uh-min) *USP.*
Use: Diagnostic aid, pernicious anemia; radioactive agent.

cyanocobalamin crystalline. *Rx-OTC.*
Use: Vitamin B_{12} supplement.
See: Cyomin.
Vitamin B_{12}.

Cyanokit. (King Pharma) Hydroxocobalamin 25 mg/mL (after reconstitution). Inj., lyophilized Pow. for Soln. 5 g kit. In two 250-mL colorless glass vials (2.5 g per vial), 2 sterile transfer spikes, 1 sterile IV infusion set. *Rx.*
Use: Detoxification agent, antidote.

Cyanover. (Research Supplies) Cyanocobalamin 100 mcg, liver injection 10 mcg, folic acid 10 mg/mL. *Lyo-layer* vial 10 mL with vial of diluent 10 mL. *Rx.*
Use: Mineral, vitamin supplement.

•**cyclacillin.** (SIGH-klah-SILL-in) *USP.*
Use: Anti-infective.

Cyclafem 1/35. (Qualitest Pharmaceuticals) Ethinyl estradiol 35 mcg, norethindrone 1 mg. Film coated. Lactose, PEG. Tab. 28s w/7 inert tablets (film coated, lactose, PEG). *Rx.*
Use: Monophasic oral contraceptive.

Cyclafem 7/7/7. (Qualitest Pharmaceuticals) **Phase 1:** Ethinyl estradiol 35 mcg, norethindrone 0.5 mg. **Phase 2:** Ethinyl estradiol 35 mcg, norethindrone 0.75 mg. **Phase 3:** Ethinyl estradiol 35 mcg, norethindrone 1 mg.Film coated. Lactose. Tab. 28s w/7 inert tablets. *Rx.*
Use: Triphasic oral contraceptive.

cyclamate sodium. Cyclohexanesulfamate dihydrate salt.

•**cyclamic acid.** (sigh-KLAM-ik) USAN.
Use: Sweetener, nonnutritive.

•**cyclazocine.** (SIGH-CLAY-zoe-seen) USAN. Under study.
Use: Analgesic.

Cyclessa. (Organon) **Phase 1:** Desogestrel 0.1 mg, ethinyl estradiol 25 mcg. 7 tabs. **Phase 2:** Desogestrel 0.125 mg, ethinyl estradiol 25 mcg. 7 tabs. **Phase 3:** Desogestrel 0.15 mg, ethinyl estradiol 25 mcg. 7 tabs. Lactose, talc. Tab. 28s with 7 inert tabs. *Rx.*
Use: Sex hormone, contraceptive hormone.

•**cyclindole.** (sigh-KLIN-dole) USAN.
Use: Antidepressant.

Cyclinex-1. (Ross) Protein 7.5 g (from carnitine, cystine, histidine, isoleucine, leucine, lysine, methionine, phenylalanine, taurine, threonine, tryptophan, tyrosine, valine), fat 27 g (from palm oil, hydrogenated coconut oil, soy oil), carbohydrate 52 g (from hydrolyzed corn starch), linoleic acid 2000 mg, Fe 10 mg, Na 215 mg, K 760 mg, Ca, vitamins A, B_1, B_2, B_3, B_5, B_6, B_{12}, C, D, E, K, biotin, choline, folic acid, inositol, Cl, Cu, I, Mg, Mn, P, Se, Zn and 515 Cal per 100 g. Nonessential amino acid free. Pow. Can 350 g. *OTC.*
Use: Nutritional supplement.

Cyclinex-2. (Ross) Protein 15 g (from carnitine, cystine, histidine, isoleucine, leucine, lysine, methionine, phenylalanine, taurine, threonine, tryptophan, tyrosine, valine), fat 20.7 g (from palm oil, hydrogenated coconut oil, soy oil), carbohydrate 40 g (from hydrolyzed cornstarch), Fe 17 mg, Na 1175 mg, K 1830 mg, Ca, vitamins A, B_1, B_2, B_3, B_5, B_6, B_{12}, C, D, E, K, biotin, choline, folic acid, inositol, Cl, Cu, I, Mg, Mn, P, Se, Zn and 480 Cal per 100 g. Nonessential amino acid free. Pow. Can 325 g. *OTC.*
Use: Nutritional supplement.

•**cycliramine maleate.** (SIGH-klih-rah-meen) USAN.
Use: Antihistamine.

Cyclivert. (Laser) Cyclizine 25 mg (as hydrochloride). Tab. 100s. *OTC.*
Use: Antiemetic/antivertigo agent, anticholinergic.

•**cyclizine.** (SIGH-klih-zeen) *USP.*
Use: Antihistamine.

•**cyclizine hydrochloride.** (SIGH-klih-zeen) *USP.*
Use: Antiemetic.
See: Bonine for Kids.
Cyclivert.
Marezine.

•**cyclizine lactate injection.** (SIGH-klih-zeen LACK-tate) *USP.*
Use: Antihistamine; antinauseant.

cyclobarbital.
Use: Central depressant.

cyclobarbital calcium.
Use: Hypnotic; sedative.

•**cyclobendazole.** (SIGH-kloe-BEN-dah-zole) USAN.
Use: Anthelmintic.

•**cyclobenzaprine hydrochloride.** (SIGH-kloe-BEN-zuh-preen) *USP.*
Use: Muscle relaxant.
See: Amrix.
Fexmid.

cyclobenzaprine hydrochloride. (Mylan) Cyclobenzaprine hydrochloride 15 mg, 30 mg. PEG, sugar spheres. ER Cap. 60s, 500s. *Rx.*
Use: Skeletal muscle relaxant, centrally acting.

cyclobenzaprine hydrochloride. (Various Mfr.) Cyclobenzaprine hydrochloride 5 mg, 10 mg. May contain lactose. Tab. Bot. 30s, 100s, 500s, 1000s, UD 30s (5 mg only). *Rx.*
Use: Muscle relaxant.

cyclobenzaprine hydrochloride. (Watson) Cyclobenzaprine hydrochloride 7.5 mg. Tab. 30s, 100s, 1000s. *Rx.*
Use: Muscle relaxant.

cyclocumarol.
Use: Anticoagulant.

•**cyclofilcon A.** (SIGH-kloe-FILL-kahn A) USAN.
Use: Contact lens material, hydrophilic.

Cyclogen. (Schwarz Pharma) Dicyclomine hydrochloride 10 mg, sodium chloride 0.9%, chlorobutanol hydrate 0.5%. Vial 10 mL, Box 12s. *Rx.*
Use: Antispasmodic.

•**cycloguanil pamoate.** (SIGH-kloe-GWAHN-ill PAM-oh-ate) USAN.
Use: Antimalarial.

Cyclogyl. (Alcon) Cyclopentolate hydrochloride 0.5%, 1%, 2%. Soln. *Droptainer* 2 mL, 5 mL, 15 mL. *Rx.*
Use: Cycloplegic; mydriatic.

•**cycloheximide.** (sigh-KLOE-HEX-ih-mid) USAN.
Use: Antipsoriatic.

•**cyclomethicone.** (sigh-kloe-METH-ih-cone) *NF.*
Use: Pharmaceutic aid, wetting agent.

cyclomethycaine and methapyrilene.
Use: Anesthetic, local.

cyclomethycaine sulfate.
Use: Anesthetic, local.

Cyclomydril. (Alcon) Phenylephrine hydrochloride 1%, cyclopentolate hydrochloride 0.2%. Droptainer 2 mL, 5 mL. *Rx.*
Use: Mydriatic.

Cyclonil. (Seatrace) Dicyclomine hydrochloride 10 mg/mL. Vial 10 mL. *Rx.*
Use: Anticholinergic; antispasmodic.

Cyclopar. (Parke-Davis) Tetracycline hydrochloride. Cap. **250 mg:** Bot. 100s, 1000s. **500 mg:** Bot. 100s, UD 100s. *Rx.*
Use: Anti-infective, tetracycline.

•**cyclopentamine hydrochloride.** (SIGH-kloe-PEN-teh-meen) *USP.*
Use: Adrenergic, vasoconstrictor.

•**cyclopenthiazide.** (SIGH-kloe-pen-THIGH-ah-zide) USAN.
Use: Antihypertensive; diuretic.

•**cyclopentolate hydrochloride.** (sigh-kloe-PEN-toe-tate) *USP.*
Use: Anticholinergic, ophthalmic.
See: AK-Pentolate.
Cyclogyl.
W/Phenylephrine Hydrochloride.
See: Cyclomydril.

cyclopentolate hydrochloride. (Various Mfr.) Cyclopentolate hydrochloride 1%, 2%. Benzalkonium chloride, EDTA, boric acid. Soln.; Ophth. 2 mL, 5 mL, 15 mL. *Rx.*
Use: Anticholinergic, ophthalmic.

8 cyclopentyl 1,3-dipropylxanthine. (SciClone)
Use: Cystic fibrosis. [Orphan Drug]

cyclopentylpropionate.
See: Depo-Testosterone.

•**cyclophenazine hydrochloride.** (SIGH-kloe-FEH-nazz-een) USAN.
Use: Antipsychotic.

•**cyclophosphamide.** (sigh-kloe-FOSS-fuh-mide) *USP.*
Use: Antineoplastic, immunosuppressant; alkylating agent; nitrogen mustard.
See: Cytoxan.

cyclophosphamide. (Baxter) Cyclophosphamide (as monohydrate) 500 mg, 1 g, 2 g. Inj., Pow. for Soln. Single-dose vial. *Rx.*
Use: Alkylating agent, nitrogen mustard.

cyclophosphamide. (Roxanne) Cyclophosphamide 25 mg, 50 mg. Lactose. Tab. 100s. *Rx.*
Use: Alkylating agent, nitrogen mustard.

cyclophosphamide. (Various Mfr.) Cyclophosphamide 25 mg, 50 mg. Cap. 100s. *Rx.*
Use: Alkylating agent, nitrogen mustard.

cycloplegic mydriatics.
See: Atropine Sulfate.
Tropicamide.

•**cyclopropane.** (sigh-kloe-PRO-pane) *USP.*
Use: Anesthetic, general.

•**cycloserine.** (sigh-kloe-SER-een) *USP.*
Tall Man: cycloSERINE
Use: Antituberculosis agent.

cycloserine. *Formerly Seromycin Pulvules.* (Various Mfr.) Cycloserine

250 mg. Cap. UD 30s.
Use: Antituberculosis agent.

l-cycloserine.
Use: Treat Gaucher disease. [Orphan Drug]

Cycloset. (Santarus) Bromocriptine mesylate 0.8 mg. Lactose. Tab. Unit of use. 200s, 600s. *Rx.*
Use: Antiparkinson agent.

cyclosporin A.
Use: Immunosuppressant.
See: Cyclosporine.

•**cyclosporine.** (SIGH-kloe-spore-EEN) *USP. Formerly Cyclosporin A.*
Tall Man: cycloSPORINE
Use: Immunosuppressant.
See: Gengraf.
Neoral.
Sandimmune.

cyclosporine. (Apotex) Cyclosporine 25 mg, 100 mg. May contain alcohol. Cap. 30s. *Rx.*
Use: Immunologic agent, immunosuppressive.

cyclosporine injection. (Bedford Labs) Cyclosporine 50 mg/mL. Inj. Amp. 5 mL. *Rx.*
Use: Immunosuppressant.

cyclosporine modified. (Ivax) Cyclosporine 50 mg. Sorbitol. Soft. Gel. Cap. UD 30s. *Rx.*
Use: Immunologic agent.

cyclosporine modified. (Various Mfr.) Cyclosporine. **Soft gelatin Cap.:** 25 mg, 100 mg. May contain alcohol. UD 30s. **Oral Soln.:** 100 mg/mL. May contain alcohol. 50 mL. *Rx.*
Use: Immunosuppressant.

cyclosporine ophthalmic.
Use: Severe keratoconjunctivitis sicca; graft rejection following keratoplasty. [Orphan Drug]

cyclosporine ophthalmic emulsion.
Use: Immunologic agent.
See: Restasis.

cyclosporine 2% ophthalmic ointment. (Allergan)
Use: Treatment of graft rejection after keratoplasty and corneal melting syndromes. [Orphan Drug]

•**cyclothiazide.** (SIGH-kloe-thigh-AZZ-ide) USAN.
Use: Antihypertensive; diuretic.

Cycofed. (Cypress) Codeine phosphate 20 mg, pseudoephedrine hydrochloride 60 mg per 5 mL. Spearmint flavor. Syr. Bot. 473 mL. *c-III.*
Use: Upper respiratory combination, antitussive, decongestant.

Cycofed Pediatric. (Cypress) Codeine phosphate 10 mg, pseudoephedrine hydrochloride 30 mg, guaifenesin 100 mg/5 mL, alcohol 6%. Syrup. Bot. 480 mL. *c-v.*
Use: Antitussive, decongestant, expectorant.

Cydec Oral. (Cypress) Pseudoephedrine hydrochloride 25 mg, carbinoxamine maleate 2 mg/mL, raspberry flavor. Drops. Bot. 30 mL. *Rx.*
Use: Upper respiratory combination, decongestant, antihistamine.

•**cyheptamide.** (sigh-HEP-tah-mid) USAN.
Use: Anticonvulsant.

Cyklokapron. (Pfizer) Tranexamic acid. Inj. 100 mg/mL. Amp. 10 mL. *Rx.*
Use: Hemostatic.

Cylex Sugar Free. (Pharmakon) Benzocaine 15 mg, cetylpyridinium chloride 5 mg, sorbitol. Loz. Pkg. 12s. *OTC.*
Use: Antiseptic; analgesic, topical.

Cylex Throat. (Pharmakon) Benzocaine 15 mg, cetylpyridinium chloride 5 mg, sorbitol. Loz. Pkg. 12s. *OTC.*
Use: Antiseptic; analgesic, topical.

Cymbalta. (Eli Lilly) Duloxetine 20 mg, 30 mg, 60 mg. Sucrose, sugar spheres. Enteric-coated pellets. DR Cap. 30s (except 20 mg), 60s (20 mg only), 90s (except 20 mg), 1,000s (except 20 mg), UD 30s (60 mg only), UD 100s (except 20 mg). *Rx.*
Use: Antidepressant.

Cynobal. (Arcum) Cyanocobalamin 10 mcg, 1000 mcg/mL. Inj. Vial 10 mL (1000 mcg only), 30 mL. *Rx.*
Use: Vitamin supplement.

•**cypenamine hydrochloride.** (sigh-PEN-ah-meen) USAN.
Use: Antidepressant.

•**cyprazepam.** (sigh-PRAY-zeh-pam) USAN.
Use: Hypnotic; sedative.

•**cyproheptadine.** (sip-row-HEP-tuh-deen) *USP.*
Use: Antihistamine, nonselective piperidine; antipruritic.

cyproheptadine. (Various Mfr.) Cyproheptadine. **Tab.:** 4 mg. Bot. 100s, 1,000s, UD 100s. **Syr.:** 2 mg/5 mL. May contain alcohol. Bot. 473 mL. *Rx.*
Use: Antihistamine, nonselective piperidine; antipruritic.

•**cyprolidol hydrochloride.** (sigh-PRO-lih-dahl) USAN.
Use: Antidepressant.

•**cyproterone acetate.** (sigh-PRO-ter-ohn) USAN.
Use: Antiandrogen.

•**cyproximide.** (sigh-PROX-ih-MIDE) USAN.
Use: Antidepressant; antipsychotic.

Cyramza. (Eli Lilly) Ramucirumab 10 mg/mL. Glycine, polysorbate 80, sodium chloride. Preservative free. Inj., Soln. Single-dose vial. 10 mL, 50 mL. *Rx.*
Use: Antineoplastic, monoclonal antibody.

Cyren A.
See: Diethylstilbestrol.

Cyronine. (Major) Liothyronine sodium 25 mcg. Tab. Bot. 100s. *Rx.*
Use: Hormone, thyroid.

Cystadane. (Rare Disease Therapeutics) Betaine anhydrous 1 g/1.7 mL. Pow. for Inj. Bot. 180 g. *Rx.*
Use: Treatment of homocystinuria.

Cystagon. (Mylan) Cysteamine bitartrate 50 mg, 150 mg. Cap. Bot. 100s, 500s. *Rx.*
Use: Urinary tract agent.

Cystamin.
See: Methenamine.

Cystamine. (Tennessee Pharmaceutic) Methenamine 2 g, phenyl salicylate 0.5 g, phenazopyridine hydrochloride 10 mg, benzoic acid ⅛ g, hyoscyamine sulfate g, atropine sulfate g. SC Tab. Bot. 100s, 1000s. *Rx.*
Use: Anti-infective, urinary.

Cystaran. (Sigma-Tau Pharmaceuticals) Cysteamine 0.44% (equiv. to cysteamine hydrochloride 6.5 mg/mL). Benzalkonium chloride. Soln.; Ophth. 15 mL. *Rx.*
Use: Cystine-depleting agent.

•**cysteamine.** (sis-TEE-ah-MEEN) USAN.
Use: Antiurolithic, cystine calculi; nephropathic cystinosis. [Orphan Drug]
See: Cystaran.
Procysbi.

•**cysteamine hydrochloride.** (sis-TEE-ah-MEEN) USAN.
Use: Antiurolithic, cystine calculi; nephropathic cystinosis.
See: Cystagon.

Cystex. (Numark) Methenamine 162 mg, sodium salicylate 162.5 mg, benzoic acid 32 mg. Tab. Bot. 40s, 100s. *OTC.*
Use: Anti-infective, urinary.

cystic fibrosis gene therapy. (Genzyme)
Use: Cystic fibrosis. [Orphan Drug]

cystic fibrosis TR gene therapy (recombinant adenovirus). (Gerac)
Use: Cystic fibrosis. [Orphan Drug]
See: AdGVCFTR 10.

•**cystine.** (SIS-TEEN) USAN.
Use: Amino acid replacement therapy, an additive for infants on TPN.

cystine-depleting agents.
See: Cysteamine.

Cysto. (Freeport) Methenamine 40.8 mg, methylene blue 5.4 mg, phenyl salicylate 18.1 mg, atropine sulfate 0.03 mg, hyoscyamine 0.03 mg, benzoic acid 4.5 mg. Tab. Bot. 1000s. *Rx.*
Use: Anti-infective, urinary.

Cystografin. (Bracco Diagnostics) Diatrizoate meglumine 300 mg, iodine 141 mg/mL. EDTA. Inj. Bot. 100 mL in 200 mL, 300 mL fill in 400 mL. *Rx.*
Use: Radiopaque agent.

Cystografin Dilute. (Bracco Diagnostics) Diatrizoate meglumine 180 mg, iodine 85 mg/mL. EDTA. Inj. Bot. 300 mL w/or without administration sets. *Rx.*
Use: Radiopaque agent.

Cysview. (GE Healthcare Inc) Hexaminolevulinate hydrochloride 100 mg (equiv. to hexaminolevulinate base 85 mg). Pow. for Soln.; intravesical. Kit w/100 mg vial, diluents (50 mg vial), and 1 *Luer-Lock* catheter adapter. *Rx.*
Use: In vivo diagnostic aid.

•**cytarabine.** (SIGH-tar-ah-bean) *USP.*
Use: Antineoplastic; antiviral.
See: DepoCyt.
Tarabine PFS.

cytarabine. (Various Mfr.) Cytarabine. **Inj.:** 20 mg/mL, 100 mg/mL. 5 mL single- and multidose vials (w/0.9% benzyl alcohol) and preservative-free 50 mL flip-top vial (pharmacy bulk package) (20 mg/mL); 20 mL single-dose vial (100 mg/mL). **Pow. for Inj.:** 100 mg, 500 mg, 1 g, 2 g. Vial. *Rx.*
Use: Antineoplastic, antimetabolite, pyrimidine analog.

•**cytarabine hydrochloride.** (SITE-ah-rah-been) USAN. *Formerly Cytosine Arabinoside Hydrochloride.*
Use: Antiviral management of acute leukemias.
See: Cytosar-U.

Cyto B2. (Solace Nutrition) Riboflavin 343 mg per 1 g. Pow. 100 g. *OTC.*
Use: Water-soluble vitamin.

CytoGam. (CSL Behring) Cytomegalovirus immune globulin IV (human) 50 ± 10 mg/mL. Sucrose 5%, human albumin 1%, preservative free, solvent/detergent treated. Soln. for Inj. Vial 20 mL, 50 mL. *Rx.*
Use: Antiviral, cytomegalovirus; immune globulin.

cytomegalovirus immune globulin (human) intravenous.
Use: Immune globulin.
See: CytoGam.

cytomegalovirus immune globulin intravenous (human). (Bayer)
Use: With ganciclovir sodium for the treatment of CMV pneumonia in bone

marrow transplant patients. [Orphan Drug]

Cytomel. (Monarch) Liothyronine sodium 5 mcg, 25 mcg, 50 mcg, sucrose. Tab. Bot. 100s. *Rx.*
Use: Hormone, thyroid.

cytoprotective agents.
See: Allopurinol sodium.
Amifostine.
Dexrazoxane.
Mesna.

cytosine arabinoside hydrochloride. Cytarabine hydrochloride.

Cytosol. (Cytosol) Calcium chloride 48 mg, magnesium chloride 30 mg, potassium chloride 75 mg, sodium acetate 390 mg, sodium chloride 640 mg, sodium citrate 170 mg/100 mL. Soln. Bot. 200 mL, 500 mL. *Rx.*
Use: Irrigant.

Cytotec. (Pfizer) Misoprostol 100 mcg, 200 mcg. Tab. Bot. UD 100s, unit-of-use 60s, 100s (200 mcg only), 120s (100 mg only). *Rx.*
Use: Prostaglandins, antiulcerative.

Cytovene. (Roche) Ganciclovir 500 mg, sodium 46 mg. Inj. (as sodium). Pow, lyophilized. Vial. 10 mL. *Rx.*
Use: Antiviral.

Cytox. (MPL) Cyanocobalamin 500 mcg, vitamins B_6 20 mg, B_1 100 mg, benzyl alcohol 2% in isotonic solution of sodium chloride/mL. Inj. Vial 10 mL. *Rx.*
Use: Vitamin supplement.

Cytra-K. (Cypress) Potassium citrate monohydrate/citric acid monohydrate. **Soln.:** 1,100 mg/334 mg per 5 mL. Parabens, PEG, propylene glycol, sorbitol, sucralose. Each mL contains potassium ion 2 mEq and is equiv. to bicarbonate 2 mEq. Cherry flavor. 473 mL. **Pow. for Soln.:** 3,300 mg/1,002 mg per packet. Saccharin. Sugar free. Fruit punch flavor. UD packets. *Rx.*
Use: Alkalinizer, systemic.

Cytra-3. (Cypress) Potassium citrate monohydrate 550 mg, sodium citrate dihydrate 500 mg, citric acid monohydrate 334 mg/5 mL. PEG, propylene glycol, saccharin, sodium benzoate, sorbitol. Each mL contains potassium ion 1 mEq and is equiv. to bicarbonate 2 mEq. Alcohol free and sugar free. Raspberry flavor. Soln. 473 mL. *Rx.*
Use: Alkalinizer, systemic.

Cytra-2. (Cypress) Sodium citrate dihydrate 500 mg, citric acid monohydrate 334 mg/5 mL. PEG, propylene glycol, saccharin, sodium benzoate, sorbitol. Each mL contains sodium ion 1 mEq and is equiv. to bicarbonate 1 mEq. Sugar free. Grape flavor. Soln. 473 mL. *Rx.*
Use: Alkalinizer, systemic.

D

DAA.
See: Dihydroxy Aluminum Aminoacetate.

DAB_{389} IL-2. (Seragen)
Use: Cutaneous T-cell lymphoma. [Orphan Drug]

•**dabigatran.** (da-bye-GAT-ran) USAN.
Use: Deep vein thrombosis; stroke prevention.

•**dabigatran etexilate.** (da-bye-GAT-ran ee-TEKS-i-late) USAN.
Use: Deep vein thrombosis; stroke prevention.
See: Pradaxa.

•**dabigatran etexilate mesylate.** (da-bye-GAT-ran ee-TEKS-i-late) USAN.
Use: Deep vein thrombosis; stroke prevention.

•**dabrafenib.** (da-BRAF-e-nib) USAN.
Use: Antineoplastic.
See: Tafinlar.

•**dabrafenib mesylate.** (da-BRAF-e-nib) USAN.
Use: Antineoplastic.

•**dabuzalgron hydrochloride.** (da-bue-ZAL-gron) USAN.
Use: Urinary agent.

•**dacarbazine.** (da-CAR-buh-zeen) *USP.*
Use: Antineoplastic.
See: DTIC-Dome.

dacarbazine. (Various Mfr.) Dacarbazine 100 mg, 200 mg. May contain mannitol. Pow. for Inj. Vials. *Rx.*
Use: Alkylating agent, antineoplastic.

Dacex-A. (Cypress) Phenylephrine hydrochloride 2 mg, carbinoxamine maleate 1 mg, dextromethorphan HBr 2 mg per 1 mL. Sugar and alcohol free. Saccharin, sorbitol. Cherry flavor. Oral Drops. Bot. 30 mL with calibrated dropper. *Rx.*
Use: Pediatric antitussive.

Dacex-DM. (Cypress) Dextromethorphan HBr 25 mg, guaifenesin 175 mg, phenylephrine hydrochloride 12.5 mg per 5 mL. Alcohol and sugar free. Saccharin, sorbitol. Strawberry flavor. Syrup. 473 mL. *Rx.*
Use: Upper respiratory combination, antitussive and expectorant combination.

Dacex-PE. (Cypress) Dextromethorphan HBr 30 mg, guaifenesin 600 mg, phenylephrine hydrochloride 10 mg. Sugar, gluten, and dye free. ER Tab. 100s. *Rx.*
Use: Antitussive and expectorant combination, upper respiratory combination.

•**daclatasvir.** (dak-LAT-as-vir) USAN.
Use: Treatment of hepatitis C.

•**daclatasvir dihydrochloride.** (dak-LAT-as-vir) USAN.
Use: Treatment of hepatitis C.

•**daclizumab.** (dac-KLYE-zue-mab) USAN.
Use: Immunosuppressant.

Dacodyl. (Major) **Tab.:** Bisacodyl 5 mg. Bot. 100s, 250s, 1000s. UD 100s. **Supp.:** Bisacodyl 10 mg. Box 12s, 100s. *OTC.*
Use: Laxative.

Dacogen. (Eisai) Decitabine 50 mg. Pow. for Inj., lyophilized. Single-dose vials. *Rx.*
Use: Antineoplastic; DNA demethylation agent.

•**dacomitinib.** (DAK-oh-MI-ti-nib) USAN.
Use: Antineoplastic.

•**dactinomycin.** (DAK-tih-no-MY-sin) *USP.*
Tall Man: DACTINomycin
Use: Antineoplastic; antibiotic.
See: Cosmegen.

dactinomycin. (Bedford Labs) Dactinomycin 500 mcg. Mannitol 20 mg. Inj., lyophilized Pow. for Soln. Single-dose vial. *Rx.*
Use: Antineoplastic antibiotic.

•**dactolisib.** (DAK-toe-LIS-ib) USAN.
Use: Antineoplastic.

•**dactolisib tosylate.** (DAK-toe-LIS-ib) USAN.
Use: Antineoplastic.

Daily Betic. (Optimum) Vitamin A (as beta carotene) 2,500 units, C 60 mg, D 200 units, E 30 units, B_1 1.5 mg, B_2 1.7 mg, B_3 20 mg, B_5 10 mg, B_6 2.5 mg, B_{12} 5 mcg, folic acid 200 mcg, biotin 75 mcg, lutein 250 mcg, alpha-lipoic acid 50 mg, Ca, Cr, I, K, Mg, Mn, Se, V, Zn. PEG. Tab. 60s. *OTC.*
Use: Multivitamin with minerals (except iron).

Daily Cleaner. (Bausch & Lomb) Isotonic solution with sodium Cl, sodium phosphate, tyloxapol, hydroxyethylcellulose, polyvinyl alcohol with thimerosal 0.004%, EDTA 0.2%. Soln. Bot. 45 mL. *OTC.*
Use: Contact lens care.

Daily Conditioning Treatment. (Blairex) Padimate O 7.5%, oxybenzone 3.5%, petrolatum. Stick 11.4 g. SPF 15. *OTC.*
Use: Lip protectant.

Daily Vitamins. (Rugby) Vitamins A 2500 units, D 400 units, E 15 units, C 60 mg, B_1 1.2 mg, B_2 1.2 mg, B_6 1.05 mg, B_{12} 4.5 mcg, niacinamide 13.5 mg/5 mL. Bot. 273 mL, 473 mL. *OTC.*
Use: Vitamin supplement.

Daily Vitamins Tablets. (Kirkman) Vitamins A 5000 units, D 400 units, C 50 mg, B_1 3 mg, B_2 2.5 mg, B_6 1 mg, B_{12} 1 mcg, niacinamide 20 mg, d-calcium pantothenate 1 mg. Tab. Bot. 100s. *OTC.*
Use: Vitamin supplement.

Daily Vitamins w/Iron. (Kirkman) Vitamins A 5000 units, D 400 units, B_1 2 mg, B_2 2.5 mg, B_6 1 mg, B_{12} 1 mcg, niacinamide 20 mg, d-calcium pantothenate 1 mg, iron 18 mg. Tab. Bot. 100s. *OTC.*
Use: Vitamin supplement.

Daily-Vite. (Rugby) Vitamins A 5,000 units, C 60 mg, D 400 units, E 30 units, B_1 1.5 mg, B_2 1.7 mg, B_3 20 mg, B_5 10 mg, B_6 2 mg, B_{12} 6 mcg, folic acid 400 mcg, Fe 18 mg. Dextrose, glyceryl, PEG, sucrose, soy. Tab. 100s, 1,000s. *OTC.*
Use: Multivitamin.

Daily-Vite w/Iron & Minerals. (Rugby) Iron 18 mg, vitamins A 5000 units, D 400 units, E 30 mg, B_1 1.5 mg, B_2 1.7 mg, B_3 20 mg, B_5 10 mg, B_6 2 mg, B_{12} 6 mcg, C 60 mg, folic acid 0.4 mg, Ca, Cl, Cr, Cu, I, K, Mg, Mn, Mo, P, Se, zinc 15 mg, biotin, vitamin K. Tab. Bot. 100s. *OTC.*
Use: Mineral, vitamin supplement.

Dairy Ease. (Blistex) Lactase 3300 FCC units, mannitol, sucrose. Tab. Bot. 60s, 100s. *OTC.*
Use: Digestive enzyme.

Dakin's Solution.
See: Sodium Hypochlorite Solution.

Dakin's Solution Full Strength. (Century) Sodium hypochlorite 0.5%. Soln. Bot. Pt, gal. *OTC.*
Use: Anti-infective, topical.

Dakin's Solution Half Strength. (Century) Sodium hypochlorite 0.25%. Soln. Bot. Pt. *OTC.*
Use: Anti-infective, topical.

•**dalantercept.** (dal-ANT-ar-sept) USAN.
Use: Antineoplastic.

d-ala-peptide T.
Use: Antiviral.

•**dalbavancin.** (dal-ba-VAN-sin) USAN.
Use: Investigational antibiotic.

•**daledalin tosylate.** (dah-LEH-dah-lin TAH-sill-ate) USAN.
Use: Antidepressant.

•**dalfampridine.** (dal-FAM-pri-deen) USAN.
Use: Potassium channel blocker.
See: Ampyra.

•**dalfopristin.** (dal-FOE-priss-tin) USAN.
Use: Anti-infective.
W/Quinupristin.
See: Synercid.

Daliresp. (Forest Pharmaceuticals) Roflumilast 500 mcg. Lactose. Tab. 30s, 90s. *Rx.*
Use: Selective phosphodiesterase 4 inhibitor.

Dallergy. (Laser) **Tab.:** Chlorcyclizine hydrochloride 25 mg, phenylephrine hydrochloride 10 mg. 100s. **Chew. Tab.:** Chlorcyclizine hydrochloride 12.5 mg, phenylephrine hydrochloride 5 mg. Mannitol, xylitol. Grape flavor. 100s. **Oral Drops:** Phenylephrine hydrochloride 2 mg, chlorpheniramine maleate 1 mg per 1 mL. Glycerin, propylene glycol, saccharin, sorbitol. Alcohol free and sugar free. Peach flavor. 30 mL with dropper. **Syrup:** Chlorcyclizine hydrochloride 12.5 mg, phenylephrine hydrochloride 5 mg per 5 mL. Glycerin, propylene glycol, sorbitol, sucralose. Grape flavor. 473 mL. *OTC.*
Use: Upper respiratory combination, decongestant and antihistamine.

Dallergy-D. (Laser) Chlorpheniramine maleate 2 mg, phenylephrine hydrochloride 5 mg/5 mL. Bot. 118 mL. *OTC.*
Use: Antihistamine, decongestant.

•**dalotuzumab.** (DAL-oh-TOOZ-oo-mab) USAN.
Use: Antineoplastic.

d'Alpha E 1000 Softgels. (Naturally) Vitamin E (as d-alpha tocopherol) 1000 IU. Cap. 30s, 60s. *OTC.*
Use: Vitamin supplement.

•**dalteparin sodium.** (dal-TEH-puh-rin) USAN.
Use: Anticoagulant; antithrombotic; low molecular weight heparin.
See: Fragmin.

•**daltroban.** (DAL-troe-ban) USAN.
Use: Platelet aggregation inhibitor; immunosuppressant.

•**dalvastatin.** (DAL-vah-STAT-in) USAN.
Use: Antihyperlipidemic.

Damacet-P. (Mason) Hydrocodone bitartrate 5 mg, acetaminophen 500 mg. Tab. Bot. 100s, 500s. *c-III.*
Use: Analgesic combination; narcotic.

Dambose.
See: Inositol.

Danatrol. (Sanofi-Synthelabo) Danazol. Cap. *Rx.*
Use: Gonadotropin inhibitor.

•**danazol.** (DAN-uh-ZOLE) *USP.*
Use: Anterior pituitary suppressant, sex hormone.

danazol. (Various Mfr.) Danazol 50 mg, 100 mg, 200 mg. Cap. Bot. 60s

(200 mg only), 100s, 500s (200 mg only). *Rx.*
Use: Anterior pituitary suppressant, sex hormone.

Dandruff Shampoo. (Walgreen) Zinc pyrithione 2 g/100 mL. Bot. 11 oz. Tube 7 oz. *OTC.*
Use: Antiseborrheic.

•**danegaptide.** (dan-e-GAP-tide) USAN.
Use: Cardiovascular agent.

•**daniplestim.** (dan-ih-PLEH-stim) USAN.
Use: Antineutropenic; hematopoietic stimulant; treatment of chemotherapy-induced bone marrow suppression.

•**danirixin.** (DAN-i-RIX-in) USAN.
Use: Treatment of chronic obstructive pulmonary disease.

Danogar Tablets. (Sanofi-Synthelabo) Danazol. *Rx.*
Use: Gonadotropin inhibitor.

Danol Capsules. (Sanofi-Synthelabo) Danazol. *Rx.*
Use: Gonadotropin inhibitor.

•**danoprevir.** (dan-OH-pre-vir) USAN.
Use: Treatment of hepatitis C.

•**danoprevir sodium.** (dan-OH-pre-vir) USAN.
Use: Treatment of hepatitis C.

Dantrium. (Procter & Gamble) Dantrolene sodium. Cap. **25 mg:** Bot. 100s, 500s, UD 100s; **50 mg:** Bot. 100s; **100 mg:** Bot. 100s, UD 100s. *Rx.*
Use: Muscle relaxant.

Dantrium IV. (Procter & Gamble) Dantrolene sodium 20 mg. Vial. 70 mL. *Rx.*
Use: Muscle relaxant.

•**dantrolene.** (dan-troe-LEEN) USAN.
Use: Muscle relaxant.

•**dantrolene sodium.** (dan-troe-LEEN) USAN.
Use: Muscle relaxant.
See: Dantrium.
Revonto.

dantrolene sodium. (Actavis Totowa) Dantrolene sodium 25 mg, 50 mg, 100 mg. Lactose. Cap. 100s, 500s, UD 100s. *Rx.*
Use: Direct acting skeletal muscle relaxants.

Dapa Extra Strength Tablets. (Ferndale) Acetaminophen 500 mg. Bot. 50s, 100s, 1000s, UD 100s. *OTC.*
Use: Analgesic.

•**dapagliflozin.** (dap-A-gli-FLOE-zin) USAN.
Use: Investigational antidiabetic agent.
See: Farxiga.

Dapco. (Schlicksup) Salicylamide 300 mg, butabarbital 15 mg. Tab. Bot. 100s, 1000s. *C-III.*
Use: Analgesic; hypnotic; sedative.

•**dapiclermin.** (DA-pi-kler-min) USAN.
Use: Dietary aid.

•**dapiprazole hydrochloride.** (DAP-ih-PRAY-zole) USAN.
Use: Alpha-adrenergic blocker; antiglaucoma agent; neuroleptic; psychotherapeutic agent.

•**dapoxetine hydrochloride.** (dap-OX-eh-teen) USAN.
Use: Antidepressant.

•**dapsone.** (DAP-sone) *USP. Formerly Diaminodiphenylsulfone.*
Use: Leprostatic; topical anti-infective.
See: Aczone.

dapsone. (Jacobus) Dapsone 25 mg, 100 mg. Tab. Bot. 100s. *Rx.*
Use: Leprostatic.

Daptacel. (Aventis Pasteur) Diphtheria toxoid 15 Lf, tetanus toxoid 5 Lf, pertussis toxoid 10 mcg, hemagglutinin 5 mcg, pertactin 3 mcg, fimbriae types 2 and 3 5 mcg/0.5 mL. Formaldehyde, phenoxyethanol. Inj. Single-dose vials. *Rx.*
Use: Immunization.

•**daptomycin.** (DAP-toe-MY-sin) USAN.
Tall Man: DAPTOmycin
Use: Anti-infective.
See: Cubicin.

Daragen. (Galderma) Collagen polypeptide, benzalkonium Cl in a mild amphoteric base. Shampoo. Bot. 8 oz. *OTC.*
Use: Dermatologic.

•**darapladib.** (dar-AP-la-dib) USAN.
Use: Lp-PLA2 inhibitor.

Daraprim. (Amedra Pharmaceuticals) Pyrimethamine 25 mg. Lactose. Tab. Bot. 100s. *Rx.*
Use: Antimalarial.

Dara Soapless Shampoo. (Galderma) Purified water, potassium coco hydrolyzed protein, sulfated castor oil, pentasodium triphosphate, sodium benzoate, sodium lauryl sulfate, fragrance. Shampoo. Bot. 8 oz, 16 oz. *OTC.*
Use: Dermatologic, scalp.

•**daratumumab.** (DAR-a-TOOM-ue-mab) USAN.
Use: Antineoplastic.

•**darbepoetin alfa.** (DAR-be-POE-e-tin) USAN.
Use: Hematopoietic agent, recombinant human erythropoietin.
See: Aranesp.

•**darbufelone mesylate.** (DAR-byoo-feh-lone) USAN.
Use: Anti-inflammatory; antiarthritic.

Darco G-60. (AstraZeneca) Activated carbon from lignite.
Use: Purifier.

•**darglitazone sodium.** (dahr-GLIH-tah-zone) USAN.
Use: Oral hypoglycemic.
•**darifenacin.** (dare-ee-FEN-a-sin) USAN.
Use: Treatment of overactive bladder.
•**darifenacin hydrobromide.** (dar-ih-FEN-ah-sin)
Use: Treatment of overactive bladder.
See: Enablex.
•**darodipine.** (DA-row-dih-PEEN) USAN.
Use: Antihypertensive; bronchodilator; vasodilator.
•**darunavir.** (dar-UE-na-vir) USAN.
Use: Antiretroviral.
darunavir ethanolate.
Use: Antiretroviral.
See: Prezista.
•**dasantafil.** (da-SAN-ta-fil) USAN.
Use: Erectile dysfunction.
•**dasatinib.** (da-SA-ti-nib) USAN.
Use: Protein-tyrosine kinase inhibitor; treatment of leukemia.
See: Sprycel.
Da-Sed. (Sheryl) Butabarbital 0.5 g. Tab. Bot. 100s. *c-III.*
Use: Hypnotic; sedative.
Dasetta 1/35. (Northstar Rx) Ethinyl estradiol 35 mcg, norethindrone 1 mg. Lactose. Tab. 28s w/7 inert tablets (lactose). *Rx.*
Use: Monophasic oral contraceptive.
Dasetta 7/7/7. (Northstar Rx) **Phase 1:** Ethinyl estradiol 35 mcg, norethindrone 0.5 mg. **Phase 2:** Ethinyl estradiol 35 mcg, norethindrone 0.75 mg. **Phase 3:** Ethinyl estradiol 35 mcg, norethindrone 1 mg.Lactose. Tab. 28s w/7 inert tablets. *Rx.*
Use: Triphasic oral contraceptive.
Dasin. (GlaxoSmithKline) Ipecac 3 mg, acetylsalicylic acid 130 mg, camphor 15 mg, caffeine 8 mg, atropine sulfate 0.13 mg. Cap. Bot. 100s, 500s. *Rx.*
Use: Analgesic; anticholinergic; antispasmodic.
•**dasiprotimut-T.** (DAS-i-PROE-ti-mut tee) USAN.
Use: Antineoplastic.
•**dasolampanel.** (DA-soe-LAM-pa-nel) USAN.
Use: Analgesic.
•**dasolampanel etibutil.** (DA-soe-LAM-pa-nel E-ti-BUE-til) USAN.
Use: Analgesic.
•**dasolampanel etibutil tosylate.** (DA-soe-LAM-pa-nel E-ti-BUE-til TOS-i-late) USAN.
Use: Analgesic.
DaTscan. (GE Healthcare) Ioflupane I 123 74 MBq (2 mCi) per mL at calibration (each mL contains ioflupane 0.07 to 0.13 mcg, acetic acid 5.7 mg, sodium acetate 7.8 mg, and ethanol 0.05 mL [5%]). Preservative free. Inj., Soln. Single-use vial. 2.5 mL. *c-II.*
Use: In vivo diagnostic aid.
daturine hydrobromide.
See: Hyoscyamine Salts.
daunorubicin citrate liposomal.
Use: Antibiotic.
See: DaunoXome.
daunorubicin citrate liposome.
Use: Treatment of advanced HIV-associated Kaposi sarcoma. [Orphan Drug]
See: DaunoXome.
•**daunorubicin hydrochloride.** (DAW-no-RUE-bih-sin) *USP.*
Tall Man: DAUNOrubicin
Use: Antineoplastic.
See: Cerubidine
daunorubicin hydrochloride. (Various Mfr.) Daunorubicin hydrochloride 20 mg, 50 mg, mannitol 100 mg (20 mg), 250 mg (50 mg). Pow. for Inj., lyophilized. Single-dose vial 10 mL (20 mg only), 20 mL (50 mg only). *Rx.*
Use: Antineoplastic.
daunorubicin hydrochloride for injection. (Various Mfr.) Daunorubicin hydrochloride for Injection 5 mg/mL (equivalent to 5.34 mg daunorubicin hydrochloride), preservative free. Single-use vial. 4 mL, 10 mL. *Rx.*
Use: Antibiotic.
DaunoXome. (Galen) Daunorubicin citrate liposomal 2 mg/mL (equivalent to daunorubicin base 50 mg). Inj. Single-use vials and single-unit packs. *Rx.*
Use: Antibiotic; treatment of advanced HIV-associated Kaposi sarcoma.
•**davalintide.** (DA-va-LIN-tide) USAN.
Use: Treatment of obesity.
•**davalintide acetate.** (DA-va-LIN-tide) USAN.
Use: Treatment of obesity.
Davosil. (Colgate Oral) Silicon carbide in glycerin base. Jar 8 oz, 10 oz. *OTC.*
Use: Agent for oral hygiene.
•**davunetide.** (dav-u-NE-tide) USAN.
Use: Alzheimer disease.
Dayalets + Iron. (Abbott) Vitamins B_1 1.5 mg, B_2 1.7 mg, B_6 2 mg, B_{12} 6 mcg, C 60 mg, A 5000 units, D 400 units, E 30 units, iron 18 mg, folic acid 0.4 mg, niacinamide 20 mg. Filmtab. Bot. 100s. *OTC.*
Use: Mineral, vitamin supplement.
Daycare. (Procter & Gamble) Pseudoephedrine hydrochloride 10 mg, dex-

tromethorphan HBr 3.3 mg, guaifenesin 33.3 mg, acetaminophen 108 mg. Alcohol 10%, saccharin. Expectorant Liq. Bot. 180 mL, 300 mL. *OTC.*
Use: Analgesic, antitussive, decongestant, expectorant.

Dayhist-1. (Major) Clemastine fumarate 1.34 mg (equivalent to clemastine 1 mg). Lactose. Tab. Pkg. 8s. *OTC.*
Use: Antihistamine, nonselective ethanolamine.

Daypro. (Searle) Oxaprozin 600 mg. Film-coated. Capl. Bot. 100s, 500s, UD 100s. *Rx.*
Use: Nonsteroidal anti-inflammatory agent.

Daypro ALTA. (Pharmacia) Oxaprozin potassium 678 mg (equivalent to 600 mg oxaprozin). Film-coated. Tab. Bot. 100s, 500s, UD 100s. *Rx.*
Use: Nonsteroidal anti-inflammatory agent.

DayQuil.
See: Vicks DayQuil.

Daysee. (Lupin Pharmaceuticals)
Phase 1: Ethinyl estradiol 30 mcg, levonorgestrel 0.15 mg. Film coated. Lactose, PEG. Tab. 84s. **Phase 2:** Ethinyl estradiol 10 mcg. Film coated. Lactose, PEG. Tab. 7s. *Rx.*
Use: Biphasic oral contraceptive.

Day Tab. (Towne) Vitamins A 5000 units, D 400 units, B_1 15 mg, B_2 10 mg, B_6 5 mg, B_{12} 5 mcg, folic acid 400 mcg, pantothenic acid 10 mg, zinc 15 mg, copper 2 mg, C 600 mg, niacinamide 20 mg. Tab. Bot. 100s, 200s. *OTC.*
Use: Mineral, vitamin supplement.

Day Tab Essential. (Towne) Vitamins A 5000 units, D 400 units, E 15 units, C 60 mg, folic acid 0.4 mg, B_1 1.5 mg, B_2 1.7 mg, B_6 2 mg, B_{12} 6 mcg, niacin 20 mg. Tab. Bot. 200s. *OTC.*
Use: Vitamin supplement.

Day Tab Plus Iron. (Towne) Iron 18 mg, vitamins A 5000 units, D 400 units, B_1 1.5 mg, B_2 1.7 mg, B_6 2 mg, B_{12} 6 mcg, pantothenic acid 10 mg, folic acid 0.1 mg, niacinamide 20 mg, C 60 mg. Tab. Bot. 100s. *OTC.*
Use: Mineral, vitamin supplement.

Day Tabs, New. (Towne) Vitamins A 5000 units, E 15 units, D 400 units, C 60 mg, folic acid 0.4 mg, B_1 1.5 mg, B_2 1.7 mg, B_6 20 mg, B_{12} 6 mcg, niacin 20 mg. Tab. Bot. 100s, 250s. *OTC.*
Use: Vitamin supplement.

Day Tabs Plus Iron, New. (Towne) Vitamins A 5000 units, E 15 units, D 400 units, C 60 mg, folic acid 0.4 mg, B_1 1.5 mg, B_2 1.7 mg, B_6 20 mg, B_{12} 6 mcg, niacin 20 mg, iron 18 mcg. Tab. Bot. 250s. *OTC.*
Use: Mineral, vitamin supplement.

Day Tab Stress Complex. (Towne) Vitamins A 5000 units, C 600 mg, B_1 15 mg, B_2 10 mg, B_6 5 mg, B_{12} 6 mcg, niacin 100 mg, D 400 units, E 30 units, folic acid 400 mcg, pantothenic acid 20 mg, iron 18 mg, zinc 15 mg, copper 2 mg. Tab. Bot. 60s. *OTC.*
Use: Mineral, vitamin supplement.

Day Tab with Iron. (Towne) Vitamins A 5000 units, D 400 units, E 15 units, C 60 mg, folic acid 1.5 mg, B_1 15 mg, B_2 1.7 mg, B_6 2 mg, B_{12} 6 mcg, niacin 20 mg, iron 18 mg. Tab. Bot. 200s. *Rx.*
Use: Mineral, vitamin supplement.

Daytime Sinus Relief Non-Drowsy Maximum Strength. (Akyma) Pseudoephedrine hydrochloride 30 mg, acetaminophen 500 mg. Tab. 24s. *OTC.*
Use: Decongestant and analgesic.

Dayto-Anase. (Dayton) Bromelains 50,000 units (protease activity). Tab. Bot. 60s. *OTC.*
Use: Enzyme.

Dayto Himbin. (Dayton) Yohimbine 5.4 mg. Tab. Bot. 60s. *Rx.*
Use: Alpha-adrenergic blocker.

Daytrana. (Noven Therapeutics) Methylphenidate 10 mg per 9 h (1.1 mg/h; 27.5 mg of total methylphenidate/patch; 12.5 cm^2), 15 mg per 9 h (1.6 mg/h; 41.3 mg of total methylphenidate/patch; 18.75 cm^2), 20 mg per 9 h (2.2 mg/h; 55 mg of total methylphenidate/patch; 25 cm^2), 30 mg per 9 h (3.3 mg/h; 82.5 mg of total methylphenidate/patch; 37.5^2). Patch; transdermal. 30s. *c-II.*
Use: Central nervous system stimulant.

•**dazadrol maleate.** (DAY-zah-drole) USAN.
Use: Antidepressant.

•**dazepinil hydrochloride.** (dahz-EH-pih-NILL) USAN.
Use: Antidepressant.

•**dazmegrel.** (DAZE-meh-grell) USAN.
Use: Inhibitor (thromboxane synthetase).

•**dazopride fumarate.** (DAY-zoe-PRIDE) USAN.
Use: Peristaltic stimulant.

•**dazoxiben hydrochloride.** (DAZE-OX-ih-ben) USAN.
Use: Antithrombotic.

Dbed. Dibenzylethylenediamine dipenicillin G.
Use: Anti-infective; penicillin.

DB Electrode Paste. (Day-Baldwin) Tube 5%.

DCA.
See: Desoxycorticosterone Acetate.
DCF.
Use: Anti-infective.
See: Nipent.
DCP. (Towne) Calcium 180 mg, phosphorus 105 mg, vitamins D 66.7 units. Tab. Bot. 100s. *OTC.*
Use: Mineral, vitamin supplement.
DC Softgels. (Ivax) Docusate calcium 240 mg. Softgel Cap. Bot. 100s, 500s. *OTC.*
Use: Laxative.
DC 240. (Ivax) Docusate calcium 240 mg. Cap. Bot. 100s, 500s. *OTC.*
Use: Laxative.
DDAVP. (Sanofi-Aventis) Desmopressin acetate. **Tab.:** 0.1 mg, 0.2 mg, lactose. 100s. **Spray Soln., Intranasal:** 0.1 mg/mL. 5 mL (50 sprays of 10 mcg). Rhinal tube delivery system. 2.5 mL w/2 applicator tubes. **Inj.:** 4 mcg/mL. Single-dose amp. 1 mL, multidose vial 10 mL. *Rx.*
Use: Posterior pituitary hormone.
ddI. Didanosine.
Use: Antiviral.
Ddrops. (J.R. Carlson Labs) Vitamin D_3 (cholecalciferol) 1,000 units per 0.03 mL, 2,000 units per 0.03 mL. Gluten free, preservative free, and sugar free. Drops. 11 mL. *OTC.*
Use: Fat-soluble vitamin.
DDS.
See: Dapsone.
DDT.
See: Chlorophenothane.
deacetyllanatoside C.
See: Deslanoside.
deadly nightshade leaf.
See: Belladonna Leaf.
1-deamino-8-d-arginine vasopressin.
Desmopressin acetate.
Use: Hormone.
See: Concentraid.
DDAVP.
deba.
See: Barbital.
Debacterol. (Epien Medical) Sulfuric acid 30%, sulfonated phenolics 50%. Liq. 1.5 mL *Rx.*
Use: Mouth and throat product.
•**debrisoquin sulfate.** (deb-RICE-oh-kwin) USAN.
Use: Antihypertensive.
Debrox. (GlaxoSmithKline) Carbamide peroxide 6.5%, glycerin, propylene glycol, sodium stannate. Drops. 30 mL with dropper. *OTC.*
Use: Otic preparation.
Deca-Bon. (Barrows) Vitamins A 3000 units, D 400 units, C 60 mg, B_1 1 mg, B_2 1.2 mg, B_6 1 mg, B_{12} 1 mcg, niacinamide 8 mg, panthenol 3 mg, biotin 30 mcg/0.6 mL. Drops. Bot. 50 mL. *OTC.*
Use: Vitamin supplement.
Decaderm. (Merck & Co.) Dexamethasone 0.1% w/isopropyl myristate gel, wood alcohols, refined lanolin alcohol, microcrystalline wax, anhydrous citric acid, anhydrous sodium phosphate dibasic. Tube 30 g. *Rx.*
Use: Corticosteroid.
Decagen. (Ivax) Iron 18 mg, vitamins A 5000 units, D 400 units, E 30 units, B_1 1.7 mg, B_2 2 mg, B_3 20 mg, B_5 10 mg, B_6 3 mg, B_{12} 6 mcg, C 60 mg, folic acid 0.4 mg, Ca, Cl, Cr, Cu, B, I, K, Mg, Mn, Mo, Ni, P, Se, Si, Sn, V, Zn 15 mg, vitamin K, biotin 30 mcg. Tab. Bot. 130s. *OTC.*
Use: Mineral, vitamin supplement.
Decalix. (Pharmed) Dexamethasone 0.5 mg/5 mL. Bot. 100 mL. *Rx.*
Use: Corticosteroid.
Decapryn. (Hoechst) Doxylamine succinate 12.5 mg. Tab. Bot. 100s. *OTC.*
Use: Antihistamine.
Decara. (Medecor Pharma) Vitamin D_3 25,000 units, 50,000 units. Glycerol, soya oil, vitamin E 14.9 units (50,000 units only). Cap. 50s (50,000 units only), 100s (25,000 units only). *OTC.*
Use: Fat-soluble vitamin.
Decasone Injection. (Forest) Dexamethasone sodium phosphate equivalent to dexamethasone phosphate 4 mg/mL. Vial 5 mL. *Rx.*
Use: Corticosteroid.
Decavac. (Aventis Pasteur) Diphtheria 2 Lf units and tetanus 5 Lf units per 0.5 mL dose. Preservative free. Inj. 0.5 mL *Luer-Lok* syringe (with not more than 0.28 mg of aluminum and trace thimerosal [up to 0.3 mcg mercury/dose]). *Rx.*
Use: Agent for active immunization.
decavitamin. (Various Mfr.) Vitamins A 4000 units, D 400 units, C 70 mg, calcium pantothenate 10 mg, B_1 2 mg, B_2 2 mg, B_6 2 mg, B_{12} 5 mcg, folic acid 100 mcg, nicotinamide 20 mg. Cap. or Tab. *OTC.*
Use: Vitamin supplement.
•**decernotinib.** (DEE-ser-NOE-ti-nib) USAN.
Use: Immunomodulator.
De-Chlor HD. (Cypress) Hydrocodone bitartrate 2.5 mg, chlorpheniramine maleate 4 mg, phenylephrine hydro-

chloride 10 mg per 5 mL. Alcohol and sugar free. Saccharin, sorbitol. Cherry flavor. Liq. 473 mL. *c-III.*
Use: Upper respiratory combination, antitussive combination.
Decholin. (Bayer Consumer Care) Dehydrocholic acid 250 mg. Tab. Bot. 100s, 500s. *OTC.*
Use: Hydrocholeretic.
Decicain. Tetracaine hydrochloride.
•**decitabine.** (deh-SIGH-tah-BEAN) USAN.
Use: Antineoplastic; DNA demethylation agent.
See: Dacogen.
decitabine. (Various Mfr.) Decitabine 50 mg. Inj., lyophilized Pow. for Soln. Single-dose vial. *Rx.*
Use: Antineoplastic, DNA demethylation agent.
declaben. (DEH-klah-BEN) *Formerly Lodelaben.*
Use: Antiarthritic; emphysema therapy adjunct.
Declomycin. (CorePharma) Demeclocycline hydrochloride 150 mg, 300 mg. Tab. Bot. 100s (150 mg only), 48s (300 mg only). *Rx.*
Use: Anti-infective; tetracycline.
Decodult. (Wesley Pharmacal) Phenylephrine hydrochloride 5 mg, chlorpheniramine maleate 2 mg, acetaminophen 300 mg. Tab. Bot. 1000s. *OTC.*
Use: Upper respiratory combination, decongestant, antihistamine, analgesic.
Decohistine DH. (Morton Grove) Pseudoephedrine hydrochloride 30 mg, chlorpheniramine maleate 2 mg, codeine phosphate 10 mg per 5 mL. Alcohol 5.8%, sugar, menthol, parabens, sorbitol, grape/honey flavor. Liq. Bot. 118 mL, 473 mL, 3.8 L. *c-v.*
Use: Upper respiratory combination, antihistamine, antitussive, decongestant.
Decolate. (Wesley) Phenylephrine hydrochloride 5 mg, chlorpheniramine maleate 4 mg, guaifenesin 100 mg. Tab. Bot. 1000s. *Rx.*
Use: Upper respiratory combination, decongestant, antihistamine, expectorant.
Deconamine. (Kenwood) Chlorpheniramine maleate 4 mg, pseudoephedrine hydrochloride 60 mg. Lactose. Tab. 100s. *Rx.*
Use: Upper respiratory combination, antihistamine and decongestant.
Deconex DM. (Poly Pharmaceuticals) Dextromethorphan HBr 30 mg, guaifenesin 900 mg, phenylephrine hydrochloride 30 mg. ER Tab. 100s. *Rx.*
Use: Antitussive and expectorant combination, upper respiratory combination.
Deconex DMX. (Poly Pharmaceuticals) Dextromethorphan HBr 15 mg, guaifenesin 380 mg, phenylephrine hydrochloride 10 mg. Maltodextrin. Cap. 60s. *OTC.*
Use: Upper respiratory combination; antitussive, expectorant, decongestant.
decongestant, analgesic, antihistamine, antitussive combinations.
Use: Upper respiratory combination.
decongestant, analgesic, antihistamine combinations.
Use: Upper respiratory combination.
decongestant, analgesic, antitussive, expectorant combinations.
Use: Upper respiratory combination.
decongestant and analgesic combinations.
Use: Upper respiratory combination.
decongestant and antihistamine combinations.
Use: Upper respiratory combination.
decongestant and expectorant combinations.
Use: Upper respiratory combination.
decongestant, anticholinergic, and antihistamine combinations.
Use: Upper respiratory combination.
decongestant, anticholinergic, antihistamine, and antitussive combinations.
Use: Upper respiratory combination.
decongestant, antihistamine, and analgesic combinations.
Use: Upper respiratory combination.
decongestant, antihistamine, and antitussive combinations.
Use: Upper respiratory combination.
decongestant, antihistamine, and expectorant combinations.
Use: Upper respiratory combination.
decongestant, antihistamine, antitussive, and expectorant combinations.
Use: Upper respiratory combination.
decongestant, antitussive, and expectorant combinations.
Use: Upper respiratory combination.
Decongestant Formula Mediquell. (Parke-Davis) Dextromethorphan HBr 30 mg, pseudoephedrine hydrochloride 60 mg. Square.
Use: Antitussive, decongestant.
decongestant, nasal.
See: Nasal Decongestants.
•**dectaflur.** (DECK-tah-flure) USAN.
Use: Dental caries agent.
Decubitex. (I.C.P. Pharmaceuticals)
Oint.: Biebrich scarlet red sulfonated 0.1%, balsam Peru, castor oil, zinc ox-

ide, starch, sodium propionate, parabens. Jar 15 g, 60 g, 120 g, lb. **Pow.:** Biebrich scarlet red sulfonated 0.1%, starch, zinc oxide, sodium propionate, parabens. Bot. 30 g, UD 1 g. *OTC.*
Use: Antipruritic; dermatologic, wound therapy; emollient.

Deep-Down Pain Relief Rub. (GlaxoSmithKline) Methyl salicylate 15%, menthol 5%, camphor 0.5%. Tube 1.25 oz, 3 oz. *OTC.*
Use: Analgesic, topical.

Deep Strength Musterole. (Schering-Plough) Methyl salicylate 30%, menthol 3%, methyl nicotinate 0.5%. Tube 1.25 oz, 3 oz. *OTC.*
Use: Analgesic, topical.

•**deferasirox.** (de-FER-a-sir-ox) USAN.
Use: Chelating agent.
See: Exjade.

•**deferiprone.** (de-FER-ip-rone) USAN.
Use: Chelating agent.
See: Ferriprox.

•**deferitazole.** (DEE-fer-IT-a-zole) USAN.
Use: Treatment of transfusional iron overload.

•**deferitazole magnesium.** (DEE-fer-IT-a-zole) USAN.
Use: Treatment of transfusional iron overload.

•**deferitrin.** (de-FER-i-trin) USAN.
Use: Chelating agent.

•**deferoxamine.** (DEE-fer-OX-ah-meen) USAN.
Use: Chelating agent (iron).

•**deferoxamine hydrochloride.** (DEE-fer-OX-ah-meen) USAN.
Use: Chelating agent for iron.

•**deferoxamine mesylate.** (DEE-fer-OX-ah-meen) *USP.*
Use: Iron depleter; antidote to iron poisoning; chelating agent.
See: Desferal.

deferoxamine mesylate. (Hospira) Deferoxamine mesylate 500 mg, 2 g. Pow. for Inj., lyophilized. Vials. *Rx.*
Use: Detoxification agent, chelating agent.

defibrotide. (Crinos International)
Use: Thrombotic thrombocytopenic purpura. [Orphan Drug]

Deficol. (Vangard Labs, Inc.) Bisacodyl 5 mg. Tab. Bot. 100s, 1000s. *OTC.*
Use: Laxative.

Definity. (Bristol-Myers Squibb) Octafluoropropane 6.52 mg/mL in lipid-coated microspheres. Preservative free. Inj. Single-use vials. 2 mL. Requires activation with a *Vialmix* (not included). *Rx.*
Use: Radiopaque agent, parenteral agent.

•**deflazacort.** (deh-FLAZE-ah-cart) USAN.
Use: Anti-inflammatory.

•**degarelix.** (DEG-a-REL-ix) USAN.
Use: Antineoplastic.

•**degarelix acetate.** (DEG-a-REL-ix) USAN.
Use: Treatment of prostate cancer.
See: Firmagon.

Dehistine. (Cypress) Phenylephrine hydrochloride 10 mg, chlorpheniramine maleate 2 mg, methscopolamine nitrate 1.25 mg/5 mL. Root beer flavor, alcohol free, sugar free. Syrup. Bot. 473 mL. *Rx.*
Use: Upper respiratory combination, decongestant, antihistamine, anticholinergic.

dehydrated alcohol. (Various Mfr.) Ethyl alcohol ≥ 98%. Preservative free. Inj., Soln. 5 mL vial; 1 mL and 5 mL ampule. *Rx.*
Use: CNS agent.

Dehydrex. (Holles)
Use: Recurrent corneal erosion. [Orphan Drug]

•**dehydrocholate sodium injection.** *USP.*
Use: Relief of liver congestion; diagnosis of cardiac failure.
See: Decholin Sodium.

7-dehydrocholesterol, activated. (Various Mfr.) Vitamin D-3.
Use: Vitamin supplement.
See: Cholecalciferol.

•**dehydrocholic acid.** (dee-HIGH-droe-KOLE-ik) *USP.*
Use: Orally, hydrocholeretic and choleretic.
See: Atrocholin.
Cholan-DH.
Decholin.
W/Bile, Homatropine Methylbromide, Pepsin.
See: Biloric.
W/Desoxycholic Acid.
See: Combichole.
W/Docusate Sodium, Phenolphthalein.
See: Bolax.

dehydrocholin.
Use: Hydrocholeretic.
See: Dehydrocholic Acid.

dehydrodesoxycholic acid.
See: Cholanic Acid.

dehydroepiandrosterone. (Genelabs Technologics, Inc.)
Use: Treatment of systemic lupus erythematosus (SLE). [Orphan Drug]

dehydroepiandrosterone sulfate sodium. (Pharmadigm)
Use: Treat serious burns; accelerate re-epithelialization of donor sites in autologous skin grafting. [Orphan Drug]

DEKA. (Dayton) Dextromethorphan hydrobromide 15 mg, guaifenesin 100 mg, pseudoephedrine hydrochloride 15 mg, dexbrompheniramine maleate 0.5 mg per 5 mL. Saccharin, sucrose, parabens. Grape flavor. Liq. 120 mL. *Rx.*
Use: Antitussive and expectorant.

DEKA Pediatric. (Dayton) Pseudoephedrine hydrochloride 12.5 mg, dextromethorphan hydrobromide 4 mg, guaifenesin 40 mg, dexbrompheniramine maleate 0.5 mg per 1 mL. Alcohol free. EDTA, parabens, saccharin, sucrose. Grape flavor. Drops. 30 mL with calibrated dropper. *Rx.*
Use: Pediatric antitussive and expectorant.

Dekasol. (Seatrace) Dexamethasone phosphate 4 mg/mL. Vial 5 mL, 10 mL. *Rx.*
Use: Corticosteroid.

Dekasol L.A. (Seatrace) Dexamethasone acetate 8 mg/mL. Vial 5 mL. *Rx.*
Use: Corticosteroid.

De-Koff. (Whiteworth Towne) Terpin hydrate w/dextromethorphan. Elix. Bot. 4 oz. *OTC.*
Use: Antitussive, expectorant.

•**delafloxacin.** (DEL-a-FLOX-a-sin) USAN.
Use: Antibacterial.

•**delafloxacin meglumine.** (DEL-a-FLOX-a-sin ME-gloo-meen) USAN.
Use: Antibacterial.

•**delamanid.** (DEL-a-MAN-id) USAN.
Use: Treatment of tuberculosis.

•**delanzomib.** (del-ANZ-oh-mib) USAN.
Use: Antineoplastic.

•**delapril hydrochloride.** (DELL-ah-prill) USAN.
Use: Antihypertensive; angiotensin-converting enzyme inhibitor.

Del Aqua-10. (Del-Ray) Benzoyl peroxide 10%. 42.5 g. *Rx.*
Use: Dermatologic, acne.

Delaquin. (Schlicksup) Hydrocortisone 0.5%, iodoquin 3%. Lot. Bot. 3 oz. *Rx.*
Use: Antifungal; corticosteroid.

Delatestadiol. (Dunhall Pharmaceuticals, Inc.) Testosterone enanthate 90 mg, estradiol valerate 4 mg/mL, chlorobutanol in sesame oil. Amp. 10 mL. *Rx.*
Use: Androgen, estrogen combination.

•**delavirdine mesylate.** (de-la-VIR-deen) USAN.
Use: Antiretroviral, non-nucleoside reverse transcriptase inhibitor.
See: Rescriptor.

Delazinc. (Mericon) Zinc oxide 25%. Mineral oil petrolatum. Oint. 454 g. *OTC.*
Use: Skin protectant.

•**delcasertib.** (DEL-ka-SER-tib) USAN.
Use: Cardiovascular agent.

•**delcasertib acetate.** (DEL-ka-SER-tib) USAN.
Use: Cardiovascular agent.

Delcid. (GlaxoSmithKline) Aluminum hydroxide 600 mg, magnesium hydroxide 665 mg/5 mL. Alcohol 0.3%, saccharin. Bot. 8 oz. *OTC.*
Use: Antacid.

Del-Clens. (Del-Ray) Soapless cleanser. Bot. 8 oz. *OTC.*
Use: Dermatologic, cleanser.

Delco-Lax. (Delco) Bisacodyl 5 mg. Tab. Bot. 1000s. *OTC.*
Use: Laxative.

Delcozine. (Delco) Phendimetrazine tartrate 70 mg. Tab. Bot. 1000s, 5000s. *c-III.*
Use: Anorexiant.

•**deldeprevir.** (del-DE-pre-vir) USAN.
Use: Treatment of hepatitis C.

•**deldeprevir sodium.** (del-DE-pre-vir) USAN.
Use: Treatment of hepatitis C.

•**deleobuvir.** (DEL-e-OH-bue-vir) USAN.
Use: Treatment of hepatitis C.

•**deleobuvir sodium.** (DEL-e-OH-bue-vir) USAN.
Use: Treatment of hepatitis C.

•**delequamine hydrochloride.** (deh-LEH-kwah-meen) USAN.
Use: Anti-impotence agent.

Delestrec. Estradiol 17-undecanoate. *Rx.*
Use: Estrogen.

Delestrogen. (JHP) Estradiol valerate. **10 mg/mL:** In sesame oil, chlorobutanol. Multidose Vial 5 mL. **20 mg/mL, 40 mg/mL:** In castor oil, benzyl benzoate, benzyl alcohol. Multidose Vial 5 mL. *Rx.*
Use: Estrogen, sex hormone.

•**deligoparin sodium.** (de-li-GOE-pa-rin) USAN.
Use: Inflammatory bowel disease.

delinal. Propenzolate hydrochloride.

•**delmadinone acetate.** (del-MAD-ih-nohn ASS-eh-tate) USAN.
Use: Antiandrogen; antiestrogen; hormone, progestin.

•**delmitide acetate.** (DEL-mi-tide) USAN.
Use: Antidiarrheal.

Del-Mycin. (Del-Ray) Erythromycin 2%, ethyl alcohol 66%. Topical Soln. Bot. 60 mL. *Rx.*
Use: Dermatologic, acne.

Delos. (Rochester Pharmaceuticals) Benzoyl peroxide 3.5%. Alcohols, aloe, caprylic/capric triglyceride, edetate disodium, glycerin, parabens, soya ste-

rols. Lot. 45 g. *Rx.*
Use: Topical anti-infective, antibiotic.

•**delparantag.** (del-PAR-an-tag) USAN.
Use: Heparin antagonist.

•**delparantag pentahydrochloride.** (del-PAR-an-tag) USAN.
Use: Heparin antagonist.

Del-Stat. (Del-Ray) Abradant cleaner. Jar. 2 oz. *OTC.*
Use: Dermatologic, acne.

Delsym. (Reckitt Benckiser) Dextromethorphan HBr (as polistirex) 30 mg/5 mL. EDTA, corn syrup, sucrose, parabens. Orange flavor, grape flavor. ER Oral Susp. Bot. 89 mL, 148 mL. *OTC.*
Use: Nonnarcotic antitussive.

Delsym Children's Night Time Cough & Cold. (Reckitt Benckiser) Diphenhydramine hydrochloride 6.25 mg, phenylephrine hydrochloride 2.5 mg per 5 mL. Acesulfame K, edetate disodium, maltitol, propylene glycol, sodium 3 mg per 5 mL, sodium benzoate. Grape flavor. Liq. 118 mL w/dosing cup. *OTC.*
Use: Upper respiratory combination, decongestant and antihistamine.

Delsym Night Time Cough & Cold. (Reckitt Benckiser) Diphenhydramine hydrochloride 6.25 mg, phenylephrine hydrochloride 2.5 mg. Acesulfame K, edetate disodium, maltitol, propylene glycol, sodium 3 mg per 5 mL, sodium benzoate. Grape flavor. Liq. 120 mL w/dosing cup. *OTC.*
Use: Upper respiratory combination, decongestant and antihistamine.

Deltacortone. Prednisone.
Use: Corticosteroid.

Delta-Cortril. Prednisolone.
Use: Corticosteroid.

Delta-D. (Freeda) Cholecalciferol (vitamin D_3) 400 IU. Sugar free. Tab. Bot. 250s, 500s. *OTC.*
Use: Vitamin supplement.

•**deltafilcon A.** (DELL-tah-FILL-kahn A) USAN.
Use: Contact lens material, hydrophilic.

•**deltafilcon B.** (DELL-tah-FILL-kahn B) USAN.
Use: Contact lens material, hydrophilic.

delta-1-cortisone.
Use: Corticosteroid.

delta-1-hydrocortisone.
Use: Corticosteroid.
See: Prednisolone.

•**deltibant.** (DELL-tih-bant) USAN.
Use: Antagonist (bradykinin).

Del-Trac. (Del-Ray) Acne lotion. Bot. 2 oz. *OTC.*
Use: Dermatologic, acne.

•**delucemine hydrochloride.** (de-LOO-se-meen) USAN.
Use: Neuroprotector.

Delysid. Lysergic acid diethylamide.
Use: Potent psychotogenic.

Delzicol. (Warner Chilcott) Mesalamine 400 mg. Lactose, PEG. Cap., delayed release. 180s. *Rx.*
Use: Gastrointestinal agent.

Demadex. (Roche) Torsemide 5 mg, 10 mg, 20 mg, 100 mg. Tab. UD 100s. *Rx.*
Use: Diuretic.

•**demcizumab.** (dem-SIZ-ue-mab) USAN.
Use: Antineoplastic.

•**demeclocycline.** (DEH-meh-kloe-SIGH-kleen) *USP.* Formerly Demethylchlortetracycline.
Use: Anti-infective.
See: Declomycin.

•**demeclocycline hydrochloride.** (DEH-meh-kloe-SIGH-kleen) *USP.*
Use: Anti-infective, tetracycline.
See: Declomycin.

demeclocycline hydrochloride. (Impax) Demeclocycline hydrochloride 150 mg, 300 mg. Lactose. Tab. 48s (300 mg only), 100s, 500s. *Rx.*
Use: Anti-infective.

demeclocycline hydrochloride and nystatin tablets.
Use: Anti-infective.

•**demecycline.** (DEH-meh-SIGH-kleen) USAN.
Use: Anti-infective.

Demerol. (Abbott) Meperidine hydrochloride 25 mg/mL, 50 mg/mL, 75 mg/mL, 100 mg/mL. Inj. Amp (preservative free). 0.5 mL (50 mg only), 1 mL (50 mg and 100 mg only); 1.5 mL and 2 mL (50 mg only). Multidose vial (contains metacresol as preservative) 20 mL (100 mg only), 30 mL (50 mg only). *Carpuject* syringe (preservative free). 1 mL. *c-II.*
Use: Opioid analgesic, narcotic agonist.

Demerol. (Sanofi-Synthelabo) Meperidine hydrochloride. **Syrup:** 50 mg/5 mL. Alcohol free. Glucose, saccharin. Banana flavor. Bot. 473 mL. **Tab.:** 50 mg, 100 mg. Bot. 100s; 500s, UD 25s (50 mg only). *c-II.*
Use: Opioid analgesic.

demethylchlortetracycline hydrochloride.
Use: Anti-infective; tetracycline.
See: Demeclocycline hydrochloride.

•**demoxepam.** (dem-OX-eh-pam) USAN.
Use: Anxiolytic.

Demser. (Aton Pharma) Metyrosine 250 mg. Cap. Bot. 100s. *Rx.*
Use: Antihypertensive.

•**denagliptin tosylate.** (den-a-GLIP-tin) USAN.
Use: Antidiabetic agent.

Denalan Denture Cleanser. (Whitehall-Robins) Sodium percarbonate 30%. Bot. 7 oz., 13 oz. *OTC.*
Use: Agent for oral hygiene.

•**denatonium benzoate.** (DEE-nah-TOE-nee-uhm BEN-zoh-ate) *NF.*
Use: Pharmaceutic aid (flavor, alcohol denaturant).

Denavir. (Prestium Pharma) Penciclovir 10 mg/g. Cream. Tube 2 g. *Rx.*
Use: Cold sores.

Denaze. (Cypress) Phenylephrine hydrochloride 10 mg, chlorpheniramine maleate 4 mg, methscopolamine nitrate 1.25 mg per 5 mL. Saccharin, sorbitol. Sugar, alcohol, and dye free. Blue raspberry flavor. Liq. 473 mL. *Rx.*
Use: Decongestant, antihistamine, and anticholinergic combination, upper respiratory combination.

Dencorub. (Last) Methyl salicylate 20%, menthol 0.75%, camphor 1%, eucalyptus oil 0.5%. Tube 1.25 oz, 2.75 oz. *OTC.*
Use: Analgesic, topical.

Dencorub Analgesic Liquid. (Last) Oleoresin capsicum suspension in aqueous vehicle. Bot. 6 oz. *OTC.*
Use: Analgesic, topical.

Dendracin Neurodendraxcin. (Physicians' Science and Nature) Capsaicin 0.0375%, methyl salicylate 30%, menthol 10%. Aloe gel, benzocaine, borage oil, cetyl alcohol, parabens, PEG 100. Lot. 60 mL. *OTC.*
Use: Topical local anesthetic.

•**denenicokin.** (DEN-en-i-KOE-kin) USAN.
Use: Antineoplastic agent.

•**denibulin hydrochloride.** (den-i-BUE-lin) USAN.
Use: Antineoplastic.

•**denileukin diftitox.** (deh-nih-LOO-kin DIFF-tih-tox) USAN.
Use: Treatment of proliferative malignant diseases and autoimmune diseases expressing interleukin 2 receptors. Biological response modifier; antineoplastic.

•**denofungin.** (DEE-no-FUN-jin) USAN.
Use: Antifungal; antibacterial.

Denorex Dual Force. (Ultimark) Pyrithione zinc 1% (use 5 days/week) and salicylic acid (use 2 days/week). Menthol, methylisothiazolinone, propylene glycol. Shampoo. 200 mL/100 mL dual bottle. *OTC.*
Use: Antiseborrheic combination, antiseborrheic shampoo.

Denorex Everyday Dandruff. (Prestige) Pyrithione zinc 2%. Propylene glycol, menthol. Shampoo. 118 mL, 240 mL. *OTC.*
Use: Dermatologic agent.

Denorex Mountain Fresh. (Prestige) Coal tar solution 9%, menthol 1.5%. Bot. 4 oz, 8 oz. *OTC.*
Use: Antiseborrheic.

Denorex with Conditioners. (Prestige) Coal tar solution 9%, menthol 1.5%. Bot 4 oz, 8 oz. *OTC.*
Use: Antiseborrheic.

•**denosumab.** (den-o-SUE-mab) USAN.
Use: Osteoporosis.
See: Prolia.
Xgeva.

Denquel. (Procter & Gamble) Potassium nitrate 5%, calcium carbonate, glycerin, flavors. Tube 1.6 oz, 3 oz, 4.5 oz. *OTC.*
Use: Dentrifice.

Denta 5000 Plus. (Rising Pharmaceuticals) Sodium fluoride 1.1%, spearmint flavor. Cream. 51 g (2s). *Rx.*
Use: Dental caries agent.

DentaGel. (Rising Pharmaceuticals) Sodium fluoride 1.1%, saccharin, parabens, sorbitol, fresh mint flavor. Gel. 56 g. *Rx.*
Use: Dental caries agent.

Dental Caries Preventive. (Colgate Oral) Fluoride ion 1.2%, alumina abrasive. 2 g Box 200s, Jar 9 oz. *Rx.*
Use: Dental caries agent.

Dentiva. (Nuvora) Eucalyptus oil, menthol, peppermint oil, sucralose, wintergreen oil, xylitol, zinc. Alcohol free and sugar free. Loz. 12s. *OTC.*
Use: Mouth and throat product.

Dent-O-Kain/20. (Geritrex) Benzocaine 20%. Benzyl alcohol, saccharin. Liq. 9 mL. *OTC.*
Use: Mouth and throat product.

Dentrol. (Block Drug) Carboxymethylcellulose, polyethylene oxide homopolymer, peppermint and spearmint in mineral oil base. Bot. 0.9 oz, 1.8 oz. *OTC.*
Use: Denture adhesive.

Dent's Dental Poultice. (C.S. Dent & Co.) Glycerin, mineral oil, polyoxyethylene sorbitan monooleate. Bot. 0.125 oz, 0.25 oz. *OTC.*
Use: Dental poultice.

Dent's Ear Wax Drops. (C.S. Dent & Co.) Glycerin, mineral oil, polyoxyethylene sorbitan monooleate. Bot. 0.125 oz, 0.25 oz. *OTC.*
Use: Otic.

Dent's Extra Strength Toothache Gum. (C.S. Dent & Co.) Benzocaine 20%.

Gum. Box. 1 g. *OTC.*
Use: Anesthetic, local.

Dent's Lotion-Jel. (C.S. Dent & Co.) Benzocaine. Lot./Gel; dental. 6 g. *OTC.*
Use: Anesthetic, local.

Dent's Maximum Strength Toothache Drops. (C.S. Dent & Co.) Benzocaine 20%. Alcohol 74%, eugenol chlorobutanol anhydrous 0.09%. Liq. 3.7 mL. *OTC.*
Use: Anesthetic, local.

Dent's Toothache Drops Treatment. (C.S. Dent & Co.) Alcohol 60%, chlorobutanol anhydrous (chloroform derivative) 0.09%, propylene glycol, eugenol. Bot. 3.75 mL. *OTC.*
Use: Anesthetic, local.

Dent's Toothache Gum. (C.S. Dent & Co.) Benzocaine, eugenol, petrolatum in base of cotton and wax. Box 1.05 g. *OTC.*
Use: Anesthetic, local.

Denture Orajel. (Del) Benzocaine 10%, saccharin. Gel. Tube. 9.45 g. *OTC.*
Use: Anesthetic, local.

Dent-Zel-Ite. (Last) Oral Mucosal Analgesic: Benzocaine 5%, alcohol, glycerin. Bot. 1.875 g. **Temporary Dental Filling:** Sandarac gum, alcohol. Bot. 1 oz. **Toothache Drops:** Eugenol 85% in alcohol. Bot. 1 oz. *OTC.*
Use: Anesthetic, local.

•**denufosol tetrasodium.** (den-ue-FOE-sol) USAN.
Use: Investigational for cystic fibrosis.

denyl sodium.
Use: Anticonvulsant.
See: Diphenylhydantoin Sodium.

deodorizers, systemic. Chlorophyll derivatives (chlorophyllin). *OTC.*
Use: Oral: Control of fecal and urinary odors in colostomy, ileostomy, or incontinence. Topical: Reduce pain and inflammation (wounds, burns, surface ulcers, skin irritation).
See: Chloresium.
Chlorophyll.
Derifil.

2′deoxycoformycin. Pentostatin.
Use: Antibiotic; antineoplastic.
See: Nipent.

deoxynojirimycin. (Pharmacia) Butyl-DNJ. *Rx.*
Use: Antiviral.

Depacon. (AbbVie) Valproate 100 mg/mL. EDTA. Preservative free. Inj., concentrate. Single-dose vials. 5 mL. *Rx.*
Use: Anticonvulsant.

Depakene. (AbbVie) Valproic acid. **Cap.:** 250 mg. Parabens, corn oil. 100s. **Soln.:** 250 mg/5 mL. Glycerin, sorbitol, parabens, sucrose. 473 mL, UD 5 mL. *Rx.*
Use: Anticonvulsant.

Depakote. (AbbVie) Divalproex sodium. **DR Tab.:** 125 mg, 250 mg, 500 mg. Talc. 100s, 500s (except 125 mg). **Sprinkle Cap.:** 125 mg. Coated particles. 100s, UD 100s. *Rx.*
Use: Anticonvulsant.

Depakote ER. (AbbVie) Divalproex sodium 250 mg, 500 mg. Lactose, polydextrose (500 mg only). ER Tab. 60s (250 mg only), 100s, 500s, UD 100s. *Rx.*
Use: Anticonvulsant.

Depa-Syrup. (Alra) Valproic acid syrup 250 mg/5 mL. Bot. 4 oz, 16 oz. *Rx.*
Use: Anticonvulsant.

•**depelestat.** (dep-EL-e-stat) USAN.
Use: Cystic fibrosis.

Depen. (Wallace) Penicillamine 250 mg. Tab. Bot. 100s. *Rx.*
Use: Chelating agent.

depepsen. Amylosulfate sodium.
Use: Digestive aid.

depGynogen. (Forest) Estradiol cypionate in cottonseed oil 5 mg/mL, cottonseed oil, chlorobutanol. Inj. Vial 10 mL. *Rx.*
Use: Estrogen.

Deplin. (Pamlab) Folic acid (as L-methylfolate) 7.5 mg, 15 mg. Gluten free, lactose free, and sugar free. Tab. 30s (7.5 mg only), 90s, 500s (7.5 mg only). *Rx.*
Use: Vitamin.

Deplin 15. (Pamlab) L-methylfolate 15 mg. Glucose, mannitol, sodium caseinate, soy, sunflower oil. Cap. 90s. *Rx.*
Use: Water-soluble vitamin.

Deplin 7.5. (Pamlab) L-methylfolate 7.5 mg. Glucose, mannitol, sodium caseinate, soy, sunflower oil. Cap. 90s. *Rx.*
Use: Water-soluble vitamin.

DepoCyt. (Sigma-Tau) Cytarabine, liposomal 10 mg/mL, preservative free, sodium chloride 0.9%. Inj. Vial. 5 mL. *Rx.*
Use: Antimetabolite.

DepoDur. (EKR Therapeutics) Morphine sulfate 10 mg/mL. ER Liposomal Inj. Single-use vials in cartons of 5. 1 mL, 1.5 mL, 2 mL. *c-II.*
Use: Opioid analgesic.

Depoestra. (Tennessee Pharmaceutic) Estradiol cypionate 5 mg/mL. Vial 10 mL. *Rx.*
Use: Estrogen.

Depo-Estradiol. (Pfizer) Estradiol cypionate 5 mg/mL. Chlorobutanol 5.4 mg, cottonseed oil. Inj. Vial 5 mL. *Rx.*
Use: Estrogen, sex hormone.

DepoGen. (Hyrex) Estradiol cypionate 5 mg/mL, cottonseed oil, chlorobutanol. Inj. Vial 10 mL. *Rx.*
Use: Estrogen.

Depo-Medrol. (Pfizer) Methylprednisolone acetate 20 mg/mL, 40 mg/mL, 80 mg/mL. Polyethylene glycol, myristyl-gamma-picolinium chloride. Inj. Vials. 1 mL (except 20 mg/mL), 5 mL, 10 mL (40 mg/mL only). *Rx.*
Use: Adrenocortical steroid, glucocorticoid.

Depo-Provera. (Pfizer) Medroxyprogesterone acetate 400 mg/mL. PEG. Inj., Susp. Vial. 2.5 mL. *Rx.*
Use: Hormone, progestin.

Depo-Provera Contraceptive Injection. (Pfizer) Medroxyprogesterone acetate 150 mg/mL. Parabens, PEG, polysorbate 80. Inj., Susp. 1 mL vial and prefilled syringe. *Rx.*
Use: Contraceptive.

Depo-Sub Q Provera 104. (Pfizer) Medroxyprogesterone acetate 104 mg per 0.65 mL. Parabens, PEG, polysorbate 80. Inj., Susp. Prefilled single-use syringes. 0.65 mL. *Rx.*
Use: Contraceptive hormone.

Depo-Testadiol. (Pfizer) Testosterone cypionate 50 mg, estradiol cypionate 2 mg/mL, chlorobutanol in cottonseed oil. Inj. (in oil). Vial 10 mL. *Rx.*
Use: Androgen, estrogen combination.

Depo-Testosterone. (Pfizer) Testosterone cypionate. Inj. Soln. **100 mg/mL:** In benzyl alcohol 9.45 mg, cottonseed oil 736 mg. Benzyl benzoate 0.1 mL. Vials. 10 mL. **200 mg/mL:** In benzyl benzoate 0.2 mL, benzyl alcohol 9.45 mg, cottonseed oil 560 mg. Vials. 1 mL, 10 mL. *c-III.*
Use: Sex hormone, androgen.

deprenyl. Selegiline hydrochloride.
See: Eldepryl.

•**depreotide.** (deh-PREE-oh-tide) USAN.
Use: Diagnostic aid.

Deproist Expectorant/Codeine. (Geneva) Pseudoephedrine hydrochloride 30 mg, codeine phosphate 10 mg, guaifenesin 100 mg/5 mL. Bot. 120 mL, 480 mL. *c-V.*
Use: Antitussive, decongestant, expectorant.

•**deprostil.** (deh-PRAHST-ill) USAN.
Use: Antisecretory, gastric.

Dequasine. (Miller Pharmacal Group) L-lysine 20 mg, l-cysteine 50 mg, DL-methionine 150 mg, N-acetyl cysteine 50 mg, vitamin C 200 mg, Ca 40 mg, Cu 1 mg, Fe 5 mg, I 0.015 mg, K 20 mg, Mg 40 mg, Mn 5 mg, Mo 150 mcg, Zn 5 mg. Tab. Bot. 100s. *OTC.*
Use: Amino acid; vitamin, mineral supplement.

•**deracoxib.** (der-ah-KOX-ib) USAN.
Use: Anti-inflammatory; analgesic.

Derifil. (Rystan) Chlorophyllin copper complex 100 mg. Tab. Bot. 30s, 100s, 1000s. *OTC.*
Use: Deodorant, oral.

Dermabase. (Paddock) Mineral oil, petrolatum, cetostearyl alcohol, propylene glycol, sodium lauryl sulfate, isopropyl palmitate, imidazolidinyl urea, methyl- and propylparabens. Cream. Jar 1 lb. *OTC.*
Use: Emollient.

Dermacort. (Solvay) Hydrocortisone. **Cream:** 0.5%, 1% in a water soluble cream of stearyl alcohol, cetyl alcohol, isopropyl palmitate, citric acid, polyoxyethylene 40 stearate, sodium phosphate, propylene glycol, water, benzyl alcohol, buffered to pH 5. 0.5% in 30 g tube, 1% in 1 lb jar. **Lot.:** 1% in lotion base, buffered to pH 5. Paraben free. Bot. 120 mL. *Rx.*
Use: Corticosteroid, topical.

Derma-Cover. (Scrip) Sulfur, salicylic acid, hyamine 10x, isopropyl alcohol 22%, in powder film forming base. Bot. 2 oz. *OTC.*
Use: Keratolytic.

Dermadrox. (Geritrex) Aluminum hydroxide gel, zinc chloride, lanolin, calcium carbonate, vitamin A in a hydrophilic ointment base. Oint. 113 g. *OTC.*
Use: Topical combination.

Derma-Guard. (Greer) Protective adhesive pow. Can w/sifter top, 4 oz. Spray Top Bot. 4 oz, pkg. 1 lb. Rings. Pkg. 5s, 10s. *OTC.*
Use: Dermatologic, protectant.

Dermal Therapy Finger Care. (Bayer) Urea 20%. Beeswax, cetyl alcohol, disodium EDTA, emulsifying wax, parabens, PEG, petrolatum, lactic acid, triethanolamine. Lot. 18 mL. *OTC.*
Use: Emollient.

Dermamycin. (Pfeiffer) **Cream:** Diphenhydramine hydrochloride 2% in a base of parabens, polyethylene glycol monostearate and propylene glycol. Tube 28.35 g. **Spray:** Diphenhydramine hydrochloride 2%, menthol 1%, alcohol, methylparaben. Bot. 60 mL. *OTC.*
Use: Antihistamine, topical.

Dermaneed. (Hanlon) Zirconium oxide 4.5%, calamine 6%, zinc oxide 4%, actamer 0.1% in bland lotionized base. Bot. 4 oz. *OTC.*
Use: Antipruritic, topical.

Derma-Pax. (Recsei) Diphenhydramine hydrochloride 0.5%. Benzyl alcohol. Lot. 118 mL. *OTC.*
Use: Antihistamine, topical; corticosteroid, topical.

Derma-Pax HC. (Recsei) Hydrocortisone 0.5%, pyrilamine maleate 0.2%, pheniramine 0.06%, benzyl alcohol 1%. Liq. Bot. 60 mL, 120 mL, 480 mL. *OTC.*
Use: Antihistamine, topical; corticosteroid, topical.

DermaPhor. (DermaRite) Petrolatum 44%, lanolin alcohol, mineral oil, paraffin wax. Oint. 228 g. *OTC.*
Use: Emollient.

Dermarest. (Del) Diphenhydramine hydrochloride 2%, resorcinol 2%, aloe vera gel, benzalkonium chloride, EDTA, menthol, methylparaben, propylene glycol. Gel. Tube 29.25 g, 56.25 g. *OTC.*
Use: Antihistamine, topical.

Dermarest Dricort. (Del) Hydrocortisone 1%, white petrolatum. Cream. Bot. 14 g. *OTC.*
Use: Corticosteroid, topical.

Dermarest Plus. (Del) **Gel:** Diphenhydramine hydrochloride 2%, menthol 1%, aloe vera gel, benzalkonium chloride, isopropyl alcohol, methylparaben, propylene glycol. Tube 15 g, 30 g. **Spray:** Diphenhydramine hydrochloride 2%, menthol 1%, aloe vera gel, benzalkonium chloride, methylparaben propylene glycol, SDA 40 alcohol, EDTA. Bot. 60 mL. *OTC.*
Use: Antihistamine, topical.

Dermasil. (Chesebrough-Ponds USA) Glycerin and dimethicone in a base containing cyclomethicone, sunflower oil, petrolatum, borage oil, lecithin, vitamin E acetate, vitamin A palmitate, vitamin D_3, corn oil, EDTA, methylparaben. Lot. Bot. 120 mL, 240 mL. *OTC.*
Use: Emollient.

Derma-Smoothe/FS Oil. (Hill Dermaceuticals) Fluocinolone acetonide 0.01%. Oil. Bot. 4 oz. *Rx.*
Use: Antipsoriatic; antiseborrheic, topical.

Derma-Smoothe Oil. (Hill Dermaceuticals) Refined peanut oil, mineral oil in lipophilic base. *OTC.*
Use: Antipruritic; dermatologic, protectant.

Derma Soap. (Ferndale) Dowicil 0.1%. 4 oz w/dispenser. *OTC.*
Use: Antiseptic.

Derma-Soft. (Vogarell) Salicylic acid, castor oil, triethanolamine. Medicated cream. Tube 3/4 oz. *OTC.*
Use: Keratolytic.

Derma-Sone 1%. (Hill Dermaceuticals) Hydrocortisone 1%, pramoxine hydrochloride 1%, cetyl alcohol, glyceryl monostearate, isopropyl myristate, potassium sorbate, furcelleran. *Rx-OTC.*
Use: Anesthetic; corticosteroid, local.

Dermasorb AF. (Crown Laboratories) Clioquinol 3%/hydrocortisone 0.5%. Alcohols, glycerin, polysorbate 80. Cream. 30 g kits w/120 mL of *Dermsorb* hydrating serum (urea, propylene glycol, glycolic acid, PEG). *Rx.*
Use: Topical corticosteroid, corticosteroid and antifungal combination.

Dermasorb HC. (Crown Laboratories) Hydrocortisone 2%. Isopropyl alcohol, propylene glycol. Lot. 29.6 mL and in kits w/*Dermasorb* shampoo and body wash (glycerin, menthol, parabens, propylene glycol, urea). 240 mL. *Rx.*
Use: Anti-inflammatory agent, topical corticosteroid.

Dermasorb TA. (Crown Laboratories) Triamcinolone acetonide 0.1%. Mineral oil, propylene glycol, wax. Cream. 85.2 g and in kits w/*Dermasorb Barrier Repair Emollient* (alcohols, glycerin, milk lipids, mineral oil, petrolatum). 180 g. *Rx.*
Use: Anti-inflammatory agent, topical corticosteroid.

Dermasorb XM. (Crown Laboratories) Urea 39%. Glycerin, wax. Cream. 227 g and kits w/*Dermasorb Extreme* moisturizer (227 g). *Rx.*
Use: Emollient.

Dermasorcin. (Lamond) Resorcin 2%, sulfur 5%. Bot. 1 oz, 2 oz, 4 oz, 8 oz, pt, 32 oz, 0.5 gal. *OTC.*
Use: Dermatologic, acne; antiseborrheic, topical.

Dermastringe. (Lamond) Bot. 4 oz, 6 oz, 8 oz, pt, 32 oz, gal. *OTC.*
Use: Dermatologic, cleanser.

Dermasul. (Lamond) Sulfur 5%. Bot. 1 oz, 2 oz, 4 oz, 8 oz, pt, 32 oz, 0.5 gal, gal. *OTC.*
Use: Dermatologic, acne; antiseborrheic, topical.

Dermathyn. (Davis & Sly) Benzyl alcohol 3%, benzocaine 3.5%, butyl-p-aminobenzoate 1%, phenylmercuric borate. Tube 1 oz. *OTC.*
Use: Anesthetic, local.

Dermatic Base. (Whorton Pharmaceuticals, Inc.) Compounding cream base. Bot. 16 oz.
Use: Pharmaceutical aid, emollient base.

Dermatol.
See: Bismuth Subgallate.

dermatologic alpha-adrenergic agonists.
See: Brimonidine Tartrate.

Dermatop. (Valeant) Prednicarbate 0.1%. **Cream:** White petrolatum, lanolin alcohols, mineral oil, cetostearyl alcohol, EDTA, lactic acid. Tube. 15 g, 60 g. **Oint.:** Glycerin. Tube. 15 g, 60 g. *Rx.*
Use: Corticosteroid, topical.

DermaVite. (GlaxoSmithKline) Vitamin A 3500 units (29% as beta carotene), E 60 units, B_2 8.5 mg, B_6 10 mg, C 120 mg, folate 400 mcg, Zn 45 mg, biotin 600 mcg, lycopene 5 mg, Ca, Cr, Cu, Mn, Se, Si, sucrose. Tab. Bot. 60s. *OTC.*
Use: Vitamin, mineral supplement.

DermaZinc. (Dermalogix) Pyrithione zinc. **Cream:** 0.25%. Aloe vera, cetyl alcohol, dimethicone, lanolin, methylparaben, mineral oil, PEG-75. 114 g. **Shampoo:** 2%. Alcohol, menthol, methylparaben. 240 mL. *OTC.*
Use: Emollient.

Dermazine. (Dermalogix) Pyrithione zinc 0.25%. Parabens. Shampoo. 240 mL. *OTC.*
Use: Dermatologic agent.

Dermed. (Holloway) Vitamins A and D with hydrogenated vegetable oil. Cream. Tube 60 g, 120 g. *OTC.*
Use: Emollient.

Dermeze. (Premo) Thenylpyramine hydrochloride 2%, benzocaine 2%, tyrothricin 0.25 mg/g. Massage Lot. Bot. 5¾ oz. *OTC.*
Use: Anesthetic; antihistamine; anti-infective.

Dermolate Anti-Itch. (Schering-Plough) Hydrocortisone 0.5% petrolatum, mineral oil, chlorocresol. Cream. Tube 15 g, 30 g. *OTC.*
Use: Corticosteroid, topical.

Dermol HC. (Dermol Pharmaceuticals, Inc.) **Cream:** Hydrocortisone 1%, 2.5%. Tube 30 g. **Oint.:** Hydrocortisone 1%. Tube 30 g. *Rx.*
Use: Anorectal preparation.

Dermolin. (Roberts) Menthol racemic, methyl salicylate, camphor, mustard oil, isopropyl alcohol 8%. Bot. 3 oz, pt, gal. *OTC.*
Use: Liniment.

Dermoplast. (Prestige) Benzocaine. **Lot.:** 8%. Aloe, glycerin, lanolin, menthol 0.5%, parabens. 90 mL. **Spray:** 20%. Aloe, lanolin, menthol 0.5%, methylparaben. 59 mL. *OTC.*
Use: Topical local anesthetic, ester local anesthetic.

Dermoplast Antibacterial. (Medtech) Benzocaine 20%. Benzethonium chloride 0.2%, menthol, methylparaben, aloe, lanolin. Spray. 59 mL. *OTC.*
Use: Topical local anesthetic, ester local anesthetic.

DermOtic. (Hill Dermaceuticals) Fluocinolone acetonide oil 0.01%. Otic Drops. 20 mL. *Rx.*
Use: Otic preparation.

Dermovan. (Galderma) Glyceryl stearate, spermaceti, mineral oil, glycerin, cetyl alcohol, butylparaben, methylparaben, propylparaben, purified water. Vanishing-type base, Jar 1 lb. *OTC.*
Use: Dermatologic, protectant.

Dermtex HC. (Pfeiffer) Hydrocortisone 0.5% in a glycerin base. Tube 15 g. *OTC.*
Use: Corticosteroid, topical.

Dermuspray. (Warner Chilcott) Trypsin 0.1 mg, balsam Peru 72.5 mg, castor oil 650 mg/0.82 mL. Aer. Bot. 120 g. *Rx.*
Use: Enzyme, topical.

DES.
See: Diethylstilbestrol.

desacchromin. A nonprotein bacterial colloidal dispersion of polysaccharide.

•**desciclovir.** (DESS-sigh-kloe-veer) USAN.
Use: Antiviral.

•**descinolone acetonide.** (DESS-SIN-ole-ohn ah-SEE-toe-nide) USAN.
Use: Corticosteroid, topical.

Desenex. (Novartis) Clotrimazole 1%. Benzyl alcohol 1%, cetostearyl alcohol. Cream. Tube. 15 g, 30 g. *OTC.*
Use: Antifungal, topical.

Desenex. (Novartis) Miconazole nitrate 2%. **Aer.:** 133 g. **Aer. Pow.:** Alcohol, aloe. 113 g. **Pow.:** Alcohol, aloe vera, talc. 85 g. *OTC.*
Use: Topical anti-infective, antifungal agent.

Desenex Foot & Sneaker Spray. (Novartis) Aluminum chlorohydrex w/alcohol 89.3%. Aerosol Can 2.7 oz. *OTC.*
Use: Foot deodorant; antiperspirant.

Desenex Jock Itch. (Novartis) Miconazole nitrate 2%. Aer. Pow. 113 g. *OTC.*
Use: Topical anti-infective, antifungal agent.

De Serpa. (de Leon) Reserpine 0.25 mg, 0.5 mg. Tab. Bot. 100s, 500s, 1000s (0.25 mg only). *Rx.*
Use: Antihypertensive.

deserpidine.
Use: Antihypertensive.
W/Methyclothiazide.
See: Enduronyl.

Desert Pure Calcium. (CalWhite Mineral Co.) Calcium (from mineral calcite) 500 mg, vitamin D 125 units. Tab. Bot. 200s. *OTC.*
Use: Mineral, vitamin supplement.

Desferal. (Novartis) Deferoxamine mesylate 500 mg/5 mL. Amp. 4s. *Rx.*
Use: Antidote.

•**desflurane.** (dess-FLEW-rane) *USP.*
Use: Anesthetic.
See: Suprane.

•**desipramine hydrochloride.** (dess-IPP-ruh-meen) *USP.*
Use: Antidepressant.
See: Norpramin.

desipramine hydrochloride. (Various Mfr.) Desipramine hydrochloride 10 mg, 25 mg, 50 mg, 75 mg, 100 mg, 150 mg. May contain lactose, PEG. Tab. 50s (150 mg only), 100s (except 150 mg). *Rx.*
Use: Antidepressant.

•**desirudin.** (deh-SIHR-uh-din) USAN.
Use: Anticoagulant.
See: Iprivask.

Desitin. (Pfizer) Cod liver oil, zinc oxide 40%, talc, petrolatum, lanolin. Oint. 30 g, 60 g, 120 g, 240 g, 270 g. *OTC.*
Use: Astringent; skin protectant.

Desitin Clear. (Pfizer) White petrolatum 60.4%. Cocoa butter, light mineral oil, mineral oil, modified lanolin, sunflower seed oil, vitamin A, vitamin D, vitamin E. Top. Oint. 50 g, 99 g. *OTC.*
Use: Diaper rash product.

Desitin Creamy. (Pfizer) Zinc oxide 10%, mineral oil, white petrolatum, parabens. Oint. Tube 57 g. *OTC.*
Use: Antifungal, topical.

Desitin with Zinc Oxide. (Pfizer) Cornstarch 88.2%, zinc oxide 10%. Pow. Bot. 28 g, 397 g. *OTC.*
Use: Diaper rash preparation.

•**deslanoside.** (dess-LAN-oh-side) *USP.*
Use: Cardiovascular agent.

•**desloratadine.** (dess-lore-AT-ah-deen) USAN.
Use: Antihistamine, peripherally selective piperidine.
See: Clarinex.
Clarinex RediTabs.
W/Pseudoephedrine Sulfate.
See: Clarinex-D 12 Hour.
Clarinex-D 24 Hour.

desloratadine. (Dr. Reddy's Laboratories) Desloratadine 2.5 mg, 5 mg. Aspartame, mannitol, lactose, phenylalanine 5 mg (2.5 mg) or 10.1 mg (5 mg). Tab., disintegrating. UD 30s. *Rx.*
Use: Antihistamine, peripherally selective piperidine.

desloratadine. (Various Mfr.) Desloratadine 5 mg. May contain PEG. Tab. 30s, 100s, 500s, 1,000s. *Rx.*
Use: Antihistamine; peripherally selective piperidine.

•**deslorelin.** (DESS-low-REH-lin) USAN.
Use: Gonadotropin inhibitor; LHRH agonist. [Orphan Drug]
See: Somagard (as acetate).

Desma. (Tablicaps) Diethylstilbestrol 25 mg. Tab. Patient dispenser 10s. *Rx.*
Use: Estrogen.

•**desmopressin acetate.** (DESS-moe-PRESS-in) USAN.
Use: Posterior pituitary hormone.
See: DDAVP.
Stimate.
W/Chlorobutanol.
See: Minirin.

desmopressin acetate. (Various Mfr.) Desmopressin acetate. **Tab.:** 0.1 mg, 0.2 mg. May contain lactose. 100s. **Inj., Soln.:** 4 mcg/mL. Single-dose Amp. 1 mL, multidose vial 10 mL. **Spray, Soln., intranasal:** 0.1 mg/mL (10 mcg/spray). Bot. 5 mL (50 sprays), rhinal tube delivery system. 2.5 mL (2 applicators per carton). *Rx.*
Use: Posterior pituitary hormone.

•**desmoteplase.** (des-moe-TE-plase) USAN.
Use: Cardiovascular agent.

Desogen. (Organon) Desogestrel 0.15 mg, ethinyl estradiol 30 mcg. Lactose. Tab. Pack. 28s with 7 inert tabs. *Rx.*
Use: Sex hormone, contraceptive hormone.

•**desogestrel.** (DESS-oh-JESS-trell) *USP.*
Use: Hormone, progestin.
W/Ethinyl Estradiol.
See: Apri.
Azurette.
Caziant.
Cesia.
Desogen.
Emoquette.
Mircette.
Ortho-Cept.
Reclipsen.
Velivet.
Viorele.

desogestrel/ethinyl estradiol. (North-Star Rx) Ethinyl estradiol 30 mcg, desogestrel 0.15 mg. Lactose, PEG. Tab. 28s (w/7 inert tablets [lactose, PEG, polydextrose]). *Rx.*
Use: Monophasic oral contraceptive.

Desonate. (Bayer HealthCare Pharmaceuticals) Desonide 0.05%. Edetate disodium dihydrate, glycerin, parabens, propylene glycol. Gel. 60 g. *Rx.*
Use: Anti-inflammatory agent, topical corticosteroid.

•**desonide.** (DESS-oh-nide) USAN.
Use: Anti-inflammatory.

See: Desonate.
Verdeso.

desonide. (Fougera) Desonide 0.05%, light mineral oil, cetyl alcohol, stearyl alcohol, parabens, EDTA. Lot. 59 mL, 118 mL. *Rx.*
Use: Anti-inflammatory; corticosteroid, topical.

desonide. (Various Mfr.) Desonide 0.05%. Oint. Cream. Tube 15 g, 60 g. *Rx.*
Use: Anti-inflammatory; corticosteroid, topical.

desonide cream. (Galderma) Desonide 0.05% in cream base. Tube 15 g, 60 g. *Rx.*
Use: Corticosteroid, topical.

DesOwen. (Galderma) Desonide 0.05%. Cream. Tube 15 g, 60 g. *Rx.*
Use: Corticosteroid, topical.

•**desoximetasone.** (dess-OX-ee-MET-ah-sone) *USP.*
Use: Anti-inflammatory; corticosteroid, topical.
See: Topicort.

desoximetasone. (Perrigo) Desoximetasone. **Gel.:** 0.05%. SD alcohol 20%, docusate sodium, EDTA, trolamine. Tubes. 15 g, 60 g. **Oint.:** 0.25%. Sorbitan sesquioleate, white petrolatum. Tubes. 15 g, 60 g. *Rx.*
Use: Anti-inflammatory; topical corticosteroid.

•**desoxycorticosterone acetate.** (dess-OX-ee-core-tih-koe-STURR-ohn) *USP.*
Use: Adrenocortical steroid (salt-regulating).

•**desoxycorticosterone pivalate.** (dess-OX-ee-core-tih-koe-STURR-ohn) *USP.*
Use: Adrenocortical steroid (salt-regulating).

•**desoxycorticosterone trimethylacetate.** (dess-OX-ee-core-tih-koe-STURR-ohn) *USP.*
Use: Adrenocortical steroid (salt-regulating).

desoxyephedrine hydrochloride. (Various Mfr.) *c-II.*
Use: CNS stimulant.
See: Methamphetamine Hydrochloride.

Desoxyn. (Recordati Rare Diseases) Methamphetamine hydrochloride 5 mg. Lactose. Tab. Bot. 100s. *c-II.*
Use: CNS stimulant, amphetamine.

desoxy norephedrine.
Use: CNS stimulant.
See: Amphetamine Hydrochloride.

desoxyribonuclease.
Use: Enzyme, topical.

Despec DM. (International Ethical) **ER Tab.:** Dextromethorphan HBr 60 mg, guaifenesin 800 mg, pseudoephedrine hydrochloride 120 mg. 100s. **Liq.:** Dextromethorphan HBr 15 mg, guaifenesin 100 mg, phenylephrine hydrochloride 5 mg per 5 mL. Saccharin, sorbitol. Grape flavor. 15 mL, 473 mL. *Rx.*
Use: Antitussive and expectorant combination.

Despec-EXP. (International Ethical) Dihydrocodeine bitartrate 7.5 mg, guaifenesin 100 mg, pseudoephedrine hydrochloride 15 mg per 5 mL. Saccharin, sorbitol. Alcohol free, dye free, and sugar free. Vanilla mint flavor. Syrup. 473 mL. *c-III.*
Use: Upper respiratory combination, antitussive and expectorant combination.

Despec NR. (International Ethical) Dextromethorphan hydrobromide 4 mg, guaifenesin 20 mg, phenylephrine hydrochloride 1.5 mg per mL. Saccharin, sorbitol. Grape flavor. Drops. 15 mL, 30 mL w/dropper. *Rx.*
Use: Upper respiratory combination; antitussive, decongestant, expectorant.

Desquam-E 5 & 10. (Westwood Squibb) Benzoyl peroxide 10%, EDTA. Gel. Tube 42.5 g. *Rx.*
Use: Dermatologic, acne.

Desquam-X 10. (Westwood Squibb) Benzoyl peroxide 10%. Lactic acid, EDTA, sorbitol. Bar 106 g. *Rx.*
Use: Dermatologic, acne.

Desquam-X Wash. (Ranbaxy Labs) Benzoyl peroxide 5%, 10%. EDTA. Liq. 150 mL. *OTC.*
Use: Topical anti-infective, antibiotic agent.

de-Stat. (Sherman Pharmaceuticals, Inc.) Surfactant cleaner, benzalkonium Cl 0.01%, EDTA 0.25%. Soln. Bot. 118 mL. *OTC.*
Use: Contact lens care.

destructive agents.
See: Chloroacetic Acids.

desvenlafaxine.
Use: Antidepressant, serotonin and norepinephrine reuptake inhibitor.
See: Khedezla.

•**desvenlafaxine succinate.** (des-VEN-la-fax-een) USAN.
Use: Antidepressant, serotonin and norepinephrine reuptake inhibitor.
See: Pristiq.

desvenlafaxine succinate. (Various Mfr.) Desvenlafaxine succinate 50 mg, 100 mg. ER Tab. 14s, 30s, 90s, 100s, 1,000s, UD 100s. *Rx.*
Use: Antidepressant, serotonin and norepinephrine reuptake inhibitor.

Detachol. (Ferndale) Bland, nonirritating liquid for removing adhesive tape. Pkg. 4 oz.
Use: Adhesive remover.

Detane. (Del) Benzocaine 7.5%. Carbomer 940, PEG 400. Gel. Tubes. 15 g. *OTC.*
Use: Topical local anesthetic.

•**deterenol hydrochloride.** (dee-TEER-eh-nahl) USAN.
Use: Adrenergic, ophthalmic.

detergents. Surface-active.
See: pHisoDerm.
pHisoHex.
Zephiran.

detigon hydrochloride.
See: Chlophedianol hydrochloride.

•**detirelix acetate.** (DEH-tih-RELL-ix) USAN.
Use: Antagonist (LHRH).

•**detomidine hydrochloride.** (deh-TOE-mih-deen) USAN.
Use: Hypnotic; sedative.

detoxification agents.
See: Antidotes.
Chelating Agents.

Detrol. (Pfizer) Tolterodine tartrate 1 mg, 2 mg. Tab. Bot. 60s, 500s, UD 140s. *Rx.*
Use: Anticholinergic.

Detrol LA. (Pfizer) Tolterodine tartrate 2 mg, 4 mg. Sucrose. ER Cap. Bot. 30s, 90s, 500s, UD blisters 100s. *Rx.*
Use: Anticholinergic.

Detussin Expectorant. (Various Mfr.) Pseudoephedrine hydrochloride 60 mg, hydrocodone bitartrate 5 mg, guaifenesin 200 mg, alcohol. Liq. Bot. 480 mL. *c-III.*
Use: Antitussive, decongestant, expectorant.

•**deuterium oxide.** (doo-TEER-ee-uhm) USAN.
Use: Radiopharmaceutical.

•**devazepide.** (dev-AZE-eh-PIDE) USAN.
Use: Antagonist (cholecystokinin); antispasmodic, gastrointestinal.

Devrom. (Parthenon) Bismuth subgallate 200 mg, lactose, sugar. Chew. Tab. Bot. 100s.
Use: Deodorant, systemic.

Dexacort Phosphate Respihaler. (Medeva) Dexamethasone sodium phosphate equivalent to 0.1 mg dexamethasone phosphate (≈ 0.084 mg dexamethasone) w/fluorochlorohydrocarbons as propellants, alcohol 2%. Aerosol for oral inhalation, 170 sprays in 12.6 g pressurized container.
Use: Bronchodilator.

Dexacort Phosphate Turbinaire. (Medeva) Dexamethasone sodium phosphate 0.1 mg equivalent to dexamethasone 0.084 mg w/fluorochlorohydrocarbons as propellants and alcohol 2%. Aerosol w/nasal applicator. Container 170 sprays; refill package without nasal applicator.
Use: Nasal corticosteroid.

Dexafed. (Roberts) Phenylephrine hydrochloride 5 mg, dextromethorphan HBr 10 mg, guaifenesin 100 mg/5 mL. Syr. Bot. 120 mL. *OTC.*
Use: Antitussive, decongestant, expectorant.

DexAlone. (DexGen) Dextromethorphan HBr 30 mg. Sorbitol. Cap., Liquid-filled. Pkg. 30s. *OTC.*
Use: Nonnarcotic antitussive.

•**dexamethasone.** (DEX-uh-METH-uh-sone) *USP.*
Use: Adrenocortical steroid, glucocorticoid; corticosteroid, topical.
See: Aeroseb-Dex.
Baycadron.
Decaderm.
Dexaport.
DexPak Jr. 10 Day TaperPak.
DexPak 6 Day TaperPak.
DexPak Taperpak.
DexPak 13 Day TaperPak.
Maxidex.
Ozurdex.
TobraDex.
Zema-Pak 10 Day.
Zema-Pak 13 Day.
W/Ciprofloxacin.
See: Ciprodex.
W/Neomycin Sulfate, Polymyxin B Sulfate.
See: Dexasporin.
Maxitrol Ointment.
Methadex.
Poly-Dex.

dexamethasone. (Roxane) Dexamethasone 1 mg, 2 mg. Tab. 100s, UD 100s. *Rx.*
Use: Adrenocortical steroid, glucocorticoid.

dexamethasone. (Steris) Dexamethasone 0.1%. Susp., Ophth. 5 mL. *Rx.*
Use: Corticosteroid, ophthalmic.

dexamethasone. (Various Mfr.) Dexamethasone. **Elix.:** 0.5 mg/5 mL. May contain alcohol. 100 mL, 237 mL. **Oral Soln.:** 0.5 mg/5 mL. May contain sorbitol. Sugar free. 500 mL, UD 5 mL, UD 20 mL, 237 mL. **Tab.:** 0.25 mg, 0.5 mg, 0.75 mg, 1.5 mg, 4 mg, 6 mg. 50s (1.5 mg, 4 mg, 6 mg only), 100s, 500s (0.75 mg, 1.5 mg, 4 mg only), 1,000s

(except 6 mg), UD 100s (except 0.25 mg). *Rx.*
Use: Adrenocortical steroid, glucocorticoid.

•**dexamethasone acefurate.** (DEX-ah-METH-ah-sone ASS-eh-fer-ate) USAN.
Use: Anti-inflammatory; topical steroid.

•**dexamethasone acetate.** (DEX-ah-METH-ah-sone) *USP.*
Use: Adrenocortical steroid (anti-inflammatory).

•**dexamethasone beloxil.** (DEX-ah-METH-ah-sone bel-OX-il) USAN.
Use: Anti-inflammatory.

•**dexamethasone dipropionate.** (DEX-ah-METH-ah-sone die-PRO-pee-oh-nate) USAN.
Use: Anti-inflammatory; steroid.

Dexamethasone Intensol. (Roxane) Dexamethasone 1 mg/mL. Alcohol 30%. Concentrated oral soln. Bot. 30 mL w/dropper. *Rx.*
Use: Glucocorticoid, adrenocortical steroid.

•**dexamethasone sodium phosphate.** (DEX-ah-METH-ah-sone) *USP.*
Use: Adrenocortical steroid (anti-inflammatory); corticosteroid, topical.
See: Solurex.

dexamethasone sodium phosphate. (Various Mfr.) Dexamethasone sodium phosphate. **Inj.: 4 mg/mL:** 1 mL, 5 mL, 10 mL, 30 mL vials and 1 mL disp. syringe and 1 mL fill in 2 mL vials. **10 mg/mL:** 1 mL and 10 mL vials and 1 mL disp. syringe. **Soln., otic:** 0.1%. Sodium citrate, sodium borate, polysorbate 80, edetate disodium dihydrate, sodium bisulfite 0.1%, phenylethyl alcohol 0.25%, benzalkonium chloride 0.02%. Bot. 5 mL. **Ophth. Soln.:** 0.1%. 5 mL. *Rx.*
Use: Adrenocortical steroid (anti-inflammatory); corticosteroid, topical; ophthalmic corticosteroid.

•**dexamisole.** (DEX-AM-ih-sole) USAN.
Use: Antidepressant.

dexamphetamine.
See: Dextroamphetamine.

Dexaphen-S.A. Tablets. (Major) Pseudoephedrine sulfate 120 mg, dexbrompheniramine maleate 6 mg. Bot. 100s, 500s. *Rx.*
Use: Antihistamine, decongestant.

Dexaport. (Freeport) Dexamethasone 0.75 mg. Tab. Bot. 1000s. *Rx.*
Use: Corticosteroid.

Dexasporin Suspension. (Various Mfr.) Dexamethasone 0.1%, neomycin sulfate equivalent to 0.35%, neomycin base and 10,000 units polymyxin B sulfate/mL, hydroxypropyl methylcellulose, polysorbate 20, benzalkonium chloride. Drops. Bot. 5 mL. *Rx.*
Use: Anti-infective; corticosteroid, ophthalmic.

Dexatrim Max Daytime Appetite Control. (Chattem) Asian ginseng root standardized extract 250 mg, Ca, caffeine 200 mg, Cr, epigallocatechin gallate 90 mg, vitamins B_1 15 mg, B_2 17 mg, B_3 20 mg, B_5 25 mg, B_6 10 mg, B_{12} 60 mcg. Film-coated. ER Tab. 60s. *OTC.*
Use: Dietary aid.

Dexatrim Natural Caffeine Free Caplets. (Chattem) Chromium 250 mcg, heartleaf 120 mg, thermonutrient blend 100 mg, vanadium 100 mcg. Box. Blister pak 30s. *OTC.*
Use: Dietary aid.

•**dexbrompheniramine maleate.** (DEX-brom-fen-IR-a-meen) *USP.*
Use: Antihistamine.
See: Ala-hist IR.
W/Acetaminophen, Phenylephrine Hydrochloride.
See: Sinadrin PE.
W/Chlophedianol Hydrochloride, Pseudoephedrine Hydrochloride.
See: Chlo Tuss.
W/Codeine Phosphate, Pseudoephedrine Hydrochloride.
See: M-End Max D.
W/Dextromethorphan Hydrobromide, Phenylephrine Hydrochloride.
See: Panatuss DXP.
Y-Cof DM.
W/Dextromethorphan Hydrobromide, Pseudoephedrine Hydrochloride.
See: M-End DMX.
W/Pseudoephedrine Sulfate.
See: Drixoral Cold & Allergy.
Drixoral Cold & Allergy Maximum Strength.

dexbrompheniramine tannate.
W/Dextromethorphan Tannate, Phenylephrine Tannate, Pyrilamine Maleate.
See: Poly Tan DM.

•**dexchlorpheniramine maleate.** (DEX-klor-fen-IR-a-meen) *USP.*
Use: Antihistamine, nonselective alkylamine.
See: Polaramine.
Polaramine Repetabs.
W/Carbetapentane Citrate, Phenylephrine Hydrochloride.
See: Corzall-PE.
W/Methscopolamine Nitrate, Phenylephrine Hydrochloride.
See: Extendryl.
Dexphen M.
Re-Drylex.

W/Methscopolamine Nitrate, Pseudoephedrine Hydrochloride.
See: CoryZa-D.
D-Hist D.
Histatab D.
W/Phenylephrine Hydrochloride.
See: Ala-Hist PE.
W/Pseudoephedrine Hydrochloride.
See: Rescon.

dexchlorpheniramine maleate. (Morton Grove) Dexchlorpheniramine maleate 2 mg/5 mL. Alcohol, orange flavor. Syrup. 473 mL. *Rx.*
Use: Antihistamine.

dexchlorpheniramine maleate. (Various Mfr.) Dexchlorpheniramine maleate 4 mg, 6 mg. ER Tab. Bot. 100s, 1000s. *Rx.*
Use: Antihistamine, non-selective alkylamine.

dexchlorpheniramine tannate.
W/Dextromethorphan Tannate, Phenylephrine Tannate.
See: Dextromethorphan Tannate, Phenylephrine Tannate, Dexchlorpheniramine Tannate.
W/Dextromethorphan Tannate, Pseudoephedrine Tannate.
See: Dur-Tann Forte.

•**dexclamol hydrochloride.** (DEX-claymahl) USAN.
Use: Hypnotic; sedative.

Dexcon-DM. (Cypress Pharmaceutical) Dextromethorphan HBr 20 mg, guaifenesin 100 mg, phenylephrine hydrochloride 10 mg per 5 mL. Sugar and alcohol free. Saccharin, sorbitol. Strawberry flavor. Syrup. 473 mL. *Rx.*
Use: Antitussive and expectorant combination.

Dexedrine Spansules. (Amedra) Dextroamphetamine sulfate 5 mg, 10 mg, 15 mg. Sugar spheres. ER. Cap. 100s. *c-II.*
Use: CNS stimulant, amphetamine.

•**dexelvucitabine.** (DEX-el-vue-SYE-tabeen) USAN.
Use: Antiretroviral.

•**dexetimide.** (dex-ETT-ih-mid) USAN.
Use: Anticholinergic; antiparkinsonian.

DexFerrum. (American Regent) Iron 50 mg/mL (as dextran). Inj. Single-dose vial. 1 mL, 2 mL. *Rx.*
Use: Hematinic, trace element.

DexFol. (Rising) Vitamin B_1 1.5 mg, B_2 1.5 mg, B_3 20 mg, B_5 10 mg, B_6 50 mg, B_{12} 1 mg, C 60 mg, FA 5 mg, biotin 300 mcg. Tab. 90s. *Rx.*
Use: Nutritional product.

Dex4 Glucose. (Can-Am Care) Glucose, lemon, orange, raspberry, grape flavors. Chew. Tab. Bot. 10s, 50s. *OTC.*
Use: Glucose-elevating agent.

Dex GG TR. (Boca Pharmacal) Dextromethorphan HBr 60 mg, guaifenesin 1000 mg. ER Tab. Bot. 100s. *Rx.*
Use: Upper respiratory combination, antitussive, expectorant.

•**dexibuprofen.** (dex-EYE-byoo-PRO-fen) USAN.
Use: Analgesic; anti-inflammatory.

•**dexibuprofen lysine.** (dex-EYE-byoo-PRO-fen LIE-seen) USAN.
Use: Analgesic (cyclooxygenase inhibitor); anti-inflammatory.

Dexilant. (Takeda Pharmaceuticals America) Dexlansoprazole 30 mg, 60 mg. PEG, sucrose, sugar spheres. Cap., delayed release. 30s, 90s (60 mg only). *Rx.*
Use: GI agent, proton pump inhibitor.

•**deximafen.** (dex-IH-mah-fen) USAN.
Use: Antidepressant.

•**dexivacaine.** (dex-IH-vah-CANE) USAN.
Use: Anesthetic.

•**dexlansoprazole.** (dex-lan-SOE-prazole) USAN.
Use: Gastrointestinal agent.
See: Dexilant.

•**dexmecamylamine.** (DEX-mek-a-MIL-ameen) USAN.
Use: Treatment of overactive bladder.

•**dexmecamylamine hydrochloride.** (DEX-mek-a-MIL-a-meen) USAN.
Use: Treatment of overactive bladder.

•**dexmedetomidine.** (DEX-meh-dih-TOE-mih-deen) USAN.
Use: Anxiolytic.

•**dexmedetomidine hydrochloride.** (DEX-meh-dih-TOE-mih-deen)
Use: Sedative/hypnotic, nonbarbiturate.
See: Precedex.

•**dexmethylphenidate hydrochloride.** (dex-meth-il-FEN-i-date) USAN.
Use: Central nervous system stimulant.
See: Focalin.
Focalin XR.

dexmethylphenidate hydrochloride. (Teva) Dexmethylphenidate hydrochloride 2.5 mg, 5 mg, 10 mg. Lactose. Tab. 100s. *c-II.*
Use: Central nervous system stimulant.

dexmethylphenidate hydrochloride. (Various Mfr.) Dexmethylphenidate hydrochloride 15 mg, 30 mg, 40 mg. May contain PEG, sugar. ER Cap. 100s. *c-II.*
Use: Central nervous system stimulant.

Dexodryl. (Dexo Pharma) **Chew Tab.:** Chlorpheniramine maleate (as chlor-

pheniramine tannate) 2 mg, methscopolamine nitrate 1.5 mg. Saccharin, sugar. 100s. **Susp.:** Chlorpheniramine maleate (as chlorpheniramine tannate) 2 mg, methscopolamine nitrate 1.5 mg per 5 mL. Parabens, sucralose. 118 mL. *Rx.*
Use: Upper respiratory combination, decongestant, antihistamine, and anticholinergic combination.

•**dexormaplatin.** (DEX-ore-mah-PLAT-in) USAN.
Use: Antineoplastic.

•**dexoxadrol hydrochloride.** (dex-OX-ah-drole) USAN.
Use: Antidepressant; stimulant (central); analgesic.

DexPak Jr. 10 Day TaperPak. (ECR) Dexamethasone 1.5 mg. Lactose. Tab. 10-day pack. 35s. *Rx.*
Use: Adrenocortical steroid, glucocorticoid.

DexPak 6 Day TaperPak. (ECR) Dexamethasone 1.5 mg. Lactose. Tab. 6-day pack. 21s. *Rx.*
Use: Adrenocortical steroid, glucocorticoid.

DexPak TaperPak. (ECR) Dexamethasone 1.5 mg. Tab. 51s. *Rx.*
Use: Adrenocortical steroid, glucocorticoid.

DexPak 13 Day TaperPak. (ECR) Dexamethasone 1.5 mg. Lactose. Tab. 13-day pack. 51s. *Rx.*
Use: Adrenocortical steroid, glucocorticoid.

•**dexpanthenol.** (DEX-PAN-theh-nahl) *USP.*
Use: Treatment of paralytic ileus and postoperative distention; cholinergic.
See: Ilopan.
Panthoderm.

•**dexpemedolac.** (dex-peh-MED-oh-lack) USAN.
Use: Analgesic.

Dexphen M. (Boca Pharmacal) Dexchlorpheniramine maleate 1 mg, methscopolamine nitrate 1.25 mg, phenylephrine hydrochloride 10 mg per 5 mL. Sorbitol. Root beer flavor. Oral Soln. 473 mL. *Rx.*
Use: Upper respiratory combination, decongestant, antihistamine, and anticholinergic combination.

•**dexpramipexole.** (DEX-pram-i-PEX-ole) USAN.
Use: Treatment of amyotrophic lateral sclerosis.

•**dexpramipexole dihydrochloride.** (DEX-pram-i-PEX-ole) USAN.
Use: Treatment of amyotrophic lateral sclerosis.

•**dexpropanolol hydrochloride.** (DEX-pro-PRAN-oh-lole) USAN.
Use: Antiadrenergic (β-receptor); cardiovascular agent (antiarrhythmic).

•**dexrazoxane.** (dex-ray-ZOX-ane) USAN.
Use: Cytoprotective agent.
See: Totect.
Zinecard

dexrazoxane. (Bedford) Dexrazoxane (as dexrazoxane hydrochloride) 250 mg, 500 mg. Pow. for Soln., Inj., lyophilized. Single-use vials with 25 mL sodium lactate injection (250 mg) or 50 mL sodium lactate injection (500 mg). *Rx.*
Use: Cytoprotective agent.

•**dexsotalol hydrochloride.** (dex-SOE-ta-lol) USAN.
Use: Cardiovascular agent (antiarrhythmic).

•**dextofisopam.** (dex-toe-FIS-oh-pam) USAN.
Use: Crohn disease

dextran adjunct. *Rx.*
Use: Plasma expander.
See: Promit.

dextran and deferoxamine.
Use: Acute iron poisoning. [Orphan Drug]
See: Bio-Rescue.

•**dextran 40.** (DEX-tran 40) USAN. Polysaccharide (m.w. 40,000) produced by the action of *Leuconostoc mesenteroides* on sucrose.
Use: Blood flow adjuvant; plasma volume extender.
See: 10% LMD.
Gentran 40.
Rheomacrodex.

dextran 40. (McGaw) Dextran 40 10% with 0.9% sodium chloride or in 5% dextrose. Inj. 500 mL. *Rx.*
Use: Plasma expander.

dextran 45. (McGaw) Polysaccharide (m.w. 45,000) produced by the action of *Leuconostoc mesenteroides* on saccharose. *Rx.*
Use: Blood volume expander.

dextranomer.
Use: Gastrointestinal agent.
W/Sodium Hyaluronate.
See: Solesta.

•**dextran 1.** (DEX-tran 1) *USP.*
Use: Plasma volume extender.

•**dextran 70.** (DEX-tran 70) USAN. Polysaccharide (m.w. 70,000) produced by the action of *Leuconostoc mesenteroides* on sucrose.

Use: Plasma volume extender.
See: Hyskon.

•**dextran 75.** (DEX-tran 75) USAN. Polysaccharide (m.w. 75,000) produced by the action of *Leuconostoc mesenteroides* on sucrose.
Use: Plasma volume extender.

dextran 6%. (Abbott) *Rx.*
See: Dextran 75.

dextran sulfate, inhaled aerosolized.
Use: Antiviral. [Orphan Drug]
See: Uendex.

dextran sulfate sodium. (Ueno Fine Chemicals Industry)
Use: AIDS drug. [Orphan Drug]

•**dextrates.** (DEX-traytz) *NF.* Mixture of sugars (≈ 92% dextrose monohydrate and 8% higher saccharides; dextrose equivalent is 95% to 97%) resulting from the controlled enzymatic hydrolysis of starch.
Use: Pharmaceutic aid (tablet binder, diluent).

•**dextrin.** *NF.*
Use: Pharmaceutic aid (suspending, viscosity-increasing agent; tablet binder; tablet, capsule diluent).

•**dextroamphetamine.** (DEX-troe-am-FET-ah-meen) USAN.
Use: Stimulant (central).

dextroamphetamine. (Various Mfr.) Dextroamphetamine sulfate. **Tab:** 5 mg, 10 mg. May contain sucrose. Bot. 100s. **ER Cap:** 5 mg, 10 mg, 15 mg. May contain sucrose. Bot. 100s. *c-II.*
Use: CNS stimulant, amphetamine.

dextroamphetamine phosphate. Monobasic d-a-methylphenethlyamine phosphate. (+)-α-Methylphenethylamine phosphate.
Use: CNS stimulant.

dextroamphetamine saccharate.
Use: CNS stimulant.
W/Amphetamine Aspartate, Amphetamine Sulfate, Dextroamphetamine Sulfate.
See: Adderall.
Adderall XR.
MAS-ER.

dextroamphetamine saccharate/ amphetamine aspartate/dextroamphetamine sulfate/amphetamine sulfate. (Barr) Dextroamphetamine saccharate/amphetamine aspartate/dextroamphetamine sulfate/amphetamine sulfate 5 mg (1.25 mg/1.25 mg/1.25 mg/ 1.25 mg), 10 mg (2.5 mg/2.5 mg/2.5 mg/ 2.5 mg), 15 mg (3.75 mg/3.75 mg/ 3.75 mg/3.75 mg), 20 mg (5 mg/5 mg/ 5 mg/5 mg), 25 mg (6.25 mg/6.25 mg/ 6.25 mg/6.25 mg), 30 mg (7.5 mg/ 7.5 mg/7.5 mg/7.5 mg). ER Cap. 100s. c-ii.
Use: Amphetamine mixture.

•**dextroamphetamine sulfate.** (DEX-troe-am-FET-uh-meen) *USP.*
Use: CNS stimulant, amphetamine.
See: Dexedrine Spansules.
Dextrostat.
LiQuadd.
ProCentra.
Zenzedi.
W/Amphetamine Aspartate, Amphetamine Sulfate, Dextroamphetamine Saccharate.
See: Adderall.
Adderall XR.
MAS-ER.

dextroamphetamine sulfate. (Various Mfr.) Dextroamphetamine sulfate 5 mg per 5 mL. May contain benzoic acid, saccharin, sorbitol. Soln. 473 mL. *c-II.*
Use: Central nervous system stimulant, amphetamine.

Dextro-Chek Calibrators. (Bayer Consumer Care) Clear liquid soln. containing measured amounts of glucose. Low calibrator contains 0.05% w/v glucose. High calibrator contains 0.3% w/v glucose.
Use: Glucometer calibration aid.

Dextro-Chek Normal Control. (Bayer Consumer Care) Clear liquid containing measured amount of glucose 0.1%.
Use: Glucometer calibration aid.

Dextro-Chlorpheniramine Maleate.
Use: Antihistamine.
See: Polaramine.

•**dextromethorphan.** (DEX-troe-meth-OR-fan) *USP.*
Use: Cough suppressant; antitussive.
See: Vicks Nature Fusion Cough.
W/Combinations.
See: DMax Pediatric.

•**dextromethorphan hydrobromide.** (DEX-troe-meth-OR-fan) *USP.*
Use: Antitussive.
See: AeroTuss 12.
Buckley's Cough.
Creomulsion Adult Formula.
Creomulsion for Children.
Creo-Terpin.
Delsym.
DexAlone.
ElixSure Children's Cough.
Formula 44 Custom Care Dry Cough Suppressant.
Hold DM.
Little Colds Cough Formula.
Long-Acting Cough Suppressant.
PediaCare Children's Long-Acting Cough.

Robitussin Children's Cough Long-Acting.
Robitussin Lingering Cold Long-Acting Cough.
Robitussin Lingering Cold Long-Acting CoughGels.
Robitussin Pediatric Cough.
Scot-Tussin Diabetes.
Scot-Tussin DM Cough Chasers.
Silphen DM.
Simply Cough.
Sucrets DM.
Sucrets DM Cough Formula.
Sucrets DM Cough Suppressant.
Theraflu Thin Strips Long Acting Cough.
Triaminic Long Acting Cough.
Vicks DayQuil Cough.
Vicks Nature Fusion Cough.

W/Acetaminophen.
See: PediaCare Children's Cough & Sore Throat.
Triaminic Cough & Sore Throat.
Tylenol Plus Children's Cough & Sore Throat.

W/Acetaminophen, Chlorpheniramine Maleate.
See: Coricidin HBP Maximum Strength Flu.
Formula 44 Custom Care Cough & Cold PM.
Triaminic Flu, Cough & Fever.
Tylenol Plus Children's Cough & Runny Nose.
Vicks Alcohol-Free NyQuil Cold & Flu Relief.
Vicks Formula 44 Custom Care Cough & Cold PM.

W/Acetaminophen, Chlorpheniramine Maleate, Phenylephrine Hydrochloride.
See: Alka-Seltzer Plus Cold & Cough.
Dimetapp Children's Multi-Symptom Cold & Flu.
Theraflu Nighttime Severe Cold.

W/Acetaminophen, Diphenhydramine.
See: Diabetic Tussin Cold & Flu.
Diabetic Tussin Night Time Formula Cold/Flu.

W/Acetaminophen, Diphenhydramine Hydrochloride, Phenylephrine Hydrochloride.
See: Respa C & C.

W/Acetaminophen, Doxylamine Succinate.
See: Tylenol Cough & Sore Throat Nighttime.
Vicks Nature Fusion Cold & Flu Nighttime Relief.
Vicks NyQuil Cold/Flu Relief.

W/Acetaminophen, Doxylamine Succinate, Phenylephrine Hydrochloride.
See: Alka-Seltzer Plus Day & Night Cold.
Alka-Seltzer Plus Night Cold.
Alka-Seltzer Plus Severe Sinus Congestion Allergy & Cough.
Tylenol Cold Multi-Symptom Nighttime.

W/Acetaminophen, Doxylamine Succinate, Pseudoephedrine Hydrochloride.
See: All-Nite.

W/Acetaminophen, Guaifenesin.
See: Comtrex Multi-Symptom Deep Chest Cold.
Phenflu G.
Sine-Off Cough/Cold.
Sudafed PE Multi-Symptom Cold and Cough.

W/Acetaminophen, Guaifenesin, Phenylephrine Hydrochloride.
See: Mucinex Children's Cold, Cough and Sore Throat.
Mucinex Fast-Max Cold, Flu and Sore Throat.
Mucinex Fast-Max Severe Congestion and Cold.

W/Acetaminophen, Guaifenesin, Pseudoephedrine Hydrochloride.
See: Duraflu.
Flutabs.
Maxiflu DM.
Maxiflu G.
Tylenol Cold Severe Congestion.

W/Acetaminophen, Phenylephrine Hydrochloride.
See: Alka-Seltzer Plus Day & Night Cold.
Alka-Seltzer Plus Day Cold.
Alka-Seltzer Plus Day Non-Drowsy Cold.
Comtrex Maximum Strength Day & Night Cold & Cough.
Mapap Cold Formula Multi-Symptom.
Theraflu Daytime Severe Cold & Cough.
Theraflu Severe Cold & Cough Daytime/Nighttime.
Theraflu Warming Relief Daytime Multi-Symptom Cold.
Tylenol Cold Head Congestion Daytime.
Tylenol Cold Multi-Symptom Daytime.
Vicks DayQuil Multi-Symptom Cold/Flu Relief.
Vicks Nature Fusion Cold & Flu Relief.

W/Acetaminophen, Pseudoephedrine Hydrochloride.
See: 666 Cold Preparation Maximum Strength.

W/Aspirin, Doxylamine Succinate, Phenylephrine Bitartrate.
See: Alka-Seltzer Plus Day & Night Cold.
Alka-Seltzer Plus Night Cold.

W/Aspirin, Phenylephrine Bitartrate.
See: Alka-Seltzer Plus Day & Night Cold.
W/Benzocaine.
See: Cēpacol Sore Throat Plus Cough Relief.
Chloraseptic Total Sore Throat + Cough.
W/Benzocaine, Glycerin.
See: Cēpacol Dual Relief Sore Throat + Cough.
W/Brompheniramine Maleate, Guaifenesin, Phenylephrine Hydrochloride.
See: Bromhist-PDX.
W/Brompheniramine Maleate, Guaifenesin, Pseudoephedrine Hydrochloride.
See: Bromhist DM Pediatric.
Histacol DM Pediatric.
Pediahist DM.
W/Brompheniramine Maleate, Phenylephrine Hydrochloride.
See: Alahist DM.
BPM-DM-PHEN.
BROM/PE/DM.
BrōveX PEB DM.
Children's Dimaphen DM.
Dimetapp Children's Cold + Cough.
LoHist-DM.
LoHist PEB DM.
TGQ 7.5PEH/4BRM/15DM.
TL-Hist DM.
W/Brompheniramine Maleate, Pseudoephedrine Hydrochloride.
See: Brometane-DX Cough.
Bromfed DM.
Bromhist-DM.
Bromhist PDX.
Brotapp DM.
BrōveX PSB.
BrōveX PSE DM.
Dimaphen DM Cough, Cold & Allergy.
DM/PSE/BPM.
Myphetane DX Cough.
Neo DM.
Pediahist DM.
Prohist DM.
Q-Tapp DM Cold and Cough.
TGQ 50PSE/3BRM/30DM.
TGQ 40PSE/4BRM/20DM.
TGQ 30PSE/3BRM/15DM.
W/Carbinoxamine Maleate, Phenylephrine Hydrochloride.
See: TriTuss-A.
W/Chlorpheniramine Maleate.
See: AMBI 20DM/4CPM.
Coricidin HBP Cough & Cold.
Dimetapp Children's Long Acting Cough Plus Cold.
Robitussin Pediatric Cough & Cold Long Acting.
Scot-Tussin DM.
Triaminic Cough & Runny Nose.
Tricodene Sugar Free.
Vicks Children's NyQuil Cold & Cough Relief.
W/Chlorpheniramine Maleate, Guaifenesin, Phenylephrine Hydrochloride.
See: Chlordex GP.
DM/CPM/PE/GG.
Donatussin.
Genelan-NF.
W/Chlorpheniramine Maleate, Phenylephrine Hydrochloride.
See: AMBI 10PEH/4CPM/20DM.
Ameritus AD.
Balamine DM.
Cardec DM.
Corfen-DM.
CP DEC-DM.
DM/PE/CPM.
Donatussin DM.
Ed-A-Hist DM.
Father John's Medicine Plus.
Maxichlor PEH DM.
Nasohist DM.
Neo DM.
PE-Hist DM.
Relahist-DM.
Rondec-DM.
Rondex-DM.
Sonahist DM.
TGQ 15DM/5PEH/2CPM.
Trigofen DM.
Virdec DM.
Z-Dex 12D.
ZoDen DM.
W/Chlorpheniramine Maleate, Pseudoephedrine Hydrochloride.
See: Allres DS.
AMBI 60PSE/4CPM/20DM.
CPM/PSE DM.
Dicel DM.
Esocor P.
KidKare Children's Cough/Cold.
Mesehist DM.
Neutrahist PDX.
Pedia Relief Cough-Cold.
Pediatric Cough & Cold.
Pediatric Cough & Cold Medicine.
Rescon DM.
Triaminic-D Children's.
W/Dexbrompheniramine Maleate, Phenylephrine Hydrochloride.
See: Panatuss DXP.
Y-Cof DM.
W/Dexbrompheniramine Maleate, Pseudoephedrine Hydrochloride.
See: M-End DMX.
W/Diphenhydramine Tannate, Phenylephrine Tannate.
See: Duratuss AC.

W/Doxylamine Succinate.
See: Vicks NyQuil Cough.
W/Doxylamine Succinate, Pseudoephedrine Hydrochloride.
See: Lortuss DM.
W/Guaifenesin.
See: Alka-Seltzer Plus Mucus & Congestion.
Biospec DMX.
Cheracol D Cough Formula.
Cheracol Plus.
Congesta DM.
Coricidin HBP Chest Congestion & Cough.
Diabetic Tussin DM.
Diabetic Tussin Maximum Strength DM.
Extra Action Cough.
Fenesin DM IR.
Formula 44 Custom Care Chesty Cough Medicine.
Geri-Tussin DM.
Guaifenesin DM.
Guaifenesin-DM NR.
Iophen DM-NR.
Mucinex Cough for Kids.
Mucinex Cough Mini-Melts for Kids.
Mucinex DM Maximum Strength.
Mucus Relief DM.
Mucinex DM.
NeoTuss.
PediaCare Children's Cough & Congestion.
Robitussin Cough & Congestion.
Robitussin Cough DM.
Robitussin Cough Sugar-Free DM.
Robitussin-DM.
Safe Tussin DM.
Scot-Tussin Senior Clear.
Siltussin-DM.
Vicks DayQuil Mucus Control Liquid DM.
Vicks Formula 44 Custom Care Chesty Cough.
Vicks Nature Fusion Cough & Chest Congestion.
Zotex-EX.
W/Guaifenesin, Phenylephrine Hydrochloride.
See: AMBI 10PEH/400GFN/20DM.
Biobron SF.
Biogil.
BioGtuss.
Bio T Pres.
Bio T Pres Pediatric.
Biotuss.
Bio-Tussi.
Bio-Tussi Pediatric.
Broncotron-D.
Brontuss DX.
Dacex DM.
Dacex PE.
Deconex DM.
Deconex DMX.
Despec NR.
Dynatuss EX.
Endacon.
ExeCof.
ExeTuss-DM.
GFN 1200/DM 20/PE 40.
Giltuss.
Giltuss Pediatric.
Giltuss TR.
Guaifen.
Maxiphen DM.
NeoTuss-D.
Phlemex Forte.
Phlemex-PE.
Robitussin Children's Cough & Cold CF.
Robitussin Pediatric Cough/Cold CF.
SINUtuss DM.
TriTuss.
TriTuss ER.
Tussi-Pres.
Tussi-Pres Pediatric.
Tusso DM.
Tusso DMR.
Tusso XR.
Vanacof DM.
Z-Dex.
Z-Dex Pediatric.
Zotex.
Zotex Pediatric.
W/Guaifenesin, Potassium Citrate
See: Sorbutuss NR.
W/Guaifenesin, Pseudoephedrine Hydrochloride.
See: Aldex GS DM.
Ambifed-G DM.
AMBI 40PSE/400GFN/20DM.
AMBI 60/580/30.
AMBI 60PSE/400GFN/20DM.
Bionel.
Bionel Pediatric.
Capmist DM.
Despec.
Donatussin DM.
Entex PAC.
Entre-Cough.
GFN 600/PSE 60/DM 30.
Liquicough DM.
Maxifed DM.
Maxifed DMX.
Medent-DMI.
Poly-Vent DM.
Pseudo Cough.
Q-Tussin CF.
Relacon DM NR.
Relasin DM.
Robafen CF.
Robitussin Cough & Cold D.

Sudafed Multi-Symptom Cold & Cough.
TGQ 30PSE/150GFN/15DM.
Tidafen DM.
TL-DEX DM.
Touro CC-LD.
Trispec PSE.
Tusnel.
Tusnel-DM Pediatric.
Tusnel Pediatric.
Z-Cof DMX.
Z-Cof 8 DM.
Z-Cof I.
W/Pheniramine Maleate, Phenylephrine Hydrochloride.
See: Theraflu Cold & Cough.
W/Phenylephrine Hydrochloride.
See: Little Colds Decongestant Plus Cough.
PediaCare Children's Multi-Symptom Cold.
Theraflu Thin Strips Daytime Cough & Cold.
Triaminic Children's Thin Strips Day Time Cold & Cough.
Triaminic Daytime Cold & Cough.
W/Phenylephrine Hydrochloride, Pyrilamine Maleate.
See: MyHist-DM.
Poly Hist DM.
Pyril DM.
W/Promethazine Hydrochloride.
See: Promethazine w/Dextromethorphan Cough.
W/Pyrilamine Maleate.
See: Capron DM.

dextromethorphan hydrobromide/benzocaine.
Use: Nonnarcotic antitussive.
See: Cēpacol Ultra Sore Throat Plus Cough.
Cough-X.
Tetra Formula.

dextromethorphan hydrobromide/guaifenesin. (URL) Dextromethorphan HBr 30 mg, guaifenesin 500 mg. Dye-free. ER Tab. 100s. *Rx.*
Use: Antitussive with expectorant, upper respiratory combination.

dextromethorphan hydrobromide, pseudoephedrine hydrochloride, chlorpheniramine maleate 30-30-4 mg. (Acella Pharmaceuticals) Chlorpheniramine maleate 4 mg, dextromethorphan hydrobromide 30 mg, pseudoephedrine hydrochloride 30 mg per 5 mL. Parabens, saccharin. Grape bubble gum flavor. Susp. 473 mL. *Rx.*
Use: Upper respiratory combination, antitussive combination.

•**dextromethorphan polistirex.** (DEX-troe-meth-OR-fan pahl-ee-STIE-rex) USAN.
Use: Antitussive.
W/Combinations.
See: Atuss-12 DM.
Atuss-12 DX.

dextromethorphan tannate.
Use: Antitussive.
W/Brompheniramine Tannate, Phenylephrine Tannate.
See: Neo DM.
W/Combinations.
See: TanaCof-DM.
Tanafed DMX.
Viravan-DM.
W/Dexbrompheniramine Tannate, Phenylephrine Tannate, Pyrilamine Maleate.
See: Poly Tan DM.
W/Dexchlorpheniramine Tannate, Pseudoephedrine Tannate.
See: Atuss DS Tannate.
Dur-Tann Forte.
W/Guaifenesin, Pseudoephedrine Tannate.
See: Z-Cof 12 DM.

dextromethorphan tannate, phenylephrine tannate, dexchlorpheniramine tannate. (River's Edge) Dexchlorpheniramine tannate 2 mg, dextromethorphan tannate 30 mg, phenylephrine tannate 20 mg per 5 mL. Saccharin. Alcohol free and sugar free. Cotton candy or strawberry flavor. Susp., Oral. 473 mL. *Rx.*
Use: Upper respiratory combination, antitussive combination.

dextromethorphan tannate, phenylephrine tannate, pyrilamine tannate. (River's Edge) Dextromethorphan tannate 25 mg, phenylephrine tannate 15.5 mg, pyrilamine tannate 15.5 mg per 5 mL. Saccharin. Alcohol free and sugar free. Cherry flavor. Susp., Oral. 473 mL. *Rx.*
Use: Upper respiratory combination, antitussive combination.

dextromoramide tartrate.
Use: Analgesic; narcotic.

dextro-pantothenyl alcohol.
See: Ilopan.
Panthenol.

dextropropoxyphene hydrochloride.
Use: Analgesic.
See: Propoxyphene Hydrochloride.

•**dextrorphan hydrochloride.** (DEX-trore-fan) USAN.
Use: Treatment of cerebral ischemia; vasospastic therapy adjunct.

•**dextrose.** (DEX-trose) *USP.*
Use: Fluid and nutrient replenisher.

W/Fructose, Phosphoric Acid.
See: Emetrol.
Nausatrol.
Nausea Relief.
Nausetrol.

dextrose and Isolyte combinations.
Use: Intravenous nutritional therapy, intravenous replenishment solution.
See: Isolyte M in 5% Dextrose.
Isolyte H in 5% Dextrose.
Isolyte P in 5% Dextrose.
Isolyte S with 5% Dextrose.
Isolyte R in 5% Dextrose.

dextrose and Normosol combinations.
Use: Intravenous nutritional therapy, intravenous replenishment solution.
See: Normosol-M and 5% Dextrose.
Normosol-R and 5% Dextrose.

dextrose and Plasmalyte combinations.
Use: Intravenous nutritional therapy, intravenous replenishment solution.
See: Plasma-Lyte 56 and 5% Dextrose.
Plasma-Lyte M and 5% Dextrose.
Plasma-Lyte 148 and 5% Dextrose.
Plasma-Lyte R and 5% Dextrose.

dextrose and Ringer's combinations.
Use: Intravenous nutritional therapy, intravenous replenishment solution.
See: Half-Strength Lactated Ringer's in 2.5% Dextrose.
Lactated Ringer's in 5% Dextrose.
Ringer's in 5% Dextrose.

dextrose-electrolyte solutions. *Rx.*
Use: Intravenous nutritional therapy, intravenous replenishment solutions.
See: Dextrose 2.5% with 0.45% Sodium Chloride.
Dextrose 3.3% and 0.3% Sodium Chloride.
Dextrose 5% and Electrolyte No. 48.
Dextrose 5% and Electrolyte No. 75.
Dextrose 5% with 0.2% Sodium Chloride.
Dextrose 5% and 0.225% Sodium Chloride.
Dextrose 5% with 0.3% Sodium Chloride.
Dextrose 5% with 0.33% Sodium Chloride.
Dextrose 5% with 0.45% Sodium Chloride.
Dextrose 5% with 0.9% Sodium Chloride.
Dextrose 10% and Electrolyte No. 48.
Dextrose 10% with 0.2% Sodium Chloride.
Dextrose 10% with 0.225% Sodium Chloride.
Dextrose 10% with 0.45 Sodium Chloride.
Dextrose 10% and 0.9% Sodium Chloride.
Dianeal Low Calcium w/4.25% Dextrose.
Dianeal Low Calcium w/1.5% Dextrose.
Dianeal Low Calcium w/2.5% Dextrose.
Dianeal PD-2 w/4.25% Dextrose.
Dianeal PD-2 w/1.5% Dextrose.
Dianeal PD-2 w/3.5% Dextrose.
Dianeal PD-2 w/2.5% Dextrose.
UltraBag Dianeal PD-2 w/4.25% Dextrose.
UltraBag Dianeal PD-2 w/1.5% Dextrose.
UltraBag Dianeal PD-2 w/2.5% Dextrose.
Half-Strength Lactated Ringer's in 2.5% Dextrose.
Ionosol B and 5% Dextrose.
Ionosol-T and 5% Dextrose.
Isolyte H in 5% Dextrose.
Isolyte M in 5% Dextrose.
Isolyte P in 5% Dextrose.
Isolyte R in 5% Dextrose.
Isolyte S with 5% Dextrose.
Lactated Ringer's in 5%% Dextrose.
Normosol-M and 5%% Dextrose.
Normosol-R and 5% Dextrose.
Plasma-Lyte 56 and 5% Dextrose.
Plasma-Lyte M and 5% Dextrose.
Plasma-Lyte 148 and 5% Dextrose.
Plasma-Lyte R and 5% Dextrose.
Potassium Chloride in 5% Dextrose and Lactated Ringer's.
Potassium Chloride in 5% Dextrose.
Potassium Chloride in 3.3% Dextrose and 0.3% Sodium Chloride.
Potassium Chloride in 5% Dextrose and 0.2% Sodium Chloride.
Potassium Chloride in 5% Dextrose and 0.33% Sodium Chloride.
Potassium Chloride in 5% Dextrose and 0.45% Sodium Chloride.
Potassium Chloride in 5% Dextrose and 0.9% Sodium Chloride.
Potassium Chloride in 10% Dextrose and 0.2% Sodium Chloride.
Ringer's in 5% Dextrose.

•**dextrose excipient.** (DEX-trose) *NF.*
Use: Pharmaceutic aid (tablet excipient).

dextrose 5% and electrolyte No. 48. (Baxter PPI) Dextrose 50 g, calories 180/L with Na^+ 25 mEq, K^+ 20 mEq, Mg^{++} 3 mEq, Cl^- 24 mEq, phosphate 3 mEq, acetate 23 mEq with osmolarity 348 mOsm/L. Soln. Bot. 250 mL. *Rx.*
Use: Intravenous nutritional therapy, intravenous replenishment.

dextrose 5% and electrolyte No. 75. (Baxter PPI) Dextrose 50 g, calories 180/L with Na^+ 40 mEq, K^+ 35 mEq, Cl^-

48 mEq, phosphate 15 mEq, and lactate 20 mEq with osmolarity 402 mOsm/L. Soln. Bot. 250 mL, 500 mL, 1000 mL. *Rx.*
Use: Intravenous nutritional therapy, intravenous replenishment.

dextrose 5% and lactated Ringer's and potassium chloride.
Use: Intravenous nutritional therapy, intravenous replenishment solution.
See: Potassium Chloride in 5% Dextrose and Lactated Ringer's.

dextrose 5% and potassium chloride.
Use: Intravenous nutritional therapy, intravenous replenishment solution.
See: Potassium Chloride in 5% Dextrose.

dextrose 5% and sodium chloride 0.45% and potassium chloride.
Use: Intravenous nutritional therapy, intravenous replenishment solution.
See: Potassium Chloride in 5% Dextrose and 0.45% Sodium Chloride.

dextrose 5% and sodium chloride 0.9% and potassium chloride.
Use: Intravenous nutritional therapy, intravenous replenishment solution.
See: Potassium Chloride in 5% Dextrose and 0.9% Sodium Chloride.

dextrose 5% and sodium chloride 0.33% and potassium chloride.
Use: Intravenous nutritional therapy, intravenous replenishment solution.
See: Potassium Chloride in 5% Dextrose and 0.33% Sodium Chloride.

dextrose 5% and sodium chloride 0.2% and potassium chloride.
Use: Intravenous nutritional therapy, intravenous replenishment solution.
See: Potassium Chloride in 5% Dextrose and 0.2% Sodium Chloride.

dextrose 5% and 0.225% sodium chloride. (Abbott) Dextrose 50 g, calories 170/L, Na^+ 38.5 mEq, Cl^- 38.5 mEq, osmolarity 329 mOsm/L. Soln. Bot. 250 mL, 500 mL, 1000 mL. *Rx.*
Use: Intravenous nutritional therapy, intravenous replenishment solution.

dextrose 5% with 0.45% sodium chloride. (Various Mfr.) Dextrose 50 g, calories 170/L, Na^+ 77 mEq, Cl^- 77 mEq, osmolarity ≈ 405 mOsm/L. Soln. Bot. 250 mL, 500 mL, 1000 mL. *Rx.*
Use: Intravenous nutritional therapy, intravenous replenishment solution.

dextrose 5% with 0.9% sodium chloride. (Various Mfr.) Dextrose 50 g, calories 170/L, Na^+ 154 mEq, Cl^- 154 mEq, osmolarity ≈ 560 mOsm/L. Soln. Bot. 250 mL, 500 mL, 1000 mL. *Rx.*
Use: Intravenous nutritional therapy, intravenous replenishment solution.

dextrose 5% with 0.3% sodium chloride. (Abbott) Dextrose 50 g, calories 170/L, Na^+ 51 mEq, Cl^- 51 mEq, osmolarity 355 mOsm/L. Soln. Bot. 250 mL, 500 mL, 1000 mL. *Rx.*
Use: Intravenous nutritional therapy, intravenous replenishment solution.

dextrose 5% with 0.33% sodium chloride. (Various Mfr.) Dextrose 50 g, calories 170/L, Na^+ 56 mEq, Cl^- 56 mEq, osmolarity 365 mOsm/L. Soln. Bot. 250 mL, 500 mL, 1000 mL. *Rx.*
Use: Intravenous nutritional therapy, intravenous replenishment solution.

dextrose 5% with 0.2% sodium chloride. (Various Mfr.) Dextrose 50 g, calories 170/L, Na^+ 34 mEq, Cl^- 34 mEq, osmolarity ≈ 320 mOsm/L. Soln. Bot. 250 mL, 500 mL, 1000 ML. *Rx.*
Use: Intravenous nutritional therapy, intravenous replenishment solution.

dextrose large volume parenterals. (Abbott Hospital Products) *Rx.*
Use: Nutritional supplement, parenteral.

dextrose small volume parenterals. (Abbott Hospital Products) **Dextrose 5%:** 50 mL, 100 mL pressurized pintop vial. **Dextrose 10%:** 5 mL amp. **Dextrose 25%:** 10 mL syringe. **Dextrose 50%:** 50 mL Abboject syringe (18 g × 1.5"), 50 mL Fliptop vial. **Dextrose 70%:** 70 mL pressurized pintop vial. *Rx.*
Use: Nutritional supplement, parenteral.

dextrose-sodium chloride injection. (Abbott) 10% dextrose and 0.225% sodium chloride. Inj. Single-dose container. 500 mL.
Use: Nutritional supplement, parenteral.

dextrose 10% and electrolyte no. 48. (Baxter Healthcare) Dextrose 100 g, calories 350/L, Na^+ 25 mEq, K^+ 20 mEq, Mg^{++} 3 mEq, Cl^- 24 mEq, phosphate 3 mEq, lactate 23 mEq, osmolarity 600 mOsm/L, sodium bisulfite Soln. Bot. 250 mL. *Rx.*
Use: Intravenous nutritional therapy, intravenous replenishment solution.

dextrose 10% and 0.9% sodium chloride. (Various Mfr.) Dextrose 100 g, calories 340/L, Na^+ 154 mEq, Cl^- 154 mEq, osmolarity 813–815 mOsm/L. Soln. Bot. 500 mL, 1000 mL. *Rx.*
Use: Intravenous nutritional therapy, intravenous replenishment solution.

dextrose 10% and 0.2% sodium chloride and potassium chloride.
Use: Intravenous nutritional therapy, intravenous replenishment solution.
See: Potassium Chloride in 10% Dextrose and 0.2% Sodium Chloride.

dextrose 10% with 0.45% sodium chloride. (B. Braun) Dextrose 100 g, calories 340/L, Na^+ 77 mEq, Cl^- 77 mEq, osmolarity 660 mOsm/L. Soln. Bot. 1000 mL. *Rx.*
Use: Intravenous nutritional therapy, intravenous replenishment solution.

dextrose 10% with 0.2% sodium chloride. (Various Mfr.) Dextrose 100 g, calories 340/L, Na^+ 34 mEq, Cl^- 34 mEq, osmolarity 575 mOsm/L. Soln. Bot. 250 mL. *Rx.*
Use: Intravenous nutritional therapy, intravenous replenishment solution.

dextrose 10% with 0.225% sodium chloride. (Abbott) Dextrose 100 g, calories 340/L, Na^+ 38.5 mEq, Cl^- 38.5 mEq, osmolarity 582 mOsm/L. Soln. Bot. 250 mL, 500 mL. *Rx.*
Use: Intravenous nutritional therapy, intravenous replenishment solution.

dextrose 3.3% and 0.3% sodium chloride. (B. Braun) Dextrose 33 g, calories 110/L, Na^+ 51 mEq, Cl^- 51 mEq, osmolarity 270 mOsm/L. Soln. Bot. 250 mL, 500 mL, 1000 mL. *Rx.*
Use: Intravenous nutritional therapy, intravenous replenishment solution.

dextrose 3.3% dextrose and 0.3% sodium chloride and potassium chloride.
Use: Intravenous nutritional therapy, intravenous replenishment solution.
See: Potassium chloride in 3.3% Dextrose and 0.3% Sodium Chloride.

dextrose 2.5% with 0.45% sodium chloride. (Various Mfr.) Dextrose 25 g, calories 85/L, Na^+ 77 mEq, Cl^- 77 mEq, osmolarity 280 mOsm/L. Soln. Bot. 500 mL, 1000 mL. *Rx.*
Use: Intravenous nutritional therapy, intravenous replenishment solution.

DextroStat. (Shire Richwood) Dextroamphetamine sulfate 5 mg, 10 mg. Sucrose, lactose, tartrazine. Tab. Bot. 100s. *c-II.*
Use: CNS stimulant, amphetamine.

Dexule. (Health for Life Brands) Vitamins A 1333 units, D 133 units, B_1 0.33 mg, B_2 0.4 mg, C 10 mg, niacinamide 3.3 mg, iron 3.3 mg, calcium 29 mg, phosphorus 15 mg, methylcellulose 100 mg, benzocaine 3 mg. Cap. Bot. 21s, 90s. *OTC.*
Use: Mineral, vitamin supplement.

Dexyl. (Pinex) Dextromethorphan HBr 15 mg, vitamin C 20 mg. Tab. Box 20s. *OTC.*
Use: Antitussive; vitamin supplement.

•**dezaguanine.** (DEH-zah-GWAHN-een) USAN.
Use: Antineoplastic.

•**dezaguanine mesylate.** (DEE-zah-GWAHN-een) USAN.
Use: Antineoplastic.

•**dezinamide.** (deh-ZIN-ah-mide) USAN.
Use: Anticonvulsant.

D-Film. (Ciba Vision) Poloxamer 407, EDTA 0.25%, benzalkonium Cl 0.025%. Gel. Tube 25 g. *OTC.*
Use: Contact lens care.

D-5000 Super Strength. (21st Century) Cholecalciferol 5,000 units. Calcium 180 mg. Gluten free. Tab. 110s. *OTC.*
Use: Fat-soluble vitamin.

DFMO. Eflornithine hydrochloride. *Rx.*
Use: Anti-infective.
See: Ornidyl.

D400. (Mason) Cholecalciferol (D_3). **Chew. Tab.:** 400 units. Fructose, sucrose, sunflower oil, xylitol. Vanilla flavor. 100s. **Cap., softgel:** 400 units. Glycerin, soybean oil. 100s. *OTC.*
Use: Vitamin, fat-soluble vitamin.

d4T.
Use: Antiviral.
See: Stavudine.

DFP. Disopropyl fluorophosphate (Various Mfr.)

d-Glucose. Dextrose. *Rx.*
Use: Nutritional supplement, parenteral.
See: D-10-W.

DHEA. (Athena Neurosciences) EL10. *Rx.*
Use: Antiviral; immunomodulator.

D.H.E. 45. (Xcel) Dihydroergotamine mesylate 1 mg/mL, alcohol 6.2%, glycerin 15%. Inj. Amp. 1 mL. *Rx.*
Use: Antimigraine, ergotamine derivative.

D-Hist D. (Midlothian) Pseudoephedrine hydrochloride 45 mg, dexchlorpheniramine maleate 3.5 mg, methscopolamine nitrate 1 mg. ER Tab. 100s. *Rx.*
Use: Upper respiratory combination, decongestant, antihistamine, and anticholinergic combination.

DHPG. Ganciclovir sodium. *Rx.*
Use: Antiviral.
See: Cytovene.

DHS Conditioning Rinse. (Person and Covey) Conditioning ingredients. Bot. 8 oz. *OTC.*
Use: Dermatologic, hair.

DHS Shampoo. (Person and Covey) Blend of cleansing surfactants and emulsifiers. Plastic bot. w/dispenser 8 oz, 16 oz. *OTC.*
Use: Dermatologic, hair, and scalp.

DHS Tar Gel Shampoo. (Person and Covey) Coal tar 0.5% Bot. 240 g. *OTC.*
Use: Antipsoriatic; antiseborrheic.

DHS Tar Shampoo. (Person and Covey) Coal tar 0.5%. Liq. Bot. 120 mL,

240 mL, 480 mL. *OTC.*
Use: Antipsoriatic; antiseborrheic.

DHS Zinc. (Person and Covey) Pyrithione zinc 2%. Shampoo. Bot. 240 mL, 360 mL. *OTC.*
Use: Dermatologic agent.

DiaBeta. (Hoechst Marion Roussel) Glyburide 1.25 mg, 2.5 mg, 5 mg. Tab. 50s (1.25 mg only), 100s (2.5 mg only), 500s (except 1.25 mg), 1000s (5 mg only). *Rx.*
Use: Antidiabetic.

Diabetic Tussin. (Health Care Products) Guaifenesin 100 mg/5 mL. Alcohol and dye free. Aspartame, menthol, methylparaben, phenylalanine 8.4 mg/5 mL. Liq. Bot. 118 mL. *Rx.*
Use: Antitussive, decongestant, expectorant.

Diabetic Tussin Cold & Flu. (Health Care Products) Acetaminophen 325 mg, dextromethorphan hydrobromide 10 mg, diphenhydramine 12.5 mg. Acesulfame K, aspartame, menthol, methylparaben, orange flavoring, PEG, phenylalanine 8.4 mg, potassium sorbate, propylene glycol. Alcohol free, dye free, and sugar free. Liq. 118 mL, 237 mL. *OTC.*
Use: Upper respiratory combination, antitussive combination.

Diabetic Tussin DM. (Health Care Products) Dextromethorphan HBr 10 mg, guaifenesin 100 mg per 5 mL. Methylparaben, menthol, aspartame, phenylalanine 8.4 mg per 5 mL. Alcohol, sugar, and dye free. Liq. Bot. 118 mL. *OTC.*
Use: Upper respiratory combination, antitussive with expectorant.

Diabetic Tussin Maximum Strength DM. (Health Care Products) Dextromethorphan HBr 10 mg, guaifenesin 200 mg per 5 mL. Aspartame, phenylalanine 8.4 mg per 5 mL, menthol, methylparaben, PEG. Sugar, alcohol, and dye free. Liq. Bot. 237 mL. *OTC.*
Use: Upper respiratory combination, antitussive with expectorant.

Diabetic Tussin Mucus Relief. (Health Care Products) Guaifenesin 400 mg. Maltodextrin. Sugar free, dye free. Tab. 50s. *OTC.*
Use: Expectorant.

Diabetic Tussin Night Time Formula Cold/Flu. (Health Care Products) Acetaminophen 325 mg, dextromethorphan hydrobromide 10 mg, diphenhydramine 12.5 mg. Acesulfame K, aspartame, menthol, methylparaben, PEG, phenylalanine 8.4 mg per 5 mL. Alcohol free, dye free, and sugar free. Liq. 118 mL. *OTC.*
Use: Upper respiratory combination, antitussive combination.

DiabetiDerm. (Health Care Products) Alcohols, benzyl alcohol, glycerin, glyceryl, lactic acid, parabens, urea, dimethicone, caprylic/capric triglyceride. Lot. 237 mL. *OTC.*
Use: Emollient.

DiabetiDerm. (Health Care Products) Undecylenic acid 10%. Aloe, cetyl alcohol, clotrimazole, disodium EDTA, glyceryl, lavender oil, parabens, PEG-100, tea tree oil, triethanolamine, urea. Cream. 42 g. *OTC.*
Use: Anti-infective, topical; antifungal agent.

diacetic acid test.
See: Acetest Reagent.

Diaceto w/Codeine. (Archer-Taylor) Codeine 0.25 g, 0.5 g. Tab. or Cap. Bot. 500s, 1000s. *c-II.*
Use: Analgesic; narcotic.

Diaceto w/Gelsemium. (Archer-Taylor) Phenobarbital 0.5 g, gelsemium 3 min. Tab. Bot. 1000s. *c-IV.*
Use: Hypnotic; sedative.

•**diacetolol hydrochloride.** (DIE-ah-SEET-oh-lahl) USAN.
Use: Antiadrenergic (β-receptor).

diacetrizoate, sodium.
See: Diatrizoate.

diacetylated monoglycerides.
Use: Pharmaceutic aid (plasticizer).

diacetylcholine chloride. Succinylcholine Cl.
See: Anectine Chloride.

diacetyl-dihydroxydiphenylisatin.
See: Oxyphenisatin Acetate.

diacetyldioxyphenylisatin.
See: Oxyphenisatin Acetate.

diacetylmorphine salts. Heroin. Illegal in USA by federal statute because of its addiction potential.

Di-Ademil.
See: Hydroflumethiazide.

diagnostic agents.
See: Aplisol.
Aplitest.
Candida Albicans Skin Test Antigen.
Candin.
Cardio-Green Disposable Unit.
Cea-Roche.
Cholecystography Agents.
Cholografin Meglumine.
Coccidioidin.
Evans Blue Dye.
EZ Detect Strep-A Test.
Fertility Tape.
First Choice.
Fluor-I-Strip.

Fluor-I-Strip A.T.
Fluress.
Hema-Combistix Reagent Strips.
Histolyn-CYL.
Histoplasmin.
HIVAB HIV-1/HIV-2 (rDNA) EIA.
Immunex CRP.
Indigo Carmine.
Kidney Function Agents.
Liver Function Agents.
Mannitol.
Mono-Latex.
Mono-Plus.
MSTA.
Mumps Skin Test Antigen.
Persantine IV.
Pharmalgen Hymenoptera Venoms.
Pharmalgen Standardized Allergenic Extracts.
Phentolamine Methanesulfonate.
Radiopaque Agents.
Rheumatex.
Rheumaton.
Spherulin.
SureCell Herpes (HSV) Test.
SureCell Strep A Test.
Tine Test.
True Test.
Tubersol.
Urography Agents.
Venomil.

diagnostic agents for urine.
See: Acetest Reagent.
Albustix Reagent Strips.
Biotel Diabetes.
Biotel U.T.I.
Chemstrip Micral.
Clinistix Reagent Strips.
Clinitest.
Fortel Midstream.
Fortel Plus.
HCG-Nostick.
Hema-Combistix Reagent Strips.
Hemastix Reagent Strips.
Hematest Reagent Strips.
Ictotest Reagent Tablets.
Ketostix Reagent Strips.
SureCell hCG-Urine Test.
Uristix.
Wampole One-Step hCG.

diallylamicol. Diallyl-diethylaminoethyl phenol di hydrochloride.

diallylbarbituric acid. Allobarbital, Allobarbitone, Curral.

dialminate. Mixture of magnesium carbonate and (aluminate) dihydroxyaluminum glycinate.

Dialyte Pattern LM w/4.25% Dextrose. (Gambro) Dextrose 42.5 g/L, Na^+ 131.5, Ca^{++} 3.5, Mg^{++} 0.5, Cl^- 94, and lactate 40 with osmolarity 485 mOsm/L. Soln. Bot. 1000 mL, 2000 mL, 4000 mL. *Rx.*
Use: Peritoneal dialysis solution.

Dialyte Pattern LM w/1.5% Dextrose. (Gambro) Dextrose 15 g/L, Na^+ 131 mEq, Ca^{++} 3.5 mEq, Mg^{++} 0.5 mEq, Cl^- 94 mEq, and lactate 40 mEq with osmolarity 345 mOsm/L. Soln. Bot. 1000 mL, 2000 mL, 4000 mL. *Rx.*
Use: Peritoneal dialysis solution.

Dialyte Pattern LM w/2.5% Dextrose. (Gambro) Dextrose 25 g/L, Na^+ 131.5 mEq, Ca^{++} 3.5 mEq, Mg^{++} 0.5 mEq, Cl^- 94 mEq, and lactate 40 mEq with osmolarity 395 mOsm/L. Soln. Bot. 1000 mL, 2000 mL, 4000 mL. *Rx.*
Use: Peritoneal dialysis solution.

Dialyvite 800 with Iron. (Hillestad) Fe 29 mg, vitamins B_1 1.5 mg, B_2 1.7 mg, B_3 20 mg, B_5 10 mg, B_6 10 mg, B_{12} 6 mcg, C 60 mg, folic acid 0.8 mg, biotin 300 mcg. Glyceryl. Tab. 100s. *OTC.*
Use: Multivitamin with iron.

Dialyvite Multi-Vitamins for Dialysis Patients. (Hillestad) Vitamin $B_6$10 mg, vitamin B_{12} 6 mcg, vitamin C 100 mg, folic acid 1 mg, d-biotin 300 mcg, pantothenic acid 10 mg, thiamine 1.5 mg, riboflavin 1.7 mg, niacinamide 20 mg. Tab. 100s. *Rx.*
Use: Nutritional combination product.

Dialyvite 3000. (Hillestad) Vitamin C 100 mg, B_1 1.5 mg, B_2 1.7 mg, B_3 20 mg, B_5 10 mg, B_6 25 mg, B_{12} 1 mg, FA 3 mg, biotin 300 mcg, E 30 units, Se 70 mcg, Zn 15 mg. Tab. 90s. *OTC.*
Use: Nutritional combination product.

Dialyvite with Zinc. (Hillestad) Vitamin B_1 1.5 mg, vitamin B_2 1.7 mg, vitamin B_3 20 mg, vitamin B_5 10 mg, vitamin B_6 10 mg, vitamin B_{12} 6 mcg, C 100 mg, d-biotin 300 mcg, folic acid 1 mg, Zn 50 mg. Tab. 100s. *Rx.*
Use: Nutritional combination, B vitamin with vitamin C.

diaminodiphenylsulfone.
Use: Antimalarial.
See: Dapsone.

diaminopropyl tetramethylene.
See: Spermine.

3,4-diaminopyridine. (Jacobus)
Use: Lambert-Eaton myasthenic syndrome. [Orphan Drug]

•**diamocaine cyclamate.** (die-AM-oh-CANE SIH-klah-mate) USAN.
Use: Anesthetic, local.

Diamox Squels. (Barr) Acetazolamide 500 mg. ER Cap. 100s. *Rx.*
Use: Diuretic, carbonic anhydrase inhibitor.

diamthazole dihydrochloride. (DYE-am-tha-ZOLE)
Use: Antifungal.

Dianeal Low Calcium w/4.25% Dextrose. (Baxter) Dextrose 4.25 g/L, Na^+132 mEq/L, Ca^{++} 2.5 mEq/L, Mg^{++} 0.5 mEq/L, Cl^- 95 mEq/L, lactate 40 mEq/L, osmolarity 483 mOsm/L. Preservative free. Inj., Soln. *AMBU-FLEX II* and *AMBU-FLEX III* containers. 2,000 mL, 2,500 mL, 3,000 mL, 5,000 mL, 6,000 mL. *Rx.*
Use: Electrolyte, peritoneal dialysis solution.

Dianeal Low Calcium w/1.5% Dextrose. (Baxter) Dextrose 1.5 g/L, Na^+ 132 mEq/L, Ca^{++} 2.5 mEq/L, Mg^{++} 0.5 mEq/L, Cl^- 95 mEq/L, lactate 40 mEq/L, osmolarity 344 mOsm/L. Preservative free. Inj., Soln. *AMBU-FLEX II* container. 2,000 mL, 2,500 mL, 3,000 mL, 5,000 mL, 6,000 mL. *Rx.*
Use: Electrolyte, peritoneal dialysis solution.

Dianeal Low Calcium w/2.5% Dextrose. (Baxter) Dextrose 2.5 g/L, Na^+ 132 mEq/L, Ca^{++} 2.5 mEq/L, Mg^{++} 0.5 mEq/L, Cl^- 95 mEq/L, lactate 40 mEq/L, osmolarity 395 mOsm/L. Preservative free. Inj., Soln. *AMBU-FLEX II* and *AMBU-FLEX III* containers. 2,000 mL, 2,500 mL, 3,000 mL, 5,000 mL, 6,000 mL. *Rx.*
Use: Electrolyte, peritoneal dialysis solution.

Dianeal 137 w/4.25% Dextrose. (Baxter) Dextrose 42.5 g/L, Na^+ 132 mEq, Ca^{++} 3.5 mEq, Mg^{++} 1.5 mEq, Cl^- 102 mEq, lactate 35 mEq with osmolarity 486 mOsm/L. Soln. 2,000 mL. *Rx.*
Use: Peritoneal dialysis solution.

Dianeal 137 w/1.5% Dextrose. (Baxter) Dextrose 15 g/L, Na^+ 132 mEq, Ca^{++} 3.5 mEq, Mg^{++} 1.5 mEq, Cl^- 102 mEq, lactate 35 mEq with osmolarity 347 mOsm/L. Soln. 2,000 mL. *Rx.*
Use: Peritoneal dialysis solution.

Dianeal PD-2 w/4.25% Dextrose. (Baxter) Dextrose 4.25 g/L, Na^+ 132 mEq/L, Ca^{++} 3.5 mEq/L, Mg^{++} 0.5 mEq/L, Cl^- 96 mEq/L, lactate 40 mEq/L, osmolarity 485 mOsm/L. Preservative free. Inj., Soln. *AMBU-FLEX II* container. 1,000 mL, 2,000 mL, 2,500 mL, 3,000 mL, 5,000 mL, 6,000 mL. *AMBU-FLEX III* container. 500 mL, 1,000 mL, 2,000 mL, 2,500 mL, 3,000 mL, 5,000 mL, 6,000 mL. *Rx.*
Use: Electrolyte, peritoneal dialysis solution.

Dianeal PD-2 w/1.5% Dextrose. (Baxter) Dextrose 1.5 g/L, Na^+ 132 mEq/L, Ca^{++} 3.5 mEq/L, Mg^{++} 0.5 mEq/L, Cl^- 96 mEq/L, lactate 40 mEq/L, osmolarity 346 mOsm/L. Preservative free. Inj., Soln. *AMBU-FLEX II* container. 1,000 mL, 2,000 mL, 2,500 mL, 3,000 mL, 5,000 mL, 6,000 mL. *AMBU-FLEX III* container. 250 mL, 500 mL, 1,000 mL, 2,000 mL, 2,500 mL, 3,000 mL, 5,000 mL, 6,000 mL. *Rx.*
Use: Electrolyte, peritoneal dialysis solution.

Dianeal PD-2 w/3.5% Dextrose. (Baxter) Dextrose 3.5 g/L, Na^+ 132 mEq/L, Ca^{++} 3.5 mEq/L, Mg^{++} 0.5 mEq/L, Cl^- 96 mEq/L, lactate 40 mEq/L, osmolarity 447 mOsm/L. Preservative free. Inj., Soln. *AMBU-FLEX III* container. 2,500 mL. *Rx.*
Use: Electrolyte, peritoneal dialysis solution.

Dianeal PD-2 w/2.5% Dextrose. (Baxter) Dextrose 2.5 g/L, Na^+ 132 mEq/L, Ca^{++} 3.5 mEq/L, Mg^{++} 0.5 mEq/L, Cl^- 96 mEq/L, lactate 40 mEq/L, osmolarity 396 mOsm/L. Preservative free. Inj., Soln. *AMBU-FLEX II* container. 1,000 mL, 2,000 mL, 2,500 mL, 3,000 mL, 5,000 mL, 6,000 mL. *AMBU-FLEX III* container. 250 mL, 500 mL, 1,000 mL, 2,000 mL, 2,500 mL, 3,000 mL, 5,000 mL, 6,000 mL. *Rx.*
Use: Electrolyte, peritoneal dialysis solution.

Dianeal peritoneal dialysis solution with 1.1% amino acid.
Use: Nutritional supplement for dialysis patients. [Orphan Drug]

Dianeal w/4.25% Dextrose. (Baxter) Dextrose 42.5 g/L, Na^+ 141 mEq, Ca^{++} 3.5 mEq, Mg^{++} 1.5 mEq, Cl^- 101 mEq, lactate 45 mEq with osmolarity 503 mOsm/L. Soln. Bot. 2000 mL. *Rx.*
Use: Peritoneal dialysis solution.

Dianeal w/1.5% Dextrose. (Baxter) Dextrose 15 g/L, Na^+ 141 mEq, Ca^{++} 3.5 mEq, Mg^{++}1.5 mEq, Cl^- 101 mEq, lactate 45 mEq with osmolarity 364 mOsm/L. Soln. Bot. 1000 mL, 2000 mL. *Rx.*
Use: Peritoneal dialysis solution.

•**dianexin.** (DYE-a-NEX-in) USAN.
Use: Prevention of ischemia reperfusion injury.

•**diapamide.** (die-APP-am-ide) USAN.
Use: Antihypertensive; diuretic.

Diapantin. (Janssen) Isopropamide bromide. *Rx.*
Use: Anticholinergic.

Diaparene. (Bayer Consumer Care) Methylbenzethonium chloride. Pow. Bot.

4 oz, 9 oz, 12.5 oz, 14 oz.
Use: Disinfectant; surface active agent.

Diaparene Ointment. (Bayer Consumer Care) Methylbenzethonium chloride 0.1% w/petrolatum, glycerin. Tube 1 oz, 2 oz, 4 oz. *OTC.*
Use: Antimicrobial, topical.

Diaparene Peri-Anal Cream. (Bayer Consumer Care) Methylbenzethonium chloride 1:1000, zinc oxide, starch, cod liver oil, white petrolatum, lanolin, calcium caseinate. Cream. Tube 1 oz, 2 oz, 4 oz. *OTC.*
Use: Antimicrobial; astringent.

Diaper Guard. (Del) Dimethicone 1%, white petrolatum 66%, cocoa butter, parabens, vitamins A, D_3, E, zinc oxide. Oint. Tube 49.6 g, 99.2 g. *OTC.*
Use: Diaper rash preparation.

Diaper Rash. (Various Mfr.) Zinc oxide, cod liver oil, lanolin, methylparaben, petrolatum, talc. Oint. Tube 113 g. *OTC.*
Use: Diaper rash preparation.

diaphenylsulfone. Dapsone.
Use: Leprostatic.

•**diaplasinin.** (dye-a-PLAS-in-in) USAN.
Use: Hematologic agent.

Di-Ap-Trol. (Foy Laboratories) Phendimetrazine tartrate 35 mg. Tab. Bot. 100s, 1000s. *c-III.*
Use: Anorexiant.

Diarrest. (Dover Pharmaceuticals) Calcium carbonate, pectin. Tab. Sugar, lactose, salt free. UD box 500s. *OTC.*
Use: Antidiarrheal.

diarrhea therapy.
See: Antidiarrheal.

Diaserp. (Major) Chlorothiazide 250 mg, 500 mg, w/reserpine. Tab. Bot. 100s. *Rx.*
Use: Antihypertensive.

Diasporal. (Doak Dermatologics) *Formerly Sulfur Salicyl Diasporal.* Sulfur 3%, salicylic acid 2%, isopropyl alcohol in diasporal base. Cream. Jar 3¾ oz. *OTC.*
Use: Antiseptic, topical.

Diastase.
See: Aspergillus oryzae enzyme.

Diastat. (Valeant Pharmaceuticals) Diazepam 2.5 mg. Benzyl alcohol 1.5%, ethyl alcohol 10%. Rectal gel. Twin pack. Includes lubricating jelly, plastic applicator with flexible, molded tip in two lengths.
Use: Anticonvulsant.

Diastat AcuDial. (Xcel) Diazepam 2.5 mg, 10 mg, 20 mg. Benzyl alcohol 1.5%, ethyl alcohol 10%. Rectal Gel. Twin packs. Includes lubricating jelly and plastic applicator. *c-IV.*
Use: Anticonvulsant; antianxiety agent.

•**diatrizoate meglumine.** (die-ah-TRIH-zoe-ate meh-GLUE-meen) *USP.*
Use: Radiopaque agent, parenteral agent.
See: Angiovist 282.
Cystografin.
Cystografin Dilute.
W/Sodium diatrizoate.
See: Renovist.

diatrizoate meglumine 52.7% and iodipamide meglumine 26.8% (38% iodine).
Use: Radiopaque agent.
See: Sinografin.

diatrizoate meglumine 66% and diatrizoate sodium 10%.
Use: Radiopaque agent, iodinated GI contrast agent.
See: Gastrografin.
Hypaque-76.
MD-76 R.
RenoCal-76.

diatrizoate methylglucamine.
Use: Diagnostic aid (radiopaque medium).
See: Diatrizoate Meglumine.

diatrizoate methylglucamine sodium.
Use: Diagnostic aid (radiopaque medium).

•**diatrizoate sodium.** (DYE-a-trye-ZOE-ate) *USP.*
Use: Diagnostic aid (radiopaque medium).
See: Hypaque.
Urovist Sodium 300.
W/Methylglucamine diatrizoate, sodium citrate, disodium ethylenediamine tetraacetate dihydrate, methylparaben, propylparaben.
See: Renovist.

diatrizoate sodium (59.87% iodine).
Use: Radiopaque agent, iodinated GI contrast agent.
See: Hypaque Sodium.

•**diatrizoate sodium I 131.** (DYE-a-trye-ZOE-ate) USAN.
Use: Radiopharmaceutical.

•**diatrizoate sodium I 125.** (DYE-a-trye-ZOE-ate) USAN.
Use: Radiopharmaceutical.

•**diatrizoic acid.** (DIE-at-rih-ZOE-ik) *USP.*
Use: Diagnostic aid (radiopaque medium).
See: Hypaque Sodium Salt.

Diatx. (Pan American) Vitamin B_1 1.5 mg, B_2 1.5 mg, B_3 20 mg, B_5 10 mg, B_6 50 mg, B_{12} 1 mg, C 60 mg, folic acid 5 mg, D-biotin 300 mcg, dye free. Tab. Bot. 90s. *Rx.*
Use: Vitamin supplement.

DiatxFe. (Pan American) Fe (as ferrous fumarate) 100 mg, B_1 1.5 mg, B_2 1.5 mg, B_3 20 mg, B_5 10 mg, B_6 50 mg, B_{12} 1 mg, C 60 mg, folic acid 5 mg, D-biotin 300 mcg, dye free. Tab. Bot. 90s. *Rx.*
Use: Vitamin supplement.

•**diaveridine.** (DIE-ah-ver-ih-deen) USAN.
Use: Anti-infective.

•**diazepam.** (DIE-aze-uh-pam) *USP.*
Use: Agent for control of emotional disturbances; anxiolytic; hypnotic; sedative.
See: Diastat.
Diastat AcuDial.
Diazepam Intensol.
Valium.

diazepam. (Roxane) Diazepam 5 mg/5 mL. Sorbitol, wintergreen spice flavor. Oral Soln. 500 mL, 5 mg patient cups, 10 mg patient cups. *c-IV.*
Use: Agent for control of emotional disturbances; anxiolytic; hypnotic; sedative; anticonvulsant.

diazepam. (Teva) Diazepam 2.5 mg, 10 mg, 20 mg. Benzyl alcohol 1.5%, ethyl alcohol 10%, benzoic acid, propylene glycol. Gel, rectal. Prefilled unit-dose rectal delivery system 2s. Includes lubricating jelly and plastic applicator with flexible, molded tip 4.4 cm (2.5 mg, 10 mg) or 6 cm (20 mg) in length. *c-IV.*
Use: Antianxiety agent, benzodiazepine.

diazepam. (Various Mfr.) **Tab.:** 2 mg, 5 mg, 10 mg. May contain lactose. Bot. 100s, 500s, 1000s, 5000s. **Inj.:** 5 mg/mL. Propylene glycol 40%, ethyl alcohol 10%, sodium benzoate 5%, benzoic acid, benzyl alcohol 1.5%. 2 mL *Carpuject* cartridges. *c-IV.*
Use: Agent for control of emotional disturbances; anxiolytic; hypnotic; sedative; anticonvulsant.

Diazepam Intensol. (Roxane) Diazepam 5 mg/mL. Alcohol 19%. Oral Soln. Concentrate. 30 mL with dropper. *c-IV.*
Use: Anxiolytic; anticonvulsant.

diazepam viscous solution for rectal administration. (Athena Neurosciences)
Use: To treat acute repetitive seizures. [Orphan Drug]

•**diaziquone.** (DIE-azz-ih-kwone) USAN.
Use: Antineoplastic.

diazomycins A, B, and C. Antibiotic obtained from *Streptomyces ambofaciens.* Under study.

•**diazoxide.** (DIE-aze-OX-ide) *USP.*
Use: Antihypertensive.
See: Proglycem.

dibasic calcium phosphate dihydrate.
Use: Replenisher (calcium); pharmaceutic aid (tablet base).
See: Diostate D.

Dibatrol. (Lexis Laboratories) Chlorpropamide 100 mg, 250 mg. Tab. Bot. 100s, 1000s. *Rx.*
Use: Antidiabetic.

dibenzapine derivatives.
Use: Antipsychotic.
See: Asenapine.
Clozapine.
Loxapine.
Olanzapine.
Quetiapine Fumarate.

•**dibenzepin hydrochloride.** (die-BEN-zeh-pin) USAN.
Use: Antidepressant.

•**dibenzothiophene.** (die-BEN-zoe-THIGH-oh-feen) USAN.
Use: Keratolytic.

Dibenzyline. (Wellspring) Phenoxybenzamine hydrochloride 10 mg. Cap. Bot. 100s. *Rx.*
Use: Pheochromocytoma agent; antihypertensive.

•**dibotermin alfa.** (dye-BOE-ter-min) USAN.
Use: Osteoinductive agent.

•**dibromsalan.** (die-BROME-sah-lan) USAN.
Use: Antimicrobial; disinfectant.

•**dibucaine.** (DIE-byoo-cane) *USP.*
Use: Topical local anesthetic, amide local anesthetic.
See: Nupercainal.
W/Sodium bisulfite.
See: Nupercainal.
W/Zinc oxide, bismuth subgallate, acetone sodium bisulfite.
See: Nupercainal.

dibucaine. (Various Mfr.) Dibucaine 1%. Oint. 30 g. *OTC.*
Use: Topical local anesthetic, amide local anesthetic.

•**dibucaine hydrochloride.** (DIE-byoo-cane) *USP.*
Use: Anesthetic, local.
W/Antipyrine, hydrocortisone, polymyxin B sulfate, neomycin sulfate.
See: Otocort.
W/Colistin sodium methanesulfonate, citric acid, sodium citrate.
See: Coly-Mycin M Parenteral.

dibutoline sulfate. Ethyl (2-hydroxyethyl)-dimethylammonium sulfate (2:1) bis (dibutyl-carbam-ate).
Use: Anticholinergic; antispasmodic.

•**dibutyl sebacate.** (dye-BUE-til SEB-a-kate) *NF.*
Use: Pharmaceutic aid (plasticizer).

Dical. (Rugby) Calcium 116 mg, vitamin

D 133 units, phosphorus 90 mg. Captab. Bot. 1000s. *OTC.*
Use: Mineral, vitamin supplement.

dicalcium phosphate. (Various Mfr.) Dibasic calcium phosphate, monocalcium phosphate. **Cap.:** 7.5 g, 10 g. **Tab.:** 7.5 g, 10 g, 15 g. **Wafer:** 15 g. *OTC.*
Use: Mineral supplement.
W/Calcium Gluconate and Vitamin D.
See: CalciCaps.

Dical-Dee. (Alpharma) Vitamin D 350 units, dibasic calcium phosphate 4.5 g, calcium gluconate 3 g. Cap. Bot. 100s, 1000s. *OTC.*
Use: Mineral, vitamin supplement.

Dicaldel. (Faraday) Dibasic calcium phosphate 300 mg, calcium gluconate 200 mg, vitamin D 33 units. Cap. Bot. 100s, 250s, 500s, 1000s. *OTC.*
Use: Mineral, vitamin supplement.

Dical-D with Vitamin C. (Abbott) Dibasic calcium phosphate containing calcium 116.7 mg, phosphorus 90 mg, vitamin D 133 units, ascorbic acid 15 mg. Cap. Bot. 100s.
Use: Mineral, vitamin supplement.

Dicaltabs. (Faraday) Dibasic calcium phosphate 108 mg, calcium gluconate 140 mg, vitamin D 35 units. Tab. Bot. 100s, 250s, 1000s. *OTC.*
Use: Mineral, vitamin supplement.

Dicarbosil. (BIRA) Calcium carbonate 500 mg (elemental calcium 200 mg). Sodium < 2 mg, ANC 10 mEq. Peppermint flavor. Chew. Tab. Roll 12s. *OTC.*
Use: Mineral supplement; antacid.

Dicel CD. (Centrix) Brompheniramine maleate 2 mg, chlophedianol hydrochloride 12.5 mg, pseudoephedrine hydrochloride 30 mg. Glycerin, grape flavoring, propylene glycol, saccharin, sorbitol. Alcohol free, dye free, and sugar free. Liq. 473 mL. *OTC.*
Use: Upper respiratory combination, antitussive combination.

Dicel DM. (Centrix) Chlorpheniramine maleate 2 mg, dextromethorphan hydrobromide 10 mg, pseudoephedrine hydrochloride 30 mg. Maltodextrin, glycyrrhizic, vegetable oil, PEG, soy lecithin, sucralose, sugar. Alcohol free. Cotton candy flavor. Chew. Tab. 20s. *Rx.*
Use: Upper respiratory combination, antitussive combination.

Di-Cet. (Sanford & Son) Methylbenzethonium Cl 24.4 g, sodium carbonate monohydrate 48.8 g, sodium nitrite 24.4 g, trisodium ethylenediamine tetraacetate monohydrate 2.4 g. Pow. Pkg. 2.4 g. Box 24s.
Use: Disinfectant.

dichloralantipyrine. Dichloralphenazone. Chloralpyrine. A complex of 2 mol. chloral hydrate with 1 mol. antipyrine. Sominat.
W/Isometheptene mucate, acetaminophen.
See: Midrin.

•**dichloralphenazone.** (die-klor-al-FEN-ah-zone) *USP.*
Use: Hypnotic; sedative.
W/Acetaminophen, Isometheptene Mucate.
See: Epidrin.
Midrin.
Migrazone.
Nodolor.

Dichloramine T. (Various Mfr.) (1% to 5% in chlorinated paraffin). P-Toluenesulfonedichloramine.
Use: Antiseptic.

dichloren.
See: Mechlorethamine Hydrochloride.

dichloroacetic acid. *Rx.*
Use: Cauterizing agent.

•**dichlorodifluoromethane.** (die-KLOR-oh-die-flure-oh-METH-ane) *NF.*
Use: Pharmaceutic aid (aerosol propellant).
W/Trichloromonofluroromethane.
See: Gebauer's Spray and Stretch.

dichlorodiphenyl trichloroethane.
See: Chlorophenothane.

dichlorophenarsine hydrochloride. (Chlorarsen, Clorarsen, Fontarsol, Halarsol).

dichlorophene. Related to hexachlorophene.

•**dichlorotetrafluoroethane.** (die-KLOR-oh-teh-trah-flur-oh-ETH-ane) *NF.*
Use: Pharmaceutic aid (aerosol propellant).
W/Ethyl Chloride.
See: Fluro-Ethyl.

•**dichlorvos.** (DIE-klor-vahs) USAN.
Use: Anthelmintic.

•**dicirenone.** (die-sigh-REN-ohn) USAN.
Use: Hypotensive; aldosterone antagonist.

Dickey's Old Reliable Eye Wash. (Dickey Drug) Berberine sulfate, boric acid, parabens. Plastic dropper bot. 8 mL, 12 mL, 1 oz. *OTC.*
Use: Counterirritant, ophthalmic.

Diclegis. (Duchesnay USA) Doxylamine succinate 10 mg/pyridoxine hydrochloride 10 mg. Film coated. PEG. Tab., delayed release. 100s. *Rx.*
Use: Antiemetic/antivertigo agent.

•**diclofenac.** (dye-KLOE-fen-ak) USAN.
Use: Analgesic.

diclofenac epolamine.
Use: Nonsteroidal anti-inflammatory agent, topical.

•**diclofenac potassium.** (die-KLOE-fen-ak) USAN.
Use: Analgesic; NSAID.
See: Cambia.
Cataflam.
Zipsor.

diclofenac potassium. (Various Mfr.) Diclofenac potassium 50 mg. Tab. Bot. 100s, 500s. *Rx.*
Use: Analgesic; NSAID.

•**diclofenac sodium.** (die-KLOE-fen-ak) *USP.*
Use: Analgesic; NSAID.
See: Solaraze.
Voltaren.
Voltaren-XR.

diclofenac sodium. (Akorn) Diclofenac sodium 0.1%. EDTA. Soln., Ophth. 2.5 mL, 5 mL. *Rx.*
Use: Nonsteroidal anti-inflammatory drug.

diclofenac sodium. (Various Mfr.) Diclofenac sodium. **ER Tab.:** 100 mg. 100s. **DR Tab.:** 25 mg, 50 mg, 75 mg. May be enteric coated. 42s (except 25 mg), 60s, 100s, 500s (except 25 mg), 1000s (except 25 mg), UD 100s (50 mg only). **Gel:** 3%. May contain benzyl alcohol, castor oil. 50 g, 100 g. *Rx.*
Use: Analgesic; NSAID.

diclofenac sodium and misoprostol.
Use: Arthritis treatment, antiulcerative.
See: Arthrotec.

diclofenac sodium/misoprostol. (Watson) Diclofenac sodium/misoprostol 50 mg/200 mcg, 75 mg/200 mcg. Castor oil, lactose. Tab., delayed release (each tablet consists of an enteric-coated core containing diclofenac sodium surrounded by an outer mantle containing misoprostol). 60s. *Rx.*
Use: Nonnarcotic analgesic combination.

diclofenac sodium ophthalmic solution 0.1%. Diclofenac sodium 0.1%, mannitol. Soln. Bot. 5 mL. *Rx.*
Use: Analgesic; NSAID, ophthalmic.

Dicloxacil. (Ivax) Dicloxacillin sodium 250 mg, 500 mg. Cap. Bot. 100s. *Rx.*
Use: Anti-infective; penicillin.

•**dicloxacillin.** (DIE-klox-uh-SILL-in) USAN.
Use: Anti-infective.
See: Dynapen.
Pathocil.

•**dicloxacillin sodium.** (DIE-klox-uh-SILL-in) *USP.*
Use: Anti-infective.

dicloxacillin sodium. (Various Mfr.) Dicloxacillin sodium 250 mg, 500 mg. Cap. Bot. 30s (500 mg only), 40s, 50s (500 mg only), 100s, 500s, UD 100s. *Rx.*
Use: Anti-infective

Dicole. (Halsey Drug) Docusate sodium 100 mg. Cap. Bot. 100s. *OTC.*
Use: Laxative.

Dicomal-DM. (Econolab) Dextromethorphan HBr 10 mg, pyrilamine maleate 8.33 mg, phenylephrine hydrochloride 5 mg per 5 mL. Menthol, saccharin, sorbitol. Alcohol, sugar, and dye free. Syrup. Bot. 473 mL. *OTC.*
Use: Upper respiratory combination, antitussive, antihistamine, decongestant.

dicophane.
Use: Pediculicide.
See: Chlorophenothane.
DDT.

•**dicumarol.** (dye-KOO-ma-role) USAN.
Use: Anticoagulant.

•**dicyclomine hydrochloride.** (die-SIGH-kloe-meen) *USP.*
Use: Anticholinergic; antispasmodic.
See: Bentyl.

dicyclomine hydrochloride. (Various Mfr.) Dicyclomine hydrochloride. **Cap.:** 10 g, 20 mg. 30s (10 mg only), 100s, 120s (10 mg only), 1000s, UD 100s (10 mg only). **Tab.:** 20 mg. 15s, 20s, 30s, 100s, 120s, 250s, 1000s, UD 100s. **Syrup:** 10 mg/5 mL. 118 mL, pt, gal. **Inj.:** 10 mg/mL. Vials. 2 mL, 10 mL. *Rx.*
Use: Gastrointestinal antispasmodic/anticholinergic.

Dicynene. (Baxter PPI) *Rx.*
Use: Hemostatic.
See: Ethamsylate.

dicysteine.
See: Cystine.

•**didanosine.** (die-DAN-oh-SEEN) USAN.
Use: Antiretroviral, nucleoside reverse transcriptase inhibitor.
See: Videx.
Videx EC.

didanosine. (Aurobindo Pharma USA) Didanosine. **Tab. for Susp.:** 100 mg, 150 mg, 200 mg. Aspartame, orange flavoring, phenylalanine 36.5 mg, sorbitol. 60s. **Pow. for Soln.:** 2 g. 100 mL (after reconstitution). *Rx.*
Use: Antiretroviral agent, nucleoside reverse transcriptase inhibitor.

didanosine. (Barr) Didanosine 125 mg, 200 mg, 250 mg, 400 mg. Dextrose, talc. Enteric-coated pellets. DR Cap. 30s, UD 1s (250 mg and 400 mg). *Rx.*
Use: Nucleoside reverse transcriptase inhibitor.

didanosine. (Mylan) Didanosine 125 mg.

Cap., delayed release. 30s, 500s. *Rx.*
Use: Antiretroviral agent, nucleoside reverse transcriptase inhibitor.

didehydrodideoxythymidine.
Use: Antiviral.
See: Stavudine.

Di-Delamine. (Del) Tripelennamine hydrochloride 0.5%, diphenhydramine hydrochloride 1%, benzalkonium chloride 0.12%. **Gel:** In clear gel. Tube 1.25 oz. **Spray:** Spray pump 4 oz. *OTC.*
Use: Antipruritic, topical.

dideoxycytidine.
Use: Antiviral.

2,3 dideoxycytidine.
Use: Antiviral (AIDS).

dideoxyinisine.
Use: Antiviral.

Didrex. (Pharmacia) Benzphetamine hydrochloride 50 mg. Lactose, sorbitol. Tab. Bot. 100s, 500s. *c-III.*
Use: CNS stimulant, anorexiant.

Didronel. (Procter & Gamble Pharm) Etidronate disodium 400 mg. Tab. 60s. *Rx.*
Use: Bisphosphonate.

•**dienestrol.** (die-en-ESS-trole) *USP.*
Use: Estrogen therapy; atrophic vaginitis.
See: D V. Cream.
Ortho Dienestrol Vaginal Cream.

dienestrol. (Ortho-McNeil) Dienestrol 0.01%. Tube 78 g w/applicator.
Use: Estrogen.

•**dienogest.** (dye-EN-oh-jest) USAN.
Use: Oral contraceptive; hormone replacement therapy.
W/Estradiol Valerate.
See: Natazia.

diet aids, nonprescription.
Use: Dietary aid.

•**diethanolamine.** (DYE-eth-a-NOL-a-meen) *NF.*
Use: Pharmaceutic acid (alkalizing agent).
See: Diolamine.

diethazine hydrochloride.
Use: Antiparkinsonian.

diethoxin. Intracaine hydrochloride.

•**diethylcarbamazine citrate.** (die-ETH-ill-car-BAM-ah-zeen) *USP.*
Use: Anthelmintic.

diethyldithiocarbamate.
Use: Trial drug for AIDS. [Orphan Drug]
See: Imuthiol.

diethylenediamine citrate. Piperazine Citrate, Piperazine Hexahydrate.

diethylmalonylurea.
See: Barbital.

•**diethyl phthalate.** (dye-ETH-il THAL-ate) *NF.*
Use: Pharmaceutic aid (plasticizer).

diethylpropion. (Various Mfr.) **Tab.:** Diethylpropion 25 mg. Bot. 100s, 500s, 1000s. **SR Tab.:** Diethylpropion 75 mg. Bot. 100s, 250s, 500s, 1000s. *c-IV.*
Use: Anorexiant.

•**diethylpropion hydrochloride.** (die-ETH-uhl-PRO-pee-ahn) *USP.*
Use: Anorexic.
See: Tepanil.
Tepanil Ten-Tab.

diethylpropion hydrochloride. (Various Mfr.) Diethylpropion hydrochloride. **Tab.:** 25 mg. Bot. 100s. **CR Tab.:** 75 mg. Bot. 100s. *c-IV.*
Use: CNS stimulant, anorexiant.

diethylstilbestrol dipropionate. (Various Mfr.) Diethylstilbestrol dipropionate. **Amp.:** In oil, 0.5 mg, 1 mg, 5 mg/mL. **Tab.:** 0.5 mg, 1 mg, 5 mg.
Use: Estrogen.

•**diethyltoluamide.** (die-ETH-ill-toe-LOO-ah-mide) *USP.*
Use: Repellent (arthropod).

n, n-diethylvanillamide.
See: Ethamivan.

Diet-Tuss. (Health for Life Brands) Dextromethorphan 30 mg, thenylpyramine hydrochloride, pyrilamine maleate 80 mg, sodium salicylate 200 mg, sodium citrate 600 mg, ammonium Cl 100 mg/fl oz. Sugar free. Bot. 4 oz. *OTC.*
Use: Analgesic, antihistamine, antitussive, expectorant.

•**difenoximide hydrochloride.** (dye-fen-OX-i-mide) USAN.
Use: Antiperistaltic.

•**difenoxin.** (DIE-fen-OX-in) USAN.
Use: Antidiarrheal; antiperistaltic.
W/Atropine sulfate.
See: Motofen.

Differin. (Galderma) Adapalene. **Gel:** 0.1%. EDTA, methylparaben. Tube. 45 g. **Cream:** 0.1%. EDTA, glycerin, parabens. Tube. 45 g. **Lot:** 0.1%. EDTA, parabens, phenoxyethanol, propylene alcohol, stearyl alcohol, triglycerides. 56.6 g. **Soln.:** 0.1%. Alcohol 30%, PEG-400. 30 mL glass bottles with applicator and 60 unit-of-use pledgets. *Rx.*
Use: Dermatologic, acne; retinoid.

Diff-Stat. (Medical Nutrition) 8.5 billion CFU blend of *S. boulardii* and *B. coagulans.* Cottonseed oil, dextrose, sugar. Pineapple/orange flavor. Chew. Tab. 30s. *OTC.*
Use: Probiotic.

Dificid. (Optimer Pharmaceuticals) Fidaxomicin 200 mg. Film coated. Poly-

vinyl alcohol, PEG. Tab. 20s, 60s, UD 100s. *Rx.*
Use: Anti-infective, macrolide.

Difil-G. (Stewart-Jackson) Dyphylline 200 mg, guaifenesin 300 mg. Tab. 100s. *Rx.*
Use: Antiasthmatic combination, xanthine combination.

Difil-G 400. (SJ Pharmaceuticals) Dyphylline 200 mg, guaifenesin 400 mg. Maltodextrin. Tab. 100s. *Rx.*
Use: Antiasthmatic combination, xanthine combination.

•**diflorasone diacetate.** (die-FLORE-ah-sone) *USP.*
Use: Anti-inflammatory, topical; antipruritic.
See: ApexiCon E.
Florone.
Maxiflor.
Psorcon E.

diflorasone diacetate. (Various Mfr.) Diflorasone diacetate 0.05%. Cream. Oint. Tube. 15 g, 30 g, 60 g. *Rx.*
Use: Anti-inflammatory, topical; antipruritic.

•**difloxacin hydrochloride.** (die-FLOX-ah-SIN) USAN.
Use: Anti-infective (DNA gyrase inhibitor).

•**difluanine hydrochloride.** (die-FLEW-an-EEN) USAN.
Use: CNS stimulant.

Diflucan. (Pfizer) Fluconazole. **Tab.:** 50 mg, 100 mg, 150 mg, 200 mg. Bot. 30s (except 150 mg), UD 100s (100 mg, 200 mg only), UD 1s (150 mg only). **Pow. for Oral Susp.:** 10 mg/mL when reconstituted, sucrose, orange flavor. Bot. 350 mg; 40 mg/mL when reconstituted, sucrose, orange flavor. Bot. 1,400 mg. *Rx.*
Use: Antifungal.

•**diflucortolone.** (die-flew-CORE-toe-lone) USAN.
Use: Corticosteroid, topical.

•**diflucortolone pivalate.** (die-flew-CORE-toe-lone) USAN.
Use: Corticosteroid, topical.

•**diflumidone sodium.** (die-FLEW-mih-DOHN) USAN.
Use: Anti-inflammatory.

•**diflunisal.** (die-FLOO-nih-sal) *USP.*
Use: Salicylate.

diflunisal. (Teva) Diflunisal 500 mg. Tab. Bot. 100s, 500s, unit-of-use 60s. *Rx.*
Use: Salicylate.

•**difluprednate.** (DIE-flew-PRED-nate) USAN.
Use: Corticosteroid, ophthalmic.
See: Durezol.

•**diftalone.** (DIFF-tah-lone) USAN.
Use: Anti-inflammatory; analgesic.

•**digalloyl trioleate.** (dye-GAL-loe-il trye-OH-lee-ate) USAN.

Di-Gel. (Schering-Plough) Aluminum hydroxide (equivalent to dried gel) 200 mg, magnesium hydroxide 200 mg, simethicone 20 mg/5 mL. Saccharin, sorbitol. Liq. Bot. 180 mL, 360 mL. *OTC.*
Use: Antacid; antiflatulent.

Di-Gel, Advanced. (Schering-Plough) Magnesium hydroxide 128 mg, calcium carbonate 280 mg, simethicone 20 mg. Tab. Bot. 30s, 60s, 90s. *OTC.*
Use: Antacid; antiflatulent.

Digestamic. (Lexis Laboratories) Pancrelipase 300 mg, pepsin 100 mg. Tab. Bot. 50s. *Rx-OTC.*
Use: Digestive aid.

Digestamic Liquid. (Lexis Laboratories) Belladonna leaf fluid extract 0.64 min/5 mL. Bot. 8 oz. *Rx-OTC.*
Use: Anticholinergic; antispasmodic.

Digestant. (Canright) Pancreatin 5.25 g, ox bile extract 2 g, pepsin 5 g, betaine hydrochloride 1 g. Tab. Bot. 100s, 1000s. *Rx-OTC.*
Use: Digestive aid.

Digestive Compound. (Thurston) Betaine hydrochloride 3.25 g, pepsin 1 g, papain 2 g, mycozyme 2 g, ox bile 2 g. 2 Tab. Bot. 100s, 500s. *Rx-OTC.*
Use: Digestive aid.

digestive enzymes.
See: Amylase.
Kutrase Capsules.
Ku-Zyme Capsules.
Lipase.
Lipram.
Pancrease.
Pancrecarb.
Pancrelipase.
Panokase Tablets.
Plaretase 800.
Protease.
Ultrase.
Viokase.

digestive products, miscellaneous.
Use: Digestive enzyme supplement.
See: Arco-Lase.
Enzobile Improved.
Ku-Zyme Capsules.

Digex NF. (Pronova) Hyoscyamine sulfate 0.0625 mg, phenyltoloxamine citrate 15 mg. Lactose. Cap. 100s. *Rx.*
Use: Gastrointestinal anticholinergic/antispasmodic, gastrointestinal anticholinergic combination.

Digibar 190. (E-Z-EM) Barium sulfate 190%. Artificial candied sugar flavoring, saccharin, sorbitol. Susp. 232 g. *Rx.*

Use: Radiopaque agent, miscellaneous gastrointestinal contrast agent.

Digidote. (Boehringer Mannheim)
Use: Antidote. [Orphan Drug]

DigiFab. (Savage) Digoxin immune Fab (ovine) 40 mg/vial, sodium acetate 2 mg, preservative free. Each vial will bind ≈ 0.5 mg digoxin. Pow. for Inj., lyophilized. Vial. *Rx.*
Use: Antidote.

•**digitalis.** (dih-jih-TAL-iss) *USP.*
Use: Cardiovascular agent.
See: Crystodigin.
Deslanoside.
Digoxin.
Lanoxin.

digitalis leaf, powdered.
Use: Cardiovascular agent.

digitalis tincture.
Use: Cardiovascular agent.

•**digoxin.** (dih-JOX-in) *USP.*
Use: Cardiovascular agent.
See: Lanoxin.

digoxin. (Elkins-Sinn) Digoxin 0.25 mg/mL, alcohol 0.1 mL, propylene glycol 0.4 mL per mL. Inj. Amp. 2 mL. *Rx.*
Use: Inotropic agent; cardiac glycoside.

digoxin. (Various Mfr.) Digoxin. **Tab.:** 0.125 mg, 0.25 mg. Bot. 1000s **Ped. Elix.:** 0.05 mg/mL. Bot. 60 mL; UD 2.5 mL, 5 mL. **Inj.:** 0.25 mg/mL, alcohol 10%, propylene glycol 40% per mL. *Tubex* or *Carpuject* 1 mL, 2 mL. *Rx.*
Use: Inotropic agent; cardiac glycoside.

digoxin antibody.
See: Digibind.

digoxin immune Fab (ovine).
Use: Antidote.
See: Digidote.
DigiFab.

digoxin injection, pediatric. (Abbott) Digoxin 0.1 mg/mL, propylene glycol 40%, alcohol 10%. Ped. Inj. Amp. 1 mL. *Rx.*
Use: Inotropic agent; cardiac glycoside.

digoxin I-125 immunoassay. (Abbott Diagnostics) Digoxin diagnostic kit for the quantitative determination of serum digoxin. 100s, 300s.
Use: Diagnostic aid.

Digoxin Riabead. (Abbott Diagnostics) Solid-phase radioimmunoassay for quantitative measurement of serum digoxin. Test kit 100s, 300s.
Use: Diagnostic aid.

•**dihexyverine hydrochloride.** (die-HEX-ih-ver-een) USAN.
Use: Anticholinergic.

Dihistine Elixir. (Various Mfr.) Phenylephrine hydrochloride 5 mg, chlorpheniramine maleate 2 mg/5 mL. Bot. Pt, gal. *OTC.*
Use: Antihistamine, decongestant.

Dihistine Expectorant. (Alpharma) Pseudoephedrine hydrochloride 30 mg, codeine phosphate 10 mg, guaifenesin 100 mg per 5 mL. Alcohol 7.5%, saccharin, sorbitol, sucrose. Liq. Bot. 473 mL. *c-v.*
Use: Upper respiratory combination, antitussive, decongestant, expectorant.

dihydan soluble.
See: Phenytoin Sodium.

dihydrocodeine. Paracodin. Drocode.
Use: Analgesic, antitussive.

•**dihydrocodeine bitartrate.** (die-high-droe-KOE-deen bye-TAR-trate) *USP.*
Use: Analgesic.
See: Hydrocodone Bitartrate.
W/Acetaminophen, Caffeine.
See: Trezix.
W/Brompheniramine Maleate, Phenylephrine Hydrochloride.
See: Poly-Tussin DHC.
W/Brompheniramine Maleate, Pseudoephedrine Hydrochloride.
See: J-Cof DHC.
W/Caffeine, Aspirin.
See: Synalgos-DC.
W/Chlorpheniramine Maleate, Phenylephrine Hydrochloride.
See: Pancof PD.
W/Combinations.
See: Novahistine DH.
Pancof.
Pancof EXP.
Tricof.
Tricof EXP.
Tricof PD.
WellTuss EXP.
W/Guaifenesin.
See: J-Max DHC.
W/Guaifenesin, Phenylephrine Hydrochloride.
See: Donatuss DC.
Poly-Tussin EX.
W/Guaifenesin, Pseudoephedrine Hydrochloride.
See: Despec-EXP.
W/Phenylephrine Hydrochloride.
See: Alahist DHC.
W/Phenylephrine Hydrochloride, Pyrilamine Maleate.
See: Poly Hist DHC.

dihydrocodeinone resin complex.
W/Phenyltoloxamine resin complex.
See: Tussionex.

dihydroergocornine. Ergot alkaline component of hydergine.

dihydroergocristine. Ergot alkaloid component of hydergine.

dihydroergocryptine. Ergot alkaloid component of hydergine.

dihydroergotamine. (Sandoz) (D.H.E. 45) Dihydroergotamine mesylate. Amp. *Rx.*
Use: Agent for migraine; antiadrenergic.

•**dihydroergotamine mesylate.** (DIE-high-droe-err-GOT-uh-meen) *USP.* Dihydroergotamine methanesulfonate.
Use: Antiadrenergic; antimigraine.
See: D.H.E. 45.
Migranal.

dihydroergotamine mesylate. (Various Mfr.) Dihydroergotamine mesylate 1 mg/mL. Alcohol 6.2%, glycerin 15%. Inj. Vial. 1 mL. *Rx.*
Use: Migraine agent.

dihydroergotoxine. Ergoloid mesylate. *Rx.*
Use: Psychotherapeutic agent.
See: Ergoloid Mesylates.
Gerimal.
Hydergine.

5,6-dihydro-5-azacytidine. (Ilex Oncology)
Use: Antineoplastic. [Orphan Drug]

dihydrofollicular hormone.
See: Estradiol.

dihydrofolliculin.
See: Estradiol.

dihydrohydroxycodeinone.
Use: Analgesic; narcotic.
See: Oxycodone. (Eucodal, Eukodal).

dihydroindolone derivatives.
Use: Antipsychotic.
See: Molindone Hydrochloride.

dihydromorphinone hydrochloride.
See: Dilaudid.

•**dihydrostreptomycin sulfate.** (die-HIGH-droe-strep-toe-MY-sin) *USP.*
Use: Anti-infective.

dihydrotachysterol. (die-HIGH-droe-tack-ISS-ter-ole)
Use: Vitamin.

dihydrotestosterone.
Use: AIDS. [Orphan Drug]
See: Androgel-DHT.

dihydrotheelin.
See: Estradiol.

dihydroxyacetone.
See: Chromelin Complexion Blender.

•**dihydroxyaluminum aminoacetate.** (die-hye-DROX-ee-ah-LOO-mi-num ah-MEE-no-ASS-eh-tate) *USP.*
Use: Antacid.

•**dihydroxyaluminum sodium carbonate.** (die-hye-DROX-ee-ah-LOO-mi-num ah-MEE-no-ASS-eh-tate) *USP.*
Use: Antacid.
See: Rolaids.

dihydroxycholecalciferol.
See: Rocaltrol.

24,25 dihydroxycholecalciferol. (Lemmon)
Use: Uremic osteodystrophy. [Orphan Drug]

dihydroxyestrin.
See: Estradiol.

dihydroxyfluorane. Fluorescein.

dihydroxyphenylisatin.
See: Oxyphenisatin Acetate.

dihydroxyphenyloxindol.
See: Oxyphenisatin Acetate.

dihydroxypropyl theophylline. Dyphylline.
See: Neothylline

•**dihydroxy (stearato) aluminum.** *NF.* Aluminum monostearate.

diiodohydroxyquin.
Use: Amebicide.
See: Iodoquinol.

diiodohydroxyquinoline.
See: Iodoquinol.

diisopromine hydrochloride. (Lab. for Pharmaceutical Development, Inc.)
See: Desquam-X.

diisopropyl phosphorofluoridate.
See: Floropryl.

diisopropyl sebacate.
Use: Moisturizing agent.

Dilacor XR. (Watson Pharma) Diltiazem hydrochloride 240 mg. Maltodextrin, PEG. ER Cap. 100s. *Rx.*
Use: Calcium channel blocker.

dilaminate. Mixture of magnesium carbide and dihydroxyaluminum glycinate. *OTC.*
Use: Antacid.

Dilantin. (Parke-Davis) Phenytoin 30 mg, 100 mg. Lactose, sugar. ER Cap. 100s, 1,000s, UD 100s. *Rx.*
Use: Anticonvulsant, hydantoin.

Dilantin Infatab. (Pfizer) Phenytoin 50 mg. Saccharin, sucrose. Chew. Tab. 100s, UD 100s. *Rx.*
Use: Anticonvulsant.

Dilantin-125. (Pfizer) Phenytoin 125 mg per 5 mL. Alcohol ≤ 0.6%, glycerin, sodium benzoate, sucrose. Orange-vanilla flavor. Susp. 240 mL. *Rx.*
Use: Anticonvulsant.

Dilantin Sodium w/Phenobarbital Kapseal. (Parke-Davis) Phenytoin sodium 100 mg, phenobarbital 16 mg, 32 mg. Cap. Bot. 100s, 1000s, UD 100s (32 mg only). *Rx.*
Use: Anticonvulsant; hypnotic; sedative.

Dilantin-30 Pediatric. (Parke-Davis) Phenytoin 30 mg/5 mL, alcohol 0.6%. Susp. Bot. 240 mL, 5 mL. *Rx.*
Use: Anticonvulsant.

Dilatrate-SR. (Actient Pharmaceuticals) Isosorbide dinitrate 40 mg. Lactose, sucrose. SR Cap. Bot. 100s. *Rx.*
Use: Vasodilator.

Dilaudid. (Purdue Pharma) Hydromorphone hydrochloride. **Inj., Soln.:** 1 mg/mL, 2 mg/mL, 4 mg/mL. Preservative free. Amps. 1 mL. **Liq.:** 1 mg/1 mL. Parabens, sucrose, glycerin. May contain sodium metabisulfite. 473 mL. **Tab.:** 2 mg, 4 mg, 8 mg (may contain sodium metabisulfite). Lactose. 100s, 500s (4 mg only), UD 100s (except 8 mg). *c-II.*
Use: Opioid analgesic.

Dilaudid-HP. (Purdue Pharma) Hydromorphone hydrochloride. **Inj. Soln., Conc.:** 10 mg/mL. Preservative free. Amps. 1 mL, 5 mL. Single-dose vials. 50 mL. **Inj., Lyophilized Pow. for Soln., Conc.:** 250 mg (10 mg/mL after reconstitution). Preservative free. Single-dose vials. *c-II.*
Use: Opioid analgesic.

•**dilevalol hydrochloride.** (DIE-LEV-ah-lole) USAN.
Use: Antihypertensive; antiadrenergic (β-receptor).

Dilex-G. (Poly) Dyphylline 100 mg, guaifenesin 100 mg per 5 mL. Alcohol free. Parabens, saccharin, sucrose, sorbitol. Menthol flavor. Syrup. 473 mL. *Rx.*
Use: Antiasthmatic combination, xanthine combination.

Dilex-G 400. (Poly) Dyphylline 200 mg, guaifenesin 400 mg. Tab. 100s. *Rx.*
Use: Antiasthmatic combination, xanthine combination.

Dilex-G 200. (Poly) Dyphylline 100 mg, guaifenesin 200 mg per 5 mL. Sugar free. Syrup. 473 mL. *Rx.*
Use: Antiasthmatic combination, xanthine combination.

dilithium carbonate. Lithium carbonate, USP.
Use: Antipsychotic.

•**dilmapimod.** (dil-MAP-i-mod) USAN.
Use: Respiratory agent.

•**dilmapimod tosylate.** (dil-MAP-i-mod) USAN.
Use: Respiratory agent.

Dilotab II. (Zee Medical) Acetaminophen 325 mg, phenylephrine hydrochloride 5 mg. Tab. 100s, 250s. *OTC.*
Use: Analgesic, decongestant, upper respiratory combination.

•**diloxanide furoate.** (dye-LOX-a-nide FUR-oh-ate) *USP.*
Use: Anti-infective.

Dilt-CD. (Apotex USA) Diltiazem hydrochloride 120 mg, 180 mg, 240 mg, 300 mg. Sucrose. ER Cap. 30s, 90s, 500s. *Rx.*
Use: Calcium channel blocker.

•**diltiazem hydrochloride.** (dill-TIE-uh-zem) *USP.*
Use: Vasodilator (coronary), calcium channel blocker.
See: Cardizem.
Cardizem CD.
Cardizem LA.
Cartia XT.
Dilacor XR.
Dilt-CD.
Dilt-XR.
Diltzac.
Matzim LA.
Taztia XT.
Tiazac.

diltiazem hydrochloride. (Various Mfr.) Diltiazem hydrochloride. **Inj.:** 5 mg/mL. Vials. 5 mL, 10 mL, 25 mL. **Tab.:** 30 mg, 60 mg, 90 mg, 120 mg. May contain lactose or methylparaben. 100s, 500s, 1,000s. **ER Tab.:** 120 mg, 180 mg, 240 mg, 300 mg, 360 mg, 420 mg. May contain PEG, polydextrose, sucrose, vegetable oil. 30s, 90s. **ER Cap.:** 60 mg, 90 mg, 120 mg, 180 mg, 240 mg, 300 mg. May contain sucrose or sugar spheres. 30s (except 60 mg, 90 mg), 90s (except 60 mg, 90 mg), 100s (except 300 mg), 500s (except 60 mg, 90 mg), 1,000s (except 60 mg, 90 mg). *Rx.*
Use: Calcium channel blocker.

•**diltiazem maleate.** (dill-TIE-ah-zem MAL-ate) USAN.
Use: Calcium channel blocker; antihypertensive.

Dilt-XR. (Apotex USA) Diltiazem hydrochloride 120 mg, 180 mg, 240 mg. ER Cap. 100s. *Rx.*
Use: Calcium channel blocker.

Diltzac. (Apotex) Diltiazem hydrochloride 120 mg, 180 mg, 240 mg, 300 mg, 360 mg. ER Cap. 30s, 90s, 100s, 500s, 1,000s (120 mg only). *Rx.*
Use: Cardiovascular agent, calcium channel blocking agent.

diluent.
See: Broncho Saline.
Sodium Chloride.
Sodium Chloride 0.45%.
Sodium Chloride 0.9%.

Dimaphen DM. (Major) Pseudoephedrine hydrochloride 15 mg, brompheniramine maleate 1 mg, dextromethorphan HBr 5 mg per 5 mL. Saccharin, sorbitol, grape flavor, alcohol free. Elix. Bot. 118 mL. *OTC.*

Use: Upper respiratory combination, antitussive combination.

•**dimefadane.** (DIE-meh-fah-dane) USAN.
Use: Analgesic.

•**dimefilcon A.** (DIE-meh-FILL-kahn A) USAN.
Use: Contact lens material (hydrophilic).

•**dimefline hydrochloride.** (DIE-meh-fleen) USAN.
Use: Respiratory.

•**dimefocon A.** (DIE-meh-FOE-kahn A) USAN.
Use: Contact lens material (hydrophobic).

Dimenest. (Forest) Dimenhydrinate 50 mg/mL. Vial 10 mL. *Rx.*
Use: Antiemetic; antivertigo.

•**dimenhydrinate.** (die-men-HIGH-drih-nate) *USP.*
Tall Man: dimenhyDRINATE
Use: Antiemetic; antihistamine.
See: Dimenest.
Dimentabs.
Dramamine.
Dymenate.
Signate.
Traveltabs.

Dimentabs. (Jones Pharma) Dimenhydrinate 50 mg. Tab. Bot. 100s. *OTC.*
Use: Antiemetic; antivertigo.

•**dimepranol acedoben.** (DIE-MEH-prah-nahl ah-SEE-doe-BEN) USAN.
Use: Immunomodulator.

•**dimercaprol.** (die-mer-CAP-role) *USP.*
Formerly BAL.
Use: Antidote to gold, arsenic, and mercury poisoning; metal complexing agent.
See: BAL in Oil.

Dimetane Decongestant. (Wyeth Consumer Healthcare) **Capl.:** Brompheniramine maleate 4 mg, phenylephrine hydrochloride 10 mg. Capl. Bot. 24s, 48s. **Elix.:** Brompheniramine maleate 2 mg, phenylephrine hydrochloride 5 mg/5 mL, alcohol 2.3%. Bot. 120 mL. *OTC.*
Use: Antihistamine, decongestant.

Dimetapp Children's Cold & Allergy. (Wyeth Consumer Healthcare) **Elix.:** Brompheniramine maleate 2 mg, phenylephrine hydrochloride 5 mg. Alcohol, saccharin, sorbitol. Grape flavor. 237 mL. **Syrup:** Brompheniramine maleate 1 mg, phenylephrine hydrochloride 2.5 mg per 5 mL. Alcohol free. Sorbitol, sucralose. Grape flavor. 237 mL with dosage cup. *OTC.*
Use: Upper respiratory combination, decongestant and antihistamine.

Dimetapp Children's Cold & Cough. (Wyeth Consumer Healthcare) Brompheniramine maleate 1 mg, dextromethorphan hydrobromide 5 mg, phenylephrine hydrochloride 2.5 mg. Propylene glycol, sodium benzoate, sorbitol, sucralose. Alcohol free. Grape flavor. Liq. 118 mL. *OTC.*
Use: Upper respiratory combination, decongestant and antihistamine.

Dimetapp Children's Long Acting Cough Plus Cold. (Wyeth Consumer Healthcare) Chlorpheniramine maleate 1 mg, dextromethorphan hydrobromide 7.5 mg. Propylene glycol, sodium 3 mg, sorbitol, sucralose. Alcohol free. Grape flavor. Syrup. 118 mL. *OTC.*
Use: Upper respiratory combination, antihistamine.

Dimetapp Children's Multi-Symptom Cold & Flu. (Wyeth Consumer Healthcare) Acetaminophen 160 mg, chlorpheniramine maleate 1 mg, dextromethorphan hydrobromide 5 mg, phenylephrine hydrochloride 2.5 mg. Glycerin, menthol, polyethylene glycol, sodium benzoate, sorbitol, sucralose. Alcohol free. Grape flavor. Liq. 118 mL. *OTC.*
Use: Upper respiratory combination; decongestant, antihistamine, and analgesic combination.

Dimetapp Children's Nighttime Cold & Congestion. (Wyeth Consumer Healthcare) Diphenhydramine hydrochloride 6.25 mg, phenylephrine hydrochloride 2.5 mg. Propylene glycol, sodium 4 mg, sorbitol, sucralose. Alcohol free. Grape flavor. Syrup. 118 mL. *OTC.*
Use: Upper respiratory combination, decongestant and antihistamine.

•**dimethadione.** (DIE-meth-ah-DIE-ohn) USAN.
Use: Anticonvulsant.

•**dimethicone.** (DIE-meth-ih-cone) *NF.*
Use: Prosthetic aid (soft tissue); component of barrier creams; lubricant; hydrophobic agent.
See: Aloe Vesta.
Aveeno Baby.
Aveeno Daily Moisturizing.
Gold Bond Medicated Triple Action Relief.
NeutrapHor Skin Protectant.
Pro-Q.
Silicone.
TheraSeal Hand Protection.

W/Pramoxine Hydrochloride.
See: Gold Bond Intensive Healing.

W/Zinc Oxide.
See: A & D Zinc Oxide Cream.
Soothe & Cool.

•**dimethicone 350.** (DIE-meth-ih-cone 350) USAN.
Use: Prosthetic aid for soft tissue.
•**dimethindene maleate.** (DIE-METH-in-deen) *USP.*
Use: Antihistamine.
•**dimethisoquin hydrochloride.** (die-meh-THIGH-so-kwin) USAN.
Use: Antibiotic, topical.
•**dimethisterone.** (DIE-meth-ISS-ter-ohn) *NF.*
Use: Hormone, progestin.
dimethoxyphenyl penicillin sodium.
Use: Anti-infective.
See: Methicillin Sodium.
dimethpyridene maleate. Dimethindene Maleate.
dimethylaminophenazone.
See: Aminopyrine.
dimethylamino pyrazine sulfate.
See: Ampyzine Sulfate.
dimethylcarbamate.
See: Mestinon.
•**dimethyl fumarate.** (dye-METH-il) USAN.
Use: Immunomodulator.
See: Tecfidera.
dimethylhexestrol dipropionate. Promethestrol Dipropionate.
dimethyl polysiloxane.
See: Dimethicone.
•**dimethyl sulfoxide.** (die-METH-uhl sull-FOX-ide) *USP.*
Use: Interstitial cystitis agent.
See: Rimso-50.
dimethyl sulfoxide. (Bioniche) Dimethyl sulfoxide in a 50% aqueous solution. 50 mL. *Rx.*
Use: Interstitial cystitis agent.
dimethyl sulfoxide. (Pharma 21)
Use: Increased intracranial pressure. [Orphan Drug]
dimethyl-tubocurarine iodide.
Use: Muscle relaxant.
dimethylurethimine.
See: Meturedepa.
•**dimoxamine hydrochloride.** (die-MOX-AH-meen) USAN.
Use: Memory adjuvant.
Dimycor. (Standard Drug Co.) Pentaerythritol tetranitrate 10 mg, phenobarbital 15 mg. Tab. Bot. 1000s. *Rx.*
Use: Antianginal; hypnotic; sedative.
•**dinaciclib.** (din-a-SYE-klib) USAN.
Use: Antineoplastic.
Dinacrin. (Sanofi-Synthelabo) Isonicotinic acid, hydrazide. *Rx.*
Use: Antituberculosal.
•**dinoprost.** (DIE-no-proste) USAN.
Use: Oxytocic; prostaglandin.
•**dinoprostone.** (DIE-no-PROSTE-ohn) *USP.*
Use: Abortifacient; agent for cervical ripening; oxytocic; prostaglandin.
See: Cervidil.
Prepidil.
Prostin E_2.
•**dinoprost tromethamine.** (DIE-no-proste troe-METH-ah-meen) *USP.*
Use: Oxytocic; prostaglandin.
Diocto. (Various Mfr.) Docusate sodium. **Syr.:** 60 mg/15 mL. Bot. 480 mL. **Liq.:** 150 mg/15 mL. Bot. 480 mL. *OTC.*
Use: Laxative.
Dioctolose. (Ivax) Docusate potassium 100 mg. Cap. Bot. 100s, 1000s.
Use: Laxative.
dioctyl calcium sulfosuccinate. (die-OCK-till SULL-foe-SUCK-sih-nate) Docusate Calcium.
Use: Laxative.
dioctyl sodium sulfosuccinate.
Use: Non-laxative fecal softener.
See: Docusate Sodium.
Dioctyn. (Dixon-Shane) Docusate sodium 100 mg. Sorbitol. Tab. 1,000s. *OTC.*
Use: Fecal softener.
diodone injection.
See: Iodopyracet injection.
•**diohippuric acid I 125.** (dye-oh-hip-YOOR-ik) USAN.
Use: Radiopharmaceutical.
•**diohippuric acid I 131.** (dye-oh-hip-YOOR-ik) USAN.
Use: Radiopharmaceutical.
Dio-Hist. (Health for Life Brands) Dextromethorphan 30 mg, thenylpyramine hydrochloride 80 mg, phenylephrine hydrochloride 20 mg, potassium tartrate 1/24 g/oz. Bot. 4 oz. *OTC.*
Use: Antihistamine.
diolamine. Diethanolamine.
diolostene.
See: Methandriol.
Dionex. (Henry Schein) Docusate sodium 100 mg, 250 mg. Cap. Bot. 100s, 250s, 1000s. *OTC.*
Use: Laxative.
dionin. Ethylmorphine hydrochloride.
Use: Cough depressant, oral; ocular lymphagogue.
Dionosil Oily. (GlaxoSmithKline) Propyliodone 60% in peanut oil. Inj. Vial 20 mL.
Use: Radiopaque agent.
diophyllin.
See: Aminophylline.
diopterin. Pteroylglutamic acid, PDGA, Pteroyl-alpha-glutamylglutamic acid.
Use: Antineoplastic.

Diorapin. (Standex) **Tab.:** Estrogenic conjugate 0.625 mg, methyltestosterone 5 mg. Bot. 100s. **Inj.:** Estrone 2 mg, testosterone 25 mg/mL. Vial 10 mL. *Rx.*
Use: Androgen, estrogen combination.

Diosmin. Buchu resin obtained from lvs. of *Barosma serratifolia* and allied Rutaceae.

Dio-Soft. (Standex) Docusate sodium 100 mg, casanthranol 30 mg. Cap. Bot. 100s. *OTC.*
Use: Laxative.

Diostate D. (Pharmacia) Vitamin D 400 units, calcium 343 mg, phosphorus 265 mg. 3 Tab. Bot. 100s. *OTC.*
Use: Mineral, vitamin supplement.

•**diotyrosine I 125.** (die-oh-TIE-row-seen) USAN.
Use: Radiopharmaceutical.

•**diotyrosine I 131.** (die-oh-TIE-row-seen) USAN.
Use: Radiopharmaceutical.

Diovan. (Novartis) Valsartan 40 mg, 80 mg, 160 mg, 320 mg. Polyethylene glycol 8000. Tab. Bot. 30s (40 mg only), 90s (except 40 mg), UD 100s (except 320 mg). *Rx.*
Use: Renin angiotensin system antagonist.

Diovan HCT. (Novartis) Valsartan/hydrochlorothiazide 80 mg/12.5 mg, 160 mg/12.5 mg, 160/25 mg, 320 mg/12.5 mg, 320 mg/25 mg. Tab. Bot. 90s, UD 100s. *Rx.*
Use: Antihypertensive.

•**dioxadrol hydrochloride.** (die-OX-ah-drole) USAN.
Use: Antidepressant.

dioxindol. Diacetylhydroxyphenylisatin.

dioxyanthranol.
See: Anthralin.

•**dioxybenzone.** (die-ox-ee-BEN-zone) *USP.*
Use: Ultraviolet screen.
W/Oxybenzone.
See: Solbar Plus 15.

dipalmitoylphosphatidylcholine. Colfosceril palmitate.
Use: Synthetic lung surfactant.

dipalmitoylphosphatidylcholine/phosphatidylglycerol.
Use: Neonatal respiratory distress syndrome. [Orphan Drug]
See: ALEC.

diparcol hydrochloride. Diethazine.

Dipegyl.
See: Nicotinamide.

Dipentum. (UCB) Olsalazine sodium 250 mg. Cap. Bot. 100s, 500s. *Rx.*
Use: Gastrointestinal agent.

dipeptidyl peptidase-4 inhibitor.
Use: Antidiabetic agent.
See: Alogliptin.
Linagliptin.
Saxagliptin.
Sitagliptin Phosphate.

diperodon hydrochloride.
Use: Anesthetic.
W/Methapyrilene Hydrochloride, Pyrilamine Maleate, Allantoin, Benzocaine, Menthol.
See: Antihistamine.

diphenadione.
Use: Anticoagulant.

Diphen AF. (Morton Grove) Diphenhydramine hydrochloride 12.5 mg/5 mL, saccharin, sugar, cherry flavor. Liq. Bot. 118 mL, 237 mL, 473 mL. *OTC.*
Use: Antihistamine, nonselective ethanolamine.

Diphenatol. (Rugby) Diphenoxylate hydrochloride 2.5 mg, atropine sulfate 0.025 mg. Tab. Bot. 100s, 500s, 1000s.
Use: Antidiarrheal.

Diphenhist. (Rugby) Diphenhydramine hydrochloride. **Cap.:** 25 mg. Benzyl alcohol, butylparaben, EDTA, lactose, parabens. 100s. **Oral Soln.:** 12.5 mg/5 mL. Saccharin sucrose. Bot. 120 mL, 473 mL. *OTC.*
Use: Antihistamine.

Diphenhist Captabs. (Rugby) Diphenhydramine hydrochloride 25 mg. Tab. Bot. 100s. *OTC.*
Use: Antihistamine, nonselective ethanolamine.

diphenhydramine. (Various Mfr.) Diphenhydramine hydrochloride 25 mg. Tab. Bot. 24s, 100s. *OTC.*
Use: Antihistamine, nonselective ethanolamine.

•**diphenhydramine citrate.** (die-fen-HIGH-druh-meen) *USP.*
Tall Man: diphenhydrAMINE
Use: Antihistamine.
W/Acetaminophen.
See: Goody's PM.
W/Aspirin.
See: Alka-Seltzer PM.

•**diphenhydramine hydrochloride.** (die-fen-HIGH-druh-meen) *USP.*
Tall Man: diphenhydrAMINE
Use: Antihistamine, nonselective ethanolamine, antitussive.
See: Altaryl Children's Allergy.
Banophen.
Banophen Allergy.
Banophen Children's Allergy.
Benadryl Allergy Dye-Free.
Benadryl Allergy KapGels.
Benadryl Allergy ULTRATAB.

Benadryl Children's Allergy.
Benadryl Children's Dye-Free Allergy.
Benadryl Itch Stopping Extra Strength.
Benahist.
Clearly CalaGel.
Dermamycin.
Dermarest.
Fenylhist.
40 Winks.
Histine.
Hydramine Cough.
Hyrexin-50.
Nighttime Sleep Aid.
Nytol Maximum Strength.
PediaCare Children's NightTime Cough.
Q-dryl.
Silphen Cough.
Simply Sleep.
Sleep-ettes D Nighttime Sleep Aid.
Snooze Fast.
Theraflu Thin Strips Multi Symptom.
Triaminic Cough & Runny Nose.
Triaminic Thin Strips Long Acting Cough.
Tusstat.
Unisom SleepGels.
Unisom SleepMelts.
ZzzQuil.
ZzzQuil Liquicaps.

W/Acetaminophen.
See: Aceta-Gesic.
Acetaminophen PM Extra Strength.
Excedrin PM.
Legatrin PM.
Pain Reliever PM Extra Strength.
Percogesic Extra Strength.
Tylenol PM.
Tylenol PM Extra Strength.
Tylenol Severe Allergy.
Tylenol Sore Throat Nighttime.
Unisom PM Pain.

W/Acetaminophen, Dextromethorphan Hydrobromide.
See: Diabetic Tussin Cold & Flu.
Diabetic Tussin Night Time Formula Cold/Flu.

W/Acetaminophen, Dextromethorphan Hydrobromide, Phenylephrine Hydrochloride.
See: Respa C & C.

W/Acetaminophen, Phenylephrine Hydrochloride.
See: Benadryl Allergy & Cold.
Benadryl Allergy & Sinus Headache.
Benadryl Severe Allergy & Sinus Headache Maximum Strength.
Sudafed PE Multi-Symptom Severe Cold.
Sudafed PE Nighttime Cold Maximum Strength.
Theraflu Nighttime Severe Cough & Cold.
Theraflu Severe Cold & Cough Daytime/Nighttime.
Theraflu Sugar-Free Nighttime Severe Cough & Cold.
Theraflu Warming Relief Flu & Sore Throat.
Tylenol Allergy Multi-Symptom Convenience Pack.
Tylenol Allergy Multi-Symptom Nighttime.
Tylenol Plus Children's Cold & Allergy.

W/Benzethonium Chloride, Zinc Acetate.
See: Calagel Maximum Strength.

W/Calamine.
See: Ivarest Maximum Strength.

W/Codeine Phosphate, Phenylephrine Hydrochloride.
See: Airacof.

W/Dextromethorphan Hydrobromide, Phenylephrine Hydrochloride.
See: Duratuss AC.

W/Hydrocortisone, Nystatin.
See: First Duke's Mouthwash.

W/Hydrocortisone, Nystatin, Tetracycline Hydrochloride.
See: First Mary's Mouthwash.

W/Ibuprofen.
See: Advil PM.

W/Naproxen Sodium.
See: Aleve PM.

W/Phenylephrine Hydrochloride.
See: Aldex-CT.
Benadryl-D Children's Allergy & Sinus.
Delsym Children's Night Time Cough & Cold.
Delsym Night Time Cough & Cold.
Dimetapp Children's Nighttime Cold & Congestion.
Robitussin Pediatric Cough & Cold Nighttime.
Sudafed PE Day & Night.
Theraflu Thin Strips Nighttime Cold & Cough.
Triaminic Children's Thin Strips Night Time Cold & Cough.
Triaminic Night Time Cold & Cough.
ZoDen PD.

W/Pseudoephedrine Hydrochloride.
See: Respa-SA.
Tekral.

W/Zinc Acetate.
See: Anti-Itch.
Benadryl Extra Strength.
Benadryl Extra Strength Itch Relief Stick.
Benadryl Extra Strength Itch Stopping Cream.
Benadryl Original Strength Itch Stopping Cream.

Benadryl ReadyMist Itch Stopping Spray.

diphenhydramine hydrochloride. (Various Mfr.) Diphenhydramine hydrochloride 25 mg, 50 mg. Cap. Bot. 24s (25 mg only), 100s, 1000s. *Rx-OTC.*
Use: Antihistamine.

diphenhydramine hydrochloride. (Various Mfr.) Diphenhydramine hydrochloride 50 mg/mL. Inj. 1 mL fill in 2 mL cartridges. *Rx.*
Use: Antihistamine.

diphenhydramine hydrochloride. (Various Mfr.) Diphenhydramine hydrochloride 25 mg, 50 mg. Tab. 24s (25 mg), 50s (50 mg), 100s (25 mg). *OTC.*
Use: Antihistamine.

diphenhydramine hydrochloride, acetaminophen, and pseudoephedrine hydrochloride combinations.
Use: Upper respiratory combination, antihistamine, analgesic, decongestant.

diphenhydramine hydrochloride, acetaminophen, dextromethorphan hydrobromide, pseudoephedrine hydrochloride combinations.
Use: Upper respiratory combination, antihistamine, analgesic, antitussive, decongestant.

diphenhydramine hydrochloride and acetaminophen combinations.
Use: Upper respiratory combination, antihistamine, analgesic.

diphenhydramine hydrochloride and pseudoephedrine hydrochloride combinations.
Use: Upper respiratory combination, antihistamine, decongestant.

•**diphenidol hydrochloride.** (die-FEN-ih-dahl) USAN.
Use: Antiemetic.

•**diphenidol pamoate.** (die-FEN-ih-dahl) USAN.
Use: Antiemetic.

•**diphenoxylate hydrochloride.** (die-fen-OX-ih-late) *USP.*
Use: Antiperistaltic to treat diarrhea.
W/Atropine.
See: Lomotil.

diphenylhydantoin. Phenytoin.
Use: Anticonvulsant.

diphenylhydantoin sodium. Phenytoin sodium.
Use: Anticonvulsant.

diphenylhydroxycarbinol. Benzhydrol hydrochloride.

diphenylisatin.
See: Oxyphenisatin Acetate.

diphosphonic acid.
See: Etidronic acid.

diphosphopyridine (DPN).
Use: Antialcoholic. Under study.

diphosphothiamin. Cocarboxylase.

diphtheria and tetanus toxoids, adult. (Merck) Diphtheria 2 Lf units, tetanus 2 Lf units/0.5 mL dose. Aluminum ≤ 0.53 mg, formaldehyde < 100 mcg (0.02%), trace thimerosal (mercury ≤ 0.3 mcg/dose). Inj., Susp. Single-dose vial. 0.5 mL. *Rx.*
Use: Active immunization, toxoid.

diphtheria and tetanus toxoids, adsorbed (for adult use).
Use: Active immunization, toxoid.
See: Decavac.
Diphtheria & Tetanus Toxoids, Adult.

diphtheria and tetanus toxoids, adsorbed (for pediatric use).
Use: Active immunization, toxoid.
See: Diphtheria & Tetanus Toxoids, Pediatric.

diphtheria and tetanus toxoids and acellular pertussis adsorbed, hepatitis B (recombinant) and inactivated poliovirus vaccine combined.
Use: Active immunization, toxoid.
See: Pediarix.

diphtheria and tetanus toxoids and acellular pertussis vaccine, adsorbed.
Use: Prevention against diphtheria, tetanus, and pertussis; immunizing agent.
See: Adacel.
Boostrix.
Daptacel.
Infanrix.

diphtheria and tetanus toxoids, pediatric. (Sanofi Pasteur) Diphtheria 25 Lf units, tetanus 5 Lf units per 0.5 mL dose. Preservative free. Inj., Susp. Single-dose vial (w/aluminum phosphate 1.5 mg, free formaldehyde < 100 mcg). 0.5 mL. *Rx.*
Use: Agent for active immunization.

diphtheria equine antitoxin. *Rx.*
Use: Prophylaxis and treatment of diphtheria.

•**diphtheria toxin for Schick Test.** (diff-THEER-ee-uh) *USP. Formerly Diphtheria Toxin, Diagnostic.*
Use: Diagnostic aid (dermal reactivity indicator).

Dipimol. (Everett) Dipyridamole 25 mg, 50 mg, 75 mg. Tab. Bot. 100s, 500s, 1000s.
Use: Antianginal.

dipivalyl epinephrine.
See: Propine Sterile Ophthalmic.

•**dipivefrin.** (die-PIHV-eh-FRIN) USAN. *Formerly Dipivalyl Epinephrine.*
Use: Adrenergic, ophthalmic.

•**dipivefrin hydrochloride.** (die-PIHV-eh-FRIN) *USP.*
Use: Antiglaucoma agent.

Diprivan. (APP Pharmaceuticals) Propofol 10 mg/mL, soybean oil 100 mg, glycerol 22.5 mg, egg lecithin 12 mg, EDTA 0.005%, ph = 7 to 8.5. Inj. Single-use amp. 20 mL. Single-use infusion vial 50 mL, 100 mL. Prefilled single-use syr. 50 mL. *Rx.*
Use: Anesthetic, general.

Diprolene. (Schering-Plough) Betamethasone dipropionate 0.05%. **Cream:** In cream base. Tube 15 g. **Oint.:** In ointment base. Tube 15 g, 45 g. *Rx.*
Use: Anti-inflammatory; antipruritic, topical.

Diprolene AF Cream. (Schering-Plough) Betamethasone dipropionate cream equivalent to 0.05% betamethasone. Tube 15 g, 45 g. *Rx.*
Use: Corticosteroid, topical.

dipropylacetic acid.
See: Valproic Acid.

Diprosone. (Schering-Plough) Betamethasone dipropionate 0.64 mg (equiv. to 0.5 mg betamethasone). **Cream:** W/mineral oil, white petrolatum, polyethylene glycol 1000 monocetyl ether, cetostearyl alcohol, phosphoric acid, monobasic sodium phosphate with 4-chloro-m-cresol as preservative. Tube 15 g, 45 g. **Lot.:** W/isopropyl alcohol (46.8%). Bot. 20 mL, 60 mL. **Oint.:** In white petrolatum and mineral oil base. Tube 15 g, 45 g. *Rx.*
Use: Corticosteroid, topical.

Diprosone Aerosol 0.1%. (Schering-Plough) Betamethasone dipropionate 6.4 mg (equiv. to 5 mg betamethasone) in vehicle of mineral oil, caprylic-capric triglyceride w/isopropyl alcohol 10%, inert hydrocarbon propellants (propane and isobutane). Can 85 g. *Rx.*
Use: Corticosteroid, topical.

•**dipyridamole.** (DIE-pih-RID-uh-mole) *USP.*
Use: Coronary vasodilator; antiplatelet agent.
See: Persantine.
W/Aspirin.
See: Aggrenox.

dipyridamole. (Various Mfr.) **Tab.:** **25 mg:** 90s, 100s, 500s, 1,000s, 5,000s, UD 100s. **50 mg, 75 mg:** 100s, 500s, 1,000s, UD 100s. **Inj.:** 5 mg/mL. 50 mg of polyethylene glycol 600, tartaric acid 2 mg. Vial. 2 mL, 10 mL. *Rx.*
Use: Coronary vasodilator; antiplatelet agent.

•**dipyrithione.** (DIE-pihr-ih-THIGH-ohn) USAN.
Use: Antifungal; anti-infective.

•**dipyrone.** (DIE-pie-rone) USAN. *Formerly Methampyrone.*
Use: Analgesic; antipyretic.

•**diquafosol tetrasodium.** (dye-kwa-FOS-ol) USAN.
Use: Dry eye.

direct factor Xa inhibitors.
See: Apixaban.

•**dirithromycin.** (die-RITH-row-MY-sin) USAN.
Use: Anti-infective, macrolide.

•**dirucotide.** (dye-RUK-oh-tide) USAN.
Use: Multiple sclerosis.

•**dirucotide acetate.** (dye-RUK-oh-tide) USAN.
Use: Multiple sclerosis.

disaccharide tripeptide glycerol dipalmitoyl.
Use: Antineoplastic. [Orphan Drug]
See: ImmTher.

Disalcid. (3M) Salsalate. **Tab.:** 500 mg, 750 mg. Bot. 100s, 500s, UD 100s. **Cap.:** 500 mg. Bot. 100s. *Rx.*
Use: Analgesic.

Discase. (Omnis Surgical) Chymopapain 5 units/2 mL. Vial 5 mL. *Rx.*
Use: Intradiscal injection for herniated lumbar intervertebral discs.

DisCoVisc. (Alcon) Sodium hyaluronate 17 mg and sodium chondroitin sulfate 40 mg per mL. Soln. Single-use disposable syringe with 27-gauge cannula and cannula locking ring delivering 0.5 mL or 1 mL packaged in a blister tray. *Rx.*
Use: Ophthalmic surgical adjunct.

Disinfecting Solution. (Bausch & Lomb) Buffered, isotonic. Sodium chloride, sodium borate, boric acid, chlorhexidine 0.005%, EDTA 0.1%, thimerosal 0.001%. Bot. 355 mL. *OTC.*
Use: Contact lens disinfection system.

•**disiquonium chloride.** (die-SIH-CONE-ee-uhm) USAN.
Use: Antiseptic.

Diskets. (Cebert) Methadone hydrochloride 40 mg. Orange-pineapple flavor. Dispersible Tab. 100s. *c-II.*
Use: Opioid analgesic.

Dismiss Douche. (Schering-Plough) Sodium Cl, sodium citrate, citric acid, cetearyl octoate, ceteareth-27, fragrance. Pow. for dilution. Pkg. 2s.
Use: Vaginal agent.

Disobrom. (Geneva) Pseudoephedrine sulfate 120 mg, dexbrompheniramine maleate 6 mg. Tab. Bot 100s, 1000s.

Rx.
Use: Antihistamine, decongestant.

•**disobutamide.** (DIE-so-BYOO-tam-ide) USAN.
Use: Cardiovascular agent (antiarrhythmic).

disodium carbonate.
See: Sodium Carbonate.

disodium chromate. Sodium Chromate Cr 51 Injection.

disodium chromoglycate.
See: Intal.
Nasalcrom.

disodium clodronate. (Discovery)
Use: Antihypercalcemic. [Orphan Drug]

disodium clodronate tetrahydrate.
Use: Increased bone resorption due to malignancy. [Orphan Drug]
See: Bonefos.

disodium edathamil.
See: Edathamil Disodium.

disodium edetate. Disodium ethylenediaminetetra acetate.
See: Edetate disodium.

disodium phosphate.
See: Sodium phosphate.

disodium phosphate heptahydrate.
See: Sodium phosphate.

disodium thiosulfate pentahydrate.
See: Sodium thiosulfate.

di-sodium versenate.
See: Edathamil Disodium.

•**disofenin.** (DIE-so-FEN-in) USAN.
Use: Diagnostic aid (carrier agent).

Disophrol. (Schering-Plough) Pseudoephedrine sulfate 60 mg, dexbrompheniramine maleate 2 mg. Tab. Bot. 100s. *OTC.*
Use: Antihistamine, decongestant.

Disophrol Chronotabs. (Schering-Plough) Dexbrompheniramine maleate 6 mg, pseudoephedrine sulfate 120 mg. SA Tab. Bot. 100s. *OTC.*
Use: Antihistamine, decongestant.

•**disopyramide.** (DIE-so-PIR-uh-mide) USAN.
Use: Cardiovascular agent (antiarrhythmic).

•**disopyramide phosphate.** (DIE-so-PIHR-ah-mide) *USP.*
Use: Cardiovascular agent; antiarrhythmic.
See: Norpace.
Norpace CR.

disopyramide phosphate. (Various Mfr.) Disopyramide phosphate. **Cap.:** 100 mg, 150 mg. Bot. 100s, 500s. **ER Cap.:** 150 mg. Bot. 100s. *Rx.*
Use: Antiarrhythmics.

•**disoxaril.** (die-SOX-ar-ILL) USAN.
Use: Antiviral.

DisperMox. (Ranbaxy) Amoxicillin 200 mg, 400 mg. Aspartame, phenylalanine 5.6 mg. Strawberry flavor. Tab. for Oral Susp. 20s, 60s, 500s (400 mg only), 1000s (200 mg only), UD 100s. *Rx.*
Use: Penicillin, aminopenicillin.

Dispos-a-Med. (Parke-Davis) Isoetharine hydrochloride 0.5%, 1%. Can of prefilled sterile tubes 0.5 mL. 50s. *Rx.*
Use: Bronchodilator.

distaquaine.
See: Penicillin V.

distigmine bromide. Hexamarium bromide.

•**disufenton sodium.** (dye-soo-FEN-ton) USAN.
Use: Neuroprotectant.

•**disulfiram.** (die-SULL-fih-ram) *USP.*
Use: Alcohol deterrent.
See: Antabuse.

disulfiram. (Various Mfr.) Disulfiram 250 mg, 500 mg. May contain lactose. Tab. 100s. *Rx.*
Use: Antialcoholic agent.

Ditate DS. (Savage) Testosterone enanthate 360 mg, estradiol valerate 16 mg, benzyl alcohol 2% in sesame oil. Syringe 2 mL. Box 10s. Vial 2 mL. *Rx.*
Use: Androgen, estrogen combination.

•**ditekiren.** (DIE-teh-KIE-ren) USAN.
Use: Antihypertensive.

dithranol.
See: Anthralin.

D.I.T.I. Creme. (Dunhall Pharmaceuticals, Inc.) Iodoquinol 100 mg, sulfanilamide 500 mg, diethylstilbestrol 0.1 mg/g. Jar. 4 oz. *Rx.*
Use: Anti-infective, vaginal.

D.I.T.I.-2 Creme. (Dunhall Pharmaceuticals, Inc.) Sulfanilamide 15%, aminacrine hydrochloride 0.2%, allantoin 2%. Tube 142 g. *Rx.*
Use: Anti-infective, vaginal.

•**ditiocade sodium.** (DIT-ee-oh-kade) USAN.
Use: Radiopharmaceutical.

Ditropan XL. (Janssen) Oxybutynin chloride 5 mg, 10 mg, 15 mg, lactose. ER Tab. Bot. 100s *Rx.*
Use: Anticholinergic.

Diulo. (Pharmacia) Metolazone 2.5 mg, 5 mg, 10 mg. Tab. Bot. 100s. *Rx.*
Use: Antihypertensive, diuretic.

diuretic combinations.
See: Alazide.
Aldactazide.
Dyazide.
Maxzide.

Maxzide-25 MG.
Moduretic.
Spironazide.
Spironolactone w/Hydrochlorothiazide.
Spirozide.
Triamterene w/Hydrochlorothiazide.

diuretics.
See: Diuretics, Loop.
Diuretics, Thiazides and Related.

diuretics, loop.
See: Bumex.
Edecrin.
Edecrin Sodium Intravenous.
Furosemide.
Lasix.
Luramide.

diuretics, osmotic.
See: Ismotic.
Mannitol.
Osmitrol.

diuretics, potassium-sparing.
See: Amiloride Hydrochloride.
Spironolactone.
Triamterene.

diuretics, thiazides and related.
See: Chlorothiazide.
Chlorthalidone.
Hydrochlorothiazide.
Indapamide.
Methyclothiazide.
Metolazone.

Diuretic Tablets. (Faraday) Buchu leaves 150 mg, uva ursi leaves 150 mg, juniper berries 120 mg, bone meal, parsley, asparagus. Bot. 100s. *Rx.*
Use: Diuretic.

Diuril. (Ovation) Chlorothiazide (as chlorothiazide sodium) 500 mg. Preservative free. Inj., Lyophilized, Pow. for Soln. Single-use vials. *Rx.*
Use: Diuretic.

Diuril. (Salix) Chlorothiazide 250 mg/ 5 mL. Alcohol 0.5%. Parabens, saccharin, sucrose. Oral Susp. 237 mL. *Rx.*
Use: Antihypertensive; diuretic.

•**divalproex sodium.** (die-VAL-pro-ex) USAN.
Use: Anticonvulsant.
See: Depakote.
Depakote ER.

divalproex sodium. (Various Mfr.) Divalproex sodium. **Tab., delayed release:** 125 mg, 250 mg, 500 mg. Enteric coated. May contain lactose, polysorbate 80, tartrazine. 100s, 300s (125 mg only), 500s, UD 80s (500 mg only), UD 100s. **ER Tab.:** 250 mg, 500 mg. 30s, 90s, 100s, 500s, UD 30s (500 mg only), UD 80s, UD 100s. **Cap., sprinkle:** 125 mg. May contain sugar. 100s, 500s, 1,000s, UD 30s, UD 80s, UD 100s. *Rx.*
Use: CNS agent, anticonvulsant.

Divigel. (Upsher-Smith) Estradiol 0.1%. Ethanol. Gel. Single-dose packets (30s). 0.25 g, 0.5 g, 1 g. *Rx.*
Use: Sex hormone, estrogen.

divinyl oxide. Vinyl ether, divinyl ether.
Use: Inhalation anesthetic.

Dizac. (Ohmeda) Diazepam 5 mg/mL, preservative free. Inj. Vial 3 mL. *c-IV.*
Use: Anxiolytic; anticonvulsant; muscle relaxant.

Dizmiss. (Jones Pharma) Meclizine hydrochloride 25 mg. Tab. Bot. 100s, 1000s. *OTC.*
Use: Antiemetic; antivertigo.

•**dizocilpine maleate.** (die-ZOE-sill-PEEN) USAN.
Use: Neuroprotective.

dl-desoxyephedrine hydrochloride.
See: dl-Methamphetamine hydrochloride.

dl-methamphetamine hydrochloride.
dl-Desoxyephedrine hydrochloride.

dl-norephedrine hydrochloride.

DMax. (Great Southern) Dextromethorphan HBr 15 mg, phenylephrine hydrochloride 8 mg, carbinoxamine maleate 4 mg per 5 mL. Berry flavor. Syrup. 30 mL, 473 mL. *Rx.*
Use: Antitussive, antihistamine, decongestant.

DMax Pediatric. (Great Southern) Dextromethorphan HBr 4 mg, phenylephrine 2 mg, carbinoxamine maleate 2 mg per 1 mL. Purple. Berry flavor. Drops. 30 mL bot. with 1 mL dropper. *Rx.*
Use: Antitussive, antihistamine, decongestant.

DM Cough. (Rosemont) Dextromethorphan HBr 10 mg/5 mL, alcohol 5%. Syrup. Bot. 120 mL, pt, gal. *OTC.*
Use: Antitussive.

DM/CPM/PE/GG. (Kylemore Pharmaceuticals) Dextromethorphan hydrobromide 15 mg, guaifenesin 100 mg, phenylephrine hydrochloride 10 mg, chlorpheniramine maleate 2 mg per 5 mL. Fruit gum flavoring, glycerin, parabens, propylene glycol, saccharin, sorbitol. Syrup. 473 mL. *Rx.*
Use: Upper respiratory combination, antitussive and expectorant combination.

DMCT. (Wyeth) Demethylchlortetracycline. *Rx.*
Use: Anti-infective; tetracycline.
See: Declomycin hydrochloride.

d-methorphan hydrobromide.
See: Dextromethorphan Hydrobromide.

d-methylphenylamine sulfate.
See: Dextroamphetamine Sulfate.

DML Dermatological Moisturizing Lotion. (Person and Covey) Purified water, petrolatum, glycerin, methyl glucose sesquisterate, dimethicone, methyl gluceth-20 sesquisterate, benzyl alcohol, volatile silicone, glyceryl stearate, stearic acid, palmitic acid, cetyl alcohol, xanthan gum, magnesium aluminum silicate carbomer 941, sodium hydroxide. Bot. 8 oz. *OTC.*
Use: Emollient.

DML Facial Moisturizer. (Person and Covey) Octyl methoxycinnamate 8%, oxybenzone 4%, benzyl alcohol, petrolatum, EDTA. SPF 15. Cream. Tube 45 g. *OTC.*
Use: Sunscreen.

DML Forte. (Person and Covey) Petrolatum, PPG-2 myristyl ether propionate, glyceryl stearate, glycerin, stearic acid, d-panthenol, DEA-cetyl phosphate, simethicone, PVP eicosene copolymer, benzyl alcohol, cetyl alcohol, silica, disodium EDTA, BHA, magnesium aluminum silicate, sodium carbomer 1342. Tube 113 g. *OTC.*
Use: Emollient.

DM/PE/CPM. (Kylemore Pharmaceuticals) Chlorpheniramine maleate 1 mg, dextromethorphan hydrobromide 3 mg, phenylephrine hydrochloride 1.5 mg. Glycerin, parabens, propylene glycol, saccharin, sorbitol. Alcohol free and sugar free. Fruit gum flavor. Drops. 30 mL w/dropper. *Rx.*
Use: Upper respiratory combination, antitussive combination.

DM/PSE/BPM. (Kylemore Pharmaceuticals) Brompheniramine maleate 3 mg, dextromethorphan hydrobromide 30 mg, pseudoephedrine hydrochloride 50 mg per 5 mL. Glycerin, parabens, propylene glycol, saccharin, sorbitol. Berry-vanilla flavor. Syrup. 473 mL. *Rx.*
Use: Upper respiratory combination, antitussive combination.

DMP 777. (DuPont)
Use: Cystic fibrosis. [Orphan Drug]

DMSO.
See: Dimethyl sulfoxide.

DNA demethylation agents.
See: Azacitidine.
Decitabine.
Nelarabine.

DNA topoisomerase inhibitors.
See: Irinotecan hydrochloride.
Topotecan.

Doak Tar. (Doak Dermatologics) **Lot.:** Tar distillate 5%. Bot. 118 mL. **Oil:** Tar distillate 2%. Mineral oil. Bot. 237 mL. **Shampoo:** Coal tar 1.2%, isopropyl alcohol. Bot. 237 mL. *OTC.*
Use: Antiseborrheic.

Doak Tar Oil Forte. (Doak Dermatologics) Tar distillate 5%. Bot. 4 oz.
Use: Antiseborrheic.

Doak Tersaseptic. (Doak Dermatologics) Liquid cleanser, pH 6.8. Bot. 4 oz, pt, gal. *OTC.*
Use: Detergent.

Doan's. (Novartis Consumer Health) Magnesium salicylate 377 mg (as tetrahydrate, equiv. to magnesium salicylate anhydrous 303.7 mg). Tab. 24s. *OTC.*
Use: Analgesic.

Doan's Backache Spray. (Novartis Consumer Health) Methyl salicylate 15%, menthol 8.4%, methyl nicotinate 0.6%. Aerosol Can 4 oz. *OTC.*
Use: Analgesic, topical.

Doan's Pills. (Novartis Consumer Health) Magnesium salicylate 325 mg. Tab. Ctn. 24s, 48s. *OTC.*
Use: Analgesic.

Doan's PM Extra Strength. (Novartis Consumer Health) Magnesium salicylate 580 mg, diphenhydramine hydrochloride 25 mg. Methylparaben, PEG. Tab. 20s. *OTC.*
Use: Sleep aid.

dobutamine. (Various Mfr.) Dobutamine hydrochloride 12.5 mg/mL. May contain sulfites. Inj., Soln., Conc. Single-use vial 20 mL, 40 mL, 100 mL pharmacy bulk packages. *Rx.*
Use: Cardiovascular agent.

•**dobutamine hydrochloride.** (doe-BYOOT-ah-meen) *USP.*
Tall Man: DOBUTamine
Use: Cardiovascular agent.

dobutamine hydrochloride in 5% dextrose injection. (Baxter) Dobutamine 250 mg per 250 mL (1 mg/mL), 500 mg per 500 mL (1 mg/mL), 500 mg per 250 mL (2 mg/mL), 1,000 mg per 250 mL (4 mg/mL). Sodium bisulfite. Preservative free. Inj., Soln. Single-use *Viaflex Plus* plastic container. 250 mL (except 500 mg/500 mL), 500 mL (500 mg/500 mL). *Rx.*
Use: Vasopressor.

•**dobutamine in dextrose for injection.** (doe-BYOOT-ah-meen) *USP.*
Tall Man: DOBUTamine
Use: Cardiovascular agent.

•**dobutamine lactobionate.** (doe-BYOOT-ah-meen) USAN.
Tall Man: DOBUTamine
Use: Cardiovascular agent.

•**dobutamine tartrate.** (doe-BYOOT-ah-meen) USAN.
Tall Man: DOBUTamine
Use: Cardiovascular agent.

•**docebenone.** (dah-SEH-beh-nohn) USAN.
Use: Inhibitor (5-lipoxygenase).

Docefrez. (Sun Pharmaceutical) Docetaxel 20 mg, 80 mg. Single-use vial (diluent contains ethanol in polysorbate 80). Inj., lyophilized Pow. for Soln. *Rx.*
Use: Antimitotic agent, taxoid.

•**docetaxel.** (doe-seh-TAX-ehl) USAN.
Tall Man: DOCEtaxel
Use: Antineoplastic, antimitotic.
See: Docefrez.
Taxotere.

docetaxel. (Winthrop) Docetaxel 20 mg/mL. Alcohol, polysorbate 80 (in 50/50 [v/v] ratio polysorbate 80/dehydrated alcohol). Inj., Soln.; concentrate. Single-use vial. *Rx.*
Use: Antimitotic agent, taxoid.

docetaxel. (Various Mfr.) Docetaxel. **Inj., Soln., concentrate:** 20 mg/mL, 40 mg/mL. May contain alcohol, polysorbate 80. Single-use vial. 0.5 mL, 2 mL (40 mg/mL); 1 mL, 4 mL, 8 mL (20 mg/mL). **Inj., Soln.:** 10 mg/mL. May contain alcohol, PEG, polysorbate 80. Multidose vial. 2 mL, 8 mL, 16 mL. *Rx.*
Use: Antimitotic agent, taxoid.

•**doconazole.** (doe-KOE-nah-zole) USAN.
Use: Antifungal.

•**docosanol.** (doe-KOE-sah-nole) USAN.
Use: Antiviral.
See: Abreva.

DocQlace. (Qualitest) Docusate sodium 100 mg. Glycerin, PEG, sodium 5 mg, sorbitol. Cap., softgel. 100s, 1,000s. *OTC.*
Use: Laxative, fecal softener/surfactant.

Doctase. (Purepac) Docusate sodium 100 mg, casanthranol 30 mg. Cap. Bot. 100s. *OTC.*
Use: Laxative.

Doctyl. (Health for Life Brands) Docusate sodium 100 mg. Tab. Bot. 40s, 100s, 1000s. *OTC.*
Use: Laxative.

Doctylax. (Health for Life Brands) Docusate sodium 100 mg, acetophenolisatin 2 mg, prune conc. ¾ mg. Tab. Bot. 40s, 100s, 1000s. *OTC.*
Use: Laxative.

Docu. (Hi-Tech Pharmacal) Docusate sodium. **Syrup:** 20 mg/5 mL, alcohol 5%. Bot. 480 mL. **Liq.:** 150 mg/15 mL. Bot. 480 mL. *OTC.*
Use: Laxative.

•**docusate calcium.** (DOCK-you-sate) *USP. Formerly Dioctyl Calcium Sulfosuccinate.*
Use: Laxative; stool softener.
See: DC Softgels.
Stool Softner.
Stool Softner DC.
Surfak Stool Softener.

docusate calcium. (Various Mfr.) Docusate calcium 240 mg. Cap. Bot. 100s, 500s, UD 100s, 300s. *OTC.*
Use: Laxative.

•**docusate potassium.** (DOCK-you-sate) *USP.*
Use: Laxative; stool softener.

•**docusate sodium.** (DOCK-you-sate) *USP. Formerly Dioctyl Sodium Sulfosuccinate.*
Use: Pharmaceutical aid (surfactant); stool softener.
See: Colace.
Coloctyl.
Diocto.
Dioctyn Softgels.
DocQlace.
Docu.
Docusoft-S.
DocuSol Mini.
DOK.
D.O.S.
D-S-S.
Dulcolax Stool Softener.
Duosol.
Easy-Lax.
Enemeez.
Enemeez Plus.
ex-lax Stool Softener.
Konsto.
Non-Habit Forming Stool Softner.
Phillips' Liqui-Gels.
Silace.
Sof-lax.
Stool Softner.
Stulex.

W/Betaine Hydrochloride, Zinc, Manganese, Molybdenum.
See: Hemaferrin.

W/Casanthranol.
See: Calotabs.
Dio-Soft.
DOK-Plus.
Easy-Lax Plus.
Laxative and Stool Softener.

W/Ferrous Fumarate, Betaine Hydrochloride, Desiccated Liver, Vitamins, Minerals.
See: Hemaferrin.

W/Phenolphthalein.
See: Feen-A-Mint Dual Formula.
Phillips' LaxCaps.

W/Phenolphthalein, Dehydrocholic Acid.
See: Bolax.

W/Polyoxyethylene-Nonyl-Phenol, Sodium Edetate, 9-Aminoacridine Hydrochloride.
See: Vagisec Plus.
W/Senna Concentrate.
See: DOK Plus.
PeriColace.
Senna Plus.
Senokot S.
W/Sennosides.
See: ex-lax Gentle Strength.
Laxacin.
Senna-S.
docusate sodium. (Roxane) Docusate sodium 50 mg/15 mL, 100 mg/30 mL, saccharin, sucrose, parabens. Syr. UD 15 mL, 30 mL (100s). *OTC.*
Use: Laxative.
docusate sodium. (UDL) Docusate sodium 50 mg. Softgel cap. Bot. 100s, UD 100s *OTC.*
Use: Laxative.
docusate sodium. (Various Mfr.) Docusate sodium. **Cap.:** 250 mg. Bot. 100s, 1000s, UD 100s. **Softgel Cap.:** 100 mg, 250 mg. Bot. 100s, 1000s, UD 100s, 300s (100 mg only). *OTC.*
Use: Laxative.
docusate with casanthranol. (Various Mfr.) Docusate sodium 100 mg, casanthranol 30 mg. Cap. Bot. 100s, 1000s, UD 100s, 300s, 600s. *OTC.*
Use: Laxative; stool softener.
Docusoft-S. (G & W Labs) Docusate sodium 100 mg. Glycerin, PEG, sorbitol. Cap. 60s. *OTC.*
Use: Laxative, fecal softener/surfactant.
DocuSol Mini. (Alliance Labs) Docusate sodium 283 mg. PEG, glycerin. Enema, rectal. 5s. *OTC.*
Use: Laxative.
•**dofetilide.** (doe-FEH-till-ide) USAN.
Use: Cardiovascular agent; antiarrhythmic.
See: Tikosyn.
Dofus. (Miller) 1 billion organism 10:1 blend of *L. acidophilus* and *L. bifidus.* Cap. 60s. *OTC.*
Use: Probiotic.
DOK. (Major) Docusate sodium 250 mg. Cap. 100s. *OTC.*
Use: Laxative.
DOK Plus. (Major) Docusate 50 mg (as sodium), senna concentrate 8.6 mg (as sennosides). PEG-400. Tab. 100s. *OTC.*
Use: Laxative combination.
Doktors Spray. (Scherer) Phenylephrine hydrochloride 0.25%, chlorobutanol, sodium bisulfite, benzalkonium chloride. Soln. Bot. 30 mL. *OTC.*
Use: Decongestant.
Dolamide Tabs. (Major) Chlorpropamide 100 mg, 250 mg. Bot. 100s, 500s, 1000s. *Rx.*
Use: Antidiabetic.
Dolamin. (Harvey) Ammonium sulfate 0.75% with sodium chloride, benzyl alcohol. Amp. 10 mL. In 12s, 25s, 100s. *Rx.*
Use: Antineuralgic.
dolantin.
See: Meperidine hydrochloride.
•**dolasetron mesylate.** (dahl-AH-set-rahn) *USP.*
Use: Antiemetic; antimigraine.
See: Anzemet.
Dolcin. (Dolcin) Aspirin 3.7 g, calcium succinate 2.8 g. Tab. Bot. 100s, 200s. *OTC.*
Use: Analgesic.
Doldram. (Dram) Salicylamide 7.5 g. Tab. Bot. 100s.
Use: Analgesic.
Dolene AP-65. (Wyeth) Propoxyphene hydrochloride 65 mg, acetaminophen 650 mg. Tab. Bot. 100s, 500s. *c-IV.*
Use: Analgesic combination; narcotic.
Dolene Compound-65. (Wyeth) Propoxyphene hydrochloride 65 mg, aspirin 389 mg, caffeine 32.4 mg. Cap. Bot. 100s, 500s. *c-IV.*
Use: Analgesic combination; narcotic.
Dolene Plain. (Wyeth) Propoxyphene hydrochloride 65 mg. Cap. Bot. 100s, 500s. *c-IV.*
Use: Analgesic; narcotic.
Dolgic. (Athlon) Acetaminophen 650 mg, butalbital 50 mg. Tab. Bot. 100s. *Rx.*
Use: Analgesic.
Dolgic LQ. (Athlon) Acetaminophen 108.3 mg, caffeine 13.3 mg, butalbital 16.6 mg/5 mL, alcohol 7.368%, orange, tropical fruit punch flavors. Soln. 473 mL. *Rx.*
Use: Analgesic, nonnarcotic.
Dolgic Plus. (Shionogi Pharma) Butalbital 50 mg, acetaminophen 750 mg, caffeine 40 mg. Film-coated. Tab. 100s. *Rx.*
Use: Nonnarcotic analgesic combination.
Dolomite. (Halsey Drug) Calcium 426 mg, magnesium 246 mg. Tab. w/guar and acacia gum. Bot. 250s. *OTC.*
Use: Mineral supplement.
Dolomite. (NBTY) Magnesium 78 mg, calcium 130 mg. Tab. Bot. 100s, 250s. *OTC.*
Use: Mineral supplement.
Dolomite Plus Capsules. (Barth's) Magnesium 37 mg, calcium 187 mg, phos-

phorus 50 mg, iodine 0.25 mg. Bot. 100s, 500s, 1000s. *OTC.*
Use: Mineral supplement.

Dolomite Tablets. (Faraday) Calcium 150 mg, magnesium 90 mg. Bot. 250s. *OTC.*
Use: Mineral supplement.

Dolonil. (Parke-Davis)
See: Pyridium Plus.

Dolono. (R.I.D.) Acetaminophen 160 mg/ 5 mL, sorbitol, sucrose, alcohol free, cherry flavor. Elixir. Bot. 120 mL. *OTC.*
Use: Analgesic.

Dolophine Hydrochloride. (Roxane) Methadone hydrochloride 5 mg, 10 mg. Tab. Bot. 100s. *c-II.*
Use: Opioid analgesic.

Dolopirona Tablets. (Sanofi-Synthelabo) Dipyrone with chlormezanone. *Rx.*
Use: Analgesic; anxiolytic; muscle relaxant.

Doloral. (Progressive Enterprises) Colchicine salicylate 0.1 mg, phenobarbital 8 mg, sodium para-aminobenzoate 15 mg, vitamins B_1 25 mg, aspirin 325 mg. Tab. Bot. 100s, 1000s. *Rx.*
Use: Antiarthritis, antigout.

dolosal.
See: Meperidine hydrochloride.

•**dolutegravir.** (DOE-loo-TEG-ra-vir) USAN.
Use: Treatment of HIV infection.
See: Tivicay.

•**dolutegravir sodium.** (DOE-loo-TEG-ra-vir) USAN.
Use: Treatment of HIV infection.

dolvanol.
Use: Analgesic; narcotic.
See: Meperidine Hydrochloride.

•**domazoline fumarate.** (DOME-AZE-oh-leen) USAN.
Use: Anticholinergic.

Domeboro Otic. (Bayer Consumer Care) Acetic acid 2% (in aluminum acetate solution). Soln. Bot. 60 mL with dropper. *Rx.*
Use: Otic.

Dome-Paste Bandage. (Bayer Consumer Care) Zinc oxide, calamine and gelatin bandage. Pkg. 4" × 10 yd. and 3" × 10 yd. impregnated gauze bandage. *OTC.*
Use: Dermatologic, wound therapy.

domestrol.
See: Diethylstilbestrol.

D.O.M.F.
Use: Antimicrobial.
See: Merbromin (Mercurochrome).

•**domiodol.** (dome-EYE-oh-DOLE) USAN.
Use: Mucolytic.

•**domiphen bromide.** (DOE-mih-fen) USAN.
Use: Antiseptic; anti-infective, topical.

Domol Bath and Shower Oil. (Bayer Consumer Care) D_1-isopropyl sebacate, isopropyl myristate with mineral oil. Bot. 240 mL. *OTC.*
Use: Emollient.

•**domperidone.** (dome-PEH-rih-dohn) USAN.
Use: Investigational antiemetic.

Donatuss DC. (Laser) Dihydrocodeine bitartrate 7.5 mg, guaifenesin 50 mg, phenylephrine hydrochloride 7.5 mg per 5 mL. Saccharin, sucrose. Alcohol free and gluten free. Grape flavor. Syr. 473 mL. *c-III.*
Use: Upper respiratory combination, antitussive and expectorant combination.

Donatussin. (Laser) Chlophedianol hydrochloride 12.5 mg, guaifenesin 120 mg, phenylephrine hydrochloride 5 mg per 5 mL. Glycerin, propylene glycol, saccharin, sorbitol, sucralose. Berry-vanilla flavor. Syrup. 473 mL. *OTC.*
Use: Upper respiratory combination, antitussive and expectorant combination.

Donatussin. (Laser) Guaifenesin 20 mg, phenylephrine hydrochloride 1.5 mg. Saccharin, sorbitol. Alcohol free and sugar free. Raspberry flavor. Drops. 30 mL with dropper. *Rx.*
Use: Upper respiratory combination, decongestant and expectorant combination.

Donatussin DM. (Laser) **Drops:** Dextromethorphan HBr 3 mg, chlorpheniramine maleate 1 mg, phenylephrine hydrochloride 1.5 mg per 1 mL. Bubble gum flavor. 30 mL with dropper. **Syrup:** Dextromethorphan HBr 15 mg, guaifenesin 150 mg, pseudoephedrine hydrochloride 30 mg per 5 mL. Alcohol and sugar free. Saccharin, sorbitol. Cool-mint flavor. 30 mL, 473 mL. *Rx.*
Use: Antitussive combination, antitussive and expectorant combination, upper respiratory combination.

Dondril. (Whitehall-Robins) Dextromethorphan HBr 10 mg, phenylephrine hydrochloride 5 mg, chlorpheniramine maleate 1 mg. Tab. Bot. 24s. *OTC.*
Use: Antihistamine; antitussive; decongestant.

donepezil. (Various Mfr.) Donepezil hydrochloride. **Tab.:** 5 mg, 10 mg, 23 mg. May contain lactose. 30s, 90s, 500s, 1,000s, 2,650s (10 mg only),

4,000s (5 mg only), UD 100s (except 23 mg). **Tab., orally disintegrating:** 5 mg, 10 mg. May contain aspartame, mannitol, phenylalanine, xylitol. UD 30s, UD 100s. *Rx.*
Use: Cholinesterase inhibitor.

donepezil. (UDL) Donepezil hydrochloride. *Rx.*
Use: Cholinesterase inhibitor.

•**donepezil hydrochloride.** (doe-NEPP-eh-zill) USAN.
Use: Treatment of mild to moderate dementia of the Alzheimer type.
See: Aricept.
Aricept ODT.

D1000. (Mason) Cholecalciferol 1,000 units. Fructose, sucrose, sunflower oil, xylitol. Preservative free. Peach vanilla flavor. Chew. Tab. 50s. *OTC.*
Use: Fat-soluble vitamin, vitamin D.

D-1000 Extra Strength. (21st Century HealthCare) Vitamin D 1,000 units, calcium 90 mg. Gluten free and preservative free. Tab. 300s. *OTC.*
Use: Nutritional combination product.

D1000 Plus. (Mason) Vitamin D_3 1,000 units, B_6 10 mg, B_{12} 200 mcg, folic acid 400 mcg. PEG. Tab. 60s. *OTC.*
Use: Multivitamin with minerals.

•**donetidine.** (doe-NEH-tih-DEEN) USAN.
Use: Antiulcerative.

Donna. (Arcum) Menthol, thymol, eucalyptol, exsiccated alum, boric acid. 4 oz, 14 oz. *Rx.*
Use: Vaginal agent.

Donnaphen. (Health for Life Brands) Phenobarbital 16.2 mg, hyoscyamine sulfate 0.1037 mg, atropine sulfate 0.0194 mg, hyoscine HBr 0.0065 mg/5 mL. Elix. Bot. Pt, gal. *Rx.*
Use: Anticholinergic; antispasmodic.

Donna-Sed Elixir. (Vortech Pharmaceuticals) Atropine sulfate 0.0194 mg, scopolamine HBr 0.0065, hyoscyamine HBr, or SO_4 0.1037 mg, phenobarbital 16.2 mg, alcohol 23%. Liq. Bot. 118 mL, gal. *Rx.*
Use: Gastrointestinal; anticholinergic.

Donnatal. (PBM Pharm) **Elix.:** Atropine sulfate 0.0194 mg, scopolamine hydrobromide 0.0065 mg, hyoscyamine hydrobromide or sulfate 0.1037 mg, phenobarbital 16.2 mg per 5 mL. Ethyl alcohol 95%, saccharin, sucrose, sorbitol. Grape flavor. 118 mL, 473 mL. **Tab.:** Atropine sulfate 0.0194 mg, scopolamine hydrobromide 0.0065 mg, hyoscyamine hydrobromide or sulfate 0.1037 mg, phenobarbital 16.2 mg. Lactose. 100s, 1,000s. *Rx.*
Use: Gastrointestinal anticholinergic combination.

Donnatal Extentabs. (PBM Pharm) Atropine sulfate 0.0582 mg, scopolamine hydrobromide 0.0195 mg, hyoscyamine sulfate 0.3111 mg, phenobarbital 48.6 mg. Lactose, polydextrose. Film-coated. ER Tab. 100s, 500s. *Rx.*
Use: Gastrointestinal anticholinergic combination.

Don't. (Del) Sucrose octa acetate 5%, isopropyl alcohol 54%. Bot. 0.45 oz. *OTC.*
Use: Nail-biting deterrent.

•**dopamantine.** (DOE-pah-MAN-teen) USAN.
Use: Antiparkinsonian.

dopamine. (AstraZeneca) Dopamine. **Amp.:** 200 mg/5 mL, Box 10s; 400 mg/10 mL, Box 5s. **Additive Syringe:** 200 mg/5 mL, Box 1s; 400 mg/10 mL, Box 1s. *Rx.*
Use: Inotropic agent.

•**dopamine hydrochloride.** (DOE-puh-meen) *USP.*
Tall Man: DOPamine
Use: Adrenergic; vasopressor.

dopamine hydrochloride. (Various Mfr.) Dopamine hydrochloride 40 mg/mL, 80 mg/mL, 160 mg/mL. May contain sodium metabisulfate. Inj. Vials. 5 mL, 10 mL (except 160 mg/mL). *Rx.*
Use: Vasopressor.

dopamine hydrochloride and dextrose injection.
Use: Adrenergic; emergency treatment of low blood pressure.

dopamine hydrochloride in dextrose 5% injection. (Various Mfr.) Dopamine 200 mg/250 mL (0.8 mg/mL), 400 mg/500 mL (0.8 mg/mL), 400 mg/250 mL (1.6 mg/mL), 800 mg/500 mL (1.6 mg/mL), 800 mg/250 mL (3.2 mg/mL). May contain sulfites. Inj., Soln. Premixed single-use container. 250 mL (200 mg/250 mL, 400 mg/250 mL, 800 mg/250 mL), 500 mL (400 mg/500 mL, 800 mg/500 mL). *Rx.*
Use: Vasopressor.

dopamine receptor agonists, nonergot.
Use: Antiparkinson agents.
See: Pramipexole Dihydrochloride.
Rotigotine.

dopaminergics.
Use: Antiparkinson agents.
See: Apomorphine Hydrochloride.
Dopamine Receptor Agonists, Nonergot.
Ropinirole Hydrochloride.

•**dopexamine.** (doe-PEX-ah-MEEN) USAN.
Use: Cardiovascular agent.

•**dopexamine hydrochloride.** (doe-PEX-ah-MEEN) USAN.
Use: Cardiovascular agent.
Dopram. (West-Ward) Doxapram hydrochloride 20 mg/mL, 0.9% benzyl alcohol. Inj. Multiple-dose vial 20 mL. *Rx.*
Use: CNS stimulant, analeptic.
Doral. (Nuro Pharma) Quazepam 7.5 mg, 15 mg. Tab. Bot. 100s, 500s, UD 100s. *c-IV.*
Use: Sedative/hypnotic, nonbarbiturate.
•**doramapimod.** (dore-a-MAP-i-mod) USAN.
Use: Crohn disease; RA; psoriasis.
•**dorastine hydrochloride.** (DAHR-ass-teen) USAN.
Use: Antihistamine.
•**doravirine.** (DOR-a-VIR-een) USAN.
Use: Antiviral agent.
•**doretinel.** (DOE-REH-tin-ell) USAN.
Use: Antikeratinizing agent.
Doribax. (Shionogi) Doripenem 250 mg, 500 mg. Preservative free. Inj., Pow. for Soln. Single-use vials. *Rx.*
Use: Carbapenem, antibiotic.
Doriglute Tabs DEA. (Major) Glutethimide 0.5 g. Tab. Bot. 100s, 250s, 1000s. *c-II.*
Use: Hypnotic.
•**doripenem.** (dore-i-PEN-em) USAN.
Use: Antibiotic, carbapenem.
See: Doribax.
Dormeer. (Taylor Pharmaceuticals) Scopolamine aminoxide HBr 0.2 mg. Cap. Bot. 100s, 1000s. *Rx.*
Use: Hypnotic; sedative.
dormethan.
See: Dextromethorphan Hydrobromide
Dormin. (Randob) Diphenhydramine hydrochloride 25 mg. Lactose. Cap. 32s, 72s. *OTC.*
Use: Antihistamine, nonselective ethanolamine.
Dormin Sleeping Caplets. (Randob) Diphenhydramine hydrochloride 25 mg. Bot. 32s. *OTC.*
Use: Sleep aid.
Dormiral.
See: Phenobarbital.
Dormonal.
See: Barbital.
Dormutol. (Health for Life Brands) Scopolamine aminoxide HBr 0.2 mg. Cap. Bot. 24s, 60s. *Rx.*
Use: Hypnotic; sedative.
•**dornase alfa.** (DOR-nace AL-fuh) USAN.
Use: Cystic fibrosis. [Orphan Drug]
See: Pulmozyme.
Doryx. (Warner Chilcott) Doxycycline hyclate 150 mg, 200 mg. Lactose. DR Tab. 60s. *Rx.*
Use: Anti-infective; tetracycline.
dorzolamide. (Prasco Laboratories) Dorzolamide 2% (as dorzolamide hydrochloride). Benzalkonium chloride 0.0075%, hydroxyethyl cellulose, sodium hydroxide, sodium citrate. Soln., Ophth. *Ocumeter Plus.* 10 mL. *Rx.*
Use: Agent for glaucoma, carbonic anhydrase inhibitor.
•**dorzolamide hydrochloride.** (dore-ZOLE-lah-mide) *USP.*
Use: Carbonic anhydrase inhibitor.
See: TruSopt.
dorzolamide hydrochloride and timolol maleate.
Use: Agents for glaucoma.
See: Cosopt.
Cosopt PF.
dorzolamide hydrochloride and timolol maleate. (Various Mfr.) Dorzolamide hydrochloride 2%, timolol maleate 0.5%. May contain benzalkonium chloride 0.0075%. Soln., Ophth. 5 mL, 10 mL. *Rx.*
Use: Agent for glaucoma.
D.O.S. (Goldline Consumer) Docusate sodium 100 mg, 250 mg, parabens. Softgel Cap. Bot. 100s, 500s (250 mg only), 1000s (100 mg only). *OTC.*
Use: Laxative.
Dosaflex. (Richwood Pharmaceuticals) Senna fruit extract, parabens, sucrose, alcohol 7%. Syrup. Bot. 237 mL. *OTC.*
Use: Laxative.
Doss Syrup. (Rosemont) Docusate sodium 20 mg/5 mL. Bot. Pt, gal. *OTC.*
Use: Laxative; stool softener.
Dotarem. (Guerbet) Gadoterate meglumine 0.5 mmol/mL. Preservative free. Inj., Soln. Prefilled syringe and vial. 10 mL, 15 mL, 20 mL. *Rx.*
Use: Miscellaneous radiopaque agent.
•**dothiepin hydrochloride.** (DOE-THIGH-eh-pin) USAN.
Use: Antidepressant.
Dotirol. (Sanofi-Synthelabo) Ampicillin trihydrate available in Cap, Susp., Inj. (IV, IM). *Rx.*
Use: Anti-infective; penicillin.
Double-Action Toothache Kit. (C.S. Dent & Co.) **Liq.; dental:** Benzocaine. Alcohol 74%, chlorobutanol anhydrous 0.09%. 3.7 mL. **Maronox Pain Relief Tablets:** Acetaminophen 325 mg. Tab. Box. 8s. *OTC.*
Use: Analgesic, topical.
Double Antibiotic. (Fougera) Polymyxin B sulfate 10,000 units, bacitracin zinc 500 units per g. Oint. Tubes. ≈ 15 g, ≈ 30 g, UD 0.9 g (144s). *OTC.*
Use: Topical anti-infective, antibiotic.

Double Sal. (Pal-Pak, Inc.) Sodium salicylate 648 mg. EC Tab. Bot. 1000s. *OTC.*
Use: Analgesic.

Double Strength Gaviscon-2. (GlaxoSmithKline) Aluminum hydroxide 160 mg, magnesium trisilicate 40 mg, alginic acid, calcium stearate, sodium bicarbonate, sucrose. Tab. Bot. 48s. *OTC.*
Use: Antacid.

Dovacet Capsules. (Pal-Pak, Inc.) Dover's powder 24.3 mg, aspirin 324 mg, caffeine 32.4 mg. Bot. 1000s.
Use: Analgesic.

Dover's Powder. Ipecac 1 part, opium 1 part, lactose 8 parts.
Use: Analgesic; diaphoretic; sedative.
W/Atropine Sulfate, A.P.C., Camphor.
See: Dasin.

Dovonex. (LeoPharma) Calcipotriene 0.005%. Cream. Tube. 30 g, 60 g, 100 g. *Rx.*
Use: Dermatologic; antipsoriatic.

Dowicil 200.
Use: Antibacterial.
See: Derma Soap.

Dow-Isoniazid. (Hoechst) Isoniazid 300 mg. Tab. Bot. 30s. *Rx.*
Use: Antituberculosal.

Doxamin. (Forest) Thiamine hydrochloride 100 mg, vitamin B_6 100 mg/mL. Vial 10 mL. *Rx.*
Use: Vitamin supplement.

Doxapap-N. (Major) Propoxyphene napsylate 100 mg, acetaminophen 650 mg. Tab. Bot. 100s, 500s. *c-iv.*
Use: Analgesic combination, narcotic.

Doxaphene Capsules. (Major) Propoxyphene hydrochloride 65 mg. Cap. Bot. 1000s. *c-iv.*
Use: Analgesic; narcotic.

Doxaphene Compound 65 Caps. (Major) Propoxyphene hydrochloride, acetaminophen. Cap. Bot. 1000s. *c-iv.*
Use: Analgesic combination, narcotic.

•**doxapram hydrochloride.** (DOX-uh-pram) *USP.*
Use: Respiratory and CNS stimulant, analeptic.
See: Dopram.

doxapram hydrochloride. (Bedford) Doxapram hydrochloride 20 mg/mL. Benzyl alcohol 0.9%. Inj. Multiple-dose vial. 20 mL.
Use: Respiratory and CNS stimulant.

•**doxaprost.** (DOX-ah-proste) USAN.
Use: Bronchodilator.

Doxate. Docusate sodium. *OTC.*
Use: Laxative.

•**doxazosin mesylate.** (DOX-uh-ZOE-sin) USAN.
Use: Antihypertensive, antiadrenergic.
See: Cardura.
Cardura XL.

doxazosin mesylate. (Various Mfr.) Doxazosin mesylate (as base) 1 mg, 2 mg, 4 mg, 8 mg. May contain lactose. Tab. Bot. 100s, 500s, 1000s, UD 100s. *Rx.*
Use: Antihypertensive, antiadrenergic.

doxepin. (Par) Doxepin hydrochloride 150 mg. Cap. 50s, 100s, 500s. *Rx.*
Use: Antidepressant.

doxepin. (Various Mfr.) Doxepin hydrochloride. **Cap.:** 10 mg, 25 mg, 50 mg, 75 mg, 100 mg. 100s, 1,000s, UD 100s (except 75 mg). **Oral Conc.:** 10 mg/mL. May contain glycerin, parabens. 120 mL. *Rx.*
Use: Antidepressant.

•**doxepin hydrochloride.** (DOX-uh-pin) *USP.*
Use: Psychotherapeutic agent; antidepressant.
See: Prudoxin.
Silenor.

•**doxercalciferol.** (dox-ehr-kal-SIFF-eh-role) USAN.
Use: Secondary hyperparathyroidism associated with end-stage renal disease.
See: Hectorol.

doxercalciferol. (Various Mfr.) Doxercalciferol. **Cap., softgel:** 0.5 mcg, 1 mcg, 2.5 mcg. May contain coconut oil. 50s. **Inj., Soln.:** 2 mcg/mL. May contain disodium edetate, ethanol. Single-use 2 mL vial. *Rx.*
Use: Fat-soluble vitamin.

Doxil. (Janssen) Doxorubicin hydrochloride 2 mg/mL. Sucrose. Preservative free. Inj., Susp., Liposomal Conc. Single-use vials. 10 mL, 30 mL. *Rx.*
Use: Antibiotic, anthracycline.

•**doxofylline.** (DOX-oh-fill-een) USAN.
Use: Bronchodilator.

•**doxorubicin.** (DOX-oh-ROO-bih-sin) USAN.
Tall Man: DOXOrubicin
Use: Antineoplastic; antibiotic, anthracycline.

•**doxorubicin hydrochloride.** (DOX-oh-ROO-bih-sin) *USP.*
Tall Man: DOXOrubicin
Use: Antineoplastic; antibiotic, anthracycline.
See: Adriamycin.
Doxil.
Lipodox.
Lipodox 50.

doxorubicin hydrochloride. (Bedford Labs) Doxorubicin hydrochloride. **Inj.,**

lyophilized, Pow. for Soln.: 10 mg, 50 mg. Single-dose flip-top vials. **Inj., Soln.:** 2 mg/mL. Vials. 5 mL, 10 mL, 25 mL, 75 mL, 100 mL. *Rx.*
Use: Antibiotic, anthracycline.

doxorubicin hydrochloride. (Caraco) Doxorubicin hydrochloride 2 mg/mL. Sucrose. Preservative free. Inj., Susp.; liposomal concentrate. Single-use vial. 10 mL, 25 mL. *Rx.*
Use: Antineoplastic antibiotic, anthracycline.

•**doxpicomine hydrochloride.** (DOX-PIH-koe-meen) USAN. *Formerly Doxpicodin Hydrochloride.*
Use: Analgesic.

•**doxycycline.** (DOX-ee-SIGH-kleen) *USP.*
Use: Anti-infective, tetracycline; mouth and throat product.
See: Avidoxy.
Doryx.
Doxy 100.
Monodox.
Oracea.

doxycycline. (Teva) Doxycycline 25 mg per 5 mL (as monohydrate). Maltodextrin, parabens, sucrose. Raspberry flavor. Pow. for Susp. 60 mL. *Rx.*
Use: Anti-infective agent, tetracycline.

•**doxycycline hyclate.** (DOX-ee-SIGH-kleen) *USP.*
Use: Anti-infective, tetracycline.
See: Alodox Convenience Kit.
Doryx.
Doxy.
Morgidox.
Ocudox Convenience Kit.
Vibramycin.

doxycycline hyclate. (Various Mfr.) Doxycycline hyclate. **Tab.:** 20 mg (may contain lactose) (film-coated), 100 mg. 30s, 50s (100 mg only); 60s (20 mg only); 100s; 500s, UD 100s (100 mg only). **Tab., delayed release:** 75 mg, 100 mg, 150 mg. Lactose. 60s (75 mg), 100s (100 mg and 150 mg only). **Cap.:** 50 mg, 100 mg. 20s (100 mg only), 50s, 500s. **Cap., coated pellets, delayed release:** 100 mg. May contain alcohol. 50s. **Pow. for Inj., lyophilized:** 100 mg. Vials. *Rx.*
Use: Anti-infective, tetracycline.

doxycycline monohydrate. (Various Mfr.) Doxycycline monohydrate. **Tab.:** 50 mg, 75 mg, 100 mg, 150 mg (polydextrose). May contain corn starch, lactose. Film coated. 30s (150 mg only), 50s (100 mg only), 100s (50 mg, 75 mg only), 250s (100 mg only). **Cap.:** 50 mg, 75 mg, 100 mg, 150 mg. 50s (50 mg, 100 mg only), 250s (100 mg only), 500s (50 mg only), 60s (150 mg only), 100s (75 mg only). *Rx.*
Use: Tetracycline.

•**doxylamine succinate.** (dox-IL-a-meen) *USP.*
Use: Antihistamine, nonselective ethanolamine.
See: Decapryn.
Doxytex.
Unisom SleepTabs.
W/Acetaminophen, Dextromethorphan Hydrobromide.
See: Tylenol Cough & Sore Throat Nighttime.
Vicks Nature Fusion Cold & Flu Nighttime Relief.
Vicks NyQuil Cold/Flu Relief.
W/Acetaminophen, Dextromethorphan Hydrobromide, Phenylephrine Hydrochloride.
See: Alka-Seltzer Plus Day & Night Cold.
Alka-Seltzer Plus Night Cold.
Alka-Seltzer Plus Severe Sinus Congestion Allergy & Cough.
Tylenol Cold Multi-Symptom Nighttime.
W/Aspirin, Dextromethorphan Hydrobromide, Phenylephrine Bitartrate.
See: Alka-Seltzer Plus Day & Night Cold.
Alka-Seltzer Plus Night Cold.
W/Dextromethorphan Hydrobromide.
See: Vicks NyQuil Cough.
W/Dextromethorphan Hydrobromide, Pseudoephedrine Hydrochloride.
See: All-Nite.
Lortuss DM.
W/Pseudoephedrine Hydrochloride.
See: Lortuss LQ.
W/Pyridoxine Hydrochloride.
See: Diclegis.

doxylamine succinate, acetaminophen, and pseudoephedrine hydrochloride combinations.
Use: Upper respiratory combination, antihistamine, analgesic, decongestant.
See: Acetaminophen, Doxylamine Succinate, and Pseudoephedrine Hydrochloride Combinations.

Doxy 100. (APP) Doxycycline hyclate 100 mg. Mannitol 300 mg. Pow. for Inj., lyophilized. Vial. *Rx.*
Use: Anti-infective; tetracycline.

Doxytex. (Centurion Labs) Doxylamine succinate 2.5 mg per 2.5 mL. Alcohol free, sugar free. Apple sauce flavor. Liq. 473 mL. *Rx.*
Use: Antihistamine; ethanolamine, nonselective.

DPPC. Colfosceril palmitate. *Rx.*
Use: Lung surfactant.
•**draflazine.** (DRAFF-lah-ZEEN) USAN.
Use: Cardioprotectant.
Dramamine. (Prestige) Dimenhydrinate 50 mg. Tab. 36s, 100s, 1,000s, blister pkg. 12s, UD 100s. *OTC.*
Use: Antiemetic; antivertigo.
Dramamine for Kids. (Prestige) Dimenhydrinate 25 mg. Phenylalanine 0.84 mg. Chew. Tab. 8s. *OTC.*
Use: Antiemetic; antivertigo.
Dramamine Less Drowsy Formula. (Prestige) Meclizine hydrochloride 25 mg, lactose. Tab. Pkg. 8s. *OTC.*
Use: Antiemetic; antivertigo.
Dramanate. (Taylor Pharmaceuticals) Dimenhydrinate 50 mg/mL. Inj. Vial 10 mL. *Rx.*
Use: Antiemetic; antivertigo.
Dramarin.
See: Dramamine.
Dramyl.
See: Dramamine.
Drawing Salve. (Whiteworth Towne) Tube oz. *OTC.*
Use: Dermatologic, wound therapy.
Drawing Salve with Triquinodin. (Whiteworth Towne) Tube 2 oz. *OTC.*
Use: Dermatologic, wound therapy.
Dr. Berry's Skin Toner. (Last) Hydroquinone 2%. Jar oz. *Rx.*
Use: Dermatologic.
Dr. Brown's Home Drug Testing System. (Personal Health and Hygiene) 1 urine specimen collection kit for detecting drugs of abuse (marijuana, cocaine, amphetamine, methamphetamine, phencyclidine, codeine, morphine, heroin). Kit 1s. *OTC.*
Use: Diagnostic aid.
DRC Peri-Anal Cream. (Xttrium) Lassar's paste 37.5%, anhydrous lanolin, 37.5%, cold cream 25%. Tube 5 oz. *OTC.*
Use: Dermatologic protectant, perianal.
Dr. Dermi-Heal. (Quality Formulations, Inc.) Zinc oxide 25%, allantoin 1%, peruvian balsam, castor oil, white petrolatum. Oint. Tube 75 g. *OTC.*
Use: Astringent.
Dr. Drake's Cough Medicine. (Last) Dextromethorphan HBr 10 mg/5 mL. Bot. 2 oz. *OTC.*
Use: Antitussive.
Dr. Edwards' Olive. (Oakhurst) Sennosides (from senna concentrate) 8.6 mg. Tab. 75s. *OTC.*
Use: Laxative.
Dri-A Caps. (Barth's) Vitamin A 10,000 units. Cap. Bot. 100s, 500s. *OTC.*
Use: Vitamin supplement.
Dri A & D Caps. (Barth's) Vitamins A 10,000 units, D 400 units. Cap. Bot. 100s, 500s. *OTC.*
Use: Vitamin supplement.
•**dribendazole.** (dry-BEN-dah-ZOLE) USAN.
Use: Anthelmintic.
Dri-E. (Barth's) Vitamin E. Cap.
100 units: Bot. 100s, 500s, 1000s.
200 units: Bot. 100s, 250s, 500s.
400 units: Bot. 100s, 250s. *OTC.*
Use: Vitamin supplement.
Dri/Ear. (Pfeiffer) Isopropyl alcohol 95%, glycerin 5%. Liq. 30 mL. *OTC.*
Use: Otic preparation.
dried aluminum hydroxide gel.
Use: Antacid.
See: Aluminum Hydroxide Gel, dried.
dried yeast.
See: Yeast, dried.
DriHist SR. (Prasco) Phenylephrine hydrochloride 20 mg, chlorpheniramine maleate 8 mg, methscopolamine nitrate 2.5 mg. ER Tab. 100s. *Rx.*
Use: Upper respiratory combination, decongestant, antihistamine, anticholinergic combination.
Driminate Tabs. (Major) Dimenhydrinate 50 mg. Tab. Bot. 100s, 1000s. *OTC.*
Use: Antiemetic; antivertigo.
•**drinidene.** (DRIH-nih-deen) USAN.
Use: Analgesic.
•**drisapersen.** (DRYE-sa-PER-sen) USAN.
Use: Treatment of Duchenne muscular dystrophy.
•**drisapersen sodium.** (DRYE-sa-PER-sen) USAN.
Use: Treatment of Duchenne muscular dystrophy.
Drisdol. (Sanofi Pharm) Ergocalciferol (Vitamin D_2). **Cap.:** 50,000 units. Tartrazine. Bot. 50s. **Drops:** 8000 units/mL in propylene glycol. Liq. Bot. 60 mL. *Rx-OTC.*
Use: Refractory rickets; hypophosphatemia; hypoparathyroidism.
Dristan Cold Multi-Symptom Formula. (Wyeth Consumer) Phenylephrine hydrochloride 5 mg, chlorpheniramine maleate 2 mg, acetaminophen 325 mg. PEG. Tab. 20s. *OTC.*
Use: Upper respiratory combination; decongestant, antihistamine, and analgesic.
Dristan 12-Hr Nasal. (Wyeth Consumer) Oxymetazoline hydrochloride 0.05%, benzalkonium chloride, benzyl alcohol,

edetate sodium, sodium chloride. Spray. 15 mL. *OTC.*
Use: Nasal decongestant, imidazoline.

Dritho-Scalp. (Summers Lab) Anthralin 0.5%. White petrolatum, cetostearyl alcohol. Cream. Tube 50 g. *Rx.*
Use: Antipsoriatic.

Drixoral. (Schering-Plough) Dexbrompheniramine maleate 6 mg, pseudoephedrine sulfate 120 mg. SA Tab. Box 10s, 20s, 40s. Bot. 48s, 100s. *OTC.*
Use: Antihistamine, decongestant.

Drixoral. (Schering-Plough) Pseudoephedrine sulfate 30 mg, brompheniramine maleate 2 mg. Sorbitol, sugar. Syrup. Bot. 118 mL. *OTC.*
Use: Antihistamine, decongestant.

Drixoral Allergy Sinus. (Schering-Plough) Pseudoephedrine sulfate 60 mg, dexbrompheniramine maleate 3 mg, acetaminophen 500 mg. Parabens. ER Tab. Pkg. 12s. *OTC.*
Use: Upper respiratory combination, decongestant, antihistamine, analgesic.

Drixoral Cold & Allergy. (Schering-Plough) Dexbrompheniramine maleate 6 mg, pseudoephedrine sulfate 120 mg. Sugar, lactose, butylparaben. Tab. Pkg. 20s. *OTC.*
Use: Upper respiratory combination, decongestant and antihistamine.

Drixoral Cold & Allergy Maximum Strength. (Schering-Plough) Dexbrompheniramine maleate 6 mg, pseudoephedrine sulfate 120 mg. Lactose, sucrose. ER Tab. 20s. *OTC.*
Use: Upper respiratory combination, decongestant and antihistamine.

Drixoral Cough & Congestion Liquid Caps. (Schering-Plough) Pseudoephedrine hydrochloride 60 mg, dextromethorphan HBr 30 mg. Cap. Pkg. 10s. *OTC.*
Use: Antihistamine, decongestant.

Drixoral Non-Drowsy Formula. (Schering-Plough) Pseudoephedrine sulfate 120 mg. Sugar. Tab. Pkg. 10s, 20s. *OTC.*
Use: Decongestant.

Drixoral Plus. (Schering-Plough) Pseudoephedrine sulfate 60 mg, dexbrompheniramine maleate 3 mg, acetaminophen 500 mg. TR Tab. Bot. 12s, 24s. *OTC.*
Use: Analgesic, antihistamine, decongestant.

Drixoral Sustained-Action. (Schering-Plough) Pseudoephedrine sulfate 120 mg, dexbrompheniramine maleate 6 mg. Sugar, lactose. Tab. Pkg. 10s. Bot. 20s, 40s. *OTC.*
Use: Antihistamine; decongestant.

•**drobuline.** (DROE-byoo-leen) USAN.
Use: Cardiovascular agent (antiarrhythmic).

•**drocinonide.** (droe-SIN-oh-nide) USAN.
Use: Anti-inflammatory.

drocode.
See: Dihydrocodeine.

•**droloxifene.** (drole-OX-ih-feen) USAN.
Use: Antineoplastic.

•**droloxifene citrate.** (drole-OX-ih-feen) USAN.
Use: Antineoplastic.

•**drometrizole.** (DROE-meh-TRY-zole) USAN.
Use: Ultraviolet screen.

•**dromostanolone propionate.** (DRAHM-oh-STAN-oh-lone) *USP.*
Use: Antineoplastic.

•**dronabinol.** (droe-NAB-ih-nahl) *USP.*
Use: Antiemetic; antivertigo.
See: Marinol.

dronabinol. (Watson) Dronabinol 2.5 mg, 5 mg, 10 mg. Sesame oil. Cap. 60s. *c-III.*
Use: Antiemetic; antivertigo.

dronedarone. (DROE-ne-da-rone)
Use: Antiarrhythmic.
See: Multaq.

drop chalk. (Various Mfr.) Calcium carbonate, prepared. Prepared chalk.

•**droperidol.** (dro-PER-i-dahl) *USP.*
Use: Antipsychotic; anxiolytic; general anesthetic.

droperidol. (Various Mfr.) Droperidol 2.5 mg/mL. Inj. Vial 2 mL. *Rx.*
Use: Anesthetic, general.

•**droprenilamine.** (droe-preh-NILL-ah-meen) USAN.
Use: Vasodilator (coronary).

•**drospirenone.** (droe-SPYE-reh-nohn) USAN.
Use: Sex hormone, contraceptive, hormone.
See: Yasmin.
W/Estradiol.
See: Angeliq.
W/Ethinyl Estradiol.
See: Gianvi.
Loryna.
Ocella.
Syeda.
Vestura.
YAZ.
Zarah.
W/Ethinyl Estradiol, Levomefolate Calcium.
See: Beyaz.

drospirenone/ethinyl estradiol. (Lupin) Drospirenone 3 mg, ethinyl estradiol

30 mcg. Film coated. Lactose, PEG. Tab. 28s (w/7 inert tablets). *Rx.*
Use: Monophasic oral contraceptive.

•**droxacin sodium.** (DROX-ah-sin) USAN.
Use: Anti-infective.

Droxia. (Bristol-Myers Squibb Oncology/Virology) Hydroxyurea 200 mg, 300 mg, 400 mg. Lactose. Cap. Bot. 60s. *Rx.*
Use: Antisickling agent.

•**droxidopa.** (droks-eye-DOE-pa) USAN.
Use: Neurogenic hypotension.
See: Northera.

•**droxifilcon A.** (DROX-ih-fill-kahn A) USAN.
Use: Contact lens material (hydrophilic).

•**droxinavir hydrochloride.** (drox-IN-ah-veer) USAN.
Use: Antiviral.

•**drozitumab.** (droe-ZIT-ue-mab) USAN.
Use: Antineoplastic.

Dr. Scholl's Advanced Pain Relief Corn Removers. (Schering-Plough) Salicylic acid 40% in a rubber-based vehicle. Disc. 6s. *OTC.*
Use: Keratolytic.

Dr. Scholl's Athlete's Foot. (Schering-Plough) **Pow.:** Tolnaftate 1%. Talc. Bot. 63 g. **Spray Liq.:** Tolnaftate 1%, alcohol 36%. Bot. 113 mL. *OTC.*
Use: Antifungal, topical.

Dr. Scholl's Athlete's Foot Cream. (Schering-Plough) Tolnaftate 1%. Tube 0.5 oz. *OTC.*
Use: Antifungal, topical.

Dr. Scholl's Callus Removers. (Schering-Plough) Salicylic acid 40% in a rubber-based vehicle. 6 pads, 4 discs. Extra thick in 4 discs. *OTC.*
Use: Keratolytic.

Dr. Scholl's Clear Away. (Schering-Plough) Salicylic acid 40% in a rubber-based vehicle. Disc 18s. *OTC.*
Use: Keratolytic.

Dr. Scholl's Clear Away One Step. (Schering-Plough) Salicylic acid 40% in a rubber-based vehicle. Strip 14s. *OTC.*
Use: Keratolytic.

Dr. Scholl's Clear Away Plantar. (Schering-Plough) Salicylic acid 40% in a rubber-based vehicle. Disc 24s. *OTC.*
Use: Keratolytic.

Dr. Scholl's Corn/Callus Remover. (Schering-Plough) Salicylic acid 12.6% in a flexible collodion, alcohol 18%, ether 55%, hydrogenated vegetable oil. Liq. 10 mL with 3 cushions. *OTC.*
Use: Keratolytic.

Dr. Scholl's Corn/Callus Salve. (Schering-Plough) Salicylic acid 15%. Tube 0.4 oz. *OTC.*
Use: Keratolytic.

Dr. Scholl's Corn Remover. (Schering-Plough) Salicylic acid 40% in a rubber-based vehicle. Discs: 6s as wrap-arounds, 9s as ultra thin, small, waterproof, regular, soft, and extra-thick. *OTC.*
Use: Keratolytic.

Dr. Scholl's Corn Salve. (Schering-Plough) Salicylic acid 15%. Jar 0.4 oz. *OTC.*
Use: Keratolytic.

Dr. Scholl's Cracked Heel Relief. (Schering-Plough) Lidocaine 2%, benzethonium chloride 0.13%. Aloe. Cream. Tubes. 89 mL. *OTC.*
Use: Anesthetic, local.

Dr. Scholl's Ingrown Toenail Reliever. (Schering-Plough) Sodium sulfide 1%. Bot. 0.33 oz. *OTC.*
Use: Foot preparation.

Dr. Scholl's Maximum Strength Tritan. (Schering-Plough) Tolnaftate 1%. **Pow.:** Talc. Bot. 56 g. **Spray Pow.:** SD alcohol 40 14%. Bot. 85 g. *OTC.*
Use: Antifungal, topical.

Dr. Scholl's Moisturizing Corn Remover Kit. (Schering-Plough) Salicylic acid 40% in a rubber-based vehicle, moisturizing cream, pain relief cushions. Disc 6s. *OTC.*
Use: Keratolytic.

Dr. Scholl's One Step Corn Removers. (Schering-Plough) Salicylic acid 40% in a rubber-based vehicle. Strips 6s. *OTC.*
Use: Keratolytic.

Dr. Scholl's Pro Comfort Jock Itch Spray. (Schering-Plough) Tolnaftate 1%. Aerosol Can 3.5 oz. *OTC.*
Use: Antifungal, topical.

Dr. Scholl's Wart Remover Kit. (Schering-Plough) Salicylic acid 17% in a flexible collodion, alcohol 17%, ether 52%. Liq. 10 mL with brush and 6 adhesive pads. *OTC.*
Use: Keratolytic.

Dr. Scholl's Zino Pads with Medicated Disks. (Schering-Plough) Salicylic acid 20%, 40%. Protective pads designed for use with and without salicylic acid-impregnated disks. *OTC.*
Use: Keratolytic.

Dr. Smith's Adult Care. (Beta Dermaceuticals) Zinc oxide 10%, petrolatum, lanolin, mineral oil, olive oil. Oint. Tube. 85 g. *OTC.*
Use: Topical protectant.

Dr. Smith's Diaper. (Beta Dermaceuticals) Zinc oxide 10%, petrolatum, lanolin, mineral oil, olive oil. Oint. Tube. 85 g. *OTC.*
Use: Topical protectant.

Drucon C R. (Standard Drug Co.) Phenylephrine hydrochloride 25 mg, chlorpheniramine maleate 4 mg. Tab. Bot. 100s. *OTC.*
Use: Antihistamine, decongestant.

Drucon with Codeine. (Standard Drug Co.) Codeine phosphate 10 mg, phenylephrine hydrochloride 10 mg, chlorpheniramine maleate 2 mg, menthol 1 mg, alcohol 5%/5 mL. Bot. Pt. *c-v.*
Use: Antihistamine, antitussive, decongestant.

Dry Eye Omega Benefits With Vitamin D-3. (Physician Recommended Nutriceuticals) Omega-3 667 mg (DHA 140 mg, EPA 420 mg, other omega-3s 107 mg), vitamin D 250 units. Soy. Dairy free, gluten free. Cap., softgel. 120s. *OTC.*
Use: Multivitamin and mineral with omega-3 polyunsaturated fatty acids.

Dry Eyes. (Bausch & Lomb) White petrolatum 94%, mineral oil 3%, lanolin. Preservative free. Oint. 3.5 g. *OTC.*
Use: Lubricant, ophthalmic.

Dry Eye Therapy. (Bausch & Lomb) Glycerin 0.3%, potassium chloride, sodium chloride, sodium citrate, sodium phosphate, zinc chloride. Drop. Single-use Bot. 0.3 mL (UD 32s). *OTC.*
Use: Ophthalmic.

drying agents.
See: Aluminum Chloride (Hexahydrate).
Formaldehyde.

DryMax. (Jaymac Pharmaceuticals) Chlorpheniramine maleate 4 mg, methscopolamine nitrate 1.25 mg, pseudoephedrine hydrochloride 30 mg. Glycerin, propylene glycol, saccharin, sucrose. Alcohol free and gluten free. Grape flavor. Syrup. 118 mL. *Rx.*
Use: Upper respiratory combination; decongestant, antihistamine, and anticholinergic combination.

DryMax AF. (JayMac Pharmaceuticals) **Tab.:** Chlophedianol hydrochloride 25 mg, chlorpheniramine maleate 4 mg, phenylephrine hydrochloride 15 mg. 20s. **Syrup:** Chlophedianol hydrochloride 25 mg, chlorpheniramine maleate 4 mg, pseudoephedrine hydrochloride 45 mg. Glycerin, grape flavoring, propylene glycol, saccharin, sorbitol. Alcohol free. 118 mL. *OTC.*
Use: Upper respiratory combination, antitussive combination.

Dryphen Multi-Symptom Formula. (Major) Phenylephrine hydrochloride 5 mg, chlorpheniramine maleate 2 mg, acetaminophen 325 mg. Tab. Bot. 40s. *OTC.*
Use: Upper respiratory combination, decongestant, antihistamine, analgesic.

Drysec. (A.G. Marin) Phenylephrine hydrochloride 20 mg, chlorpheniramine maleate 8 mg, methscopolamine nitrate 2.5 mg. ER Tab. 100s. *Rx.*
Use: Decongestant, antihistamine, and anticholinergic combination, upper respiratory combination.

Dry Skin Creme. (Gordon Laboratories) Cetyl alcohol, lubricating oils in a water-soluble base. Jar 2 oz, 1 lb, 5 lb. *OTC.*
Use: Emollient.

Drysol. (Person & Covey) Aluminum chloride hexahydrate 20% in 93% SD alcohol 40. Bot. 37.5 mL; 35 mL, 60 mL w/*Dab-O-Matic* applicator. *Rx.*
Use: Drying agent.

Drysum Shampoo. (Summers) Alcohol 15%, acetone 6%. Plastic bot. 4 oz. *OTC.*
Use: Dermatologic, hair.

Drytergent. (C & M Pharmacal) TEA-dodecylbenzenesulfonate, boric acid, lauramide DEA, propylene glycol, tartrazine, purified water, color, fragrance. Liq. Bot. 240 mL, 480 mL. *OTC.*
Use: Dermatologic, acne.

Drytex. (C & M Pharmacal) Salicylic acid 2%, benzalkonium chloride 0.1%, acetone 10%, isopropyl alcohol 40%, tartrazine. Lot. Bot. 240 mL. *OTC.*
Use: Dermatologic, acne.

DSS. (Dioctyl sodium sulfosuccinate) Docusate sodium. *OTC.*
Use: Laxative.
See: Colace.
Docusate Sodium.
DOK.
DOS.
D-S-S.

D-S-S. (Magno-Humphries) Docusate sodium 100 mg. Cap. Bot. 100s. *OTC.*
Use: Laxative; stool softener.

DST. Dihydrostreptomycin.
See: Dihydrostreptomycin Sulfate.

D-10-W. (Various Mfr.) Dextrose in water injection 10% (amps 3 mL); vials 250 mL, 500 mL, 1000 mL; 17 mL fill in 20 mL, 500 mL fill in 1000 mL, 1000 mL fill in 2000 mL vials. *Rx.*
Use: Carbohydrate supplement.

D-3. D vitamin.
See: Cholecalciferol.

D_3. (Mason) Cholecalciferol 2,000 units. Vitamin E. Peppermint flavor. Spray. 30 mL. *OTC.*
Use: Fat-soluble vitamin.

D_3 Dots. (VitaMed MD) Cholecalciferol (D_3) 2,000 units. Mannitol, xylitol. Tan-

gerine flavor. Tab. 100s. *OTC.*
Use: Fat-soluble vitamin.

D3-50. (Bio-Tech) Vitamin D_3 50,000 units. Dye free, preservative free, sugar free, yeast free. Cap. 100s. *OTC.*
Use: Fat-soluble vitamin.

D_3 Healthy Kids. (Mason Vitamins) Vitamin D_3 400 units. Fructose, sucrose, sunflower oil. Chew. Tab. 60s. *OTC.*
Use: Fat-soluble vitamin.

DTIC. Dacarbazine.
Use: Antineoplastic.
See: DTIC-Dome.

DTIC-Dome. (Bayer) Dacarbazine 100 mg, 200 mg. May contain mannitol. Inj. Vials. *Rx.*
Use: Antineoplastic.

DTP. Diphtheria and tetanus toxoids and pertussis vaccine, adsorbed. *Rx.*
Use: Immunization.
See: Infanarix.
Tripedia.

D-2. D vitamin.
See: Ergocalciferol.

Duac. (Stiefel) Benzoyl peroxide 5%, clindamycin phosphate 1%. Dimethicone, edetate disodium, glycerin, methylparaben. Gel. 45 g. *Rx.*
Use: Acne product.

Duac CS. (GlaxoSmithKline) Benzoyl peroxide 5%, clindamycin 1%, EDTA, glycerin, methylparaben. Gel 45 g. *Formerly Duac. Rx.*
Use: Anti-infective, topical.

Dual Action Complete. (Major Pharmaceuticals) Calcium carbonate 800 mg, famotidine 10 mg, magnesium hydroxide 165 mg. Aspartame, dextrates, lactose, phenylalanine 2.2 mg. Chew Tab. 25s. *OTC.*
Use: Histamine H_2 antagonist combination.

Dual-Wet. (Alcon) Polyvinyl alcohol, duasorb water-soluble polymetric system, benzalkonium chloride 0.01%, disodium edetate 0.05%. Bot. 2 oz. *OTC.*
Use: Contact lens care.

Duavee. (Pfizer) Conjugated estrogens 0.45 mg/bazedoxifene 20 mg (equiv. to bazedoxifene acetate 22.6 mg). Lactose, maltitol, PEG, polydextrose, sucrose. Tab. UD 30s. *Rx.*
Use: Sex hormone, estrogen-selective estrogen receptor modulator combination.

•**duazomycin.** (doo-AZE-oh-MY-sin) USAN. Antibiotic isolated from broth filtrates of *Streptomyces ambofaciens.*
Use: Antineoplastic.

duazomycin A. *Name used for Duazomycin.*
Use: Antineoplastic.

duazomycin B. *Name used for Azotomycin.*
Use: Antineoplastic.

duazomycin C. *Name used for Ambomycin.*
Use: Antineoplastic.

Duetact. (Takeda) Pioglitazone hydrochloride/glimepiride 30 mg/2 mg, 30 mg/4 mg. Lactose. Tab. 30s, 90s. *Rx.*
Use: Antidiabetic combination.

Duet DHA. (Eckson Labs) Folic acid 1 mg, Ca 200 mg, Fe 25 mg, vitamins A 2,800 units, D 820 units, E 3 units, B_1 1.8 mg, B_2 4 mg, B_3 20 mg, B_6 50 mg, B_{12} 12 mcg, C 120 mg. Cu, I, Mg, Zn. **Cap., softgel:** Omega-3 fatty acids (as DHA and EPA) 430 mg, glycerin. Gluten free. 30s. **Tab.:** PEG. 30s. *Rx.*
Use: Prenatal vitamin with minerals.

Duet DHA Balanced. (Eckson Labs) Folic acid 1 mg, calcium 215 mg, iron 25 mg, vitamins A 2,800 units, D 640 units, E 22.5 units, B_1 1.5 mg, B_2 2 mg, B_3 20 mg, B_6 50 mg, B_{12} 12 mcg, C 120 mg, Cu, I, Mg, Se, Zn, choline 55 mg. **Tab.:** PEG. Gluten free. UD 30s. **Cap., softgels:** Omega fatty acids (as DHA, EPA, DPA, ALA) 267 mg. Glycerin, rice bran oil. Gluten free. UD 30s. *Rx.*
Use: Prenatal vitamin with minerals.

Duet DHA 400. (Eckson Labs) Folic acid 1 mg, calcium 200 mg, iron 25 mg, vitamins A 2,800 units, D 820 units, E 4.1 units, B_1 1.8 mg, B_2 4 mg, B_3 20 mg, B_6 50 mg, B_{12} 12 mcg, C 120 mg, Cu, I, Mg, Zn. **Tab.:** PEG. Gluten free. 30s. **Cap., softgel:** Omega-3 fatty acids (as DHA and EPA) 400 mg. Glycerin. Gluten free. 30s. *Rx.*
Use: Prenatal vitamin with minerals.

Duet DHA 430. (Eckson Labs) Folic acid 1 mg, calcium 200 mg, iron 25 mg, vitamins A 2,800 units, D 820 units, E 4.5 units, B_1 1.8 mg, B_2 4 mg, B_3 20 mg, B_6 50 mg, B_{12} 12 mcg, C 120 mg, Cu, I, Mg, Zn. **Tab.:** PEG. Gluten free. 30s. **Cap., softgel:** Omega-3 fatty acids (as DHA and EPA) 430 mg. Glycerin. Gluten free. 30s. *Rx.*
Use: Prenatal vitamin with minerals.

Duexis. (Horizon Pharma) Ibuprofen 800 mg/famotidine 26.6 mg. Film coated. Lactose, PEG. Tab. 90s. *Rx.*
Use: Nonnarcotic analgesic combination.

•**dulaglutide.** (DOO-la-GLOO-tide) USAN.
Use: Antidiabetic agent.

Dulcagen Suppositories. (Ivax) Bisacodyl 10 mg. Box 12s, 100s. *OTC.*
Use: Laxative.

Dulcolax. (Boehringer Ingelheim) **EC Tab.:** Bisacodyl 5 mg, lactose, sucrose,

parabens. Bot. 10s, 25s, 50s, 100s. **Liq.:** Magnesia (magnesium hydroxide) 400 mg per 5 mL. Original flavor. Sugar free. 355 mL. *OTC.*
Use: Laxative; antacid.

Dulcolax Balance. (Boehringer Ingelheim) PEG 3350 17 g. Pow. for Soln. 238 g. *OTC.*
Use: Laxative, bowel evacuant.

Dulcolax Bowel Prep Kit. (Boehringer Ingelheim) Bisacodyl. **Tab., delayed release:** 5 mg. Docusate sodium, lactose, parabens, sucrose. 4s. **Supp.:** 10 mg. Hydrogenated vegetable oil. 1s. *OTC.*
Use: Laxative.

Dulcolax Stool Softener. (Boehringer Ingelheim) Docusate sodium 100 mg. Glycerin, sorbitol. Soft Gel Cap. 25s. *OTC.*
Use: Laxative.

DuLeek-Dp 15. (Seton Pharmaceuticals) Folate 15 mg. Tab. 90s. *Rx.*
Use: Water-soluble vitamin.

DuLeek-Dp 7.5. (Seton Pharmaceuticals) Folate 7.5 mg. Tab. 30s, 90s. *Rx.*
Use: Water-soluble vitamin.

Dulera. (Schering) Mometasone furoate/formoterol fumarate 100 mcg/5 mcg, 200 mcg/5 mcg per actuation. Aer. Canister w/actuator. 13 g. *Rx.*
Use: Respiratory inhalant combination.

Dull-C. (Freeda) Ascorbic acid 1060 mg/¼ tsp. Sugar free. Pow. Bot. 120 g, 1 lb. *OTC.*
Use: Vitamin supplement.

•**duloxetine.** (doo-LOX-eh-teen) USAN.
Tall Man: DULoxetine
Use: Antidepressant.
See: Cymbalta.

duloxetine. (Various Mfr.) Duloxetine 20 mg, 30 mg, 60 mg. May contain lactose, sucrose. Cap., delayed release (contains enteric-coated pellets). 30s, 60s (20 mg only), 90s, 100s (except 60 mg), 500s, 1,000s, UD 30s (20 mg only), UD 100s (except 20 mg). *Rx.*
Use: Antidepressant, serotonin and norepinephrine reuptake inhibitor.

Dulphalac. (Solvay) Lactulose 10 g/5 mL. Syr. Bot. 240 mL, 480 mL, 960 mL, UD 30 mL. *Rx.*
Use: Laxative.

Duo. (GlaxoSmithKline) Tube 0.5 oz.
Use: Adhesive.

Duocaine. (Amphastar) Lidocaine hydrochloride 10 mg/mL, bupivacaine hydrochloride 3.75 mg/mL. Preservative free. Inj. 10 mL single-dose vials. Cartons of 25. *Rx.*
Use: Anesthetic, injectable local.

DuoDERM. (ConvaTec) **Sterile dressing:** 10 cm × 10 cm. Pack 5s. 20 cm × 20 cm. Pack 3s. **Sterile gran.:** Packet 4 g. Pack 5s. *OTC.*
Use: Dermatologic, wound therapy.

DuoDERM Extra Thin. (ConvaTec) Flexible hydroactive sterile dressings. 4" × 4", 6" × 6". Pck. 10s. *OTC.*
Use: Dressing, topical.

DuoDote. (Survival Technology) Atropine 2.1 mg/0.7 mL, pralidoxime chloride 600 mg/2 mL. Benzyl alcohol 40 mg. Inj. Soln. Single-use dual chamber prefilled auto-injectors. *Rx.*
Use: Antidote.

Duofer. (Breckenridge Pharmaceutical) Elemental Fe 28 mg (as heme iron polypeptide 6 mg, polysaccharide iron complex 22 mg). Film coated. Mineral oil, sodium lauryl sulfate, soy. Tab. 30s. *OTC.*
Use: Trace element.

Duofilm. (Stiefel) Salicylic acid 16.7%, lactic acid 16.7% in flexible collodion. Bot. 15 mL w/applicator. *OTC.*
Use: Keratolytic.

Duo-Flow. (Ciba Vision) Poloxamer 188, benzalkonium Cl 0.013%, EDTA 0.25%. Soln. Bot. 120 mL. *OTC.*
Use: Contact lens care.

Duo-K. (Various Mfr.) Potassium 20 mEq, chloride 3.4 mEq/15 mL (from potassium gluconate and potassium chloride). Bot. Pt, gal. *Rx.*
Use: Mineral supplement.

Duolube. (Bausch & Lomb) White petrolatum, mineral oil. Sterile, preservative and lanolin free. Oint. Tube 3.5 g. *OTC.*
Use: Lubricant, ophthalmic.

Duonate-12. (URL) Phenylephrine tannate 5 mg, pyrilamine tannate 30 mg/5 mL. Susp. Unit of use 118 mL w/oral syr. *Rx.*
Use: Upper respiratory combination, decongestant, antihistamine.

DuoNeb. (Dey) Ipratropium bromide 0.5 mg, albuterol sulfate 3 mg (equivalent to albuterol base 2.5 mg). Inhalation soln. Unit-dose vial 3 mL. Box 30s, 60s. *Rx.*
Use: Bronchodilator, anticholinergic.

•**duoperone fumarate.** (DOO-oh-per-OHN) USAN.
Use: Neuroleptic.

DuoPlant. (Stiefel) Salicylic acid 27%, alcohol 50%, flexible collodion, hydroxypropyl cellulose, lactic acid. Liq. Bot. 14 g. *OTC.*
Use: Ketatolytic (wart removal).

Duosol. (Kirkman) Docusate sodium 100 mg, 250 mg. Cap. Bot. 100s, 1000s. *OTC.*
Use: Laxative.

Duotal. (Health for Life Brands) **1.5 g.:** Secobarbital sodium ¾ g, amobarbital g. Cap. **3 g.:** Secobarbital sodium 1.5 g, amobarbital 1.5 g. Cap. Bot. 100s, 500s, 1000s. *c-II.*
Use: Hypnotic; sedative.

duotal.
See: Guaiacol Carbonate.

Duotan PD. (Scientific Laboratories) Pseudoephedrine tannate 75 mg, dexchlorpheniramine tannate 2.5 mg per 5 mL. Methylparaben, saccharin, sucrose. Strawberry-banana flavor. Susp. 118 mL, 473 mL. *Rx.*
Use: Pediatric decongestant and antihistamine.

Duotrate 45. (Jones Pharma) Pentaerythritol tetranitrate 45 mg. SR Cap. Bot. 100s. *Rx.*
Use: Antianginal.

Duotrate 30. (Jones Pharma) Pentaerythritol tetranitrate 30 mg. SR Cap. Bot. 100s. *Rx.*
Use: Antianginal.

Duovin-S. (Spanner) Estrone 2.5 mg, progesterone 25 mg/mL. Vial 10 mL. *Rx.*
Use: Estrogen, progestin combination.

Duo-WR, No. 1 & No. 2. (Whorton Pharmaceuticals, Inc.) **No. 1:** Salicylic acid, compound tincture benzoin. **No. 2:** Compound tincture benzoin, formaldehyde. Bot. 0.25 oz. *OTC.*
Use: Keratolytic.

•**dupilumab.** (doo-PIL-ue-mab) USAN.
Use: Treatment of atopic diseases.

Duplast. (Beiersdorf) Adhesive coated elastic cloth. 8" × 4" Strip. Box 10s. 10" × 5" Strip. Box 8s, 10s.

Duplex Shampoo. (C & M Pharmacal) Sodium lauryl sulfate 15%, lauramide DEA, purified water. Bot. Pt, gal. *OTC.*
Use: Dermatologic.

duponol.
See: Gardinol type detergents (Sodium Lauryl Sulfate).

Durabac. (Poly Pharmaceuticals) Acetaminophen 325 mg, caffeine 50 mg, phenyltoloxamine citrate 20 mg, salicylamide 250 mg. Cap. 100s. *Rx.*
Use: Nonnarcotic analgesic combination.

Durabac Forte. (Poly Pharmaceuticals) Acetaminophen 500 mg, magnesium salicylate 500 mg, caffeine 50 mg, phenyltoloxamine citrate 20 mg. Tab. 100s. *Rx.*
Use: Nonnarcotic analgesic.

DURAcare. (Blairex) Buffered hypertonic salt solution, non-ionic detergents with thimerosal 0.004%, EDTA 0.1%. Soln. Bot. 30 mL. *OTC.*
Use: Contact lens care.

Duraclon. (Bioniche Pharma) Clonidine hydrochloride 100 mcg/mL, 500 mcg/mL. Preservative free. Inj. Vials. 10 mL. *Rx.*
Use: Analgesic.

DuraDEX. (ProEthic Pharmaceuticals) Dextromethorphan HBr 20 mg, guaifenesin 1200 mg. Dye free. ER Tab. 100s. *Rx.*
Use: Antitussive with expectorant.

Duradryl. (Breckenridge Pharm.) Phenylephrine hydrochloride 10 mg, chlorpheniramine maleate 2 mg, methscopolamine nitrate 1.25 mg/5mL. Alcohol and sugar free. Sorbitol. Cherry flavor. Syrup. Bot. 473 mL. *Rx.*
Use: Upper respiratory combination, decongestant, antihistamine, anticholinergic.

Dura-Estrin. (Roberts) Estradiol cypionate in oil 5 mg/mL. Inj. Vial 10 mL. *Rx.*
Use: Estrogen.

Duraflex Comfort. (Trimarc Labs) Aloe, capsicum, glucosamine, menthol, methyl salicylate, methyl sulfonyl methane, methylparaben, sorbitol, urea. Gel. 59.14 g. *OTC.*
Use: Rub and liniment.

Duraflu. (Poly Pharmaceuticals) Dextromethorphan HBr 20 mg, guaifenesin 200 mg, pseudoephedrine hydrochloride 60 mg, acetaminophen 500 mg. Dye free. Tab. 100s. *OTC.*
Use: Upper respiratory combination, antitussive and expectorant combination.

Duragen. (Roberts) Estradiol valerate in oil 20 mg, 40 mg/mL. Inj. Vial 10 mL. *Rx.*
Use: Estrogen.

Duragesic-50. (Janssen) Fentanyl 8.4 mg (50 mcg/h). Transdermal System. UD 5s. *c-II.*
Use: Opioid analgesic.

Duragesic-100. (Janssen) Fentanyl 16.8 mg (100 mcg/h). Transdermal System. UD 5s. *c-II.*
Use: Opioid analgesic.

Duragesic-75. (Janssen) Fentanyl 12.6 mg (75 mcg/h). Transdermal System. UD 5s. *c-II.*
Use: Opioid analgesic.

Duragesic-12. (Janssen) Fentanyl 2.1 mg (12.5 mcg/h). Transdermal System. UD 5s. *c-II.*
Use: Opioid analgesic.

Duragesic-25. (Janssen) Fentanyl 4.2 mg (25 mcg/h). Transdermal System. UD 5s. *c-II.*
Use: Opioid analgesic.

Duralex. (American Urologicals, Inc.) Pseudoephedrine hydrochloride 120 mg, chlorpheniramine maleate 8 mg. SR Cap. Bot. 100s, 1000s. *Rx.*
Use: Antihistamine, decongestant.

Dura-Meth. (Foy Laboratories) Methylprednisolone 40 mg/mL. Vial 5 mL, 10 mL. *Rx.*
Use: Corticosteroid.

Duramist Plus 12-Hr Decongestant. (Pfeiffer) Oxymetazoline hydrochloride 0.05%, benzalkonium chloride, EDTA, sodium chloride. Spray. Bot. 15 mL. *OTC.*
Use: Nasal decongestant, imidazoline.

Duramorph. (West-Ward) Morphine sulfate 0.5 mg/mL, 1 mg/mL. Inj. Single-use amp. 10 mL. *c-II.*
Use: Opioid analgesic.

Durapam. (Major) Flurazepam hydrochloride 15 mg, 30 mg. Cap. Bot. 100s, 500s. *c-IV.*
Use: Hypnotic; sedative.

•**durapatite.** (der-APP-ah-tite) USAN.
Use: Prosthetic aid.

Duraphen Forte. (ProEthic Laboratories) Dextromethorphan HBr 30 mg, guaifenesin 1200 mg, phenylephrine hydrochloride 30 mg. Dye free. ER Tab. 100s. *Rx.*
Use: Antitussive and expectorant combination.

Duraphen II DM. (ProEthic Laboratories) Dextromethorphan HBr 20 mg, guaifenesin 800 mg, phenylephrine hydrochloride 20 mg. Dye free. ER Tab. 100s. *Rx.*
Use: Antitussive and expectorant combination.

DuraProxin. (Pharmaceutica North America) Camphor 3%, menthol 1.25%. Disodium ethylenediaminetertraacetate, glycerin, polysorbate 80. Patch. 30s. *OTC.*
Use: Rub and liniment, patch.

DuraProxin ES. (Pharmaceutica North America) Camphor 3%, menthol 1.25%, methyl salicylate 10%. Disodium ethylenediaminetertraacetate, glycerin, polysorbate 80. Patch. 30s. *OTC.*
Use: Rub and liniment, patch.

Duraquin. (Parke-Davis) Quinidine gluconate 330 mg. SR Tab. Bot. 100s, UD 100s. *Rx.*
Use: Cardiovascular agent.

Durasal II. (Prasco) Pseudoephedrine hydrochloride 60 mg, guaifenesin 600 mg. SR Tab. 100s. *Rx.*
Use: Upper respiratory combination, decongestant, expectorant.

DuraScreen. (Schwarz Pharma) SPF 30. Octyl methoxycinnamate, octyl salicylate, oxybenzone, 2-phenylbenzimidazole-sulfonic acid, titanium dioxide, cetearyl alcohol, diazolidinyl urea, parabens, shea butter. Lot. Bot. 105 mL. *OTC.*
Use: Sunscreen.

DuraScreen SPF 15. (Schwarz Pharma) SPF 15. Ethylhexyl p-methoxycinnamate, 2-ethylhexyl salicylate, oxybenzone, parabens, titanium dioxide. Lot. Bot. 105 mL. *OTC.*
Use: Sunscreen.

Dura-Tap/PD. (Dura) Pseudoephedrine hydrochloride 60 mg, chlorpheniramine maleate 4 mg. Cap. Bot. 100s. *Rx.*
Use: Antihistamine, decongestant.

Duratears Naturale. (Alcon) White petroleum, anhydrous liquid lanolin, mineral oil. Oint. Tube 3.5 g. *OTC.*
Use: Lubricant, ophthalmic.

Duration. (Schering-Plough) Oxymetazoline hydrochloride 0.05%, benzalkonium chloride, EDTA. Soln. Spray Bot. 30 mL. *OTC.*
Use: Nasal decongestant, imidazoline.

Duration Mentholated Vapor Spray. (Schering-Plough) Oxymetazoline hydrochloride 0.05%, aromatics. Squeeze bot. 15 mL. *OTC.*
Use: Decongestant.

Duration Mild Nasal Spray. (Schering-Plough) Phenylephrine hydrochloride 0.5%. Bot. 15 mL. *OTC.*
Use: Decongestant.

Duratuss DA. (Victory) Chlorpheniramine maleate 12 mg, pseudoephedrine hydrochloride 100 mg. Sugar. Cap. 100s. *Rx.*
Use: Upper respiratory combination, decongestant and antihistamine.

Duravent. (Auriga) Chlorpheniramine maleate 2 mg, methscopolamine nitrate 1.25 mg, phenylephrine hydrochloride 10 mg. Mannitol, sugar. Root beer flavor. Chew. Tab. 100s. *Rx.*
Use: Upper respiratory combination; decongestant, antihistamine, and anticholinergic combination.

Duravent-DA. (Auriga) Chlorpheniramine maleate 8 mg, methscopolamine nitrate 2.5 mg, phenylephrine hydrochloride 20 mg. ER Tab. 100s. *Rx.*
Use: Upper respiratory combination; decongestant, antihistamine, and anticholinergic combination.

Duraxin. (Portal) Phenyltoloxamine citrate 25 mg, acetaminophen 325 mg, salicylamide 200 mg. Cap. 30s. *Rx.*
Use: Antihistamine and analgesic.

Durazyme. (Blairex) Nonionic detergent preserved w/thimerosal 0.004%, EDTA

0.1% in sterile buffered hypertonic salt soln. Bot. 30 mL. *OTC.*
Use: Contact lens care.

Durezol. (Alco Vision) Difluprednate 0.05%. Sodium EDTA, boric acid, glycerin, polysorbate 80, sodium acetate, sodium hydroxide, sorbic acid 0.1%. Ophth. Emulsion. Bot. 2.5 mL, 5 mL. *Rx.*
Use: Corticosteroid, ophthalmic.

Dur-Tann Forte. (Midlothian) Dextromethorphan tannate 30 mg, dexchlorpheniramine tannate 3.5 mg, pseudoephedrine tannate 45 mg per 5 mL. Methylparaben, saccharin, sucrose. Grape flavor. Susp. 473 mL. *Rx.*
Use: Upper respiratory combination, antitussive combination.

•**dusigitumab.** (DOO-si-GIT-ue-mab) USAN.
Use: Antineoplastic.

Dusotal. (Harvey) Sodium amobarbital ¾ g, sodium secobarbital g. Cap. Bot. 1000s. (3 g) Bot. 1000s. *c-II.*
Use: Hypnotic; sedative.

•**dusting powder, absorbable.** *USP.*
Use: Lubricant.

dusting powder, surgical.
See: B-F-I.

•**dutasteride.** (doo-TASS-teer-ide) USAN.
Use: Benign prostatic hyperplasia, sex hormone, androgen hormone inhibitor.
See: Avodart.
W/Tamsulosin.
See: Jalyn.

dutch oil. Oil of turpentine, sulfurated.

•**dutogliptin.** (DOO-toe-GLIP-tin) USAN.
Use: Antidiabetic.

•**dutogliptin tartrate.** (DOO-toe-GLIP-tin) USAN.
Use: Antidiabetic.

Dutoprol. (AstraZeneca) Hydrochlorothiazide/metoprolol tartrate 12.5 mg/25 mg (equiv to metoprolol succinate 23.75 mg ER), 12.5 mg/50 mg (equiv. to metoprolol succinate 47.5 mg ER), 12.5 mg/100 mg (equiv. to metoprolol succinate 95 mg ER). Film coated. PEG. ER Tab. 30s. *Rx.*
Use: Antihypertensive combination.

•**duvelisib.** (DOO-ve-LIS-ib) USAN.
Use: Antineoplastic.

•**duvoglustat.** (due-voe-GLUE-stat) USAN.
Use: Treatment of Pompe disease.

•**duvoglustat hydrochloride.** (due-voe-GLUE-stat) USAN.
Use: Treatment of Pompe disease.

D V Cream. (Hoechst) Dienestrol 0.01% w/lactose, propylene glycol, stearic acid, diglycol stearate, TEA, benzoic acid, butylated hydroxytoluene, disodium edetate, buffered w/lactic acid to an acid pH. Tube 3 oz, w/applicator. *Rx.*
Use: Estrogen.

D-Vita. (Major) Cholecalciferol (D_3) 400 units/mL. Glycerin, polysorbate 80, potassium sorbate, propylene glycol, sodium benzoate. Alcohol free, gluten free, lactose free, and sugar free. Fruit flavor. Soln., concentrate. 50 mL w/dropper. *OTC.*
Use: Fat-soluble vitamin.

Dwelle. (Dakryon Pharmaceuticals) EDTA 0.09%, sodium chloride, potassium chloride, boric acid, povidone, NPX 0.001%. Drop. Bot. 15 mL. *OTC.*
Use: Artificial tears.

DX 114 Foot Powder. (Amlab) Zinc undecylenate 1%, salicylic acid 1%, benzoic acid 1%, ammonium alum 5%, boric acid 10.5% w/zinc stearate, chlorophyll, talc, kaolin, starch, calcium silicate, oil of wormwood. Cont. 2 oz. *OTC.*
Use: Antifungal, topical.

Dyantoin Caps. (Major) Phenytoin sodium 100 mg. Cap. Bot. 100s, 1000s. *Rx.*
Use: Anticonvulsant.

Dyazide. (GlaxoSmithKline) Triamterene 37.5 mg, hydrochlorothiazide 25 mg. Cap. Bot. 1000s, UD 100s, Patient Pack 100s. *Rx.*
Use: Antihypertensive; diuretic.

Dycill. (GlaxoSmithKline) Dicloxacillin sodium 250 mg, 500 mg. Cap. Bot. 100s. *Rx.*
Use: Anti-infective; penicillin.

•**dyclonine hydrochloride.** (DIE-kloe-neen) *USP.*
Use: Anesthetic, topical.
See: Sucrets Children's Formula.
Sucrets Complete.
Sucrets Maximum Strength Sore Throat.
Sucrets Original Formula Sore Throat.
Sucrets Throat.
W/Benzethonium Chloride.
See: Skin Shield.

Dycomene. (Hance) Hydrocodone bitartrate ⅙ g, pyrilamine maleate 1 g/fl. oz. Bot. 3 oz, gal. *c-III.*
Use: Antitussive; sleep aid.

•**dydrogesterone.** (DIE-droe-JESS-ter-ohn) *USP.*
Use: Hormone, progestin.

dyes.
See: Antiseptic, Dyes.

Dyflex-G. (Econo Med) Dyphylline 200 mg, guaifenesin 200 mg. Tab. Bot. 100s, 1000s. *Rx.*

Use: Antiasthmatic combination, xanthine combination.

Dyflex-200 Tablets. (Econo Med) Dyphylline 200 mg. Bot. 100s, 1000s. *Rx.*
Use: Bronchodilator.

Dy-G. (Cypress) Dyphylline 100 mg, guaifenesin 100 mg/5 mL. Alcohol free. Mint flavor. Liq. Bot. 473 mL. *Rx.*
Use: Antiasthmatic combination, xanthine combination.

dylate. Clonitrate.
Use: Coronary vasodilator.

Dylix. (Lunsco) Dyphylline 100 mg per 15 mL. Alcohol 20%. Elix. 473 mL. *Rx.*
Use: Bronchodilator.

•**dymanthine hydrochloride.** (DIE-man-theen) USAN.
Use: Anthelmintic.

Dymenate. (Keene Pharmaceuticals) Dimenhydrinate 50 mg/mL. Vial 10 mL. *Rx.*
Use: Antiemetic; antivertigo.

Dymista. (Meda Pharmaceuticals) Azelastine hydrochloride 137 mcg, fluticasone propionate 50 mcg per spray. Alcohol, polysorbate 80. Spray, Susp.; intranasal. 23 g (120 metered sprays) w/metered-dose pump and nasal adapter. *Rx.*
Use: Intranasal steroid.

Dynacin. (Par) Minocycline hydrochloride (as base) 50 mg, 75 mg, 100 mg. Film coated. Lactose. Tab. 50s (100 mg only), 100s (except 100 mg). *Rx.*
Use: Anti-infective; tetracycline.

Dynafed Asthma Relief. (BDI) Ephedrine hydrochloride 25 mg, guaifenesin 200 mg. Tab. Bot. 60s. *OTC.*
Use: Upper respiratory combination, decongestant, expectorant.

Dynafed Plus, Maximum Strength.
See: Maximum Strength Dynafed Plus.

Dyna-Hex Skin Cleanser. (Western Medical) Chlorhexidine gluconate 4%, isopropyl alcohol 4%. Liq. Bot. 120 mL, 240 mL, 480 mL, gal. *OTC.*
Use: Antimicrobial; antiseptic.

Dyna-Hex 2 Skin Cleanser. (Western Medical) Chlorhexidine gluconate 2%, isopropyl alcohol 4%. Liq. Bot. 120 mL, 240 mL, 480 mL, gal. *OTC.*
Use: Antimicrobial; antiseptic.

dynamine. (Mayo Foundation)
Use: Antispasmodic, Lambert-Eaton myasthenic syndrome, hereditary motor and sensory neuropathy type I (Charcot-Marie-Tooth Disease). [Orphan Drug]

Dynapen. (Apothecon) Dicloxacillin sodium. **Cap.:** 125 mg, 250 mg, 500 mg. Bot. 24s (except 500 mg), 50s (500 mg only), 100s (except 500 mg). **Pow. for Oral Susp.:** 62.5 mg/5 mL. Bot. 100 mL, 200 mL. *Rx.*
Use: Anti-infective; penicillin.

Dynaplex. (Alton) Vitamin B complex. Bot. 100s, 1000s. *OTC.*
Use: Vitamin supplement.

Dynatuss EX. (Breckenridge) Dextromethorphan HBr 30 mg, guaifenesin 200 mg, phenylephrine hydrochloride 10 mg per 5 mL. PEG, saccharin, sorbitol. Syrup. 473 mL. *Rx.*
Use: Upper respiratory combination, antitussive and expectorant combination.

Dy-O-Derm. (Galderma) Purified water, isopropyl alcohol, acetone, dihydroxyacetone, FD&C yellow No. 6, FD&C blue No. 1, FD&C red No. 33. Bot. 4 oz.
Use: Dermatologic, vitiligo stain.

Dy-Phyl-Lin. (Foy Laboratories) Dyphylline 250 mg/mL with benzyl alcohol. Inj. Vial 10 mL. *Rx.*
Use: Bronchodilator.

•**dyphylline.** (DIE-fih-lin) *USP.*
Use: Vasodilator; bronchodilator.
See: Dylix.
Lufyllin.
Lufyllin-400.
W/Guaifenesin.
See: Difil-G.
Difil-G 400.
Dilex-G.
Dilex-G 400.
Dilex-G 200.
Dyflex-G.
Dy-G Liquid.
Dyphylline and Guaifenesin.
Dyphylline-GG.
Dyphylline GG ES.
Jay-Phyl.
Lufyllin-GG.
Panfil G.

•**dyphylline and guaifenesin.** (DIE-fih-lin and GWIE-fen-ah-sin) *USP.*
Use: Antiasthmatic combination, xanthine combination.

dyphylline and guaifenesin. (Various Mfr.) Dyphylline 200 mg, guaifenesin 200 mg. May contain dextrose. Tab. Bot. 100s. *Rx.*
Use: Antiasthmatic combination, xanthine combination.

Dyphylline GG Elixir. (Various Mfr.) Dyphylline 33.3 mg, guaifenesin 33.3 mg per 5 mL. Alcohol 17%, saccharin, sucrose. Elix. Bot. 473 mL. *Rx.*
Use: Bronchodilator.

Dyphylline GG ES. (Breckenridge) Dyphylline 200 mg, guaifenesin 300 mg. Maltodextrin, saccharin, vanilla flavoring.

Tab. 100s. *Rx.*
Use: Antiasthmatic combination, xanthine combination.

Dyprotex. (Blairex) Micronized zinc oxide 40%, petrolatum 37.6%, dimethicone 2.5%, cod liver oil, aloe extract, zinc stearate. Pad. Pkg. 3s (9 applications). *OTC.*
Use: Astringent.

Dyrenium. (GlaxoSmithKline) Triamterene 50 mg, 100 mg. Cap. Bot. 100s, 1000s (100 mg only), UD 100s. *Rx.*
Use: Diuretic.

Dyretic. (Keene Pharmaceuticals) Furosemide 10 mg/mL. Vial 10 mL. *Rx.*
Use: Diuretic.

Dyrexan-OD. (Trimen Laboratories, Inc.) Phendimetrazine tartrate 105 mg. SR Cap. Bot. 100s. *c-III.*
Use: Anorexiant.

Dyspel. (Dover Pharmaceuticals) Acetaminophen, ephedrine sulfate, atropine sulfate. Sugar, lactose, salt free. Tab. UD Box 500s. *Rx.*
Use: Analgesic.

Dysport. (Tercica) AbobotulinumtoxinA 300 units, 500 units (1 unit corresponds to the calculated median lethal intraperitoneal dose in mice). Albumin (human) 125 mg, lactose 2.5 mg. Preservative free. Inj., lyophilized powder for Soln. Single-use vial. *Rx.*
Use: Botulinum toxin.

E

EACA. (Wyeth) Epsilon aminocaproic acid. *Rx.*
Use: Antifibrinolytic.
See: Amicar.

Ear-Dry. (Scherer) Isopropyl alcohol, boric acid 2.75%. Dropper bot. 30 mL. *OTC.*
Use: Otic preparation.

Earex Ear Drops. (Health for Life Brands) Benzocaine 0.15 g, antipyrine 0.7 g/ 0.5 oz. Bot. 0.5 oz. *Rx.*
Use: Otic.

Ear-Gesic. (Qualitest Pharmaceuticals) Antipyrine 5%, benzocaine 5%, phenylephrine hydrochloride 0.25%. Sodium metabisulfite. Soln., Otic. 15 mL. *Rx.*
Use: Ophthalmic and otic agent, otic preparation.

Earocol Ear Drops. (Roberts) Benzocaine 1.4%, antipyrine 5.4%, glycerin, oxyquinoline sulfate. Soln. Dropper bot. 15 mL. *Rx.*
Use: Otic preparation.

EarSol-HC. (Parnell) Hydrocortisone 1%, alcohol 44%, propylene glycol, *Dermprotective Factor* yerba santa, benzyl benzoate. Soln. 30 mL. *OTC.*
Use: Miscellaneous otic preparation.

earthnut oil. Peanut oil.

Ease. (NeuroGenesis/Matrix Tech.) D, L-phenylalanine 500 mg, L-glutamine 15 mg, L-tyrosine 25 mg, L-carnitine 10 mg, L-arginine pyroglutamate 10 mg, L-ornithine/L-aspartate 10 mg, Cr 0.033 mg, Se 0.012 mg, B_1 0.33 mg, B_2 5 mg, B_3 3.3 mg, B_5 0.33 mg, B_6 0.33 mg, B_{12} 1 mcg, E 5 units, biotin 0.05 mg, FA 0.066 mg, Fe 1 mg, Zn 2.5 mg, Ca 35 mg, I 0.25 mg, Cu 0.33 mg, Mg 25 mg. Cap. Bot. 42s. *OTC.*
Use: Nutritional supplement.

Easprin. (Parke-Davis) Aspirin 15 g. EC Tab. Bot. 100s. *Rx.*
Use: Analgesic.

East-A. (Eastwood) Therapeutic lotion. Bot. 16 oz. *OTC.*
Use: Emollient.

Easy-Lax. (Walgreen) Docusate sodium 100 mg. Cap. Bot. 60s. *OTC.*
Use: Laxative; stool softener.

Easy-Lax Plus. (Walgreen) Docusate sodium 100 mg, casanthranol 30 mg. Cap. Bot. 60s. *OTC.*
Use: Laxative; stool softener.

Eazol. (Roberts) Fructose, dextrose, orthophosphoric acid with controlled hydrogen ion concentration. Bot. 473 mL. *OTC.*
Use: Antinauseant.

•**ebanicline tosylate.** (EE-ba-ni-kleen) USAN.
Use: Analgesic.

E-Base. (Barr) Erythromycin. **Cap.:** 333 mg. Bot. 100s, 500s, 1000s. **Tab.:** 333 mg, 500 mg. Bot. 100s, 500s. *Rx.*
Use: Anti-infective; erythromycin.

•**ebastine.** (EBB-ass-teen) USAN.
Use: Antihistamine.

EBV-VCA. (Wampole) Epstein-Barr virus, viral capsid antigen antibody test. Qualitative and semi-quantitative detection of EBV antibody in human serum. Test 100s.
Use: Diagnostic aid.

EBV-VCA Ig. (Wampole) Epstein-Barr virus, viral capsid antigen Ig antibody. Qualitative and semiqualitative detection of EBV-VCA Ig antibody in human serum. Test 50s.
Use: Diagnostic aid.

•**ecadotril.** (ee-CAD-oh-trill) USAN.
Use: Antihypertensive.

•**ecalcidene.** (ee-KAL-si-deen) USAN.
Use: Psoriasis.

•**ecallantide.** (ee-KAL-lan-tide) USAN.
Use: Hematological agent.
See: Kalbitor.

•**ecamsule.** (eh-KAM-sool) USAN.
Use: Sunscreen.
W/Avobenzone, Octocrylene.
See: Anthelios SX.
UV Protective.
W/Avobenzone, Octocrylene, Titanium Dioxide.
See: Capital Soleil 20.

Ecee Plus. (Edwards) Vitamin E 165 mg, ascorbic acid 100 mg, magnesium sulfate 70 mg, zinc sulfate 80 mg. Tab. Bot. 100s. *OTC.*
Use: Mineral, vitamin supplement.

echinacea angustifolia. (EK-i-NAY-sha)
Use: Dietary supplement.

echinacea pallida. (EK-i-NAY-sha)
Use: Dietary supplement.

echinacea purpurea. (EK-i-NAY-sha)
Use: Dietary supplement.

echinocandins.
Use: Antifungal.
See: Anidulafungin.
Caspofungin Acetate.

•**echothiophate iodide.** (eck-oh-THIGH-oh-fate EYE-oh-dide) *USP.*
Use: Glaucoma agent.

•**eclanamine maleate.** (eh-KLAN-ah-MEEN) USAN.
Use: Antidepressant.

•**eclazolast.** (eh-CLAY-zole-AST) USAN.
Use: Antiallergic; inhibitor (mediator release).

Eclipse After Sun. (Novartis) Petrolatum, glycerin, oleth-3 phosphate, carbomer-934, imidazolidinyl urea, benzyl alcohol, cetyl esters wax. Lot. Bot. 180 mL. *OTC.*
Use: Emollient.

Eclipse Lip and Face Protectant. (Novartis) Padimate O, oxybenzone. Stick 4.5 g. *OTC.*
Use: Lip protectant.

Eclipse Original Sunscreen. (Novartis) Padimate O, glyceryl PABA. Lot. Bot. 120 mL. *OTC.*
Use: Sunscreen.

Eclipse Suntan, Partial. (Novartis) Padimate O. Lot. Bot. 120 mL. *OTC.*
Use: Sunscreen.

EC-Naprosyn. (Roche) Naproxen 375 mg, 500 mg. Enteric coated. DR Tab. Bot. 100s. *Rx.*
Use: Nonsteroidal anti-inflammatory agent.

•**econazole.** (ee-CON-uh-zole) USAN.
Use: Antifungal.

•**econazole nitrate.** (ee-CON-uh-zole) *USP.*
Use: Antifungal.
See: Ecoza.

econazole nitrate. (Various Mfr.) Econazole nitrate 1%. Cream. 15 g, 30 g, 85 g. *Rx.*
Use: Antifungal agent, topical anti-infective.

Econo B & C. (Vangard Labs, Inc.) Vitamins B_1 15 mg, B_2 10.2 mg, B_3 50 mg, B_5 10 mg, B_6 5 mg, C 300 mg. Cap. Bot. 100s, UD 100s. *OTC.*
Use: Vitamin supplement.

•**ecopipam hydrochloride.** (E-koe-pi-pam) USAN.
Use: Addiction disorders.

•**ecopladib.** (ek-oh-PLA-dib) USAN.
Use: Analgesic.

Ecotrin Low Strength. (GlaxoSmithKline) Aspirin 81 mg. EDTA, parabens. EC Tab. 45s. *OTC.*
Use: Analgesic.

Ecotrin Maximum Strength. (GlaxoSmithKline) Acetylsalicylic acid 500 mg. **Tab.:** Bot. 60s, 150s. **Cap.:** Bot. 60s. *OTC.*
Use: Analgesic.

Ecotrin Regular Strength. (GlaxoSmithKline) Aspirin 325 mg. EC Tab. Bot. 100s, 250s, 1000s. *OTC.*
Use: Analgesic.

Ecoza. (Quinnova) Econazole nitrate 1%. Glycerin, propylene glycol, trolamine. Aer., foam. 70 g. *Rx.*
Use: Topical anti-infective, antifungal agent.

•**ecraprost.** (E-kra-prost) USAN.
Use: Peripheral arterial occlusive disease.

•**ecromeximab.** (e-KROE-mek-si-mab) USAN.
Use: Monoclonal antibody.

•**eculizumab.** (ek-yoo-LYE-zyoo-mab) USAN.
Use: Monoclonal antibody.
See: Soliris.

•**edaglitazone sodium.** (ED-a-GLI-ta-zone) USAN.
Use: Antidiabetic agent.

Ed A-Hist. (Edwards) Chlorpheniramine maleate 4 mg, phenylephrine hydrochloride 10 mg. **Tab.:** Tartrazine. 100s. **Liq.:** Sugar free. Alcohol 5%. Grape flavor. 473 mL. *Rx.*
Use: Upper respiratory combination, decongestant and antihistamine.

Ed A-Hist DM. (Edwards) Phenylephrine hydrochloride 10 mg, chlorpheniramine maleate 4 mg, dextromethorphan 15 mg per 5 mL. Parabens, potassium citrate, potassium sorbate, propylene glycol, sorbitol, sucralose. Gluten free and sugar free. Banana flavor. Liq. 473 mL. *OTC.*
Use: Upper respiratory combination, antitussive combination.

Ed A-Hist PSE. (Edwards) Pseudoephedrine hydrochloride 60 mg, triprolidine hydrochloride 2.5 mg. Tartrazine. Tab. 100s. *Rx.*
Use: Upper respiratory combination, decongestant and antihistamine.

Ed-Apap Children's. (Edwards) Acetaminophen 160 mg/5 mL. Alcohol free. Sorbitol. Cherry flavor. Oral Soln. 236 mL. *OTC.*
Use: Analgesic.

Edarbi. (Arbor Pharmaceuticals) Azilsartan medoxomil 40 mg (equiv. to azilsartan kamedoxomil 42.68 mg), 80 mg (equiv. to azilsartan kamedoxomil 85.36 mg). Mannitol. Tab. 30s, 90s. *Rx.*
Use: Renin angiotensin system antagonist, angiotensin II receptor antagonist.

Edarbyclor. (Takeda Pharmaceuticals) Azilsartan medoxomil/chlorthalidone 40 mg/12.5 mg, 40 mg/25 mg (equiv. to azilsartan kamedoxomil 42.68 mg). Film coated. Mannitol, PEG. Tab. 30s, 90s. *Rx.*
Use: Antihypertensive combination.

edathamil. Edetate ethylenediamine tetraacetic acid.

edathamil calcium-disodium. Calcium disodium ethylenediamine tetraacetate.

edathamil disodium. Disodium salt of ethylenediamine tetraacetic acid.
See: Endrate.

•**edatrexate.** (EE-dah-TREX-ate) USAN.
Use: Antineoplastic.

Ed-Bron G. (Edwards) Theophylline 50 mg, guaifenesin 33.3 mg per 5 mL. Sugar free. Liq. 473 mL. *Rx.*
Use: Antiasthmatic combination, xanthine combination.

Ed-Bron GP. (Edwards) Guaifenesin 100 mg, phenylephrine hydrochloride 5 mg per 5 mL. Parabens, potassium citrate, potassium sorbate, propylene glycol, sorbitol, sucralose. Alcohol free, dye free, and sugar free. Orange flavor. Liq. 473 mL. *OTC.*
Use: Upper respiratory combination, decongestant and expectorant combination.

Ed ChlorPed. (Edwards) Chlorpheniramine maleate 2 mg/mL. Propylene glycol, saccharin, sorbitol. Cotton candy flavor. Liq. 60 mL. *OTC.*
Use: Antihistamine, nonselective alkylamine.

Ed ChlorPed D. (Edwards) Chlorpheniramine maleate 2 mg, phenylephrine hydrochloride 5 mg. Glycerin, parabens, potassium citrate, potassium sorbate, propylene glycol, sucralose. Alcohol free, gluten free, and sugar free. Applesauce flavor. Drops. 60 mL w/dropper. *Rx.*
Use: Upper respiratory combination, decongestant and antihistamine.

Ed ChlorPed Jr. (Edwards) Chlorpheniramine maleate 2 mg per 5 mL. Parabens, potassium sorbate, propylene glycol, sorbitol, sucralose. Alcohol free and sugar free. Cherry flavor. Syrup. 473 mL. *Rx.*
Use: Antihistamine, nonselective alkylamine.

Ed-Chlortan. (Edwards) Chlorpheniramine maleate 4 mg. Tab. 100s. *OTC.*
Use: Antihistamine, nonselective alkylamine.

Ed-Chlor-Tan. (Edwards) Chlorpheniramine tannate 8 mg. Tab. 100s. *Rx.*
Use: Antihistamine, nonselective alkylamine.

Edecrin. (Valeant) Ethacrynic acid 25 mg. Lactose. Tab. 100s. *Rx.*
Use: Diuretic.

Edecrin Sodium Intravenous. (Valeant) Ethacrynate sodium equivalent to 50 mg ethacrynic acid w/mannitol 62.5 mg. Inj., Pow. for Soln. Vial. 50 mL for reconstitution. *Rx.*
Use: Diuretic.

•**edetate calcium disodium.** (E-de-tate) *USP. Formerly Edathamil.*
Use: Chelating agent (metal).
See: Calcium Disodium Versenate.

•**edetate dipotassium.** (E-de-tate) USAN.
Use: Pharmaceutic aid (chelating agent).

•**edetate disodium.** (E-de-tate) *USP.*
Use: Chelating agent (metal); pharmaceutic aid (chelating agent).

•**edetate sodium.** (E-de-tate) USAN.
Use: Chelating agent.
See: Vagisec Plus.

•**edetate trisodium.** (E-de-tate) USAN.
Use: Chelating agent.

•**edetic acid.** (ED-eh-tic) *NF.*
Use: Pharmaceutic aid (chelating agent).

•**edetol.** (eh-deh-TOLE) USAN.
Use: Pharmaceutic aid (alkalinizing agent).

Edex. (Actient Pharmaceuticals) Alprostadil. **Inj.:** 10 mcg, 20 mcg, 40 mcg (after reconstitution), lactose. Inj. Single-dose vial or kit containing prefilled syringe (with 1.2 mL of 0.9% sodium chloride), plunger rod, 2 one-half inch needles (one 27-gauge and one 30-gauge), 2 alcohol swabs, tape. **Pow. for Inj., lyophilized:** 10 mcg, 20 mcg, 40 mcg. Lactose. Single-dose, dual-chamber cartridges for use with reusable injection device. *Rx.*
Use: Anti-impotence agent.

Ed-Flex. (Edwards) Phenyltoloxamine citrate 20 mg, acetaminophen 300 mg, salicylamide 200 mg. Cap. Bot. 30s, 100s. *Rx.*
Use: Upper respiratory combination, antihistamine, analgesic.

•**edifoligide sodium.** (e-dif-oh-LIG-ide) USAN.
Use: Graft-vs-host disease.

•**edifolone acetate.** (EH-DIH-fah-LONE) USAN.
Use: Cardiovascular agent (antiarrhythmic).

edithamil.
See: Edathamil.

•**edivoxetine.** (E-di-VOX-e-teen) USAN.
Use: CNS agent.

•**edivoxetine hydrochloride.** (E-di-VOX-e-teen) USAN.
Use: CNS agent.

Edluar. (Meda Pharmaceuticals) Zolpidem tartrate 5 mg, 10 mg. Mannitol, saccharin. Sublingual Tab. UD 30s. *c-IV.*
Use: Sedative and hypnotic, nonbarbiturate; imidazopyridine.

•**edobacomab.** (eh-dah-BACK-ah-mab) USAN.
Use: Antiendotoxin monoclonal antibody.

•**edodekin alfa.** (e-DOE-de-kin AL-fa) USAN.
Use: Antiasthmatic.

•**edonetan.** (ed-ON-en-tan) USAN.
Use: Heart failure.

•**edotecarin.** (ed-oh-TEK-ar-in) USAN.
Use: Antineoplastic.

•**edotreotide.** (ed-oh-TREE-oh-tide) USAN.
Use: Tumor staging.

•**edoxaban.** (e-DOX-a-ban) USAN.
Use: Cardiovascular agent.

•**edoxaban tosylate.** (e-DOX-a-ban) USAN.
Use: Cardiovascular agent.

•**edoxudine.** (e-DOX-ue-deen) USAN.
Use: Antiviral.

•**edratide.** (ED-ra-tide) USAN.
Use: Lupus erythematosus.

•**edrecolomab.** (E-dre-KOL-oh-mab) USAN.
Use: Monoclonal antibody (antineoplastic adjuvant).

edrofuradene. *Name used for Nifurdazil.*

•**edrophonium chloride.** (eh-droe-FOE-nee-uhm) *USP.*
Use: Antidote to curare principles; diagnostic aid, myasthenia gravis.
See: Reversol.

ED-Spaz. (Edwards) Hyoscyamine sulfate 0.125 mg. Mannitol. Tab., disintegrating. 100s. *Rx.*
Use: Anticholinergic/antispasmodic, belladonna alkaloids.

EDTA.
See: Edathamil.

Edurant. (Tibotec) Rilpivirine 25 mg (equiv. to rilpivirine hydrochloride 27.5 mg). Film coated. Lactose. Tab. 30s. *Rx.*
Use: Antiretroviral agent, nonnucleoside reverse transcriptase inhibitor.

E.E.S. 400. (Arbor Pharmaceuticals) Erythromycin ethylsuccinate (as base). **Tab.:** 400 mg. Sugar. Film-coated. 100s, 500s. **Susp.:** 400 mg/5 mL. Parabens, sucrose. Orange flavor. Bot. 100 mL, 473 mL. *Rx.*
Use: Anti-infective; erythromycin.

E.E.S. Granules. (Arbor Pharmaceuticals) Erythromycin ethylsuccinate (as base) 200 mg/5 mL when reconstituted. Sucrose. Cherry flavor. Pow. for Oral Susp. Bot. 100 mL, 200 mL. *Rx.*
Use: Anti-infective; erythromycin.

•**efalizumab.** (e-fa-li-ZOO-mab) USAN.
Use: Humanized anti-CD11a monoclonal antibody; immunosuppressive.

•**efaproxiral.** (ef-a-PROKS-ir-al) USAN.
Use: Investigational hemoglobin modifier.

efavirenz.
Use: Antiretroviral agent, nonnucleoside reverse transcriptase inhibitor.
See: Sustiva.
W/Emtricitabine, Tenofovir Disoproxil Fumarate.
See: Atripla.

Efedron Nasal. (Hyrex) Ephedrine hydrochloride 0.6%, chlorobutanol 0.5% w/sodium chloride, menthol, and cinnamon oil in a water-soluble jelly base. Tube 20 g. *OTC.*
Use: Decongestant.

Efed-II. (Alto) Ephedrine sulfate 25 mg. Cap. Box 24s. *OTC.*
Use: Decongestant.

•**efegatran sulfate.** (EH-feh-GAT-ran) USAN.
Use: Antithrombotic.

E-Ferol. (Forest) **Spray:** Alpha tocopherol equivalent to 30 units vitamin E/mL. Can 6 oz. **Vanishing Cream:** Alpha tocopherol. Jar 2 oz. *OTC.*
Use: Emollient.

E-Ferol Succinate. (Forest) d-alpha tocopherol acid succinate, equivalent to Vitamin E. **Cap. 100 units, 400 units:** Bot. 100s, 500s, 1000s. **Cap. 200 units:** Bot. 50s, 100s, 500s, 1000s. **Tab. 50 units:** Bot. 100s, 500s, 1000s. *OTC.*
Use: Vitamin supplement.

Effaclar Duo. (LaRoche-Posay) Benzoyl peroxide 5.5% micronized. Micro-exfoliating LHA 0.4%, disodium EDTA, glycerin, isostearyl alcohol. Soln. 40 mL. *OTC.*
Use: Topical anti-infective, antibiotic agent.

Effectin Tablets. (Sanofi-Synthelabo) Bitolterol mesylate. *Rx.*
Use: Bronchodilator.

Effective Strength Cough Formula. (Alra) Chlorpheniramine maleate 2 mg, dextromethorphan HBr 15 mg, alcohol 10%. Liq. Bot. 240 mL. *OTC.*
Use: Antihistamine, antitussive.

Effective Strength Cough w/Decongestant. (Alra) Pseudoephedrine hydrochloride 20 mg, dextromethorphan HBr 10 mg, alcohol 10%. Liq. Bot. 240 mL. *OTC.*
Use: Antitussive, decongestant.

Effer-K. (Nomax) Potassium (as bicarbonate and citrate). **10 mEq:** Sucralose (flavored only), dextrose, maltodextrin.

Unflavored and cherry vanilla flavor. 30s. **20 mEq:** Sucralose (flavored only), dextrose, maltodextrin. Unflavored and orange cream flavor. 30s. **25 mEq:** Saccharin. Orange or lime flavors. 30s, 100s, 250s. Effervescent Tab. *Rx.*
Use: Electrolyte, potassium replacement product.

Effexor XR. (Wyeth Pharmaceuticals) Venlafaxine hydrochloride 37.5 mg, 75 mg, 150 mg. ER Cap. Bot. 15s, 30s, 90s, *Redipak* 100s. *Rx.*
Use: Antidepressant.

Effient. (Eli Lilly and Company) Prasugrel 5 mg, 10 mg. Film coated. Mannitol. Tab. 7s (5 mg only), 30s, UD 90s (10 mg only). *Rx.*
Use: Antiplatelet agent, aggregation inhibitor.

Efidac 24 Chlorpheniramine. (Hogil) Chlorpheniramine maleate 16 mg. ER Tab. Pkg. 6s. *OTC.*
Use: Antihistamine.

•**efinaconazole.** (EF-in-a-KON-a-zole) USAN.
Use: Antifungal agent.

•**efletirizine dihydrochloride.** (ef-le-TI-ra-zeen) USAN.
Use: Antihistaminic.

•**eflornithine hydrochloride.** (ee-FLAHR-nih-THEEN) USAN.
Use: Antineoplastic; antiprotozoal.
See: Vaniqa.

•**efungumab.** (ef-UN-gue-mab) USAN.
Use: Anti-infective.

•**egaptivon pegol.** (e-GAP-ti-von PEG-ol) USAN.
Use: Treatment of platelet dysfunction disorders.

•**eglumegad.** (e-GLUE-me-gad) USAN.
Use: Anti-anxiety agent; smoking cessation.

egraine. A protein binder from oats.

Egrifta. (EMD Serono) Tesamorelin 2 mg (equiv. to tesamorelin acetate 2.2 mg). Mannitol 100 mg. Preservative free. Inj., lyophilized Pow. for Soln. Single-use vial w/diluent. *Rx.*
Use: Endocrine and metabolic agent, growth hormone-releasing factor.

•**egtazic acid.** (egg-TAY-zik) USAN.
Use: Pharmaceutic aid.

EHDP.
See: Etidronate Disodium.

8-MOP. (ICN Pharmaceuticals) Methoxsalen 10 mg. Cap. 50s. *Rx.*
Use: Pigmenting agent.

•**elacridar hydrochloride.** (eh-LACK-rih-dahr) USAN.
Use: Potentiation of chemotherapy in cancer (multidrug resistance inhibitor in cancer); antineoplastic (adjunct).

•**elacytarabine.** (EL-a-sye-TAYR-a-been) USAN.
Use: Antineoplastic.

•**elagolix.** (el-a-GOE-lix) USAN.
Use: Endometriosis.

•**elagolix sodium.** (el-a-GOE-lix) USAN.
Use: Endometriosis.

•**elantrine.** (EL-an-treen) USAN.
Use: Anticholinergic.

Elaprase. (Shire Human Genetic Therapies) Idursulfase 2 mg/mL. Sodium chloride 24 mg, sodium phosphate monobasic monohydrate 6.75 g, sodium phosphate dibasic heptahydrate 2.97 mg. Preservative free. Soln. for Inj. Singe-use vials. 5 mL. *Rx.*
Use: Hunter syndrome.

•**elarofiban.** (el-a-roe-FYE-ban) USAN.
Use: Thrombotic disorders.

•**elastofilcon A.** (ee-LASS-toe-FILL-kahn A) USAN.
Use: Contact lens material, hydrophilic.

•**elbasvir.** (EL-bas-vir) USAN.
Use: Antiviral, treatment of hepatitis C.

elcatonin. (Innapharma, Inc.)
Use: Intrathecal treatment of intractable pain. [Orphan Drug]

•**eldacimibe.** (ell-DASS-ih-mibe) USAN.
Use: Antiatherosclerotic; antihyperlipidemic.

Eldec Kapseals. (Parke-Davis) Elemental iron 3.3 mg, Vitamins A 1667 units, E 10 mg, B_1 10 mg, B_2 0.9 mg, B_3 17 mg, B_5 10 mg, B_6 0.7 mg, B_{12} 2 mcg, C 67 mg, folic acid 0.3 mg, calcium iodine. Cap. Bot. 100s. *OTC.*
Use: Mineral, vitamin supplement.

Eldecort. (AstraZeneca) Hydrocortisone 2.5%, light mineral oil, propylene glycol, allantoin. Cream. Tube 15 g, 30 g. *Rx.*
Use: Corticosteroid, topical.

•**eldelumab.** (el-DEL-ue-mab) USAN.
Use: Immunologic agent.

Eldepryl. (Dey) Selegiline hydrochloride 5 mg, lactose. Cap. Bot. 60s. *Rx.*
Use: Antiparkinsonian.

Eldercaps. (Merz) Vitamins A 4000 units, D 400 units, E 25 units, B_1 10 mg, B_2 5 mg, B_3 25 mg, B_5 10 mg, B_6 2 mg, C 200 mg, folic acid 1 mg, Zn 15.8 mg, Mg, Mn. Cap. Bot. 100s. *Rx.*
Use: Mineral, vitamin supplement.

Eldertonic. (Merz) Vitamins B_1 0.17 mg, B_2 0.19 mg, B_3 2.22 mg, B_5 1.11 mg, B_6 0.22 mg, B_{12} 0.67 mcg, alcohol 13.5%, Mg, Mn, zinc 1.7 mg/5 mL. Bot. 473 mL. *OTC.*
Use: Mineral, vitamin supplement.

Eldisine. (Eli Lilly)
See: Vindesine sulfate.
Eldo-B & C. (Canright) Vitamins C 250 mg, B_1 25 mg, B_2 10 mg, B_6 5 mg, niacinamide 150 mg, d-calcium pantothenate 20 mg. Tab. Bot. 100s, 1000s. *OTC.*
Use: Mineral, vitamin supplement.
Eldofe. (Canright) Ferrous fumarate 225 mg. Chew. Tab. Bot. 100s, 1000s. *OTC.*
Use: Mineral supplement.
Eldofe-C. (Canright) Ferrous fumarate 225 mg, ascorbic acid 50 mg. Tab. Bot. 100s. *OTC.*
Use: Mineral, vitamin supplement.
Eldopaque. (Valeant) Hydroquinone 2% with sunblock. Cream. Tube. 14.2 g, 28.4 g. *OTC.*
Use: Dermatologic.
Eldopaque Forte. (Valeant) Hydroquinone 4% in a sunblock base. Talc, light mineral oil, EDTA, sodium metabisulfite. Cream. Tube. 28.4 g. *Rx.*
Use: Dermatologic.
Eldoquin Forte. (Valeant) Hydroquinone 4% in vanishing base. Light mineral oil, propylparaben, sodium metabisulfite. Cream. Tube. 28.4 g. *Rx.*
Use: Dermatologic.
Elecal. (Western Research) Calcium 250 mg, magnesium 15 mg. Tab. Bot. 1000s. *OTC.*
Use: Mineral supplement.
electrolyte and invert sugar solutions.
Use: Intravenous nutritional therapy, intravenous replenishment solution.
See: Invert Sugar-Electrolyte Solutions.
electrolyte concentrates, combined.
Use: Intravenous nutritional therapy, intravenous replenishment solution.
See: Hyperlyte CR.
Lypholyte.
Lypholyte-II.
Multilyte-40.
Multilyte-20.
Nutrilyte.
Nutrilyte II.
TPN Electrolytes.
TPN Electrolytes III.
TPN Electrolytes II.
electrolyte-dextrose solutions.
Use: Intravenous nutritional therapy, intravenous replenishment solution.
See: Dextrose-Electrolyte Solutions.
electrolyte No. 48 and dextrose 10%.
Use: Intravenous nutritional therapy, intravenous replenishment solution.
See: Dextrose 10% and Electrolyte No. 48.
electrolyte No. 48 injection.
Use: Intravenous nutritional therapy, intravenous replenishment solution.
See: Dextrose 5% and Electrolyte No. 48.
electrolyte No. 75 and 5% dextrose.
Use: Intravenous nutritional therapy, intravenous replenishment solution.
See: Dextrose 5% and Electrolyte No. 75.
electrolytes.
Use: Nutritional therapy.
See: Potassium Chloride.
Potassium Salts.
Sodium Chloride.
electrolyte solutions, combined.
Use: Intravenous nutritional therapy, intravenous replenishment solution.
See: Isolyte S pH 7.4.
Lactated Ringer's.
Normosol-M.
Normosol-R.
Normosol-R pH 7.4.
Plasma-Lyte A pH 7.4.
Plasma-Lyte 148.
Plasma-Lyte R.
Potassium Chloride in 0.9% Sodium Chloride.
Ringer's.
Elegen-G. (Grafton) Amitriptyline 10 mg, 25 mg, 50 mg. Tab. Bot. 100s, 1000s. *Rx.*
Use: Antidepressant, tricyclic.
Elelyso. (Pfizer) Taliglucerase alfa 200 units. Mannitol, polysorbate 80. Preservative free. Inj., lyophilized Pow. for Soln. Single-use vial. *Rx.*
Use: Endocrine and metabolic agent.
elesclomol.
Use: Investigational antineoplastic agent.
Elestat. (Allergan) Epinastine hydrochloride 0.05%. Benzalkonium chloride 0.01%, EDTA. Soln., Ophthalmic. 8 mL, 15 mL. *Rx.*
Use: Ophthalmic antihistamine.
Elestrin. (Azur Pharma) Estradiol 0.06% (estradiol 0.52 mg per 0.87 g unit dose). EDTA. Top. Gel. 144 g metered-dose pump. *Rx.*
Use: Sex hormone, estrogen.
Eletone. (Mission) Cetostearyl alcohol, mineral oil, parabens, petrolatum. Cream. 100 g. *Rx.*
Use: Emollient.
•**eletriptan hydrobromide.** (all-eh-TRIP-tan HIGH-droe-BROE-mide)
Use: Antimigraine agent, serotonin 5-HT receptor agonist.
See: Relpax.

•**eleuthero.** *NF.*
Use: Dietary supplement.

Elevites. (Barth's) Vitamins A 6000 units, D 400 units, B_1 1.5 mg, B_2 3 mg, B_{12} 10 mcg, C 60 mg, niacin 1 mg, E 10 units, malt diastase 15 mg, iron 15 mg, calcium 381 mg, phosphorus 0.172 mg, citrus bioflavonoid complex 15 mg, rutin 15 mg, nucleic acid 3 mg, red bone marrow 30 mg, peppermint leaves 10 mg, wheat germ 30 mg. Tab. or Cap. Bot. 100s, 500s, 1000s. *Rx.*
Use: Mineral, vitamin supplement.

Elidel. (Valeant) Pimecrolimus 1%. Benzyl alcohol, cetyl alcohol, oleyl alcohol, stearyl alcohol. Cream. Tube. 30 g, 60 g, 100 g. *Rx.*
Use: Topical immunomodulator.

Eligard. (Sanofi-Synthelabo) Leuprolide acetate **Pow. for Inj., lyophilized:** 7.5 mg. Single-use kit w/ 2-syringe mixing system and 20-gauge, ½-inch needle. **Inj.:** 22.5 mg (3-month depot), 30 mg (4-month depot), 45 mg (6-month depot). Single-use kit with 2-syringe mixing system and 20-gauge, ½-inch needle (22.5 mg only). Single-use kit w/ 2-syringe mixing system and syringe containing *Atrigel* (30 mg, 45 mg only). *Rx.*
Use: Antineoplastic.

Eligard 22.5 mg. (Sanofi-Synthelabo) Leuprolide acetate 22.5 mg. Inj. Single-use kit w/2-syringe mixing system and 20-gauge, ½-inch needle. *Rx.*
Use: Antineoplastic.

•**eliglustat.** (EL-i-GLOO-stat) USAN.
Use: Treatment of lysosomal storage disorders.

•**eliglustat tartrate.** (EL-i-GLOO-stat) USAN.
Use: Treatment of lysosomal storage disorders.

Elimite. (Allergan) Permethrin 5%. Lanolin alcohols, coconut oil, mineral oil. Cream. Tube 60 g. *Rx.*
Use: Scabicide; pediculicide.

Elinest. (Northstar) Ethinyl estradiol 30 mcg, norgestrel 0.3 mg. Lactose, PEG. Tab. 28s w/7 inert tablets (lactose, PEG). *Rx.*
Use: Monophasic oral contraceptive.

•**elinogrel.** (el-IN-oh-grel) USAN.
Use: Antithrombotic agent.

•**elinogrel potassium.** (el-IN-oh-grel) USAN.
Use: Antithrombotic agent.

Eliphos. (Hawthorn) Calcium acetate 667 mg. Elemental calcium 169 mg, PEG-8000. Tab. 200s. *Rx.*
Use: Mineral, calcium.

Eliquis. (Bristol-Myers Squibb) Apixaban 2.5 mg, 5 mg. Film coated. Lactose. Tab. 60s, 180s, UD 100s. *Rx.*
Use: Anticoagulant, direct factor Xa inhibitor.

Elitek. (Sanofi-Synthelabo) Rasburicase 1.5 mg/vial (mannitol 10.6 mg), 7.5 mg (mannitol 53 mg). Pow. for Inj., lyophilized. Single-use vials with 1 mL amps of diluent (1.5 mg only). Single-use vials with 5 mL of diluent (7.5 mg only). *Rx.*
Use: Antimetabolite.

Elixicon. (Berlex) Theophylline 100 mg/5 mL with methylparabens and propylparabens. Susp. Bot. 237 mL. *Rx.*
Use: Bronchodilator.

Elixiral. (Vita Elixir) Phenobarbital 16.2 mg, hyoscyamine sulfate 0.1037 mg, atropine sulfate 0.194 mg, hyoscine HBr 0.0065 mg/5 mL. Liq. Pt, gal. *Rx.*
Use: Anticholinergic; antispasmodic; hypnotic; sedative.

Elixophyllin. (Caraco) Theophylline 80 mg/15 mL. Alcohol 20%. Saccharin. Mixed fruit flavor. Elix. 473 mL, 946 mL, 3,785 mL. *Rx.*
Use: Bronchodilator.

ElixSure Children's Congestion. (Taro Consumer) Pseudoephedrine 15 mg per 5 mL. Glycerin, propylparaben, sucralose. Bubble gum, cherry, and grape flavors. Syr. 118 mL. *OTC.*
Use: Nasal decongestant.

ElixSure Children's Cough. (Taro Consumer) Dextromethorphan hydrobromide 7.5 mg per 5 mL. Propylparaben, sorbitol, sucralose. Cherry and bubble gum flavors. Syrup. 118 mL. *OTC.*
Use: Nonnarcotic antitussive.

ElixSure Children's Fever Reducer/ Pain Reliever. (Alterna) Acetaminophen 160 mg/5 mL. Butylparaben, sucralose. Cherry flavor. Oral Soln. 120 mL. *OTC.*
Use: Analgesic.

Ella. (Afaxys) Ulipristal acetate 30 mg. Lactose. Tab. UD 1s. *Rx.*
Use: Sex hormone, contraceptive hormone.

Ellence. (Pharmacia & Upjohn) Epirubicin hydrochloride 2 mg/mL. Preservative free. Inj. Soln. Single-use vial 25 mL, 100 mL. *Rx.*
Use: Antibiotic, anthracycline.

Ellesdine. (Janssen) Pipenperone. *Rx.*
Use: Anxiolytic.

Elliotts B. (QOL Medical) Dextrose 8 g/L, sodium 149 mEq/L, potassium 4 mEq/L, calcium 2.7 mEq/L, magnesium 2.4 mEq/L, chloride 132 mEq/L, phos-

phate 1.5 mEq/L, osmolarity 288 mOsm/L. Preservative free. Soln., intrathecal Inj. Amp. 10 mL. *Rx.*
Use: Dextrose-electrolyte solution.

Elliot's B Solution. (Orphan Medical)
Use: Acute lymphatic leukemias and acute lymphoblastic lymphomas. [Orphan Drug]

•**elm.** *USP.* Dried inner bark of *Ulmus rubra* Muhlenberg (*Ulmus fulva* Michaux).
Use: Pharmaceutic aid (suspending agent); demulcent.

Elmiron. (Janssen) Pentosan polysulfate sodium 100 mg. Cap. Bot. 100s. *Rx.*
Use: Relief of bladder pain associated with interstitial cystitis.

•**elobixibat.** (EL-oh-BIX-i-bat) USAN.
Use: Laxative.

Elocon Cream. (Schering-Plough)
Cream: Mometasone furoate 0.1%, hexylene glycol, phosphoric acid, propylene glycol stearate, stearyl alcohol, ceteareth-20, titanium dioxide, aluminum starch octenyl succinate, white wax, white petrolatum. Tube 15 g, 45 g. **Lot.:** Mometasone furoate 0.1%. Bot. 30 mL, 60 mL. **Oint.:** Mometasone furoate 0.1%, hexylene glycol, propylene glycol stearate, white wax, white petrolatum. Tube 15 g, 45 g. *Rx.*
Use: Corticosteroid, topical.

Elon Barrier Protectant. (Dartmouth) Paraffinum, liquidum, isopropyl palmitate, cetearyl alcohol, polyglyceryl-2, dipolyhydroxystearate, propylene glycol, cetearyl glucoside, C12-15 alkyl benzoate, stearic acid, bisabalol, petrolatum, phenoxyethanol, PEG-30 dipolyhydroxystearate, PEG-40 stearate, parabens, *Hamamelis virginiana*, denatured alcohol. Liq. 28 g. *OTC.*
Use: Protectant.

Elon Dual Defense Antifungal Formula. (Dartmouth) Undecylenic acid 25%. Alcohol. Soln. 30 mL. *OTC.*
Use: Antifungal agent.

•**elosulfase alfa.** (EL-oh-SUL-fase) USAN.
Use: Treatment of Morquio syndrome.
See: Vimizim.

•**elotuzumab.** (EL-oh-TOOZ-ue-mab) USAN.
Use: Antineoplastic.

Eloxatin. (Sanofi Aventis) Oxaliplatin 5 mg/mL. Preservative free. Inj.; Soln, Conc. Single-use vial. 10 mL, 20 mL, 40 mL. *Rx.*
Use: Antineoplastic agent, platinum coordination complex.

•**elpetrigine.** (EL-pe-TRI-gine) USAN.
Use: CNS agent.

Elphemet. (Canright) Phendimetrazine tartrate 35 mg. Tab. Bot. 100s, 1000s. *c-III.*
Use: Anorexiant.

Elprecal. (Canright) Vitamins A 5000 units, D 400 units, B_1 3 mg, B_2 2 mg, B_6 0.1 mg, B_{12} 1 mcg, C 50 mg, E 2 units, calcium pantothenate 2.5 mg, niacinamide 15 mg, inositol 5 mg, choline 5 mg, calcium lactate 500 mg, ferrous sulfate 50 mg, Cu 1 mg, Mn 1 mg, Mg 2 mg, K 2 mg, Zn 0.5 mg, sulfur 1 mg. Cap. Bot. 100s. *OTC.*
Use: Mineral, vitamin supplement.

•**elsamitrucin.** (els-AM-ih-TRUE-sin) USAN.
Use: Antineoplastic.

Elserpine. (Canright) Reserpine 0.25 mg. Tab. Bot. 100s, 1000s. *Rx.*
Use: Antihypertensive.

•**elsibucol.** (el-si-BUE-kol) USAN.
Use: Immunosuppressive.

Elta SilverGel. (Swiss-American) Silver 55 ppm. Gel. 30 mL, 45 mL, 236 mL, 473 mL. 2" × 2" and 4" × 4" dressings. 10s. *OTC.*
Use: Dermatological agent, wound healing agent.

EL 10. (Elan) *Rx.*
Use: Antiviral; immunomodulator.

•**eltrombopag olamine.** (el-TROM-boe-pag) USAN.
Use: Hematopoietic agent.
See: Promacta.

•**elubrixin.** (EL-ue-BRIX-in) USAN.
Use: Treatment of cystic fibrosis, chronic obstructive pulmonary disease.

•**elubrixin tosylate.** (EL-ue-BRIX-in) USAN.
Use: Treatment of cystic fibrosis, chronic obstructive pulmonary disease.

•**elucaine.** (eh-LOO-cane) USAN.
Use: Anticholinergic, gastric.

•**eluxadoline.** (EL-ux-AD-oh-leen) USAN.
Use: Antidiarrheal.

Elvanol. (DuPont) Polyvinyl alcohol. *Rx.*
Use: Pharmaceutical aid.

•**elvitegravir.** (EL-vi-TEG-ra-vir) USAN.
Use: Treatment of HIV infections.
W/Cobicistat, Emtricitabine, Tenofovir Disoproxil Fumarate.
See: Stribild.

•**elvucitabine.** (el-vue-SYE-ta-been) USAN.
Use: Hepatitis B; HIV.

•**elzasonan citrate.** (el-za-SONE-an) USAN.
Use: Antidepressant.

•**elzasonan hydrochloride.** (el-za-SONE-an) USAN.
Use: Antidepressant.

Emadine. (Alcon) Emedastine difumarate 0.05% (0.5 mg/mL), benzalkonium chloride 0.01%. Ophth. Soln. Dispenser 5 mL. *Rx.*
Use: Antihistamine, ophthalmic.

embechine. Aliphatic chloroethylamine.
Use: Antineoplastic.

Embrex 600. (Andrx) Ca 240 mg, Fe (as carbonyl iron) 90 mg, vitamin A 3500 units, D_3 400 units, E (dl-alpha tocopherol acetate) 30 units, B_1 2 mg, B_2 3 mg, B_6 3 mg, B_{12} 12 mg, C 60 mg, folic acid 1 mg, Zn 20 mg, Cu, Mg, dioctylsulfosuccinate sodium 50 mg. Chew. Tab. Blister pack 35s, 91s. *Rx.*
Use: Vitamin, mineral supplement.

Emcodeine Tabs. (Major) Aspirin with codeine as #2, #3, #4. Bot. 100s, 500s. *c-III.*
Use: Analgesic combination; narcotic.

Emcyt. (Pharmacia) Estramustine phosphate sodium equivalent to 140 mg estramustine phosphate. Cap. Bot. 100s. *Rx.*
Use: Antineoplastic; hormone, alkylating agent.

Emdol. (Health for Life Brands) Salicylamide, para-aminobenzoic acid, sodium calcium succinate, vitamin D-1250. Bot. 100s, 1000s. *OTC.*
Use: Analgesic combination.

•**emedastine difumarate.** (eh-meh-DASS-teen die-FEW-mah-rate) *USP.*
Use: Management of allergic conjunctivitis; antiasthmatic; antiallergic; antihistamine (H_1-receptor).
See: Emadine.

Emend. (Merck) **Cap.:** Aprepitant 40 mg, 80 mg, 125 mg. Sucrose. Unit-of-use 1s, UD 5s (40 mg); unit-of-use bipack of 2, UD 6s (80 mg); UD 6s, unit-of-use tripack containing one 125 mg capsule and two 80 mg capsules. **Inj., lyophilized Pow. for Soln.:** Fosaprepitant 150 mg (equiv. to fosaprepitant dimeglumine 245.3 mg). Lactose, edetate disodium, polysorbate 80. Single-dose vial. *Rx.*
Use: Antiemetic/antivertigo agent.

•**emepepimut-S.** (EM-e-PEP-i-mut-es) USAN.
Use: Antineoplastic.

emergency contraceptives.
See: Next Choice One Dose.
Plan B.
Plan B One.

emergency kits.
See: Cyanide Antidote Package.

Emeroid. (Delta Pharmaceutical Group) Zinc oxide 5%, diperodon hydrochloride 0.25%, bismuth subcarbonate 0.2%, pyrilamine maleate 0.1%, phenylephrine hydrochloride 0.25%, in a petrolatum base containing cod liver oil. Tube 1.25 oz. *OTC.*
Use: Anorectal preparation.

Emerson 1% Sodium Fluoride Dental Gel. (Emerson) Red and plain. Bot. 2 oz. *Rx.*
Use: Dental caries agent.

emetics.
See: Ipecac.

•**emetine hydrochloride.** (EM-eh-teen) *USP.*
Use: Antiamebic.

Emetrol. (Wellspring Pharmaceutical) Dextrose 1.87 g, fructose 1.87 g, phosphoric acid 21.5 mg, methylparaben, lemon, mint, or cherry flavor. Soln. Bot. 118 mL, 236 mL, 473 mL. *OTC.*
Use: Antiemetic.

EMF. (Wesley Pharmacal) Alanine, arginine, aspartic acid, cysteine, glutamic acid, glycine, histidine, hydroxylysine, hydroxyproline, isoleucineline, leucine, lysine, methionine, phenylalanine, proline, serine, threonine, tyrosine, valine, protein 15 g, sorbitol, saccharin, cherry flavor. Liq. Bot. Qt. *OTC.*
Use: Amino acid.

Emgel. (GlaxoSmithKline) Erythromycin 2%. Alcohol 77%. Gel. Tubes. 27 g, 50 g. *Rx.*
Use: Topical anti-infective, antibiotic.

EM-GG. (Econo Med Pharmaceuticals) Guaifenesin 100 mg/5 mL. Bot. Pt. *OTC.*
Use: Expectorant.

•**emicerfont.** (em-eye-SER-font) USAN.
Use: CNS agent.

•**emilium tosylate.** (EE-MILL-ee-uhm TAH-sill-ate) USAN.
Use: Cardiovascular agent (antiarrhythmic).

Emitrip Tabs. (Major) Amitriptyline. Tab. **10 mg, 25 mg:** Bot. 100s, 250s, 1000s, UD 100s. **50 mg:** Bot. 100s, 250s, 1000s, UD 100s. **75 mg:** Bot. 100s, 250s, UD 100s. **100 mg:** Bot. 100s, 250s, 1000s, UD 100s. **150 mg:** Bot. 100s, 250s. *Rx.*
Use: Antidepressant, tricyclic.

•**emivirine.** (e-mi-VYE-rene) USAN.
Use: HIV-1 infection.

•**emixustat.** (em-IX-ue-stat) USAN.
Use: Dry age-related macular degeneration.

•**emixustat hydrochloride.** (em-IX-ue-stat) USAN.

Use: Dry age-related macular degeneration.

EMLA. (Akorn) Lidocaine 2.5%, prilocaine 2.5%. Preservative free. Cream. 5 g, 30 g. *Rx.*
Use: Topical local anesthetic.

Emollia-Creme. (Gordon Laboratories) Cetyl alcohol, lubricating oils in water-soluble base. Jar 4 oz, 5 lb. *OTC.*
Use: Emollient.

Emollia-Lotion. (Gordon Laboratories) Water-dispersable waxes, lubricating bland oils in a water-soluble lotion base. Bot. 1 oz, 4 oz, gal. *OTC.*
Use: Emollient.

Emoquette. (Qualitest Pharmaceuticals) Ethinyl estradiol 30 mcg, desogestrel 0.15 mg. Film coated. Lactose, PEG. Tab. 28s w/7 inert tablets (lactose, PEG). *Rx.*
Use: Monophasic oral contraceptive.

•**empagliflozin.** (EM-pa-gli-FLOE-zin) USAN.
Use: Antidiabetic agent.

Empirin Aspirin. (GlaxoSmithKline) Aspirin 325 mg. Tab. Bot. 50s, 100s, 250s. *OTC.*
Use: Analgesic.

Empirin w/Codeine. (GlaxoSmithKline) Aspirin 325 mg with codeine phosphate 15 mg, 30 mg, 60 mg. Tab. **No. 2:** Codeine phosphate 15 mg. Bot. 100s. **No. 3:** Codeine phosphate 30 mg. Bot. 100s, 500s, 1000s, *Dispenserpak* 25s. **No. 4:** Codeine phosphate 60 mg. Bot. 100s, 500s, *Dispenserpak* 25s. *c-III.*
Use: Analgesic combination; narcotic.

Emsam. (Dey Labs) Selegiline hydrochloride 6 mg/24 hr (20 mg/20 cm^2), 9 mg/24 hr (30 mg/30 cm^2), 12 mg/24 hr (40 mg/40 cm^2). Patch; transdermal system. Box. 30s. *Rx.*
Use: Antiparkinson agent.

•**emtricitabine.** (em-try-SIGH-tah-bean) USAN.
Use: Antiviral.
See: Emtriva.
W/Cobicistat, Elvitegravir, Tenofovir Disoproxil Fumarate.
See: Stribild.
W/Efavirenz, Tenofovir Disoproxil Fumarate.
See: Atripla.
W/Rilpivirine, Tenofovir Disoproxil Fumarate.
See: Complera.
W/Tenofovir Disoproxil.
See: Truvada.

Emtriva. (Gilead) Emtricitabine. **Cap.:** 200 mg. 30s. **Oral Soln.:** 10 mg/mL. Xylitol, parabens. Cotton-candy flavor. 170 mL with dosing cup. *Rx.*
Use: Antiviral.

Emulave. (Rydelle)
See: Aveenobar Oilated.

Emulsion SB. (PruGen) Capric acid, disodium EDTA, glycerin, glyceryl, linoleic acid, PEG, petrolatum, squalane, wax. Emulsion; topical. 90 g. *Rx.*
Use: Miscellaneous topical combination.

Emulsoil. (Paddock) Castor oil 95% w/emulsifying agents, butylparaben. Emulsion. Bot. 63 mL. *OTC.*
Use: Laxative.

E-Mycin. (Pharmacia) Erythromycin 250 mg, 333 mg. EC Tab. Bot. 40s (250 mg only), 100s, 500s, UD 100s. *Rx.*
Use: Anti-infective; erythromycin.

Enablex. (Novartis) Darifenacin 7.5 mg, 15 mg. Lactose. ER Tab. 30s, 90s, UD 100s. *Rx.*
Use: Treatment of overactive bladder.

•**enadoline hydrochloride.** (en-AHD-ole-en) USAN.
Use: Analgesic; severe head injury. [Orphan Drug]

•**enalaprilat.** (EH-NAL-uh-prill-at) *USP.*
Use: Renin angiotensin system antagonist, angiotensin-converting enzyme inhibitor.

enalaprilat. (Various Mfr.) Enalaprilat 1.25 mg/mL. Inj. Vial 1 mL, 2 mL. *Rx.*
Use: Renin angiotensin system antagonist, angiotensin-converting enzyme inhibitor.

•**enalapril maleate.** (EH-NAL-uh-prill) *USP.*
Use: Renin angiotensin system antagonist, angiotensin-converting enzyme inhibitor.
See: Epaned.
Vasotec.
W/Diltiazem maleate.
See: Teczem.
W/Hydrochlorothiazide.
See: Enalapril Maleate/Hydrochlorothiazide.
Vaseretic.

enalapril maleate. (Various Mfr.) Enalapril maleate 2.5 mg, 5 mg, 10 mg, 20 mg. Tab. 30s, 100s, 500s (2.5 mg and 20 mg only), 1,000s, 5,000s (except 2.5 mg), UD 100s. *Rx.*
Use: Renin angiotensin system antagonist, angiotensin-converting enzyme inhibitor.

enalapril maleate/hydrochlorothiazide. (Eon) Hydrochlorothiazide/enalapril maleate 12.5 mg/5 mg, 25 mg/10 mg.

Lactose. Tab. Bot. 100s, 1000s. *Rx.*
Use: Antihypertensive.

•**enalkiren.** (en-al-KIE-ren) USAN.
Use: Antihypertensive.

•**enavatuzumab.** (EN-a-va-TOOZ-oo-mab) USAN.
Use: Antineoplastic.

•**enazadrem phosphate.** (eh-NAZZ-ah-drem) USAN.
Use: Antipsoriatic; inhibitor (5-lipoxygenase).

Enbrel. (Amgen) Etanercept. **Inj. Soln.:** 25 mg, 50 mg. Preservative free. Sucrose, sodium chloride, sodium phosphate. Single-use prefilled syringes. Single-use prefilled *Sure-Click* autoinjectors (50 mg only). **Inj., Lyophilized, Pow. for Soln.:** 25 mg. Preservative free. Mannitol, sucrose. Multiple-use vial. Diluent contains benzyl alcohol 0.9%. *Rx.*
Use: Immunologic agent, immunomodulator.

•**encaleret.** (en-KAL-er-et) USAN.
Use: Treatment of osteoporosis.

•**encaleret sulfate.** (en-KAL-er-et) USAN.
Use: Treatment of osteoporosis.

encapsulated porcine islet preparation.
Use: Type 1 diabetes. [Orphan Drug]
See: BetaRx.

•**enciprazine hydrochloride.** (en-SIH-PRAH-zeen) USAN.
Use: Anxiolytic.

•**enclomiphene.** (en-KLOE-mih-FEEN) USAN. Formerly Cisclomiphene.

•**encyprate.** (en-SIGH-prate) USAN.
Use: Antidepressant.

EndaCof-C. (Larken) Codeine phosphate 10 mg, chlorpheniramine maleate 2 mg. Saccharin, sodium benzoate, sorbitol. Alcohol free, dye free, and sugar free. Cotton candy flavor. Liq. 473 mL. *c-v.*
Use: Upper respiratory combination, antitussive combination.

EndaCof-DC. (Larken) Codeine phosphate 10 mg, pseudoephedrine hydrochloride 30 mg. Saccharin, sodium benzoate, sorbitol. Alcohol free, dye free, and sugar free. Fruit gum flavor. Liq. 473 mL. *c-v.*
Use: Upper respiratory combination, antitussive combination.

Endacon. (Allegis) Dextromethorphan hydrobromide 20 mg, guaifenesin 100 mg, phenylephrine hydrochloride 10 mg. Benzoic acid, edetate disodium, glycerin, propylene glycol, sorbitol. Alcohol free and sugar free. Strawberry flavor. Liq. 473 mL. *Rx.*
Use: Upper respiratory combination, antitussive and expectorant combination.

Endafed. (Forest) Pseudoephedrine hydrochloride 120 mg, brompheniramine maleate 12 mg. SR Cap. Bot. 100s. *Rx.*
Use: Antihistamine, decongestant.

EndaRoid. (Larken) Hydrocortisone acetate 1%, pramoxine hydrochloride 1%. Cream. 28 g. *Rx.*
Use: Anorectal preparation, steroid-containing product.

Endep. (Roche) Amitriptyline hydrochloride 10 mg, 25 mg, 50 mg, 75 mg, 100 mg, 150 mg. Tab. **10 mg:** Bot. 100s, *Tel-E-Dose* 100s. **25 mg:** Bot. 100s, 500s, *Tel-E-Dose* 100s. **50 mg:** Bot. 100s, 500s, *Tel-E-Dose* 100s. **75 mg:** Bot. 100s, *Tel-E-Dose* 100s. **100 mg:** Bot. 100s, *Tel-E-Dose* 100s. **150 mg:** Bot 100s. *Rx.*
Use: Antidepressant, tricyclic.

endobenziline bromide.
Use: Anticholinergic.

endocaine. Pyrrocaine.
Use: Anesthetic, local.

Endocet. (Endo) Oxycodone hydrochloride/acetaminophen 5 mg/325 mg, 7.5 mg/325 mg, 7.5 mg/500 mg, 10 mg/325 mg, 10 mg/650 mg. Tab. Bot. 100s, 500s. *c-II.*
Use: Analgesic; narcotic.

endocrine and metabolic agents.
See: Cysteamine.
Elosulfase Alfa.
Growth Hormone-Releasing Factors.
Ivacaftor.
Sodium Phenylbutyrate.
Vasopressin Receptor Antagonists.
Velaglucerase Alfa.

Endometrin. (Ferring Pharmaceuticals) Progesterone 100 mg. Vaginal Insert, Micronized. UD with 21 vaginal applicators. *Rx.*
Use: Sex hormone, progestin.

endomycin. A new antibiotic obtained from cultures of *Streptomyces endus.* Under study.

endophenolphthalein. (Roche) Diacetyldioxyphenylisatin-isacen-bisatin. *OTC.*
Use: Laxative.

endothelin receptor antagonists.
Use: Vasodilator.
See: Ambrisentan.
Bosentan.
Macitentan.

•**endralazine mesylate.** (en-DRAL-ah-zeen MEH-sih-late) USAN.
Use: Antihypertensive.

•**endrysone.** (EN-drih-sone) USAN.
Use: Anti-inflammatory, topical; ophthalmic.

Enduron. (Abbott) Methyclothiazide 5 mg. Tab. Bot. 100s, 1000s, 5000s, *Abbo-Pac* 100s. *Rx.*
Use: Diuretic.

Enecat CT. (Mallinckrodt) Barium sulfate 5%. Simethicone, sorbitol. Conc. Susp. Bot. 110 mL w/480 mL bot. for dilution w/flexible tubing, clamp, enema tip. *Rx.*
Use: Radiopaque agent, GI contrast agent.

Enemark. (Lafayette) Rectal marker. 85% w/v liquid barium. Case of 12 kits.
Use: Rectal marker during radiation therapy.

enemas.
See: Docusol Mini-Enema.
Fleet.
Fleet Bisacodyl.
Fleet Mineral Oil.
Therevac-Plus.
Therevac-SB.

Enemeez. (Alliance Labs) Docusate sodium 283 mg per 5 mL. Glycerin, PEG. Enema; rectal. 30s. *OTC.*
Use: Laxative, enema.

Enemeez Plus. (Alliance Labs) Docusate sodium 283 mg, benzocaine 20 mg in PEG, glycerin per 5 mL. Enema; rectal. 30s. *OTC.*
Use: Laxative, enema.

Enerjets. (Chilton) Caffeine 75 mg, sugar, coffee, mocha mint, and butterscotch flavors. Loz. Pkg. 10s. *OTC.*
Use: CNS stimulant, analeptic.

Eneset 1. (Lafayette) Barium sulfate suspension 300 mL/air contrast examination kit. Unit-of-use kit. Case 12s.
Use: Radiopaque agent.

Eneset 600. (Lafayette) Barium sulfate suspension 600 mL/air contrast examination kit. Unit-of-use kit. Case 12s.
Use: Radiopaque agent.

Eneset 2. (Lafayette) Barium sulfate suspension 450 mL/contrast examination kit. Unit-of-use kit. Case 12s.
Use: Radiopaque agent.

EnfaCare. (Mead Johnson Nutritionals) Protein (nonfat milk, whey protein concentrate, taurine, L-carnitine) 2.8 g, carbohydrate (maltodextrin, lactose) 10.7 g, fat (high oleic sunflower oil, soy oil, medium chain triglycerides, coconut oil, monoglycerides and diglycerides, soy lecithin) 5.3 g/100 cal, vitamins A, B_1, B_2, B_3, B_5, B_6, B_{12}, C, D, E, K, folic acid 26 mcg/100 cal, biotin, choline, inositol, linoleic acid, Ca, chloride, Cu, Fe 1.8 mg, I, Mg, Mn, P, Se, Zn, Na 35 mg, K 105 mg/100 cal, 22 cal/oz. Liq. Pow. *Nursette* bot. 3 oz. (Liq. only). Can 14 oz (Pow. only). *OTC.*
Use: Enteral nutritional therapy.

Enfamil. (Mead Johnson Nutritionals) Vitamins A 2000 units, D 400 units, E 20 units, C 52 mg, B_1 0.5 mg, B_2 1 mg, B_6 0.4 mg, B_{12} 1.5 mcg, niacin 8 mg, Ca 440 mg, P 300 mg, folic acid 100 mcg, pantothenic acid 3 mg, inositol 30 mg, biotin 15 mcg, K-1 55 mcg, choline 100 mg, Fe 1.4 mg, K 650 mg, Cl 400 mg, Cu 0.6 mg, I 65 mcg, Na 175 mg, Mg 50 mg, Zn 5 mg, Mn 100 mg. Qt. Concentrated Liq. 13 fl oz, Instant Pow. lb. *OTC.*
Use: Nutritional supplement.

Enfamil D•Vi•Sol. (Mead Johnson Nutritionals) Cholecalciferol (D_3) 400 units/mL. Glycerin, polysorbate 80. Gluten free, lactose free, and sugar free. Liq., concentrate. 50 mL w/dropper. *OTC.*
Use: Nutritional supplement.

Enfamil Fer-In-Sol. (Mead Johnson Nutritionals) Iron 15 mg per mL. Alcohol, sorbitol, sugar. Drops. 50 mL. *OTC.*
Use: Trace element, iron-containing product.

Enfamil Human Milk Fortifier. (Mead Johnson Nutritionals) Whey protein, casein, corn syrup solids, lactose, protein 0.7 g, carbohydrate 2.7 g, fat 0.04 g, calories 14. Pow. Packet 0.95 g, Box 100s. *OTC.*
Use: Nutritional supplement.

Enfamil LactoFree LIPIL. (Mead Johnson Nutritionals) Protein 2.1 g, fat 5.3 g, carbohydrate 10.9 g, calories 100/serving, linoleic acid 860 mg, A 300 units, D 60 units, E 2 units, K 8 mcg, B_1 80 mcg, B_2 140 mcg, B_3 1000 mcg, B_5 500 mcg, B_6 60 mcg, B_{12} 0.3 mcg, folic acid 16 mcg, biotin 3 mcg, C 12 mg, choline 12 mg, inositol (liquid only) 17 mg, inositol (powder only) 6 mg, Ca 82 mg, P 55 mg, Mg 8 mg, Fe 1.8 mg, Zn 1 mg, Mn 15 mcg, Cu 75 mcg, I 15 mcg, Se 2.8 mcg, Na 30 mg, K 110 mg, Cl 67 mg. Liq., Liq. Conc., Pow. Bot. 397 g (pow.), 384 mL (liq. conc.), 946 mL (liq.). *OTC.*
Use: Nutritional therapy, enteral.

Enfamil LIPIL with Iron. (Mead Johnson Nutritionals) Protein (reduced minerals, whey, nonfat milk, taurine) 2.1 g, fat (vegetable oil [palm olein, soy, coconut, and high-oleic sunflower oils], and less than 1% mortierella alpina oil, crypthecodinium cohnii oil, mono- and diglycerides, soy, lecithin) 5.3 g, carbohydrate (lactose) 10.9 g/100 cal, A, B_1, B_2, B_3, B_5, B_6, B_{12}, C, D, E, K, folic acid

16 mg/cal, biotin, chloride, choline, inositol, linoleic acid, Ca, Cu, Fe, I, Mg, Mn, P, Se, Zn, Na 27 mg and K 108 mg/100 cal. 20 cal/oz. **Liq.:** *Nursette* bottles 3 oz, 6 oz. **Liq. Conc.:** Cans 13 oz. **Pow.:** Cans. 12.9 oz, 25.7 oz. *OTC.*
Use: Nutritional therapy.

Enfamil Natalins Rx. (Mead Johnson Nutritionals) Ca 100 mg, Fe 27 mg, vitamin A 2000 units, D 200 units, E 7.5 units, B_1 0.75 mg, B_2 0.8 mg, B_3 8.5 mg, B_5 3.5 mg, B_6 2 mg, B_{12} 1.25 mcg, C 40 mg, folate 0.5 mg, biotin 15 mcg, Zn 12.5 mg, Cu, Mg. TR Tab. Bot. 200s. *Rx.*
Use: Vitamin, mineral supplement.

Enfamil Next Step. (Mead Johnson Nutritionals) Protein 17.3 g, carbohydrates 74 g, fat 33.3 g/liter, with appropriate vitamins and minerals. **Liq.:** 390 mL concentrate, 1 qt ready-to-use. **Pow.:** 360 g, 720 g. *OTC.*
Use: Nutritional supplement.

Enfamil Nursette. (Mead Johnson Nutritionals) Ready-to-feed *Enfamil* 20 kcal/fl oz, 4 fl oz, 6 fl oz and 8 fl oz. 4 bottles per sealed carton. W/Iron. Ready to use. Bot. 6 fl oz 4s, 24s. *OTC.*
Use: Nutritional supplement.

Enfamil Premature Formula. (Mead Johnson Nutritionals) Nonfat milk, whey protein concentrate, corn syrup solids, lactose, coconut oil, corn oil, medium chain triglycerides, soy lecithin. Protein 2.8 g, carbohydrate 10.7 g, fat 4.9 g, calories 96. Pow. *Nursettes* 120 mL. *OTC.*
Use: Nutritional supplement.

Enfamil Ready To Use. (Mead Johnson Nutritionals) Ready-to-use *Enfamil* infant formula 20 kcal/fl oz. Can 8 fl oz, 6-can pack; 32 fl oz, 6 cans per case. *OTC.*
Use: Nutritional supplement.

Enfamil with Iron. (Mead Johnson Nutritionals) Iron 12 mg. Qt. Pkg. Con. Liq. 13 fl oz. 24s. Pow. 1 lb. 6s. *OTC.*
Use: Nutritional supplement.

Enfamil with Iron Ready to Use. (Mead Johnson Nutritionals) Ready-to-use infant formula 20 kcal/fl oz. Can 8 fl oz, 6-can pack; 32 fl oz, 6 cans per case. *OTC.*
Use: Nutritional supplement.

•**enflurane.** (EN-flew-rane) *USP.*
Use: Anesthetic, inhalation.
See: Compound 347.
Ethrane.

enflurane. (Abbott) Enflurane 125 mL and 250 mL/Inhalation. *Rx.*
Use: Anesthetic, inhalation.

•**enfuvirtide.** (en-FYOO-veer-tide) USAN.
Use: Antiretroviral.
See: Fuzeon.

Engerix-B. (GlaxoSmithKline) Hepatitis B surface antigen 20 mcg/mL, thimerosal (mercury < 1 mcg), preservative free. Inj. Single-dose vial, prefilled syringe. *Rx.*
Use: Active immunization, viral vaccine.

•**englitazone sodium.** (EN-GLIH-tah-zone) USAN.
Use: Antidiabetic.

Enhancer. (Mallinckrodt) Barium sulfate 98%. Simethicone, sorbitol, sucrose, lemon-vanilla flavor. Susp. UD 312 g. *Rx.*
Use: Radiopaque agent, GI contrast agent.

•**enilconazole.** (EE-nill-KOE-nah-zole) USAN.
Use: Antifungal.

•**eniluracil.** (en-ill-YOUR-ah-sill) USAN.
Use: Potentiator of antineoplastic activity of fluorouracil (uracil reductase inhibitor); antineoplastic (adjunct).

•**enisoprost.** (en-EYE-so-prahst) USAN.
Use: Antiulcerative.

Enisyl. (Person and Covey) L-Lysine monohydrochloride 334 mg, 500 mg. Tab. Bot. 100s, 250s. *OTC.*
Use: Nutritional supplement.

Enjuvia. (Barr/Duramed) Synthetic conjugated estrogens, B, 0.3 mg, 0.45 mg, 0.625 mg, 1.25 mg. EDTA, PEG, lactose. Film-coated. Tab. 100s. *Rx.*
Use: Sex hormone, estrogen.

•**enlimomab.** (en-LIE-moe-mab) USAN.
Use: Anti-inflammatory; monoclonal antibody.

Enlive!. (Abbott) Protein (whey protein isolate) 10 g, carbohydrates (maltodextrin, sucrose) 65 g, fat 0 g, Na 65 mg, K 40 mg/L. H_2O 840 mOsm/kg, 1.25 cal/mL. Vitamin A, B_1, B_2, B_3, B_5, B_6, B_{12}, C, D, E, K, biotin, chlorine, Ca, Cl, Cu, Cr, Fe, I, Mg, Mo, P, Se, Zn. Gluten-free. Apple and peach flavors. Liq. 240 mL. *OTC.*
Use: Enteral nutrition therapy.

•**enloplatin.** (en-LOW-PLAT-in) USAN.
Use: Antineoplastic.

Ennds. (Oakhurst) Sodium copper chlorophyllin 10 mg. Lactose, peppermint flavoring, saccharin, sugar. Tab. 100s. *OTC.*
Use: Gastrointestinal agent, systemic deodorizer.

Ennex Ointment. (Ennex) Aloe vera extract 37.5%. **Skin Oint.:** Zinc oxide

12.5%, coal tar 1.5%, alcohol 4.5%. Tube oz. **Hemorrhoidal Oint.:** Tube oz. *OTC.*
Use: Anti-inflammatory; astringent; antipruritic.

•**enobosarm.** (EN-oh-BOE-sarm) USAN.
Use: Nonsteroidal androgen receptor agonist.

•**enofelast.** (EE-no-fell-ast) USAN.
Use: Antiasthmatic.

•**enokizumab.** (EN-oh-KIZ-oo-mab) USAN.
Use: Asthma.

•**enolicam sodium.** (ee-NO-lih-kam) USAN.
Use: Anti-inflammatory; antirheumatic.

Enovid-E 21. (Pharmacia) Norethynodrel 2.5 mg, mestranol 0.1 mg. Tab. Compack disp. 21s, 6 × 21. Refill 21s, 12 × 21. *Rx.*
Use: Estrogen, progestin combination.

Enovil. (Roberts) Amtriptyline hydrochloride 10 mg/mL. Vial 10 mL. *Rx.*
Use: Antidepressant.

•**enoxacin.** (en-OX-ah-SIN) USAN.
Use: Anti-infective.

•**enoxaparin sodium.** (ee-NOX-ah-PAR-in) USAN.
Use: Anticoagulant.
See: Lovenox.

enoxaparin sodium. (Sandoz) Enoxaparin sodium 30 mg per 0.3 mL, 40 mg per 0.4 mL, 60 mg per 0.6 mL, 80 mg per 0.8 mL, 100 mg/mL, 120 mg per 0.8 mL, 150 mg/mL. Preservative free. Inj., Soln. Single-dose prefilled syringe with 27-gauge × ½-inch needle. *Rx.*
Use: Anticoagulant, low molecular weight heparin.

enoxaparin sodium. (Sanofi-Aventis) Enoxaparin sodium 300 mg per 3 mL. Benzyl alcohol 15 mg/mL. Inj., Soln. Multidose vial. 3 mL. *Rx.*
Use: Anticoagulant, low molecular weight heparin.

•**enoximone.** (EN-ox-ih-MONE) USAN.
Use: Cardiovascular agent.

•**enpiroline phosphate.** (en-PIHR-oh-LEEN) USAN.
Use: Antimalarial.

Enpresse. (Barr) **Phase 1:** Levonorgestrel 0.05 mg, ethinyl estradiol 30 mcg. 6 tab. **Phase 2:** Levonorgestrel 0.075 mg, ethinyl estradiol 40 mcg. 5 tab. **Phase 3:** Levonorgestrel 0.125 mg, ethinyl estradiol 30 mcg. 10 tab. Lactose. Box. 28s with 7 inert tabs. *Rx.*
Use: Sex hormone, contraceptive hormone.

•**enprofylline.** (en-PRO-fih-lin) USAN.
Use: Bronchodilator.

•**enpromate.** (EN-pro-mate) USAN.
Use: Antineoplastic.

•**enprostil.** (en-PRAHS-till) USAN.
Use: Antisecretory; antiulcerative.

Enrich. (Ross) Liquid food with fiber providing complete, balanced nutrition as a full liquid diet, liquid supplement, or tube feeding. One serving provides 5 g dietary fiber. 1100 calories/L. 1530 calories provides 100% US RDA for vitamins and minerals. Ready-to-Use: Can 8 fl oz (vanilla, chocolate). *OTC.*
Use: Nutritional supplement, enteral.

Ensidon. (Novartis) Opipramol hydrochloride. *Rx.*
Use: Antidepressant.

•**ensituximab.** (EN-si-TUX-i-mab) USAN.
Use: Antineoplastic.

•**ensulizole.** (en-SUL-i-zole) *USP.* Formerly phenylbenzimidazole sulfonic acid.
Use: Sunscreen.

Ensure. (Ross) Liquid food providing 1.06 calories/mL. Can be used as a full liquid diet, liquid supplement or tube feeding. Two quarts (2000 calories) provides 100% US RDA for vitamins and minerals for adults and children over 4 yrs. **Ready-to-Use:** Bot. 8 fl oz (vanilla). Can 8 fl oz (chocolate, black walnut, coffee, strawberry, eggnog, vanilla), 32 fl oz (vanilla, chocolate). **Pow.:** Can 14 oz (400 g) (vanilla). *OTC.*
Use: Nutritional supplement.

Ensure High Protein. (Ross) Protein 50.4 g, carbohydrate 129.4 g, fat 25.2 g, < 21 mg cholesterol, Na 1218 mg, K 2100 mg, vitamin A 5250 units, D 420 units, E 47.5 units, K 84 mcg, C 125 mg, folic acid 420 mg, B_1 1.6 mg, B_2 1.8 mg, B_3 21 mg, B_5 10.5 mg, B_6 2.1 mg, B_{12} 6.3 mcg, biotin 315 mcg, Ca 1050 mg, Cl, P, Mg, I, Mn, Cu, Zn 24 mg, Fe 19 mg, Se, Cr, Mo, 945 calories per 237 mL. Liq. Bot. 237 mL. *OTC.*
Use: Nutritional supplement.

Ensure HN. (Ross) High nitrogen low residue liquid food providing complete, balanced nutrition as tube feeding or oral supplement with 1.06 calories/mL. Provides 100% US RDA for vitamins and minerals for adults and children over 4 yrs. 1400 calories (1321 mL). Ready-to-Use: Can 8 fl oz (vanilla). *OTC.*
Use: Nutritional supplement.

Ensure Osmolite. (Ross)
See: Osmolite.

Ensure Plus. (Ross) High-calorie liquid food w/caloric density of 1500 calories/L. Six servings (8 oz and 2130 calories each) provides 100% US RDA for vitamins and minerals for adults and children. Ready-to-Use: Bot. 8 fl oz (vanilla). Can 8 fl oz (chocolate, vanilla, eggnog, coffee, strawberry). *OTC.*
Use: Nutritional supplement.

Ensure Plus HN. (Ross) High-calorie, high-nitrogen liquid food providing 1.5 calories/mL; 1420 calories provides 100% US RDA for vitamins and minerals for adults and children. Calorie/nitrogen ratio is 150:1. Can 8 fl oz (vanilla). *OTC.*
Use: Nutritional supplement.

Ensure Pudding. (Ross) Protein 6.8 g (nonfat milk), carbohydrate 34 g (sucrose, modified food starch), fat 9.7 g (partially hydrogenated soybean oil), vitamin A 850 units, D 68 units, E 7.7 units, K 12 mcg, C 15.4 mg, folic acid 68 mcg, B_1 0.25 mg, B_2 0.29 mg, B_3 3.4 mg, B_5 1.7 mg, B_6 0.34 mg, B_{12} 1.1 mcg, choline, biotin, Na 240 mg, K 330 mg, Cl 220 mg, Ca 200 mg, P, Mg, I, Mn, Cu, Zn 3.83 mg, Fe 3.06 mg, 250 calories/Can. Pudding. 150 g. *OTC.*
Use: Nutritional supplement.

Entab 650. (Merz) Aspirin 650 mg. EC tab. Bot. 100s. *OTC.*
Use: Analgesic.

•**entacapone.** (en-TACK-ah-pone) USAN.
Use: Antidyskinetic; antiparkinsonian.
See: Comtan.
W/Carbidopa and Levodopa.
See: Stalevo 50.
Stalevo 100.
Stalevo 150.
Stalevo 125.
Stalevo 75.
Stalevo 200.

entacapone. (Wockhardt USA) Entacapone 200 mg. Glycerol, mannitol, sucrose, vegetable oil. Tab. 100s, 500s. *Rx.*
Use: Antiparkinson agent.

•**entecavir.** (en-TE-ka-vihr) USAN.
Use: Antiviral.
See: Baraclude.

Entereg. (Cubist Pharmaceuticals) Alvimopan 12 mg. PEG. Cap. UD 30s. *Rx.*
Use: Gastrointestinal agent.

Enterogenic Concentrate. (Integrative Therapeutics) 150 mg blend of *L. acidophilus, B. bifidum, B. infantis, E. faecium.* Gluten free, preservative free, and sugar free. Cap. 120s. *OTC.*
Use: Probiotic.

Entero-Test. (HDC) Cap. to identify duodenal parasites; to diagnose and locate upper GI bleeding, pH disorders, achlorhydria, and esophageal reflux. Bot. 10s, 25s.
Use: Diagnostic aid.

Entero-Test Pediatric. (HDC) To identify duodenal parasites; to diagnose and locate upper GI bleeding, pH disorders, achlorhydria, and esophageal reflux. Cap. Bot. 10s, 25s.
Use: Diagnostic aid.

Enterotube. (Roche) Culture-identification method for Enterobacteriaceae ACA. Test kit 25s.
Use: Diagnostic aid.

Entero VU. (E-Z-EM) Barium sulfate 13%, 24%. Saccharin, sorbitol. Susp. 600 mL. *Rx.*
Use: GI contrast agent.

Entertainer's Secret. (KLI Corp.) Sodium carboxymethylcellulose, potassium chloride, dibasic sodium phosphate, aloe vera gel, glycerin, parabens. Soln. Bot. 60 mL spray. *OTC.*
Use: Saliva substitute.

Entex ER. (Andrx) Phenylephrine hydrochloride 10 mg, guaifenesin 300 mg. Maltodextrin, sucrose, parabens. ER Cap. 30s, 100s. *Rx.*
Use: Decongestant and expectorant.

Entex LQ. (WraSer) Guaifenesin 100 mg, phenylephrine hydrochloride 10 mg. Benzoic acid, edetate disodium, glycerin, propylene glycol, sorbitol. Alcohol free and sugar free. Strawberry flavor. Liq. 473 mL. *OTC.*
Use: Upper respiratory combination, decongestant and expectorant combination.

Entex PAC. (Wraser) Kit w/*Entex T* tablets and *Entex S* liquid. **Liq.:** Dextromethorphan hydrobromide 20 mg. Benzoic acid, edetate disodium, propylene glycol, saccharin, sorbitol. Strawberry flavor. 118 mL. **Tab.:** Guaifenesin 375 mg, pseudoephedrine hydrochloride 60 mg. 30s. *OTC.*
Use: Upper respiratory combination, antitussive and expectorant combination.

Entex T. (Wraser) Guaifenesin 375 mg, pseudoephedrine hydrochloride 60 mg. Tab. 100s. *OTC.*
Use: Upper respiratory combination, decongestant and expectorant combination.

•**entinostat.** (en-tin-OH-stat) USAN.
Use: Antineoplastic agent.

Entocort EC. (AstraZeneca) Budesonide 3 mg (micronized), sugar spheres. Cap.

Bot. 100s. *Rx.*
Use: Adrenocortical steroid, glucocorticoid.

Entolase HP. (Wyeth) Lipase 8000 units, protease 50,000 units, amylase 40,000 units. Cap. (enteric coated microbeads). Bot. 100s, 250s. *Rx.*
Use: Digestive enzyme.

•**entolimod.** (en-TOL-i-mod) USAN.
Use: Countermeasure for total body irradiation, cancer therapeutic.

Entre-B. (Acella Pharmaceuticals) Brompheniramine maleate 6 mg, phenylephrine hydrochloride 10 mg. Benzoic acid, glycerin, parabens, propylene glycol, saccharin. Bubble gum flavor. Susp. 118 mL. *OTC.*
Use: Upper respiratory combination, decongestant and antihistamine.

Entre-Cough. (Acella Pharmaceuticals) Dextromethorphan hydrobromide 15 mg, guaifenesin 175 mg, pseudoephedrine hydrochloride 30 mg. Acesulfame K, aspartame, glycerin, methylparaben, phenylalanine, sodium benzoate. Cherry flavor. Susp. 473 mL. *OTC.*
Use: Upper respiratory combination, antitussive and expectorant combination.

Entre-Hist PSE. (Acella Pharmaceuticals) Pseudoephedrine hydrochloride 10 mg, triprolidine hydrochloride 0.938 mg. Cotton candy flavoring, glycerin, methylparaben, sucralose, xylitol. Soln., concentrate drops. 30 mL. *OTC.*
Use: Upper respiratory combination, decongestant and antihistamine.

Entrition Half Strength. (Biosearch Medical Products) Calcium and sodium caseinates, maltodextrin, corn oil, soy lecithin, monoglycerides and diglycerides, protein 17.5 g, carbohydrate 68 g, fat 17.5 g, Na 350 mg, K 600 mg, calories 0.5/mL, osmolarity 120 mOsm/kg, water, vitamins A, B_1, B_2, B_3, B_5, B_6, B_{12}, C, D, E, K, Ca, P, Mg, I, Fe, Zn, Mn, Cu, Cl, biotin, choline, folic acid. Pouch 1 liter. *OTC.*
Use: Nutritional supplement.

Entrition HN Entri-Pak. (Biosearch Medical Products) Sodium and calcium caseinates, soy protein isolate, maltodextrin, corn oil, soy lecithin, monoglycerides and diglycerides, vitamins A, B_1, B_2, B_3, B_5, B_6, B_{12}, C, D, E, K, folic acid, biotin, choline, Ca, Cl, Cu, Fe, I, Mg, Mn, P, Zn. Pouch 1 liter. *OTC.*
Use: Nutritional supplement.

Entrobag Set. (Lafayette) Enteroclysis set. Case 6 sets.
Use: Enteroclysis of the small intestine.

Entrobar. (Mallinckrodt) Barium sulfate 50%. Simethicone. Susp. Bot. 500 mL w/ or w/out kit. *Rx.*
Use: Radiopaque agent, GI contrast agent.

Entrokit. (Lafayette) Barium sulfate susp. (*Entrobar*), methylcellulose (*Entrolcel*). Case 4 kits.
Use: Radiopaque agent.

Entrolcel. (Lafayette) Methylcellulose 1.8% w/w concentrate for dilution at time of use. Bot. 500 mL, case 24 Bot.
Use: Diagnostic aid.

Entsol. (Pharmaderm) Sodium chloride. **Gel, intranasal:** Aloe, benzalkonium chloride, disodium EDTA, propylene glycol, glycerin, triethanolamine, vitamin E. Preservative free. 20 g. **Soln., intranasal:** Spray. 29.6 mL. *OTC.*
Use: Nasal decongestant.

•**entsufon sodium.** (ENT-sue-fahn) USAN.
Use: Detergent.

Entuss-D Junior. (Roberts) Pseudoephedrine hydrochloride 30 mg, hydrocodone bitartrate 2.5 mg, guaifenesin 100 mg w/alcohol 5%, saccharin, sorbitol, sucrose. Liq. Bot. 120 mL, pt. *c-III.*
Use: Antitussive, expectorant combination.

Entuss-D Liquid. (Roberts) Hydrocodone bitartrate 5 mg, pseudoephedrine 30 mg/5 mL. 473 mL. *c-III.*
Use: Antitussive, decongestant.

Entuss-D Tablets. (Roberts) Pseudoephedrine 30 mg, hydrocodone bitartrate 5 mg, guaifenesin 300 mg. Tab. Bot. 100s. *c-III.*
Use: Antitussive, decongestant, expectorant.

Enuclene. (Alcon) Tyloxapol 0.25%. Soln. *Drop-tainer* 15 mL. *OTC.*
Use: Artificial eye care.

Enulose. (Alra) Lactulose 10 g, (galactose < 1.6 g, lactose < 1.2 g, other sugars ≤ 1.2 g). Soln. Bot. 473 mL, 1.89 L. *Rx.*
Use: Laxative.

•**enviradene.** (en-VIE-rah-DEEN) USAN.
Use: Antiviral.

Enviro-Stress. (Vitaline) Vitamins B_1 50 mg, B_2 50 mg, B_3 100 mg, B_5 50 mg, B_6 50 mg, B_{12} 25 mcg, C 600 mg, E 30 units, folic acid 0.4 mg, zinc 30 mg, Mg, Se, PABA. SR Tab. Bot. 90s, 1000s. *OTC.*
Use: Mineral, vitamin supplement.

•**enviroxime.** (en-VIE-rox-eem) USAN.
Use: Antiviral.

Envisan Treatment Multipack. (Hoechst) Dextranomer with PEG 3000 and PEG

600. Paste 10 g packets with nylon net and semi-occlusive film. *OTC.*
Use: Dermatologic, wound therapy.

•**enzacamene.** (en-za-KAM-een) USAN.
Use: Sunscreen.

•**enzalutamide.** (EN-za-LOO-ta-mide) USAN.
Use: Antineoplastic.
See: Xtandi.

•**enzastaurin hydrochloride.** (en-za-STORE-in) USAN.
Use: Antineoplastic.

Enzest. (Barth's) Seven natural enzymes, calcium carbonate 250 mg. Tab. Bot. 100s, 250s, 500s. *OTC.*
Use: Digestive enzymes; antacid.

Enzobile Improved. (Roberts) Pancreatic enzyme concentrate 100 mg, ox bile extract 100 mg, cellulase 10 mg in inner core and pepsin 150 mg in outer layer. EC Tab. Bot. 100s. *Rx-OTC.*
Use: Digestive enzymes.

Enzone. (Forest) Hydrocortisone acetate 1%, pramoxine hydrochloride 1% in hydrophilic base w/stearic acid, aquaphor, isopropyl palmitate, polyoxyl 40, stearate, triethanolamine lauryl sulfate. Cream. Tube 30 g w/rectal applicator. *Rx.*
Use: Corticosteroid combination.

enzyme combinations, injectable.
Use: Collagenase Clostridium Histolyticum.

enzyme combinations, topical.
See: Accuzyme.
Ethezyme.
Ethezyme 830.
Gladase.
GranulDerm.
Granulex.
Panafil.
Papain.
Papain-Urea-Chlorophyllin.

Enzyme Formula #E-2. (Barth's) Amylase 30 mg, lipase 25 mg, bile salts 1 g, wilzyme 10 mg, pepsin 2 g, pancreatin 0.5 g, calcium carbonate 4 g. Tab. Bot. 100s, 250s. *Rx-OTC.*
Use: Digestive aid.

enzyme preparations.
See: Collagenase.
Enzyme Combinations, Injectable.
Enzyme Combinations, Topical.

enzymes.
See: Asparaginase.
Coenzyme Q10.
Lactase.
Pegaspargase.

enzymes, digestive.
See: Pancreatin.

E-Oil. (Nature's Bounty) Vitamin E 100 units per 0.25 mL. Corn oil, lemon oil, sesame oil, soybean oil, wheat germ oil. Oil, Top. 74 mL. *OTC.*
Use: Emollient.

E-Oil. (Nature's Bounty) Vitamin E 100 units (as d-alpha tocopheryl acetate) per 0.25 mL. Corn oil, lemon oil, sesame oil, soybean oil, wheat germ oil. Soln., Conc. 74 mL. *OTC.*
Use: Fat-soluble vitamin.

EPA. (NBTY) N-3 fat content (mg) EPA 180 mg, DHA 120 mg, vitamin E 1 units. Cap. Bot. 50s, 100s. *OTC.*
Use: Nutritional supplement.

Epaned. (Silvergate) Enalapril maleate 1 mg/mL (after reconstitution). Glycerin, mannitol, parabens, saccharin, sorbitol. Pow. for Soln. 150 mL w/diluent. *Rx.*
Use: Renin angiotensin system antagonist, angiotensin-converting enzyme inhibitor.

•**epelsiban.** (e-PEL-si-ban) USAN.
Use: Oxytocin antagonist for treatment of premature ejaculation.

•**epelsiban besylate.** (e-PEL-si-ban) USAN.
Use: Oxytocin antagonist for treatment of premature ejaculation.

•**eperezolid.** (eh-per-EH-zoe-lid) USAN.
Use: Anti-infective.

•**epetirimod.** (E-pe-TIR-i-mod) USAN.
Use: Antiviral; antineoplastic.

•**epetirimod esylate.** (E-pe-TIR-i-mod ES-i-late) USAN.
Use: Antiviral, antineoplastic.

•**ephedrine.** (eh-FED-rin) *USP.*
Tall Man: ePHEDrine
Use: Adrenergic (bronchodilator); vasopressor.

•**ephedrine hydrochloride.** (eh-FED-rin) *USP.*
Tall Man: ePHEDrine
Use: Bronchodilator.
W/Guaifenesin.
See: Broncholate.
Primatene.

ephedrine hydrochloride. (Various Mfr.) Ephedrine hydrochloride. Cryst. Box 0.25 oz, 4 oz.
Use: Bronchodilator.

ephedrine hydrochloride nasal jelly.
See: Efedron Nasal.

•**ephedrine sulfate.** (eh-FED-rin) *USP.*
Tall Man: ePHEDrine
Use: Bronchodilator, sympathomimetic; vasopressor.
See: Pretz-D.
W/Guaifenesin.
See: Bronkaid Dual Action.

W/Zinc Oxide.
See: Pazo Hemorrhoid.
ephedrine sulfate. (Hospira) Ephedrine sulfate 50 mg/mL. Preservative free. Inj. Single-dose amps. 1 mL. *Rx.*
Use: Vasopressor.
ephedrine sulfate. (West-Ward) Ephedrine sulfate 25 mg. Cap. Bot. 100s. *OTC.*
Use: Bronchodilator, sympathomimetic; vasopressor.
ephedrine sulfate. (Various Mfr.) Ephedrine sulfate 50 mg/mL. Inj. Single-dose vials. *Rx.*
Use: Bronchodilator, sympathomimetic.
ephedrine sulfate and phenobarbital.
Use: Bronchodilator; hypnotic; sedative.
Ephenyllin. (CMC) Theophylline 130 mg, ephedrine hydrochloride 24 mg, phenobarbital 8 mg. Tab. Bot. 100s, 500s, 1000s. *Rx.*
Use: Bronchodilator; decongestant; hypnotic; sedative.
Epi-C. (Mallinckrodt) Barium sulfate 150%. Simethicone, spearmint flavor. Susp. Bot. 450 mL. *Rx.*
Use: Radiopaque agent, GI contrast agent.
•**epicillin.** (EH-pih-SILL-in) USAN.
Use: Anti-infective.
EpiCream. (PuraCap) Disodium EDTA, glycerin, glyceryl stearate, hydroxypropyl bispalmitamide MEA (ceramide), PEG-100, petrolatum. Emulsion, Top. 90 g. *Rx.*
Use: Topical combination, miscellaneous.
epidermal growth factor (human). (Chiron Therapeutics)
Use: Accelerate corneal healing. [Orphan Drug]
epidermal growth factor receptor inhibitors.
See: Erlotinib.
Epi-Derm Balm. (Pedinol Pharmacal) Methyl salicylate, menthol, propylene glycol, alcohol. Bot. Gal. *OTC.*
Use: Analgesic, topical.
Epidrin. (Excellium) Acetaminophen 325 mg, dichloralphenazone 100 mg, isometheptene mucate 65 mg. Cap. 100s, 250s. *c-iv.*
Use: Agent for migraine, migraine combination.
Epiduo. (Galderma) Adapalene 0.1%, benzoyl peroxide 2.5%. Edetate disodium, glycerin. Gel. 45 g. *Rx.*
Use: Acne product, combination.
Epifoam. (Meda Pharmaceuticals) Hydrocortisone acetate 1%, pramoxine hydrochloride 1% in base of propylene glycol, cetyl alcohol, PEG-100 stearate, glyceryl stearate, laureth-23, polyoxyl 40 stearate, methylparaben, propylparaben, trolamine, or hydrochloric acid to adjust pH, purified water, butane, propane inert propellant. Aerosol container 10 g. *Rx.*
Use: Corticosteroid, topical.
Epiform-HC. (Delta Pharmaceutical Group) Hydrocortisone 1%, iodohydroxyquin 3% in cream base. Tube 20 g. *Rx.*
Use: Antifungal; corticosteroid, topical.
Epilyt. (GlaxoSmithKline) Propylene glycol, glycerin, oleic acid, quaternium-26, lactic acid, BHT. Lotion. Bot. 118 mL. *OTC.*
Use: Emollient.
•**epimestrol.** (EH-pih-MESS-trole) USAN.
Use: Anterior pituitary activator.
epinastine. (Cypress) Epinastine 0.05%. Benzalkonium chloride 0.01%, edetate disodium. Soln., Ophth. 5 mL. *Rx.*
Use: Ophthalmic antihistamine.
•**epinastine hydrochloride.** (epp-ih-NAS-teen) USAN.
Use: Ophthalmic antihistamine.
See: Elestat.
epinephran.
See: Epinephrine.
•**epinephrine.** (epp-ih-NEFF-rin) *USP.*
Tall Man: EPINEPHrine
Use: Bronchodilator, sympathomimetic, vasopressor.
See: Adrenaclick.
Adrenalin Chloride
AsthmaNefrin.
EpiPen.
EpiPen Jr.
Nephron.
Racepinephrine Hydrochloride.
S2.
W/Lidocaine hydrochloride.
See: Ardecaine 1 w/epinephrine.
Ardecaine 2 w/epinephrine.
Lidocaine and Epinephrine.
Lidocaine Hydrochloride.
Lidocaine Hydrochloride and Epinephrine.
Lidosite Topical System.
Octocaine.
Xylocaine MPF.
Xylocaine w/epinephrine.
epinephrine. (Adamis Labs) Epinephrine 1:1,000 (0.3 mg per 0.3 mL) May contain sodium metabisulfite. Inj., Soln. Prefilled single-dose syringe. *Rx.*
Use: Vasopressor used in shock.
epinephrine. (Greenstone) Epinephrine 1:1,000 (0.15 mg per 0.15 mL). May

contain chlorobutanol, sodium bisulfite. Inj., Soln. Single-dose injector. *Rx.*
Use: Vasopressor used in shock.

epinephrine. (Various Mfr.) Epinephrine 1:1000 (1 mg/mL as hydrochloride), 1:10,000 (0.1 mg/mL as hydrochloride). Soln. Inj. Amp. 1 mL (1:1000 only) (may contain sulfites). Prefilled syringe and vial. 10 mL (1:10,000 only) vial. 30 mL (1:1,000). *Rx.*
Use: Bronchodilator, sympathomimetic; vasopressor.

•**epinephrine bitartrate.** (epp-ih-NEFF-rin) *USP.*
Tall Man: EPINEPHrine
Use: Adrenergic, ophthalmic.
See: Primatene Mist.

epinephrine borate.
Use: Adrenergic, ophthalmic.
See: Epinal.

epinephrine hydrochloride.
See: Adrenalin Cl.
EpiPen.
EpiPen Jr.
Vaponefrin.

epinephrine hydrochloride. (Ciba Vision) Epinephrine hydrochloride 0.1%. Soln. 1 mL Dropperettes (12s). *Rx.*
Use: Adrenergic, ophthalmic. Emergency kit, anaphylaxis.

epinephrine, racemic.
See: AsthmaNefrin.

epinephrine-related compounds.
See: Sympathomimetic agents.

•**epinephryl borate ophthalmic solution.** (EPP-ih-NEFF-rill) *USP.*
Use: Adrenergic.

EpiPen. (Dey) Epinephrine 1:1,000 (0.3 mg per 0.3 mL). Latex free. Sodium metabisulfite Inj., Soln. Single-dose auto-injector. 0.3 mL (contains a total of epinephrine 2 mL). *Rx.*
Use: Emergency kit; vasopressor.

EpiPen Jr. (Dey) Epinephrine 1:2,000 (0.15 mg per 0.3 mL). Sodium metabisulfite. Latex free. Inj., Soln. Single-dose autoinjector. 0.3 mL (contains a total of 2 mL of epinephrine injection solution). *Rx.*
Use: Emergency kit; vasopressor.

epipodophyllotoxins.
See: Podophyllotoxin Derivatives.

•**epipropidine.** (EPP-ih-PRO-pih-deen) USAN.
Use: Antineoplastic.

EpiQuin Micro. (SkinMedica) Hydroquinone 4%, vitamin A, E, and C, cetyl alcohol, benzyl alcohol, EDTA, glycerin, methylparaben, sodium metabisulfite. Cream. 30 g. *Rx.*
Use: Dermatologic, pigment agent.

epirenan.
See: Epinephrine.

•**epirizole.** (eh-PEER-IH-zole) USAN.
Use: Analgesic; anti-inflammatory.

•**epirubicin hydrochloride.** (EH-pih-ROO-bih-sin) USAN.
Use: Antineoplastic; antibiotic; anthracycline.
See: Ellence.

epirubicin hydrochloride. (Bedford) Epirubicin hydrochloride 2 mg/mL. Preservative free. Inj. Soln. Single-use vials. 25 mL, 100 mL. *Rx.*
Use: Antibiotic, anthracycline.

epirubicin hydrochloride. (Mayne) Epirubicin hydrochloride 50 mg, 200 mg. Lactose. Inj., Lyophilized, Pow. for Soln. Single-use vials. *Rx.*
Use: Antibiotic; anthracycline.

Episil. (Cangene bioPharma) Glycerol, soy lecithin, ethanol, propylene glycol, polysorbate 80, peppermint oil. Liq. 10 mL w/metering pump (65 applications). *Rx.*
Use: Mouth and throat product.

•**epitetracycline hydrochloride.** (epp-ih-TEH-trah-SIGH-kleen HIGH-droe-KLOR-ide) *USP.*
Use: Anti-infective.

•**epithiazide.** (EH-pih-THIGH-azz-ide) USAN.
Use: Antihypertensive; diuretic.

Epitol. (Teva) Carbamazepine 200 mg. Lactose. Tab. 100s, 3,000s. *Rx.*
Use: Anticonvulsant.

Epivir. (GlaxoSmithKline) Lamivudine. **Tab.:** 150 mg, 300 mg. PEG. Film-coated. Bot. 30s (300 mg only), 60s (150 mg only). **Oral Soln.:** 10 mg/mL. Parabens, sucrose 200 mg/mL, strawberry-banana flavor. Bot. 240 mL. *Rx.*
Use: Antiretroviral agent, nucleoside reverse transcriptase inhibitor.

Epivir-HBV. (GlaxoSmithKline) Lamivudine. **Tab.:** 100 mg. Film-coated. Bot. 60s. **Oral Soln.:** 5 mg/mL. Parabens, sucrose 200 mg/mL, parabens, strawberry-banana flavor. Bot. 240 mL. *Rx.*
Use: Antiretroviral agent, nucleoside reverse transcriptase inhibitor.

•**eplerenone.** (eh-PLER-en-ohn) USAN.
Use: Antihypertensive, aldosterone antagonist, renin angiotensin system antagonist.
See: Inspra.

eplerenone. (Apotex) Eplerenone 25 mg, 50 mg. Film coated. Tab. 30s, 90s, 500s (25 mg only), 1,000s, blister 100s. *Rx.*
Use: Renin angiotensin system antago-

nist, selective aldosterone receptor antagonist.

•**eplivanserin.** (EP-li-VAN-ser-in) USAN.
Use: Treatment of insomnia.

•**eplivanserin fumarate.** (EP-li-VAN-ser-in) USAN.
Use: Treatment of insomnia.

EPO.
See: Epogen.
Procrit.

•**epoetin alfa, recombinant.** (eh-POE-eh-tin) USAN.
Use: Antianemic; hematinic; hematopoietic.
See: Epogen.
Procrit.

•**epoetin beta.** (eh-POE-eh-tin) USAN.
Use: Hematopoietic; hematinic; antianemic. [Orphan Drug]

•**epoetin delta.** (eh-POE-eh-tin) USAN.
Use: Antianemic.

Epogen. (Amgen) Epoetin alfa (Erythropoietin; EPO) 2,000 units/mL, 3,000 units/mL, 4,000 units/mL, 10,000 units/mL, 20,000 units/mL. Preservative free w/2.5 mg albumin (human) per mL. Single-dose vials. 1 mL (except 20,000 units/mL). Multidose vials. 1 mL (20,000 units/mL only), 2 mL (10,000 units/mL only) (benzyl alcohol 1%). *Rx.*
Use: Hematopoietic.

•**epoprostenol.** (EH-poe-PROSTE-eh-nole) USAN. *Formerly Prostacyclin, PGI_2, Prostaglandin I_2, Prostaglandin X, PGX.*
Use: Peripheral vasodilator.

•**epoprostenol sodium.** (EH-poe-PROSTE-eh-nole) USAN.
Use: Peripheral vasodilator.
See: Flolan.
Veletri.

epoprostenol sodium. (Teva Parenteral Medicines) Epoprostenol sodium 0.5 mg, 1.5 mg. Sodium chloride. Inj., Pow. for Soln. Vials. 10 mL. *Rx.*
Use: Vasodilator, peripheral.

•**epostane.** (EH-poe-stain) USAN.
Use: Interceptive.

epothilones.
Use: Antimitotic agents.
See: Ixabepilone.

epoxytropine tropate methylbromide.
See: Methscopolamine Bromide.

•**epristeride.** (eh-PRISS-the-ride) USAN.
Use: Inhibitor (alpha reductase).

eprodisate.
Use: Investigational amyloid fibrinogenesis inhibitor.

Epromate. (Major) Aspirin 325 mg, meprobamate 200 mg Tab. Bot. 100s, 500s. *c-IV.*
Use: Analgesic; anxiolytic.

•**eprosartan.** (eh-pro-SAHR-tan) USAN.
Use: Antihypertensive.

eprosartan. (Mylan) Eprosartan mesylate 400 mg, 600 mg. Film coated. Lactose, PEG. Tab. 30s (600 mg only), 60s (400 mg only), 90s (600 mg only), 120s (400 mg only), 500s. *Rx.*
Use: Renin angiotensin system antagonist, angiotensin II receptor antagonist.

eprosartan and hydrochlorothiazide.
Use: Antihypertensive.
See: Teveten HCT.

•**eprosartan mesylate.** (eh-pro-SAHR-tan) USAN.
Use: Antihypertensive.
See: Teveten.

•**eprosidate disodium.** (e-PROE-di-sate) USAN.
Use: Amyloidosis.

Epsal. (Press Chem. & Pharm Labs) Saturated soln. of Epsom salts 80% in ointment form. Jar 0.5 oz, 2 oz. *OTC.*
Use: Drawing ointment.

Epsivite Forte. (Standex) Vitamin E 1000 units. Cap. Bot. 100s. *OTC.*
Use: Vitamin supplement.

Epsivite 400. (Standex) Vitamin E 400 units. Cap. Bot. 100s. *OTC.*
Use: Vitamin supplement.

Epsivite 100. (Standex) Vitamin E 100 units. Cap. Bot. 100s. *OTC.*
Use: Vitamin supplement.

Epsivite 200. (Standex) Vitamin E 200 units. Cap. Bot. 100s. *OTC.*
Use: Vitamin supplement.

Epsom salt. (Various Mfr.) Magnesium sulfate. Gran. Bot. 120 g, 1 lb., 4 lb. *OTC.*
Use: Laxative.
See: Magnesium Sulfate.

eptifibatide.
Use: Antiplatelet agent, glycoprotein IIb/IIIa inhibitor.
See: Integrilin.

eptoin.
See: Phenytoin Sodium.

e.p.t. Stick Test. (Parke-Davis) Reagent in-home kit for urine testing. Pregnancy test. Kit 1s. *OTC.*
Use: Diagnostic aid.

Epulor. (VistaPharm) **Liq.:** Fat 31 g, carbohydrate 5 g, protein 4 g, calories 315/serving, biotin 100 mcg, B 50 mcg, Ca 333 mg, chloride 12 mg, Cr 40 mcg, Cu 200 mcg, folic acid 133 mcg, I 50 mcg, Fe 6 mg, Mg 133 mg, Mn 667 mcg, Mo

25 mcg, P 333 mg, K 35 mg, Se 23 mcg, Si 667 mcg, Na 7 mg, Sn 3 mcg, V 3 mcg, vitamin A 1667 units, B_1 500 mcg, B_2 567 mcg, B_3 7 mg, B_5 3 mg, B_6 667 mcg, B_{12} 2 mcg, Ni 2 mcg, C 20 mg, D 133 units, E 58 units, K 8 mcg, Zn 5 mg. Pkg. 24s. **Pow.:** Protein (milk protein, isoleucine, leucine, lysine, methionine/cystine, phenylalanine/tyrosine, threonine, trytophan, valine) 89 g, fat (soybean oil) 755 g/L, vitamin A, B_1, B_2, B_3, B_5, B_6, B_{12}, C, D, E, K, biotin, folate, B, Ca, chloride, Cr, Cu, Fe, I, Mg, Mn, Mo, Ni, P, Se, Si, Sn, V, Zn, lemon flavor, 7.1 cal/mL. Pouch. 1.5 oz. *OTC.*
Use: Nutritional therapy, enteral.

Epzicom. (GlaxoSmithKline) Abacavir (as sulfate) 600 mg/lamivudine 300 mg. Film-coated. Tab. 30s. *Rx.*
Use: Antiretroviral, nucleoside analog reverse transcriptase inhibitor combination.

Equagesic. (Leitner) Aspirin 325 mg, meprobamate 200 mg. Tab. 100s. *c-IV.*
Use: Nonnarcotic analgesic.

Equal. (Nutrasweet) Aspartame. **Packet:** 0.035 oz. (1 g). Box 50s, 100s, 200s. **Tab.:** Bot. 100s. *OTC.*
Use: Artificial sweetener.

Equalactin. (Numark) Calcium polycarbophil 625 mg (equivalent to 500 mg polycarbophil), citrus acid flavor. Chew. Tab. Bot. 24s, 48s. *OTC.*
Use: Antidiarrheal; laxative.

Equazine M. (Rugby) Aspirin 325 mg, meprobamate 200 mg, tartrazine. Tab. Bot. 100s, 500s. *c-IV.*
Use: Analgesic; anxiolytic.

Equetro. (Shire) Carbamazepine 100 mg, 200 mg, 300 mg. Lactose, PEG. ER Cap. 120s. *Rx.*
Use: Anticonvulsant.

Equilet. (Mission) Calcium carbonate 500 mg (elemental calcium 200 mg). Sodium up to 35 mg. Chew. Tab. 150s. *OTC.*
Use: Mineral supplement.

•**equilin.** (EK-wi-lin) *USP.*
Use: Estrogen.

Equipertine. (Sanofi-Synthelabo) Oxypertine. Cap. *Rx.*
Use: Anxiolytic.

Eradacil. (Sanofi-Synthelabo) Rosoxacin. Cap. *Rx.*
Use: Antigonococcal agent.

Eramycin. (Wesley) Erythromycin FC Tab. Bot. 100s, 500s. *Rx.*
Use: Anti-infective; erythromycin.

•**eravacycline.** (ER-a-va-SYE-kleen) USAN.
Use: Antibiotic.

•**eravacycline dihydrochloride.** (ER-a-va-SYE-kleen) USAN.
Use: Antibiotic.

Eraxis. (Roerig) Anidulafungin 50 mg, 100 mg. Preservative free. Pow. for Inj., lyophilized. Single-use vial with diluent. *Rx.*
Use: Antifungal agent.

Erbitux. (Bristol-Myers Squibb) Cetuximab 2 mg/mL. Preservative-free. Sodium chloride 8.48 mg/mL, sodium phosphate dibasic heptahydrate 1.88 mg/mL, sodium phosphate monobasic monohydrate 0.41 mg/mL. Inj., Soln. Single-use vials. 50 mL, 100 mL. *Rx.*
Use: Monoclonal antibody.

•**erbulozole.** (ehr-BYOO-low-zole) USAN.
Use: Radiosensitizer; antineoplastic (adjunct).

Ergo Caff. (Rugby) Ergotamine tartrate 1 mg, caffeine 100 mg. Tab. Bot. 100s. *Rx.*
Use: Antimigraine.

•**ergocalciferol.** (ehr-go-kal-SIFF-eh-role) *USP. Formerly Oleovitamin D, Synthetic; Calciferol.*
Use: Treatment of refractory rickets; familial hypophosphatemia; hypoparathyroidism, vitamin (antirachitic).
See: Calciferol.
Drisdol.
Ergocalciferol Drops.

ergocalciferol. (Winthrop) Ergocalciferol 50,000 units. Parabens, soybean oil. Cap. 50s. *Rx.*
Use: Fat-soluble vitamin, vitamin D.

Ergocalciferol Drops. (County Line Pharmaceuticals) Ergocalciferol (D_2) 8,000 units/mL. Liq. 60 mL w/dropper in propylene glycol. *OTC.*
Use: Fat-soluble vitamin.

ergocornine. (Various Mfr.) Ergot alkaloid. *Rx.*
Use: Peripheral vascular disorders.

ergocristine. (Various Mfr.) Ergot alkaloid. *Rx.*
Use: Vascular disorders.

ergocryptine. (Various Mfr.) Ergot alkaloid. *Rx.*
Use: Peripheral vascular disorders.

•**ergoloid mesylates.** (err-GO-loyd) *USP. Formerly Dihydroergotoxine Mesylate; Dihydroergotoxine Methanesulfonate; Dihydrogenated Ergot Alkaloids, Hydrogenated Ergot Alkaloids.*
Use: Psychotherapeutic; cognition adjuvant.
See: Hydergine.

Ergomar. (Rosedale Therapeutics) Ergotamine tartrate 2 mg. Saccharin. Peppermint flavor. Sublingual Tab. Pkg. 20s. *Rx.*
Use: Antimigraine.
ergometrine maleate.
See: Ergonovine.
•**ergonovine maleate.** (ehr-go-NO-veen) *USP.*
Use: Oxytocic.
ergosterol, activated, or irradiated.
See: Ergocalciferol.
ergostetrine.
See: Ergonovine.
Ergot Alkalside Dihydrogenated.
See: Ergoloid Mesylates.
ergotamine derivatives.
See: Dihydroergotamine Mesylate.
Ergotamine Tartrate.
•**ergotamine tartrate.** (ehr-GOT-ah-mean) *USP.*
Use: Analgesic (specific in migraine).
See: Ergomar.
W/Bellafoline, Caffeine, Pentobarbital.
See: Cafergot P-B Suppositories.
W/Bellafoline, Caffeine, Pentobarbital Sodium.
See: Cafergot P-B Tablets.
W/Caffeine.
See: Cafergot Tablets.
ergotamine tartrate and caffeine. (West-Ward) Ergotamine tartrate 1 mg, caffeine 100 mg. Sugar. Tab. 30s, 100s, 500s. *Rx.*
Use: Migraine combination.
ergotamine tartrate and caffeine suppositories.
Use: Vascular headache; analgesic (specific in migraine).
See: Cafergot.
ergotamine tartrate and caffeine tablets.
Use: Vascular headache; analgesic (specific in migraine).
ergot, fluid extract. (Various Mfr.) Ergot 1 g/mL Bot. 4 oz, pt.
ergotocine.
See: Ergonovine.
ergot-related products.
See: Cafergot.
Cafergot P-B.
D.H.E. 45.
Ergonovine.
Ergotamine.
Ergotrate.
Hydergine.
Hydro-Ergot.
•**eribaxaban.** (ER-i-BAX-a-ban) USAN.
Use: Thromboembolic disorders.
•**eribulin mesylate.** (er-e-BU-lin) USAN.
Use: Halichondrin B analog.
See: Halaven.
eriodictyon. Flext., aromatic syrup.
Use: Pharmaceutic aid (flavor).
•**erismodegib.** (er-IS-moe-DEG-ib) USAN.
Use: Antineoplastic.
•**eritoran tetrasodium.** (ER-i-TORE-an) USAN.
Use: Endotoxin antagonist.
Erivedge. (Genentech) Vismodegib 150 mg. Lactose. Cap. 28s. *Rx.*
Use: Antineoplastic.
•**erlotinib.** (er-LOE-tye-nib) USAN.
Use: Epidermal growth factor receptor inhibitor.
See: Tarceva.
E•R•O Ear. (Scherer) Carbamide peroxide 6.5%, anhydrous glycerin. Drops. 15 mL. *OTC.*
Use: Otic preparation.
Errin. (Barr) Norethindrone 0.35 mg. Lactose. Tab. Box. 28s. *Rx.*
Use: Sex hormone, contraceptive hormone.
•**ersofermin.** (EER-so-FEER-min) USAN.
Use: Dermatologic, wound therapy.
Ertaczo. (Valeant) Sertaconazole nitrate 2%. Light mineral oil, methylparaben. Cream. Tube. 60 g. *Rx.*
Use: Antifungal agent, topical anti-infective.
•**ertapenem sodium.** (er-ta-PEN-em) USAN.
Use: Antibacterial; carbapenem.
See: Invanz.
•**erteberel.** (er-TEB-er-el) USAN.
Use: Treatment of prostate diseases.
Ertine. (Health for Life Brands) Hexachlorophene, benzocaine, cod liver oil, allantoin, boric acid, lanolin. Tube 1.5 oz. *Rx.*
Use: Burn and first aid remedy.
•**ertiprotafib.** (er-ti-PROE-ta-fib) USAN.
Use: Antidiabetic.
•**ertugliflozin.** (er-TOO-gli-FLOE-zin) USAN.
Use: Antidiabetic agent.
erwina L-asparaginase.
Use: Acute lymphocytic leukemia.
Erwinaze. (EUSA Pharma) Asparaginase 10,000 units. Glucose 5 mg. Derived from *Erwinia chrysanthemi.* Inj., lyophilized Pow. for Soln. Single-dose vial. *Rx.*
Use: Antineoplastic, enzyme.
Eryc. (Warner-Chilcott) Erythromycin 250 mg. Lactose. Contains enteric-coated pellets. Cap., delayed release. 75,000s. *Rx.*
Use: Anti-infective, macrolide.

Erycette. (Ortho-McNeil) Erythromycin 2%. Pkg. 60 pledgets. *Rx.*
Use: Dermatologic, acne.

Eryderm 2%. (Abbott) Erythromycin 2%. Alcohol 77%. Top. Soln. 60 mL with applicator. *Rx.*
Use: Topical anti-infective, antibiotic.

Erygel. (Merz Pharmaceuticals) Erythromycin 2%. Alcohol 92%. Top. Gel. 30 g. *Rx.*
Use: Topical anti-infective, antibiotic.

Erymax. (Allergan) Erythromycin 2%. Soln. 59 mL, 118 mL. *Rx.*
Use: Dermatologic, acne.

Ery Pads. (Perrigo) Erythromycin 2%. Alcohol 60.5%. Pledgets. 60s. *Rx.*
Use: Topical anti-infective, antibiotic.

Erypar. (Parke-Davis) Erythromycin stearate. Filmseal. **250 mg:** Bot. 100s, 500s. **500 mg:** Bot. 100s. *Rx.*
Use: Anti-infective; erythromycin.

EryPed Drops. (Abbott) Erythromycin ethylsuccinate (as base) 100 mg/2.5 mL. Sucrose, fruit flavor. Susp. Bot. 50 mL. *Rx.*
Use: Anti-infective; erythromycin.

EryPed 400. (Abbott) Erythromycin ethylsuccinate (as base) 400 mg/5 mL when reconstituted. Sucrose, banana flavor. Pow. for Oral Susp. 100 mL, 200 mL, UD 5 mL (100s). *Rx.*
Use: Anti-infective; erythromycin.

EryPed 200. (Abbott) Erythromycin ethylsuccinate (as base) 200 mg/5 mL when reconstituted. Sucrose, fruit flavor. Pow. for Oral Susp. 100 mL, 200 mL. *Rx.*
Use: Anti-infective; erythromycin.

Ery-Tab. (Arbor Pharmaceuticals) Erythromycin enteric coated 250 mg, 333 mg, 500 mg. DR Tab. 100s, 500s (except 500 mg). *Rx.*
Use: Anti-infective; erythromycin.

•**erythorbic acid.** (ER-i-THOR-bik) *NF.*
Use: Pharmaceutic aid.

•**erythritol.** (e-RITH-ri-tol) *NF.*
Use: Pharmaceutic aid; sweetening agent.

•**erythrityl tetranitrate, diluted.** (eh-RITH-rih-till TEH-trah-NYE-trate) *USP. Formerly Erythrol Tetranitrate.*
Use: Coronary vasodilator.
See: Cardilate.

erythrityl tetranitrate tablets. (Various Mfr.) Erythritol, erythrol tetranitrate, nitroerythrite, tetranitrin, tetranitrol.
Use: Coronary vasodilator.

Erythrocin. (Arbor Pharmaceuticals) Erythromycin stearate (as base) 250 mg, 500 mg. Film-coated. Tab. Bot. 100s, 500s (250 mg only). *Rx.*
Use: Anti-infective.

Erythrocin Lactobionate. (Hospira) Erythromycin lactobionate (as base) 500 mg, 1 g. May contain benzyl alcohol. Pow. for Inj., lyophilized. Vials. *Rx.*
Use: Anti-infective; erythromycin.

•**erythromycin.** (eh-RITH-row-MY-sin) *USP.*
Use: Anti-infective.
See: Akne-Mycin.
A/T/S.
Del-Mycin.
E-Base.
Emgel.
E-Mycin.
Eryderm 2%.
Erygel.
Erymax.
Ery Pads.
Erythromycin.
Erythromycin Base.
Erythromycin Ethylsuccinate.
Erythromycin Lactobionate.
Erythromycin Stearate.
Ilotycin.
Robimycin.

erythromycin. (Arbor) Erythromycin base 250 mg, 500 mg. Film-coated. Tab. 100s, 500s (250 mg only). *Rx.*
Use: Anti-infective; erythromycin.

erythromycin. (Various Mfr.) Erythromycin base. **DR Cap.:** 250 mg. Enteric-coated pellets. 100s, 500s. **Gel:** 2%. Contains alcohol. 30 g, 60 g. **Oint.:** 0.5%. 3.5 g. **Top. Soln.:** 2%. Contains alcohol. 60 mL. *Rx.*
Use: Anti-infective.

•**erythromycin acistrate.** (eh-RITH-row-MY-sin ass-IH-strate) USAN.
Use: Anti-infective.

erythromycin base.
Use: Anti-infective.
See: Ery-Tab.
PCE Dispertab.

erythromycin-benzoyl peroxide. (Various Mfr.) Erythromycin 3%, benzoyl peroxide 5%. Gel. 23 g, 46 g. *Rx.*
Use: Anti-infective.

•**erythromycin estolate.** (eh-RITh-row-MY-sin ESS-toe-late) *USP. Formerly Erythromycin Propionate Lauryl Sulfate.*
Use: Anti-infective; erythromycin.

•**erythromycin ethylsuccinate.** (eh-RITH-row-MY-sin ETH-il-SUX-i-nate) *USP.*
Use: Anti-infective; erythromycin.
See: E.E.S.
EryPed.

erythromycin ethylsuccinate. (Arbor) Erythromycin ethylsuccinate (as base). **Tab.:** 400 mg. Sugar. 100s, 500s.

Susp.: 200 mg/5 mL, 400 mg/5 mL. Parabens, sucrose. 473 mL. *Rx.*
Use: Anti-infective.

•**erythromycin ethylsuccinate and sulfisoxazole acetyl for oral suspension.** (eh-RITH-row-MY-sin Eth-ill-SUCK-sih-nate and sull-fih-SOX-ah-zole ASS-eh-till) *USP.*
Use: Anti-infective.

erythromycin gel. (Glades) Erythromycin 2%, alcohol 95%. Gel. Tube 30 g, 60 g. *Rx.*
Use: Dermatologic, acne.

•**erythromycin gluceptate, sterile.** (eh-RITH-row-MY-sin glue-SEP-tate) *USP.*
Use: Anti-infective; erythromycin.
See: Ilotycin Gluceptate.

•**erythromycin lactobionate.** (eh-RITH-row-MY-sin lack-toe-BYE-oh-nate) *USP.*
Use: Anti-infective; erythromycin.
See: Erythrocin Lactobionate.

erythromycin ointment. (Various Mfr.) Erythromycin 0.5%. Oint. Tube 3.5 g. *Rx.*
Use: Anti-infective, topical.

•**erythromycin pledgets.** *USP.*
Use: Anti-infective; erythromycin.

Erythromycin Pledgets. (Glades) Erythromycin 2%, alcohol 68.5%. Pledgets. Bot. 60s. *Rx.*
Use: Anti-infective; erythromycin.

•**erythromycin propionate.** (eh-RITH-row-MY-sin) USAN.
Use: Anti-infective.

erythromycin propionate lauryl sulfate.
Use: Anti-infective; erythromycin.
See: Erythromycin Estolate.
Ilosone.

•**erythromycin salnacedin.** (eh-RITH-row-MY-sin sal-NAH-seh-din) USAN.
Use: Dermatologic, acne.

•**erythromycin stearate.** (eh-RITH-row-MY-sin STEE-ah-rate) *USP.*
Use: Anti-infective; erythromycin.

erythromycin sulfate.
Use: Anti-infective; erythromycin.

erythromycin tablets. (Various Mfr.) Erythromycin 100 mg, 250 mg. Tab. Bot. 25s (250 mg only,) 100s. *Rx.*
Use: Anti-infective.

erythromycin topical. (Various Mfr.) Erythromycin. **Gel:** 2%. Contains alcohol. Tube 30 g, 60 g. **Soln.:** 2%. Contains alcohol. Bot. 60 mL. *Rx.*
Use: Dermatologic, acne.

•**erythromycin 2-propionate dodecyl sulfate.** (e-RITH-roe-MYE-sin PROE-pee-oh-nate) *USP.* Erythromycin Estolate.
Use: Anti-infective; erythromycin.

erythropoiesis-stimulating agents.
See: Peginesatide.

erythropoietin receptor activator, continuous.
Use: Investigational hematopoietic agent.

erythrosine sodium. *USP.*
Use: Diagnostic aid (dental disclosing agent).

•**escitalopram oxalate.** (ESS-sigh-TAL-oh-pram)
Use: Antidepressant, serotonin reuptake inhibitor.
See: Lexapro.

esclabron. Guaithylline.
Use: Antiasthmatic.

Eserdine Forte Tabs. (Major) Methyclothiazide, reserpine 0.5 mg. Bot. 100s. *Rx.*
Use: Antihypertensive; diuretic.

Eserdine Tabs. (Major) Methyclothiazide, reserpine 0.25 mg. Bot. 100s, 250s. *Rx.*
Use: Antihypertensive; diuretic.

Eserine. Physostigmine as alkaloid, salicylate or sulfate salt. *Rx.*
Use: Antiglaucoma.

Eserine Salicylate. (Alcon) Physostigmine 0.5%. Soln. 2 mL. *Rx.*
Use: Antiglaucoma.

Eserine Sulfate Sterile Ophthalmic Ointment. (Ciba Vision) Physostigmine sulfate 0.25%. Tube 3.5 g. *Rx.*
Use: Antiglaucoma.

Esgic. (Gilbert Laboratories.) Butalbital 50 mg, caffeine 40 mg, acetaminophen 325 mg. Cap. Tab. Bot. 100s. *Rx.*
Use: Analgesic; hypnotic; sedative.

Esgic-Plus. (Forest) Acetaminophen 500 mg, butalbital 50 mg, caffeine 40 mg. Tab. Bot. 100s, 500s. Cap. Bot. 20s, 100s, 500s. *Rx.*
Use: Analgesic; hypnotic; sedative.

Eskalith CR. (GlaxoSmithKline) Lithium carbonate 450 mg. CR Tab. Bot. 100s. *Rx.*
Use: Antipsychotic.

•**esketamine.** (es-KET-a-meen) USAN.
Use: Antidepressant.

•**esketamine hydrochloride.** (es-KET-a-meen) USAN.
Use: Antidepressant.

•**eslicarbazepine.** (ES-lye-kar-BAY-ze-peen) USAN.
Use: Anticonvulsant.

•**eslicarbazepine acetate.** (ES-lye-kar-BAY-ze-peen) USAN.
Use: Anticonvulsant.
See: Aptiom.

•**esmirtazapine maleate.** (es-mir-TAZ-a-peen) USAN.
Use: Serotonin receptor antagonist.

•**esmolol hydrochloride.** (ESS-moe-lahl) USAN.
Use: Antiadrenergic/sympatholytic, beta-adrenergic blocking agent.
See: Brevibloc.

esmolol hydrochloride. (Baxter) Esmolol hydrochloride 10 mg/mL. Preservative-free. Inj. Vials. 10 mL. *Rx.*
Use: Antiadrenergic/sympatholytic, beta-adrenergic blocking agent.

Esocor P. (Acella) Chlorpheniramine maleate 4 mg, dextromethorphan hydrobromide 30 mg, pseudoephedrine hydrochloride 30 mg per 5 mL. Benzoic acid, glycerin, parabens, propylene glycol, saccharin. Grape bubble gum flavor. Susp. 473 mL. *Rx.*
Use: Upper respiratory combination, antitussive combination.

•**esomeprazole magnesium.** (ES-oh-MEP-ra-zole) USAN.
Use: Proton pump inhibitor.
See: Nexium.
Nexium I.V.

•**esomeprazole potassium.** (ES-oh-MEP-ra-zole) USAN.
Use: Gastrointestinal agent.

•**esomeprazole sodium.** (ES-oh-MEP-ra-zole) USAN.
Use: Proton pump inhibitor.

•**esomeprazole strontium.** (ES-oh-MEP-ra-zole STRON-shee-um) USAN.
Use: Gastrointestinal agent.

esomeprazole strontium. (Various Mfr.) Esomeprazole strontium 24.65 mg (equiv. to esomeprazole 20 mg), 49.3 mg (equiv. to esomeprazole 40 mg). Sugar. Cap., delayed release. 30s. *Rx.*
Use: Gastrointestinal agent, proton pump inhibitor.

•**esorubicin hydrochloride.** (ESS-oh-ROO-bih-sin) USAN.
Use: Antineoplastic.

Esoterica Dry Skin Treatment Lotion. (GlaxoSmithKline) Bot. 13 fl oz. *OTC.*
Use: Emollient.

Esoterica Facial. (Medicis) Hydroquinone 2%, octyldimethyl PABA, benzophone, stearyl alcohol, sodium bisulfite, parabens, EDTA. Cream. Tube 90 g. *OTC.*
Use: Dermatologic.

Esoterica Fade Cream. (Medicis) Hydroquinone 2%. Padimate O 3.3%, oxybenzone 2.5%, alcohol, edetate disodium, glyceryl, parabens, propylene glycol, sodium metabisulfite. Cream. 70 g. *OTC.*
Use: Pigment agent.

Esoterica Regular. (Medicis) Hydroquinone 2%, light mineral oil, stearyl alcohol, parabens, sodium bisulfite, EDTA. Cream. Jar 90 g. *OTC.*
Use: Dermatologic.

Esoterica Sunscreen. (Medicis) Hydroquinone 2%, padimate O 3.3%, oxybenzone 2.5%, mineral oil, parabens, sodium bisulfite, EDTA. Cream. Jar 85 g. *OTC.*
Use: Dermatologic.

•**esoxybutynin chloride.** (es-ox-i-BUE-ti-nin) USAN.
Use: Antispasmodic, anticholinergic.

•**esproquin hydrochloride.** (ESS-pro-kwin) USAN.
Use: Adrenergic.

Essentia. (Theralogix) Vitamins A 3,000 units, C 100 mg, D_3 2,000 units, E 60 units, K 100 mcg, B_1 10 mg, B_2 10 mg, B_3 25 mg, B_5 10 mg, B_6 6 mg, B_{12} 25 mcg, folate 400 mcg, Ca 100 mg, Fe 18 mg, biotin, choline, I, Mg, Zn, Se, Cu, Mn, Cr, Mo, B, V. Tab. 180s. *Rx.*
Use: Multivitamin with minerals.

Essential-8. Liquid amino acid protein supplement.
Use: Protein supplement.
See: Vivonex, Standard.
Vivonex T.E.N.

Essential ProPlus. (NutriSoy) Protein 16.3 g, fat 0.2 g, carbohydrates 6.4 g, Na 242.5 mg, K 112.5 mg, Ca 70 mg, Mg 31.3 mg, Fe 3 mg, P 187.5 mg, Cu 0.4 mg, Zn 0.5 mg, I 12.9 mcg, B_1 0.1 mg, B_3 0.2 mg, folic acid 0.1 mg/25 g. Pow. Cont. 2 lb. *OTC.*
Use: Nutritional supplement.

Essential Protein. (NutriSoy) Protein 16 g, fat 0.3 g, carbohydrates 5.6 g, sodium 5 mg, K 750 mg, Ca 97.5 mg, Mg 80 mg, Fe 2.5 mg, P 202.5 g, Cu 0.4 mg, Zn 0.8 mg, I 10 mcg, B_1 0.1 mg, B_3 0.2 mg, B_6 0.1 mg, folic acid 0.1 mg/25 g. Pow. Cont. 2 lb. *OTC.*
Use: Nutritional supplement.

Estarylla. (Sandoz) Ethinyl estradiol 35 mcg, norgestimate 0.25 mg. Lactose. Tab. 28s w/7 inert tablets (with lactose). *Rx.*
Use: Monophasic oral contraceptive.

•**estazolam.** (ess-TAZZ-OH-lam) USAN.
Use: Sedative/hypnotic, nonbarbiturate.

estazolam. (Zenith-Goldline) Estazolam 1 mg, 2 mg Tab. Bot. 30s, 100s, 500s, 1000s. *Rx.*
Use: Sedative/hypnotic, nonbarbiturate.

Ester-C Plus 500 mg Vitamin C. (Solgar) Vitamin C 500 mg, citrus bioflavonoids 25 mg, acerola 10 mg, rutin 5 mg, rose hips 10 mg, calcium 62 mg. Sugar and sodium free. Cap. Bot. 250s. *OTC.*
Use: Water-soluble vitamin.

Ester-C Plus Multi-Mineral. (Solgar) Vitamin C 425 mg, citrus bioflavonoid complex 50 mg, acerola 12.5 mg, rose hips 12.5 mg, rutin 5 mg, calcium 25 mg, magnesium 13 mg, potassium 12.5 mg, zinc 2.5 mg. Sugar and sodium free. Cap. Bot. 60s, 90s. *OTC.*
Use: Water-soluble vitamin.

Ester-C Plus 1000 mg Vitamin C. (Solgar) Vitamin C 1000 mg, citrus bioflavonoid complex 200 mg, acerola 25 mg, rutin 25 mg, rose hips 25 mg, calcium 125 mg. Sugar and sodium free. Tab. Bot. 90s. *OTC.*
Use: Water-soluble vitamin.

esterified estrogens.
See: Estrogens, esterified.

esterified estrogens and methyltestosterone. (Various Mfr.) Esterified estrogens/methyltestosterone 1.25 mg/ 2.5 mg. May contain lactose. Tab. 100s, 1000s. *Rx.*
Use: Sex hormone, estrogen and androgen combination.

esterified estrogens and methyltestosterone H.S. (Various Mfr.) Esterified estrogens 0.625 mg/methyltestosterone 1.25 mg. May contain lactose. Tab. 100s, 1000s. *Rx.*
Use: Sex hormone, estrogen and androgen combination.

•**esterifilcon A.** (ess-TER-ih-FILL-kahn A) USAN.
Use: Contact lens material, hydrophilic.

ester local anesthetics.
Use: Injectable local anesthetic, topical local anesthetic.
See: Benzocaine.
Cocaine.
Chloroprocaine Hydrochloride.
Procaine Hydrochloride.
Tetracaine Hydrochloride.

Estilben.
See: Diethylstilbestrol Dipropionate.

Estinyl. (Schering-Plough) Ethinyl estradiol. **Tab., coated. 0.02 mg, 0.05 mg:** Bot. 100s, 250s; **Tab. 0.5 mg:** Bot. 100s. *Rx.*
Use: Estrogen.

Estrace. (Warner Chilcott) Estradiol micronized 0.5 mg, 1 mg, 2 mg. Tartrazine (2 mg only), lactose. Tab. Bot. 100s, 500s (except 0.5 mg). *Rx.*
Use: Estrogen, sex hormone.

Estrace Vaginal. (Warner Chilcott) Estradiol 0.1 mg/g in a nonliquefying base. EDTA, methylparaben, steryl alcohol. Cream. Tube w/calibrated applicator 42.5 g. *Rx.*
Use: Estrogen, sex hormone.

Estracon. (Freeport) Conjugated estrogens 1.25 mg. Tab. Bot. 1000s. *Rx.*
Use: Estrogen.

Estraderm. (Novartis) Estradiol 4 mg (0.05 mg/day), 8 mg (0.1 mg/day). Calendar packs of 8 and 24 systems. *Rx.*
Use: Estrogen, sex hormone.

•**estradiol.** (ESS-truh-DIE-ole) *USP.* The form now known to be physiologically active is the β form rather than the α.
Use: Estrogen, sex hormone.
See: Alora.
Climara.
Divigel.
Elestrin.
Estrace.
Estraderm.
Estring.
EstroGel.
Evamist.
FemPatch.
Minivelle.
Vivelle-Dot.
W/Drospirenone.
See: Angeliq.
W/Estrone, estriol.
See: Sanestro.
W/Levonorgestrel.
See: ClimaraPro.
W/Norethindrone acetate.
See: CombiPatch.
Mimvey.
W/Norgestimate.
See: Prefest.
W/Testosterone and chlorobutanol in cottonseed oil.
See: Depo-Testadiol.
Estraderm.

estradiol. (Various Mfr.) Micronized estradiol 0.5 mg, 1 mg, 2 mg. May contain lactose. Tab. Bot. 100s, 500s (except 0.5 mg). *Rx.*
Use: Estrogen, sex hormone.

•**estradiol acetate.** (ESS-trah-DIE-ole) USAN.
Use: Estrogen.

estradiol benzoate.
Use: Estrogen.

•**estradiol cypionate.** (ESS-trah-DIE-ole SIP-ee-oh-nate) *USP.*
Use: Estrogen, sex hormone.
See: Depo-Estradiol.
W/Chlorobutanol, cottonseed oil
See: depGynogen.
DepoGen.
W/Testosterone cypionate.
See: Menoject, L.A.
W/Testosterone cypionate, chlorobutanol.
See: Depo-Testadiol.

estradiol cypionate. (Various Mfr.) Estradiol cypionate 5 mg/mL, cottonseed oil

w/chlorobutanol. Inj. Vial. 10 mL. *Rx.*
Use: Estrogen.
estradiol dipropionate.
Use: Estrogen.
•**estradiol enanthate.** (ESS-trah-DIE-ole eh-NAN-thate) USAN.
Use: Estrogen.
estradiol, ethinyl.
See: Ethinyl Estradiol.
estradiol hemihydrate.
Use: Estrogen.
See: Estrasorb.
See: Vagifem.
estradiol, micronized.
Use: Estrogen.
See: Estrace.
estradiol/norethindrone acetate. (Breckenridge) Estradiol 1 mg, norethindrone acetate 0.5 mg. May contain lactose. Tab. Blister packs. 28s. *Rx.*
Use: Sex hormone.
estradiol, oral. (Teva) Micronized estradiol 0.5 mg, 1 mg, 2 mg. Tab. Bot. 100s. *Rx.*
Use: Estrogen.
estradiol, topical emulsion.
Use: Sex hormone.
estradiol transdermal system.
Use: Estrogen, sex hormone.
See: Alora.
Climara.
Esclim.
Estraderm.
Menostar.
Vivelle.
Vivelle-Dot.
W/Levonorgestrel.
See: ClimaraPro.
W/Norethindrone Acetate.
See: CombiPatch.
estradiol transdermal system. (Mylan) Estradiol 0.97 mg (0.025 mg/day), 1.46 mg (0.0375 mg/day), 1.94 mg (0.05 mg/day), 2.33 mg (0.06 mg/day), 2.91 mg (0.075 mg/day), 3.88 mg (0.1 mg/day). Patch. 4s. *Rx.*
Use: Estrogen, sex hormone.
•**estradiol undecylate.** (ESS-trah-DIE-ole UHN-DEH-sill-ate) USAN.
See: Delestrec.
estradiol vaginal cream.
Use: Estrogen.
•**estradiol valerate.** (ESS-trah-DIE-ole VAL-eh-rate) *USP.*
Use: Estrogen.
See: Ardefem 10, 20.
Delestrogen.
Duragen.
Estra-L.
Valergen.
W/Dienogest.
See: Natazia.
W/Testosterone enanthate.
See: Ardiol 90/4, 180/8.
Delatestadiol.
Estra-Testrin.
Teev.
Tesogen LA.
Valertest.
estradiol valerate. (Sandoz) Estradiol valerate 10 mg/mL, 20 mg/mL, 40 mg/mL. Sesame oil (10 mg/mL only); benzyl alcohol, benzyl benzoate, castor oil (20 mg, 40 mg only). Inj. Multidose vial. 5 mL. *Rx.*
Use: Estrogen, sex hormone.
estradiol valerate. (Various Mfr.) Estradiol valerate 20 mg/mL, 40 mg/mL. Inj. Vial 10 mL. 40 mg/mL. Vial 10 mL. *Rx.*
Use: Estrogen.
Estra-L. (Taylor Pharmaceuticals) Estradiol valerate in oil 40 mg/mL. Vial 10 mL. *Rx.*
Use: Estrogen.
•**estramustine.** (ESS-truh-muss-TEEN) USAN.
Use: Antineoplastic.
•**estramustine phosphate sodium.** (ESS-truh-muss-TEEN) USAN.
Use: Antineoplastic, alkylating agent.
See: Emcyt.
Estrasorb. (Medicis) Estradiol hemihydrate 2.5 mg/g. Soybean oil, ethanol. Top. Emulsion. 1.74 g pouches. *Rx.*
Use: Sex hormone; estrogen.
Estratab. (Solvay) Esterified estrogens 0.3 mg, 0.625 mg, 2.5 mg. Tab. Bot. 100s, 1000s (0.625 mg only). *Rx.*
Use: Estrogen.
•**estrazinol hydrobromide.** (ESS-trazz-ih-nahl) USAN.
Use: Estrogen.
estrin.
See: Estrone.
Estrinex. (Pharmacia)
See: Toremifene.
Estring. (Pharmacia) Estradiol 2 mg. Releases estradiol 7.5 mcg/24 hours over 90 days. Vaginal ring. Single packs. *Rx.*
Use: Estrogen, sex hormone.
•**estriol.** (ESS-tree-ole) *USP.*
Use: Estrogen.
Estrobene DP.
See: Diethylstilbestrol Dipropionate.
Estrofem. (Taylor Pharmaceuticals) Estradiol cypionate 5 mg/mL in oil. Inj. Vial 10 mL.
Use: Estrogen.
•**estrofurate.** (ESS-troe-FYOOR-ate) USAN.
Use: Estrogen.

Estrogel. (Ascend) Estradiol 0.06% (estradiol 0.75 mg/1.25 g unit dose). Alcohol. Gel. Pump. 93 g. Tube. 80 g. *Rx.*
Use: Sex hormone, estrogen.

estrogen and androgen combinations.
Use: Sex hormone.
See: Covaryx.
Covaryx H.S.
Estratest.
Estratest H.S.

estrogen-androgen therapy.
See: Androgen-estrogen therapy.

estrogenic substance aqueous. (Various Mfr.) Estrogenic substance or estrogens (mainly estrone) 2 mg/mL. Inj. Vial 10 mL, 30 mL. *Rx.*
Use: Estrogen.

estrogenic substances, conjugated. (Water-soluble) A mixture containing the sodium salts of the sulfate esters of the estrogenic substances, principally estrone and equilin that are of the type excreted by pregnant mares. *Rx.*
See: Ces.
Estroquin.
Prelestrin.
Premarin.
W/Meprobamate.
See: PMB 400.
PMB 200.

estrogenic substances in aqueous suspension. (Wyeth) Sterile estrone suspension 2 mg/mL. Vial 10 mL. *Rx.*
Use: Estrogen.

estrogenic substances mixed. May be a crystalline or an amorphous mixture of the naturally occurring estrogens obtained from the urine of pregnant mares. **Aqueous Susp.:** Inj. **Cap.:** W/Androgen therapy, vitamins, iron, d-desoxyephedrine hydrochloride.

estrogen/nitrogen mustard.
Use: Alkylating agent.
See: Estramustine Phosphate Sodium.

estrogens.
Use: Sex hormones.
See: Conjugated Estrogens.
Esterified Estrogens.
Estradiol.
Estradiol Cypionate.
Estradiol Topical Emulsion.
Estradiol Transdermal System.
Estradiol Valerate in Oil.
Estropipate.
Estrogens, Miscellaneous, Vaginal.
Synthetic Conjugated Estrogens, A.
Synthetic Conjugated Estrogens, B.
Topical Estrogens, Miscellaneous.

estrogens and progestins combined.
Use: Sex hormone.
See: Activella.
Alesse.
Angeliq.
Apri.
Aviane.
Brevicon.
ClimaraPro.
CombiPatch.
Desogen.
Estrostep Fe.
Femhrt.
Jenest-28.
Levora.
Loestrin Fe 1/20.
Loestrin Fe 1.5/30.
Loestrin 21 1/20.
Loestrin 21 1.5/30.
Lo/Ovral.
Low-Ogestrel.
Microgestin Fe 1/20.
Microgestin Fe 1.5/30.
Mircette.
Modicon.
MonoNessa.
Necon 1/50.
Necon 1/35.
Necon 10/11.
Necon 0.5/35.
Nordette.
Norinyl 1 + 50.
Norinyl 1 + 35.
Nortrel 1/35.
Nortrel 0.5/35.
Ogestrel.
Ortho-Cept.
Ortho-Cyclen.
Ortho-Novum 1/50.
Ortho-Novum 1/35.
Ortho-Novum 7/7/7.
Ortho-Novum 10/11.
Ortho Tri-Cyclen.
Ovcon-50.
Ovcon-35.
Ovral-28.
Prefest.
Premphase.
Prempro.
Tri-Norinyl.
Triphasil.
Trivora-28.
Yasmin.
Yaz.
Zovia 1/50E.
Zovia 1/35E.

•**estrogens, conjugated.** (ESS-truh-janz KAHN-juh-gay-tuhd) *USP.*
Use: Estrogen.
See: Conest.
Ganeake.
PMB.
Premarin.

Premarin Intravenous.
W/Bazedoxifene.
See: Duavee.
W/Meprobamate.
See: PMB.
estrogens, conjugated and medroxyprogesterone acetate.
Use: Sex hormone.
See: Premphase.
Prempro.
estrogens equine.
See: Estrogen.
•**estrogens, esterified.** (ESS-troe-jenz, ess-TER-ih-fide) *USP.*
Use: Estrogen.
See: Estratab.
Menest.
W/Methyltestosterone.
See: Covaryx.
Covaryx H.S.
estrogens, esterified and androgens.
Use: Estrogen, androgen supplement.
See: Covaryx.
Covaryx H.S.
Estratab.
Estratest.
Estratest H.S.
Menest.
estrogens, miscellaneous topical.
Use: Sex hormone, estrogen.
See: Divigel.
Elestrin.
Estrasorb.
Estrogel.
Evamist.
estrogens, miscellaneous, vaginal.
Use: Estrogen, sex hormone.
See: Estrace Vaginal.
Estring.
Femring.
Premarin Vaginal.
Vagifem.
estrogens, natural.
Use: Estrogen.
See: Depogen.
Estradiol.
Estrogenic Substance.
Estrone.
PMB.
Premarin.
estrogens, synthetic conjugated A.
See: Cenestin.
estrogens, synthetic conjugated B.
See: Enjuvia.
Estrogestin A. (Harvey) Estrogenic substance 1 mg, progesterone 10 mg/mL in peanut oil. Vial 10 mL. *Rx.*
Use: Estrogen, progestin combination.
Estrogestin C. (Harvey) Estrogenic substance 1 mg, progesterone 12.5 mg/mL in peanut oil. Vial 10 mL. *Rx.*
Use: Estrogen, progestin combination.
•**estrone.** (ESS-trone) *USP.*
Use: Estrogen.
See: Bestrone.
Estrogenic Substances in Aqueous Susp.
Foygen.
Kestrone 5.
Par-Supp.
Propagon-S.
W/Estrogens.
See: Estrogenic Substances.
W/Progesterone.
See: Duovin-S.
W/Testosterone.
See: Andesterone.
estrone aqueous. (Various Mfr.) Estrone aqueous 5 mg/mL. Inj. Vial 10 mL. *Rx.*
Use: Estrogen.
estrone sulfate, piperazine.
See: Ogen.
estrone sulfate, potassium.
See: Estrogen.
•**estropipate.** (ESS-troe-PIH-pate) *USP.* *Formerly Piperazine Estrone Sulfate.*
Use: Estrogen, sex hormone.
estropipate. (Various Mfr.) Estropipate 0.75 mg (sodium estrone sulfate 0.625 mg), 1.5 mg (sodium estrone sulfate 1.25 mg), 3 mg (sodium estrone sulfate 2.5 mg), 6 mg (sodium estrone sulfate 5 mg). Tab. Bot. 30s, 100s, 500s. *Rx.*
Use: Estrogen, sex hormone.
Estroquin. (Sheryl) Purified conjugated estrogens 1.25 mg. Tab. Bot. 100s. *Rx.*
Use: Estrogen.
Estrostep Fe. (Warner Chilcott) **Phase 1:** Norethindrone acetate 1 mg, ethinyl estradiol 20 mcg. 5 tabs. **Phase 2:** Norethindrone acetate 1 mg, ethinyl estradiol 30 mcg. 7 tabs. **Phase 3:** Norethindrone acetate 1 mg, ethinyl estradiol 35 mcg. 9 tabs. Lactose, sucrose. Box. 28s with 7 brown tabs. with ferrous fumarate 75 mg per tab. *Rx.*
Use: Sex hormone, contraceptive hormone.
•**eszopiclone.** (es-zoe-PIK-lone) USAN.
Use: Sedative and hypnotic, nonbarbiturate.
See: Lunesta.
eszopiclone. (Various Mfr.) Eszopiclone 1 mg, 2 mg, 3 mg. May contain lactose, PEG. Tab. 30s (1 mg only), 100s, 500s (2 mg and 3 mg only), 1,000s, UD 98s. *c-iv.*
Use: Nonbarbiturate sedative and hypnotic.
•**etafedrine hydrochloride.** (EH-tah-FED-rin) USAN.
Use: Bronchodilator; adrenergic.

•**etafilcon A.** (EH-tah-FILL-kahn A) USAN.
Use: Contact lens material, hydrophilic.

Etalent. (Roger) Ethaverine hydrochloride 100 mg. Cap. Bot. 50s, 500s. *Rx.*
Use: Vasodilator.

•**etalocib.** (e-TAL-oh-kib) USAN.
Use: Antineoplastic.

•**etanercept.** (et-a-NER-sept) USAN.
Use: Immunologic agent, immunomodulator.
See: Enbrel.

•**etanidazole.** (ETT-ah-NIDE-ah-zole) USAN.
Use: Antineoplastic (hypoxic cell radiosensitizer).

•**etarotene.** (ett-AHR-oh-teen) USAN.
Use: Keratolytic.

•**etazolate hydrochloride.** (eh-TAY-zoe-late) USAN.
Use: Antipsychotic.

•**eteplirsen.** (e-TEP-lir-sen) USAN.
Use: Treatment of Duchenne muscular dystrophy.

Eterna 27. (Revlon) Pregnenolone acetate 0.5% in cream base. *OTC.*
Use: Emollient.

•**eterobarb.** (ee-TEER-oh-barb) USAN.
Use: Anticonvulsant.

•**ethacrynate sodium for injection.** (ETH-ah-KRIN-ate) *USP.*
Use: Diuretic.
See: Edecrin Sodium I.V.

•**ethacrynic acid.** (eth-uh-KRIN-ik) *USP.*
Use: Diuretic.
See: Edecrin.

•**ethambutol hydrochloride.** (eth-AM-byoo-tahl) *USP.*
Use: Anti-infective (tuberculostatic).
See: Myambutol.

ethambutol hydrochloride. (Heritage) Ethambutol hydrochloride 100 mg, 400 mg. Sorbitol, sucrose. Film-coated. Tab. 100s. *Rx.*
Use: Antituberculosis agent.

Ethamicort.
See: Hydrocortamate.

•**ethamivan.** (eth-AM-ih-van) USAN.
Use: Stimulant (central and respiratory).

Ethamolin. (Questcor) Ethanolamine oleate 5%. Inj. Amp. 2 mL. *Rx.*
Use: Sclerosing agent.

•**ethamsylate.** (ETH-AM-sill-ate) USAN.
Use: Hemostatic.

ethanol. (Various Mfr.) Alcohol, anhydrous.

ethanolamine. Olamine.

•**ethanolamine oleate.** (ETH-ah-nahl-ah-MEEN OH-lee-ate) USAN.
Use: Sclerosing agent.
See: Ethamolin.

ethanolamines, nonselective.
Use: Antihistamine.
See: Carbinoxamine Maleate.
Clemastine Fumarate.
Diphenhydramine Hydrochloride.
Doxylamine Succinate.

ethenol, homopolymer. Polyvinyl alcohol.

•**ether.** (EE-ther) *USP.*
Use: Anesthetic, general; inhalation.

•**ethinyl estradiol.** (ETH-in-ill ess-trah-DIE-ole) *USP.*
Use: Estrogen.
See: Amethia.
Camrese.
Estinyl.
Feminone.
Menolyn.
W/Desogestrel.
See: Azurette.
Caziant.
Emoquette.
Viorele.
W/Drospirenone.
See: Gianvi.
Loryna.
Ocella.
Syeda.
Vestura.
Yaz.
Zarah.
W/Drospirenone, Levomefolate Calcium.
See: Beyaz.
W/Levonorgestrel.
See: Altavera.
Amethia.
Amethia Lo.
Amethyst.
Camrese.
Camrese Lo.
Daysee.
Falmina.
Introvale.
Levonest.
LoSeasonique.
Marlissa.
Myzilra.
Orsythia.
W/Norelgestromin.
See: Xulane.
W/Norethindrone.
See: Alyacen 1/35.
Alyacen 7/7/7.
Briellyn.
Cyclafem 1/35.
Cyclafem 7/7/7.
Dasetta 1/35.
Dasetta 7/7/7.
Generess Fe.
Gildagia.
Lo Loestrin Fe.
Nortrel 7/7/7.

Philith.
Pirmella 1/35.
Pirmella 7/7/7.
Tri-Legest Fe.
Wera.
Wymzya Fe.
Zenchent.
W/Norethindrone Acetate.
See: Femhrt.
Gildess Fe 1.5/30.
Gildess 1.5/30.
Gildess 1/20.
Gildess 1/20 Fe.
Jinteli.
Larin Fe 1.5/30.
Larin Fe 1/20.
Larin 1/20.
Lomedia 24 Fe.
Microgestin 1/20.
Minastrin 24 Fe.
Tilia Fe.
Tri-Legest Fe.
W/Norgestimate.
See: Estarylla.
Previfem.
Tri-Linyah.
W/Norgestrel.
See: Elinest.

ethinyl estradiol. (Bio-Technology General)
Use: Turner syndrome. [Orphan Drug]

ethinyl estradiol and dimethisterone tablets.
Use: Estrogen, progestin combination.

ethinyl estradiol with combinations.
See: Alesse.
Apri.
Aranelle.
Aviane.
Balziva.
Brevicon.
Cesia.
Desogen.
Estrostep Fe.
Femcon Fe.
GenCept.
Jenest-28.
Jolessa.
Junel Fe 1/20.
Junel Fe 1.5/30.
Junel 21 Day 1.5/30.
Junel 21 Day 1/20.
Kelnor 1/35.
Leena.
Levora.
Loestrin 21 1/20.
Loestrin 21 1.5/30.
Loestrin Fe 1/20.
Loestrin Fe 1.5/30.
Loestrin 24 Fe.
Low-Ogestrel.
Lutera.
Microgestin Fe 1/20.
Microgestin Fe 1.5/30.
Mircette.
Modicon.
MonoNessa.
Nelulen.
Norinyl 1 + 35.
Norlestrin.
Norlestrin Fe.
NuvaRing.
Ortho-Cept.
Ortho-Cyclen.
Ortho-Evra.
Ortho-Novum 1/35, 7/7/7.
Ortho Tri-Cyclen.
Ovcon-35.
Ovlin.
Previfem.
Quasense.
Reclipsen.
Seasonique.
Solia.
Sronyx.
Tri-Norinyl.
Tri-Previfem.
Trivora.
Velivet.
Yasmin.
Zovia 1/50E.
Zovia 1/35E.

ethinyl estrenol.
See: Lynestrenol.

•**ethiodized oil injection.** (eth-EYE-oh-dized) *USP.*
Use: Radiopaque agent.

•**ethiodized oil I 131.** (eth-EYE-oh-dized) USAN.
Use: Antineoplastic; radiopharmaceutical.

•**ethionamide.** (eh-THIGH-ohn-ah-mide) *USP.*
Use: Antituberculosis agent.
See: Trecator.

ethisterone.
See: Anhydrohydroxyprogesterone.

Ethocaine.
See: Procaine Hydrochloride.

ethodryl.
See: Diethylcarbamazine Citrate.

ethohexadiol. Used in Comp. dimethyl phthalate.
Use: Insect repellent.

•**ethonam nitrate.** (ETH-oh-nam NYE-trate) USAN.
Use: Antifungal.

•**ethosuximide.** (ETH-oh-SUX-ih-mide) *USP.*
Use: Anticonvulsant.
See: Zarontin.

ethosuximide. (Copley) Ethosuximide

250 mg/5 mL, saccharin, sucrose, raspberry flavor. Syr. Bot. 483 mL. *Rx.*
Use: Anticonvulsant.
ethosuximide. (Sidmark) Ethosuximide 250 mg. Cap. 100s. *Rx.*
Use: Anticonvulsant.
•**ethotoin.** (ETH-oh-toyn) *USP.*
Use: Anticonvulsant.
See: Peganone.
ethovan. Ethyl Vanillin.
•**ethoxazene hydrochloride.** (eth-OX-ah-zeen) USAN.
Use: Analgesic.
ethoxzolamide.
Use: Carbonic anhydrase inhibitor.
Ethrane. (Baxter Healthcare) Enflurane. Volatile Liq. Bot. 125 mL, 250 mL. *Rx.*
Use: Anesthetic, general.
•**ethybenztropine.** (ETH-ih-BENZ-troe-peen) USAN.
Use: Anticholinergic.
•**ethyl acetate.** (ETH-ill) *NF.*
Use: Pharmaceutic aid, flavoring; solvent.
ethyl aminobenzoate. Anesthesin, anesthrone, benzocaine, parathesin.
Use: Anesthetic, local.
See: Benzocaine.
ethyl bromide. (Various Mfr.) Bromoethane. *Rx.*
Use: Anesthetic, general.
ethyl carbamate.
See: Urethan.
•**ethylcellulose.** (eth-il-SEL-yoo-lose) *NF.*
Use: Tablet binder; pharmaceutic aid.
ethylcellulose aqueous dispersion.
Use: Tablet binder; pharmaceutic aid.
ethyl chaulmoograte.
Use: Hansen disease; sarcoidosis.
•**ethyl chloride.** (ETH-ill) *USP.*
Use: Anesthetic, topical.
W/Dichlorotetrafluoroethane.
See: Fluro-Ethyl.
•**ethyl dibunate.** (ETH-ill DIE-byoo-nate) USAN.
Use: Cough suppressant; antitussive.
ethyl diiodobrassidate. Iodobrassid. Lipoiodine.
ethyldimethylammonium bromide.
See: Ambutonium Bromide.
ethylene. (Various Mfr.) Ethene. *Rx.*
Use: Anesthetic, general.
•**ethylenediamine.** (eth-ih-leen-DIE-ah-meen) *USP.*
Use: Component of aminophylline injection.
ethylenediamine solution. (67% w/v).
Use: Solvent (Aminophylline Inj.).
ethylenediaminetetraacetate.
See: Endrate Disodium.
ethylenedinitrilotetraacetate disodium.
See: Edathamil.
EDTA.
ethylenimines/methylmelamines.
Use: Alkylating agents.
See: Altretamine.
Mechlorethamine Derivative.
Thiotepa.
•**ethylestrenol.** (ETH-ill-ESS-tree-nahl) USAN.
Use: Anabolic.
ethylhydrocupreine hydrochloride.
Use: Antiseptic.
ethylmorphine hydrochloride.
Use: Narcotic.
ethyl nitrite spirit. Ethyl nitrite. Sweet Spirit of Niter. Spirit of Nitrous Ether.
•**ethyl oleate.** (ETH-ill) *NF.*
Use: Pharmaceutic aid (vehicle).
ethyl oxide; ethyl ether.
Use: Solvent.
•**ethylparaben.** (eth-ill-PAR-ah-ben) *NF.*
Use: Pharmaceutic aid (antifungal preservative).
ethylstibamine. Astaril, neostibosan.
Use: Antimony therapy.
•**ethyl vanillin.** (ETH-ill) *NF.*
Use: Pharmaceutic aid (flavor).
•**ethynerone.** (eth-EYE-ner-ohn) USAN.
Use: Hormone, progestin.
•**ethynodiol diacetate.** (eh-THIN-oh-die-ole die-ASS-eh-tate) *USP.*
Use: Progesterone, progestin.
W/Ethinyl estradiol.
See: Estrostep Fe.
Kelnor 1/35.
Nelulen.
Ovulen.
Zovia.
W/Mestranol.
See: Ovulen.
ethynodiol diacetate and ethinyl estradiol tablets.
Use: Contraceptive.
ethynodiol diacetate and mestranol tablets.
Use: Contraceptive.
ethynylestradiol.
See: Ethinyl Estradiol.
Mestranol.
Ethyol. (MedImmune Oncology) Amifostine 500 mg (as amifostine trihydrate). Inj., Pow. for Soln. Single-use vials. 10 mL. *Rx.*
Use: Cytoprotective agent.
•**etibendazole.** (eh-tie-BEN-dah-ZOLE) USAN.
Use: Anthelmintic.
Eticylol. (Novartis) Ethinyl estradiol. *Rx.*
Use: Estrogen.

•**etidocaine.** (eh-TIE-doe-cane) USAN.
Use: Anesthetic, local.

•**etidronate disodium.** (eh-TIH-DROE-nate) *USP.*
Use: Bisphosphonate.
See: Didronel.

etidronate disodium. (Genpharm) Etidronate disodium 200 mg, 400 mg. Tab. 60s. *Rx.*
Use: Bisphosphanate.

•**etidronic acid.** (eh-tih-DRAH-nik) USAN.
Use: Calcium regulator.

•**etifenin.** (EH-tih-FEN-in) USAN.
Use: Diagnostic aid.

•**etiguanfacine.** (E-ti-GWAHN-fa-seen) USAN.
Use: Treatment of attention deficit hyperactivity disorder.

•**etilevodopa.** (et-il-ee-voe-DOE-a) USAN.
Use: Parkinson disease.

•**etintidine hydrochloride.** (ett-IN-tih-DEEN) USAN.
Use: Antiulcerative.

etiocholanedoine. (SuperGen)
Use: Aplastic anemia; Prader-Willi syndrome. [Orphan Drug]

•**etiprednol dicloacetate.** (e-ti-PRED-nole dye-KLOE-a-se-tate) USAN.
Use: Anti-inflammatory; corticosteroid.

•**etirinotecan pegol.** (ET-eye-ri-noe-TEE-kan PEG-ol) USAN.
Use: Antineoplastic.

•**etirinotecan pegol tetrahydrochloride.** (ET-eye-ri-noe-TEE-kan PEG-ol) USAN.
Use: Antineoplastic.

•**etirinotecan pegol tetratriflutate.** (ET-eye-ri-noe-TEE-kan PEG-ol) USAN.
Use: Antineoplastic.

•**etocrylene.** (EH-toe-KRIH-leen) USAN.
Use: Ultraviolet screen.

•**etodolac.** (EE-toe-DOE-lak) *USP.*
Use: Analgesic; NSAID.

etodolac. (Various Mfr.) Etodolac **Tab.:** 400 mg, 500 mg. Bot. 100s, 500s, 1000s (500 mg only). **Cap.:** 200 mg, 300 mg. Bot. 100s, 500s, 1000s. **ER Tab.:** 400 mg, 500 mg, 600 mg. Bot. 100s, 500s (400 mg only). *Rx.*
Use: Analgesic; NSAID.

•**etofenamate.** (EH-toe-FEN-am-ate) USAN.
Use: Analgesic; anti-inflammatory.

•**etoformin hydrochloride.** (EH-toe-FORE-min) USAN.
Use: Antidiabetic.

•**etomidate.** (eh-TAHM-ih-date) USAN.
Use: Hypnotic; sedative.
See: Amidate.

etomidate. (Parenta) Etomidate 2 mg/mL. Inj., Soln. Single-dose vials. 10 mL, 20 mL. *Rx.*
Use: Hypnotic; sedative.

etomide hydrochloride. Bandol. Carbiphene hydrochloride.

•**etonogestrel.** (ETT-oh-no-JESS-trell) USAN.
Use: Hormone, progestin.
See: Implanon.
Nexplanon.
W/Ethinyl estradiol.
See: NuvaRing.

•**etoperidone hydrochloride.** (EH-toe-PURR-ih-dohn) USAN.
Use: Antidepressant.

Etopophos. (Bristol-Myers Squibb) Etoposide phosphate100 mg. Lyophilized Pow. for Inj. Vial. Single dose. *Rx.*
Use: Antineoplastic.

•**etoposide.** (EH-toe-POE-side) *USP.*
Use: Antineoplastic.
See: Etopophos.
Toposar.
Vepesid.

etoposide. (Various Mfr.) Etoposide. **Cap.:** 50 mg. Blister pack. 10s. **Inj.:** 20 mg/mL. May contain alcohol, benzyl alcohol, polysorbate 80, PEG, citric acid. Vial. 5 mL, 12.5 mL, 25 mL, 50 mL. *Rx.*
Use: Epipodophyllotoxin; antineoplastic.

•**etoposide phosphate.** (ee-toe-POE-side) USAN.
Use: Antineoplastic.
See: Etopophos.

•**etoprine.** (ETT-oh-preen) USAN.
Use: Antineoplastic.

•**etoricoxib.** (e-TOR-i-KOX-ib) USAN.
Use: Anti-inflammatory.

etoval.
See: Butethal.

•**etoxadrol hydrochloride.** (eh-TOX-ah-drole) USAN.
Use: Anesthetic.

•**etozolin.** (EAT-oh-zoe-lin) USAN.
Use: Diuretic.

Etrafon-A (4-10). (Schering-Plough) Perphenazine 4 mg, amitriptyline hydrochloride 10 mg. Tab. Bot. 100s, UD 100s. *Rx.*
Use: Psychotherapeutic combination.

Etrafon Forte (4-25). (Schering-Plough) Perphenazine 4 mg, amitriptyline hydrochloride 25 mg. Tab. Bot. 100s, 500s, UD 100s. *Rx.*
Use: Psychotherapeutic combination.

Etrafon (2-25). (Schering-Plough) Perphenazine 2 mg, amitriptyline hydrochloride 25 mg. Tab. Bot. 100s, 500s,

UD 100s. *Rx.*
Use: Psychotherapeutic combination.
•**etravirine.** (ET-ra-VIR-een) USAN.
Use: Antiretroviral, non-nucleoside reverse transcriptase inhibitor.
See: Intelence.
•**etretinate.** (eh-TRETT-ih-nate) USAN.
Use: Antipsoriatic.
•**etrolizumab.** (ET-roe-LIZ-oo-mab) USAN.
Use: Gastrointestinal agent.
etrynit. Propatyl nitrate.
Use: Cardiovascular agent.
•**etryptamine acetate.** (ee-TRIP-tah-meen) USAN.
Use: Central stimulant.
E.T.S.-2%. (Paddock) Erythromycin topical 2%. Soln. Bot. 60 mL. *Rx.*
Use: Dermatologic, acne.
ettriol trinitrate.
See: Propatyl nitrate.
etybenzatropine. Ethybenztropine.
etynodiol acetate. Ethynodiol diacetate.
eubasin.
See: Sulfapyridine.
eucaine hydrochloride. (Novartis) Menthol 8%, eucalyptus oil, SD 3A alcohol. Gel. Tube 60 g. *OTC.*
Use: Liniment.
Eucalyptamint. (Novartis) Menthol 8%, eucalyptus oil, SD 3A alcohol. Gel 60 g. *OTC.*
Use: Liniment.
Eucalyptamint Maximum Strength. (Novartis) Menthol 16%, lanolin, eucalyptus oil. Oint. Tube 60 mL. *OTC.*
Use: Liniment.
•**eucalyptol.** (yoo-ka-LIP-tol) USAN.
Use: Pharmaceutic aid (flavor); antitussive; decongestant, nasal.
See: Vicks Sinex.
eucalyptus oil.
Use: Flavor; antitussive; decongestant, nasal; expectorant; analgesic, topical.
See: Victors.
W/Camphor, Menthol.
See: Vicks VapoRub.
•**eucatropine hydrochloride.** (you-CAT-troe-peen) *USP.*
Use: Pharmaceutical necessity for ophthalmic dosage form; anticholinergic, ophthalmic.
eucatropine hydrochloride. (Glogau) Crystal, Bot. g.
Use: Pharmaceutical necessity for ophthalmic dosage form; anticholinergic, ophthalmic.
Eucerin. (Beiersdorf) Unscented moisturizing formula. **Creme:** Jar 120 g, lb. **Lot.:** Bot. 240 mL, 480 mL. *OTC.*
Use: Emollient.
Eucerin Cleansing. (Beiersdorf) Sodium laureth sulfate, cocoamphocarboxyglycinate, cocamidopropyl betaine, cocamide MEA, PEG-7 glyceryl cocoate, PEG-5 lanolate, PEG-120 methyl glucose dioleate, lanolin alcohol, imidazolidinyl urea. Soap free. Lot. Bot. 240 mL. *OTC.*
Use: Dermatologic, cleanser.
Eucerin Dry Skin Care Daily Facial. (Beiersdorf) Ethylhexyl p-methoxycinnamate, titanium dioxide, 2-phenylbenzimidazole-5-sulfonic acid, 2-ethylhexyl salicylate, mineral oil, cetearyl alcohol, castor oil, lanolin alcohol, EDTA. SPF 20. Lot. Bot. 120 mL. *OTC.*
Use: Sunscreen.
Eucerin Itch-Relief Moisturizing. (Beiersdorf) Menthol 0.15%, glycerin, mineral oil, cetyl alcohol, *Oenothera biennis* (evening primrose oil). Spray. 200 mL. *OTC.*
Use: Emollient.
Eucerin Moisturizing Face. (Beiersdorf) Alcohols, castor oil, dimethicone, EDTA, ensulizole 2%, glycerin, glyceryl, lactic acid, octinoxate 7.5%, ocitasalate 4.5%, PEG, titanium dioxide 2.38%, zinc oxide 4.85%. SPF 30. Fragrance free. Lot. 118 mL. *OTC.*
Use: Emollient.
Eucerin Plus. (Beiersdorf) Mineral oil, hydrogenated castor oil, sodium lactate 5%, urea 5%, glycerin, lanolin alcohol. Lot. Bot. 177 mL. *OTC.*
Use: Emollient.
eucodal.
See: Oxycodone.
eucupin dihydrochloride. Isoamylhydrocupreine dihydrochloride.
Eudal-SR. (Forest) Pseudoephedrine 120 mg, guaifenesin 400 mg. SR Tab. Bot. 100s. *Rx.*
Use: Decongestant, expectorant.
euflavine.
See: Acriflavine.
Euflexxa. (Ferring) Sodium hyaluronate 10 mg/mL. Inj. Prefilled syringes. 2 mL. *Rx.*
Use: Physical adjunct.
•**eugenol.** (you-jeh-nole) *USP.*
Use: Dental analgesic; oral anesthetic.
See: Benzodent.
eukadol.
See: Dihydrohydroxycodeinone.
Eulcin. (Leeds) Methscopolamine bromide 2.5 mg, butabarbital sodium 10 mg, aluminum hydroxide gel, dried, 250 mg, magnesium trisilicate 250 mg. Tab. Bot. 100s. *Rx.*
Use: Antacid; anticholinergic; antispasmodic; hypnotic; sedative.

Eumydrin Drops. (Sanofi-Synthelabo) Atropine methonitrate. *Rx.*
Use: Anticholinergic; antispasmodic.
euneryl.
See: Phenobarbital.
Euphorbia Compound. (Sherwood Davis & Geck) *Euphorbia pilulifera* fluid extract 1.5 mL, lobelia tincture 2.2 mL, nitroglycerin spirit 0.29 mL, sodium iodide 1.04 g, sodium bromide 1.04 g, alcohol 24%/30 mL. Bot. Pt, gal. *Rx.*
Use: Expectorant; hypnotic; sedative.
euphorbia pilulifera.
W/Phenyl salicylate and various oils.
See: Rayderm.
Eupractone. (Baxter PPI) Dimethadione.
•**euprocin hydrochloride.** (YOU-pro-sin) USAN.
Use: Anesthetic, local.
euquinine. Quinine ethyl carbonate.
Use: Antimalarial; antipyretic.
Eurax. (Bristol-Myers Squibb) Crotamiton. **Cream:** 10% in vanishing base. Cetyl alcohol. Tube 60 g. **Lotion:** 10% in emollient base. Cetyl alcohol. Bot. 60 g, 454 g. *Rx.*
Use: Scabicide; pediculicide.
•**evabotulinumtoxinA.** (E-va-BOT-ue-LYE-num TOX-in-AY) USAN.
Use: Botulinum toxin.
Evac. (Burgin-Arden) **Supp.:** Sodium bicarbonate, sodium biphosphate, dioctyl sodium sulfosuccinate 50 mg. Supp. **Tab.:** Guar gum 300 mg, danthron 50 mg, sodium 100 mg. Tab. *OTC.*
Use: Laxative.
•**evacetrapib.** (E-va-SET-ra-pib) USAN.
Use: Cardiovascular agent.
Evactol. (Delta Pharmaceutical Group) Docusate sodium 100 mg, sodium carboxymethyl cellulose 200 mg. Cap. Pkg. 10s. Bot. 10s, 30s, 100s. *OTC.*
Use: Laxative.
Evac-U-Gen. (Lee Pharmaceuticals) Sennosides 10 mg. Sugar. Chew. Tab. 35s. *OTC.*
Use: Laxative.
Evamist. (Ther-Rx) Estradiol 1.53 mg. Alcohol, octisalate. Spray Soln. 8.1 mL (56 sprays of 90 mcL). *Rx.*
Use: Estrogen, sex hormone.
Evans Blue. *USP.*
Use: Diagnostic aid (blood volume determination).
Evans Blue Dye. (New World Trading Corp.) Evans blue dye 5 mL. Inj. *Rx.*
Use: Diagnostic aid.
Evarrest. (Ethicon) Fibrinogen 7.8 mg and thrombin (human) 31.5 units per cm^2. Albumin (human). Preservative free. Patch; topical. 10.2 × 10.2 cm. 1s. *Rx.*
Use: Fibrin sealant, human.
•**evatanepag.** (EV-a-ta-NEP-ag) USAN.
Use: Treatment of fracture.
•**evatanepag sodium.** (EV-a-ta-NEP-ag) USAN.
Use: Treatment of fracture.
•**evernimicin.** (E-ver-ni-MYE-sin) USAN.
Use: Antibacterial.
•**everolimus.** (e-ver-OH-li-mus) USAN.
Use: Immunosuppressant.
See: Afinitor.
Afinitor Disperz.
Evicyl Tablets. (Sanofi-Synthelabo) Inositol hexanicotinate. *Rx.*
Use: Hypolipidemic; peripheral vasodilator.
Eviron. (Delta Pharmaceutical Group) Ferrous fumarate 160 mg, copper 1 mg, ascorbic acid 75 mg. Tab. *OTC.*
Use: Mineral, vitamin supplement.
Evista. (Eli Lilly) Raloxifene 60 mg, lactose. Tab. Unit-of-use. 30s, 100s, 2000s. *Rx.*
Use: Osteoporosis prevention; sex hormone, selective estrogen receptor modulator.
E-Vital Creme. (Taylor Pharmaceuticals) Vitamins E 100 units, A 250 units, D 100 units, d-panthenol 0.2%, allantoin 0.1%/g. Jar 2 oz, lb. *OTC.*
Use: Emollient.
Evithrom. (J & J Wound Management) Thrombin (human origin) 800 to 1,200 units/mL. Soln., frozen; topical. Single-use vial. 2 mL, 5 mL, 20 mL. *Rx.*
Use: Topical hemostatic.
Evoclin. (GlaxoSmithKline) Clindamycin 1%. Cetyl alcohol, dehydrated alcohol (ethanol 58%), stearyl alcohol. Foam. 50 g (pressurized with a hydrocarbon [propane/butane] propellant). *Rx.*
Use: Anti-infective, topical.
•**evodenoson.** (E-voe-DEN-oh-son) USAN.
Use: Agent for glaucoma.
•**evolocumab.** (E-voe-LOK-ue-mab) USAN.
Use: Treatment of hyperlipidemia.
Evoxac. (Daiichi) Cevimeline hydrochloride 30 mg, lactose. Cap. Bot. 100s, 500s. *Rx.*
Use: Sjögran syndrome; dry mouth.
Exalgo. (Alza) Hydromorphone hydrochloride 8 mg, 12 mg, 16 mg, 32 mg. BHT, lactose, PEG. ER Tab. 100s. *c-II.*
Use: Opioid analgesic.
Exall-D. (Hawthorn) Carbetapentane citrate 10 mg, guaifenesin 100 mg,

pseudoephedrine hydrochloride 30 mg. Saccharin, sorbitol. Alcohol free, dye free, and sugar free. Fruit gum flavor. Liq. 473 mL. *Rx.*
Use: Upper respiratory combination, antitussive and expectorant combination.

•**exametazime.** (EX-ah-MET-ah-zeem) USAN.
Use: Diagnostic aid (regional cerebral perfusion imaging).

•**exaprolol hydrochloride.** (EX-ah-PRO-lahl) USAN.
Use: Antiadrenergic (β-receptor).

•**exatecan mesylate.** (ex-a-TE-can) USAN.
Use: Antineoplastic.

Ex-Caloric Wafers. (Eastern Research) Carboxymethylcellulose 181 mg, methylcellulose 272 mg. Bot. 100s, 500s, 5000s. *OTC.*
Use: Dietary aid.

Excedrin Back & Body Extra Strength. (Novartis Consumer Health) Acetaminophen 250 mg, buffered aspirin 250 mg. Tab. 24s. *OTC.*
Use: Nonnarcotic analgesic.

Excedrin Extra Strength. (Novartis Consumer Health) Acetaminophen 250 mg, aspirin 250 mg, caffeine 65 mg, saccharin. **Cap.:** Bot. 24s, 50s, 100s, 175s, 275s. **Tab.:** Bot. 24s, 50s, 100s, 175s, 275s. **Geltab.:** Bot. 24s, 40s, 80s. *OTC.*
Use: Analgesic combination.

Excedrin Migraine. (Novartis Consumer Health) Acetaminophen 250 mg, aspirin 250 mg, caffeine 65 mg. Tab. Bot. 50s, 100s. *OTC.*
Use: Analgesic combination.

Excedrin P.M. (Novartis Consumer Health) **Tab.:** Acetaminophen 500 mg, diphenhydramine citrate 38 mg. Parabens, mineral oil. 24s, 50s, 100s. **Cap.:** Acetaminophen 500 mg, diphenhydramine citrate 38 mg. 24s, 50s, 100s. **Liq.:** Acetaminophen 167 mg, diphenhydramine hydrochloride 8.3 mg per 5 mL; acetaminophen 1,000 mg, diphenhydramine hydrochloride 50 mg per 30 mL. Alcohol 10%, sucrose. Wild berry flavor. 180 mL. *OTC.*
Use: Analgesic; sleep aid.

Excedrin Sinus Headache. (Novartis Consumer Health) Phenylephrine hydrochloride 5 mg, acetaminophen 325 mg. Film-coated. Tab. 24s. *OTC.*
Use: Upper respiratory combination, decongestant and analgesic.

Excedrin Tension Headache. (Novartis Consumer Health) Acetaminophen 500 mg, caffeine 65 mg. Parabens. Caplets, Geltabs. 50s, 100s. *OTC.*
Use: Nonnarcotic analgesic combination.

Excita Extra. (Durex) Nonoxynol-9 8% Ribbed Condom. Box 3s, 12s, 36s. *OTC.*
Use: Condom with spermicide.

ExeCof. (Larken) Dextromethorphan HBr 60 mg, guaifenesin 1000 mg, phenylephrine hydrochloride 40 mg. Dye free. ER Tab. 100s. *Rx.*
Use: Upper respiratory combination, antitussive and expectorant.

ExeFen-IR. (Larken) Guaifenesin 400 mg, pseudoephedrine hydrochloride 60 mg. Tab. 100s. *OTC.*
Use: Upper respiratory combination, decongestant and expectorant combination.

Exelderm. (Ranbaxy) Sulconazole nitrate 1%. Cream: Tube. 15 g, 30 g, 60 g. Soln.: 30 mL. *Rx.*
Use: Anti-infective, antifungal agent.

Exelon. (Novartis) Rivastigmine. **Cap.:** As rivastigmine tartrate. 1.5 mg, 3 mg, 4.5 mg, 6 mg. 60s. **Transdermal Patch:** 4.6 mg/24 h (rivastigmine 9 mg per transdermal system, 5 cm^2), 9.5 mg/24 h (rivastigmine 18 mg per transdermal system, 10 cm^2), 13.3 mg/24 h (rivastigmine 27 mg per transdermal system, 15 cm^2). 30s. *Rx.*
Use: Cholinesterase inhibitor.

•**exemestane.** (ex-e-MES-tane) USAN.
Use: Antineoplastic.
See: Aromasin.

exemestane.
Use: Hormonal therapy of metastatic breast carcinoma. [Orphan Drug]

exemestane. (Various Mfr.) Exemestane 25 mg. May contain mannitol, methylparaben, PEG, polydextrose, sucrose. Tab. 30s. *Rx.*
Use: Hormone, aromatase inhibitor.

•**exenatide.** (ex-EN-a-tide) USAN.
Use: Antidiabetic agent, incretin mimetic agent.
See: Bydureon.
Byetta.

ExeTuss-DM. (Larken) Dextromethorphan hydrobromide 25 mg, guaifenesin 600 mg, phenylephrine hydrochloride 20 mg. Dye free and sugar free. ER Tab. 100s. *Rx.*
Use: Upper respiratory combination, antitussive and expectorant combination.

Exforge. (Novartis) Amlodipine besylate/valsartan 5 mg/160 mg, 5 mg/320 mg, 10 mg/160 mg, 10 mg/320 mg. Film-

coated. Tab. 30s, 90s, UD 100s. *Rx.*
Use: Antihypertensive combination.

Exforge HCT. (Novartis) Hydrochlorothiazide/amlodipine/valsartan. 12.5 mg/5 mg/160 mg, 12.5 mg/10 mg/160 mg, 25 mg/5 mg/160 mg, 25 mg/10 mg/160 mg, 25 mg/10 mg/320 mg. Film coated. Tab. 30s, 90s. *Rx.*
Use: Antihypertensive combination.

Exidine-4 Scrub. (Xttrium) Chlorhexidine gluconate 4%, isopropyl alcohol 4%. Soln. Bot. 120 mL, 240 mL, 480 mL, 887 mL, gal. *OTC.*
Use: Antiseptic; antimicrobial.

Exidine Skin Cleanser. (Xttrium) Chlorhexidine gluconate 4%, isopropyl alcohol 4%. Bot. 120 mL, 240 mL, 16 oz, 32 oz, gal. *OTC.*
Use: Antiseptic; antimicrobial.

Exidine-2 Scrub. (Baxter PPI) Chlorhexidine gluconate 2%, isopropyl alcohol 4%. Soln. Bot. 120 mL. *OTC.*
Use: Antiseptic; antimicrobial.

exisulind.
Use: Investigational apoptotic antineoplastic drug.

Exjade. (Novartis) Deferasirox 125 mg, 250 mg, 500 mg. Lactose. Tab. for Oral Susp. 30s. *Rx.*
Use: Chelating agent.

ex-lax. (Novartis Consumer Health) Sennosodes 15 mg, sucrose. Tab. Pkg. 8s, 30s, 60s. *OTC.*
Use: Laxative.

ex-lax Chocolated. (Novartis Consumer Health) Sennosides 15 mg, sugar, oil, dry milk, chocolated. Tab. Pkg. 6s, 18s, 48s. *OTC.*
Use: Laxative.

ex-lax Gentle Strength. (Novartis Consumer Health) Docusate sodium 65 mg, sennosides 10 mg, lactose, methylparaben, polydextrose. Tab. Box. 24s. *OTC.*
Use: Laxative.

ex-lax, Maximum Relief. (Novartis Consumer Health) Sennosides 25 mg, sucrose. Tab. Pkg. 24s, 48s. *OTC.*
Use: Laxative.

ex-lax Stool Softener. (Novartis Consumer Health) Docusate sodium 100 mg, methylparabens. Tab. Bot. 40s. *OTC.*
Use: Laxative.

ex-lax Ultra. (Novartis Consumer Health) Bisacodyl 5 mg. Lactose, methylparaben. Coated. Tab. 24s. *OTC.*
Use: Irritant or stimulant laxative.

Exoderm. (A.G. Marin Pharmaceuticals) Salicylic acid 3%, sulfur 10%. Soap. 91.67 mL. *OTC.*
Use: Topical anti-infective, antifungal combination.

Exoten-C Pain Relief. (MedChem) Capsaicin 0.001%, menthol 10%, methyl salicylate 20%, alcohol, glycerin, trolamine, vitamin E. Lot. 113.4 mL. *OTC.*
Use: Rub and liniment.

Exparel. (Pacira Pharmaceuticals) Bupivacaine liposome 13.3 mg/mL (1.3%). Preservative free. Inj., Susp. Single-use vial. 10 mL, 20 mL. *Rx.*
Use: Injectable local anesthetic, amide local anesthetic.

expectorant and antitussive combinations.
Use: Upper respiratory combination.

expectorant and decongestant combinations.
Use: Upper respiratory combination.

expectorant, antihistamine, and decongestant combinations.
Use: Upper respiratory combination.

expectorant, antitussive, and decongestant combinations.
Use: Upper respiratory combination.

Expectorant DM Cough Syrup. (Weeks & Leo) Dextromethorphan HBr 15 mg, guaifenesin 100 mg/5 mL, alcohol 7.125%. Bot. 6 oz. *OTC.*
Use: Antitussive, expectorant.

expectorants.
See: Guaifenesin.

Expendable Blood Collection Unit ACD. (Baxter PPI) Citric acid 540 mg, sodium citrate 1.49 g, dextrose 1.65 g/67.5 mL. *Rx.*
Use: Anticoagulant.

Exratuss. (Midlothian) Carbetapentane tannate 30 mg, chlorpheniramine tannate 4 mg, phenylephrine tannate 12.5 mg per 5 mL. Methylparaben, saccharin, sucrose. Strawberry flavor. Susp. 118 mL. *Rx.*
Use: Antitussive.

Extavia. (Novartis) Interferon beta-1b 0.3 mg. Human albumin 15 mg, mannitol 15 mg per vial. Preservative free. Single-use 3 mL capacity vial with 1.2 mL prefilled syringe of diluents (sodium chloride 0.54%), alcohol prep pads, and vial adaptor w/attached needle for each drug vial. Blister unit 15s. *Rx.*
Use: Immunologic agent, immunomodulator.

extended-spectrum penicillins.
Use: Anti-infective.

Extendryl. (Auriga) **Chew. Tab.:** Chlorpheniramine maleate 2 mg, phenylephrine hydrochloride 10 mg, methscopolamine nitrate 1.25 mg. Mannitol, sugar. Root beer flavor. Chew. Tab. Bot. 100s. **Syrup:** Dexchlorpheniramine

maleate 1 mg, phenylephrine hydrochloride 10 mg, methscopolamine nitrate 1.25 mg per 5 mL. Sorbitol, sugar. Root beer flavor. Bot. 473 mL. *Rx.*
Use: Upper respiratory combination, decongestant, antihistamine, and anticholinergic combination.

Extendryl GCP. (Auriga) Carbetapentane citrate 15 mg, guaifenesin 100 mg, phenylephrine hydrochloride 5 mg per 5 mL. Alcohol free. Maltitol, saccharin, sorbitol. Strawberry flavor. Oral Soln. 473 mL. *Rx.*
Use: Upper respiratory combination, antitussive combination.

Extendryl PEM. (Auriga) Methscopolamine nitrate 1.25 mg, phenylephrine hydrochloride 30 mg. ER Tab. 100s. *Rx.*
Use: Upper respiratory combination, decongestant, antihistamine, and anticholinergic combination.

Exten Strone 10. (Schlicksup) Estradiol valerate 10 mg/mL. Vial 10 mL. *Rx.*
Use: Estrogen.

Extenzyme Soflens Protein Cleaner. (Allergan) Papain, sodium chloride, sodium carbonate, sodium borate, edetate disodium. Vial w/Tab. 24s. Refill 36s. *OTC.*
Use: Contact lens care.

Extina. (Prestium Pharma) Ketoconazole 2%. Cetyl alcohol, ethanol 58%, stearyl alcohol. Foam. 50 g, 100g. *Rx.*
Use: Topical anti-infective, antifungal agent.

Extra Action Cough. (Rugby) Dextromethorphan hydrobromide 10 mg, guaifenesin 100 mg. Cherry flavoring, corn syrup, glycerin, menthol, saccharin, sodium benzoate. Syrup. 473 mL. *OTC.*
Use: Upper respiratory combination, antitussive with expectorant.

Extraneal. (Baxter) Icodextrin 75 g, Na 132 mEq, Ca 3.5 mEq, Mg 0.5 mEq, Cl 96 mEq, lactate 40 mEq/L, osmolarity 282 to 286 mOsm/L. Soln. *Ultrabag* and *Ambu-Flex* 1.5, 2, 2.5 L. *Rx.*
Use: Peritoneal dialysis solution.

extraocular irrigating solutions.
Use: Ophthalmic nonsurgical adjuncts.
See: AK-Rinse.
Collyrium for Fresh Eyes Wash.
Eye Stream.
Eye Irrigating Solution.
Irrigate Eye Wash.
Optigene.

Extra Strength Adprin-B. (Pfeiffer) Aspirin 500 mg, calcium carbonate, magnesium carbonate, magnesium oxide. Tab, coated. Bot. 130s. *OTC.*
Use: Analgesic.

Extra Strength Alka-Seltzer Effervescent. (Bayer Consumer Care) Sodium bicarbonate (heat-treated) 1985 mg, aspirin 500 mg, citric acid 1000 mg, sodium 588 mg. Tab. Bot. 12s and 24s. *OTC.*
Use: Antacid.

Extra Strength Aspirin Capsules. (Walgreen) Aspirin 500 mg. Bot. 80s. *OTC.*
Use: Analgesic.

Extra Strength Bayer Enteric 500 Aspirin. (Bayer) Aspirin 500 mg. Tab. Enteric coated. Bot. 60s. *OTC.*
Use: Analgesic.

Extra Strength Bayer Plus. (Bayer) Aspirin 500 mg with calcium carbonate, magnesium carbonate, magnesium oxide. Tab. Bot. 30s, 60s. *OTC.*
Use: Salicylate, aspirin, buffered.

Extra Strength Excedrin. (Bristol-Myers Squibb) Acetaminophen 250 mg, aspirin 250 mg, caffeine 65 mg. Cap. Bot. 24s, 50s, 80s. Tab. Bot. 30s, 60s, 100s, 165s, 225s, Pkg. 12s. *OTC.*
Use: Analgesic combination.

Extra Strength 5 mg Biotin Forte. (Vitaline) Vitamins B_1 10 mg, B_2 10 mg, B_3 40 mg, B_5 10 mg, B_6 25 mg, B_{12} 10 mcg, C 100 mg, biotin 5 mg, FA 800 mcg. Tab. Bot. 60s, 1000s. *OTC.*
Use: Mineral, vitamin supplement.

Extra Strength Gas-X. (Novartis) Simethicone 125 mg. Tab. Pkg. 18s. *OTC.*
Use: Antiflatulent.

Extra-Virt Plus DHA. (Virtus Pharmaceuticals) Folic acid 1.25 mg, calcium 160 mg, iron 29 mg, vitamins D 800 units, E 30 units, B_6 25 mg, C 28 mg, biotin 250 mcg, DHA 350 mg, docusate calcium 55 mg. Beeswax, glycerin, soy lecithin. Cap.; softgel. 30s. *Rx.*
Use: Prenatal vitamin with minerals.

Extreme Cold Formula. (Major) Pseudoephedrine hydrochloride 30 mg, chlorpheniramine maleate 1 mg, dextromethorphan HBr 15 mg, acetaminophen 500 mg. Cap. Bot. 10s. *OTC.*
Use: Analgesic, antihistamine, antitussive, decongestant.

Eye, Face, and Body Wash Station. (Lavoptik) Sodium chloride 0.49 g, sodium biphosphate 0.4 g, sodium phosphate 0.45 g/100 mL, benzalkonium chloride 0.005%. Bot. 32 oz. *OTC.*
Use: Emergency wash.

Eye Irrigating Solution. (Rugby) Sodium chloride, sodium phosphate mono- and dibasic, benzalkonium chloride, EDTA. Soln. Bot. 118 mL. *OTC.*
Use: Irrigant, ophthalmic.

Eye Mo. (Sanofi-Synthelabo) Boric acid, benzalkonium chloride, phenylephrine hydrochloride, zinc sulfate. *OTC.*
Use: Astringent, ophthalmic.

Eye Stream. (Alcon) Sodium chloride 0.64%, potassium chloride 0.075%, magnesium chloride hexahydrate 0.03%, calcium chloride dihydrate 0.048%, sodium acetate trihydrate 0.39%, sodium citrate dihydrate 0.17%, benzalkonium chloride 0.013%. Bot. 30 mL, 118 mL. *OTC.*
Use: Irrigant, ophthalmic.

Eye Wash. (Bausch & Lomb) Boric acid, potassium chloride, EDTA, sodium carbonate, benzalkonium chloride 0.01%. Soln. Bot. 118 mL. *OTC.*
Use: Irrigant, ophthalmic.

Eye Wash. (Goldline) Boric acid, potassium chloride, EDTA, anhydrous sodium carbonate, benzalkonium chloride 0.1%. Soln. Bot. 118 mL. *OTC.*
Use: Irrigant, ophthalmic.

Eye Wash. (Lavoptik) Sodium chloride 0.49%, sodium biphosphate 0.4%, sodium phosphate 0.45%, benzalkonium chloride 0.005%. Soln. Bot. 180 mL with eye cup. *OTC.*
Use: Irrigant, ophthalmic.

Eylea. (Regeneron Pharmaceuticals Inc) Aflibercept 40 mg/mL. Preservative free. Soln.; Inj. Single-use vial. *Rx.*
Use: Selective vascular endothelial growth factor antagonist.

EZ Char. (Paddock) Activated charcoal 25 g. Bentonite, magnesium 35 mg, potassium 18 mg, sodium 57 mg. Pellets for Susp. 25 g. *OTC.*
Use: Detoxification agent, antidote.

EZ Detect. (Biomerica) Occult blood screening test. Kit 3s.
Use: Diagnostic aid.

EZ Detect Strep-A Test. (Biomerica) Coated stick test for detection of group A streptococci taken directly from a throat swab.
Use: Diagnostic aid.

Eze Pain. (Halsey Drug) Acetaminophen 2.5 g, salicylamide, caffeine. Cap. Bot. 21s. *OTC.*
Use: Analgesic combination.

•**ezetimibe.** (ezz-ET-ih-mibe) USAN.
Use: Antihyperlipidemic.
See: Zetia.
W/Atorvastatin.
See: Liptruzet.
W/Simvastatin.
See: Vytorin.

EzFe Forte. (R.A. McNeil) Folic acid 1 mg, iron 155 mg, vitamins B_1 1.5 mg, B_2 1.7 mg, B_3 20 mg, B_5 10 mg, B_6 25 mg, B_{12} 1,000 mcg, C 45 mg, biotin 150 mcg. Cap. 90s. *Rx.*
Use: Prenatal vitamin with minerals.

EZFE 200. (R.A. McNeil) Iron 200 mg. Cap. 100s. *OTC.*
Use: Dietary supplement.

E-Z Gas II. (EZ EM) Citric acid 1,530 mg, simethicone 40 mg, sodium bicarbonate 2,210 mg. Saccharin. Orange flavor. Effervescent Gran. 4 g packet. 50s. *OTC.*
Use: Antacid combination.

E-Z-HD. (EZ EM) Barium sulfate 98%. Parabens, simethicone, sorbitol. Strawberry-vanilla flavor. Susp. 340 g. *Rx.*
Use: Radiopaque agent, miscellaneous gastrointestinal contrast agent.

Ezide. (Econo Med Pharmaceuticals) Hydrochlorothiazide 50 mg. Tab. Bot. 100s, 1000s. *Rx.*
Use: Diuretic.

•**ezlopitant.** (ez-LOE-pi-tant) USAN.
Use: Emesis; pain; inflammation.

•**ezogabine.** (e-ZOG-a-been) USAN.
Use: Antiepileptic.
See: Potiga.

Ezol. (Stewart-Jackson Pharmacal) Butalbital 50 mg, caffeine 40 mg, acetaminophen 325 mg. Bot. 100s. *Rx.*
Use: Analgesic; hypnotic; sedative.

Ezol #3. (Stewart-Jackson Pharmacal) Acetaminophen 650 mg, codeine 30 mg. Bot. 100s. *c-III.*
Use: Analgesic combination; narcotic.

E-Z-Paque. (EZ EM) Barium sulfate 96%. Saccharin, simethicone, sorbitol. Strawberry-lemon flavor. Susp. 176 g, 285 g, 1,200 g. *Rx.*
Use: Radiopaque agent, miscellaneous gastrointestinal contrast agent.

E-Z-Paque Liquid. (EZ EM) Barium sulfate 60%. Saccharin, simethicone, sodium benzoate, sorbitol. Susp. 355 mL, 1,900 mL. *Rx.*
Use: Radiopaque agent, miscellaneous gastrointestinal contrast agent.

E-Z-Paste. (EZ EM) Barium sulfate 60%. Parabens, saccharin, simethicone, sorbitol. Vanilla flavor. Cream. 454 g. *Rx.*
Use: Radiopaque agent, miscellaneous gastrointestinal contrast agent.

F

Fabior. (Stiefel Laboratories) Tazarotene 0.1%. Lt. mineral oil. Foam; topical. 50 g, 100 g. *Rx.*
Use: Retinoid.

Fabrase.
Use: Immunomodulator Fabry disease. [Orphan Drug]

Fabrazyme. (Genzyme) Agalsidase beta. **5.5 mg:** 5 mg/mL when reconstituted. Mannitol 33 mg, sodium phosphate monobasic monohydrate 3 mg, sodium phosphate dibasic heptahydrate 8.8 mg. Preservative free. Pow. for Inj., lyophilized. Single-use vials. 5 mL. **37 mg (5 mg/mL when reconstituted):** Mannitol 222 mg, sodium phosphate monobasic monohydrate 20.4 mg, sodium phosphate dibasic heptahydrate 59.2 mg/vial. Preservative free. Pow. for Inj., lyophilized. Single-use vials. 20 mL. *Rx.*
Use: Fabry disease.

Face CÔTZ. (Fallene) Titanium dioxide 8%, zinc oxide 3.8%, dimethicone, PEG. SPF 40. Lot. 45 mL. *OTC.*
Use: Sunscreen.

Faces Only Moisturizing Sunblock by Coppertone. (Schering-Plough) Ethylhexyl p-methoxycinnamate, oxybenzone. SPF 15. Lot. Bot. 55.5 mL. *OTC.*
Use: Sunscreen.

Fact Home Pregnancy Test. (Johnson & Johnson) Accurate test for pregnancy in 45 minutes, for use as early as 3 days after a missed period. Test kit 1s.
Use: Diagnostic aid.

Factive. (Oscient) Gemifloxacin mesylate 320 mg, film-coated. Tab. Unit of use 5s, 7s. *Rx.*
Use: Fluoroquinolone.

factor VIII.
See: Antihemophilic factor.

factor IX, coagulation.
See: Coagulation Factor IX.

•**factor IX complex.** (FAK-tor) *USP.*
Use: Hemostatic.
See: Alpha Nine SD.
Konyne 80.
Mononine.
Profilnine SD.

factor IX complex, vapor heated Bebulin VH immuno. (Immuno U.S.) Purified, sterile, stable freeze-dried concentrate of coagulation Factor IX (Christmas Factor), Factors II (prothrombin) and X (Stuart Prower), low amounts of Factor VII, ≤ 0.15 International Units (units) heparin/units Factor IX. Pow. for Inj. Single-dose vial w/Sterile Water for Injection, double-ended needle, filter needle. *Rx.*
Use: Hemostatic.

factor IX concentrates. (FAK-tor)
Use: Antihemophilic agents.
See: AlphaNine SD.
Bebulin VH.
BeneFIX.
Mononine.
Profilnine SD.

factor IX (recombinant).
See: Rixubis.

factor XIII concentrate. (FAK-tor)
Use: Antihemophilic agent.
See: Corifact.

Fact Plus. (Johnson & Johnson) Reagent in-home kit for urine testing. Pregnancy test. Kit 1s, 2s.
Use: Diagnostic aid.

•**fadolmidine hydrochloride.** (fa-DOL-mid-ine) USAN.
Use: Analgesic (spinal).

•**fadrozole hydrochloride.** (FAHD-rah-ZOLE) USAN.
Use: Antineoplastic.

•**faldaprevir.** (fal-DA-pre-vir) USAN.
Use: Treatment of chronic hepatitis C.

•**faldaprevir sodium.** (fal-DA-pre-vir) USAN.
Use: Treatment of chronic hepatitis C.

Falgos. (Sanofi-Synthelabo) Acetylsalicylic acid. Tab. *OTC.*
Use: Analgesic.

•**falimarev (CEA, MUC-1, fowlpox virus).** (fa-LIM-a-rev) USAN.
Use: Antineoplastic.

Falmina. (NorthStar) Ethinyl estradiol 20 mcg, levonorgestrel 0.1 mg. Lactose, PEG. Tab. 28s w/7 inert tablets (lactose, polydextrose, PEG). *Rx.*
Use: Oral monophasic contraceptive.

Falmonox. (Sanofi-Synthelabo) Teclozan. Susp., Tab. *Rx.*
Use: Amebicide.

•**famciclovir.** (fam-SIGH-kloe-veer) USAN.
Use: Antiviral agent, antiherpes virus agent.
See: Famvir.

famciclovir. (Teva) Famciclovir 125 mg, 250 mg, 500 mg. May contain lactose, PEG. Tab. 30s. *Rx.*
Use: Antiviral agent, antiherpes virus agent.

•**famotidine.** (fah-MOE-tih-den) *USP.*
Use: Histamine H_2 antagonist.
See: Heartburn Relief Max Strength.
Pepcid.
Pepcid AC.
Pepcid AC Maximum Strength.
Pepcid AC Maximum Strength EZ Chews.

Pepcid RPD.
W/Calcium Carbonate, Magnesium Hydroxide.
See: Acid Reducer + Antacid.
Dual Action Complete.
Pepcid Complete Dual Action.
Tums Dual Action.
W/Ibuprofen.
See: Duexis.

famotidine. (Baxter) Famotidine 20 mg/50 mL. Inj. (premixed). Single-dose *Galaxy* containers. 50 mL. *Rx.*
Use: Histamine H_2 antagonist.

famotidine. (Ivax) Famotidine 10 mg. Tab. Bot. 18s, 30s, 50s, 70s. *OTC.*
Use: Histamine H_2 antagonist.

famotidine. (Various Mfr.) Famotidine. **Tab.:** 20 mg, 40 mg. May contain lactose. Bot. 30s, 100s, 500s, 1000s, UD 100s; *Robot–Ready* 25s (20 mg only). **Pow. for Susp.:** 40 mg per 5 mL. May contain parabens, sodium benzoate, sucrose, sugar. 50 mL. **Inj.:** 10 mg/mL. May contain mannitol or benzyl alcohol. Single-dose vials. 1 mL, 2 mL. Multidose vials. 4 mL, 20 mL, 50 mL. *Rx.*
Use: Histamine H_2 antagonist.

famotidine, calcium carbonate, and magnesium hydroxide combinations.
Use: Histamine H_2 antagonist.
See: Dual Action Complete.
Pepcid Complete.

•**famotine hydrochloride.** (FAM-oh-teen) USAN.
Use: Antiviral.

•**fampridine.** (FAHM-prih-DEEN) USAN.
Use: Symptomatic treatment of multiple sclerosis.

Famvir. (Novartis) Famciclovir 125 mg, 250 mg, 500 mg. Lactose. Film-coated. Tab. Bot. 30s, UD 50s (500 mg only). *Rx.*
Use: Management of acute herpes zoster (shingles).

•**fananserin.** (fan-AN-ser-in) USAN.
Use: Antipsychotic; antischizophrenic (dual dopamine D_4 and serotonin 5-HT_2 receptor antagonist).

Fanapt. (Novartis) Iloperidone 1 mg, 2 mg, 4 mg, 6 mg, 8 mg, 10 mg, 12 mg. Lactose. Tab. 60s, titration pack (two 1 mg tablets, two 2 mg tablets, two 4 mg tablets, two 6 mg tablets) (1 mg, 2 mg, 4 mg, 6 mg). *Rx.*
Use: Antipsychotic agent, benzisoxazole derivative.

•**fandosentan potassium.** (fan-doe-SEN-tan) USAN.
Use: Pulmonary hypertension.

•**fanetizole mesylate.** (fan-EH-tih-zole) USAN.
Use: Immunoregulator.

•**fantridone hydrochloride.** (FAN-trih-dohn) USAN.
Use: Antidepressant.

Faramals. (Faraday) Vitamins A 10,000 units, D 2000 units, B_1 6 mg, B_2 4 mg, B_6 0.5 mg, folic acid 0.1 mg, C 100 mg, calcium pantothenate 5 mg, niacinamide 30 mg, E 5 units, B_{12} 3 mcg. Tab. Bot. 100s, 250s, 500s, 1000s. *OTC.*
Use: Mineral, vitamin supplement.

Faramals-M. (Faraday) Faramals plus calcium 103 mg, cobalt 0.1 mg, Cu 1 mg, I 0.15 mg, Fe 10 mg, Mg 6 mg, Mo 0.2 mg, P 80 mg, K 5 mg, Zn 1.2 mg. Tab. Bot. 100s, 250s, 500s, 1000s. *OTC.*
Use: Mineral, vitamin supplement.

Faramins. (Faraday) Vitamins B_1 20 mg, B_2 6 mg, C 40 mg, niacinamide 20 mg, calcium pantothenate 3 mg, B_6 0.5 mg, powdered whole dried liver 125 mg, dried debittered yeast 125 mg, choline dihydrogen citrate 20 mg, inositol 20 mg, dl-methionine 20 mg, folic acid 0.1 mg, B_{12} 10 mcg, ferrous gluconate 30 mg, dicalcium phosphate 250 mg, copper sulfate 5 mg, magnesium sulfate 10 mg, manganese sulfate 5 mg, cobalt sulfate 0.2 mg, potassium Cl 2 mg, potassium iodide 0.15 mg. Tab. Bot. 100s, 250s, 500s, 1000s. *OTC.*
Use: Mineral, vitamin supplement.

Faratol. (Faraday) Vitamins A 12,500 units, D 1000 units, B_1 20 mg, B_2 6 mg, B_6 0.5 mg, B_{12} 15 mcg, folic acid 0.1 mg, niacinamide 10 mg, calcium pantothenate 3 mg, C 60 mg, E 5 units, choline dihydrogen citrate 20 mg, inositol 20 mg, dl-methionine 20 mg, whole dried liver 100 mg, dried debittered yeast 100 mg, dicalcium phosphate 200 mg, ferrous gluconate 30 mg, potassium iodide 0.2 mg, magnesium sulfate 7.2 mg, copper sulfate 5 mg, manganese sulfate 3.4 mg, cobalt sulfate 0.2 mg, potassium Cl 1.3 mg, zinc sulfate 2 mg, molybdenum 0.2 mg in a base of alfalfa. Tab. Bot. 100s, 250s, 500s, 1000s. *OTC.*
Use: Mineral, vitamin supplement.

Farbee with Vitamin C. (Major) Vitamins B_1 15 mg, B_2 10.2 mg, B_3 50 mg, B_5 10 mg, B_6 5 mg, C 300 mg. Capl. Bot. 100s, 130s, 1000s. *OTC.*
Use: Vitamin supplement.

Farbital. (Major) Butalbital. Tab. Bot. 100s. *c-III.*
Use: Hypnotic; sedative.

Farbital Compound. (Major) Butalbital, caffeine, aspirin. Cap. Bot. 100s. *c-III.*
Use: Analgesic; hypnotic; sedative.

Farbital Compound with Codeine #3. (Major) Butalbital, caffeine, aspirin, codeine 30 mg. Bot. 1000s. *c-III.*
Use: Analgesic; hypnotic; sedative.

Fareston. (ProStrakan) Toremifene citrate 60 mg. Lactose. Tab. Bot. 30s, 100s. *Rx.*
Use: Antiestrogen, hormone.

•**farletuzumab.** (FAR-le-TOOZ-oo-mab) USAN.
Use: Antineoplastic.

•**faropenem medoxomil.** (FAR-oh-PEN-em) USAN.
Use: Anti-infective.

Farxiga. (Bristol-Myers Squibb Company) Dapagliflozin propanediol 5 mg, 10 mg. Film coated. Lactose. Tab. 30s, 90s, 500s, UD 100s. *Rx.*
Use: Antidiabetic agent, sodium-glucose cotransporter 2 inhibitor.

•**fasiglifam.** (FA-si-GLI-fam) USAN.
Use: Antidiabetic.

•**fasinumab.** (fa-SIN-ue-mab) USAN.
Use: Analgesic.

Faslodex. (AstraZeneca) Fulvestrant 50 mg/mL. Alcohol, benzyl alcohol, castor oil. Inj. Prefilled Syringe. 5 mL. *Rx.*
Use: Hormone, antiestrogen.

Fastlene. (BDI) Caffeine 200 mg. Cap. Bot. 100s, 500s. *OTC.*
Use: CNS stimulant, analeptic.

fat emulsion, intravenous.
See: Intralipid 30%.
Intralipid 20%.
Liposyn 10%.
Liposyn 20%.
Liposyn II 10%.
Liposyn II 20%.
Travamulsion 10%.
Travamulsion 20%.

•**fat, hard.** *NF.*
Use: Pharmaceutic aid (suppository base).

Father John's Medicine Plus. (Oakhurst Co.) Phenylephrine hydrochloride 1.67 mg, chlorpheniramine maleate 0.67 mg, dextromethorphan HBr 1.67 mg per 5 mL. Alcohol free. Liq. Bot. 118 mL. *OTC.*
Use: Upper respiratory combination, antitussive combination.

fat soluble vitamins.
See: Beta-carotene.
Calcifediol.
Calciferol.
Calcijex.
Calcitriol.
Cholecalciferol.
d' ALPHA E 400 Softgels.
d' ALPHA E 1000 Softgels.
Delta-D.
Doxercalciferol.
Drisdol.
Ergocalciferol.
Hectorol.
Mephyton.
Mixed E 400 Softgels.
Mixed E 1000 Softgels.
Palmitate-A 5000.
Paricalcitol.
Phytonadione.
Vita-Plus E.
Vitamin A.
Vitamin D_3.
Vitamin E.
Vitamin E with Mixed Tocopherols.
Vitamin K.
Zemplar.

Fattibase. (Paddock) Preblended fatty acid suppository base composed of triglycerides of coconut oil and palm kernel oil. Jar 1 lb, 5 lb.
Use: Pharmaceutical aid, suppository base.

•**faxeladol.** (FAX-el-a-dole) USAN.
Use: Analgesic.

FazaClo. (Jazz Pharmaceuticals) Clozapine 12.5 mg (phenylalanine 0.87 mg), 25 mg (phenylalanine 1.74 mg), 100 mg (phenylalanine 6.96 mg), 150 mg (phenylalanine 10.44 mg), 200 mg (phenylalanine 13.92 mg). Aspartame, mannitol. Mint flavor. Orally Disintegrating Tab. UD 48s (25 mg, 100 mg, 150 mg, 200 mg), 100s. *Rx.*
Use: Antipsychotic.

fazadinium bromide.
Use: Neuromuscular blocking agent.

•**fazarabine.** (fah-ZAY-rah-BEAN) USAN.
Use: Antineoplastic.

FE Aspartate. (Miller) Ferrous aspartate 112 mg (elemental iron 18 mg)/aspartic acid 85 mg. Tab. 90s. *OTC.*
Use: Mineral supplement.

Feberin. (Arcum) Ferrous gluconate 3 g, vitamins C 25 mg, B_1 2 mg, B_2 1 mg, B_6 1 mg, niacinamide 5 mg. Tab. Bot. 100s, 1000s. *OTC.*
Use: Mineral, vitamin supplement.

febrile antigens. (Laboratory Diagnostics) Group O antigens (somatic) are dyed blue and group H antigens (flagellars) are dyed red for clear identification for detection of bacterial agglutinins, bacterial infections. Vial 5 mL.
Use: Diagnostic aid.

Febrinol. (Eon Labs) Acetaminophen

325 mg. Tab. Bot. 100s, 1000s. *OTC.*
Use: Analgesic.

Fe-Brone. (Forest) Vitamins B_{12} 1 units, folic acid 1 mg, ferrous sulfate exsiccated (powdered) 200 mg, ferrous sulfate exsiccated (timed) 200 mg, C acid 100 mg, B_6 0.5 mg, B_1 2 mg, B_2 1 mg, copper 0.9 mg, zinc 0.5 mg, manganese 0.3 mg. Cap. Bot. 30s, 100s, 1000s. *Rx.*
Use: Mineral, vitamin supplement.

•**febuxostat.** (feb-UX-oh-stat) USAN.
Use: Hyperuricemia; xanthine oxidase/dehydrogenase inhibitor.
See: Uloric.

fecal softeners/surfactants.
See: Colace.
DC Softgels.
Diocto.
Docu.
Docusate Calcium.
Docusate Sodium.
D.O.S.
D-S-S.
ex-lax Stool Softener.
Genasoft.
Modane Soft.
Non-Habit Forming Stool Softener.
Phillips Liqui-Gels.
Regulax SS.
Silace.
Stool Softener.
Stool Softener DC.
Surfak Liquigels.

Fedahist Expectorant. (Schwarz Pharma) Guaifenesin 200 mg, pseudoephedrine hydrochloride 20 mg/5 mL, sorbitol. Alcohol free. *OTC.*
Use: Antihistamine, decongestant.

Fedahist Gyrocaps. (Schwarz Pharma) Pseudoephedrine hydrochloride 65 mg, chlorpheniramine maleate 10 mg. SR Cap. Bot. 100s. *Rx.*
Use: Antihistamine; decongestant.

Fedahist Tablets. (Schwarz Pharma) Pseudoephedrine hydrochloride 60 mg, chlorpheniramine maleate 4 mg, sorbitol (alcohol and sugar free). Tab. Bot. 100s. *Rx.*
Use: Antihistamine; decongestant.

Fedahist Timecaps. (Schwarz Pharma) Pseudoephedrine hydrochloride 120 mg, chlorpheniramine maleate 8 mg. SR Cap. Bot. 100s. *Rx.*
Use: Antihistamine; decongestant.

•**fedratinib.** (fe-DRA-ti-nib) USAN.
Use: Antineoplastic.

Feen-a-Mint. (Schering-Plough) Bisacodyl 5 mg, talc, lactose, sugar. EC Tab. Pkg. 30s. *OTC.*
Use: Laxative.

Feen-a-Mint Dual Formula. (Schering-Plough) Docusate sodium 100 mg, yellow phenolphthalein 65 mg. Tab. Box 15s, 30s, 60s. *OTC.*
Use: Laxative.

Feen-a-Mint Gum. (Schering-Plough) Yellow phenolphthalein 97.2 mg. Chewing gum. Tab. Box 5s, 16s, 40s. *OTC.*
Use: Laxative.

Feg-I. (Western Research) Ferrous gluconate 300 mg. Tab. Handicount 28s (36 bags of 28 tab.). *OTC.*
Use: Mineral supplement.

Feiba NF. (Baxter) Anti-inhibitor coagulant complex 500 units/vial, 1,000 units/vial, 2,500 units/vial. Dry natural rubber latex, sodium chloride 8 mg/mL, trisodium citrate 4 mg/mL. Nanofiltered and vapor heated. Heparin free. Inj., lyophilized Pow. for Soln. Single-dose vial w/*Baxject* needleless transfer device w/20 mL or 50 mL of diluent. *Rx.*
Use: Antihemophilic agent.

•**felbamate.** (FELL-buh-MATE) USAN.
Use: Antiepileptic; treatment of Lennox-Gastaut syndrome [Orphan Drug]
See: Felbatol.

felbamate. (Various Mfr.) Felbamate. **Tab.:** 400 mg, 600 mg. May contain lactose. 30s, 90s, 100s, 180s (600 mg only), 270s, 500s. **Susp.:** 600 mg per 5 mL. May contain glycerin, parabens, polysorbate 80, saccharin, sorbitol. 240 mL, 473 mL, 946 mL. *Rx.*
Use: Adjuvant anticonvulsant.

Felbatol. (Wallace) Felbamate. **Tab.:** 400 mg, 600 mg, lactose. Bot. 100s, UD 100s. **Susp.:** 600 mg/5 mL, sorbitol, parabens, saccharin. Bot. 240 mL, 960 mL. *Rx.*
Use: Antiepileptic. It has been recommended that use of this drug be discontinued if aplastic anemia or hepatic failure occurs unless, in the judgment of the physician, continued therapy is warranted. For further information contact Wallace Labs at 609-655-6000.

•**felbinac.** (FELL-bih-nak) USAN.
Use: Anti-inflammatory.

Feldene. (Pfizer) Piroxicam 10 mg, 20 mg. Lactose. Cap. Bot. 100s. *Rx.*
Use: Nonsteroidal anti-inflammatory agent.

Fellobolic. (Forest) Methandriol dipropionate 50 mg/mL. Inj. Vial 10 mL. *Rx.*

•**felodipine.** (feh-LOW-dih-peen) *USP.*
Use: Vasodilator, calcium channel blocker.

felodipine. (Mutual) Felodipine 2.5 mg,

5 mg, 10 mg. Film-coated. ER Tab. 30s, 90s, 100s, 250s, 500s, 1000s. *Rx.*
Use: Vasodilator, calcium channel blocker.

felodipine and enalapril maleate.
Use: Antihypertensive.

•**felvizumab.** (fell-VYE-zoo-mab) USAN.
Use: Antiviral (systemic), monoclonal antibody.

•**felypressin.** (fell-ih-PRESS-in) USAN.
Use: Vasoconstrictor.

Femagene. (Tennessee Pharmaceutic) Boric acid, sodium borate, lactic acid, menthol, methylbenzethonium Cl, parachlorometaxylenol, lactose, surface-active agents. Pow. 6 oz. *OTC.*
Use: Feminine hygiene.

Femara. (Novartis) Letrozole 2.5 mg. Lactose. Film-coated. Tab. Bot. 30s. *Rx.*
Use: Hormone; aromatase inhibitor.

Femazole. (Major) Metronidazole 250 mg, 500 mg. Tab. **250 mg:** Bot. 100s, 250s, 500s. **500 mg:** Bot. 50s, 100s. *Rx.*
Use: Anti-infective.

Femcaps. (Buffington) Acetaminophen, caffeine, ephedrine sulfate, atropine sulfate. Tab. Sugar, lactose, and salt free. Dispens-a-Kit 500s, Aidpaks 100s. *Rx.*
Use: Analgesic; anticholinergic; antispasmodic; bronchodilator.

Femcon Fe. (Warner Chilcott) Ethinyl estradiol/norethindrone 35 mcg/0.4 mg. Lactose, maltodextrin, sucralose. Spearmint flavor. Chew. Tab. 21s with 7 brown tablets (ferrous fumarate 75 mg). *Rx.*
Use: Oral contraceptive.

Femergin.
See: Ergotamine Tartrate.

Femhrt. (Warner Chilcott) Ethinyl estradiol/norethindrone acetate 2.5 mcg/0.5 mg. Lactose. Tab. 90s, blister card 28s. *Rx.*
Use: Sex hormone, estrogens and progestins combined.

Femidyn.
See: Estrone.

Feminone. (Pharmacia) Ethinyl estradiol 0.05 mg. Tab. Bot. 100s. *Rx.*
Use: Estrogen.

Femiron. (Menley & James Labs, Inc.) Ferrous fumarate 63 mg (iron 20 mg). Tab. Bot. 40s, 120s. *OTC.*
Use: Mineral supplement.

Femotrone. (Bluco) Progesterone in oil 50 mg/mL. Vial 10 mL. *Rx.*
Use: Hormone, progestin.

FemPatch. (Parke-Davis) Estradiol 10.3 mg (0.025 mg/day). Patch. Box. 4s. *Rx.*
Use: Estrogen.

Fem ph. (Pharmics) Glacial acetic acid 0.9%, oxyquinoline sulfate 0.025%, glycerin, PEG 4500. Vaginal jelly. 50 g w/applicator. *OTC.*
Use: Vaginal preparation.

Femring. (Warner Chilcott) Estradiol acetate 0.05 mg/day, 0.1 mg/day. Vaginal Ring. Single packs. *Rx.*
Use: Estrogen, sex hormone.

•**fenalamide.** (fen-AL-am-IDE) USAN.
Use: Muscle relaxant.

fenamisal. Phenyl aminosalicylate.

•**fenamole.** (FEN-ah-mole) USAN.
Use: Anti-inflammatory.

Fenaprin. (Sanofi-Synthelabo) Aspirin, chlormezanone. Tab. *Rx.*
Use: Analgesic; anxiolytic.

Fenarol. (Sanofi-Synthelabo) Chlormezanone 100 mg, 200 mg. Tab. Bot. 100s.
Use: Anxiolytic.

fenarsone.
See: Carbarsone.

•**fenbendazole.** (FEN-BEND-ah-zole) USAN.
Use: Anthelmintic.

•**fenbufen.** (FEN-byoo-fen) USAN.
Use: Anti-inflammatory.

•**fencibutirol.** (fen-sih-BYOO-tih-role) USAN.
Use: Choleretic.

•**fenclofenac.** (FEN-kloe-fen-ACK) USAN.
Use: Anti-inflammatory.

•**fenclonine.** (fen-KLOE-neen) USAN. Under study by Pfizer.
Use: Serotonin inhibitor.

•**fenclorac.** (FEN-kloe-rack) USAN.
Use: Anti-inflammatory.

Fend. (Mine Safety Appliances) **A-2:** Water-soluble cream which forms a physical barrier to water-insoluble irritants. Tube 3 oz, Jar lb. **E-2:** This cream combines the functions of the water-soluble Fend A-2 and water-insoluble Fend I-2 creams. Tube 3 oz, Jar lb. **I-2:** Water-insoluble cream which forms a physical barrier to water-soluble irritants. Tube 3 oz, Jar lb. **S-2:** A silicone cream which forms a barrier against a combination of water-soluble and water-insoluble irritants Tube 3 oz, Jar lb. **X:** Industrial cold cream which rubs well into the skin and serves as a skin conditioner. Tube 3 oz, Jar lb. *OTC.*
Use: Skin protectant.

Fendol. (Buffington) Salicylamide, caffeine, acetaminophen, phenylephrine hydrochloride. Sugar, lactose and salt free. Tab. Dispens-A-Kit 500s. Bot. 100s. *OTC.*
Use: Analgesic combination.

•**fendosal.** (FEN-doe-sal) USAN.
Use: Anti-inflammatory.

Fenesin DM IR. (Pharma Medica) Dextromethorphan HBr 15 mg, guaifenesin 400 mg. Tab. 100s. *OTC.*
Use: Upper respiratory combination, antitussive with expectorant.

•**fenestrel.** (feh-NESS-trell) USAN. Under study.
Use: Estrogen.

•**fenethylline hydrochloride.** (FEN-ETH-ill-in) USAN.
Use: Stimulant (central).

•**fenfluramine hydrochloride.** (fen-FLUR-a-meen) USAN.
Use: Used as anorexic agent before withdrawal from US market.

•**fengabine.** (FEN-GAH-bean) USAN.
Use: Mood regulator.

•**fenimide.** (FEN-ih-mid) USAN.
Use: Anxiolytic; antipsychotic.

FE 90 Plus. (Acella) Iron 90 mg, vitamins B_{12} 12 mcg, C 120 mg, folic acid 1 mg, docusate sodium 50 mg. Tab. 90s. *Rx.*
Use: Trace element.

•**fenisorex.** (fen-EYE-so-rex) USAN.
Use: Anorexigenic; anorexic.

•**fenmetozole hydrochloride.** (FEN-MET-oh-zole) USAN.
Use: Antidepressant; antagonist (to narcotics).

•**fenmetramide.** (fen-MEH-trah-mide) USAN.
Use: Antidepressant.

•**fennel oil.** (FEN-el) *NF.*
Use: Pharmaceutic aid (flavor).

•**fenobam.** (FEN-oh-bam) USAN.
Use: Hypnotic; sedative.

•**fenoctimine sulfate.** (fen-OCK-tih-MEEN) USAN.
Use: Gastric antisecretory.

•**fenofibrate.** (FEN-oh-FYE-brate) *USP.*
Use: Antihyperlipidemic, fibric acid derivative.
See: Antara.
Fenoglide.
Fibricor.
Lipofen.
Lofibra.
TriCor.
Triglide.
Trilipix.

fenofibrate. (Global Pharmaceuticals) Fenofibrate 160 mg. Polydextrose. Film coated. Tab. 90s, 100s, 500s, 1,000s. *Rx.*
Use: Antihyperlipidemic, fibric acid derivative.

fenofibrate. (Lupin Pharmaceuticals) Fenofibrate 48 mg, 145 mg. Lactose, PEG, sucrose. Tab. 90s, 500s, 1,000s (145 mg only). *Rx.*
Use: Antihyperlipidemic, fibric acid derivative.

fenofibrate. (Various Mfr.) Fenofibrate. **Cap. (micronized):** 43 mg, 67 mg, 130 mg, 134 mg, 200 mg. 30s (43 mg and 130 mg only), 90s (except 43 mg), 100s (except 43 mg and 130 mg), 500s (134 mg and 200 mg only), UD 30s (200 mg only). **Tab.:** 48 mg, 54 mg, 145 mg, 160 mg. 90s, blister pack 1s (except 54 mg), UD 30s (except 54 mg). *Rx.*
Use: Antihyperlipidemic, fibric acid derivative.

fenofibric acid. (Various Mfr.) Fenofibrate (as choline fenofibrate) 45 mg, 135 mg. Cap., delayed release. 90s. *Rx.*
Use: Antihyperlipidemic agent, fibric acid derivative.

Fenoglide. (Santarus) Fenofibrate 40 mg, 120 mg. Lactose. Tab. 90s. *Rx.*
Use: Antihyperlipidemic agent, fibric acid derivative.

•**fenoldopam mesylate.** (feh-NAHL-doe-pam) *USP.*
Use: Antihypertensive; dopamine agonist.
See: Corlopam.

fenoldopam mesylate. (Baxter) Fenoldopam mesylate 10 mg/mL. Sodium metabisulfite. Inj. Single-dose amps. 1 mL, 2 mL. *Rx.*
Use: Antihypertensive.

•**fenoprofen.** (FEN-oh-PRO-fen) USAN.
Use: Anti-inflammatory; analgesic.

fenoprofen. (Qualitest) Fenoprofen 200 mg, 300 mg. Cap. Bot. 100s. *Rx.*
Use: Anti-inflammatory; analgesic.

fenoprofen. (Various Mfr.) Fenoprofen calcium. **Cap.:** 200 mg, 300 mg. 100s. **Tab.:** 600 mg. May contain PEG. 100s. *Rx.*
Use: Anti-inflammatory; analgesic, NSAID.

•**fenoprofen calcium.** (FEN-oh-PRO-fen) *USP.*
Use: Anti-inflammatory; analgesic.
See: Nalfon.

•**fenoterol hydrobromide.** (FEN-oh-TER-ahl) USAN.
Use: Investigational bronchodilator.

•**fenpipalone.** (FEN-PIP-ah-lone) USAN.
Use: Anti-inflammatory.

•**fenprinast hydrochloride.** (fen-PRIH-nast) USAN.
Use: Bronchodilator, antiallergic.

•**fenprostalene.** (FEN-PRAHST-ah-leen) USAN.
Use: Luteolysin.

•**fenquizone.** (FEN-kwih-zone) USAN.
Use: Diuretic.

•**fenretinide.** (fen-RET-ih-nide) USAN.
Use: Investigational antineoplastic.

•**fenspiride hydrochloride.** (FEN-spi-ride) USAN.
Use: Bronchodilator; antiadrenergic (α-receptor).

•**fentanyl.** (FEN-ta-nil) USAN.
Tall Man: fentaNYL
Use: Opioid analgesic.
See: Abstral.
Actiq.
Fentora.
Sublimaze.
Subsys.

fentanyl. (Watson Laboratories) Fentanyl citrate 100 mcg, 200 mcg, 400 mcg, 600 mcg, 800 mcg. Mannitol. Tab.; buccal. UD 28s. *c-II.*
Use: Opioid analgesic.

•**fentanyl citrate.** (FEN-tuh-nill) *USP.*
Tall Man: fentaNYL
Use: Opioid analgesic.
See: Lazanda.
Onsolis.

fentanyl citrate. (Various Mfr.) Fentanyl citrate (as base) 50 mcg/mL. Inj. Amp. 2 mL, 5 mL, 10 mL, 20 mL. Single-dose vials. 30 mL, 50 mL. *c-II.*
Use: Opioid analgesic.

•**fentanyl citrate injection.** (FEN-tuh-nill) *USP.*
Use: Opioid analgesic.

fentanyl citrate nasal spray.
Use: Opioid analgesic.
See: Lazanda.

fentanyl citrate transmucosal. (Various Mfr.) Fentanyl citrate (as base) 200 mcg, 400 mcg, 600 mcg, 800 mcg, 1200 mcg, 1600 mcg. Sugar. Berry flavor. Loz. on a Stick. 30s with carton blister packs. *c-II.*
Use: Opioid analgesic.

fentanyl citrate transmucosal system.
Use: Opioid analgesic.
See: Actiq.

fentanyl transdermal system.
Use: Opioid analgesic.
See: Duragesic-12.
Duragesic-50.
Duragesic-100.
Duragesic-75.
Duragesic-25.

fentanyl transdermal system. (Sandoz) Fentanyl 1.25 mg (12.5 mcg/h). Transdermal System. Cartons containing 5 individually packaged systems. *c-II.*
Use: Opioid analgesic.

fentanyl transdermal system. (Various Mfr.) Fentanyl 1.28 to 2.1 mg (12 mcg/h), 2.1 mg (12 mcg/h), 2.5 to 4.2 mg (25 mcg/h), 4.2 mg (25 mcg/h), 5 to 8.4 mg (50 mcg/h), 8.4 mg (50 mcg/h), 7.5 to 12.6 mg (75 mcg/h), 12.6 mg (75 mcg/h), 10 to 16.8 mg (100 mcg/h), 16.8 mg (100 mcg/h). Transdermal system. UD 5s. *c-II.*
Use: Opioid analgesic.

•**fentiazac.** (fen-TIE-azz-ACK) USAN.
Use: Anti-inflammatory.

•**fenticlor.** (FEN-tih-Klor) USAN.
Use: Antifungal; antiseptic, topical.

•**fenticonazole nitrate.** (FEN-tih-KOE-nah-zole) USAN.
Use: Antifungal.

Fenton. (Sanofi-Synthelabo) Ferrous gluconate. Elix. *OTC.*
Use: Mineral supplement.

Fentora. (Cephalon) Fentanyl citrate (as base) 100 mcg, 200 mcg, 400 mcg, 600 mcg, 800 mcg. Mannitol. Tab. Blister cards. 28s. *c-II.*
Use: Opioid analgesic.

Fenylhist. (Roberts) Diphenhydramine hydrochloride 25 mg, 50 mg. Cap. Bot. 1000s. *OTC.*
Use: Antihistamine.

fenyramidol hydrochloride. Phenyramidol hydrochloride.

•**fenyripol hydrochloride.** (FEH-nee-rih-pahl) USAN.
Use: Muscle relaxant.

Feocyte Injectable. (Oxypure) Peptonized iron 15 mg, vitamin B_{12} 200 mcg, liver injection, beef 10 units, sodium citrate 10 mg, benzyl alcohol 2%/mL. Inj. Vial 10 mL. *Rx.*
Use: Mineral, vitamin supplement.

Feocyte Tablets. (Oxypure) Iron 110 mg, vitamins C 100 mg, B_6 2 mg, B_{12} 50 mcg, copper sulfate, folic acid 0.8 mg, desiccated liver 15 mg. Prolonged Action Tab. Bot. 100s. *Rx.*
Use: Mineral, vitamin supplement.

FeoGen. (Rising) Fe 66 mg (as elemental iron), vitamin B_{12} 10 mcg, desiccated stomach substance 100 mg, C 250 mg. Cap. UD 100s. *Rx.*
Use: Vitamin, mineral supplement.

FeoGen Forte. (Rising) Fe 15 mg, B_{12} 10 mcg, C 60 mg, folic acid 1 mg. Softgel Cap. 100s. *Rx.*
Use: Vitamin, mineral supplement.

Feosol Natural Release. (Meda Pharmaceuticals) Carbonyl iron 45 mg. Tab. 30s, 60s. *OTC.*
Use: Mineral supplement.

Feosol Original. (Meda Pharmaceuticals) Ferrous sulfate exsiccated (dried)

200 mg (iron 65 mg), 325 mg (65 mg). Glucose (200 mg only); lactose, PEG, polydextrose, sorbitol (325 mg only). Tab. 100s (200 mg), 125s (325 mg). *OTC.*
Use: Mineral supplement.

Feosol Elixir. (Various Mfr.) Ferrous sulfate (44 mg iron) 220 mg/5 mL. Alcohol 5%. Elix. 16 oz. *OTC.*
Use: Mineral supplement.

FE-Plus Protein. (Miller Pharmacal Group) Iron (as an iron-protein complex) 50 mg. Tab. Bot. 100s. *OTC.*
Use: Mineral supplement.

Feraheme. (AMAG Pharmaceuticals) Ferumoxytol. Elemental iron 30 mg/mL. Mannitol 44 mg. Preservative free. Single-use vial. *Rx.*
Use: Trace element.

Feratab. (Upsher-Smith) Ferrous sulfate 300 mg (60 mg iron). Exsiccated. Tab. UD 100s. *OTC.*
Use: Trace element.

Ferate-C. (Pal-Pak, Inc.) Ferrous fumarate 150 mg, ascorbic acid 200 mg, docusate sodium 25 mg. Tab. Bot. 100s, 1000s. *OTC.*
Use: Mineral, vitamin supplement; stool softener.

Ferate Tabs. (Major) Ferrous gluconate 246 mg (iron 28 mg). Sodium < 5 mg. Gluten free, lactose free, and preservative free. Tab. 100s. *OTC.*
Use: Trace element.

Fergon. (Bayer) Ferrous gluconate 225 mg (iron 27 mg). Tab. Bot. 100s. *OTC.*
Use: Mineral supplement.

Fer-Iron. (Rugby) Ferrous sulfate 15 mg of iron per mL. Alcohol 0.2%, lemon flavoring, sorbitol, sucrose. Drops. 50 mL. *OTC.*
Use: Trace element, iron-containing product.

FeRiva. (Avion Pharmaceuticals) Iron 75 mg, vitamins B_{12} 12 mcg, C 152 mg, folic acid 1 mg, biotin 300 mcg, docusate sodium 25 mg. Olive oil. Cap. 30s. *Rx.*
Use: Multivitamin with iron.

FeRivaFA with Quatrefolic. (Avion Pharmaceuticals) Iron 110 mg, vitamins B_{12} 12 mcg, C 175 mg, folate 1 mg, Cu, biotin, docusate sodium. Cap. 30s. *Rx.*
Use: Multivitamin with minerals.

Ferocyl. (Arco) Ferrous fumarate 150 mg (iron 50 mg), docusate sodium 100 mg. TR Cap. Bot. 100s. *OTC.*
Use: Mineral supplement; stool softener.

Fero-Folic 500. (Abbott) Ferrous sulfate controlled-release (equivalent to 105 mg iron), vitamin C 500 mg, folic acid 0.8 mg. Filmtab. Bot. 100s, 500s. *Rx.*
Use: Mineral, vitamin supplement.

Fero-Grad-500. (Abbott) Sodium ascorbate 500 mg, ferrous sulfate equivalent to 105 mg iron. Castor oil. CR Tab. Blister pack 30s. *OTC.*
Use: Mineral supplement.

Ferolix. (Century) Ferrous sulfate 5 g, alcohol 5%/10 mL Elix. Bot. 8 oz, pt, gal. *OTC.*
Use: Mineral supplement.

Ferosan. (Sandia) Ferrous fumarate 91.2 mg, B_1 10 mg, B_6 3 mg, B_{12} 25 mcg/5 mL. Syr. Bot. 16 oz, gal. *OTC.*
Use: Mineral, vitamin supplement.

Ferosan Forte. (Sandia) Ferrous fumarate 300 mg, liver-stomach concentrate 150 mg, vitamin B_{12} w/intrinsic factor concentrate 7.5 mcg, intrinsic factor concentrate 150 mg, B_{12} 7.5 mcg, ascorbic acid 75 mg, folic acid 1 mg, sorbitol 50 mg. Tab. Bot. 100s. *Rx.*
Use: Mineral, vitamin supplement.

Ferospace. (Hudson Corp.) Ferrous sulfate 250 mg (iron 50 mg). TR Cap. Bot. 100s. *OTC.*
Use: Mineral supplement.

FeroSul. (Major) Ferrous sulfate 325 mg (iron 65 mg). Tab. 100s, 1,000s. *OTC.*
Use: Mineral supplement.

Ferotrinsic. (Rugby) Iron 110 mg (from ferrous fumarate), vitamins B_{12} 15 mcg, C 75 mg, intrinsic factor (as concentrate or from stomach preparations) 240 mg, folic acid 0.5 mg. Cap. 100s, 500s, 1000s. *Rx.*
Use: Mineral, vitamin supplement.

Feroweet. (Barth's) Vitamins B_1 6 mg, B_2 12 mg, niacin 4 mg, iron 30 mg, B_{12} 10 mcg, B_6 95 mcg, pantothenic acid 50 mcg. 3 Cap. Bot. 100s, 500s, 1000s. *OTC.*
Use: Mineral, vitamin supplement.

Ferracomp. (Roberts) Liver 2 mcg, vitamins B_{12} 15 mcg, B_1 10 mg, B_2 5 mg, B_6 1 mg, calcium pantothenate 1 mg, niacinamide 10 mg, iron 31.3 mg/mL. Vial 30 mL. *OTC.*
Use: Mineral, vitamin supplement.

Ferralet 90. (Mission Pharmacal) Iron 90 mg (as carbonyl iron), folic acid 1 mg, vitamin B12 12 mcg, vitamin C 120 mg, docusate sodium 50 mg. Film coated. Tab. 90s. *Rx.*
Use: Nutritional agent, trace element.

Ferralet Plus. (Mission Pharmacal) Ferrous gluconate equivalent to 46 mg

iron, C 400 mg, folic acid 0.8 mg, vitamin B_{12} 25 mcg. Tab. Bot. 60s. *OTC.*
Use: Mineral, vitamin supplement.

Ferrets. (Pharmics) Ferrous fumarate 325 mg, iron 106 mg. Polydextrose. Film-coated. Tab. Bot. 60s. *OTC.*
Use: Mineral supplement.

Ferrex 150. (Breckenridge) Iron (as polysaccharide-iron complex) 150 mg. Cap. UD 100s. *OTC.*
Use: Mineral supplement.

Ferrex 150 Forte. (Breckenridge) Iron 150 mg (as polysaccharide-iron complex), folic acid 1 mg, B_{12} 25 mcg. Cap. UD 100s. *Rx.*
Use: Vitamin, mineral supplement.

Ferrex 150 Forte Plus. (Breckenridge) Iron sucrose 150 mg (as elemental iron). Succinic acid 50 mg, PEG. Cap. 90s. *Rx.*
Use: Trace element.

Ferrex 150 Plus. (Breckenridge) Fe (from polysaccharide iron and ferrous bisglycinate) 150 mg, ascorbic acid 50 mg. Cap. UD 100s. *OTC.*
Use: Mineral, vitamin supplement.

Ferrex PC. (Breckenridge) Iron 60 mg (as polysaccharide-iron complex), folic acid 1 mg, C 50 mg, B_{12} 3 mcg, A 4000 units, D 400 units, B_1 3 mg, B_2 3 mg, B_6 2 mg, niacinamide 10 mg, Ca 25 mg, Zn 18 mg. Tab. UD 100s. *Rx.*
Use: Vitamin, mineral supplement.

Ferrex PC Forte. (Breckenridge) Vitamins A 5000 units, C 80 mg, Ca 250 mg, iron 60 mg (as polysaccharide-iron complex), D 400 units, E (as dl-alpha-tocopheryl acetate) 30 units, B_1 3 mg, B_2 3.4 mg, niacinamide 20 mg, B_6 4 mg, folic acid 1 mg, B_{12} 12 mcg, I, Mg, Zn 25 mg, Cu. Tab. UD 100s. *Rx.*
Use: Vitamin, mineral supplement.

•**ferric ammonium citrate.** (FER-ik) *USP.* Ammonium iron (Fe^{+++}) citrate.
Use: Mineral supplement.

•**ferric ammonium citrate for oral solution.** (FER-ik) *USP.*
Use: Mineral supplement.

ferric ammonium sulfate. (Various Mfr.)
Use: Astringent.

ferric ammonium tartrate. (Various Mfr.)
Use: Mineral supplement.

ferric cacodylate. (Various Mfr.)
Use: Leukemias; hematinic.

ferric carboxymaltose.
Use: Trace element, iron.
See: Injectafer.

ferric chloride. (Various Mfr.)
Use: Astringent.

•**ferric chloride Fe 59.** (FER-ik) USAN.
Use: Radiopharmaceutical.

ferric citrochloride tincture. Iron (Fe^{+++}) chloride citrate.
Use: Hematinic.

•**ferric fructose.** (FER-ik FRUKE-tose) USAN.
Use: Hematinic.

ferric glycerophosphate. Glycerol phosphate iron (Fe^{+++}) salt.
Use: Pharmaceutic necessity.

ferric hypophosphate. Iron (Fe^{+++}) phosphonate.
Use: Pharmaceutic necessity.

•**ferriclate calcium sodium.** (fer-ih-KLATE) USAN.
Use: Hematinic.

•**ferric oxide.** (FER-ik) *NF.*
Use: Pharmaceutic aid (color).

ferric oxide, yellow.
Use: Pharmaceutic aid (color).

ferric "peptonate". (Various Mfr.)
See: Iron Peptonized.

ferric pyrophosphate, soluble. Iron (Fe^{+++}) citrate pyrophosphate.

ferric quinine citrate, "green". (Various Mfr.)
Use: Mineral supplement.

•**ferric subsulfate.** (FER-ik) *USP.*
Use: Local use on the skin.
See: AstrinGyn.

•**ferric sulfate.** (FER-ik) *USP.*
Use: Compounding agent.

Ferriprox. (ApoPharma USA) Deferiprone 500 mg. Film coated. Tab. 100s. *Rx.*
Use: Detoxification agent, chelating agent.

•**ferristene.** (FER-ih-steen) USAN.
Use: Diagnostic aid, paramagnetic.

Ferrizyme. (Abbott Diagnostics) Enzyme immunoassay for qualitative determination of ferritin in human serum or plasma. Test kit 100s.
Use: Diagnostic aid, paramagnetic.

Ferrlecit. (Sanofi Pharmaceuticals) Sodium ferric gluconate complex 62.5 mg/5 mL (12.5 mg/mL of elemental iron). Benzyl alcohol 9 mg/mL, sucrose 195 mg/mL. Inj., Soln. Vial. 5 mL. *Rx.*
Use: Iron-containing product.

ferrocholate.
See: Ferrocholinate.

ferrocholinate. Ferrocholate. Ferrocholine. A chelate prepared by reacting equimolar quantities of freshly precipitated ferric hydroxide with choline dihydrogen citrate.
Use: Mineral supplement.

ferrocholine.
See: Ferrocholinate.

Ferro-Cyte. (Spanner) Iron peptonate

20 mg, liver injection (20 mg/mL) 0.25 mL, vitamins B_1 22 mg, B_2 0.5 mg, B_6 2.5 mg, B_{12} 30 mcg, niacinamide 25 mg, panthenol 1 mg/mL. Inj. Multiple-dose vial 10 mL. *Rx.*
Use: Mineral, vitamin supplement.

Ferro-Docusate TR. (Parmed Pharmaceuticals, Inc.) Ferrous fumarate 150 mg (iron 50 mg), docusate sodium 100 mg. TR Cap. Bot. 100s. *OTC.*
Use: Mineral supplement; stool softener.

Ferro-Dok TR. (Major) Ferrous fumarate 150 mg (iron 50 mg), docusate sodium 100 mg. TR Cap. Bot. 100s. *OTC.*
Use: Mineral supplement; stool softener.

Ferrodyl Chewable Tablets. (Arcum) Ferrous fumarate 320 mg, vitamin C 200 mg. Bot. 100s, 1000s. *OTC.*
Use: Mineral, vitamin supplement.

Ferromar. (Marnel) Ferrous fumarate 201.5 mg (iron 65 mg), vitamin C 200 mg. SR Capl. Bot. 100s. *OTC.*
Use: Mineral supplement.

Ferroneed. (Hanlon) Ferrous gluconate 300 mg, ascorbic acid 60 mg. Cap. Bot. 100s. *OTC.*
Use: Mineral, vitamin supplement.

Ferroneed T-Caps. (Hanlon) Ferrous fumarate 250 mg, thiamine hydrochloride 5 mg, ascorbic acid 50 mg. TD Cap. Bot. 100s. *OTC.*
Use: Mineral, vitamin supplement.

Ferronex. (Taylor Pharmaceuticals) Iron from ferrous gluconate 2.9 mg, vitamins B_{12} equivalent 1 mcg, B_2 0.75 mg, B_3 50 mg, B_5 1.25 mg, B_{12} 15 mcg, procaine 2%/mL. Inj. Vial 30 mL. *Rx.*
Use: Mineral, vitamin supplement.

Ferro-Sequels. (Can-Am/Access) Ferrous fumarate 150 mg (iron 50 mg), sodium docusate 100 mg, lactose. TR Tab. Bot. 30s, 90s. *OTC.*
Use: Mineral supplement.

Ferrospan. (Imperial Lab) Ferrous fumarate 200 mg, ascorbic acid 100 mg. Tab. Bot. 100s, 1000s. *OTC.*
Use: Mineral, vitamin supplement.

Ferrosyn Injection. (Standex) Cyanocobalamin 30 mcg, liver 2 mcg, ferrous gluconate 100 mg, riboflavin 1.5 mg, panthenol 2.5 mg, niacinamide 100 mg, procaine 2%. Inj. Vial 30 mL. *Rx.*
Use: Mineral, vitamin supplement.

Ferrosyn S.C. (Standex) Iron 60 mg, vitamin B_{12} 5 mcg, magnesium 0.6 mg, copper 0.3 mg, manganese 0.1 mg, potassium 0.5 mg, zinc 0.15 mg. Tab. Bot. 100s, 1000s. *OTC.*
Use: Mineral, vitamin supplement.

Ferrosyn See. (Standex) Iron 34 mg, ascorbic acid 60 mg. Tab. Bot. 100s, 1000s. *OTC.*
Use: Mineral, vitamin supplement.

Ferrosyn Tablets. (Standex) Fe 60 mg, vitamin B_{12} 5 mcg, Mg 0.6 mg, Cu 0.3 mg, Mn 0.1 mg, K 0.5 mg, Zn 0.15 mg. Tab. Bot. 100s. *OTC.*
Use: Mineral, vitamin supplement.

ferrous aspartate.
Use: Mineral supplement.
See: FE Aspartate.

ferrous carbonate mass. Vallet's mass. (Various Mfr.)
Use: Mineral supplement.

ferrous carbonate, saccharated. (Various Mfr.)
Use: Mineral supplement.

•**ferrous citrate Fe 59.** (FER-uhs) USAN.
Use: Radiopharmaceutical.

Ferrous Drops. (Major) Ferrous sulfate 15 mg/mL. Sugar, sorbitol, sodium metabisulfite. Gluten free. Fruit flavor. Drops. 50 mL w/dosing syringe. *OTC.*
Use: Trace element.

•**ferrous fumarate.** (FER-uhs) *USP.*
Use: Hematinic.
See: Albafort.
Ferretts.
Ferro-Sequels.
Hemocyte.
W/Ascorbic Acid.
See: Eldofe-C.
Ferrodyl.
Ferromar.
W/Ascorbic Acid and Folic Acid.
See: Fer-Regules.
Ferro-Docusate TR.
Ferro Dok TR.
Ferro-DSS SR.
Ferro-Sequels.
W/Norethindrone, Mestranol.
See: Ortho Novum Fe-28.
W/Polysaccharide Iron Complex
See: Tandem.
W/Vitamins and Minerals.
See: Stuartnatal 1 + 1.
Stuart Prenatal.

ferrous fumarate. (Mission) Ferrous fumarate 90 mg (iron 29.5 mg). Sugar. Tab. Bot. 100s. *OTC.*
Use: Mineral supplement.

ferrous fumarate. (Various Mfr.) Ferrous fumarate 324 mg (iron 106 mg). Tab. 100s. *OTC.*
Use: Mineral supplement.

ferrous fumarate and docusate sodium.
Use: Mineral supplement.

•**ferrous gluconate.** (FER-uhs) *USP.*
Use: Hematinic.
See: Ferate Tabs.
Fergon.

ferrous gluconate. (Various Mfr.) Ferrous gluconate 225 mg (iron 27 mg), 324 mg (iron 38 mg), 325 mg (iron 36 mg). Tab. Bot. 100s (except 325 mg), 1,000s (325 mg only). *OTC.*
Use: Mineral supplement.

ferrous iodide. (Various Mfr.)
Use: In chronic tuberculosis.

ferrous iodide syrup. (Various Mfr.)
Use: In chronic tuberculosis.

ferrous lactate. (Various Mfr.)
Use: Mineral supplement.

•**ferrous sulfate.** (FER-uhs) *USP.*
Use: Hematinic.
See: Enfamil Fer-In-Sol.
Feosol.
Feratab.
Fer-Iron.
Ferolix.
FeroSul.
Ferrous Drops.
Irospan.
W/Ascorbic Acid.
See: Fero-Grad-500.
W/Ascorbic Acid, Folic Acid.
See: Fero-Folic-500.

ferrous sulfate. (Hi-Tech) Iron 15 mg/mL. Alcohol 0.2%, sodium bisulfite, sorbitol, sucrose. Gluten free and lactose free. Drops. 50 mL w/dropper. *OTC.*
Use: Trace element, iron.

ferrous sulfate. (Ivax) Ferrous sulfate 325 mg (elemental iron 65 mg). Tab. Bot. 100s. *OTC.*
Use: Mineral supplement.

ferrous sulfate. (Magnus-Humphries Labs) Ferrous sulfate 27 mg. PEG. Tab. 100s. *OTC.*
Use: Trace element.

ferrous sulfate. (Pharmaceutical Associates) Ferrous sulfate 300 mg per 5 mL (60 mg iron per 5 mL). Sucrose. Cinnamon flavor. Liq. UD 100s of 5 mL each. *OTC.*
Use: Dietary supplement.

ferrous sulfate. (Qualitest) Ferrous sulfate 75 mg per 0.6 mL (iron 15 mg per 0.6 mL). Alcohol 0.2%. Drops. 50 mL. *OTC.*
Use: Trace element.

ferrous sulfate. (Rugby) **SR Tab.:** Ferrous sulfate exsiccated (dried) 160 mg (iron 50 mg). Blisterpack 60s. **ER Cap.:** Ferrous sulfate 140 mg (iron 45 mg). Film coated. Glyceryl, maltodextrin, PEG. UD 30s, UD 60s. *OTC.*
Use: Mineral supplement.

ferrous sulfate. (Various Mfr.) Ferrous sulfate. **Tab.:** 325 mg (iron 65 mg). 100s, 1,000s, UD 100s. **Elix.:** 220 mg/5 mL (iron 44 mg/5 mL). May contain alcohol. Bot. 473 mL. *OTC.*
Use: Mineral supplement.

•**ferrous sulfate, dried.** (FER-uhs) *USP.*
Use: Antianemic.
See: Feosol.
Fer-In-Sol.
Slow Fe.

ferrous sulfate exsiccated (dried).
Use: Mineral supplement.
See: Feosol.
Slow FE.
Slow Release Iron.

•**ferrous sulfate Fe 59.** (FER-uhs) USAN.
Use: Radiopharmaceutical.

Fertility Tape. (Weston Labs.) Regular, extrasensitive, less-sensitive. W/Fertility Testor, cervical glucose test. Pkg. test 60s.
Use: Diagnostic aid.

•**ferucarbotran.** (fur-you-CAR-boe-tran) USAN.
Use: Diagnostic aid (paramagnetic).

•**ferumoxides.** (feh-roo-MOX-ides) USAN.
Use: Radiopaque agent.

•**ferumoxtran-10.** (fur-you-MOX-tran 10) USAN.
Use: Diagnostic aid (paramagnetic).

•**ferumoxytol.** (fer-yoo-MOX-i-tole) USAN.
Use: Diagnostic aid (MRI); iron deficiency.
See: Feraheme.

Ferusal. (Eon Labs) Ferrous sulfate 325 mg. Tab. *OTC.*
Use: Mineral supplement.

•**fesoterodine fumarate.** (FES-oh-TER-oh-deen) USAN.
Use: Treatment of overactive bladder.
See: Toviaz.

Festalan. (Hoechst) Lipase 6000 units, amylase 30,000 units, protease 20,000 units, atropine methylnitrate 1 mg. EC Tab. Bot. 100s, 1000s. *Rx.*
Use: Digestive enzyme.

Fetinic. (Roberts) Iron 3.6 mg, vitamins B_{12} equivalent to 2 mcg, B_1 10 mg, B_2 0.5 mg, B_3 10 mg, B_5 1 mg, B_6 1 mg, B_{12} 15 mcg, chlorobutanol 0.5%, benzyl alcohol 2%/mL. Vial 30 mL. *Rx.*
Use: Mineral, vitamin supplement.

Fetinic-MW. (Roberts) Iron 66 mg (from ferrous fumarate), vitamins B_{12} 5 mcg, C 60 mg. SR Cap. Bot. 100s. *OTC.*
Use: Mineral, vitamin supplement.

Fe-Tinic 150 Forte. (Ethex) Iron 150 mg (as polysaccharide-iron complex), folic acid 1 mg, B_{12} 25 mcg. Cap. UD 100s. *Rx.*
Use: Vitamin, mineral supplement.

•**fetoxylate hydrochloride.** (fee-TOX-ih-LATE) USAN.
Use: Muscle relaxant.

Fetzima. (Forest) Levomilnacipran 20 mg, 40 mg, 80 mg, 120 mg. Sugar spheres. ER Cap. 30s, 90s (except 20 mg), UD 100s, titration pack (20 mg and 40 mg). *Rx.*
Use: Antidepressant, serotonin and norepinephrine reuptake inhibitor.

FeverAll. (Actavis) Acetaminophen 650 mg. Hydrogenated vegetable oil. Supp. 50s. *OTC.*
Use: Analgesic.

FeverAll Children's. (Actavis) Acetaminophen 120 mg. Hydrogenated vegetable oil. Supp. Pkg. 6s, 50s. *OTC.*
Use: Analgesic.

FeverAll Infants. (Actavis) Acetaminophen 80 mg. Hydrogenated vegetable oil. Supp. Pkg. 6s, 50s. *OTC.*
Use: Analgesic.

FeverAll Junior Strength. (Actavis) Acetaminophen 325 mg. Hydrogenated vegetable oil. Supp. Pkg. 12s, 50s. *OTC.*
Use: Analgesic.

•**feverfew.** (FEE-ver-fyoo) *NF.*
Use: Dietary supplement.

Fexmid. (Shionogi Pharma) Cyclobenzaprine hydrochloride 7.5 mg. Film-coated. Tab. 100s. *Rx.*
Use: Skeletal muscle relaxant.

•**fexofenadine hydrochloride.** (fex-oh-FEN-ah-deen) USAN.
Use: Antihistamine, peripherally selective piperidine.
See: Allegra Allergy.
Allegra Children's Allergy.
W/Pseudoephedrine Hydrochloride.
See: Allegra-D 12 Hour Allergy & Congestion.
Allegra-D 24 Hour Allergy & Congestion.

fexofenadine hydrochloride. (Various Mfr.) Fexofenadine hydrochloride 30 mg, 60 mg, 180 mg. May contain lactose. Tab. 30s, 60s (60 mg only), 100s, 500s, UD 100s. *Rx.*
Use: Antihistamine, peripherally selective piperidine.

fexofenadine hydrochloride/pseudoephedrine hydrochloride. (Various Mfr.) Fexofenadine hydrochloride 180 mg, pseudoephedrine hydrochloride 240 mg. May contain PEG, vegetable oil. ER Tab. UD 10s. *OTC.*
Use: Upper respiratory combination, decongestant and antihistamine.

•**fezakinumab.** (FEZ-a-KIN-ue-mab) USAN.
Use: Anti-inflammatory.

•**fezolamine fumarate.** (feh-ZOLE-ah-MEEN) USAN.
Use: Antidepressant.

fgn-1. (Cell Pathways, Inc.)
Use: Treatment of adenomatous polyposis coli. [Orphan Drug]

•**fiacitabine.** (fih-AH-sit-ah-BEEN) USAN.
Use: Antiviral.

•**fialuridine.** (fie-al-YOUR-ih-deen) USAN.
Use: Antiviral.

FIAU. (Oclassen)
Use: Antiviral, hepatitis B. [Orphan Drug]

fiber.
Use: Laxative.
See: Benefiber.
Benefiber Drink Mix.
Benefiber for Children.
Benefiber Plus Calcium.
Benefiber Plus Heart Health.
Benefiber Sticks.
Benefiber Ultra.

Fiberall Natural Flavor. (Novartis) **Pow.:** Psyllium hydrophilic mucilloid 3.4 g, wheat bran, sodium < 10 mg, potassium 60 mg, calories 6/5.9 g, saccharin. Can 150 g, 300 g, 450 g. **Wafer:** Psyllium hydrophilic mucilloid 3.4 g, wheat bran, oats, sucrose. Box 14s. *OTC.*
Use: Laxative.

Fiberall Orange Flavor. (Heritage Consumer) Psyllium hydrophilic mucilloid 3.5 g/dose, aspartame. Pow. Can 480 g. *OTC.*
Use: Laxative.

Fiberall Tropical Fruit Flavor. (Heritage Consumer) Psyllium hydrophilic mucilloid 3.5 g/dose, aspartame. Pow. Can. 454 g, UD 10 g packets. *OTC.*
Use: Laxative.

FiberCon. (Wyeth) Calcium polycarbophil 625 mg (equiv. to 500 mg polycarbophil). Tab. 36s, 60s, 90s, 150s. *OTC.*
Use: Laxative.

Fiber Guard. (Wyeth) All natural high-fiber supplement 530 mg. Tab. Bot. 100s, 200s. *OTC.*
Use: Fiber supplement.

Fiberlan. (Elan) Protein 50 g, fat 40 g, carbohydrates 160 g, Na 920 mg, K 1.56 g, fiber 14 g/per L. With vitamins A, C, B, B_2, B_3, D, E, B_5, B_6, B_{12}, K, Ca, Fe, folic acid, P, I, Mg, Zn, Cu, biotin, Mn, choline, Cl, Se, Cr, Mo. Liq. Bot. 237 mL. *OTC.*
Use: Nutritional supplement.

Fiber-Lax. (Rugby) Calcium polycarbophil 625 mg (equiv. to 500 mg poly-

carbophil). Tab. Bot. 60s, 90s, 500s. *OTC.*
Use: Laxative.

Fibermed High-Fiber Snacks. (Purdue) One serving (15 snacks) contains 5 g dietary fiber. Box 8 oz. Packs of 24 × 1.3 oz. *OTC.*
Use: Fiber supplement.

Fibermed High-Fiber Supplement. (Purdue) Each supplement contains 5 g dietary fiber. Box 14s. Institutional pack, Box 144s of two supplements. *OTC.*
Use: Fiber supplement.

FiberNorm. (G & W) Polycarbophil 625 mg. Tab. Bot. 60s, 90s. *OTC.*
Use: Laxative.

Fiber Therapy Original Texture. (Major) Psyllium husk ≈3.4 g, carbohydrates 6 g, sodium 3 mg, 25 calories per dose. Sugar. Pow. 538 g. *OTC.*
Use: Bulk-producing laxative.

•**fiboflapon.** (FYE-boe-FLAP-on) USAN.
Use: Treatment of asthma and chronic obstructive pulmonary disease.

•**fiboflapon sodium.** (FYE-boe-FLAP-on) USAN.
Use: Treatment of asthma and chronic obstructive pulmonary disease.

Fibre Trim. (Schering-Plough) Grain and citrus fruit concentrated dietary fiber. Tab. Bot. 100s, 250s. *OTC.*
Use: Dietary aid.

Fibre Trim w/Calcium. (Schering-Plough) Grain and citrus fruit concentrated dietary fiber w/calcium. Tab. Bot. 90s, 225s. *OTC.*
Use: Dietary aid.

fibric acid derivatives.
Use: Antihyperlipidemic.
See: Fenofibrate.
Gemfibrozil.

Fibricor. (Caraco) Fenofibrate 35 mg, 105 mg. Tab. 30s, 60s, 90s, 100s, 250s, 500s, 1,000s. *Rx.*
Use: Antihyperlipidemic agent, fibric acid derivative.

fibrin agents.
See: Fibrin Sealant (Human).

fibrinogen concentrate (human).
See: RiaSTAP.

fibrinogen (human). (Alpha Therapeutic) Partially purified fibrinogen prepared by fractionation from normal human plasma.
Use: Coagulant, clotting factor. [Orphan Drug]

•**fibrinogen I 125.** (FIE-BRIN-oh-jen) USAN.
Use: Diagnostic aid (vascular patency); radiopharmaceutical.

fibrinogen sealant (human). (fye-BRIN-oh-jen)
See: TachoSil.
W/Thrombin (human)
See: Evarrest.

fibrinolysis inhibitor.
See: Amicar.
W/Calcium Chloride, Fibrin Sealant (Human), Protein, Thrombin (Human).
See: Tisseel.

fibrin sealant (human).
Use: Fibrin agent.
See: Artiss.
W/Calcium Chloride, Fibrinolysis Inhibitor, Protein, Thrombin (Human).
See: Tisseel.

Fibrogammin P. (Aventis Behring)
Use: Congenital Factor XIII deficiency. [Orphan Drug]

•**ficlatuzumab.** (FYE-kla-TOOZ-ue-mab) USAN.
Use: Antineoplastic.

•**fidaxomicin.** (fye-DAX-oh-MYE-sin) USAN.
Use: Anti-infective.
See: Dificid.

•**fidexaban.** (fye-DEX-a-ban) USAN.
Use: Anticoagulant.

•**fiduxosin hydrochloride.** (fi-DUX-oe-sin) USAN.
Use: Benign prostatic hyperplasia.

50+ Companion Women's. (Theralogix) Vitamins A 3,500 units, C 100 mg, E 30 units, B_1 5 mg, B_2 5 mg, B_3 20 mg, B_5 10 mg, B_6 5 mg, B_{12} 30 mcg, folic acid 400 mcg, Ca, I, Mg, Zn, Se, Mn, Cu, Cr, Mo, choline 100 mg, biotin 30 mcg, B, V. Tab. 180s. *OTC.*
Use: Multivitamin with minerals.

•**figitumumab.** (FIG-i-TOOM-ue-mab) USAN.
Use: Antineoplastic.

•**filaminast.** (fih-LAM-in-ast) USAN.
Use: Antiasthmatic (selective phosphodiesterase IV inhibitor).

Filaxis. (Amlab) Vitamins A 25,000 units, D 1250 units, C 150 mg, E 5 units, B_1 12 mg, B_2 5 mg, B_6 0.5 mg, B_{12} 5 mcg, calcium pantothenate 5 mg, niacinamide 100 mg, Fe 15 mg, I 0.15 mg, Mg 10 mg, K 5 mg, Ca 75 mg, P 60 mg. Tab. Bot. 30s, 100s. Available w/B_{12}. Bot. 30s, 60s, 100s. *OTC.*
Use: Mineral, vitamin supplement.

•**filgrastim.** (fill-GRAH-stim) USAN.
Use: Biological response modifier; antineoplastic adjunct; antineutropenic; hematopoietic stimulant. [Orphan Drug]
See: Neupogen.

•**filibuvir.** (fil-i-BUE-vir) USAN.
Use: Anti-infective.
•**filipin.** (FIH-lih-pin) USAN.
Use: Antifungal.
•**filorexant.** (FYE-loe-REX-ant) USAN.
Use: Treatment of insomnia.
Finac. (C & M Pharmacal) Salicylic acid 2%, isopropyl alcohol 22.5%, propylene glycol, acetone in lotion base. Bot. 60 mL. *OTC.*
Use: Dermatologic, acne.
Finacea. (Bayer) Azelaic acid 15%, EDTA, benzoic acid. Gel. 30 g. *Rx.*
Use: Anti-inflammatory.
•**finasteride.** (fih-NASS-teer-ide) *USP.*
Use: Benign prostatic hypertrophy therapy; antineoplastic; antineutropenic; inhibitor (alpha-reductase); androgen hormone inhibitor.
See: Propecia.
Proscar.
finasteride. (Dr. Reddy's Laboratories) Finasteride 1 mg. May contain docusate sodium, lactose, PEG. Tab. 30s, 90s, 180s, 500s. *Rx.*
Use: Sex hormone, androgen hormone inhibitor.
finasteride. (Various Mfr.) Finasteride 5 mg. Lactose. Film-coated. Tab. 30s, 100s, 500s. *Rx.*
Use: Androgen hormone inhibitor.
Finevin. (Berlex) Azelaic acid 20%, glycerin, cetearyl alcohol. Cream. Tube. 30 g. *Rx.*
Use: Anti-infective, antibiotic, topical.
•**fingolimod hydrochloride.** (fin-GOLE-i-mod) USAN.
Use: Immunomodulator.
See: Gilenya.
Fioricet. (Actavis) **Tab.:** Acetaminophen 325 mg, butalbital 50 mg, caffeine 40 mg. 100s, 500s, UD 100s. **Cap.:** Acetaminophen 300 mg, butalbital 50 mg, caffeine 40 mg. 100s. *c-III.*
Use: Analgesic; hypnotic; sedative.
Fioricet with Codeine. (Actavis) Codeine phosphate 30 mg, acetaminophen 300 mg, caffeine 40 mg, butalbital 50 mg. Cap. 100s. *c-III.*
Use: Narcotic analgesic combination.
Fiorinal. (Actavis) Butalbital 50 mg, caffeine 40 mg, aspirin 325 mg, benzyl alcohol, parabens, EDTA. Cap. Bot. 100s, 500s, UD 25s. *c-III.*
Use: Analgesic; hypnotic; sedative.
Fiorinal with Codeine No. 3. (Actavis) Butalbital 50 mg, caffeine 40 mg, aspirin 325 mg, codeine phosphate 30 mg. Cap. Bot. 100s. *Control Pak* 25s. *c-III.*
Use: Analgesic combination; hypnotic; sedative.
Firazyr. (Shire) Icatibant acetate 10 mg/mL. Sodium chloride. Preservative free. Inj., Soln. Single-use, prefilled syringe. *Rx.*
Use: Hematological agent, bradykinin inhibitor.
fire ant venom, allergenic extract, imported.
Use: Dermatologic aid-skin test; immunotherapy. [Orphan Drug]
Firmagon. (Ferring) Degarelix acetate 80 mg, 120 mg. Mannitol 200 mg. Inj., lyophilized Pow. for Soln. Vial. *Rx.*
Use: Sex hormone, gonadotropin-releasing hormone antagonist.
Firmdent. (Moyco Union Broach Division) *Formerly Moy.* Karaya gum 94.6%, sodium borate 5.36%. Pkg. 3 oz. *OTC.*
Use: Denture adhesive.
•**firocoxib.** (fir-oh-KOX-ib) USAN.
Use: Analgesic, anti-inflammatory.
First Aid Cream. (Johnson & Johnson) Cetyl alcohol, glyceryl stearate, isopropyl palmitate, stearyl alcohol, synthetic beeswax. Tube 0.8 oz, 1.5 oz, 2.5 oz. *OTC.*
Use: Antiseptic; dermatologic, protectant.
First Aid Cream. (Walgreen) Benzocaine 3%, allantoin 0.2%, benzyl alcohol 4%, phenol 0.25%. Tube 1.5 oz. *OTC.*
Use: Anesthetic; antiseptic.
First BXN Mouthwash. (Cutis Pharma) Diphenhydramine hydrochloride 0.2 g, lidocaine hydrochloride 1.6 g, nystatin 1.6 g. Alcohol, benzyl alcohol, FD&C yellow #5, propylparaben, saccharin, sorbitol. Susp. Compounding kit. *Rx.*
Use: Mouth and throat product.
First Duke's Mouthwash. (Cutis Pharma) Diphenhydramine hydrochloride 0.525 g, hydrocortisone 0.06 g, nystatin 0.6 g. Benzyl alcohol, propylene glycol, propylparabens, saccharin, sorbitol. Susp. 237 mL compounding kit. *Rx.*
Use: Mouth and throat product.
First Mary's Mouthwash. (Cutis Pharma) Diphenhydramine hydrochloride 0.45 g, hydrocortisone 0.06 g, nystatin 1.2 g, tetracycline hydrochloride 1.5 g. Benzyl alcohol, propylene glycol, propylparabens, saccharin, sorbitol. Susp. 237 mL compounding kit. *Rx.*
Use: Mouth and throat product.
First Mouthwash BLM. (Cutis Pharma) Diphenhydramine hydrochloride 0.2 g, lidocaine hydrochloride 1.6 g, aluminum hydroxide 3.15 g, magnesium hydroxide 3.15 g, simethicone 0.315 g. Benzyl alcohol, parabens, saccharin, sorbitol. Susp. Compounding kit. *Rx.*
Use: Mouth and throat product.

First Response Ovulation Predictor. (Tambrands, Inc.) Monoclonal antibody-based enzyme immunoassay test for hLH in urine. Test kit 1s. *OTC.*
Use: Diagnostic aid.

First Response Pregnancy Test. (Tambrands, Inc.) Reagent in-home kit for urine testing. Test kit 1s. *OTC.*
Use: Diagnostic aid.

•**firtecan pegol.** (fir-TEE-kan PEG-ol) USAN.
Use: Antineoplastic.

fish oil concentrate, natural. Natural fish oil concentrate containing EPA (Eicosanoic acid) and DHA (Docosahexaenoic acid).
Use: Nutritional supplement.
See: Animi-3 With Vitamin D.

Fish Oil + D_3. (Nature's Bounty) Fish oil 1,200 mg (omega-3 360 mg as DHA, EPA, and other fatty acids), vitamin D 1,000 units. Gluten free, lactose free, preservative free. Glycerin. Cap., softgel. 90s. *OTC.*
Use: Multivitamin and mineral with omega-3 polyunsaturated fatty acids.

•**fispemifene.** (fis-PEM-i-feen) USAN.
Use: Selective estrogen antagonist.

Fitness Tabs for Men. (MDR Fitness Corp.) **AM:** Iron 8 mg, calcium 225 mg, vitamins A 3,000 units, D 400 units, E 60 units, B_1 5 mg, B_2 5 mg, B_3 33 mg, B_5 15 mg, B_6 5 mg, B_{12} 12 mcg, C 150 mg, folic acid 0.3 mg, Cr, Cu, Mg, Mn, Se, Zn, biotin, garlic. PEG. Sugar free. Tab. 60s. **PM:** Iron 2 mg, calcium 275 mg, vitamins A 1,500 units, D 400 units, E 40 units, B_1 2 mg, B_2 1.2 mg, B_3 7 mg, B_5 5 mg, B_6 2 mg, B_{12} 6 mcg, C 150 mg, folic acid 0.1 mg, Cr, Cu, Mg, Mn, Se, Zn, biotin, garlic. PEG. Sugar free. Tab. 60s. *OTC.*
Use: Multivitamin with minerals.

Fitness Tabs for Women. (MDR Fitness Corp.) **AM:** Iron 12 mg, calcium 220 mg, vitamins A 3,000 units, D 400 units, E 70 units, B_1 4 mg, B_2 5 mg, B_3 33 mg, B_5 15 mg, B_6 6 mg, B_{12} 12 mcg, C 150 mg, folic acid 0.3 mg, Cr, Cu, Mg, Mn, Se, Zn, biotin, garlic. Sugar free. Tab. 60s. **PM:** Iron 3 mg, calcium 345 mg, vitamins A 1,000 units, D 400 units, E 30 units, B_1 3 mg, B_2 2 mg, B_3 7 mg, B_5 5 mg, B_6 2 mg, B_{12} 6 mcg, C 100 mg, folic acid 0.1 mg, Cr, Cu, Mg, Mn, Se, Zn, biotin, garlic. PEG. Sugar free. Tab. 60s. *OTC.*
Use: Multivitamin with minerals.

FIV-ASA. (Paddock) 5-aminosalicylic acid 500 mg. Supp. Bot. 30s. *Rx.*
Use: Gastrointestinal agent.

5-FC.
See: Flucytosine

5-FU.
See: Fluorouracil.

5-HT_{1A} receptor agonists.
See: Vilazodone Hydrochloride.

523. (Enzyme Process) Pancreatin 200 mg, tryspin, chymotrypsin, amylase, lipase enzymes from pancreatin, raw beef pancreas. Tab. Bot. 100s, 250s.
Use: Digestive enzyme.

Fixodent. (Procter & Gamble) Calcium sodium poly (vinyl methyl ether-maleate), carboxymethylcellulose sodium in a petrolatum base. Tube 0.75 oz, 1.5 oz, 2.5 oz. *OTC.*
Use: Denture adhesive.

FK506.
See: Prograf.

FK-565.
Use: Immunomodulator.

Flagyl. (Pfizer) Metronidazole 250 mg, 500 mg. Film coated. PEG. 50s, 100s. *Rx.*
Use: Anti-infective.

Flagyl ER. (Pfizer) Metronidazole 750 mg. Film coated. Lactose, PEG. ER Tab. 30s. *Rx.*
Use: Anti-infective.

Flagyl 375. (Pfizer) Metronidazole 375 mg. Cap. 50s, UD 100s. *Rx.*
Use: Anti-infective.

Flanders Buttocks Ointment. (Flanders) Zinc oxide, castor oil, balsam peru, boric acid in an emollient base. Tube. 60 g. *OTC.*
Use: Dermatologic, counterirritant.

•**flanvotumab.** (flan-VOT-ue-mab) USAN.
Use: Antineoplastic.

Flarex. (Alcon) Fluorometholone acetate 0.1%. Benzalkonium chloride 0.01%, EDTA, hydroxyethylcellulose, tyloxapol, sodium chloride, monobasic sodium phosphate. Ophth. Susp. Bot. 2.5 mL, 5 mL, 10 mL *Drop-Tainers. Rx.*
Use: Corticosteroid, ophthalmic; anti-inflammatory.

Flatulence. (Pal-Pak, Inc.) Nux vomica 16.2 mg, cascara sagrada extract 64.8 mg, ginger 48.6 mg, capsicum 16.2 mg, asafetida. Tab. Bot. *OTC.*
Use: Antiflatulent; laxative.

Flatulex. (Dayton) Simethicone 40 mg/0.6 mL. Drops. 30 mL with calibrated dropper. *OTC.*
Use: Antiflatulent.

Flatus. (Foy Laboratories) Nux vomica extract 0.25 g, cascara extract 1 g, ginger ¾ g, capsicum g, w/asfetida qs. Tab. Bot. 1000s. *OTC.*
Use: Antiflatulent; laxative.

Flav-A-D. (Kirkman) Vitamins A 5000 units, D 1000 units, C 100 mg. Tab. Bot. 100s, 1000s. Also w/fluoride. Bot. 100s, 1000s. *Rx-OTC.*
Use: Vitamin supplement.

flavine.
See: Acriflavine Hydrochloride.

Flavinoid-C. (Barth's) **Tab.:** Vitamin C 150 mg, hesperidin complex 10 mg, citrus bioflavonoid 50 mg, rutin 20 mg. Bot. 100s, 500s, 1000s. **Liq.:** Vitamin C 100 mg, bioflavonoid complex 100 mg/5 mL. Bot. 4 oz. *OTC.*
Use: Vitamin supplement.

flavocoxid.
Use: Oral nutritional supplement.
See: Limbrel.

•**flavodilol maleate.** (FLAY-voe-DILL-ole) USAN.
Use: Antihypertensive.

flavolutan.
See: Progesterone.

flavonoid compounds.
See: Bio-Flavonoid Compounds; Vitamin P.

Flavons. (Freeda) Bioflavonoids 500 mg (also contains calcium carbonate, calcium stearate). Sugar free. Tab. Bot. 100s, 250s. *OTC.*
Use: Water-soluble vitamin.

Flavons-500. (Freeda) Citrus bioflavonoids 500 mg. Sugar free. Tab. Bot. 100s, 250s. *OTC.*
Use: Water-soluble vitamin.

flavored diluent. (Roxane) Flavored vehicle for the immediate administration of crushed tablet or capsule product. Bot. 500 mL, UD 15 mL × 100.
Use: Flavored vehicle.

•**flavoxate hydrochloride.** (flay-VOKES-ate) USAN.
Tall Man: flavoxATE
Use: Antispasmodic, urinary; muscle relaxant; anticholinergic.
See: Urispas.

flavoxate hydrochloride. (Global) Flavoxate hydrochloride 100 mg. Film coated. Tab. 100s. *Rx.*
Use: Anticholinergic.

flavurol. Merbromin.
Use: Antiseptic.

•**flazalone.** (FLAY-zah-lone) USAN.
Use: Anti-inflammatory.

Flebogamma 5% DIF. (Grifols Biologicals) Immune globulin (human) 5% (50 mg/mL). D-sorbitol 5 g, polyethylene glycol ≤ 3 mg/mL. Preservative free. Inj., Soln. Vial. 10 mL, 50 mL, 100 mL, 200 mL, 400 mL. *Rx.*
Use: Immune globulin.

Flebogamma 10% DIF. (Grifols Biologicals) Immune globulin (human) 10% (100 mg/mL). D-sorbitol 5 g, polyethylene glycol ≤ 6 mg/mL. Preservative free. Inj., Soln. Vial. 50 mL, 100 mL, 200 mL. *Rx.*
Use: Immune globulin.

•**flecainide acetate.** (fleh-CANE-ide) *USP.*
Use: Antiarrhythmic agent.
See: Tambocor.

flecainide acetate. (Various Mfr.) Flecainide acetate 50 mg, 100 mg, 150 mg. Tab. 100s. *Rx.*
Use: Antiarrhythmic agent.

Fleet. (Fleet) Dibasic sodium phosphate 7 g, monobasic sodium phosphate 19 g/118 mL delivered dose (sodium 4.4 g/dose). Disp. enema. Squeeze bot. Pediatric 66 mL, Adult 133 mL. *OTC.*
Use: Laxative, enema.

Fleet Babylax. (Fleet) Glycerin 2.8 g. 4 mL per applicator. Liq.; rectal. App. 6s. *OTC.*
Use: Laxative.

Fleet Bagenema. (Fleet) Castile soap or Fleets bisacodyl prep. *OTC.*
Use: Laxative.

Fleet Bisacodyl. (Fleet) Bisacodyl 10 mg/30 mL delivered dose. Disp. enema. Squeeze bot. 37 mL. *OTC.*
Use: Laxative, enema.

Fleet Enema. (Fleet) Sodium biphosphate 19 g, sodium phosphate 7 g/118 mL. Bot. w/rectal tube 4.5 oz. Pediatric size 67.5 mL, 135 mL. *OTC.*
Use: Laxative.

Fleet Glycerin Suppositories. (Fleet) Glycerin 2 g. Supp.; rectal. 12s, 24s, 50s, 100s. *OTC.*
Use: Laxative.

Fleet Laxative. (Fleet) Bisacodyl. **EC Tab.:** 5 mg, sucrose. Bot. 25s, 100s. **Supp.:** 10 mg. Box 4s, 12s, 50s, 100s. *OTC.*
Use: Laxative.

Fleet Liquid Glycerin Suppositories. (Fleet) Glycerin 5.4 g. Liq.; rectal. 4s w/applicator (7.8 mL per applicator). *OTC.*
Use: Laxative.

Fleet Medicated Wipes. (Fleet) Hamamelis water 50%, alcohol 7%, glycerin 10%, benzalkonium Cl, methylparaben. Rectal pads. 100s. *OTC.*
Use: Perianal hygiene.

Fleet Mineral Oil. (Fleet) Mineral oil. Squeeze bot. 133 mL. *OTC.*
Use: Laxative, enema.

Fleet Pain Relief. (Fleet) Pramoxine hydrochloride 1%, glycerin 12%. Pads. 100s. *OTC.*
Use: Anorectal preparation.

Fleet Pedia-Lax. (Fleet) Glycerin 2.8 g. Liq.; rectal. 6s w/applicator (4 mL per applicator). *OTC.*
Use: Laxative.

Fleet Pedia-Lax Glycerin Suppositories. (Fleet) Glycerin 1 g. Supp.; rectal. 12s. *OTC.*
Use: Laxative.

Fleet Prep Kit 3. (Fleet) *Phospho-Soda* 45 mL (monobasic sodium phosphate 21.6 g, dibasic sodium phosphate 8.1 g), 4 bisacodyl tablets (5 mg each), bisacodyl enema 30 mL (10 mg). *OTC.*
Use: Laxative, enema.

•**fleroxacin.** (fler-OX-ah-SIN) USAN.
Use: Anti-infective.

•**flestolol sulfate.** (FLESS-toe-lahl) USAN.
Use: Antiadrenergic (β-receptor).

•**fletazepam.** (FLET-AZE-eh-pam) USAN.
Use: Muscle relaxant.

Fletcher's Castoria. (Mentholatum Co.) Senna concentrate 33.3 mg/mL, alcohol free, sucrose, parabens. Liq. Bot. 74 mL, 150 mL. *OTC.*
Use: Laxative.

Fletcher's Castoria for Children. (Mentholatum Co.) Senna 6.5%, alcohol 3.5%. Liq. Bot. 74 mL, 150 mL. *OTC.*
Use: Laxative.

Flexall. (Chattem) Menthol 7%. Aloe leaf juice, eucalyptus oil, glycerin, peppermint oil, methyl salicylate, SD-alcohol, thyme oil, triethanolamine, tocopherol. Gel. 113.3 g. *OTC.*
Use: Rub and liniment.

Flexall 454. (Chattem) Menthol 7%, alcohol, allantoin, aloe vera gel, boric acid, carbomer 940, diazolidinyl urea, eucalyptus oil, glycerin, iodine, parabens, methyl salicylate, peppermint oil, polysorbate 60, potassium iodide, propylene glycol, thyme oil, triethanolamine. Gel. Tube. 240 g. *OTC.*
Use: Analgesic, topical.

Flexall 454, Maximum Strength. (Chattem) Menthol 16%, aloe vera gel, eucalyptus oil, methylsalicylate, SD alcohol 38-B, thyme oil. Gel. Tube. 90 mg. *OTC.*
Use: Analgesic, topical.

Flex Anti-Dandruff Shampoo. (Revlon) Zinc pyrithione 1% in liquid shampoo. *OTC.*
Use: Antiseborrheic.

Flex Anti-Dandruff Styling Mousse. (Revlon) Zinc pyrithione 0.1%. Aerosol foam. *OTC.*
Use: Antiseborrheic.

Flexgen. (Kramer Novis) Vitamin C 500 mg, citrus bioflavonoids 50 mg, hawthorn berry extract 25 mg, horse chestnut extract 25 mg, hesperidin complex 25 mg, rutin 40 mg, witch hazel extract 25 mg. PEG. Tab. 60s. *OTC.*
Use: Water-soluble vitamin.

flexible hydroactive dressings/granules.
See: DuoDerm.
Intra Site.
Shur-Clens.
Sorbsan.

FlexiGel Strands. (Smith-Nephew) Single-use absorbent matrix. 6 g unit. Absorbent wound dressing. 10s. *OTC.*
Use: Dressing.

Flexitol Heel Balm. (LaCorium Health USA) Urea 25%. Aloe vera, benzyl alcohol, cetearyl alcohol, glyceryl, glycolic acid, lanolin, mineral oil, panthenol, paraffin, PEG, shea butter, tea tree oil, tocopheryl acetate. Oint. 28 g, 56 g, 70 g, 112 g. *OTC.*
Use: Emollient.

Flex Omega Benefits With Vitamin D-3. (Physician Recommended Nutriceuticals) Omega-3 667 mg (DHA 140 mg, EPA 420 mg, other omega-3s 107 mg), vitamin D 250 units. Soy. Dairy free, gluten free. Cap., softgel. 120s, 180s. *OTC.*
Use: Multivitamin and mineral with omega-3 polyunsaturated fatty acids.

Flexon. (Various Mfr.) Orphenadrine citrate 30 mg/mL. Inj. Vial 10 mL. *Rx.*
Use: Muscle relaxant.

Flex-Power Performance Sports. (Flex-Power) Trolamine salicylate 10%. Cetyl alcohol, EDTA, parabens, glycerols, stearyl alcohol, sodium metabisulfite. Cream. Citrus light and clean scents. 120 g. *OTC.*
Use: Rub and liniment.

Flexsol. (Alcon) Sterile, buffered, isotonic aqueous soln. of sodium Cl, sodium borate, boric acid, adsorbobase. Bot. 6 oz. *OTC.*
Use: Contact lens care.

•**flibanserin.** (flib-AN-ser-in) USAN.
Use: Antidepressant.

•**flindokalner.** (flin-doe-KAL-ner) USAN.
Use: Neuroprotectant.

Flintstones Children's. (Bayer Consumer Care) Vitamin A 2500 units, E 15 mg, C 60 mg, folic acid 0.3 mg, B_1 1.05 mg, B_2 1.2 mg, B_3 13.5 mg, B_6 1.05 mg, B_{12} 4.5 mcg, D 400 units. Chew. Tab. Bot. 60s, 100s. *OTC.*
Use: Vitamin supplement.

Flintstones Complete. (Bayer Consumer Care) Elemental iron 18 mg, vitamins A 5000 units, D 400 units, E 30 mg, B_1

1.5 mg, B_2 1.7 mg, B_3 20 mg, B_5 10 mg, B_6 2 mg, B_{12} 6 mcg, C 60 mg, folic acid 0.4 mg, biotin 40 mcg, Ca, Cu, I, Mg, P, zinc 15 mg. Chew. Tab. Bot. 60s, 120s. *OTC.*
Use: Mineral, vitamin supplement.

Flintstones Plus Calcium. (Bayer Consumer Care) Vitamin A 2500 units, D units 400, E 15 units, C 60 mg, folic acid 0.3 mg, B_1 1.05 mg, B_2 1.2 mg, B_3 13.5 mg, B_6 1.05 mg, B_{12} 4.5 mcg, Ca 200 mg. Chew. Tab. Bot. 60s. *OTC.*
Use: Mineral, vitamin supplement.

Flintstones Plus Extra C Children's. (Bayer Consumer Care) Vitamins A 2500 units, D 400 units, E 15 mg, C 250 mg, folic acid 0.3 mg, B_1 1.05 mg, B_2 1.2 mg, niacin 13.5 mg, B_6 1.05 mg, B_{12} 4.5 mcg. Tab. Bot. 60s, 100s. *OTC.*
Use: Vitamin supplement.

Flintstones Plus Iron Multivitamins. (Bayer Consumer Care) Vitamins A 2500 units, E 15 mg, C 60 mg, folic acid 0.3 mg, $B_1$1.05 mg, B_2 1.2 mg, niacin 13.5 mg, B_6 1.05 mg, B_{12} 4.5 mcg, D 400 units, iron 15 mg. Chew. Tab. Bot. 60s, 100s. *OTC.*
Use: Mineral, vitamin supplement.

Flo-Coat. (Mallinckrodt) Barium sulfate 100%. Simethicone. Susp. Bot. 1850 mL. *Rx.*
Use: Radiopaque agent, GI contrast agent.

Flocor. (SynthRx Corp.) Poloxamer 188.
Use: Treatment of sickle cell crisis. [Orphan Drug]

•**floctafenine.** (FLOCK-tah-FEN-een) USAN.
Use: Analgesic.

Flolan. (Gilead) Epoprostenol sodium 0.5 mg, 1.5 mg. Mannitol, sodium chloride. Pow. for Reconstitution. 17 mL. *Rx.*
Use: Antihypertensive; vasodilator.

Flomax. (Boehringer Ingelheim) Tamsulosin hydrochloride 0.4 mg. Cap. Bot. 100s, 1000s. *Rx.*
Use: Benign prostatic hyperplasia treatment, antiadrenergic.

Flonase. (GlaxoSmithKline) Fluticasone propionate 50 mcg/actuation. Dextrose, polysorbate 80, benzalkonium chloride 0.02% w/w, phenylethyl alcohol w/w 0.25%. Spray Susp. Intranasal. Amber glass bot. w/meterizing atomizer pump and nasal adapter. 16 g (120 actuations). *Rx.*
Use: Respiratory inhalant, intranasal steroid.

Flo-Pred. (Taro Pharmaceuticals) Prednisolone 15 mg/5 mL (equiv. to prednisolone acetate 16.7 mg). Butylparaben, disodium edetate, glycerin, propylene glycol, sorbitol, sucralose. Cherry flavor. Oral Susp. 52 mL, 65 mL. *Rx.*
Use: Adrenocortical steroid, glucocorticoid.

Florajen Acidophilus. (American Lifeline) *L. acidophilus* > 20 billion live cultures. Rice maltodextrin. Gluten free, preservative free, and sugar free. Cap. 30s, 60s. *OTC.*
Use: Probiotic.

Florajen Bifidoblend. (American Lifeline) *B. bifidum* > 9 billion live cultures, *B. longum* > 1 billion live cultures. Rice maltodextrin. Gluten free, preservative free, and sugar free. Cap. 60s. *OTC.*
Use: Probiotic.

Florajen 4 Kids. (American Lifeline) 6 billion live culture blend of *B. lactis*, *B. bifidum*, *L. acidophilus*, *L. rhamnosus*. Glucose, rice maltodextrin. Gluten free and preservative free. Cap. 30s. *OTC.*
Use: Probiotic.

Florajen 3. (American Lifeline) *L. acidophilus* 7.5 billion, *B. lactis* 6 billion, *B. longum* 1.5 billion. Rice maltodextrin. Gluten free, preservative free, and sugar free. Cap. 60s. *OTC.*
Use: Probiotic.

Floranex. (Rising) Mixed culture of *Lactobacillus acidophilus* and *L. bulgaricus*. **Chew. Tab.:** 1 million CFU. Lactose, nonfat dried milk, sucrose. 50s. **Gran.:** 100 million CFU. 1 g packets. 12s. *OTC.*
Use: Nutritional supplement.

Flora-Q. (PharmaDerm) 8 billion CFU blend of *L. acidophilus*, *Bifidobacterium*, *L. paracasei*, *S. thermophilus*. Maltodextrin. Gluten free, lactose free, and preservative free. Cap. 30s. *OTC.*
Use: Probiotic.

Flora-Q2. (PharmaDerm) 16 billion CFU blend of *L. acidophilus*, *Bifidobacterium*, *L. paracasei*, *S. thermophilus*. Maltodextrin. Gluten free, lactose free, and preservative free. Cap. 30s. *OTC.*
Use: Probiotic.

Florastor. (Biocodex) *Saccharomyces boulardil lyo* 250 mg. Lactose. Cap. 10s, 50s. *OTC.*
Use: Oral nutritional supplement.

Florastor Kids. (Biocodex) *Saccharomyces boulardil lyo* 250 mg. Tutti-frutti flavor. Oral Pow. 10s. *OTC.*
Use: Oral nutritional supplement.

•**florbenazine F 18.** (flor-BEN-a-zeen) USAN.
Use: Diagnostic imaging agent.

•**florbetaben F18.** (flor-BAY-ta-BEN) USAN.
Use: Diagnostic radiopharmaceutical.

•**florbetapir F 18.** (flor-BAY-ta-pir) USAN.
Use: Diagnostic imaging agent.

Flor-D Chewable Tab. (Derm Pharm.) Fluoride 1 mg, vitamins A 4000 units, D 400 units, C 75 mg, B_1 1.5 mg, B_2 1.8 mg, niacinamide 15 mg, B_6 1 mg, B_{12} 3 mcg, calcium pantothenate 10 mg. Chew. Tab. Bot. 100s. *Rx.*
Use: Mineral, vitamin supplement.

Flor-D Drops. (Derm Pharm.) Fluoride 0.5 mg, vitamins A 3000 units, D 400 units, C 60 mg, B_1 1 mg, B_2 1.2 mg, niacinamide 8 mg/0.6 mL. Drops. Bot. 60 mL. *Rx.*
Use: Mineral, vitamin supplement.

•**flordipine.** (FLORE-dih-peen) USAN.
Use: Antihypertensive.

Florical. (Mericon) Ca 145 mg (calcium content expressed in mg elemental calcium), fluoride 3.75 mg (fluoride content expressed in mg elemental fluoride). Tab. 100s, 500s. *OTC.*
Use: Nutritional supplement, multimineral.

Florida Foam. (Hill Dermaceuticals) Benzalkonium Cl, aluminum subacetate, boric acid 2%. Bot. 8 oz. *OTC.*
Use: Soap substitute; antiseborrheic; antifungal; dermatologic-acne.

Florida Sunburn Relief. (Pharmacel Laboratory, Inc.) Benzyl alcohol 3%, phenol 0.4%, camphor 0.2%, menthol 0.15%. Lot. Bot. 60 mL. *OTC.*
Use: Sunburn relief.

Florinef Acetate. (Monarch) Fludrocortisone acetate, 0.1 mg, lactose. Tab. Bot. 100s. *Rx.*
Use: Corticosteroid.

Florone Cream. (Dermik) Diflorasone diacetate 0.5 mg/g (0.05%) w/stearic acid, sorbitan mono-oleate, polysorbate 60, sorbic acid, citric acid, propylene glycol, purified water. Cream. Tube 15 g, 30 g, 60 g. *Rx.*
Use: Corticosteroid, topical.

Florone E. (Dermik) Diflorasone diacetate 0.5 mg. Tube 15 g, 30 g, 60 g. *Rx.*
Use: Corticosteroid, topical.

Florone Ointment. (Dermik) Diflorasone diacetate 0.5 mg/g (0.05%), polyoxypropylene 15-stearyl ether, stearic acid, lanolin alcohol, white petrolatum. Oint. Tube 15 g, 30 g, 60 g. *Rx.*
Use: Corticosteroid, topical.

Floropryl. (Merck & Co.) Isoflurophate 0.025% in sterile ophthalmic ointment in polyethylene-mineral oil gel. Tube 3.5 g. *Rx.*
Use: Agent for glaucoma.

Florvite Drops. (Everett) Fluoride 0.25 mg, 0.5 mg, A 1500 units, D 400 units, E 5 units, B_1 0.5 mg, B_2 0.6 mg, B_3 8 mg, B_6 0.4 mg, B_{12} 2 mcg, C 35 mg. Bot. 50 mL. *Rx.*
Use: Mineral, vitamin supplement; dental caries agent.

Florvite Half Strength. (Everett) Elemental fluoride 0.5 mg, vitamins A 2500 units, D 400 units, E 15 mg, B_1 1.05 mg, B_2 1.2 mg, B_3 13.5 mg, B_6 1.05 mg, B_{12} 4.5 mcg, C 60 mg, folic acid 0.3 mg. Chew. Tab. Bot. 100s. *Rx.*
Use: Mineral, vitamin supplement; dental caries agent.

Florvite Pediatric Drops. (Everett) Elemental fluorine, 0.25 mg/mL, 0.5 mg/mL, Vitamins A 1500 units, D 400 units, E 5 mg, B_1 0.5 mg, B_2 0.6 mg, B_3 8 mg, B_6 0.4 mg, B_{12} 2 mcg, C 35 mg/mL. Bot. 50 mL *Rx.*
Use: Mineral, vitamin supplement; dental caries agent.

Florvite + Iron Chewable. (Everett) Fluoride 1 mg, iron 12 mg, vitamins A 2500 units, D 400 units, E 15 mg, B_1 1.05 mg, B_2 1.2 mg, B_3 13.5 mg, B_6 1.05 mg, B_{12} 4.5 mcg, C 60 mg, folic acid 0.3 mg, Cu, Zn 10 mg, sucrose. Chew. Tab. Bot. 100s. *Rx.*
Use: Mineral, vitamin supplement; dental caries agent.

Florvite + Iron Drops. (Everett) Elemental fluorine 0.25 mg, 0.5 mg, Vitamins A 1500 units, D 400 units, E 5 mg, B_1 0.5 mg, B_2 0.6 mg, B_3 8 mg, B_6 0.4 mg, C 35 mg, iron 10 mg/mL. Liq. Bot. 50 mL. *Rx.*
Use: Mineral, vitamin supplement; dental caries agent.

Florvite Tablets. (Everett) Fluoride 1 mg, vitamins A 2500 units, D 400 units, E 15 mg, B_1 1.05 mg, B_2 1.2 mg, B_3 13.5 mg, B_6 1.05 mg, B_{12} 4.5 mcg, C 60 mg, folic acid 0.3 mg. Chew. Tab. Bot. 100s, 1000s. *Rx.*
Use: Mineral, vitamin supplement; dental caries agent.

•**flosequinan.** (flow-SEH-kwih-NAHN) USAN.
Use: Antihypertensive (vasodilator).

Flovent Diskus. (GlaxoSmithKline) Fluticasone propionate 50 mcg/actuation, 100 mcg/actuation, 250 mcg/actuation. Lactose. Pow., Inhal. Inhalation device containing 60 blisters. *Rx.*
Use: Respiratory inhalant, corticosteroid.

Flovent HFA. (GlaxoSmithKline) Fluticasone propionate/actuation 44 mcg, 110 mcg, 220 mcg. Aerosol. Susp. Inh. Canister with actuator. 10.6 g (120 metered inhalations) (44 mcg only), 12 g

(120 metered inhalations) (110 mcg and 220 mcg only). *Rx.*
Use: Respiratory inhalant, corticosteroid.

•**floxacillin.** (FLOX-ah-SILL-in) USAN.
Use: Anti-infective.

Floxin. (Ortho-McNeil) Ofloxacin, 200 mg, 300 mg, 400 mg. Lactose. Tab. Bot. 50s (except 400 mg), 100s (400 mg only); UD 6s (200 mg only), 100s. *Rx.*
Use: Anti-infective, fluoroquinolone.

Floxin Otic. (Daiichi) Ofloxacin 3 mg/mL. Benzalkonium chloride 0.0025%. Otic Soln. Dropper Bot. 5 mL, 10 mL. *Rx.*
Use: Otic antibiotic.

•**floxuridine.** (flox-YOUR-ih-deen) *USP.*
Use: Antiviral; antineoplastic.
See: FUDR.

floxuridine. (Bedford) Floxuridine 500 mg. Pow. for Inj., lyophilized. Vial 5 mL. *Rx.*
Use: Antiviral; antineoplastic.

Fluarix. (GlaxoSmithKline) Hemagglutinin 15 mcg each of A/Christchurch/16/2010 NIB-74XP (H1N1) (an A/California/7/2009-like virus), A/Texas/50/2012 NYMC X-223A (H3N2) (an A/Victoria/361/2011-like virus), and B/Massachusetts/2/2012 NYMC BX-51B per 0.5 mL. Each 0.5 mL dose also contains octoxynol-10 ≤ 0.085 mg, alpha-tocopheryl hydrogen succinate ≤ 0.1 mg, and ≤ 0.415 mg polysorbate 80. Each dose also may contain residual amounts of hydrocortisone ≤ 0.0016 mcg, gentamicin sulfate ≤ 0.15 mcg, ovalbumin ≤ 0.05 mcg, formaldehyde ≤ 5 mcg, and sodium deoxycholate ≤ 50 mcg. Preservative free. Inj., Susp. (purified split-virus). 0.5 mL prefilled, single-dose syringes (the tip caps of the prefilled syringes may contain natural latex rubber; the rubber plungers do not contain latex). *Rx.*
Use: Viral vaccine.

Fluarix Quadrivalent. (GlaxoSmithKline) Hemagglutinin 15 mcg each of A/Christchurch/16/2010 NIB-74XP (H1N1) (an A/California/7/2009-like virus), A/Texas/50/2012 NYMC X-223A (H3N2) (an A/Victoria/361/2011-like virus), B/Massachusetts/2/2012 NYMC BX-51B, and B/Brisbane/60/2008 per 0.5 mL. Each 0.5 mL dose also contains octoxynol-10 ≤ 0.115 mg, alpha-tocopheryl hydrogen succinate ≤ 0.135 mg, and ≤ 0.55 mg of polysorbate 80. Each dose also may contain residual amounts of hydrocortisone ≤ 0.0016 mcg, gentamicin sulfate ≤ 0.15 mcg, ovalbumin ≤ 0.05 mcg, formaldehyde ≤ 5 mcg, and sodium deoxycholate ≤ 65 mcg. Preservative free. Inj., Susp. (purified split virus). 0.5 mL prefilled, single-dose syringe (the tip caps of the prefilled syringes may contain natural latex rubber; the rubber plungers do not contain latex). *Rx.*
Use: Viral vaccine.

•**fluazacort.** (flew-AZE-ah-kort) USAN.
Use: Anti-inflammatory.

•**flubanilate hydrochloride.** (flew-BAN-ill-ate) USAN.
Use: Antidepressant; CNS stimulant.

•**flubendazole.** (FLEW-BEN-dah-zole) USAN.
Use: Antiprotozoal.

Flublok. (Protein Sciences Corporation) Hemagglutinin 45 mcg each of A/California/7/2009 (H1N1), A/Texas/50/2012 (H3N2), B/Massachusetts/2/2012 per 0.5 mL. Latex free and preservative free. Inj., Soln. Single-dose vial. 0.5 mL. Each 0.5 mL dose may also contain residual amounts of baculovirus and host cell proteins (≤ 28.5 mcg), baculovirus and cellular DNA (≤ 10 ng), and *Triton X-100* (≤ 100 mcg). *Rx.*
Use: Viral vaccine.

Flucaine. (Altaire) Proparacaine hydrochloride 0.5%, fluorescein sodium 0.25%. Soln. 5 mL. *Rx.*
Use: Ophthalmic local anesthetic.

flucarbril.
Use: Muscle relaxant; analgesic.

Flucelvax. (Novartis Vaccines) Hemagglutinin 15 mcg each of A/Brisbane/10/2010 (H1N1) (an A/California/7/2009-like virus), A/Texas/50/2012 NYMC X-223A (H3N2) (an A/Victoria/361/2011-like virus), and B/Massachusetts/2/2012 per 0.5 mL. Each 0.5 mL dose may contain residual amounts of Madin Darby Canine Kidney (MDCK) cell protein (≤ 8.4 mcg), protein other than hemagglutinin (≤ 120 mcg), MDCK cell DNA (≤ 10 ng), polysorbate 80 (≤ 1,125 mcg), cetyltrimethylammonium bromide (≤ 13.5 mcg), and beta-propiolactone (≤ 0.5 mcg). Inj., Susp. (purified split-virus). Preservative free. 0.5 mL prefilled, single-dose syringe (the tip caps of the prefilled syringes may contain natural latex rubber; the rubber plungers do not contain latex). *Rx.*
Use: Viral vaccine.

•**fluciclatide F 18.** (floo-SIK-la-tide) USAN.
Use: Radiopharmaceutical.

•**flucindole.** (flew-SIN-dole) USAN.
Use: Antipsychotic.

•**flucloronide.** (flew-KLOR-oh-nide) USAN.
Use: Corticosteroid, topical.

Flu, Cold & Cough Medicine. (Major) Pseudoephedrine hydrochloride 60 mg, chlorpheniramine 4 mg, dextromethorphan HBr 20 mg, acetaminophen 500 mg. Pow. Pck. 6s. *OTC.*
Use: Analgesic; antihistamine; antitussive; decongestant.

•**fluconazole.** (flew-KOE-nuh-sole) *USP.*
Use: Antifungal.
See: Diflucan.

fluconazole. (Various Mfr.) Fluconazole. **Tab.:** 50 mg, 100 mg, 150 mg, 200 mg. 30s, 100s, UD 12s (150 mg only), UD 30s (200 mg only). **Pow. for Susp.:** 10 mg/mL, 40 mg/mL when reconstituted. May contain sodium benzoate, sucrose. 35 mL. *Rx.*
Use: Antifungal agent, triazole antifungal.

fluconazole in dextrose. (Various Mfr.) Fluconazole 2 mg/mL. Contains dextrose 56 mg/mL. Inj., Soln. Flexible container. 100 mL, 200 mL. *Rx.*
Use: Antifungal agent, triazole antifungal.

fluconazole in sodium chloride 0.9%. (Various Mfr.) Fluconazole 2 mg/mL. Contains sodium chloride 9 mg/mL. Inj., Soln. 50 mL vial; 100 and 200 mL vial and flexible container. *Rx.*
Use: Antifungal agent, triazole antifungal.

•**flucrylate.** (FLEW-krih-late) USAN.
Use: Surgical aid (tissue adhesive).

•**flucytosine.** (flew-SITE-oh-seen) *USP.*
Use: Antifungal.
See: Ancobon.

flucytosine. (Oceanside Pharmaceuticals) Flucytosine 250 mg, 500 mg. Lactose. Cap. 100s. *Rx.*
Use: Anti-infective, antifungal.

•**fludalanine.** (flew-DAL-AH-neen) USAN.
Use: Anti-infective.

•**fludarabine phosphate.** (flew-DAR-uh-BEAN) USAN.
Use: Antineoplastic. [Orphan Drug]

fludarabine phosphate. (Various Mfr.) Fludarabine phosphate. **Inj., Lyophilized, Cake:** 50 mg. Preservative free. Single-dose vials. **Inj.:** 25 mg/mL. Preservative free. Mannitol 25 mg/mL, sodium hydroxide. Single-dose vial. 2 mL. *Rx.*
Use: Antimetabolite.

•**fludazonium chloride.** (FLEW-dazz-OH-nee-uhm) USAN.
Use: Anti-infective, topical.

•**fludeoxyglucose F 18 injection.** (FLEW-dee-OX-ee-GLUE-kose) *USP.*
Use: Diagnostic aid (brain disorders, thyroid disorders, liver disorders, cardiac disease, and neoplastic disease); radiopharmaceutical.

•**fludorex.** (FLEW-doe-rex) USAN.
Use: Anorexic; antiemetic.

•**fludrocortisone acetate.** (flew-droe-CORE-tih-sone) *USP.*
Use: Adrenocortical steroid (salt-regulating).
See: Florinef Acetate.

fludrocortisone acetate. (Various Mfr.) Fludrocortisone acetate 0.1 mg. Tab. Bot. 100s. *Rx.*
Use: Adrenocortical steroid.

•**flufenamic acid.** (FLEW-fen-AM-ik) USAN.
Use: Anti-inflammatory.

•**flufenisal.** (flew-FEN-ih-sal) USAN.
Use: Analgesic.

Fluidex. (Columbia) Natural botanical ingredients. Tab. Bot. 36s, 72s.
Use: Diuretic.

Flu-Imune. (Wyeth) Influenza virus vaccine. Vial 5 mL (10 doses). (Purified surface antigen.) *Rx.*
Use: Immunization.

fluitran. Trichlormethiazide.

FluLaval. (GlaxoSmithKline) Hemagglutinin 15 mcg each of A/California/7/2009 NYMC X-179A (H1N1), A/Texas/50/2012 NYMC X-223A (H3N2) (an A/Victoria/361/2011-like virus), and B/Massachusetts/2/2012 NYMC BX-51B per 0.5 mL. Mercury ≤ 25 mcg/dose, thimerosal. Each dose may also contain residual amounts of ovalbumin ≤ 0.3 mcg, formaldehyde ≤ 25 mcg, and sodium deoxycholate ≤ 50 mcg. Inj., Susp. (purified split virus). Multidose vial. 5 mL. *Rx.*
Use: Viral vaccine.

FluLaval Quadrivalent. (GlaxoSmithKline) Hemagglutinin 15 mcg each of A/California/7/2009 NYMC X-179A (H1N1), A/Texas/50/2012 NYMC X-223A (H3N2) (an A/Victoria/361/2011-like virus), B/Massachusetts/02/2012 NYMC BX-51B, and B/Brisbane/60/2008 per 0.5 mL. Each 0.5 mL dose contains thimerosal 50 mcg (mercury < 25 mcg), alpha-tocopheryl hydrogen succinate (≤ 320 mcg), and polysorbate 80 (≤ 887 mcg). Each 0.5 mL dose may also contain residual amounts of ovalbumin (≤ 0.3 mcg), formaldehyde (≤ 25 mcg), and sodium deoxycholate (≤ 50 mcg) from the manufacturing process. Inj., Susp. (purified split virus). Multidose vial. 5 mL. *Rx.*
Use: Viral vaccine.

Flumadine. (Caraco) Rimantadine hydrochloride 100 mg. Film-coated. Tab. 100s. *Rx.*
Use: Antiviral.

•**flumazenil.** (flew-MAZ-ah-nil) USAN.
Use: Antagonist (to benzodiazepine), antidote.
See: Romazicon.

flumazenil. (Various Mfr.) Flumazenil 0.1 mg/mL. May contain EDTA, parabens, sodium chloride. Inj. Multidose vials. 5 mL, 10 mL. *Rx.*
Use: Antidote.

•**flumequine.** (FLEW-meh-kwin) USAN.
Use: Anti-infective.

•**flumeridone.** (FLEW-MER-ih-dohn) USAN.
Use: Antiemetic.

•**flumethasone.** (FLEW-meth-ah-zone) USAN.
Use: Corticosteroid, topical.

•**flumethasone pivalate.** (FLEW-meth-ah-zone PIH-vah-late) *USP.*
Use: Corticosteroid, topical.

flumethiazide.
Use: Diuretic.

•**flumetramide.** (flew-MEH-trah-mide) USAN.
Use: Muscle relaxant.

•**flumezapine.** (FLEW-MEZZ-ah-peen) USAN.
Use: Antipsychotic; neuroleptic.

•**fluminorex.** (flew-MEE-no-rex) USAN.
Use: Anorexic.

FluMist Quadrivalent. (MedImmune Vaccines) Fluorescent focus units $10^{6.5\text{-}7.5}$ of A/California/7/2009 (H1N1), A/Texas/50/2012 (H3N2) (an A/Victoria/361/2011-like virus), B/Massachusetts/2/2012 (B/Yamagata/16/88 lineage), and B/Brisbane/60/2008 (B/Victoria/2/87 lineage) per 0.2 mL actuation. Each 0.2 mL dose also contains monosodium glutamate 0.188 mg, hydrolyzed porcine gelatin 2 mg, arginine 2.42 mg, sucrose 13.68 mg, dibasic potassium phosphate 2.26 mg, and monobasic potassium phosphate 0.96 mg. Each dose contains residual amounts of ovalbumin (< 0.25 mcg) and may contain residual amounts of gentamicin sulfate (< 0.015 mcg/mL) ethylenediaminetetraacetic acid (< 0.37 mcg). Preservative free, latex free. Spray, Soln.; intranasal. Prefilled, single-dose sprayer. 0.2 mL. *Rx.*
Use: Viral vaccine.

•**flumizole.** (FLEW-mih-zole) USAN.
Use: Anti-inflammatory.

•**flumoxonide.** (flew-MOX-OH-nide) USAN.
Use: Adrenocortical steroid.

flunarizine.
Use: Alternating hemiplegia. [Orphan Drug]
See: Sibelium.

•**flunarizine hydrochloride.** (flew-NAR-ih-zeen) USAN.
Use: Vasodilator.

•**flunidazole.** (FLEW-nih-dah-ZOLE) USAN.
Use: Antiprotozoal.

•**flunisolide.** (flew-NIH-sole-ide) *USP.*
Use: Corticosteroid, topical, respiratory inhalant.
See: Aerospan.

flunisolide. (Bausch & Lomb) Flunisolide 0.025% (25 mcg/actuation), propylene glycol, polyethylene glycol 3350, EDTA, benzalkonium chloride. Soln. 25 mL nasal pump dispenser (200 sprays/bot). *Rx.*
Use: Respiratory inhalant, intranasal steroid.

•**flunisolide acetate.** (flew-NIH-sole-ide) USAN.
Use: Anti-inflammatory.

•**flunitrazepam.** (flew-NYE-TRAY-zeh-pam) USAN.
Use: Hypnotic; sedative.

•**flunixin.** (flew-NIX-in) USAN.
Use: Analgesic; anti-inflammatory.

•**flunixin meglumine.** (flew-NIX-in meh-GLUE-meen) *USP.*
Use: Analgesic; anti-inflammatory.

Fluocet. (Alra) Fluocinolone acetonide 0.025%, 0.01%. Cream. Tube 15 g, 60 g. *Rx.*
Use: Corticosteroid, topical.

fluocinolide. (flew-oh-SIN-oh-lide)
See: Fluocinonide.

•**fluocinolone acetonide.** (flew-oh-SIN-oh-lone ah-SEE-toe-nide) *USP.*
Use: Corticosteroid, topical; corticosteroid, ophthalmic.
See: Fluocinolone Acetonide Body.
Fluocinolone Acetonide Scalp.
Fluonid.
Retisert.
Synalar.
Synalar TS Kit.
W/Hydroquinone, Tretinoin.
See: Tri-Luma.

fluocinolone acetonide. (Amneal) Fluocinolone acetonide 0.01%. Isopropyl alcohol, lt. mineral oil, peanut oil. Oil; otic. 20 mL w/dropper. *Rx.*
Use: Otic corticosteroid.

fluocinolone acetonide body. (Amneal) Fluocinolone acetonide 0.01%. Isopro-

pyl alcohol, lt. mineral oil, peanut oil. Oil. 118 mL. *Rx.*
Use: Anti-inflammatory agent, topical corticosteroid.

fluocinolone acetonide scalp. (Amneal) Fluocinolone acetonide 0.01%. Isopropyl alcohol, lt. mineral oil, peanut oil. Oil. 118 mL w/2 shower caps. *Rx.*
Use: Anti-inflammatory agent, topical corticosteroid.

•**fluocinonide.** (FLEW-oh-SIN-oh-nide) *USP. Formerly Fluocinolide.*
Use: Corticosteroid, topical.
See: Lidex.
Lidex-E.
Vanos.

fluocinonide. (Various Mfr.) Fluocinonide. **Cream:** 0.05%, 0.1%. May contain glycerin, glyceryl, PEG, propylene glycol. 15 g (0.05% only), 30 g, 60 g, 120 g. **Oint.:** 0.05%. 15 g, 30 g, 60 g. **Soln.:** 0.05%. 60 mL. **Gel:** 0.05%. 60 g.
Use: Corticosteroid, topical.

•**fluocortin butyl.** (FLEW-oh-CORE-tin BYOO-tuhl) USAN.
Use: Anti-inflammatory.

•**fluocortolone.** (FLEW-oh-CORE-toe-lone) USAN.
Use: Corticosteroid, topical.

•**fluocortolone caproate.** (FLEW-oh-CORE-toe-lone) USAN.
Use: Corticosteroid, topical.

Fluonex. (AstraZeneca) Fluocinonide 0.05%. Cream. Tube. 15 g, 30 g. *Rx.*
Use: Corticosteroid, topical.

Fluonid. (Allergan) Fluocinolone acetonide 0.01%. Soln. Bot. 20 mL, 60 mL. *Rx.*
Use: Corticosteroid, topical.

Fluoracaine. (Akorn) Proparacaine hydrochloride 0.5%, fluorescein sodium 0.25%. Glycerin, povidone, polysorbate 80, thimerosal 0.01%, boric acid, sodium hydroxide and/or hydrochloric acid. Soln. 5 mL. *Rx.*
Use: Anesthetic, local; ophthalmic.

Fluor-A-Day. (Arbor Pharmaceuticals) Fluoride 0.25 mg (from 0.55 mg of sodium fluoride), 0.5 mg (from 1.1 mg of sodium fluoride), 1 mg (from 2.2 mg of sodium fluoride). Maltodextrin, sorbitol, xylitol. Sugar free. Raspberry flavor. Chew. Tab. 120s. *Rx.*
Use: Trace element, fluoride.

•**fluorescein.** (FLURE-eh-seen) *USP.*
Use: Diagnostic aid (corneal trauma indicator).
See: Fluorescite.

Fluorescein Injection Lite. (HUB) Fluorescein sodium 10%. Inj., Soln. Single-dose vials. 5 mL. *Rx.*
Use: Ophthalmic diagnostic product.

•**fluorescein sodium.** (FLURE-eh-seen) *USP. Formerly Fluorescein, soluble.*
Use: Diagnostic aid, corneal trauma indicator.
See: AK-Fluor.
Fluorescein Injection Lite.
Fluorescite.
Fluorets.
Fluor-I-Strips.
Ful-Glo.
Funduscein.
Ophthifluor.
W/Benoxinate Hydrochloride.
See: Altafluor.
Fluress.
Flurox.
W/Proparacaine Hydrochloride.
See: Flucaine.
Fluoracaine.

fluorescein sodium/benoxinate hydrochloride. (Bausch & Lomb) Benoxinate hydrochloride 0.4%, fluorescein sodium 0.25%. Povidone, boric acid, chlorobutanol 1%. Soln., Ophth. 5 mL w/dropper. *Rx.*
Use: Ophthalmic local anesthetic.

fluorescein sodium intravenous.
See: Fluorescite.

fluorescein sodium/sodium hyaluronate.
See: Sodium Hyaluronate and Fluorescein Sodium Healon Yellow.

fluorescein sodium 2%. (Ciba Vision) Sterile aqueous solution containing fluorescein sodium 2%. *Dropperette* 1 mL, Box 12s.
Use: Diagnostic aid, ophthalmic.

fluorescein sodium 2% solution. (Alcon) *Drop-Tainer* 15 mL, *Steri-Unit* 2 mL 12s.
Use: Diagnostic aid, ophthalmic.

fluorescein sodium with proparacaine hydrochloride. (Various Mfr.) Proparacaine hydrochloride 0.5%, fluorescein sodium 0.25%. Povidone, glycerin, EDTA, thimerosal 0.01%. Soln. Bot. 5 mL with dropper. *Rx.*
Use: Anesthetic, local; diagnostic aid, ophthalmic.

Fluorescite. (Alcon) Fluorescein sodium 10%. Inj. Amp. 5 mL with syringes. *Rx.*
Use: Diagnostic aid, ophthalmic.

Fluoresoft 0.35%. (Various Mfr.) Fluorexon 0.35%. Preservative free. Soln. 0.35 mL ampules. 20s. *OTC.*
Use: Diagnostic aid, ophthalmic.

Fluorets. (Bausch & Lomb) Fluorescein sodium 1 mg. Strip. Box 100s. *OTC.*
Use: Diagnostic aid, ophthalmic.

fluorexon.
Use: Ophthalmic diagnostic product.
See: Fluoresoft 0.35%.
fluorexon disodium.
Use: Ophthalmic local anesthetic.
See: FluraSafe.
fluoride. (Kirkman) Fluoride 1 mg (sodium fluoride 2.21 mg). Tab. Bot. 1000s. *Rx.*
Use: Dental caries agent.
Fluoride Loz. (Kirkman) Fluoride 1 mg (sodium fluoride 2.21 mg). Bot. 1000s. *Rx.*
Use: Dental caries agent.
fluoride sodium.
See: Ludent.
ReNaf.
Sodium Fluoride.
fluoride therapy.
See: Cari-Tab.
ControlRx.
Coral.
Fluor-A-Day.
Fluorineed.
Fluorinse.
Monocal.
Mulvidren-F.
OrthoWash.
PerioMed.
Point Two.
Poly-Vi-Flor.
SF 5000 Plus.
SF 1.1%.
SodiPhluor.
Soluvite-F.
Tri-Vi-Flor.
Fluoridex Daily Defense Sensitivity Relief. (Discus Dental) Sodium fluoride 1.1%, potassium nitrate 5%. Saccharin, sorbitol. Mint flavor. Dental paste. 112 g. *Rx.*
Use: Mouth and throat product, preparation for sensitive teeth.
Fluorigard. (Colgate Oral) Fluoride 0.02% (from sodium fluoride 0.05%), alcohol 6%, tartrazine. Bot. 180 mL, 300 mL, 480 mL. *Rx.*
Use: Dental caries agent.
Fluorineed. (Hanlon) Fluoride 1 mg. Chew. Tab. Bot. 100s, 1000s. *Rx.*
Use: Dental caries agent.
Fluorinse. (Oral-B) Fluoride 0.09% from sodium fluoride 0.2%. Bot. 480 mL. *Rx.*
Use: Dental caries agent.
Fluorinse. (Pacemaker) Fluoride mouthwash. Pack. Fluoride ion level 0.05%, 0.2%. UD Bot. 32 oz. Concentrate 1 oz, 4 oz, gal. *Rx.*
Use: Dental caries agent.
Fluoritab. (Fluoritab) Sodium fluoride 2.2 mg equivalent to 1 mg of fluorine (as fluoride ion) w/inert organic filler 75.8 mg. Tab. 100s; Liq. Dropper Bot. Fluoride 0.125 mg from sodium fluoride 0.275 mg. Drop 30 mL. *Rx.*
Use: Dental caries agent.
5-fluorocytosine.
See: Ancobon.
•**fluorodopa F 18 injection.** (FLEW-roe-DOE-pah) *USP.*
Use: Diagnostic aid (brain imaging); radiopharmaceutical.
fluorogestone acetate.
Use: Hormone, progestin.
fluorohydrocortisone acetate.
9-α-Fluorohydrocortisone.
•**fluorometholone.** (flure-oh-METH-oh-lone) *USP.*
Use: Corticosteroid, ophthalmic.
See: Flarex.
FML.
fluorometholone. (Various Mfr.) Fluorometholone 0.1%. Benzalkonium chloride 0.004%, EDTA, polysorbate 80, polyvinyl alcohol 1.4%. Ophth. Susp. Bot. 5 mL, 10 mL, 15 mL. *Rx.*
Use: Corticosteroid, ophthalmic; anti-inflammatory.
•**fluorometholone acetate.** (flure-oh-METH-oh-LONE) USAN.
Use: Corticosteroid, ophthalmic; anti-inflammatory.
fluorophene.
Use: Antiseptic.
Fluoroplex. (Aqua Pharmaceuticals) Fluorouracil 1%. Benzyl alcohol, emulsifying wax, mineral oil. Cream. Tube 30 g. *Rx.*
Use: Pyrimidine antagonist, topical.
fluoroquinolones.
Use: Anti-infective.
See: Ciprofloxacin.
Enoxacin.
Gemifloxacin Mesylate.
Levofloxacin.
Lomefloxacin Hydrochloride.
Moxifloxacin Hydrochloride.
Norfloxacin.
•**fluorosalan.** (FLEW-oh-row-SAH-lan) USAN.
Use: Antiseptic; disinfectant.
fluorothyl.
See: Flurothyl.
•**fluorouracil.** (FLURE-oh-YOUR-uh-sill) *USP.*
Use: Antimetabolite; antineoplastic; pyrimidine antagonist, topical.
See: Adrucil.
Carac.
Fluoroplex.
fluorouracil. (Mylan) Fluorouracil 5%.

Parabens, stearyl alcohol, white petrolatum. Cream. 40 g. *Rx.*
Use: Pyrimidine antagonist, topical.

fluorouracil. (Taro) Fluorouracil 2%, 5%. Soln. Dropper bot. 10 mL. *Rx.*
Use: Pyrimidine antagonist, topical.

fluorouracil. (Various Mfr.) Fluorouracil 50 mg/mL. Vial 10 mL, 20 mL, 100 mL. Amp. 10 mL. *Rx.*
Use: Antineoplastic; antimetabolite.

•**fluotracen hydrochloride.** (FLEW-oh-TRAY-sen) USAN.
Use: Antipsychotic; antidepressant.

•**fluoxetine hydrochloride.** (flew-OX-eh-teen) *USP.*
Tall Man: FLUoxetine
Use: Antidepressant, selective serotonin reuptake inhibitor.
See: Prozac.
Prozac Weekly.
Sarafem.
Selfemra.
W/Olanzapine.
See: Symbyax.

fluoxetine hydrochloride. (Various Mfr.) Fluoxetine hydrochloride. **Cap.:** 10 mg, 20 mg, 40 mg. 28s (except 40 mg) 30s, 84s (except 40 mg), 100s, 500s, 1,000s, UD 100s. **Cap., delayed release:** 90 mg. May contain isopropyl alcohol, PEG, sugar. UD 4s. **Tab.: 10 mg:** May contain lactose, PEG. 30s, 100s, 1,000s. **20 mg:** 30s, 90s, 100s, 1,000s. **60 mg:** May contain glycerol, mannitol, sucrose. Film coated. 30s. **Oral Soln.:** 20 mg/5 mL. May contain alcohol, sucrose. 120 mL. *Rx.*
Use: Antidepressant, selective serotonin reuptake inhibitor.

•**fluoxymesterone.** (flew-ox-ee-MESS-teh-rone) *USP.*
Use: Sex hormone, androgen.
See: Androxy.

fluoxymesterone. (Various Mfr.) Fluoxymesterone 10 mg. Tab. Bot. 100s. *c-III.*
Use: Sex hormone, androgen.

•**fluparoxan hydrochloride.** (flew-pah-ROX-an) USAN.
Use: Antidepressant.

•**fluperamide.** (flew-purr-ah-mide) USAN.
Use: Antiperistaltic.

•**fluperolone acetate.** (FLEW-per-oh-lone) USAN.
Use: Corticosteroid, topical.

•**fluphenazine decanoate.** (flew-FEN-uh-zeen) *USP.*
Tall Man: fluPHENAZine
Use: Antipsychotic.

fluphenazine decanoate. (Various Mfr.) Fluphenazine decanoate 25 mg/mL, may contain sesame oil and benzyl alcohol. Inj. Multidose vials 5 mL. *Rx.*
Use: Antipsychotic.

•**fluphenazine enanthate.** (flew-FEN-uh-zeen) *USP.*
Tall Man: fluPHENAZine
Use: Antipsychotic; anxiolytic.

•**fluphenazine hydrochloride.** (flew-FEN-uh-zeen) *USP.*
Tall Man: fluPHENAZine
Use: Antipsychotic; anxiolytic.

fluphenazine hydrochloride. (American Pharmaceutical Partners) Fluphenazine hydrochloride. **Elix.:** 2.5 mg/mL. May contain alcohol 14% and sucrose. 60 mL, 473 mL. **Inj.:** 2.5 mg/mL. Parabens. Vial. 10 mL. *Rx.*
Use: Antipsychotic.

fluphenazine hydrochloride. (Pharmaceutical Associates) Fluphenazine hydrochloride 5 mg/mL. Alcohol 14%. Oral Soln., concentrated. 120 mL with safety-cap dropper calibrated at 0.1 mL and in 0.2 mL increments. *Rx.*
Use: Antipsychotic agent.

fluphenazine hydrochloride. (Various Mfr.) Fluphenazine hydrochloride. **Tab.:** 1 mg, 2.5 mg, 5 mg, 10 mg. Bot. 50s, 100s, 500s, 1000s, UD 100s. **Elixir:** 2.5 mg/mL. May contain alcohol 14% and sucrose. 60 mL, 473 mL. *Rx.*
Use: Antipsychotic.

•**flupirtine maleate.** (flew-PIHR-teen) USAN.
Use: Investigational analgesic.

•**fluprednisolone.** (FLEW-pred-NIH-so-lone) USAN.
Use: Corticosteroid, topical.

•**fluprednisolone valerate.** (FLEW-pred-NIH-so-lone VAL-eh-rate) USAN.
Use: Corticosteroid, topical.

•**fluproquazone.** (FLEW-PRO-kwah-zone) USAN.
Use: Analgesic.

•**fluprostenol sodium.** (flew-PROSTE-een-ole) USAN.
Use: Prostaglandin.

•**fluquazone.** (FLEW-kwah-zone) USAN.
Use: Anti-inflammatory.

•**fluradoline hydrochloride.** (FLURE-ade-OLE-een) USAN.
Use: Analgesic.

Flura-Drops. (Kirkman) Fluoride. **Drops:** 0.25 mg (from 0.55 mg sodium fluoride). Bot. 30 mL. **Rinse:** 0.02% (from 0.05% sodium fluoride). Bot. 480 mL. *Rx.*
Use: Dental caries agent.

•**fluralaner.** (FLUR-a-LAN-er) USAN.
Use: Treatment of animal flea and tick infestations.

Flura-Loz. (Kirkman) Sodium fluoride 2.2 mg providing 1 mg fluoride. Loz. Bot. 100s, 1000s. *Rx.*
Use: Dental caries agent.

•**flurandrenolide.** (FLURE-an-DREEN-oh-lide) *USP.* Cream; Ointment, USP. *Formerly Flurandrenolone.*
Use: Corticosteroid, topical.
See: Cordran.

flurandrenolone. (FLURE-an-DREE-nahl-ohn)
Use: Corticosteroid, topical.

FluraSafe. (Altaire) Benoxinate hydrochloride 0.4%, fluorexon disodium 0.35%. Soln.; Ophth. 6 mL w/dropper (w/povidone, boric acid, chlorobutanol 0.5%, polysorbate 80, PEG-400). *Rx.*
Use: Ophthalmic local anesthetic.

Flura-Tablets. (Kirkman) Sodium fluoride 2.21 mg, equivalent to 1 mg fluoride ion. Tab. Bot. 100s, 1000s. *Rx.*
Use: Dental caries agent.

•**flurazepam hydrochloride.** (flure-AZE-uh-pam) *USP.*
Use: Anticonvulsant; hypnotic; muscle relaxant; sedative/hypnotic, nonbarbiturate.

flurazepam hydrochloride. (Various Mfr.) Flurazepam hydrochloride 15 mg, 30 mg. Cap. 100s. *c-iv.*
Use: Sedative/hypnotic, nonbarbiturate.

•**flurbiprofen.** (FLURE-bih-PRO-fen) *USP.*
Use: Analgesic; anti-inflammatory.

flurbiprofen. (Various Mfr.) Flurbiprofen 50 mg, 100 mg. Tab. 100s, 500s (100 mg only). *Rx.*
Use: Analgesic, NSAID.

•**flurbiprofen sodium.** (FLURE-bih-PRO-fen) *USP.*
Use: Analgesic, NSAID; prostaglandin synthesis inhibitor.
See: Ocufen.

flurbiprofen sodium. (Various Mfr.) Flurbiprofen sodium 0.03%. Polyvinyl alcohol 1.4%, thimerosal 0.005%, EDTA. Ophth. Soln. Bot. 2.5 mL. *Rx.*
Use: Analgesic, NSAID.

Fluress. (Akorn) Fluorescein sodium 0.25%, benoxinate hydrochloride 0.4%. Povidone, boric acid, chlorobutanol 1%, sodium hydroxide and/or hydrochloric acid. Bot. 5 mL. *Rx.*
Use: Local anesthetic, ophthalmic.

•**fluretofen.** (flure-EH-TOE-fen) USAN.
Use: Anti-inflammatory; antithrombotic.

flurfamide. (FLURE-fah-MIDE)
See: Flurofamide.

•**flurocitabine.** (FLEW-row-SIGH-tah-bean) USAN.
Use: Antineoplastic.

Fluro-Ethyl. (Gebauer) Ethyl chloride 25%, dichlorotetrafluoroethane 75%. Aer. Spray. 270 mL. *Rx.*
Use: Anesthetic, topical.

•**flurofamide.** (FLEW-row-fah-MIDE) USAN. *Formerly Flurfamide.*
Use: Enzyme inhibitor (urease).

•**flurogestone acetate.** (FLEW-row-JEST-ohn) USAN.
Use: Hormone, progestin.

•**flurothyl.** (FLURE-oh-thill) USAN.
Use: Stimulant (central).

Flurox. (Ocusoft) Benoxinate hydrochloride 0.4%, fluorescein sodium 0.25%. Soln. 5 mL. *Rx.*
Use: Ophthalmic local anesthetic.

•**fluroxene.** (flure-OX-een) USAN.
Use: General inhalation anesthetic.

•**flurpiridaz F 18.** (flur-PIR-i-daz) USAN.
Use: Diagnostic imaging agent.

Flush-Free Niacin. (Integrative Therapeutics) Niacin (B_3) 590 mg. Gluten free, preservative free. Cap. 60s. *OTC.*
Use: Water-soluble vitamin.

•**fluspiperone.** (FLEW-spih-per-OHN) USAN.
Use: Antipsychotic.

•**fluspirilene.** (flew-SPIRE-ih-leen) USAN.
Use: Antipsychotic; anxiolytic.

Flutabs. (Breckenridge) Dextromethorphan HBr 20 mg, guaifenesin 200 mg, pseudoephedrine hydrochloride 60 mg, acetaminophen 500 mg. Dye free. Tab. 100s. *Rx.*
Use: Upper respiratory combination, antitussive and expectorant combination.

•**flutamide.** (FLEW-tuh-mide) *USP.*
Use: Hormone, antiandrogen.

flutamide. (Various Mfr.) Flutamide 125 mg, may contain lactose. Cap. Bot. 100s, 180s, 500s, UD 100s. *Rx.*
Use: Hormone, antiandrogen.

•**flutemetamol F 18.** (FLOO-te-MET-a-mol) USAN.
Use: Imaging agent.

•**fluticasone furoate.** (floo-TICK-a-sone FUR-oh-ate) USAN.
Use: Anti-inflammatory, intranasal steroid, corticosteroid, respiratory inhalant.
See: Veramyst.
W/Vilanterol.
See: Breo Ellipta.

•**fluticasone propionate.** (flew-TICK-ah-SONE) USAN.
Use: Anti-inflammatory, respiratory inhalant, intranasal steroid, corticosteroid.
See: Cutivate.

Flonase.
Flovent Diskus.
Flovent HFA.
Veramyst.
W/Azelastine Hydrochloride.
See: Dymista.
W/Salmeterol
See: Advair Diskus.
Advair HFA.

fluticasone propionate. (Fougera) Fluticasone propionate 0.005%. Oint. Tubes. 15 g, 30 g, 60 g. *Rx.*
Use: Anti-inflammatory agent.

fluticasone propionate. (Glenmark Pharmaceuticals) Fluticasone propionate 0.05%. Cetostearyl alcohol, dimethicone, lt. mineral oil, parabens, propylene glycol. Lot. 60 mL. *Rx.*
Use: Anti-inflammatory agent, topical corticosteroid.

fluticasone propionate. (Par) Fluticasone propionate 50 mcg/actuation. Dextrose, polysorbate 80, 0.02% w/w benzalkonium chloride, 0.25% w/w phenylethyl alcohol. Spray. Susp. Intranasal. Amber glass bot. 16 g (120 actuations) with metering atomizing pump and nasal adapter. *Rx.*
Use: Intranasal steroid, respiratory inhalant.

fluticasone propionate. (Sandoz) Fluticasone propionate 0.05%. Cetostearyl alcohol, mineral oil. Cream. Tubes. 15 g, 30 g, 60 g. *Rx.*
Use: Anti-inflammatory agent.

fluticasone propionate. (Various Mfr.) Fluticasone propionate 0.05%. Cetostearyl alcohol, mineral oil. Cream. 15 g, 30 g, 60 g. *Rx.*
Use: Anti-inflammatory agent.

Flutra. Trichlormethiazide.
Use: Diuretic.

•**flutroline.** (FLEW-troe-LEEN) USAN.
Use: Antipsychotic.

•**fluvastatin sodium.** (FLEW-vah-STAT-in) USAN.
Use: Antihyperlipidemic inhibitor, HMG-CoA reductase inhibitor.
See: Lescol.
Lescol XL.

fluvastatin sodium. (Sandoz) Fluvastatin sodium 80 mg. Film coated. PEG. ER Tab. 30s, 100s. *Rx.*
Use: Antihyperlipidemic agent, HMG-CoA reductase inhibitor.

fluvastatin sodium. (Various Mfr.) Fluvastatin sodium 20 mg, 40 mg. Cap. 30s, 90s, 100s. *Rx.*
Use: Antihyperlipidemic agent, HMG-CoA reductase inhibitor.

Fluvirin. (Novartis Vaccines) Hemagglutinin 15 mcg each of A/Christchurch/16/2010 NIB-74 (H1N1) (an A/California/7/2009-like virus), A/Texas/50/2012 NYMC X-223 (H3N2) (an A/Victoria/361/2011-like virus), and B/Massachusetts/2/2012 per 0.5 mL. Inj., Susp. (purified split virus). Preservative-free, 0.5 mL prefilled single-dose syringe (tip caps of the prefilled syringes may contain natural latex rubber; rubber plungers do not contain latex; formulated without preservative; however, thimerosal is used during manufacturing and is removed by subsequent purification steps to a trace amount [mercury ≤ 1 mcg per 0.5 mL dose]). 5 mL multidose vials (mercury ≤ 25 mcg/dose; may also contain residual amounts of ovalbumin [≤ 1 mcg], polymyxin [≤ 3.75 mcg], neomycin [≤ 2.5 mcg], betapropiolactone [≤ 0.5 mcg], and nonylphenol ethoxylate [≤ 0.015%]) with preservative (thimerosal). *Rx.*
Use: Viral vaccine.

•**fluvoxamine maleate.** (flew-VOX-ah-meen) USAN.
Tall Man: fluvoxaMINE
Use: Antidepressant; selective serotonin reuptake inhibitor.
See: Luvox.
Luvox CR.

fluvoxamine maleate. (Par Pharmaceutical) Fluvoxamine maleate 100 mg, 150 mg. May contain sugar. ER Cap. 30s, 750s (150 mg only), 1,000s (100 mg only). *Rx.*
Use: Antidepressant, selective serotonin reuptake inhibitor.

fluvoxamine maleate. (Various Mfr.) Fluvoxamine maleate 25 mg, 50 mg, 100 mg. Tab. 100s, 500s. *Rx.*
Use: Antidepressant, selective serotonin reuptake inhibitor.

•**fluzinamide.** (flew-ZIN-ah-mide) USAN.
Use: Anticonvulsant.

Fluzone. (Sanofi Pasteur) Hemagglutinin 7.5 mcg (0.25 mL dose) or 15 mcg (0.5 mL dose) each of A/California/07/2009 NYMC X-179A (H1N1), A/Texas/50/2012 X-223A (H3N2), and B/Massachusetts/02/2012 per 0.25 or 0.5 mL. Mercury ≤ 25 mcg/dose. Each 0.5 mL dose contains formaldehyde (≤ 100 mcg), octylphenol ethoxylate (≤ 150 mcg), and gelatin (0.05%); each 0.25 mL dose contains formaldehyde (≤ 50 mcg), octylphenol ethoxylate (≤ 75 mcg), and gelatin (0.05%). Inj., Susp. (purified split virus). Preservative-free, 0.25 and 0.5 mL prefilled single-dose syringe; preservative-free, 0.5 mL

single-dose vial; 5 mL multidose vial with preservative (thimerosal). *Rx.*
Use: Viral vaccine.

Fluzone High-Dose. (Sanofi Pasteur) Hemagglutinin 60 mcg each of A/California/07/2009 NYMC X-179A (H1N1), A/Texas/50/2012 X-223A (H3N2), and B/Massachusetts/02/2012 per 0.5 mL. Each 0.5 mL dose contains formaldehyde (≤ 100 mcg) and octylphenol ethoxylate (≤ 250 mcg). Preservative free. Inj., Susp. (purified split virus). Prefilled, single-dose syringe. 0.5 mL. *Rx.*
Use: Viral vaccine.

Fluzone Intradermal. (Sanofi Pasteur) Hemagglutinin 9 mcg each of A/California/07/2009 NYMC X-179A (H1N1), A/Texas/50/2012 X-223A (H3N2), and B/Massachusetts/02/2012 per 0.1 mL. Each 0.1 mL dose contains formaldehyde (≤ 20 mcg) and octylphenol ethoxylate (≤ 50 mcg). Preservative free. Inj., Susp. (purified split virus). Single-dose, prefilled microinjection system. 0.1 mL. *Rx.*
Use: Viral vaccine.

Fluzone Quadrivalent. (Sanofi Pasteur) Hemagglutinin 15 mcg each of A/California/07/2009 X-179A (H1N1), A/Texas/50/2012 X-223A (H3N2) (an A/Victoria/361/2011-like virus), B/Massachusetts/02/2012 (B Yamagata lineage), and B/Brisbane/60/2008 (B Victoria lineage) per 0.5 mL. Preservative free. Inj., Susp. (purified split virus). 0.25 and 0.5 mL single-dose, prefilled syringes and 0.5 mL single-dose vials. Each 0.5 mL dose contains formaldehyde (≤ 100 mcg) and octylphenol ethoxylate (≤ 250 mcg); each 0.25 mL dose contains formaldehyde (≤ 50 mcg) and octylphenol ethoxylate (≤ 125 mcg). *Rx.*
Use: Viral vaccine.

FML. (Allergan) Fluorometholone 0.1%. Benzalkonium chloride 0.004%, EDTA, polysorbate 80, polyvinyl alcohol 1.4%, sodium chloride, sodium phosphate. Ophth. Susp. Bot. 5 mL, 10 mL, 15 mL. *Rx.*
Use: Corticosteroid, ophthalmic; anti-inflammatory.

FML Forte. (Allergan) Fluorometholone 0.25%. Benzalkonium chloride 0.005%, EDTA, polysorbate 80, polyvinyl alcohol 1.4%, sodium chloride, sodium phosphate. Ophth. Susp. Bot. 5 mL, 10 mL, 15 mL. *Rx.*
Use: Corticosteroid, ophthalmic; anti-inflammatory.

FML S.O.P. (Allergan) Fluorometholone 0.1%. Phenylmercuric acetate 0.0008%, white petrolatum, mineral oil, lanolin alcohol. Ophth. Oint. Tube 3.5 g. *Rx.*
Use: Corticosteroid, ophthalmic; anti-inflammatory.

Focalin. (Novartis) Dexmethylphenidate hydrochloride 2.5 mg, 5 mg, 10 mg. Lactose. Tab. Bot. 100s. *c-II.*
Use: Central nervous system stimulant.

Focalin XR. (Novartis) Dexmethylphenidate hydrochloride 5 mg, 10 mg, 15 mg, 20 mg, 25 mg, 30 mg, 35 mg, 40 mg. Sugar spheres. ER Cap. 100s. *c-II.*
Use: Central nervous system stimulant.

•**focofilcon A.** (FOE-koe-FILL-kahn) USAN.
Use: Contact lens material (hydrophilic).

•**fodipir.** (FO-di-pir) USAN.
Use: Excipient.

Foillecort. (Blairex) Hydrocortisone acetate 0.5%. Cream. Tube 3.5 g. *OTC.*
Use: Corticosteroid, topical.

Foille Medicated First Aid. (Blistex) **Oint.:** Benzocaine 5% with chloroxylenol 0.1%, benzyl alcohol, EDTA in a corn oil base. 3.5 g, 28 g. **Aerosol:** Benzocaine 5% with chloroxylenol 0.6%, benzyl alcohol in corn oil. 92 mL. *OTC.*
Use: Topical local anesthetic, ester local anesthetic.

Folacin.
See: Folic acid.

Folastin. (Acella Pharmaceuticals) Vitamins B_6 25 mg, B_{12} 2,000 mcg, folic acid 2.5 mg. Tab. 90s. *Rx.*
Use: Multivitamin.

folate.
Use: Water-soluble vitamin.
See: DuLeek-DP 7.5.
DuLeek-DP 15.

Folbic RF. (Breckenridge Pharmaceutical) Vitamins B_6 25 mg, B_{12} 2,000 mcg, folate 1.13 mg. Tab. 90s. *Rx.*
Use: Multivitamin.

Folcal DHA. (Midlothian) Folic acid 1.25 mg, calcium 160 mg, iron 27 mg, vitamins D 400 units, E 30 units, B_6 25 mg, C 28 mg, DHA 300 mg, docusate sodium 55 g. Beeswax, glycerin, lecithin, sorbitol, soybean oil. Cap. 30s. *Rx.*
Use: Prenatal vitamin with minerals.

Folcaps Omega 3. (Midlothian) Folic acid 1 mg, calcium 150 mg, iron 27 mg, vitamins D 170 units, E 30 units, B_6 25 mg, C 25 mg, omega-3 fatty acids 330 mg (DHA 260 mg, EPA 40 mg, ALA 30 mg) and linoleic acid 30 mg. Beeswax, corn oil, glycerin, soy lecithin. Cap. 30s. *Rx.*
Use: Prenatal vitamin with minerals.

Folgard. (Upsher-Smith) B_6 10 mg, B_{12} 115 mcg, folic acid 0.8 mg. Tab. Bot. 60s. *OTC.*
Use: Vitamin, mineral supplement.

Folgard Rx. (Upsher-Smith) B_6 25 mg, B_{12} 500 mcg, folic acid 2.2 mg. Tab. Bot. 100s. *Rx.*
Use: Vitamin, mineral supplement.

•**folic acid.** (FOLE-ik) *USP.*
Use: Anemia; vitamin (hematopoietic).
See: Deplin.
W/Iron.
See: Tandem F.

folic acid. (Fujisawa Healthcare) Folic acid 5 mg/mL w/benzyl alcohol 1.5%, EDTA. Inj. Vials 10 mL. *Rx.*
Use: Vitamin supplement.

folic acid. (Various Mfr.) Folic acid. Tab. **0.4 mg, 0.8 mg:** Bot. 100s. **1 mg:** Bot. 30s, 100s, 1000s, UD 100s. *Rx.*
Use: Vitamin supplement.

folic acid antagonists.
See: Daraprim.
Methotrexate.
Pemetrexed.
Pralatrexate.
Pyrimethamine.

folinic acid. Leucovorin Calcium, USP.

Fol-Li-Bee. (Foy Laboratories) Liver inj. equivalent to cyanocobalamin 10 mcg, folic acid 1 mg, cyanocobalamin 100 mcg/mL, phenol 0.5% pH adjusted w/sodium hydroxide and/or hydrochloride. Vial 10 mL multi-dose, Monovials. *Rx.*
Use: Anemia.

follicle-stimulating hormone, human. Menotropins.

Follicormon.
See: Estradoil Benzoate.

follicular hormones.
See: Estrone.

Follistim AQ. (Organon) Follicle-stimulating hormone 75 units per 0.5 mL, 150 units per 0.5 mL. Sucrose 25 mg, sodium 7.35 mg. Inj. Single-use vials. *Rx.*
Use: Ovulation stimulant.

Follistim AQ Cartridge. (Organon) Follitropin beta 175 units per 0.2 mL (150 units follicle-stimulating hormone), 350 units per 0.42 mL (300 units follicle-stimulating hormone), 650 units per 0.78 mL (600 units follicle-stimulating hormone), 975 units per 1.17 mL (900 units follicle-stimulating hormone). Benzyl alcohol 10 mg/mL, sodium 14.7 mg/mL, sucrose 50 mg/mL. Inj. Cartridges with *BD* micro-fine pen needles. *Rx.*
Use: Ovulation stimulants.

follitropin alfa.
Use: Sex hormone, ovulation stimulant.
See: Gonal-F.
Gonal-f RFF Pen.

follitropin beta.
Use: Sex hormone, ovulation stimulant.
See: Follistim AQ.
Follistim AQ Cartridge.

Folotyn. (Allos Therapeutics Inc) Pralatrexate 20 mg/mL. Preservative free. Inj., Soln. Single-use vial. 1 mL, 2 mL. *Rx.*
Use: Antimetabolite, folic acid antagonist.

Folpace. (Alaven) Vitamin B_6 25 mg, vitamin B_{12} 425 mcg, FA 2.05 mg, E 100 units, Mg 100 mg. Tab. 90s. *Rx.*
Use: Nutritional product.

Foltanx RF. (Breckenridge Pharmaceutical) Vitamins B_6 35 mg, B_{12} 2,000 mcg, folate 3 mg, algae-S powder 90.314 mg. Cap. 90s. *Rx.*
Use: Multivitamin.

Foltrin. (Eon Labs) Liver and stomach concentrate 240 mg, B_{12} 15 mcg, iron 110 mg, C 75 mg, folic acid 0.5 mg. Cap. Bot. 100s, 1000s. *Rx.*
Use: Mineral, vitamin supplement.

FOLTX. (PAMLAB) B_{12} 2,000 mcg, B_6 25 mg, folate 1.13 mg. Film coated. Gluten free, lactose free, and sugar free. Tab. 90s. *Rx.*
Use: Vitamin, mineral supplement.

•**fomepizole.** (foe-MEH-pih-ZOLE) USAN.
Use: Antidote (alcohol dehydrogenase inhibitor).
See: Antizol.

fomepizole. (X-Gen) Fomepizole 1 g/mL. Preservative free. Inj., Soln. Vials. 1.5 mL. *Rx.*
Use: Antidote.

Fonatol.
See: Diethylstilbestrol.

•**fonazine mesylate.** (FAH-nazz-een) USAN.
Use: Serotonin inhibitor.

•**fondaparinux sodium.** (fon-da-PAR-in-ux) USAN.
Use: Anticoagulant, selective factor Xa inhibitor.
See: Arixtra.

fondaparinux sodium. (Apotex) Fondaparinux sodium 2.5 mg per 0.5 mL, 5 mg per 0.4 mL, 7.5 mg per 0.6 mL, 10 mg per 0.8 mL. Preservative free. Inj., Soln. Single-dose, prefilled syringe w/27-gauge needle. *Rx.*
Use: Anticoagulant, selective factor Xa inhibitor.

fontarsol.
See: Dichlorophenarsine Hydrochloride.

•**fontolizumab.** (fon-toe-LIZ-oo-mab) USAN.
Use: Immunoregulator.

Foradil Aerolizer. (Schering) Formoterol fumarate 12 mcg. Lactose. Inh. Pow. in Cap. Blister Pack 12s, 60s w/*Aerolizer Inhaler. Rx.*
Use: Bronchodilator, sympathomimetic.

Foralicon Plus. (Forbes) Vitamins B_{12} 16.7 mcg, B_6 4 mg, iron 200 mg (equivalent to elemental iron 24 mg), niacinamide 40 mg, folic acid 0.8 mg, sorbitol soln. q.s./15 mL. Elix. Bot. 8 oz, 16 oz. *Rx.*
Use: Mineral, vitamin supplement.

Forane. (Baxter Healthcare) Isoflurane. Gas. Volume 100 mL. *Rx.*
Use: Anesthetic, general.

•**forasartan.** (far-ah-SAHR-tan) USAN.
Use: Antihypertensive.

Fordustin. (Sween) Cornstarch based powder with deodorizing action. Bot. 3 oz, 8 oz. *OTC.*
Use: Powder, topical.

•**foretinib.** (for-e-TIN-ib) USAN.
Use: Antineoplastic.

Forfivo XL. (Edgemont Pharmaceuticals) Bupropion hydrobromide 450 mg. Film coated. PEG. ER Tab. 30s. *Rx.*
Use: Antidepressant.

•**forigerimod.** (FOR-eye-JIR-i-mod) USAN.
Use: Treatment of systemic lupus erythematosus.

•**forigerimod acetate.** (FOR-eye-JIR-i-mod) USAN.
Use: Treatment of systemic lupus erythematosus.

Formadon. (Gordon Laboratories) Formalin 3.7% to 4% (10% of USP strength) in an aqueous perfumed base. Soln. Bot. 1 oz, 4 oz, 0.5 gal, 1 gal. *Rx.*
Use: Bromhidrosis, hyperhidrosis agent.

Formalaz. (River's Edge) Formaldehyde 10%. Liq. Roll-on plastic bot. 85.05 g. *Rx.*
Use: Drying agent.

•**formaldehyde.** (for-MAL-deh-hide) *USP.*
Use: Drying agent.
See: Formalyde 10.
Lazer Formalyde.

formaldehyde. (Rochester Pharmaceuticals) Formaldehyde 10%. Soln., topical. 90 mL roll-on plastic bottle. *Rx.*
Use: Dermatological agent, drying agent.

Formalin.
See: Formaldehyde.

Formalyde-10. (Pedinol) Formaldehyde 10%, SD-40 alcohol. Spray. Bot. 60 mL. *Rx.*
Use: Drying agent.

Forma-Ray. (Gordon Laboratories) Formalin 7.4% to 8% (20% of USP strength) in aqueous, scented, tinted solution. Soln. Bot. 1.5 oz, 4 oz. *OTC.*
Use: Drying.

•**formocortal.** (FORE-moe-CORE-tal) USAN.
Use: Corticosteroid, topical.

•**formofilcon A.** (FOR-moe-FIL-kon) USAN.
Use: Contact lens polymer.

•**formofilcon B.** (FOR-moe-FIL-kon) USAN.
Use: Contact lens polymer.

•**formoterol fumarate.** (fore-MOE-ter-ole) USAN.
Use: Bronchodilator, sympathomimetic.
See: Foradil Aerolizer.
Perforomist.
W/Budesonide.
See: Symbicort.
W/Mometasone Furoate.
See: Dulera.

Formula B. (Major) Vitamins B_1 15 mg, B_2 15 mg, B_3 100 mg, B_5 18 mg, B_6 4 mg, B_{12} 5 mcg, C 500 mg, folic acid 0.5 mg. Tab. Bot 250 g. *Rx.*
Use: Vitamin supplement.

Formula B Plus. (Major) Iron 27 mg, A 5000 units, E 30 units, B_1 20 mg, B_2 20 mg, B_3 100 mg, B_5 25 mg, B_6 25 mg, B_{12} 50 mcg, C 500 mg, folic acid 0.8 mg, biotin 0.15 mg, Cr, Cu, Mg, Mn, Zn. Tab. Bot 100s, 500s. *Rx.*
Use: Mineral, vitamin supplement.

Formula EM. (Major) Dextrose 1.87 g, fructose 1.87 g, phosphoric acid 21.5 mg/5 mL. Methylparaben. Cherry-flavor. Soln. 118 mL. *OTC.*
Use: Antiemetic, antivertigo agent.

Formula 405. (Doak Dermatologics) **Bar:** Sodium tallowate, sodium cocoate, Doak Additive A, PPF-20 methyl glucose ether, titanium dioxide, trochlorocarbanilide, pentasodium pentatate, EDTA. 100 g. **Cream:** Coconut oil, beeswax, PEG-40, petrolatum, mineral oil, lanolin alcohol, isopropyl palmitate, sweet almond oil, ceresin, stearyl alcohol, lanolin, vitamin E, urea parabens. 56.7 g. *OTC.*
Use: Dermatologic, cleanser.

Formula 44 Custom Care Chesty Cough Medicine. (Proctor & Gamble) Dextromethorphan hydrobromide 20 mg, guaifenesin 200 mg. High fructose corn syrup, propylene glycol, saccharin sodium, sodium benzoate, sodium citrate. Liq. 177 mL. *OTC.*
Use: Upper respiratory combination, antitussive with expectorant.

Formula 44 Custom Care Cough & Cold PM. (Proctor & Gamble) Acetaminophen 650 mg, chlorpheniramine maleate 4 mg, dextromethorphan hydrobromide 30 mg. Acesulfame potassium, high fructose corn syrup, polyethylene glycol, propylene glycol, saccharin sodium, sodium benzoate, sodium citrate, sucralose. Liq. 177 mL. *OTC.*
Use: Upper respiratory combination, antitussive combination.

Formula 44 Custom Care Dry Cough Suppressant. (Proctor & Gamble) Dextromethorphan hydrobromide 30 mg. High fructose corn syrup, propylene glycol, saccharin sodium, sodium benzoate, sodium citrate. Liq. 177 mL. *OTC.*
Use: Nonnarcotic antitussive.

Formula No. 81. (Fellows) Liver (beef) 1 mcg, ferrous gluconate 100 mg, niacinamide 100 mg, B_2 1.5 mg, panthenol 2.5 mg, B_{12} 3 mcg, procaine hydrochloride 25 mg/2 mL. Inj. Vial 30 mL. *OTC.*
Use: Mineral, vitamin supplement.

Formula 1207. (Thurston) Iodine, liver fraction No. 2, caseinates. Tab. Bot. 100s, 250s. *OTC.*
Use: Mineral supplement.

Formulation R. (G & W Labs) **Cream:** Glycerin 12%, petrolatum 18%, phenylephrine hydrochloride 0.025%. Tube. 52 g. **Oint.:** Petrolatum 71.9%, mineral oil 14%, phenylephrine hydrochloride 0.25%, parabens. Tube. 28.4 g, 56.8 g. *OTC.*
Use: Anorectal preparation.

Formula VM-2000. (Solgar) Iron 5 mg, A 12,500 units, D 200 units, E 100 units, B_1 50 mg, B_2 50 mg, B_3 50 mg, B_5 50 mg, B_6 50 mg, B_{12} 50 mcg, C 150 mg, folic acid 0.2 mg, B, Ca, Cr, Cu, I, K, Mg, Mn, Mo, Se, Zn 7.5 mg, betaine, biotin 50 mcg, choline, bioflavonoids, amino acids, hesperidin, inositol, l-glutethione, PABA, rutin. Tab. Bot. 30s, 60s, 90s, 180s. *OTC.*
Use: Mineral, vitamin supplement.

formyl tetrahydropteroylglutamic acid. Leucovorin Calcium.

•**forodesine.** (FORE-oh-de-seen) USAN.
Use: Antineoplastic.

•**forodesine hydrochloride.** (fore-OH-de-seen) USAN.
Use: Antineoplastic.

Forta Drink. (Ross) Whey protein concentrate, sucrose, vitamins A, B_1, B_2, B_3, B_5, B_6, B_{12}, C, D, E, folic acid, biotin, Ca, Cu, Fe, I, Mg, Mn, P, Zn. Pow. Can. 482 g. *OTC.*
Use: Nutritional supplement.

Forta-Flora. (Barth's) Whey-lactose 90%, pectin. Pow. Jar lb. Wafer. Bot. 100s. *OTC.*

Forta Instant Cereal. (Ross) Lactose-free oat or bran cereal provides 6.25 g dietary fiber/serving. Can 1 lb 1 oz. *OTC.*
Use: Nutritional supplement.

Forta Instant Pudding. (Ross) Lactose-free in pudding base. Can 1 lb 12 oz. Vanilla, chocolate, butterscotch flavors. *OTC.*
Use: Nutritional supplement.

Fortamet. (First Horizon) Metformin hydrochloride 500 mg, 1000 mg. Film-coated. ER Tab. 60s. *Rx.*
Use: Antidiabetic agent, biguanide.

Forta Pudding Mix. (Ross) Milk protein isolate, sucrose, hydrolyzed cornstarch, modified tapioca starch, partially hydrogenated soybean oil, vitamins A, B_1, B_2, B_3, B_5, B_6, B_{12}, C, D, E, folic acid, biotin, Ca, Fe, P, I, Mg, Zn, Cu, Mn, tartrazine. Can 794 g. *OTC.*
Use: Nutritional supplement.

Forta Shake Powder. (Ross) Nonfat dry milk, sucrose, vitamins A, B_1, B_2, B_3, B_5, B_6, B_{12}, C, D, E, folic acid, biotin, Ca, Cu, Fe, I, Mg, Mn, P, Zn, tartrazine. Can lb, pkt. 1.4 oz. Can 1 lb 2.7 oz, pkt. 1.6 oz. *OTC.*
Use: Nutritional supplement.

Forta Soup Mix. (Ross) Milk protein isolate, sodium and calcium caseinate, hydrolyzed cornstarch, modified tapioca starch, powdered shortening (partially hydrogenated coconut oil), vitamins A, B_1, B_2, B_3, B_5, B_6, B_{12}, C, D, E, folic acid, biotin, Ca, Cu, Fe, I, Mg, Mn, P, Zn. Chicken flavor. Can. 454 g. *OTC.*
Use: Nutritional supplement.

Fortaz. (Covis) Ceftazidime Pow. for Inj. Sodium 2.3 mEq/g. **500 mg:** Vial. **1 g:** Vial, *ADD-Vantage* vial, Infusion Pack. **2 g:** Vial, *ADD-Vantage* vial, Infusion Pack. **6 g:** Bulk Pkg. **Inj.:** 1 g (dextrose hydrous 2.2 g), 2 g (dextrose hydrous 1.6 g). Vial 50 mL, premixed, frozen. *Rx.*
Use: Anti-infective, cephalosporin.

Forte L.I.V. (Foy Laboratories) Cyanocobalamin 15 mcg liver injection equivalent to vitamin B_{12} activity 1 mcg, ferrous gluconate 50 mg, B_2 0.75 mg, panthenol 1.25 mg, niacinamide 50 mg, citric acid 8.2 mg, sodium citrate 118 mg/mL, procaine hydrochloride 2%. Bot. 30 mL. *OTC.*
Use: Mineral, vitamin supplement.

Fortel Midstream. (Biomerica) Reagent in-home urine test for pregnancy. 1 test stick per kit.
Use: Diagnostic aid, pregnancy.

Fortel Ovulation. (Biomerica) Monoclonal antibody-based home test to predict ovulation. Kit 1s.
Use: Diagnostic aid.

Fortel Plus. (Biomerica) Reagent in-home urine pregnancy test. Kit contains urine collection cup, dropper, test device.
Use: Diagnostic aid, pregnancy.

Forteo. (Lilly) Teriparatide 250 mcg/mL, mannitol 45.4 mg. Inj. Prefilled pen delivery device 2.4 mL (20 mcg of teriparatide per dose). *Rx.*
Use: Parathyroid hormone.

Fortesta. (Endo Pharmaceuticals Inc) Testosterone 10 mg per 0.5 g. Ethanol, propylene glycol. Gel. 60 g metered-dose pumps (each metered-dose pump delivers 120 metered 10 mg doses). *c-III.*
Use: Sex hormone, androgen.

Fortical. (Upsher-Smith) Calcitonin-salmon 200 units per activation (0.09 mL/dose). Sodium chloride, benzyl alcohol, phenylethyl alcohol. Nasal spray. Metered-dose, glass bot. with pump. 3.7 mL. *Rx.*
Use: Antihypercalcemic.

Fortral. (Sanofi-Synthelabo) Pentazocine as solution and tablets. *c-IV.*
Use: Analgesic, narcotic.

Fortramin. (Thurston) Vitamins E 200 units, A 6000 units, D 600 units, B_1 4.5 mg, B_2 4.5 mg, B_6 4.5 mg, B_{12} 5 mcg, C 2.75 mg, rutin 8 mg, hesperidin complex 10 mg, lemon bioflavonoids 15 mg, d-calcium pantothenate 50 mg, para-aminobenzoic acid 7.5 mg, biotin 10 mg, folic acid 24 mcg, niacinamide 20 mg, desiccated liver 25 mg, iron 3 mg, calcium 75 mg, phosphorus 34 mg, manganese 10 mg, copper 0.5 mg, zinc 0.5 mg, iodine 0.375 mg, potassium 500 mg, magnesium 5 mg. Tab. Bot. 100s, 250s. *OTC.*
Use: Mineral, vitamin supplement.

.44 Magnum. (BDI) Caffeine 200 mg. Cap. Bot. 100s, 500s. *OTC.*
Use: CNS stimulant, analeptic.

40 Winks. (Roberts) Diphenhydramine hydrochloride 50 mg. Cap. Bot. 30s. *OTC.*
Use: Sleep aid.

Fosamax. (Merck) Alendronate 70 mg (equiv. to alendronate sodium 91.37 mg). Lactose. Tab. UD 4s. *Rx.*
Use: Bisphosphonate.

Fosamax Plus D. (Merck) Alendronate/vitamin D_3 70 mg/70 mcg (equiv. to vitamin D 2800 units), 70 mg/140 mcg (equiv. to vitamin D 5600 units). Lactose, sucrose. Tab. Unit-of-use blisters of 4, UD 20s. *Rx.*
Use: Bisphosphonate.

•**fosamprenavir calcium.** (FOSS-am-PREN-ah-veer) USAN.
Use: Antiretroviral agents.
See: Lexiva.

•**fosamprenavir sodium.** (FOSS-am-PREN-ah-veer) USAN.
Use: Antiviral.

•**fosaprepitant dimeglumine.** (FOS-ap-RE-pi-tant)
Use: Antiemetic/antivertigo agent.
See: Emend.

•**fosarilate.** (FOSS-ah-RILL-ate) USAN.
Use: Antiviral.

•**fosazepam.** (foss-AZZ-eh-pam) USAN.
Use: Hypnotic; sedative.

•**fosbretabulin disodium.** (fos-BRE-ta-BUE-lin) USAN.
Use: Antineoplastic.

•**fosbretabulin tromethamine.** (fos-BRE-ta-BUE-lin troe-METH-a- meen) USAN.
Use: Antineoplastic.

•**foscarnet sodium.** (foss-CAR-net) USAN.
Use: Antiviral.

foscarnet sodium. (Hospira) Foscarnet sodium 24 mg per mL. Inj. 250 mL, 500 mL. *Rx.*
Use: Antiviral agent.

•**fosdevirine.** (FOS-de-VIR-een) USAN.
Use: Antiviral.

•**fosfomycin.** (foss-foe-MY-sin) USAN.
Use: Anti-infective.
See: Monurol.

•**fosfomycin tromethamine.** (foss-foe-MY-sin troe-METH-ah-meen) USAN.
Use: Anti-infective.
See: Monurol.

•**fosfonet sodium.** (FOSS-foe-net) USAN.
Use: Antiviral.

Fosfree. (Mission Pharmacal) Iron 14.5 mg, A 1500 units, D_3 150 units, B_1 4.5 mg, B_2 2 mg, B_3 10.5 mg, B_5 1 mg, B_6 2.5 mg, B_{12} 2 mcg, C 50 mg, Ca 175.5 mg, sugar. Tab. Bot. 120s. *OTC.*
Use: Mineral, vitamin supplement.

fosinopril. (FAH-sen-oh-PRIL)
Use: Angiotensin-converting enzyme inhibitor; antihypertensive.
See: Monopril.

•**fosinoprilat.** (fah-SIN-oh-prill-at) USAN.
Use: Antihypertensive.

•**fosinopril sodium.** (FAH-sen-oh-PRIL) USAN.
Use: Renin angiotensin system antagonist, angiotensin-converting enzyme inhibitor.
See: Monopril.

W/Hydrochlorothiazide.
See: Monopril-HCT.

fosinopril sodium. (Teva) Fosinopril sodium 10 mg, 20 mg, 40 mg. Isopropyl alcohol, lactose. Tab. 90s, 1,000s. *Rx.*
Use: Renin angiotensin system antagonist, angiotensin-converting enzyme inhibitor.

fosinopril sodium and hydrochlorothiazide. (Ranbaxy) Hydrochlorothiazide/fosinopril sodium 12.5 mg/10 mg, 12.5 mg/20 mg. Lactose. Tab. 30s, 100s, 1,000s. *Rx.*
Use: Antihypertensive combination.

•**fosphenytoin sodium.** (FOSS-FEN-ih-toe-in) USAN.
Use: Anticonvulsant.
See: Cerebyx.

fosphenytoin sodium. (Various Mfr.) Fosphenytoin sodium 75 mg/mL (equiv. to phenytoin sodium 50 mg/mL). Inj., Soln.; concentrate. Vial. 2 mL, 10 mL. *Rx.*
Use: Anticonvulsant, hydantoin.

•**fospropofol disodium.** (fos-proe-POE-fol) USAN.
Use: Sedative/hypnotic agent.

•**fosquidone.** (FOSS-kwih-dohn) USAN.
Use: Antineoplastic.

Fosrenol. (Shire) Lanthanum carbonate 500 mg, 750 mg, 1000 mg. Chew. Tab. 90s. *Rx.*
Use: Phosphate binder.

•**fostamatinib.** (FOS-tam-A-ti-nib) USAN.
Use: Immunomodulator.

•**fostamatinib disodium.** (FOS-tam-A-ti-nib) USAN.
Use: Immunomodulator.

•**fostedil.** (FOSS-teh-dill) USAN.
Use: Vasodilator, calcium channel blocker.

Fostex. (Bristol-Myers Squibb) Benzoyl peroxide 10%, EDTA, urea. Bar. 106 g. *OTC.*
Use: Dermatologic, acne.

Fostex Acne Cleansing Cream. (Bristol-Myers Squibb) Salicylic acid 2%, EDTA, stearyl alcohol. Cream. Bot. 118 g. *OTC.*
Use: Dermatologic, acne.

Fostex Acne Medication Cleansing Bar. (Bristol-Myers Squibb) Salicylic acid 2%, EDTA. Bar. 106 g. *OTC.*
Use: Dermatologic, acne.

•**fostriecin sodium.** (FOSS-try-eh-SIN) USAN.
Use: Antineoplastic.

•**fosveset.** (FOS-ve-set) USAN.
Use: Ligant excipient.

Fototar. (ICN Pharm) Coal tar extract (equiv. to 2% coal tar) in emollient moisturizing cream base. Cream. Tube 85 g, 454 g. *OTC.*
Use: Dermatologic.

4 Hair Softgel. (Marlyn Nutraceuticals) Iron 2.5 mg, A 1250 units, E 10 units, B_3 5 mg, B_5 2.5 mg, B_6 1.5 mg, B_{12} 44 mcg, C 25 mg, folic acid 33.3 mg, biotin 250 mcg, I, Mg, Cu, Zn 7.5 mg, choline bitartrate, inositol, Mn, methionine, PABA, B_1, L-cysteine, tyrosine, Si. Cap. Bot 60s. *OTC.*
Use: Mineral, vitamin supplement.

4 Nails Softgel. (Marlyn Nutraceuticals) Ca 167 mg, iron 3 mg, A 833 units, D 67, E 10 mg, B_1 3.3 mg, B_2 1.7 mg, B_3 8.3 mg, B_5 8.3 mg, B_6 8.3 mg, B_{12} 8.3 mcg, C 10 mg, folic acid 33.3 mg, biotin 8.3 mcg, P, I, Mg, Cu, Zn 3.3 mg, Cr, Mn, methionine, inositol, choline bitartrate, Se, PABA, protein isolate, gelatin, lecithin, unsaturated fatty acid, predigested protein L-cysteine, B mucopolysaccharides, silicon amino acid chelate, Si. Cap. Bot. 60s. *OTC.*
Use: Mineral, vitamin supplement.

4-N-1. (DermaRite) Dimethicone 1%, alcohols, parabens, PEG. Latex free. Cream. 114 g. *OTC.*
Use: Miscellaneous protectant.

4 Trace Elements. (Hospira) Chromium (as chloride) 6 mcg, copper (as chloride) 0.42 mg, manganese (as chloride) 0.37 mg, zinc (as chloride) 1.67 mg. Vial. 5 mL. *Rx.*
Use: Intravenous nutritional therapy.

4-Way Fast Acting Nasal Spray. (Novartis Consumer Health) Phenylephrine hydrochloride 1%, benzalkonium chloride, boric acid, sodium borate. Soln. Spray Bot. 30 mL. *OTC.*
Use: Nasal decongestant, arylalkylamine.

4-Way Menthol. (Novartis Consumer Health) Phenylephrine hydrochloride 1%. Menthol. Nasal Spray. 14.8 mL. *OTC.*
Use: Nasal decongestant, arylalkylamine.

4-Way Moisturizing Relief. (Novartis Consumer Health) Xylometazoline hydrochloride 0.1%. Benzalkonium chloride, edetate disodium. Spray, Soln. Intranasal. 14.8 mL. *c-v.*
Use: Nasal decongestant, imidazoline.

Fowler's Solution. Potassium Arsenite Solution.

Foxalin. (Standex) Digitoxin 0.1 mg, sodium carboxymethylcellulose. Cap. Bot. 100s. *Rx.*
Use: Cardiovascular agent.

foxglove.
See: Digitalis.

Foygen Aqueous. (Foy Laboratories) Estrogenic substance or estrogens 2 mg/mL with sodium carboxymethylcellulose, povidone, benzyl alcohol, methyl and propyl parabens. Inj. Vial 10 mL. *Rx.*
Use: Estrogen.

Foyplex. (Foy Laboratories) Sterile injectable soln. of nine water-soluble vitamins. Packaged as 2 separate solutions for extemporaneous combination. Inj. *Rx.*
Use: Nutritional supplement, parenteral.

Fragmin. (Eisai) Dalteparin sodium 2,500 units/0.2 mL (16 mg/0.2 mL), 5,000 units/0.2 mL (32 mg/0.2 mL), 7,500 units/0.3 mL (48 mg/0.3 mL), 10,000 units/mL (64 mg/mL), 10,000 units/0.4 mL (64 mg/0.4 mL), 12,500 units/0.5 mL (80 mg/0.5 mL), 15,000 units/0.6 mL (96 mg/0.6 mL), 18,000 units/0.72 mL (115.2 mg/0.72 mL), 95,000 units/3.8 mL (160 mg/mL). Preservative free (except 95,000 units/3.8 mL). Anti-Factor Xa International Units. Inj. Soln. Single-dose prefilled syringe 0.2 mL with 27-gauge × ½-inch needle (2,500 units/0.2 mL, 5,000 units/0.2 mL only), single-dose prefilled syringe 0.3 mL with 27-gauge × ½-inch needle (7,500 units/0.3 mL only), single-dose prefilled syringe 0.4 mL with 27-gauge × ½-inch needle (10,000 units/0.4 mL only), single-dose graduated syringes 1 mL with 27-gauge × ½-inch needle (10,000 units/mL only), single-dose prefilled syringes 0.5 mL with 27-gauge × ½-inch needle (12,500 units/0.5 mL only), single-dose prefilled syringes 0.6 mL with 27-gauge × ½-inch needle (15,000 units/0.6 mL only), single-dose prefilled syringes 0.72 mL with 27-gauge × ½-inch needle (18,000 units/0.72 mL only), multidose vials 3.8 mL with benzyl alcohol 14 mg/mL (95,000 units/3.8 mL only). *Rx.*
Use: Anticoagulant.

FreAmine HBC 6.9%. (B. Braun) High branched 6.9% amino acid formulation for hypercatabolic patients. Bot. 1000 mL. *Rx.*
Use: Nutritional supplement, parenteral.

FreAmine III. (B. Braun) Amino acid 8.5%, 10%. Bot. 500 mL, 1000 mL. *Rx.*
Use: Nutritional supplement, parenteral.

FreAmine III 3% w/Electrolytes. (B. Braun) Amino acid 3% with electrolytes. Bot. 1000 mL. *Rx.*
Use: Nutritional supplement, parenteral.

Free & Clear. (Pharmaceutical Specialties) Ammonium laureth sulfate, disodium cocamide MEA sulfosuccinate, cocamidopropyl hydroxysultaine, cocamide DEA, PEG-120 methyl glucose dioleate, EDTA, potassium sorbate, citric acid. Shampoo. Bot. 240 mL. *OTC.*
Use: Dermatologic, cleanser.

Freedavite. (Freeda) Iron 10 mg (from ferrous fumarate), vitamins A 5000 units, D 400 units, E 3 units, B_1 5 mg, B_2 3 mg, B_3 25 mg, B_5 5 mg, B_6 2 mg, B_{12} 2 mcg, C 60 mg, choline, inositol, potassium iodide, Ca, Cu, K, Mg, Mn, Se, Zn 0.2 mg. Bot. 100s, 250s. *OTC.*
Use: Mineral, vitamin supplement.

Freedox. (Pharmacia) Tirilazad.
Use: A 21 aminosteroid antioxidant.

•**frentizole.** (FREN-tih-zole) USAN.
Use: Immunoregulator.

Fresenius Propoven. (APP Pharmaceutical) Propofol 10 mg/mL. Glycerol, oleic acid, purified egg phosphatides, soybean oil, medium chain triglycerides. Inj., Emuls. Single-use ampule, 20 mL. Single-use vial, 20 mL, 50 mL, 100 mL. *Rx.*
Use: General anesthetic.

FreshBurst Listerine. (Warner Lambert) Thymol 0.064%, eucalyptol 0.092%, methyl salicylate 0.06%, menthol 0.042%, alcohol 21.6%. Rinse. Bot. 250 mL. *OTC.*
Use: Mouthwash.

FreshKote. (Focus Labs) Polyvinyl alcohol 2.7%, polyvinyl pyrrolidone 2%, boric acid, disodium EDTA, polixetonium, potassium chloride, sodium chloride. Soln., Ophth. 15 mL. *OTC.*
Use: Artificial tear solution.

Fresh n' Feminine. (Walgreen) Benzethonium Cl 0.2% Bot. 8 oz. *OTC.*
Use: Vaginal agent.

•**fresolimumab.** (FRE-soe-LIM-ue-mab) USAN.
Use: Monoclonal antibody.

Frova. (Endo Pharmaceuticals) Frovatriptan succinate 2.5 mg. Film coated. Lactose, PEG. UD 9s. *Rx.*
Use: Agent for migraine, serotonin 5-HT_1 receptor agonist.

•**frovatriptan succinate.** (froe-va-TRIP-tan) USAN.
Use: Antimigraine, serotonin 5-HT_1 receptor agonist.
See: Frova.

•**fructose.** (FRUK-tose) *USP.*
Use: Nutritional supplement.
See: Frutabs.
W/Dextrose, Phosphoric Acid.
See: Emetrol.
Nausatrol.

Nausea Relief.
Nausetrol.

fructose. (Various Mfr.) Fructose 10%. Soln. Bot. 1000 mL.
Use: Nutritional supplement.

fructose and sodium chloride injection.
Use: Electrolyte, fluid, nutrient replacement.

Fruit C 500. (Freeda) Vitamin C 500 mg (as calcium ascorbate and ascorbic acid). Rose hips. Sugar free. Chew. Tab. Bot. 100s, 250s. *OTC.*
Use: Water-soluble vitamin.

Fruit C 100. (Freeda) Vitamin C 100 mg (as calcium ascorbate and ascorbic acid). Sugar free. Chew. Tab. Bot. 250s. *OTC.*
Use: Water-soluble vitamin.

Fruit C 200. (Freeda) Vitamin C 200 mg (as calcium ascorbate and ascorbic acid). Rose hips. Sugar free. Chew. Tab. Bot. 100s, 250s. *OTC.*
Use: Water-soluble vitamin.

Fruity Chews. (Ivax) Vitamins A 2500 units, D 400 units, E 15 mg, B_1 1.05 mg, B_2 1.2 mg, B_3 13.5 mg, B_6 1.05 mg, B_{12} 4.5 mcg, C (as sodium ascorbate and ascorbic acid) 60 mg, folic acid 0.3 mg. Chew. Tab. Bot. 100s. *OTC.*
Use: Mineral, vitamin supplement.

Fruity Chews w/Iron. (Ivax) Elemental iron 12 mg, vitamins A 2500 units, D 400 units, E 15 mg, B_1 1.05 mg, B_2 1.2 mg, B_3 13.5 mg, B_6 1.05 mg, B_{12} 4.5 mcg, C (as sodium ascorbate and ascorbic acid) 60 mg, folic acid 0.3 mg, zinc 8 mg. Chew. Tab. Bot. 100s. *OTC.*
Use: Mineral, vitamin supplement.

Frutabs. (Pfanstiehl) Fructose 2 g. Tab. Bot. 100s. *OTC.*
Use: Carbohydrate supplement.

FS Shampoo. (Hill Dermaceuticals) *OTC.*
See: Capex.

FTA-ABS. (Wampole) Fluorescent treponemal antibody-absorbed test in vitro for confirming a positive reagent test for syphilis. Test 100s.
Use: Diagnostic aid.

FTA-ABS/DS. (Wampole) Fluorescent treponemal antibody-absorbed test in vitro for confirming a positive reagent test for syphilis. Test 100s.
Use: Diagnostic aid.

•**fuchsin, basic.** (FYOO-sin) *USP.*
Use: Anti-infective, topical.

FUDR. (Roche) Floxuridine 500 mg. Pow. for Inj., lyophilized. Vial 5 mL. *Rx.*
Use: Antineoplastic; antimetabolite.

Ful-Glo. (Akorn) Fluorescein sodium 0.6 mg. Strip. Box 300s. *OTC.*
Use: Diagnostic aid, ophthalmic.

Fuller. (Birchwood) Pkg. 1 shield.
Use: Anorectal preparation.

Full Spectrum B. (National Vitamin) Vitamin B_1 1.5 mg, B_2 1.7 mg, B_3 20 mg, B_5 10 mg, B_6 10 mg, B_{12} 6 mcg, C 60 mg, FA 800 mcg, biotin 3 mg. Preservative-free. Tab. 100s. *OTC.*
Use: Nutrition combination product.

•**fulranumab.** (ful-RAN-ue-mab) USAN.
Use: Treatment of pain.

•**fulvestrant.** (ful-VES-trant)
Use: Hormone, antiestrogen.
See: Faslodex.

Fulyzaq. (Salix Pharmaceuticals Inc) Crofelemer 125 mg. Tab., delayed release. 60s. *Rx.*
Use: Antidiarrheal.

•**fumaric acid.** (fyoo-MAR-ik) *NF.*
Use: Acidifier.

•**fumoxicillin.** (fyoo-MOX-ih-SILL-in) USAN.
Use: Antibacterial.

Fungatin. (Major) Tolnaftate 1%. Cream. Tube 15 g. *OTC.*
Use: Antifungal, topical.

fungicides.
See: Amphotericin B.
Ancobon.
Asterol.
Desenex.
Diflucan.
Fluconazole.
Griseofulvin Ultramicrosize.
Gris-PEG.
Itraconazole.
Miconazole Nitrate.
Mycostatin.
Nifuroxime.
Nilstat.
Nizoral.
Nystatin.
Sporanox.
Undecylenic Acid.

Fungi Cure Intensive. (Alva-Amco) Clotrimazole 1%. Alcohol. Spray, Soln. Pump spray. 60 mL. *OTC.*
Use: Topical anti-infective, antifungal agent.

Fungi Cure Maximum Strength. (Alva-Amco) Undecylenic acid 25%. Aloe vera, isopropyl alcohol 70%. Liq., topical. 30 mL. *OTC.*
Use: Topical anti-infective.

•**fungimycin.** (FUN-jih-MY-sin) USAN.
Use: Antifungal.

Fungi-Nail. (Kramer) Resorcinol 1%, salicylic acid 2%, parachlorometaxylenol 2%, benzocaine 0.5%, acetic acid 2.5%,

propylene glycol, hydroxypropyl methylcellulose, alcohol 0.5%. Bot. 30 mL. *OTC.*
Use: Antifungal, topical.

Fungizone for Laboratory Use in Tissue Culture. (Bristol-Myers Squibb) Amphotericin B 50 mg, sodium desoxycholate 41 mg. Vial 20 mL.
Use: Diagnostic aid.

Fungoid-HC Creme. (Pedinol) Miconazole nitrate 2%, hydrocortisone 1%. Cream. In 56.7 g, 1 g dual packets. *Rx.*
Use: Antifungal, topical.

Fungoid Tincture. (Pedinol) Miconazole nitrate 2%. Alcohol. Soln. Bot. with brush applicator 7.39 mL, 29.57 mL. *Rx.*
Use: Antifungal agent, topical anti-infective.

Furadantin. (Shionogi) Nitrofurantoin 25 mg per 5 mL. Glycerin, parabens, saccharin, sorbitol. Oral Susp. Bot. 60 mL, 470 mL. *Rx.*
Use: Anti-infective, urinary.

furalazine hydrochloride.
Use: Antimicrobial compound.

Furanite. (Major) Nitrofurantoin 50 mg, 100 mg. Tab. Bot. 100s. *Rx.*
Use: Anti-infective, urinary.

•**furaprofen.** (FYOOR-ah-PRO-fen) USAN. *Formerly Enprofen.*
Use: Anti-inflammatory.

•**furazolidone.** (fyoor-ah-ZOE-lih-dohn) *USP.*
Use: Antiprotozoal.

•**furazolium chloride.** (FYOOR-ah-zoe-lee-uhm) USAN.
Use: Anti-infective.

•**furazolium tartrate.** (FYOOR-ah-ZOE-lee-uhm) USAN.
Use: Anti-infective.

•**furazosin hydrochloride.** (FYOOR-ah-zoe-sin) Under study.
Use: Antihypertensive.

•**furegrelate sodium.** (fyoor-eh-GRELL-ate) USAN.
Use: Inhibitor (thromboxane synthetase).

•**furobufen.** (FER-oh-BYOO-fen) USAN.
Use: Anti-inflammatory.

•**furodazole.** (fyoor-OH-dah-zole) USAN.
Use: Anthelmintic.

Furonatal FA. (Lexis Laboratories) Vitamins A 8000 units, D 400 units, E 30 units, C 60 mg, folic acid 1 mg, B_1 2 mg, B_2 2.8 mg, B_6 2.5 mg, B_{12} 8 mcg, niacinamide 20 mg, iron 65 mg, calcium 125 mg. Tab. Bot. 100s, 1000s. *Rx.*
Use: Mineral, vitamin supplement.

•**furosemide.** (fyu-ROH-se-mide) *USP.* Oral Solution, USP.
Use: Diuretic.

furosemide. (Roxane) Furosemide. **10 mg/mL:** Soln. Dropper bot. 60 mL. **40 mg/5 mL:** Soln. Bot. 5 mL, 10 mL, 500 mL. *Rx.*
Use: Diuretic.

furosemide. (Various Mfr.) **Tab.:** 20 mg, 40 mg, 80 mg. Bot. 60s (40 mg only), 100s, 500s, 1000s, UD 100s. **Oral Soln.:** 10 mg/mL Bot. 60 mL, 120 mL. **Inj.:** 10 mg/mL Vial 10 mL; single-dose vial 2 mL, 10 mL; partial fill single-dose vial 4 mL. *Rx.*
Use: Diuretic.

•**fursalan.** (FYOOR-sal-an) USAN. Under study.
Use: Disinfectant.

•**fusidate sodium.** (FEW-sih-DATE) USAN.
Use: Anti-infective.

•**fusidic acid.** (few-SIH-dik) USAN.
Use: Anti-infective.

Fusilev. (Spectrum Pharmaceuticals) *Formerly levoleucovorin.* Levoleucovorin. **Inj., lyophilized, Pow. for Soln.:** 50 mg (equiv. to levoleucovorin calcium 64 mg). Mannitol 50 mg. Single-use vial. **Inj., Soln.:** 10 mg/mL (as levoleucovorin calcium). Sodium chloride 8.3 mg. Preservative free. Single-use vial. 17.5 mL, 25 mL. *Rx.*
Use: Water-soluble vitamin.

•**futuximab.** (fue-TUX-i-mab) USAN.
Use: Antineoplastic.

Fuzeon. (Hoffman-LaRoche) Enfuvirtide 108 mg. Pow. for Inj., lyophilized. Convenience Kit with single-use vials, syringes, diluent, alcohol wipes. *Rx.*
Use: Anti-infective, tetracycline.

Fycompa. (Eisai Inc) Perampanel 2 mg, 4 mg, 6 mg, 8 mg, 10 mg, 12 mg. Film coated. Lactose, PEG. Tab. 30s, 90s. *c-III.*
Use: Anticonvulsant.

G

•**gabapentin.** (GAB-uh-PEN-tin) USAN.
Use: Anticonvulsant; amyotrophic lateral sclerosis agent.
See: Gabarone.
Gralise.
Horizant.
Neurontin.

gabapentin. (Various Mfr.) Gabapentin. **Tab.:** 600 mg, 800 mg. May contain lactose. 100s, 500s; 1,000s, UD 100s, UD 300s (600 mg only). **Cap.:** 100 mg, 300 mg, 400 mg. 30s (300 mg only), 60s (300 mg only), 90s, 100s, 180s, 270s, 500s, 1,000s, 2,500s (400 mg only), 3,500s (300 mg only), 8,500s (100 mg), UD 50s, UD 100s. *Rx.*
Use: Anticonvulsant.

•**gabapentin enacarbil.** (GAB-uh-PEN-tin EN-a-KAR-bil) USAN.
Use: Treatment of neuropathic pain and restless legs syndrome.
See: Horizant.

Gabarone. (Ivax) Gabapentin 100 mg, 300 mg, 400 mg. Lactose. Tab. 100s, 500s, 1000s (400 mg only), 2,000s (300 mg only), 5,000s (100 mg only), UD 100s. *Rx.*
Use: Anticonvulsant.

Gabbromicina. Aminosidine.
Use: Anti-infective. [Orphan Drug]

Gabitril Filmtabs. (Cephalon) Tiagabine hydrochloride 2 mg, 4 mg, 12 mg, 16 mg. Lactose. Tab. 30s. *Rx.*
Use: Anticonvulsant.

Gablofen. (CNS Therapeutics) Baclofen 0.05 mg/mL, 10 mg/20 mL, 10 mg/5 mL. Preservative free. Inj., Soln.; intrathecal. Single-use syringe. *Rx.*
Use: Skeletal muscle relaxant, centrally acting.

•**gaboxadol.** (gab-OX-a-dol) USAN.
Use: Insomnia.

Gacid. (Arcum) Magnesium trisilicate 500 mg, aluminum hydroxide 250 mg. Tab. Bot. 100s, 1000s. *OTC.*
Use: Antacid.

Gadavist. (Bayer Health Care) Gadobutrol 1 mmol/mL (equiv. to gadobutrol 604.72 mg/mL). Preservative free. Inj., Soln. Single-dose vial and prefilled syringe. 7.5 mL, 10 mL, 15 mL. *Rx.*
Use: Miscellaneous radiopaque agent.

•**gadobenate dimeglumine.** (gad-oh-BEN-ate die-meh-GLUE-meen) USAN.
Use: Radiopaque agent.
See: MultiHance.

•**gadobutrol.** (GAD-oh-BUE-trol) USAN.
Use: Miscellaneous radiopaque agent.
See: Gadavist.

•**gadodiamide.** (GAD-oh-DIE-ah-mide) *USP.*
Use: Radiopaque agent, parenteral.
W/Caldiamide.
See: Omniscan.

•**gadofosveset trisodium.** (gad-oh-FOS-ve-set) USAN.
Use: Diagnostic contrast agent.
See: Ablavar.

•**gadopentetate dimeglumine.** (GAD-oh-PEN-teh-tate die-meh-GLUE-meen) *USP.*
Use: Radiopaque agent, parenteral.
See: Magnevist.

•**gadoterate meglumine.** (GAD-oh-TER-ate MEG-loo-meen) USAN.
Use: Radiopaque agent.
See: Dotarem.

•**gadoteridol.** (GAD-oh-TER-ih-dahl) *USP.*
Use: Radiopaque agent, parenteral.
See: ProHance.

•**gadoversetamide.** (gad-oh-ver-SET-ah-mide) *USP.*
Use: Radiopaque agent, parenteral.
See: OptiMARK.

•**gadoxanum.** (gad-oh-ZAN-uhm) USAN.
Use: Diagnostic aid.

•**gadoxetate disodium.** (gad-OX-e-tate) USAN.
Use: Contrast agent.

•**gadozelite.** (gad-oh-ZEH-lite) USAN.
Use: Diagnostic aid.

•**galantamine.** (ga-LAN-ta-meen) USAN.
Use: Alzheimer disease; cholinesterase inhibitor.

galantamine hydrobromide.
Use: Cholinesterase inhibitor; Alzheimer disease.
See: Razadyne.
Razadyne ER.

galantamine hydrobromide. (Roxane) Galantamine 4 mg/mL. May contain parabens, saccharin. Soln. 100 mL w/calibrated pipette. *Rx.*
Use: Cholinesterase inhibitor.

galantamine hydrobromide. (Various Mfr.) Galantamine hydrobromide. **Tab.:** 4 mg, 8 mg, 12 mg. May contain lactose. 60s, UD 30s. **ER Cap.:** 8 mg, 16 mg, 24 mg. May contain sugar. 30s. *Rx.*
Use: Cholinesterase inhibitor.

Galardin. (Glycomed, Inc.) Matrix metalloproteinase inhibitor.
Use: Corneal ulcers. [Orphan Drug]

•**galasomite.** (GAL-ah-som-ite) USAN.
Use: Verocytotoxogenic *E. coli* infections.

•**galdansetron hydrochloride.** (gahl-DAN-seh-trahn) USAN.
Use: Antiemetic.
•**galeterone.** (ga-LE-ter-one) USAN.
Use: Antineoplastic.
•**galiximab.** (gal-IX-i-mab) USAN.
Use: Psoriasis.
•**gallamine triethiodide.** (GAL-ah-meen try-eth-EYE-oh-dide) *USP.*
Use: Neuromuscular blocker.
•**gallium citrate Ga 67 injection.** (GAL-ee-uhm SIH-trate) *USP.*
Use: Diagnostic aid (radiopaque medium); radiopharmaceutical.
•**gallium nitrate.** (GAL-ee-uhm NYE-trate) USAN.
Use: Calcium regulator; antihypercalcemic.
gallochrome.
See: Merbromin.
gallotannic acid.
See: Tannic Acid.
gallstone solubilizing agents.
See: Chenodiol.
Ursodiol.
•**galsulfase.** (gal-SUL-fase) USAN.
Use: Mucopolysaccharidosis VI.
See: Naglazyme.
•**galunisertib.** (gal-UE-ni-SER-tib)) USAN.
Use: Antineoplastic.
Galzin. (Gate Pharmaceuticals) Zinc 25 mg, 50 mg. Cap. 250s. *Rx.*
Use: Trace element; Wilson disease.
GamaSTAN S/D. (Grifols Therapeutics) Immune globulin (human) 15% to 18% protein, glycine 0.21 to 0.32 M, solvent/detergent treated, preservative free. Soln. for Inj. Single-dose vial 2 mL, 10 mL; single-dose syringe 2 mL. *Rx.*
Use: Immune globulin.
Gamazole Tabs. (Major) Sulfamethoxazole 500 mg. Tab. Bot. 100s, 500s, 1000s. *Rx.*
Use: Anti-infective; sulfonamide.
•**gamfexine.** (gam-FEX-ine) USAN.
Use: Antidepressant.
gamma benzene hexachloride.
See: Lindane.
Gammagard S/D. (Baxter Healthcare) Immune globulin (human) 2.5 g, 5 g, 10 g. Sodium chloride 0.85% (sodium 3.34 mg/mL), albumin (human) 3 mg/mL, glycine 22.5 mg/mL, glucose 20 mg/mL, PEG 2 mg/mL, polysorbate 80 100 mcg/mL in a 5% solution. Preservative free. Inj., lyophilized Pow. for Soln. Single-use bottle (w/diluent, transfer device, administration set, and filter). *Rx.*
Use: Immune globulin.
Gammagard S/D Less IgA. (Baxter Healthcare) Immune globulin (human) 5 g, 10 g. Sodium chloride 0.85% (sodium 3.34 mg/mL), albumin (human) 3 mg/mL, glycine 22.5 mg/mL, glucose 20 mg/mL, PEG 2 mg/mL, polysorbate 80 100 mcg/mL in a 5% solution, immunoglobulin A < 1 mcg/mL. Preservative free. Inj., lyophilized Pow. for Soln. Single-use bottle (w/diluent, transfer device, administration set, and filter). *Rx.*
Use: Immune globulin.
gamma globulin.
See: Immune Globulin Intramuscular.
Immune Globulin Intravenous.
Immune Globulin Subcutaneous.
gamma-hydroxybutyrate. (Biocraft)
Use: Narcolepsy. [Orphan Drug]
gamma-hydroxybutyric acid. Under study.
Use: Anesthetic adjuvant, sleep disorders. [Orphan Drug]
gamma interferon.
See: Actimmune.
Gammaked. (Kedrion Biopharma) Immune globulin (human) IV/subcutaneous 10% (100 mg/mL) Glycine. Preservative free. Single-use vial (each consists of protein 9% to 11% and glycine 0.16 to 0.24 M). 10 mL, 25 mL, 50 mL, 100 mL, 200 mL. *Rx.*
Use: Immune globulin.
gammalinolenic acid.
Use: Juvenile rheumatoid arthritis. [Orphan Drug]
Gammaplex. (BPL) Immune globulin (human) 5% (50 mg/mL). Normal human immunoglobulin ≈ 5 g, D-sorbitol 5 g, glycine 0.6 g, sodium acetate 0.2 g, sodium chloride 0.3 g, polysorbate 80 ≈ 5 mg per 100 mL. Preservative free. Inj., Soln. Single-use vial. 50 mL, 100 mL, 200 mL. *Rx.*
Use: Immune globulin.
Gamunex-C. (Talecris Biotherapeutics) Immune globulin (human) 10% (100 mg/mL) (each vial consists of 9% to 11% protein in 0.16 to 0.24 M of glycine). Preservative free. Inj., Soln. Single-use vial. 10 mL, 25 mL, 50 mL, 100 mL, 200 mL. *Rx.*
Use: Immune globulin.
ganaxolone. (Cocensys, Inc.)
Use: Infantile spasms; epilepsy; migraine. [Orphan Drug]
•**ganciclovir.** (gan-SIGH-kloe-VIHR) *USP.*
Use: Antiviral.
See: Cytovene.
Zirgan.
ganciclovir. (APP) Ganciclovir sodium

500 mg. Sodium 46 mg. Inj., lyophilized Pow. for Soln. Vial. 10 mL. *Rx.*
Use: Anti-infective, antiviral agent.

•**ganciclovir sodium.** (gah-SIGH-kloe-VIHR) USAN.
Use: Antiviral.
See: Cytovene.

•**gandotinib.** (gan-DOE-ti-nib) USAN.
Use: Antineoplastic.

Ganeake. (Geneva) Conjugated Estrogens, 0.625 mg, 1.25 mg, 2.5 mg. Tab. Bot. 100s, 1000s. *Rx.*
Use: Estrogen.

ganeden BC30.
See: Ganeden Sustenex.

Ganeden Sustenex. (Ganeden) Ganeden BC30 2 billion cells. Lactose free. Cap. 30s. *OTC.*
Use: Oral nutritional supplement, probiotic.

•**ganetespib.** (ga-NET-es-pib) USAN.
Use: Antineoplastic.

ganglionic blocking agents.
See: Dibenzyline Hydrochloride.
Hexamethonium Chloride and Bromide.
Hydergine.
Priscoline Hydrochloride.
Regitine.

Ganidin NR. (Cypress) Guaifenesin 100 mg/5 mL. Liq. 473 mL. *Rx.*
Use: Expectorant.

•**ganirelix acetate.** (ga-ni-REL-ix) USAN.
Use: Sex hormone.

ganirelix acetate. (Organon) Ganirelix acetate 250 mcg/0.5 mL. Inj. Prefilled disp. syr. 1 mL. Box 1s, 5s, 50s. *Rx.*
Use: Sex hormone.

•**ganitumab.** (ga-NIT-ue-mab) USAN.
Use: Antineoplastic.

•**gantenerumab.** (GAN-te-NER-ue-mab) USAN.
Use: Alzheimer disease.

Garamycin. (Fera) Gentamicin 0.3% (as gentamicin sulfate). **Soln.; Ophth.:** Benzalkonium chloride. 5 mL dropper bottle. **Oint.; Ophth.:** Mineral oil, white petrolatum. 3.5 g. *Rx.*
Use: Ophthalmic antibiotic.

Gardasil. (Merck) Approximately 20 mcg of human papillomavirus (HPV) 6 L1 protein, 40 mcg of HPV 11 L1 protein, 40 mcg of HPV 16 L1 protein, 20 mcg of HPV 18 L1 protein per 0.5 mL. Preservative free. Soln. for Inj. Single-dose vials. 0.5 mL. *Rx.*
Use: Active immunization; viral vaccine.

gardinol type detergents. Aurinol, cyclopon, dreft, drene, duponol, lissapol, maprofix, modinal, orvus, sandopan, sadipan.
Use: Detergent.

gardol. Sodium lauryl sarcosinate.

•**garenoxacin mesylate.** (gar-en-OX-a-sin) USAN.
Use: Antibacterial.

Garfield's Tea. (Last) Senna leaf powder 68.3%. Bot. 2 oz. *OTC.*
Use: Laxative.

Garimide. (Rochester Pharmaceuticals) Sodium sulfacetamide 9%, sulfur 4.5%. Alcohols, aloe, BHT, disodium EDTA, glyceryl, green tea, parabens, PEG. Soap. 454 g. *Rx.*
Use: Acne product.

Garitabs. (Halsey Drug) Iron 50 mg, vitamins B_1 5 mg, B_2 5 mg, B_5 2 mg, B_6 0.5 mg, B_{12} 3 mcg, C 75 mg, niacinamide 30 mg. Bot. 1000s. *OTC.*
Use: Mineral, vitamin supplement.

Gari-Tonic Hematinic. (Halsey Drug) Vitamins B_1 5 mg, B_2 5 mg, B_6 1 mg, B_{12} 6 mcg, pantothenic acid 4 mg, niacinamide 100 mg, choline bitartrate 100 mg, iron 100 mg/30 mL Bot. 16 oz. *OTC.*
Use: Mineral, vitamin supplement.

•**garlic.** (GAR-lik) *NF.* Allium.
Use: Antispasmodic.

garlic capsules. (Miller Pharmacal Group) Garlic 166 mg. Cap. Bot. 100s. *OTC.*
Use: Antispasmodic.

garlic oil.
See: Natural Garlic Oil.

garlic oil capsules. (Kirkman) Bot. 100s. *OTC.*

•**garnocestim.** (gar-no-SES-tim) USAN.
Use: Chemotherapeutic aid.

Gas Ban. (Roberts) Calcium carbonate 300 mg, simethicone 40 mg. Tab. Bot. UD 8s, 1000s. *OTC.*
Use: Antacid.

Gas Ban DS. (Roberts) Aluminum hydroxide 400 mg, magnesium hydroxide 400 mg, simethicone 40 mg/5 mL. Liq. Bot. 150 mL. *OTC.*
Use: Antacid.

Gas Permeable Lens Starter System. (PBH Wesley Jessen) **Daily cleanser:** Bot. 3 mL **Wetting and soaking soln.:** Bot. 60 mL.*Hydra-Mat II* spin cleansing unit. Kit. *OTC.*
Use: Contact lens care.

Gas Permeable Wetting & Soaking Solution. (PBH Wesley Jessen) Sterile aqueous, isotonic soln. of low viscosity, buffered to physiological pH. Bot. 60 mL, 120 mL. *OTC.*
Use: Contact lens care.

Gas Relief. (Rugby) Simethicone. **Chew.**

Tab.: 80 mg, 125 mg. 60s (125 mg only), 100s (80 mg only). **Soln., concentrate:** 20 mg per 0.3 mL. Mannitol, sodium benzoate. Dye free. 30 mL w/dropper. *OTC.*
Use: Antiflatulent.

gastric acidifiers.
See: Glutamic Acid Hydrochloride.

Gastroccult. (SmithKline Diagnostics) Occult blood screening test. In 40s.
Use: Diagnostic aid.

Gastrocrom. (Celltech) Cromolyn sodium 100 mg/5 mL. Oral Conc. 8 UD Amps/foil pouch. *Rx.*
Use: Antiasthmatic.

Gastrografin. (Bracco Diagnostics) Diatrizoate meglumine 660 mg, diatrizoate sodium 100 mg, iodine 367 mg/mL. EDTA, polysorbate 80, saccharin, simethicone, lemon flavor. Soln. Bot. 120 mL. *Rx.*
Use: Radiopaque agent, GI contrast agent.

gastrointestinal agents.
See: Antidiarrheals.
Antiflatulents.
Helicobacter Pylori Agents.
Linaclotide.
Mesalamine.
Proton Pump Inhibitors.
Sucralfate.
Sulfasalazine.
Systemic Deodorizers.

gastrointestinal anticholinergics/antispasmodics.
See: Belladonna Alkaloids.
Quaternary Anticholinergics.

gastrointestinal contrast agents (iodinated).
Use: Radiopaque agent.
See: Diatrizoate Meglumine and Diatrizoate Sodium.
Diatrizoate Sodium.

gastrointestinal contrast agents (miscellaneous).
Use: Radiopaque agent.
See: Barium Sulfate.
Radiopaque Polyvinyl Chloride.
Sodium Bicarbonate and Tartaric Acid.

gastrointestinal function tests.
See: Secretin.
Simethicone-coated Cellulose Suspension.
Sincalide.

gastrointestinal stimulants.
See: Maxolon.
Metoclopramide.
Metoclopramide Hydrochloride.
Octamide.
Reclomide.
Reglan.

gastrointestinal tests.
See: Entero-Test.
Gastro-Test.

Gastrosed. (Roberts) Hyoscyamine sulfate. **Soln.:** 0.125 mg/mL. Dropper Bot. 5 mL. Alcohol free. **Tab.:** 0.125 mg. Bot. 100s. *Rx.*
Use: Anticholinergic; antispasmodic.

Gastro-Test. (HDC) To determine stomach pH and to diagnose and locate gastric bleeding. Test 25s.
Use: Diagnostic aid.

Gas-X. (Novartis) Simethicone 80 mg. Softgel Cap. Pkg. 12s, 30s. *OTC.*
Use: Antiflatulent.

Gas-X, Extra Strength. (Novartis) Simethicone 125 mg, sorbitol. Softgel Cap. Box 30s, 100s. *OTC.*
Use: Antiflatulent.

Gas-X Thin Strips. (Novartis) Simethicone 62.5 mg. Maltodextrin, menthol, sorbitol, sucralose. Orally Disintegrating Strips. 18s. *OTC.*
Use: Antiflatulent.

Gas-X with Maalox Extra Strength. (Novartis) Calcium carbonate 500 mg, simethicone 125 mg. Dextrose, mannitol. Orange and wild berry flavors. Chew. Tab. 8s, 24s. *OTC.*
Use: Antacid.

•**gataparsen.** (GAT-a-PAR-sen) USAN.
Use: Antineoplastic.

•**gataparsen sodium.** (GAT-a-PAR-sen) USAN.
Use: Antineoplastic.

•**gatifloxacin.** (gat-ih-FLOX-ah-sin) USAN.
Use: Fluoroquinolone, antibiotic.
See: Zymar.

gatifloxacin. (Lupin) Gatifloxacin 0.3%, 0.5%. Benzalkonium chloride, EDTA. Soln., Ophth. 2.5 mL, 5 mL (0.3%); 2.5 mL dropper bottle (0.5%). *Rx.*
Use: Ophthalmic antibiotic.

Gattex. (NPS Pharmaceuticals) Teduglutide 5 mg. Mannitol. Preservative free. Inj., lyophilized Pow. for Soln. Single-use vial w/diluent (sterile water for injection 0.5 mL in prefilled syringe). *Rx.*
Use: Glucagon-like peptide-2 analog.

•**gauze, absorbent.** (gawz) *USP.*
Use: Surgical aid.

•**gauze, petrolatum.** (gawz PET-roe-LAY-tum) *USP.*
Use: Surgical aid.

•**gavestinel.** (ga-VE-sti-nel) USAN.
Use: Stroke.

GaviLAX. (Gavis) 17 g of PEG 3350. Pow. for oral Soln. 238 g, 510 g. *OTC.*
Use: Laxative, bowel evacuant.

GaviLyte-C. (Gavis Pharmaceuticals)

240 g of PEG 3350, sodium bicarbonate 6.72 g, sodium chloride 5.84 g, sodium sulfate 22.72 g, potassium chloride 2.98 g. Pow. for Soln. 4 L w/lemon flavor pack. *Rx.*
Use: Laxative, bowel evacuant.

GaviLyte-G. (Gavis Pharmaceuticals) 236 g of PEG 3350, sodium bicarbonate 6.74 g, sodium chloride 5.86 g, sodium sulfate 22.74 g, potassium chloride 2.97 g. Pow. for Soln. 4 L w/lemon flavor pack. *Rx.*
Use: Laxative, bowel evacuant.

GaviLyte-N. (Gavis Pharmaceuticals) 420 g of PEG 3350, sodium bicarbonate 5.72 g, sodium chloride 11.2 g, potassium chloride 1.48 g. Pow. for Soln. 4 L w/lemon flavor pack. *Rx.*
Use: Laxative, bowel evacuant.

Gaviscon. (GlaxoSmithKline) Aluminum hydroxide 80 mg. Magnesium 5 mg, magnesium trisilicate 14.2 mg, alginic acid, sodium bicarbonate, sucrose. Chew. Tab. 100s. *OTC.*
Use: Antacid.

Gaviscon Extra Strength Antacid. (GlaxoSmithKline) Aluminum hydroxide 160 mg, magnesium carbonate 105 mg. Acesulfame K, alginic acid, corn syr., mannitol, sodium bicarbonate, sucrose, calcium stearate, sodium 19 mg. Cherry flavor. Chew. Tab. 30s, 100s. *OTC.*
Use: Antacid.

Gaviscon Extra Strength Relief Formula. (GlaxoSmithKline) Aluminum hydroxide 254 mg, magnesium carbonate 237.5 mg. Parabens, EDTA, saccharin, sorbitol, simethicone, sodium alginate/5 mL. Liq. Bot. 355 mL. *OTC.*
Use: Antacid.

Gaviscon Liquid. (GlaxoSmithKline) Aluminum hydroxide 31.7 mg, magnesium carbonate 119.3 mg/5 mL. Bot. 177 mL, 355 mL. *OTC.*
Use: Antacid.

Gaviscon-2, Double Strength Tablets. (GlaxoSmithKline) Aluminum hydroxide 160 mg, magnesium trisilicate 40 mg, alginic acid, sodium bicarbonate, sucrose. Chew. Tab. Bot. 48s. *OTC.*
Use: Antacid.

Gazyva. (Genentech) Obinutuzumab 25 mg/mL. Preservative free. Inj., Soln., concentrate. Single-use vial. 40 mL. *Rx.*
Use: Monoclonal antibody.

GBA.
See: Gamma Hydroxybutyrate.

G-BID DM TR. (Boca Pharmacal) Dextromethorphan HBr 60 mg, guaifenesin 1200 mg. ER Tab. 100s. *Rx.*
Use: Antitussive with expectorant.

G.B.S. (Forest) Dehydrocholic acid 125 mg, phenobarbital 8 mg, homatropine methylbromide 2.5 mg. Tab. 100s, 1000s. *Rx.*
Use: Hydrocholeretic.

G-CSF. Granulocyte Colony-Stimulating Factor.
See: Neupogen.

Gebauer's Ethyl Chloride. (Gebauer) Chloroethane. Aer. spray. *Spra-Pak.* 105 mL (fine, medium, and coarse spray). *Formerly Ethyl Chloride. Rx.*
Use: Anesthetic, local.

Gebauer's 114. (Gebauer) Dichlorotetrafluoroethane 100%. Can 8 oz.
Use: Anesthetic, local.

Gebauer's Spray and Stretch. (Gebauer) Tetrafluoroethane and pentafluoropropane. Spray. 103.5 mL. *Rx.*
Use: Local anesthetic, topical.

•**gefitinib.** (ge-FI-tye-nib) USAN.
Use: Antineoplastic.

Geladine. (Barth's) Gelatin, protein, vitamin D. Cap. Bot. 100s, 500s. *OTC.*

Gelamal. (Halsey Drug) Magnesium-aluminum hydroxide gel. Bot. 12 oz. *OTC.*
Use: Antacid.

•**gelatin.** (JEL-a-tin) *NF.*
Use: Pharmaceutic aid (encapsulating, suspending agent, tablet binder, tablet coating agent).

•**gelatin film, absorbable.** (JEL-a-tin) *USP.*
Use: Local hemostatic.
See: Gelfilm.

gelatin film, sterile.
See: Neupogen.

gelatin powder, sterile.
See: Gelfoam.

gelatin sponge.
See: Gelfilm.

•**gelatin sponge, absorbable.** (JEL-a-tin) *USP.*
Use: Hemostatic, local.
See: Gelfoam.

gelatin, zinc.
See: Zinc Gelatin.

Gelclair. (Dara BioSciences) Glycyrrhetinic acid, polyvinylpyrrolidone, sodium hyaluronate. Benzalkonium chloride, castor oil, disodium edetate, hydroxyethylcellulose, maltodextrin, potassium sorbate, propylene glycol, saccharin, sodium benzoate. Gel. Single-use packet. 15 mL. *Rx.*
Use: Mouth and throat product.

Gel-Clean. (PBH Wesley Jessen) Gel formulated with nonionic surfactant. Tube 30 g. *OTC.*
Use: Contact lens care.

G-11. (Givaudan) Hexachlorophene Pow. for Mfg.
See: Hexachlorophene.

Gelfilm. (Pharmacia) Sterile, absorbable gelatin film. Envelope 1s. 100 mm × 125 mm. Also available as Ophth. Sterile 25 × 50 mm. Box 6s. *Rx.*
Use: Hemostatic, topical.

Gelfoam Dental Pack. (Pharmacia) Size 4, 20 mm × 20 mm × 7 mm. Jar 15 sponges. *Rx.*
Use: Hemostatic, topical.

Gelfoam Powder. (Pharmacia) Sterile Jar 1 g. *Rx.*
Use: Hemostatic, topical.

Gelfoam Prostatectomy Cones. (Pharmacia) Prostatectomy cones (for use with Foley catheter) 13 cm, 18 cm in diameter. Box 6s. *Rx.*
Use: Hemostatic.

Gelhist Pediatric Suspension. (Econolab) Phenylephrine tannate 5 mg, chlorpheniramine tannate 2 mg, pyrilamine tannate 12.5 mg/5 mL, methylparaben, saccharin, sucrose. Susp. Bot. 118 mL, 473 mL. *Rx.*
Use: Antihistamine, decongestant.

Gel Jet Gelatin Capsules. (Kirkman) Bot. 100s, 250s.

Gel-Kam. (Colgate Oral) **Gel:** Fluoride 0.1% (stannous fluoride 0.4%). Mint, fruit, berry, bubble gum, cinnamon flavors. Bot. w/applicator tip. 4.3 oz, 7 oz. **Rinse:** Sodium fluoride 0.04%. Mint, fruit and berry, bubblegum, and cinnamon flavors. 4.3 oz, 7 oz. **Rinse Concen.:** Stannous fluoride 0.63%. Glycerin. Cinnamon and mint flavors. 283 g. *Rx-OTC.*
Use: Dental caries agent.

Gelnique 10%. (Watson) Oxybutynin chloride 10%. Alcohol. Gel. Sachet. 1 g. *Rx.*
Use: Renal and genitourinary agent, anticholinergic.

Gelnique 3%. (Watson) Oxybutynin chloride 3%. Alcohol, BHT, propylene glycol. Gel. Metered pump dispenser. 92 g. *Rx.*
Use: Renal and genitourinary agent, urinary anticholinergic.

Gelocast. (Beiersdorf) Unna's Boot medicated bandage: Semi-rigid cast impregnated with zinc oxide mixtures. Box 4 inches × 10 yd, 3 inches × 10 yd.
Use: Unna's cast dressing.

Gel-One. (Zimmer) Hyaluronate (cross-linked) 10 mg/mL. Sodium chloride. Inj., gel. Prefilled syringe. 3 mL. *Rx.*
Use: Physical adjunct.

gelsemium. (Various Mfr.) Pkg. oz.
Use: Neuralgia.
W/A.P.C.
See: APC Combinations.
W/Combinations
See: UB.
Urisan-P.

gelsolin, recombinant human. (Biogen)
Use: Cystic fibrosis. [Orphan Drug]

Gel-Tin. (Young Dental) Fluoride 0.1% (from stannous fluoride 0.4%). Gel Bot. 57 g, 623 g. *Rx.*
Use: Dental caries agent.

•**gemcabene calcium.** (JEM-ka-been) USAN.
Use: Atherosclerosis.

•**gemcadiol.** (JEM-kah-DIE-ole) USAN.
Use: Antihyperlipoproteinemic.

•**gemcitabine.** (jem-SYE-ta-been) USAN.
Use: Antineoplastic.

gemcitabine. (Hospira) Gemcitabine hydrochloride 38 mg/mL. Inj., Soln.; concentrate. Single-use vial. 5.26 mL, 26.3 mL, 52.6 mL. *Rx.*
Use: Antimetabolite, pyrimidine analog.

gemcitabine. (Various Mfr.) Gemcitabine hydrochloride 200 mg, 1 g, 2 g. May contain mannitol. Inj., lyophilized Pow. for Soln. Single-use vial. *Rx.*
Use: Antimetabolite, pyrimidine analog.

•**gemcitabine elaidate.** (jem-SYE-ta-been el-ay-i-date) USAN.
Use: Antineoplastic.

•**gemcitabine hydrochloride.** (jem-SYE-ta-been) *USP.*
Use: Antineoplastic; antimetabolite.
See: Gemzar.

•**gemeprost.** (JEH-meh-PRAHST) USAN.
Use: Prostaglandin.

•**gemfibrozil.** (gem-FIE-broe-ZILL) *USP.*
Use: Antihyperlipidemic.
See: Lopid.

gemfibrozil. (Various Mfr.) Gemfibrozil 600 mg. Tab., Bot. 60s, 500s; blister-pack 25s; UD 100s. *Rx.*
Use: Antihyperlipidemic.

•**gemifloxacin mesylate.** (jeh-mih-FLOKS-ah-sin MEH-sih-LATE) USAN.
Use: Fluoroquinolone.
See: Factive.

•**gemopatrilat.** (ge-moe-PA-tril-at) USAN.
Use: Hypertension; congestive heart failure.

•**gemtuzumab ozogamicin.** (jem-TOOZ-ue-mab OH-zoe-ga-MYE-sin) USAN.
Use: Monoclonal antibody.

Gemzar. (Eli Lilly) Gemcitabine hydrochloride 200 mg, 1 g. Mannitol. Pow. for Inj., lyophilized. Single-use vials. 10 mL (200 mg only), 50 mL (1 g only). *Rx.*
Use: Antineoplastic.

Genac. (Ivax) Triprolidine hydrochloride 2.5 mg, pseudoephedrine hydrochloride 60 mg. Lactose. Tab. Bot. 24s, 48s. *OTC.*
Use: Upper respiratory combination, antihistamine, and decongestant.

Genacol. (Ivax) Pseudoephedrine hydrochloride 30 mg, chlorpheniramine maleate 2 mg, dextromethorphan HBr 10 mg, acetaminophen 325 mg. Tab. Bot. 50s. *OTC.*
Use: Analgesic, antihistamine, antitussive, decongestant.

Genacol Maximum Strength Cold & Flu Relief. (Ivax) Dextromethorphan HBr 15 mg, chlorpheniramine maleate 2 mg, pseudoephedrine hydrochloride 30 mg, acetaminophen 500 mg. Tab. Bot. 50s. *OTC.*
Use: Upper respiratory combination, antitussive, antihistamine, decongestant, analgesic.

Genagesic. (Ivax) Propoxyphene hydrochloride 165 mg, acetaminophen 650 mg. Tab. Bot. 100s, 500s. *c-IV.*
Use: Analgesic combination, narcotic.

Genahist. (Goldline) Diphenhydramine hydrochloride. **Liq.:** 12.5 mg/5 mL, cherry flavor. Bot. 118 mL. **Tab.:** 25 mg. 24s. **Cap.:** 25 mg, lactose, parabens. 100s. *OTC.*
Use: Antihistamine.

Genallerate. (Ivax) Chlorpheniramine maleate 4 mg, lactose. Tab. Bot. 24s. *OTC.*
Use: Antihistamine.

Genapap. (Ivax) Acetaminophen 325 mg. Tab. Bot. 100s. *OTC.*
Use: Analgesic.

Genapap Children's. (Ivax) Acetaminophen 80 mg. Grape flavor. Chew. Tab. Bot. 30s. *OTC.*
Use: Analgesic.

Genapap Extra Strength. (Ivax) Acetaminophen 500 mg. Tab., Rapid Release. 100s. *OTC.*
Use: Analgesic.

Genapax. (Key) Gentian violet 5 mg. Tampon. Box 12s.
Use: Antifungal, vaginal.

Genaphed. (Ivax) Pseudoephedrine hydrochloride 30 mg, lactose. Tab. Bot. 24s. *OTC.*
Use: Nasal decongestant, arylalkylamine.

Genasal. (Goldline) Oxymetazoline hydrochloride 0.05%, benzalkonium chloride, edetate disodium, PEG 1450. Soln. Spray Bot. 15 mL, 30 mL. *OTC.*
Use: Nasal decongestant, arylalkylamine.

Genasyme. (Ivax) Simethicone 80 mg. Tab. Bot. 100s. *OTC.*
Use: Antiflatulent.

Genaton. (Ivax) Aluminum hydroxide 80 mg, magnesium trisilicate 20 mg, alginic acid, sodium bicarbonate, sodium 18.4 mg, sucrose, sugar. Chew. Tab. Bot. 100s. *OTC.*
Use: Antacid.

Genaton, Extra Strength. (Ivax) Aluminum hydroxide 160 mg, magnesium carbonate 105 mg, alginic acid, sodium bicarbonate, sodium 29.9 mg, sucrose, calcium stearate. Chew. Tab. Bot. 100s. *OTC.*
Use: Antacid.

Genaton Liquid. (Ivax) Aluminum hydroxide 31.7 mg, magnesium carbonate 137.3 mg, sodium alginate, sodium 13 mg, EDTA, saccharin, sorbitol/5 mL. Bot. 355 mL. *OTC.*
Use: Antacid.

genatropine hydrochloride. (jen-AT-row-peen) Atropine-N-oxide hydrochloride. Aminoxytropine tropate hydrochloride.
See: X-tro.

Gen-bee with C. (Ivax) Vitamins B_1 15 mg, B_2 10.2 mg, B_3 50 mg, B_5 10 mg, B_6 5 mg, C 300 mg. Cap. Bot. 130s, 1000s. *OTC.*
Use: Vitamin supplement.

Gencept. (Gencon) **0.5/35:** Norethindrone 0.5 mg, ethinyl estradiol, 35 mcg. Tab (with 7 inert tabs). Pkgs 21s and 28s. **1/35:** Norethindrone 1 mg, ethinyl estradiol 35 mcg. Tab (with 7 inert tabs). Pkgs 21s and 28s. **10/11:** Norethindrone 0.5 mg and 1 mg, ethinyl estradiol 35 mcg. Tab (with 7 inert tabs). Pkg 21s and 28s. *Rx.*
Use: Contraceptive.

Gendecon. (Ivax) Phenylephrine hydrochloride 5 mg, chlorpheniramine maleate 2 mg, acetaminophen 325 mg. Tab. Bot. 50s. *OTC.*
Use: Analgesic, antihistamine, decongestant.

Genebrom-DM. (PGD) Dextromethorphan HBr 10 mg, brompheniramine maleate 2 mg, pseudoephedrine hydrochloride 30 mg per 5 mL. Alcohol free. Parabens, sugar, saccharin. Cherry flavor. Liq. 473 mL. *Rx.*
Use: Antitussive combination.

Genelan-NF. (PGD) Dextromethorphan HBr 15 mg, guaifenesin 100 mg, phenylephrine hydrochloride 10 mg, chlorpheniramine maleate 2 mg per 5 mL. Sugar, alcohol, and dye free. Parabens, aspartame, phenylalanine. Liq. 473 mL. *Rx.*

Use: Antitussive and expectorant combination.

general anesthetics.
Use: Anesthetics, general.
See: Barbiturates.
Fospropofol Disodium.

Generess Fe. (Watson) Ethinyl estradiol 25 mcg, norethindrone 0.8 mg. Lactose, mannitol, spearmint flavoring, sucralose. Chew. Tab. 28s w/4 inert Chew. Tab. (ferrous fumarate 75 mg, sucralose; spearmint flavoring). *Rx.*
Use: Monophasic oral contraceptive.

Generet-500. (Ivax) Iron 105 mg, Vitamins B_1 6 mg, B_2 6 mg, B_3 30 mg, B_5 10 mg, B_6 5 mg, B_{12} 25 mcg, C (as sodium ascorbate) 500 mg. TR Tab. Bot. 60s. *OTC.*
Use: Mineral, vitamin supplement.

Generix-T. (Ivax) Iron 15 mg, vitamins A 10,000 units, D 400 units, E 5.5 mg, B_1 15 mg, B_2 10 mg, B_3 100 mg, B_5 10 mg, B_6 2 mg, B_{12} 7.5 mcg, C 150 mg, Cu, I, Mg, Mn, zinc 1.5 mg. Tab. Bot. 100s. *OTC.*
Use: Mineral, vitamin supplement.

Generlac. (Morton Grove Pharmaceuticals) Lactulose 10 g per 15 mL. Soln., Oral and Rectal. 473 mL, 1,892 mL. *Rx.*
Use: Laxative, hyperosmotic agent.

Gene-T-Press. (PGD) Dextromethorphan HBr 15 mg, guaifenesin 200 mg, phenylephrine hydrochloride 5 mg per 5 mL. Sugar and alcohol free. Parabens, aspartame, phenylalanine. Cherry flavor. Liq. 473 mL. *Rx.*
Use: Antitussive and expectorant combination.

Genfiber. (Goldline Consumer) Psyllium hydrophilic mucilloid fiber 3.4 g, 14 cal/dose, dextrose. Pow. Can 595 g. *OTC.*
Use: Laxative.

Genfiber, Orange Flavor. (Goldline Consumer) Psyllium hydrophilic mucilloid fiber 3.4 g/dose, sucrose, orange flavor. Pow. Can 397 g. *OTC.*
Use: Laxative.

Gengraf. (Abbott) Cyclosporine. **Cap.:** 25 mg, 100 mg, alcohol 12.8%, castor oil. UD 30s. **Oral Soln.:** 100 mg/mL. Castor oil. 50 mL. *Rx.*
Use: Immunosuppressant.

genital herpes treatment.
See: Acyclovir.
Zovirax.

Genite. (Ivax) Pseudoephedrine hydrochloride 10 mg, doxylamine succinate 1.25 mg, dextromethorphan HBr 5 mg, acetaminophen 167 mg, alcohol 25%/5 mL. Bot. 177 mL. *OTC.*
Use: Analgesic, antihistamine, antitussive, decongestant.

genitourinary irrigants.
See: Acetic Acid for Irrigation.
Glycine (Aminoacetic Acid) for Irrigation.
Hexitol Irrigants.
Neosporin G.U. Irrigant.
Renacidin.
Sodium Chloride for Irrigation.
Sorbitol.
Sorbitol-Mannitol.
Sterile Water for Irrigation.
Suby's Solution G.

Gen-K. (Ivax) **Pow.:** Potassium chloride. Bot. 20 mEq. Pkt. Box 30s. **Tab.:** Effervescent potassium. Bot. 30s. *Rx.*
Use: Electrolyte supplement.

Genna Tablets. (Ivax) Senna concentrate 217 mg. Bot. 100s, 1000s. *OTC.*
Use: Laxative.

Gennin. (Ivax) Buffered aspirin 5 g. Tab. Bot. 100s. *OTC.*
Use: Analgesic.

genophyllin.
See: Aminophylline.

Genotropin. (Pfizer) Somatropin 5 mg, 12 mg. Glycine, mannitol, metacresol. Inj., lyophilized Pow. for Soln. 2-chamber cartridge. *Rx.*
Use: Growth hormone.

Genotropin MiniQuick. (Pfizer) Somatropin 0.2 mg (≈ 0.6 units), 0.4 mg (≈ 1.2 units), 0.6 mg (≈ 1.8 units), 0.8 mg (≈ 2.4 units), 1 mg (≈ 3 units), 1.2 mg (≈ 3.6 units), 1.4 mg (≈ 4.2 units), 1.6 mg (≈ 4.8 units), 1.8 mg (≈ 5.4 units), 2 mg (≈ 6 units) per cartridge. Glycine 0.23 mg, mannitol 13.74 mg, preservative free. Pow. for Inj., lyophilized. Single-use syringe w/2-chamber cartridge. Box 7s. *Rx.*
Use: Growth hormone.

Genprep Ointment. (Ivax) Live yeast cell derivative supplying 2000 units skin respiratory factor/oz of ointment w/shark liver oil 3%, phenylmercuric nitrate 1:10,000. Tube 2 oz. *OTC.*
Use: Anorectal preparation.

Genprin. (Ivax) Aspirin 325 mg. Tab. 100s. *OTC.*
Use: Analgesic.

gensalate sodium.
Use: Analgesic.

Gentafair. (Bausch & Lomb) **Oint.:** Gentamicin 3 mg/g with liquid lanolin, white petrolatum, mineral oil, parabens. Tube 3.75 g, 15 g. **Soln.:** Gentamicin 3 mg/mL, polyoxyl 40 stearate, polyethylene glycol. Dropper bot. 5 mL, 15 mL. *Rx.*
Use: Anti-infective, ophthalmic.

Gentak. (Akorn) Gentamicin 0.3% (as gentamicin sulfate). **Soln.; Ophth.:** Benzalkonium chloride. 5 mL dropper bottle. **Oint.; Ophth.:** Mineral oil, parabens, white petrolatum. 3.5 g. *Rx.*
Use: Ophthalmic antibiotic.

gentamicin. (Various Mfr.) Gentamicin sulfate. **Oint.:** 0.1% (as base), may contain white petrolatum, parabens. 15 g. **Cream:** 0.1% (as base), may contain propylene glycol, parabens. 15 g. *Rx.*
Use: Anti-infective, topical.

gentamicin and prednisolone acetate ophthalmic suspension.
Use: Anti-infective; anti-inflammatory.

gentamicin impregnated PMMA beads on surgical wire.
Use: Chronic osteomyelitis. [Orphan Drug]

gentamicin liposome injection.
Use: Mycobacterium avium-intracellulare infection. [Orphan Drug]

gentamicin ophthalmic. (Various Mfr.) Gentamicin sulfate 3 mg/mL. Soln. 5 mL, 15 mL. *Rx.*
Use: Antibiotic.

•**gentamicin sulfate.** (JEN-tuh-MY-sin) *USP.*
Use: Anti-infective.
See: Garamycin.
Gentak.
W/Combinations.
See: Pred-G.
Pred-G Ophthalmic Suspension.

gentamicin sulfate. (Fera) Gentamicin 0.3%. May contain mineral oil, white petrolatum. Oint.; Ophth. 3.5 g. *Rx.*
Use: Ophthalmic antibiotic.

gentamicin sulfate. (Various Mfr.) Gentamicin 0.3%. May contain benzalkonium chloride. Soln.; Ophth. 5 mL, 15 mL. *Rx.*
Use: Ophthalmic antibiotic.

gentamicin sulfate. (Various Mfr.) Gentamicin sulfate 10 mg/mL, 40 mg/mL. May contain EDTA, parabens, sulfites. Inj., Soln.; concentrate. *ADD-Vantage* 60 mg, 80 mg, 100 mg vials and 2 mL vial (10 mg/mL); 2 mL and 20 mL vials (40 mg/mL). *Rx.*
Use: Anti-infective, parenteral aminoglycoside.

gentamicin sulfate in 0.9% sodium chloride. (Various Mfr.) Gentamicin sulfate (as gentamicin base) 0.6 mg/mL, 0.8 mg/mL, 0.9 mg/mL, 1 mg/mL, 1.2 mg/mL, 1.4 mg/mL, 1.6 mg/mL, 2 mg/mL. Sodium chloride 0.9%. Inj. Single-dose flexible containers. 50 mL (1.2 mg/mL, 1.4 mg/mL, 1.6 mg/mL, 2 mg/mL only), 100 mL (0.6 mg/mL, 0.8 mg/mL, 0.9 mg/mL, 1 mg/mL only). *Rx.*
Use: Aminoglycoside.

gentamicin sulfate, pediatric. (APP) Gentamicin (as sulfate) 10 mg/mL. Preservative free. Inj. Vial. 2 mL. *Rx.*
Use: Anti-infective.

GenTeal Mild. (Novartis) Hypromellose 0.2%, boric acid, phosphonic acid, potassium chloride, sodium chloride, sodium perborate. Preservative free. Soln., Ophth. 25 mL. *OTC.*
Use: Artificial tear solution.

GenTeal Mild to Moderate. (Novartis) Hypromellose 0.3%, boric acid, phosphonic acid, potassium chloride, sodium chloride, sodium perborate. Preservative free. Soln., Ophth. 25 mL. *OTC.*
Use: Artificial tear solution.

GenTeal Moderate to Severe. (Novartis) Carboxymethylcellulose sodium 0.25%, hypromellose 0.3%, boric acid, sodium perborate, magnesium chloride, phosphonic acid, potassium chloride, sodium chloride. Preservative free. Soln., gel forming; Ophth. 25 mL. *OTC.*
Use: Artificial tear solution.

GenTeal PM. (Novartis) Mineral oil 15%, white petrolatum 85%. Oint.; Ophth. 3.5 mL. *OTC.*
Use: Ocular lubricant.

GenTeal Severe Eye Relief. (Novartis) Hypromellose 0.3%, phosphonic acid, sodium hydroxide, sodium perborate. Preservative free. Gel; Ophth. 10 g. *OTC.*
Use: Ocular lubricant.

Gentex 30. (Gentex) Carbetapentane citrate 30 mg, guaifenesin 200 mg, phenylephrine hydrochloride 8 mg per 5 mL. EDTA, parabens, saccharin. Cherry flavor. Liq. 118 mL. *Rx.*
Use: Upper respiratory combination, antitussive, and expectorant combination.

•**gentian violet.** (JEN-shun) *USP. Formerly Methylrosaniline Chloride.*
Use: Topical anti-infective, antifungal agent.

gentian violet. (Various Mfr.) Gentian violet 1%, 2%. Top. Soln. Bot. 30 mL. *OTC.*
Use: Anti-infective; antifungal, topical.

gentisic acid ethanolamide.
Use: Pharmaceutic aid, complexing agent.

Gentle Cream. (Geritrex) Mineral oil, cetearyl alcohol, petrolatum, castor oil, lanolin, triethanolamine, propylene glycol, EDTA, zinc oxide, vitamins A, D, & E, aloe vera oil. Cream. 120 g. *OTC.*
Use: Emollient.

Gentle Iron. (Nature's Bounty) Fe 28 mg (as ferrous bisglycinate), vitamin B_{12} 8 mcg, C 60 mg, FA 0.4 mg. Cap. 90s. *OTC.*
Use: Vitamin.

Gentle Nature Natural Vegetable Laxative. (Novartis) Sennosides A and B as calcium salts. 20 mg. Tab. Box 16s, 32s. *OTC.*
Use: Laxative.

Gentle Shampoo. (Ulmer Pharmacal) Bot. 4 oz, gal. *OTC.*
Use: Dermatologic, hair.

Gentran 40. (Baxter PPI) Dextran 40 10% w/sodium chloride 0.9% or Dextran 40 10% w/dextrose 5%. Inj. Plastic Bot. 500 mL. *Rx.*
Use: Plasma expander.

Gentran 75. (Baxter PPI) Dextran 75 6% in sodium chloride 0.9%. Inj. Bot. 500 mL. *Rx.*
Use: Plasma expander.

Gentrasul. (Bausch & Lomb) Gentamicin. **Oint.:** 3 mg. **Soln.:** 3.5 g. Dropper bot. 5 mL. *Rx.*
Use: Anti-infective, ophthalmic.

Genuine Bayer Aspirin. (Bayer Consumer Care) Aspirin 325 mg. FC Tab. Bot. 12s, 24s, 50s, 200s, 300s. *OTC.*
Use: Analgesic.

Geodon. (Pfizer) **Cap.:** Ziprasidone hydrochloride 20 mg, 40 mg, 60 mg, 80 mg. Lactose. Bot. 60s, UD 80s. **Pow. for Inj.:** Ziprasidone mesylate 20 mg. Vials. Single use. *Rx.*
Use: Antipsychotic; benzisoxazole derivative.

Geopen. (Roerig) Carbenicillin disodium. Inj. **Vial:** 1 g, 2 g, 5 g. Pkg. 10s. **Piggyback Vial:** 2 g, 5 g, 10 g. **Bulk Pharmacy Pack:** 30 g. *Rx.*
Use: Anti-infective, penicillin.

•**gepirone hydrochloride.** (jeh-PIE-rone) USAN.
Use: Anxiolytic; antidepressant.

Gera Plus. (Towne) Iron 50 mg, vitamins B_1 5 mg, B_2 5 mg, B_6 0.5 mg, B_{12} 3 mcg, C 75 mg, niacinamide 30 mg, calcium pantothenate 2 mg. Tab. Bot. 100s. *OTC.*
Use: Mineral, vitamin supplement.

Geravim. (Major) Vitamins B_1 0.83 mg, B_2 0.42 mg, B_3 8.3 mg, B_5 1.67 mg, B_6 0.17 mg, B_{12} 0.17 mg, I, Fe 2.5 mg, Zn 0.3 mg, choline, Mn, alcohol 18%. Liq. Bot. Pt, gal. *OTC.*
Use: Mineral, vitamin supplement.

Geravite. (Roberts) Vitamins B_1 0.3 mg, B_2 0.4 mg, B_3 33.3 mg, B_{12} 3.3 mcg, L-lysine, alcohol 15%, parabens, sorbitol, sucrose. Elix. Bot. 480 mL. *OTC.*
Use: Mineral, vitamin supplement.

Gerber Baby Formula Low Iron Formula. (Bristol-Myers Squibb) Protein (from non-fat milk) 14.7 g, carbohydrate (from lactose) 71.3 g, fat (from palm olein, soy, coconut, and high oleic sunflower oils) 36 g, linoleic acid 5.9 g, vitamins A, D, E, K, C, B_1, B_2, B_3, B_5, B_6, B_{12}, folic acid, biotin, choline, inositol, Ca, P, Mg, Fe 3.4 mg, Zn, Mn, Cu, I, Na 220 mg, K 720 mg, Cl, taurine, calories per L 666.7. **Ready to use liq.:** Bot. 943 mL. **Concentrated liq.:** Bot. 433 mL. **Pow.:** Can 457 g and 914 g. *OTC.*
Use: Nutritional supplement.

Gerber Soothe Colic. (Nestle Infant Nutrition) 100 million colony-forming units of *L. reuteri* protectis per 5 drops. Medium chain triglyceride oil, sunflower oil. Soln., concentrate. 5 mL. *OTC.*
Use: Probiotic.

Geri-All-D. (Barth's) Vitamins A 10,000 units, D 400 units, B_1 7 mg, B_2 14 mg, B_6 0.35 mg, B_{12} 25 mcg, C 200 mg, niacin 4.17 mg, E 50 units, pantothenic acid 0.63 mg, trace minerals, and other factors. 2 Cap. Bot. 1 mo., 3 mo., and 6 mo. supply of Geri-All regular and Geri-All-D. *OTC.*
Use: Mineral, vitamin supplement.

geriatric supplements with multivitamins/minerals.
See: Geravite.
Gerimed.
Geriot.
Geri-Plus.
Geritol Complete.
Gerivite.
Gerix.
Hep-Forte.
Mega VM-80.
Optivite P.M.T.
Strovite Plus.
Ultra Freeda.
Ultra Freeda Iron Free.
Vigortol.
Viminate.
Vita-Plus G.

Geriatroplex. (Morton Grove) Cyanocobalamin 30 mcg, liver inj. 0.1 mL, vitamins B_2 1.5 mg, B_{12} activity 2 mcg, ferrous gluconate 50 mg, calcium pantothenate 2.5 mg, niacinamide 100 mg, citric acid 16.4 mg, sodium citrate 23.6 mg/2 mL. Vial 30 mL. *OTC.*
Use: Mineral, vitamin supplement.

Geri-Derm. (Barth's) Vitamins A 400,000 units, D 40,000 units, E 200 units, panthenol 800 mg/4 oz. Jar 4 oz. *OTC.*
Use: Skin supplement.

Geridium. (Goldline) Phenazopyridine hydrochloride 100 mg, 200 mg. Sugar coated. Tab. Bot. 100s, 1000s (100 mg only). *Rx.*
Use: Analgesic; anti-infective, urinary.

Geri-Hydrolac. (Geritrex) **Cream:** Ammonium lactate (equiv. to 12% lactic acid), light mineral oil, petrolatum, propylene glycol, glycerin, cetyl alcohol, parabens. Cream. 140 g. **Lot.:** Lactic acid buffered 5%, ammonium hydroxide, cetyl alcohol, dimethicone, EDTA, glycerin, parabens, petrolatum. 237 mL. *OTC.*
Use: Emollient.

Geri-Hydrolac 12. (Geritrex Corp) Ammonium lactate 12%, cetyl alcohol, glycerin, mineral oil, parabens, PEG-100, propylene glycol. Lot. 225 g, 400 g. *OTC.*
Use: Emollient.

Gerilets. (Abbott) Vitamins A 5000 units, D 400 units, E 45 units, C 90 mg (from sodium ascorbate), folic acid 0.4 mg, B_1 2.25 mg, B_2 2.6 mg, niacin 30 mg, B_6 3 mg, B_{12} 9 mcg, biotin 0.45 mg, pantothenic acid 15 mg, iron 27 mg (from ferrous sulfate). Tab. Bot. 100s. *OTC.*
Use: Mineral, vitamin supplement.

Gerimal. (Rugby) Ergoloid mesylates. **Sublingual Tab.:** 0.5 mg, 1 mg. Bot. 100s, 500s, 1000s. **Oral Tab.:** 1 mg. Bot. 100s, 500s, 1000s. *Rx.*
Use: Psychotherapeutic agent.

Gerimed. (Fielding) Vitamins A 5000 units, D 400 units, E 30 mg, B_1 3 mg, B_2 3 mg, B_3 25 mg, B_6 2 mg, B_{12} 6 mcg, C 120 mg, calcium 370 mg, zinc 15 mg, Mg, P. Tab. Bot. 60s. *OTC.*
Use: Mineral, vitamin supplement.

Geri-Mucil. (Geri-Care) Psyllium husk 3.4 g. Sodium 10 mg, 14 calories/dose, dextrose. Pow. 368 g. *OTC.*
Use: Laxative, bulk-producing laxative.

Geriot. (Ivax) Vitamins A 6000 units, D 400 units, E 30 units, B_1 1.5 mg, B_2 1.7 mg, B_3 20 mg, B_5 10 mg, B_6 2 mg, B_{12} 6 mcg, C 60 mg, folic acid 0.4 mg, iron 50 mg (from ferrous sulfate), biotin 45 mcg, Ca, Cl, Cr, Cu, I, K, Mg, Mn, Mo, Ni, P, Se, Si, Sn, V, Zn, vitamin K. Tab. Bot. 100s. *OTC.*
Use: Mineral, vitamin supplement.

Geri-Plus. (Health for Life Brands) **Cap.:** Vitamins A 12,500 units, D 1200 units, B_1 15 mg, B_2 10 mg, B_6 0.5 mg, B_{12} 15 mcg, C 75 mg, niacinamide 30 mg, calcium pantothenate 2 mg, E 5 units, Brewer's yeast 10 mg, iron 11.58 mg, desiccated liver 15 mg, choline bitartrate 30 mg, inositol 30 mg, Ca 59 mg, P 45 mg, Zn 0.68 mg, francium dicalcium phosphate 200 mg, Mn, enzymatic factors, amino acids. Cap. Bot. 50s, 100s, 1000s. **Elix.:** Vitamins B_1 25 mg, B_2 10 mg, B_6 1 mg, B_{12} 20 mcg, niacinamide 100 mg, calcium pantothenate 5 mg, iron ammonium citrate 100 mg, choline 200 mg, inositol 100 mg, magnesium chloride 2 mg, manganese citrate 2 mg, zinc acetate 2 mg, amino acids/fl oz. Bot. Pt. *OTC.*
Use: Mineral, vitamin supplement.

Geri-Silk Bath Oil. (Geritrex) Mineral oil, PEG-4 dilaurate, lanolin oil. Oil. 237 mL. *OTC.*
Use: Emollient.

Geri-Soft. (Geritrex) Mineral oil, propylene glycol, cetearyl alcohol, sorbitol, petrolatum, dimethicone, lanolin, castor oil, stearic acid, parabens, stearyl alcohol, EDTA, lemon oil. Lot. 240 g. *OTC.*
Use: Emollient.

Geri SS. (Geritrex) Mineral oil, propylene glycol, cetearyl alcohol, petrolatum, glycerin, dimethicone, colloidal oatmeal, hydrogenated castor oil, parabens, stearyl alcohol, EDTA, lemon oil, tocopheryl acetate. Lot. 240 g. *OTC.*
Use: Emollient.

Geritol Complete. (Meda Pharmaceuticals) **Complete:** Vitamins A 6000 units, E 30 units, C 60 mg, folic acid 400 mcg, B_1 1.5 mg, B_2 1.7 mg, B_3 20 mg, B_5 10 mg, B_6 2 mg, B_{12} 6 mcg, D 400 units, K, biotin 45 mcg, iron 18 mg, Ca, Cl, Cr, Cu, I, K, Mg, Mn, Mo, Ni, P, Se, Si, Sn, V, Zn, vitamin K. Tab. Bot. 14s, 40s, 100s, 180s. **Extended:** Iron 10 mg, vitamins A 3333 units, D 200 units, E 15 units, B_1 1.2 mg, B_2 1.4 mg, B_3 15 mg, B_6 2 mg, B_{12} 2 mg, C 60 mg, folic acid 0.2 mg, vitamin K, Ca, I, Mg, Se, Zn 15 mg. Capl. Bot. 40s, 100s. **Tonic Liq.:** Iron 18 mg, vitamins B_1 2.5 mg, B_2 2.5 mg, B_3 50 mg, B_5 2 mg, B_6 0.5 mg, methionine 25 mg, choline bitartrate 50 mg/15 mL, alcohol 12%. Bot. 120 mL, 360 mL. *OTC.*
Use: Mineral, vitamin supplement.

Geri-Tussin DM. (Geri-Care) Dextromethorphan hydrobromide 10 mg, guaifenesin 100 mg. Fructose, glucose, saccharin. Alcohol free. Liq. 473 mL. *OTC.*
Use: Upper respiratory combination, antitussive with expectorant.

Gerivite. (Ivax) Vitamins B_1 0.8 mg, B_2 0.4 mg, B_3 8.3 mg, B_5 1.7 mg, B_6 0.2 mg, B_{12} 0.2 mcg, iron 0.3 mg, Zn 0.3 mg, choline, I Mg, Mn, alcohol 18%, methylparaben, sorbitol. Liq. Bot.

473 mL. *OTC.*
Use: Mineral, vitamin supplement.

Gerix. (Abbott) Vitamins B_1 6 mg, B_2 6 mg, B_6 1.6 mg, niacin 100 mg, iron 15 mg, cyanocobalamin 6 mcg, alcohol 20%/30 mL. Elix. Bot. 480 mL. *OTC.*
Use: Mineral, vitamin supplement.

germanin. (Centers for Disease Control & Prevention) *Rx.*
Use: Anti-infective.
See: Suramin Sodium (Naphuride Sodium).

Germicin. (CMC) Benzalkonium chloride 50%. Bot. Pt, gal. *OTC.*
Use: Antiseptic; antimicrobial.

Ger-O-Foam. (Roberts) Methyl salicylate 30%, benzocaine 3%, volatile oils. Aerosol Can 4 oz. *OTC.*
Use: Analgesic; anesthetic.

Geroton Forte. (Kenwood) Vitamin B_1 1.7 mg, B_2 1.9 mg, B_3 2.22 mg, B_5 1.11 mg, B_6 0.22 mg, B_{12} 0.67 mcg, Zn 1.7 mg, Mg, Mn, alcohol 13%. Liq. Bot. 473 mL. *OTC.*
Use: Mineral, vitamin supplement.

Gerterol Depo. (Fellows) Medroxyprogesterone acetate 50 mg, 100 mg/mL. Vial 5 mL. *Rx.*
Use: Hormone, progestin.

Gesic. (Lexalabs) Aspirin 226.8 mg, caffeine 32.4 mg, codeine 32.4 mg. Tab. Bot. 100s. *c-III.*
Use: Analgesic combination, narcotic.

•**gestaclone.** (JEST-ah-klone) USAN.
Use: Hormone, progestin.

•**gestodene.** (JEST-oh-deen) USAN.
Use: Hormone, progestin.

Gestoneed. (Hanlon) Calcium lactate 1069 mg, vitamins C 100 mg, nicotinic acid 18 mg, B_1 1.8 mg, B_2 2.4 mg, B_6 9 mg, D 500 units, A 6000 units. Cap. Bot. 100s. *OTC.*
Use: Mineral, vitamin supplement.

•**gestonorone caproate.** (jess-TOE-nore-ohn CAP-row-ate) USAN.
Use: Hormone, progestin.

•**gestrinone.** (JESS-trih-nohn) USAN.
Use: Hormone, progestin.

Get Better Bear Sore Throat Pops. (Whitehall-Robins) Pectin 19 mg, corn syr., sucrose, parabens. Loz. on a stick. Pkg. 10s. *OTC.*
Use: Mouth and throat product.

Gets-It. (Oakhurst) Salicylic acid, zinc chloride, collodion in ether ≈ 35%, alcohol ≈ 28%. Liq. Bot. 12 mL. *OTC.*
Use: Keratolytic.

•**gevokizumab.** (JEV-oh-KIZ-oo-mab) USAN.
Use: Treatment of diabetes, inflammatory disorders.

•**gevotroline hydrochloride.** (jeh-VOE-troe-LEEN) USAN.
Use: Antipsychotic.

Gevrabon. (Wyeth) Vitamins B_1 0.83 mg, B_2 0.42 mg, B_3 8.3 mg, B_5 1.67 mg, B_6 0.17 mg, B_{12} 0.17 mcg, Fe 2.5 mg, choline, I, Mg, Mn, Zn 0.3 mg, alcohol 18%. Liq. Bot. 480 mL. *OTC.*
Use: Mineral, vitamin supplement.

Gevral. (Wyeth) Vitamins A 5000 units, B_1 1.5 mg, B_2 1.7 mg, B_3 20 mg, B_6 2 mg, B_{12} 6 mcg, folic acid 0.4 mg, C 60 mg, E 30 mg, Ca, P, iron 18 mg, Mg, I, lactose, parabens, sucrose. Tab. Bot. 100s. *OTC.*
Use: Mineral, vitamin supplement.

GFN 1000/DM 50. (Cypress) Dextromethorphan HBr 50 mg, guaifenesin 1000 mg. ER Tab. 100s. *Rx.*
Use: Antitussive, expectorant.

GFN 1200/DM 60/PSE 120. (Cypress) Dextromethorphan HBr 60 mg, guaifenesin 1200 mg, pseudoephedrine hydrochloride 120 mg, dye free. SR Tab. Bot. 100s. *Rx.*
Use: Upper respiratory combination, antitussive, expectorant, decongestant.

GFN 1200/DM 20/PE 40. (Cypress) Dextromethorphan HBr 20 mg, guaifenesin 1200 mg, phenylephrine hydrochloride 40 mg. Dye free. ER Tab. 100s. *Rx.*
Use: Upper respiratory combination, antitussive and expectorant combination.

GFN 600/PSE 60/DM 30. (Cypress) Dextromethorphan HBr 30 mg, guaifenesin 600 mg, pseudoephedrine hydrochloride 60 mg. Dye free. ER Tab. 100s. *Rx.*
Use: Upper respiratory combination, antitussive and expectorant combination.

G-4.
See: Dichlorophene.

Gianvi. (Teva) Ethinyl estradiol 20 mcg, drospirenone 3 mg. Film coated. Lactose, PEG, polysorbate 80. Tab. 24s w/4 white, round, inert tablets. Blister pack. 28s. *Rx.*
Use: Oral contraceptive.

Gildagia. (Qualitest Pharmaceuticals) Ethinyl estradiol 35 mcg, norethindrone 0.4 mg. Lactose, PEG. Tab. 28s w/7 inert tablets (lactose, PEG). *Rx.*
Use: Monophasic oral contraceptive.

Gildess FE 1.5/30. (Qualitest Pharmaceuticals) Ethinyl estradiol 30 mcg, norethindrone acetate 1.5 mg. Film coated. Lactose, PEG, sugar. Tab. 21s w/7 tablets (ferrous fumarate 75 mg per tablet). *Rx.*
Use: Monophasic oral contraceptive.

Gildess 1.5/30. (Qualitest Pharmaceuticals) Ethinyl estradiol 30 mcg, norethindrone acetate 1.5 mg. Film coated. Lactose, PEG. Tab. 21s. *Rx.*
Use: Monophasic oral contraceptive.

Gildess 1/20. (Qualitest Pharmaceuticals) Ethinyl estradiol 20 mcg, norethindrone acetate 1 mg. Film coated. Lactose, PEG, sugar. Tab. 21s. *Rx.*
Use: Monophasic oral contraceptive.

Gildess 1/20 Fe. (Qualitest Pharmaceuticals) Ethinyl estradiol 20 mcg, norethindrone acetate 1 mg. Film coated. Lactose, PEG, sugar. Tab. 21s w/7 tablets (ferrous fumarate 75 mg per tablet). *Rx.*
Use: Monophasic oral contraceptive.

Gilenya. (Novartis) Fingolimod 0.5 mg (equiv. to fingolimod hydrochloride 0.56 mg). Mannitol. Cap. UD 7s, 28s. *Rx.*
Use: Immunologic agent, immunomodulator.

Gilotrif. (Boehringer Ingelheim) Afatinib 20 mg (equiv. to afatinib dimaleate 29.56 mg), 30 mg (equiv. to afatinib dimaleate 44.34 mg), 40 mg (equiv. to afatinib dimaleate 59.12 mg). Lactose. Film coated. Tab. 30s. *Rx.*
Use: Antineoplastic, kinase inhibitor, tyrosine kinase inhibitor.

Giltuss. (GIL) Dextromethorphan HBr 15 mg, guaifenesin 300 mg, phenylephrine hydrochloride 10 mg per 5 mL. Alcohol and sugar free. Phenylalanine 3.75 mg/5 mL. Grape flavor. Liq. 473 mL. *Rx.*
Use: Upper respiratory combination, antitussive and expectorant combination.

Giltuss Ped-C. (GIL) Codeine phosphate 3 mg, guaifenesin 50 mg, phenylephrine hydrochloride 25 mg per 5 mL. Alcohol and sugar free. Phenylalanine 0.6 mg/mL. Strawberry-banana flavor. Liq. 60 mL. *Rx.*
Use: Upper respiratory combination, antitussive and expectorant combination.

Giltuss Pediatric. (GIL) Dextromethorphan HBr 5 mg, guaifenesin 50 mg, phenylephrine hydrochloride 2.5 mg per 5 mL. Alcohol and sugar free. Grape flavor. Liq. 60 mL. *Rx.*
Use: Upper respiratory combination, antitussive, and expectorant combination.

Giltuss TR. (GIL) **Cap.:** Dextromethorphan HBr 14 mg, guaifenesin 288 mg, phenylephrine hydrochloride 7 mg. Maltodextrin. Sugar free. 100s, 500s, 1000s. **Tab.:** Dextromethorphan HBr 30 mg, guaifenesin 600 mg, phenylephrine hydrochloride 20 mg. Dye, sugar, and preservative free. 100s, 1000s. *Rx.*
Use: Upper respiratory combination, antitussive and expectorant combination.

•**giminabant.** (ji-MIN-a-bant) USAN.
Use: Treatment of obesity.

•**ginger.** *NF.*
Use: Dietary supplement.

•**ginseng, American.** *NF.*
Use: Dietary supplement.

•**ginseng, Asian.** *NF.*
Use: Dietary supplement.

•**ginseng extract.** *NF.*
Use: Dietary supplement.

•**girentuximab.** (JIR-en-TUK-see-mab) USAN.
Use: Antineoplastic.

•**giripladib.** (jir-IP-la-dib) USAN.
Use: Analgesic.

•**gisadenafil.** (JEES-a-DEN-a-fil) USAN.
Use: Genitourinary agent.

•**gisadenafil besylate.** (JEES-a-DEN-a-fil) USAN.
Use: Genitourinary agent.

glandubolin.
See: Estrone.

Glassia. (Baxter Healthcare) Alpha-1 proteinase inhibitor (human) 1 g. Preservative free and latex free. Inj., Soln. Single-use vial w/filter needle. *Rx.*
Use: Respiratory enzyme.

•**glatiramer acetate.** (glah-TEER-ah-mer ASS-eh-tate) USAN.
Use: Multiple sclerosis; immunosuppressant.
See: Copaxone.

Glauber's salt.
See: Sodium Sulfate.

glaucoma, agents for.
See: Brimonidine Tartrate/Brinzolamide.
Brimonidine Tartrate/Timolol.
Brinzolamide.
Carbonic Anhydrase Inhibitors.
Dorzolamide Hydrochloride.
Dorzolamide Hydrochloride/Timolol Maleate.
Echothiophate Iodide.
Latanoprost.
Miotics, Cholinesterase Inhibitors.
Ophthalmic Alpha Adrenergic Agonists.
Prostaglandin Agonists.
Unoprostone Isopropyl.

•**glaze, pharmaceutical.** *NF.*
Use: Pharmaceutic aid (tablet coating agent).

Gleevec. (Novartis) Imatinib mesylate 100 mg, 400 mg. Film-coated. Tab. Bot. 30s (400 mg only), 100s (100 mg only). *Rx.*
Use: Protein-tyrosine kinase inhibitor.

•**glemanserin.** (gleh-MAN-ser-in) USAN.
Use: Anxiolytic.

•**glembatumumab.** (GLEM-ba-TOOM-oo-mab) USAN.
Use: Antineoplastic.

•**glembatumumab vedotin.** (GLEM-ba-TOOM-oo-mab ve-DOE-tin) USAN.
Use: Antineoplastic.

Gliadel. (Arbor Pharmaceuticals) Carmustine (BCNU) 7.7 mg, preservative free. Wafer. Single-dose treatment box with 8 individually pouched wafers. *Rx.*
Use: Alkylating agent.

•**gliamilide.** (glie-AM-ih-lide) USAN.
Use: Antidiabetic.

glibenclamide.
See: Glyburide.

•**glibornuride.** (glie-BORN-you-ride) USAN.
Use: Oral hypoglycemic agent; antidiabetic.

•**glicetanile sodium.** (glie-SET-AH-nile) USAN. *Formerly Glydanile Sodium.*
Use: Antidiabetic.

•**gliflumide.** (GLIH-flew-mide) USAN.
Use: Antidiabetic.

glim.
See: Gardinol Type Detergents.

•**glimepiride.** (GLIE-meh-pie-ride) USAN.
Use: Hypoglycemic; antidiabetic.
See: Amaryl.
W/Pioglitazone Hydrochloride.
See: Duetact.
W/Rosiglitazone Maleate.
See: Avandaryl.

glimepiride. (Various Mfr.) Glimepiride 1 mg, 2 mg, 4 mg. May contain lactose. Tab. 30s, 100s, 250s, (4 mg only), 500s, 1000s, UD 100s (except 1 mg). *Rx.*
Use: Antidiabetic agent.

•**glipizide.** (GLIP-ih-zide) *USP.*
Tall Man: glipiZIDE
Use: Antidiabetic.
See: Glucotrol.
Glucotrol XL.
W/Metformin Hydrochloride.
See: Metaglip.

glipizide. (Various Mfr.) Glipizide 5 mg, 10 mg. Tab. 100s, 500s, 1000s, UD 100s. *Rx.*
Use: Antidiabetic.

glipizide ER. (Watson) Glipizide 5 mg, 10 mg. Film-coated. ER Tab. 100s. *Rx.*
Use: Antidiabetic.

glipizide extended-release. (Andrx) Glipizide 2.5 mg. ER Tab. 30s. *Rx.*
Use: Antidiabetic.

glipizide extended-release. (Various Mfr.) Glipizide 5 mg, 10 mg. ER Tab. 100s, 500s. *Rx.*
Use: Antidiabetic.

glipizide/metformin hydrochloride. (Various Mfr.) Glipizide/metformin hydrochloride 2.5 mg/250 mg, 2.5 mg/500 mg, 5 mg/500 mg. Tab. 100s. *Rx.*
Use: Antidiabetic combination.

globulin, cytomegalovirus immune.
See: CytoGam.

globulin, gamma.
See: Immune Globulin Intramuscular.
Immune Globulin Intravenous.

globulin, hepatitis B immune.
See: BayHep B.
H-BIG.

•**globulin, immune.** (GLAH-byoo-lin) *USP. Formerly Globulin, Immune Human Serum.*
Use: IM, measles prophylactic and polio; immunization.

globulin, immune, intravenous.
Use: Immunodeficiency; immune thrombocytopenia purpura; Kawasaki syndrome.
See: Gamimune N.
Gammagard S/D.
Iveegam.
Polygam S/D.
Sandoglobulin.
Venoglobulin-I.
Venoglobulin-S.

globulin, rabies immune.
Use: Immunization.
See: Imogam Rabies.

globulin, Rh_o(D) immune.
Use: Prevention of Rh isoimmunization; immune thrombocytopenic purpura.
See: BayRho D.
Gamulin Rh.
MICRhoGAM.
Mini-Gamulin Rh.
RhoGAM.
WinRho SD.

•**globulin serum, anti-human.** (GLOB-ue-lin) *USP.*
Use: Immunization.

globulin, tetanus immune.
Use: Immunization.
See: Baytet.

globulin, vaccinia immune.
Use: Immunization.

globulin, varicella-zoster immune.
Use: Immunization.
See: Varicella-zoster Immune Globulin.

•**gloximonam.** (GLOX-ih-MOE-nam)

USAN.
Use: Anti-infective.
GL-7 Skin Adherent. (Gordon Laboratories) Plastic material which may be used full strength or diluted with 3 to 10 parts 99% isopropyl alcohol, acetone or naphtha. Pkg. Pt, qt, gal. *OTC.*
GL-2 Skin Adherent. (Gordon Laboratories) Ready-to-use. Bot. Pt, qt, gal. *OTC.*
GlucaGen. (Bedford Laboratories) Glucagon 1 mg (1 unit), lactose 107 mg. Pow. for Inj. Vials with 1 mL diluent. *Rx.*
Use: Glucose-elevating agent, diagnostic aid, emergency kit.
GlucaGen HypoKit. (Novo Nordisk) Glucagon 1 mg (1 unit). Lactose 107 mg. Pow. for Inj. Disposable syringe w/1 mL diluent. *Rx.*
Use: Glucose-elevating agent.
•**glucagon.** (GLUE-kuh-gahn) *USP.*
Use: Emergency treatment of hypoglycemia; antidiabetic.
See: GlucaGen.
Glucagon Diagnostic Kit.
Glucagon Emergency Kit.
glucagon. (Eli Lilly) 1 unit/mL w/diluent. 10 units w/10 mL diluent. Glucagon hydrochloride 1 mg, 10 mg w/diluent; soln. contains lactose, glycerin 1.6% w/phenol 0.2% as a preservative. Vial. *Rx.*
Use: Hypoglycemic shock; antidiabetic.
Glucagon Diagnostic Kit. (Bedford) Glucagon 1 mg (1 unit), lactose 107 mg. Pow. for Inj. Vial w/1 mL syringe diluent. *Rx.*
Use: Glucose-elevating agent.
Glucagon Emergency Kit. (Eli Lilly) Glucagon 1 mg (1 unit), lactose 49 mg, glycerin 12 mg/mL. Pow. for Inj. Vial w/1 mL syr. diluent. *Rx.*
Use: Glucose-elevating agent.
glucagon-like peptide 1 receptor agonists.
See: Albiglutide.
Exenatide.
Liraglutide.
glucagon-like peptide-2 analogs.
See: Teduglutide.
Glucamide. (Teva) Chlorpropamide 100 mg, 250 mg. Tab. Bot. 100s, 250s, 500s, 1000s, UD 100s. *Rx.*
Use: Antidiabetic.
glucarpidase.
Use: Detoxification agent, antidote.
See: Voraxaze.
•**gluceptate sodium.** (GLUE-sep-tate) USAN.
Use: Pharmaceutic aid.
Glucerna. (Ross) Protein 41 g (amino acids), carbohydrate 93 g (hydrolyzed cornstarch, fructose, soy fiber), fat 55 g (high oleic safflower oil, soy oil, soy lecithin), sodium 917 mg (40 mEq), potassium 1542 mg (40 mEq), vitamins A, B_1, B_2, B_3, B_5, B_6, B_{12}, C, D, E, K, folic acid, Cl, Ca, P, Mg, I, Mn, Cu, Zn, Fe, Se, Cr, Mo, biotin, choline. Liq. Can 240 mL, Cont. 1 L. Ready-to-use. *OTC.*
Use: Nutritional supplement.
Glucerna Select. (Abbott) Protein (sodium and calcium caseinates, soy protein isolate) 50 g, carbohydrates (fructose, fructooligosaccharides, maltodextrin, soy fiber, sugar alcohols) 95.7 g, fat (canola oil, high oleic safflower oil, soy lecithin) 54.4 g, Na 940 mg, 1810 mg K/L. H_2O 470 mOsm/kg, 1 cal/mL. Vitamin A, B_1, B_2, B_3, B_5, B_6, B_7, B_9, B_{12}, C, D, E, K, choline, Ca, Cl, Cu, Cr, Fe, I, Mg, Mn, Mo, P, Se, Zn. Gluten-free. Vanilla flavor. Liq. 240 mL, 1000 mL, 1500 mL. *OTC.*
Use: Enteral nutrition therapy.
Glucerna Weight Loss Shake. (Abbott) Protein (sodium and calcium caseinates, soy protein isolate) 54.6 g, carbohydrates (fructose, fructooligosaccharides, maltodextrin, soy fiber, sugar alcohols) 163.8 g, fat (canola oil, high oleic safflower oil, soy lecithin) 46.2 g, Na 1176 mg, K 2100 mg. 0.89 cal/mL. Vitamin A, B_1, B_2, B_3, B_5, B_6, B_{12}, FA, C, D, E, K, biotin, choline, Ca, Cl, Cu, Cr, Fe, I, Mg, Mn, Mo, P, Se, Zn. Gluten-free. Vanilla, chocolate, banana, peach, dulce de leche flavors. Liq. 325 mL. *OTC.*
Use: Enteral nutrition therapy.
glucocerebrosidase-beta-glucosidase.
Use: Treatment of Gaucher disease.
See: Ceredase.
glucocerebrosidase (PEG).
See: PEG-glucocerebrosidase.
glucocerebrosidase, recombinant retroviral vector. (Genetic Therapy)
Use: Treatment for Gaucher disease. [Orphan Drug]
glucocorticoids.
See: Betamethasone.
Betamethasone Sodium Phosphate and Betamethasone Acetate.
Budesonide.
Cortical Hormone Products.
Cortisone.
Dexamethasone.
Dexamethasone Acetate.
Dexamethasone Sodium Phosphate.
Dexamethasone Sodium Phosphate with Lidocaine Hydrochloride.
Hydrocortisone.
Hydrocortisone Acetate.

Hydrocortisone Cypionate.
Hydrocortisone Sodium Phosphate.
Hydrocortisone Sodium Succinate.
Methylprednisolone.
Methylprednisolone Acetate.
Methylprednisolone Sodium Succinate.
Prednisolone.
Prednisolone Acetate.
Prednisolone Sodium Phosphate.
Prednisolone Tebutate.
Prednisone.
Triamcinolone.
Triamcinolone Acetonide.
Triamcinolone Hexacetonide.

Glucolet Automatic Lancing Device. (Bayer Consumer Care) To obtain sample for blood glucose testing. Automatic spring-loaded lancing device.
Use: Diagnostic aid.

Glucolet Endcaps. (Bayer Consumer Care) To obtain sample for blood glucose testing. Controls depth of lancet penetration. Regular or super puncture.
Use: Diagnostic aid.

Glucometer II Blood Glucose Meter. (Bayer Consumer Care) Electronic meter for blood glucose testing. *OTC.*
Use: Diagnostic aid.

d-gluconic acid, calcium salt. Calcium gluconate.

gluconic acid salts.
See: Calcium Gluconate.
Ferrous Gluconate.
Magnesium Gluconate.
Potassium Gluconate.

•**gluconolactone.** (glue-koe-no-LACK-tone) *USP.*
Use: Chelating agent.

Glucophage. (Bristol-Myers Squibb) Metformin hydrochloride 500 mg, 850 mg, 1000 mg. Film-coated. Tab. Bot. 100s, 500s (500 mg only). *Rx.*
Use: Antidiabetic, biguanide.

Glucophage XR. (Bristol-Myers Squibb) Metformin hydrochloride 500 mg, 750 mg. ER Tab. Bot. 100s. *Rx.*
Use: Antidiabetic, biguanide.

•**glucosamine.** (glue-KOSE-ah-meen) USAN.
Use: Pharmaceutic aid.
W/Tetracycline.
See: Tetracyn.

glucose.
See: Glutose.
Insta-Glucose.

glucose and ketone urine test. (Major) Reagent test for glucose and ketones in urine. Bot. 100s.
Use: Diagnostic aid.

glucose-elevating agents.
See: B-D Glucose.
Glucagon.
Glutose.
Insta-Glucose.
Insulin Reaction.
Proglycem.

glucose enzymatic test strip.
Use: Diagnostic aid (in vitro, reducing sugars in urine).

glucose (HK) reagent strips. Reagent strip test for detection of glucose in serum or plasma. Bot. 50s.
Use: Diagnostic aid.

•**glucose, liquid.** (GLUE-kose) *NF.*
Use: As a 5% to 50% solution as nutrient; for acute hepatitis and dehydration; to increase blood volume; pharmaceutic aid (tablet binder, tablet-coating agent).

d-glucose, monohydrate. Dextrose.

•**glucose oxidase.** (GLOO-kose OX-i-dase) USAN.
Use: Anti-infective.

glucose polymers.
See: Polycose.

glucose reagent strips. (Bayer Consumer Care) A quantitative strip test for glucose in serum or plasma. Seralyzer reagent strips. Bot. 50s.
Use: Diagnostic aid.

glucose test.
See: Combistix.
First Choice.
Glucose Reagent.

Glucostix Reagent Strips. (Bayer Consumer Care) Cellulose strip containing glucose oxidase and indicator system. Bot. 50s, 100s, UD 25s. *OTC.*
Use: Diagnostic aid.

glucosulfone sodium, injection.
See: Sodium Glucosulfone.

Gluco System Lancets. (Bayer Consumer Care) Disposable lancets for use in Miles diagnostic autolet or glucolet.
Use: Diagnostic aid.

Glucotrol. (Pfizer) Glipizide 5 mg, 10 mg. Lactose. Tab. Bot. 100s, 500s, UD 100s. *Rx.*
Use: Antidiabetic.

Glucotrol XL. (Pfizer) Glipizide 2.5 mg, 5 mg, 10 mg. ER Tab. Bot. 30s (2.5 mg only); 100s, 500s (except 2.5 mg). *Rx.*
Use: Antidiabetic.

Glucovance. (Bristol-Myers Squibb) Glyburide/metformin hydrochloride 1.25 mg/250 mg, 2.5 mg/500 mg, 5 mg/500 mg. Film-coated. Tab. Bot. 100s. *Rx.*
Use: Antidiabetic combination.

Glucovite. (Pal-Pak, Inc.) Ferrous gluconate 260 mg, vitamins B_1 1 mg, B_2

0.5 mg, C 10 mg. Tab. Bot. 1000s, 5000s. *OTC.*
Use: Mineral, vitamin supplement.

glucurolactone. Gamma lactone of glucofuranuronic acid.

glufanide disodium. (GLOO-fa-nide)
See: Oglufanide Disodium.

Glu-K. (Western Research) Potassium gluconate 486 mg. Tab. Bot. 1000s. *OTC.*
Use: Electrolyte supplement.

Glumetza. (Santarus) Metformin hydrochloride 500 mg, 1000 mg. Film-coated. ER Tab. 90s (1000 mg), 100s (500 mg). *Rx.*
Use: Antidiabetic agent.

gluside.
See: Saccharin.

•**glutamic acid.** (gloo-TAM-ik AS-id) *USP.*
Use: Nutritional supplement.

glutamic acid hydrochloride. Acidogen, aciglumin, glutasin. *OTC.*
Use: Gastric acidifier.

glutamic acid salts.
See: Calcium Glutamate.

•**glutamine.** (GLOO-ta-meen) *USP.*
Use: Dietary supplement; treatment of short bowel syndrome. [Orphan Drug]
See: NutreStore.

•**glutaral concentrate.** (GLUE-tah-ral) *USP.*
Use: Disinfectant.
See: Cidex.

glutaraldehyde.
Use: Sterilizing, disinfecting agent.
See: Cidex.
Cidex Plus.
Cidex-7.

Glutarex-1. (Ross) Protein 15 g, fat 23.9 g, carbohydrates 46.3 g, linoleic acid 1800 mg, Fe 9 mg, Na 190 mg, K 675 mg, Ca, vitamins A, B_1, B_2, B_3, B_5, B_6, B_{12}, C, D, E, K, biotin, choline, folic acid, inositol, Cl, Cu, I, Mg, Mn, P, Se, Zn, and 480 Cal per 100 g, lysine and tryptophan free. Pow. Can 350 g. *OTC.*
Use: Nutritional supplement.

Glutarex-2. (Ross) Protein 30 g, fat 15.5 g, carbohydrates 30 g, Fe 13 mg, Na 880 mg, K 1370 mg, Ca, vitamins A, B_1, B_2, B_3, B_5, B_6, B_{12}, C, D, E, K, biotin, choline, folic acid, inositol, Cl, Cu, I, Mg, Mn, P, Se, Zn, and 410 Cal per 100 g, lysine and tryptophan free. Pow. Can 325 g. *OTC.*
Use: Nutritional supplement.

l-glutathione, reduced.
Use: Treatment of AIDS-associated cachexia. [Orphan Drug]
See: Cachexon.

Glutofac. (Kenwood) Vitamins A 500 units, E 30 units, B_1 15 mg, B_2 10 mg, B_3 50 mg, B_5 20 mg, B_6 50 mg, C 300 mg, Zn 5 mg, Ca, Cr, Cu, Fe, K, Mg, Mn, P, Se. Capl. Bot. 90s. *OTC.*
Use: Mineral, vitamin supplement.

Glutol. (Paddock) Dextrose 100 g/180 mL. Bot. 180 mL.
Use: Diagnostic aid.

Glutose. (Paddock) Liquid glucose (40% dextrose). Concentrated glucose for insulin reactions. Gel. Bot. 60 g. *OTC.*
Use: Hyperglycemic.

•**glyburide.** (glie-BYOO-ride) *USP.*
Tall Man: glyBURIDE
Use: Antidiabetic.
See: DiaBeta.
Glynase PresTab.
W/Metformin Hydrochloride.
See: Glucovance.

glyburide. (Various Mfr.) Glyburide. Tab. **1.25 mg:** Bot. 50s, 100s, 500s. **1.5 mg (micronized):** Bot. 100s, 500s, 1000s, UD 100s. **2.5 mg & 5 mg:** Bot. 90s, 100s, 500s, 1000s, UD 100s; Blister pack 25s, 100s, 600s. **3 mg (micronized):** Bot. 100s, 500s, 1000s, UD 100s. **4.5 mg (micronized):** Bot. 100s, 500s, 1000s. **6 mg (micronized):** 100s, 500s, 1000s. *Rx.*
Use: Antidiabetic.

glyburide/metformin hydrochloride. (PAR) Glyburide/metformin hydrochloride 1.25 mg/250 mg, 2.5 mg/500 mg, 5 mg/500 mg. Film-coated. Tab. 100s. *Rx.*
Use: Antidiabetic combination.

glyburide, micronized. (Various Mfr.) Micronized glyburide 1.5 mg, 3 mg, 4.5 mg, 6 mg. Tab. Bot. 100s, 500s (except 4.5 mg), 1000s, UD 100s (1.5 mg and 3 mg only). *Rx.*
Use: Antidiabetic.

Glycate. (Nuro Pharma) Glycopyrrolate 1.5 mg. Lactose. Tab. 100s. *Rx.*
Use: Gastrointestinal anticholinergic/antispasmodic, quaternary anticholinergic.

Glycate Chewables. (Forest) Glycine 150 mg, calcium carbonate 300 mg. Chew. Tab. Bot. 1000s. *OTC.*
Use: Antacid.

•**glycerin.** (GLIH-suh-rin) *USP.*
Use: Pharmaceutic aid (humectant, solvent).
See: Colace.
Colace Infant/Child.
Corn Huskers.
Fleet Babylax.
Fleet Glycerin Suppositories.
Gleet Liquid Glycerin Suppositories.
Fleet Pedia-Lax.

Fleet Pedia-Lax Glycerin Suppositories.
Sani-Supp.
W/Antipyrine, Benzocaine, Zinc Acetate Dihydrate.
See: Otozin.
W/Benzocaine.
See: Cēpacol Dual Relief Sore Throat + Coating Spray.
W/Benzocaine, Dextromethorphan Hydrobromide.
See: Cēpacol Dual Relief Sore Throat + Cough.
W/Carboxymethylcellulose Sodium.
See: Clear Eyes for Dry Eyes.
Dermasil.
Optive.
W/Polysorbate 80.
See: Refresh Dry Eye Therapy.

glycerin suppositories. (Various Mfr.) Glycerin. **Adults:** Box 10s, 12s, 25s, 50s, 100s. **Pediatric:** 10s, 12s, 25s. *OTC.*
Use: Rectal evacuant, cathartic.

glycerol.
See: Glycerin.

•**glycerol, iodinated.** (GLIH-ser-ole EYE-oh-dih-nay-tehd) USAN.
Use: Expectorant.

•**glycerol phenylbutyrate.** (GLIS-er-ol FEN-il-BUE-ti-rate) USAN.
Use: Endocrine and metabolic agent.
See: Ravicti.

•**glyceryl behenate.** (GLIS-er-il be-HEN-ate) *NF.*
Use: Pharmaceutic aid (tablet/capsule lubricant).

glyceryl guaiacolate.
Use: Expectorant.
See: Guaifenesin.

glyceryl guaiacolate carbamate. Methocarbamol.
See: Robaxin.
Robaxin 750.

glyceryl guaiacol ether.
See: Guaifenesin.

•**glyceryl monostearate.** (GLIS-ir-il mon-oh-STEER-ate) *NF.*
Use: Pharmaceutic aid (emulsifying agent).

glyceryl triacetate.
See: Triacetin.

glyceryl triacetin. (Various Mfr.) Triacetin.
See: Fungacetin.

glyceryl trierucate.
Use: Adrenoleukodystrophy. [Orphan Drug]

glyceryl trinitrate ointment.
See: Nitrol.

glyceryl trinitrate tablets.
See: Nitroglycerin.
Nitroglyn.

glyceryl trioleate.
Use: Adrenoleukodystrophy. [Orphan Drug]

Glycets-Antacid Tablets. (Weeks & Leo) Calcium carbonate 350 mg, simethicone 25 mg. Chew. Tab. Bot. 100s. *OTC.*
Use: Antacid; antiflatulent.

glycinato dihydroxyaluminum hydrate.
See: Dihydroxyaluminum Aminoacetate.

•**glycine.** (GLIE-seen) *USP. Formerly Aminoacetic Acid.*
Use: Myasthenia gravis treatment, irrigating solution.
W/Aluminum Hydroxide-Magnesium Carbonate Coprecipitated Gel.
See: Glycogel.
W/Calcium Carbonate.
See: Antacid No. 6.
Glycate Chewables.
Titralac.
W/Glutamic Acid, Alanine.
See: Prostall.

glycine, aluminum salt.
See: Dihydroxyaluminum Aminoacetate.

glycine hydrochloride. (Various Mfr.)
Use: Gastric acidifier.

glycobiarsol.
Use: Amebiasis, *Trichomonas vaginalis*, *Monilia albicans.*

glycocoll. Glycine.
See: Aminoacetic Acid.

glycocyamine. Guanidoacetic acid.

Glycofed. (Pal-Pak, Inc.) Pseudoephedrine 30 mg, guaifenesin 100 mg. Tab. Bot. 1000s. *OTC.*
Use: Decongestant, expectorant.

GlycoLax. (Kremers Urban) PEG 3350 17 g in 14 single-dose packets, 255 g in 16 oz with dosing cup. Pow. for Oral Soln. *Rx.*
Use: Laxative.

•**glycol distearate.** (GLIE-kole dih-STEE-ah-rate) USAN.
Use: Pharmaceutic aid (thickening agent).

glycol monosalicylate.
W/Oil of Mustard, Camphor, Menthol, Methyl Salicylate.
See: Musterole.

glycophenylate bromide.
See: Mepenzolate Methylbromide.

glycoprotein.
Use: Antiplatelet agent.
See: Kogenate FS.

glycoprotein IIb/IIIa inhibitors.
Use: Antiplatelet agent.
See: Abciximab.

Eptifibatide.
Tirofiban Hydrochloride.

•**glycopyrrolate.** (glie-koe-PIE-row-late) *USP.*
Use: Anticholinergic.
See: Cuvposa.
Glycate.
Robinul.
Robinul Forte.

glycopyrrolate. (Nexgen Pharma) Glycopyrrolate 1.5 mg. Lactose. Tab. 100s. *Rx.*
Use: Quaternary anticholinergic.

glycopyrrolate. (Rising) Glycopyrrolate 1 mg, 2 mg. Lactose. Tab. 100s, 1000s. *Rx.*
Use: Gastrointestinal anticholinergic/antispasmodic.

glycopyrrolate. (Various Mfr.) Glycopyrrolate 0.2 mg/mL. May contain benzyl alcohol. Inj. Vials. 1 mL, 2 mL, 5 mL, 20 mL. *Rx.*
Use: Quaternary anticholinergic.

Glycotuss. (Pal-Pak, Inc.) Guaifenesin 100 mg. Tab. Bot. 100s, 1000s. *OTC.*
Use: Expectorant.

Glycotuss-DM. (Pal-Pak, Inc.) Guaifenesin 100 mg, dextromethorphan HBr 10 mg. Tab. Bot. 100s, 1000s. *OTC.*
Use: Antitussive, expectorant.

glycylclines.
See: Tigecycline.

glycyrrhiza. Pure extract, fluid extract. Licorice root.
Use: Flavoring agent.

glycyrrhiza extract, pure.
Use: Flavoring agent.

glycyrrhiza fluid extract.
Use: Flavoring agent.

glydanile sodium. (GLIE-dah-neel SO-dee-uhm)
See: Glicetanile Sodium.

•**glyhexamide.** (glie-HEX-ah-mid) USAN.
Use: Antidiabetic.

Glylorin. (Cellegy) Monolaurin.
Use: Congenital primary ichthyosis. [Orphan Drug]

•**glymidine sodium.** (GLIE-mih-deen) USAN.
Use: Oral hypoglycemic agent; antidiabetic.

glymol.
See: Petrolatum Liquid.

Glynase PresTab. (Pharmacia & Upjohn) Glyburide. Tab., micronized. Lactose. **1.5 mg:** Tab. Bot. 100s, UD 100s. **3 mg:** Tab. Bot. 100s, 500s, 1000s, UD 100s. **6 mg:** Tab. Bot. 100s, 500s. *Rx.*
Use: Antidiabetic.

•**glyoctamide.** (glie-OCKT-am-id) USAN.
Use: Hypoglycemic agent; antidiabetic.

Gly-Oxide Liquid. (GlaxoSmithKline) Carbamide peroxide 10%. Soln. Bot. 15 mL, 60 mL. *OTC.*
Use: Mouth and throat product.

glyoxyldiureide.
See: Allantoin.

•**glyparamide.** (glie-PAR-am-ide) USAN.
Use: Oral hypoglycemic agent; antidiabetic.

Glypressin. (Ferring) Terlipressin.
Use: Bleeding esophageal varicies. [Orphan Drug]

Glyquin. (ICN) Hydroquinone 4%, padimate O, oxybenzone, octyl methoxycinnamate, methylparaben. SPF 15. In a vanishing base. Cream. Tube. 28 g. *Rx.*
Use: Pigment agent.

Glyquin-XM. (ICN) Hydroquinone 4%. Octocrylene, oxybenzone, avobenzone, vitamin E, methylparaben, EDTA, SPF 15. In a vanishing base. Cream. 28 g. *Rx.*
Use: Pigment agent.

Glyset. (Bayer Consumer Care) Miglitol 25 mg, 50 mg, 100 mg. Tab. Bot. 100s, 1000s (except 25 mg), UD 100. *Rx.*
Use: Antidiabetic.

GM-CSF. Granulocyte macrophage colony-stimulating factor.
See: Leukine.

gododiamide.
Use: Diagnostic aid.

Golacol. (Arcum) Codeine sulfate 30 mg, papaverine hydrochloride 30 mg, emetine hydrochloride 2 mg, ephedrine hydrochloride 15 mg, q.s./30 mL, alcohol 6.25%. Syr. Bot. 4 oz, 16 oz, gal. Orange flavor. *c-III.*
Use: Antitussive; bronchodilator.

Gold Alka-Seltzer Effervescent. (Bayer Consumer Care) Sodium bicarbonate (heat treated) 958 mg, citric acid 832 mg, potassium bicarbonate 312 mg. Tab. Bot. 20s, 36s. *OTC.*
Use: Antacid.

Gold Bond Antiseptic First Aid Quick Spray. (Chattem) Benzethonium chloride 0.13%, menthol 1%. Glycerin, parabens, SD alcohol 40, urea. Spray. 60 mL. *OTC.*
Use: Anti-infective, topical; antiseptic and germicide.

Gold Bond Foot Pain Relieving. (Chattem) Menthol 16%, aloe, benzyl alcohol, capsaicin, cetyl alcohol, cetearyl alcohol, disodium EDTA, SD alcohol, stearyl alcohol, urea. Cream. 113 g. *OTC.*
Use: Emollient.

Gold Bond Intensive Healing. (Chattem) Dimethicone 6%, pramoxine hydrochloride 1%. Aloe, cetearyl alcohol, cetyl alcohol, EDTA, glycerin, glyceryl stearate, parabens, petrolatum, propylene glycol, stearyl alcohol, urea. Cream. 28 g. *OTC.*
Use: Topical local anesthetic.

Gold Bond Medicated Triple Action Relief. (Chattem) Dimethicone 5%, menthol 0.15%, aloe, alcohols, EDTA, glycerin, parabens, petrolatum. Lot. 236 mL. *OTC.*
Use: Emollient.

Gold Bond Pain Relieving Foot Roll-On. (Chattem) Menthol 16%. Capsaicin, glycerin, propylene glycol, SD alcohol, triethanolamine. Liq., topical. 73 mL. *OTC.*
Use: Rub and liniment.

gold compounds.
See: Gold Sodium Thiosulfate.
Ridaura.
Solganal.

•**goldenseal.** (GOLD-n-seal) *NF.*
Use: Dietary supplement.

Golden-West Compound. (Golden-West) Gentian root, licorice root, cascara sagrada, damiana leaves, senna leaves, psyllium seed, buchu leaves, crude pepsin. Box 1.5 oz. *OTC.*
Use: Laxative.

Goldicide Concentrate. (Pedinol Pharmacal) Bot. oz. Ctn. 10s.
Use: Disinfectant.

Gold Seal Calcium 600. (Walgreen) Calcium 1200 mg. Tab. Bot. 60s. *OTC.*
Use: Mineral supplement.

Gold Seal Calcium 600 with Vitamin D. (Walgreen) Calcium 1200 mg, vitamin D. Tab. Bot. 60s. *OTC.*
Use: Mineral supplement.

Gold Seal Chewable Vitamin C. (Walgreen) Ascorbic acid 250 mg, 500 mg. Tab. Bot. 100s. *OTC.*
Use: Vitamin supplement.

Gold Seal Ferrous Gluconate. (Walgreen) Iron 37 mg. Tab. Bot. 100s. *OTC.*
Use: Mineral supplement.

Gold Seal Ferrous Sulfate. (Walgreen) Ferrous sulfate 325 mg. Tab. Bot. 100s, 1000s. *OTC.*
Use: Mineral supplement.

Gold Seal Time Release Ferrous Sulfate. (Walgreen) Iron 50 mg. Tab. Bot. 100s. *OTC.*
Use: Mineral supplement.

•**gold sodium thiomalate.** (gold SO-dee-uhm thigh-oh-MAL-ate) *USP.*
Use: Antirheumatic.
See: Aurolate.

gold sodium thiomalate. (Parenta) Gold sodium thiomalate 50 mg/mL. Benzyl alcohol 0.5%. Inj. 1 mL single-dose and 10 mL multidose vials. *Rx.*
Use: Antirheumatic agent.

gold sodium thiosulfate. Sterile, auricidine, aurocidin, aurolin, auropin, aurosan, novacrysin, solfocrisol, thiochrysine.
Use: Antirheumatic.

gold thioglucose.
See: Aurothioglucose.

•**golimumab.** (goe-li-MUE-mab) USAN.
Use: Monoclonal antibody.
See: Simponi.
Simponi Aria.

•**golnerminogene pradenovec.** (GOL-ner-MIN-oh-jeen PRA-den-oh-vek) USAN.
Use: Antineoplastic.

•**golotimod.** (goe-LOE-ti-mod) USAN.
Use: Anti-infective agent.

•**golvatinib.** (gol-VA-ti-nib) USAN.
Use: Antineoplastic.

•**golvatinib tartrate.** (gol-VA-ti-nib) USAN.
Use: Antineoplastic.

GoLYTELY. (Braintree) **Disp. Jug:** PEG 3350 236 g, sodium sulfate 22.74 g, sodium bicarbonate 6.74 g, sodium chloride 5.86 g, potassium chloride 2.97 g. Pow. for Oral Soln. **Packet:** PEG 3350 227.1 g, sodium sulfate 21.5 g, sodium bicarbonate 6.36 g, sodium chloride 5.53 g, potassium chloride 2.82 g. *Rx.*
Use: Bowel evacuant.

•**gomiliximab.** (goe-mi-LIX-i-mab) USAN.
Use: Allergic asthma.

gonacrine.
See: Acriflavine.

•**gonadorelin acetate.** (goe-NAD-oh-REL-in) *USP.*
Use: Ovulation induction [Orphan Drug].

•**gonadorelin hydrochloride.** (goe-NAD-oh-REL-in) USAN. *Formerly Luteinizing Hormone-releasing Factor Dihydrochloride.*
Use: In vivo diagnostic aid.

gonadotropic substance.
See: Gonadotropin Chorionic.

•**gonadotropin, chorionic.** (go-NAD-oh-TROE-pin, core-ee-AHN-ik) *USP.*
Use: Gonad-stimulating principle. In women: Chronic cystic mastitis, functional sterility, dysmenorrhea, premenstrual tension, threatened abortion. In men: Cryptorchidism, hypogenitalism, dwarfism, impotency, enuresis.
See: A.P.L.

Chorex-10.
Choron 10.
Gonic.
Pregnyl.
Profasi.

gonadotropin, pituitary anterior lobe. Extracted from anterior lobe of equine pituitaries (not pregnant mare urine) (rat unit = 1 Fevold-Hisaw unit).

gonadotropin-releasing hormone analogs.
See: Goserelin Acetate.
Histrelin Acetate.
Leuprolide Acetate.
Leuprolide Acetate/Norethindrone Acetate.
Triptorelin Pamoate.

gonadotropin-releasing hormone antagonists.
Use: Sex hormone.
See: Abarelix.
Cetrorelix Acetate.
Degarelix.
Ganirelix Acetate.

gonadotropin-releasing hormones.
Use: Sex hormone.
See: Nafarelin Acetate.

gonadotropins.
Use: Ovulation stimulant.
See: Lutropin Alfa.
Menotropins.
Pergonal.

gonadotropins, follitropin alfa.
Use: Sex hormone, ovulation stimulant.
See: Gonal-f.
Gonal-f RFF Pen.

gonadotropins, follitropin beta.
Use: Sex hormone, ovulation stimulant.
See: Follistim.

gonadotropins, menotropins.
Use: Sex hormone, ovulation stimulant.
See: Pergonal.
Repronex.

gonadotropins, urofollitropin.
Use: Sex hormone, ovulation stimulant.
See: Bravelle.

Gonak. (Akorn) Hydroxypropyl methylcellulose 2.5%. Soln. Bot. 15 mL. *OTC.*
Use: Ophthalmic.

Gonal-f. (Serono) Follitropin alfa 600 units (to deliver 450 units), 1,200 units (to deliver 1,050 units) FSH activity, sucrose 30 mg. Pow. for Inj., lyophilized. Multidose vial with prefilled syringes of bacteriostatic water (with 0.9% benzyl alcohol) for injection as diluent and 6 syringes (600 units) or 10 syringes (1,200 units). *Rx.*
Use: Sex hormone, ovulation stimulant.

Gonal-f RFF Pen. (Serono) Follitropin alfa 415 units (to deliver ≥ 300 units/0.5 mL), 568 units (to deliver ≥ 450 units/0.75 mL), 1026 units (to deliver ≥ 900 units/1.5 mL) FSH activity. Inj. Prefilled pens with needles with benzyl alcohol 0.9%. *Rx.*
Use: Ovulation stimulant.

gonioscopic hydroxypropyl methylcellulose.
See: Goniosol.

Goniosoft. (Ocusoft) Hydroxypropyl methylcellulose 2.5%. Benzalkonium chloride 0.01%, EDTA. Ophth. Soln. 15 mL. *OTC.*
Use: Ophthalmic and otic agent, ophthalmic surgical adjunct.

Goniosol. (Novartis Ophthalmics) Gonioscopic hydroxypropyl methylcellulose 2.5%. Bot. 15 mL. *OTC.*
Use: Ophthalmic.

Gonodecten Test Kit. (United States Packaging) Tube test for urethral discharge from males, for detection of *Neisseria gonorrhoeae.* Test kit 10s, 25s.
Use: Diagnostic aid.

gonorrhea tests.
See: Biocult-GC.
Gonodecten Test Kit.
Gonozyme.
Isocult for *Neisseria gonorrhoeae.*
MicroTrak *Neisseria gonorrhoeae* Culture Test.

Gonozyme. (Abbott Diagnostics) Enzyme immunoassay for detection of *Neisseria gonorrhoeae* in urogenital swab specimens. Test kit 100s.
Use: Diagnostic aid.

Good Samaritan Ointment. (Good Samaritan) Tube 1.25 oz. *OTC.*
Use: Counterirritant.

Good Sense Maximum Strength Dose Sinus. (Perrigo) Pseudoephedrine hydrochloride 30 mg, chlorpheniramine maleate 2 mg, acetaminophen 500 mg. Tab. Pkg. 24s. *OTC.*
Use: Upper respiratory combination, decongestant, antihistamine, analgesic.

Good Sense Maximum Strength Pain Relief Allergy Sinus. (Perrigo) Pseudoephedrine hydrochloride 30 mg, chlorpheniramine maleate 2 mg, acetaminophen 500 mg. Gelcap. Pkg. 24s. *OTC.*
Use: Upper respiratory combination, decongestant, antihistamine, analgesic.

Goody's Body Pain Powder. (Prestige) Acetaminophen 325 mg, aspirin 500 mg, lactose. Pow. Pkg. 6s, 24s. *OTC.*
Use: Analgesic.

Goody's Cool Orange. (Prestige) Acetaminophen 325 mg, aspirin 500 mg, caffeine 65 mg. Mannitol, sucralose. Orange flavor. Pow. 2s, 6s, 24s. *OTC.*

Use: Nonnarcotic analgesic combination.

Goody's Extra Strength. (Prestige) Acetaminophen 250 mg, aspirin 250 mg, caffeine 65 mg. Maltodextrin, polydextrose. Tab. 24s, 100s. *OTC.*
Use: Nonnarcotic analgesic combination.

Goody's Extra Strength Headache. (Prestige) Acetaminophen 260 mg, aspirin 500 mg, caffeine 32.5 mg. Lactose, potassium 60 mg. Pow., Oral. 2s, 6s, 24s, 50s. *OTC.*
Use: Nonnarcotic analgesic.

Goody's Migraine Relief. (Prestige) Acetaminophen 250 mg, aspirin 250 mg, caffeine 65 mg. Saccharin. Tab. 100s. *OTC.*
Use: Nonnarcotic analgesic combination.

Goody's PM. (Prestige) Diphenhydramine citrate 38 mg, acetaminophen 500 mg. Docusate sodium, lactose, potassium 55 mg, sodium benzoate. Pow. Packets. 6s, 16s. *OTC.*
Use: Nonprescription sleep aid.

Gordobalm. (Gordon Laboratories) Chloroxylenol, methyl salicylate, menthol, camphor, thymol, eucalyptus oil, isopropyl alcohol 16%, fast-drying gum base. Bot. 4 oz, gal. *OTC.*
Use: Analgesic, topical.

Gordochom. (Gordon Laboratories) Undecylenic acid 25%, chloroxylenol in an oily base. Soln. Bot. 30 mL. *OTC.*
Use: Antifungal, topical.

Gordofilm. (Gordon Laboratories) Salicylic acid 16.7%, lactic acid 16.7% in flexible colloidan. Bot. 15 mL. *OTC.*
Use: Keratolytic.

Gordogesic Cream. (Gordon Laboratories) Methyl salicylate 10% in absorption base. Jar 2.5 oz, 1 lb. *OTC.*
Use: Analgesic, topical.

Gordomatic. (Gordon Laboratories) **Crystals:** Sodium borate, sodium bicarbonate, sodium chloride, thymol, menthol, eucalyptus oil. Jar 8 oz, 7 lb. **Lot.:** Menthol, camphor, propylene glycol, isopropyl alcohol. Bot. 1 oz, 4 oz, gal. **Pow.:** Menthol, thymol camphor, eucalyptus oil, salicylic acid, alum bentonite, talc. Shaker can 3.5 oz. Can 1 lb, 5 lb. *OTC.*
Use: Counterirritant.

Gordon's Urea. (Gordon Laboratories) Urea 22%, 40%. Lanolin, petrolatum, wax. Oint. 30 g. *Rx-OTC.*
Use: Emollient.

Gordophene. (Gordon Laboratories) Neutral coconut oil soap 15%, glycerin with Septi-Chlor (trichlorohydroxy diphenyl ether) broad-spectrum antimicrobial and bacteriostatic agent. Bot. 4 oz, gal.
Use: Dermatologic, cleanser.

Gordo-Vite A. (Gordon Laboratories) **Creme:** Vitamin A 100,000 units/oz. in water-soluble base. Jar 0.5 oz, 2.5 oz, 4 oz, lb, 5 lb. **Lot.:** Vitamin A 100,000 units/oz. Plastic bot. 4 oz, gal. *OTC.*
Use: Emollient.

Gordo-Vite E Creme. (Gordon Laboratories) Vitamin E 1500 units/oz in water-soluble base. Jar 2.5 oz, lb. *OTC.*
Use: Emollient.

Gormel Cream. (Gordon Laboratories) Urea 20% in emollient base. Jar 0.5 oz, 2.5 oz, 4 oz, 1 lb, 5 lb. *OTC.*
Use: Emollient.

•**goserelin.** (GO-suh-REH-lin) USAN.
Use: LHRH agonist.
See: Zoladex.

goserelin acetate.
Use: Gonadotropin-releasing hormone analog.
See: Zoladex.

•**gosogliptin.** (goe-soe-GLIP-tin) USAN.
Use: Antidiabetic.

gossypol.
Use: Antineoplastic. [Orphan Drug]

gotamine. (Vita Elixir) Ergotamine tartrate 1 mg, caffeine 100 mg. Tab. *Rx.*
Use: Antimigraine.

gout, agents for.
See: Allopurinol.
Colchicine.
Lesinurad.
Lesinurad Sodium.
Pegloticase.
Probenecid.
Probenecid with Colchicine.
Sulfinpyrazone.

•**govafilcon A.** (GO-vaff-ILL-kahn A) USAN.
Use: Contact lens material, hydrophilic.

•**goxalapladib.** (gox-a-LAP-la-dib) USAN.
Use: Atherosclerosis.

G Phen. (Boca Pharmacal) Dextromethorphan HBr 60 mg, guaifenesin 600 mg, phenylephrine hydrochloride 40 mg. Film-coated. ER Tab. 100s. *Rx.*
Use: Antitussive and expectorant combination.

gp100 adenoviral gene therapy. (Genzyme)
Use: Antineoplastic. [Orphan Drug]

G/P 1200/60. (Cypress) Pseudoephedrine hydrochloride 60 mg, guaifenesin 1200 mg. SR Tab. Bot. 100s. *Rx.*

Use: Upper respiratory combination, decongestant, expectorant.

Grafco. (Graham-Field) Potassium nitrate 25%, silver nitrate 75%. Swab, topical. 100s. *Rx.*
Use: Topical antiseptic, antiseptic and germicide.

Gralise. (Depomed) Gabapentin 300 mg, 600 mg. Tab. 30s (300 mg only), 90s (600 mg only), 30-day starter packs (contains 78 tablets: 9 × 300 mg and 69 × 600 mg tablets). *Rx.*
Use: Anticonvulsant.

•**gramicidin.** (gram-ih-SIH-din) *USP.*
Use: Anti-infective.
W/Neomycin.
See: Spectrocin.
W/Benzocaine, Neomycin Sulfate, Polymyxin B Sulfate.
See: Mycolog Cream.
W/Hydrocortisone Acetate, Neomycin Sulfate, Polymyxin B Sulfate.
See: Cortisporin.
W/Neomycin Sulfate, Polymyxin B Sulfate.
See: AK-Spore.
Neosporin.
Neosporin-G.
Ocutricin.
W/Neomycin Sulfate, Polymyxin B Sulfate, Thimerosal.
See: AK-Spore Ophthalmic Solution.
Neo-Polycin.
Neosporin Ophthalmic Solution.

Grandpa's Wonder Pin Tar Conditioner. (Grandpa Brands) Pin tar oil. Cetearyl alcohol, glyceryl, sunflower seed oil. Liq. 237 mL. *OTC.*
Use: Miscellaneous tar-containing product.

•**granisetron.** (gran-IH-SEH-trahn) USAN.
Use: Antiemetic/antivertigo agent, 5-HT_3 receptor antagonist.
See: Sancuso.

granisetron. (Bedford Laboratories) Granisetron 0.1 mg/mL. Preservative free. May contain sodium chloride. Inj., Soln. Single-dose vial. *Rx.*
Use: Antiemetic/antivertigo agent, 5-HT_3 receptor antagonist.

•**granisetron hydrochloride.** (gran-IH-SEH-trahn) USAN.
Use: Antiemetic/antivertigo agent, 5-HT_3 receptor antagonist.
See: Granisol.
Kytril.

granisetron hydrochloride. (Various Mfr.) Granisetron. **Inj., Soln.:** 0.1 mg/mL (may contain sodium chloride), 1 mg/mL (may contain benzyl alcohol, parabens, sodium chloride). Single-use vials. 1 mL. Multiple-use vials (1 mg/mL only). 4 mL. **Tab.:** 1 mg. May contain lactose. 20s, 100s, blister 2s, blister 20s. *Rx.*
Use: Antiemetic/antivertigo agent, 5-HT_3 receptor antagonist.

Granisol. (PediatRx) Granisetron 1 mg per 5 mL. Sorbitol. Orange flavor. Oral Soln. 30 mL. *Rx.*
Use: Antiemetic/antivertigo agent, 5-HT_3 receptor antagonist.

Granix. (Teva Pharmaceuticals USA) Filgrastim (as tbo-filgrastim) 300 mcg/0.5 mL, 480 mcg/0.8 mL. Polysorbate 80. Preservative free. Inj., Soln. Single-use prefilled syringe. 0.5 mL (300 mcg/0.5 mL), 0.8 mL (480 mcg/0.8 mL). *Rx.*
Use: Granulocyte colony-stimulating factor.

Granulex. (Bertek) Trypsin 0.12 mg, balsam Peru 87 mg, castor oil 788 mg/g. Aerosol. 113.4 g. *Rx.*
Use: Enzyme preparation, topical.

granulocyte colony-stimulating factor.
See: Filgrastim.
tbo-Filgrastim.

granulocyte macrophage colony-stimulating factor.
See: Leukine.

•**grapiprant.** (GRA-pi-prant) USAN.
Use: Anti-inflammatory, antirheumatic agent.

grass pollen allergen extract.
Use: Allergenic extract.
See: Grastek.

Grastek. (Merck & Co) Grass pollen allergen extract (Timothy grass) 2,800 bioequivalent allergy units. Mannitol. Tab., sublingual. UD 30s. *Rx.*
Use: Allergenic extract.

gratus strophanthin. Ouabain.

Gravineed. (Hanlon) Vitamins C 100 mg, E 10 units, B_1 3 mg, B_2 2 mg, B_6 10 mg, B_{12} 5 mcg, A 4000 units, D 400 units, niacin 10 mg, folic acid 0.1 mg, iron fumarate 40 mg, calcium 67 mg. Cap. Bot. 100s. *OTC.*
Use: Mineral, vitamin supplement.

•**grazoprevir.** (graz-OH-pre-vir) USAN.
Use: Antiviral.

Green Glo. (Hub Pharmaceuticals) Lissamine green 1.5 mg. Strip, Ophth. 100s. *Rx.*
Use: Ophthalmic diagnostic product.

Green Mint. (Block Drug) Urea, glycine, polysorbate 60, sorbitol, alcohol 12.2%, peppermint oil, menthol, chlorophyllin-copper complex. Bot. 7 oz, 12 oz. *OTC.*
Use: Mouth and throat preparation.

green soap.
Use: Detergent.

Green Throat Spray. (Clay-Park Labs) Phenol 1.4%. Glycerin, saccharin. Alcohol-free. Throat spray. 473 mL. *OTC.*
Use: Mouth and throat product.

•**grepafloxacin hydrochloride.** (grep-ah-FLOX-ah-sin) USAN.
Use: Antibacterial.

Grifulvin V. (Ortho) Griseofulvin microsize 500 mg. Tab. 100s, 500s. *Rx.*
Use: Antifungal.

•**griseofulvin.** (griss-ee-oh-FULL-vin) *USP.*
Use: Antifungal.
See: Fulvicin P/G.
Fulvicin U/F.
Grifulvin V.
Griseofulvin Ultramicrosize.
Gris-PEG.

griseofulvin. (Various Mfr.) Griseofulvin 165 mg, 330 mg. Tab. Bot. 100s. *Rx.*
Use: Antifungal.

griseofulvin microsize.
Use: Antifungal.
See: Grifulvin V.

griseofulvin microsize. (Various Mfr.) Griseofulvin microsize 125 mL per 5 mL. Alcohol, menthol, parabens, saccharin, sucrose. Susp. 118 mL, 120 mL. *Rx.*
Use: Antifungal.

griseofulvin ultramicrosize.
Use: Antifungal.
See: Gris-PEG.

griseofulvin ultramicrosize. (Various Mfr.) Griseofulvin (ultramicrosize) 125 mg, 250 mg. May contain parabens. Tab. 100s. *Rx.*
Use: Antifungal.

Gris-PEG. (Pedinol) Griseofulvin (ultramicrosize) 125 mg, 250 mg. Film coated. Lactose (125 mg only), methylparaben, PEG. Tab. 100s. *Rx.*
Use: Antifungal.

growth hormone. Extract of human pituitaries containing predominantly growth hormone.
See: Crescormon.
Somatropin.

growth hormone-releasing factor. (ICN)
Use: Long-term treatment of growth failure. [Orphan Drug]
See: Tesamorelin.

GRx Dyne. (Geritrex) Povidone iodine 10%. Glycerin. **Soln.; topical:** 118 mL, 237 mL, 472 mL. **Swab; topical:** 1s. *OTC.*
Use: Antiseptic and germicide, iodine compound.

GRx Dyne Scrub. (Geritrex) Povidone iodine 7.5%. Glycerin. Soap. 118 mL. *OTC.*
Use: Antiseptic and germicide, iodine compound.

GRx HiCort 25. (Geritrex) Hydrocortisone acetate 25 mg (in a hydrogenated cocoglyceride base). Supp.; rectal. 12s, 24s, 50s, 100s. *Rx.*
Use: Gastrointestinal agent, anorectal preparation, steroid-containing product.

GRx Vitamin E. (Geritrex) Tocopheryl acetate 1,000 units. Cetyl alcohol, dimethicone, disodium EDTA, glycerin, mineral oil, parabens, triethanolamine. Cream. 112 g. *OTC.*
Use: Emollient.

g-strophanthin. Ouabain.

guaiacol carbonate. (Various Mfr.) Duotal.
Use: Expectorant.

guaiacol glyceryl ether.
See: Guaifenesin.

guaiacol potassium sulfonate.
See: Bronchial.
W/Ammonium Chloride, Sodium Citrate, Benzyl Alcohol, Carbinoxamine Maleate.
See: Clistin Expectorant.
W/Dextromethorphan Hydrobromide.
See: Bronchial DM.
W/Pheniramine Maleate, Pyrilamine Maleate, Codeine Phosphate.
See: Tritussin.

guaianesin.
Use: Expectorant.
See: Guaifenesin.

•**guaiapate.** (GWIE-ah-pate) USAN.
Use: Antitussive.

Guaifed Syrup. (Muro) Pseudoephedrine hydrochloride 30 mg, guaifenesin 200 mg/5 mL, EDTA, menthol, saccharin, sorbitol, sucrose, cherry flavor, alcohol free. Syr. Bot. 473 mL. *OTC.*
Use: Upper respiratory combination, decongestant, expectorant.

Guaifen DM. (Breckenridge) Dextromethorphan HBr 20 mg, guaifenesin 1200 mg, phenylephrine hydrochloride 40 mg. Dye free. ER Tab. 100s. *Rx.*
Use: Upper respiratory combination, antitussive and expectorant combination.

•**guaifenesin.** (GWIE-fen-ah-sin) *USP.* *Formerly Glyceryl Guaiacolate.* Synonyms: Glyceryl guaiacolate, glyceryl guaiacol ether, guaianesin, guaifylline, guayanesin.
Tall Man: guaiFENesin
Use: Expectorant.
See: AMBI.
Bidex-400.
Buckley's Chest Congestion.
Consin-GG.
Diabetic Tussin.
Diabetic Tussin EX.

Diabetic Tussin Mucus Relief.
Duratuss-G.
GG-Cen.
Glycotuss.
G-100.
G-Tussin.
Guiatuss.
Humibid Maximum Strength.
Liquibid.
Liquituss GG.
Monafed.
Mucinex.
Mucinex Children's.
Mucinex for Kids.
Mucinex Mini-Melts Children's.
Mucinex Mini-Melts Junior Strength.
Muco-Fen-LA.
Mucus Relief.
Organ-I NR.
Pheunomist.
Robitussin Mucus + Chest Congestion.
Scot-Tussin Expectorant.
Siltussin.
Tusibron.
2/G.

W/Acetaminophen.
See: Comtrex Multi-Symptom Deep Chest Cold.
Theraflu Chest Congestion.
Tylenol Chest Congestion.

W/Acetaminophen, Dextromethorphan Hydrobromide, Phenylephrine Hydrochloride.
See: Mucinex Children's Cold, Cough and Sore Throat.
Mucinex Fast-Max Cold, Flu and Sore Throat.
Mucinex Fast-Max Severe Congestion and Cold.
Phenflu G.
Sine-Off Cough/Cold.
Sudafed PE Multi-Symptom Cold and Cough.

W/Acetaminophen, Dextromethorphan Hydrobromide, Pseudoephedrine Hydrochloride.
See: Duraflu.
Flutabs.
Maxiflu DM.
Maxiflu G.
Tylenol Cold Severe Congestion.

W/Acetaminophen, Phenylephrine Hydrochloride.
See: Mucinex Fast-Max Cold and Sinus.
Tylenol Sinus Severe Congestion & Pain Severe Daytime.

W/Acetaminophen, Pseudoephedrine Hydrochloride.
See: Tylenol Sinus Severe Congestion.

W/Brompheniramine Maleate, Dextromethorphan Hydrobromide, Phenylephrine Hydrochloride.
See: Bromhist-PDX.

W/Brompheniramine Maleate, Dextromethorphan Hydrobromide, Pseudoephedrine Hydrochloride.
See: Bromhist DM Pediatric.
Histacol DM Pediatric.
Pediahist DM.

W/Carbetapentane Citrate.
See: Allfen C.
XPect-AT.

W/Carbetapentane Citrate, Phenylephrine Hydrochloride.
See: Albatussin.
Carbatab-12.
Carbatuss.
Extendryl GCP.
Gentex 30.
Levall.
Phencarb GG.
Zinx GCP.

W/Carbetapentane Citrate, Pseudoephedrine Hydrochloride.
See: Exall-D.

W/Chlophedianol Hydrochloride.
See: Chlo Tuss Ex.

W/Chlophedianol Hydrochloride, Phenylephrine Hydrochloride.
See: Vanacof GPE.

W/Chlophedianol Hydrochloride, Pseudoephedrine Hydrochloride.
See: Certuss-D.
Vanacof DX.

W/Chlorpheniramine Maleate, Dextromethorphan Hydrobromide, Phenylephrine Hydrochloride.
See: Chlordex GP.
DM/CPM/PE/GG.
Donatussin.
Genelan-NF.
Qual-Tussin.

W/Chlorpheniramine Maleate, Hydrocodone Bitartrate, Pseudoephedrine Hydrochloride.
See: Tussend.
ZTuss Expectorant.

W/Codeine Phosphate.
See: Allfen CDX.
Brontex.
CGU WC.
Cheracol Cough.
Cheratussin AC Expectorant Cough Suppressant.
Iophen C-NR.
Iophen DM-NR.
Mar-Cof-CG.
M-Clear.
M-Clear WC.
Tussi-Organidin-S NR.

Virtussin A/C.
W/Codeine Phosphate, Phenylephrine Hydrochloride.
See: Giltuss Ped-C.
Tridal.
W/Codeine Phosphate, Pseudoephedrine Hydrochloride.
See: Ambifed CD.
Ambifed CDX.
Cheratussin DAC.
Guiatuss DAC.
Lortuss EX.
Novagest Expectorant with Codeine.
Sudatuss-2 DF.
Tusnel C.
Zodryl DEC 80.
Zodryl DEC 50.
Zodryl DEC 40.
Zodryl DEC 60.
Zodryl DEC 30.
Zodryl DEC 35.
Zodryl DEC 25.
Z-Tuss E.
W/Dexbrompheniramine Maleate, Dextromethorphan Hydrobromide, Pseudoephedrine Hydrochloride.
See: DEKA.
DEKA Pediatric.
W/Dextromethorphan Hydrobromide.
See: Alka-Seltzer Plus Mucus & Congestion.
Atuss-12 DX.
Biospec DMX.
Cheracol D Cough Formula.
Cheracol Plus.
Congesta DM.
Coricidin HBP Chest Congestion & Cough.
Diabetic Tussin DM.
Diabetic Tussin Maximum Strength DM.
Extra Action Cough.
Fenesin DM IR.
Formula 44 Custom Care Chesty Cough Medicine.
Geri-Tussin DM.
Guaifenesin DM.
Mucinex Cough for Kids.
Mucinex Cough Mini-Melts for Kids.
Mucinex DM.
Mucinex DM Maximum Strength.
Mucus Relief DM.
NeoTuss.
PediaCare Children's Cough & Congestion.
Phanatuss DM.
Pulexn DM.
Robitussin Cough & Congestion.
Robitussin Cough DM.
Robitussin Cough Sugar-Free DM.
Robitussin DM.
Safe Tussin DM.
Scot-Tussin Senior Clear.
Siltussin DM.
Vicks DayQuil Mucus Control Liquid DM.
Vicks Formula 44 Custom Care Chesty Cough.
Vicks Nature Fusion Cough & Chest Congestion.
Zotex-EX.
W/Dextromethorphan Hydrobromide, Phenylephrine Hydrochloride.
See: AMBI 10PEH/400GFN/20DM.
Biobron SF.
Biogil.
BioGtuss.
Bio T Pres.
Bio T Pres Pediatric.
Biotuss.
Bio-Tussi.
Bio-Tussi Pediatric.
Broncotron-D.
Brontuss DX.
Dacex PE.
Deconex DM.
Deconex DMX.
Despec DM.
Despec NR.
Dynatuss EX.
Endacon.
ExeCof.
ExeTuss-DM.
Gene-T-Pres.
GFN 1200/DM 20/PE 40.
Giltuss.
Giltuss Pediatric.
Giltuss TR.
Guaifen.
Maxiphen DM.
NeoTuss-D.
Phlemex Forte.
Phlemex-PE.
Phenydex Pediatric.
Robitussin Children's Cough & Cold CF.
Robitussin Pediatric Cough/Cold CF.
SINUtuss DM.
TriTuss.
TriTuss ER.
Tussi-Pres.
Tussi-Pres Pediatric.
Tusso DMR.
Tusso XR.
Vanacof DM.
Z-Dex.
Z-Dex Pediatric.
Zotex.
Zotex Pediatric.
W/Dextromethorphan Hydrobromide, Phenylephrine Hydrochloride, Pyrilamine Maleate.
See: Phenydex.

W/Dextromethorphan Hydrobromide, Potassium Citrate.
See: Sorbutuss NR.
W/Dextromethorphan Hydrobromide, Pseudoephedrine Hydrochloride.
See: Aldex GS DM.
Ambifed-G DM.
AMBI 40PSE/400GFN/20DM.
AMBI 60/580/30.
AMBI 60PSE/400GFN/20DM.
Bionel.
Bionel Pediatric.
Capmist DM.
Despec.
Donatussin DM.
Entex PAC.
Entre-Cough.
GFN 600/PSE 60/DM 30.
Iophen NR.
Liquicough DM.
Maxifed DM.
Maxifed DMX.
Medent DMI.
PanMist-DM.
Poly-Vent DM.
Pseudo Cough.
Q-Tussin CF.
Relacon DM NR.
Relasin DM.
Robaben CF.
Robitussin Cough & Cold D.
Sudafed Multi-Symptom Cold & Cough.
TGQ 30PSE/150GFN/15DM.
Tidafen DM.
TL-DEX DM.
Touro CC-LD.
Trispec PSE.
Tusnel.
Tusnel-DM Pediatric.
Tusnel Pediatric.
Z-Cof DMX.
Z-Cof 8 DM.
Z-Cof I.
W/Dihydrocodeine Bitartrate.
See: J-Max DHC.
W/Dihydrocodeine Bitartrate, Phenylephrine Hydrochloride.
See: Donatuss DC.
Poly-Tussin EX.
W/Dihydrocodeine Bitartrate, Pseudoephedrine Hydrochloride.
See: Despec-EXP.
W/Dyphylline.
See: Difil-G.
Difil-G 400.
Dilex-G.
Dilex-G 400.
Dilex-G 200.
Dyflex-G.
Dy-G.
Dyphylline-GG.
Dyphylline GG ES.
Ed-Bron G.
Jay-Phyl.
Lufyllin-GG.
W/Ephedrine Hydrochloride.
See: Primatene.
W/Ephedrine Sulfate.
See: Broncholate.
Bronkaid Dual Action.
W/Hydrocodone Bitartrate.
See: ZTuss ZT.
W/Phenylephrine Hydrochloride.
See: Donatussin.
ED Bron GP.
Entex LQ.
ExeTuss GP.
J-Max.
Liquibid D-R.
Liquibid PD-R.
Lusair.
MucaphEd.
Mucinex Children's Stuffy Nose & Cold.
MucusRelief Sinus.
Nu-COPD.
PhenaVent LA.
Reese's OneTab Congestion & Cough.
Refenesen PE.
Rescon GG.
SINUtab PE.
Sudafed PE Non-Drying Sinus.
TG 10PEH/380GFN.
Triaminic Chest & Nasal Congestion.
ZoDen.
W/Pseudoephedrine Hydrochloride.
See: Aldex GS.
Altarussin-PE.
Congestac.
Entex T.
ExeFen-IR.
Mucinex D.
Poly-Vent IR.
Respaire-30.
Rydex G.
Sudafed Maximum Strength Non-Drowsy Non-Drying Sinus.
Tenar PSE.
TG 45PSE/400GFN.
Zephrex.
W/Pseudoephedrine Hydrochloride, Theophylline.
See: Broncomar.

guaifenesin. (AvKARE) Guaifenesin 400 mg. Maltodextrin. Tab. 30s, 60s. *OTC.*
Use: Expectorant.

guaifenesin. (URL) Guaifenesin 400 mg. Dye-free. Tab. 50s, 100s. *OTC.*
Use: Expectorant.

guaifenesin. (Various Mfr.) Guaifenesin.

ER Tab.: 600 mg. Bot. 100s, **SR Tab.:** 1000 mg. Bot. 100s. **Syr.:** 100 mg/5 mL. Bot. 473 mL. **Tab.:** 200 mg. 100s. *Rx-OTC.*
Use: Expectorant.

guaifenesin and codeine phosphate. (Boca Pharmacal) Codeine phosphate 10 mg, guaifenesin 100 mg. Alcohol 3.5%, cherry flavoring, disodium edetate, glycerin, saccharin, sodium 4 mg per 5 mL, sodium benzoate, sorbitol. Liq. Soln. 473 mL. *c-v.*
Use: Upper respiratory combination, antitussive with expectorant.

•**guaifenesin and codeine phosphate oral solution.** (GWIE-fen-ah-sin and KOE-deen) *USP.*
Use: Antitussive, expectorant.

guaifenesin and phenylephrine hydrochloride. (River's Edge) Phenylephrine hydrochloride 30 mg, guaifenesin 900 mg. Dye free. SR Tab. 100s. *Rx.*
Use: Decongestant and expectorant.

Guaifenesin DAC. (Cypress) Codeine phosphate 10 mg, pseudoephedrine hydrochloride 30 mg, guaifenesin 100 mg/5 mL, alcohol 1.9%, saccharin, sorbitol. Liq. Bot. 480 mL. *OTC.*
Use: Antitussive, decongestant, expectorant.

Guaifenesin DM. (UDL) Dextromethorphan HBr 10 mg, guaifenesin 100 mg per 5 mL. Saccharin, sorbitol, alcohol free. Syr. UD 5 mL, 10 mL. *OTC.*
Use: Upper respiratory combination, antitussive with expectorant.

Guaifenesin-DM NR. (Silarx) Dextromethorphan HBr 10 mg, guaifenesin 100 mg per 5 mL. Methylparaben, saccharin, sorbitol, raspberry flavor, alcohol free, sugar free. Liq. Bot. 118 mL, 473 mL, 3785 mL. *Rx.*
Use: Upper respiratory combination, antitussive with expectorant.

Guaifenesin NR. (Silarx) Guaifenesin 100 mg/5 mL. Raspberry flavor. Liq. 473 mL. *Rx.*
Use: Expectorant.

guaifenesin 1000 mg and dextromethorphan HBr 60 mg. (URL Laboratories) Dextromethorphan HBr 60 mg, guaifenesin 1000 mg. LA Tab. Bot. 100s. *Rx.*
Use: Upper respiratory combination, antitussive, expectorant.

guaifenesin/pseudoephedrine hydrochloride. (Major) Pseudoephedrine hydrochloride 60 mg, guaifenesin 600 mg. SR Tab. Bot. 100s. *Rx.*
Use: Upper respiratory combination, decongestant, expectorant.

guaifenesin/pseudoephedrine hydrochloride/codeine phosphate syrup. (Schein) Pseudoephedrine hydrochloride 30 mg, codeine phosphate 10 mg, guaifenesin 100 mg, alcohol 1.4%/5 mL. Bot. 473 mL. *c-v.*
Use: Antitussive, decongestant, expectorant.
See: Guaifenesin DAC.

guaifenesin/pseudoephedrine hydrochloride/dextromethorphan HBr 800/90/60. (Medicosa) Dextromethorphan HBr 60 mg, guaifenesin 800 mg, pseudoephedrine hydrochloride 90 mg. ER Tab. 100s. *Rx.*
Use: Antitussive and expectorant combination.

GuaiMist DM. (Scientific Laboratories) Dextromethorphan hydrobromide 15 mg, guaifenesin 100 mg, pseudoephedrine hydrochloride 40 mg per 5 mL. Sugar, alcohol, and dye free. Syr. 473 mL. *Rx.*
Use: Antitussive and expectorant combination.

Guaipax PSE. (Eon) Pseudoephedrine hydrochloride 120 mg, guaifenesin 600 mg. SR Tab. Bot. 100s, 250s, 500s. *Rx.*
Use: Upper respiratory combination, decongestant, expectorant.

Guaiphotol. (Foy Laboratories) Iodine 1/30 g, calcium creosote 4 g. Tab. Bot. 1000s. *Rx.*
Use: Expectorant.

Guaitab. (Muro) Pseudoephedrine hydrochloride 60 mg, guaifenesin 400 mg, lactose. Tab. Bot. 100s. *OTC.*
Use: Decongestant; expectorant.

Guaitex PSE. (Rugby) Pseudoephedrine hydrochloride 120 mg, guaifenesin 500 mg. Tab. Bot. 100s. *Rx.*
Use: Decongestant, expectorant.

•**guaithylline.** (GWIE-thill-in) USAN.
Use: Bronchodilator; expectorant.

Guaivent. (Ethex) Guaifenesin 250 mg, pseudoephedrine hydrochloride 120 mg, parabens, EDTA, sucrose. Cap. Bot. 100s, 500s. *Rx.*
Use: Decongestant, expectorant.

Guaivent PD. (Ethex) **300:** Guaifenesin 300 mg, pseudoephedrine hydrochloride 60 mg, parabens, sucrose. Cap. Bot. 100s, 500s. **600:** Guaifenesin 600 mg, pseudoephedrine hydrochloride 60 mg, parabens, EDTA, sucrose. Cap. Bot. 100s, 500s. *Rx.*
Use: Decongestant, expectorant.

guamide.
See: Sulfaguanidine.

•**guanabenz.** (GWAHN-uh-benz) USAN.
Use: Antihypertensive.

•**guanabenz acetate.** (GWAHN-uh-benz) *USP.*
Use: Antihypertensive.

•**guanacline sulfate.** (GWAHN-ah-kleen) USAN.
Use: Antihypertensive.

•**guanadrel sulfate.** (GWAHN-uh-drell) *USP.*
Use: Antihypertensive.

•**guancydine.** (GWAHN-sigh-deen) USAN.
Use: Antihypertensive.

•**guanethidine sulfate.** (gwahn-ETH-ih-deen) USAN.
Use: Antihypertensive.
See: Ismelin.
W/Hydrochlorothiazide.
See: Esimil.

•**guanfacine hydrochloride.** (GWAHN-fay-seen) *USP.*
Tall Man: guanFACINE
Use: Antihypertensive.
See: Intuniv.
Tenex.

guanfacine hydrochloride. (Various Mfr.) Guanfacine 1 mg, 2 mg. May contain lactose. Tab. 100s, 500s. *Rx.*
Use: Antiadrenergic/sympatholytic; antiadrenergic agent, centrally acting.

guanidine hydrochloride. (Key) Guanidine hydrochloride 125 mg. Mannitol. Tab. Bot. 100s. *Rx.*
Use: Muscle stimulant.

•**guanisoquin sulfate.** (GWAHN-eye-so-kwin) USAN.
Use: Antihypertensive.

•**guanoclor sulfate.** (GWAHN-oh-klahr) USAN.
Use: Antihypertensive.

•**guanoctine hydrochloride.** (GWAHN-ock-teen) USAN.
Use: Antihypertensive.

•**guanoxabenz.** (gwahn-OX-ah-benz) USAN.
Use: Antihypertensive.

•**guanoxan sulfate.** (GWAHN-ox-an) USAN.
Use: Antihypertensive.

•**guanoxyfen sulfate.** (GWAHN-OX-eh-fen) USAN.
Use: Antihypertensive; antidepressant.

Guaphenyl II. (River's Edge) Phenylephrine hydrochloride 20 mg, guaifenesin 375 mg. Maltodextrin, sucrose. Cap. 100s. *Rx.*
Use: Decongestant and expectorant combination.

Guardal. (Morton Grove) Vitamins A 10,000 units, B_1 20 mg, B_2 8 mg, B_6 0.5 mg, B_{12} 8 mcg, C 50 mg, niacinamide 10 mg, calcium d-pantothenate 5 mg, iron 10 mg, dried whole liver 100 mg, yeast 100 mg, choline bitartrate 30 mg, mixed tocopherols 5 mg, dicalcium phosphate anhydrous 150 mg, magnesium sulfate dried 7.2 mg, sodium 1 mg, potassium chloride 1.3 mg. Tab. Bot. 100s. *OTC.*
Use: Mineral, vitamin supplement.

Guardex. (Archer-Taylor) Tube 4 oz, 1 lb, 4.5 lb. *OTC.*
Use: Emollient.

•**guar gum.** *NF.*
Use: Pharmaceutic aid (tablet binder; tablet disintegrant).
See: Benefiber.
W/Danthron, Docusate Sodium.
See: Guarsol.
W/Standardized Senna Concentrate.
See: Gentlax B.

guayanesin.
Use: Expectorant.
See: Guaifenesin.

Guiadrine DM. (Breckenridge Pharmaceutical) Dextromethorphan HBr 30 mg, guaifenesin 600 mg. SR Tab. Bot. 100s, 250s. *Rx.*
Use: Upper respiratory combination, antitussive, expectorant.

Guiamid Expectorant. (Vangard Labs, Inc.) Guaifenesin 100 mg/5 mL, alcohol 3.5%. Bot. Pt, gal. *OTC.*
Use: Expectorant.

Guiaphed. (Various Mfr.) Theophylline 45 mg, ephedrine sulfate 36 mg, guaifenesin 150 mg, phenobarbital 12 mg, alcohol 19%/15 mL. Elix. Bot. 480 mL. *Rx.*
Use: Antiasthmatic combination.

Guiatex PSE. (Rugby) Pseudoephedrine hydrochloride, guaifenesin 500 mg. Tab. Bot. 100s. *Rx.*
Use: Decongestant, expectorant.

Guiatuss. (Various Mfr.) Guaifenesin 100 mg/5 mL, may contain saccharin, menthol, corn syr. Syr. Bot. 118 mL. *OTC.*
Use: Expectorant.

Guiatuss DAC. (Various Mfr.) Pseudoephedrine hydrochloride 30 mg, codeine phosphate 10 mg, guaifenesin 100 mg per 5 mL. Alcohol 1.9%, menthol, saccharin, sodium 4 mg/5 mL, sorbitol. Syr. Bot. 473 mL. *c-v.*
Use: Upper respiratory combination, antitussive and expectorant combination.

Guiatussin/Codeine Expectorant. (Rugby) Codeine phosphate 10 mg,

guaifenesin 100 mg/5 mL, alcohol 3.5%. Syr. Bot. 120 mL, pt, gal. *c-v.*
Use: Antitussive, expectorant.

Guiatussin/Dextromethorphan. (Rugby) Dextromethorphan HBr 15 mg, guaifenesin 100 mg, alcohol 1.4%/5 mL. Liq. Bot. 480 mL. *OTC.*
Use: Antitussive, expectorant.

Guiatuss Syrup. (Various Mfr.) Guaifenesin 100 mg/5 mL. Syr. Bot. 120 mL, 240 mL, pt, gal. *OTC.*
Use: Expectorant.

Guistrey Fortis. (Jones Pharma) Guaifenesin 100 mg, phenylephrine hydrochloride 10 mg, chlorpheniramine maleate 1 mg. Tab. Bot. 1000s. *OTC.*
Use: Antihistamine, decongestant, expectorant.

Gulfasin. (Major) Sulfisoxazole 500 mg. Tab. Bot. 100s, 250s, 1000s.
Use: Anti-infective, sulfonamide.

guncotton, soluble. Pyroxylin.

•**guselkumab.** (gus-ELK-ue-mab) USAN.
Use: Treatment of inflammatory diseases, psoriasis.

gusperimus.
Use: Acute renal graft-rejection episodes.

•**gusperimus trihydrochloride.** (guss-PURR-ih-muss try-HIGH-droe-KLOR-ide) USAN.
Use: Immunosuppressant.

Gustalac. (Roberts) Calcium carbonate 300 mg, defatted skim milk pow. 200 mg. Tab. Bot. 100s, 250s, 1000s. *OTC.*
Use: Antacid; calcium supplement.

•**gutta percha.** (GUT-a-PER-cha) *USP.*
Use: Dental restoration agent.

G-vitamin.
See: Riboflavin.

Gynecort 10, Extra Strength. (Combe) Hydrocortisone acetate 1%, parabens, zinc pyrithione. Cream. Tube 15 g. *OTC.*
Use: Corticosteroid, topical.

Gyne-Lotrimin 3. (Schering-Plough) Clotrimazole. **Vag. Supp.:** 200 mg. Pkg. 3s w/applicator. **Vag. Cream:** 2%, benzyl alcohol. Tube 21 g w/3 disp. applicators. *OTC.*
Use: Antifungal, vaginal.

Gyne-Lotrimin 3 Combination Pack. (Schering-Plough) **Vaginal Supp.:** Clotrimazole 200 mg, lactose. Pkg. 3s w/applicator. **Topical Cream:** Clotrimazole 1%, benzyl alcohol, cetyl stearyl alcohol. Tube 7 g. *OTC.*
Use: Antifungal, vaginal.

gynergon.
See: Estradiol.

Gynogen L.A. (Forest) **10:** Estradiol valerate in sesame oil 10 mg/mL. Vial 10 mL. **20:** Estradiol valerate in castor oil 20 mg/mL. Inj. Multi-dose Vial 10 mL. **40:** Estradiol valerate in castor oil 40 mg/mL. Inj. Vial 10 mL. *Rx.*
Use: Estrogen.

Gyno-Petraryl. (Janssen) Econazole nitrate. *Rx.*
Use: Antifungal, vaginal.

Gynovite Plus. (Optimox) Vitamins A 833 units, D 67 units, E 67 mg (as d-alpha tocopheryl acid succinate), B_1 1.7 mg, B_2 1.7 mg, B_3 3.3 mg, B_5 1.7 mg, B_6 3.3 mg, B_{12} 21 mcg, C 30 mg, calcium 83 mg, iron 3 mg, folic acid 0.07 mg, boron, betaine, biotin, Cr, Cu, hesperidin, I, inositol, Mg, Mn, PABA, pancreatin, rutin, Se, Zn 2.5 mg. Tab. Bot. 100s. *OTC.*
Use: Mineral, vitamin supplement.

H

Habitrol. (Basel Pharm.) Nicotine transdermal system. Dose absorbed in 24 hours. Patch 21 mg, 14 mg, 7 mg. Box 30 systems. *OTC.*
Use: Smoking deterrent, nicotine.

Haemophilus b conjugate vaccine.
Use: Agent for active immunization, bacterial vaccine.
See: ActHIB.
Hiberix.
Liquid PedvaxHIB.
W/DTP vaccine.
See: ActHIB/DTP.

Haemophilus b conjugate vaccine with hepatitis B vaccine.
Use: Agent for active immunization, bacterial vaccine.
See: Comvax.

Haemophilus influenzae type b conjugate vaccine (DTaP-HIB).
Use: Active immunization, toxoid.

Hair Booster Vitamin. (NBTY) Vitamin B_3 35 mg, B_5 100 mg, B_{12} 6 mcg, folic acid 0.4 mg, zinc 15 mg, Cu, iron 18 mg, I, Mn, choline bitartrate, inositol, PABA, protein. Tab. Bot. 60s. *OTC.*
Use: Mineral, vitamin supplement.

Halac Kit. (Acella) Halobetasol propionate 0.05%. Beeswax, petrolatum, propylene glycol. Kit. 50 g w/225 g of ammonium lactate lotion 12%. *Rx.*
Use: Anti-inflammatory agent, topical corticosteroid.

Halaven. (Eisai) Eribulin mesylate 0.5 mg/mL. Ethanol. Inj., Soln. Single-use vial. 2 mL. *Rx.*
Use: Antimitotic agent, halichondrin B analog.

•**halazone.** (HAL-ah-zone) *USP.*
Use: Disinfectant.

•**halcinonide.** (hal-SIN-oh-nide) *USP.*
Use: Corticosteroid, topical; anti-inflammatory.
See: Halog.

Halcion. (Upjohn) Triazolam 0.25 mg. Tab. 500s. *c-IV.*
Use: Sedative/hypnotic, nonbarbiturate.

Haldol. (McNeil) Haloperidol 5 mg (as lactate)/mL. Inj. Amp. 1 mL. *Rx.*
Use: Antipsychotic, phenylbutylpiperadine derivative.

Haldol Decanoate 100. (McNeil) Haloperidol 100 mg/mL (141.04 mg decanoate), sesame oil, benzyl alcohol 1.2%. Amp. 1 mL. *Rx.*
Use: Antipsychotic.

Haldrone. (Eli Lilly) Paramethasone acetate 1 mg, 2 mg. Tab. Bot. 100s. *Rx.*
Use: Corticosteroid.

Halercol. (Roberts) Vitamins A 5000 units, D 400 units, E 1.36 mg, B_1 1.5 mg, B_2 2 mg, B_3 20 mg, B_5 1 mg, B_6 0.1 mg, B_{12} 1 mcg, C 37.5 mg. Cap. Bot. 100s. *OTC.*
Use: Vitamin supplement.

Haley's M-O. (Bayer Consumer Care) Magnesium hydroxide ≈ 900 mg, mineral oil 3.75 mL/15 mL, saccharin (vanilla creme only). Regular or vanilla creme. Liq. Bot. 360 mL, 780 mL (vanilla creme only). *OTC.*
Use: Laxative.

Halfort-T. (Halsey Drug) Vitamins C 300 mg, B_1 15 mg, B_2 10 mg, niacin 100 mg, B_6 5 mg, B_{12} 4 mcg, pantothenic acid 20 mg. Tab. Bot. 100s. *OTC.*
Use: Vitamin supplement.

Halfprin 81. (Kramer) Aspirin 81 mg. EC Tab. Bot. 90s. *OTC.*
Use: Analgesic.

Half Strength Entrition Entri-Pak. (Biosearch Medical Products) Protein 17.5 g (Na and Ca caseinates), carbohydrate 68 g (maltodextrin), fat 17.5 g (corn oil, soy lecithin, monoglycerides and diglycerides), sodium 350 mg, potassium 600 mg, mOsm/120 kg H_2O, calories 0.5/mL, vitamins A, B_1, B_2, B_3, B_5, B_6, B_{12}, C, D, E, K, P, Ca, Mg, I, Fe, Zn, Mn, Cu, Cl, biotin, choline, folic acid. Liq. Pouch 1 L. *OTC.*
Use: Nutritional supplement.

Half Strength Florvite with Iron. (Everett) Fluoride 0.5 mg, Vitamins A 2500 units, D 400 units, E 15 units, B_1 1.05 mg, B_2 1.2 mg, B_3 13.5 mg, B_6 1.05 mg, B_{12} 4.5 mcg, C 60 mg, folic acid 0.3 mg, Cu, iron 12 mg, Zn 10 mg, sucrose. Tab. Bot. 100s. *Rx.*
Use: Mineral, vitamin supplement; dental caries agent.

Half Strength Introlan. (Elan) Protein 22.5 g, fat 18 g, carbohydrates 70 g, Na 345 mg, K 585 mg/L. Vitamins A, C, B_1, B_2, B_3, B_5, B_6, B_{12}, D, E, K, Ca, Fe, folic acid, P, I, Mg, Zn, Cu, biotin, Mn, choline, Cl, Se, Cr, Mo. Liq. In 1,000 mL *New Pak* closed systems with and without color check. *OTC.*
Use: Nutritional supplement.

Half-Strength Lactated Ringer's in 2.5% Dextrose. (Various Mfr.) Dextrose 25 g/L, calories 85 to 89/L, Na^+ ≈ 65.5 mEq, K^+ 2 mEq, Ca^{++} ≈ 1.5 mEq, Cl^- ≈ 55 mEq, lactate 14 mEq/L, osmolarity ≈ 264 mOsm/L. Soln. Bot. 250 mL, 500 mL, 1,000 mL. *Rx.*
Use: Intravenous nutritional therapy, intravenous replenishment solution.

Hali-Best. (Barth's) Vitamins A

10,000 units, D 400 units. Cap. Bot. 100s, 500s. *OTC.*
Use: Vitamin supplement.

halibut liver oil.
Use: Vitamin supplement.

halichondrin B analogs.
See: Eribulin Mesylate.

haliver oil.
See: Halibut Liver Oil.

Hall's Defense. (Warner Lambert) Ascorbic acid 60 mg. Glucose, sugar. Assorted citrus flavors. Loz. 30s. *OTC.*
Use: Water-soluble vitamin, vitamin C.

Hall's Mentho-Lyptus Cough Lozenges. (Warner Lambert) Menthol and eucalyptus oil in varying amounts and flavors. *Stick-Pack* 9s. Bag 30s. *OTC.*
Use: Mouth and throat preparation.

Hall's Mentho-Lyptus Sugar Free. (Warner Lambert) Menthol 5 mg, 6 mg, eucalyptus oil 2.8 mg. Tab. Pkg. 25s. *OTC.*
Use: Mouth and throat preparation.

Hall's-Plus Maximum Strength. (Warner Lambert) Menthol 10 mg, corn syrup, sugar. Cherry, honey-lemon, and regular flavors. Tab. Pkg. 10s, 25s. *OTC.*
Use: Mouth and throat preparation.

Hall's Zinc Defense. (Warner Lambert) Zinc acetate 5 mg, sugar, cherry, or peppermint flavor. Loz. 24s. *OTC.*
Use: Mineral supplement.

•**halobetasol propionate.** (hal-oh-BEH-tah-sahl) USAN.
Use: Anti-inflammatory; corticosteroid, topical.
See: Halac Kit.
Halonate.
Ultravate.
Ultravate X.

halobetasol propionate. (Various Mfr.) Halobetasol propionate. **Cream:** 0.05%. May contain cetyl alcohol, glycerin, diazolidinyl urea. 15 g, 50 g. **Oint.:** 0.05%. May contain petrolatum. 15 g, 50 g. *Rx.*
Use: Anti-inflammatory.

Halofed. (Halsey Drug) **Tab.:** Pseudoephedrine hydrochloride 30 mg, 60 mg. Bot. 100s, 1000s. **Syr.:** Pseudoephedrine hydrochloride 30 mg/5 mL. Bot. 120 mL, 240 mL, pt, gal. *OTC.*
Use: Decongestant.

•**halofenate.** (HAY-low-FEN-ate) USAN.
Use: Antihyperlipoproteinemic; uricosuric.

•**halofuginone hydrobromide.** (HAY-low-FOO-jin-ohn) USAN.
Use: Antiprotozoal.

Halog. (Ranbaxy) Halcinonide. **Cream:** 0.1%, in specially formulated cream base consisting of glyceryl monostearate, cetyl alcohol, myristyl stearate, isopropyl palmitate, polysorbate 60, propylene glycol, purified water. Tube 15 g, 30 g, 60 g. Jar 240 g. **Oint.:** Halcinonide 0.1%, in *Plastibase* (plasticized hydrocarbon gel), PEG 400, PEG 6000 distearate, PEG 300, PEG 1540, butylated hydroxy toluene. Tube 15 g, 30 g, 60 g. Jar 240 g. **Sol.:** 0.1%, EDTA, PEG 300, purified water, butylated hydroxy toluene as preservative. Bot. 20 mL, 60 mL. *Rx.*
Use: Corticosteroid, topical.

Halonate. (Innocutis Holdings) Halobetasol propionate 0.05%. Beeswax, petrolatum propylene glycol. Oint. 50 g w/120 mL of ammonium lactate mousse 12%. *Rx.*
Use: Topical corticosteroid.

•**halopemide.** (hal-OH-pe-mide) USAN.
Use: Antipsychotic.

•**haloperidol.** (HAY-low-PURR-ih-dahl) *USP.*
Use: Antipsychotic; tranquilizer; antidyskinetic (in Gilles de la Tourette disease).
See: Haldol.

haloperidol. (Various Mfr.) Haloperidol. **Tab.:** 0.5 mg, 1 mg, 2 mg, 5 mg, 10 mg, 20 mg. Tab. Bot. 100s, 1000s (except 0.5 mg and 20 mg), UD 100s (except 20 mg). **Conc.:** 2 mg/mL. Bot. 15 mL, 120 mL, and 5 mL, UD 100s. **Inj.:** 5 mg/mL. May contain parabens. Vial 1 mL, 2 mL, 10 mL. *Rx.*
Use: Antipsychotic.

•**haloperidol decanoate.** (HAY-low-PURR-ih-dahl deh-KAN-oh-ate) USAN.
Use: Antipsychotic.
See: Haldol Decanoate.

haloperidol decanoate. (Various Mfr.) Haloperidol 50 mg/mL (70.5 mg decanoate), 100 mg/mL (141.04 mg decanoate), may contain sesame oil, benzyl alcohol 1.2%. Inj. Single-dose vial. 1 mL. Multidose vial. 5 mL. *Rx.*
Use: Antipsychotic.

•**halopredone acetate.** (HAY-low-PREH-dohn) USAN.
Use: Anti-inflammatory, topical.

•**haloprogesterone.** (HAL-oh-pro-jeh-STEE-rone) USAN.
Use: Hormone, progestin.

•**halothane.** (HAL-oh-thane) *USP.*
Use: General anesthetic, inhalation.

Halotussin. (Halsey Drug) Guaifenesin 100 mg/5 mL. Bot. 4 oz, 8 oz, pt, gal. *OTC.*
Use: Expectorant.

•**halquinols.** (HAL-kwin-oles) USAN.
Use: Anti-infective, topical; antimicrobial.

HAMA. Hydroxyaluminum magnesium aminoacetate.

hamamelis water.
See: Witch Hazel.
Tucks.

•**hamycin.** (HAY-MY-sin) USAN.
Use: Antifungal.

Hang-Over-Cure. (Silvers) Calcium carbonate, glycine, thiamine hydrochloride, pyridoxine hydrochloride, aspirin. Cont. Tab. 6 g. *OTC.*
Use: Antacid; analgesic combination.

Haniform. (Hanlon) Vitamins A 25,000 units, D 1000 units, B_1 10 mg, B_2 5 mg, C 150 mg, niacinamide 150 mg. Cap. Bot. 100s. *OTC.*
Use: Vitamin supplement.

Haniplex. (Hanlon) Vitamins B_1 20 mg, B_2 10 mg, B_6 1 mg, B_{12} 5 mcg, calcium pantothenate 10 mg, niacin 20 mg, liver concentrate 50 mg, C 150 mg. Cap. Bot. 100s. *OTC.*
Use: Mineral, vitamin supplement.

Harbolin. (Arcum) Hydralazine hydrochloride 25 mg, hydrochlorothiazide 15 mg, reserpine 0.1 mg. Tab. Bot. 100s, 1000s. *Rx.*
Use: Antihypertensive combination.

hard fat.
Use: Pharmaceutic necessity.

hartshorn. Ammonium carbonate.

Haugase. (Madland) Trypsin, chymotrypsin. Bot. 50s, 250s.
Use: Enzyme preparation.

Havab. (Abbott Diagnostics) Radioimmunoassay or enzyme immunoassay for detection of antibody to hepatitis A virus. Test kit 100s.
Use: Diagnostic aid.

Havab EIA. (Abbott Diagnostics) Enzyme immunoassay for the detection of antibody to hepatitis A virus.
Use: Diagnostic aid.

Havab-M. (Abbott Diagnostics) Radioimmunoassay for the detection of specific Ig antibody to hepatitis A virus. Test kit 100s.
Use: Diagnostic aid.

Havab-M EIA. (Abbott Diagnostics) Enzyme immunoassay for the detection of Ig antibody to hepatitis A virus.
Use: Diagnostic aid.

Havrix. (GlaxoSmithKline) Hepatitis A vaccine, inactivated. **Adult:** 1440 ELU (ELISA [enzyme-linked immunosorbent assay] units) of viral antigen per mL. Inj. Single-dose vial; prefilled syringe. **Pediatric:** 720 ELU of viral antigen per 0.5 mL. Inj. Single-dose vial; prefilled syringe. *Rx.*
Use: Immunization, viral vaccine.

Hawaiian Tropic Aloe Paba Sunscreen. (Tanning Research Labs) Padimate O, oxybenzone. Cream. Bot. 120 g. *OTC.*
Use: Sunscreen.

Hawaiian Tropic Baby Faces. (Tanning Research Labs) SPF 20. Octyl methoxycinnamate, octocrylene, benzophenone-3, menthyl anthranilate, PABA free, waterproof. Gel. Tube 120 g. *OTC.*
Use: Sunscreen.

Hawaiian Tropic Baby Faces Sunblock. (Tanning Research Labs) Octyl methoxycinnamate, benzophenone-3, octyl salicylate, titanium dioxide, octocrylene, PABA free, waterproof. **SPF 35:** Lot. Bot. 60 mL, 120 mL, 300 mL. **SPF 50:** Lot. Bot. 120 mL. *OTC.*
Use: Sunscreen.

Hawaiian Tropic Cool Aloe with I.C.E. (Tanning Research Labs) Lidocaine, menthol, aloe, SD alcohol 40, diazolidinyl urea, EDTA, vitamins A and E, tartrazine. Gel. Jar 360 g. *OTC.*
Use: Emollient.

Hawaiian Tropic Dark Tanning. (Tanning Research Labs) **Gel:** Phenylbenzimidazole sulfonic acid. SPF 2. Bot. 240 mL. **Oil:** 2-ethylhexyl methoxycinnamate, octyl dimethyl, PABA, waterproof. Bot. 240 mL. *OTC.*
Use: Sunscreen.

Hawaiian Tropic Dark Tanning with Sunscreen. (Tanning Research Labs) **Oil:** Ethylhexyl p-methoxycinnamate, octyl dimethyl, PABA, waterproof. SPF 4. Bot. 240 mL. **Gel:** Phenylbenzimidazole, sulfonic acid. PABA free. SPF 4. Tube 240 g. *OTC.*
Use: Sunscreen.

Hawaiian Tropic 8 Plus. (Tanning Research Labs) Octyl methoxycinnamate, benzophenone-3, menthyl anthranilate, PABA free, waterproof. SPF 8+. Gel. Tube 120 g. *OTC.*
Use: Sunscreen.

Hawaiian Tropic 15 Plus. (Tanning Research Labs) Octyl methoxycinnamate, octocrylene, benzophenone-3, menthyl anthranilate, PABA free, waterproof. Gel. Tube 120 g. *OTC.*
Use: Sunscreen.

Hawaiian Tropic 15 Plus Sunblock. (Tanning Research Labs) Menthyl anthranilate, octyl methoxycinnamate, benzophenone-3, PABA free, waterproof. Lot. Bot. 7.5 mL, 15 mL, 60 mL, 120 mL, 240 mL, 300 mL. *OTC.*
Use: Sunscreen.

Hawaiian Tropic 15 Plus Sunblock Lip Balm. (Tanning Research Labs) Padimate O, oxybenzone. SPF 15, waterproof. Stick 4.2 g. *OTC.*
Use: Sunscreen.

Hawaiian Tropic 45 Plus Sunblock Lip Balm. (Tanning Research Labs) Octyl methoxycinnamate, benzophenone-3, octyl salicylate, titanium dioxide, menthyl anthranilate, PABA free, waterproof. SPF 45+. Lip balm 4.2 g. *OTC.*
Use: Sunscreen.

Hawaiian Tropic Just for Kids Sunblock. (Tanning Research Labs)
SPF 30: Homosalate, octyl methoxycinnamate, benzophenone-3, menthyl anthranilate, octyl salicylate, PABA free, waterproof. Lot. Bot. 88.7 mL. **SPF 45:** Octyl methoxycinnamate, benzophenone-3, octyl salicylate, octocrylene, titanium dioxide, PABA free, waterproof. Lot. Bot. 88.7 mL. *OTC.*
Use: Sunscreen.

Hawaiian Tropic Lip Balm Sunblock. (Tanning Research Labs) Padimate O, oxybenzone. Stick 4 g. *OTC.*
Use: Sunscreen.

Hawaiian Tropic Protective Tanning. (Tanning Research Labs) Titanium dioxide, PABA free, waterproof. SPF 6. Lot. Bot. 240 mL. *OTC.*
Use: Sunscreen.

Hawaiian Tropic Protective Tanning Dry. (Tanning Research Labs) SPF 6. **Oil:** 2-ethylhexyl p-methoxycinnamate, homosalate, menthyl anthranilate, waterproof. Bot. 180 mL. **Gel:** Phenylbenzimidazole, sulfonic acid, benzophenone-4. Tube 180 g. *OTC.*
Use: Sunscreen.

Hawaiian Tropic Self Tanning Sunblock. (Tanning Research Labs) Octyl methoxycinnamate, benzophenone-3, aloe, cetyl alcohol, stearyl alcohol, cocoa butter, parabens, vitamin E, PABA free. SPF 15. Cream. Tube 93.75 mL. *OTC.*
Use: Sunscreen.

Hawaiian Tropic Sport Sunblock. (Tanning Research Labs) SPF 15, SPF 30. Methoxycinnamate, octocrylene, benzophenone-3, octyl salicylate, titanium dioxide, PABA free, waterproof. Lot. Bot. 88.7 mL. *OTC.*
Use: Sunscreen.

Hawaiian Tropic Sunblock. (Tanning Research Labs) Titanium dioxide, octyl methoxycinnamate, benzophenone-3, octyl salicylate, octocrylene, PABA free, waterproof. **SPF 30+:** Lot. Bot. 120 mL. **SPF 45+:** Lot. Bot. 120 mL, 300 mL. *OTC.*
Use: Sunscreen.

Hawaiian Tropic Swim 'n' Sun. (Tanning Research Labs) Padimate O, oxybenzone. Lot. Bot. 120 mL. *OTC.*
Use: Sunscreen.

Hawaiian Tropic 10 Plus. (Tanning Research Labs) Octyl methoxycinnamate, benzophenone-3, menthyl anthranilate, PABA free, waterproof. SPF 10+. Gel. Tube 120 g. *OTC.*
Use: Sunscreen.

•**hawthorne leaf with flower.** (HAW-thorn) *NF.*
Use: Dietary supplement.

Hayfebrol Liquid. (Scot-Tussin) Pseudoephedrine hydrochloride 30 mg, chlorpheniramine 2 mg. Syr. Bot. 118 mL. *OTC.*
Use: Antihistamine; decongestant.

1% HC. (C & M Pharmacal) Hydrocortisone 1%, petrolatum base. Oint. Tube 15, 20, 30, 60, 120, 240 g, lb. *OTC.*
Use: Corticosteroid, topical.

HC Derma-Pax. (Recsei) Hydrocortisone 0.5% in liquid base. Dropper Bot. 2 oz. *OTC.*
Use: Corticosteroid, topical.

HCG.
See: Chorionic Gonadotropin.

HCG-Nostick. (Organon Teknika) Sol Particle Immunoassay (SPIA) for detection of hCG in urine. Stick 30s.
Use: Diagnostic aid, pregnancy.

HC Pram 1%. (River's Edge) Hydrocortisone acetate 1%, pramoxine hydrochloride 1%. Cetearyl alcohol, glycerin, phenoxyethanol, safflower seed oil, stearyl alcohol, tetrasodium EDTA. Cream. 30 g. *Rx.*
Use: Anti-inflammatory agent, topical corticosteroid.

HC Pram 2.5%. (River's Edge) Hydrocortisone acetate 2.5%, pramoxine hydrochloride 1%. Cetearyl alcohol, glycerin, phenoxyethanol, safflower seed oil, stearyl alcohol, tetrasodium EDTA. Cream. 4 g (UD 12s and UD 30s), 30 g. *Rx.*
Use: Anti-inflammatory agent, topical corticosteroid.

HC Pramoxine. (Veracity) Hydrocortisone acetate 2.5%, pramoxine hydrochloride 1%. Cetyl alcohol. Cream. 28 g. *Rx.*
Use: Anorectal preparations.

HD 85. (Mallinckrodt) Barium sulfate 85%. Simethicone, saccharin, Raspberry flavor. Susp. Kits. 150 mL, 450 mL. Bot. 1900 mL. *Rx.*
Use: Radiopaque agent, GI contrast agent.

HD 200 Plus. (Mallinckrodt) Barium sulfate 98%. Simethicone, sorbitol, sucrose. Strawberry flavor. Pow. for Susp. UD 312 g. *Rx.*
Use: Radiopaque agent, GI contrast agent.

Head & Shoulders. (Procter & Gamble) Pyrithione zinc 1%. **Cream:** Tube 51 g, 75 g, 120 g, 210 g. **Lot.:** Bot. 120 mL, 210 mL, 330 mL, 450 mL. **Shampoo:** Cetyl and benzyl alcohol. Normal to oily and normal to dry formulas. 200 mL, 400 mL, 750 mL. *OTC.*
Use: Dermatologic agent.

Head & Shoulders Conditioner. (Procter & Gamble) Pyrithione zinc 0.3%. Bot. 4 oz, 11 oz. *OTC.*
Use: Antiseborrheic.

Head & Shoulders Dry Scalp. (Procter & Gamble) Pyrithione zinc 1%. Cetyl and benzyl alcohol, regular and conditioning formulas. Shampoo. Bot. 200 mL, 400 mL, 750 mL, 1000 mL. *OTC.*
Use: Dermatologic agent.

Head & Shoulders Intensive Treatment. (Procter & Gamble) Selenium sulfide 1%. Lotion/Shampoo. Bot. 400 mL. *OTC.*
Use: Antiseborrheic.

Healon. (Abbott) Sodium hyaluronate 10 mg/mL. Inj. Syringe 0.4 mL, 0.55 mL, 0.85 mL, 2 mL. *Rx.*
Use: Ophthalmic surgical adjunct.

Healon Endocoat. (Abbott) Sodium hyaluronate 30 mg/mL (w/sodium chloride 5 mg/mL). Inj. Disposable syringe w/cannula. 0.85 mL. *Rx.*
Use: Ophthalmic surgical adjunct.

Healon5. (Abbott) Sodium hyaluronate 23 mg/mL. Sodium chloride 8.5 mg/mL. Inj. Disposable syringe. 0.6 mL. *Rx.*
Use: Ophthalmic surgical adjunct.

Healon GV. (Abbott) Sodium hyaluronate 14 mg/mL. Inj. Syringe 0.55 mL, 0.85 mL. *Rx.*
Use: Surgical aid, ophthalmic.

Healthbreak. (Lemar Labs) Silver acetate 6 mg. Chewing gum. Pack 24s. *OTC.*
Use: Smoking deterrent.

Healthy Colon. (Major) ≥ 3 billion cells blend of *L. acidophilus*, *B. bifidum*, *B. longum*. Cap. 30s. *OTC.*
Use: Probiotic.

Healthy Heart Complex. (Mason) Vitamins B_6 100 mg, B_{12} 200 mcg, folic acid 800 mcg, coenzyme Q10 100 mg, proprietary fruit and veggie blend 80 mg. Maltodextrin, soy lecithin. Tab. 60s. *OTC.*
Use: Multivitamin.

Heartburn Antacid. (Walgreen) Aluminum hydroxide dried gel 80 mg, magnesium trisilicate 60 mg. Tab. Bot. 100s. *OTC.*
Use: Antacid.

Heartburn Relief Max Strength. (Major) Famotidine 20 mg. Tab. 50s, UD 25s. *OTC.*
Use: Histamine H_2 antagonist.

Heartline. (BDI) Aspirin 81 mg. EC Tab. Bot. 36s. *OTC.*
Use: Anti-inflammatory.

Heather. (Glenmark Generics) Norethindrone 0.35 mg. Lactose. Tab. 28s. *Rx.*
Use: Oral contraceptive, progestin.

heavy metal poisoning, antidote.
See: BAL.
Calcium Disodium Versenate.

Hectorol. (Genzyme) Doxercalciferol. **Cap.:** 0.5 mcg, 1 mcg, 2.5 mcg. Ethanol (1 mcg and 2.5 mcg only). Peach flavor (1 mcg). Bot. 50s. **Inj.:** 2 mcg/mL. 100% ethanol 0.05 mL, disodium edetate 1.1 mg, sodium chloride 1.5 mg, sodium phosphate dibasic, sodium phosphate monobasic. Amps. 2 mL. *Rx.*
Use: Hyperparathyroidism.

Heet Liniment. (Whitehall-Robins Laboratories) Methyl salicylate 15%, camphor 3.6%, oleoresin capsicum 0.025%, alcohol 70%. Bot. 2⅓ oz, 5 oz. *OTC.*
Use: Analgesic-topical.

•**hefilcon A.** (heh-FILL-kahn A) USAN.
Use: Contact lens material (hydrophilic).

•**hefilcon B.** (heh-FILL-kahn B) USAN.
Use: Contact lens material (hydrophilic).

•**hefilcon C.** (heh-FILL-kahn C) USAN.
Use: Contact lens material (hydrophilic).

Helicobacter pylori agents.
See: Omeprazole/Amoxicillin/Clarithromycin.

Helidac. (Prometheus) **Chew Tab.:** Bismuth subsalicylate 262.4 mg. **Tab.:** Metronidazole 250 mg. **Cap.:** Tetracycline 500 mg.14 blister cards of 4s (Cap. and Tab. only), 8s (Chew. Tab. only). *Rx.*
Use: Antiulcerative.

Helistat. (Hoechst) Absorbable collagen hemostatic sponge. 1" × 2" and 3" × 4" in 10s, 9" × 10" in 5s. *Rx.*
Use: Hemostatic.

•**helium.** (HEE-lee-uhm) *USP.*
Use: Diluent for gases.

Helixate. (Aventis) Concentrated recombinant hemophilic factor. After reconstitution, also contains glycine 10 to 30 mg, imidazole ≤ 500 mcg/1000 units, polysorbate 80 H 600 mcg/1000 units,

Calcium Cl 2 to 5 mM, sodium 100 to 130 mEq/L, chloride 100 to 130 mEq/L, albumin (human) 4 to 10 mg/mL. units 250, 500, 1000. *Rx.*
Use: Antihemophilic.

Helixate FS. (CSL Behring) Recombinant antihemophilic factor 250 units, 500 units, 1,000 units, 2,000 units. Glycine, histidine, sodium, sucrose. Preservative free and albumin free. Solvent/detergent treated. Inj., lyophilized Pow. for Soln. Single-dose Bot. and diluent (2.5 mL sterile water for injection). *Rx.*
Use: Antihemophilic agent.

Hemabate. (Pharmacia) Carboprost tromethamine equivalent to 250 mcg carboprost, tromethamine 83 mcg/mL. Inj. Amp. 1 mL. *Rx.*
Use: Abortifacient.

Hema-Chek Slides. (Bayer Consumer Care) Fecal occult blood test containing slide tests, developer, and applicators. Pkg. 100s, 300s, 1000s.
Use: Diagnostic aid.

Hema-Combistix Reagent Strips. (Seimans Medical) Four-way strip test for urinary pH, glucose, protein, and occult blood. Strip. Bot. 100s.
Use: Diagnostic aid.

Hemaferrin. (Western Research) Ferrous fumarate 150 mg, desiccated liver 50 mg, docusate sodium 25 mg, betaine hydrochloride 100 mg, folic acid 0.4 mg, vitamins C 50 mg, B_6 2 mg, B_{12} 5 mcg, Mn 2 mg, Cu 1 mg, Zn 2 mg, Mo 0.4 mg. Tab. 28s. Pack 1000s. *OTC.*
Use: Mineral, vitamin supplement; stool softener.

Hemafolate. (Canright) Ferrous gluconate 293 mg, liver fraction II 250 mg, gastric substance 100 mg, vitamins C 50 mg, B_{12} 10 mcg. Tab. Bot. 100s, 1000s. *OTC.*
Use: Mineral, vitamin supplement.

Hemalive. (Barth's) **Liq.:** Vitamins B_1 3.15 mg, B_2 3.33 mg, B_6 0.81 mg, B_{12} 6 mcg, biotin 3.6 mcg, iron 60 mg, choline, inositol, liver fraction No. 1, niacin 22.5 mg, pantothenic acid/15 mL. Bot. 8 oz, 24 oz. **Tab.:** Vitamins B_1 2.5 mg, B_2 5 mg, B_6, B_{12} 25 mcg, iron 75 mg, niacin 1.4 mg, C 30 mg, liver 240 mg, pantothenic acid, aminobenzoic acid, choline, inositol, biotin, Mg, Mn, Cu. Tab. Bot. 100s, 500s, 1000s. *OTC.*
Use: Mineral, vitamin supplement.

Hemaneed. (Hanlon) Hematinic B_{12}, intrinsic factor, Fe. Cap. Bot. 100s. *OTC.*
Use: Mineral, vitamin supplement.

Hemangeol. (Pierre Fabre Pharmaceuticals) Propranolol hydrochloride 4.28 mg/mL. Saccharin. Alcohol free, sugar free. Strawberry/vanilla flavor. Soln. 120 mL w/oral dosing syringe. *Rx.*
Use: Antiadrenergic/sympatholytic, beta-adrenergic blocking agent.

Hemastix Reagent Strips. (Bayer Consumer Care) Cellulose strip, impregnated with a peroxide and orthotolidine for detection of hematuria and hemoglobinuria. Strip Bot. 50s.
Use: Diagnostic aid.

Hematest Reagent Tablets. (Bayer Consumer Care) Reagent Tab. for blood in the feces. Bot. 100s.
Use: Diagnostic aid.

hematin.
Use: Porphyria.
See: Panhematin.

Hematinic. (Cypress) Ferrous fumarate 106 mg, folic acid 1 mg. Tab. Bot. 100s. *Rx.*
Use: Mineral, vitamin supplement.

Hematinic Plus. (Cypress) Ferrous fumarate 106 mg, vitamin B_1 10 mg, B_2 6 mg, B_3 30 mg, B_6 5 mg, B_{12} 15 mcg, C 200 mg, folic acid 1 mg, pantothenic acid, Cu, Mg, Mn, Zn 18.2 mg. Tab. 100s. *Rx.*
Use: Mineral, vitamin supplement.

hematinics.
See: Iron Products.
Ferric Compounds.
Ferrous Compounds.
Liver Products.
Vitamin B_{12}.
Vitamin Products.

hematological agents.
See: Antihemophilic Combinations.
Bradykinin Inhibitors.
Hemostatics, Systemic.
Hemostatics, Topical.
Kallikrein Inhibitors.
Protein C1 Inhibitors.

hematopoietic agents.
See: Colony Stimulating Factors.
Erythropoiesis-Stimulating Agents.
Interleukins.
Recombinant Human Erythropoietin.
Stem Cell Mobilizers.
Thrombopoietin Receptor Agonists.

Hematrin. (Towne) Iron 50 mg, vitamins B_1 10 mg, B_2 10 mg, B_6 2 mg, B_{12} 10 mcg, C 150 mg, copper 2 mg, niacinamide 50 mg, calcium pantothenate 5 mg, desiccated liver 200 mg. Captab. Bot. 60s, 100s. *OTC.*
Use: Mineral, vitamin supplement.

Hemax. (Pronova) Fe 150 mg (from carbonyl iron), folic acid 1 mg, intrinsic factor as concentrate, vitamins B_{12} 60 mcg, C 500 mg, E 30 units, Cu, bio-

tin 150 mg, docusate sodium 50 mg. French vanilla flavoring, maltodextrin, mineral oil, PEG, sodium benzoate. Cap. 90s. *Rx.*
Use: Multivitamin with iron.

heme arginate.
Use: Acute porphyria; myelodysplastic syndromes. [Orphan Drug]

Hemenatal OB. (WH Nutritionals) Folic acid 1 mg, Fe 34 mg, vitamins D_3 400 units, E 10 units, B_1 1.5 mg, B_2 1.6 mg, B_3 17 mg, B_5 10 mg, B_6 50 mg, B_{12} 12 mcg, biotin 30 mcg. Cu, I, Se, Zn. PEG. Tab. 90s. *Rx.*
Use: Prenatal vitamin with minerals.

Hemenatal OB + DHA. (WH Nutritionals) Folic acid 1 mg, Fe 34 mg, vitamins D_3 400 units, E 10 units, B_1 1.5 mg, B_2 1.6 mg, B_3 17 mg, B_5 10 mg, B_6 50 mg, B_{12} 12 mcg, biotin 30 mcg. Cu, Se, I, Zn. **Cap., softgel:** Omega-3 fatty acids (DHA 200 mg, ALA 0.5 mg, DPA 2.5 mg), glycerin, rice bran oil. 30s. **Tab.:** PEG. 30s. *Rx.*
Use: Prenatal vitamin with minerals.

HemeSelect. (SmithKline Diagnostics) Occult blood screening test. Box 40 test kits.
Use: Diagnostic aid, fecal.

HemeTab. (WH Nutritionals) Iron 28 mg (as polysaccharide iron complex 22 mg and heme iron polypeptide 6 mg), vitamin B_{12} 25 mcg, folic acid 1 mg. PEG. Tab. 90s. *Rx.*
Use: Multivitamin with iron.

Hemex. (Vogarell) Oint. Tube 1.25 oz. Supp. Box 12s.
Use: Anorectal preparation.

Hemex. Hemin and zinc mesoporphyrin.
Use: Acute porphyric syndromes. [Orphan Drug]

Hemiacidrin. Citric acid, glucono-delta-lactone, magnesium carbonate.
Use: Genitourinary irrigant.
See: Renacidin.

hemin.
Use: Acute intermittent porphyria. [Orphan Drug]
See: Panhematin.

hemin and zinc mesoporphyrin.
Use: Acute porphyric syndromes. [Orphan Drug]
See: Hemex.

hemisine.
See: Epinephrine.

Hemoccult SENSA. (SmithKline Diagnostics) Occult blood screening tests.
Use: Diagnostic aid, fecal.

Hemoccult Slides. (SmithKline Diagnostics) Occult blood detection (fecal). In 100s, 1000s, and tape dispensers (test 100s).
Use: Diagnostic aid.

Hemoccult II. (SmithKline Diagnostics) Occult blood detection (fecal). In 102s, kit 100s.
Use: Diagnostic aid.

Hemocitrate. (Hemotec Medical Products) Trisodium citrate concentrate.
Use: Leukapheresis procedures. [Orphan Drug]

Hemocyte. (US Pharmaceutical Corp.) Ferrous fumarate 324 mg (iron 106 mg). Tab. Bot. 30s, 100s. *OTC.*
Use: Mineral supplement.

Hemocyte-F. (US Pharmaceutical Corp.) **Elix.:** Fe (as polysaccharide-iron complex) 100 mg, B_{12} 25 mcg, folic acid 1 mg/5 mL, alcohol 10%, parabens, saccharin, sorbitol, sherry wine flavor. 473 mL. **Tab.:** Iron 106 mg (from ferrous fumarate), folic acid 1 mg. 100s. *Rx.*
Use: Mineral supplement.

Hemocyte Plus. (US Pharmaceutical Corp.) Iron 106 mg (from ferrous fumarate), sodium ascorbate 200 mg, vitamins B_1 10 mg, B_2 6 mg, B_3 30 mg, B_5 10 mg, B_6 5 mg, B_{12} 15 mcg, folic acid 1 mg, zinc 18.2 mg, Mg, Mn sulfate, Cu. Tab. Bot. 100s. *Rx.*
Use: Mineral, vitamin supplement.

Hemocyte Plus Elixir. (US Pharmaceutical Corp.) Polysaccharide iron complex 12 mg, vitamin B_3 13.3 mg, B_5 3.3 mg, B_6 1.3 mg, B_{12} 4 mcg, folic acid 0.33 mg, zinc 5 mg, Mn 1.3 mg/15 mL. Bot. 473 mL. *Rx.*
Use: Mineral, vitamin supplement.

Hemofil M. (Baxter PPI) Antihemophilic factor (human) (factor VIII; AHF) 250 units, 500 units, 1,000 units, 1,700 units. Method M, monoclonal antibody purified, solvent/detergent treated. Albumin (human) ≤ 12.5 mg/mL, glycine, histidine, PEG, ≤ 0.1 ng of mouse protein per AHF unit. Inj., lyophilized Pow. for Soln. Kits with single-dose bottles and diluent (sterile water for injection). *Rx.*
Use: Antihemophilic agent.

Hemofil T. (Baxter PPI) Antihemophilic factor (human), method four, dried, heat-treated 225 to 375 units/10 mL; 450 to 650 units/20 mL; 675 to 999 units/30 mL; 1000 to 1600 units/30 mL. *Rx.*
Use: Antihemophilic.

•**hemoglobin crosfumaril.** (HEE-moe-GLOBE-in CROSS-FEW-mah-ril) USAN.
Use: Red cell substitute; treatment of prefusion deficit disorders.

•**hemoglobin raffimer.** (HEE-moe-GLOBE-in RAF-fi-mer) USAN.
Use: Blood substitute.

Hemoglobin Reagent Strips. (Bayer Consumer Care) Seralyzer reagent strips. Bot. 50s. Quantitative strip test for hemoglobin in whole blood.
Use: Diagnostic aid.

Hemopad. (AstraZeneca) Fibrous absorbable collagen hemostat. 2.5 cm × 5 cm, 5 cm × 8 cm, 8 cm × 10 cm. *Rx.*
Use: Hemostatic.

Hemorid for Women. (Thompson Medical) **Lotion:** Mineral oil, petrolatum, diazolidinyl urea, cetyl alcohol, glycerin, parabens. Bot. 118 mL. **Cream:** White petrolatum 30%, mineral oil 20%, pramoxine hydrochloride 1%, phenylephrine hydrochloride 0.25%, aloe vera gel, parabens, cetyl and stearyl alcohols. Tube 28.3 g. **Supp.:** Zinc oxide 11%, phenylephrine hydrochloride 0.25%, hard fat 88.25%, aloe vera. Box 12s. *OTC.*
Use: Perianal hygiene.

hemorrheologic agent.
See: Pentoxifylline.

Hemorrhoidal HC. (Various Mfr.) Hydrocortisone acetate 25 mg. Supp. Box 12s, 24s, 50s, 100s, UD 12s. *Rx.*
Use: Anorectal preparation.

Hemorrhoidal Ointment. (Ivax) Live yeast cell derivative supplying skin respiratory factor 2000 units/oz of ointment w/shark liver oil 3%, phenyl mercuric nitrate 1:10,000. *OTC.*
Use: Anorectal preparation.

Hemorrhoidal Suppositories. (Geritrex Corporation) Phenylephrine hydrochloride 0.25%, cocoa butter 85.5%, parabens, shark liver oil. Supp.; rectal. 12s. *OTC.*
Use: Anorectal preparation.

Hemorrhoidal Uniserts. (Upsher-Smith) Bismuth subgallate 2.25%, bismuth resorcin compound 1.75%, benzyl benzoate 1.2%, balsam Peru 1.8%, zinc oxide 11%. Supp. Carton 12s, 50s. *OTC.*
Use: Anorectal preparation.

hemostatics, local.
See: Absorbable Gelatin Sponge.
Gelfilm.
Helistat.
Oxidized Cellulose.
Thrombin.

hemostatics, systemic.
See: Amicar.
Aminocaproic Acid.
Fibrinogen Concentrate (Human).
Prothrombin Complex Concentrate (Human).
Tranexamic Acid.

hemostatics, topical. Thrombin.
See: Ferric Subsulfate.
Fibrinogen Sealant (Human).
Thrombin.
Thrombinar.
Thrombostat.

hemostatin.
See: Epinephrine.

Hemovit. (Dayton) Vitamin B_1 1.5 mg, B_2 1.7 mg, B_3 20 mg, B_5 10 mg, B_6 10 mg, B_{12} 6 mcg, C 60 mg, folic acid 1 mg, d-biotin 300 mcg, dye free. Tab. Blister 100s. *Rx.*
Use: Nutritional product.

Hemozyme Elixir. (Barrows) Vitamins B_1 5 mg, B_2 5 mg, B_6 1 mg, panthenol 4 mg, niacinamide 100 mg, B_{12} 3 mcg, iron 100 mg, choline bitartrate 100 mg, dl-methionine 100 mg, yeast extract, alcohol 12%/fl oz. Bot. 12 oz. *OTC.*
Use: Mineral, vitamin supplement.

Hem-Prep. (G & W) Phenylephrine hydrochloride 0.25%, zinc oxide 11%. Supp. Bot. 12s. *OTC.*
Use: Anorectal preparation.

Hem-Prep Ointment. (G & W) Phenylephrine hydrochloride 0.025%, zinc oxide 11%, white petrolatum. Oint. 42.5 g. *OTC.*
Use: Anorectal preparation.

Hemril-HC Uniserts. (Upsher-Smith) Hydrocortisone acetate 25 mg. Supp. 12s. *Rx.*
Use: Anorectal preparation.

Hemril Uniserts. (Upsher-Smith) Bismuth subgallate 2.25%, bismuth resorcin compound 1.75%, benzyl benzoate 1.2%, balsam Peru 1.8%, zinc oxide 11%. Supp. Box 12s, 50s. *OTC.*
Use: Anorectal preparation.

henbane.
See: Hyoscyamus.

Henydin-M. (Arcum) Thyroid desiccated pow. 0.5 g, vitamins B_1 1 mg, B_2 0.5 mg, B_6 0.5 mg, niacinamide 2.5 mg. Tab. Bot. 100s, 1000s. *Rx.*
Use: Vitamin supplement.

Henydin-R. (Arcum) Thyroid desiccated pow. 1 g, vitamins B_1 2 mg, B_2 1 mg, B_6 1 mg, niacinamide 5 mg. Tab. Bot. 100s, 1000s. *Rx.*
Use: Vitamin supplement.

HepaGam B. (Cangene Biopharma) Hepatitis B immune globulin. Protein 5% (50 mg/mL). Solvent/detergent treated. Maltose 10%, polysorbate 80 0.03%. Preservative free. Soln. for Inj. Single-dose vials. 1 mL, 5 mL. *Rx.*
Use: Immune globulin.

heparin.
Use: Anticoagulant.
See: Heparin Sodium and Sodium Chloride.
Heparin Sodium Injection.
Heparin Sodium Lock Flush Solution.

heparin antagonist.
Use: Coagulant.
See: Protamine Sulfate.

•**heparin calcium.** (HEP-uh-rin) *USP.*
Use: Anticoagulant.

Heparin I.V. Flush. (Medefil) Heparin 1 unit/mL, 10 units/mL, 100 units/mL. Inj., Soln. 1 mL, 2 mL, 2.5 mL, 3 mL, 5 mL, 10 mL prefilled syringes. *Rx.*
Use: Anticoagulant.

heparin lock flush. (Various Mfr.) Heparin sodium. Inj., Soln. May contain benzyl alcohol or parabens. **10 units/mL:** 1 mL, 2 mL, 3 mL, 5 mL, 10 mL. **100 units/mL:** 1 mL, 2 mL, 3 mL, 5 mL. *Rx.*
Use: Anticoagulant.

•**heparin sodium.** (HEP-uh-rin) *USP.*
Use: Anticoagulant. Note: Protamine sulfate is antidote.
See: Hepflush-10.
Monoject PreFill Advanced.

heparin sodium. (Various Mfr.) Heparin sodium. Inj., Soln. **1,000 units/mL:** 1 mL vial. **2,000 units/2 mL:** 2 mL vial. **10,000 units/10 mL:** 10 mL vial. **30,000 units/30 mL:** 30 mL vial. **10,000 units/5 mL:** 5 mL vial. **25,000 units/10 mL:** 10 mL vial. **5,000 units/mL:** 1 mL vial. **50,000 units/10 mL:** 10 mL vial. **10,000 units/mL:** 1 mL vial. **40,000 units/4 mL:** 4 mL vial. **50,000 units/5 mL:** 5 mL vial. **20,000 units/mL:** 1 mL vial. *Rx.*
Use: Anticoagulant.

heparin sodium and sodium chloride 0.9%. (Baxter PPI) Heparin sodium 1,000 units in 500 mL, 2,000 units in 1,000 mL. Inj, Soln. *Rx.*
Use: Anticoagulant.

heparin sodium in dextrose 5%. (Various Mfr.) Heparin sodium in dextrose. Inj., Soln. **20,000 units/500 mL:** 500 mL container. **12,500 units/250 mL:** 250 mL container. **25,000 units/500 mL:** 500 mL container. **25,000 units/250 mL:** 250 mL container. *Rx.*
Use: Anticoagulant.

heparin sodium in sodium chloride 0.45%. (Hospira) Heparin sodium 12,500 units/250 mL, 25,000 units/500 mL, 25,000 units/250 mL. Inj., Soln. 250 mL (12,500 units/250 mL, 25,000 units/250 mL), 500 mL (25,000 units/500 mL). *Rx.*
Use: Anticoagulant.

heparin sodium lock flush solution. *Rx.*
Use: Anticoagulant.
See: Heparin Lock Flush.
Hepflush-10.

heparin, 2-0-desulfated.
Use: Cystic fibrosis. [Orphan Drug]
See: Aeropin.

HepatAmine. (McGaw) Amino acid 8%. Inj. Bot. 500 mL. *Rx.*
Use: Nutritional supplement, parenteral.

hepatitis A, inactivated and hepatitis B, recombinant vaccine.
Use: Active immunization, viral vaccine.
See: Twinrix.

hepatitis A vaccine, inactivated. *Rx.*
Use: Immunization, active.
See: Havrix.
Vaqta.

hepatitis B and Haemophilus type b vaccine, combined.
See: Comvax.

•**hepatitis B immune globulin.** (hep-uh-TIGHT-iss B ih-myoon GLAH-byoo-lin) *USP.*
Use: Immunization.
See: HepaGam B.
HyperHEP B S/D.
Nabi-HB.

hepatitis B immune globulin intravenous (human).
Use: Prophylaxis against hepatitis B virus reinfection in liver transplant patients. [Orphan Drug]
See: Nabi-HB.

hepatitis B vaccine, recombinant.
Use: Immunization.
See: Engerix-B.
Recombivax HB.

hepatitis B vaccine (recombinant) and inactivated poliovirus vaccine combined, diphtheria and tetanus toxoids and acellular pertussis adsorbed.
Use: Active immunization, toxoid.
See: Diphtheria and tetanus toxoids and acellular vaccine adsorbed and hepatitis B vaccine (recombinant) and inactivated poliovirus vaccine combined.

•**hepatitis B virus vaccine inactivated.** (hep-uh-TIGHT-iss B vak-SEEN) *USP.*
Use: Immunization.

Hepflush-10. (American Pharmaceutical Partners) Heparin sodium 10 units/mL, preservative free. Inj. Single-dose vial 10 mL. *Rx.*
Use: Catheter patency agent.

Hepfomin R Injection. (Keene Pharmaceuticals) Liver inj. equivalent to cyano-

cobalamin 10 mcg, folic acid 0.4 mg, cyanocobalamin 100 mcg. Vial 10 mL. *Rx.*
Use: Nutritional supplement, parenteral.

Hep-Forte. (Marlyn Nutraceuticals) Vitamins A 1200 units, E 10 mg, B_1 1 mg, B_2 1 mg, B_3 10 mg, B_5 2 mg, B_6 0.5 mg, B_{12} 1 mcg, C 10 mg, folic acid 0.06 mg, zinc 0.5 mg, choline, inositol, biotin, dl-methionine, desiccated liver, liver concentrate, liver fraction No. 2. Cap. Bot. 100s, 300s, 500s. *OTC.*
Use: Vitamin, liver supplement.

Hepsera. (Gilead Sciences) Adefovir dipivoxil 10 mg. Lactose. Tab. Bot. 30s. *Rx.*
Use: Antiviral.

Herbal Cellulex. (NBTY) Vitamin C 83 mg, K 33 mg, iron 9 mg. Tab. Bot. 90s. *OTC.*
Use: Vitamin supplement.

Herceptin. (Genentech) Trastuzumab 440 mg. Pow. for Inj., lyophilized. Preservative free. Vials. Diluent 20 mL vial of Bacteriostatic Water for Inj. w/1.1% benzyl alcohol. *Rx.*
Use: Monoclonal antibody.

Hermal Bath Oil. (Healthpoint Medical) Soybean oil-based bath oil. Bot. 8 oz, 32 oz. *OTC.*
Use: Emollient.

Herpecin-L. (Chattem Consumer Products) Dimethicone 1%, meradimate 5%, octinoxate 7.5%, octisalate 5%, oxybenzone 6%. *Helianthus annuus* (hybrid sunflower) oil, petrolatum mineral oil, talc, titanium dioxide. Lip balm stick. 1 tube per package. *OTC.*
Use: Cold sores.

herpes simplex virus gene. (Genetic Therapy)
Use: Antineoplastic. [Orphan Drug]

Herrick Lacrimal Plug. (Lacrimedics) Silicone plug 0.3 mm, 0.5 mm Pkg. 2 plugs. *Rx.*
Use: Punctal plug.

HES. Hetastarch.
Use: Plasma expander.
See: Hespan.

Hespan. (B. Braun Medical) Hetastarch 6 g, sodium Cl 0.9%/100 mL. Inj. Bot. 500 mL. *Rx.*
Use: Plasma volume expander.

hesperidin.
Use: Capillary fragility and permeability; hemorrhage.
See: Vitamin P; also Rutin.
W/Combinations.
See: A.C.N.
Hesper Bitabs.
Nialex.
Vita Cebus.

hesperidin methyl chalcone.
Use: Vitamin P supplement.

Hesperidin w/C. (Various Mfr.)
Use: Vitamin supplement.

•**hetacillin.** (HET-ah-SILL-in) USAN.
Use: Anti-infective.

•**hetacillin potassium.** (HET-ah-SILL-in) *USP.*
Use: Anti-infective.

•**hetaflur.** (HEH-tah-flure) USAN.
Use: Dental caries prophylactic.

•**hetastarch.** (HET-uh-starch) USAN.
Use: Plasma volume expander.
See: Hespan.
Hextend.
6% Hetastarch.

6% hetastarch. (Various Mfr.) Hetastarch 6 g per 100 mL in sodium chloride 0.9%. Inj., Soln. 500 mL single-dose container. *Rx.*
Use: Plasma volume expander.

•**heteronium bromide.** (HET-er-oh-nee-uhm) USAN.
Use: Anticholinergic.

Hetlioz. (Vanda Pharmaceuticals) Tasimelteon 20 mg. Lactose. Cap. 30s. *Rx.*
Use: Sedative and hypnotic, nonbarbiturate; melatonin receptor agonist.

Hexabamate #1. (Rugby) Tridihexethyl Cl 25 mg, meprobamate 200 mg. Tab. Bot. 100s, 500s. *Rx.*
Use: Anticholinergic combination.

Hexabamate #2. (Rugby) Tridihexethyl Cl 25 mg, meprobamate 400 mg. Tab. Bot. 100s, 500s. *Rx.*
Use: Anticholinergic combination.

Hexa-Betalin. (Eli Lilly) Pyridoxine hydrochloride. Inj. Vial 100 mg/mL. Ctn. 10s, vial 10 mL. *Rx.*
Use: Vitamin supplement.

•**hexachlorophene.** (hex-ah-KLOR-oh-feen) *USP.*
Use: Anti-infective, topical; antiseptic; detergent.
See: Derl.
Gamophen, Leaves.
pHisoHex.

hexachlorophene cleansing emulsion.
Use: Anti-infective, topical detergent.

hexachlorophene liquid soap, detergent liquid.
Use: Anti-infective, topical detergent.
See: pHisoHex.

hexacose. Mixture of C-6 alcohols derived from oxidation of tetracosane $C_{24}H_{50}$.

hexadecadrol.
See: Dexamethasone.

hexadienol. Hexacose.

Hexafed. (Alaven Pharmaceuticals)

Pseudoephedrine hydrochloride 60 mg, dexchlorpheniramine maleate 4 mg. Sugar free. Film-coated. ER Tab. 100s. *Rx.*
Use: Decongestant and antihistamine.

•**hexafluorenium bromide.** (HEK-sah-flure-EE-nee-uhm) USAN.
Use: Muscle relaxant, synergist (succinylcholine).

hexafluorodiethyl ether. *Name used for Flurothyl.*

hexahydroxycyclohexane.
See: Inositol.

hexakose. Mixture of tetracosanes and oxidation products.

Hexalen. (EISAI) Altretamine 50 mg. Lactose. Cap. 100s. *Rx.*
Use: Antineoplastic.

hexamethonium chloride. (Various Mfr.) Hexamethylene (bistrimethylammonium) chloride.

hexamethylamine.
Use: Hypotensive.
See: Hexastat.

hexamethylenamine.
See: Methenamine.

hexamethylenetetramine.
See: Methenamine.

hexamethylmelamine. Altretamine.
Use: Antineoplastic.
See: Hexalen.

hexamethylpararosaniline chloride.
See: Bismuth Violet.

hexamethylrosaniline chloride.
See: Gentian Violet.

hexamine.
See: Methenamine.

•**hexaminolevulinate hydrochloride.** (hex-a-MIN-oh-le-VUE-lin-ate) USAN.
Use: Diagnostic agent, bladder cancer.
See: Cysview.

hexapradol hydrochloride.
Use: CNS stimulant.

Hexate. (Davis & Sly) Atropine sulfate 1/2000 g, extract of hyoscyamus 0.25 g, methylene blue g, methenamine 0.5 g, benzoic acid 0.5 g, salol 0.5 g. Tab. Bot. 1000s. *Rx.*
Use: Anti-infective, urinary.

Hexavitamin SC. (Halsey Drug)
Use: Vitamin supplement.

Hexavitamin Tablets. (Various Mfr.) Vitamins A 5000 units, B_1 2 mg, B_2 3 mg, B_3 20 mg, C 75 mg, D 400 units. Bot. 100s, 1000s, UD 100s. *OTC.*
Use: Vitamin supplement.

•**hexedine.** (HEX-eh-deen) USAN.
Use: Anti-infective.

hexene-ol. Hexacose.

hexenol. Hexacose.

hexitol irrigants.
Use: Irrigant, genitourinary.
See: Sorbitol.
Sorbitol-mannitol.

hexobarbital. *Name previously used Hexobarbitone.*

•**hexobendine.** (HEX-oh-BEN-deen) USAN.
Use: Vasodilator.

Hexopal. (Bayer Consumer Care) Inositol hexanicotinate. *Rx.*
Use: Hypolipidemic; peripheral vasodilator.

•**hexoprenaline sulfate.** (hex-oh-PREN-ah-leen) USAN.
Use: Tocolytic.

Hextend. (Hospira) Hetastarch 6 g per 100 mL in lactated electrolytes. (Each 100 mL contains sodium chloride 672 mg, sodium lactate 317 mg, dextrose 99 mg, calcium chloride 37 mg, potassium chloride 22 mg, magnesium chloride 9 mg. Electrolyte composition is sodium 143 mEq/L, chloride 124 mEq/L, lactate 28 mEq/L, calcium 5 mEq/L, potassium 3 mEq/L, and magnesium 0.9 mEq/L. The solution contains no bacteriostatic or antimicrobial agent and is intended only for single-dose injection.) Preservative free. Inj., Soln. 500 mL single-dose container. *Rx.*
Use: Plasma expander.

•**hexylene glycol.** (HEX-il-een-GLYE-kol) *NF.*
Use: Pharmaceutic aid (humectant, solvent).

•**hexylresorcinol.** (hex-ill-reh-SORE-sih-nole) *USP.*
Use: Anthelmintic (intestinal roundworms and trematodes); throat preparation.
See: Sucrets Original Formula Sore Throat.

H-F Gel. (Paddock) Calcium gluconate gel 2.5%.
Use: Emergency burn treatment. [Orphan Drug]

H.H.R. (Geneva) Hydralazine hydrochloride 25 mg, hydrochlorothiazide 15 mg, reserpine 0.1 mg. Tab. Bot. 100s, 1000s. *Rx.*
Use: Antihypertensive.

Hiberix. (GlaxoSmithKline) Purified haemophilus B capsular polysaccharide 10 mcg, tetanus toxoid 25 mcg per 0.5 mL. Lactose. Preservative free. Single-dose vial w/*Tip-Lok* syringe containing 0.7 mL of saline diluent. *Rx.*
Use: Agent for active immunization, bacterial vaccine.

Hibistat. (J & J Merck Consumer Pharm.) Chlorhexidine gluconate 0.5%. **Liq.:** Isopropyl alcohol 70%, emollients. Bot. 4 oz, 8 oz. **Towelettes:** Unit-of-use pocket-size towelette impregnated with 5 mL. *OTC.*
Use: Antimicrobial; antiseptic.

Hibplex. (Standex) Vitamins B_1 100 mg, B_2 2 mg, B_3 100 mg, panthenol 2 mg/mL. Vial 30 mL. *Rx.*
Use: Vitamin supplement.

Hi B with C. (Towne) Vitamin C 300 mg, B_1 15 mg, B_2 10.2 mg, B_6 5 mg, niacin 50 mg, pantothenic acid 10 mg. Cap. Bot. 100s. *Rx.*
Use: Vitamin supplement.

Hicon. (DRAXIMAGE) Sodium iodide I-131 1000 mCi/mL. Disodium edetate dihydrate < 2 mg. Oral Soln. In 0.25 mL, 0.5 mL, 1 mL kits with 10 capsules of dibasic sodium phosphate 300 mg and 10 empty large hard gelatin capsules. *Rx.*
Use: Radiopharmaceutical.

Hi-Cor 1.0. (C & M Pharmacal) Hydrocortisone 1%% in a nonionic, ester-free, salt-free, paraben-free washable base. Tube 30 g. Jar 60 g, lb. *Rx.*
Use: Corticosteroid, topical.

Hi-Cor 2.5. (C & M Pharmacal) Hydrocortisone 2.5% in a nonionic, ester-free, salt-free, paraben-free washable base. Tube 30 g. Jar 60 g. *Rx.*
Use: Corticosteroid, topical.

hiestrone.
See: Estrone.

High B12. (Barth's) Vitamin B_{12}, desiccated liver. Cap. Bot. 100s, 500s. *OTC.*
Use: Vitamin supplement.

High Potency Acidophilus. (21st Century) 175 mg blend of *L. acidophilus, L. salivarius, B. bifidum, S. thermophilus*. Cap. 100s. *OTC.*
Use: Probiotic.

High Potency Chewable Acidophilus. (Nature's Blend) 1 billion *Lactobacillus acidophilus*. Sucrose. Gluten free and preservative free. Raspberry flavor. Chew. Tab. 100s. *OTC.*
Use: Probiotic.

High Potency Cold Cap. (Weeks & Leo) Salicylamide 325 mg, chlorpheniramine maleate 4 mg, dextromethorphan HBr 15 mg, caffeine 16.2 mg. Tab. Bot. 18s. *OTC.*
Use: Analgesic; antihistamine; antitussive.

High Potency D-1000. (Nature's Bounty) Cholecalciferol 1,000 units. Glycerin, soybean oil. Cap., softgel. 200s. *OTC.*
Use: Fat-soluble vitamin.

high potency insulin.
Use: Antidiabetic.
See: Humulin R Regular U-500 (Concentrated).
Insulin Injection Concentrated.

High Potency N-Vites. (Nion Corp.) Vitamins B_1 15 mg, B_2 10 mg, B_3 100 mg, B_5 20 mg, B_{12} 10 mcg, C 500 mg. Tab. Bot. 100s. *OTC.*
Use: Vitamin supplement.

High Potency Pain Relievers. (Weeks & Leo) Acetaminophen 300 mg, salicylamide 300 mg. Cap. Bot. 20s, 40s. *OTC.*
Use: Analgesic.

High Potency Vitamins and Minerals. (Burgin-Arden) Vitamins A 25,000 units, D 400 units, B_1 10 mg, B_2 5 mg, B_6 1 mg, B_{12} 5 mcg, C 150 mg, niacinamide 100 mg, calcium 103 mg, phosphorus 80 mg, iron 10 mg, magnesium 5.5 mg, manganese 1 mg, potassium 5 mg, zinc 1.4 mg. Tab. Bot. 100s. *OTC.*
Use: Mineral, vitamin supplement.

•**hilafilcon A.** (high-lah-FILL-kahn A) USAN.
Use: Contact lens material (hydrophilic).

•**hilafilcon B.** (high-lah-FILL-kahn B) USAN.
Use: Contact lens material (hydrophilic).

Hill-Shade Lotion. (Hill Dermaceuticals) Para-aminobenzoic acid, alcohol 65%. SPF 22. *OTC.*
Use: Sunscreen.

•**hioxifilcon A.** (high-ock-sih-FILL-kahn A) USAN.
Use: Contact lens material (hydrophilic).

Hipotest. (Marlop) Ca 53.5 mg, iron 50 mg, vitamins A 10,000 units, D 400 units, E 2.5 mg, B_1 25 mg, B_2 25 mg, B_3 50 mg, B_5 13 mg, B_6 15 mg, B_{12} 50 mcg, C 150 mg, choline, betaine, PABA, rutin, bioflavonoids, biotin 1 mg, desiccated liver, bone meal, Cu, Mg, Mn, Zn 2.2 mg, I, P, lecithin. Tab. Bot. 100s. *OTC.*
Use: Mineral, vitamin supplement.

Hi-Po-Vites Tablets. (Hudson Corp.) Iron 6 mg, vitamins A 10,000 units, D 400 units, E 13 mg, B_1 25 mg, B_2 25 mg, B_3 50 mg, B_5 12.5 mg, B_6 15 mg, B_{12} 50 mcg, C 150 mg, folic acid 0.4 mg, Ca, Cr, Cu, I, K, Mg, Mn, Mo, P, Se, Zn 5 mg, biotin 1 mg, bioflavonoids, bone meal, PABA, choline bitartrate, betaine, inositol, lecithin, desiccated liver, rutin. Tab. Bot. 100s. *OTC.*
Use: Mineral, vitamin supplement.

hippramine.
See: Methenamine Hippurate.

hipputope. (Bristol-Myers Squibb) Radio-

iodinated sodium iodohippurate (^{131}I) Inj. Bot. 1 m Ci, 2 m Ci.
Use: Diagnostic aid.

Hiprex. (Hoechst) Methenamine hippurate 1 g. Tab. Bot. 100s. *Rx.*
Use: Anti-infective, urinary.

Histacol DM Pediatric. (Breckenridge) Pseudoephedrine hydrochloride 15 mg, brompheniramine maleate 1 mg, dextromethorphan HBr 4 mg per 1 mL. Sugar and alcohol free. Sorbitol. Grape flavor. Drops 30 mL with 1 mL dropper. *Rx.*
Use: Upper respiratory combination, antitussive and expectorant combination.

Histade. (Breckenridge) Pseudoephedrine hydrochloride 120 mg, chlorpheniramine maleate 12 mg, sucrose. SR Cap. Bot. 100s. *Rx.*
Use: Upper respiratory combination, antihistamine, decongestant.

Histagesic Modified Tablets. (Jones Pharma) Phenylephrine hydrochloride 10 mg, chlorpheniramine maleate 4 mg, acetaminophen 324 mg. Tab. Bot. 1000s. *OTC.*
Use: Analgesic, antihistamine, decongestant.

Histalet. (Solvay) Pseudoephedrine hydrochloride 45 mg, chlorpheniramine maleate 3 mg/5 mL. Syr. Bot. 473 mL. *Rx.*
Use: Antihistamine, decongestant.

Histalet X. (Solvay) **Syr.:** Pseudoephedrine hydrochloride 45 mg, guaifenesin 200 mg/5 mL, alcohol 15%. Bot. 480 mL. **Tab.:** Pseudoephedrine hydrochloride 120 mg, guaifenesin 400 mg. Tab. Bot. 100s. *Rx.*
Use: Decongestant, expectorant.

•**histamine dihydrochloride.** (HISS-tah-meen die-HIGH-droe-KLOR-ide) *USP.*
Use: Analgesic, topical.

histamine H_2 antagonists.
See: Cimetidine.
Famotidine.
Nizatidine.
Ranitidine Hydrochloride.

Histatab. (Breckenridge) Chlorpheniramine maleate 8 mg, methscopolamine nitrate 1.25 mg, pseudoephedrine hydrochloride 60 mg. ER Tab. 100s. *Rx.*
Use: Upper respiratory combination; decongestant, antihistamine, and anticholinergic combination.

Histatab D. (Breckenridge) Dexchlorpheniramine maleate 3.5 mg, methscopolamine nitrate 1 mg, pseudoephedrine hydrochloride 45 mg. Tab. 100s. *Rx.*
Use: Upper respiratory combination, decongestant, antihistamine, and anticholinergic combination.

Histatab Plus. (Century) Phenylephrine hydrochloride 5 mg, chlorpheniramine maleate 2 mg. Tab. Bot. 30s, 100s, 1000s. *OTC.*
Use: Upper respiratory combination, decongestant, antihistamine.

Histatrol. (Center) 2.75 mg/mL histamine phosphate, equivalent to 1 mg/mL histamine base, in 50% glycerin w/v, 5 mL vial; available in a Multitest dosage form or dropper bottle; 0.275 mg/mL histamine phosphate, equivalent to 0.1 mg/mL histamine base, 5 mL vial.
Use: Diagnostic aid, skin test control.

Histenol-Forte. (Zee Medical) Acetaminophen 325 mg, pseudoephedrine hydrochloride 30 mg, dextromethorphan HBr 10 mg. Tab. 24s. *OTC.*
Use: Antitussive combination.

Histex CT. (Teamm) Carbinoxamine maleate 8 mg. Film-coated. TR Tab. Bot. 30s, 100s. *Rx.*
Use: Antihistamine, nonselective ethanolamine.

Histex I/E. (Teamm) Carbinoxamine maleate 10 mg. ER Cap. 60s. *Rx.*
Use: Antihistamine.

Histex Pd. (Teamm) Carbinoxamine maleate 4 mg/5 mL. Dye, alcohol, and sugar free. Saccharin, sorbitol, gum fruit flavor. Liq. Bot. 473 mL. *Rx.*
Use: Antihistamine.

•**histidine.** (HISS-tih-deen) *USP.*
Use: Amino acid.
W/Combinations.
See: Monarc-M.

histidine monohydrochloride.
Use: I.M., peptic and jejunal ulcers.

Histine-8. (Freeport) Chlorpheniramine maleate 8 mg. TR Tab. Bot. 1000s. *OTC.*
Use: Antihistamine.

Histine-50. (Freeport) Diphenhydramine hydrochloride 50 mg. Cap. Bot. 1000s. *OTC.*
Use: Antihistamine, antitussive; anticholinergic; antiemetic; sedative.

Histine-4. (Freeport) Chlorpheniramine maleate 4 mg. Tab. Bot. 1000s. *OTC.*
Use: Antihistamine.

Histine-1. (Freeport) Diphenhydramine hydrochloride 10 mg, alcohol 12% to 14%/4 mL. Bot. 4 oz. *OTC.*
Use: Antihistamine, antitussive; anticholinergic; antiemetic; sedative.

Histine-12. (Freeport) Chlorpheniramine maleate 12 mg. TR Tab. Bot. 1000s. *OTC.*
Use: Antihistamine.

Histine-25. (Freeport) Diphenhydramine hydrochloride 25 mg. Cap. Bot. 1000s. *OTC.*
Use: Antihistamine, antitussive; anticholinergic; antiemetic; sedative.

Histine-2. (Freeport) Diphenhydramine hydrochloride 12.5 mg/5 mL w/alcohol 5%. Bot. 4 oz. *OTC.*
Use: Antihistamine, antitussive; anticholinergic; antiemetic; sedative.

histone deacetylase inhibitors.
Use: Antineoplastic agents.
See: Vorinostat.

•**histoplasmin.** (hiss-toe-PLAZZ-min) *USP.* (Parke-Davis) An aqueous solution containing standardized sterile culture filtrate of *Histoplasma capsulatum* grown on liquid synthetic medium.
Use: Diagnostic aid (dermal reactivity indicator).
See: Histoplasmin, Diluted.

histoplasmin, diluted. (Parke-Davis) 1:100 w/v. Standardized sterile filtrate from cultures of *Histoplasma capsulatum*, 0.5% phenol, polysorbate 80. 1 mL. Inj. *Rx.*
Use: Diagnostic aid.

Hist-PSE. (Cypress) Pseudoephedrine hydrochloride 10 mg, triprolidine hydrochloride 0.938 mg. Glycerin, propylene glycol, saccharin, sorbitol. Alcohol free and sugar free. Cotton candy flavor. Drops. 30 mL. *OTC.*
Use: Upper respiratory combination, decongestant and antihistamine.

•**histrelin.** (hiss-TRELL-in) USAN.
Use: LHRH agonist; treatment of porphyria. [Orphan Drug]
See: Supprelin.

histrelin acetate.
Use: Hormone, gonadotropin-releasing hormone analog.
See: Supprelin LA.
Vantas.

Hitone. (Lafayette) Barium sulfate suspension 125% w/v. Bot. 2000 mL. Case 4s.
Use: Radiopaque agent.

Hi-Tor. (Barth's) B_1 6 mg, B_2 12 mg, B_6 54 mcg, Vitamins B_{12} 15 mcg, niacin 1.5 mg, pantothenic acid 150 mcg, choline 3.75 mg, inositol 5.25 mg. Tab. Bot. 100s, 500s, 1000s. *OTC.*
Use: Vitamin supplement.

Hi-Tor 900. (Barth's) Vitamins B_1 13.5 mg, B_2 5.2 mg, B_6 0.6 mg, B_{12} 2.5 mcg, niacin 15 mg, pantothenic acid 1.2 mg, biotin, iron 0.9 mg, protein 7.5 g, inositol 50 mg, choline 40 mg, aminobenzoic acid 0.15 to 2.4 mg/15 g. Bot. 1 lb, 3 lb. *OTC.*
Use: Mineral, vitamin supplement.

HIVAG HIV-1/HIV-2 (rDNA) EIA. (Abbott) Enzyme immunoassay for qualitative detection of antibodies to human immunodeficiency virus type 1 or type 2 in human serum or plasma. Test kits 100s, 1000s, 5000s.
Use: Diagnostic aid.

Hi-Vegi-Lip Tablets. (Freeda) Lipase 4,800 units, protease 60,000 units, amylase 60,000 units. Mannitol. Gluten free, lactose free, and sugar free. Tab. 100s, 250s. *OTC.*
Use: Digestive aid.

Hivig. (NABI) Human immunodeficiency virus immune globulin.
Use: Antiviral, HIV. [Orphan Drug]

Hiwolfia. (Jones Pharma) Rauwolfia 25 mg, 50 mg, 100 mg. Tab. Bot. 100s, 1000s.
Use: Antihypertensive.

Hizentra. (CSL Behring LLC) Immune globulin (human) subcutaneous 20% protein (200 mg/mL) (contains L-proline 210 to 290 mmol/L and polysorbate 80 10 to 30 mg/L). Preservative free. Inj., Soln. Single-use vial. 5 mL, 10 mL, 20 mL. *Rx.*
Use: Immune globulin.

HMG-CoA reductase inhibitors.
Use: Antihyperlipidemic agents.
See: Atorvastatin.
Fluvastatin.
Lovastatin.
Pitavastatin.
Pravastatin Sodium.
Rosuvastatin Calcium.
Simvastatin.

HMM.
See: Hexamethylmelamine.

HN_2. Mechlorethamine hydrochloride.
Use: Antineoplastic.
See: Mustargen.

H 9600. (Cypress) Pseudoephedrine hydrochloride 90 mg, guaifenesin 600 mg, dye free. SR Tab. Bot. 100s. *Rx.*
Use: Upper respiratory combination, decongestant, expectorant.

•**hofocon A.** (hoe-FOE-kon) USAN.
Use: Hydrophobic.

H_2 OEX. (Fellows) Benzthiazide 50 mg. Tab. Bot. 100s, 1000s. *Rx.*
Use: Diuretic.

Hold. (GlaxoSmithKline) Dextromethorphan HBr 5 mg. Loz. Plastic tube 10 oz. *OTC.*
Use: Antitussive.

Hold DM. (B.F. Ascher) Dextromethorphan HBr 5 mg. Corn syrup, sucrose. Original and cherry flavor. Loz. Pkg. 10s.

OTC.
Use: Nonnarcotic antitussive.
holocaine hydrochloride. (Various Mfr.) Phenacaine hydrochloride.
Use: Anesthetic, local.
homarylamine hydrochloride. N-Methyl-3,4-methylenedioxyphenethylamine hydrochloride.
•**homatropine hydrobromide.** (hoe-MA-troe-peen) *USP.*
Use: Anticholinergic, ophthalmic; mydriatic, cycloplegic.
See: Isopto Homatropine.
Murocoll.
W/Hydrocodone Bitartrate.
See: Tussigon.
homatropine hydrobromide. (Various Mfr.) Homatropine HBr 5%. Soln. Bot. 1 mL, 2 mL, 5 mL. *Rx.*
Use: Mydriatic, cycloplegic.
homatropine hydrochloride.
Use: Anticholinergic, topical; mydriatic, cycloplegic.
•**homatropine methylbromide.** (hoe-MA-troe-peen) *USP.*
Use: Anticholinergic.
W/Combinations.
See: Hydromide.
Hydropane.
Panitol H.M.B.
Spasmatol.
Tapuline.
W/Hydrocodone Bitartrate.
See: Hydromet.
homatropine methylbromide and phenobarbital combinations.
Use: Anticholinergic.
See: Gustase Plus.
Hominex-1. (Ross) Protein 15 g, fat 23.9 g, carbohydrate 46.3 g, linoleic acid 1800 mg, Fe 9 mg, Na 190 mg, K 675 mg, Ca, vitamins A, B_1, B_2, B_3, B_5, B_6, B_{12}, C, D, E, K, biotin, choline, folic acid, inositol, Cl, Cu, I, Mg, Mn, P, Se, Zn and 480 Cal per 100 g. Methionine free. Pow. Can 350 g. *OTC.*
Use: Nutritional supplement.
Hominex-2. (Ross) Protein 30 g, fat 15.5 g, carbohydrate 30 g, Fe 13 mg, Na 880 mg, K 1370 mg, Ca, vitamins A, B_1, B_2, B_3, B_5, B_6, B_{12}, C, D, E, K, biotin, choline, folic acid, inositol, Cl, Cu, I, Mg, Mn, P, Se, Zn and 410 Cal per 100 g. Methionine free. Pow. Can 325 g. *OTC.*
Use: Nutritional supplement.
Homogene-S. (Spanner) Testosterone 25 mg/mL, 50 mg/mL, 100 mg/mL. Vial 10 mL. *c-III.*
Use: Androgen.
•**homosalate.** (hoe-moe-SAL-ate) USAN.
Formerly Homomenthyl Salicylate.
Use: Ultraviolet screen.
W/Avobenzone, Octisalate, Octocrylene, Oxybenzone.
See: Neutrogena Ultra Sheer Dry-Touch Sunblock.
W/Combinations.
See: Coppertone.
honey bee venom.
See: Albay.
Pharmalgen.
Venomil.
•**hoquizil hydrochloride.** (HOE-kwih-zill) USAN.
Use: Bronchodilator.
Horizant. (XenoPort) Gabapentin 300 mg, 600 mg (as gabapentin enacarbil). ER Tab. 30s. *Rx.*
Use: Anticonvulsant.
hormofollin.
See: Estrone.
hormones.
See: Androgens.
Antiandrogens.
Antiestrogens.
Aromatase Inhibitors.
Cetrorelix Acetate.
Choriogonadotropin Alfa.
Clomiphene Citrate.
Estrogen/Nitrogen Mustard.
Estrogens.
Ganirelix Acetate.
Gonadotropin-Releasing Hormone Analog.
Intrauterine Progesterone Contraceptive System.
Levonorgestrel-Releasing Intrauterine System.
Medroxyprogesterone Acetate/Estradiol Cypionate.
Medroxyprogesterone Contraceptive Injection.
Progestins.
Raloxifene.
hormones, contraceptive.
Use: Contraceptive hormones.
See: Etonogestrel.
hormones, growth.
Use: Growth hormones.
hormones, posterior pituitary.
Use: Posterior pituitary hormones.
hormones, sex.
Use: Sex hormones.
hornet venom.
See: Albay.
Pharmalgen.
Venomil.
•**horse chestnut.** *NF.*
Use: Anti-inflammatory.
Hospital Foam Cleaner. (Health & Medical Techniques) 0-phenylphenol 0.1%,

4-chloro-2-cyclopentyl-phenol 0.08%, lauric diethanolamide 0.2%, triethanolamine dodecylbenzenesulfonate 0.3%. Aerosol spray 19 oz.
Use: Antimicrobial; disinfectant.

Hospital Lotion. (Paddock) Diisobutylcresoxyethoxy-ethyl dimethyl benzyl ammonium chloride, menthol, lanolin, mineral and vegetable oils. Bot. 4 oz, 8 oz, gal. *OTC.*
Use: Emollient.

H.P. Acthar. (Questcor) Repository corticotropin injection 80 units/mL, gelatin 16%. Multidose vial 5 mL. *Rx.*
Use: Corticosteroid.

HPR Plus. (PruGen Pharmaceuticals) **Cream:** Glycerin, alcohol, propylene glycol, petrolatum, parabens, disodium EDTA, dimethicone, sodium hyaluronate. 100 g, 450 g. **Aer. Foam:** Alcohol, dimethicone, disodium EDTA, glycerin, parabens, petrolatum, propylene glycol, sodium hyaluronate. 100 g, 150 g. *Rx.*
Use: Emollient.

HRC-Tylaprin. (Cenci, H.R. Labs, Inc.) Acetaminophen 120 mg, alcohol 7%/5 mL. Elix. Bot. 2 oz, 4 oz. *OTC.*
Use: Analgesic.

H-R Lubricating Jelly. (Wallace) Hydroxypropyl methylcellulose, parabens. Jelly 150 g. *OTC.*
Use: Lubricant.

H.S. Need. (Hanlon) Chloral hydrate 3¾ g, 7.5 g. Cap. Bot. 100s. *Rx.*
Use: Sedative.

HSV-1. (Wampole) Herpes simplex virus type 1 test system. For the qualitative and semi-quantitative detection of HSV-1 antibody in human serum. Test 100s.
Use: Diagnostic aid.

HSV-2. (Wampole) Herpes simplex virus type 2 antibody test. For the qualitative and semi-quantitative detection of HSV-2 antibody in human serum. Test 100s.
Use: Diagnostic aid.

H.T. Factorate. (Centeon) Antihemophilic factor (human) dried, heat treated for IV administration only. Single-dose vial w/diluent and needles. *Rx.*
Use: Antihemophilic.

H.T. Factorate Generation II. (Centeon) Antihemophilic factor (human) dried, heat treated for IV administration only. Single-dose vial w/diluent and needles. *Rx.*
Use: Antihemophilic.

HTSH EIA. (Abbott Diagnostics) Enzyme immunoassay for the quantitative determination of human thyroid-stimulating hormone (TSH) in human serum or plasma.
Use: Diagnostic aid.

HTSH RIAbead. (Abbott Diagnostics) Immunoradiometric assay for the quantitative measurement of human thyroid-stimulating hormone (TSH) in serum.
Use: Diagnostic aid.

5-HT$_3$ receptor antagonists.
See: Alosetron Hydrochloride.
Dolasetron Mesylate.
Granisetron Hydrochloride.
Ondansetron Hydrochloride.
Palonosetron Hydrochloride.

H-Tuss-D. (Cypress) Hydrocodone bitartrate 5 mg, pseudoephedrine hydrochloride 60 mg/5 mL, Liq. Bot. 473 mL. *Rx.*
Use: Expectorant.

Humalog. (Lilly) Human insulin lispro 100 units/mL. Inj. Vials. 10 mL. Cartridges. 5 × 1.5 mL, 5 × 3 mL. Disp. pen insulin delivery devices. 5 × 3 mL. *Rx.*
Tall Man: HumaLOG
Use: Antidiabetic, insulin.

Humalog Mix 50/50. (Lilly) Insulin lispro (human) 100 units/mL. Metacresol 2.2 mg/mL, protamine sulfate 0.19 mg/mL. Contains 50% insulin lispro protamine (rDNA origin) suspension and 50% insulin lispro (rDNA origin) injection. Inj., Susp. Vial. 10 mL. Disposable pen and *KwikPen* insulin delivery device. 5 × 3 mL. *Rx.*
Tall Man: HumaLOG
Use: Antidiabetic agent, insulin.

Humalog Mix 75/25. (Lilly) Human insulin lispro 100 units/mL. Protamine sulfate 0.28 mg. Contains 75% insulin lispro protamine suspension and 25% insulin lispro injection (rDNA). Inj. Disp. pen insulin delivery devices. 5 × 3 mL. Vials. 10 mL. *Rx.*
Tall Man: HumaLOG
Use: Antidiabetic, insulin.

human albumin grifols. (Grifols) Human albumin 25%. Inj. 50 mL, 100 mL. *Rx.*
Use: Plasma expander.

human antihemophilic factor.
See: Antihemophilic.

human B-type natriuretic peptide.
Use: Vasodilator.
See: Nesiritide.

human growth hormone function test.
See: R-Gene 10.

•**human insulin.** *USP.* Insulin human.
Use: Hypoglycemic.
See: Humulin.

humanized anti-Tac.
Use: Immunosuppressant. [Orphan Drug]
See: Zenapax.

•**human papillomavirus recombinant vaccine, bivalent.**
Use: Cervarix.

human papillomavirus recombinant vaccine, quadrivalent.
Use: Active immunization; viral vaccine.
See: Gardasil.

human protein C.
Use: Thrombolytic agent.
See: Drotrecogin Alfa (Activated). Protein C Concentrate (Human).

human serum albumin.
See: Albumotope.

human T-lymphotropic virus type III Gp 160 antigens.
Use: AIDS. [Orphan Drug]
See: Vaxsyn HIV-1.

Humate-P. (CSL Behring) Antihemophilic factor and von Willebrand factor: Ristocetin cofactor (vWF/RCo) 250 units/ 600 units per vial, 500 units/1200 units per vial, 1000 units/2400 units per vial. When reconstituted, each milliliter contains Factor VIII activity 40 to 80 units, vWF/RCo activity 72 to 224 units, glycine 15 to 33 mg, sodium citrate 3.5 to 9.3 mg, sodium chloride 2 to 5.3 mg, albumin (human) 8 to 16 mg, other proteins 2 to 14 mg, total proteins 10 to 30 mg. Contains anti-A and anti-B blood group isoagglutinins. Heat-treated. Pow. for Inj., Soln. Lyophilized. Single-dose vials with 5 mL (250 units/600 units), 10 mL (500 units/1200 units), 15 mL (1000 units/2400 units) diluent, filter transfer set for reconstitution, and a vented filter spike for withdrawal. *Rx.*
Use: Antihemophilic agent.

Humatin. (Parke-Davis) Paromomycin sulfate 250 mg. Cap. Bot. 16s. *Rx.*
Use: Amebicide.

Humatrope. (Eli Lilly) Somatropin 5 mg, 6 mg, 12 mg, 24 mg. Glycine, mannitol. Inj., lyophilized Pow. for Soln. Vial w/diluent (metacresol, glycerin) (5 mg only); cartridge w/prefilled syringe of diluent (metacresol, glycerin) (except 5 mg). *Rx.*
Use: Growth hormone.

Humibid CS. (Cornerstone Biopharma) Dextromethorphan HBr 20 mg, guaifenesin 400 mg. Saccharin. Tab. 24s. *OTC.*
Use: Antitussive with expectorant.

Humibid DM. (Carolina Pharmaceuticals) Dextromethorphan HBr 50 mg, guaifenesin 400 mg, potassium guaiacolsulfonate 200 mg. Sucrose. ER Cap. Bot. 30s, 100s. *Rx.*
Use: Upper respiratory combination, antitussive and expectorant combination.

Humibid Maximum Strength. (Adams) Guaifenesin 1,200 mg. ER Tab. 100s. *OTC.*
Use: Expectorant.

Humira. (AbbVie) Adalimumab 20 mg/ 0.4 mL, 40 mg/0.8 mL. Preservative free. Inj. Soln. Single-use prefilled syringes. Single-use prefilled pens (40 mg/ 0.8 mL only). Each dose tray consists of a single-use syringe or pen with a fixed 27-gauge ½-inch needle. *Rx.*
Use: Immunomodulator.

HuMist. (Scherer) Sodium Cl 0.65%, chlorobutanol. Soln. Bot. 45 mL. *OTC.*
Use: Nasal decongestant.

Humulin N. (Lilly) Human insulin (rDNA) 100 units/mL. Inj. Disp. pen insulin delivery device 5 × 3 mL, Vials. 10 mL. *OTC.*
Tall Man: HumuLIN
Use: Antidiabetic, insulin.

Humulin R. (Lilly) Regular insulin (rDNA) 100 units/mL. Inj. Vials. 10 mL. *OTC.*
Tall Man: HumuLIN
Use: Antidiabetic, insulin.

Humulin R Regular U-500 (Concentrated). (Lilly) Insulin concentrate regular 500 units/mL. M-cresol 2.5 mg, glycerin 16 mg/mL. Inj. Vials. 20 mL. *Rx.*
Tall Man: HumuLIN
Use: Antidiabetic, insulin.

Humulin 70/30. (Lilly) Human insulin (rDNA) 100 units/mL. Inj. Disp. pen insulin delivery devices. 5 × 3 mL. Vials. 10 mL. *OTC.*
Tall Man: HumuLIN
Use: Antidiabetic, insulin.

Hurricaine. (Beutlich) Benzocaine 20%. **Gel; dental:** Alcohol 60%, saccharin. 7 g. **Spray:** Cherry flavor. 60 mL. **Swab:** PEG, saccharin. 72s. *OTC.*
Use: Topical local anesthetic, ester local anesthetic.

Hurricaine ONE. (Beutlich) Benzocaine 20%. PEG, saccharin. Wild cherry flavor. Spray; dental. UD 0.5 mL. *OTC.*
Use: Topical local anesthetic, ester local anesthetic.

Hurricaine Topical Anesthetic Spray Kit. (Beutlich) Benzocaine 20%. Kit: Aerosol 60 g plus 200 disposable extension tubes. *OTC.*
Use: Anesthetic, topical.

HVS 1 & 2. (Chemi-Tech Laboratories) Benzalkonium Cl in a specially formulated base. Soln. Bot. 15 mL. *OTC.*
Use: Cold sores, fever blisters, herpes virus.

Hyacide. (Niltig) Benzethonium chloride 0.1%, sodium nitrite 0.55%. Soln. Bot. oz. *OTC.*
Use: Antiseptic.

Hyalex. (Miller Pharmacal Group) Magnesium salicylate 260 mg, magnesium p-aminobenzoate 163 mg, vitamins A 1500 units, C 30 mg, D 100 units, E 3 units, B_{12} 2 mcg, pantothenic acid 5 mg, zinc 0.7 mg. Tab. Bot. 100s. *OTC.*
Use: Mineral, vitamin supplement.

Hyalgan. (Fidia Farmaceutica) Sodium hyaluronate 10 mg/mL. Prefilled syringes and vials. 2 mL. Prefilled Syringe. *Rx.*
Use: Antiarthritic.

hyalidase.
See: Hyaluronidase.

hyaluronan.
See: Monovisc.
Ocean Nasal Moisturizer.
Orthovisc.

hyaluronic acid derivatives.
Use: Physical adjunct, correction of facial wrinkles and folds.
See: Bionect.
Euflexxa.
Gel-One.
Hyalgan.
Hylaform.
Hylira.
Juvederm 30.
Juvederm 30HV.
Juvederm 24HV.
Juvederm Ultra.
Juvederm Ultra Plus.
Juvederm Ultra Plus XC.
Juvederm Ultra XC.
Juvederm Voluma XC.
Orthovisc.
Perlane.
Perlane-L.
Restylane.
Restylane-L.
Sodium Hyaluronate.
Supartz.
Synvisc.
Synvisc-One.

•**hyaluronidase.** (hye-al-ur-ON-i-dase) *USP.*
Use: Physical adjunct.
See: Amphadase.
Hylenex.
Vitrase.

•**hyaluronidase (human recombinant).** (hye-al-ur-ON-i-dase) USAN.
Use: Spreading agent.

•**hyaluronidase injection.** (high-uhl-yur-AHN-ih-dase) *USP.* Hyalidase, Hydase Enzymes which depolymerize hyaluronic acid. Hyalase, Rondase.
Use: Hypodermoclyses, promotion of diffusion, spreading agent.
See: Wydase.

•**hyaluronidase ovine.** (hye-al-ur-ON-i-dase) USAN.
Use: Spreading agent.

hyamagnate. Hydroxy-Aluminum-Magnesium-Aminoacetate, Sodium-free.

Hybec Forte. (Amlab) Vitamins B_1 100 mg, B_2 20 mg, B_6 2.5 mg, B_{12} 10 mcg, niacinamide 25 mg, C 200 mg, calcium pantothenate 5 mg, iron 10 mg, choline bitartrate 24 mg, inositol 10 mg, biotin 5 mcg, liver 50 mg, yeast 100 mg. Tab. Bot. 30s, 100s. *OTC.*
Use: Mineral, vitamin supplement.

Hycamtin. (GlaxoSmithKline) Topotecan (as topotecan hydrochloride). **Cap.:** 0.25 mg, 1 mg. Hydrogenated vegetable oil. 10s. **Inj., Lyophilized. Pow. for Soln.:** 4 mg. Preservative free. Single-dose vials. *Rx.*
Use: Antineoplastic; DNA topoisomerase inhibitor.

•**hycanthone.** (HIGH-kan-thone) USAN.
Use: Antischistosomal.

Hycet. (Eclat Pharmaceuticals) Hydrocodone bitartrate 2.5 mg/acetaminophen 108 mg per 5 mL. Alcohol 7%, glycerin, parabens, saccharin, sorbitol, sucrose. Oral Soln. 473 mL. *c-III.*
Use: Analgesic, narcotic.

Hyclorite. *USP.* Sodium hypochlorite soln.

HycoClear Tuss. (Ethex) Hydrocodone bitartrate 5 mg, guaifenesin 100 mg/5 mL. Alcohol, dye, sugar free. Syrup. Bot. 118 mL, 473 mL. *c-III.*
Use: Antitussive, expectorant.

Hycort. (Everett) **Cream:** Hydrocortisone 1% in a cream base. Tube oz. **Oint.:** Hydrocortisone 1% in ointment base. Tube oz. *Rx.*
Use: Corticosteroid, topical.

Hycortole. (Teva) Hydrocortisone. **Cream:** 0.5%: 5 g, 20 g; 1%: 5 g, 20 g, 4 oz; 2.5%: Tube 5 g, 20 g. **Oint.:** 1%, 2.5%. Tube 5 g, 20 g.
Use: Corticosteroid, topical.

Hycosin Expectorant. (Alpharma) Hydrocodone bitartrate 5 mg, guaifenesin 100 mg per 5 mL. Alcohol 10%, parabens, saccharin, sorbitol, sucrose, butterscotch flavor. Syr. Bot. 473 mL. *c-III.*
Use: Upper respiratory combination, antitussive, expectorant.

hydantoin derivatives.
Use: Anticonvulsant.
See: Dilantin.
Diphenylhydantoin Sodium.
Mesantoin.
Phenantoin.

hydantoins.
See: Ethotoin.
Fosphenytoin Sodium.

Phenytoin.

Hydergine. (Novartis) **Liq.:** Equal parts of dihydroergocornine, dihydroergocristine, dihydroergocryptine (Ergoloid Mesylates). 1 mg/mL. Bot. 100 mL w/dropper. **Oral:** Equal parts of dihydroergocornine, dihydroergocristine, dihydroergocryptine (Ergoloid Mesylates). 1 mg. Tab. Bot. 100s, 500s. *SandoPak* (UD) 100s, 500s. **Sublingual:** Equal parts of dihydroergocornine, dihydroergocristine, dihydroergocryptine (Ergoloid Mesylates). 0.5 mg, 1 mg. Tab. Bot. 100s, 1000s, *SandoPak* (UD) 100s. *Rx.*
Use: Psychotherapeutic agent.

Hydoril. (Cenci, H.R. Labs, Inc.) Hydrochlorothiazide 25 mg, 50 mg. Tab. Bot. 100s, 1000s. *Rx.*
Use: Diuretic.

hydrabamine phenoxymethyl penicillin.
See: Penicillin V Hydrabamine.

hydracrylic acid beta lactone.
See: Propiolactone.

hydralazine. (Solopak Pharmaceuticals, Inc.) Hydralazine hydrochloride 20 mg/mL Inj. Vial 1 mL. *Rx.*
Use: Antihypertensive.

•**hydralazine hydrochloride.** (high-DRAL-uh-zeen) *USP.*
Tall Man: hydrALAZINE
Use: Antihypertensive.
See: Apresoline.
W/Hydrochlorothiazide.
See: Apresoline-Esidrix.
Hydralazide.
Hydroserpine Plus.
W/Isosorbide Dinitrate.
See: BiDil.
W/Reserpine.
See: Dralserp.
Serpasil-Apresoline.
W/Reserpine, hydrochlorothiazide.
See: Harbolin.

hydralazine hydrochloride. (Various Mfr.) Hydralazine hydrochloride 10 mg, 25 mg, 50, mg 100 mg. Tab. Bot. 100s, 1000s, UD 100s (except 100 mg).
Use: Antihypertensive.

•**hydralazine polistirex.** (high-DRAL-ah-zeen pahl-ee-STIE-rex) USAN.
Tall Man: hydrALAZINE
Use: Antihypertensive.

Hydra Mag Tablets. (Pal-Pak, Inc.) Aluminum hydroxide gel, dried, 195 mg, magnesium trisilicate 195 mg, kaolin 162 mg. Tab. Bot. 1000s. *OTC.*
Use: Antacid.

Hydramine Cough. (Various Mfr.) Diphenhydramine hydrochloride 12.5 mg/mL, may contain alcohol. Syr. Bot. 473 mL. *Rx-OTC.*
Use: Antitussive.

Hydraserp. (Geneva) Hydrochlorothiazide 25 mg, 50 mg, reserpine 0.1 mg. Tab. Bot. 100s, 1000s. *Rx.*
Use: Antihypertensive combination.

hydrastine hydrochloride. (Penick) Pow. Bot. oz.
Use: Hemostatic.

Hydrazide. (Ivax) **25/25:** Hydrochlorothiazide 25 mg, hydralazine 25 mg. Cap. **50/50:** Hydrochlorothiazide 50 mg, hydralazine 50 mg. Cap. Bot. 100s. *Rx.*
Use: Antihypertensive.

Hydra-Zide. (Par Pharmaceuticals) Hydralazine hydrochloride 50 mg, hydrochlorothiazide 50 mg. Cap. Bot. 100s, 500s, 1000s. *Rx.*
Use: Antihypertensive.

hydrazone.
Use: Pulmonary tuberculosis.
See: Rimactane.

Hydrea. (Bristol-Myers Squibb) Hydroxyurea 500 mg, lactose. Cap. Bot. 100s. *Rx.*
Use: Antineoplastic.

hydriodic acid. (Various Mfr.)
Use: Expectorant.

hydriodic acid therapy.
See: Aminoacetic Acid Hydrochloride.

Hydrisalic. (Pedinol) Salicylic acid 6%. Alcohol. Gel. 28.35 g. *OTC.*
Use: Keratolytic agent.

Hydrisinol. (Pedinol Pharmacal) Sulfonated hydrogenated castor oil. **Cream:** Spout Cap Jar 4 oz, lb. **Lot.:** Bot. 8 oz. *OTC.*
Use: Emollient.

Hydro-Ban. (Whiteworth Towne) Juniper oil 10 mg, uva ursi 50 mg, buchu extract 50 mg, parsley piert extract 50 mg, iron 6 mg. Cap. Bot. 42s. *OTC.*
Use: Diuretic.

Hydrocare Cleaning and Disinfecting. (Allergan) Buffered, isotonic. Tris (2-hydroxyethyl) tallow ammonium Cl, thimerosal 0.002%, bis (2-hydroxyethyl) tallow ammonium Cl, sodium bicarbonate, sodium phosphates, hydrochloric acid, propylene glycol, polysorbate 80, polyhema. Soln. Bot. 240 mL, 360 mL. *OTC.*
Use: Contact lens care, disinfective.

Hydrocare Preserved Saline. (Allergan) Isotonic, buffered, NaCl, sodium hexametaphosphate, boric acid, sodium borate, EDTA 0.01%, thimerosal 0.001%. Soln. Bot. 240 mL, 360 mL. *OTC.*
Use: Contact lens care, rinsing/storage solution.

Hydrocerin. (Geritrex) **Cream:** Petrolatum, mineral oil, mineral wax, ceresin,

lanolin alcohol, parabens. 480 g. **Lotion:** EDTA, lanolin alcohol, parabens, PEG-40 sorbitan, peroleate, propylene glycol, sorbitol, water. 240 g. *OTC.*
Use: Emollient.

hydrochlorate. Same as Hydrochloride.

•**hydrochloric acid.** (HYE-droe-KLOR-ik) *NF.*
Use: Well diluted, achlorhydria; pharmaceutic aid (acidifying agent).

hydrochloric acid. (Various Mfr.) Muriatic acid, Absolute 38%. Diluted 10%.

hydrochloric acid therapy.
Use: Well diluted, achlorhydria; pharmaceutic aid (acidifying agent); gastric acidifier.
See: Betaine Hydrochloride.
Glutamic Acid Hydrochloride.
Glycine Hydrochloride.

Hydrochloroserpine. (Freeport) Hydralazine hydrochloride 25 mg, hydrochlorothiazide 15 mg, reserpine 0.1 mg. Tab. Bot. 1000s.
Use: Antihypertensive combination.

•**hydrochlorothiazide.** (high-droe-klor-oh-THIGH-uh-zide) *USP.*
Use: Diuretic.
See: Ezide.
HydroDiuril.
Hydro-Par.
Microzide.
W/Aliskiren.
See: Tekturna HCT.
W/Aliskiren Hemifumarate, Amlodipine Besylate.
See: Amturnide.
W/Amlodipine/Valsartan.
See: Exforge HCT.
W/Benazepril.
See: Lotensin HCT.
W/Bisoprolol.
See: Ziac.
W/Candesartan Cilexetil.
See: Atacand HCT.
W/Enalapril Maleate.
See: Vaseretic.
W/Eprosartan.
See: Teveten HCT.
W/Fosinopril Sodium.
See: Monopril-HCT.
W/Hydralazine Hydrochloride.
See: Apresoline-Esidrix.
W/Irbesartan.
See: Avalide.
W/Lisinopril.
See: Prinzide.
Zestoretic.
W/Losartan Potassium.
See: Hyzaar.
W/Metoprolol Tartrate.
See: Lopressor HCT.
W/Moexipril Hydrochloride.
See: Uniretic.
W/Olmesartan Medoxomil.
See: Benicar HCT.
W/Quinapril Hydrochloride.
See: Accuretic.
Quinaretic.
W/Telmisartan.
See: Micardis HCT.
W/Triamterene.
See: Dyazide.
W/Valsartan.
See: Diovan HCT.

hydrochlorothiazide. (Various Mfr.) Hydrochlorothiazide. **Cap.:** 12.5 mg. Bot. 100s, 500s. **Tab.:** 12.5 mg (100s, 1000s), 25 mg (30s, 100s, 500s, 1000s, 5000s, UD 32s, UD 100s), 50 mg (30s, 100s, 500s, 1000s, 5000s, UD 100s), 100 mg (30s, 100s, 250s, 500s, 1000s, UD 100s). *Rx.*
Use: Diuretic.

hydrochlorothiazide/amiloride.
See: Amiloride Hydrochloride and Hydrochlorothiazide.

hydrochlorothiazide and benazepril hydrochloride.
See: Benazepril Hydrochloride/Hydrochlorothiazide.

hydrochlorothiazide/metoprolol tartrate.
See: Metoprolol Tartrate/Hydrochlorothiazide.

hydrocholeretic combinations.
See: G.B.S.

hydrocholeretics.
See: Bile Salts.
Dehydrocholic Acid.
Ox Bile Extract.

Hydrocil Instant. (Numark) Psyllium hydrophilic mucilloid 3.5 g/dose. Pow. Jar 250 g. *OTC.*
Use: Laxative.

•**hydrocodone bitartrate.** (HIGH-droe-KOE-dohn by-TAR-TRATE) *USP.* Dihydrocodeinone bitartrate.
Tall Man: HYDROcodone
Use: Antitussive, analgesic, narcotic.
W/Acetaminophen.
See: Anexsia 7.5/650.
Anexsia 10/660.
Co-Gesic.
Hycet.
Hydrogesic.
Liquicet.
Lorcet Plus.
Lorcet 10/650.
Lortab.
Margesic H.
Maxidone.
Norco.

Norco 5/325.
Stagesic.
T-Gesic.
Vicodin.
Xodol.
Zamicet.
Zohydro ER.
Zolvit.
Zydone.

W/Chlorpheniramine Maleate.
See: TussiCaps Full Strength.
TussiCaps Half Strength.
Vituz.

W/Chlorpheniramine Maleate, Guaifenesin, Pseudoephedrine Hydrochloride.
See: ZTuss Expectorant.

W/Chlorpheniramine Maleate, Phenylephrine Hydrochloride.
See: Neo HC.
Notuss-Forte.
Relacon-HC.

W/Chlorpheniramine Maleate, Phenylephrine Hydrochloride, Pseudoephedrine Hydrochloride, Pyrilamine Maleate.
See: Statuss Green.

W/Chlorpheniramine Maleate, Pseudoephedrine Hydrochloride.
See: Notuss-Forte.

W/Chlorpheniramine Polistirex.
See: Tussionex Pennkinetic.

W/Guaifenesin.
See: ZTuss ZT.

W/Homatropine Hydrobromide.
See: Tussigon.

W/Ibuprofen.
See: Ibudone.
Reprexain.
Vicoprofen.

W/Methylbromide.
See: Hydromet.

W/Phenylephrine Hydrochloride, Pyrilamine Maleate.
See: Tussplex.

hydrocodone bitartrate/acetaminophen. (Boca Pharmacal) Hydrocodone bitartrate 5 mg, acetaminophen 300 mg. Tab. 100s. *c-III.*
Use: Opioid analgesic combination.

hydrocodone bitartrate and acetaminophen. (KLE 2) Hydrocodone bitartrate 2.5 mg, acetaminophen 325 mg. Tab. 100s. *c-III.*
Use: Opioid analgesic combination.

hydrocodone bitartrate and acetaminophen. (Qualitest) Hydrocodone bitartrate 2.5 mg, acetaminophen 500 mg. Sucrose. Tab. 100s, 500s, 1,000s. *c-III.*
Use: Narcotic analgesic.

hydrocodone bitartrate and acetaminophen. (Various Mfr.) **Caplets:** Hydrocodone bitartrate 7.5 mg, acetaminophen 650 mg. 100s, 500s. **Capsules:** Hydrocodone bitartrate 5 mg, acetaminophen 500 mg. 100s, 500s. **Elixir:** Hydrocodone bitartrate 2.5 mg, acetaminophen 167 mg/5 mL, alcohol 7%. 473 mL. **Soln.:** Hydrocodone bitartrate 2.5 mg, acetaminophen 108 mg per 5 mL. May contain alcohol 7%, glycerin, parabens, propylene glycol, saccharin, sorbitol, sucrose. 118 mL, 473 mL. **Tab.:** Hydrocodone bitartrate/acetaminophen 5 mg/300 mg, 7.5 mg/300 mg, 10 mg/300 mg, 2.5 mg/325 mg, 5 mg/325 mg, 7.5 mg/325 mg, 10 mg/325 mg, 5 mg/500 mg, 7.5 mg/500 mg, 7.5 mg/650 mg, 7.5 mg/750 mg, 10 mg/500 mg, 10 mg/650 mg, 10 mg/660 mg, 10 mg/750 mg. 30s (5 mg/325 mg), 60s (10 mg/325 mg), 90s (5 mg/325 mg, 7.5 mg/325 mg, 10 mg/325 mg), 100s (except 7.5 mg/500 mg, 7.5 mg/750 mg, 10 mg/500 mg), 120s (5 mg/325 mg, 7.5 mg/325 mg, 10 mg/325 mg), 150s (10 mg/325 mg), 180s (5 mg/325 mg), 240s (10 mg/325 mg), 500s (except 7.5 mg/650 mg, 7.5 mg/750 mg, 10 mg/750 mg), 1,000s (5 mg/325 mg, 7.5 mg/325 mg, 10 mg/325 mg), UD 90s (5 mg/500 mg), UD 100s (5 mg/325 mg, 7.5 mg/325 mg, 10 mg/325 mg, 5 mg/500 mg, 7.5 mg/750 mg, 10 mg/500 mg, 10 mg/650 mg, 10 mg/660 mg), UD 750s (5 mg/500 mg). *c-III.*
Use: Analgesic combination, narcotic.

hydrocodone bitartrate and homatropine methylbromide. (Alpharma) Hydrocodone bitartrate 5 mg, homatropine methylbromide 1.5 mg per 5 mL. Methylparaben, saccharin, sucrose. Cherry flavor. Syrup. 473 mL, 3785 mL. *c-III.*
Use: Antitussive combination.

hydrocodone bitartrate and ibuprofen. (Amneal Pharmaceuticals) Hydrocodone bitartrate/ibuprofen 2.5 mg/200 mg, 5 mg/200 mg. Film coated. PEG, polydextrose. Tab. 100s. *c-III.*
Use: Opioid analgesic combination.

hydrocodone bitartrate and ibuprofen. (Various Mfr.) Hydrocodone bitartrate/ibuprofen 7.5 mg/200 mg, 10 mg/200 mg. Film coated. May contain PEG, polydextrose. Tab. 10, 100s, 500s (7.5 mg/200 mg only), 1000s. *c-III.*
Use: Narcotic analgesic.

hydrocodone bitartrate/chlorpheniramine maleate/pseudoephedrine hydrochloride. (Various Mfr.) Hydrocodone bitartrate 5 mg, chlorpheniramine maleate 4 mg, pseudoephedrine hydrochloride 60 mg per 5 mL. May contain glycerin, parabens, propylene glycol, saccharin, sucrose. Soln. 480 mL. *c-III.*

Use: Upper respiratory combination, antitussive combination.

hydrocodone bitartrate 5 mg/pseudoephedrine hydrochloride 30 mg/carbinoxamine maleate 2 mg. (URL) Hydrocodone bitartrate 5 mg, carbinoxamine maleate 2 mg, pseudoephedrine hydrochloride 30 mg per 5 mL. Alcohol free. Liq. Bot. 473 mL. *c-III.*

Use: Upper respiratory combination, antitussive, antihistamine, decongestant.

hydrocodone bitartrate/homatropine methylbromide. (Pharmaceutical Associates) Hydrocodone bitartrate 5 mg, homatropine methylbromide 1.5 mg. Alcohol < 0.1%, glycerin, parabens, sorbitol, sugar. Cherry flavor. Syr. UD 5 mL. *c-III.*

Use: Upper respiratory combination, antitussive combination.

hydrocodone bitartrate, phenylephrine hydrochloride, chlorpheniramine maleate. (Cypress) Hydrocodone bitartrate 1.67 mg, phenylephrine hydrochloride 5 mg, chlorpheniramine maleate 2 mg/5 mL. Syr. Bot. Pt, gal. *c-III.*

Use: Decongestant, antihistamine, antitussive.

•**hydrocodone bitartrate tablets.** (hye-droe-KOE-done) *USP.*

Tall Man: HYDROcodone

Use: Analgesic, narcotic.

hydrocodone comp. syrup. (Various Mfr.) Hydrocodone bitartrate 5 mg, homatropine methylbromide 1.5 mg. Bot. 473 mL, gal. *c-III.*

Use: Antitussive.

Hydrocodone CP. (Morton Grove) Hydrocodone bitartrate 2.5 mg, phenylephrine hydrochloride 5 mg, chlorpheniramine maleate 2 mg per 5 mL. Saccharin, sorbitol, fruit flavor, alcohol free. Syr. Bot. 237 mL, 473 mL. *c-III.*

Use: Upper respiratory combination, antitussive, antihistamine, decongestant.

Hydrocodone GF. (Morton Grove Pharmaceuticals) Hydrocodone bitartrate 5 mg, guaifenesin 100 mg per 5 mL. Saccharin, sorbitol, fruit flavor. Alcohol, sugar, and dye free. Syrup. Bot. 237 mL, 473 mL. *c-III.*

Use: Upper respiratory combination, antitussive, expectorant.

Hydrocodone HD. (Morton Grove) Hydrocodone bitartrate 1.67 mg, phenylephrine hydrochloride 5 mg, chlorpheniramine maleate 2 mg per 5 mL. Sugar, menthol, parabens, cherry flavor, alcohol free. Liq. Bot. 236 mL, 473 mL. *c-III.*

Use: Upper respiratory combination, antihistamine, decongestant, antitussive.

•**hydrocodone polistirex.** (high-droe-KOE-dohn pahl-ee-STIE-rex) USAN.

Tall Man: HYDROcodone

Use: Antitussive.

W/Chlorpheniramine Maleate.

See: Tussionex Pennkinetic.

hydrocodone resin complex.

Use: Antitussive.

W/Phenyltoloxamine Resin Complex.

See: Tussionex.

Hydrocof-HC. (Morton Grove) Hydrocodone bitartrate 3 mg, chlorpheniramine maleate 2 mg, pseudoephedrine hydrochloride 15 mg per 5 mL. Sugar, alcohol, and dye free. Saccharin, sorbitol. Grape flavor. Liq. 473 mL. *c-III.*

Use: Antitussive combination.

hydrocortamate hydrochloride. 17-Hydroxycorticosterone-21-diethylaminoacetate hydrochloride.

Use: Anti-inflammatory, topical.

•**hydrocortisone.** (HIGH-droe-CORE-tih-sone) *USP.*

Use: Anti-inflammatory, topical; corticosteroid, topical.

See: Acticort Lotion 100.

Aveeno Active Naturals Hydrocortisone.

Balneol For Her.Caldecort.

Cetacort.

Colocort.

Cort-Dome.

Cortef.

Cortisone•10 Anti-Itch.

Cortisone•10 Children's Cooling Cream.

Cortisone•10 Cooling Relief Anti-Itch.

Cortisone•10 Easy Relief Applicatory Anti-Itch.

Cortisone•10 Hydratensive Anti-Itch.

Cortisone•10 Intensive Healing Eczema.

Cortisone•10 Intensive Healing Formula Anti-Itch.

Cortisone•10 Plus Ultra Moisturizing.

Cortisone•10 Poison Ivy Relief Pads.

Cortizone-10 Quickshot.

Dermacort.

Dermasorb HC.

Dermolate.

Dermol HC.

Eldecort.

HC Derma-Pax.

Hi-Cor 1.0.

Hi-Cor 2.5.

Hycort.

Hycortole.

Hydroskin.
Hytone.
Ivy Soothe.
Ivy Stat.
Noble Formula HC.
Proctocort.
Recort Plus.
Scalacort.
Scalpicin.
Synacort.
Texacort.
T/Scalp.
W/Acyclovir.
See: Xerese.
W/Benzalkonium Chloride, Chloroxylenol, Pramoxine Hydrochloride.
See: Cortic-ND.
Mediotic-HC.
W/Benzoyl Peroxide.
See: Vanoxide-HC.
W/Chloroxylenol, Pramoxine Hydrochloride.
See: Oto-End 10.
Otomar-HC.
Pramoxine-HC.
Zoto-HC.
W/Ciprofloxacin.
See: Cipro HC Otic.
W/Clioquinol.
See: Dermasorb AF.
Hysone.
W/Clioquinol, Pramoxine Hydrochloride.
See: 1 + 1-F Creme.
W/Colistin, Neomycin, Thonzonium.
See: Coly-Mycin S Otic.
Cortisporin-TC Otic.
W/Diphenhydramine Hydrochloride, Nystatin.
See: First Duke's Mouthwash.
W/Diphenhydramine Hydrochloride, Nystatin, Tetracycline Hydrochloride.
See: First Mary's Mouthwash.
W/Ketoconazole.
See: Xolegel CorePak.
W/Oxytetracycline Hydrochloride.
See: Terra-Cortril.
W/Pramoxine Hydrochloride.
See: Cortane-B.

hydrocortisone. (Major) Hydrocortisone 10 mg. Tab. 100s. *Rx.*
Use: Adrenocortical steroid, glucocorticoid.

hydrocortisone. (Pharmacia) Micronized nonsterile powder for prescription compounding.
Use: Anti-inflammatory, topical; corticosteroid, topical.

hydrocortisone. (Various Mfr.) Hydrocortisone 2.5%, may contain stearyl alcohol, cetyl alcohol, light mineral oil. Lot. Bot. 59 mL. *Rx.*
Use: Anti-inflammatory, corticosteroid, topical.

hydrocortisone. (Various Mfr.) Hydrocortisone 5 mg, 20 mg. May contain lactose. Tab. **5 mg:** 10s, 50s, 100s, 1,000s. **20 mg:** 100s. *Rx.*
Use: Adrenocortical steroid, glucocorticoid.

•**hydrocortisone acetate.** (HYE-droe-KOR-ti-sone) *USP.*
Use: Glucocorticoid.
See: AlcortinA.
Anucort-HC.
Anuprep HC.
Anusol-HC.
Cortifoam.
Gynecort.
Hemril-HC Uniserts.
Keratol HC.
NuCort.
Proctocort.
Rectacort-HC.
Tucks Ointment.
U-cort.
W/Bacitracin Zinc, Neomycin Sulfate, Polymyxin B Sulfate.
See: Coracin.
W/Benzocaine, Chloroxylenol.
See: TriOxin.
W/Colistin Sulfate, Neomycin Sulfate, Thonzonium Bromide.
See: Coly-Mycin S.
Cortisporin-TC.
W/Iodoquinol.
See: Hydro-Iodoquinol 2-1.
Vytone.
W/Lidocaine.
See: Lida-Mantle HC.
LidoCort.
Xyralid.
Xyralid RC.
W/Neomycin Sulfate, Polymyxin B Sulfate.
See: Cortisporin.
W/Pramoxine Hydrochloride.
See: Analpram-E.
EndaRoid.
Epifoam.
HC Pram 1%
HC Pramoxine.
HC Pram 2.5%.
Novacort.
PramCort.
Pram-HCA.
Pramosone.
Pramosone E.
ProCort.
Proctofoam-HC.
Zypram.
W/Urea.
See: Carmol HC.

hydrocortisone acetate. (Pharmacia) Micronized nonsterile powder for prescription compounding.
Use: Anti-inflammatory, topical; corticosteroid, topical.

hydrocortisone acetate. (Various Mfr.) Hydrocortisone acetate 25 mg. Supp. 12s, 24s. *Rx.*
Use: Anorectal preparation.

hydrocortisone acetate maximum strength. (Clay-Park) Hydrocortisone acetate 1% (equiv. to hydrocortisone 10 mg/g), aloe extract, white petrolatum. Oint. Tube 28 g. *OTC.*
Use: Anti-inflammatory, corticosteroid, topical.

hydrocortisone acetate/pramoxine hydrochloride. (Various Mfr.) Hydrocortisone acetate 2.5%, pramoxine hydrochloride 1%. Alcohols, mineral oil, parabens, triethanolamine, PEG, potassium sorbate, white petrolatum. Cream. 28 g, 57 g. *Rx.*
Use: Topical corticosteroid combination.

hydrocortisone acetate 2.5% with pramoxine hydrochloride 1%. (Brookstone) Hydrocortisone acetate 2.5%, pramoxine hydrochloride 1%. Cetostearyl alcohol, lanolin alcohol, mineral oil, parabens, PEG-40, white petrolatum. Cream. 4 g. *Rx.*
Use: Topical corticosteroid, corticosteroid combination.

hydrocortisone acetate with aloe. (River's Edge) Hydrocortisone acetate 2%. Aloe, benzyl alcohol, camphor, cetyl alcohol, dimethicone, glycerin, menthol, PEG-7, triethanolamine. Lot. 59.14 mL. *Rx.*
Use: Anti-inflammatory agent, topical corticosteroid.

hydrocortisone and acetic acid. (Taro) Hydrocortisone 1%, acetic acid 2%, propylene glycol diacetate 3%, sodium acetate 0.015%, benzethonium chloride 0.02%. Citric acid 0.2%. Otic Soln. 10 mL dropper tip bottle. *Rx.*
Use: Otic preparation.

hydrocortisone and acetic acid otic solution.
Use: Anti-inflammatory, otic.

hydrocortisone and iodoquinol 1%. (Various Mfr.) Hydrocortisone 1%, iodoquinol 1%, may contain cetearyl alcohol, EDTA. Cream. Tube 30 g. *Rx.*
Use: Anti-inflammatory, corticosteroid, topical.

•**hydrocortisone butyrate.** (HIGH-droe-CORE-tih-sone) *USP.*
Use: Corticosteroid, topical.
See: Locoid.

hydrocortisone butyrate. (Taro) Hydrocortisone butyrate. **Cream:** 0.1%. 5 g, 10 g, 15 g, 30 g, 45 g. **Oint.:** 0.1%. 5 g, 10 g, 15 g, 30 g, 45 g. **Soln.:** 0.1%. Isopropyl alcohol 50%, glycerin. 20 mL, 60 mL. *Rx.*
Use: Anti-inflammatory agent.

•**hydrocortisone cypionate.** (HIGH-droe-CORE-tih-sone) *USP.* Oral Susp.
Use: Corticosteroid, topical.

hydrocortisone diethylaminoacetate hydrochloride.
See: Hydrocortamate.

•**hydrocortisone hemisuccinate.** (HIGH-droe-CORE-tih-sone hem-ih-SUCK-sih-nate) *USP.*
Use: Adrenocortical steroid.

hydrocortisone intravenous.
See: A-Hydro Cort.
Solu-Cortef.

hydrocortisone/iodochlorhydroxyquin. (Various Mfr.) **Cream:** Hydrocortisone 0.5%, 3%, iodochlorhydroxyquin 3%. 15 g, 30 g, 480 g. **Oint.:** Hydrocortisone 1%, iodochlorhydroxyquin 3%. 20 g, 30 g. *Rx-OTC.*
Use: Corticosteroid, topical.

hydrocortisone-neomycin. (Various Mfr.) Hydrocortisone 1%, neomycin sulfate 0.5%. Oint. 20 g. *Rx-OTC.*
Use: Corticosteroid, topical.

hydrocortisone phosphate.
See: Hydrocortone Phosphate.

•**hydrocortisone probutate.** (HYE-droe-KOR-ti-sone proe-BUE-tate) USAN.
Use: Atopic dermatitis (glucocorticoid).
See: Pandel.

•**hydrocortisone sodium phosphate.** (HIGH-droe-CORE-tih-sone) *USP.*
Use: Adrenocortical steroid (anti-inflammatory); corticosteroid, topical.

•**hydrocortisone sodium succinate.** (HIGH-droe-CORE-tih-sone) *USP.*
Use: Adrenocortical steroid (anti-inflammatory); corticosteroid, topical.
See: A-hydroCort.
Solu-Cortef.

•**hydrocortisone valerate.** (HIGH-droe-CORE-tih-sone VAL-eh-rate) *USP.*
Use: Corticosteroid, topical.
See: Westcort.

hydrocortisone valerate. (Copley) Hydrocortisone valerate 0.2% in hydrophilic base, white petrolatum, alcohol. Cream. Tube 15 g, 45 g, 60 g. *Rx.*
Use: Corticosteroid, topical.

hydrocortisone valerate. (Taro) Hydrocortisone valerate 0.2% in hydrophilic base, white petrolatum, alcohol, mineral

oil. Oint. Tube 15 g, 45 g, 60 g. *Rx.*
Use: Corticosteroid, topical.

hydrocortisone with aloe. (G & W Labs) Hydrocortisone 1%. Aloe, mineral oil, white petrolatum, parabens. Oint. 28.4 g. *OTC.*
Use: Anti-inflammatory agent.

Hydrocream Base. (Paddock) Petrolatum, mineral oil, woolwax alcohol, imidazolidinyl urea, methyl- and propylparabens. Cream. Jar lb.
Use: Emollient.

HydroDIURIL. (Merck) Hydrochlorothiazide 25 mg. Lactose. Tab. Bot. 100s, 1000s. *Rx.*
Use: Diuretic.

Hydro-D Tablets. (Halsey Drug) Hydrochlorothiazide. 25 mg, 50 mg. Tab. Bot. 1000s. *Rx.*
Use: Diuretic.

Hydro-Ergot. (Henry Schein) Hydrogenated ergot alkaloids 0.5 mg, 1 mg. Tab. Bot. 100s. *Rx.*
Use: Psychotherapeutic agent.

•**hydrofilcon A.** (HIGH-droe-FILL-kahn A) USAN.
Use: Contact lens material (hydrophilic).

•**hydroflumethiazide.** (HIGH-droe-flew-meth-EYE-ah-zide) *USP.*
Use: Antihypertensive; diuretic.

Hydro 40. (Quinnova) Urea 40%. Glycerin, parabens. Aerosol Foam. 70 g. *Rx.*
Use: Emollient.

hydrogen dioxide.
See: Hydrogen Peroxide.

hydrogen iodide.
Use: Expectorant.
See: Hydriodic Acid.

•**hydrogen peroxide concentrate.** (HIGH-droe-jen per-OX-ide) *USP.*
Use: Anti-infective, topical.

hydrogen peroxide solution 30%. Perhydrol, hydrogen peroxide. Bot. 0.25 lb, 0.5 lb, 1 lb.
Use: Dentistry, preparing the 3% solution.

hydrogen peroxide topical solution. (Various Mfr.) Hydrogen peroxide (3%). Bot. 4 oz, 8 oz, pt.
Use: Anti-infective, topical.

Hydrogesic. (Edwards) Hydrocodone bitartrate 5 mg, acetaminophen 500 mg. Cap. Bot. 100s. *c-III.*
Use: Analgesic combination, narcotic.

Hydro-Iodoquinol 2-1. (Seton Pharmaceuticals) Hydrocortisone acetate 2%, iodoquinol 1%. Aloe polysaccharide 1%, amino methylpropanol 95%, benzyl alcohol, glycerin, glyceryl, propylene glycol, SD alcohol. Gel. Packettes. 2 g. *Rx.*
Use: Anti-inflammatory agent, topical corticosteroid.

Hydroloid-G Sublingual. (Major) Ergoloid mesylates 0.5 mg, 1 mg. Tab. Bot. 100s, 250s, 500s (0.5 mg only), 1000s (1 mg only), UD 100s. *Rx.*
Use: Psychotherapeutic agent.

Hydroloid-G Tabs. (Major) Ergoloid mesylates 1 mg. Tab. Bot. 100s, 250s, 1000s, UD 100s. *Rx.*
Use: Psychotherapeutic agent.

Hydromet. (Alpharma) Hydrocodone bitartrate 5 mg, homatropine methylbromide 1.5 mg per 5 mL. Saccharin, sucrose, methylparaben, cherry flavor. Syr. Bot. 473 mL, 3.8 L. *c-III.*
Use: Upper respiratory combination, antitussive combination.

Hydromide. (Major) Hydrocodone bitartrate 5 mg, homatropine methylbromide 1.5 mg per 5 mL. Alcohol < 0.1%, cherry flavor. Syrup. Bot. 473 mL. *c-III.*
Use: Upper respiratory combination, antitussive combination.

hydromorphone. *c-II.*
Tall Man: HYDROmorphone
Use: Analgesic, narcotic.

•**hydromorphone hydrochloride.** (HIGH-droe-MORE-phone) *USP. Formerly Dihydromorphinone Hydrochloride.*
Tall Man: HYDROmorphone
Use: Opioid analgesic.
See: Dilaudid.
Dilaudid-HP.

hydromorphone hydrochloride. (Paddock) Hydromorphone hydrochloride 3 mg. May contain cocoa butter. Supp. Box 6s. *c-II.*
Use: Opioid analgesic.

hydromorphone hydrochloride. (Various Mfr.) Hydromorphone hydrochloride. **Tab.:** 2 mg, 4 mg, 8 mg. 100s, 500s (4 mg only), UD 100s (except 8 mg). **Inj., Soln.:** 1 mg/mL, 2 mg/mL, 4 mg/mL. Preservative free. 1 mL amp. 1 mL and 20 mL vials (2 mg/mL only). 1 mL single-dose prefilled syringe (except 4 mg/mL). **Inj., Soln., Conc.:** 10 mg/mL. Preservative free. Single-dose vials. 1 mL, 5 mL, 50 mL. 1 mL and 5 mL amps. **Liq.:** 1 mg/1 mL. May contain parabens, saccharin, sodium metabisulfite. 473 mL. *c-II.*
Use: Opioid analgesic.

hydromorphone sulfate.
Use: Analgesic, narcotic.

Hydropane. (Watson) Hydrocodone bitartrate 5 mg, homatropine methylbromide 1.5 mg per 5 mL. Parabens, sucrose, cherry flavor. Syrup. Bot. 473 mL, 3.8 L.

c-III.
Use: Upper respiratory combination, antitussive combination.

Hydro-Par. (Parmed) Hydrochlorothiazide 25 mg, 50 mg. Tab. 1000s, 5000s (50 mg only). *Rx.*
Use: Diuretic.

Hydropel. (C & M Pharmacal) Silicone 30%, hydrophobic starch derivative 10%, petrolatum. Jar 2 oz, lb. *OTC.*
Use: Emollient.

Hydrophed. (Rugby) Theophylline 130 mg, ephedrine sulfate 25 mg, hydroxyzine hydrochloride 10 mg. Tab. Bot. 100s, 1000s. *Rx.*
Use: Antiasthmatic combination.

hydrophilic ointment. (E. Fougera) Stearyl alcohol, white petrolatum, propylene glycol, sodium lauryl sulfate, water. Jar lb.
Use: Pharmaceutic aid, ointment base.

hydrophilic ointment base. (Emerson) Oil in water emulsion bases. 1 lb.
Use: Pharmaceutic aid, ointment base.
See: Aquaphilic.
Cetaphil.
Dermovan.
Lanaphilic.
Polysorb.
Unibase.

Hydrophor. (Geritrex) Petrolatum 42%, lanolin alcohol, mineral oil, wax. Oint. 228 g. *OTC.*
Use: Skin protectant.

Hydropine. (Rugby) Hydroflumethiazide 25 mg, reserpine 0.125 mg. Tab. Bot. 100s. *Rx.*
Use: Antihypertensive combination.

Hydropine H.P. Tablets. (Rugby) Hydroflumethiazide 50 mg, reserpine 0.125 mg. Bot. 100s, 500s, 1000s. *Rx.*
Use: Antihypertensive combination.

•**hydroquinone.** (high-DROE-KWIN-ohn) *USP.*
Use: Depigmentor.
See: Aclaro PD.
Artra Skin Tone, Cream.
Black and White Bleaching.
Eldopaque.
Eldopaque Forte.
Eldoquin Forte.
EpiQuin Micro.
Esoterica.
Glyquin.
Lustra.
Lustra-AF.
Melpaque HP.
Melquin HP.
Nuquin HP.
Solaquin.

W/Fluocinolone Acetonide, Tretinoin.
See: Tri-Luma.

hydroquinone. (Glades) Hydroquinone. **Gel:** 3%, 4%. Padimate O, dioxybenzone, EDTA, sodium metabisulfite, alcohol (4% only), hydroalcoholic base. 30 g (3% only), 28.35 g (4% only). **Soln.:** 3%, SD Alcohol 40-B, isopropyl alcohol. 29 mL with applicator. *Rx.*
Use: Depigmentor.

hydroquinone. (River's Edge) Hydroquinone 4%. Benzyl alcohol, cetyl alcohol, EDTA. Emulsion, Top. 48 g. *Rx.*
Use: Depigmentor.

hydroquinone. (Various Mfr.) Hydroquinone 4%. May contain EDTA, parabens, mineral oil, sodium metabisulfite. Cream 28.35 g. *Rx.*
Use: Depigmentor.

hydroquinone monobenzyl ether.
See: Benoquin.

hydroquinone with sunscreen. (Various Mfr.) Hydroquinone 4%. May contain padimate O, dioxybenzone, oxybenzone, octyl methoxycinnamate, octyl dimethyl-p-aminobenzoate, cetearyl alcohol, vitamin E, parabens, mineral oil, stearyl alcohol, lactic acid, EDTA, sodium metabisulfite. Cream 28.35 g. *Rx.*
Use: Depigmentor.

Hydrosal. (Hydrosal Co.) Aluminum acetate 5%. **Susp.:** Bot. 16 oz, gal. **Oint.:** 54 g, 113.4 g, Jar 54 g, 454 g. *OTC.*
Use: Astringent.

Hydrosine 50. (Major) Hydrochlorothiazide 50 mg, reserpine 0.125 mg. Tab. Bot. 100s. *Rx.*
Use: Antihypertensive combination.

Hydrosine 25. (Major) Hydrochlorothiazide 25 mg, reserpine 0.125 mg. Tab. Bot. 100s. Tartrazine. *Rx.*
Use: Antihypertensive combination.

HydroSKIN. (Rugby) Hydrocortisone 1%. **Cream:** Mineral oil, lanolin alcohol, cetyl alcohol, parabens. 113.4 g. **Lot.:** Cetyl alcohol, parabens. 118 mL. *OTC.*
Use: Anti-inflammatory, corticosteroid, topical.

Hydro-T. (Major) Hydrochlorothiazide 25 mg, 50 mg, 100 mg. Tab. Bot. 100s, 250s (100 mg only), 1000s, UD 100s. *Rx.*
Use: Diuretic.

Hydrotensin. (Merz) Hydrochlorothiazide 50 mg, reserpine 0.125 mg. Tab. Bot. 100s, 1000s. *Rx.*
Use: Antihypertensive combination.

Hydro 35. (Quinnova) Urea 35%. Dimethicone, glycerin, lactic acid, parabens. Aer. Foam. 150 g. *Rx.*
Use: Emollient.

Hydro-12. (Table Rock) Crystalline hydroxocobalamin 1000 mcg/mL. Pkg. 10 mL. *Rx.*
Use: Vitamin supplement.

•**hydroxocobalamin.** (high-DROX-oh-koe-BAL-ah-meen) *USP.*
Use: Treatment of megaloblastic anemia; vitamin (hematopoietic); detoxification agent, antidote.
See: Cyanokit.

•**hydroxyamphetamine hydrobromide.** (high-DROX-ee-am-FET-uh-meen) *USP.*
Use: Adrenergic (ophthalmic); mydriatic.

2-hydroxybenzamide.
See: Salicylamide.

hydroxy bis (acetato-O) aluminum. Aluminum Subacetate.

hydroxy bis (salicylato) aluminum diacetate.
See: Aluminum Aspirin.

hydroxybutyrate, sodium/gamma.
See: Sodium Gamma-Hydroxybutyrate Acid.

•**hydroxychloroquine sulfate.** (high-drox-ee-KLOR-oh-kwin) *USP.*
Use: Antimalarial; lupus erythematosus suppressant; antirheumatic agent.
See: Plaquenil.

hydroxychloroquine sulfate. (Various Mfr.) Hydroxychloroquine sulfate 200 mg. Tab. 100s, 180s, 500s, UD 100s. *Rx.*
Use: Antirheumatic agent.

hydroxycholecalciferol. (D_3).
Use: Antihypocalcemia.
See: Calcifediol.

•**hydroxyethyl cellulose.** (high-drox-ee-ETH-ill SELL-you-lohs) *NF.*
Use: Pharmaceutic aid (suspending, viscosity-increasing agent).

•**hydroxyethyl starch 130/0.4.** (hye-DROX-ee-ETH-il stahrch) USAN.
Use: Plasma volume expander; prevention of hypervolemia.
See: Hespan.
Voluven.

hydroxyisoindolin. Under study.
Use: Antihypertensive.

hydroxymagnesium aluminate.
Use: Antacid.
See: Magaldrate.

hydroxymycin. An antibiotic substance obtained from cultures of *Streptomyces paucisporogenes.*

•**hydroxyphenamate.** (high-DROX-ee-FEN-ah-mate) USAN.
Use: Anxiolytic.

4-hydroxyphenylpyruvate dioxygenase inhibitor.
Use: Tyrosinemia.
See: Nitisinone.

•**hydroxyprogesterone caproate.** (hye-DROX-ee-proe-JES-ter-one KAP-roe-ate) *USP.*
Use: Sex hormone, progestin.
See: Makena.

•**hydroxypropyl cellulose.** (high-drox-ee-PRO-pill SELL-you-lohs) *NF.*
Use: Topical protectant; pharmaceutic aid, emulsifying tablet-coating agent.

hydroxypropyl methylcellulose.
See: Goniosoft.
Hypromellose.

•**hydroxypropyl methylcellulose phthalate.** (high-drox-ee-PRO-pill) *NF.*
Use: Pharmaceutic aid (coating agent).
See: Hypromellose Phthalate.

hydroxypropyl methylcellulose phthalate 200731.
Use: Pharmaceutic aid (coating agent).

hydroxypropyl methylcellulose phthalate 220824.
Use: Pharmaceutic aid (coating agent).

hydroxystearin sulfate. Sulfonate hydrogenated castor oil.

L-5-hydroxytryptophan. (Circa) L-5HTP.
Use: Postanoxic intention myoclonus. [Orphan Drug]

•**hydroxyurea.** (high-DROX-ee-you-REE-uh) *USP.*
Use: Antineoplastic; sickle cell disease.
See: Droxia.
Hydrea.

hydroxyurea. (Various Mfr.) Hydroxyurea 500 mg. Cap. Bot. 100s, UD 100s. *Rx.*
Use: Antineoplastic.

•**hydroxyzine.** (high-DROX-ih-zeen) *USP.*
Tall Man: hydrOXYzine
Use: Anxiolytic; antihistamine, nonselective piperazine.
See: Vistaril.
W/Ephedrine Sulfate, Theophylline.
See: Marax.
Marax DF.
Theo-Drox.

hydroxyzine. (Various Mfr.) Hydroxyzine. **Tab.:** 10 mg, 25 mg, 50 mg. Bot. 100s, 500s, 1000s. **Syrup:** 10 mg/5 mL. May contain alcohol. 118 mL, 473 mL. *Rx.*
Use: Antihistamine, nonselective piperazine; anxiolytic.

hydroxyzine hydrochloride. (Various Mfr.) Hydroxyzine hydrochloride 25 mg/mL, 50 mg/mL. May contain benzyl alcohol. Vials. 1 mL, 2 mL, 10 mL (50 mg/mL only). *Rx.*
Use: Antihistamine.

•**hydroxyzine pamoate.** (hye-DROX-i-zeen PAM-oh-ate) *USP.*
Tall Man: hydrOXYzine

Use: Tranquilizer (minor); antihistamine.
See: Vistaril.

hydroxyzine pamoate. (Various Mfr.) Hydroxyzine pamoate 25 mg, 50 mg, 100 mg (equivalent to hydrochloride). Cap. 100s, 500s, 1000s, UD 100s (except 100 mg). *Rx.*
Use: Antihistamine, nonselective piperazine; anxiolytic.

Hydro-Z-50. (Merz) Hydrochlorothiazide 50 mg. Tab. Bot. 100s, 1000s. *Rx.*
Use: Diuretic.

Hy-Flow Solution. (Ciba Vision) Polyvinyl alcohol with hydroxyethylcellulose, benzalkonium Cl, EDTA. Bot. 60 mL. *OTC.*
Use: Contact lens care.

HyGel. (Aletheia) Sodium hyaluronate 0.2%. Parabens. Spray; topical. 340 mL. *Rx.*
Use: Physical adjunct; hyaluronic acid derivative, dermal.

Hygienic Cleansing. (Rugby) Witch hazel 50%, glycerin, benzalkonium Cl, methylparaben. Pads 100s. *OTC.*
Use: Anorectal preparation.

hylan polymers.
See: Synvisc.
Synvisc-One.

Hylase Wound. (ECR Pharmaceuticals) Sodium hyaluronate 2.5%. Methylparaben, PEG. Gel. 75 g. *Rx.*
Use: Physical adjunct; hyaluronic acid derivative, dermal.

Hylatopic. (Onset Dermatologics) Cetearyl alcohol, disodium EDTA, glycerin, petrolatum, parabens, theobroma gradiflorum seed butter. Foam. 100 g. *Rx.*
Use: Emollient.

Hylatopic Plus. (Onset Dermatologics) Cetearyl alcohol, dimethicone, disodium EDTA, glycerin, parabens, petrolatum, propylene glycol, sodium hyaluronate. Cream. 100 g. *Rx.*
Use: Emollient.

Hylenex. (Baxter Anesthesia) Hyaluronidase (recombinant human) 150 units/mL. Sodium chloride 8.5 mg, sodium phosphate dibasic dihydrate 1.8 mg, sodium hydroxide 4.2 mg, human serum albumin 1 mg, EDTA 1 mg, calcium chloride dihydrate 0.4 mg. Soln. for Inj. Single-dose vials. 1 mL. *Rx.*
Use: Physical adjunct.

Hylidone. (Major) Chlorthalidone. Tab. **25 mg, 50 mg:** Bot. 100s, 250s, 1000s, UD 100s. **100 mg:** Bot. 100s, 250s, 500s, 1000s. *Rx.*
Use: Diuretic.

Hylira. (Hawthorn) Hyaluronic acid 0.2%. Parabens. Top. Spray. 113 g, 340 g. *Rx.*
Use: Physical adjunct.

Hyliver Plus. (Hyrex) Folic acid 0.4 mg, liver 10 mcg, vitamin B_{12} 100 mcg/mL. Vial 10 mL with phenol. *Rx.*
Use: Vitamin supplement.

•**hymecromone.** (HIGH-meh-KROE-mone) USAN.
Use: Choleretic.

hymenoptera venom/venom protein. Purified venoms of honeybee, wasp, white faced hornet, yellow hornet, yellow jacket, and mixed vespids (both hornets and yellow jackets). *Rx.*
Use: Allergenic extract.
See: Albay.
Venomil.

•**hymetellose.** (hye-ME-tel-lose) *NF.*
Use: Pharmaceutic aid.

HY-N.B.P. Ointment. (Jones Pharma) Bacitracin zinc 400 units, neomycin sulfate 5 mg, polymyxin B sulfate 10,000 units/g. Tube ⅛ oz. *Rx.*
Use: Anti-infective, topical.

HyoMax. (Aristos) Hyoscyamine sulfate 0.125 mg. Lactose, mannitol. Tab. 100s. *Rx.*
Use: Gastrointestinal anticholinergic/antispasmodic, belladonna alkaloid.

Hyomax-DT. (Aristos) Hyoscyamine sulfate 0.375 mg (biphasic tablet formulated to release hyoscyamine 0.125 mg as immediate release and hyoscyamine 0.25 mg as extended release). Lactose. ER Tab. 90s. *Rx.*
Use: Gastrointestinal anticholinergic/antispasmodic, belladonna alkaloid.

HyoMax-FT. (Aristos) Hyoscyamine sulfate 125 mg. Lactose, mannitol. Mint flavor. Tab. 100s. *Rx.*
Use: Gastrointestinal anticholinergic/antispasmodic, belladonna alkaloid.

Hyomax-SL. (Aristos) Hyoscyamine sulfate 0.125 mg. Lactose, mannitol. Peppermint flavor. Tab., sublingual. 100s. *Rx.*
Use: Gastrointestinal anticholinergic/antispasmodic, belladonna alkaloid.

Hyomax-SR. (Aristos) Hyoscyamine sulfate 0.375 mg. Lactose. ER Tab. 100s. *Rx.*
Use: Gastrointestinal anticholinergic/antispasmodic, belladonna alkaloid.

Hyophen. (BioComp Pharma) Benzoic acid 9 mg, hyoscyamine sulfate 0.12 mg, methenamine 81.6 mg, methylene blue 10.8 mg, phenyl salicylate 36.2 mg. PEG. Tab. 100s. *Rx.*
Use: Anti-infective, methenamine combination.

hyoscine hydrobromide. Scopolamine HBr.

Use: Antispasmodic.
W/Combinations.
See: Phenazopyridine Plus.
Pyridium Plus.
W/Butalbital, Phenazopyridine Hydrochloride.
See: PhenazoForte Plus.
•**hyoscyamine.** (high-oh-SIGH-ah-meen) *USP.*
Use: Anticholinergic.
See: Cystospaz.
hyoscyamine-atropine-hyoscine.
Use: Anticholinergic.
See: Atropine w/hyoscyamine w/hyoscine.
•**hyoscyamine hydrobromide.** (HYE-oh-SYE-a-meen) *USP.*
Use: Anticholinergic.
W/Atropine Sulfate, Phenobarbital, Scopolamine Hydrobromide.
See: PB-Hyos.
Se-Donna PB Hyos.
W/Butabarbital, Phenazopyridine Hydrochloride.
See: Phenazopyridine Plus.
hyoscyamine hydrochloride. (Various Mfr.)
hyoscyamine salts.
Use: Anticholinergic.
W/Atropine salts.
See: Atropine w/hyoscyamine.
•**hyoscyamine sulfate.** (HYE-oh-SYE-a-meen) *USP.*
Use: Anticholinergic.
See: ED-Spaz.
HyoMax.
HyoMax-DT.
HyoMax-FT.
HyoMax-SL.
HyoMax-SR.
Hyosyne.
Levbid.
Levsin.
Levsin/SL.
Mar-Spas.
NuLev.
Oscimin.
Oscimin SR.
Symax Duotab.
Symax FasTab.
Symax-SL.
Symax-SR.
W/Atropine Sulfate, Benzoic Acid, Methenamine, Methylene Blue, Phenyl Salicylate.
See: Uritact DS.
W/Atropine Sulfate, Chlorpheniramine Maleate, Phenylephrine Hydrochloride, Scopolamine Hydrobromide.
See: Bellahist-D LA.
W/Atropine Sulfate, Chlorpheniramine Maleate, Pseudoephedrine Hydrochloride, Scopolamine Hydrobromide.
See: Stahist.
W/Atropine Sulfate, Phenobarbital, Scopolamine Hydrobromide.
See: Antispasmodic.
Donnatal.
Donnatal Extentabs.
PB-Hyos.
Quadrapax.
Se-Donna PB Hyos.
W/Benzoic Acid, Methenamine, Methylene Blue, Phenyl Salicylate.
See: Hyophen.
W/Methenamine, Methylene Blue, Phenyl Salicylate, Sodium Biphosphate.
See: Urimax.
W/Methenamine, Methylene Blue, Phenyl Salicylate, Sodium Phosphate Monobasic.
See: Phosphasal.
Uticap.
Ultrona-C.
W/Methenamine, Methylene Blue, Sodium Phosphate Monobasic.
See: Uryl.
W/Phenyltoloxamine Citrate.
See: Digex NF.
hyoscyamine sulfate. (Ethex) Hyoscyamine sulfate 0.375 mg. ER Cap. Bot. 100s. *Rx.*
Use: Anticholinergic.
hyoscyamine sulfate. (Franklin Pharmaceuticals) Hyoscyamine sulfate 0.125 mg. Lactose, mannitol. Tab. 100s. *Rx.*
Use: Gastrointestinal anticholinergic/antispasmodic, belladonna alkaloid.
hyoscyamine sulfate. (Goldline) Hyoscyamine sulfate 0.125 mg/mL, alcohol 5%. Soln. Bot. with dropper. 15 mL. *Rx.*
Use: Anticholinergic.
hyoscyamine sulfate. (River's Edge Pharmaceuticals) Hyoscyamine sulfate 0.125 mg (immediate release), hyoscyamine 0.25 mg (controlled release). Tab. 90s. *Rx.*
Use: Gastrointestinal anticholinergic/antispasmodic, belladonna alkaloid.
hyoscyamine sulfate. (Various Mfr.) Hyoscyamine sulfate. **Tab.:** 0.125 mg. May contain mannitol, sucralose, xylitol. 100s. **ER Tab.:** 0.375 mg. May contain lactose. 100s. **Sublingual Tab.:** 0.125 mg. May contain mannitol, sucralose, xylitol. 100s. **Tab., disintegrating:** 0.125 mg. May contain mannitol, sucralose, xylitol. 100s. **Elix.:** 0.125 mg per 5 mL. May contain alcohol, glycerin, sorbitol, sucrose. 473 mL. **Soln.:** 0.125 mg/mL. May contain alcohol, pro-

pylene glycol, saccharin. 15 mL bottle w/calibrated dropper. *Rx.*
Use: Anticholinergic.

hyoscyamine sulfate. (Vision Pharma) Hyoscyamine sulfate 0.125 mg. Aspartame, mannitol, phenylalanine 2.2 mg. Mint flavor. Tab. 90s, 100s. *Rx.*
Use: Gastrointestinal anticholinergic/antispasmodic, belladonna alkaloid.

hyoscyamine sulfate ODT. (Various Mfr.) Hyoscyamine sulfate 0.125 mg. May contain lactose, mannitol. Tab., chewable/dispersible. 100s, 500s. *Rx.*
Use: Gastrointestinal anticholinergic/antispasmodic, belladonna alkaloid.

hyoscyamus extract.
W/A.P.C.
See: Valacet Junior.
W/A.P.C., gelsemium extract.
See: Valacet.

hyoscyamus products and phenobarbital combinations.
Use: Anticholinergic, sedative.
See: Anaspaz PB.
Donnatal.
Elixiral.

Hyosophen Elixir. (Rugby) Atropine sulfate 0.0194 mg, scopolamine HBr 0.0065 mg, hyoscyamine HBr or sulfate 0.1037 mg, phenobarbital 16.2 mg, alcohol 23%, sugar, sorbitol. Bot. 120 mL, pt, gal. *Rx.*
Use: Gastrointestinal, anticholinergic.

Hyosophen Tablets. (Rugby) Atropine sulfate 0.0194 mg, scopolamine HBr 0.0065 mg, hyoscyamine HBr or SO_4 0.1037 mg, phenobarbital 16.2 mg. Bot. 1000s. *Rx.*
Use: Anticholinergic combination.

Hyosyne. (Silarx) Hyoscyamine sulfate 0.125 mg/mL. Alcohol 5%, glycerin, sodium benzoate, sorbitol, sucrose. Orange flavor. **Elix.:** 473 mL. **Soln.:** 15 mL bottle w/calibrated dropper. *Rx.*
Use: Gastrointestinal anticholinergic/antispasmodic, belladonna alkaloid.

Hypaque-M 90%. (Sanofi-Synthelabo) Diatrizoate meglumine 60%, diatrizoate sodium 30%, EDTA. Vial 50 mL.
Use: Radiopaque agent.

Hypaque-M 75%. (Sanofi-Synthelabo) Diatrizoate meglumine 50%, diatrizoate sodium 25%, iodine 38.5%, EDTA. Vial 20 mL, 50 mL.
Use: Radiopaque agent.

Hypaque Oral. (Sanofi-Synthelabo) **Pow.:** Diatrizoate sodium oral pow. containing iodine 600 mg/g. Can 250 g, Bot. 10 g. **Liq.:** Soln. 41.66%. Bot. 120 mL.
Use: Radiopaque agent.

Hypaque-76. (Nycomed) Diatrizoate meglumine 660 mg, diatrizoate sodium 100 mg, iodine 370 mg/mL. EDTA. Inj. Vials. 50 mL. Bot. 200 mL. 100 mL and 150 mL in 200 mL dilution bot. *Rx.*
Use: Radiopaque agent, parenteral.

HyperHEP B S/D. (Grifols Therapeutics) Hepatitis B immune globulin (human) 15% to 18% protein. 0.21 to 0.32 M glycine, solvent/detergent treated, preservative free. Soln. for Inj. Single-dose vials. 1 mL, 5 mL. Neonatal single-dose syringes. 0.5 mL. Single-dose syringes. 1 mL. *Rx.*
Use: Immune globulin.

hypericin. (VIMRxyn Pharm/NIH) *Rx.*
Use: Antiviral.

hyperlipidemia, agents for.
See: Atromid-S.
Choloxin.
Clofibrate.
Colestid.
Lescol.
Lopid.
Lorelco.
Mevacor.
Pravachol.
Questran.
Questran Light.
Zocor.

Hyperlyte. (B. Braun) Sodium 25 mEq, potassium 40.5 mEq, calcium 5 mEq, magnesium 8 mEq, chloride 33.5 mEq, acetate 40.6 mEq, gluconate 5 mEq, 6050 mOsm/L. Inj. Vial 25 mL fill in 50 mL. *Rx.*
Use: Nutritional supplement, parenteral.

Hyperlyte CR. (B. Braun) Sodium 25 mEq, potassium 20 mEq, calcium 5 mEq, magnesium 5 mEq, chloride 30 mEq, acetate 30 mEq, 5500 mOsm/L. Inj. Pharmacy bulk packaging. *Super-vial* 250 mL. *Rx.*
Use: Intravenous nutritional therapy, intravenous replenishment solution.

Hyperlyte R. (B. Braun) Sodium 25 mEq, potassium 20 mEq, calcium 5 mEq, magnesium 5 mEq, chloride 30 mEq, acetate 25 mEq, 4200 mOsm/L. Inj. Vial 25 mL fill in 50 mL. *Rx.*
Use: Nutritional supplement, parenteral.

Hypermune RSV. (MedImmune) Respiratory syncytial virus immune globulin, human.
Use: Respiratory syncytial virus treatment. [Orphan Drug]

Hyperopto 5%. (Professional Pharmacal) Sodium Cl 5%. Oint. Tube 3.5 g. *OTC.*
Use: Ophthalmic.

Hyperopto Ointment. (Professional Pharmacal) Sodium hydrochloride 50 mg, D.I. water 150 mg, anhydrous

lanolin 150 mg, liquid petrolatum 50 mg, white petrolatum 599 mg, methylparaben 7 mg, propylparaben 3 mg/g. Tube 3.5 g. *OTC.*
Use: Ophthalmic.

hyperosmotic agents.
Use: Laxative.
See: Cephulac.
Cholac.
Chronulac.
Colace.
Constulose.
Duphalac.
Enulose.
Fleet Babylax.
Glycerin.
Lactulose.
Sani-Supp.

HyperRab S/D. (Grifols Therapeutics) Rabies immune globulin, human, 150 units/mL. Preservative free. Glycine 0.21 to 0.32 M. Solvent/detergent treated. Inj. Single-dose vials. 2 mL, 10 mL. *Rx.*
Use: Immune globulin.

HyperRHO S/D Full Dose. (Talecris Biotherapeutics) Rh_o(D) immune globulin 15% to 18% protein (≥ 1,500 units). Glycine 0.21 to 0.32 M. Solvent/detergent treated. Preservative free. Inj., Soln. Single-dose syringe w/attached needle. 1s. *Rx.*
Use: Biologic and immunological agent, immune globulin.

HyperRHO S/D Mini-Dose. (Talecris Biotherapeutics) Rh_o(D) immune globulin micro-dose 15% to 18% protein (≥ 250 units). Glycine 0.21 to 0.32 M. Solvent/detergent treated. Preservative free. Inj., Soln. Single-dose syringe. 10s. *Rx.*
Use: Immune globulin.

hypertensive emergency agents.
See: Diazoxide.
Fenoldopam Mesylate.
Nitroprusside Sodium.

HyperTET S/D. (Talecris Biotherapeutics) Tetanus immune globulin (human) 250 units (solvent/detergent treated). Preservative free. Inj., Soln. Prefilled syringe. *Rx.*
Use: Immune globulin.

Hyphylline. Dyphylline. *Rx.*
See: Neothylline.

hypnogene.
See: Barbital.

Hypnomidate. (Janssen) Etomidate. *Rx.*
Use: Anesthetic, general.

hypnotics.
See: Sedative/Hypnotic Agents.

"hypo".
See: Sodium thiosulfate.

Hypo-Bee. (Towne) Vitamins B_1 50 mg, B_2 20 mg, B_6 5 mg, B_{12} 15 mcg, niacinamide 25 mg, calcium pantothenate 5 mg, C 300 mg, E 200 units, iron 10 mg. Tab. Bot. 30s, 100s. *OTC.*
Use: Mineral, vitamin supplement.

hypochlorite preps.
See: Antiformin.
Dakin's.
Hyclorite.

Hypoclear. (Bausch & Lomb) Isotonic soln. with sodium Cl 0.9%. Aerosol soln. 240 mL, 300 mL. *OTC.*
Use: Contact lens care.

hypoglycemic agents.
See: Chlorpropamide.
Diabeta.
Diabinese.
Dymelor.
Glucotrol.
Glynase.
Micronase.
Orinase.
Phenformin Hydrochloride.
Tolbutamide.
Tolinase.

α-hypophamine. Oxytocin.

•**hypophosphorous acid.** (high-poe-FOSS-for-uhs) *NF.*
Use: Pharmaceutic aid (antioxidant).

HypoTears Ophthalmic Liquid. (Novartis Ophthalmics) Polyvinyl alcohol 1%, PEG-400, dextrose 1%, benzalkonium Cl 0.01%, EDTA. Bot. 15 mL, 30 mL. *OTC.*
Use: Lubricant, ophthalmic.

HypoTears Ophthalmic Ointment. (Novartis Ophthalmics) White petrolatum, light mineral oil. Tube 3.5 g. *OTC.*
Use: Lubricant, ophthalmic.

hypotensive agents.
See: Antihypertensives.

•**hypromellose.** (hye-PROE-me-lose) *USP. Formerly hydroxypropyl methylcellulose.*
Use: Pharmaceutical aid (suspending agent), tablet excipient, viscosity-increasing agent.
See: Bion Tears.
Goniosol.
Gonak.
OcuCoat.
Tears Naturale Free.
Tears Naturale II.
Tears Renewed.
W/Combinations.
See: Clear Eyes Plus Redness Relief.
Isopto Plain.
Isopto Tears.
Lacril.
Tearisol.

Tears Naturale.
Ultra Tears.

Hyrexin-50. (Hyrex) Diphenhydramine hydrochloride 50 mg/mL, benzethonium chloride. Vial 10 mL. Amp. 1 mL. *Rx.*
Use: Antihistamine.

Hyscorbic Plus Tablets. (Sanofi-Synthelabo) Vitamins E 45 units, C 600 mg, folic acid 400 mcg, B_1 20 mg, B_2 10 mg, niacinamide 100 mg, B_6 10 mg, B_{12} 25 mcg, pantothenic acid 25 mg, copper 3 mg, zinc 23.9 mg. Tab. Bot. 60s. *OTC.*
Use: Mineral, vitamin supplement.

HySept. (Partrin Pharma) Sodium hypochlorite 0.25%, 0.5%. Soln.; topical. 473 mL. *OTC.*
Use: Topical anti-infective, antiseptic and germicide.

Hyserp. (Freeport) Reserpine alkaloid 0.25 mg. Tab. Bot. 1000s. *Rx.*
Use: Antihypertensive.

Hyskon. (Pharmacia) Dextran 70 32% in 10% w/v dextrose. Bot. 100 mL, 250 mL. *Rx.*
Use: Diagnostic aid. For distending the uterine cavity and irrigating and visualizing its surfaces.

Hysone. (Roberts) Clioquinol 30 mg, hydrocortisone 10 mg/g. Cream. Tube 20 g. *OTC.*
Use: Antifungal; corticosteroid, topical.

hysteroscopy fluid.
Use: Diagnostic aid.
See: Hyskon.

Hytone Cream. (Dermik) Hydrocortisone in cream base. **1%:** 1 oz. Jar 4 oz. **2.5%:** Tube 1 oz, 2 oz. *Rx-OTC.*
Use: Corticosteroid, topical.

Hytone Lotion. (Dermik) Hydrocortisone 2.5% (25 mg/mL) in lotion base. Bot. 60 mL. *Rx.*
Use: Corticosteroid, topical.

Hytone Ointment. (Dermik) Hydrocortisone in ointment base, mineral oil, white petrolatum. **1%:** Tube 28.3 g, 113.4 g. **2.5%:** Tube 28.3 g. *Rx.*
Use: Corticosteroid, topical.

Hytone Spray. (Dermik) Hydrocortisone 1%. 45 mL. *Rx.*
Use: Corticosteroid, topical.

Hytrin. (Abbott) Terazosin hydrochloride 1 mg, 2 mg, 5 mg, 10 mg, parabens. Cap. Bot. 100s, UD 100s. *Rx.*
Use: Antihypertensive, antiadrenergic.

Hyzaar. (Merck) Losartan potassium/hydrochlorothiazide 50 mg/12.5 mg (potassium 4.24 mg), 100 mg/12.5 mg (potassium 8.48 mg), 100 mg/25 mg (potassium 8.48 mg). Lactose. Tab. Bot. 30s, 90s, 1000, 5000s (except 100 mg/25 mg), 4000s (100 mg/25 mg only), UD 100s. *Rx.*
Use: Antihypertensive.

Hyzine-50. (Hyrex) Hydroxyzine hydrochloride 50 mg as hydrochloride/mL. Vial 10 mL. *Rx.*
Use: Anxiolytic.

I

•**ibafloxacin.** (ih-BAH-FLOX-ah-sin) USAN.
Use: Anti-infective.
•**ibalizumab.** (I-ba-LIZ-oo-mab) USAN.
Use: Treatment of HIV/AIDS.
ibandronate. (Various Mfr.) Ibandronate. **Inj., Soln.:** 1 mg/mL (as ibandronate sodium 3.375 mg). Single-use vial. 3 mL. **Tab.:** 150 mg (as ibandronate sodium 168.75 mg). May contain lactose, PEG. UD 1s. *Rx.*
Use: Bisphosphonate.
•**ibandronate sodium.** (ih-BAN-droe-nate) USAN.
Use: Bone resorption inhibitor; antihypercalcemic; bisphosphonate.
See: Boniva.
ibenzmethyzin. *Name used for Procarbazine Hydrochloride.*
•**iboctadekin.** (ib-OK-ta-DE-kin) USAN.
Use: Immunologic mediator.
•**ibopamine.** (EYE-BOE-pah-meen) USAN.
Use: Dopaminergic (peripheral).
•**ibritumomab tiuxetan.** (ib-ri-TYOO-momab tye-UX-e-tan) USAN.
Use: Monoclonal antibody.
See: Zevalin.
•**ibrolipim.** (ib-ROE-li-pim) USAN.
Use: Antiatherogenic; anti-obesity; antidyslipidemia; anticachexia; antidiabetes agent.
•**ibrutinib.** (eye-BROO-ti-nib) USAN.
Use: Antineoplastic.
See: Imbruvica.
Ibudone. (ProEthic Pharmaceuticals) Hydrocodone bitartrate/ibuprofen 5 mg/200 mg, 10 mg/200 mg. PEG. Film-coated. Tab. 100s. *c-III.*
Use: Narcotic analgesic.
•**ibufenac.** (eye-BYOO-feh-nak) USAN.
Use: Antirheumatic; anti-inflammatory; analgesic; antipyretic.
•**ibuprofen.** (eye-BYOO-pro-fen) *USP.*
Use: Anti-inflammatory; analgesic.
See: Advil.
Advil Migraine.
Caldolor.
Children's Advil.
Children's Motrin.
Dynafed IB.
Ibuprin.
Ibutab.
Infants' Motrin.
Junior Strength Motrin.
Menadol.
Midol Cramp & Body Aches.
Midol Maximum Strength Cramp Formula.
Motrin IB.
Motrin, Junior Strength.
Motrin Migraine Pain.
PediaCare Children's Pain Reliever Fever Reducer IB.
PediaCare Infants' Pain Reliever Fever Reducer IB.
Pediatric Advil.
Saleto.
W/Diphenhydramine Hydrochloride.
See: Advil PM.
W/Famotidine.
See: Duexis.
W/Hydrocodone Bitartrate.
See: Ibudone.
Reprexain.
Vicoprofen.
W/Pseudoephedrine Hydrochloride.
See: Advil Children's Cold.
Advil Cold & Sinus.
Children's Ibuprofen Cold.
Children's Motrin Cold.
W/Pseudoephedrine Hydrochloride, Chlorpheniramine Maleate.
See: Advil Allergy Sinus.
ibuprofen. (Perrigo) Ibuprofen 40 mg/mL. Oral Drops. Bot. 15 mL. *OTC.*
Use: Analgesic; NSAID.
ibuprofen. (Various Mfr.) Ibuprofen. **Tab.:** 200 mg, 400 mg, 600 mg, 800 mg. Bot. **200 mg:** 24s, 50s, 100s, 250s, 1000s, UD 100s. **400 mg, 600 mg, 800 mg:** 100s, 270s (600 mg, 800 mg only), 360s (400 mg only), 500s, UD 100s, UD 300s, unit-of-use 100s, *Robot* ready 25s, *Emergi-script* 60s. **Susp.:** 100 mg/5 mL. Bot. 118 mL. *Rx-OTC.*
Use: Analgesic; NSAID.
•**ibuprofen aluminum.** (eye-BYOO-profen ah-LOO-min-uhm) USAN.
Use: Anti-inflammatory.
•**ibuprofen lysine.** (EYE-bue-PROE-fen LYE-seen) USAN.
Use: Anti-inflammatory.
See: NeoProfen.
•**ibuprofen piconol.** (eye-BYOO-pro-fen PIK-oh-nahl) USAN.
Use: Anti-inflammatory, topical.
•**ibuprofen sodium.** (EYE-bue-PROE-fen) USAN.
Use: Treatment of pain, fever, and rheumatic disorders.
ibuprofen suspension. (Various Mfr.) Ibuprofen 100 mg/5 mL. UD 50s. *Rx.*
Use: Analgesic; NSAID.
Ibutab. (Zee Medical) Ibuprofen 200 mg. Tab. 24s. *OTC.*
Use: Analgesic; NSAID.
•**ibutilide fumarate.** (ih-BYOO-tih-lide) USAN.

Use: Cardiac depressant (antiarrhythmic).
See: Corvert.
ibutilide fumarate. (Bioniche Pharma Group) Ibutilide fumarate 0.1 mg/mL (equiv. to ibutilide 0.087 mg). Inj., Soln. Single-dose vial. 10 mL. *Rx.*
Use: Antiarrhythmic agent.
ICAPS Plus. (Ciba Vision) Vitamin A 6000 units, C 200 mg, E 60 units, B_2 20 mg, Zn 14.25 mg, Cu, Se, Mn. Sugar free. Tab. Bot. 60s, 120s. *OTC.*
Use: Mineral, vitamin supplement.
ICAPS Time Release. (Ciba Vision) Vitamin A 7000 units, C 200 mg, E 100 units, B_2 20 mg, Zn 14.25 mg, Cu, Se. Sugar free. Tab. Bot. 60s, 120s. *OTC.*
Use: Mineral, vitamin supplement.
Icar. (Hawthorn) Carbonyl iron. **Chew. Tab.:** 15 mg. Sorbitol, grape flavor. 60s. **Susp.:** 15 mg/1.25 mL. Fructose, parabens, grape and lemon flavors. Bot. 118 mL. *OTC.*
Use: Mineral supplement.
•**icatibant acetate.** (eye-CAT-ih-bant) USAN.
Use: Bradykinin antagonist.
See: Firazyr.
Ice Mint. (Bristol-Myers Squibb) Stearic acid, synthetic cocoa butter, lanolin oil, camphor, menthol, beeswax, mineral oil, sodium borate, aromatic oils, emulsifiers. Jar 4 oz. *OTC.*
Use: Emollient; counterirritant.
IC-Green. (Akorn) Indocyanine green 25 mg. Pow. for Inj. Vials with 10 mL amps of aqueous solvent. 6s. *Rx.*
Use: Ophthalmic diagnostic product.
I-Chlor 0.5%. (Akorn) Chloramphenicol 5 mg/mL. Bot. 7.5 mL, 15 mL. *Rx.*
Use: Anti-infective, ophthalmic.
•**ichthammol.** (ICK-thah-mole) *USP.*
Use: Anti-infective, topical.
W/Aluminum Hydroxide, Phenol, Zinc Oxide, Camphor, Eucalyptol.
See: Boil-Ease Anesthetic Drawing Salve.
W/Hydrocortisone Acetate, Benzocaine, Oxyquinoline Sulfate, Ephedrine Hydrochloride.
See: Derma Medicone-HC.
W/Naftalan, Calamine, Amber Pet.
See: Naftalan.
ichthammol. (Allan Pharmaceutical) Ichthammol 20%. Lanolin, mineral oil, petrolatum. Oint. 30 g. *OTC.*
Use: Dermatological agent, miscellaneous topical combination.
ichthammol. (Alra) Ichthammol 10%, 20% in a lanolin-petrolatum base. Oint. Tube 28.4 g. *OTC.*
Use: Antiseptic.
ichthammol. (Eli Lilly) Ichthammol 10%, 20% Oint. *OTC.*
Use: Antiseptic.
ichthynate.
See: Ichthammol.
•**iclaprim.** (EYE-kla-prim) USAN.
Use: Anti-infective agent.
•**iclaprim mesylate.** (EYE-kla-prim) USAN.
Use: Anti-infective agent.
Iclusig. (ARIAD Pharmaceuticals) Ponatinib hydrochloride 15 mg, 45 mg. Film coated. Lactose. Tab. 30s (45 mg), 60s (15 mg), 90s (45 mg), 180s (15 mg). *Rx.*
Use: Kinase inhibitor, tyrosine kinase inhibitor.
•**icodextrin.** (eye-koe-DEX-trin) USAN.
Use: Osmotic.
•**icopezil maleate.** (eye-KOE-peh-zill) USAN.
Use: Alzheimer disease treatment (cognition enhancer); cognition adjuvant; acetylcholinesterase inhibitor.
•**icosapent ethyl.** (eye-KOE-sa-pent eth-il) USAN.
Use: Treatment of hypertriglyceridemia.
See: Vascepa.
•**icotidine.** (eye-KOE-tih-DEEN) USAN.
Use: Antagonist (to histamine H_2 and H_1 receptors).
•**icrucumab.** (ey-KROO-kue-mab) USAN.
Use: Antineoplastic.
•**ictasol.** (IK-tah-sahl) USAN.
Use: Disinfectant.
Ictotest Reagent Tablets. (Bayer Consumer Care) Reagent Tab. for urinary bilirubin. Bot. 100s.
Use: Diagnostic aid.
Icy Hot Back Pain Relief. (Chattem) Menthol 5%, glycerin. Patch. 5s. *OTC.*
Use: Rub and liniment.
Icy Hot Balm. (Chattem) Methyl salicylate 29%, menthol 7.6%. Jar 3.5 oz, 7 oz. *OTC.*
Use: Analgesic, topical.
Icy Hot Chill Stick. (Chattem) Methyl salicylate 30%, menthol 10%, hydrogenated castor oil, stearyl alcohol. Stick. 49 g. *OTC.*
Use: Rub and liniment.
Icy Hot Cream. (Chattem) Methyl salicylate 30%, menthol 10%. Tube 0.25 oz, 1.25 oz, 3 oz. *OTC.*
Use: Analgesic, topical.
Icy Hot Extra Strength. (Chattem) **Cream:** Methyl salicylate 30%, menthol 10%, carbomer, cetyl esters wax, emul-

sifying wax, triethanolamine. 35.4 g. **Stick:** Methyl salicylate 30%, menthol 10%, ceresin, cyclomethicone, hydrogenated castor oil, PEG-150 distearate, propylene glycol, stearic acid, stearyl alcohol. 52.5 g. *OTC.*
Use: Rub and liniment.

Icy Hot Pain Relieving Gel. (Chattem) Menthol 2.5%. Alcohol 15%, aloe, parabens, triethanolamine. Gel. 70.8 g. *OTC.*
Use: Rub and liniment, gel.

Icy Hot PM. (Chattem) Capsaicin 0.025%. Menthol 5%, benzyl alcohol, disodium EDTA. Patch. 6s. *OTC.*
Use: Dermatological agent, counterirritant.

Icy Hot PM Medicated. (Chattem) Menthol 7.5%. Aloe, benzyl alcohol, capsaicin, cetearyl alcohol, cetyl alcohol, disodium EDTA, ethanol, PEG-2, stearyl alcohol. Lot. 113 g. *OTC.*
Use: Rub and liniment, lotion and liniment.

Icy Hot Pop & Peel. (Chattem) Menthol 5%, glycerin. Patch. 5s. *OTC.*
Use: Rub and liniment.

Icy Hot Pro-Therapy. (Chattem) Menthol 5%. Diazolidinyl urea, parabens. Top. Pad. 4s. *OTC.*
Use: Rubs and liniments.

Icy Hot Roll. (Chattem) Menthol 7.5%. Mineral oil. Patch. 3s. *OTC.*
Use: Rub and liniment.

I.D.A. Capsules. (Ivax) Isometheptene mucate 65 mg, dichloralphenazone 100 mg, acetaminophen 324 mg. Bot. 100s. *Rx.*
Use: Analgesic.

Idamycin PFS. (Pfizer) Idarubicin hydrochloride 1 mg/mL. Preservative free. Inj. Single-use vials. 5 mL, 10 mL, 20 mL. *Rx.*
Use: Antibiotic, anthracycline.

•**idarubicin hydrochloride.** (eye-DUH-RUE-bih-sin) *USP.*
Tall Man: IDArubicin
Use: Antineoplastic; antibiotic, anthracycline.
See: Idamycin PFS.

idarubicin hydrochloride. (GensiaSicor) Idarubicin hydrochloride 1 mg/mL. Preservative free. Inj. Single-use vials. 5 mL, 10 mL, 20 mL. *Rx.*
Use: Antibiotic, anthracycline.

•**idelalisib.** (eye-DEL-a-LIS-ib) USAN.
Use: Antineoplastic.

•**idoxifene.** (ih-dox-ih-feen) USAN.
Use: Antineoplastic; hormone replacement therapy (estrogen receptor antagonist); osteoporosis treatment and prevention.

•**idronoxil.** (id-roe-NOX-il) USAN.
Use: Antineoplastic agent.

I-Drops. (Akorn) Tetrahydrozoline hydrochloride 0.5%. Ophthalmic Soln. Bot. 0.5 oz. *Rx.*
Use: Mydriatic, vasoconstrictor.

•**idursulfase.** (eye-dur-SUL-fase) USAN.
Use: Hunter syndrome.
See: Elaprase.

iFerex 150. (Nnodum Pharmaceuticals) Iron 150 mg. Cap. 100s. *OTC.*
Use: Trace element.

iFerex 150 Forte. (Nnodum Pharmaceuticals) Fe 150 mg, B_{12} 25 mcg, folic acid 1 mg. Cap. 100s. *Rx.*
Use: Trace element.

•**ifetroban.** (ih-FEH-troe-ban) USAN.
Use: Antithrombotic.

•**ifetroban sodium.** (ih-FEH-troe-ban) USAN.
Use: Antithrombotic.

Ifex. (Baxter) Ifosfamide 1 g, 3 g. Pow. for Inj. Vial single dose. *Rx.*
Use: Antineoplastic.

•**ifosfamide.** (eye-FOSS-fuh-MIDE) *USP.*
Use: Antineoplastic.
See: Ifex.

ifosfamide. (American Pharmaceutical Partners) Ifosfamide 1 g, 3 g. Pow. for Inj., lyophilized. Vials. Single-dose. *Rx.*
Use: Antineoplastic.

I-Gent. (Akorn) Gentamicin sulfate 3 mg/mL. Ophthalmic soln. Bot. 5 mL. *Rx.*
Use: Anti-infective, ophthalmic.

Igepal Co-880. (General Aniline & Film) Nonoxynol-30. *OTC.*
Use: Contraceptive, spermicide.

Igepal Co-430. (General Aniline & Film) Nonoxynol-4. *OTC.*
Use: Contraceptive, spermicide.

Igepal Co-730. (General Aniline & Film) Nonoxynol-15. *OTC.*
Use: Contraceptive, spermicide.

IgG monoclonal anti-CD4.
See: Chimeric m-t412 (Human-Murine) IgG Monoclonal Anti-CD4.

IGIV. (Various Mfr.) Immune globulin intravenous. *Rx.*
Use: Immunomodulator (Phase II/III pediatric HIV), immunization.
See: Immune Globulin Intravenous

•**igmesine hydrochloride.** (IGG-meh-seen) USAN.
Use: Antidepressant.

I-Homatrine 5%. (Akorn) Homatropine hydrobromide 5%. Ophth. Soln. Bot. 5 mL. *Rx.*
Use: Cycloplegic; mydriatic.

Ilaris. (Novartis) Canakinumab 180 mg. Preservative free. Inj., lyophilized Pow.

for Soln. Single-use vial. 6 mL. *Rx.*
Use: Immunologic agent, immunomodulator.

•**ilepcimide.** (eye-LEPP-sih-mide) USAN. *Formerly antiepilepsirine.*
Use: Anticonvulsant.

Iletin I. (Eli Lilly) Regular and modified insulin products from beef and pork. **Regular:** 100 units/mL. Bot. 10 mL. **Lente:** 100 units/mL. Bot. 10 mL. **NPH:** 100 units/mL. Bot. 10 mL. *OTC.*
Use: Antidiabetic.

Iletin II Concentrated. (Eli Lilly) Purified pork regular insulin 500 units/mL. Vial 20 mL. *Rx.*
Use: Antidiabetic.

Iletin II Regular. (Eli Lilly) Insulin 100 units/mL purified pork. Inj. Vial 10 mL. *OTC.*
Use: Antidiabetic.

Ilevro. (Alcon) Nepafenac 0.3%. Susp.; Ophth. 1.7 mL dropper bottle (w/benzalkonium chloride 0.005%, boric acid, carboxymethylcellulose, edetate disodium, propylene glycol, sodium chloride, sodium hydroxide and/or hydrochloric acid). *Rx.*
Use: Ophthalmic nonsteroidal anti-inflammatory drug.

•**ilmofosine.** (ill-MOE-fose-een) USAN.
Use: Antineoplastic.

•**ilomastat.** (eye-LOW-mah-stat) USAN.
Use: Corneal ulcers; inflammatory conditions; cancers.

•**ilonidap.** (ile-OHN-ih-dap) USAN.
Use: Anti-inflammatory.

Ilopan. (Pharmacia) Dexpanthenol 250 mg/mL. Disp. syringe 2 mL. *Rx.*
Use: Gastrointestinal stimulant.

•**iloperidone.** (ill-oh-PURR-ih-dohn) USAN.
Use: Antipsychotic.
See: Fanapt.

•**iloprost.** (EYE-loe-prost) USAN.
Use: Treatment of pulmonary arterial hypertension.
See: Ventavis.

•**ilorasertib.** (eye-LOR-a-SER-tib) USAN.
Use: Antineoplastic.

Ilosone. (Eli Lilly) Erythromycin estolate. **Tab.:** 500 mg, Bot. 50s. **Susp.:** 125 mg, 250 mg/5 mL. Bot. 100 mL (250 mg only), 480 mL. *Rx.*
Use: Anti-infective, erythromycin.

Ilosone Pulvules. (Eli Lilly) Erythromycin estolate 250 mg. Cap. Bot. 100s. *Rx.*
Use: Anti-infective, erythromycin.

Ilotycin. (Fera Pharmaceuticals) Erythromycin 0.5%. Mineral oil, white petrolatum. Oint., Ophth. 1 g. *Rx.*
Use: Ophthalmic and otic agent, ophthalmic antibiotic.

Ilotycin Gluceptate. (Eli Lilly) Erythromycin gluceptate 1 g. Inj. Vial 30 mL. *Rx.*
Use: Anti-infective, erythromycin.

Ilozyme. (Pharmacia) Pancrelipase equivalent to lipase 11,000 units, protease 30,000 units, amylase 30,000 units. Tab. Bot. 250s. *Rx.*
Use: Digestive enzymes.

IL-2. (Various Mfr.) Interleukin-2. *Rx.*
Use: Immunomodulator.
See: Proleukin.

•**imafen hydrochloride.** (IH-mah-fen) USAN.
Use: Antidepressant.

•**imagabalin.** (IM-a-GAB-a-lin) USAN.
Use: CNS agent.

•**imagabalin hydrochloride.** (IM-a-GAB-a-lin) USAN.
Use: CNS agent.

Imager ac. (Mallinckrodt) Barium sulfate 100%. Simethicone, sorbitol, sodium benzoate. Susp. Bot. 650 mL w/enema tip-tubing assemblies w/kit, 1900 mL bot. *Rx.*
Use: Radiopaque agent, gastrointestinal contrast agent.

•**imatinib mesylate.** (im-AT-in-ib MES-i-late) USAN.
Use: Protein-tyrosine kinase inhibitor.
See: Gleevec.

•**imazodan hydrochloride.** (ih-MAY-zoe-DAN) USAN.
Use: Cardiovascular agent.

Imbruvica. (Pharmacyclics) Ibrutinib 140 mg. Cap. 90s, 120s. *Rx.*
Use: Kinase inhibitor, tyrosine kinase inhibitor.

•**imciromab pentetate.** (im-SIHR-ah-mab) USAN.
Use: Monoclonal antibody (antimyosin). [Orphan Drug]
See: Myoscint.

Imdur. (Key) Isosorbide mononitrate 30 mg, 60 mg, 120 mg. ER Tab. Bot. 100s, UD 100s. *Rx.*
Use: Vasodilator.

Imenol. (Sigma-Tau) Guaiacol 0.1 g, eucalyptol 0.08 g, iodoform 0.02 g, camphor 0.05 g/mL. Vial 30 mL. *Rx.*
Use: Expectorant.

•**imetelstat.** (im-e-TEL-stat) USAN.
Use: Antineoplastic.

•**imetelstat sodium.** (im-e-TEL-stat) USAN.
Use: Antineoplastic.

l-methorphinan levorphanol.
See: Levo-Dromoran.

•**imexon.** (eye-MEX-on) USAN.
Use: Antineoplastic.
Imexon. (Amplimed) DM 06.002.
Use: Multiple myeloma. [Orphan Drug]
Imferon. (Medeva) An iron-dextran complex containing iron 50 mg/mL. Amp. 2 mL. Box 10s. Vial (w/phenol 0.5%) 10 mL. Box 2s. *Rx.*
Use: Mineral supplement.
•**imgatuzumab.** (IM-ga-TOOZ-ue-mab) USAN.
Use: Antineoplastic.
imidazole antifungal.
Use: Antifungal agent.
See: Ketoconazole.
Miconazole.
imidazole carboxamide.
Use: Antineoplastic.
See: Dacarbazine.
DTIC-Dome.
imidazolines.
Use: Nasal decongestant.
See: Afrin No-Drip Sinus with Vapornase.
Afrin Sinus with Vapornase.
Benzedrex.
Dristan Fast Acting Formula.
Dristan 12-Hr Nasal.
Duramist Plus 12-Hr Decongestant.
Duration.
Genasal.
Naphazoline Hydrochloride.
Nasal Decongestant Combinations.
Nasal Decongestant Inhalers.
Nasal Decongestant, Maximum Strength.
Nasal Relief.
Neo-Synephrine 12-Hour.
Neo-Synephrine 12-Hour Extra Moisturizing.
Nōstrilla 12-Hour.
Otrivin.
Otrivin Pediatric Nasal.
Oxymetazoline Hydrochloride.
Privine.
Tetrahydrozoline Hydrochloride.
12 Hour Nasal.
Twice-A-Day 12-Hour Nasal.
Tyzine.
Tyzine Pediatric.
Xylometazoline Hydrochloride.
imidazopyridines.
Use: Sedative/hypnotic nonbarbiturate.
See: Zolpidem Tartrate.
imidazotetrazine derivatives.
Use: Antineoplastic agents.
See: Temozolomide.
•**imidecyl iodine.** (IH-mih-DEH-sill EYE-uh-dine) USAN.
Use: Anti-infective, topical.
•**imidocarb hydrochloride.** (ih-MIH-doe-KARB) USAN.
Use: Antiprotozoal (Babesia).
•**imidoline hydrochloride.** (im-ID-oh-leen) USAN.
Use: Anxiolytic; antipsychotic.
•**imidurea.** (ih-mid-your-EE-ah) *NF.*
Use: Antimicrobial.
•**imiglucerase.** (ih-mih-GLUE-ser-ACE) USAN.
Use: Enzyme replenisher; treatment for Gaucher disease (glucocerebrosidase). [Orphan Drug]
See: Cerezyme.
•**imilecleucel-T.** (IM-i-lek-LOO-sel-tee) USAN.
Use: Cellular immunotherapy for treatment of multiple sclerosis.
•**imiloxan hydrochloride.** (ih-mill-OX-ahn) USAN.
Use: Antidepressant.
imipemide.
Use: Anti-infective.
See: Imipenem.
•**imipenem.** (ih-mih-PEN-em) *USP. Formerly imipemide.*
Use: Anti-infective.
W/Cilastatin for Injection.
See: Primaxin.
imipenem/cilastatin. (Various Mfr.) Imipenem/cilastatin. Inj. Pow. for Soln. **250 mg/250 mg:** As cilastatin sodium 18.8 mg, sodium bicarbonate 10 mg. Single-dose vial. **500 mg/500 mg:** As cilastatin sodium 37.5 mg, sodium bicarbonate 20 mg. Single-dose vial. *Rx.*
Use: Anti-infective, carbapenem.
•**imipramine hydrochloride.** (im-IPP-ruh-meen) *USP.*
Use: Antidepressant.
See: Tofranil.
imipramine hydrochloride. (Various Mfr.) Imipramine hydrochloride 10 mg, 25 mg, 50 mg. Tab. Bot. 50s (50 mg only), 100s, 250s, 500s, 1000s, UD 20s (50 mg only). *Rx.*
Use: Antidepressant.
imipramine pamoate.
Use: Antidepressant.
See: Tofranil-PM.
imipramine pamoate. (Mallinckrodt) Imipramine pamoate 75 mg, 100 mg, 125 mg, 150 mg. Parabens. Cap. 30s. *Rx.*
Use: Antidepressant.
•**imiquimod.** (ih-mih-KWIH-mahd) USAN.
Use: Immunomodulator.
See: Aldara.
Zyclara.
imiquimod. (Fougera) Imiquimod 5%.

May contain benzyl alcohol, cetyl alcohol, parabens, stearyl alcohol, white petrolatum. Cream. Single-use packet. 24s. *Rx*.
Use: Topical immunomodulator.

Imitrex. (GlaxoSmithKline) Sumatriptan. **Inj. Soln.:** As sumatriptan succinate. 4 mg/0.5 mL (sodium chloride 3.8 mg/mL), 6 mg/0.5 mL (sodium chloride 3.5 mg/mL). **4 mg/0.5 mL:** 4 mg *STATdose System* (2 prefilled single-dose syringe cartridges, 1 *STATdose Pen*, and instructions for use), injection cartridge pack. Contains 2 prefilled syringe cartridges for refill of *STATdose System* only. **6 mg/0.5 mL:** 6 mg single-dose vials and*STATdose System* (2 prefilled single-dose syringes, 1 *STATdose Pen* and instructions for use) injection cartridge pack. Contains 2 prefilled syringe cartridges for refill of *STATdose System* only. **Soln. Intranasal:** 5 mg, 20 mg. Unit-dose spray device. 100 mcL. Box 6s. **Tab.:** 25 mg (equiv. to sumatriptan succinate 35 mg), 50 mg (equiv. to sumatriptan succinate 70 mg), 100 mg (equiv. to sumatriptan succinate 140 mg). Blister pack 9s. *Rx*.
Use: Antimigraine, serotonin 5-HT_1 receptor agonist.

Imodium A-D. (McNeil Consumer) Loperamide hydrochloride. Liq. **1 mg per 5 mL:** Alcohol 5.25%. Cherry/licorice flavor. 60 mL, 90 mL, 120 mL. **1 mg per 7.5 mL:** Glycerin, propylene glycol, simethicone, sodium 4 mg, sodium benzoate, sucralose. 120 mL. *OTC*.
Use: Antidiarrheal.

ImmTher. (Immuno Therapeutics) Disaccharide tripeptide glycerol dipalmitoyl.
Use: Antineoplastic. [Orphan Drug]

Immun-Aid. (McGaw) A custard flavored liquid containing 18.5 g protein, 60 g carbohydrate, 11 g fat, sodium 290 mg, potassium 530 mg per liter. 1 calorie/mL. With appropriate vitamins and minerals. Pow. Packets 123 g. 24s. *OTC*.
Use: Nutritional supplement, enteral.

immune globulin. (ih-MYOON GLAH-byoo-lin) Immune Serum Globulin Human. Gamma-globulin fraction of normal human plasma. Vial 10 mL. Tubex 1 mL, 2 mL w/thimerosal 1:10,000. *Rx*.
Use: Modification of active measles; prophylaxis of hepatitis A; treatment of immune deficiencies; prevention of infection associated with bone marrow transplantation (BMT); decrease frequency of certain pediatric HIV-related infections and conjunctive therapy for Kawasaki syndrome.

immune globulin, antithymocyte (rabbit).
Use: Immunization.
See: Thymoglobulin.

immune globulin, cytomegalovirus.
See: CytoGam.

immune globulin, hepatitis B.
See: BayHep B.
H-BIG.
Nabi-HB.

immune globulin (human).
See: Bivigam.
GamaSTAN S/D.
Gammagard S/D.
Gammagard S/D Less IgA.
Gammaplex.
Privigen.

immune globulin intramuscular.
Use: Immunization.

immune globulin intravenous.
Use: Immunization.
See: BayGam.
Carimune NF.
Flebogamma 5% DIF.
Flebogamma 10% DIF.
GamaSTAN S/D.
Gammagard.
Gammaked.
Gamunex-C.
Privigen.
Rho_o(D) Immune Globulin IV (Human).
Sandoglobulin.
Venoglobulin-I.
WinRho SDF.

immune globulin intravenous, botulism.
Use: Infant botulism.
See: BabyBIG.

•**immune globulin intravenous pentetate.** (ih-MYOON GLAH-byoo-lin in-trah-VEE-nuhs) USAN.
Use: Diagnostic aid.

immune globulin intravenous/subcutaneous.
See: Gamunex-C.

immune globulin intravenous, vaccinia.
Use: Immunization.

immune globulin, lymphocyte, antithymocyte (equine).
Use: Immunization.
See: Atgam.

immune globulin, rabies.
Use: Immunization.
See: Imogam Rabies-HT.

immune globulin, Rh_o(D).
See: BayRho D Full Dose.
BayRho D Mini Dose.
MICRhoGAM.
RhoGAM.
WinRho SDF.

immune globulins.
See: Antithymocyte Globulin (Rabbit).

Botulism Immune Globulin IV.
Cytomegalovirus Immune Globulin Intravenous, Human.
Hepatitis B Immune Globulin (Human).
Immune Globulin (Human).
Immune Globulin Intravenous.
Immune Globulin Subcutaneous (Human).
Lymphocyte Immune Globulin, Antithymocyte Globulin (Equine).
Rabies Immune Globulin, Human.
Rho_o(D) Immune Globulin.
Rho_o(D) Immune Globulin IV Human.
Rho_o(D) Immune Globulin Micro-Dose.
Respiratory Syncytial Virus Immune Globulin Intravenous (Human).
Tetanus Immune Globulin (Human).
Vaccinia Immune Globulin IV.

immune globulin subcutaneous (human).
Use: Immune globulin.
See: Gammaked.
Hizentra.

immune globulin, tetanus.
Use: Immunization.
See: BayTet.

immune globulin, varicella-zoster.
Use: Immunization.
See: Varicella-Zoster Immune Globulin (Human).

immune serum (animal).
See: Botulism Antitoxin.
Diphtheria Antitoxin.

immune serums.
See: Cytomegalovirus Immune Globulin Intravenous (Human).
Hepatitis B Immune Globulin.
Immune Globulin Intramuscular.
Immune Globulin Intravenous.
Immune Serum Globulin (Human).
Rabies Immune Globulin.
Rho_o(D) Immune Globulin.
Tetanus Immune Globulin.
Vaccinia Immune Globulin.
Varicella-Zoster Immune Globulin.

Immunex C-RP. (Wampole) Two-minute latex agglutination slide test for the qualitative detection of C-Reactive protein in serum. Kit 100s.
Use: Diagnostic aid.

Immunicare. (MedChem) Vitamins E 15 units, C 15 mg, Se, ARA-6 10 mg, beta-glucan 50 mg, cat's claw powder 10 mg, curcumin 50 mg, garlic 10 mg, grape seed 50 mg, graviola 150 mg, green tea 100 mg, *Herbal Complex* 50 mg, Korean ginseng 10 mg, lycopene 1 mg, *Mushroom Complex* 40 mg, olive leaf extract 25 mg, pine bark 50 mg, pomegranate 25 mg, quercetin 25 mg, red raspberry juice extract 100 mg. Soy. Cap. 60s. *OTC.*
Use: Multivitamin with minerals (except iron).

immunization, active.
See: Toxoids.
Vaccines, Bacterial.
Vaccines, Viral.

Immuno-C. (Biomune Systems, Inc.) Bovine Whey Protein Concentrate.
Use: Cryptosporidiosis treatment. [Orphan Drug]

Immunocal. (Immunotech Research) Protein (from milk protein isolate) 9 g/10 g, vitamin A, Ca, chloride, Fe, MG, P, Na 25 mg, K 30 mg/10 g, 37 cal/10 g. Pow. Pouch. 10 g. *OTC.*
Use: Enteral nutritional therapy.

Immunocal. (Immunotech Research) Protein (from milk protein isolate) 9 g/10 g, sodium 25 mg, potassium 30 mg, calcium 60 mg, magnesium 9 mg, P 21 mg, calories 37/pkt. Pow. Pkt. 10 g (30s). *OTC.*
Use: Nutritional supplement.

immunologic agents.
See: Immunomodulators.
Immunostimulants.
Immunosuppressives.

immunomodulators.
See: Abatacept.
Adalimumab.
Anakinra.
Apremilast.
Canakinumab.
Certolizumab Pegol.
Dimethyl Fumarate.
Etanercept.
Fingolimod.
Golimumab.
Imiquimod.
Infliximab.
Interferon alfacon-1.
Interferon alfa-2b, Recombinant.
Interferon beta-1a.
Interferon beta-1b.
Interferon gamma-1b.
Lenalidomide.
Mitoxantrone Hydrochloride.
Natalizumab.
Peginterferon alfa-2a.
Peginterferon alfa-2b.
Pimecrolimus.
Pomalidomide.
Rilonacept.
Teriflunomide.
Thalidomide.
Tocilizumab.
Ustekinumab.

immunomodulators, topical.
See: Imiquimod.

Ingenol Mebutate.
Pimecrolimus.
Tacrolimus.

Immunorex. (Antigen Laboratories) Allergenic extracts, various. Vial. *Rx.*
Use: Allergen desensitization.

immunostimulants.
See: Pegademase Bovine.

immunosuppressives.
See: Alefacept.
Azathioprine.
Basiliximab.
Belatacept.
Cylcosporine.
Daclizumab.
Efalizumab.
Glatiramer Acetate.
Muromonab-CD3.
Mycophenolate Mofetil.
Mycophenolate Sodium.
Mycophenolic Acid.
Sirolimus.
Tacrolimus.

ImmuRAID. (Immunomedics) Technetium Tc-99M murine monoclonal antibody to hCG and human AFP.
Use: Diagnostic aid. [Orphan Drug]

ImmuRAIT. (Immunomedics) Iodine I^{131} murine monoclonal antibody IgG2a to B cell.
Use: Antineoplastic, investigational.

Imodium Capsules. (Janssen) Loperamide 2 mg. Cap. Bot. 100s, 500s, UD 100s. *Rx.*
Use: Antidiarrheal.

Imodium Multi-Symptom Relief. (McNeil Consumer) Loperamide hydrochloride 2 mg, simethicone 125 mg. **Tab. Chew.:** Calcium 50 mg, saccharin, sorbitol, sugar. Mint flavor. 18s, 42s. **Tab.:** Acesulfame K, calcium 165 mg, sodium 4 mg. 12s, 18s, 30s, 42s. *OTC.*
Use: Antidiarrheal combination product.

Imogam Rabies-HT. (Sanofi Pasteur) Rabies immune globulin (human) (RIG) 150 units/mL. Preservative free, glycine 0.3 M, heat treated. Vials. 2 mL, 10 mL. *Rx.*
Use: Immunization, rabies.

Imovax Rabies Vaccine (Human Diploid Cell). (Aventis Pasteur) Rabies antigen ≥ 2.5 IU/mL. Freeze-dried suspension of Wistar rabies virus strain PM-1503-3M grown in human diploid cell cultures (inactivated whole virus). Human albumin < 100 mg, neomycin sulfate < 150 mcg, phenol red indicator 20 mcg. Inj., Lyophilized Pow. for Reconstitution. In single-dose vial with disposable needle and syringe containing diluent and disposable needle for administration. *Rx.*
Use: Active immunization, viral vaccine.

Impact Advanced Recovery. (Nestle Nutrition) Protein 18.1 g (caseinate, L-arginine), carbohydrate 44.7 g (sucrose), fat 9.2 g (corn oil, medium chain triglycerides), sodium 350 mg, potassium 450 mg. Fiber 3.3 g, vitamins A, B_1, B_2, B_3, B_5, B_6, B_{12}, C, D, E, K, Ca, Cl, Cr, Cu, Fe, I, Mg, Mn, Mo, P, Se, Zn, biotin, choline, folic acid. Lactose free. Chocolate and vanilla flavors. Liq. 273 mL. *OTC.*
Use: Defined formula diet, lactose-free product.

Impavido. (Paladin) Miltefosine 50 mg. Lactose. Cap. UD 28s. *Rx.*
Use: Anti-infective agent, antiprotozoal.

Implanon. (Organon) Etonogestrel 68 mg. Implant. Preloaded needle with disposable applicator. *Rx.*
Use: Contraceptive hormone.

imported fire ant venom, allergenic extract. (ALK)
Use: Allergy testing. [Orphan Drug]

impotence agents.
See: Alprostadil.
Phosphodiesterase Type 5 Inhibitors.
Sildenafil Citrate.
Tadalafil.
Vardenafil Hydrochloride.
Yohimbine Hydrochloride.

Impromen. (Janssen) Bromperidol decanoate. *Rx.*
Use: Antipsychotic.

Impromen Decanoate. (Janssen) Bromperidol decanoate. *Rx.*
Use: Antipsychotic.

•**impromidine hydrochloride.** (im-PRAH-mid-deen) USAN.
Use: Diagnostic aid (gastric secretion indicator).

Improved Congestant Tablets. (Rugby) Chlorpheniramine maleate 2 mg, acetaminophen 325 mg. Tab. Bot. 100s, 1000s. *OTC.*
Use: Antihistamine, analgesic.

Imreg-1. (Imreg) *Rx.*
Use: Immunomodulator.

Imreg-2. (Imreg) *Rx.*
Use: Immunomodulator.

Imuran. (Prometheus) Azathioprine 50 mg. Tab. Bot. 100s, UD 100s. *Rx.*
Use: Immunosuppressant.

Imuthiol. (Aventis Pasteur) Diethyldithiocarbamate. *Rx.*
Use: Immunomodulator.

Imuvert. (Celltech) *Serratia marcescens* extract (polyribosomes).
Use: Primary brain malignancies. [Orphan Drug]

•**inalimarev (CEA, MUC-1, vaccinia virus).** (in-a-LIM-a-rev) USAN.
Use: Antineoplastic.

•**inamrinone.** (eye-NAM-ri-none) *USP. Formerly Amrinone.*
Use: Cardiovascular agent.

•**inamrinone lactate.** (eye-NAM-ri-none) *USP. Formerly Amrinone Lactate.*
Use: Cardiovascular agent.

Incivek. (Vertex) Telaprevir 375 mg. Film coated. PEG. Tab. 168s, UD 168s. *Rx.*
Use: Anti-infective, antiviral agent.

•**inclacumab.** (in-KLAK-ue-mab) USAN.
Use: Cardiovascular agent.

•**incobotulinumtoxinA.** (IN-koe-BOT-ue-LYE-num-TOX-in-AY) USAN.
Use: Botulinum toxin.
See: Xeomin.

Increlex. (Tercica) Mecasermin (rDNA origin) 10 mg/mL. Benzyl alcohol 9 mg/mL, sodium chloride 5.84 mg/mL, polysorbate 20 2 mg/mL, acetate 0.5 M. Inj. Multiple-dose vials. 40 mL. *Rx.*
Use: Insulin-like growth factor.

incretin mimetic agents.
Use: Antidiabetic agent.
See: Exenatide.

•**incyclinide.** (in-SYE-kli-nide) USAN.
Use: Anti-inflammatory.

•**indacaterol.** (in-da-KAT-er-ol) USAN.
Use: Treatment of COPD.
See: Arcapta Neohaler.

•**indacaterol maleate.** (in-da-KAT-er-ol) USAN.
Use: Treatment of COPD.

•**indacrinone.** (IN-dah-KRIH-nohn) USAN.
Use: Antihypertensive, diuretic.

indalone.
See: Butopyronoxyl.

indandione derivative.
Use: Anticoagulant.
See: Anisindione.

•**indapamide.** (IN-DAP-uh-mide) *USP.*
Use: Diuretic.

indapamide. (Mylan) Indapamide 2.5 mg. Lactose. Film-coated. Tab. 100s, 1000s. *Rx.*
Use: Diuretic.

indapamide. (Various Mfr.) Indapamide 1.25 mg. Tab. Bot. 100s, 500s, 1000s. *Rx.*
Use: Diuretic.

•**indeglitazar.** (IN-de-GLIT-a-zar) USAN.
Use: Antidiabetic agent.

•**indeloxazine hydrochloride.** (in-DELL-OX-ah-zeen) USAN.
Use: Antidepressant.

Inderal LA. (Akrimax) Propranolol hydrochloride 60 mg, 80 mg, 120 mg, 160 mg. ER Cap. 100s. *Rx.*
Use: Antiadrenergic/sympatholytic; beta-adrenergic blocker.

Inderal XL. (Mist Pharmaceutical) Propranolol hydrochloride 80 mg, 120 mg. Contains sustained-release beads. PEG, sugar. ER Cap. 30s, 100s. *Rx.*
Use: Antiadrenergic/sympatholytic, beta-adrenergic blocking agent.

indian gum.
See: Karaya Gum.

indigo carmine. (Akorn) Sodium indigotindisulfonate 8 mg/mL. Amp. 5 mL. Box. 10s, 100s.
Use: Diagnostic aid.
See: Sodium Indigotindisulfonate.

indigo carmine solution. (Becton Dickinson & Co.) Indigotindisulfonate sodium (0.8% aqueous soln. sodium salt of indigotindisulfonic acid) 40 mg/5 mL. Inj. Amp. 5 mL, 10s.
Use: Diagnostic aid.

•**indigotindisulfonate sodium.** (IN-dih-go-tin-die-SULL-foe-nate) *USP.* Indigo Carmine.
Use: Diagnostic aid (cystoscopy).
See: Sodium Indigotindisulfonate.

•**indinavir.** (in-DIN-ah-veer) USAN.
Use: Antiviral (HIV-protease inhibitor).

•**indinavir sulfate.** (in-DIN-ah-veer) USAN.
Use: Antiretroviral, protease inhibitor.
See: Crixivan.

•**indiplon.** (IN-di-plon) USAN.
Use: Sedative, hypnotic.

•**indisulam.** (IN-di-SOO-lam) USAN.
Use: Antineoplastic.

•**indium chlorides In 113m.** (IN-dee-uhm) USAN.
Use: Radiopharmaceutical.

Indium DTPA In 111. (GE Healthcare) Pentetate indium disodium In 111 37 MBq (1 mCi) per mL at calibration. Inj. Single-dose vials. 1.5 mL. *Rx.*
Use: In vivo diagnostic aid.

•**indium In 111 chloride solution.** (IN-dee-uhm) *USP.*
Use: Radiopharmaceutical.

•**indium In 111 ibritumomab tiuxetan injection.** (IN-dee-uhm) *USP.*
Use: Radiopharmaceutical.

indium In 111 murine monoclonal antibody fab to myosin.
Use: Diagnostic aid in myocarditis. [Orphan Drug]
See: Myoscint.

•**indium In 111 oxyquinoline solution.** (IN-dee-uhm OX-ee-KWIN-oh-lin) *USP.*
Use: Radiopharmaceutical, diagnostic aid.

•**indium In 111 pentetate injection.** (IN-dee-uhm) *USP.*
Use: Diagnostic aid (radionuclide cisternography), radiopharmaceutical.

•**indium In 111 pentetreotide.** (IN-dee-uhm In 111 pen-teh-TREE-oh-tide) *USP.*
Use: Diagnostic aid, radiopharmaceutical.

•**indium In 111 satumomab pendetide.** (IN-dee-uhm sat-YOU-mah-mab PEN-deh-TIDE) USAN.
Use: Radiodiagnostic monoclonal antibody (ovarian and colorectal carcinoma), radiopharmaceutical.

Indocin. (Iroko) Indomethacin. **Oral Susp.:** 25 mg/5 mL. Alcohol 1%. Sorbitol. Pineapple, coconut, and mint flavor. Bot. 237 mL. **Supp.:** 50 mg. 30s. *Rx.*
Use: Analgesic; nonsteroidal anti-inflammatory drug.

Indocin I.V. (Lundbeck) Indomethacin sodium trihydrate equivalent to 1 mg indomethacin/Vial. Vial single-dose. *Rx.*
Use: Arterial patency agent.

•**indocyanine green.** (in-doe-SIGH-ah-neen) *USP.*
Use: Diagnostic aid (cardiac output determination, hepatic function determination); ophthalmic diagnostic product.
See: Cardio-Green.
IC-Green.

Indogesic. (Century) Acetaminophen 32.5 mg, butalbital 50 mg. Tab. Bot. 100s, 1000s. *Rx.*
Use: Analgesic; hypnotic, sedative.

Indoklon. Hexafluorodiethyl ether. Flurothyl. Bis-(2,2,2-trifluorethyl) ether. *Rx.*
Use: Shock-inducing agent (convulsant).

•**indolapril hydrochloride.** (in-DAHL-ah-PRILL) USAN.
Use: Antihypertensive.

•**indolidan.** (in-DOE-lih-DAN) USAN.
Use: Cardiovascular agent.

Indometh. (Major) Indomethacin. Cap. **25 mg:** Bot. 100s, 1000s. **50 mg:** Bot. 100s, 500s. *Rx.*
Use: Nonsteroidal anti-inflammatory agent.

•**indomethacin.** (in-doe-METH-ah-sin) *USP.*
Use: Nonsteroidal anti-inflammatory agent.
See: Indocin.
Tivorbex.

indomethacin. (Bedford Labs) Indomethacin sodium 1 mg. Inj., lyophilized Pow. for Soln. Single-dose vial. Rx.
Use: Agent for patent ductus arteriosus.

indomethacin. (G & W Laboratories) Indomethacin 50 mg. Rectal Supp. 30s. *Rx.*
Use: Nonsteroidal anti-inflammatory agent.

indomethacin. (Various Mfr.) Indomethacin sodium 1 mg. Inj., lyophilized Pow. for Soln. Single-dose vial. *Rx.*
Use: Agent for patent ductus arteriosus.

indomethacin. (Various Mfr.) Indomethacin 25 mg, 50 mg. Cap. Bot. 50s (25 mg only), 100s, 500s, 1000s, UD 100s, *Robot* ready 25s. *Rx.*
Use: Nonsteroidal anti-inflammatory agent.

indomethacin extended-release. (Inwood) Indomethacin 75 mg. Sucrose, parabens. SR Cap. Bot. 60s, 100s. *Rx.*
Use: Nonsteroidal anti-inflammatory agent.

•**indomethacin sodium.** (in-doe-METH-ah-sin) *USP.*
Use: Nonsteroidal anti-inflammatory agent.

indomethacin sodium trihydrate. *Rx.*
Use: Arterial patency agent.
See: Indocin I.V.

indomethacin SR. (Various Mfr.) Indomethacin 75 mg. SR Cap. Bot. 60s, 100s, 500s. *Rx.*
Use: Nonsteroidal anti-inflammatory agent.

•**indoprofen.** (in-doe-PRO-fen) USAN.
Use: Analgesic; anti-inflammatory.

•**indoramin.** (in-DAHR-ah-min) USAN.
Use: Antihypertensive.

•**indoramin hydrochloride.** (in-DAHR-ah-min) USAN.
Use: Antihypertensive.

•**indorenate hydrochloride.** (in-DAHR-en-ATE) USAN.
Use: Antihypertensive.

•**indoxole.** (IN-dox-OLE) USAN.
Use: Antipyretic; anti-inflammatory.

•**indriline hydrochloride.** (IN-drih-leen) USAN.
Use: Stimulant, central.

I-Neocort. (American Pharmaceutical) Neomycin sulfate 5 mg, hydrocortisone acetate 15 mg/5 mL. Ophth. Susp. Bot. 5 mL. *Rx.*
Use: Anti-infective; corticosteroid.

I-Neospor. (American Pharmaceutical) Polymyxin B sulfate, gramicidin, neomycin sulfate. Ophth. Soln. Bot. 10 mL. *Rx.*
Use: Anti-infective, ophthalmic.

Infalyte Oral Solution. (Bristol-Myers Squibb) Electrolyte mixture with 30 g/L rice syrup solids containing 4.2 calo-

ries/fl. oz. In 1 liter. *OTC.*
Use: Nutritional supplement.

Infanate Balance. (Acella) Folic acid 1 mg, calcium 104 mg, iron 29 mg, vitamins D 400 units, E 30 units, B_6 25 mg, DHA 265 mg, docusate sodium 50 mg. Glycerin, sorbitol, soy lecithin, soybean oil. Cap., softgel. 30s. *Rx.*
Use: Prenatal vitamin with minerals.

Infanrix. (GlaxoSmithKline) Diphtheria toxoid 25 Lf units, tetanus toxoid 10 Lf units, inactivated pertussis toxin 25 mcg, filamentous hemagglutinin 25 mcg, pertactin 8 mcg/0.5 mL. Formaldehyde, sodium chloride, phenoxyethanol. Inj. Single-dose Vials and disposable *Tip-Lok* syringes. *Rx.*
Use: Immunization, active toxoid.

Infantaire. (Altaire) Acetaminophen 100 mg/mL. Soln., Conc., Oral. 15 mL, 30 mL with 0.8 mL dropper. *OTC.*
Use: Analgesic.

infant foods.
Use: Nutritional supplement.
See: Enfamil.
Enfamil Human Milk Fortifier.
Enfamil Premature 20 Formula.
RCF.
Similac.
Similac PM 60/40.
Similac Sensitive for Fussiness & Gas.
Similac Sensitive for Spit-Up.

infant foods, hypoallergenic.
Use: Nutritional supplement.
See: Isomil.
Isomil SF.
I-Soyalac.
Nutramigen.
Pregestimil.
ProSobee.
Similac Soy Isomil.
Soyalac.

Infants' Motrin. (McNeil) Ibuprofen 40 mg/mL. Sorbitol, sucrose, berry flavor. Oral drops. Bot. 15 mL w/dropper. *OTC.*
Use: Anti-inflammatory; analgesic.

Infants' No-Aspirin Drops. (Walgreen) Acetaminophen 80 mg/0.8 mL. Nonalcoholic. Bot. 15 mL. *OTC.*
Use: Analgesic.

Infants' Silapap. (Silarx) Acetaminophen 80 mg/0.8 mL. Drops. Bot. 15 mL. Alcohol free. *OTC.*
Use: Analgesic; antipyretic.

Infarub Cream. (Whitehall-Robins Laboratories) Methyl salicylate 35%, menthol 10% in vanishing cream base. Tube 1.25 oz, 3.5 oz. *OTC.*
Use: Analgesic, topical.

Infasurf. (ONY) Phospholipids 35 mg/mL suspended in 0.9% sodium chloride solution, 0.65 mg proteins. Intratracheal Susp. Single-use vial 6 mL. *Rx.*
Use: Lung surfactant.

Infectrol Ointment. (Bausch & Lomb) Dexamethasone 0.1%, neomycin sulfate equivalent to 0.35% neomycin base, 10,000 units polymyxin B sulfate/g. White petrolatum, lanolin, mineral oil, parabens. Tube 3.5, 3.75 g. *Rx.*
Use: Anti-infective, corticosteroid, topical.

Infectrol Suspension. (Bausch & Lomb) Dexamethasone 0.1%, neomycin sulfate equivalent to 0.35% neomycin base, 10,000 units polymyxin B sulfate/mL. Hydroxypropyl methylcellulose, polysorbate 20, benzalkonium chloride. Drop. Bot. 5 mL. *Rx.*
Use: Anti-infective; corticosteroid, ophthalmic.

INFeD. (Schein) Iron 50 mg/mL (as dextran), sodium chloride approximately 0.9%. Inj. Single-dose Vial 2 mL. *Rx.*
Use: Mineral supplement.

Infergen. (Three Rivers) Interferon alfacon-1 9 mcg, 15 mcg, preservative free. Inj. Single-dose vial. 0.3 mL (9 mcg), 0.5 mL (15 mcg). *Rx.*
Use: Immunologic, immunomodulator.

•**infliximab.** (in-FLIX-i-mab) USAN.
Tall Man: inFLIXimab
Use: Immunologic agent; immunomodulator.
See: Remicade.

Influenza A (H5N1) virus vaccine, adjuvanted. (GlaxoSmithKline) Hemagglutinin 3.75 mcg of A/Indonesia/05/2005 (H5N1) per 0.5 mL. Thimerosal. Multidose vial (each 0.5 mL dose contains thimerosal 5 mcg, a mercury derivative, as a preservative [less than 2.5 mcg of mercury], squalene 10.69 mg, DL-α-tocopherol 11.86 mg, polysorbate 80 4.86 mg; each 0.5 mL dose may also contain residual amounts of ovalbumin [0.083 mcg or less], formaldehyde [12.5 mcg or less], and sodium deoxycholate [3.75 mcg or less] from the manufacturing process) with adjuvant. *Rx.*
Use: Viral vaccine.

Influenza A virus vaccine, H5N1. (Sanofi Pasteur) Hemagglutinin 90 mcg of strain A/Vietnam/1203/2004 (H5N1, clade 1) per mL. Thimerosal (each 1 mL dose is formulated to contain not more than 98.2 mcg of thimerosal [approximately 50 mcg mercury per dose]). Inj., Susp. (purified split virus). 5 mL multidose vial (each dose may also contain

residual amounts of formaldehyde [not more than 200 mcg], polyethylene glycol p-isooctylphenyl ether [not more than 0.05%], and sucrose [not more than 2%]). *Rx.*
Use: Viral vaccine.

•**influenza virus vaccine.** (in-flew-EN-zuh) *USP.*
Use: Immunization.
See: Afluria.
Agriflu.
Fluarix.
Flucelvax.
FluLaval.
FluMist.
Fluvirin.
Fluzone.
Fluzone High-Dose.
Fluzone Intradermal.

Infumorph 500. (West-Ward) Morphine sulfate 25 mg/mL. Soln. for Inj. Amp. 20 mL (500 mg). *c-II.*
Use: Opioid analgesic.

Infumorph 200. (West-Ward) Morphine sulfate 10 mg/mL. Inj. Amp. 20 mL (200 mg). *c-II.*
Use: Opioid analgesic.

Infuvite Adult. (West-Ward) Vitamin A 2300 units, D_3 200 units, E (dl-alpha tocopheryl acetate) 10 units, B_1 6 mg, B_2 3.6 mg, B_3 40 mg, B_5 15 mg, B_6 6 mg, B_{12} 5 mcg, C 200 mg, K 150 mcg, biotin 60 mcg, folic acid 600 mcg/10 mL (after combining vials), polysorbate 80. Inj. Vials. 2.5 mL. *Rx.*
Use: Nutritional supplement.

Infuvite Pediatric. (Baxter) Vitamin A 2300 units, D_3 400 units, E (dl-alpha tocopheryl acetate) 7 units, B_1 1.2 mg, B_2 14 mg, B_3 17 mg, B_5 15 mg, B_6 1 mg, B_{12} 1 mcg, C 80 mg, K 0.2 mg, biotin 20 mcg, folic acid 140 mcg/5 mL (after combining vials), polysorbate 80. Inj. 2 vials (4 mL and 1 mL). *Rx.*
Use: Nutritional supplement.

Ingadine Tabs. (Major) Guanethidine sulfate 10 mg, 25 mg. Bot. 100s, 1000s. *Rx.*
Use: Antihypertensive.

•**ingenol mebutate.** (IN-jen-ol me-BUE-tate) USAN.
Use: Antineoplastic agent.
See: Picato.

•**ingliforib.** (in-gli-FOE-rib) USAN.
Use: Antidiabetic.

INH. (Novartis) Isoniazid 300 mg. Tab. *Rx.*
Use: Antituberculosis agent.

Inhal-Aid. (Key)
Use: Respiratory drug delivery system.

Inhibace. (Roche) Cilazapril. *Rx.*
Use: Antihypertensive.

•**iniparib.** (in-i-PAR-ib) USAN.
Use: Antineoplastic.

injectable local anesthetics.
See: Anesthetics, Injectable Local.

Injectafer. (American Regent) Ferric carboxymaltose 750 mg (50 mg of elemental iron/mL). Inj., Soln. Single-use vial. 15 mL. *Rx.*
Use: Trace element.

Inlyta. (Pfizer) Axitinib 1 mg, 5 mg. Film coated. Lactose. Tab. 60s (5 mg), 180s (1 mg). *Rx.*
Use: Kinase inhibitor, tyrosine kinase inhibitor.

Innerclean Herbal Laxative. (Last) Senna leaf powder, psyllium seed, buckthorne, anise seed, fennel seed. Bot. 1 oz, 2 oz. *OTC.*
Use: Laxative.

Innertabs. (Last) Senna leaf powder and psyllium seed tablets. Bot. 80s, 200s. *OTC.*
Use: Laxative.

InnoPran XL. (Akrimax) Propranolol hydrochloride 80 mg, 120 mg, sugar spheres. ER Cap. 30s, 100s. *Rx.*
Use: Antiadrenergic/sympatholytic, beta-adrenergic blocking agent.

Inocor Lactate. (Sanofi-Synthelabo) Amrinone lactate (base equivalent) 5 mg/mL, sodium metabisulfite 0.25 mg. Inj. Amp. 20 mL. Box 5s. *Rx.*
Use: Inotropic.

•**inocoterone acetate.** (ih-NO-koe-ter-ohn) USAN.
Use: Dermatologic, acne.

INOmax. (INO Therapeutics) Nitric oxide 100 ppm, 800 ppm. Gas. 353 L (delivered volume 344 L), 1963 L (delivered volume 1918 L). *Rx.*
Use: Respiratory inhalant.

inophylline.
See: Aminophylline.

inosine pranobex. Isoprinosine.
Use: Antiviral. [Orphan Drug]
See: Isoprinosine.

Inosiplex. (Newport Pharmaceuticals) Isoprinosine. *Rx.*
Use: Antiviral.

inosit.
See: Inositol.

Inositech. (Bio-tech) Inositol 324 mg. Cap. 100s. *OTC.*
Use: Lipotropic product.

inositol.
Use: Lipotropic.
See: Inositech.

•**inositol niacinate.** (in-OH-sih-tole NIE-ah-sin-ate) USAN.
Use: Vasodilator.

inositol nicotinate.
See: Inositol Niacinate.

inotropic agents.
See: Digitek.
Digoxin.
Digoxin Injection, Pediatric.
Inamrinone Lactate.
Lanoxin.
Milrinone Lactate.
Primacor.

Inova Easy Pad. (JSJ Pharmaceuticals) Benzoyl peroxide 4%, 8%. Disodium EDTA, glycerin, methylparaben. Pad. Kit w/30 pads and 28 tocopherol 5% topical capsules. *Rx.*
Use: Anti-infective, topical; antibiotic agent.

Inova 8/2 Acne Control Therapy. (JSJ Pharmaceuticals) Benzoyl peroxide 8%, salicylic acid 2%, tocopherol 5%. Disodium EDTA, glycerin, methylparaben. Pad. Kit w/30 benzoyl peroxide pads, 30 salicylic acid pads, and 28 tocopherol 5% topical capsules. *Rx.*
Use: Acne product combination

Inova 4/1 Acne Control Therapy. (JSJ Pharmaceuticals) Benzoyl peroxide 4%, salicylic acid 1%, tocopherol 5%. Disodium EDTA, glycerin, methylparaben. Pad. Kit w/30 benzoyl peroxide pads, 30 salicylic acid pads, and 28 tocopherol 5% topical capsules. *Rx.*
Use: Acne product combination.

InspirEase. (Key) *Rx.*
Use: Respiratory drug delivery system.

Inspra. (Searle) Eplerenone 25 mg, 50 mg, lactose. Tab. Bot. 30s, 90s, unit doses (25 mg only). *Rx.*
Use: Renin angiotensin system antagonist.

Insta-Char. (Kerr Drug) **Regular:** Aqueous suspension activated charcoal 50 g/8 oz. **Pediatric:** Aqueous suspension activated charcoal 15 g/4 oz. *OTC.*
Use: Antidote.

Insta-Glucose. (ICN) Undiluted USP glucose. UD tube containing liquid glucose 31 g. *OTC.*
Use: Hyperglycemic.

Inst-E-Vite. (Barth's) Vitamin E 100 units, 200 units. Cap. **100 units:** Bot 100s, 500s, 1000s. **200 units:** Bot. 100s, 250s, 500s. *OTC.*
Use: Vitamin supplement.

•**insulin.** (IN-suh-lin) *USP.*
Use: Antidiabetic.
See: Insulin Analog.
Insulin Detemir.
Insulin Glargine.
Insulin Glulisine.
Insulin Human (Inhalation).
Insulin Injection Concentrated.
Insulin Injection (Regular).
Insulin Regular Concentrate.
Insulin Zinc Suspension, Extended (Ultralente).
Insulin Zinc Suspension (Lente).
Isophane Insulin Suspension (NPH).
Isophane Insulin Suspension (NPH) and Insulin Injection (Regular).

insulin analog.
Use: Antidiabetic.
See: Humalog.
Humalog Mix 75/25.
NovoLog.

•**insulin aspart.** (IN-suh-lin ASS-part) USAN.
Use: Antidiabetic.

•**insulin, dalanated.** (IN-suh-lin dah-LAHN-ate-ed) USAN.
Use: Antidiabetic.

•**insulin degludec.** (IN-su-lin de-GLOO-dek) USAN.
Use: Antidiabetic.

•**insulin detemir.** (IN-suh-lin DEHT-ih-meer) USAN.
Use: Antidiabetic.
See: Levemir.

•**insulin glargine.** (IN-suh-lin GLAHR-gine) USAN.
Use: Antidiabetic.
See: Lantus.

•**insulin glulisine.** (IN-suh-lin gloo-LIS-een) USAN.
Use: Antidiabetic.
See: Apidra.

•**insulin human.** (IN-suh-lin) *USP.*
Use: Antidiabetic.
See: Humulin.

•**insulin human, isophane, suspension.** (IN-suh-lin hue-man EYE-so-fane) *USP.*
Use: Antidiabetic.

•**insulin human zinc, extended, suspension.** (IN-suh-lin) *USP.*
Use: Antidiabetic.

•**insulin human zinc suspension.** (IN-suh-lin) *USP.*
Use: Antidiabetic.

insulin inhaled.
Use: Investigational antidiabetic agent.

insulin injection, concentrated.
Use: Antidiabetic.
See: Humulin R Regular U-500 (Concentrated).

insulin injection (regular).
Use: Antidiabetic.
See: Humulin R.
Novolin R.
Novolin R PenFill.
Novolin R Prefilled.

•**insulin, isophane, suspension.** (IN-suh-lin EYE-so-fane) *USP.*
Use: Antidiabetic.
See: NPH.

•**insulin I 131.** (IN-suh-lin) USAN.
Use: Radiopharmaceutical.

•**insulin I 125.** (IN-suh-lin) USAN.
Use: Radiopharmaceutical.

insulin-like growth factor.
See: Mesermin.
Mecasermin Rinfabate.

insulin-like growth factor-1, recombinant.
Use: Amyotrophic lateral sclerosis. [Orphan Drug]

•**insulin lispro.** (IN-suh-lin LICE-pro) *USP.*
Use: Antidiabetic.
See: Humalog.
Humalog Mix 50/50.
Humalog Mix 75/25.

•**insulin, neutral.** (IN-suh-lin) USAN.
Use: Antidiabetic.

insulin Novo rapitard. Biphasic Insulin.

•**insulin peglispro.** (IN-sul-in peg-LIS-pro) USAN.
Use: Antidiabetic agent.

•**insulin, protamine zinc suspension.** (IN-suh-lin PRO-tah-meen zingk) *USP.* 40 units, 100 units/mL. Vials 10 mL.
Use: Antidiabetic.

insulin, regular.
Use: Antidiabetic.
See: Humulin BR.
Humulin R.
Novolin R.
Novolin R PenFill.
Velosulin.
Velosulin (Pork).

insulin, regular concentrate.
Use: Antidiabetic.
See: Humulin R.
Regular U-500 (Concentrated).

insulin suspension, isophane.
Use: Antidiabetic.
See: Humulin 70/30.
Novolin 70/30.
Novolin 70/30 PenFill.

insulin suspension, lente.
Use: Antidiabetic.
See: Lente Insulin.
Lente Insulin (Beef).
Lente L.
Lente Iletin II (Beef).
Lente Purified Pork Insulin.
Novolin L.

insulin suspension, NPH.
Use: Antidiabetic.
See: Beef NPH Iletin II.
Humulin N.
Novolin N.
Novolin N PenFill.
NPH Iletin I (Beef and Pork).
NPH Insulin (Beef).
NPH-N Purified (Pork).

insulin suspension, PZI. *OTC.*
Use: Antidiabetic.

insulin suspension semilente. *OTC.*
Use: Antidiabetic.

insulin suspension, ultralente. *OTC.*
Use: Antidiabetic.
See: Ultralente Insulin (Beef).

•**insulin zinc, prompt, suspension.** (IN-suh-lin) *USP.*
Use: Antidiabetic.

•**insulin zinc, suspension, extended (ultralente).** (IN-suh-lin) *USP.*
Use: Antidiabetic.

•**insulin zinc suspension (lente).** (IN-suh-lin) *USP.*
Use: Antidiabetic.

Intal. (King) Cromolyn sodium 800 mcg/actuation. Aerosol. 8.1 g (≥ 112 metered sprays), 14.2 g (≥ 200 metered sprays). *Rx.*
Use: Antiasthmatic.

Integra F. (US Pharmaceutical) Iron 125 mg, vitamins B_3 3 mg, C 40 mg, folate 1 mg, *ProAscorb C* 324 mg. Cap. 30s, 90s. *Rx.*
Use: Multivitamin with iron.

Integra Plus. (US Pharmaceutical) Iron 125 mg, vitamins B_1 5 mg, B_2 5 mg, B_3 20 mg, B_5 7 mg, B_6 25 mg, B_{12} 10 mcg, C 210 mg, folate 1 mg, biotin 300 mcg, *ProAscorb C* 324 mg. Cap. 30s, 90s. *Rx.*
Use: Multivitamin with iron.

integrase inhibitors.
Use: Antiretroviral agents.
See: Dolutegravir.
Raltegravir.

Integrilin. (Schering) Eptifibatide 0.75 mg/mL, 2 mg/mL. Inj. for Soln. Vial 10 mL (2 mg/mL only), 100 mL. *Rx.*
Use: Antiplatelet, glycoprotein IIb/IIIa inhibitor.

Integrin Caps. (Sanofi-Synthelabo) Oxypertine. *Rx.*
Use: Anxiolytic.

Intelence. (Centocor Ortho Biotech) Etravirine 25 mg, 100 mg, 200 mg. Lactose (except 200 mg). Tab. 60s (200 mg), 120s (25 mg and 100 mg). *Rx.*
Use: Antiretroviral agent, non-nucleoside reverse transcriptase inhibitors.

Intensol. (Roxane) A system of concentrated solutions of drugs w/calibrated dropper: Chlorpromazine hydrochloride 30 mg/mL, 100 mg/mL; dexamethasone 1 mg/mL; dihydrotachysterol 0.2 mg/mL;

hydrochlorothiazide 100 mg/mL; prednisone 5 mg/mL; thioridazine hydrochloride 30 mg/mL, 100 mg/mL.

interferon. A family of naturally occurring, small protein molecules with molecular weights of approximately 15,000 to 21,000 daltons. They are formed by the interaction of animal cells with viruses capable of conferring on animal cells' resistance to virus infection. Three major classes of interferons have been identified: alpha, beta, and gamma. Interferon was first derived from human white blood cells and originally used in Finland.
Use: Antineoplastic, antiviral; treatment of breast cancer lymphoma, multiple melanoma, and malignant melanoma.
See: Actimmune.
Avonex.
Betaseron.
Intron A.

interferon alfacon-1.
Use: Immunologic, immunomodulator.
See: Infergen.

•**interferon alfa-n1.** (IN-ter-FEER-ahn AL-fuh) USAN.
Use: Antineoplastic, antiviral; biological response modifier. [Orphan Drug]

•**interferon alfa-2a, recombinant.** (IN-ter-FEER-ahn AL-fuh-2a ree-KAHM-bih-nent) USAN.
Use: Antineoplastic, antiviral; biological response modifier; immunomodulator. [Orphan Drug]

•**interferon alfa-2b, recombinant.** (IN-ter-FEER-ahn AL-fuh-2b) USAN.
Use: Antineoplastic, antiviral; biological response modifier; immunomodulator.
See: Intron A.

interferon, beta.
Use: Immunomodulator; treatment of multiple sclerosis.
See: Avonex.
Betaseron.

•**interferon beta-1a.** (in-ter-FEER-ohn BAY-tuh-1a) USAN.
Use: Biological response modifier; immunologic agent, immunomodulator.
See: Avonex.
Rebif.

•**interferon beta-1b.** (IN-ter-FEER-ahn BAY-tuh-1b) USAN.
Use: Immunologic agent, immunomodulator.
See: Betaseron.
Extavia.

•**interferon gamma-1b.** (IN-ter-FEER-ahn GAM-uh-1b) USAN.
Use: Antineoplastic, antiviral; immunoregulator, biological response modifier; immunomodulator.
See: Actimmune.

interleukin-1 receptor antagonist, human recombinant.
Use: Juvenile rheumatoid arthritis; graft-vs-host disease in transplant patients. [Orphan Drug]
See: Antril.

interleukins.
Use: Hematopoietic.
See: Oprelvekin.

interleukin-3, human recombinant. (Novartis) *Rx.*
Use: Immunomodulator. [Orphan Drug]

interleukin-2.
Use: Immunomodulator; antineoplastic. [Orphan Drug]
See: Proleukin.
Teceleukin.

interleukin-2 PEG. (Cetus) *Rx.*
Use: Immunomodulator.

interleukin-2, recombinant liposome encapsulated.
Use: Antineoplastic. [Orphan Drug]

Intermezzo. (Purdue Pharma) Zolpidem tartrate 1.75 mg, 3.5 mg. Mannitol, sorbitol, sucralose. Sublingual Tab. UD 1s, UD 30s. *c-IV.*
Use: Nonbarbiturate sedative/hypnotic, imidazopyridine.

interstitial cystitis agents.
See: Dimethyl Sulfoxide.
Interstitial Cystitis Combinations.
Pentosan Polysulfate Sodium.
Phenazopyridine Hydrochloride.

interstitial cystitis combinations.
See: Phenazopyridine Hydrochloride, Hyoscyamine Hydrobromide, Butabarbital.

Intestinex. (A.G. Marin) *Lactobacillus acidophilus* 700 million units. Lactose. Preservative free and sugar free. Cap. 30s. *OTC.*
Use: Nutritional supplement.

•**intetumumab.** (IN-te-TUM-ue-mab) USAN.
Use: Antineoplastic.

Intralipid 30%. (Baxter) Soybean oil 30%, egg yolk phospholipids 1.2%, glycerin 1.7%. 200 mOsmol/L. 3 kcal/mL. Inj., Emulsion. Pharmacy bulk packages. 500 mL. *Rx.*
Use: Intravenous fat emulsion, lipid, intravenous nutritional therapy.

Intralipid 20% I.V. Fat Emulsion. (Baxter) IV fat emulsion containing soybean oil 20%, egg yolk phospholipids 1.2%, glycerin 2.25%, water for injection. I.V. Flask 50 mL, 100 mL, 250 mL, 500 mL. *Rx.*
Use: Nutritional supplement, parenteral.

intranasal steroids.
See: Beclomethasone Dipropionate.
Budesonide.
Ciclesonide.
Flunisolide.
Fluticasone.
Mometasone Furoate Monohydrate.
Triamcinolone Acetonide.

IntraSite. (Smith & Nephew) Graft T starch copolymer 2%, water 8%, propylene glycol 20%. Sterile amorphous interactive hydrogel dressing. 25 g. *Rx.*
Use: Dermatologic, wound therapy.

intraval sodium.
See: Pentothal Sodium.

intravenous nutritional therapy.
See: Combined Electrolyte Concentrates.
Combined Electrolyte Solutions.
Dextrose 2.5% with 0.45% Sodium Chloride.
Dextrose 3.3% and 0.3% Sodium Chloride.
Dextrose 5% and Electrolyte No. 48.
Dextrose 5% and Electrolyte No. 75.
Dextrose 5% with 0.2% Sodium Chloride.
Dextrose 5% and 0.225% Sodium Chloride.
Dextrose 5% with 0.3% Sodium Chloride.
Dextrose 5% with 0.33% Sodium Chloride.
Dextrose 5% with 0.45% Sodium Chloride.
Dextrose 5% with 0.9% Sodium Chloride.
Dextrose 10% and Electrolyte No. 48.
Dextrose 10% with 0.2% Sodium Chloride.
Dextrose 10% with 0.225% Sodium Chloride.
Dextrose 10% with 0.45% Sodium Chloride.
Dextrose 10% and 0.9% Sodium Chloride.
Electrolytes.
Half-Strength Lactated Ringer's in 2.5% Dextrose.
Hyperlyte CR.
Invert Sugar-Electrolyte Solutions.
Isolyte H in 5% Dextrose.
Isolyte M in 5% Dextrose.
Isolyte P in 5% Dextrose.
Isolyte R in 5% Dextrose.
Isolyte S pH 7.4.
Isolyte S with 5% Dextrose.
Lactated Ringer's.
Lactated Ringer's in 5% Dextrose.
Lypholyte.
Lypholyte-II.
Magnesium.
Minerals.
Multilyte-20.
Multilyte-40.
Multiple Electrolytes and 5% Travert.
Multiple Electrolytes and 10% Travert.
Normosol-M.
Normosol-M and 5% Dextrose.
Normosol-R.
Normosol-R and 5% Dextrose.
Normosol-R pH 7.4.
Nutrilyte.
Nutrilyte II.
Phosphate.
Plasma-Lyte A pH 7.4.
Plasma-Lyte 56 and 5% Dextrose.
Plasma-Lyte 148.
Plasma-Lyte 148 and 5% Dextrose.
Plasma-Lyte R.
Plasma-Lyte R and 5% Dextrose.
Potassium Chloride in 0.9% Sodium Chloride.
Potassium Chloride in 3.3% Dextrose and 0.3% Sodium Chloride.
Potassium Chloride in 5% Dextrose.
Potassium Chloride in 5% Dextrose and Lactated Ringer's.
Potassium Chloride in 5% Dextrose and 0.2% Sodium Chloride.
Potassium Chloride in 5% Dextrose and 0.33% Sodium Chloride.
Potassium Chloride in 5% Dextrose and 0.45% Sodium Chloride.
Potassium Chloride in 5% Dextrose and 0.9% Sodium Chloride.
Potassium Chloride in 10% Dextrose and 0.2% Sodium Chloride.
Potassium Salts.
Ringer's.
Ringer's in 5% Dextrose.
Sodium Chloride.
TPN Electrolytes.
TPN Electrolytes II.
TPN Electrolytes III.

intravenous replenishment solutions.
Use: Intravenous nutritional therapy.
See: Intravenous Nutritional Therapy.

•**intrazole.** (IN-trah-zole) USAN.
Use: Anti-inflammatory.

•**intriptyline hydrochloride.** (in-TRIP-tih-leen) USAN.
Use: Antidepressant.

Introlite. (Ross) Protein 22.2 g, carbohydrate 70.5 g, fat 18.4 g, Na 930 mg, K 1570 mg/L with 200 mOsm/kg water, with appropriate vitamins and minerals, 0.53 Cal/mL. Liq. *OTC.*
Use: Nutritional supplement.

Intron A. (Schering) Interferon alfa-2b, recombinant. **Inj., Pow. for Soln.:**

10 million, 18 million, 50 million units/vial. Each mL contains human albumin 1 mg, glycine 20 mg, sodium phosphate dibasic 2.3 mg, sodium phosphate monobasic 0.55 mg. Vials w/1 mL diluent vial. Diluent is sterile water for injection. **Inj. Soln.:** 3 million, 5 million, 10 million, 18 million, 25 million units/vial. Each mL contains sodium chloride 7.5 mg, sodium phosphate dibasic 1.8 mg, sodium phosphate monobasic 1.3 mg, EDTA 0.1 mg, polysorbate 80 0.1 mg, m-cresol 1.5 mg as preservative. Vials. Pak-10 (6 vials, 6 B-D *Safety-Lok* syringes) (10 million). Multidose vials. 22.8 million units/3.8 mL (18 million units). Multidose vials. 32 million units/3.2 mL (25 million units). Multidose pens (6 doses) with needles. 22.5 million units/1.5 mL/pen (3 million units), 37.5 million units/1.5 mL/pen (5 million units), 75 million units/1.5 mL/pen (10 million units). *Rx.*
Use: Immunologic agent, immunomodulator.

Intropaque Liquid. (Lafayette) Barium sulfate 60% w/v suspension. Bot. Gal. Case 4s.
Use: Radiopaque agent.

Intropaste. (Mallinckrodt) Barium sulfate 70%. Simethicone, sorbitol, saccharin, parabens. Paste. Tube 454 g. *Rx.*
Use: Radiopaque agent, GI contrast agent.

Introvale. (Sandoz) Ethinyl estradiol 30 mcg, levonorgestrel 0.15 mg. Film coated. Lactose, PEG. Tab. 91s w/7 inert tablets (lactose, PEG). *Rx.*
Use: Monophasic oral contraceptive.

Intuniv. (Shire) Guanfacine 1 mg, 2 mg, 3 mg, 4 mg. Lactose. ER Tab. 100s. *Rx.*
Use: Antiadrenergic/sympatholytic; antiadrenergic agent, centrally acting.

•**inulin.** (IN-you-lin) *USP.*
Use: Diagnostic aid (renal function determination).

inulin. (DuPont) Purified inulin 5 g/50 mL sodium Cl 0.9%, sodium hydroxide to adjust pH. Amp. 50 mL.
Use: Diagnostic aid.

Invanz. (Merck) Ertapenem sodium 1.046 g (equivalent to ertapenem 1 g). Sodium bicarbonate 175 mg, sodium 6 mEq. Pow., for Inj., lyophilized. Single-dose vials. *Rx.*
Tall Man: INVanz
Use: Anti-infective.

Invega. (Janssen) Paliperidone 3 mg (lactose), 6 mg, 9 mg. ER Tab. 30s, 350s, UD 100s. *Rx.*
Use: Antipsychotic agent.

Invega Sustenna. (Janssen) Paliperidone 39 mg, 78 mg, 117 mg, 156 mg, 234 mg. PEG 4000. Kit w/prefilled syringe and 2 safety needles. *Rx.*
Use: Antipsychotic agent, benzisoxazole derivative.

invert sugar. (Abbott) 10%. Soln. Bot. 1000 mL. *Rx-OTC.*
Use: Nutritional supplement, parenteral.
See: Travert.

invert sugar-electrolyte solutions. *Rx.*
Use: Nutritional supplement, parenteral.
See: 5% Travert and Electrolyte No. 2.
10% Travert and Electrolyte No. 2.
Multiple Electrolytes and 5% Travert.
Multiple Electrolytes and 10% Travert.
Multiple Electrolyte 2 w/5% Invert Sugar.
Multiple Electrolyte 2 w/10% Invert Sugar.

invert sugar injection.
Use: Fluid, nutrient replacement.

Invirase. (Roche) Saquinavir mesylate. **Cap.:** 200 mg. Lactose. Bot. 270s. **Tab.:** 500 mg. Lactose. 120s. *Rx.*
Use: Antiviral.

Invites Rx. (Breckenridge Pharmaceuticals) Vitamin C 60 mg, B_1 1.5 mg, B_2 1.7 mg, B_3 20 mg, B_6 10 mg, B_{12} 6 mcg, folic acid 1 mcg, biotin 300 mcg, Zn. Film-coated. Tab. 100s. *Rx.*
Use: Multivitamin with minerals.

in vivo diagnostic aids.
See: Benzylpenicilloyl Polylysine.
Capromab Pendetide.
Gadofosveset Trisodium.
Gastrointestinal Function Tests.
Gonadorelin Hydrochloride.
Hexaminolevulinate Hydrochloride.
Ioflupane I 123.
Methacholine Chloride.
Metyrapone.
Pentetate Indium Disodium In 111.
Regadenoson.
Technetium Tc 99m Tilmanocept.
Tolbutamide Sodium.
Thyroid Function Tests.
Tuberculin Purified Protein Derivative.

Invokana. (Janssen Pharmaceuticals) Canagliflozin 100 mg, 300 mg. Film coated. Lactose. Tab. 30s, 90s, 500s, UD 100s. *Rx.*
Use: Antidiabetic agent, sodium-glucose cotransporter 2 inhibitor.

•**iobenguane I 131.** (EYE-oh-BEN-gwane) USAN.
Use: Diagnostic aid; radiopharmaceutical.

•**iobenguane I 123 injection.** (EYE-oh-BEN-gwane) *USP.*
Use: Radiopharmaceutical.
See: AdreView.

•**iobenguane sulfate I 131.** (EYE-oh-BEN-gwane) USAN.
Use: Diagnostic aid; radiopharmaceutical.

•**iobenguane sulfate I 123.** (EYE-oh-BEN-gwane) USAN.
Use: Diagnostic aid, radioactive, adrenomedullary disorders, and neuroendocrine tumors; radiopharmaceutical.

•**iobenzamic acid.** (EYE-oh-ben-ZAM-ik) USAN.
Use: Diagnostic aid (radiopaque medium, cholecystographic).

•**iocanlidic acid I 123.** (eye-oh-kan-LIH-dik) USAN.
Use: Diagnostic aid (radioactive, cardiac disease) for assessment of viable myocardium.

Iocare Balanced Salt Solution. (Novartis Ophthalmic) Sodium Cl 0.64%, potassium Cl 0.075%, magnesium Cl 0.03%, calcium Cl 0.048%, sodium acetate 0.39%, sodium citrate 0.17%, sodium hydroxide or hydrochloric acid. Soln. Bot. 15 mL. *Rx.*
Use: Irrigant, ophthalmic.

•**iocarmate meglumine.** (EYE-oh-KAR-mate meh-GLUE-meen) USAN.
Use: Diagnostic aid (radiopaque medium).

•**iocarmic acid.** (EYE-oh-KAR-mik) USAN.
Use: Diagnostic aid (radiopaque medium).

•**iocetamic acid.** (eye-oh-seh-TAM-ik) *USP.*
Use: Diagnostic aid (radiopaque medium).

i-octadecanol.
See: Stearyl Alcohol.

•**iodamide.** (EYE-oh-dah-MIDE) USAN.
Use: Diagnostic aid (radiopaque medium).

•**iodamide meglumine.** (EYE-oh-dah-MIDE meh-GLUE-meen) USAN.
Use: Diagnostic aid (radiopaque medium).
W/Combinations.
See: Renovue-Dip.
Renovue-65.

Iodex. (Lee) Iodine 4.7% in petrolatum ointment base. 28.35 g. *OTC.*
Use: Antimicrobial; antiseptic.

Iodex with Methyl Salicylate. (Lee) Iodine 4.7%, methyl salicylate 4.8%. Oleic acid, paraffin, petrolatum. Oint. 28 g. *OTC.*
Use: Antiseptic; analgesic, topical.

iodide, sodium, I-131 capsules.
Use: Antineoplastic; diagnostic aid (thyroid function determination); radiopharmaceutical.
See: Iodotope.

iodide, sodium, I-131 solution.
Use: Antineoplastic; diagnostic aid (thyroid function determination); radiopharmaceutical.
See: Iodotope.

iodide, sodium, I-125 capsules.
Use: Diagnostic aid (thyroid function determination); radiopharmaceutical.

iodide, sodium, I-125 solution.
Use: Diagnostic aid (thyroid function determination), radiopharmaceutical.

iodide, sodium, I-123 capsules.
Use: Diagnostic aid (thyroid function determination).

iodide, sodium, I-123 tablets.
Use: Diagnostic aid (thyroid function determination).

iodinated glycerol and codeine phosphate liquid. (Various Mfr.) Codeine phosphate 10 mg, iodinated glycerol 30 mg. Liq. Bot. Pt, gal. *c-v.*
Use: Antitussive, expectorant, narcotic.

iodinated human serum albumin.
See: Albumotope.

iodinated I-131 albumin aggregated injection.
Use: Radiopharmaceutical.
See: Albumin, Aggregated Iodinated I-131 serum.

iodinated I-131 albumin injection.
Use: Diagnostic aid (blood volume determination and intrathecal imaging); radiopharmaceutical.
See: Albumin, Iodinated I-131.

iodinated I-125 albumin injection.
Use: Diagnostic aid (blood volume determination); radiopharmaceutical.
See: Albumin, Iodinated I-125.

•**iodine.** (EYE-uh-dine) *USP.*
Use: Anti-infective, topical; source of iodine.
See: Curity Sponge Sticks.
Curity Wet Skin Scrub Pack.
Iodex.
Iodoflex.
Iodosorb.
Kelp.
W/Methyl Salicylate
See: Iodex with Methyl Salicylate.
W/Potassium Iodide.
See: Strong Iodine Solution (Lugol's Solution).

iodine cacodylate, colloidal. Cacodyne Iodine.

iodine combination.
See: Calcidrine.
iodine-iodophor.
See: Betadine.
iodine I 131 murine monoclonal antibody IgG2a to B cell.
Use: Antineoplastic. [Orphan Drug]
See: Immurait.
iodine I 131 murine monoclonal antibody to alpha-fetoprotein. (Immunomedics)
Use: Antineoplastic. [Orphan Drug]
iodine I 131 murine monoclonal antibody to hCG. (Immunomedics)
Use: Antineoplastic. [Orphan Drug]
iodine I 131 6b-iodomethyl-19-norcholesterol.
Use: Diagnostic aid. [Orphan Drug]
iodine I 131 tositumomab and tositumomab.
Use: Antineoplastic.
•**iodine I 124 girentuximab.** (JIR-en-TUX-i-mab) USAN.
Use: Diagnostic agent.
iodine I 123 murine monoclonal antibody to alpha-fetoprotein. (Immunomedics)
Use: Diagnostic aid. [Orphan Drug]
iodine I 123 murine monoclonal antibody to hCG. (Immunomedics)
Use: Diagnostic aid. [Orphan Drug]
iodine 131: capsules diagnostic-capsules therapeutic-solution therapeutic oral.
See: Iodotope.
•**iodine povacrylex.** (poe-va-KREYE-lex) USAN.
Use: Topical antiseptic.
iodine povidone.
See: Iodophor.
Mallisol.
iodine products, anti-infective.
See: Anayodin.
Betadine.
Chiniofon.
Diiodohydroxyquinoline.
Prepodyne.
Quinoxyl.
Surgidine.
Vioform.
iodine products, diagnostic.
See: Chloriodized Oil.
Ethyl Iodophenylundecylate.
Iodoalphionic Acid.
Iodobrassid.
Iodohippurate Sodium.
Iodopanoic Acid.
Iodophthalein Sodium.
Iodopyracet.
Methiodal Sodium.
Optiray 350.
Pantopaque.
Sodium Acetrizoate.
Sodium Iodomethamate.
Telepaque.
iodine products, nutritional.
See: Calcium Iodobehenate.
Entodon.
Hydriodic Acid.
Iodobrassid.
iodine ration. (Barth's) Iodine (from kelp) 0.15 mg, trace minerals. Tab. Bot. 90s, 180s, 360s. *OTC.*
Use: Mineral supplement.
iodine ration. (Nion Corp.) Iodine (from kelp) 0.15 mg. 3 Tab. Bot. 175s, 500s. *OTC.*
Use: Mineral supplement.
iodine surface active complex.
See: Ioprep.
iodine tincture, strong.
Use: Anti-infective, topical.
•**iodipamide.** (eye-oh-DIH-pah-mide) *USP.*
Use: Pharmaceutic necessity for Iodipamide Meglumine Injection.
•**iodipamide meglumine 52%.** (eye-oh-DIH-pah-mide meh-GLUE-meen) *USP.*
Use: Radiopaque agent, parenteral.
See: Cholografin Meglumine.
iodipamide methylglucamine. Also sodium salt injection.
W/Diatrizoate Methylglucamine.
See: Sinografin.
iodipamide sodium injection.
See: Cholografin Sodium.
•**iodipamide sodium I 131.** (eye-oh-DIH-pah-mide) USAN.
Use: Radiopharmaceutical.
iodipamide 26.8% and diatrizoate meglumine 52.7%.
Use: Radiopaque agent.
See: Diatrizoate Meglumine 52.7% and Iodipamide Meglumine 26.8% (38% Iodine).
•**iodixanol.** (EYE-oh-DIX-an-ole) *USP.*
Use: Radiopaque agent, parenteral.
See: Visipaque 270.
Visipaque 320.
iodoalphionic acid. Biliselectan dikol, pheniodol.
•**iodoantipyrine I 131.** (EYE-oh-doe-ANN-tee-PI-reen) USAN.
Use: Radiopharmaceutical.
iodobehenate calcium. Calcium iodododocosanoate.
Use: Antigoitrogenic.
iodobrassid. Ethyl Diiodobrassidate. Lipoiodine.
•**iodocetylic acid I 123.** (eye-OH-doe-SEE-till-ik) USAN.
Use: Diagnostic aid; radiopharmaceutical.

iodochlorhydroxyquin.
Use: Antiamebic; anti-infective, topical.
See: Clioquinol.

•**iodocholesterol I 131.** (EYE-oh-DOE-koe-LESS-teh-role) USAN.
Use: Radiopharmaceutical.

Iodo Cream. (Day-Baldwin) Clioquinol 3%. Tube 1 oz, Jar 1 lb. *OTC.*
Use: Antifungal, topical.

•**iodofiltic acid I 123.** (eye-oh-doe-FIL-tic) USAN.
Use: Metabolic imaging agent.

Iodoflex. (Smith & Nephew) Iodine 0.9% w/w iodine (equiv. to cadexomer iodine 600 mg per g). PEG. Pads, Gel; Top. 5 g (4 cm × 6 cm), 10 g (6 cm × 8 cm) packet. *Rx.*
Use: Antiseptic and germicide, iodine compound.

•**iodoform.** (EYE-oh-doe-form) *USP.*

Iodo H-C. (Day-Baldwin) Clioquinol 3%, hydrocortisone 1%. **Oint.:** Tube 20 g, Jar 1 lb. **Cream:** Tube 20 g, Jar 1 lb. *Rx.*
Use: Antifungal; corticosteroid.

•**iodohippurate, sodium I 131 injection.** (EYE-oh-doe-HIP-you-rate) *USP.*
Use: Diagnostic aid (renal function determination); radiopharmaceutical.
See: Hipputope.

•**iodohippurate sodium I 125.** (EYE-oh-doe-HIP-you-rate) USAN.
Use: Radiopharmaceutical.
See: Hipputope I 125.

•**iodohippurate sodium I 123 injection.** (EYE-oh-doe-HIP-you-rate) *USP.*
Use: Radiopharmaceutical; diagnostic aid (renal function determination).

iodohippuric acid.
See: Hipputope.

Iodo Ointment. (Day-Baldwin) Clioquinol 3%. Tube 1 oz, Jar 1 lb. *Rx.*
Use: Antifungal, topical.

Iodo-Pak. (SoloPak Pharmaceuticals, Inc.) Iodine 100 mcg/mL. Inj. Vial 10 mL. *Rx.*
Use: Nutritional supplement, parenteral.

iodopanoic acid.
Use: Diagnostic aid (radiopaque medium).

Iodopen. (American Pharmaceutical Partners) Sodium iodide 118 mcg/mL. Inj. 10 mL. *Rx.*
Use: Nutritional supplement, parenteral.

iodophene. Iodophthalein.

iodophene sodium.
See: Iodophthalein Sodium.

iodophor.
See: Betadine.

iodophthalein sodium. Tetraiodophenolphthalein Sodium, Tetraiodophthalein Sodium, Tetiothalein Sodium (Antinosin, Cholepulvis, Cholumbrin, Foriod, Iodophene, Iodorayoral, Nosophene Sodium, Opacin, Photobiline, Piliophen, Radiotetrane).
Use: Radiopaque agent.

iodopropylidene glycerol.
See: Organidin.

iodopyracet compound. Diodrast.

iodopyracet concentrated. Diodrast.

iodopyracet injection. Diatrast, Diodone, Iopyracil, Neo-Methiodal, NeoSkiodan.
Use: Radiopaque medium.

•**iodopyracet I 131.** (EYE-oh-doe-peer-ah-set) USAN.
Use: Radiopharmaceutical.

•**iodopyracet I 125.** (EYE-oh-doe-peer-ah-set) USAN.
Use: Radiopharmaceutical.

iodopyrine. Antipyrine iodide.
Use: Iodides, analgesic.

•**iodoquinol.** (EYE-oh-doe-KWIH-nole) *USP. Formerly Diiodohydroxyquin.*
Use: Antiamebic.
See: Floraquin.
Sebaquin.
Yodoxin.
W/9-Aminoacridine Hydrochloride.
See: Vagitric.
Yodoxin.
W/Hydrocortisone Acetate.
See: Hydro-Iodoquinol 2-1.
Vytone.
W/Hydrocortisone, Coal Tar Solution.
See: Gynben.
Gynben Insufflate.
W/Surfactants.
See: Lycinate.
W/Sulfanilamide, Diethylstilbestrol.
See: Amide V/S.
D.I.T.I.

Iodosorb. (Smith & Nephew) Iodine 0.9% w/w iodine (equiv. to cadexomer iodine 500 mg per g). PEG. Oint. 10 g, 40 g. *Rx.*
Use: Antiseptic and germicide, iodine compound.

•**iodoxamate meglumine.** (EYE-oh-DOX-ah-mate meh-GLUE-meen) USAN.
Use: Diagnostic aid (radiopaque medium).

•**iodoxamic acid.** (EYE-oh-dox-AM-ik) USAN.
Use: Diagnostic aid (radiopaque medium).

iodoxyl.
See: Sodium Iodomethamate.

Iofed. (Iomed) Brompheniramine maleate 12 mg, pseudoephedrine hydrochloride

120 mg. ER Cap. Bot. 100s. *Rx.*
Use: Antihistamine, decongestant.

Iofed PD. (Iomed) Brompheniramine maleate 6 mg, pseudoephedrine hydrochloride 60 mg. ER Cap. Bot. 100s. *Rx.*
Use: Antihistamine, decongestant.

•**iofetamine hydrochloride I 123.** (EYE-oh-FET-ah-meen) USAN.
Use: Diagnostic aid; radiopharmaceutical.

•**ioflubenzamide I 131.** (EYE-oh-floo-BEN-za-mide) USAN.
Use: Radiotherapeutic agent.

•**ioflupane I 123.** (EYE-oh-FLOO-pane) USAN.
Use: Imaging agent.
See: DaTscan.

•**iofolastat I 123.** (EYE-oh-FOL-a-stat)
Use: Diagnostic agent.

•**ioforminol.** (EYE-oh-FOR-mi-nol) USAN.
Use: Contrast medium.

•**ioglicic acid.** (eye-oh-GLIH-sick) USAN.
Use: Diagnostic aid (radiopaque medium).

•**ioglucol.** (EYE-oh-GLUE-kahl) USAN.
Use: Diagnostic aid (radiopaque medium).

•**ioglucomide.** (EYE-oh-GLUE-koe-mide) USAN.
Use: Diagnostic aid (radiopaque medium).

•**ioglycamic acid.** (EYE-oh-glie-KAM-ik) USAN.
Use: Diagnostic aid (radiopaque medium, cholecystographic).

•**iogulamide.** (EYE-oh-GULL-ah-mide) USAN.
Use: Diagnostic aid (radiopaque medium).

•**iohexol.** (EYE-oh-HEX-ole) *USP.*
Use: Radiopaque agent, parenteral.
See: Omnipaque 140.
Omnipaque 300.
Omnipaque 350.
Omnipaque 240.

•**iomeprol.** (EYE-oh-MEH-prole) USAN.
Use: Diagnostic aid (radiopaque medium).

•**iomethin I 131.** (EYE-oh-METH-in) USAN.
Use: Diagnostic aid (neoplasm); radiopharmaceutical.

•**iomethin I 125.** (EYE-oh-METH-in) USAN.
Use: Diagnostic aid (neoplasm); radiopharmaceutical.

•**iometopane I 123.** (eye-oh-meh-TOE-pane) USAN.
Use: Diagnostic aid.

Ionax Astringent Cleanser. (Galderma) Isopropyl alcohol 48%, acetone, salicylic acid. Bot. 240 mL. *OTC.*
Use: Dermatologic, acne.

Ionax Foam. (Galderma) Benzalkonium Cl, propylene glycol. Aerosol Can 150 mL. *OTC.*
Use: Dermatologic, acne.

Ionax Scrub. (Galderma) SD alcohol 40, benzalkonium Cl. Tube 60 g, 120 g. *OTC.*
Use: Dermatologic, acne.

ion-exchange resins.
See: Polyamine Methylene Resin.
Resins, Sodium-Removing.

Ionil Plus Shampoo. (Galderma) Salicylic acid 2%, sodium laureth sulfate, lauramide DEA, quaternium-22, talloweth-60 myristyl glycol, laureth-23, TEA lauryl sulfate, glycol disterate, laureth-4, TEA-abietoyl hydrolyzed collagen, DMDM hydantoin, tetrasodium EDTA, sodium hydroxide, FD&C blue No. 1. Bot. 4 oz, 8 oz. *OTC.*
Use: Antiseborrheic.

Ionil Rinse. (Galderma) Conditioners with benzalkonium Cl in water base. Bot. 16 oz. *OTC.*
Use: Dermatologic, hair.

Ionil Shampoo. (Galderma) Salicylic acid, benzalkonium Cl, alcohol 12%, polyoxyethylene ethers. Plastic bot. w/dispenser cap 4 oz, 8 oz, 16 oz, 32 oz. *OTC.*
Use: Antiseborrheic.

Ionil T. (Valeant) Coal tar solution 1%. Alcohols, benzalkonium chloride, EDTA. Shampoo. 237 mL, 473 mL. *OTC.*
Use: Antiseborrheic.

Ionosol B and 5% Dextrose. (Hospira) Dextrose 50 g, Na^+ 57 mEq, K^+ 25 mEq, Mg^{++} 5 mEq, Cl^- 49 mEq, phosphate 7 millimoles, lactate 25 mEq, 426 mOsm per L. Inj. Single-dose containers. 500 mL, 1000 mL. *Rx.*
Use: Intravenous nutritional therapy.

Ionosol D-CM. (Abbott Hospital Products) Sodium Cl 516 mg, potassium Cl 89.4 mg, calcium Cl anhydrous 27.8 mg, magnesium Cl anhydrous 14.2 mg, sodium lactate 560 mg/100 mL. Bot. 1000 mL. *Rx.*
Use: Nutritional supplement, parenteral.

Ionosol-T and 5% Dextrose. (Hospira) Dextrose 50 g, sodium 40 mEq, potassium 35 mEq, chloride 40 mEq, phosphate 15 mM, lactate 20 mEq, 432 mOsm per L. Inj., Soln. 500 mL, 1000 mL. *Rx.*
Use: Intravenous nutritional therapy, intravenous replenishment solutions.

•**iopamidol.** (EYE-oh-PAM-ih-dahl) *USP.*
Use: Radiopaque agent, parenteral.
See: Isovue-M 300.
Isovue-M 200.
Isovue 300.
Isovue 370.
Isovue-200.
Isovue-250.

•**iopentol.** (EYE-oh-PEN-tole) USAN.
Use: Diagnostic aid (radiopaque medium).

Iophen-C. (Various Mfr.) Codeine phosphate 10 mg, iodinated glycerol 30 mg/5 mL. Liq. Bot. Pt, gal. *c-v.*
Use: Antitussive, expectorant.

Iophen C-NR. (Qualitest) Codeine phosphate 10 mg, guaifenesin 100 mg per 5 mL. Glycerin, propylene glycol, raspberry flavoring, saccharin, sodium benzoate, sorbitol. Liq. 473 mL. *c-v.*
Use: Upper respiratory combination, antitussive with expectorant.

Iophen-DM. (Various Mfr.) Dextromethorphan HBr, iodinated glycerol 30 mg/5 mL. Liq. Bot. 120 mL, pt, gal. *Rx.*
Use: Antitussive, expectorant.

Iophen DM-NR. (Qualitest) Dextromethorphan hydrobromide 10 mg, guaifenesin 100 mg. Glycerin, propylene glycol, raspberry flavoring, saccharin, sodium benzoate, sorbitol. Liq. 473 mL. *OTC.*
Use: Upper respiratory combination, antitussive with expectorant.

iophendylate injection. Ethiodan, Myodil. Ethyl Iodophenylundecylate.
Use: Diagnostic aid (radiopaque medium).
See: Pantopaque.

Iophen NR. (Qualitest) Guaifenesin 100 mg per 5 mL. Glycerin, propylene glycol, raspberry flavoring, saccharin, sodium 2 mg, sodium benzoate, sorbitol. Liq. 473 mL. *OTC.*
Use: Expectorant.

Iopidine. (Alcon) Apraclonidine 0.5%, 1%, benzalkonium Cl 0.01%. Dispenser Bot. 0.25 mL (1%), *Drop-Tainer* 5 mL (0.5%). *Rx.*
Use: Antiglaucoma agent.

iopodate sodium.
See: Ipodate Sodium.

Ioprep. (Johnson & Johnson) Nonylphenoxypolyethyleneoxy (4) ethanol and nonylphenoxypolyethyleneoxy (15) ethanol iodine complex 5.5%, nonylphenoxypolyethyleneoxy (30) ethanol 10%. Solution provides 1% available iodine. Plastic bot. Gal.
Use: Antiseptic.

•**ioprocemic acid.** (EYE-oh-pro-SEH-mik acid) USAN.
Use: Diagnostic aid (radiopaque medium).

•**iopromide.** (eye-oh-PRO-mide) *USP.*
Use: Radiopaque agent, parenteral.
See: Ultravist 150.
Ultravist 300.
Ultravist 370.
Ultravist 240.

•**iopronic acid.** (eye-oh-PRO-nik acid) USAN.
Use: Diagnostic aid (radiopaque medium, cholecystographic).

•**iopydol.** (eye-oh-PIE-dahl) USAN.
Use: Diagnostic aid (radiopaque medium, bronchographic).

•**iopydone.** (eye-oh-PIE-dohn) USAN.
Use: Diagnostic aid (radiopaque medium, bronchographic).

Iosat. (Anbex) Potassium iodide 130 mg. Tab. 14s. *OTC.*
Use: Thyroid drug.

•**iosefamic acid.** (EYE-oh-seh-FAM-ik) USAN.
Use: Diagnostic aid; radiopaque medium.

•**ioseric acid.** (eye-oh-SEH-rik) USAN.
Use: Diagnostic aid (radiopaque medium).

•**iosimenol.** (EYE-oh-SIM-e-nol) USAN.
Use: Iodinated x-ray contrast agent.

Iosopan. (Ivax) Magaldrate 540 mg/5 mL. Liq. Bot. 355 mL. *OTC.*
Use: Antacid.

Iosopan Plus. (Ivax) Magaldrate 540 mg, simethicone 40 mg/5 mL. Liq. Bot. 355 mL. *OTC.*
Use: Antacid.

•**iosulamide meglumine.** (eye-oh-SULL-ah-mide meh-GLUE-meen) USAN.
Use: Diagnostic aid (radiopaque medium).

•**iosumetic acid.** (eye-oh-sue-MEH-tick) USAN.
Use: Diagnostic aid (radiopaque medium).

•**iotasul.** (EYE-oh-tah-sull) USAN.
Use: Diagnostic aid (radiopaque medium).

•**iotetric acid.** (eye-oh-TEH-trick) USAN.
Use: Diagnostic aid (radiopaque medium).

iothalamate meglumide and iothalmate sodium injection.
Use: Diagnostic aid (radiopaque medium).

•**iothalamate meglumine.** (eye-oh-THAL-am-ate MEG-loo-meen) *USP.*
Use: Radiopaque agent.
See: Conray.

Conray 43.
Conray 30.

•**iothalamate sodium injection.** (eye-oh-THAL-am-ate) *USP.*
Use: Diagnostic aid (radiopaque medium).
See: Conray.

•**iothalamate sodium I 131.** (eye-oh-THAL-am-ate) USAN.
Use: Radiopharmaceutical.

•**iothalamate sodium I 125 injection.** (eye-oh-THAL-am-ate) *USP.*
Use: Radiopharmaceutical.

•**iothalamic acid.** (eye-oh-THAL-am-ik) *USP.*
Use: Diagnostic aid (radiopaque medium).

iothiouracil sodium. Sodium salt of 5-iodo-2-thiouracil.

•**iotrolan.** (EYE-oh-TRAHL-an) USAN.
Formerly Iotrol.
Use: Diagnostic aid (radiopaque medium).

•**iotroxic acid.** (EYE-oh-TRAHK-sick) USAN.
Use: Diagnostic aid (radiopaque medium).

•**iotyrosine I 131.** (eye-oh-TYE-roe-seen) USAN.
Use: Radiopharmaceutical.

•**ioversol.** (EYE-oh-ver-sole) *USP.*
Use: Radiopaque agent, parenteral.
See: Optiray 160.
Optiray 300.
Optiray 350.
Optiray 320.
Optiray 240.

ioversol 74%.
Use: Radiopaque agent, parenteral.
See: Optiray 350.

ioversol 68%.
Use: Radiopaque agent, parenteral.
See: Optiray 320.

ioversol 64%.
Use: Radiopaque agent, parenteral.
See: Optiray 300.

ioversol 34%.
Use: Radiopaque agent, parenteral.
See: Optiray 160.

•**ioxaglate meglumine.** (eye-ox-AGG-late meh-GLUE-meen) USAN.
Use: Diagnostic aid (radiopaque medium).

•**ioxaglate sodium.** (eye-ox-AGG-late) USAN.
Use: Diagnostic aid (radiopaque medium).

•**ioxaglic acid.** (eye-ox-AGG-lick) *USP.*
Use: Diagnostic aid (radiopaque medium).

•**ioxilan.** (eye-OX-ee-lan) USAN.
Use: Diagnostic aid.

•**ioxotrizoic acid.** (eye-OX-oh-TRY-zoe-ik) USAN.
Use: Diagnostic aid (radiopaque medium).

•**ipatasertib.** (eye-PAT-a-SER-tib) USAN.
Use: Antineoplastic.

•**ipazilide fumarate.** (ih-PAZZ-ih-LIDE) USAN.
Use: Cardiovascular agent.

•**ipecac.** (IPP-uh-kak) *USP.*
Use: Emetic.
W/Combinations.
See: Ipsatol.
Mallergan.

ipecac. (Various Mfr.) Ipecac alcohol 1.5% to 1.75%, 2%. Syrup. Bot. 15 mL, 30 mL. *OTC.*
Use: Antidote.

•**ipexidine mesylate.** (eye-PEX-ih-DEEN) USAN.
Use: Dental caries agent.

•**ipilimumab.** (i-pi-LIM-ue-mab) USAN.
Use: Antineoplastic.
See: Yervoy.

I-Pilopine. (Akorn) Pilocarpine hydrochloride 1%. Ophthalmic soln. Bot. 15 mL. *Rx.*
Use: Antiglaucoma agent.

•**ipodate calcium.** (EYE-poe-date) *USP.*
Use: Diagnostic aid (radiopaque medium).
See: Oragrafin Calcium.

•**ipodate sodium.** (EYE-poe-date) *USP.*
Use: Diagnostic aid (radiopaque medium).

IPOL. (Sanofi Pasteur) Suspension of 3 types of poliovirus (Types 1, 2, and 3) grown in monkey kidney cell cultures. Each dose contains 2-phenoxyethanol 0.5%, formaldehyde 0.02% (maximum), streptomycin ≤ 200 ng, polymyxin B 25 ng, neomycin 5 ng. Inj. Single-dose syringe with integrated needle. 0.5 mL. *Rx.*
Use: Immunization.

Ipran. (Major) Propranolol hydrochloride 10 mg, 20 mg, 40 mg, 60 mg, 80 mg, 90 mg. Tab. **10 mg, 20 mg, 40 mg:** Bot. 100s, 250s, 1000s, UD 100s. **60 mg:** Bot. 100s, 500s. **80 mg:** Bot. 100s, 500s, 1000s, UD 100s. **90 mg:** Bot. 100s, 500s. *Rx.*
Use: Beta-adrenergic blocker.

•**ipratropium bromide.** (IH-pruh-TROE-pee-uhm) USAN.
Use: Bronchodilator.
See: Atrovent.
Atrovent HFA.

W/Albuterol Sulfate.
See: Combivent.
Combivent Respimat.
DuoNeb.

ipratropium bromide. (Dey) Ipratropium bromide 0.02%. Soln. for Inhal. Vial. 2.5 mL (UD 25s, UD 30s, UD 60s). *Rx.*
Use: Anticholinergic.

ipratropium bromide. (Various Mfr.) Ipratropium bromide 0.03% (21 mcg/spray), 0.06% (42 mcg/spray). Nasal Spray. 30 mL with spray pump (345 sprays) (0.03% only), 15 mL with spray pump (165 sprays) (0.06% only). *Rx.*
Use: Anticholinergic.

ipratropium bromide and albuterol sulfate. (Sandoz) Albuterol sulfate 3 mg (equiv. to 2.5 mg base), ipratropium bromide 0.5 mg/3 mL. Inh. Soln. 3 mL unit-dose vials. 30s, 60s. *Rx.*
Use: Bronchodilator, anticholinergic.

I-Pred. (Akorn) Prednisolone sodium phosphate 0.5%, 1%. Ophth. Soln. Bot. 5 mL. *Rx.*
Use: Corticosteroid, ophthalmic.

•**iprindole.** (IH-prin-dole) USAN.
Use: Antidepressant.

Iprivask. (Aventis) Desirudin 15 mg, preservative free. Pow. for Inj., lyophilized. Single-use vials with diluent (mannitol 0.6 mL [3%] in water for injection). *Rx.*
Use: Anticoagulant, antithrombin agent.

•**iprofenin.** (IH-pro-FEN-in) USAN.
Use: Diagnostic aid (hepatic function determination).

•**ipronidazole.** (ih-pro-NIH-dah-zole) USAN.
Use: Antiprotozoal *Histomonas.*

•**iproplatin.** (IH-pro-PLAT-in) USAN.
Use: Antineoplastic.

iproveratril. *Name used for Verapamil.*

•**iproxamine hydrochloride.** (IH-PROX-ah-meen) USAN.
Use: Vasodilator.

•**ipsapirone hydrochloride.** (ipp-sah-PIE-rone) USAN.
Use: Anxiolytic.

IPV.
Use: Immunization.
See: IPOL.
Polio Virus Vaccine, Inactivated.

Iquix. (Vistakon) Levofloxacin 1.5%. Glycerin. Ophth. Soln. 5 mL. *Rx.*
Use: Antibiotic.

•**iratumumab.** (IR-a-TOOM-ue-mab) USAN.
Use: Antineoplastic.

•**irbesartan.** (ihr-beh-SAHR-tan) *USP.*
Use: Renin angiotensin system antagonist, angiotensin II receptor antagonist.
See: Avapro.
W/Hydrochlorothiazide.
See: Avalide.

irbesartan. (Teva Pharmaceuticals) Irbesartan 75 mg, 150 mg, 300 mg. Tab. 30s, 90s, 500s (except 75 mg). *Rx.*
Use: Renin angiotensin system antagonist, angiotensin II receptor antagonist.

irbesartan. (Various Mfr.) Irbesartan 75 mg, 150 mg, 300 mg. May contain lactose, PEG. Tab. 30s, 90s, 500s (except 75 mg). *Rx.*
Use: Renin angiotensin system antagonist, angiotensin II receptor antagonist.

irbesartan/hydrochlorothiazide. (Various Mfr.) Irbesartan/hydrochlorothiazide 150 mg/12.5 mg, 300 mg/12.5 mg. May contain lactose, PEG. Tab. 30s, 90s, 500s, UD 30s, UD 90s. *Rx.*
Use: Antihypertensive combination.

Ircon. (Kenwood) Iron (as carbonyl iron) 66 mg. Tab. Blister Pack 100s. *OTC.*
Use: Mineral supplement.

•**irdabisant.** (ir-DAB-i-sant) USAN.
Use: CNS agent.

•**irdabisant hydrochloride.** (ir-DAB-i-sant) USAN.
Use: CNS agent.

Irgasan CF3. Cloflucarban.
Use: Antiseptic, topical.

•**iridium Ir 192.** (ih-RID-ee-uhm) USAN.
Use: Radioactive agent.

•**irinotecan hydrochloride.** (eye-rih-no-TEE-can) USAN.
Use: DNA topoisomerase inhibitor.
See: Camptosar.

irinotecan hydrochloride. (Various Mfr.) Irinotecan 20 mg. May contain sorbitol. IV Inj. Vials. 2 mL, 5 mL. *Rx.*
Use: DNA topoisomerase inhibitor.

•**irinotecan sucrosofate.** (EYE-ri-noe-TEE-kan soo-KROE-soe-fate) USAN.
Use: Antineoplastic.

irisin. A polysaccharide found in several species of iris.

irocaine.
See: Procaine Hydrochloride.

Irodex. (Keene Pharmaceuticals) Iron dextran complex 50 mg/mL. Vial 10 mL. *Rx.*
Use: Mineral supplement.

Iromin-G. (Mission Pharmacal) Ferrous gluconate 260 mg (iron 30 mg), vitamins B_{12} (crystalline on resin) 2 mcg, C 100 mg, A acetate 4000 units, D

400 units, B_1 5 mg, B_2 2 mg, B_3 10 mg, B_5 1 mg, B_6 20.6 mg, folic acid 0.8 mg, Ca. Tab. Bot. 100s. *OTC.*
Use: Mineral, vitamin supplement.

iron.
See: Carbonyl Iron.
Duofer.
Ferrous Fumarate.
Ferrous Gluconate.
Ferrous Sulfate.
Ferrous Sulfate Exsiccated (Dried).
Iron Dextran.
Iron Sucrose.
Iron with Vitamin C.
Polysaccharide-Iron Complex.
Sodium Ferric Gluconate Complex.

iron carbonate complex.
See: Polyferose.

Iron Chews. (Midlothian) Carbonyl iron 15 mg. Sorbitol, grape flavor. Chew. Tab. 60s. *OTC.*
Use: Nutritional supplement.

Ironco-B. (Pal-Pak, Inc.) Ferrous sulfate 120.4 mg, manganese sulfate 21.6 mg, dicalcium phosphate 129.6 mg, vitamins B_1 1 mg, B_2 1 mg, niacin 6 mg, D 100 units. Tab. Bot. 100s, 1000s. *OTC.*
Use: Mineral, vitamin supplement.

iron complex. (Integrative Therapeutics) Ferrous succinate 25 mg, vitamin B_{12} 100 mcg, chlorophyll 10 mg, liquid liver fractions 250 mg, vitamin C 60 mg, folic acid 0.2 mg. Glycerin, soy, soybean oil. Gluten free, preservative free. Cap., softgel. 90s. *Rx.*
Use: Iron with vitamin B_{12} and intrinsic factor.

•**iron dextran.** (iron DEX-tran) *USP.*
Use: Hematinic.
See: DexFerrum.
Ferumoxytol.
INFeD.

Iron-Folic 500. (Major) Ferrous sulfate 105 mg, B_1 6 mg, B_2 6 mg, B_3 30 mg, B_5 10 mg, B_{12} 25 mcg, C 500 mg, folic acid 0.8 mg. Tab. Bot. 100s, 500s. *OTC.*
Use: Mineral, vitamin supplement.

iron/liver combination, injection.
See: Hemocyte.
Liver-Iron B Complex w/Vitamin B_{12}.

iron/liver combination, oral.
See: Feocyte.
Liquid Geritonic.

Iron 100 Plus. (Cypress Pharmaceutical) Iron 100 mg, vitamins B_{12} 25 mcg, C 250 mg, folic acid 1 mg. Mineral oil, PEG. Tab. 100s. *OTC.*
Use: Multivitamin with iron.

iron oxide mixture with zinc oxide. Calamine, USP.

iron, parenteral.
See: DexFerrum.
Ferumoxytol.
INFeD.

iron products, injection.
See: INFeD.

•**iron sorbitex injection.** (SORE-bih-tex) *USP.*
Use: Hematinic.

•**iron sucrose.** (EYE-urn-SOO-krose) *USP.*
Use: Trace element.
See: Venofer.

iron (2+) fumarate. Ferrous Fumarate, USP.

iron (2+) gluconate.
See: Ferrous Gluconate, USP.

iron with vitamin B_{12} and IFC.
See: Albafort.
Contrin.
Chromagen.
Fergon Plus.
Ferotrinsic.
Livitrinsic-f.
Multigen.
Pronemia Hematinic.
TriHEMIC 600.
Trinsicon.
Vitagen Advance.

iron with vitamin C.
See: Fero-Grad-500.
Ferrex 150 Plus.
Niferex-150.
Vitelle Irospan.
Vitron-C.

iron with vitamins.
See: Gentle Iron.
Tandem F.

Irospan. (Fielding) Ferrous sulfate 65 mg, vitamin C 150 mg. Cap. Bot. 60s. Tab. Bot. 100s. *OTC.*
Use: Mineral, vitamin supplement.

•**irosustat.** (IR-oh-SOO-stat) USAN.
Use: Antineoplastic.

irradiated ergosterol.
See: Calciferol.

irrigating solutions, physiological.
Use: Irrigant.
See: Lactated Ringer's Irrigation.
Physiolyte.
PhysioSol.
Tis-U-Sol.

irrigating solutions, urinary.
Use: Irrigant.
See: Acetic Acid.
Glycine (Aminoacetic acid).
Neosporin G.U. Irrigant.
Renacidin.
Resectisol.
Sodium Chloride.

Sorbitol-Mannitol.
Sterile Water.

irritant or stimulant laxatives.
See: Agoral.
Aromatic Cascara Fluid Extract.
Bisac-Evac.
Bisacodyl.
Bisacodyl Uniserts.
Black-Draught.
Caroid.
Cascara Aromatic.
Cascara Sagrada.
Correctol.
Dulcolax.
ex-lax.
ex-lax chocolated.
Feen-a-mint.
Fleet Laxative.
Fletcher's Castoria.
Maximum Relief ex-lax.
Modane.
Reliable Gentle Laxative.
Senexon.
Senna-Gen.
Sennosides.
Senokot.
Senokot XTRA.
Women's Gentle Laxative.

•**irtemazole.** (ihr-TEH-mah-zole) USAN.
Use: Uricosuric.

isacen.
See: Oxyphenisatin.

•**isamoxole.** (eye-SAH-MOX-ole) USAN.
Use: Antiasthmatic.

•**isatoribine.** (eye-sah-TORE-ih-been) USAN.
Use: Immunomodulator.

•**isavuconazonium.** (EYE-sa-vue-KON-a-ZOE-nee-um) USAN.
Use: Antifungal agent.

•**isavuconazonium sulfate.** (EYE-sa-vue-KON-a-ZOE-nee-um) USAN.
Use: Antifungal agent.

Iscador. (Weleda) Mistletoe.
Use: Cancer (not FDA-approved).

•**iscotrizinol.** (IS-koe-TRIZ-i-nol) USAN.
Use: Sunscreen.

•**iseganan hydrochloride.** (eye-se-GAN-an) USAN.
Use: Antimicrobial.

Isentress. (Merck) Raltegravir. **Tab.:** 400 mg (equiv. to raltegravir potassium 434.4 mg). Lactose. Film coated. 60s. **Chew. Tab.:** 25 mg (equiv. to raltegravir potassium 27.16 mg), 100 mg (equiv. to raltegravir potassium 108.6 mg). Aspartame, fructose, mannitol, phenylalanine, saccharin, sorbitol, sucralose. Orange-banana flavor. 60s. **Pow. for Susp.:** 100 mg. Fructose, maltodextrin, mannitol, sorbitol, sucralose, sucrose. Banana flavor. Single-use packet. *Rx.*
Use: Antiretroviral agent, integrase inhibitor.

•**isepamicin.** (eye-SEP-ah-MY-sin) USAN.
Use: Antibacterial (aminoglycoside).

ISG. Immune globulin intramuscular. *Rx.*
Use: Immunization.

Ismo. (Reddy Pharmaceuticals) Isosorbide mononitrate 20 mg. Lactose. Tab. Bot. 100s, UD 100s. *Rx.*
Use: Vasodilator.

•**ismomultin alpha.** (IZ-moe-MUL-tin) USAN.
Use: Rheumatoid arthritis.

iso-alcoholic elixir.
Use: Vehicle.

isoamylhydrocupreine dihydrochloride.
See: Eucupin Dihydrochloride.

isoamyl methoxycinnamate.
See: Amiloxate.

isoamyl nitrate.
See: Amyl Nitrite.

isoamyne.
See: Amphetamine.

Iso-B. (Tyson) Vitamins B_1 25 mg, B_2 25 mg, B_3 75 mg, B_5 125 mg, B_6 50 mg, B_{12} 100 mcg, FA 0.2 mg, pyridoxal 5 phosphate 2.5 mg, PABA 50 mg, inositol 50 mg, choline bitartrate 125 mg, biotin 100 mcg. Cap. Bot. 120s. *OTC.*
Use: Mineral, vitamin supplement.

isobornyl thiocyanoacetate, technical.
Use: Pediculicide.
See: Barc.
W/Docusate Sodium and Related Terpenes.
See: Barc.

•**isobucaine hydrochloride.** (eye-so-BYOO-kane) *USP.*
Use: Anesthetic, local.

•**isobucaine hydrochloride and epinephrine injection.** (eye-so-BYOO-kane HIGH-droe-KLOR-ide & epp-ih-NEFF-rin) *USP.*
Use: Anesthetic, local.

•**isobutamben.** (EYE-so-BYOO-tam-ben) USAN.
Use: Anesthetic, local.

•**isobutane.** (eye-so-BYOO-tane) *NF.*
Use: Aerosol propellant.

isobutylallylbarbituric acid.
W/Aspirin, Phenacetin, Caffeine.
See: Buff-A-Comp.
Fiorinal.
Palgesic.
Tenstan.
W/Codeine Phosphate.
See: Fiorinal w/Codeine.

isobutyl p-aminobenzoate.
See: Isobutamben, USAN.

isobutyramide. (Vertex)
Use: Sickle cell disease; beta-thalassemia. [Orphan Drug]

isobutyramide oral solution. (Alpha Therapeutic)
Use: Sickle call disease; beta-thalassemia. [Orphan Drug]

isocaine. Isobutamben.

Isocal. (Bristol-Myers Squibb) Lactose-free isotonic liquid containing as a percentage of the calories protein 13% as caseinate and soy protein; fat 37% as soy oil and medium chain triglycerides; carbohydrate 50% as corn syrup solids w/vitamins and minerals for the tube-fed patient. Bot. 8 fl oz, 12 fl oz, 32 fl oz. *OTC.*
Use: Nutritional supplement.

Isocal HCN. (Bristol-Myers Squibb) High calorie nitrogen nutritionally complete food. Protein 15%, fat 45%, carbohydrate 40%. Can 8 fl oz. *OTC.*
Use: Nutritional supplement.

Isocal HN. (Bristol-Myers Squibb) $\approx$ 1 Kcal/mL with protein 44 g, fat 45 g, carbohydrates 124 g/L. In 237 mL. *OTC.*
Use: Nutritional supplement.

•**isocarboxazid.** (eye-so-car-BOX-ah-zid) *USP.*
Use: Antidepressant.
See: Marplan.

Isoclor Expectorant. (Medeva) Codeine phosphate 10 mg, pseudoephedrine hydrochloride 30 mg, guaifenesin 100 mg/5 mL, alcohol 5%. Bot. Pt. *c-v.*
Use: Antitussive, decongestant, expectorant.

isococaine. Pseudococaine.

Isocom. (Nutripharm Laboratories, Inc.) Isometheptene mucate 65 mg, dichloralphenazone 100 mg, acetaminophen 325 mg. Cap. Bot. 50s, 100s, 250s. *Rx.*
Use: Antimigraine.

•**isoconazole.** (EYE-so-CONE-ah-zole) USAN.
Use: Anti-infective; antifungal.

isoephedrine hydrochloride. d-Isoephedrine hydrochloride.
See: Pseudoephedrine Hydrochloride.

d-isoephedrine sulfate.
See: Pseudoephedrine Sulfate.

•**isoetharine.** (EYE-so-ETH-uh-reen) USAN.
Use: Bronchodilator.

•**isoetharine hydrochloride.** (EYE-so-ETH-uh-reen) *USP.*
Use: Bronchodilator, sympathomimetic.

•**isoetharine mesylate.** (EYE-so-ETH-uh-reen) *USP.*
Use: Bronchodilator.
See: Bronkometer.

•**isoflupredone acetate.** (eye-so-FLEW-PREH-dohn) USAN.
Use: Anti-inflammatory.

•**isoflurane.** (EYE-so-FLEW-rane) *USP.*
Use: Anesthetic, general.
See: Terrell.

•**isoflurophate.** (eye-so-FLURE-oh-fate) *USP.*
Use: Cholinergic, ophthalmic.
See: Floropryl.

iso-iodeikon.
See: Phentetiothalein Sodium.

Isoject. (Roerig) A purified, sterile, disposable injection system.
Use: Injection system.
See: Permapen (Benzathine Penicillin G) Aqueous Soln. 1,200,000 units/2 mL. 10s.

Isolan. (Elan) Protein 40 g, fat 36 g, carbohydrates 144 g, Na 690 g, K 1.17 g/L, with appropriate vitamins and minerals. Lactose free. Liq. In 237 mL Tetra Pak containers and 1000 mL New Pak closed systems with and without Color Check. *OTC.*
Use: Nutritional supplement.

Isolate Compound Elixir. (Various Mfr.) Theophylline 45 mg, ephedrine sulfate 12 mg, isoproterenol hydrochloride 2.5 mg, potassium iodide 150 mg, phenobarbital 6 mg/15 mL, alcohol 19%. Elix. Bot. Pt, gal. *Rx.*
Use: Antiasthmatic combination.

•**isoleucine.** (EYE-so-LOO-seen) *USP.*
Use: Amino acid.

isoleucine. (Pfaltz & Bauer) Pow. 10 g.
Use: Amino acid.

Isolyte G with Dextrose. (McGaw) Sodium 65 mEq, potassium 17 mEq, chloride 150 mEq, NH_4 70 mEq, dextrose 50 g, 170 Cal, 555 mOsm/L. Bot. 1000 mL. *Rx.*
Use: Nutritional supplement, parenteral.

Isolyte H in 5% Dextrose. (B. Braun) Dextrose 50 g/L, calories 170 Cal/L, Na^+ 39 mEq, K^+ 13 mEq, Mg^{++} 3 mEq, Cl^- 44 mEq, acetate 16 mEq/L, osmolarity 360 mOsm/L. Inj. Soln. 1000 mL. *Rx.*
Use: Intravenous nutritional therapy, intravenous replenishment solution.

Isolyte M in 5% Dextrose. (B. Braun) Dextrose 50 g/L, calories 170 cal/L, Na^+ 36 mEq, K^+ 35 mEq, Cl^- 49 mEq, phosphate 15 mEq, acetate 20 mEq/L, osmolarity 390 mOsm/L. Inj. Soln. 500 mL, 1000 mL. *Rx.*

Use: Intravenous nutritional therapy, intravenous replenishment solution.

Isolyte P in 5% Dextrose. (B. Braun) Dextrose 50 g/L, calories 170 Cal/L, Na^+ 23 mEq, K^+ 20 mEq, Mg^{++} 3 mEq, Cl^- 29 mEq, phosphate 3 mEq, acetate 23 mEq/L, osmolarity 340 mOsm/L. Inj. Soln. 250 mL, 500 mL, 1000 mL. *Rx.*
Use: Intravenous nutritional therapy, intravenous replenishment solution.

Isolyte R in 5% Dextrose. (B. Braun) Sodium 39 mEq, potassium 16 mEq, calcium 5 mEq, magnesium 3 mEq, chloride 46 mEq, acetate 24 mEq, dextrose 50 g, 170 Cal, 375 mOsm/L. Inj. Soln. 1000 mL. *Rx.*
Use: Intravenous nutritional therapy, intravenous replenishment solution.

Isolyte S pH 7.4. (B. Braun) Sodium 141 mEq, potassium 5 mEq, magnesium 3 mEq, chloride 98 mEq, acetate 27 mEq, gluconate 23 mEq, phosphate 1 mEq, 295 mOsm/L, preservative free. Inj. Bot. Soln. 500 mL, 1000 mL. *Rx.*
Use: Intravenous nutritional therapy, intravenous replenishment solution.

Isolyte S with 5% Dextrose. (B. Braun) Sodium 140 mEq, potassium 5 mEq, magnesium 3 mEq, chloride 106 mEq, acetate 27 mEq, gluconate 23 mEq, dextrose 50 g, Cal 170, 550 mOsm/L. Inj. Soln. 1000 mL. *Rx.*
Use: Intravenous nutritional therapy, intravenous replenishment solution.

•**isomazole hydrochloride.** (eye-SO-mah-ZOLE) USAN.
Use: Cardiovascular agent.

isomeprobamate.
See: Carisoprodol.

•**isomerol.** (EYE-so-MER-ole) USAN. *Formerly Parahydrecin.*
Use: Antiseptic.

isometheptene/caffeine/acetaminophen. (Women's Choice Pharmaceuticals) Acetaminophen 500 mg, caffeine 20 mg, isometheptene mucate 130 mg. Tab. 50s. *Rx.*
Use: Agent for migraine.

•**isometheptene/dichloralphenazone/acetaminophen.** (eye-so-meth-EPP-teen/die-klor-uhl-FEN-uh-zone/A-SEET-a-MIN-oh-fen) *USP.*
Use: Antimigraine.
See: Epidrin.
Midrin.
Migrazone.

isometheptene/dichloralphenazone/acetaminophen. (Various Mfr.) Isometheptene 65 mg, dichloralphenazone 100 mg, acetaminophen 325 mg. Cap. 50s, 100s, 250s, 500s. *c-iv.*
Use: Antimigraine.

•**isometheptene mucate.** (eye-so-meth-EPP-teen MYOO-kate) *USP.*
See: Midrin.
W/Acetaminophen, Caffeine.
See: MigraTen.
Prodrin.
W/Acetaminophen, Dichloralphenazone.
See: Nodolor.

Isomil. (Ross) Soy protein isolate infant formula containing 20 calories/fl oz. **Pow.:** Can 14 oz. **Concentrated Liq.:** Can 13 fl oz. **Ready-to-feed:** Can 32 fl oz. **Nursing Bottles:** Hospital use. Bot. 8 fl oz. *OTC.*
Use: Nutritional supplement.

Isomil DF. (Ross) Protein 17.9 g, carbohydrates 67.3 g, fat 36.7 g, Fe 12 mg, Na 293 mg, K 720 mg, with appropriate vitamins and minerals. 676 cal/L. Lactose free. Liq. 960 mL prediluted, ready-to-use cans. *OTC.*
Use: Nutritional supplement.

Isomil SF. (Ross) Low osmolar sucrose-free soy protein isolate infant formula containing 20 calories/fl oz. **Concentrated Liq.:** Can 13 fl oz. **Ready-to-feed:** Can 32 fl oz. **Nursing Bottles:** Hospital use. Bot. 8 fl oz. *OTC.*
Use: Nutritional supplement, enteral.

Isomune-CK. (Roche) Rapid immunochemical separation method of the heart specific CK-MB isoenzyme for quantitating when used with an appropriate CK substrate reagent. Test kit 100s, 250s.
Use: Diagnostic aid.

Isomune-LD. (Roche) Rapid immunochemical separation method of the heart specific LD-1 isoenzyme for quantitating when used with an appropriate LD substrate reagent. Test kit 40s, 100s.
Use: Diagnostic aid.

•**isomylamine hydrochloride.** (EYE-so-MILL-ah-meen) USAN.
Use: Muscle relaxant.

isomyn.
See: Amphetamine.

IsonaRif. (VersaPharm) Rifampin 300 mg, isoniazid 150 mg. Lactose. Cap. 60s. *Rx.*
Use: Antituberculosis agent.

Isonate Sublingual. (Major) Isosorbide 2.5 mg, 5 mg. Sublingual Tab. Bot. 100s, 1000s, UD 100s. *Rx.*
Use: Antianginal.

Isonate Tablets. (Major) Isosorbide. **5 mg, 10 mg:** Bot. 100s, 1000s, UD 100s. **20 mg, 30 mg:** Bot. 100s, 1000s. *Rx.*
Use: Antianginal.

Isonate TD-Caps. (Major) Isosorbide 40 mg. Bot. 100s, 1000s. *Rx.*
Use: Antianginal.
Isonate T.R. Tabs. (Major) Isosorbide 40 mg. Bot. 100s, 1000s. *Rx.*
Use: Antianginal.
•**isoniazid.** (eye-so-NYE-uh-zid) *USP.*
Use: Antituberculosis agent.
See: Calpas-INH.
Dow-Isoniazid.
INH.
Laniazid.
Nydrazid.
W/Calcium P-Aminosalicylate, Vitamin B_6.
See: Calpas-INAH-6.
Calpas Isoxine.
W/Pyridoxine Hydrochloride (Vitamin B_6).
See: Niadox.
Pasna, Tri-Pack 300.
Teebaconin w/B_6.
W/Rifampin.
See: IsonaRif.
Rifater.
isoniazid. (Carolina Medical Products) Isoniazid 50 mg/5 mL, sorbitol, orange flavor. Syr. Bot. Pt. *Rx.*
Use: Antituberculosis agent.
isoniazid. (Sandoz) Isoniazid 100 mg/mL. Inj., Soln. Vials. 10 mL. *Rx.*
Use: Antituberculosis agent.
isoniazid. (Various Mfr.) Isoniazid 100 mg, 300 mg. Tab. Bot. 30s, 60s (300 mg only), 100s, 200s (300 mg only), 1000s. *Rx.*
Use: Antituberculosis agent.
isoniazid combinations.
Use: Antituberculous agent.
See: Rifamate.
Rifater.
isonicotinic acid hydrazide.
See: Isoniazid.
isonicotinyl hydrazide.
See: Isoniazid.
isonipecaine hydrochloride.
See: Meperidine Hydrochloride.
isonoradrenaline.
See: Isoproterenol.
isopentaquine.
Use: Antimalarial.
isophane insulin suspension (NPH).
Use: Antidiabetic.
See: Humulin N.
Novolin N.
Novolin N PenFill.
Novolin N Prefilled.
isophane insulin suspension (NPH)/ insulin injection (regular).
Use: Antidiabetic.
See: Humulin 50/50.
Humulin 70/30.
Novolin 70/30.
Novolin 70/30 Penfill.
Novolin 70/30 Prefilled.
isopregnenone.
See: Dydrogesterone.
Isoprinosine. (Newport Pharmaceuticals) Inosine pranobex.
Use: Antiviral; immunomodulator.
•**isopropamide iodide.** (EYE-soe-PROE-pa-mide EYE-oh-dide) *USP.*
Use: Anticholinergic.
isopropanol.
Use: Antiseptic.
W/Combinations.
See: Ivy-Dry.
Ivy-Dry Super.
isoprophenamine hydrochloride. *Name used for Clorprenaline Hydrochloride.*
isopropicillin potassium.
Use: Anti-infective.
•**isopropyl alcohol.** (eye-so-PRO-pill AL-koe-hahl) *USP.*
Use: Topical anti-infective; pharmaceutic aid (solvent).
isopropyl alcohol spray. (Morton Grove) Isopropyl alcohol w/propellant. Aer. Can 6 oz. *OTC.*
Use: Anti-infective.
isopropylarterenol hydrochloride.
Use: Asthma; vasoconstrictor, allergic states.
isopropylarterenol sulfate.
See: Isoproterenol Sulfate.
•**isopropyl myristate.** (eye-so-PRO-pill mih-RIST-ate) *NF.*
Use: Pharmaceutic aid (emollient).
isopropyl-noradrenaline hydrochloride.
See: Isoproterenol Hydrochloride.
•**isopropyl palmitate.** (eye-so-PRO-pill pal-mih-tate) *NF.*
Use: Pharmaceutic aid (oleaginous vehicle).
See: Versa PLO20.
W/Lecithin.
See: SaltStable LO.
isopropyl phenazone. 4-Isopropyl antipyrine. Larodon.
isopropyl rubbing alcohol.
Use: Rubefacient, solvent.
isoproterenol. (Various Mfr.) Isoproterenol 1:5000 solution (0.2 mg/mL with sodium metabisulfite). Inj. Vials. 5 mL, 10 mL. *Rx.*
Use: Vasopressor.
•**isoproterenol hydrochloride.** (eye-so-pro-TER-uh-nahl) *USP.*
Use: Bronchodilator; vasoconstrictor.
See: Isuprel.
isoproterenol hydrochloride. (Abbott) Isoproterenol hydrochloride 0.02 mg/mL (1:50,000), sodium metabisulfite. Inj.

Prefilled syr. 10 mL. *Rx.*
Use: Bronchodilator, sympathomimetic.

isoproterenol hydrochloride. (ESI Lederle) Isoproterenol hydrochloride 0.2 mg/mL (1:5000 solution), sodium bisulfite. Inj. Amp. 5 mL. *Rx.*
Use: Bronchodilator, sympathomimetic.

•**isoproterenol sulfate.** (eye-so-pro-TER-uh-nahl) *USP.*
Use: Bronchodilator.
See: Medihaler-Iso.
W/Calcium Iodide (Anhydrous), Alcohol.
See: Norisodrine.

Isoptin SR. (FSC Laboratories) Verapamil hydrochloride 120 mg, 180 mg, 240 mg. Film-coated. ER Tab. Bot. 100s, 500s (240 mg only). *Rx.*
Use: Calcium channel blocker.

Isopto Alkaline. (Alcon) Hydroxypropyl methylcellulose 1%, benzalkonium Cl 0.01%. Sterile ophthalmic soln. Dropper bot. 15 mL. *OTC.*
Use: Artificial tears.

Isopto Carbachol. (Alcon) Carbachol 1.5%, 3%. Benzalkonium chloride 0.005%, hydroxypropyl methylcellulose 1%, sodium chloride, boric acid, sodium borate. Soln. *Drop-Tainer* 15 mL, 30 mL. *Rx.*
Use: Antiglaucoma agent.

Isopto Carpine. (Alcon) Pilocarpine hydrochloride 1%, 2%, 4%, 6%. Soln. Bot. 15 mL, 30 mL. *Rx.*
Use: Antiglaucoma agent.

Isopto Frin. (Alcon) Phenylephrine hydrochloride 0.12% in a methylcellulose Soln. *Drop-Tainer* 15 mL. *Rx.*
Use: Mydriatic; vasoconstrictor.

Isopto Homatropine. (Alcon) Homatropine HBr 2%, 5%. Soln. *Drop-Tainer* 5 mL, 15 mL. *Rx.*
Use: Cycloplegic; mydriatic.

Isopto Hyoscine. (Alcon) Hyoscine HBr 0.25%. Soln. *Drop-Tainer* 5 mL, 15 mL. *Rx.*
Use: Cycloplegic; mydriatic.

Isopto Plain. (Alcon) Hydroxypropyl methylcellulose 2910 0.5%, benzalkonium Cl 0.01%, sodium Cl, sodium phosphate, sodium citrate. *Drop-Tainer* 15 mL. *OTC.*
Use: Artificial tears.

Isopto Tears. (Alcon) Hydroxypropyl methylcellulose 0.5%, benzalkonium Cl 0.01%, sodium Cl, sodium phosphate, sodium citrate. Bot. *Drop-Tainer* 15 mL, 30 mL. *OTC.*
Use: Artificial tears.

Isordil Sublingual. (Wyeth) Isosorbide dinitrate. Tab. **2.5 mg, 5 mg:** Bot. 100s, 500s, *Redi-pak* 100s. **10 mg:** Bot. 100s. *Rx.*
Use: Antianginal.

Isordil Titradose. (Valeant) Isosorbide dinitrate 5 mg, 10 mg, 20 mg, 30 mg, 40 mg. Lactose. Tab. Bot. 100s, 500s (20 mg only), 1000s (5 mg, 10 mg only). *Rx.*
Use: Vasodilator.

Isorgen-G. (Grafton) Isosorbide 5 mg, 10 mg. Tab. Bot. 1000s. *Rx.*
Use: Antianginal.

•**isosorbide concentrate.** (EYE-sos-ORE-bide) *USP.*
Use: Diuretic.

•**isosorbide dinitrate.** (EYE-sos-ORE-bide die-NYE-trate dye-LOOT-ed) *USP.*
Use: Vasodilator, nitrate.
See: Dilatrate-SR.
Isordil.
W/Hydralazine Hydrochloride.
See: BiDil.

isosorbide dinitrate. (Rising Pharmaceuticals) Isosorbide dinitrate 40 mg. Lactose. ER Tab. 100s. *Rx.*
Use: Vasodilator, nitrate.

isosorbide dinitrate. (Various Mfr.) Isosorbide dinitrate. **Sublingual Tab.:** 2.5 mg, 5 mg. May contain lactose. Bot. 100s, 1000s, UD 100s. **Tab.:** 5 mg, 10 mg, 20 mg, 30 mg. 100s, 500s (except 20 mg), 1000s, UD 100s. *Rx.*
Use: Vasodilator, nitrate.

•**isosorbide mononitrate.** (EYE-sos-ORE-bide MAH-no-NYE-trate) USAN.
Use: Coronary vasodilator.
See: Imdur.
ISMO.
Monoket.

isosorbide mononitrate. (Teva) Isosorbide mononitrate 20 mg, lactose. Tab. Bot. 100s, 500s. *Rx.*
Use: Coronary vasodilator.

isosorbide mononitrate. (Various Mfr.) Isosorbide mononitrate. **ER Tab.:** 30 mg, 60 mg, 120 mg. May contain lactose. ER Tab. Bot. 100s, 1000s. **Tab.:** 10 mg, 20 mg. May contain lactose. 100s, 500s (20 mg only). *Rx.*
Use: Coronary vasodilator.

isosorbide oral solution.
Use: Diuretic.

Isosource. (Novartis) Protein (Ca and Na caseinate, soy protein isolate) 43.2 g, carbohydrate (maltodextrin) 1755 g, fat (MCT, canola oil, lecithin) 443.9 g, Na 760 mg, K 1182 mg, mOsm/kg H_2O 390, Cal/mL 1.2, vitamins A, B_1, B_2, B_3, B_5, B_6, B_{12}, C, D, E, K, FA, biotin, choline, Ca, Cl, Cu, Fe, I, Mg, Mn, P, Zn, Se, Cr, Mo. Liq. Bot. 250 mL, 1000 mL.

OTC.
Use: Nutritional supplement.

Isosource HN. (Novartis) Protein (Ca and Na caseinate, soy protein isolate) 56.1 g, carbohydrate (maltodextrin) 165 g, fat (MCT, canola oil, lecithin) 43.9 g, Na 760 mg, K 1772 mg, mOsm/kg H_2O 390, Cal/mL 1.2, vitamins A, B_1, B_2, B_3, B_5, B_6, B_{12}, C, D, E, K, FA, biotin, choline, Ca, P, I, Fe, Mg, Cu, Zn, Cl, Mn, Se, Cr, Mo. Liq. Bot. 250 mL, 1000 mL. *OTC.*
Use: Nutritional supplement.

Isosource 1.5 Cal. (Nestle Nutrition) Protein 68 g (L-carnitine, sodium caseinate, taurine), carbohydrate 170 g (maltodextrin), fat 65 g (canola oil, medium chain triglycerides), sodium 1,290 mg, potassium 2,250 mg. Fiber 8 g, vitamins A, B_1, B_2, B_3, B_5, B_6, B_{12}, C, D, E, K, Ca, Cl, Cr, Cu, Fe, I, Mg, Mn, Mo, P, Se, Zn, biotin, choline, folic acid. Lactose free. Liq. 250 mL, 1,000 mL, 1,500 mL. *OTC.*
Use: Defined formula diet, lactose-free product.

Isosource VHN. (Nestle Nutrition) Protein 62.7 g (Ca caseinate, Na caseinate, L-carnitine, soy fiber, taurine), carbohydrate 126.7 g (maltodextrin), fat 28.7 g (canola oil, medium chain triglycerides, soy lecithin), Na 1,346.7 mg, K 1,800 mg, vitamin A, B_1, B_2, B_3, B_5, B_6, B_{12}, C, D, E, K, Ca, Cl, Cu, Fe, I, Mg, Mn, P, Se, Zn, folic acid, biotin, choline, folic acid, biotin, choline. Methylparaben. Lactose free. Vanilla flavor. Liq. 250 mL, 1 L, 1.5 L. *OTC.*
Use: Defined formula diet, supplemental nutritional formula.

•**isostearyl alcohol.** (EYE-so-STEE-rill AL-koe-hahl) USAN.
Use: Pharmaceutic aid (emollient, solvent).

•**isosulfan blue.** (EYE-so-SULL-fan) USAN.
Use: Radiopaque agent, parenteral.
See: Lymphazurin 1%.

isosulfan blue 1%. (Bioniche Pharma) Isosulfan blue 10 mg/mL. Preservative free. Inj., Soln. Single-use vial. 5 mL. *Rx.*
Use: Radiopaque agent.

Isotein HN. (Novartis) Vanilla Flavor. Maltodextrin, delactosed lactalbumin, partially hydrogenated soy oil with BHA, fructose, medium chain triglycerides, artificial flavor, sodium caseinate, monoglycerides and diglycerides, sodium Cl, vitamins, minerals. Pow. Packet 2.75 oz. *OTC.*
Use: Nutritional supplement.

•**isotiquimide.** (eye-so-TIH-kwih-MIDE) USAN.
Use: Antiulcerative.

Isotrate ER. (Apothecon) Isosorbide mononitrate 60 mg, lactose. ER Tab. Bot. 100s, 500s. *Rx.*
Use: Coronary vasodilator.

•**isotretinoin.** (EYE-so-TREH-tin-NO-in) *USP.*
Tall Man: ISOtretinoin
Use: Retinoid, first generation.
See: Absorica.
Amnesteem.
Claravis.
Myorisan.
Sotret.
Zenatane.

•**isotretinoin anisatil.** (eye-so-TRETT-ih-noyn ah-NIH-sah-till) USAN.
Use: Dermatologic, acne.

•**isovaleramide.** (EYE-soe-val-ER-a-mide) USAN.
Use: Agent for migraine.

Isovorin. (Wyeth) L-leucovorin.
Use: Antineoplastic. [Orphan Drug]

Isovue-M 300. (Bracco Diagnostics) Iopamidol 612 mg, iodine 300 mg/mL. EDTA. Inj. Vials. 15 mL. For intrathecal use *Rx.*
Use: Radiopaque agent, parenteral.

Isovue-M 200. (Bracco Diagnostics) Iopamidol 408 mg, iodine 200 mg/mL. EDTA. Inj. Vials. 10 mL, 20 mL. For intrathecal use. *Rx.*
Use: Radiopaque agent, parenteral.

Isovue-300. (Bracco Diagnostics) Iopamidol 612 mg, iodine 300 mg/mL. EDTA. Inj. Vials. 30 mL, 50 mL. Bot. 75 mL, 100 mL, 150 mL w/wo administration sets. Power injector syringes. 100 mL, 150 mL. *Rx.*
Use: Radiopaque agent, parenteral.

Isovue-370. (Bracco Diagnostics) Iopamidol 755 mg, iodine 370 mg/mL. EDTA. Inj. Vials. 20 mL, 30 mL, 50 mL. Bot. 50 mL, 75 mL, 100 mL, 125 mL, 150 mL, 175 mL, 200 mL. Power injector syringes. 75 mL, 100 mL. *Rx.*
Use: Radiopaque agent, parenteral.

Isovue-200. (Bracco Diagnostics) Iopamidol 408 mg, iodine 200 mg/mL. EDTA. Inj. Vials. 50 mL. Bot. 100 mL, 200 mL w/infusion set. *Rx.*
Use: Radiopaque agent, parenteral.

Isovue-250. (Bracco Diagnostics) Iopamidol 510 mg, iodine 250 mg/mL. EDTA. Inj. Vials. 50 mL. Bot. 100 mL, 150 mL, 200 mL. Power injector syringes. 150 mL. *Rx.*
Use: Radiopaque agent, parenteral.

•**isoxepac.** (EYE-SOX-eh-pack) USAN.
Use: Anti-inflammatory.
•**isoxicam.** (eye-SOX-ih-kam) USAN.
Use: Anti-inflammatory.
•**isoxsuprine hydrochloride.** (eye-SOX-you-preen) *USP.*
Use: Vasodilator.
See: Vasodilan.
Voxsuprine.
isoxsuprine hydrochloride. (Various Mfr.) Isoxsuprine hydrochloride 10 mg, 20 mg. Tab. 60s, 100s, 500s, 1000s, UD 100s. *Rx.*
Use: Vasodilator.
I-Soyalac. (Mt. Vernon Foods, Inc.) P-soy protein isolate, l-methionine, CHO-sucrose, tapioca dextrin. F-soy oil, soy lecithin. Corn free. Protein 20.2 g, carbohydrate 63.4 g, fat 35.5 g, iron 12 mg, 640 Cal/serving (1 qt). Concentrate 390 mL, ready-to-use 1 qt. *OTC.*
Use: Nutritional supplement.
•**ispinesib mesylate.** (is-PIN-es-ib) USAN.
Use: Antineoplastic.
•**ispronicline.** (eyes-PRON-i-kleen) USAN.
Use: CNS agent, Alzheimer disease.
•**isradipine.** (iss-RAHD-ih-peen) *USP.*
Use: Calcium channel blocker; antagonist (calcium channel).
isradipine. (Various Mfr.) Isradipine 2.5 mg, 5 mg. Cap. 100s. *Rx.*
Use: Calcium channel blocker.
Istalol. (Ista Pharmaceuticals) Timolol maleate 0.5%, benzalkonium chloride 0.005%, monobasic sodium phosphate monohydrate, potassium sorbate 0.47%, sodium hydroxide. Soln. 5 mL. *Rx.*
Use: Agents for glaucoma.
Istodax. (Celgene) Romidepsin 10 mg. Povidone 20 mg. Inj. Kit w/single-use vial and diluent. *Rx.*
Use: Cutaneous T-cell lymphoma.
•**istradefylline.** (iz-TRA-de-fye-leen) USAN.
Use: Parkinson disease.
I-Sulfacet. (American Pharmaceutical) Sulfacetamide sodium 10%, 15%, 30% ophthalmic soln. Bot. 2 mL, 5 mL, 15 mL. *Rx.*
Use: Anti-infective, ophthalmic.
Isuprel. (Marathon) Isoproterenol hydrochloride 0.2 mg/mL (1:5000). Edetate disodium. Inj., Soln. Amp. 1 mL, 5 mL. *Rx.*
Use: Bronchodilator; sympathomimetic.
isuprene.
See: Isoproterenol.
•**itasetron.** (eye-tah-SEH-trahn) USAN.
Use: Antidepressant; antiemetic; anxiolytic.
•**itazigrel.** (ih-TAY-zih-GRELL) USAN.
Use: Platelet aggregation inhibitor.
Itchaway. (Moyco Union Broach Division) Zinc undecylenate 20%, undecylenic acid 2%. Pow. Can 1.5 oz. *OTC.*
Use: Antifungal, topical.
Itch Relief Gel Spritz. (Band-Aid) Camphor 0.5%, benzyl alcohol, glycerin SD alcohol 40 B (43%). Spray. 56 g. *OTC.*
Use: Poison ivy treatment.
Itch-X. (Ascher & Co.) Pramoxine hydrochloride 1%. **Gel:** Benzyl alcohol 10%, aloe vera gel, diazolidinyl urea, SD alcohol 40, parabens. 35.4 g. **Foam:** Hydrocortisone 1%. Cetyl alcohol, mineral oil, parabens, white petrolatum. 88.7 mL. **Spray:** Benzyl alcohol 10%, aloe vera gel, SD alcohol 40. In 60 mL. *OTC.*
Use: Topical local anesthetic.
itobarbital.
W/Acetaminophen.
See: Panitol.
•**itraconazole.** (ih-truh-KAHN-uh-zole) USAN.
Use: Antifungal, triazole.
See: Onmel.
Sporanox.
itraconazole. (Various Mfr.) Itraconazole 100 mg. Cap. 28s, 30s, 100s, 500s, UD 28s, UD 30s. *Rx.*
Use: Antifungal agent.
•**ivacaftor.** (EYE-va-KAF-tor) USAN.
Use: Treatment of cystic fibrosis.
See: Kalydeco.
I-Valex-1. (Ross) Protein 15 g, fat 23.9 g, carbohydrates 46.3 g, linoleic acid 1800 mg, Fe 9 mg, Na 190 mg, K 675 mg, with appropriate vitamins and minerals. 480 Cal/100 g. Leucine free. Pow. Can 350 g. *OTC.*
Use: Nutritional supplement.
I-Valex-2. (Ross) Protein 30 g, fat 15.5 g, carbohydrates 30 g, Na 880 mg, K 1370 mg, with appropriate vitamins and minerals. 410 Cal/100 g. Leucine free. Pow. Can 325 g. *OTC.*
Use: Nutritional supplement.
Ivarest. (Blistex) Menthol 1%, castor oil, disodium EDTA, glycerin, PEG, triclosan. Foam. 177 mL. *OTC.*
Use: Topical poison ivy product.
Ivarest Maximum Strength. (Blistex) Calamine 14%, diphenhydramine hydrochloride 2%, lanolin oil, petrolatum, propylene glycol. Cream. Tube. 56 g. *OTC.*
Use: Poison ivy product, topical.

•**ivermectin.** (eye-VER-MEK-tin) *USP.*
Use: Anthelmintic.
See: Stromectol.

I-Vite Protect. (Rugby) Vitamins A 7,160 units, E 100 units, C 113 mg, Cu, Na, Zn. Glucose, lactose, PEG, sodium benzoate. Tab. 120s. *OTC.*
Use: Multivitamin with minerals (except iron).

Ivocort. (Roberts) Micronized hydrocortisone alcohol 0.5%, 1%. Bot. 4 oz. *OTC.*
Use: Corticosteroid, topical.

Ivy Block. (EnviroDerm) Bentoquatam 5%, benzyl alcohol, methylparaben, SDA 40 denatured alcohol. Lot. 118 mL. *OTC.*
Use: Poison ivy treatment.

Ivy Cleanse. (EnviroDerm) Isopropyl alcohol, cetyl alcohol. Wipes. Packets of 12 individually wrapped towelettes. *OTC.*
Use: Poison ivy treatment.

Ivy-Dry. (Ivy Corp.) Zinc acetate 2%, isopropanol 12.5%. Glycerin, methylparaben. Lot. Bot. 118 mL. *OTC.*
Use: Poison ivy product, topical.

Ivy-Dry Super. (Ivy Corp.) Zinc acetate 2%, benzyl alcohol 10%, isopropanol 35%, menthol, camphor. Glycerin, parabens. Lot. Bot. 177 mL. *OTC.*
Use: Poison ivy product, topical.

Ivy-Rid. (Medique Products) Benzocaine 5%, benzethonium chloride 0.15%. Alcohol. Spray. 85 g. *OTC.*
Use: Poison ivy product.

Ivy Soothe. (Enviroderm) Hydrocortisone 1%, parabens, cetyl alcohol, glycerin, white petrolatum. Cream. 28 g. *OTC.*
Use: Poison ivy treatment.

Ivy Stat. (Tec Labs) Hydrocortisone 1%, propylene glycol, menthol, SD alcohol 40-B. Gel. 89 mL. *OTC.*
Use: Poison ivy treatment.

Ivy Wash. (Humco) Pramoxine hydrochloride 1%. Disodium EDTA, glycerin, nonoxynol-9, parabens, propylene glycol, urea. Wash. 177 mL. *OTC.*
Use: Poison ivy product.

I-Wash. (Akorn) Phosphate buffered saline soln. Bot. 4 oz, 8 oz. *OTC.*
Use: Irrigant, ophthalmic.

I-White. (Akorn) Phenylephrine 0.12%, polyvinyl alcohol, hydroxyethyl cellulose. Soln. Bot. 15 mL. *OTC.*
Use: Mydriatic; vasoconstrictor.

•**ixabepilone.** (ix-ab-EP-i-lone) USAN.
Use: Antimitotic, epothilone.
See: Ixempra.

•**ixazomib.** (ix-AZ-oh-mib) USAN.
Use: Antineoplastic.

•**ixazomib citrate.** (ix-AZ-oh-mib) USAN.
Use: Antineoplastic.

•**ixekizumab.** (IX-e-KIZ-ue-mab) USAN.
Use: Treatment of autoimmune diseases.

Ixempra. (Bristol-Myers Squibb) Ixabepilone 15 mg, 45 mg. Inj., Lyophilized Pow. for Soln., Conc. Single-use kits. Kit contains 1 vial of ixabepilone and 1 vial of diluent. Diluent contains purified polyoxyethylated castor oil 52.8%, dehydrated alcohol 39.8%. *Rx.*
Use: Antimitotic agent, epothilone.

Ixiaro. (Novartis) Japanese encephalitis virus vaccine 6 mcg per 0.5 mL (contains ≈ 6 mcg of purified inactivated Japanese encephalitis virus proteins and aluminum hydroxide 250 mcg). Each 0.5 mL dose contains formaldehyde ≤ 200 ppm, bovine serum albumin ≤ 100 ng/mL, host cell DNA ≤ 200 pg/mL, sodium metabisulfite ≤ 200 ppm, host cell proteins ≤ 300 ng/mL, protamine sulfate ≤ 1 mcg/mL. Preservative free. Single-dose prefilled syringes. 0.5 mL. *Rx.*
Use: Agent for active immunization, viral vaccine.

•**ixmyelocel-T.** (IX-mye-EL-oh-sel-tee) USAN.
Use: Cardiovascular agent.

Izonid. (Major) Isoniazid 300 mg. Tab. Bot. 100s. *Rx.*
Use: Antituberculosis agent.

J

Jakafi. (Incyte Corporation) Ruxolitinib phosphate 5 mg, 10 mg, 15 mg, 20 mg, 25 mg. Lactose. Tab. 60s. *Rx.*
Use: Kinase inhibitor, janus-associated kinase inhibitor.

Jalovis.
See: Hyaluronidase.

Jalyn. (GlaxoSmithKline) Dutasteride 0.5 mg/tamsulosin hydrochloride 0.4 mg. Glycerin. Cap. 30s, 90s. *Rx.*
Use: Androgen hormone inhibitor, benign prostatic hyperplasia combination.

Jantoven. (Upsher-Smith) Warfarin sodium 1 mg, 2 mg, 2.5 mg, 3 mg, 4 mg, 5 mg, 6 mg, 7.5 mg, 10 mg. Lactose. Dye free (10 mg only). Tab. 100s, 500s (7.5 mg, 10 mg only), 1000s (except 7.5 mg, 10 mg), UD 100s. *Rx.*
Use: Anticoagulant.

Janumet. (Merck) Sitagliptin (as sitagliptin phosphate)/metformin hydrochloride 50 mg/500 mg, 50 mg/1000 mg. Film-coated. Tab. 60s, 180s, 1000s, UD 50s. *Rx.*
Use: Antidiabetic combination.

Janumet XR. (Merck) Sitagliptin/metformin hydrochloride extended release 50 mg (equiv. to sitagliptin phosphate 64.25 mg)/500 mg, 50 mg (equiv. to sitagliptin phosphate 64.25 mg)/1,000 mg, 100 mg (equiv. to sitagliptin phosphate 128.5 mg)/1,000 mg. Film coated. ER Tab. 30s (100 mg/1,000 mg only), 60s (50 mg/500 mg and 50 mg/1,000 mg only), 90s (100 mg/1,000 mg only), 180s (50 mg/500 mg and 50 mg/1,000 mg only), 1,000s. *Rx.*
Use: Antidiabetic combination.

Janus-associated kinase inhibitors.
See: Ruxolitinib Phosphate.
Tofacitinib.

Januvia. (Merck) Sitagliptin phosphate 25 mg, 50 mg, 100 mg. Film-coated. Tab. 30s, 90s, 500s (100 mg only), 1000s (100 mg only), UD blister pack 100s. *Rx.*
Use: Antidiabetic agent.

Japan agar.
See: Agar.

Japanese encephalitis virus vaccine.
Use: Agent for active immunization, viral vaccine.
See: Ixiaro.

Japan gelatin.
See: Agar.

Japan isinglass.
See: Agar.

Jay-Phyl. (Jaymac) Dyphilline 100 mg, guaifenesin 50 mg per 5 mL. Alcohol and sugar free. Vanilla flavor. Syr. 473 mL. *Rx.*
Use: Antiasthmatic combination, xanthine combination.

J-COF DHC. (JayMac Pharmaceuticals) Brompheniramine maleate 3 mg, dihydrocodeine bitartrate 7.5 mg, pseudoephedrine hydrochloride 15 mg per 5 mL. Alcohol free, dye free, and sugar free. Saccharin, sorbitol. Grape flavor. Liq. 473 mL. *c-III.*
Use: Upper respiratory combination, antitussive combination.

Jencycla. (Lupin) Norethindrone 0.35 mg. Lactose. Tab. 28s. *Rx.*
Use: Oral contraceptive.

Jenest-28. (Organon) 7 white tablets norethindrone 0.5 mg, ethinyl estradiol 35 mcg; 14 peach tablets norethindrone 1 mg, ethinyl estradiol 35 mcg; 7 inert tablets. Lactose. *Cyclic Tablet dispenser* 28s. *Rx.*
Use: Sex hormone, contraceptive hormone.

Jenloga. (UPM Inc) Clonidine hydrochloride 0.1 mg (equiv. to 0.087 mg of clonidine base). Lactose. Tab., Modified release. 60s, 180s. *Rx.*
Use: Antiadrenergic/sympatholytic; antiadrenergic agent, centrally acting.

Jentadueto. (Boehringer Ingelheim) Linagliptin/metformin hydrochloride 2.5 mg/500 mg, 2.5 mg/850 mg, 2.5 mg/1,000 mg. Film coated. Tab. 60s, 180s, 2,000s. *Rx.*
Use: Antidiabetic combination.

Jeri-Bath. (Dermik) Concentrated moisturizing bath oil. Plastic Bot. 8 oz. *OTC.*
Use: Dermatologic.

Jetrea. (ThromboGenics) Ocriplasmin 2.5 mg/mL. Mannitol. Preservative free, latex free. Inj., Soln., concentrate; intravitreal. Single-use vial. 0.2 mL. *Rx.*
Use: Ophthalmic proteolytic enzyme.

Jets. (Freeda) L-lysine 300 mg, vitamins C 25 mg, B_{12} 25 mcg, B_6 5 mg, B_1 10 mg. Chew. Tab. Bot. 100s. *OTC.*
Use: Vitamin supplement; amino acid.

Jevity. (Ross) Calcium and sodium caseinates, soy fiber, hydrolyzed cornstarch, MCT (fractionated coconut oil), soy oil, corn oil, soy lecithin, vitamins A, B_1, B_2, B_3, B_5, B_6, B_{12}, C, D, E, K, folic acid, biotin, choline, Ca, P, Mg, Fe, Mn, Cu, Zn, I, Cl. Liq. Bot. 240 mL. *OTC.*
Use: Nutritional supplement.

Jevity 1.5 Cal. (Ross) Protein 63.4 g, carbohydrate 214.2 g, fat 49.6 g/L. Na 1386 mg/L, K 1848 mg/L, cal 1.5/mL. Vitamins A, B_1, B_2, B_3, B_5, B_6, B_{12}, C, D,

E, K, Ca, Cu, Fe, I, Mg, Mn, Mo, P, Se, Zn, biotin, chloride, choline, folic acid. Liq. Can. 237 mL. Ready-to-hang containers 1 L, 1.5 L. *OTC.*
Use: Enteral nutrition therapy.

Jevtana. (Sanofi-Aventis) Cabazitaxel 60 mg per 1.5 mL. Polysorbate 80. Inj., Soln., concentrate. Single-use vial w/diluents (ethanol 13% in water for injection). *Rx.*
Use: Antimitotic agent, taxoid.

Jiffy. (Block Drug) Benzocaine, menthol, eugenol in glycerin-water base with SD alcohol 38-B 76%. Bot. 0.125 oz. *OTC.*
Use: Anesthetic, local.

Jinteli. (Teva) Ethinyl estradiol 5 mcg/ norethindrone acetate 1 mg. Lactose. Tab. 90s, blister card 28s. *Rx.*
Use: Sex hormone, estrogen/progestin combination.

J-Liberty. (J Pharmacal) Chlordiazepoxide hydrochloride 5 mg, 10 mg, 25 mg. Cap. *c-IV.*
Use: Anxiolytic.

J-Max. (JayMac Pharmaceuticals) Phenylephrine hydrochloride 5 mg, guaifenesin 200 mg per 5 mL. Dye and gluten free. Aspartame, parabens. Strawberry cream flavor. Syrup. 473 mL. *Rx.*
Use: Decongestant and expectorant combination, upper respiratory combination.

J-Max DHC. (JayMac Pharmaceuticals) Dihydrocodeine bitartrate 7.5 mg, guaifenesin 100 mg per 5 mL. Menthol, saccharin, sorbitol. Alcohol free. Grape flavor. Liq. 473 mL. *c-III.*
Use: Upper respiratory combination

Johnson's Baby. (Johnson & Johnson) Dimethicone 2%. Cream. Jar 4 oz, 6 oz; Tube 2 oz. *OTC.*
Use: Dermatologic protectant.

Johnson's Baby Sunblock Extra Protection. (Johnson & Johnson) Octyl methoxycinnamate, octyl salicylate, titanium dioxide, oxybenzone, C12-15 alcohols benzoate, cetyl alcohol, EDTA, vitamin E. Lot. Bot. 120 mL. *OTC.*
Use: Sunscreen.

Johnson's Baby Sunblock SPF 15. (Johnson & Johnson) Octyl methoxycinnamate, octyl salicylate, oxybenzone, titanium dioxide, benzyl alcohol, cetyl alcohol. PABA free. Waterproof. **Cream:** Tube. 60 g. **Lot.:** Bot. 60 g. *OTC.*
Use: Sunscreen.

Johnson's Baby Sunblock SPF 30. (Johnson & Johnson) Benzophenone-3, octyl methoxycinnamate, octyl salicylate, titanium dioxide. PABA free. Waterproof. Lot. Bot. 120 mL.
Use: Sunscreen.

Johnson's Medicated. (Johnson & Johnson) Bentonite, kaolin, talc, zinc oxide. Pow. Bot. Small, Medium, Large. *OTC.*
Use: Diaper rash preparation.

Johnson's Shea & Cocoa Butter Baby Lotion. (Johnson & Johnson) *Butyrospermum parkii* (shea butter), glycerin, mineral oil, parabens, stearyl alcohol, theobroma cacao. Lot. 798 mL. *OTC.*
Use: Emollient.

Jolessa. (Barr) Ethinyl estradiol 30 mcg, levonorgestrel 0.15 mg. Lactose. Film-coated. Tab. 91s with 7 inert tablets (lactose). *Rx.*
Use: Contraceptive hormone, sex hormone.

Jolivette. (Watson) Norethindrone 0.35 mg. Lactose. Tab. 28s. *Rx.*
Use: Contraceptive hormone, sex hormone.

•**josamycin.** (JOE-sah-MYsin) USAN.
Use: Anti-infective.

J-Tan. (Jaymac) Brompheniramine tannate 4 mg. Strawberry cream flavor. Oral Susp. 473 mL. *Rx.*
Use: Antihistamine.

J-Tan D PD. (JayMac) Pseudoephedrine hydrochloride 7.5 mg, brompheniramine maleate 1 mg per 1 mL. Alcohol, sugar, and dye free. Saccharin, sorbitol. Strawberry-banana flavor. Drops. 30 mL with dropper. *Rx.*
Use: Upper respiratory combination, decongestant and antihistamine.

J-Tan PD. (JayMac) Brompheniramine maleate 1 mg/mL. Glycerin, propylene glycol, saccharin, sorbitol. Alcohol free, dye free, sugar free. Strawberry-banana flavor. Liq. 30 mL. *OTC.*
Use: Antihistamine, nonselective alkylamine.

Junel Fe 1/20. (Barr) Norethindrone acetate 1 mg, ethinyl estradiol 20 mcg. Tab. 28s with 7 brown tablets (ferrous fumarate 75 mg/tab). *Rx.*
Use: Contraceptive hormone, sex hormone.

Junel Fe 1.5/30. (Barr) Norethindrone acetate 1.5 mg, ethinyl estradiol 30 mcg. Tab. 28s with 7 brown tablets (ferrous fumarate 75 mg/tab). *Rx.*
Use: Contraceptive hormone, sex hormone.

Junel 21 Day 1.5/30. (Barr) Ethinyl estradiol 30 mcg, norethindrone acetate 1.5 mg. Lactose, sugar. Tab. 21s. *Rx.*
Use: Contraceptive hormone, sex hormone.

Junel 21 Day 1/20. (Barr) Ethinyl estradiol 20 mcg, norethindrone acetate 1 mg. Lactose, sugar. Tab. 21s. *Rx.*
Use: Contraceptive hormone, sex hormone.

Junior Strength Motrin. (McNeil) Ibuprofen. **Chew. Tab.:** 100 mg. Aspartame, phenylalanine 6 mg. Orange flavor. 24s. **Tab.:** 100 mg. Bot. 24s. *OTC.*
Use: Analgesic, NSAID.

Junior Strength Panadol. (Bayer Consumer Care) Acetaminophen 160 mg. Capl. Bot. 30s. *OTC.*
Use: Analgesic.

•**juniper tar.** (JOO-nih-per tar) *USP.*
Use: Local antieczematic, pharmaceutic necessity.

Junyer-All. (Barth's) Vitamins A 6000 units, D 400 units, B_1 3 mg, B_2 6 mg, C 120 mg, niacin 1 mg, E 12 units, B_{12} 10 mcg, calcium 217 mg, phosphorus 97.5 mg, red bone marrow 10 mg, organic iron 15 mg, iodine 0.1 mg, beef peptone 20 mg/2 Cap. Bot. 10 month, 3 month, 6 month supply. *OTC.*
Use: Vitamin, mineral supplement.

Just For Kids. (3M ESPE) Stannous fluoride 0.4%. Bubble gum flavor. Dental gel. 121.9 g. *OTC.*
Use: Nutritional agent, trace element.

Juvederm Ultra. (Allergan) Hyaluronic acid 24 mg/mL. Gel; intradermal. Single-use, prefilled syringe w/30-gauge needle. *Rx.*
Use: Physical adjunct, dermal hyaluronic acid derivative.

Juvederm Ultra Plus. (Allergan) Hyaluronic acid 24 mg/mL. Gel; intradermal. Single-use, prefilled syringe w/27-gauge needle. *Rx.*
Use: Physical adjunct, dermal hyaluronic acid derivative.

Juvederm Ultra Plus XC. (Allergan) Hyaluronic acid 24 mg/mL, lidocaine 0.3%. Gel; intradermal. Single-use syringe. *Rx.*
Use: Physical adjunct, dermal hyaluronic acid derivative.

Juvederm Ultra XC. (Allergan) Hyaluronic acid 24 mg/mL, lidocaine 0.3%. Gel; intradermal. Single-use, prefilled syringe w/30-gauge needle. *Rx.*
Use: Physical adjunct, dermal hyaluronic acid derivative.

Juvederm Voluma XC. (Allergan) Hyaluronic acid 20 mg/mL. Lidocaine 0.3%. Inj., Gel. Single-use, prefilled syringes w/25-gauge or 27-gauge needles. *Rx.*
Use: Physical adjunct, dermal hyaluronic acid derivative.

Juvisync. (Merck & Co) Sitagliptin/simvastatin 50 mg/10 mg, 50 mg/20 mg, 50 mg/40 mg (equiv. to sitagliptin phosphate 64.25 mg); 100 mg/10 mg, 100 mg/20 mg, 100 mg/40 mg (equiv. to sitagliptin phosphate 128.5 mg). Film coated. Lactose. Tab. 30s, 90s, 1,000s (100 mg/10 mg, 100 mg/20 mg, and 100 mg/40 mg). *Rx.*
Use: Antidiabetic combination product.

Juvocaine.
See: Procaine Hydrochloride.

Juxtapid. (Aegerion) Lomitapide mesylate 5 mg, 10 mg, 20 mg. Lactose. Cap. 28s. *Rx.*
Use: Antihyperlipidemic agent.

K

Kadcyla. (Genentech) Ado-trastuzumab emtansine 100 mg, 160 mg. Sucrose. Preservative free. Inj., lyophilized Pow. for Soln. Single-use vial. *Rx.*
Use: Antineoplastic.

Kadian. (Actavis) Morphine sulfate 10 mg, 20 mg, 30 mg, 40 mg, 50 mg, 60 mg, 70 mg, 80 mg; 100 mg, 130 mg, 150 mg, 200 mg (for use only in opioid-tolerant patients). PEG, sucrose. ER Pellet Cap. 100s. *c-II.*
Use: Opioid analgesic.

Kaergona.
See: Menadione.

Kala. (Freeda) Soy-based acidophilus 2 million units. Tab. Bot. 100s, 250s, 500s. *OTC.*
Use: Nutritional supplement.

•**kalafungin.** (kal-ah-FUN-jin) USAN.
Use: Antifungal.

Kalbitor. (Dyax Corp) Ecallantide 10 mg/mL (produced in Pichia pastoris yeast cells by recombinant DNA technology). Disodium hydrogen orthophosphate (dihydrate) 0.76 mg, monopotassium phosphate 0.2 mg, potassium chloride 0.2 mg, sodium chloride 8 mg. Preservative free. Inj., Soln. Single-use vial. *Rx.*
Use: Hematological agent, kallikrein inhibitor.

Kaletra. (AbbVie) **Oral Soln.:** Lopinavir 80 mg, ritonavir 20 mg/mL. Alcohol 42.4%, menthol, acesulfame K, corn syrup, saccharin, peppermint and castor oils, cotton candy or vanilla flavor. Bot. with dosing cup. 160 mL. **Tab.:** Lopinavir/ritonavir. 100 mg/25 mg, 200 mg/50 mg. Film-coated. 60s (100 mg/25 mg only), 120s (200 mg/50 mg only). *Rx.*
Use: Antiretroviral, protease inhibitor combination.

Kallikrein inhibitors.
See: Ecallantide.

Kaltostat. (GlaxoSmithKline) Calcium-sodium alginate fiber, 3" × 4¾" sterile dressing. In 1s. *OTC.*
Use: Dressing, hydroactive.

Kaltostat Forte. (GlaxoSmithKline) Calcium-sodium alginate fiber, 4" × 4" sterile dressing. In 1s. *OTC.*
Use: Dressing, hydroactive.

Kalydeco. (Vertex Pharmaceuticals) Ivacaftor 150 mg. Film coated. Lactose. Tab. 60s, UD 56s. *Rx.*
Use: Endocrine and metabolic agent.

Kamfolene. (Wade) Camphor, menthol, methyl salicylate, turpentine and eucalyptus oils, carbolic acid 2%, calamine, zinc oxide in lanolin base. Jar 2 oz, lb. *OTC.*
Use: Antiseptic.

•**kanamycin sulfate.** (kan-uh-MY-sin) *USP.*
Use: Anti-infective.

Kank-A Mouth Pain. (Blistex) Benzocaine 20%. Alcohols, benzyl alcohol, benzoin tincture, PEG, propylene glycol, castor seed oil, saccharin, tannic acid. Liq.; dental. 9.75 mL. *OTC.*
Use: Topical local anesthetic, ester local anesthetic.

Kank-A Soothing Beads. (Blistex) Benzocaine 3 mg per bead. Caprylic/capric triglyceride, eugenol, glycerin, PEG, polysorbate 80, sorbitol, sucralose, sucrose. Bead; topical. 15 5-bead doses. *OTC.*
Use: Topical local anesthetic, ester local anesthetic.

Kaochlor-Eff. (Pharmacia) Elemental potassium 20 mEq, chloride 20 mEq. Tab. Supplied by: Potassium Cl 0.6 g, potassium citrate 0.22 g, potassium bicarbonate 1 g, betaine hydrochloride 1.84 g, saccharin 20 mg, artificial fruit flavor, tartrazine (color). Tab. Sugar free. Carton 60s. *Rx.*
Use: Electrolyte supplement.

Kaodene Non-Narcotic. (Pfeiffer) Kaolin 3.9 g, pectin 194.4 mg/30 mL, bismuth subsalicylate. Alcohol free. Liq. Bot. 120 mL. *OTC.*
Use: Antidiarrheal.

Kaodene with Codeine. (Pfeiffer) Codeine phosphate 32.4 mg, kaolin 3.9 g, pectin 194.4 mg, sodium carboxymethylcellulose, bismuth subsalicylate/30 mL. Susp. Bot. 120 mL. *OTC.*
Use: Antidiarrheal.

•**kaolin.** (KAY-oh-lin) *USP.*
Use: Adsorbent.
W/Cornstarch, camphor, zinc oxide, eucalyptus oil.
See: Mexsana Medicated Powder.
W/Furazolidone, pectin.
See: Furoxone.
W/Pectin.
See: Kapectin.
W/Pectin, paregoric (equivalent).
See: Kapectin.

kaolin with pectin. (Various Mfr.) Kaolin 90 g, pectin 2 g/30 mL. Susp. Bot. 180 mL, pt, UD 30 mL. *OTC.*
Use: Antidiarrheal combination.

Kaon Cl. (Savage) Potassium Cl 500 mg, FD&C Yellow No. 5. CR Tab. Bot. 100s, 250s, 1000s. *Rx.*
Use: Electrolyte supplement.

Kaon Cl-10. (Savage) Potassium Cl 750 mg. CR Tab. Bot. 100s, 500s, 1000s. *Stat-Pak* 100s. *Rx.*
Use: Electrolyte supplement.

Kaon Cl 20%. (Savage) Potassium and chloride 40 mEq (to potassium Cl 3 g)/ 15 mL, saccharin, flavoring, alcohol 5%. Bot. Pt. *Rx.*
Use: Electrolyte supplement.

Kaon Elixir. (Savage) Elemental potassium 20 mEq (as potassium gluconate 4.68 g)/15 mL, aromatics, grape and lemon-lime flavors, alcohol 5%, saccharin. Elix. Unit pkg. Pt, gal. *Rx.*
Use: Electrolyte supplement.

Kaon Tablets. (Savage) Elemental potassium 5 mEq obtained from potassium gluconate 1.17 g. SC Tab. Bot. 100s, 500s. *Rx.*
Use: Electrolyte supplement.

Kaopectate. (Chattem) Bismuth subsalicylate 262 mg. Tab. 12s, 20s. *OTC.*
Use: Antidiarrheal.

Kaopectate, Children's. (Chattem) Bismuth subsalicylate 87 mg/5 mL, sucrose, cherry flavor. Liq. 177 mL. *OTC.*
Use: Antidiarrheal combination.

Kaopectate Extra Strength. (Chattem) Bismuth subsalicylate 175 mg/5 mL, sucrose, peppermint flavor. Liq. 236 mL. *OTC.*
Use: Antidiarrheal.

Kaophen. (Pal-Pak, Inc.) Phenobarbital 6.5 mg, belladonna extract 0.1 mg, kaolin 388.8 mg. Tab. Bot. 100s, 1000s. *OTC.*
Use: Antidiarrheal.

Kao-Spen. (Century) Kaolin 5.2 g, pectin 260 mg/30 mL. Susp. Bot. 120 mL, pt, gal. *OTC.*
Use: Antidiarrheal.

Kao-Tin. (Major) Bismuth subsalicylate 262 mg per 15 mL. Saccharin, sorbitol. Liq. 236 mL, 473 mL. *OTC.*
Use: Antidiarrheal.

Kapectin. (Health for Life Brands) Kaolin 90 g, pectin 2 g/oz. Bot. Gal. *OTC.*
Use: Antidiarrheal.

Ka-Pek. (A.P.C.) Kaolin 90 g, pectin 4.5 g/ fl oz. Bot. 6 oz, gal. *OTC.*
Use: Antidiarrheal.

kapilin.
See: Menadione.

Kapvay. (Shionogi Pharma) Clonidine hydrochloride 0.1 mg (equiv. to clonidine base 0.087 mg), 0.2 mg (equiv. to clonidine base 0.174 mg). Lactose. ER Tab. 60s, 180s. *Rx.*
Use: Antiadrenergic/sympatholytic; antiadrenergic agent, centrally acting.

karaya gum. (Penick) Indian Gum. Sterculia Gum.

karaya powder. (Sween) Bot. 3 oz.
Use: Deodorant, ostomy.

Karbinal ER. (FSC Laboratories) Carbinoxamine maleate 4 mg per 5 mL. Corn syrup, glycerin, parabens, polysorbate 80, sodium metabisulfite, sucrose. Strawberry-banana flavor. ER Susp. 480 mL. *Rx.*
Use: Antihistamine, nonselective ethanolamine.

Kareon.
See: Menadione.

Karidium. (Young Dental) **Tab.:** Sodium fluoride 2.21 mg, sodium Cl 94.49 mg, disintegrant 0.5 mg. Bot. 180s, 1000s. **Liq.:** Sodium fluoride 2.21 mg, sodium Cl 10 mg, purified water q.s./8 drops. Bot. 30 mL, 60 mL. *Rx.*
Use: Dental caries agent.

Karigel. (Young Dental) Fluoride ion 0.5%, pH 5.6. Gel. Bot. 30 mL, 130 mL, 250 mL. *Rx.*
Use: Dental caries agent.

Karigel-N. (Young Dental) Fluoride ion 0.5% in neutral pH gel. Bot. 24 mL, 125 mL. *Rx.*
Use: Dental caries agent.

Kariva. (Barr) **Phase 1:** Desogestrel 0.15 mg, ethinyl estradiol 20 mcg. 21 tabs. **Phase 2:** Ethinyl estradiol 10 mcg. 5 tabs. Lactose. Tab. Blister card. 28s with 2 inert tabs. *Rx.*
Use: Sex hormone, contraceptive update.

•**kasal.** (KAY-sal) USAN. Approximately $Na_8Al_2(OH)_2(PO_4)_4$ with ≈ 30% of dibasic sodium phosphate; sodium aluminum phosphate, basic.
Use: Food additive.

kasugamycin. Under study.
Use: Anti-infective.

Kaviton.
See: Menadione, USP.

Kayexalate. (Covis) Sodium polystyrene sulfonate (sodium content ≈ 100 mg/ g). Jar 1 lb. *Rx.*
Use: Potassium-removing resin.

Kazano. (Takeda) Alogliptin (equiv. to alogliptin benzoate 17 mg)/metformin hydrochloride 12.5 mg/500 mg, 12.5 mg/1,000 mg. Film coated. Mannitol. Tab. 60s, 180s, 500s. *Rx.*
Use: Antidiabetic combination product.

K-Bicarb. (Bio-Tech) Potassium bicarbonate 99 mg. Dye free and preservative free. Cap. 100s. *OTC.*
Use: Electrolyte.

K-C. (Century) **Susp.:** Kaolin 5.2 g, pectin 260 mg, bismuth subcarbonate 260 mg/30 mL. Bot. 120 mL, pt, gal. **Liq.:** Kaolin 5.2 g, pectin 260 mg, bis-

muth subcarbonate 260 mg/oz. Bot. 4 oz, pt, gal. *OTC.*
Use: Antidiarrheal.

Kcentra. (CSL Behring) Factors II, VII, IX, and X, and antithrombotic proteins C and S 500 units (400 to 620 units), 1,000 units (800 to 1,240 units). Prothrombin complex concentrate potency is defined by factor IX content; actual units of potency for each coagulation factor and proteins C and S is stated on the carton. Albumin (human), heparin, sodium. Preservative free. Inj., lyophilized Pow. for Soln. Kit containing single-use vial w/20 mL (500 units) or w/40 mL vial (1,000 units) vial of sterile water for injection. *Rx.*
Use: Systemic hemostatic.

KCl-20. (Western Research) Potassium Cl 1.5 g (potassium 20 mEq, chloride 20 mEq) Packet. Box 30s. *Rx.*
Use: Electrolyte supplement.

K-Dur 10 & 20. (Key) **10:** Potassium Cl 750 mg (10 mEq). SR Tab. **20:** Potassium Cl 1500 mg (20 mEq). SR Tab. Bot. 100s. *Rx.*
Use: Electrolyte supplement.

KE.
See: Cortisone Acetate.

Kedbumin. (Kedrion Biopharma) Albumin (human) 25%. Aluminum ≤ 200 mcg, sodium ion 130 to 160 mEq. Preservative free. Inj. Single-dose vial. 50 mL. *Rx.*
Use: Plasma expander, plasma protein fraction.

Keelamin. (Mericon Industries) Zinc 20 mg, manganese 5 mg, copper 3 mg. Tab. Bot. 100s. *OTC.*
Use: Mineral supplement.

Keep Alert. (Magno-Humphries Labs) Caffeine 200 mg. Tab. Bot. 60s. *OTC.*
Use: CNS stimulant, analeptic.

Keep Going. (Block Drug) Caffeine 200 mg. Tab. Pkg. 4s. *OTC.*
Use: CNS stimulant, analeptic.

Keflex. (Shionogi Pharma) **Cap.:** Cephalexin 250 mg, 333 mg, 500 mg, 750 mg. Bot. 20s, 100s (250, 500 mg only); 50s (333 mg, 750 mg only). **Pow. for Oral Susp.:** Cephalexin 125 mg/5 mL, 250 mg/5 mL. Sucrose. Bot. 100 mL, 200 mL. *Rx.*
Use: Anti-infective, cephalosporin.

Kell E. (Canright) dl-α Tocopheryl 100 units, 200 units, 400 units. Tab. Bot. 100s. *OTC.*
Use: Vitamin supplement.

Kellogg's Tasteless Castor Oil. (GlaxoSmithKline) Castor oil 100%. Bot. 2 oz. *OTC.*
Use: Laxative.

Kelnor 1/35. (Barr) Ethinyl estradiol 35 mcg, ethynodiol diacetate 1 mg. Tab. 28s with 7 inert tablets. *Rx.*
Use: Contraceptive hormone, sex hormone.

Kelp. (Arcum) Tab. Bot. 100s, 1000s. *OTC.*
Use: Supplement.

Kelp. (Faraday) Iodine from kelp 0.15 mg. Tab. Bot. 100s. *OTC.*
Use: Supplement.

Kelp Plus. (Barth's) Iodine from kelp plus 16 trace minerals. Tab. Bot. 100s, 500s, 1000s. *OTC.*
Use: Supplement.

Kenac. (Alra) Triamcinolone acetonide. **Cream:** 0.025%, 0.1%. Tube 15 g, 60 g, 80 g; Jar 240 g. **Oint.:** 0.1%. Tube 15 g, 80 g. *Rx.*
Use: Corticosteroid, topical.

Kenakion. (Harriett Lane Home of Johns Hopkins Hospital) Vitamin K-1 oxide. *Rx.*
Use: Vitamin K-induced kernicterus.

Kenalog. (Bristol-Myers Squibb) Triamcinolone acetonide. 0.1% (w/base of polyethylene, mineral oil). Oint. Tubes. 15 g, 60 g, 80 g. Jars. 240 g. *Rx.*
Use: Corticosteroid, topical.

Kenalog. (Ranbaxy) Aer. 6.6 mg/100 g, alcohol 10.3%. Cans. 23 g, 63 g.

Kenalog-40. (Bristol-Myers Squibb) Triamcinolone acetonide 40 mg/mL. Benzyl alcohol 0.9%, carboxymethylcellulose, polysorbate 80. Inj., Susp. Vials. 1 mL, 5 mL, 10 mL. *Rx.*
Use: Adrenocortical steroid, glucocorticoid.

Kenalog-10. (Bristol-Myers Squibb) Triamcinolone acetonide 10 mg/mL. Benzyl alcohol 0.9%, carboxymethylcellulose, polysorbate 80. Inj., Susp. Vials. 5 mL. *Rx.*
Use: Adrenocortical steroid, glucocorticoid.

Kenalog 0.025%. (Bristol-Myers Squibb) Triamcinolone acetonide. **Cream:** Tube 15 g, 80 g; Jar 240 g. **Oint.:** Plastibase (w/base of polyethylene and mineral oil gel). Tube 15 g, 80 g, 240 g. *Rx.*
Use: Corticosteroid, topical.

Kendall's "Compound E".
See: Cortisone Acetate.

Kendall's "Desoxy Compound B".
See: Desoxycorticosterone Acetate.

Kenwood Therapeutic. (Kenwood) Vitamins A 3333 units, D 133 units, E 1.5 units, C 50 mg, B_1 2 mg, B_2 1 mg, B_3 20 mg, B_5 2 mg, B_6 0.33 mg, Ca, K,

Mg, Mn, P per 5 mL. Liq. Bot. 240 mL. *OTC.*
Use: Mineral, vitamin supplement.

Kepivance. (Biovitrum AB) Palifermin 6.25 mg. Sucrose. Preservative free. Pow. for Inj. Single-use vials. *Rx.*
Use: Keratinocyte growth factor.

Keppra. (UCB) Levetiracetam. **Inj. Conc.:** 100 mg/mL. Sodium 45 mg. 5 mL single-use vials. **Oral Soln.:** 100 mg/mL. Dye-free. Acesulfame K, ammonium glycyrrhizinate, glycerin, parabens, maltitol. Grape flavor. 480 mL. **Tab.:** 250 mg, 500 mg, 750 mg, 1,000 mg. Film coated. PEG. 60s (1,000 mg only), 120s (except 1,000 mg). *Rx.*
Use: Anticonvulsant.

Keppra XR. (UCB) Levetiracetam 500 mg, 750 mg. Film coated. PEG. ER Tab. 60s. *Rx.*
Use: Anticonvulsant.

Keradan. (Medimetriks Pharmaceuticals) Alcohols, caprylic/capric triglyceride, glycerin, petrolatum, paraffin, silicone gel, cholesterol, beeswax, methylparaben, olive oil, linoleic acid, triethanolamine, edetate disodium, tocopheryl acetate, wax, olive fruit oil, linolenic acid, sodium hyaluronate, tocopherol. Fragrance free. Cream. 255 g. *OTC.*
Use: Emollient.

Kerafoam. (Onset Therapeutics) Urea 30%. Cetyl alcohol, parabens. Foam. 60 g. *Rx.*
Use: Emollient.

Kerafoam 42. (Onset Therapeutics) Urea 42%. Cetearyl alcohol, edetate disodium, parabens. Aer. Foam. 60 g. *Rx.*
Use: Emollient.

Keralac. (Brava) Urea 47%. Alcohol, camphor, disodium EDTA, eucalyptus oil, menthol. Cream. 142 g. *Rx.*
Use: Emollient.

Keralyt. (Summers) Salicylic acid 3%, 6%. Alcohol 21%, propylene glycol. Gel. 28.4 g. *OTC.*
Use: Keratolytic agent.

Kerasal AL. (Taro Consumer) Ammonium lactate, light mineral oil, glycerin, propylene glycol, cetyl alcohol, glyceryl monostearate, polyoxyethylene 100 stearate, magnesium aluminum silicate, methylcellulose, polyoxyl 40 stearate, laureth-4, parabens. May contain ammonium hydroxide and lactic acid. Cream. 42 g. *OTC.*
Use: Emollient.

Kerasal Ultra 20. (Alterna) Ammonium lactate 5%, urea 20%, cetyl alcohol, disodium EDTA, glycerin, glyceryl, mineral oil, parabens, PEG-100, petrolatum, propylene glycol. Cream. 56.8 g. *OTC.*
Use: Emollient.

keratinocyte growth factors.
See: Palifermin.

Keratol HC. (Breckenridge) Hydrocortisone acetate 1%. Cetyl alcohol, disodium edetate, urea 10%. Cream. 28.3 g, 95 g. *Rx.*
Use: Anti-inflammatory agent; corticosteroid, topical.

keratolytic agents.
See: Acne Products, Combinations.
Masoprocol.
Podophyllum Resin.
Salicylic Acid.
Sulfur Preparations.

Keri. (Novartis Consumer Health) Mineral oil, lanolin oil, water, propylene glycol, glyceryl stearate, PEG-100 stearate, PEG 40 stearate, PEG-4 dilaurate, laureth-4, parabens, docusate sodium, triethanolamine, quaternium 15, carbomer 934. Lot. Bot. 6.5 oz, 13 oz, 20 oz. *OTC.*
Use: Emollient.

Keri Advanced. (Novartis Consumer Health) Glycerin, petrolatum, cetyl alcohol, aloe, tocopheryl acetate, dimethicone, PEG-100 stearate, parabens, EDTA, diazolidinyl urea. Oil free. Lot. 241 g. *OTC.*
Use: Emollient.

Keri Age Defy & Protect. (Novartis Consumer Health) Octinoxate 7.5%, oxybenzone 2%, cetearyl alcohol, glycerin, ammonium lactate, dimethicone, tocopheryl, EDTA. SPF +15. Lot. 425 g. *OTC.*
Use: Emollient.

Keri Deep Conditioning Overnight. (Novartis Consumer Health) Castor oil, cetyl alcohol, cetearyl alcohol, disodium EDTA, glycerin, glyceryl, parabens, PEG-8, shea butter, vitamins A, C, and E. Lt. 425 g. *OTC.*
Use: Emollient, miscellaneous.

Keri Facial Soap. (Novartis Consumer Health) Sodium tallowate, sodium cocoate, mineral oil, octyl hydroxystearate, fragrance, glycerin, titanium dioxide, PEG-75, lanolin oil, docusate sodium, PEG-4 dilaurate, propylparaben, PEG-40 stearate, glyceryl monostearate, PEG-100 stearate, sodium Cl, BHT, EDTA. Bar 3.25 oz. *OTC.*
Use: Dermatologic cleanser.

Keri Long Lasting. (Novartis Consumer Health) Cetearyl alcohol, polysorbate 60, mineral oil, cetyl alcohol, caprylic/carpic triglycerides, propylene glycol,

dimethicone, parabens, tocopheryl acetate, disodium EDTA. Cream, Top. 113 g. *OTC.*
Use: Emollient, miscellaneous.

Keri Nourishing Shea Butter. (Novartis Consumer Health) Mineral oil, glycerin, shea butter, vitamin E acetate, parabens, sunflower seed oil, EDTA, aloe. Lot. 425 g. *OTC.*
Use: Emollient.

Keri Original. (Novartis Consumer Health) Mineral oil, glycerin, PEG-40 stearate, glyceryl stearate, PEG-100 stearate, PEG-4 dilaurate, laureth-4, aloe, sunflower seed oil, tocopheryl acetate, parabens, EDTA. Scented and unscented. Lot. 241 g. *OTC.*
Use: Emollient.

Keri Renewal Milk Body. (Novartis Consumer Health) Caprylic/carpic triglyceride, sunflower oil, glycerin, PEG-20, methyl glucose sesquistearate, laureth-7, C-13-14 isoparaffin, polyacrylamide, parabens, phenoxyethanol, dimethicone, cera alba, sodium pyruvate, tocopheryl acetate, borage oil, lactic acid, propylene glycol, hydrolyzed fibronectin, bifida fermen lysate, carbomer, sodium hydroxide, acrylates/C10-30 alkyl acrylate, crosspolymer, allantoin, disodium EDTA, citric acid, glyceryl oleate, glyceryl stearate, ascorbyl palmitate, BHT, glycosphingolipids, phospholipids, cholesterol, whey protein. Top. Lot. 241 g. *OTC.*
Use: Emollient, miscellaneous.

Keri Renewal Skin Firming. (Novartis Consumer Health) Cetyl alcohol, ceteareth-20, isostearyl isostearate, hydrolyzed fibronectin, propylene glycol, glyceryl stearate, steareth-20, PEG-6 stearate, dimethicone, tocopheryl acetate, sodium pyruvate, collagen, hydrolyzed elastin, methyl silanol, sodium mannuronate, parabens, phenoxyethanol, carbomer, sodium hydroxide, madecassicoside. Top. Lot. 119 g. *OTC.*
Use: Emollient, miscellaneous.

Keri Sensitive Skin. (Novartis Consumer Health) Glycerin, hydrogenated polyisobutane, petrolatum, cetyl alcohol, aloe, barbadensis gel, vitamin E acetate, EDTA, parabens. Lot. 241 g. *OTC.*
Use: Emollient.

Keri Shave Minimizing. (Novartis Consumer Health) Glycerin, cetearyl alcohol, mineral oil, petrolatum, SD alcohol 40-B, glyceryl dilaurate, dimethicone, parabens, hydrolyzed soy protein. Lot. 425 g. *OTC.*
Use: Emollient.

Kerlone. (Sanofi) Betaxolol hydrochloride 10 mg, 20 mg. Lactose. Film-coated. Tab. Bot. 100s. *Rx.*
Use: Antiadrenergic/sympatholytic, beta-adrenergic blocker.

Kerocaine.
See: Procaine hydrochloride.

Kerodex. (Wyeth) **No. 51:** Water-miscible. Tube 4 oz, Jar lb. **No. 71:** Water-repellent Tube 4 oz, Jar lb. *OTC.*
Use: Emollient.

kerohydric. A de-waxed, oil-soluble fraction of lanolin.
Use: Emollient, cleanser.
See: Alpha-Keri.
Keri.

W/Docusate Sodium, Sodium Alkyl Polyether Sulfonate, Sodium Sulfoacetate, Sulfur, Salicylic Acid, Hexachlorophene.
See: Sebulex with Conditioners.

Kerr Insta-Char. (VistaPharma) Activated charcoal. **Regular:** 50 g. Glycerin, propylene glycol, sodium benzoate, sucrose. Regular and cherry flavors. Susp. 240 mL w/drinking straw. **Pediatric:** 25 g. Glycerin, propylene glycol, sodium benzoate, sucrose. Cherry flavor. Susp. 120 mL w/drinking straw. *OTC.*
Use: Detoxification agent, antidote.

Kerr Triple Dye. (Kerr Drug) Gentian violet, proflavine hemisulfate, brilliant green in water. Dispensing bot. 15 mL. Single Use *Dispos-A-Swab* 0.65 mL, Box 10s, Case 10 × 50 Box. *OTC.*
Use: Antiseptic.

Kestrone 5. (Hyrex) Estrone 5 mg/mL, sodium carboxymethylcellulose, povidone, benzyl alcohol, propylparabens Inj. Multi-dose vial 10 mL. *Rx.*
Use: Estrogen.

Ketalar. (JHP Pharmaceuticals) Ketamine hydrochloride 10 mg, 50 mg, 100 mg/mL. Inj. Vial 20 mL (10 mg), 10 mL (50 mg), 5 mL (100 mg). Ctn. 10s. *c-III.*
Use: Anesthetic.

•**ketamine hydrochloride.** (KEET-uh-MEEN) *USP.*
Use: Anesthetic.
See: Ketalar.

•**ketanserin.** (KEET-AN-ser-in) USAN.
Use: Serotonin antagonist.

•**ketazocine.** (key-TAY-zoe-seen) USAN.
Use: Analgesic.

•**ketazolam.** (keet-AZE-oh-lam) USAN.
Use: Anxiolytic.

Ketek. (Sanofi-Aventis) Telithromycin 300 mg, 400 mg. Cornstarch (400 mg only), lactose. Film-coated. Tab. 20s (300 mg only); 60s, *Ketek Pak*, blister

pack 10s (400 mg only). *Rx.*
Use: Anti-infective.

•**kethoxal.** (KEY-thox-al) USAN.
Use: Antiviral.

•**ketipramine fumarate.** (key-TIH-prah-MEEN) USAN.
Use: Antidepressant.

KetoCare. (Home Diagnostics) Reagent strips for urine tests. 50s. *OTC.*
Use: Diagnostic aid.

•**ketoconazole.** (KEY-toe-KOE-nuh-zole) *USP.*
Use: Antifungal agent, topical anti-infective.
See: Extina.
Ketodan.
Nizoral A-D.
Xolegel.
Xolegel CorePak.
W/Pyrithione Zinc.
See: Xolegel Duo Convenience Pack.

ketoconazole. (Various Mfr.) Ketoconazole. **Tab.:** 200 mg. 30s, 50s, 100s, 250s, 500s, 1,000s; blister pack 10s, 30s, 50s, 100s. **Cream:** 2%. Cetyl alcohol, stearyl alcohol, sodium sulfite. Tube. 15 g, 30 g, 60 g. **Shampoo:** 2%. 120 mL. **Foam:** 2%. Alcohols, ethanol 58%, propylene glycol. 50 g, 100 g. *Rx.*
Use: Antifungal agent, topical anti-infective.

Ketodan. (Medimetriks) Ketoconazole 2%. Alcohols, ethanol 58%, propylene glycol. Foam. 100 g and in kits w/*Rehyla Wash* in 454 g (alcohols, betaine, chamomile flower extract, cholesterol, edetate disodium, glycerin, phenoxyethanol, propylene glycol, salicylic acid, sodium hyaluronate). *Rx.*
Use: Topical anti-infective, antifungal.

Ketodestrin.
See: Estrone.

ketohydroxyestratriene.
See: Estrone.

ketohydroxyestrin.
See: Estrone.

ketolides.
Use: Anti-infectives.
See: Telithromycin.

ketone tests.
Use: Diagnostic aid.
See: Acetest Reagent.
Chemstrip K.

Ketonex-1. (Ross) Protein 15 g, fat 23.9 g, carbohydrates 46.3 g, linoleic acid 1800 mg, Fe 9 mg, Na 190 mg, K 675 mg. With appropriate vitamins and minerals. 480 Cal/100 g. Isoleucine, leucine, and valine free. Pow. Can 350 g. *OTC.*
Use: Nutritional supplement.

Ketonex-2. (Ross) Protein 30 g, fat 15.5 g, carbohydrates 30 g, Fe 13 mg, Na 880 mg, K 1370 mg. With appropriate vitamins and minerals. 410 Cal/100 g. Isoleucine, leucine and valine free. Pow. Can 325 g. *OTC.*
Use: Nutritional supplement.

•**ketoprofen.** (KEY-to-pro-fen) *USP.*
Use: Nonsteroidal anti-inflammatory agent.

ketoprofen. (Andrx) Ketoprofen 100 mg, 150 mg, 200 mg. ER Cap. Bot. 100s, 1000s. *Rx.*
Use: Nonsteroidal anti-inflammatory agent.

ketoprofen. (Various Mfr.) Ketoprofen 50 mg, 75 mg. Cap. Bot. 100s, 500s (75 mg only). *Rx.*
Use: Nonsteroidal anti-inflammatory agent.

•**ketorfanol.** (key-TAR-fan-AHL) USAN.
Use: Analgesic.

•**ketorolac tromethamine.** (KEY-TOR-oh-lak tro-METH-uh-meen) *USP.*
Use: Analgesic, NSAID, ophthalmic.
See: Acular.
Acular LS.
Acuvail.
Sprix.

ketorolac tromethamine. (Apotex) Ketorolac tromethamine. **0.4%:** EDTA 0.015%, benzalkonium chloride 0.006%, sodium chloride, hydrochloric acid, and/or sodium hydroxide. **0.5%:** Benzalkonium chloride 0.01%, EDTA disodium 0.1%, octoxynol 40, sodium chloride, hydrochloric acid, and/or sodium hydroxide.Soln., Ophth. 5 mL, 10 mL. *Rx.*
Use: Ophthalmic and otic agent, nonsteroidal anti-inflammatory agent.

ketorolac tromethamine. (Bedford) Ketorolac tromethamine 15 mg/mL, 30 mg/mL. Inj. Vial 1 mL (15 mg/mL only). Single dose vial 1 mL, 2 mL; multiple-dose vial 10 mL (30 mg/mL only). *Rx.*
Use: Nonsteroidal anti-inflammatory agent.

ketorolac tromethamine. (Various Mfr.) Ketorolac tromethamine 10 mg. Tab. Bot. 100s, 500s. *Rx.*
Use: Nonsteroidal anti-inflammatory agent.

•**ketotifen fumarate.** (KEY-toe-TIE-fen) USAN.
Use: Antiasthmatic.
See: Alaway.
Alaway Children's.
Claritin Eye.

Visine All Day Eye Itch.
Zaditor.
Zyrtec Itchy Eye.

ketotifen fumarate. (Various Mfr.) Ketotifen fumarate 0.025%. Benzalkonium chloride 0.01%, glycerol, sodium hydroxide and/or hydrochloric acid. Soln., Ophth. 5 mL. *Rx.*
Use: Ophthalmic decongestant agent.

K-4. Menadiol sodium diphosphate.
Use: Vitamin K.

K-G Elixir. (Geneva) Potassium (as potassium gluconate) 20 mEq/15 mL, alcohol 5%. Elix. Bot. Pt. *Rx.*
Use: Electrolyte supplement.

Khedezla. (Par) Desvenlafaxine 50 mg, 100 mg. Film coated. ER Tab. 30s, 90s. *Rx.*
Use: Antidepressant, serotonin and norepinephrine reuptake inhibitor.

khellin.
Use: Coronary vasodilator.

Kiddie Powder. (Gordon Laboratories) Pure fine Italian talc. Can. 3.5 oz. *OTC.*
Use: Antifungal.

Kiddi-Vites, Improved. (Geneva) Vitamins A 5000 units, D 500 units, B_1 1 mg, B_2 1.5 mg, B_{12} 2 mcg, C 50 mg, B_6 1 mg, pantothenate 2 mg, niacinamide 10 mg. Tab. Bot. 100s, 1000s. *OTC.*
Use: Vitamin supplement.

Kid Kare. (Rugby) Pseudoephedrine hydrochloride 7.5 mg/0.8 mL, sorbitol, sugar, cherry flavor, alcohol free. Drops. Bot. 30 mL w/dropper. *OTC.*
Use: Nasal decongestant, arylalkylamine.

Kid Kare Children's Cough/Cold. (Rugby) Pseudoephedrine hydrochloride 15 mg, chlorpheniramine maleate 1 mg, dextromethorphan HBr 5 mg per 5 mL. Sorbitol, corn syrup, cherry flavor, alcohol free. Liq. Bot. 118 mL. *OTC.*
Use: Upper respiratory combination, antitussive combination.

kidney function agents.
See: Indigo Carmine.
Inulin.
Iodohippurate Sodium.
Methylene Blue.

KIE. (Laser) Potassium iodide 150 mg, ephedrine hydrochloride 8 mg/5 mL, saccharin, sorbitol, sucrose, cherry flavor. Syr. Bot. 473 mL. *Rx.*
Use: Upper respiratory combination, decongestant, expectorant.

kinase inhibitors.
See: BRAF Inhibitors.
Janus-Associated Kinase Inhibitors.
MEK Inhibitors.
MTOR Inhibitors.
Tyrosine Kinase Inhibitors.

kinate. Hexahydrotetra hydroxybenzoate salt, quinic acid salt.

Kindercal. (Mead Johnson Nutritionals) Protein 13%, carbohydrate 50%, fat 37%, 30 cal/oz, sucrose, vanilla flavor, lactose free, 30 cal/oz. Liq. Can. 8 oz. *OTC.*
Use: Nutritional supplement.

Kinerase Intensive Eye Cream. (Valeant) Kinetin 0.125%, safflower seed oil, cetyl alcohol, urea, parabens. Cream. 20 g. *OTC.*
Use: Emollient.

Kineret. (Amgen) Anakinra 100 mg/0.67 mL. Sodium chloride, EDTA, preservative free. Inj. Single-use Prefilled syringe 1 mL w/27-gauge needle. *Rx.*
Use: Immunologic, immunomodulator.

Kinevac. (Bracco Diagnostics) Sincalide 5 mcg/vial. Pow. for Inj., lyophilized. Vials. *Rx.*
Use: Diagnostic aid, gastrointestinal function test.

Kinrix. (GlaxoSmithKline) Diphtheria toxoid 25 Lf, tetanus toxoid 10 Lf, inactivated pertussis toxin 25 mcg, filamentous hemagglutinin 25 mcg, pertactin 8 mcg, type 1 poliovirus (Mahoney) 40 D-antigen units, type 2 poliovirus (MEF-1) 8 D-antigen units, type 3 poliovirus (Saukett) 32 D-antigen units per 0.5 mL. Sodium chloride 4.5 mg, aluminum adjuvant (≤ 0.6 mg aluminum by assay), residual formaldehyde ≤ 100 mcg, polysorbate 80 (*Tween 80*) ≤ 100 mcg, neomycin ≤ 0.05 ng, polymyxin B ≤ 0.01 ng per dose. Preservative free. Inj., Susp. 0.5 mL single-dose vial, prefilled *Tip-Lok* syringe. *Rx.*
Use: Vaccine combination, diphtheria toxoid/tetanus toxoid/acellular pertussis, adsorbed/inactivated poliovirus combination vaccine.

Kin White. (Whiteworth Towne) Triamcinolone acetonide. **Cream:** 0.025%, 1%. Tube 15 g, 80 g. **Oint.:** 1%. Tube 15 g, 80 g. *OTC.*
Use: Corticosteroid, topical.

Kionex. (Paddock) **Pow. for Susp.:** Finely ground sodium polystyrene sulfonate (4 level tsp ≈ 15 g), sodium content ≈ 100 mg (4.1 mEq)/g. 454 g. **Susp.:** Sodium polystyrene sulfonate 15 g per 60 mL. Alcohol 0.2%, parabens, propylene glycol, saccharin, sodium 1.5 g (65 mEq) per 60 mL, sorbitol 19.3 g per 60 mL. Raspberry flavor. 480 mL, UD 60 mL. *Rx.*
Use: Potassium-removing resin.

•**kitasamycin.** (kit-ah-sah-MY-sin) USAN. An antibiotic substance obtained from cultures of *Streptomyces kitasatoensis.* Under study.
Use: Anti-infective.

Klaron. (Valeant Pharmaceuticals) Sulfacetamide sodium 10%. EDTA, methylparaben, PEG, propylene glycol, simethicone, sodium metabisulfite. Lot. 118 mL. *Rx.*
Use: Topical anti-infective, antibiotic.

Klavikordal. (US Ethicals) Nitroglycerin 2.6 mg. SR Tab. Bot. 100s, 1000s. *Rx.*
Use: Antianginal.

KLB6. (NBTY) Vitamin B_6 3.5 mg, soya lecithin 100 mg, kelp 25 mg, cider vinegar 80 mg Softgels. Bot. 100s. *OTC.*
Use: Vitamin supplement.

KLB6 Complete. (NBTY) Vitamins A 833.3 units, E 5 mg (as units), B_3 3.3 mg, C 10 mg, soya lecithin 200 mg, kelp 25 mg, cider vinegar 40 mg, wheat bran 83.3 mg, D 66.7 units, FA 0.067 mg, B_1 0.25 mg, B_2 0.28 mg, B_6 8.3 mg, B_{12} 1 mcg, biotin 0.05 mg. Tab. Bot. 100s. *OTC.*
Use: Vitamin supplement.

Kleer Improved. (Scrip) Atropine sulfate 0.2 mg, chlorpheniramine maleate 5 mg/mL. *Rx.*
Use: Anticholinergic; antihistamine.

Klerist-D. (Nutripharm Laboratories, Inc.) **Cap. SR:** Pseudoephedrine hydrochloride 120 mg, chlorpheniramine maleate 8 mg. Bot. 100s, 500s. **Tab.:** Pseudoephedrine hydrochloride 60 mg, chlorpheniramine maleate 4 mg. Bot. 24s, 100s. *Rx.*
Use: Antihistamine; decongestant.

Kler-Ro. (Ulmer Pharmacal) Surgical cleanser and laboratory detergent. **Liq.:** Bot. Gal. **Pow.:** Can 2 lb, Bot. 6 lb. *Rx.*
Use: Antiseptic.

Klonopin. (Genentech) Clonazepam 0.5 mg, 1 mg, 2 mg. Lactose. Tab. 100s. *c-IV.*
Tall Man: KlonoPIN
Use: Anticonvulsant; antianxiety agent.

K-Lor. (Abbott) Potassium Cl equivalent to potassium 20 mEq and Cl 20 mEq/2.6 g for oral soln. w/saccharin. Pkg. 30s, 100s. 15 mEq/2 g Pkg. 100s. *Rx.*
Use: Electrolyte supplement.

Klor-Con 8. (Upsher-Smith) Potassium Cl 8 mEq. ER Tab. Bot. 100s, 500s. *Rx.*
Use: Electrolyte supplement.

Klor-Con M15. (Upsher-Smith) Potassium 15 mEq (from potassium chloride 1125 mg). ER Tab. Bot. 100s, 1000s, UD 100s. *Rx.*
Use: Electrolyte supplement.

Klor-Con M10. (Upsher-Smith) Potassium 10 mEq (from potassium chloride 750 mg). ER Tab. Bot. 90s, 100s, 1000s, UD 100s. *Rx.*
Use: Electrolyte supplement.

Klor-Con M20. (Upsher-Smith) Potassium 20 mEq (from potassium chloride 1500 mg). ER Tab. Bot. 90s, 100s, 500s, 1000s, UD 100s. *Rx.*
Use: Electrolyte supplement.

Klor-Con 10. (Upsher-Smith) Potassium Cl 10 mEq. ER Tab. Bot. 100s, 500s. *Rx.*
Use: Electrolyte supplement.

Klorvess. (Novartis) **Liq.:** Potassium Cl 1.5 g (20 mEq)/15 mL, alcohol 0.75%. Bot. pt. **Effervescent Granules:** Potassium 20 mEq, Cl 20 mEq supplied by potassium Cl 1.125 g, potassium bicarbonate 0.5 g, L-lysine monohydrochloride 0.913 g. Pkt. w/saccharin. Box 30s. **Effervescent Tablets:** Potassium Cl 1.125 g, potassium bicarbonate 0.5 g, L-lysine hydrochloride 0.913 g. Sodium and sugar free, saccharin. Pkg. 60s, 1000s. *Rx.*
Use: Electrolyte supplement.

Klotrix. (Bristol-Myers Squibb) Potassium Cl 10 mEq. SR Tab. Bot. 100s, 1000s, UD 100s. *Rx.*
Use: Electrolyte supplement.

Klout. (PediaMed) Acetic acid, isopropanol, sodium laureth sulfate. Parabens. Shampoo. 118.3 mL with comb. *OTC.*
Use: Scabicide/pediculicide.

K-Lyte. (Bristol-Myers Squibb) Potassium bicarbonate and citrate 25 mEq, saccharin. Lime and orange flavors. Effervescent Tab. Pkg. 30s, 100s, 250s. *Rx.*
Use: Electrolyte supplement.

K-Lyte/Cl. (Bristol-Myers Squibb) Potassium Cl 25 mEq, saccharin. Citrus and fruit punch flavor. Bulk powder 225 g Can. *Rx.*
Use: Electrolyte supplement.

K-Lyte/Cl 50. (Bristol-Myers Squibb) Potassium Cl 50 mEq, saccharin. Citrus and fruit punch flavors. Pkg. 30s, 100s. *Rx.*
Use: Electrolyte supplement.

K-Lyte DS. (Bristol-Myers Squibb) Potassium bicarbonate and citrate 50 mEq, saccharin. Lime and orange flavor. Effervescent Tab. Pkg. 30s, 100s. *Rx.*
Use: Electrolyte supplement.

Koate-DVI. (Kedrion BioPharma) Human antihemophilic factor 250 units, 500 units, 1000 units. Albumin (human) ≤ 10 mg/mL, aluminum ≤ 1 mcg/mL,

glycine, histidine, PEG. Solvent/detergent treated, heat treated. Inj., lyophilized Pow. for Soln. Single-dose Bot. and sterile water for injection. *Rx.*
Use: Antihemophilic agent.

Kodonyl Expectorant. (Halsey Drug) Bromodiphenhydramine hydrochloride 3.75 mg, diphenhydramine hydrochloride 8.75 mg, ammonium Cl 80 mg, potassium guaiacolsulfonate 80 mg, menthol 0.5 mg/5 mL. Bot. 16 oz. *OTC.*
Use: Antihistamine; expectorant.

Kof-Eze. (Roberts) Menthol 6 mg. Loz. Pkg. 4s, Bot. 500s. *OTC.*
Use: Mouth and throat preparation.

Kogenate. (Bayer) Concentrate of AHF (recombinant). When reconstituted, contains glycine 10 to 30 mg/mL, imidazole ≤ 500 mcg/1000 units, CaCl 2 to 5 mM, chloride 100 to 130 mEq/L, human albumin 4 to 10 mg/mL, monoclonal purified, Na 100 to 130 mEq/L. Preservative free. Inj., lyophilized. Single-dose bottles (actual number of AHF units indicated on bottles) with diluent, double-ended needle, filter needle, administration set. *Rx.*
Use: Antihemophilic.

Kogenate FS. (Bayer) Recombinant antihemophilic factor 250 units, 500 units, 1,000 units, 2,000 units, 3,000 units, 4,000 units. Glycine, histidine, polysorbate 80, sodium, sucrose. Preservative free and albumin free. Solvent/detergent treated, monoclonal antibody purified. Inj., lyophilized Pow. for Soln. Kit w/single-use vial and diluent (2.5 mL sterile water for injection [250 unit, 500 unit, 1,000 unit], 5 mL sterile water for injection [2,000 unit, 3,000 unit]). *Rx.*
Use: Antihemophilic agent.

•**kolfocon A.** (KAHL-FOE-kahn A) USAN.
Use: Contact lens material (hydrophobic).

•**kolfocon B.** (KAHL-FOE-kahn B) USAN.
Use: Contact lens material (hydrophobic).

•**kolfocon C.** (KAHL-FOE-kahn C) USAN.
Use: Contact lens material (hydrophobic).

•**kolfocon D.** (KAHL-FOE-kahn D) USAN.
Use: Contact lens material (hydrophobic).

Kombiglyze XR. (Bristol-Myers Squibb) Saxagliptin/metformin hydrochloride 5 mg/500 mg (equiv. to saxagliptin hydrochloride 5.58 mg), 5 mg/1,000 mg (equiv. to saxagliptin hydrochloride 5.58 mg), 2.5 mg/1,000 mg (equiv. to saxagliptin hydrochloride 2.79 mg). Film coated. ER Tab. 30s (5 mg/500 mg); 30s, 90s, 500s (5 mg/1,000 mg); 60s, 500s (2.5 mg/1,000 mg). *Rx.*
Use: Antidiabetic combination product.

Kondon's Nasal Jelly. (Kondon) Tube 20 g w/ephedrine alkaloid. *OTC.*
Use: Decongestant.

Kondremul. (Insight Pharmaceuticals) Mineral oil, Irish moss, acacia, glycerin. Emulsion Bot. 480 mL. **W/Cascara:** 0.66 g/15 mL. Bot. 14 oz. *OTC.*
Use: Laxative.

K-1. Phytonadione.
Use: Vitamin K.
See: Aqua MEPHYTON.
Mephyton.

Konsto. (Freeport) Docusate sodium 100 mg. Cap. Bot. 1000s. *OTC.*
Use: Laxative.

Konsyl. (Konsyl) Psyllium 6 g. Pow. Canister 300 g, 450 g, UD Packet 6 g. *OTC.*
Use: Laxative.

Konsyl-D. (Konsyl) Psyllium 3.4 g, 14 cal/tsp, dextrose. Pow. Canister 325 g, 500 g, UD 6.5 g. *OTC.*
Use: Laxative.

Konsyl Easy Mix Formula. (Konsyl) Psyllium 6 g, Na 4.4 mg, Ca 48 mg, P 4 mg, Zn 0.06 mg, K 42 mg, carbohydrates 0.35 g, 4 cal/5 mL. Pow. Can. 200 g, Packets. *OTC.*
Use: Laxative

Konsyl Fiber. (Konsyl) Polycarbophil 500 mg Tab. Bot. 90s. *OTC.*
Use: Laxative.

Konsyl Orange Sugar Free. (Konsyl) Psyllium 3.5 g/tsp. Aspartame, calcium 6 mg, maltodextrin, phenylalanine 21 mg, potassium 32 mg, sodium 3 mg. Sugar free. Orange flavor. Pow. 450 g. *OTC.*
Use: Laxative, bulk-producing laxative.

Korlym. (Corcept Therapeutics) Mifepristone 300 mg. Film coated. Tab. 28s, 280s. *Rx.*
Use: Uterine-active agent, abortifacient.

Koro-Flex. (Holland-Rantos) Improved contouring-spring, natural latex diaphragm 60 mm to 95 mm. *OTC.*
Use: Contraceptive.

Korum. (Geneva) Acetaminophen 5 g. Tab. Bot. 1000s. *OTC.*
Use: Analgesic.

Kotabarb. (Wesley) Phenobarbital ¼ g. Tab. Bot. 1000s. *Rx.*
Use: Hypnotic, sedative.

Kovitonic. (Freeda) Iron 42 mg, vitamins B_1 5 mg, B_6 10 mg, B_{12} 30 mcg, folic acid 0.1 mg, l-lysine 10 mg/15 mL. Liq. Bot. 120 mL, 240 mL. *OTC.*
Use: Mineral, vitamin supplement.

K-P. (Century) Kaolin 5.2 g, pectin 260 mg/oz. Susp. Bot. Gal. *OTC.*
Use: Antidiarrheal.

K-PAX Immune Support. (K-PAX) Fe 1.125 mg, Ca 50 mg, vitamin A 1,250 units, D_3 25 units, E 25 units, B_1 3.75 mg, B_2 3.75 mg, B_3 3.75 mg, B_5 3.75 mg, B_6 12.5 mg, B_{12} 0.16 mcg, C 125 mg, folate 0.05 mg, B, Cr, Cu, I, K, Mg, Mn, Mo, Se, Z. N-acetyl-L-cysteine, acetyl-L-carnitine HCl, alpha lipoic acid, betaine HCl, biotin, choline, citrus bioflavonoid complex, inositol (from soy), L-glutamic acid, mixed tocopherol blend. Cap. 240s (60 packets of 8 capsules). *OTC.*
Use: Multivitamin with minerals.

K-PAX Immune Support Protein Blend Powder. (K-PAX) Protein 20 g (from brown rice protein, N-acetyl-cysteine, L-glutamine), carbohydrate 7 g (as sugar), fat < 1 g, vitamin K 50 mg, A, B_1, B_2, B_3, B_5, B_6, B_{12}, C, D, E, alpha lipoic acid, betaine HCl, biotin, choline, citrus bioflavonoid complex, folic acid, inositol, mixed tocopherols, B, Ca, Cr, Cu, I, Mg, Mn, Mo, Se, Zn. Vegetarian formula. Pow. 505 g. *OTC.*
Use: Enteral nutritional therapy, defined formula diet.

K-PAX Protein Blend Powder. (K-PAX) Protein 10 g (from acetyl-L-carnitine HCl, N-acetyl-L-cysteine, L-glutamic acid), carbohydrate 16 g (as sugar), fat < 1 g, vitamin K 25 mg, A, B_1, B_2, B_3, B_5, B_6, B_{12}, C, D, E, alpha lipoic acid, betaine HCl, biotin, choline, citrus bioflavonoid complex, folic acid, inositol, mixed tocopherol blend, B, Ca, Cr, Cu, I, Mg, Mn, Mo, Se, Zn. Pow. 908 g. *OTC.*
Use: Enteral nutritional therapy, defined formula diet.

K-Pek II. (Rugby) Loperamide hydrochloride 2 mg, lactose. Tab, Pkg. 12s. *OTC.*
Use: Antidiarrheal.

K-Phos Neutral. (Beach) Phosphorus 250 mg, potassium 45 mg, sodium 298 mg. Film-coated. Tab. 100s, 500s. *Rx.*
Use: Mineral supplement.

K-Phos No. 2. (Beach) Potassium acid phosphate 305 mg, sodium acid phosphate, anhydrous 700 mg. Tab. Bot. 100s, 500s. *Rx.*
Use: Acidifier, urinary.

K-Phos Original. (Beach) Potassium acid phosphate 500 mg. Tab. Bot. 100s, 500s. *Rx.*
Use: Urinary acidifier; electrolyte supplement.

K + 10. (Edwards) Potassium Cl 10 mEq. Tab. Bot. 100s, 500s, 1000s. *Rx.*
Use: Electrolyte supplement.

K.P.N. (Freeda) Vitamins C 333 mg, Fe 11 mg, A 2667 units, D 133 units, E 10 mg, B_1 2 mg, B_2 2 mg, B_3 10 mg, B_5 3.3 mg, B_6 0.83 mg, B_{12} 2 mcg, C 33 mg, FA 0.27 mg, I, Cu, Mn, K, Mg, Zn 6.7 mg, bioflavonoids. Tab. Bot. 100s, 250s, 500s. *OTC.*
Use: Mineral, vitamin supplement.

Kristalose. (Bertek) Lactulose (galactose and lactose < 0.3 g/10 g). Crystals for reconstitution. Pack 10 g, 20 g. Box. 30s. *Rx.*
Use: Laxative, hyperosmotic agent.

Kronofed-A. (Ferndale) Pseudoephedrine hydrochloride 120 mg, chlorpheniramine maleate 8 mg. SR Cap. Bot. 100s, 500s. *Rx.*
Use: Upper respiratory combination, antihistamine, decongestant.

Kronofed-A Jr. (Ferndale) Pseudoephedrine hydrochloride 60 mg, chlorpheniramine maleate 4 mg. SR Cap. Bot. 100s, 500s. *Rx.*
Use: Upper respiratory combination, antihistamine, decongestant.

•**krypton clathrate Kr 85.** (KRIPP-tahn KLATH-rate) USAN.
Use: Radiopharmaceutical.

•**krypton Kr 81m.** (KRIP-tahn Kr 81 m) *USP.*
Use: Radiopharmaceutical.

Krystexxa. (Crealta) Pegloticase 8 mg/mL (as uricase protein [recombinant]). Inj., Soln., Conc. Single-use vial. 2 mL. *Rx.*
Use: Agent for gout.

K-Tab. (Abbott) Potassium Cl (10 mEq) 750 mg. ER Tab. Bot. 100s, 1000s, UD 100s. *Rx.*
Use: Electrolyte supplement.

K 34. Hexachlorophene.

K.T.V. (Knight) Vitamin B_{12}, minerals. Tab. Bot. 50s. *OTC.*
Use: Mineral, vitamin supplement.

kunecatechins. (koo-ne-KAT-e-kins)
Use: Treatment of external genital and perianal warts.
See: Veregen.

Kurvelo. (Lupin) Ethinyl estradiol 30 mcg, levonorgestrel 0.15 mg. Lactose. Tab. Blister pack 28s w/7 inert tablets. *Rx.*
Use: Oral monophasic contraceptive.

Kuvan. (BioMarin Pharmaceuticals) Sapropterin dihydrochloride 100 mg (equiv. to sapropterin base 76.8 mg). **Tab.:** Mannitol. 30s, 120s. **Pow. for Soln.:** Mannitol, potassium citrate, sucralose. UD 30s. *Rx.*
Use: Phenylketonuria agent.

K-Vescent Potassium Chloride. (Major) Potassium and chloride 20 mEq from potassium chloride 1.5 g, saccharin. Pow. Pkt. 30s, 100s. *Rx.*
Use: Potassium replacement product.

Kwikderm. (Alra) Tolnaftate 1%. **Cream:** Tube. 15 g. **Soln.:** Bot. 10 mL. *OTC.*
Use: Antifungal, topical.

Kwildane. (Major) Gamma benzene hexachloride 1%. Shampoo. Bot. 60 mL, pt, gal. *OTC.*
Use: Pediculicide.

K-Y. (Johnson & Johnson) Glycerin, methylparaben, hydroxyethylcellulose. Sterile or regular. Jelly. Tube. 12 g, 60 g, 120 g. *OTC.*
Use: Lubricant.

Kynamro. (Genzyme) Mipomersen sodium 200 mg/mL. Preservative free. Inj., Soln. Single-use 1 mL vial and prefilled syringe. *Rx.*
Use: Antihyperlipidemic agent.

Kyodex Reagent Strips. (Kyoto) A disposable plastic reagent strip for determination of glucose in whole blood. Vial 25s.
Use: Diagnostic aid.

Kyotest UGK Reagent Strip. (Kyoto) Disposable reagent strip for measurement of glucose and ketones in the urine. Vial 50s, 100s.
Use: Diagnostic aid.

Kyotest UG Reagent Strips. (Kyoto) Reagent strips for glucose and ketones in urine.
Use: Diagnostic aid.

Kyotest UK Reagent Strips. (Kyoto) Reagent strip for ketones in urine. Vial 50s.
Use: Diagnostic aid.

KY Plus. (Johnson & Johnson) Nonoxynol-9 2%, methylparaben. Nongreasy. 113 g. *OTC.*
Use: Lubricant.

Kyprolis. (Onyx Pharmaceuticals) Carfilzomib 60 mg. Preservative free. Inj., lyophilized Pow. for Soln. Single-use vial. *Rx.*
Use: Proteasome inhibitor.

Kytril. (Roche) Granisetron hydrochloride. **Inj.:** 0.1 mg/mL (0.112 mg/mL as hydrochloride), 1 mg/mL (1.12 mg/mL as hydrochloride) (benzyl alcohol 10 mg, sodium chloride 9 mg/mL). Preservative free. Single-use vials. 1 mL (0.1 mg/mL). Multidose vials. 4 mL (1 mg/mL). **Oral Soln.:** 1 mg/mL (1.12 mg/5 mL as hydrochloride). Sorbitol, orange flavor. Bot. 30 mL. *Rx.*
Use: Antiemetic (cancer therapy).

L

•**labetalol hydrochloride.** (la-BET-ul-lahl) *USP.*
Use: Alpha/beta-adrenergic blocking agent; antiadrenergic/sympatholytic.
See: Trandate.

labetalol hydrochloride. (Various Mfr.) Labetalol hydrochloride. **Inj.:** 5 mg/mL, EDTA 0.1 mg, methylparaben 0.8 mg, propylparaben 0.1 mg, dextrose. Multidose vial 20 mL, 40 mL. **Tab.:** 100 mg, 200 mg, 300 mg. Bot. 30s, 100s, 250s, 500s, 1000s. *Rx.*
Use: Antiadrenergic/sympatholytic; alpha/beta-adrenergic blocker.

•**labetuzumab.** (la-be-too-zoo-mab) USAN.
Use: Monoclonal antibody.

•**labradimil.** (la-BRAY-da-mil) USAN.
Use: Adjuvant.

Labstix Reagent Strips. (Siemans Medical) Urine screening test. Bot. 100s.
Use: Diagnostic aid.

Lac-Dose. (Rugby) Lactase 3,000 FCC units. Dextrose, mannitol, sodium 4 mg. Tab. 50s. *OTC.*
Use: Enzyme.

Lac-Hydrin Cream. (Ranbaxy) Ammonium lactate 12%. Cetyl alcohol, glycerin, glyceryl stearate, light mineral oil, parabens. Cream. 280 g, 385 g. *Rx.*
Use: Emollient.

Lac-Hydrin Five. (Ranbaxy) Lactic acid, glycerin, petrolatum, squalane, steareth-2, PCE-21-stearyl ether, propylene glycol dioctanoate, dimethicone, cetyl palmitate, diazolidinyl urea. Unscented. Lot. 120 mL, 240 mL. *OTC.*
Use: Emollient.

Lac-Hydrin Lotion. (Ranbaxy) Lactic acid 12% neutralized w/ammonium hydroxide, light mineral oil, cetyl alcohol, parabens. Tube 150 mL, 360 mL. *Rx.*
Use: Emollient.

•**lacidipine.** (lah-SIH-dih-PEEN) USAN.
Use: Antihypertensive.

Laclede Cleaner. (Laclede) Container. 2 lb. *OTC.*
Use: Detergent.

Laclede Disclosing Swab. (Laclede) Swabs 6". 100s, 500s, 1000s. *OTC.*
Use: Dentrifice.

Laclede Topi-Fluor A.P.F. Topical Cream. (Laclede) Fluoride ion 1.23% (from sodium fluoride) in orthophosphoric acid 0.98%. Jar 50 mL, 500 mL, 1000 mL, 2000 mL. *Rx.*
Use: Dental caries agent.

LAC-Lotion. (Paddock) Ammonium lactate 12% (12% lactic acid neutralized with ammonium hydroxide), mineral oil, cetyl alcohol, parabens, glycerin. Lotion. 225 g, 400 g. *Rx.*
Use: Emollient.

lacosamide.
Use: Investigational anticonvulsant.
See: Vimpat.

Lacotein. (Christina) Protein digest 5% w/preservatives. Vial 30 mL (w/iodochin), vial 30 mL. *Rx.*
Use: Protein supplement.

Lacril. (Allergan) Hydroxypropyl methylcellulose 0.5%, gelatin A 0.01%, chlorobutanol 0.5%, polysorbate 80, dextrose, magnesium Cl, sodium borate, sodium chloride. Soln. Dropper bot. 15 mL. *OTC.*
Use: Lubricant; ophthalmic.

Lacri-Lube NP. (Allergan) White petrolatum 55.5%, mineral oil 42.5%, petrolatum/lanolin alcohol 2%. Oint. 0.7 g. *OTC.*
Use: Lubricant; ophthalmic.

Lacri-Lube S.O.P. (Allergan) White petrolatum 56.8%, mineral oil 41.5%, lanolin alcohols, chlorobutanol. Tube 3.5 g, 7 g. *OTC.*
Use: Lubricant; ophthalmic.

Lacrisert. (Aton Pharma) Hydroxypropyl cellulose 5 mg/insert. Pkg. 60s w/applicators. *Rx.*
Use: Artificial tears.

Lactaid. (Ortho-McNeil) **Liq.:** Beta-D-galactosidase derived from Kluyveromyces lactis yeast (1000 Neutral Lactase units/5 drop dosage) in carrier of glycerol 50%, water 30%, inert yeast dry matter 20%. Units of 4, 12, 30, 75 one-quart dosages at 5 drops/dose. **Tab.:** Beta-D-galactosidase from Aspergillus oryzae (3300 FCC lactase units/Tab.). In 12s, 100s. *OTC.*
Use: Digestive aid.

lactalbumin hydrolysate.
See: Aminonat.

•**lactase.** (LAK-tase) USAN.
Use: Digestive aid.
See: Dairy Ease.
Lac-Dose.
Lactaid.
Lactase Fast Acting.
Lactrase.
SureLac.

Lactase Fast Acting. (Major) Lactase 9,000 FCC units. Dextrose, fructose, sugar. Tab. 32s. *OTC.*
Use: Nutritional agent, lactase enzyme.

lactated Ringer's. (Various Mfr.) Na^+ 130 mEq, K^+ 4 mEq, $Ca^{++} \approx 3$ mEq, $Cl^- \approx 109$ mEq, lactate 28 mEq, osmolarity ≈ 274 mOsm/L. Soln. Inj. Bot.

250 mL, 500 mL, 1000 mL. *Rx.*
Use: Intravenous nutritional therapy, intravenous replenishment solution.

lactated Ringer's in 5% dextrose. (Various Mfr.) Dextrose 50 g, calories 170, Na^+ 130 mEq, K^+ 4 mEq, Ca^{++} $\approx$ 3 mEq, Cl^- 109–112 mEq, lactate 28 mEq, osmolarity 525–530 mOsm/L. Soln. Bot. 250 mL, 500 mL, 1000 mL. *Rx.*
Use: Intravenous nutritional therapy, intravenous replenishment solution.

lactated Ringer's irrigation. (Hospira) Sodium chloride 600 mg, anhydrous sodium lactate 310 mg, potassium chloride 30 mg, calcium chloride dihydrate 20 mg per 100 mL. Soln. 300 mL. *Rx.*
Use: Irrigating solution.

•**lactic acid.** (LACK-tick) *USP.*
Use: Pharmaceutic necessity for sodium lactate injection.
See: Lactic Acid E.
Lactrex 12%.
Penecare.
W/Sodium Pyrrolidone Carboxylate.
See: Lactinol.

Lactic acid E. (Stratus Pharmaceutical) Lactic acid 10%, vitamin E, cetyl alcohol, disodium EDTA, glycerin, glyceryl, PEG-40, PEG-100, parabens. Cream. 113.4 g. *Rx.*
Use: Emollient.

lactic acid, lyophilized.
See: VSL#3 The Living Shield.
VSL#3 DS Double Strength.

lactic acid 10% E. (Sonar Products) Lactic acid 10%, vitamin E 3500 units per 30 g. Cetyl alcohol, EDTA, glycerin, parabens. Cream. 113.4 g, 226.8 g. *Rx.*
Use: Emollient.

Lactinex. (Becton Dickinson) *Lactobacillus acidophilus* & *Lactobacillus bulgaricus* mixed culture. **Tab.:** 1 million CFU. Glucose, lactose, mineral oil, sucrose. Gluten free. 50s. **Gran.:** 100 million CFU. Glucose, lactose, sucrose. Gluten free. 1 g pkt. 12s. *OTC.*
Use: Antidiarrheal; nutritional supplement.

Lactinol. (Pedinol Pharmacal) Lactic acid 10%. Lot. Bot. 237 mL. *Rx.*
Use: Emollient.

Lactobacillin Acidophilus. (Nature's Blend) *Lactobacillus acidophilus* 25 million units. Lactose. Cap. 100s. *OTC.*
Use: Nutritional supplement, probiotic.

Lactobacillus acidophilus. Preparation made from acid-producing bacterium.
Use: Antidiarrheal; nutritional supplement.
See: Acidophilus.
Acidophilus Lactobacilli.
Acidophilus Lactobacillin Freeze-Dried.
Acidophilus Probiotic.
Acidophilus With Goat Milk.
Acidophilus With Pectin.
Dofus.
Florajen Acidophilus.
High Potency Chewable Acidophilus.
Intestinex.
Kala.
Lactobacillin Acidophilus.
Lacto-Key-100.
Lacto-Key-600.
Megadophilus.
Megadophilus Dairy Free.
Mega Vegi-Dophilus.
More Dophilus.
Pro-Bionate.
Probiotic Acidophilus.
Probiotic Gold Extra Strength Acidophilus.
Ultimate Probiotic Formula Acidophilus.
W/Bifidobacterium Longum.
See: Acidophilus Pearls.
W/Lactobacillus Bifidus.
See: Acidophilus with Bifidus.

Lactobacillus acidophilus and bulgaricus mixed culture.
See: Floranex.
Lactinex.

Lactobacillus acidophilus, viable culture.
See: Dofus.

Lactobacillus and Bifidobacterium.
See: ReZyst IM.

Lactobacillus bifidus.
Use: Nutritional supplement.
See: Lacto-Bifidus-100.
W/Lactobacillus Acidophilus.
See: Acidophilus with Bifidus.

Lactobacillus bulgaricus.
Use: Antidiarrheal.
See: Bacid.
More Dophilus.

Lactobacillus GG.
See: Culturelle Kids.
Culturelle with Lactobacillus GG.

Lactobacillus reuteri Protectis.
Use: Nutritional supplement.
See: BioGaia.
BioGaia Probiotic Drops.
BioGaia Probiotic Straws.
BioGaia ProTectus Baby.
Gerber Soothe Colic.

Lactobacillus rhamnosus.
Use: Probiotic.
See: Culturelle Dairy Free.
Culturelle Digestive Health.
Culturelle Natural Health and Wellness.

Lacto-Bifidus-100. (Key Company) *Lactobacillus bifidus* ≥ 1 billion CFU. Cap. 60s. *OTC.*
Use: Probiotic.

lactoflavin.
See: Riboflavin.

Lacto-Key-100. (Key) *Lactobacillus acidophilus* ≥ 1 billion CFU. Cap. 60s. *OTC.*
Use: Nutritional supplement.

Lacto-Key-600. (Key) *Lactobacillus acidophilus* ≥ 6 billion CFU. Cap. 60s. *OTC.*
Use: Nutritional supplement.

Lacto-Pectin. (Bio-Tech) 35 billion CFU blend of *L. acidophilus, L. casei, B. lactis, B. longum, B. bifidum, L. rhamnosus, L. bulgaricus, L. plantarum.* Maltodextrin. Preservative free and sugar free. Cap. 100s. *OTC.*
Use: Probiotic.

lactose. Milk sugar.
Use: Pharmaceutic aid (tablet and capsule diluent).
See: Natur-Aid.

•**lactose anhydrous.** (LAK-tose an-HIGH-druss) *NF.*
Use: Pharmaceutic aid (tablet and capsule diluent).

•**lactose monohydrate.** (LAK-tose) *NF.*
Use: Pharmaceutic aid (tablet and capsule diluent).

Lacto-Tri Blend. (Key Company) 10 billion CFU blend of *L. acidophilus, L. bifidus, L. bulgaricus* per ¼ tsp. Pow. 2 oz. *OTC.*
Use: Probiotic.

Lacto-Tri Blend-100. (Key Company) 1 billion CFU blend of *L. acidophilus, L. bifidus, L. bulgaricus.* Cap. 120s. *OTC.*
Use: Probiotic.

Lacto-Tri Blend-600. (Key Company) 6 billion CFU blend of *L. acidophilus, L. bifidus, L. bulgaricus.* Cap. 120s. *OTC.*
Use: Probiotic.

Lactrase. (Aventis) Standardized enzyme lactase (β-D-galactosidase) 125 mg dispersed in maltodextrins. Cap. Bot. 100s. *OTC.*
Use: Nutritional supplement.

Lactrodectus Mactans Antivenin. (Merck & Co.) Antivenin 6000 units per vial (with 1:10,000 thimerosal), supplied with a 2.5 mL vial of Sterile Water for Injection and a 1 mg vial (with 1:10,000 thimerosal) of normal horse serum (1:10 dilution) for sensitivity testing. *Rx.*
Use: Antivenin (Black Widow spider).
See: Antivenin (Lactrodectus Mactans).

lactulose.
Use: Laxative.
See: Cephulac.
Constulose.
Enulose.
Generlac.
Kristalose.

lactulose. (Various Mfr.) Lactulose 10 g/15 mL (galactose < 1.6 g, lactose 1.2 g, other sugars 1.2 g). Soln. Bot. 237 mL, 473 mL, 960 mL, 1873 mL. *Rx.*
Use: Laxative.

•**lactulose concentrate.** (LAK-tyoo-lohs) *USP.*
Use: Laxative, treatment of hepatic coma and chronic constipation.
See: Cephulac.
Chronulac.

ladakamycin.
Use: Refractory acute myelogenous leukemia (AML) agent.
See: Azacitidine.

Ladogal. (Sanofi-Synthelabo) Danazol. *Rx.*
Use: Androgen.

Ladogar. (Sanofi-Synthelabo) Danazol. *Rx.*
Use: Androgen.

•**ladostigil.** (LAD-oh-STIJ-il) USAN.
Use: Alzheimer disease.

Lady Esther. (Menley & James Labs, Inc.) Mineral oil. Cream. 120 g. *OTC.*
Use: Emollient.

L.A.E. 40. (Seatrace) Estradiol valerate 40 mg/mL. Inj. Vial 10 mL. *Rx.*
Use: Estrogen.

L.A.E. 20. (Seatrace) Estradiol valerate 20 mg/mL. Inj. Vial 10 mL. *Rx.*
Use: Estrogen.

•**lambrolizumab.** (LAM-broe-LIZ-ue-mab) USAN.
Use: Antineoplastic.

Lamictal. (GlaxoSmithKline) Lamotrigine. **Chew. Dispersible Tab.:** 2 mg, 5 mg, 25 mg. Saccharin. Black currant flavor. 30s (2 mg only), 100s (except 2 mg). **Tab.:** 25 mg, 100 mg, 150 mg, 200 mg. Lactose. 60s (150 mg, 200 mg), 100s (25 mg, 100 mg). **Orally disintegrating Tab.:** 25 mg, 50 mg, 100 mg, 200 mg. Mannitol, sucralose. Cherry flavor. 30s. *Rx.*
Tall Man: LaMICtal
Use: Anticonvulsant.

Lamictal ODT Patient Titration Kit. (GlaxoSmithKline) Lamotrigine. Tab., orally disintegrating. **Blue ODT kit:** 25 mg, 50 mg. Mannitol, sucralose. Cherry flavor. (Titration kits contain 21 of the 25 mg tablets and 7 of the 50 mg tablets.) **Green ODT kit:** 50 mg, 100 mg. Mannitol, sucralose. Cherry flavor. (Titration kits contain 42 of the

50 mg tablets and 14 of the 100 mg tablets.) **Orange ODT kit:** 25 mg, 50 mg, 100 mg. Mannitol, sucralose. Cherry flavor. (Titration kits contain 14 of the 25 mg tablets, 14 of the 50 mg tablets, and 7 of the 100 mg tablets.) *Rx.*
Tall Man: LaMICtal
Use: Anticonvulsant.

Lamictal Starter Kit. (GlaxoSmithKline) Lamotrigine 25 mg, 100 mg. Lactose. Tab. Blue kit (contains 35 of the 25 mg tablets), green kit (contains 84 of the 25 mg tablets and 14 of the 100 mg tablets), orange kit (contains 42 of the 25 mg tablets and 7 of the 100 mg tablets). *Rx.*
Tall Man: LaMICtal
Use: Anticonvulsant.

Lamictal XR. (GlaxoSmithKline) Lamotrigine 25 mg, 50 mg, 100 mg, 200 mg, 250 mg, 300 mg. Film coated. Lactose, PEG. ER Tab. 30s. *Rx.*
Tall Man: LaMICtal
Use: Anticonvulsant.

Lamictal XR Patient Titration Kit. (GlaxoSmithKline) Lamotrigine. ER Tab. **Blue XR kit:** 25 mg, 50 mg. Film coated. Lactose. (Titration kits contain 21 of the 25 mg ER tablets and 7 of the 50 mg ER tablets.) **Orange XR kit:** 25 mg, 50 mg, 100 mg. Film coated. Lactose. (Titration kits contain 14 of the 25 mg ER tablets, 14 of the 50 mg ER tablets, and 7 of the 100 mg ER tablets.) **Green XR kit:** 50 mg, 100 mg, 200 mg. Film coated. Lactose. (Titration kits contain 14 of the 50 mg ER tablets, 14 of the 100 mg ER tablets, and 7 of the 200 mg ER tablets.) *Rx.*
Tall Man: LaMICtal
Use: Anticonvulsant.

•**lamifiban.** (la-mih-FIE-ban) USAN.
Use: Antithrombotic; platelet aggregation inhibitor; fibrinogen receptor antagonist.

Lamisil. (Novartis) Terbinafine hydrochloride. **Gran.:** 125 mg/packet, 187.5 mg/packet. Film-coated. Cartons. 14s, 42s. **Tab.:** 250 mg. Tab. Bot. 30s, 100s. *Rx.*
Tall Man: LamISIL
Use: Antifungal, allyamine.

Lamisil AF Defense. (Novartis) Tolnaftate 1%. **Pow.; Top.:** Talc. 113 g. **Aer., Pow.; Top.:** Alcohol 11%, talc. 133 g. *OTC.*
Tall Man: LamISIL
Use: Topical anti-infective, antifungal agent.

Lamisil AT. (Novartis) Terbinafine hydrochloride. **Cream:** 1%. Benzyl alcohol, cetyl alcohol, stearyl alcohol. 15 g, 30 g. **Gel:** 1%. Benzyl alcohol. 6 g, 12 g. **Spray:** 1%, ethanol, propylene glycol. Bot. 30 mL. *OTC.*
Tall Man: LamISIL
Use: Antifungal.

Lamisil AT Jock Itch. (Novartis) Terbinafine 1%. Benzyl alcohol, cetyl alcohol, stearyl alcohol. Cream. 12 g. *OTC.*
Use: Topical anti-infective, antifungal.

•**lamivudine.** (la-MIH-view-deen) USAN.
Tall Man: lamiVUDine
Use: Antiretroviral, nucleoside reverse transcriptase inhibitor.
See: Epivir.
Epivir-HBV.
W/Abacavir.
See: Epzicom.
W/Zidovudine.
See: Combivir.

lamivudine. (Various Mfr.) Lamivudine 100 mg, 150 mg, 300 mg. May contain lactose, PEG. Tab. 30s (300 mg), 60s (except 300 mg), UD 30s (150 mg only). *Rx.*
Use: Antiretroviral, nucleoside reverse transcriptase inhibitor.

lamivudine and zidovudine.
Use: Antiretroviral; AIDS.
See: Combivir.

lamivudine/zidovudine. (Teva) Lamivudine 150 mg/zidovudine 300 mg. Film coated. PEG. Tab. 60s. *Rx.*
Use: Antiretroviral agent, nucleoside analog reverse transcriptase inhibitor combination.

•**lamotrigine.** (lah-MOE-trih-JEEN) USAN.
Tall Man: lamoTRIgine
Use: Anticonvulsant; Lennox-Gastaut syndrome. [Orphan Drug]
See: Lamictal.
Lamictal ODT Patient Titration Kit.
Lamictal Starter Kit.
Lamictal XR.
Lamictal XR Patient Titration Kit.

lamotrigine. (Various Mfr.) Lamotrigine. **Tab.:** 25 mg, 100 mg, 150 mg, 200 mg. May contain lactose. 25s (25 mg only), 30s, 60s, 90s, 100s, 500s, 1,000s, 1,500s (200 mg only), 2,000 (150 mg only), 3,000 (100 mg only), UD 100s. **Chew. Dispersible Tab.:** 5 mg, 25 mg. May contain mannitol, saccharin, and/or sucralose. 30s, 90s, 100s, 500s, 1,000s, UD 100s. **ER Tab.:** 25 mg, 50 mg, 100 mg, 200 mg, 300 mg. May contain lactose, PEG. 30s, 90s (300 mg only), 100s (250 mg only), 500s. *Rx.*
Use: Anticonvulsant.

lamotrigine. (ZyGenerics) Lamotrigine 50 mg, 250 mg. May contain lactose. Tab. 60s (250 mg), 90s, 100s (50 mg),

500s, 1,000s (50 mg). *Rx.*
Use: Anticonvulsant.

lamotrigine starter kit. (Various Mfr.) Lamotrigine 25 mg, 100 mg. May contain lactose. Tab. Blue kit (contains 35 of the 25 mg tablets), green kit (contains 84 of the 25 mg tablets and 14 of the 100 mg tablets), orange kit (contains 42 of the 25 mg tablets and 7 of the 100 mg tablets). *Rx.*
Use: Anticonvulsant.

•**lampalizumab.** (LAM-pa-LIZ-ue-mab) USAN.
Use: Treatment of geographic atrophy secondary to age-related macular degeneration.

Lampit. (Bayer) Nifurtimox.
Use: Anti-infective.

Lanabiotic. (Combe) Polymyxin B sulfate 10,000 units, neomycin (as sulfate) 3.5 mg, bacitracin zinc 500 units, lidocaine 40 mg. Aloe, lanolin, mineral oil, petrolatum. Oint. Tubes. 28 g. *OTC.*
Use: Anti-infective; antibiotic, topical; anesthetic, local.

Lanacane. (Combe) **Spray:** Benzocaine 20%. Benzethonium chloride 0.1%, ethanol 36%, aloe extract. 113 mL. **Cream:** Benzocaine 6%. Benzethonium chloride 0.1%, aloe, parabens, castor oil, glycerin, isopropyl alcohol. 28 g, 56 g. *OTC.*
Use: Anesthetic, local.

Lanacort. (Combe) Hydrocortisone acetate 0.5%. Cream. Tube 0.5 oz, 1 oz. *OTC.*
Use: Corticosteroid, topical.

Lanacort 10. (Combe) Hydrocortisone acetate 1%. **Cream:** Tube 15, 30 g. **Oint.:** Tube 15 g. *OTC.*
Use: Corticosteroid, topical.

Lanaphilic. (Medco Lab) Sorbitol, isopropyl palmitate, stearyl alcohol, white petrolatum, lanolin oil, sodium lauryl sulfate, propylene glycol, methylparaben, propylparaben. Oint. Jar 16 oz. Also available w/urea 10% or 20%. *OTC.*
Use: Emollient.

Lanaphilic w/Urea 10%. (Medco Lab) Urea, stearyl alcohol, white petrolatum, isopropyl palmitate, propylene glycol, sorbitol, sodium lauryl sulfate, lactic acid, parabens. Oint. Jar 1 lb. *OTC.*
Use: Emollient.

•**lanimostim.** (LAN-i-MOE-stim) USAN.
Use: Antineoplastic agent.

•**lanolin.** (LAN-oh-lin) *USP. Formerly Anhydrous lanolin.*
Use: Pharmaceutic aid (ointment base, absorbent).
See: Kerohydric.
Lan-O-Soothe.
Lansinoh.
Lantiseptic Daily Care Skin Protectant.
Lantiseptic Therapeutic.

W/Diiosbutylcresoxyethoxyethyl, Dimethyl Benzyl Ammonium Chloride, Menthol.
See: Hospital Lotion.

•**lanolin alcohols.** (LAN-oh-lin) *NF.*
Use: Pharmaceutic aid (emulsifying agent).

Lanoline. (GlaxoSmithKline) Perfumed emollient. Oint. Tube 1.75 oz. *OTC.*
Use: Pharmaceutic aid; ointment base; absorbent; emollient.

•**lanolin, modified.** (LAN-oh-lin) *USP.*
Use: Pharmaceutic aid (ointment base, absorbent).

Lano-Lo Bath Oil. (Whorton Pharmaceuticals, Inc.) 8 oz. *OTC.*

Lanolor. (Numark) Lanolin oil, glyceryl stearates, propylene glycol, sodium lauryl sulfate, simethicone, polyoxyl 40 stearate, cetyl esters wax, methylparaben. Cream Jar 60 g, 240 g. *OTC.*
Use: Emollient.

Lan-O-Smooth. (Geritrex) Lanolin 100%. Oint. 56 g. *OTC.*
Use: Emollient.

•**lanoteplase.** (lan-OH-teh-place) USAN.
Use: Thrombolytic; plasminogen activator.

Lanoxin. (Covis Pharmaceuticals) Digoxin. **Tab.:** 0.0625 mg, 0.125 mg, 0.1875 mg, 0.25 mg. Lactose. 100s, 1,000s, UD 100s (0.125 mg and 0.25 mg only). **Inj.:** (w/propylene glycol 40%, alcohol 10%). Amp. 2 mL. **Pediatric Inj.:** 0.1 mg/mL (w/propylene glycol 40%, alcohol 10%). Amp. 1 mL. *Rx.*
Use: Inotropic agent; cardiac glycoside.

•**lanreotide acetate.** (lan-REE-oh-tide) USAN.
Use: Antineoplastic.
See: Somatuline Depot.

Lansinoh. (Lansinoh) Lanolin 100%. Oint. 59 g. *OTC.*
Use: Emollient.

Lansinoh Diaper Rash. (Lansinoh) Lanolin 15.5%, zinc oxide 5.5%, dimethicone 5%. Beeswax, petrolatum. Oint. 90 g. *OTC.*
Use: Diaper rash product.

•**lansoprazole.** (lan-SO-pruh-zole) *USP.*
Use: Proton pump inhibitor.
See: Prevacid.
Prevacid 24 Hour.

W/Amoxicillin and clarithromycin.
See: Prevpac.

lansoprazole. (Various Mfr.) Lansoprazole. **Cap., delayed release:** 15 mg,

30 mg (contain enteric-coated granules). May contain PEG, sugar spheres, sucrose. 30s (30 mg only), 90s, 100s (30 mg only), 500s (30 mg only), 1,000s, UD 30s (15 mg only), UD 80s (30 mg only), UD 100s. **Tab., delayed release:** 15 mg. May contain PEG, sugar spheres, sucrose. 14s, 28s, 42s. *Rx.*
Use: Proton pump inhibitor.

•**lanthanum carbonate.** (LAN-tha-num KAR-bo-nate)
Use: Phosphate binder.
See: Fosrenal.

lanthanum carbonate. (Various Mfr.) Lanthanum carbonate 500 mg, 750 mg, 1,000 mg. May contain dextrates. Chew. Tab. 90s. *Rx.*
Use: Renal and genitourinary agent, phosphate binder.

Lantiseptic Daily Care Skin Protectant. (Summit) Lanolin 30%. Disodium EDTA, lanolin alcohol, mineral oil, petrolatum, beeswax. Oint. 5 g, 14.2 g, 113 g, 400 g, single-use packet. *OTC.*
Use: Emollient.

Lantiseptic Multi-Purpose. (Summit) Menthol 0.45%, zinc oxide 20%, beeswax, calamine, disodium EDTA, glycerin, lanolin, mineral oil, petrolatum, parabens. Oint. 5 g, 113 g. *OTC.*
Use: Skin protectant.

Lantiseptic Therapeutic. (Summit) Lanolin 37%. Beeswax, HEEDTA, lanolin alcohol, mineral oil, petrolatum. Cream. 113 g. *OTC.*
Use: Emollient.

Lanturil. (Sanofi-Synthelabo) Oxypertine. *Rx.*
Use: Anxiolytic.

Lantus. (Aventis) Insulin glargine 100 units/mL. Inj. Vials. 10 mL. Cartridge system for use with *OptiClik.* 3 mL. *Rx.*
Use: Antidiabetic, insulin.

lanum. (Various Mfr.) Lanolin. *OTC.*
Use: Pharmaceutic aid.

lapatinib.
Use: Antineoplastic, tyrosine kinase inhibitor.
See: Tykerb.

•**lapatinib ditosylate.** (la-PA-tin-ib) USAN.
Use: Antineoplastic; tyrosine kinase inhibitor.

•**lapuleucel-T.** (LA-pul-OO-sel) USAN.
Use: Antineoplastic.

•**lapyrium chloride.** (LAH-pihr-ee-uhm KLOR-ide) USAN.
Use: Pharmaceutic aid (surfactant).

•**larazotide.** (lar-a-ZOE-tide) USAN.
Use: Immunomodulator.

Larin Fe 1.5/30. (NorthStar Rx) Ethinyl estradiol 30 mcg, norethindrone acetate 1.5 mg. Lactose, PEG, soy lecithin. Tab. 28s (w/7 tablets [ferrous fumarate 75 mg per tablet; PEG, soy lecithin]). *Rx.*
Use: Monophasic oral contraceptive.

Larin Fe 1/20. (Northstar Rx) Ethinyl estradiol 20 mcg, norethindrone acetate 1 mg. Lactose, PEG, soy lecithin. Tab. 28s (w/7 tablets [ferrous fumarate 75 mg per tablet; PEG, soy lecithin]). *Rx.*
Use: Monophasic oral contraceptive.

Larin 1/20. (Northstar Rx) Ethinyl estradiol 20 mcg, norethindrone acetate 1 mg. Lactose, PEG, soy lecithin. Tab. 21s. *Rx.*
Use: Monophasic oral contraceptive.

•**laronidase.** (lare-AHN-ih-dase) USAN.
Use: Enzyme replacement in Mucopolysaccharidosis.
See: Aldurazyme.

Larotid. (GlaxoSmithKline) Amoxicillin. **Cap.: 250 mg:** Bot. 100s, 500s, UD 100s, unit-of-use 18s. **500 mg:** Bot. 50s, 500s. **Oral Susp.:** 125 mg, 250 mg (as trihydrate)/5 mL. Bot. 80 mL, 100 mL, 150 mL. **Pediatric drops:** 50 mg (as trihydrate)/mL. Bot. 15 mL. *Rx.*
Use: Anti-infective, penicillin.

Larynex. (Dover Pharmaceuticals) Benzocaine. Sugar, lactose and salt free. Loz. UD Box 500s. *OTC.*
Use: Anesthetic, local.

Lasix. (Aventis) Furosemide 20 mg, 40 mg, 80 mg. Tab. 50s (80 mg), 100s (20 mg and 40 mg), 500s, 1,000s (20 mg and 40 mg), UD 100s. *Rx.*
Use: Diuretic.

•**lasmiditan.** (las-MID-i-tan) USAN.
Use: Agent for migraine.

•**lasmiditan succinate.** (las-MID-i-tan) USAN.
Use: Agent for migraine.

•**lasofoxifene tartrate.** (la-soe-FOX-i-feen) USAN.
Use: Osteoporosis; breast cancer.

Lassar's paste.
See: Zinc Oxide Paste.

Lastacaft. (Vistakon Pharmaceuticals) Alcaftadine 0.25%. Benzalkonium chloride 0.005%, edetate disodium. Soln., Ophth. 3 mL. *Rx.*
Use: Ophthalmic and otic agent, ophthalmic antihistamine.

•**latanoprost.** (lah-TAN-oh-prahst) USAN.
Use: Antiglaucoma agent.
See: Xalatan.

latanoprost. (Various Mfr.) Latanoprost 0.005%. May contain benzalkonium

chloride 0.02%, sodium chloride. Soln., Ophth. 2.5 mL. *Rx.*
Use: Agent for glaucoma, prostaglandin agonist.

•**latanoprostene bunod.** (la-TAN-oh-PROS-teen BUE-nod) USAN.
Use: Agent for glaucoma.

Latest-CRP Kit. (Fischer) Measures C-reactive protein in serum. Kit 1s.
Use: Diagnostic aid.

Latisse. (Allergan) Bimatoprost 0.03%. Benzalkonium chloride. Soln., Ophth. 60 disposable applicators. 3 mL. *Rx.*
Use: Agent for glaucoma, prostaglandin agonist.

•**latrepirdine.** (la-TRE-pir-deen) USAN.
Use: CNS agent.

•**latrepirdine dihydrochloride.** (la-TRE-pir-deen) USAN.
Use: CNS agent.

Latrix XM. (Stratus) Urea 45%. Caprylic/capric triglycerides, cetyl alcohol, EDTA disodium, glycerin, lactic acid, linoleic acid, PEG 300, titanium dioxide. Emuls. 240 mL. *Rx.*
Use: Emollient.

Latuda. (Sunovion) Lurasidone hydrochloride 20 mg, 40 mg, 60 mg, 80 mg, 120 mg. Mannitol. Tab. 30s, 90s, 500s, UD 100s. *Rx.*
Use: Antipsychotic agent, benzoisothiazol derivative.

•**laureth 4.** (LAH-reth 4) USAN.
Use: Pharmaceutic aid (surfactant).

•**laureth 9.** (LAH-reth 9) USAN.
Use: Pharmaceutical aid (surfactant); emulsifier; spermicide.

•**laureth 10.** (LAH-reth 10) USAN.
Use: Spermaticide.

•**laurocapram.** (LAHR-oh-KAH-pram) USAN.
Use: Pharmaceutic aid (excipient).

lauromacrogol 400. Laureth 9.

•**lauryl isoquinolinium bromide.** (LAH-rill EYE-so-KWIN-oh-lih-nee-uhm) USAN.
Use: Anti-infective.

lauryl sulfoacetate.
See: Lowila Cake.

Lavacol. (Parke-Davis) Ethyl alcohol 70%. Bot. Pt.
Use: Anti-infective, topical.

Lavatar. (Doak Dermatologics) Coal tar distillate 25.5% in a bath oil base. Liq. Bot. 4 oz, pt. *OTC.*
Use: Antipsoriatic; antipruritic.

Lavoclen-8. (Prasco Laboratories) Benzoyl peroxide 8%. Castor oil, cetearyl alcohol, glycerin, lactic acid, methylparaben, mineral oil, PEG. Soap. 170.1 g. Also in kit w/soap-free cleanser lotion (106.6 mL). *Rx.*
Use: Topical anti-infective, antibiotic agent.

Lavoclen-4. (Prasco Laboratories) Benzoyl peroxide 4%. Castor oil, cetearyl alcohol, glycerin, lactic acid, methylparaben, mineral oil, PEG. Soap. 170.1 g. Also in kit w/soap-free cleanser lotion (106.6 mL). *Rx.*
Use: Topical anti-infective, antibiotic agent.

•**lavoltidine succinate.** (lahv-OLE-tih-DEEN) USAN. *Formerly Loxotidine.*
Use: Antiulcerative (histamine H_2-receptor blocker).

Lavoptik Emergency Wash. (Lavoptik) Eye, face, body wash. 32 oz/emergency station. *OTC.*
Use: Emergency wash.

Lavoptik Eye Wash. (Lavoptik) Sodium Cl 0.49%, sodium biphosphate 0.4%, sodium phosphate 0.45%/100 mL w/benzalkonium Cl 0.005%. Bot. 6 oz. *OTC.*
Use: Irrigant; ophthalmic.

Lavoris. (Procter & Gamble) Zinc Cl, glycerin, poloxamer 407, saccharin, polysorbate 80, flavors, clove oil, alcohol, citric acid, water. Bot. 6 oz, 12 oz, 18 oz, 24 oz. *OTC.*
Use: Mouthwash.

Laxacin. (Alexso) Docusate sodium 50 mg, senna concentrate (as sennosides) 8.6 mg. Calcium 20 mg, dextrose, PEG, sodium 4 mg, sodium benzoate. Tab. 100s. *OTC.*
Use: Laxative combination.

Laxative & Stool Softener. (Rugby) Docusate sodium 100 mg, casanthranol 30 mg, parabens, sorbitol. Softgel. Cap. Bot. 100s. *OTC.*
Use: Laxative.

Laxative Caps. (Weeks & Leo) Docusate sodium 100 mg, casanthranol 30 mg. Cap. Bot. 30s, 60s. *OTC.*
Use: Laxative.

laxatives.
See: Aloe.
Aloin.
Bile Salts.
Bisacodyl.
Bisacodyl Tannex.
Bowel Evacuants.
Bulk-Producing Laxatives.
Carboxymethylcellulose Sodium.
Casanthranol.
Cascara.
Cascara Sagrada.
Castor Oil.
Citrucel.
Correctol.

Docusate Sodium.
Emulsoil.
Enemas.
ex-lax.
Fecal Softeners/Surfactants.
Feen-a-Mint.
Fleet Prep Kit 1.
Fleet Prep Kit 2.
Fleet Prep Kit 3.
Hyperosmotic Agents.
Irritant or Stimulant Laxatives.
Karaya Gum.
Laxacin.
Liquid Petrolatum Emulsion.
Magnesia Magma.
Maltsupex.
Methylcellulose.
Mucilloid of Psyllium Seed W/Dextrose.
Nature's Remedy.
Neoloid.
Oxyphenisatin Acetate.
PEG-3350 & Electrolytes.
Petrolatum.
Phenolphthalein.
Plantago Ovata, Coating.
Poloxalkol.
Senna Conc., Standardized.
Senna Fruit Extract, Standardized.
Sodium Biphosphate.
Sodium Phosphate.
Suclear.
Tridrate Bowel Cleansing System.
Unifiber.
X-Prep.
X-Prep Bowel Evacuant Kit-1.

W/Choline Base, Cephalin, Lipositol.
See: Alcolec.

W/CO_2-Releasing Suppositories.
See: Ceo-Two.

W/Polycarbophil.
See: Bulk Forming Fiber Laxative.
Cephulac.
Cholac.
Chronulac.
Citrucel Sugar Free.
Colace.
Constulose.
DC Softgels.
Diocto.
Docu.
Docusate Calcium.
D.O.S.
D-S-S.
Duphalac.
Enulose.
Equalactin.
ex-lax Stool Softener.
FiberCon.
Fiber-Lax.
FiberNorm.
Fleet.
Fleet Babylax.
Fleet Bisacodyl.
Fleet Mineral Oil.
Genasoft.
Glycerin.
Kondremul Plain.
Konsyl Fiber.
Mineral Oil.
Non-Habit Forming Stool Softener.
Phillips' Liqui-Gels.
Regulax SS.
Sani-Supp.
Silace.
Stool Softener.
Stool Softener DC.
Surfak.
Therevac-Plus.
Therevac-SB.

W/Polyethylene Glycol-Electrolyte.
See: CoLyte.
Concentrated Milk of Magnesia-Cascara.
DOK-Plus.
Emulsoil.
Evac-Q-Kwik.
Fleet Prep Kit 1.
Fleet Prep Kit 2.
Fleet Prep Kit 3.
GoLYTELY.
Haley's M-O.
Liqui-Doss.
MiraLax.
Neoloid.
NuLYTELY.
OCL.
Perdiem Overnight Relief.
Tridrate Bowel Cleansing System.
X-Prep.
X-Prep Bowel Evacuant Kit-1.
X-Prep Bowel Kit-2.

W/Psyllium.
See: Fiberall Orange Flavor.
Fiberall Tropical Fruit Flavor.
Genfiber.
Genfiber, Orange Flavor.
Hydrocil Instant.
Konsyl.
Konsyl-D.
Konsyl Easy Mix Formula.
Konsyl-Orange.
Konsyl Orange Sugar Free.
Metamucil.
Metamucil, Orange Flavor, Original Texture.
Metamucil Orange Flavor, Smooth Texture.
Metamucil, Original Texture.
Metamucil, Sugar Free, Orange Flavor, Smooth Texture.
Metamucil, Sugar Free, Smooth Texture.

Natural Fiber Laxative.
Perdiem Fiber Therapy.
Reguloid.
Reguloid, Orange.
Reguloid, Sugar Free Orange.
Reguloid, Sugar Free Regular.
Serutan.
Syllact.
W/Saline Laxatives.
See: Aromatic Cascara Fluid Extract.
Cascara Aromatic.
Epsom Salt.
Fleet Phospho-soda.
Magnesium Citrate.
Milk of Magnesia.
Milk of Magnesia-Concentrated.
Phillips' Milk of Magnesia.
Phillips' Milk of Magnesia, Concentrated.
W/Sennosides.
See: Agoral.
Bisac-Evac.
Bisacodyl Uniserts.
Black Draught.
Caroid.
Doxidan.
Dulcolax.
ex-lax Chocolated.
Fleet Laxative.
Fletcher's Castoria.
Maximum Relief ex•lax.
Modane.
Nature's Remedy.
Peri-Colace.
Reliable Gentle Laxative.
Senexon.
Senna-Gen.
Senokot.
Senokot-S.
SenokotxTRA.
Women's Gentle Laxative.
W/Vitamins.
See: Lec-E-Plex.

Laxinate 100. (Roberts) Dioctyl sodium sulfosuccinate 100 mg. Cap. Bot. 100s, 1000s.
Use: Laxative.

Lax Pills. (G & W Labs) Sennosides 15 mg, 25 mg, EDTA, parabens, sucrose. Tab. Blister pack 24s, 48s (25 mg only); 30s, 60s (15 mg only). *OTC.*
Use: Laxative.

layor carang.
See: Agar.

•**lazabemide.** (lazz-AH-bem-ide) USAN.
Use: Antiparkinsonian.

•**lazabemide hydrochloride.** (lazz-AH-bem-ide) USAN.
Use: Antiparkinsonian.

Lazanda. (Depomed) Fentanyl citrate 100 mcg, 400 mcg. Alcohol, mannitol, propylparaben, sucrose. Spray, Soln.; intranasal. 5.3 mL glass bottle containing eight 100 mcL sprays w/metered-dose nasal spray pump. *c-II.*
Use: Opioid analgesic.

Lazer Creme. (Pedinol) Vitamins E 3500 units, A 100,000 units/oz. Cream. Jar 2 oz. *OTC.*
Use: Emollient.

Lazer Formalyde. (Pedinol) Formaldehyde 10%. Soln. Bot. 90 mL. *Rx.*
Use: Drying agent.

LazerSporin-C. (Pedinol) Neomycin sulfate 5 mg, polymyxin B sulfate 10,000 units, hydrocortisone 1%. Soln. Bot. 10 mL with dropper. *Rx.*
Use: Anti-infective combination, topical.

L-baclofen.
Use: Antispasmodic. [Orphan Drug]

L-Caine E. (Century) Lidocaine hydrochloride 1%, 2%, epinephrine 1:100,000/mL. Inj. 20 mL, 50 mL. *Rx.*
Use: Anesthetic, local.

L-Caine Viscous. (Century) Lidocaine hydrochloride 2% with sodium carboxymethylcellulose. Soln. Bot. 100 mL. *Rx.*
Use: Anesthetic, local.

l-carnitine. (Freeda Vitamins) Levocarnitine 500 mg. Tab. Bot. 50s, 100s. *OTC.*
Use: Amino acid.

l-carnitine. (Various Mfr.) Amino acid derivative 250 mg. Cap. Bot. 30s, 60s, 100s. *OTC.*
Use: Amino acid.

L.C.D. (Almay) Alcohol extractions of crude coal tar. Cream, soln. Bot. 4 oz, pt. *OTC.*
Use: Antipsoriatic; antipruritic; topical.
See: Coal Tar Topical Solution.

LC-5. (TriMarc Laboratories) Lidocaine hydrochloride 5%. Aloe, cetyl alcohol, jojoba seed oil, lecithin. Cream. 45 g. *OTC.*
Use: Topical local anesthetic, amide local anesthetic.

LC-4. (TriMarc Laboratories) Lidocaine hydrochloride 4%. Aloe, cetyl alcohol, jojoba seed oil, lecithin. Cream. 45 g. *OTC.*
Use: Topical local anesthetic, amide local anesthetic.

LCR. *Rx.*
Use: Antineoplastic.
See: Vincristine sulfate.

LCx Neisseria gonorrhoeae Assay. (Abbott) Reagent kit for the detection of *Neisseria gonorrhoeae* in female endocervical, male urethral, and urine swab specimens. Kit. 96s. *Rx.*
Use: Diagnostic aid.

l-cycloserine.
Use: Gaucher disease. [Orphan Drug]

l-cysteine. (Tyson)
Use: Erythropoietic protoporphyria. [Orphan Drug]

l-cysteine hydrochloride. (Various Mfr.) Cysteine hydrochloride 50 mg/mL. Inj., Soln., concentrate. Single-dose syringe. 10 mL. *Rx.*
Use: Protein substrate.

L-deprenyl.
See: Selegiline hydrochloride.

LDH Reagent Strip. (Bayer Consumer Care) A quantitative strip test for LDH in serum or plasma. *Seralyzer* reagent strip. Bot. 25s. *Rx.*
Use: Diagnostic aid.

Leber Tabulae. (Paddock) Aloe 0.09 g, extract of rhei 0.03 g, myrrh 0.01 g, frangula 5 mg, galbanum 2 mg, olibanum 3 mg. Tab. Bot. 100s, 500s, 1000s. *OTC.*

•**lebrikizumab.** (LEB-ri-KIZ-ue-mab) USAN.
Use: Respiratory agent.

Lec-E-Plex. (Barth's) Vitamin E 100 units, 200 units, 400 units. Cap. w/lecithin. Bot. 100s, 500s, 1000s. *OTC.*
Use: Vitamin E supplement.

•**lecimibide.** (leh-SIM-ih-bide) USAN.
Use: Antihyperlipidemic.

•**lecithin.** (LESS-ih-thin) *NF.*
Use: Pharmaceutic aid (emulsifying agent).
W/Isopropyl Palmitate.
See: SaltStable LO.

lecithin. (Arcum) Lecithin 1200 mg. Cap. Bot. 100s, 1000s; Gran. Bot. 8 oz; Pow. Bot. 4 oz. (Barth's) 8 gr. Cap. Bot. 100s, 500s, 1000s; Gran. Can 8 oz, 16 oz; Pow. Can 10 oz. (Cavendish) Tab. (0.5 g) Bot. 500s. (Quality Formulations, Inc.) 1200 mg, Cap. 100s. (De Pree) Cap. Bot 100s. (Pfanstiehl) 25 g, 100 g, 500 g Pkg.
Use: Pharmaceutic aid (emulsifying agent).

lecithin. (Various Mfr.) Lecithin. **Cap.:** 520 mg. Bot. 100s, 250s, 1000s; 650 mg. Bot. 90s, 100s, 250s, 500s. **Pow.:** 120 g, kg, lb. *OTC.*
Use: Nutritional supplement.

•**lecozotan hydrochloride.** (le-KOE-zoe-tan) USAN.
Use: 5-HT_{1A} receptor antagonist; Alzheimer disease.

•**ledipasvir.** (LED-i-PAS-vir) USAN.
Use: Treatment of chronic hepatitis C.

•**ledoxantrone trihydrochloride.** (led-OX-an-trone try-HIGH-droe-KLOR-ide) USAN.
Use: Antineoplastic.

Leena. (Watson) **Phase 1:** Norethindrone 0.5 mg, ethinyl estradiol 35 mcg. 7 tabs. **Phase 2:** Norethindrone 1 mg, ethinyl estradiol 35 mcg. 9 tabs. **Phase 3:** Norethindrone 0.5 mg, ethinyl estradiol 35 mcg. 5 tabs. Lactose. Tab. 28s with 7 inert tabs. *Rx.*
Use: Contraceptive hormone, sex hormone.

•**leflunomide.** (le-FLOO-noe-mide) USAN.
Use: Antirheumatic agent.
See: Arava.

leflunomide. (Various Mfr.) Leflunomide 10 mg, 20 mg. May contain lactose. Tab. 30s. *Rx.*
Use: Antirheumatic agent.

Legatrin PM. (Columbia) Acetaminophen 500 mg, diphenhydramine hydrochloride 50 mg. Tab. 30s, 50s. *OTC.*
Use: Sleep aid.

•**lemon oil.** *NF.*
Use: Pharmaceutic aid (flavor).

•**lemon tincture.** *NF.*
Use: Pharmaceutic aid (flavor).

Lemotussin-DM. (Seneca) Dextromethorphan HBr 7.5 mg, guaifenesin 50 mg, potassium guaiacolsulfonate 50 mg, pseudoephedrine hydrochloride 10 mg, chlorpheniramine maleate 2 mg per 5 mL. Parabens, saccharin, sorbitol, alcohol free. Liq. 473 mL. *Rx.*
Use: Antitussive and expectorant combination.

•**lenalidomide.** (le-na-LID-oh-mide) USAN.
Use: Immunomodulator.
See: Revlimid.

•**lenefilcon A.** (len-e-FIL-kon A) USAN.
Use: Hydrophilic.

•**lenercept.** (LEH-ner-sept) USAN.
Use: Treatment of septic shock, multiple sclerosis, inflammatory bowel disease, rheumatoid arthritis.

lenetran. Mephenoxalone.
Use: Anxiolytic.

•**leniquinsin.** (LEN-ih-KWIN-sin) USAN. Under study.
Use: Antihypertensive.

Lenium Medicated Shampoo. (Sanofi-Synthelabo) Selenium sulfide. *OTC.*
Use: Antiseborrheic.

•**lenograstim.** (leh-no-GRAH-stim) USAN.
Use: Antineutropenic; hematopoietic stimulant; immunomodulator (granulocyte colony-stimulating factor).

•**lenperone.** (LEN-per-OHN) USAN.
Use: Antipsychotic.

Lens Clear. (Allergan) Sterile, isotonic solution surfactant cleaner w/sorbic acid

0.1%, edetate disodium 0.2%. Bot. 15 mL. *OTC.*
Use: Contact lens care.

Lensept Disinfecting Solution. (Ciba Vision) Micro-filtered hydrogen peroxide with sodium stannate 3%, sodium nitrate, phosphate buffers. Soln. Bot. 237, 355 mL. *OTC.*
Use: Disinfecting solution.

Lensept Rinse and Neutralizer. (Ciba Vision) Sodium chloride, sodium borate decahydrate, boric acid, bovine catalase, sorbic acid, EDTA. Soln. Bot. 237 mL. System includes lens cup and holder. *OTC.*
Use: Contact lens care, rinsing, neutralizing.

Lens Fresh. (Allergan) Sterile, buffered, isotonic aqueous soln., hydroxyethyl cellulose, sodium Cl, boric acid, sodium borate, sorbic acid 0.1%, edetate disodium 0.2%. Bot. 0.5 oz. *OTC.*
Use: Contact lens care.

Lensine Extra Strength. (Ciba Vision) Cleaning agent with benzalkonium Cl 0.01%, EDTA 0.1%. Soln. Bot. 45 mL. *OTC.*
Use: Contact lens care.

Lens Plus. (Allergan) Isotonic soln. w/sodium Cl 0.9%. Aerosol 3 oz, 8 oz, 12 oz. Preservative free. *OTC.*
Use: Contact lens care.

Lens Plus Oxysept Disinfecting Solution. (Allergan) Hydrogen peroxide with sodium stannate 3%, sodium nitrate, phosphate buffer. Soln. Bot. 240 mL. *OTC.*
Use: Contact lens care.

Lens Plus Oxysept Rinse and Neutralizer. (Allergan) Isotonic with sodium chloride, mono- and dibasic sodium phosphates, catalytic neutralizing agent, EDTA. Soln. Bot. 15 mL. *OTC.*
Use: Contact lens care.

Lens Plus Oxysept 2 Neutralizing. (Allergan) Catalase with buffering agents used to neutralize the Lens Plus Oxysept 1 disinfecting solution in a chemical lens care system. For soft contact lens. Tabs. Box 12s. Bot. 36s. *OTC.*
Use: Contact lens care.

Lens Plus Preservative Free. (Allergan) Isotonic sodium chloride 9%. Soln. Bot. 90 mL, 240 mL, 360 mL. *OTC.*
Use: Contact lens care.

Lens Plus Sterile Saline. (Allergan) Sodium Cl, boric acid, nitrogen. Soln. Bot. 90 mL, 240 mL, 360 mL. Aerosol. *OTC.*
Use: Contact lens care.

Lensrins. (Allergan) Sterile preserved saline for heat disinfection, rinsing and storage of soft (hydrophilic) contact lenses, rinsing solution for chemical disinfection. Soln. Bot. 8 oz. *OTC.*
Use: Contact lens care.

Lens-Wet. (Allergan) Isotonic, buffered soln. of polyvinyl alcohol, thimerosal 0.002%, EDTA 0.01%. Bot. 0.5 fl oz. *OTC.*
Use: Contact lens care.

lente insulin. (Novo/Nordisk) Insulin zinc susp. 100 units/mL Beef. Inj. Vial 10 mL. *OTC.*
Use: Antidiabetic.

lentinan. (Lenti-Chemico Pharmaceuticals)
Use: Immunomodulator.

•**lenvatinib.** (len-VA-ti-nib) USAN.
Use: Antineoplastic.

•**lenvatinib mesylate.** (len-VA-ti-nib) USAN.
Use: Antineoplastic.

LenzaGel. (Pharmaceutica North America) Lidocaine hydrochloride 4%, menthol 1%. Aloe, arnica, green tea extract, glycerin, PEG, polysorbate 80, tartrazine, triethanolamine. Gel. 120 g. *OTC.*
Use: Topical local anesthetic.

LenzaPatch. (Pharmaceutica North America) Lidocaine hydrochloride 4%, menthol 1%. Aloe, arnica, green tea extract, glycerin, PEG, polysorbate 80, tartrazine, triethanolamine. Patch. 5s. *OTC.*
Use: Topical local anesthetic.

lepromin. (Louisiana State University) Lepromin, 30 to 40 million acid-fast bacilli/mL. Vial 5 mL, 10 mL, 20 mL, 50 mL.

leprostatics.
Use: Bactericidal.
See: Dapsone.

•**lercanidipine hydrochloride.** (ler-can-i-DIP-een) USAN.
Use: Antihypertensive; calcium channel blocker.

•**lergotrile.** (LER-go-trill) USAN.
Use: Enzyme inhibitor (prolactin).

•**lergotrile mesylate.** (LER-go-trill) USAN.
Use: Enzyme inhibitor (prolactin).

•**leridistim.** (ler-ID-i-stim) USAN.
Use: Treatment of chemotherapy-induced neutropenia.

•**lersivirine.** (ler-si-VIR-een) USAN.
Use: Antiretroviral.

Lerton Ovules. (Vita Elixir) Caffeine 250 mg. Cap. *OTC.*
Use: CNS stimulant.

Lescol. (Novartis) Fluvastatin 20 mg, 40 mg. May contain benzyl alcohol, parabens, EDTA. Cap. Bot. 30s, 100s. *Rx.*
Use: Antihyperlipidemic, HMG-CoA reductase inhibitor.

Lescol XL. (Novartis) Fluvastatin 80 mg. Film-coated. ER Tab. Bot. 30s, 100s. *Rx.*
Use: Antihyperlipidemic, HMG-CoA reductase inhibitor.

•**lesinurad.** (le-SIN-ure-ad) USAN.
Use: Treatment of gout.

•**lesinurad sodium.** (le-SIN-ure-ad) USAN.
Use: Treatment of gout.

Lessina. (Barr) Levonorgestrel 0.1 mg, ethinyl estradiol 20 mcg. Lactose. Film-coated. Tab. Packs. 21s, 28s with 7 inert tabs. *Rx.*
Use: Sex hormone, contraceptive hormone.

•**lestaurtinib.** (le-STOR-tin-ib) USAN.
Use: Antineoplastic agent.

Lesterol. (Dram) Nicotinic acid 500 mg. Tab. Bot. 250s. *OTC.*
Use: Antihyperlipidemic.

Letairis. (Gilead) Ambrisentan 5 mg, 10 mg. Lactose (10 mg only). Film-coated. Tab. UD 30s. *Rx.*
Use: Vasodilator, endothelin receptor antagonist.

•**letaxaban.** (le-TAX-a-ban) USAN.
Use: Anticoagulant.

•**leteprinim potassium.** (leh-TEPP-rin-nim) USAN.
Use: Central neurodegenerative disease; Alzheimer disease; spinal cord injury; stroke.

•**letimide hydrochloride.** (LET-ih-mide) USAN.
Use: Analgesic.

•**letrozole.** (let-ROW-zahl) *USP.*
Use: Antineoplastic, hormone, aromatase inhibitor.
See: Femara.

letrozole. (Mylan) Letrozole 2.5 mg. Film coated. Lactose, PEG, polydextrose. Tab. 30s, 500s. *Rx.*
Use: Hormone, aromatase inhibitor.

•**leucine.** (LOO-SEEN) *USP.*
Use: Amino acid.

•**leucovorin calcium.** (loo-koe-VORE-in) *USP.*
Use: Antianemic; folate-deficiency; antidote to folic acid antagonists.

leucovorin calcium. (American Regent) Leucovorin calcium 10 mg/mL. Inj. Single-dose vial 5 mg. 25s (10 mg/mL only). *Rx.*
Use: Antianemic; folate-deficiency; antidote to folic acid antagonists.

leucovorin calcium. (Various Mfr.) Leucovorin calcium. **Tab.:** 5 mg, 15 mg, 25 mg (as calcium). 30s, 100s, UD 50s (5 mg); 12s, 24s, UD 50s (15 mg); 25s (25 mg). **Inj., Soln.; lyophilized:** 50 mg/vial, 100 mg/vial, 200 mg/vial, 350 mg/vial. Preservative free. *Rx.*
Use: Antineoplastic agent, cytoprotective agent.

Leukeran. (GlaxoSmithKline) Chlorambucil 2 mg. Film-coated. Tab. Bot. 50s. *Rx.*
Use: Antineoplastic; alkylating agent.

Leukine. (Genzyme) Sargramostim. Mannitol 40 mg, sucrose 10 mg, tromethamine 1.2 mg/mL. **Liq.:** 500 mcg/mL. Benzyl alcohol 1.1%. Multiple-dose vial. **Pow. for Inj., lyophilized:** 250 mcg. Preservative free. Vial. *Rx.*
Use: Hematopoietic, colony stimulating factor.

leukocyte protease inhibitor, secretory.
Use: Bronchopulmonary dysplasia. [Orphan Drug]

leukocyte typing serum. (LOO-koe-site)
Use: Diagnostic aid, blood, in vitro.

leukotriene formation inhibitor.
Use: Antiasthmatic.
See: Zileuton.

leukotriene receptor antagonists.
Use: Antiasthmatic.
See: Montelukast Sodium.
Zafirlukast.

leupeptin. (Neuromuscular Agents)
Use: Adjunct to nerve repair. [Orphan Drug]

•**leuprolide acetate.** (loo-PRO-lide) USAN.
Use: Antineoplastic; LHRH agonist; central precocious puberty.
See: Eligard.
Lupron Depot.
Lupron Depot-4 Month.
Lupron Depot-Ped.
Lupron Depot-3 Month.
Lupron for Pediatric Use.
W/Norethindrone Acetate.
See: Lupaneta Pack 1-Month.
Lupaneta Pack 3-Month.

leuprolide acetate. (Various Mfr.) Leuprolide acetate 5 mg/mL. Benzyl alcohol 9 mg/mL, sodium chloride. Inj. Multiple-dose vial. 2.8 mL. *Rx.*
Use: Antineoplastic; hormone; gonadotropin-releasing hormone analog.

leuprolide acetate pediatric. (Various Mfr.) Leuprolide acetate 5 mg/mL. May contain benzyl alcohol. Inj., Soln. Multiple-dose vial. 2.8 mL. *Rx.*

Use: Hormone, gonadotropin-releasing hormone analog.

leurocristine.
See: Vincristine Sulfate.

leurocristine sulfate (1:1) (salt). Vincristine Sulfate, USP.
Use: Antineoplastic.

Levacet. (Pharmakon) Phenyltoloxamine citrate 50 mg, acetaminophen 400 mg, salicylamide 150 mg, aspirin 400 mg, caffeine 40 mg. Tab. 50s. *Rx.*
Use: Narcotic analgesic.

levalbuterol. (Mylan) Levalbuterol hydrochloride 1.25 mg per 0.5 mL. Preservative free. Soln.; Conc., Inhal. Vial. UD 0.5 mL. *Rx.*
Use: Bronchodilator, sympathomimetic.

•**levalbuterol hydrochloride.** (lev-al-BYOO-ter-ole) USAN.
Use: Bronchodilator, sympathomimetic.
See: Xopenex.

levalbuterol hydrochloride. (Watson Pharma) Levalbuterol hydrochloride 0.31 mg per 3 mL, 0.63 mg per 3 mL, 1.25 mg per 3 mL. Sulfuric acid. Preservative free. Soln.; Inhal. UD 3 mL vial. *Rx.*
Use: Bronchodilator, sympathomimetic.

•**levalbuterol sulfate.** (lev-al-BYOO-ter-ole) USAN.
Use: Bronchodilator, antiasthmatic.

•**levalbuterol tartrate.** (lev-al-BYOO-ter-ole) USAN.
Use: Bronchodilator.
See: Xopenex HFA.

Levall. (Auriga) Carbetapentane citrate 15 mg, guaifenesin 100 mg, phenylephrine hydrochloride 5 mg per 5 mL. Maltitol, saccharin, sorbitol. Strawberry flavor, alcohol free. Liq. Bot. 473 mL. *Rx.*
Use: Upper respiratory combination, antitussive and expectorant combination.

•**levamfetamine succinate.** (LEV-am-FET-ah-meen) USAN.
Use: Anorexic.

Levaquin. (Ortho-McNeil) Levofloxacin. **Tab.:** 250 mg, 500 mg, 750 mg. Film-coated. Bot. 20s (750 mg only), 50s (except 750 mg), UD 100s, *Leva-Pak* 5s (750 mg only). **Oral Soln.:** 25 mg/mL. Benzyl alcohol, sucralose, sucrose. 480 mL. **Inj., Soln.:** 250 mg (5 mg/mL), 500 mg (5 mg/mL), 750 mg (5 mg/mL). Preservative free. Flex. Cont 50 mL (250 mg only), 100 mL (500 mg only), 150 mL (750 mg only) w/dextrose solution 5%. *Rx.*
Use: Fluoroquinolone.

levarterenol.
See: Norepinephrine Bitartrate.

Levatol. (Actient Pharmaceuticals) Penbutolol sulfate 20 mg. Tab. Bot. 100s. *Rx.*
Use: Antiadrenergic/sympatholytic, beta-adrenergic blocker.

Levbid. (Meda Pharmaceuticals) Hyoscyamine sulfate 0.375 mg. Lactose. ER Tab. 100s, 500s. *Rx.*
Use: Anticholinergic; antispasmodic.

•**levcromakalim.** (lev-KROE-mah-KAY-lim) USAN.
Use: Antihypertensive; antiasthmatic.

•**levcycloserine.** (LEV-sigh-kloe-SER-een) USAN.
Use: Enzyme inhibitor (Gaucher disease).

•**levdobutamine lactobionate.** (LEV-dah-BYOOT-ah-meen LACK-toe-BYE-oh-nate) USAN.
Use: Cardiovascular agent.

Levemir. (Novo Nordisk) Insulin detemir 100 units/mL. Inj. Vials. 10 mL. *PenFill* cartridges. 3 mL. Prefilled syringes (use with *FlexPen*). 3 mL. *Rx.*
Use: Antidiabetic, insulin.

•**levetiracetam.** (lee-ve-tye-RA-se-tam) USAN.
Tall Man: levETIRAcetam
Use: Antiepileptic.
See: Keppra.
Keppra XR.

levetiracetam. (Various Mfr.) Levetiracetam. **Tab.:** 250 mg, 500 mg, 750 mg, 1,000 mg. Film coated. May contain PEG. 30s (1,000 mg only), 60s, 80s (250 mg only), 90s (except 1,000 mg), 100s (250 mg only), 120s, 180s, 250s, 500s, UD 25s (500 mg only), UD 30s (500 mg only), UD 50s (750 mg and 1,000 mg only), UD 100s, UD 300s (500 mg only). **ER Tab.:** 500 mg, 750 mg. May contain PEG. 60s, 500s. **Soln.:** 100 mg/mL. May contain acesulfame K, ammonium glycyrrhizinate, glycerin, maltitol, parabens. 118 mL, 473 mL, 500 mL, UD 5 mL. **Inj., Soln.:** 100 mg/mL. Single-use vial. 5 mL. *Rx.*
Use: Anticonvulsant.

levetiracetam in sodium chloride injection. (Mylan) Levetiracetam 500 mg per 100 mL, 1,000 mg per 100 mL, 1,500 mg per 100 mL. Sodium chloride. Inj., Soln. Single-use bag. *Rx.*
Use: Anticonvulsant.

Leviron. (Health for Life Brands) Desiccated liver 7 gr, iron and ammonium citrate 3 gr, vitamins B_1 1 mg, B_2 0.5 mg,

B_6 0.5 mg, calcium pantothenate 0.3 mg, niacinamide 2.5 mg, B_{12} 1 mcg. Cap. Bot. 100s, 1000s. *OTC.*
Use: Mineral, vitamin supplement.

Levitra. (Schering-Plough) Vardenafil hydrochloride 2.5 mg, 5 mg, 10 mg, 20 mg. Film-coated. Tab. 30s. *Rx.*
Use: Impotence agents.

levmetamfetamine.
Use: Nasal decongestant.
See: Vicks Vapor Inhaler.

•**levoamphetamine.** (lee-voe-am-FET-uh-meen) *USP.*
Use: Nasal decongestant.

levo-amphetamine. Alginate (l-isomer) alpha-2-phenylaminopropane succinate.

•**levobetaxolol hydrochloride.** (LEE-voe-beh-TAX-oh-lahl) USAN.
Use: Antiadrenergic, β-receptor.

•**levobunolol hydrochloride.** (LEE-voe-BYOO-no-lahl) *USP.*
Use: Antiadrenergic, β-receptor.
See: AK-Beta.
Betagan Liquifilm.

levobunolol hydrochloride. (Various Mfr.) Levobunolol hydrochloride 0.25%, 0.5% Ophth. Soln. Bot. 5 mL, 10 mL, 15 mL (0.5% only). *Rx.*
Use: Antiglaucoma agent; beta-adrenergic blocker.

•**levocarnitine.** (LEE-voe-KAR-nih-teen) *USP.*
Tall Man: levOCARNitine
Use: Amino acid.
See: Carnitor.
L-Carnitine.
Vitacarn.

levocarnitine. (Rising) Levocarnitine. **Soln.:** 100 mg/mL. Sucrose, parabens. Cherry flavor. 118 mL. **Tab.:** 330 mg. Blisters of 90. *Rx.*
Use: Amino acid.

levocarnitine. (Various Mfr.) Levocarnitine 200 mg/mL. Inj. Single-dose vial. *Rx.*
Use: Amino acid.

•**levocarnitine propionate hydrochloride.** (lee-voe-KAR-ni-teen) USAN.
Use: Peripheral arterial disease.

•**levocetirizine.** (LEE-vo-se-TIR-a-zeen) USAN.
Use: Antihistamine.

levocetirizine. (Winthrop US) Levocetirizine dihydrochloride 0.5 mg/mL. May contain glycerin, maltitol, parabens, saccharin. Soln. 150 mL. *Rx.*
Use: Antihistamine; piperazine, peripherally selective.

levocetirizine. (Various Mfr.) Levocetirizine dihydrochloride 5 mg. May contain lactose. Tab. 30s, 90s. *Rx.*
Use: Antihistamine; piperazine, peripherally selective.

•**levocetirizine dihydrochloride.** (LEE-vo-se-TIR-a-zeen) USAN.
Use: Antihistamine.
See: Xyzal.

•**levodopa.** (LEE-voe-DOE-puh) *USP.*
Use: Antiparkinsonian.
W/Carbidopa.
See: Parcopa.
Sinemet CR.
Sinemet 10/100.
Sinemet 25/100.
Sinemet 25/250.
W/Carbidopa, Entacapone.
See: Stalevo 50.
Stalevo 100.
Stalevo 150.
Stalevo 125.
Stalevo 75.
Stalevo 200.

•**levofloxacin.** (lee-voe-FLOX-ah-sin) USAN.
Use: Anti-infective, fluoroquinolone.
See: Iquix.
Levaquin.
Quixin.

levofloxacin. (Pack Pharmaceuticals) Levofloxacin 0.5%. Benzalkonium chloride 0.005%. Soln., Ophth. 5 mL. *Rx.*
Use: Ophthalmic and otic agent, ophthalmic antibiotic.

levofloxacin. (Sagent Pharmaceuticals) Levofloxacin 5 mg/mL. Preservative free. Inj., Soln. 50 mL, 100 mL, and 150 mL premix flexible containers in dextrose 5% solution. *Rx.*
Use: Anti-infective, fluoroquinolone.

levofloxacin. (Various Mfr.) Levofloxacin. **Tab.:** 250 mg, 500 mg, 750 mg. May contain lactose, PEG, polydextrose, propylene glycol. 20s, 50s, 100s, 500s, 1,000s (except 750 mg), UD 100s. **Inj., Soln., concentrate:** 25 mg/mL. May be preservative free. Single-use vial. 20 mL, 30 mL. *Rx.*
Use: Anti-infective, fluoroquinolone.

•**levofuraltadone.** (LEE-voe-fer-AL-tah-dohn) USAN.
Use: Anti-infective; antiprotozoal.

•**levoglucose.** (LEE-voe-GLOO-kose) USAN.
Use: Colon cleansing before colonoscopy.

•**levoleucovorin calcium.** (LEE-voe-loo-koe-VORE-in) USAN.
Use: Antidote to folic acid antagonist; water-soluble vitamin.
See: Fusilev.
Isovorin.

•**levomefolate calcium.** (LEE-voe-FOE-late) USAN.
Use: Nutritional agent.
W/Drospirenone, Ethinyl Estradiol.
See: Beyaz.

Levomefolate DHA. (Zerxis) L-methylfolate 1.53 mg, Ca 75 mg, Fe 27 mg, vitamins E 30 units, B_6 25 mg, B_{12} 1,000 mcg, C 40 mg. Algal oil and soy lecithin blend 687 mg. Glycerin, soy. Cap. 30s. *Rx.*
Use: Prenatal vitamin with minerals.

•**levomefolic acid.** (LEE-voe-me-FOE-lik) USAN.
Use: Nutritional agent.

•**levomepromazine.** (LEE-voe-me-PROE-ma-zeen) USAN.
Use: Analgesic.

•**levomepromazine hydrochloride.** (LEE-voe-me-PROE-ma-zeen) USAN.
Use: Analgesic.

•**levomepromazine maleate.** (LEE-voe-me-PROE-ma-zeen) USAN.
Use: Analgesic.

•**levomethadyl acetate hydrochloride.** (LEE-voe-METH-uh-dill) USAN.
Use: Analgesic; narcotic. [Orphan Drug]

•**levomilnacipran.** (LEE-voe-mil-NA-si-pran) USAN.
Use: Antidepressant.
See: Fetzima.

•**levomilnacipran hydrochloride.** (LEE-voe-mil-NA-si-pran) USAN.
Use: Antidepressant.

•**levonantradol hydrochloride.** (LEE-voe-NAN-trah-DAHL) USAN.
Use: Analgesic.

Levonest. (Northstar) **Phase 1:** Ethinyl estradiol 30 mcg, levonorgestrel 0.05 mg. Lactose, PEG. 6s. **Phase 2:** Ethinyl estradiol 40 mcg, levonorgestrel 0.075 mg. 5s. **Phase 3:** Ethinyl estradiol 30 mcg, levonorgestrel 0.125 mg. 10s. Tab. 28s w/7 inert tablets. *Rx.*
Use: Triphasic oral contraceptive.

•**levonordefrin.** (lee-voe-nore-DEFF-rin) *USP.*
Use: Adrenergic, vasoconstrictor.
W/Mepivacaine Hydrochloride.
See: Scandonest L.

•**levonorgestrel.** (LEE-voe-nor-JESS-truhl) *USP.*
Use: Hormone, progestin.
See: Alesse.
Levora.
My Way.
Next Choice One Dose.
Plan B.
Plan B One-Step.
Skyla.
W/Estradiol.
See: ClimaraPro.
W/Ethinyl Estradiol.
See: Altavera.
Amethia.
Amethia Lo.
Amethyst.
Aviane.
Camrese.
Camrese Lo.
Chateal.
Daysee.
Falmina.
Introvale.
Jolessa.
Kurvelo.
Levonest.
Levora.
LoSeasonique.
Lutera.
Marlissa.
Myzilra.
Orsythia.
Plan B.
Quasense.
Seasonique.
Sronyx.
Trivora.

levonorgestrel. (Perrigo Pharmaceuticals) Levonorgestrel 0.75 mg. Lactose. Tab. UD 2s. *OTC.*
Use: Emergency contraceptive.

levonorgestrel-ethinyl estradiol. (Lupin Pharmaceuticals) **Phase 1:** Ethinyl estradiol 20 mcg, levonorgestrel 0.1 mg. Film coated. Lactose, PEG. Tab. 84s. **Phase 2:** Ethinyl estradiol 10 mcg. Film coated. Lactose, PEG. Tab. 7s. *Rx.*
Use: Biphasic oral contraceptive.

levonorgestrel/ethinyl estradiol. (Lupin Pharmaceuticals) Ethinyl estradiol/levonorgestrel. **30 mcg/0.15 mg.:** Film coated. Lactose, PEG. Tab. 91s w/7 inert tablets (w/lactose). **20 mcg/0.1 mg:** May contain lactose. Tab. 28s w/7 inert tablets (may contain lactose). *Rx.*
Use: Monophasic oral contraceptive.

levonorgestrel/ethinyl estradiol. (Mylan Pharmaceuticals) Ethinyl estradiol 30 mcg, levonorgestrel 0.15 mg. Lactose. Tab. 28s w/7 inert tablets (lactose). *Rx.*
Use: Monophasic oral contraceptive.

levonorgestrel-releasing intrauterine system.
Use: Sex hormone, contraceptive system.
See: Mirena.

Levophed. (Hospira) Norepinephrine bitartrate (as base) 1 mg/mL. Metabisulfite ≤ 2 mg. Inj. Amp. 4 mL. *Rx.*
Use: Vasoconstrictor.

•**levopropoxyphene napsylate.** (lee-voe-pro-POX-ee-feen NAP-sih-late) *USP.*
Use: Antitussive.

•**levopropylcillin potassium.** (lee-voe-pro-pihl-SILL-in) USAN.
Use: Anti-infective.

Levora. (Watson) Ethinyl estradiol 30 mcg, levonorgestrel 0.15 mg. Lactose. Tab. Pkt. 28s with 7 inert tabs. *Rx.*
Use: Sex hormone, contraceptive hormone.

levorenine.
See: Epinephrine.

Levoroxine. (Bariatric) Sodium levothyroxine 0.05 mg, 0.1 mg, 0.2 mg, 0.3 mg. Tab. Bot. 100s, 500s. *Rx.*
Use: Hormone, thyroid.

•**levorphanol tartrate.** (lee-VORE-fah-nole) *USP.*
Use: Opioid analgesic.

levorphanol tartrate. (Roxane) Levorphanol tartrate 2 mg. Lactose. Tab. Bot. 100s. *c-II.*
Use: Opioid analgesic.

•**levosimendan.** (lee-voe-sih-MEN-dan) USAN.
Use: Investigational for congestive heart failure.

Levo-T. (Wyeth) Levothyroxine sodium 0.025 mg, 0.05 mg, 0.075 mg, 0.1 mg, 0.125 mg, 0.15 mg, 0.2 mg, 0.3 mg. Tab. Bot. 100s (all strengths), 1000s (0.05, 0.1, 0.15, 0.2 mg only). *Rx.*
Use: Hormone, thyroid.

Levothroid. (Forest) Levothyroxine sodium. **Tab.:** 0.025 mg, 0.05 mg, 0.075 mg, 0.088 mg, 0.1 mg, 0.112 mg, 0.125 mg, 0.150 mg, 0.175 mcg, 0.2 mg, 0.3 mg. Bot. 100s, 1000s. *Rx.*
Use: Hormone, thyroid.

•**levothyroxine sodium.** (lee-voe-thigh-ROX-een) *USP.*
Use: Hormone, thyroid.
See: Levothroid.
Levoxyl.
Synthroid.
Unithroid.
W/Mannitol.
See: Synthroid.
W/Sodium liothyronine.
See: Thyrolar.

levothyroxine sodium. (Sandoz) Levothyroxine sodium (T_4, L-thyroxine) 0.137 mg. Tab. 100s. *Rx.*
Use: Hormone, thyroid.

levothyroxine sodium. (Various Mfr.) Levothyroxine sodium. **Pow. for Inj.:** 100 mcg, 200 mcg, 500 mcg. Single-use vial. 10 mL. **Tab.:** 0.025 mg, 0.05 mg, 0.075 mg, 0.088 mg, 0.1 mg, 0.112 mg, 0.125 mg, 0.15 mg, 0.175 mg, 0.2 mg, 0.3 mg. 100s. *Rx.*
Use: Hormone, thyroid.

•**levotofisopam.** (LEV-oh-toe-FIS-oh-pam) USAN.
Use: Anxiolytic agent.

•**levoxadrol hydrochloride.** (lev-OX-ah-drole) USAN.
Use: Anesthetic, local; muscle relaxant.

Levoxyl. (Jones Pharma) Levothyroxine sodium 0.025 mg, 0.05 mg, 0.075 mg, 0.088 mg, 0.1 mg, 0.112 mg, 0.125 mg, 0.137 mg, 0.15 mg, 0.175 mg, 0.2 mg, 0.3 mg. Tab. Bot. 100s, 1000s, UD 100s. *Rx.*
Use: Hormone, thyroid.

Levsin. (Meda Pharmaceuticals) Hyoscyamine sulfate. **Tab.:** 0.125 mg. Lactose, mannitol. 100s, 500s. **Inj., Soln.:** 0.5 mg/mL. Amp. 1 mL. *Rx.*
Use: Anticholinergic; antispasmodic.

Levsin/SL. (Meda Pharmaceuticals) Hyoscyamine sulfate 0.125 mg. Lactose, mannitol. Tab., sublingual. 100s, 500s. *Rx.*
Use: Anticholinergic; antispasmodic.

Levulan Kerastick. (DUSA) Aminolevulinic acid hydrochloride 20% (354 mg), ethanol v/v 48%, isopropyl alcohol. Top. Soln. Applicator (2 glass Amp, applicator tip. One amp 1.5 mL soln. vehicle, other amp aminolevulinic acid hydrochloride 354 mg). Box 4s, 6s, 12s. *Rx.*
Use: Photochemotherapy.

levulose. Fructose.

levulose-dextrose.
See: Invert Sugar.

Lexapro. (Forest) Escitalopram oxalate. **Tab.:** 5 mg, 10 mg, 20 mg. Film-coated. Bot. 100s, UD 100s (except 5 mg). **Oral Soln.:** 1 mg/mL. Sorbitol, parabens, peppermint flavor. Bot. 240 mL. *Rx.*
Use: Antidepressant, selective serotonin reuptake inhibitor.

•**lexatumumab.** (LEX-a-TOO-moo-mab) USAN.
Use: Antineoplastic.

•**lexibulin.** (LEX-i-BUE-lin) USAN.
Use: Antineoplastic.

•**lexipafant.** (lex-IH-pah-fant) USAN.
Use: Platelet-activating factor (PAP) antagonist.

Lexiscan. (Astellas Pharma) Regadenoson 0.4 mg/5 mL. Preservative free. Edetate disodium dihydrate. Inj., Soln. 5-mL single-use vials and single-use prefilled syringes. *Rx.*
Use: In vivo diagnostic aid.

•**lexithromycin.** (lex-ith-row-MY-sin) USAN.
Use: Anti-infective.

Lexiva. (GlaxoSmithKline) Fosamprenavir calcium. **Susp.:** 50 mg/mL (equiv. to amprenavir 43 mg/mL). Parabens, sucralose. Grape-bubblegum-peppermint flavor. 225 mL. **Tab.:** 700 mg (equiv. to amprenavir 600 mg). Film-coated. 60s. *Rx.*
Use: Antiretroviral agent, protease inhibitor.

Lextron. (Eli Lilly) Liver-stomach concentrate 50 mg, iron 30 mg, vitamins B_1 1 mg, B_2 0.25 mg, B_{12} (activity equivalent) 2 mcg, other factors of vitamin B complex present in the liver-stomach concentrate. Pulv. Bot. 84s. *OTC.*
Use: Mineral; vitamin supplement.

Lexuss 210. (Centurion) Codeine phosphate 10 mg, chlorpheniramine maleate 2 mg. Alcohol 0.1%, parabens, potassium citrate, potassium sorbate, sucralose, sorbitol. Sugar free. Vanilla cream flavor. Liq. 473 mL. *c-v.*
Use: Upper respiratory combination, antitussive combination.

L-5-hydroxytryptophan. (Circa)
Use: Postanoxic intention myoclonus. [Orphan Drug]

L'Homme. (Armenpharm Ltd.) Vitamins A 4000 units, D 400 units, B_1 1 mg, B_2 1.2 mg, B_3 10 mg, B_{12} 2 mcg, calcium pantothenate 5 mg, C 30 mg, Ca 100 mg, P 76 mg, Fe 10 mg, Mn 1 mg, Mg 1 mg, Zn 1 mg. Bot. 100s. *OTC.*
Use: Mineral, vitamin supplement.

•**liafensine.** (LYE-a-FEN-seen) USAN.
Use: Antidepressant.

Lialda. (Shire US) Mesalamine 1.2 g. Film-coated. DR Tab. 120s. *Rx.*
Use: Treatment of chronic inflammatory bowel disease.

•**liarozole fumarate.** (lie-AHR-oh-zole) USAN.
Use: Antipsoriatic.

•**liarozole hydrochloride.** (lie-AHR-oh-zole) USAN.
Use: Antineoplastic.

Li Ban. (Pfizer) Synthetic pyrethroid 0.5%, related compounds 0.065%, aromatic petroleum hydrocarbons 0.664%. Spray. Bot. 5 oz, Box 6s. *OTC.*
Use: Pediculicide, inanimate objects. (Not to be used on humans or animals).

•**libenzapril.** (lie-BENZ-ah-prill) USAN.
Use: ACE inhibitor.

Librax. (Valeant) Clidinium bromide 2.5 mg, chlordiazepoxide hydrochloride 5 mg. Lactose, parabens. Cap. Bot. 100s. *Rx.*
Use: Gastrointestinal anticholinergic combination.

Lice Treatment. (Goldline) Pyrethrins 0.33%, piperonyl butoxide. Benzyl alcohol. Shampoo. 59 mL, 118 mL with comb. *OTC.*
Use: Pediculicide.

Licide Complete Lice Treatment Kit. (Reese Chemical) Piperonyl butoxide 4%, pyrethrins 0.33%. Castor oil, PEG-25, SD alcohol. Shampoo. Kit w/gel, comb, and lice control spray. 118 mL. *OTC.*
Use: Scabicide/pediculicide.

•**licorice.** (LIK-o-ris) *NF.*
Use: Pharmaceutic aid (flavor).

•**licostinel.** (li-KOS-ti-nel) USAN.
Use: Treatment of stroke (NMDA receptor antagonist, glycine site).

•**licryfilcon A.** (lih-krih-FILL-kahn A) USAN.
Use: Contact lens material (hydrophilic).

•**licryfilcon B.** (lih-krih-FILL-kahn B) USAN.
Use: Contact lens material, hydrophilic.

LidaMantle HC. (Doak Dermatologics) Lidocaine hydrochloride 3%, hydrocortisone acetate 0.5%. Cetyl alcohol, mineral oil, methylparaben, petrolatum. Lot. 177 mL. *Rx.*
Use: Corticosteroid, topical.

LidaMantle HC Cream. (Doak Dermatologics) Lidocaine 3%, hydrocortisone acetate 0.5% in cream base. Tube 1 oz. *Rx.*
Use: Corticosteroid; anesthetic, local.

•**lidamidine hydrochloride.** (LIE-DAM-ih-deen) USAN.
Use: Antiperistaltic.

Lidex. (Roche) Fluocinonide 0.05%. **Cream:** Tube 15 g, 30 g, 60 g, 120 g. **Oint.:** Tube 15 g, 30 g, 60 g, 120 g. **Soln.:** Bot. 20 mL, 60 mL. *Rx.*
Use: Corticosteroid, topical.

Lidex-E. (Roche) Fluocinonide 0.05% in aqueous emollient base. Tube 15 g, 30 g, 60 g, 120 g. *Rx.*
Use: Corticosteroid, topical.

•**lidocaine.** (LIE-doe-cane) *USP.*
Use: Anesthetic, local.
See: AneCream5.
Lidoderm.
L-M-X5.
RectiCare.
W/Benzalkonium Chloride.
See: Bactine Pain Relieving Cleansing.
Medi-First With Lidocaine.
W/Benzethonium Chloride.
See: Dr. Scholl's Cracked Heel Relief.
W/Hyaluronic Acid.
See: Juvederm Ultra Plus XC.
Juvederm Ultra XC.

W/Phenol.
See: Skeeter Stik.
W/Polymyxin B Sulfate, Neomycin Sulfate, Bacitracin Zinc.
See: Lanabiotic.
W/Prilocaine.
See: EMLA.
EMLA Anesthetic.
Oraqix.
W/Tetracaine.
See: Pliaglis.
Synera.

lidocaine. (Watson Pharma) Lidocaine 5%. Edetate disodium, glycerin, parabens, polyvinyl alcohol, propylene glycol, urea. Patch; topical (10 × 14 cm). 30s. *Rx.*
Use: Topical local anesthetic, amide local anesthetic.

lidocaine and epinephrine. (Abbott) Lidocaine 0.5%, epinephrine 1:200,000, methylparaben, sodium metabisulfite. Inj. Multidose vial 50 mL. Lidocaine 1%, epinephrine 1:100,000, methylparaben, sodium metabisulfite. Inj. Multidose vial 20 mL, 30 mL, 50 mL. Lidocaine 1%, epinephrine 1:200,000, sodium metabisulfite. Inj. Single-dose amp. 30 mL. Lidocaine 1.5%, epinephrine 1:200,000. Inj. Single-dose amp. 5 mL, 30 mL. Single-dose vial 30 mL (sodium metabisulfite). Lidocaine 2%, epinephrine 1:200,000, sodium metabisulfite. Inj. Single-dose vial 20 mL. *Rx.*
Use: Injectable local anesthetic, amide.

lidocaine and epinephrine. (Various Mfr.) Lidocaine 2%, epinephrine 1:100,000. Inj. Cart. 1.8 mL. Multidose vial 20 mL, 30 mL, 50 mL (may contain sodium metabisulfite and methylparaben) *Rx.*
Use: Injectable local anesthetic, amide.

•**lidocaine hydrochloride.** (LIE-doe-cane) *USP.*
Use: Cardiovascular agent; antiarrhythmic agent; anesthetic, local.
See: AneCream.
Anestacon.
Ardecaine 1%, 2%.
Burn-o-Jel.
L-Caine.
LC-5.
LC-4.
Lidoderm.
LidoPen Auto-Injector.
L-M-X4.
LTA 360 Kit.
Numby Stuff.
Octocaine.
Regenecare HA.
Regenecare Wound.
Solarcaine Aloe Extra Burn Relief.
Topicaine.
Topicaine 5.
Xolido.
Xylocaine.
Xylocaine MPF.
W/Benzalkonium Chloride.
See: Bactine Antiseptic Anesthetic.
Medi-Quik.
W/Benzethonium Hydrochloride.
See: StaphAseptic.
W/Camphor.
See: TheraPatch Cold Sore.
W/Capsaicin, Menthol, Methyl Salicylate.
See: Terocin.
W/Epinephrine.
See: Lidocaine and Epinephrine.
Lidocaine Hydrochloride.
Lidosite Topical System.
Xylocaine.
Xylocaine MPF.
W/Epinephrine, Methyl Parasept.
See: L-Caine-E.
W/Hydrocortisone.
See: LidaMantle HC.
LidoCort.
W/Hydrocortisone Acetate.
See: Xyralid.
Xyralid RC.
W/Menthol.
See: LenzaGel.
LenzaPatch.
W/Methyl Parasept.
See: L-Caine.
W/Povidone Iodine.
See: ProTech First-Aid Stik.

lidocaine hydrochloride. (Abbott) Lidocaine hydrochloride. Inj. **1.5%:** With 1:200,000 epinephrine. Amp. 5 mL, 30 mL. Single-dose vial 30 mL (with sodium metabisulfite). With 7.5% dextrose. Amp. 2 mL **4%:** Single-dose amp. 5 mL. **5%:** With 7.5% dextrose. Single-dose amp. *Rx.*
Use: Injectable local anesthetic, amide.

lidocaine hydrochloride. (Moore) Lidocaine hydrochloride 5%. Oint. 50 g. *Rx.*
Use: Topical local anesthetic.

lidocaine hydrochloride. (River's Edge) Lidocaine hydrochloride 3%. Alcohols, aluminum sulfate, glycerin, light mineral oil, parabens, petrolatum. Cream. 28.35 g, 85 g. *Rx.*
Use: Local anesthetic, topical.

lidocaine hydrochloride. (Various Mfr.) Lidocaine hydrochloride. **Inj.: 0.5%:** May contain methylparaben. Single-dose vial 50 mL; multidose vial 50 mL. **1%:** Amp. 2 mL, 5 mL. Vial 5 mL (preservative free). Single-dose vial 30 mL. Multidose vial 20 mL, 30 mL, 50 mL

(may contain methylparaben). Syr. 5 mL. Cartridge. **1.5%:** Amp. 20 mL. **2%:** Amp. 2 mL, 10 mL. Vial 5 mL (preservative free). Single-dose vial 10 mL. Multidose vial 20 mL, 50 mL (may contain methylparaben). Syr. 5 mL **Top. Soln.:** 4%. May contain parabens. 50 mL. **Jelly:** 2%. May contain parabens. 5 mL, 30 mL, and UD 5, 10, and 20 mL single-use vials. 25s. *Rx.*
Use: Local anesthetic.

lidocaine hydrochloride and epinephrine. (Eastman Kodak) Lidocaine 2%, epinephrine 1:50,000, sodium metabisulfite. Dental cart. 1.8 mL *Rx.*
Use: Injectable local anesthetic, amide.

lidocaine hydrochloride cream. (River's Edge) Lidocaine hydrochloride 3%. Alcohols, aluminum sulfate, glycerin, light mineral oil, parabens, petrolatum. Cream. 28.35 g, 85 g. *Rx.*
Use: Local anesthetic, topical.

lidocaine hydrochloride for cardiac arrhythmias. (Abbott) Lidocaine hydrochloride. **1%:** 10 mg/mL. Inj. (for direct IV administration). Amps. 5 mL. Vials. 20 mL, 30 mL, 50 mL. *Abboject* syringes. 5 mL. **10%:** 100 mg/mL. Inj. (for IV admixture). Additive vials. 10 mL. **20%:** 200 mg/mL. Inj. (for IV admixture). Syringes. 5 mL, 10 mL. Vials. 10 mL. *Rx.*
Use: Antiarrhythmic agent.

lidocaine hydrochloride for cardiac arrhythmias. (Various Mfr.) Lidocaine hydrochloride. **2%:** 20 mg/mL. Inj. (for direct IV administration). Vials. 5 mL, 10 mL. 20 mL, 30 mL, 50 mL. Syringes. 5 mL. **4%:** 40 mg/mL. Inj. (for IV admixtures). Amps. 5 mL. Vials. 25 mL, 50 mL. *Rx.*
Use: Antiarrhythmic agent.

lidocaine hydrochloride in 5% dextrose. (Various Mfr.) Lidocaine hydrochloride 0.2% (2 mg/mL), 0.4% (4 mg/mL), 0.8% (8 mg/mL). Inj. (for IV infusion). 250 mL (except 0.2%), 500 mL, 1,000 mL (0.2% only). *Rx.*
Use: Antiarrhythmic agent.

lidocaine hydrochloride monohydrate.
Use: Topical local anesthetic, amide local anesthetic.
See: Zingo.

lidocaine hydrochloride 3%-hydrocortisone acetate 2.5%. (River's Edge) Hydrocortisone acetate 25 mg, lidocaine hydrochloride 30 mg per g. Cetyl alcohol, mineral oil, parabens, petrolatum, stearyl alcohol, urea. Rectal Gel. 20 single-use 7 g tubes with applicators and cleansing wipes. *Rx.*
Use: Anorectal preparation.

lidocaine/hydrocortisone cream. (River's Edge) Hydrocortisone acetate 0.5%, lidocaine hydrochloride 3%. Aluminum sulfate, alcohols, glycerin, light mieral oil, parabens, petrolatum. Cream. 28.5 g, 85 g. *Rx.*
Use: Topical corticosteroid.

lidocaine/hydrocortisone rectal. (River's Edge) Hydrocortisone acetate 0.5%, lidocaine hydrochloride 3%. Aluminum sulfate, alcohols, glycerin, light mineral oil, parabens, petrolatum. Cream. Single-use units with applicator. 7 g. *Rx.*
Use: Anorectal preparation.

lidocaine/prilocaine. (Various Mfr.) Lidocaine 2.5%, prilocaine 2.5%. Cream. 5 g, 15 g, 30 g. *Rx.*
Use: Local anesthetic, topical.

lidocaine 2% viscous. (Various Mfr.) Lidocaine hydrochloride 2%. May contain parabens, saccharin. Soln. 50 mL, 100 mL, UD 20 mL. *Rx.*
Use: Anesthetic, local.

LidoCort. (Aristos) Hydrocortisone acetate 2.5%, lidocaine 3%. Mineral oils, parabens, petrolatum. Gel, Rectal. 20 single-use 7 g tube w/applicators and cleansing wipes. *Rx.*
Use: Anorectal preparation, steroid-containing product.

Lidoderm. (Endo) Lidocaine 5%. EDTA, glycerin, parabens, polyvinyl alcohol. Patch. 10 × 14 cm. 5s. *Rx.*
Use: Anesthetic, local topical.

•**lidofenin.** (LIE-doe-FEN-in) USAN.
Use: Diagnostic aid (hepatic function determination).

•**lidofilcon A.** (lih-DAH-FILL-kahn A) USAN.
Use: Contact lens material (hydrophilic).

•**lidofilcon B.** (lih-DAH-FILL-kahn B) USAN.
Use: Contact lens material (hydrophilic).

•**lidoflazine.** (LIE-dah-FLAY-zeen) USAN.
Use: Coronary vasodilator.

Lidopen Auto-Injector. (Survival Technical) Lidocaine hydrochloride 300 mg/3 mL. EDTA, methylparaben. Inj. (for IM administration). Automatic-injection device. *Rx.*
Use: Antiarrhythmic.

LidoPro. (Terrain Pharmaceuticals) Capsaicin 0.0325%, lidocaine 4.5%, menthol 10%, methyl salicylate 27.5%, aloe, cetyl alcohol, disodium EDTA, glycerin, glyceryl, inulin, PEG, triethanolamine. Oint. 121 g. *OTC.*
Use: Rub and liniment.

•**lidorestat.** (lye-DOE-res-tat) USAN.

Use: Selective aldose reductase inhibitor.

Lidox Caps. (Major) Chlordiazepoxide hydrochloride 10 mg, clidinium bromide 2.5 mg. Cap. Bot. 100s, 500s, 1000s, UD 100s. *Rx.*
Use: Anticholinergic combination.

Lidoxide. (Henry Schein) Chlordiazepoxide hydrochloride 5 mg, clidinium bromide 2.5 mg. Tab. Bot. 100s, 500s. *Rx.*
Use: Anticholinergic combination.

lid scrubs.
Use: Cleanser, ophthalmic.
See: Eye Scrub.
OCuSOFT.

•**lifarizine.** (lih-FAR-ih-ZEEN) USAN.
Use: Cerebral anti-ischemic; platelet aggregation inhibitor.

Life-Line. (National Vitamin) Docusate calcium 240 mg. Sorbitol. Cap., softgel. 100s. *OTC.*
Use: Laxative, fecal softener/surfactant.

Lifer-B. (Burgin-Arden) Cyanocobalamin 30 mcg, liver inj. 0.1 mL, ferrous gluconate 100 mg, riboflavin 1.5 mg, panthenol 2.5 mg, niacinamide 100 mg, citric acid 16.4 mg, sodium citrate 23.6 mg/mL. Vial 30 mL. *Rx.*
Use: Mineral; vitamin supplement.

Life Saver Kit. (Whiteworth Towne) Ipecac syr. two 1 oz bottles, activated charcoal pow. 1 oz, poison treatment instruction booklet. *OTC.*
Use: Antidote; poisons.

Life Spanner. (Spanner) Vitamins A 12,500 units, D 400 units, E 5 units, B_1 10 mg, B_2 5 mg, B_6 2 mg, B_{12} 5 mcg, niacinamide 50 mg, calcium pantothenate 10 mg, biotin 10 mcg, C 100 mg, hesperidin complex 10 mg, rutin 20 mg, choline bitartrate 40 mg, inositol 30 mg, betaine anhydrous 15 mg, l-lysine monohydrochloride 25 mg, Fe 30 mg, Cu 1 mg, Mn 1 mg, K 5 mg, Ca 105 mg, P 82 mg, Mg 5.56 mg, Zn 1 mg. Cap. Bot. 100s. *OTC.*
Use: Mineral; vitamin supplement.

•**lifibrate.** (lih-FIE-brate) USAN.
Use: Antihyperlipoproteinemic.

•**lifibrol.** (lie-FIB-rahl) USAN.
Use: Hypercholesterolemic.

•**lifitegrast.** (LIF-i-TEG-rast) USAN.
Use: Treatment of ocular inflammatory diseases.

•**lifitegrast sodium.** (LIF-i-TEG-rast) USAN.
Use: Treatment of ocular inflammatory diseases.

Lifol-B. (Burgin-Arden) Liver inj. 10 mcg, folic acid 1 mg, cyanocobalamin 100 mcg, phenol 0.5%/mL. Inj. Vial 10 mL. *Rx.*
Use: Nutritional supplement.

Lifolex. (Taylor Pharmaceuticals) Liver 10 mcg, cyanocobalamin 100 mcg, folic acid 5 mg/mL. Inj. Vial 10 mL. *Rx.*
Use: Nutritional supplement.

Lilly Bulk Products. (Eli Lilly) The following products are supplied by Eli Lilly under the USP, NF, or chemical name as a service to the health professions:
See: Amyl Nitrite.
Analgesic Balm.
Apomorphine Hydrochloride.
Aromatic Elix.
Atropine Sulfate.
Bacitracin.
Belladonna Tincture.
Benzoin.
Boric Acid.
Caffeine Citrated.
Calcium Gluconate.
Calcium Hydroxide.
Calcium Lactate.
Carbarsone.
Cascara Fluid Extract, Aromatic.
Cascara Sagrada Fluid Extract.
Cocaine Hydrochloride.
Codeine Phosphate.
Codeine Sulfate.
Colchicine.
Diethylstilbestrol Dipropionate.
Ephedrine Sulfate.
Ferrous Gluconate.
Ferrous Sulfate.
Folic Acid.
Glucagon.
Green Soap.
Heparin Sodium.
Ipecac.
Isoniazid.
Isopropyl Alcohol.
Liver.
Magnesium Sulfate.
Mercuric Oxide Ophthalmic Ointment, Yellow.
Methadone Hydrochloride.
Methyltestosterone.
Milk of Bismuth.
Morphine Sulfate.
Neomycin Sulfate.
Niacin.
Niacinamide.
Nitroglycerin.
Opium Tincture, Deodorized.
Ox Bile Extract.
Pancreatin.
Papaverine Hydrochloride.
Paregoric.
Penicillin G Potassium.

Phenobarbital.
Phenobarbital Sodium.
Potassium Chloride.
Potassium Iodide.
Progesterone.
Propylthiouracil.
Protamine Sulfate.
Pyridoxine Hydrochloride.
Quinidine Gluconate.
Quinidine Sulfate.
Quinine Sulfate.
Riboflavin.
Silver Nitrate.
Sodium Bicarbonate.
Sodium Chloride.
Sodium Salicylate.
Streptomycin Sulfate.
Sulfadiazine.
Sulfapyridine.
Sulfur.
Terpin Hydrate Oral Solution.
Terpin Hydrate and Codeine Oral Solution.
Testosterone Propionate.
Thiamine Hydrochloride.
Thyroid.
Tylosterone.
Whitfield's Ointment.
Wild Cherry Syrup.
Zinc Oxide.

Limbitrol. (Valeant) Chlordiazepoxide 5 mg, amitriptyline hydrochloride 12.5 mg. Film-coated. Tab. 100s. *c-IV.*
Use: Psychotherapeutic agent.

Limbitrol DS. (Valeant) Chlordiazepoxide 10 mg, amitriptyline hydrochloride 25 mg. Film-coated. Tab. Bot. 100s. *c-IV.*
Use: Psychotherapeutic agent.

Limbrel. (Primus) Flavocoxid 250 mg, 500 mg. Maltodextrin. Cap. 60s. *Rx.*
Use: Nutrition supplement.

•**lime.** *USP.*
Use: Pharmaceutical necessity.

•**lime solution, sulfurated.** *USP.*
Use: Scabicide.

lime sulfur solution. Calcium polysulfide, calcium thiosulfate.
Use: Wet dressing.

•**linaclotide.** (LIN-a-KLOE-tide) USAN.
Use: Gastrointestinal agent.
See: Linzess.

•**linaclotide acetate.** (LIN-a-KLOE-tide) USAN.
Use: Gastrointestinal agent.

•**linagliptin.** (LIN-a-GLIP-tin) USAN.
Use: Antidiabetic agent.
See: Tradjenta.
W/Metformin Hydrochloride.
See: Jentadueto.

•**linarotene.** (lin-AHR-oh-teen) USAN.
Use: Antikeratolytic.

Lincocin. (Pfizer) Lincomycin hydrochloride 300 mg/mL. Benzyl alcohol 9.45 mg/mL. Inj. Vial 2 mL, 10 mL. *Rx.*
Use: Anti-infective.

•**lincomycin.** (LIN-koe-MY-sin) *USP.* Antibiotic produced by *Streptomyces lincolnensis* variant.
Use: Anti-infective; infections due to gram-positive organisms.

•**lincomycin hydrochloride.** (LIN-koe-MY-sin) *USP.*
Use: Anti-infective.
See: Lincocin.
Lincorex.

Lincorex. (Hyrex) Lincomycin hydrochloride 300 mg/mL. Benzyl alcohol 9.45 mg/mL. Inj. Vial 10 mL. *Rx.*
Use: Anti-infective.

lincosamides.
Use: Anti-infective.
See: Clindamycin.
Lincomycin.

•**lindane.** (LIN-dane) *USP.* Gamma-benzene-hexachloride; hexachlorocyclohexane.
Use: Pediculicide, scabicide.

lindane. (Various Mfr.) Lindane. **Lot.:** 1%. 30 mL, 59 mL, pharmacy-size only pint. **Shampoo:** 1%. 30 mL, 59 mL, pharmacy-size only pint. *Rx.*
Use: Pediculicide, scabicide.

Lindora. (Bristol-Myers Squibb) Sodium laureth sulfate, cocamide DEA, sodium Cl, lactic acid, tetra sodium EDTA, benzophenone-4, FD&C Blue No. 1. Bot. 8 oz. *OTC.*
Use: Dermatologic, cleanser.

•**linezolid.** (lin-EH-zoe-lid) USAN.
Use: Anti-infective, oxalodinone.
See: Zyvox.

•**linifanib.** (lin-i-FAN-ib) USAN.
Use: Antineoplastic.

Linodil. (Sanofi-Synthelabo) Inositol hexanicotinate. Cap. *Rx.*
Use: Hyperlipidemic; peripheral vasodilator.

•**linogliride.** (LIN-oh-GLYE-ride) USAN.
Use: Antidiabetic.

•**linogliride fumarate.** (LIN-oh-GLYE-ride) USAN.
Use: Antidiabetic.

•**linopirdine.** (lih-no-PIHR-deen) USAN.
Use: Treatment of Alzheimer disease (cognition enhancer).

•**linsitinib.** (lin-SYE-ti-nib) USAN.
Use: Antineoplastic.

Linzess. (Forest Pharmaceuticals) Linaclotide 145 mcg, 290 mcg. Cap. 30s. *Rx.*
Use: Gastrointestinal agent.

Lioresal. (Novartis) Baclofen 10 mg, 20 mg. Tab. Bot. 100s, UD 100s. *Rx.*
Use: Muscle relaxant.

Lioresal Intrathecal. (Medtronic) Baclofen 0.05 mg/mL (50 mcg/mL), 10 mg/20 mL (500 mcg/mL), 10 mg/5 mL (2000 mcg/mL), preservative free. Single-use amps. 1 amp refill kit (10 mg/20 mL only), 2 and 4 amp refill kits (10 mg/5 mL only). *Rx.*
Use: Muscle relaxant.

•**liothyronine I 131.** (lie-oh-THIGH-row-neen) USAN.
Use: Radiopharmaceutical.

•**liothyronine I 125.** (lie-oh-THIGH-row-neen) USAN.
Use: Radiopharmaceutical.

•**liothyronine sodium.** (lie-oh-THIGH-row-neen) *USP.*
Use: Hormone, thyroid.
See: Cytomel.
Triostat.

liothyronine sodium. (Various Mfr.) Liothyronine sodium 5 mcg, 25 mcg, 50 mcg. May contain sucrose. Tab. 100s, 1000s. *Rx.*
Use: Thyroid hormone.

liothyronine sodium. (X-Gen) Liothyronine sodium 10 mcg. Alcohol 6.8%, ammonia 2.19 mg. Inj. Vials. 1 mL. *Rx.*
Use: Thyroid hormone.

liothyronine sodium injection.
Use: Myxedema coma/precoma. [Orphan Drug]

•**liotrix.** (LIE-oh-trix) *USP.*
Use: Hormone, thyroid.
See: Thyrolar.

lipase.
Use: Digestive enzyme.
W/Alpha-Amylase W-100, Proteinase W-300, Cellase W-100, Estrone, Testosterone, Vitamins, Minerals.
See: Kutrase.
Ku-Zyme.
W/Amylase, Bile Salts, Pepsin, Pancreatin, Calcium.
See: Enzymes.
W/Amylase, Protease.
See: Bio-Zyme.
Creon.
Palcaps 10.
Pancreatin Quadruple Strength.
Pancreaze.
Pancrelipase.
Pertzye.
Tri-Pase 8.
Tri-Pase 16.
Tyler Panplex 2-Phase.
Tyler Similase Jr.
Ultresa.
Viokace.
Zenpep.
W/Amylolytic, Proteolytic, Cellulolytic Enzymes.
See: Arco-Lase.

lipase inhibitors.
See: Orlistat.

•**lipegfilgrastim.** (LYE-peg-fil-GRA-stim) USAN.
Use: Hematological agent.

lipid/DNA human cystic fibrosis gene. (Genzyme)
Use: Cystic fibrosis. [Orphan Drug]

lipids.
Use: Intravenous nutritional therapy.
See: Clinolipid.
Intralipid 30%.
Intralipid 20%.
Liposyn II.
Liposyn III.

Lipisorb. (Bristol-Myers Squibb) Protein 35 g/L, fat 48 g/L, carbohydrates 115 g/L, Na 733.3 mg/L, K 1250 mg/L, H_2O 320 mOsm/kg. With appropriate vitamins and minerals. 1 calorie/mL. Vanilla flavored. Pow. Can 1 lb. *OTC.*
Use: Nutritional supplement.

Lipitor. (Pfizer) Atorvastatin 10 mg, 20 mg, 40 mg, 80 mg. Lactose. Film-coated. Tab. Bot. 90s, 500s (40 mg, 80 mg only), 5000s (10 mg, 20 mg only), UD 100s (10 mg, 20 mg only). *Rx.*
Use: Antihyperlipidemic; HMG-CoA reductase inhibitor.

Lipkote by Coppertone. (Schering-Plough) Padimate O, oxybenzone. SPF 15. Lip balm 4.2 g. *OTC.*
Use: Sunscreen.

Lipkote SPF 15 Ultra Sunscreen Lipbalm. (Schering-Plough) Tube 0.15 oz. *OTC.*
Use: Sunscreen.

Lip Medex. (Blairex) Petrolatum, camphor 1%, phenol 0.54%, cocoa butter, lanolin. Oint. 210 g. *OTC.*
Use: Fever blisters; lip protectant.

lipocholine.
See: Choline dihydrogen citrate.

Lipodox. (Sun Pharmaceutical) Doxorubicin hydrochloride 2 mg/mL. Preservative free. Inj., Susp.; liposomal concentrate. Single-use vial. 5 mL, 10 mL. *Rx.*
Use: Antineoplastic antibiotic, anthracycline.

Lipodox 50. (Sun Pharmaceutical) Doxorubicin hydrochloride 2 mg/mL. Preservative free. Inj., Susp.; liposomal concentrate. Single-use vial. 25 mL. *Rx.*
Use: Antineoplastic antibiotic, anthracycline.

lipodystrophy agents.
See: Metreleptin.

Lipofen. (Kowa Pharmaceuticals) Fenofibrate 50 mg, 150 mg. Cap. 90s. *Rx.*
Use: Antihyperlipidemic agent, fibric acid derivative.

Lipoflavonoid. (Numark) Vitamins C 100 mg, B_1 0.33 mg, B_2 0.33 mg, B_3 3.33 mg, B_5 1.66 mg, B_6 0.33 mg, B_{12} 1.66 mcg, choline 111 mg, bioflavonoids 100 mg, inositol 111 mg. Capl. Bot. 100s, 500s. *OTC.*
Use: Vitamin supplement.

Lipogen. (Ivax) Choline 111 mg, inositol 111 mg, vitamins B_1 0.33 mg, B_2 0.33 mg, B_3 3.33 mg, B_5 1.7 mg, B_6 0.33 mg, B_{12} 1.7 mcg, C 20 mg, A 1667 units, E 10 units, Zn 30 mg, Cu, Se. Capl. Bot. 60s. *OTC.*
Use: Mineral, vitamin supplement.

Lipogen. (Various Mfr.) Choline 111 mg, inositol, vitamins B_1 0.33 mg, B_2 0.33 mg, B_3 3.33 mg, B_5 1.7 mg, B_6 0.33 mg, B_{12} 1.7 mcg, C 100 mg. Cap. Bot. 60s. *OTC.*
Use: Vitamin supplement.

lipoglycopeptides.
Use: Anti-infective.
See: Telavancin.

•**lipoic acid, alpha.** (li-POE-ik) *NF.*
Use: Dietary supplement.

Lipo-Nicin/100 mg. (ICN Pharm) Niacin 100 mg, niacinamide 75 mg, vitamins C 150 mg, B_1 25 mg, B_2 2 mg, B_6 10 mg. Tab. Bot. 100s. *Rx.*
Use: Vasodilator combination.

Lipo-Nicin/300 mg. (ICN Pharm) Niacin 300 mg, vitamin C 150 mg, B_1 25 mg, B_2 2 mg, B_6 10 mg. TR Cap. 100s. *Rx.*
Use: Vasodilator.

Liponol. (Rugby) Choline, inositol 83 mg, methionine 110 mg, vitamins B_1 3 mg, B_2 3 mg, B_3 10 mg, B_5 2 mg, B_6 2 mg, B_{12} 2 mcg, desiccated liver 56 mg, liver concentrate 30 mg, sorbitol, lecithin. Cap. Bot. 60s. *OTC.*
Use: Nutritional supplement.

lipopeptides.
Use: Anti-infectives.
See: Daptomycin.

liposomal amphotericin B.
Use: Antifungal. [Orphan Drug]
See: AmBisome.

liposomal doxorubicin.
See: Doxorubicin Hydrochloride.

liposome encapsulated recombinant interleukin-2. (Biomerica)
Use: Antineoplastic. [Orphan Drug]

Liposyn. (Abbott Hospital Products) Intravenous fat emulsion containing safflower oil 10%, egg phosphatides 1.2%, glycerin 2.5% in water for inj. **10%:** Single-dose container 50 mL, 100 mL, 200 mL, 500 mL; Syringe Pump Unit 50 mL single-dose. **20%:** Single-dose container 200 mL, 500 mL Syringe Pump Unit 25 mL, 50 mL single-dose. *Rx.*
Use: Nutritional supplement, parenteral.

Liposyn II. (Hospira) Intravenous fat emulsion 10%. Safflower oil 5%, soybean oil 5%. 100 mL, 200 mL, 500 mL. *Rx.*
Use: Nutritional supplement, parenteral.

Liposyn III. (Hospira) **10%:** Soybean oil 10%, linoleic acid 54.5%, oleic acid 22.4%, palmitic acid 10.5%, linolenic acid 8.3%, stearic acid 4.2%, egg phosphatides 1.2%, glycerin 2.5%, 1.1 kcal/mL, 284 mOsmol/L. 100, 200, 500 mL. **20%:** Soybean oil 10%, linoleic acid 54.5%, oleic acid 22.4%, palmitic acid 10.5%, linolenic acid 8.3%, stearic acid 4.2%, egg phosphatides 1.2%, glycerin 2.5%, 2 kcal/mL, 292 mOsmol/L. 200, 500 mL. **30%:** Soybean oil 10%, linoleic acid 54.5%, oleic acid 22.4%, palmitic acid 10.5%, linolenic acid 8.3%, stearic acid 4.2%, egg phosphatides 1.8%, glycerin 2.5%, 2.9 kcal/mL, 293 mOsmol/L. 500 mL. *Rx.*
Use: Nutritional supplement, parenteral.

Lipo-Tears. (Spectra Pharmaceuticals) Mineral oil, petrolatum, preservative free. Drops. Bot. 1 mL. 30s. *OTC.*
Use: Lubricant, ophthalmic.

Lipotriad. (Numark) Zn 30 mg, vitamin A 5000 units, C 60 mg, E 30 units, Cu, Se, B_3 20 mg, B_1 1.5 mg, B_2 1.7 mg, B_6 2 mg, B_{12} 6 mcg, B_5 10 mg, choline bitartrate, inositol. Capl. Bot. 60s. *OTC.*
Use: Mineral, vitamin supplement.

lipotropics with vitamins.
Use: Nutritional supplement.
See: Cholidase.
Cholinoid.
Lipoflavonoid.
Lipogen.
Liponol.
Lipotriad.
Methatropic.

Lipoxide. (Major) Chlordiazepoxide hydrochloride 5 mg, 10 mg, 25 mg. Cap. Bot. 100s, 500s, 1000s. *c-IV.*
Use: Anxiolytic.

•**liprotamase.** (li-PROE-tam-ase) USAN.
Use: Treatment of malabsorption.

Liptruzet. (Merck) Ezetimibe/atorvastatin 10 mg/10 mg (equiv. to atorvastatin calcium 10.34 mg), 10 mg/20 mg (equiv. to atorvastatin calcium 20.68 mg), 10 mg/40 mg (equiv. to atorvastatin cal-

cium 41.37 mg), 10 mg/80 mg (equiv. to atorvastatin calcium 82.73 mg). Film coated. Lactose. Tab. UD 30s, UD 90s. *Rx*.
Use: Antihyperlipidemic combination product.

LiQuadd. (Auriga) Dextroamphetamine sulfate 5 mg per 5 mL. Saccharin, sorbitol. Bubble gum flavor. Soln. 473 mL. *c-II*.
Use: CNS stimulant, amphetamine.

Liqua-Gel. (Paddock) Boric acid, glycerine, propylene glycol, methylparaben, propylparaben, Irish moss extract, methylcellulose. Bot. 4 oz, 16 oz. *OTC*.
Use: Lubricant.

Liquibid. (Capellon) Guaifenesin 400 mg. Tab. 100s. *Rx*.
Use: Expectorant.

Liquibid D-R. (Capellon) Guaifenesin 400 mg, phenylephrine hydrochloride 10 mg. Tab. 90s. *OTC*.
Use: Upper respiratory combination, decongestant and expectorant combination.

Liquibid PD-R. (Capellon) Guaifenesin 200 mg, phenylephrine hydrochloride 5 mg. Tab. 90s. *OTC*.
Use: Upper respiratory combination, expectorant, decongestant.

Liquicet. (Mallinckrodt) Hydrocodone bitartrate/acetaminophen 3.3 mg/167 mg, 10 mg/500 mg. Saccharin, sorbitol, sucrose. Raspberry flavor. Soln. 473 mL. *c-III*.
Use: Narcotic analgesic.

Liqui-Char. (Jones Pharma) Activated charcoal. **Liq. Bot.:** 12.5 g/60 mL, 15 g/75 mL. **Squeeze container:** 25 g/120 mL, 50 g/240 mL, 30 g/120 mL. *OTC*.
Use: Antidote.

Liqui-Coat HD. (Mallinckrodt) Barium sulfate 210%. Simethicone, sorbitol, saccharin, sodium benzoate, vanilla-raspberry flavor. Susp. UD Bot. 150 mL. *Rx*.
Use: Radiopaque agent, GI contrast agent.

Liquicough DM. (Breckenridge) Dextromethorphan hydrobromide 15 mg, guaifenesin 175 mg, pseudoephedrine hydrochloride 32 mg per 5 mL. Alcohol free. Saccharin, sorbitol, acesulfame K. Grape flavor. Sugar free. Liq. 473 mL. *Rx*.
Use: Upper respiratory combination, antitussive and expectorant combination.

Liquid Barosperse. (Mallinckrodt) Barium sulfate 60%. Simethicone, vanilla flavor. Susp. Bot. 355 mL, 1900 mL. *Rx*.
Use: Radiopaque agent, GI contrast agent.

Liquid Calcium with D_3 Maximum Strength. (Mason) Vitamin D_3 1,000 units, calcium carbonate 600 mg. Beeswax, glycerin, sorbitol, soy, soybean oil. Gluten free and preservative free. Softgels. 60s. *OTC*.
Use: Nutritional supplement.

Liquid Geritonic. (Roberts) Fe 105 mg, liver fraction 1 375 mg, B_1 3 mg, B_2 3 mg, B_3 30 mg, B_6 0.3 mg, B_{12} 9 mcg, inositol 60 mg, glycine 180 mg, yeast concentrate 375 mg, Ca, I, K, Mg, Mn, P, alcohol 20%. Liq. Bot. 240 mL, gal. *OTC*.
Use: Nutritional supplement.

Liquid Lather. (Ulmer Pharmacal) Gentle wash for hands, body, face, hair. Bot. 8 oz, gal. *OTC*.
Use: Cleanser.

Liquid PedvaxHIB. (Merck) *Haemophilus* b PRP 7.5 mcg, *Neisseria meningitidis* OMPC 125 mcg, aluminum hydroxide 225 mcg/0.5 mL. Inj. Single-dose vials. *Rx*.
Use: Agent for active immunization, bacterial vaccine.

liquid petrolatum emulsion.
See: Mineral Oil.

Liquid Polibar. (E-Z-EM) Barium sulfate 100%. Potassium sorbate, saccharin, simethicone, sodium benzoate, sorbitol. Orange flavoring. Susp. (oral and rectal). 1,900 mL. *Rx*.
Use: Radiopaque agent, miscellaneous gastrointestinal contrast agent.

Liquid Polibar Plus. (EZ EM) Barium sulfate 105%. PEG, saccharin, sorbitol. Susp. 1,900 mL. *Rx*.
Use: Radiopaque agent, miscellaneous gastrointestinal contrast agent.

Liquifilm Forte. (Allergan) Polyvinyl alcohol 3%, thimerosal 0.002%, EDTA, sodium Cl. Soln. Bot. 15 mL, 30 mL. *OTC*.
Use: Artificial tears.

Liquimat. (Galderma) Sulfur 5%, SD alcohol 40 22%, cetyl alcohol in drying makeup base. Plastic Bot. 45 mL. *OTC*.
Use: Dermatologic, acne.

Liquipake. (Lafayette) Barium sulfate suspension 100% w/v for dilution. Bot. 1850 mL, Case 4s.
Use: Radiopaque agent.

Liquituss GG. (Capellon Pharmaceuticals) Guaifenesin 200 mg per 5 mL. Glycerin, parabens, potassium citrate, potassium sorbate, propylene glycol, raspberry flavoring, saccharin. Alcohol

free and sugar free. Liq. 118 mL, 473 mL. *OTC.*
Use: Expectorant.

liquor carbonis detergens.
See: Coal Tar Topical Solution.

•**liraglutide.** (lir-A-gloo-tide) USAN.
Use: Antidiabetic agent.
See: Victoza.

•**lirilumab.** (lir-IL-ue-mab) USAN.
Use: Antineoplastic.

•**lisadimate.** (liss-AD-ih-mate) USAN.
Use: Sunscreen.

•**lisdexamfetamine dimesylate.** (lis-DEX-am-FET-a-meen) USAN.
Use: CNS stimulant, amphetamine.
See: Vyvanse.

•**lisinopril.** (lie-SIN-oh-pril) *USP.*
Use: Renin angiotensin system antagonist, angiotensin-converting enzyme inhibitor.
See: Prinivil.
Zestril.
W/Hydrochlorothiazide.
See: Prinzide.
Zestoretic.

lisinopril. (Various Mfr.) Lisinopril 2.5 mg, 5 mg, 10 mg, 20 mg, 30 mg, 40 mg. Tab. 30s, 100s, 500s (except 20 mg), 1000s, UD 25s (10 mg, 40 mg only), UD 100s (except 20 mg, 30 mg), UD 300s (5 mg, 10 mg only). *Rx.*
Use: Renin angiotensin system antagonist, angiotensin-converting enzyme inhibitor.

lisinopril/hydrochlorothiazide. (Various Mfr.) Lisinopril/hydrochlorothiazide 10 mg/12.5 mg, 20 mg/12.5 mg, 20 mg/25 mg. Tab. 100s, 500s, 1000s, UD 100s. *Rx.*
Use: Antihypertensive combination.

•**lisofylline.** (lie-SO-fih-lin) USAN.
Use: Immunomodulator.

lissamine green. (Rose Stone Enterprises) Lissamine green 1.5 mg. Strip, Ophth. 100s. *Rx.*
Use: Ophthalmic diagnostic product.
See: Green Glo.

Listerine Antiseptic. (Johnson & Johnson) Thymol 0.06%, eucalyptol 0.09%, methyl salicylate 0.06%, menthol 0.04%. Alcohol 26.9% (regular flavor), 21.6% (cool mint flavor), sorbitol, saccharin. Bot. 90 mL, 180 mL, 360 mL, 540 mL, 720 mL, 960 mL, 1440 mL. *OTC.*
Use: Mouthwash, antiseptic.

Listerine, Natural Citrus. (Johnson & Johnson) Thymol 0.064%, eucalyptol 0.092%, methyl salicylate 0.06%, menthol 0.042%. Alcohol 21.6%, sorbitol, sucralose. Mouthwash. 250 mL, 500 mL, 1 L, 1.5 L. *OTC.*
Use: Mouth and throat product.

Listerine, Tartar Control. (Johnson & Johnson) Thymol 0.064%, eucalyptol 0.092%, methyl salicylate 0.06%, menthol 0.042%. Alcohol 21.6%, sorbitol, sucralose. Wintermint flavor. Mouthwash. 250 mL, 500 mL, 1 L, 1.5 L. *OTC.*
Use: Mouth and throat product.

Listerine Tooth Defense. (Johnson and Johnson) Sodium fluoride 0.0221% (fluoride 0.01%). Alcohol 21.6%, sorbitol, sucralose. Mint flavor. Dental Liq. Rinse. 500 mL. *OTC.*
Use: Fluoride.

Listermint Arctic Mint Mouthwash. (Warner Lambert) Glycerin, poloxamer 335, PEG 600, sodium lauryl sulfate, sodium benzoate, benzoic acid, zinc chloride, saccharin. Liq. 946 mL. *OTC.*
Use: Antiseptic, mouthwash.

Lite Pred. (Horizon) Prednisolone sodium phosphate 0.125%. Soln. Bot. 5 mL. *Rx.*
Use: Corticosteroid, ophthalmic.

lithium. (Roxane) Lithium 8 mEq (equiv. to lithium carbonate 300 mg) per 5 mL. Alcohol, sorbitol. Soln., Oral. Patient cups. 5 mL. Bot. 500 mL. *Rx.*
Use: Antipsychotic agent.

lithium. (Various Mfr.) Lithium carbonate 300 mg (lithium 8.12 mEq). May contain sorbitol. ER Tab. 100s, 500s. *Rx.*
Use: Antipsychotic agent.

•**lithium carbonate.** (LITH-ee-uhm CAR-boe-nate) *USP.*
Use: Antipsychotic, manic-depressive state; antidepressant.
See: Eskalith CR.
Lithonate.
Lithotabs.

lithium carbonate. (Roxane) Lithium carbonate. **ER Tab.:** 450 mg. 100s. **Tab.:** 300 mg. Bot. 100s, 1000s, UD 100s. **Cap.:** 150 mg, 300 mg, 600 mg. Bot. 100s, 1000s, UD 100s. *Rx.*
Use: Antipsychotic, manic-depressive state; antidepressant.

•**lithium citrate.** (LITH-ee-uhm) *USP.*
Use: Antimanic.

lithium citrate. (Various Mfr.) Lithium citrate 8 mEq (equivalent to 300 mg lithium carbonate)/5 mL. Syr. Bot. 480 mL, 500 mL, UD 5 mL, 10 mL. *Rx.*
Use: Antipsychotic.

•**lithium hydroxide.** (LITH-ee-uhm high-DROX-ide) *USP.*
Use: Antipsychotic, manic-depressive state; antidepressant.

Lithonate. (Solvay) Lithium carbonate

300 mg. Cap. Bot. 100s, 1000s, UD 100s. *Rx.*
Use: Antipsychotic.

Lithostat. (Mission Pharmacal) Acetohydroxamic acid 250 mg. Tab. Bot. 100s. *Rx.*
Use: Anti-infective; urinary.

Lithotabs. (Solvay) Lithium carbonate 300 mg. Tab. Bot. 100s, 1000s, UD 100s. *Rx.*
Use: Antipsychotic.

•**litronesib.** (lit-ron-NES-ib) USAN.
Use: Antineoplastic.

Little Colds Cough Formula. (Vetco) Dextromethorphan hydrobromide 7.5 mg per mL. Glycerin, corn syr. Natural grape flavor. Soln., Conc., Oral. 30 mL. *OTC.*
Use: Nonnarcotic antitussive.

Little Colds Decongestant Plus Cough. (Medtech) Dextromethorphan hydrobromide 5 mg, phenylephrine hydrochloride 2.5 mg. Corn syrup, glycerin, sodium benzoate, sucralose. Gluten free. Grape flavor. Soln., concentrate. 30 mL w/dropper. *OTC.*
Use: Upper respiratory combination, antitussive combination.

Little Colds for Infants and Children. (Vetco) Phenylephrine hydrochloride 0.25%, sorbitol, sucralose, grape flavor, alcohol free. Soln. Oral Drops. Bot. 30 mL w/dropper. *OTC.*
Use: Nasal decongestant, arylalkylamine.

Little Fevers. (Little Remedies) Acetaminophen 80 mg/mL. Corn syrup, sucralose. Alcohol free. Soln., concentrate. 30 mL. *OTC.*
Use: Analgesic.

Little Noses Sterile Saline Nasal Mist. (Little Remedies) Sodium chloride. Alcohol free and preservative free. Mist pump. 59 mL. *OTC.*
Use: Nasal decongestant.

Little Remedies for Fevers Children's. (Medtech) Acetaminophen 160 mg per 5 mL. Glycerin, potassium sorbate, propylene glycol, sucralose, sucrose. Alcohol free, dye free, gluten free. Cherry flavor. Liq. 118 mL. *OTC.*
Use: CNS agent.

Little Remedies for Fevers Infant. (Medtech) Acetaminophen 160 mg per 5 mL. Glycerin, potassium sorbate, propylene glycol, sucralose, sucrose. Alcohol free, dye free, gluten free. Berry and grape flavors. Liq. 59 mL w/dosing syringe. *OTC.*
Use: CNS agent.

Little Tummys Laxative. (Vetco) Sennosides 8.8 mg/mL. Alcohol free. Methylparaben, sorbitol. Drops, Oral. 30 mL with dropper. *OTC.*
Use: Laxative.

Livalo. (Kowa Pharmaceuticals America) Pitavastatin 1 mg, 2 mg, 4 mg. Film-coated. Tab. 90s. *Rx.*
Use: Antihyperlipidemic agent, HMG-COA reductase inhibitor.

Livec. (Enzyme Process) Vitamins A 5000 units, B_1 1.5 mg, B_2 1.7 mg, niacin 20 mg, C 60 mg, B_6 2 mg, pantothenic acid 10 mg, E 30 units, B_{12} 6 mcg, Ca 250 mg, Fe 5 mg, D 400 units, folacin 0.075 mg/3 Tab. Bot. 100s, 300s. *OTC.*
Use: Mineral, vitamin supplement.

Liverbex. (Spanner) Liver 2 mcg, vitamins B_1, B_2, B_6, B_{12}, niacinamide, pantothenate/mL. Vial 30 mL. *OTC.*
Use: Nutritional supplement.

liver desiccated. Desiccated liver substance.

liver extract. Dry liver extract w/Vitamin B_{12}, folic acid.

liver function agents.
See: Sulfobromophthalein Sodium.

Livergran. (Rawl) Desiccated whole liver 9 g, vitamins B_1 18 mg, B_2 36 mg, niacinamide 90 mg, choline bitartrate 216 mg, B_6 3.6 mg, calcium pantothenate 3.6 mg, inositol 90 mg, biotin 6 mcg, vitamins B_{12} 5.4 mcg, methionine 198 mg, arginine 242 mg, cysteine 72 mg, glutamic acid 675 mg, histidine 99 mg, isoleucine 333 mg, leucine 495 mg, lysine 297 mg, phenylalanine 189 mg, threonine 333 mg, tryptophan 45 mg, tyrosine 180 mg, valine 306 mg/3 Tsp. Bot. 15 oz. *OTC.*
Use: Nutritional supplement.

liver injection. (Arcum; Lederle Laboratories) Vitamin B_{12} 20 mcg/mL. Vial 10 mL. *Rx.*
Use: Nutritional supplement.

liver injection. (Various Mfr.) Liver extract for parenteral use. *Rx.*
Use: Parenteral liver supplement.

liver injection, crude. (Eli Lilly and Co.) 2 mcg/mL. Vial 30 mL; (Medwick) 2 mcg/mL. Vial 30 mL. *Rx.*
Use: Liver supplement.

Liver Iron Vitamins. (Arcum) Liver inj. (10 mcg B_{12} activity/mL) 0.1 mL, crude liver inj. (2 mcg B_{12} activity/mL) 0.125 mL, green ferric ammonium citrate 20 mg, niacinamide 50 mg, vitamin B_6 0.3 mg, B_2 0.3 mg, procaine hydrochloride 0.5%, phenol 0.5%/2 mL. Inj. Vial 30 mL. *Rx.*
Use: Nutritional supplement.

•**liver, refined.** (Medwick) 20 mcg/mL. Vial 10 mL, 30 mL. *Rx.*
Use: Nutritional supplement.

Livifol. (Oxypure) Vitamin B_{12} activity from liver inj. equivalent to cyanocobalamin 10 mcg, folic acid 1 mg, cyanocobalamin 100 mcg/mL. Vial 10 mL. *Rx.*
Use: Vitamin supplement.

•**lixazinone sulfate.** (lix-AZE-ih-NOHN) USAN.
Use: Cardiotonic (phosphodiesterase inhibitor).

•**lixisenatide.** (LIX-i-SEN-a-tide) USAN.
Use: Antidiabetic agent.

•**lixivaptan.** (lix-i-VAP-tan) USAN.
Use: Nonhypovolemic hyponatremia.

Lixoil. (Lixoil Labs.) Sulfonated fatty oils and one or more esters of higher fatty acids. Bot. 16 oz. *OTC.*
Use: Dermatologic.

LKV-Drops. (Freeda) Vitamins A 5000 units, D 400 units, E 2 mg, B_1 1.5 mg, B_2 1.5 mg, B_3 10 mg, B_5 2 mg, B_6 2 mg, B_{12} 6 mcg, C 50 mg, biotin 50 mcg/0.6 mL. Bot. 60 mL. *OTC.*
Use: Vitamin supplement.

LKV Infant Drops. (Freeda) Vitamins A 2500 units, D 400 units, E 5 units, B_1 1 mg, B_2 1 mg, B_3 10 mg, B_5 3 mg, B_6 1 mg, B_{12} 4 mcg, C 50 mg, biotin 75 mcg/0.5 mL. Bot. 60 mL. *OTC.*
Use: Vitamin supplement.

lld factor.
See: Vitamin B_{12}.

L-leucovorin.
Use: Antineoplastic.
See: Isovorin.

L-Lysine. (Various Mfr.) L-lysine 312 mg, 500 mg. Tab. Bot. 100s. 1000 mg. Tab. Bot. 60s. 500 mg. Cap. Bot. 100s, 250s. *OTC.*
Use: Dietary supplement; amino acid.

LMD. (Hospira) Dextran 40 10%. 500 mL. With 0.9% sodium chloride or in 5% dextrose. *Rx.*
Use: Plasma volume expander.

L-Methyl-B6-B12. (Virtus) Vitamins B_6 35 mg, B_{12} 2,000 mcg, folate 3 mg. Film coated. PEG. Tab. 90s, 500s. *Rx.*
Use: Multivitamin.

L-Methyl-MC. (Virtus) Vitamins B_2 5 mg, B_6 50 mg, B_{12} 1,000 mcg, folate 6 mg. Film coated. Tab. 90s. *Rx.*
Use: Multivitamin.

L-Methyl-MC NAC. (Virtus) L-methylfolate calcium 6 mg, vitamin B_{12} 2,000 mcg, N-acetylcysteine 600 mg. Tab. 90s. *Rx.*
Use: Multivitamin.

LM-427. Ribabutin.
Use: CDC anti-infective agent.

LMTHF/Pyridoxine HCl/Cyanocobalamin. (Zerxis) Vitamins B_{12} (as cyanocobalamin) 2,000 mcg, B_6 25 mg, folate (as L-methylfolate calcium) 1.13 mg. Gluten free, lactose free, sugar free. Tab. 90s. *Rx.*
Use: Multivitamin.

LMWD-Dextran 40. (Pharmachemie USA, Inc.) Normal saline 0.9%, dextrose 10%. *Rx.*
Use: Plasma volume expander.

L-M-X5 Anorectal. (Sebela) Lidocaine 5%. Benzyl alcohol, cholesterol, polysorbate 80, propylene glycol, trolamine. Cream; rectal. 15 g, 30 g. *OTC.*
Use: Topical local anesthetic, amide local anesthetic.

L-M-X4. (Sebela) Lidocaine hydrochloride 4% (40 mg/g), benzyl alcohol. Cream. 15 g, 30 g. *OTC.*
Use: Topical local anesthetic, amide local anesthetic.

Lobak. (Sanofi-Synthelabo) Chlormezanone 250 mg, acetaminophen 300 mg. Tab. 40s, 100s, 1000s. *Rx.*
Use: Anxiolytic; analgesic.

Lobana Body. (Ulmer Pharmacal) Mineral oil, triethanolamine stearate, stearic acid, lanolin, cetyl alcohol, potassium stearate, propylene glycol, parabens. Lot. Bot. 120, 240 mL, gal. *OTC.*
Use: Emollient.

Lobana Body Shampoo. (Ulmer Pharmacal) Chloroxylenol. Bot. 240 mL, gal. *OTC.*
Use: Dermatologic, hair and skin.

Lobana Conditioning Shampoo. (Ulmer Pharmacal) Bot. 8 oz, gal. *OTC.*
Use: Dermatologic, hair and scalp.

Lobana Derm-Ade. (Ulmer Pharmacal) Vitamin A, D, E. Cream Jar 2 oz, 8 oz. *OTC.*
Use: Dermatologic; counterirritant.

Lobana Liquid Lather. (Ulmer Pharmacal) Sodium laureth sulfate, sodium lauroyl sarcosinate, sodium myristyl sarcosonate, lauramide DEA, linoleamide DEA, octyl hydroxystearate, polyquaternium 7, tetrasodium EDTA, quaternium 15, sodium chloride, citric acid. Liq. Bot. 240 mL, gal. *OTC.*
Use: Cleanser.

Lobana Peri-Gard. (Ulmer Pharmacal) Water-resistant ointment containing vitamins A & D. Oint. Jar 2 oz, 8 oz. *OTC.*
Use: Dermatologic, protectant.

Lobana Perineal Cleanser. (Ulmer Pharmacal) Sprayer 4 oz, 8 oz. Bot. Gal. *OTC.*
Use: Urine and fecal cleanser.

•**lobenzarit sodium.** (low-BENZ-ah-RIT) USAN.
Use: Antirheumatic.

Lobidram. (Dram) Lobeline sulfate 2 mg. Tab. Pkg. 15s, 30s. *OTC.*
Use: Smoking cessation aid.

•**lobucavir.** (lah-BYOO-kah-vihr) USAN.
Use: Antiviral.

LoCalnesium-C. (MedChem) Vitamin C 166.7 mg, Ca, Mg. Tab. 90s. *OTC.*
Use: Multivitamin with minerals (except iron).

Locoid. (Onset Dermatologics) **Cream:** Hydrocortisone butyrate 0.1%. Tube 15 g, 45 g. **Lot.:** Hydrocortisone butyrate 0.1%. Cetostearyl alcohol, light mineral oil, parabens, safflower oil, white petrolatum. 60 mL, 120 mL. **Oint.:** Hydrocortisone butyrate 0.1%. Tube 15 g, 45 g. **Soln.:** Hydrocortisone butyrate 0.1%, isopropyl alcohol 50%, glycerin, povidone. Bot. 20 mL, 60 mL. *Rx.*
Use: Corticosteroid, topical.

Locoid Lipocream. (Onset Dermatologics) Hydrocortisone butyrate 0.1%. Alcohol, mineral oil, parabens, white petrolatum. Cream. 15 g, 45 g. *Rx.*
Use: Anti-inflammatory agent.

•**lodelaben.** (low-DELL-ah-ben) USAN.
Formerly Declaben.
Use: Antiarthritic; emphysema therapy adjunct.

•**lodenosine.** (loh-DEN-oh-seen) USAN.
Use: Antiviral (HIV reverse transcriptase inhibitor).

Lodosyn. (Valeant) Carbidopa 25 mg. Tab. Bot. 100s. *Rx.*
Use: Antiparkinsonian.

•**lodoxamide ethyl.** (low-DOX-ah-mide ETH-uhl) USAN.
Use: Antiasthmatic, antiallergic, bronchodilator.

•**lodoxamide tromethamine.** (low-DOX-ah-mide troe-METH-ah-meen) USAN.
Use: Antiasthmatic, antiallergic, bronchodilator; vernal keratoconjunctivitis.
See: Alomide.

Lodrane D. (ECR Pharmaceuticals) Brompheniramine maleate 4 mg, pseudoephedrine hydrochloride 60 mg. Lactose. Cap. 60s. *OTC.*
Use: Upper respiratory combination, decongestant and antihistamine.

Lodrane LD. (ECR Pharmaceuticals) Brompheniramine maleate 6 mg, pseudoephedrine hydrochloride 60 mg, dye free. Cap. Bot. 100s. *Rx.*
Use: Upper respiratory combination, antihistamine, decongestant.

Lodrane 12 Hour. (ECR Pharmaceuticals) Brompheniramine maleate 6 mg. Dye free. ER Tab. 100s. *Rx.*
Use: Antihistamine.

Loestrin Fe 1/20. (Teva) Norethindrone acetate 1 mg, ethinyl estradiol 20 mcg. Lactose, sugar (active tablets), sucrose (inert tablets), ferrous fumarate 75 mg per tab. (brown tab. only). Tab. Pack 28s. *Rx.*
Use: Sex hormone, contraceptive hormone.

Loestrin Fe 1.5/30. (Teva) Norethindrone acetate 1.5 mg, ethinyl estradiol 30 mcg. Lactose, sugar (active tablets), sucrose (inert tablets), ferrous fumarate 75 mg per tab. (brown tab. only). Tab. Pack 28s. *Rx.*
Use: Sex hormone, contraceptive hormone.

Loestrin 24 Fe. (Warner Chilcott) Ethinyl estradiol 20 mcg, norethindrone acetate 1 mg. Sugar, lactose, ferrous fumarate 75 mg per tab. (brown tab. only). Tab. 28s. *Rx.*
Use: Contraceptive hormone, sex hormone.

Loestrin 21 1/20. (Teva) Norethindrone acetate 1 mg, ethinyl estradiol 20 mcg. Lactose, sugar. Tab. Packs 21s. *Rx.*
Use: Sex hormone, contraceptive hormone.

Loestrin 21 1.5/30. (Teva) Norethindrone acetate 1.5 mg, ethinyl estradiol 30 mcg. Lactose, sugar. Tab. Packs 21s. *Rx.*
Use: Sex hormone, contraceptive hormone.

•**lofemizole hydrochloride.** (low-FEM-ih-ZOLE) USAN.
Use: Anti-inflammatory; analgesic; antipyretic.

•**lofentanil oxalate.** (low-FEN-tah-NILL OX-ah-late) USAN.
Use: Analgesic, narcotic.

•**lofepramine hydrochloride.** (low-FEH-prah-MEEN) USAN.
Use: Antidepressant.

•**lofexidine hydrochloride.** (low-FEX-ih-DEEN) USAN.
Use: Treatment of opioid withdrawal symptoms.

Lofibra. (Gate) **Cap.:** Fenofibrate (micronized) 67 mg, 134 mg, 200 mg. Lactose. 100s. **Tab.:** Fenofibrate 54 mg, 160 mg. Lactose. Film-coated. 90s. *Rx.*
Use: Antihyperlipidemic agent, fibric acid derivative.

Logen. (Ivax) Diphenoxylate hydrochloride, atropine sulfate. **Liq.:** Bot. 2 oz.

Tab.: Bot. 100s, 500s, 1000s. *c-v.*
Use: Antidiarrheal.

LoHist. (Larken Labs) Chlorpheniramine maleate 1 mg, phenylephrine hydrochloride 2.5 mg. Glycerin, parabens, potassium sorbate, propylene glycol, sucralose. Alcohol free, dye free, gluten free, and sugar free. Cherry flavor. Drops. 59.2 mL. *OTC.*
Use: Upper respiratory combination, decongestant and antihistamine.

LoHist-D. (Larken Labs) Chlorpheniramine maleate 2 mg, pseudoephedrine hydrochloride 30 mg. Saccharin, sorbitol. Alcohol free and dye free. Peach flavor. Liq. 473 mL. *Rx.*
Use: Upper respiratory combinations, decongestant and antihistamine.

LoHist-DM. (Larken Labs) Brompheniramine maleate 2 mg, dextromethorphan hydrobromide 10 mg, phenylephrine hydrochloride 5 mg per 5 mL. Parabens, saccharin, sorbitol. Strawberry flavor. Syr. 473 mL. *Rx.*
Use: Upper respiratory combination, antitussive combination.

LoHist PEB. (Larken Labs) Brompheniramine maleate 4 mg, phenylephrine hydrochloride 10 mg. Benzoic acid, edetate disodium, glycerin, propylene glycol, saccharin, sorbitol. Alcohol free, dye free, and sugar free. Bubble gum flavor. Liq. 118 mL. *OTC.*
Use: Upper respiratory combination, decongestant and antihistamine.

LoHist PEB DM. (Larken Labs) Brompheniramine maleate 4 mg, dextromethorphan hydrobromide 20 mg, phenylephrine hydrochloride 10 mg. Benzoic acid, edetate disodium, propylene glycol, saccharin, sorbitol. Alcohol free, sugar free. Strawberry flavor. Liq. 473 mL. *OTC.*
Use: Upper respiratory combination, antitussive combination.

LoHist PSB. (Larken Labs) Brompheniramine maleate 4 mg, pseudoephedrine hydrochloride 20 mg. Benzoic acid, glycerin, PEG, saccharin, sorbitol. Alcohol free, dye free, and sugar free. Cherry flavor. Liq. 473 mL. *OTC.*
Use: Upper respiratory combination, decongestant and antihistamine.

Lo Loestrin Fe. (Warner Chilcott) Tab. Blister card 28s w/2 brown tablets (ferrous fumarate 75 mg per tablet). **Phase 1:** Ethinyl estradiol 10 mcg (24 blue tablets), norethindrone 1 mg. Lactose, mannitol. **Phase 2:** Ethinyl estradiol 10 mcg (2 white tablets). *Rx.*
Use: Oral biphasic contraceptive.

Lomanate. (Various Mfr.) Diphenoxylate hydrochloride 2.5 mg, atropine sulfate 0.025 mg/5 mL. Bot. 60 mL. *c-v.*
Use: Antidiarrheal.

Lomedia 24 Fe. (Amneal) Ethinyl estradiol 20 mcg, norethindrone acetate 1 mg. Lactose. Tab. 28s (w/4 tablets [ferrous fumarate 75 mg per tablet; lactose]). *Rx.*
Use: Oral contraceptive.

•**lomefloxacin.** (low-MEH-FLOX-ah-sin) USAN.
Use: Anti-infective, fluoroquinolone.

•**lomefloxacin hydrochloride.** (low-MEH-FLOX-ah-sin) USAN.
Use: Anti-infective, fluoroquinolone.

•**lomefloxacin mesylate.** (low-MEH-FLOX-ah-sin) USAN.
Use: Anti-infective.

•**lometraline hydrochloride.** (low-MET-rah-LEEN) USAN.
Use: Antipsychotic; antiparkinsonian.

•**lometrexol sodium.** (LOW-meh-TREX-ole) USAN.
Use: Antineoplastic.

•**lomibuvir.** (loe-MI-bue-vir) USAN.
Use: Treatment of hepatitis C.

Lo Minastrin Fe. (Warner Chilcott) **Phase 1:** Ethinyl estradiol 10 mcg, norethindrone 1 mg (24 tablets). Lactose, mannitol, sucralose. **Phase 2:** Ethinyl estradiol 10 mcg (2 white tablets). Lactose, mannitol. With 2 inert tablets. Ferrous fumarate 75 mg, mannitol, sucralose, spearmint flavoring. *Rx.*
Use: Biphasic oral contraceptive.

•**lomitapide.** (lom-i-TA-pide) USAN.
Use: Treatment of hypercholesterolemia and hypertriglyceridemia.

•**lomitapide mesylate.** (lom-i-TA-pide) USAN.
Use: Treatment of hypercholesterolemia and hypertriglyceridemia.
See: Juxtapid.

•**lomofungin.** (low-moe-FUN-jin) USAN.
Use: Antifungal.

Lomotil. (Pfizer) Diphenoxylate hydrochloride 2.5 mg, atropine sulfate 0.025 mg. Tab. or 5 mL. **Tab.:** Bot. 100s, 500s, 1000s, 2500s, UD 100s. **Liq.:** Bot. w/dropper 2 oz. *c-v.*
Use: Antidiarrheal.

•**lomustine.** (LOW-muss-teen) USAN.
Use: Antineoplastic, alkylating agent.
See: CeeNu.

•**lonafarnib.** (loe-na-FAR-nib) USAN.
Use: Chemotherapeutic.

Lonalac. (Bristol-Myers Squibb) Protein as casein 21%, fat as coconut oil 49%,

carbohydrate as lactose 30%, vitamins A 1440 units, B_1 0.6 mg, B_2 2.6 mg, niacin 1.2 mg, Ca 1.69 g, P 1.5 g, Cl 750 mg, K 1.88 g, Na 38 mg, Mg 135 mg/qt. Pow. Can 16 oz. *OTC.*
Use: Nutritional supplement.

•**lonapalene.** (loe-NA-pa-leen) USAN.
Use: Antipsoriatic.

•**lonaprisan.** (loe-na-PRIS-an) USAN.
Use: Progesterone receptor antagonist; antineoplastic.

Long-Acting Cough Suppressant. (Major) Dextromethorphan hydrobromide 15 mg per 5 mL. Corn syrup, edetate disodium, glycerin, PEG, propylene glycol, sucralose, sucrose. Alcohol free. Orange flavor. Liq. 118 mL. *OTC.*
Use: Nonnarcotic antitussive.

Long Acting Nasal Spray. (Weeks & Leo) Oxymetazoline hydrochloride 0.05%. Soln. Bot. 0.75 oz. *OTC.*
Use: Decongestant.

Lonox. (Sandoz) Diphenoxylate hydrochloride 2.5 mg, atropine sulfate 0.025 mg. Tab. Bot. 100s, 500s, 1000s, UD 100s. *c-v.*
Use: Antidiarrheal.

•**lontucirev.** (lon-TOO-si-rev) USAN.
Use: Antineoplastic agent.

loperamide. (Geri-Care) Loperamide hydrochloride 2 mg. Tab. 24s. *OTC.*
Use: Antidiarrheal.

loperamide. (Various Mfr.) Loperamide hydrochloride. **Cap.:** 2 mg. 100s, 500s, 1,000s. **Tab.:** 2 mg. 24s. **Liq.:** 1 mg per 5 mL, 1 mg per 7.5 mL (may contain glycerin, propylene glycol, simethicone, sodium benzoate, sucralose). 60 mL, 118 mL (1 mg per 5 mL); 120 mL, UD 7.5 mL, UD 15 mL (1 mg per 7.5 mL). *OTC.*
Use: Antidiarrheal.

•**loperamide hydrochloride.** (low-PURR-ah-mide) *USP.*
Use: Antiperistaltic.
See: Imodium.
K-Pek II.
Neo-Diaral.
Vaprino A-D.
W/Simethicone.
See: Imodium Multi-Symptom Relief.

Lopid. (Parke-Davis) Gemfibrozil 600 mg, parabens. Tab. Bot. 60s, 500s, UD 100s. *Rx.*
Use: Antihyperlipidemic; fibric acid derivative.

lopinavir and ritonavir.
Use: Antiretroviral; protease inhibitor combination.
See: Kaletra.

Lopressor. (Novartis) Metoprolol 50 mg, 100 mg. Lactose. Tab. 100s, 1000s, UD 100s (50 mg only). *Rx.*
Use: Antiadrenergic/sympatholytic, beta-adrenergic blocking agent.

Lopressor HCT. (Novartis) Metoprolol tartrate/hydrochlorothiazide. 50/25 mg, 100/25 mg, 100/50 mg. Lactose, sucrose. Tab. Bot. 100s. *Rx.*
Use: Antihypertensive combination.

Loprox. (Valeant) Ciclopirox. **Gel:** 0.77%. Isopropyl alcohol. 30 g, 45 g, 100 g. **Shampoo:** 1%. 120 mL. *Rx.*
Use: Topical antifungal, anti-infective.

Lopurin. (Knoll) Allopurinol 100 mg, 300 mg. Tab. Bot. 100s, 1000s, UD 100s. *Rx.*
Use: Antigout agent.

•**loracarbef.** (LOW-ra-CAR-beff) *USP.*
Use: Anti-infective.

•**lorajmine hydrochloride.** (lahr-AZH-meen) USAN.
Use: Cardiovascular agent.

•**loratadine.** (lor-AT-uh-DEEN) *USP.*
Use: Antihistamine, peripherally-selective piperidine.
See: Alavert.
Alavert Children's.
Children's Loratadine.
Claritin.
Claritin Children's Allergy.
Claritin Hives Relief.
Claritin Non-Drowsy Liqui-Gels.
Claritin RediTabs.
Claritin 24-Hour Allergy.
Clear-Atadine.
Clear-Atadine Children's.
Loratadine Hives Relief.
Non-Drowsy Allergy Relief.
Non-Drowsy Allergy Relief for Kids.
Triaminic AllerChews.
W/Pseudoephedrine Sulfate.
See: Alavert Allergy & Sinus D-12 Hour.
Allergy Relief & Nasal Decongestant.
Claritin-D 12 Hour.
Claritin-D 24 Hour.
Clear-Atadine D.
Loratadine D.

loratadine. (Ranbaxy) Loratadine 5 mg per 5 mL. Sucrose. Fruit flavor. Syr. 480 mL. *OTC.*
Use: Antihistamine, peripherally selective piperidine.

loratadine. (Various Mfr.) Loratadine 10 mg. May contain lactose. Tab. 30s, 100s. *OTC.*
Use: Antihistamine, peripherally selective piperidine.

Loratadine D. (Major) Loratadine 10 mg, pseudoephedrine sulfate 240 mg. Lac-

tose, PEG, sodium 10 mg. ER Tab. 10s, 15s. *OTC.*
Use: Upper respiratory combination, decongestant and antihistamine.

Loratadine Hives Relief. (Silarx) Loratadine 5 mg per 5 mL. Glycerin, propylene glycol, sodium benzoate, sucralose. Alcohol free, dye free, and sugar free. Grape flavor. Syrup. 120 mL. *OTC.*
Use: Antihistamine; piperidine, peripherally selective.

•**lorazepam.** (lor-AZ-e-pam) *USP.*
Tall Man: LORazepam
Use: Anxiolytic; anticonvulsant.
See: Alzapam.
Ativan.

lorazepam. (Hospira) Lorazepam 2 mg/mL, 4 mg/mL. PEG 400, propylene glycol, benzyl alcohol 2%. Inj. Prefilled syringe. 1 mL. Single-dose vials. 1 mL. Multidose vials. 10 mL. *c-iv.*
Use: Anxiolytic; hypnotic; sedative.

lorazepam. (Pharmaceutical Associates) Lorazepam 2 mg/mL. PEG, propylene glycol. Soln., concentrate. 30 mL w/dropper. *c-iv.*
Use: Antianxiety agent, benzodiazepine.

lorazepam. (Various Mfr) Lorazepam 0.5 mg, 1 mg, 2 mg. Tab. Bot. 100s, 500s, 1000s. *c-iv.*
Use: Anxiolytic; hypnotic; sedative.

Lorazepam Intensol. (Roxane) Lorazepam 2 mg/mL. Alcohol and dye free. Concentrated oral soln. Dropper Bot. 10 mL, 30 mL. *c-iv.*
Use: Anxiolytic; hypnotic; sedative.

•**lorbamate.** (lore-BAM-ate) USAN.
Use: Muscle relaxant.

•**lorcainide hydrochloride.** (lahr-CANE-ide) USAN.
Use: Cardiovascular agent; antiarrhythmic.

•**lorcaserin hydrochloride.** (lor-ca-SER-in) USAN.
Use: Anorexiant; obesity.
See: Belviq.

Lorcet Plus. (Forest) Hydrocodone bitartrate 7.5 mg, acetaminophen 650 mg. Tab. Bot. 100s, 500s, UD 100s. *c-iii.*
Use: Analgesic combination, narcotic.

Lorcet 10/650. (Forest) Hydrocodone bitartrate 10 mg, acetaminophen 650 mg. Tab. Bot. 20s, 100s, UD 100s. *c-iii.*
Use: Analgesic combination, narcotic.

•**lorcinadol.** (LORE-sin-ah-dole) USAN.
Use: Analgesic.

•**loreclezole.** (lahr-EH-kleh-zole) USAN.
Use: Antiepileptic.

Lorelco. (Hoechst) Probucol 250 mg. Tab. Bot. 120s. *Rx.*
Use: Antihyperlipidemic.

•**lormetazepam.** (lor-me-TAZ-e-pam) USAN.
Use: Hypnotic, sedative.

•**lornoxicam.** (lore-NOX-ih-kam) USAN.
Use: Anti-inflammatory; analgesic.

Lortab. (ECR Pharmaceuticals) Hydrocodone bitartrate 2.5 mg, acetaminophen 167 mg/5 mL, alcohol 7%, parabens, saccharin, sorbitol, sucrose. Elix. Bot. pt. *c-iii.*
Use: Analgesic combination, narcotic.

•**lortalamine.** (lahr-TAHL-ah-MEEN) USAN.
Use: Antidepressant.

Lortuss EX. (Poly Pharmaceuticals) Codeine phosphate 10 mg, guaifenesin 100 mg, pseudoephedrine hydrochloride 22.5 mg per 5 mL. Glycerin, propylene glycol, saccharin, sorbitol. Alcohol free, dye free, and sugar free. Cotton candy flavor. Susp. 473 mL. *c-v.*
Use: Upper respiratory combination, antitussive and expectorant combination.

Lortuss DM. (Poly Pharmaceuticals) Dextromethorphan hydrobromide 15 mg, doxylamine succinate 6.25 mg, pseudoephedrine hydrochloride 30 mg per 5 mL. Glycerin, propylene glycol, saccharin, sorbitol. Alcohol free, dye free, and sugar free. Candy apple flavor. Liq. 473 mL. *Rx.*
Use: Upper respiratory combination, antitussive combination.

Lortuss LQ. (Poly Pharmaceuticals) Doxylamine succinate 6.25 mg, pseudoephedrine hydrochloride 30 mg. Glycerin, propylene glycol, saccharin, sorbitol. Alcohol free, dye free, and sugar free. Grape flavor. Liq. 473 mL. *OTC.*
Use: Upper respiratory combination, decongestant and antihistamine.

•**lorvotuzumab mertansine.** (LOR-voe-TOOZ-oo-mab) USAN.
Use: Antineoplastic.

Loryna. (Sandoz) Drospirenone 3 mg, ethinyl estradiol 20 mg. Film coated. Lactose, PEG. Tab. Blister pack 28s (w/4 white, round inert tablets). *Rx.*
Use: Oral contraceptive.

•**lorzafone.** (LAHR-zah-FONE) USAN.
Use: Anxiolytic.

Lorzone. (Vertical) Chlorzoxazone 375 mg, 750 mg. Lactose, sodium benzoate. Tab. 100s. *Rx.*
Use: Skeletal muscle relaxant, centrally acting.

•**losartan potassium.** (low-SAHR-tan) *USP.*
Use: Renin angiotensin system antagonist, angiotensin II receptor antagonist.
See: Cozaar.
W/Hydrochlorothiazide and Potassium.
See: Hyzaar.

losartan potassium. (Various Mfr.) Losartan potassium 25 mg, 50 mg, 100 mg. May contain lactose; PEG; potassium 2.12 mg (25 mg), 4.24 mg (50 mg), 8.48 mg (100 mg). Tab. 30s (except 25 mg), 90s, 1000s. *Rx.*
Use: Renin angiotensin system antagonist, angiotensin II receptor antagonist.

losartan potassium. (ZyGenerics) Losartan potassium 25 mg, 50 mg, 100 mg. May contain lactose; PEG; potassium 2.12 mg (25 mg), 4.24 mg (50 mg), 8.48 mg (100 mg). Tab. 30s, 90s, 100s, 1000s, 5000s (except 50 mg), 10,000s (except 100 mg). *Rx.*
Use: Renin angiotensin system antagonist, angiotensin II receptor antagonist.

losartan potassium/hydrochlorothiazide. (Various Mfr.) Losartan potassium/hydrochlorothiazide 50 mg/12.5 mg, 100 mg/12.5 mg, 100 mg/25 mg. May contain lactose; PEG; potassium 4.24 mg (50 mg/12.5 mg), 8.48 mg (100 mg/12.5 mg and 100 mg/25 mg). Tab. 20s, 90s, 500s, 1000s. *Rx.*
Use: Antihypertensive combination.

losartan potassium/hydrochlorothiazide. (ZyGenerics) Losartan potassium/hydrochlorothiazide 50 mg/12.5 mg, 100 mg/12.5 mg, 100 mg/25 mg. May contain lactose; potassium 4.24 mg (50 mg/12.5 mg), 8.48 mg (100 mg/12.5 mg and 100 mg/25 mg). Tab. 30s, 90s, 1000s, 5000s. *Rx.*
Use: Antihypertensive combination.

LoSeasonique. (Teva) **Phase 1:** Ethinyl estradiol 0.02 mg, levonorgestrel 0.1 mg. Lactose. Tab. 84s. **Phase 2:** Ethinyl estradiol 0.01 mg. Lactose, PEG. Tab. 7s. *Rx.*
Use: Oral contraceptive, biphasic contraceptive.

Losec.
See: Prilosec.

•**losmapimod.** (los-MAP-i-mod) USAN.
Use: CNS agent.

LoSo Prep Bowel Cleansing System. (E-Z-EM) Magnesium citrate 18 g. Pow. for Soln. W/4 bisacodyl 5 mg tablets and 1 bisacodyl 10 mg suppository. *OTC.*
Use: Laxative, bowel evacuant.

Losotron Plus. (Various Mfr.) Magaldrate 540 mg, simethicone 20 mg/5 mL. Liq. Bot. 360 mL. *OTC.*
Use: Antacid; antiflatulent.

•**losoxantrone hydrochloride.** (low-SOX-an-trone) USAN.
Use: Antineoplastic.

•**losulazine hydrochloride.** (low-SULL-ah-zeen) USAN.
Use: Antihypertensive.

Lotawin. (Sanofi-Synthelabo) Oxypertine. Cap. *Rx.*
Use: Anxiolytic.

Lotemax. (Bausch & Lomb) Loteprednol etabonate 0.5%. **Ophth. Susp.:** EDTA, benzalkonium chloride 0.01%, glycerin, povidone. 2.5 mL, 5 mL, 10 mL, 15 mL. **Oint., Ophth.:** Mineral oil, white petrolatum. 3.5 g. **Gel; Ophth.:** Benzalkonium chloride 0.003%, boric acid, edetate disodium, glycerin, propylene glycol, tyloxapol. 10 mL. *Rx.*
Use: Ophthalmic corticosteroid.

Lotensin. (Novartis) Benazepril hydrochloride 5 mg, 10 mg, 20 mg, 40 mg. Castor oil (except 40 mg), lactose. Tab. 100s. *Rx.*
Use: Renin angiotensin system antagonist, angiotensin-converting enzyme inhibitor.

Lotensin HCT. (Novartis) Hydrochlorothiazide/benazepril 12.5 mg/10 mg, 12.5 mg/20 mg, 25 mg/20 mg. Lactose. Tab. 100s. *Rx.*
Use: Antihypertensive.

•**loteprednol etabonate.** (low-TEH-PRED-nole ET-a-BOE-nate) USAN.
Use: Ophthalmic corticosteroid.
See: Alrex.
Lotemax.
W/Tobramycin.
See: Zylet.

lotio alba. White lotion. *OTC.*
Use: Antiseborrheic; dermatologic, acne.

lotio alsulfa. (Doak Dermatologics) Colloidal sulfur 5%. Bot. 4 oz. *OTC.*
Use: Antiseborrheic; dermatologic, acne.

Lotion-Jel. (C.S. Dent & Co.) Benzocaine in gel base. Tube 0.2 oz. *OTC.*
Use: Anesthetic, local.

•**lotrafiban hydrochloride.** (low-TRAFF-ih-ban) USAN.
Use: Antiplatelet.

•**lotrafilcon A.** (lo-tra-FIL-kon A) USAN.
Use: Contact lens material.

•**lotrafilcon B.** (lo-tra-FIL-kon B) USAN.
Use: Contact lens material.

Lotrel. (Novartis) Amlodipine/benazepril hydrochloride 2.5 mg/10 mg, 5 mg/10 mg, 5 mg/20 mg, 5 mg/40 mg, 10 mg/20 mg, 10 mg, 40 mg. Lactose (5 mg/40 mg, 10 mg/20 mg, 10 mg/40 mg only). Cap. Bot. 100s. *Rx.*
Use: Antihypertensive combination.

Lotrimin AF. (Schering-Plough) Clotrimazole 1%. Benzyl alcohol, cetearyl alcohol. Cream. Tube. 12 g, 24 g. *OTC.*
Use: Antifungal, topical.

Lotrimin AF. (Schering-Plough) Miconazole nitrate. **Pow.:** 2%. Talc. 90 g. **Spray Liq.:** 2%. SD alcohol 40 17%. 113 mL. **Aer. Pow.:** 2%. SD alcohol 40 10%. 100 g. *OTC.*
Use: Topical anti-infective, antifungal agent.

Lotrimin Ultra. (Schering-Plough) Butenafine hydrochloride 1%. Benzyl alcohol, cetyl alcohol, glycerin, white petrolatum. Cream. 12 g, 24 g. *OTC.*
Use: Antifungal, topical anti-infective.

Lotrisone. (Schering) Betamethasone (as dipropionate) 0.05%, clotrimazole 1%. Alcohols, hydrophilic, mineral oil, white petrolatum. Lot. 30 mL. *Rx.*
Use: Antifungal, topical.

Lotronex. (Promethus) Alosetron hydrochloride (as base) 0.5 mg, 1 mg. Lactose. Film-coated. Tab. Bot. 30s. *Rx.*
Use: Antiemetic; antivertigo.

Lo-Trop. (Vangard Labs, Inc.) Diphenoxylate hydrochloride 2.5 mg, atropine sulfate 0.025 mg. Tab. Bot. 100s, 1000s. *c-v.*
Use: Antidiarrheal.

•**lovastatin.** (LOW-vuh-STAT-in) *USP. Formerly Mevinolin.*
Use: Antihypercholesterolemic; antihyperlipidemic, HMG-CoA reductase inhibitor.
See: Altoprev.
Mevacor.

lovastatin. (Various Mfr.) Lovastatin 10 mg, 20 mg, 40 mg. May contain lactose. Tab. 60s, 90s (except 10 mg), 100s, 500s, 1,000s, 5,000s (except 10 mg), UD 100s. *Rx.*
Use: Antihypercholesterolemic; antihyperlipidemic; HMG-CoA reductase inhibitor.

lovastatin/niacin.
Use: Antihyperlipidemic.
See: Advicor.

Lovaza. (GlaxoSmithKline) Omega-3 fatty acids 900 mg (EPA 465 mg and DHA 375 mg). Soybean oil, partially hydrogenated vegetable oils. Cap. 60s, 120s. *Rx.*
Use: Fish oil.

Love Longer. (Durex) Benzocaine 7.5% in water-soluble lubricant base. Tube 0.5 oz. *OTC.*
Use: Anesthetic, local.

Lovenox. (Sanofi-Aventis) Enoxaparin sodium. 30 mg/0.3 mL, 40 mg/0.4 mL, 60 mg/0.6 mL, 80 mg/0.8 mL, 100 mg/1 mL, 120 mg/0.8 mL, 150 mg/1 mL, 300 mg/3 mL. Benzyl alcohol 15 mg/15 mL (300 mg/3 mL only). Preservative free (except 300 mg/3 mL). Approximate anti-factor Xa activity of 1000 units (30 mg/0.3 mL, 40 mg/0.4 mL, 60 mg/0.6 mL, 80 mg/0.8 mL, 100 mg/mL, 300 mg/3 mL), 1500 units (120 mg/0.8 mL, 150 mg/1 mL) (with reference to the WHO First International Low Molecular Weight Heparin Reference Standard). Inj. **30 mg/0.3 mL:** Single-dose prefilled syringes w/27-gauge ×½-inch needle. **40 mg/0.4 mL:** Single-dose prefilled syringes with a 27-gauge ×½-inch needle. **60 mg/0.6 mL, 80 mg/0.8 mL, 100 mg/1 mL, 120 mg/0.8 mL, 150 mg/mL:** Graduated single-dose prefilled syringes with a 27-gauge ×½-inch needle. **300 mg/3 mL:** 3 mL multidose vial. *Rx.*
Use: Anticoagulant, low-molecular-weight heparin (LMWH).

•**loviride.** (LOW-vihr-ide) USAN.
Use: Antiviral for chronic oral treatment of HIV-seropositive patients (non-nucleoside reverse transcriptase inhibitor).

Lowila Cake. (Bristol-Myers Squibb) Sodium lauryl sulfoacetate, dextrin, boric acid, urea, sorbitol, mineral oil, PEG 14 M, lactic acid, cellulose gum, docusate sodium. Cake 112.5 g. *OTC.*
Use: Dermatologic, cleanser.

low-molecular-weight heparins. LMWH.
Use: Anticoagulant.
See: Dalteparin Sodium.
Enoxaparin Sodium.
Tinzaparin Sodium.

Low-Ogestrel. (Watson) Ethinyl estradiol 30 mcg, norgestrel 0.3 mg. Lactose. Tab. Pack 28s (with 7 inert tabs.). *Rx.*
Use: Sex hormone, contraceptive hormone.

Low-Quel. (Halsey Drug) Diphenoxylate hydrochloride 2.5 mg, atropine sulfate 0.025 mg. Tab. Bot. 100s. *c-v.*
Use: Antidiarrheal.

Lowsium. (Rugby) Magaldrate 540 mg/5 mL. Susp. Bot. 360 mL. *OTC.*
Use: Antacid.

Lowsium Plus. (Rugby) **Tab.:** Magaldrate 480 mg, simethicone 20 mg. Bot. 60s. **Susp.:** Magaldrate 540 mg, simethicone

40 mg/5 mL. Bot. 360 mL. *OTC.*
Use: Antacid; antiflatulent.

•**loxapine.** (LOX-ah-peen) USAN.
Use: Anxiolytic; antipsychotic, dibenzapine derivative.
See: Adasuve.
Loxitane.

loxapine hydrochloride.
Use: Anxiolytic.
See: Loxitane.

•**loxapine succinate.** (LOX-ah-peen) *USP.*
Use: Anxiolytic; antipsychotic, dibenzapine derivative.
See: Loxitane.

loxapine succinate. (Various Mfr.) Loxapine 5 mg (loxapine succinate 6.8 mg), 10 mg (loxapine succinate 13.6 mg), 25 mg (loxapine succinate 34 mg), 50 mg (loxapine succinate 68.1 mg). Cap. Bot. 100s, 1000s (5 mg only). *Rx.*
Use: Antipsychotic, dibenzapine derivative.

Loxitane. (Watson) Loxapine 5 mg (loxapine succinate 6.8 mg). Lactose. Cap. 100s. *Rx.*
Use: Antipsychotic, dibenzapine derivative.

•**loxoribine.** (LOX-ore-ih-BEAN) USAN.
Use: Immunostimulant; vaccine adjuvant.

L-PAM.
See: Melphalan.

LTA 360 Kit. (Hospira) Lidocaine hydrochloride 4%. Preservative free. Soln., Top. Single-use 4 mL prefilled vial. *Rx.*
Use: Topical local anesthetic.

L-2-oxothiazolidine-4-carboxylic acid.
Use: Treatment of adult respiratory distress syndrome. [Orphan Drug]
See: Procysteine.

•**lubabegron.** (LOO-ba-BEG-ron) USAN.
Use: Reduces environmental gas emissions per unit of beef yield.

•**lubabegron fumarate.** (LOO-ba-BEG-ron) USAN.
Use: Reduces environmental gas emissions per unit of beef yield.

Lubafax. (GlaxoSmithKline) Surgical lubricant, sterile, water-soluble, nonstaining. Foil wrapper 2.7 g, 5 g. Box 144s.
Use: Lubricant.

Lubath. (Warner Lambert) Mineral oil, PPG-15, stearyl ether, oleth-2, nonoxynol 5, fragrance, FD&C Green No. 6. Bot. 4 oz, 8 oz, 16 oz. *OTC.*
Use: Emollient.

•**lubazodone hydrochloride.** (LOO-ba-zoe-done) USAN.
Use: Antidepressant; SSRI.

•**lubeluzole.** (loo-BELL-you-zole) USAN.
Use: Stroke treatment.

Lubinol. (Purepac) Light, heavy, and extra heavy mineral oil. Bot. Pt, qt, gal. (Extra heavy Bot.) 8 oz, pt, qt, gal. *OTC.*
Use: Emollient.

•**lubiprostone.** (loo-bi-PROS-tone) USAN.
Use: Treatment of chronic constipation.
See: Amitiza.

Lubraseptic Jelly. (Guardian Laboratories) Water-soluble amyl phenyl phenol complex 0.12%, phenylmercuric nitrate, 0.007%. Bellows-type tube 10 g, 24s.
Use: Genitourinary aid.

Lubricating Jelly. (Taro) Glycerin, propylene glycol. Tube. 60 g, 125 g. *OTC.*
Use: Vaginal agent.

Lubriderm. (Johnson & Johnson) Mineral oil, petrolatum, sorbitol, lanolin, lanolin alcohol, stearic acid, TEA, cetyl alcohol, fragrance (if scented), butylparaben, methylparaben, propylparaben, sodium Cl. Lot. Bot. (scented), 4 oz, 8 oz, 16 oz; (unscented) 8 oz, 16 oz. *OTC.*
Use: Emollient.

Lubriderm Daily Moisture with SPF 15. (Johnson & Johnson) Octinoxate 7.5%, octisalate 4%, oxybenzone 3%. Lot. 100 mL, 177 mL, 296 mL, 473 mL. *OTC.*
Use: Emollient.

Lubriderm Intense Skin Repair. (Johnson & Johnson) Avena sativa (oat), kernel flour, benzaldehyde (shea butter), benzalkonium chloride, C12-15 alkyl benzoate, carbomer, ceteareth-6, cetyl alcohol, citric acid, dimethicone, glycerin, glyceryl stearate, glycine soja (soybean) sterols, hydrolyzed milk protein, hydrolyzed soy protein, mineral oil, parabens, petrolatum, stearyl alcohol, tetrasodium EDTA. Cream. 141.7 g. *OTC.*
Use: Dermatological agent.

Lubriderm Skin Nourishing with Sea Kelp Extract. (Johnson & Johnson) Glycerin, glyceryl stearate SE, cetyl alcohol, emulsifying wax, petrolatum, caprylic/capric triglyceride, castor oil, octyldodecanol, dimethicone, diazolidinyl urea, propylene glycol, xanthan gum, disodium EDTA, fragrance, giant kelp leaf extract, iodopropynyl butylcarbamate. Lot. 100 mL, 177 mL, 473 mL. *OTC.*
Use: Emollient.

LubriFresh P.M.. (Major) White petrolatum 83%, mineral oil 15%, lanolin oil. Preservative free. Oint. 3.5 g. *OTC.*
Use: Ocular lubricant.

Lubrin. (Kenwood) Glycerin, caprylic/capric triglyceride. Inserts. Pkg. 5s, 12s.

OTC.
Use: Lubricant.

Lubriskin. (Geritrex) Mineral oil, petrolatum, lanolin, lanolin alcohol, cetearyl alcohol, castor oil, triethanolamine, stearyl alcohol, propylene glycol, parabens, EDTA. Lot. 240 g. *OTC.*
Use: Emollient.

•**lucanthone hydrochloride.** (LOO-kan-thone) USAN.
Use: Antischistosomal.

•**lucatumumab.** (LOO-ka-TOOM-oo-mab) USAN.
Use: Treatment of cancer.

Lucentis. (Genentech) Ranibizumab 0.3 mg per 0.05 mL, 0.5 mg per 0.05 mL. Preservative free. Inj., Soln.; intravitreal. Single-use vial (w/one 5-micron 19-gauge × 1½-filter needle, and one 30-gauge × ½-injection needle). *Rx.*
Use: Macular degeneration.

•**lucinactant.** (loo-sin-AK-tant) USAN.
Use: Respiratory distress syndrome.
See: Surfaxin.

Ludent. (Sancilio) Fluoride 0.25 mg (from sodium fluoride 0.55 mg), 0.5 mg (from sodium fluoride 1.1 mg), 1 mg (from sodium fluoride 2.2 mg). Sucralose, xylitol. Dye free and sugar free. Orange flavor. Chew. Tab. 30s, 90s, blister pack 30s. *Rx.*
Use: Trace element, fluoride.

•**lufironil.** (loo-FIHR-ah-nill) USAN.
Use: Collagen inhibitor.

Lufyllin. (Medpointe) Dyphylline 200 mg. Tab. 100s. *Rx.*
Use: Bronchodilator.

Lufyllin-400. (Medpointe) Dyphylline 400 mg. Tab. 100s. *Rx.*
Use: Bronchodilator.

Lufyllin-GG. (Medpointe) Dyphylline 33.3 mg, guaifenesin 33.3 mg per 5 mL. Alcohol 17%, saccharin, sucrose. Wine flavor. Elix. Bot. 473 mL, 3785 mL. *Rx.*
Use: Antiasthmatic combination, xanthine combination.

Lugol's Solution. (Lyne) Iodine 5 g, potassium iodide 10 g, in purified water to make 100 mL. Soln. Bot. 15 mL. (Wisconsin Pharmacal Co.) Bot. Pt. *Rx-OTC.*
Use: Antithyroid; antiseptic, topical.

•**luliconazole.** (LOO-li-KON-a-zole) USAN.
Use: Antifungal agent.
See: Luzu.

•**lumacaftor.** (LOO-ma-KAF-tor) USAN.
Use: Treatment of cystic fibrosis.

•**lumefantrine.** (lue-mee-FAN-treen) USAN.
Use: Antimalarial.

Lumicain. (Premier Dental Products) Aluminum chloride 250 mg/g. Soln. 60 mL. *Rx.*
Use: Miscellaneous topical combination.

Lumigan. (Allergan) Bimatoprost 0.01%, 0.03%. Benzalkonium chloride 0.05 mg/mL. Soln. 2.5 mL, 5 mL, 7.5 mL. *Rx.*
Use: Antiglaucoma; prostaglandin agonist.

•**lumiliximab.** (loo-mil-IX-i-mab) USAN.
Use: Monoclonal antibody.

Luminal Sodium. (Hospira) Phenobarbital 60 mg, 130 mg. Alcohol 10%, propylene glycol 67.8%. Inj. 1 mL *Carpuject* with *Luer Lock. c-IV.*
Use: Hypnotic, sedative.

•**lumiracoxib.** (lue-mye-ra-KOX-ib) USAN.
Use: Rheumatoid arthritis; osteoarthritis.

Lumitene. (Tishcon Corp) Beta-carotene 30 mg. Glucose. Cap. 100s. *OTC.*
Use: Vitamin, fat-soluble vitamin.

Lumizyme. (Genzyme Corp) Alglucosidase alfa 50 mg. Mannitol 210 mg, 0.5 mg of polysorbate 80. Preservative free. Inj., lyophilized Pow. for Soln. Single-use vial. 20 mL. *Rx.*
Use: Endocrine and metabolic agent.

Lumopaque Capsules. (Sanofi-Synthelabo) Tyropanoate sodium.
Use: Radiopaque agent.

•**lunacalcipol.** (LOO-na-KAL-si-pol) USAN.
Use: Treatment of secondary hyperparathyroidism.

Lunesta. (Sunovion) Eszopiclone 1 mg, 2 mg, 3 mg. Lactose. Film-coated. Tab. 100s, cartons of 90s (except 1 mg). *c-IV.*
Use: Sedative/hypnotic, nonbarbiturate.

lung surfactants.
Use: Surfactant replacement therapy in neonatal respiratory distress syndrome.
See: Beractant.
Calfactant.
Lucinactant.
Poractant Alfa.

Lupaneta Pack (1-Month). (AbbVie) **Tab.:** Norethindrone acetate 5 mg. Lactose. 30s. **Inj., lyophilized microspheres for Susp.:** Leuprolide acetate 3.75 mg. Mannitol, polysorbate 80. Preservative free. Kit containing 1 prefilled dual-chamber syringe. *Rx.*
Use: Gonadotropin-releasing hormone analog, progestin combination.

Lupaneta Pack (3-Month). (AbbVie) **Tab.:** Norethindrone acetate 5 mg. Lactose. 90s. **Inj., lyophilized microspheres for Susp.:** Leuprolide acetate

11.25 mg. Mannitol, polysorbate 80. Preservative free. Kit containing 1 prefilled dual-chamber syringe. *Rx.*
Use: Gonadotropin-releasing hormone analog, progestin combination.

Lupron Depot. (AbbVie) Leuprolide acetate. **1-month:** 3.75, 7.5 mg. Mannitol, preservative free. Lyophilized microspheres for injection. Single kits, multipacks, prefilled dual-chamber syringe. **3-month:** 11.25 mg, 22.5 mg. Mannitol, preservative free. Microspheres for Inj., lyophilized. Single-use Kit, w/diluent 1.5 mL and in prefilled dual-chamber syringe. **4-month:** 30 mg. Mannitol, preservative free. Microspheres for injection, lyophilized. Single-use kit w/diluent 1.5 mL and in prefilled dual-chamber syringe. **6-month:** 45 mg. Mannitol, polysorbate 80. Preservative free. Kit containing 1 prefilled dual-chamber syringe. *Rx.*
Use: Hormone, gonadotropin-releasing hormone analog.

Lupron Depot-Ped. (AbbVie) Leuprolide acetate. **1-month:** 7.5 mg, 11.25 mg, 15 mg. Mannitol. Preservative free. Microspheres for Inj., lyophilized. Single-dose kit, prefilled dual-chamber syringe. **3-month:** 11.25 mg, 30 mg. Mannitol, polysorbate 80. Preservative free. Single-dose kit w/1 prefilled dual-chamber syringe. *Rx.*
Use: Hormone, gonadotropin-releasing hormone analog.

Lupron Injection. (TAP) Leuprolide acetate 1 mg/0.2 mL. Vial 2.8 mL. *Rx.*
Use: Antineoplastic.

Luramide. (Major) Furosemide 20 mg, 40 mg, 80 mg. Tab. Bot. 100s, 1000s. *Rx.*
Use: Diuretic.

•**lurasidone hydrochloride.** (loo-RAS-i-done) USAN.
Use: Antipsychotic.
See: Latuda.

Luride Drops. (Colgate Oral) Sodium fluoride equivalent to 0.5 mg of fluoride. Plastic dropper bot. 50 mL. *Rx.*
Use: Dental caries agent.

Luride-F Lozi Tablets. (Colgate Oral) Sodium fluoride in Lozi base tab. available as fluoride. **0.25 mg:** Bot. 120s; **0.5 mg:** Bot. 120s, 1200s; **1 mg:** Bot. 120s, 1000s, 5000s. *Rx.*
Use: Dental caries agent.

Luride Gel. (Colgate Oral) Fluoride (from sodium fluoride and hydrogen fluoride) 1.2%. Tube 7 g. *Rx.*
Use: Dental caries agent.

Luride Lozi-Tabs. (Colgate Oral Pharmaceuticals) Sodium fluoride 0.25 mg Chew. Tab. Sugar free. Bot. 120s. *Rx.*
Use: Dental caries agent.

Luride Prophylaxis Paste. (Colgate Oral Pharmaceuticals) Acidulated phosphate sodium fluoride containing 0.4% fluoride ion w/silicon dioxide abrasive. UD 3 g, Jar 50 g. *OTC.*
Use: Dentrifice.

Luride-SF Lozi Tablets. (Colgate Oral Pharmaceuticals) Sodium fluoride equivalent to 1 mg. Bot. 120s. *Rx.*
Use: Dental caries agent.

Luride Topical Gel. (Colgate Oral Pharmaceuticals) Fluoride 1.2%. Tube 7 g. *Rx.*
Use: Dental caries agent.

Luride Topical Solution. (Colgate Oral Pharmaceuticals) Acidulated phosphate sodium fluoride w/pH 3.2. Bot. 250 mL. *OTC.*
Use: Dental caries agent.

Lurline PMS. (Fielding) Acetaminophen 500 mg, pamabrom 25 mg, pyridoxine 50 mg. Tab. Bot. 24s, 50s. *OTC.*
Use: Analgesic combination.

•**lurosetron mesylate.** (loo-ROW-set-rahn) USAN.
Use: Antiemetic.

Lurotin Caps. (BASF) Beta-carotene 25 mg. Cap. Bot. 100s. *OTC.*
Use: Nutritional supplement.

•**lurtotecan dihydrochloride.** (lure-toe-TEE-kan die-HIGH-droe-KLOR-ide) USAN.
Use: Antineoplastic (DNA topoisomerase I inhibitor).

Lusair. (Centurion) Guaifenesin 200 mg, phenylephrine hydrochloride 7.5 mg. Parabens, sorbitol, sucralose. Sugar free, alcohol free, dye free, and gluten free. Strawberry flavor. Liq. 473 mL. *Rx.*
Use: Upper respiratory combination, decongestant and expectorant combination.

•**luspatercept.** (lus-PAT-er-sept) USAN.
Use: Hematological agent.

Lustra. (Medicis) Hydroquinone 4%, glycerin, alcohol, cetyl alcohol, cetearyl alcohol, benzyl alcohol, sodium metabisulfite, EDTA. Cream. Tube. 28.4 g. *Rx.*
Use: Depigmentor.

Lustra-AF. (Medicis) Hydroquinone 4%, glycerin, alcohol, cetyl alcohol, cetearyl alcohol, benzyl alcohol, sodium metabisulfite, EDTA, octyl methoxycinnamate, arobenzone. Cream. Tube. 28.4 g. *Rx.*
Use: Depigmentor.

•**lusutrombopag.** (LOO-soo-TROM-boe-pag) USAN.
Use: Treatment of thrombocytopenia.

luteogan.
See: Progesterone.
luteosan.
See: Progesterone.
Lutera. (Watson) Ethinyl estradiol 20 mcg, levonorgestrel 0.1 mg. Lactose. Tab. 28s. 7 inert tablets. *Rx.*
Use: Contraceptive hormone, sex hormone.
lutocylol. (Novartis) Ethisterone.
Lutolin-F. (Spanner) Progesterone 25 mg, 50 mg/mL. Vial 10 mL. *Rx.*
Use: Hormone, progestin.
Lutolin-S. (Spanner) Progesterone 25 mg/mL. Vial 10 mL. *Rx.*
Use: Hormone, progestin.
•**lutrelin acetate.** (loo-TRELL-in) USAN.
Use: LHRH agonist.
lutren.
See: Progesterone.
•**lutropin alfa.** (LOO-troe-pin alfa) USAN.
Use: Ovulation stimulant.
Luvox. (Jazz Pharmaceuticals) Fluvoxamine maleate 25 mg, 50 mg, 100 mg. Mannitol, PEG. Film-coated. Tab. 100s. *Rx.*
Use: Antidepressant, selective serotonin reuptake inhibitor.
Luvox CR. (Jazz Pharmaceuticals) Fluvoxamine maleate 100 mg, 150 mg. Sugar spheres. Gluten free. ER Cap. 30s. *Rx.*
Use: Antidepressant, selective serotonin reuptake inhibitor.
Luxiq. (GlaxoSmithKline) Betamethasone valerate 1.2 mg/g, cetyl alcohol, stearyl alcohol. Foam. Can. 100 g. *Rx.*
Use: Anti-inflammatory.
Luzu. (Medicis) Luliconazole 1%. Benzyl alcohol, alcohol, methylparaben, propylene glycol. Cream. 30 g, 60 g. *Rx.*
Use: Topical anti-infective, antifungal.
•**lyapolate sodium.** (lie-APP-oh-late) USAN.
Use: Anticoagulant.
See: Peson.
Lycelle Head Lice Removal Kit. (Mission) Citric acid, *Cytanyl 5,* isopropanol, methyl salicylate, methylparaben, sodium laureth sulfate. Gel. 100 mL w/comb. *Rx.*
Use: Scabicide/pediculicide.
•**lycetamine.** (lie-SEET-ah-meen) USAN.
Use: Antimicrobial, topical.
lycine hydrochloride.
See: Betaine hydrochloride.
Lydia E. Pinkham Herbal Compound. (Numark) Vitamin C, iron. Liq. Bot. 8 fl oz, 16 fl oz.
Lydia E. Pinkham Tablets. (Numark) Vitamin C, iron, calcium. Bot. 72s, 150s. *OTC.*
•**lydimycin.** (lie-dih-MY-sin) USAN.
Use: Antifungal.
Lymphazurin 1%. (United States Surgical Corp.) Isosulfan blue 10 mg/mL. Preservative free. Inj. Vials. 5 mL. *Rx.*
Use: Radiopaque agent, parenteral.
lymphocyte immune globulin antithymocyte globulin (equine).
Use: Immune globulin.
See: Atgam.
LymphoScan. (Immunomedics) Technetium TC-99M murine monoclonal antibody (IgG2a) to B-cell.
Use: Diagnostic aid. [Orphan Drug]
Lymphoseek. (Navidea Biopharmaceuticals) Technetium Tc 99m tilmanocept 250 mcg. Glycine. Inj., lyophilized Pow. for Soln. Kit w/5 tilmanocept vials and 5 diluent (4.5 mL of saline) vials. *Rx.*
Use: In vivo diagnostic aid.
•**lynestrenol.** (lin-ESS-tree-nahl) *USP.*
Use: Hormone, progestin.
Lyphocin P. (Fujisawa Healthcare) Vancomycin hydrochloride 500 mg. Vial 10 mL. *Rx.*
Use: Anti-infective.
Lypholyte. (American Pharmaceutical Partners) Na^+ 25 mEq, K^+ ≈ 40 mEq, Ca^{++} 5 mEq, Mg^{++} 8 mEq, Cl^- ≈ 33 mEq, acetate ≈ 41 mEq, gluconate 5 mEq, osmolarity ≈ 7562/20 mL or 25 mL after dilution. Conc. Single-dose vial 20 mL, 40 mL, *Maxivial* (pharmacy bulk packaging) 100 mL, 200 mL. *Rx.*
Use: Intravenous nutritional therapy, intravenous replenishment solution.
Lypholyte II. (American Pharmaceutical Partners) Na^+ 35 mEq, K^+ 20 mEq, Ca^{++} 4.5 mEq, Mg^{++} 5 mEq, Cl 35 mEq, acetate 29.5 mEq, osmolarity ≈ 6200/ 20 mL or 25 mL after dilution. Single-dose vial 20 mL, 40 mL; *Maxivial* (pharmacy bulk packaging) 100 mL, 200 mL. *Rx.*
Use: Intravenous nutritional therapy, intravenous replenishment solution.
•**lypressin nasal solution.** (LIE-PRESS-in) *USP.*
Use: Antidiuretic; vasoconstrictor.
Lyrica. (Pfizer) **Cap.:** Pregabalin 25 mg, 50 mg, 75 mg, 100 mg, 150 mg, 200 mg, 225 mg, 300 mg. Lactose. 90s, UD 100s (50 mg, 75 mg, 100 mg, 150 mg only). **Soln.:** Pregabalin 20 mg/ mL. Parabens, sucralose. Strawberry flavor. 473 mL. *c-v.*
Use: Anticonvulsant.
lysidin. Methyl glyoxalidin.

•**lysine.** (LIE-SEEN) USAN.
Use: Nutrient; rapid weight gain; amino acid.

•**lysine acetate.** (LIE-SEEN) *USP.*
Use: Amino acid.

•**lysine hydrochloride.** (LIE-SEEN) *USP.*
Use: Amino acid.
See: Enisyl.

Lysodase. (Enzon) PEG-glucocerebrosidase.
Use: Gaucher disease. [Orphan Drug]

Lysodren. (Bristol-Myers Squibb Oncology) Mitotane 500 mg. Tab. Bot. 100s. *Rx.*
Use: Antineoplastic.

•**lysostaphin.** (LIE-so-STAFF-in) USAN. Enzyme produced by *Staphylococcus staphylolyticus.*
Use: Antibiotic; antibacterial enzyme.

Lysteda. (Ferring) Tranexamic acid 650 mg. Tab. 30s, 100s, 500s, UD 30s. *Rx.*
Use: Hematological agent; hemostatic, systemic.

Lytren. (Bristol-Myers Squibb) Dextrose, sodium citrate, citric acid, sodium Cl, potassium citrate. Ready-to-use Bot. 8 fl. oz. *OTC.*
Use: Electrolyte, fluid replacement.

M

Maagel. (Health for Life Brands) Aluminum and magnesium hydroxide. Bot. 12 oz, gal. *OTC.*
Use: Antacid.

Maalox Advanced Maximum Strength. (Novartis Consumer Health) **Chew. Tab.:** Calcium carbonate 1,000 mg, simethicone 60 mg. Dextrose, maltodextrin, mannitol. Assorted fruit flavor. 35s. **Liq.:** Aluminum hydroxide 400 mg, magnesium hydroxide 400 mg, simethicone 40 mg per 5 mL. Potassium 5 mg, parabens, saccharin, sorbitol. Mint flavor. 355 mL. *OTC.*
Use: Mineral supplement; antacid.

Maalox Advanced Regular Strength. (Novartis Consumer Health) Aluminum hydroxide 200 mg, magnesium hydroxide 200 mg, simethicone 20 mg. Potassium 5 mg, parabens, saccharin sodium, sorbitol. Mint flavor. Liq. 140 mL, 355 mL, 473 mL. *OTC.*
Use: Antacid.

Maalox Children's. (Novartis Consumer Health) Calcium carbonate 400 mg (elemental calcium 160 mg). Aspartame, dextrose, maltodextrin, mannitol, phenylalanine 0.3 mg. Wild berry flavor. Chew. Tab. 32s. *OTC.*
Use: Mineral supplement.

Maalox Junior. (Novartis Consumer Health) Calcium carbonate 400 mg (elemental calcium 160 mg), simethicone 24 mg. Dextrose, maltodextrin, mannitol. Wild berry flavor. Chew. Tab. 24s. *OTC.*
Use: Antacid.

Maalox Regular Strength. (Novartis Consumer Health) Calcium carbonate 600 mg (elemental calcium 240 mg). Aspartame, dextrose, maltodextrin, mannitol. Wild berry flavor. Chew. Tab. 150s. *OTC.*
Use: Mineral supplement; antacid.

Maalox Total Relief. (Novartis Consumer Health) Bismuth subsalicylate 525 mg per 15 mL. Sodium 6 mg, parabens, sorbitol, sucralose, xanthan gum, ethyl alcohol. Strawberry flavor. Liq. 140 mL, 355 mL, 473 mL. *OTC.*
Use: Antidiarrheal.

•**macimorelin.** (MA-si-moe-REL-in) USAN.
Use: Diagnostic agent for adult growth hormone deficiency.

•**macimorelin acetate.** (MA-si-moe-REL-in) USAN.
Use: Diagnostic agent for adult growth hormone deficiency.

•**macitentan.** (MA-si-TEN-tan) USAN.
Use: Vasodilator, endothelin receptor antagonist.
See: Opsumit.

Macnatal CN DHA. (Macoven) Folic acid 1 mg, Ca 100 mg, Fe 28 mg, vitamins D_3 400 units, E 30 units, B_6 25 mg, DHA 250 mg, docusate sodium 50 mg. Glycerin, soybean oil. Cap., softgels. 30s. *Rx.*
Use: Prenatal vitamin with minerals.

MacPac. (Procter & Gamble) Nitrofurantoin macrocrystals 50 mg, 100 mg. Cap. UD 28s. *Rx.*
Use: Anti-infective, urinary.

macroaggregated albumin. (Bristol-Myers Squibb) Albumotope I-131.

Macrobid. (Almatica) Nitrofurantoin (as monohydrate/macrocrystals) 100 mg. Lactose, talc. Cap. Bot. 100s. *Rx.*
Use: Anti-infective, urinary.

Macrodantin. (Almatica) Nitrofurantoin macrocrystals 25 mg, 50 mg, 100 mg. Lactose, talc. Cap. Bot. 100s, 1000s. *Rx.*
Use: Anti-infective, urinary.

macrogol stearate 2000. Polyoxyl 40 Stearate.

macrolides.
Use: Anti-infective.
See: Azithromycin.
Clarithromycin.
Erythromycin.
Fidaxomicin.

Macrotec. (Bristol-Myers Squibb) Technetium Tc 99m Medronate kit. Vial Kit 10s.
Use: Radiopaque agent.

Macugen. (Eyetech) Pegaptanib sodium 0.3 mg (equiv. to 1.6 mg or 3.2 mg when expressed as the sodium salt form). Inj. Glass syringes. 1 mL with 27-gauge needle and shield. *Rx.*
Use: Treatment of age-related macular degeneration.

Macular Vitamin Benefit. (PRN Physician Recommended Nutriceuticals) Vitamins E 200 units, B_1 25 mg, B_2 25 mg, B_3 25 mg, B_5 25 mg, B_6 25 mg, B_{12} 500 mcg, C 250 mg, folic acid 0.5 mg, Cu, Zn, biotin 25 mcg. Film coated. Gluten free. Tab. 60s. *OTC.*
Use: Multivitamin with minerals (except iron).

MacuTrition. (Advanced Vision Research) **Cap., softgels.:** Fish oil 0.8 g (DHA 149 mg, EPA 283.5 mg), mixed tocopherol 8.5 mg, tocotrienols 6 mg, phytosterol 0.45 mg, plant squaiane 1.25 mg, vitamin D3 1,332.5 units, vitamin E 76.5 units. 60s. **Tab.:** Cu 0.25 mg, green tea leaf extract 171 mg, lutein 8 mg, vitamin C 500 mg, zea-

xanthin 2 mg, Zn 9 mg. Dextrose, maltodextrose, polydextrose. 30s. *OTC.*
Use: Nutritional supplement.

•**maduramicin.** (mad-UHR-ah-MY-sin) USAN.
Use: Anticoccidal.

•**mafenide.** (MAY-feh-NIDE) USAN.
Use: Anti-infective.

•**mafenide acetate.** (MAY-feh-NIDE) *USP.*
Use: Anti-infective, topical.
See: Sulfamylon.

mafenide acetate solution.
Use: Prevent graft loss on burn wounds. [Orphan Drug]

•**mafilcon A.** (MAY-fill-kahn) USAN.
Use: Contact lens material (hydrophilic).

•**mafodotin.** (MA-foe-DOE-tin) USAN.
Use: Antineoplastic.

Mafylon Cream. (Sanofi-Synthelabo) Mafenide acetate.
Use: Burn therapy.

•**magaldrate.** (MAG-al-drate) *USP.* Monalium Hydrate. Aluminum Magnesium Hydroxide.
Use: Antacid.
See: Lowsium.
Monalium Hydrate.
W/Simethicone.
See: Lowsium Plus.
Riopan Plus.

Magan. (Pharmacia) Magnesium salicylate (anhydrous) 545 mg. Tab. Bot. 100s, 500s. *Rx.*
Use: Analgesic.

Mag-Cal Mega. (Freeda) Mg 800 mg, Ca 400 mg, kosher, sugar free. Tab. Bot. 100s, 250s. *OTC.*
Use: Mineral, vitamin supplement.

Mag-Caps. (Genesis) Magnesium oxide ≈ 140 mg (elemental magnesium 85 mg). Cap. 100s. *OTC.*
Use: Dietary supplement.

Magdrox. (Vita Elixir) Magnesium hydroxide, aluminum hydroxide. *OTC.*
Use: Antacid.

Mag-G. (Cypress) Magnesium gluconate dihydrate 500 mg (elemental magnesium 27 mg). Tab. Bot. 100s. *OTC.*
Use: Mineral supplement.

Maginex. (Health Care Products) Magnesium L-aspartate hydrochloride 615 mg (elemental magnesium 61 mg). Enteric coated. Sugar free. Tab. Blister pack 100s, UD 100s, robot-ready 100s. *OTC.*
Use: Mineral.

Maginex DS. (Health Care Products) Magnesium L-aspartate hydrochloride 1,230 mg (elemental magnesium 122 mg/packet). Sucrose. Preservative free. Lemon flavor. Pow. 30s, robot-ready 30s. *OTC.*
Use: Mineral.

Magmalin. (Pal-Pak, Inc.) Magnesium hydroxide 0.2 g, aluminum hydroxide gel, dried 0.2 g/Loz. Bot. 1000s. *OTC.*
Use: Antacid.

Magnacal Liquid. (Biosearch Medical Products) Protein (from calcium, sodium caseinate), carbohydrate (from maltodextrin, sucrose), fat (partially hydrogenated from soy oil, lecithin, mono- and diglycerides). 1.5 Cal/mL, 590 mOsm/kg H_2O. Protein 70 g, CHO 250 g, fat 80 g, Na 1000 mg, K 1250 mg/L. Can 120 mL, 240 mL. *OTC.*
Use: Nutritional supplement.

Magnalum. (Global Source) Magnesium hydroxide 3.75 g, aluminum hydroxide 2 g. Tab. Bot. 1000s. *OTC.*
Use: Antacid.

MagneBind 400 Rx. (Nephro-Tech) Magnesium carbonate 400 mg, calcium carbonate 200 mg, folic acid 1 mg. Tab. Bot. 150s. *Rx.*
Use: Mineral supplement.

MagneBind 300. (Nephro-Tech) Magnesium carbonate 300 mg, calcium carbonate 250 mg. Tab. Bot. 150s. *OTC.*
Use: Mineral supplement.

MagneBind 200. (Nephro-Tech) Magnesium carbonate 200 mg, calcium carbonate 400 mg. Tab. Bot. 150s. *OTC.*
Use: Mineral supplement.

magnesia tablets.
Use: Antacid.

magnesia and alumina oral suspension. (Roxane) Oral Susp. 6 fl oz. 25s.
Use: Antacid.

•**magnesia, milk of.** (mag-NEE-zee-uh) *USP.*
Use: Antacid; laxative.

magnesium.
Use: Mineral.
See: Magnesium Citrate.
Magnesium Gluconate.
Magonate Natal.
Mag-Tab SR.
Mag-200.
Slow-Mag.
W/Calcium, Chloride.
See: Slow Magnesium Chloride With Calcium.

magnesium. (21st Century) Magnesium oxide 250 mg. Calcium 47 mg. Gluten free and preservative free. Tab. 110s. *OTC.*
Use: Antacid.

magnesium. (Various Mfr.) Elemental magnesium 30 mg. Tab. Bot. 100s. *OTC.*
Use: Mineral.

magnesium acetylsalicylate. Apyron, Magnespirin, Magisal, Novacetyl.
Use: Analgesic.

magnesium aluminate hydrated.
Use: Antacid.
See: Riopan.

•**magnesium aluminometasilicate.** (mag-NEE-zee-uhm ah-LOO-mihn-oh-met-uh-sill-ih-CATE) *NF.*

•**magnesium aluminosilicate.** (mag-NEE-zee-uhm ah-LOO-mihn-oh-sill-ih-CATE) *NF.*

magnesium aluminum hydroxide.
Use: Antacid.
See: Medalox Gel.

•**magnesium aluminum silicate.** (mag-NEE-zee-uhm ah-LOO-mihn-num sill-ih-CATE) *NF.*
Use: Pharmaceutic aid; suspending agent.

magnesium aspartate/potassium aspartate. (The Key Co.) Magnesium 90 mg (magnesium content expressed in mg elemental magnesium), potassium 90 mg. Sugar free. Cap. 100s. *OTC.*
Use: Nutritional supplement, multimineral.

•**magnesium carbonate.** (mag-NEE-zee-uhm kar-BAHN-ate) *USP.*
Use: Antacid.
W/Aluminum Hydroxide.
See: Acid Gone.
Gaviscon Extra Strength Antacid.
W/Aspirin, Calcium Carbonate, Magnesium Oxide.
See: Bayer Plus, Extra Strength.
Bufferin.
Bufferin Extra Strength.
W/Calcium Carbonate.
See: Antacid #2.
MagneBind 400 Rx.
MagneBind 300.
MagneBind 200.
Marblen.

•**magnesium chloride.** (mag-NEE-zee-uhm) *USP.*
Use: Electrolyte replacement; pharmaceutical necessity for hemodialysis and peritoneal dialysis.
See: Chloromag.

magnesium chloride. (Various Mfr.) Magnesium chloride 20% (200 mg/mL) (equiv. to elemental magnesium 1.97 mEq/mL). May contain benzyl alcohol, sodium chloride, aluminum. Inj., Soln., concentrate. Multiple-dose vial. 50 mL. *Rx.*
Use: Intravenous nutritional therapy, mineral.

•**magnesium citrate.** (mag-NEE-zee-uhm) *USP.*
Use: Cathartic; laxative.
See: LoSo Prep Bowel Cleansing System.

magnesium citrate. (Various Mfr.) Elemental magnesium 100 mg. Tab. Bot. 100s, 250s. *OTC.*
Use: Mineral.

magnesium citrate solution. (Humco Holding Group) Magnesium citrate 1.75 g/30 mL, saccharine, cherry, lemon flavors. Soln. Bot. 2% mL. *OTC.*
Use: Laxative.

•**magnesium gluconate.** (mag-NEE-zee-um glu-ca-nate) *USP.*
Use: Vitamin supplement, replacement.
See: Mag-G.
Magonate.
Magtrate.

magnesium gluconate. (Various Mfr.) Elemental magnesium 27.5 mg. Tab. Bot. 100s, 500s. *OTC.*
Use: Mineral.

magnesium hydroxide. (mag-NEE-zee-uhm) *USP.*
Use: Antacid; cathartic; laxative.
See: Dulcolax.
Magnesia Magma.
Milk of Magnesia.
Pedia-Lax.
Phillips' Chewable.
Phillips' Milk of Magnesia.
W/Aluminum Hydroxide.
See: Aludrox.
Delcid.
Maagel.
W/Aluminum Hydroxide, Aspirin.
See: Ascriptin.
W/Aluminum Hydroxide, Aspirin, Calcium Carbonate.
See: Ascriptin Maximum Strength.
W/Aluminum Hydroxide, Simethicone.
See: Di-Gel.
Gas Ban DS.
Maalox Advanced Maximum Strength.
Maalox Advanced Regular Strength.
Mi-Acid Maximum Strength.
Mintox.
Trial AG.
W/Calcium Carbonate.
See: Rolaids.
Rolaids Calcium Rich.
Rolaids Extra Strength.
W/Calcium Carbonate, Famotidine.
See: Acid Reducer + Antacid.
Dual Action Complete.
Pepcid Complete Dual Action.
Tums Dual Action.
W/Calcium Carbonate, Simethicone.
See: Rolaids Multi-Symptom.

magnesium-L-aspartate.
Use: Mineral.
See: Maginex.
Maginex DS.

•**magnesium oxide.** (mag-NEE-zee-uhm) *USP.*
Use: Pharmaceutic aid (sorbent).
See: Mag-Caps.
Mag-Ox 400.
Niko-Mag.
Phillips'.
Uro-Mag.
W/Aspirin, Calcium Carbonate, Magnesium Carbonate.
See: Bufferin.
Bufferin Extra Strength.
Bayer Plus, Extra Strength.
W/Citric Acid, Sodium Picosulfate.
See: Prepopik.

magnesium oxide. (Manne) Magnesium oxide 420 mg. Tab. Bot. 250s, 1000s. *OTC.*
Use: Mineral.

magnesium oxide. (Stanlabs) Magnesium oxide 10 g. Tab. Bot. 100s, 1000s. *OTC.*
Use: Mineral.

magnesium oxide. (Various Mfr.) Magnesium oxide 400 mg (elemental magnesium 241.3 mg). Tab. 120s, 400s. *OTC.*
Use: Dietary supplement.

•**magnesium phosphate.** (mag-NEE-zee-uhm) *USP.*
Use: Antacid.

•**magnesium salicylate.** (mag-NEE-zee-uhm suh-LIH-sih-late) *USP.*
Use: Analgesic; antipyretic; antirheumatic.
See: Doan's.
Magan.
W/Acetaminophen.
See: Painaid Back Relief Formula.
W/Acetaminophen, Caffeine.
See: Back Pain-Off.
W/Acetaminophen, Caffeine, Phenyltoloxamine Citrate.
See: Durabac Forte.
W/Diphenhydramine Hydrochloride.
See: Doan's PM Extra Strength.

magnesium salicylate tetrahydrate.
Use: Nonnarcotic analgesic.
See: Backache Maximum Strength Relief.
Bayer Select Maximum Strength Backache.
Momentum Muscular Backache Formula.
Painaid BRF Back Relief Formula.

•**magnesium silicate.** (mag-NEE-zee-uhm sill-IH-cate) *NF.*
Use: Pharmaceutic aid (tablet excipient).

•**magnesium stearate.** (mag-NEE-zee-uhm STEER-ate) *NF.*
Use: Pharmaceutic aid (tablet and capsule lubricant).

•**magnesium sulfate.** (mag-NEE-zee-uhm) *USP.*
Use: Anticonvulsant; electrolyte replacement; laxative.
W/Potassium Sulfate, Sodium Sulfate.
See: Suclear.
Suprep Bowel Prep.

magnesium sulfate. (Various Mfr.) Magnesium sulfate. Inj., Soln. **4% (40 mg/mL):** Equiv. to elemental magnesium 0.325 mEq/mL. Single-dose container. 50 mL, 100 mL, 500 mL, 1,000 mL. **8% (80 mg/mL):** Equiv. to elemental magnesium 0.65 mEq/mL. Single-dose container. 50 mL. **50% (500 mg/mL):** Equiv. to elemental magnesium 4 mEq/mL. May contain aluminum. Preservative free. Single-dose vial. 10 mL, 20 mL. *Rx.*
Use: Intravenous nutritional therapy, mineral.

magnesium sulfate in dextrose 5%. (Hospira) Magnesium sulfate. Inj., Soln. **1% (10 mg/mL):** Equiv. to elemental magnesium 0.081 mEq/mL. Dextrose 5 g. Single-dose container. 100 mL. **2% (20 mg/mL):** Equiv. to elemental magnesium 0.162 mEq/mL. Dextrose 5 g. Single-dose container. 500 mL, 1,000 mL. *Rx.*
Use: Intravenous nutritional therapy, mineral.

•**magnesium trisilicate.** (mag-NEE-zee-uhm try-SILL-ih-cate) *USP.*
Use: Antacid.
See: Banacid.
W/Aluminum hydroxide gel.
See: Gacid.
Gaviscon.
Maracid 2.

Magnevist. (Bayer Healthcare Pharma) Gadopentetate dimeglumine 469.01 mg/mL. Preservative free. Inj. Pharmacy bulk pkg. 100 mL. *Rx.*
Use: Radiopaque agent, parenteral.

Magonate. (Valeant) **Tab.:** Magnesium gluconate dihydrate 500 mg (elemental magnesium 27 mg), Ca 87.5 mg, P 66 mg (dibasic calcium phosphate dihydrate 376 mg). Bot. 1000s. **Liq.:** Magnesium gluconate dihydrate 1000 mg/5 mL (elemental magnesium 54 mg/5 mL), sorbitol, magnesium carbonate, melon flavored. Bot. 473 mL. *OTC.*
Use: Mineral supplement.

Magonate Natal. (Valeant) Elemental magnesium 3.52 mg (as gluconate)/mL. Liq. Bot. 480 mL. *OTC.*
Use: Mineral.

Mag-Ox 400. (Blaine) Magnesium oxide 400 mg (elemental magnesium 241.3 mg). Tab. Bot. 120s, 1000s, UD 100s. *OTC.*
Use: Antacid; vitamin, mineral supplement.

Mag-Tab SR. (Niche) Elemental magnesium (as L-lactate dihydrate) 84 mg. SR Tab. 60s, 100s, 1000s. *OTC.*
Use: Mineral supplement.

Magtrate. (Mission) Magnesium gluconate 500 mg (elemental magnesium 29 mg). Tab. Bot. 100s. *OTC.*
Use: Mineral supplement.

Mag-200. (Optimox) Elemental magnesium (as oxide) 200 mg, PABA 300 mg. Tab. Bot. 120s. *OTC.*
Use: Mineral supplement.

Maintenance Vitamin Formula w/Minerals. (Towne) Vitamins A palmitate 10,000 units, D 400 units, B_1 5 mg, B_2 2.5 mg, C 75 mg, niacinamide 40 mg, B_6 1 mg, calcium pantothenate 4 mg, B_{12} 2 mcg, E 2 units, choline bitartrate 31.4 mg, inositol 15 mg, Ca 75 mg, P 58 mg, Fe 30 mg, Mg 3 mg, Mn 0.5 mg, K 2 mg, Zn 0.5 mg. Cap. Bot. 100s. *OTC.*
Use: Mineral, vitamin supplement.

majeptil. Thioproperazine. Psychopharmacologic agent; pending release.

Major-gesic. (Major) Phenyltoloxamine citrate 30 mg, acetaminophen 325 mg. Tab. Bot. 100s, 1000s. *OTC.*
Use: Upper respiratory combination, antihistamine, analgesic.

Makena. (Ther-Rx) Hydroxyprogesterone caproate 250 mg/mL. Benzyl alcohol, benzyl benzoate, castor oil. Inj., Soln. Multidose vial. 5 mL. *Rx.*
Use: Sex hormone, progestin.

Malaraquin. (Sanofi-Synthelabo) Chloroquine phosphate. *Rx.*
Use: Antimalarial.

Malarone. (GlaxoSmithKline) Atovaquone 250 mg, proguanil hydrochloride 100 mg. Film-coated. Tab. Bot. 100s, UD 24s. *Rx.*
Use: Antimalarial.

Malarone Pediatric. (GlaxoSmithKline) Atovaquone 62.5 mg, proguanil hydrochloride 25 mg. Film-coated. Tab. Bot. 100s. *Rx.*
Use: Antimalarial.

•**malathion.** (mal-ah-THIGH-ahn) *USP.*
Use: Pediculicide.

malathion. (Various Mfr.) Malathion 0.5% (in a vehicle of isopropyl alcohol 78%, terpineol, dipentene, and pine needle oil). Lot. 59 mL. *Rx.*
Use: Dermatological agent, scabicide/pediculicide.

•**malic acid.** (MAL-ik) *NF.*
Use: Pharmaceutic aid (acidifying agent).

Mallergan-VC w/Codeine Syrup. (Roberts) Phenylephrine hydrochloride 5 mg, promethazine hydrochloride 6.25 mg, codeine phosphate 10 mg/5 mL, alcohol 7%. Syrup. Bot. 120 mL. *c-v.*
Use: Antihistamine, antitussive, decongestant.

Malogen Cyp. (Forest) Testosterone cypionate in oil 100 mg, 200 mg/mL. Inj. Vial 10 mL. *c-III.*
Use: Androgen.

Malogen Injection Aqueous. (Forest) Testosterone. **25 mg/mL:** 10 mL, 30 mL. **50 mg/mL:** 10 mL. **100 mg/mL:** 10 mL. *c-III.*
Use: Androgen.

Malogen 100 L.A. in Oil. (Forest) Testosterone enanthate 100 mg/mL. Inj. 10 mL. *c-III.*
Use: Androgen.

Malogen 200 L.A. in Oil. (Forest) Testosterone enanthate 200 mg/mL. Inj. 10 mL. *c-III.*
Use: Androgen.

malonal. (Various Mfr.) Barbital.

•**malotilate.** (mal-OH-tih-LATE) USAN.
Use: Liver disorder treatment.

Malotrone Aqueous Injection. (Bluco) Testosterone, USP 25 mg, 50 mg/mL in aqueous susp. Vial 10 mL. *c-III.*
Use: Androgen.

•**maltitol solution.** (MAL-tih-tahl) *NF.*
Use: Sweetener.

•**maltodextrin.** (MAWL-toe-DEX-trin) *NF.*
Use: Pharmaceutic aid (coating agent, tablet binder, tablet and capsule diluent, viscosity-increasing agent).

•**maltose.** (MAWL-toes) *NF.*
Use: Pharmaceutic aid.

Maltsupex. (Wallace) Malt soup extract 8 g/level scoop. Pow. Can. 227 g, 454 g. *OTC.*
Use: Laxative.

Mammol Ointment. (Abbott) Bismuth subnitrate 40%, castor oil 30%, anhydrous lanolin 22%, ceresin wax 7%, balsam Peru 1%. Tube ⅞ oz. Ctn. 12s. *OTC.*
Use: Dermatologic; protectant; emollient.

mandameth. (Major) Methenamine

mandelate 0.5 g. EC Tab. Bot. 1000s. *Rx.*
Use: Anti-infective, urinary.

mandelic acid.
Use: Anti-infective, urinary.

mandelic acid salts. (Various Mfr.) Calcium mandelate.

mandelyltropeine. (Various Mfr.) Homatropine Salts.

•**mangafodipir trisodium.** (man-gah-FOE-dih-pihr try-SO-dee-uhm) *USP.*
Use: Radiopaque agent, parenteral.

manganese.
Use: Dietary supplement.
See: Chelated Manganese.
Mangimin.

•**manganese chloride.** (MANG-ah-neese) *USP.* For Oral Solution.
Use: Manganese deficiency treatment; trace mineral supplement.

•**manganese gluconate.** (MANG-ah-neese GLOO-kahn-ate) *USP.*
Use: Manganese deficiency; trace mineral supplement.

manganese glycerophosphate. Glycerol phosphate manganese salt.
Use: Pharmaceutical necessity.

manganese hypophosphite. Manganese^{++} phosphinate.
Use: Pharmaceutical necessity.

•**manganese sulfate.** (MANG-ah-neese) *USP.*
Use: Trace mineral supplement.

Manga-Pak. (SoloPak Pharmaceuticals, Inc.) Manganese 0.1 mg/mL. Inj. Vial 10 mL, 30 mL. *Rx.*
Use: Nutritional supplement, parenteral.

Mangimin. (The Key Company) Manganese 10 mg. Tab. 100s. *OTC.*
Use: Nutrient and nutritional agent, trace element.

•**mangofilcon A.** (MAN-goe-FIL-kon) USAN.
Use: Contact lens polymer.

Maniron. (Jones Pharma) Ferrous fumarate 3 mg. Tab. Bot. 100s, 1000s, 5000s. *OTC.*
Use: Mineral supplement.

Mannan. (Rugby) Purified glucomannan 500 mg. Cap. Bot. 90s. *OTC.*
Use: Nutritional supplement.

Mann Astringent Mouth Wash Concentrate. (Manne) Bot. 4 oz, qt, 0.5 gal, gal. Mint flavored. Bot. 4 oz, qt, 0.5 gal, gal. *OTC.*
Use: Mouthwash.

manna sugar. (Various Mfr.) Mannitol.

Mann Body Deodorant. (Manne) Bot. 4 oz, 8 oz, pt, qt. *OTC.*
Use: Deodorant.

Mann Breath Deodorant. (Manne) Bot. 1 oz, 4 oz, 8 oz, pt, qt, 0.5 gal. *OTC.*
Use: Mouthwash.

Mann Emollient. (Manne) Jar. 100 g. *OTC.*
Use: Emollient.

Mannest. (Manne) Conjugated estrogens 0.625 mg, 1.25 mg, or 2.5 mg. Tab. Bot. 100s, 200s. *Rx.*
Use: Estrogen.

Mann Eugenol U.S.P. Extra. (Manne) 0.06 lb, 0.13 lb, 0.25 lb, 0.5 lb, 1 lb. *OTC.*
Use: Dermatologic, protectant.

Mann Germicidal Solution. (Manne) **Regular:** Bot. Gal, 4 gal. **Conc.:** 12.8%. Bot. Pt, qt, 0.5 gal, gal. *OTC.*
Use: Antimicrobial.

Mann Hand Lotion. (Manne) Twin pack, gal. *OTC.*
Use: Emollient.

Mann Hemostatic. (Manne) Bot. 1 oz, 4 oz, 8 oz, pt, qt. *OTC.*
Use: Hemostatic.

mannite.
See: Mannitol.

•**mannitol.** (MAN-ih-tole) *USP.*
Use: Diagnostic aid.
See: Osmitrol.

mannitol. (B. Braun McGaw) Mannitol 5 g per 100 mL in distilled water (275 mOsm/L). Soln. 2,000 mL. *Rx.*
Use: Osmotic diuretic.

mannitol. (Various Mfr.) Mannitol 10%, 15%, 20%, 25%. Inj. 150 mL, 500 mL (15%); 250 mL, 500 mL (20%); 1,000 mL (10%); 50 mL vial and syringe (25%). *Rx.*
Use: Osmotic diuretic.

mannitol and sorbitol.
See: Sorbitol-Mannitol.

mannitol hexanitrate.
Use: Coronary vasodilator.
See: Vascunitol.
W/Phenobarbital.
See: Manotensin.
Vascused.

mannitol hexanitrate and phenobarbital tablets. (Jones Pharma) Mannitol hexanitrate 0.5 g, phenobarbital 0.25 g. Tab. Bot. 1000s. *c-IV.*
Use: Vasodilator.

mannitol injection. (Abbott) Mannitol 15%, 20%. *Abbo-Vac* single-dose container 500 mL.
Use: Diagnostic aid (renal function determination); diuretic.

mannitol in sodium chloride injection.
Use: Diuretic.

Mann Liquid Soap. (Manne) Concentrated cococastile. Bot. Qt, 0.5 gal, gal.

OTC.
Use: Emollient.
Mann Lubricant and Cleanser. (Manne) Bot. Pt, qt. *OTC.*
Use: Emollient.
Mann Superfatted Bar Soap. (Manne) Rich in lanolin. Cake. 12s. *OTC.*
Use: Emollient.
Mann Talbot's Iodine. (Manne) Glycerin base. Bot. 1 oz, 4 oz, 8 oz, pt, qt. *OTC.*
Use: Antiseptic.
Mann Topical Anesthetic. (Manne) Bot. 1 oz, 4 oz, 8 oz, pt. W/stain to indicate area treated. Bot. 1 oz, 4 oz, 8 oz. *OTC.*
Use: Anesthetic, local.
Manotensin. (Oxypure) Mannitol hexanitrate 32 mg, phenobarbital 16 mg. Tab. Bot. 100s, 1000s. *c-IV.*
Use: Vasodilator.
Mantoux Test.
Use: Tuberculin test.
manvene.
Use: Antineoplastic.
MAOI.
See: Monoamine Oxidase Inhibitors.
Maox 420. (Manne) Magnesium oxide 420 mg. Tab. 250s, 1,000s. *OTC.*
Use: Antacid.
Mapap. (Major) Acetaminophen. **Cap.:** 500 mg. 24s, 50s, 100s, 175s, 500s, 1,000s. **Tab.:** 500 mg. Tab. 24s, 50s, 100s, 175s, 500s, 1,000s. **Tab., Rapid Release:** 500 mg. 24s, 50s, 100s, 175s, 500s, 1,000s. **Susp.:** 160 mg per 5 mL. Butylparaben, corn syrup, glycerin, propylene glycol, sodium borate, sorbitol, sucralose. Alcohol free and dye free. Cherry flavor. 59 mL. *OTC.*
Use: Analgesic.
Mapap Arthritis Pain. (Major) Acetaminophen 650 mg. ER Tab. 100s. *OTC.*
Use: Analgesic.
Mapap Children's. (Major) **Chew. Tab.:** Acetaminophen 80 mg. Aspartame, mannitol, phenylalanine 3 mg, sucrose. Grape, fruit, and bubble gum flavors. 30s. **Elix.:** Acetaminophen 160 mg/ 5 mL. Alcohol free. Sorbitol, sucrose. Cherry flavor. Bot. 118 mL. *OTC.*
Use: Analgesic.
Mapap Cold Formula Multi-Symptom. (Major) Acetaminophen 325 mg, phenylephrine hydrochloride 5 mg, dextromethorphan HBr 10 mg. Polyvinyl alcohol, sucralose. Tab. Pkg. 24s. *OTC.*
Use: Upper respiratory combination, antitussive combination.
Mapap Extra Strength. (Major) Acetaminophen 166.67 mg per 5 mL. Corn syrup, PEG, propylene glycol, saccharin, sodium benzoate, sorbitol. Cherry flavor. Liq. 237 mL. *OTC.*
Use: Analgesic.
Mapap Infants'. (Major) Acetaminophen 160 mg per 5 mL. Corn syrup, glycerin, propylene glycol, sodium benzoate, sorbitol, sucralose. Alcohol free, dye free. Cherry flavor. Susp. 59 mL w/dosing syringe. *OTC.*
Use: CNS agent.
Mapap Junior Strength. (Major) Acetaminophen 160 mg. Grape flavor. Chew. Tab. 24s. *OTC.*
Use: Analgesic.
Mapap Regular Strength. (Major) Acetaminophen 325 mg. Tab. Bot. 100s, 1000s, UD 100s. *OTC.*
Use: Analgesic.
Mapap Sinus Congestion and Pain Maximum Strength. (Major) Phenylephrine hydrochloride 5 mg, acetaminophen 325 mg. Acesulfame K. Tab. 24s. *OTC.*
Use: Upper respiratory combination, decongestant and analgesic combination.
Mapap Sinus Maximum Strength. (Major) Pseudoephedrine hydrochloride 30 mg, acetaminophen 500 mg. PEG. Tab. Pkg. 24s. *OTC.*
Use: Upper respiratory combination, decongestant, analgesic.
•**mapatumumab.** (MAP-a-TOOM-ue-mab) USAN.
Use: Antineoplastic.
•**mapracorat.** (MAP-ra-KOR-at) USAN.
Use: Dermatological agent.
Maprofix.
See: Gardinol Type Detergents.
•**maprotiline.** (map-ROW-tih-leen) USAN.
Use: Antidepressant.
•**maprotiline hydrochloride.** (map-ROW-tih-leen) *USP.*
Use: Antidepressant, tetracyclic compound.
maprotiline hydrochloride. (Mylan) Maprotiline hydrochloride 25 mg, 50 mg, 75 mg. PEG, polydextrose. Film coated. Tab. 100s. *Rx.*
Use: Antidepressant, tetracyclic compound.
•**maraciclatide.** (MAR-a-SIK-la-tide) USAN.
Use: Diagnostic agent.
Maracid 2. (Marlin Industries) Magnesium trisilicate 150 mg, aluminum hydroxide dried gel 90 mg, aminoacetic acid 75 mg. Tab. Bot. *OTC.*
Use: Antacid; adsorbent.
maraviroc. (mah-RAV-er-rock)
Use: Antiretroviral, cellular chemokine

receptor antagonist.
See: Selzentry.

Marbaxin 750. (Vortech Pharmaceuticals) Methocarbamol 750 mg. Tab. Bot. 500s. *Rx.*
Use: Muscle relaxant.

Marblen. (Fleming & Co.) Calcium carbonate 520 mg, magnesium carbonate 400 mg per 5 mL. **Tab.:** 100s, 1,000s. **Liq.:** 473 mL. *OTC.*
Use: Antacid.

Marcaine. (Eastman-Kodak) Bupivacaine 0.5%, epinephrine 1:200,000, sodium metabisulfite, EDTA 0.1 mg/mL. Inj. Dental Cart. 1.8 mL. *Rx.*
Use: Anesthetic, local amide.

Marcaine. (Hospira) Bupivacaine hydrochloride. Multiple-dose vial also contains methylparaben 1 mg/mL as preservative. **0.25%:** Single-dose amp. 50 mL. Single-dose vial 10 mL, 30 mL. Multiple-dose vial 50 mL. **0.5%:** Single-dose amp. 30 mL. Single-dose vial 10 mL, 30 mL. Multiple-dose vial 50 mL. **0.75%:** Single-dose amp. 30 mL. Single-dose vial 10 mL, 30 mL. **0.25% with epinephrine 1:200,000:** Sodium metabisulfite 0.5 mg, edetate calcium disodium 0.1 mg. Amp. 50 mL, 5s. Vial 10 mL, 30 mL, 50 mL (methylparaben 1 mg/mL). **0.5% with epinephrine 1:200,000:** Sodium metabisulfite 0.5 mg, edetate calcium disodium 0.1 mg. Single-dose amp. 3 mL, 30 mL. Single-dose vial 10 mL, 30 mL. **0.75% with epinephrine 1:200,000:** Sodium metabisulfite 0.5 mg, edetate calcium disodium 0.1 mg. Amp. 30 mL. Inj. *Rx.*
Use: Anesthetic, local amide.

Marcaine Spinal. (Hospira) Bupivacaine hydrochloride 0.75% in dextrose 8.25%. Preservative free. Inj., Soln. 2 mL amp. *Rx.*
Use: Injectable local anesthetic, amide local anesthetic.

Marcillin. (Marnel) Ampicillin trihydrate 500 mg. Cap. Bot. 100s. *Rx.*
Use: Anti-infective; penicillin.

Mar-Cof BP. (Marnel Pharmaceutical) Brompheniramine maleate 2 mg, codeine phosphate 7.5 mg, pseudoephedrine hydrochloride 30 mg. Magnasweet, saccharin, sorbitol. Alcohol free and sugar free. Liq. 473 mL. *c-v.*
Use: Upper respiratory combination, antitussive combination.

Mar-Cof-CG. (Marnel) Codeine phosphate 7.5 mg, guaifenesin 225 mg per 5 mL. PEG, saccharin, sorbitol. Alcohol free and sugar free. Liq. 473 mL. *c-v.*
Use: Upper respiratory combination, antitussive with expectorant.

Mardon. (Armenpharm Ltd.) Propoxyphene hydrochloride. Cap. **32 mg:** Bot. 100s, 1000s. **65 mg:** Bot. 100s, 500s, 1000s. *c-IV.*
Use: Analgesic; narcotic.

Mardon Compound. (Armenpharm Ltd.) Propoxyphene compound 65 mg, aspirin 3.5 g, phenacetin 2.5 g, caffeine 0.5 g. Cap. Bot. 100s, 500s, 1000s. *c-IV.*
Use: Analgesic combination; narcotic.

Marezine. (Himmel) Cyclizine hydrochloride 50 mg. Tab. Bot. 100s. Box 12s. *OTC.*
Use: Anticholinergic.

Margesic. (Marnel) Butalbital 50 mg, acetaminophen 325 mg, caffeine 40 mg. Cap. Bot. 100s. *Rx.*
Use: Analgesic; hypnotic; sedative.

Margesic H. (Marnel) Hydrocodone bitartrate 5 mg, acetaminophen 500 mg. Cap. Bot. 100s. *c-III.*
Use: Analgesic combination; narcotic.

Margesic No. 3. (Marnel) Codeine phosphate 30 mg, acetaminophen 300 mg. Tab. Bot. 100s. *c-III.*
Use: Analgesic combination; narcotic.

•**margetuximab.** (MAR-jee-TIX-i-mab) USAN.
Use: Antineoplastic.

•**marimastat.** (mah-RIH-mah-stat) USAN.
Use: Antineoplastic (matrix metalloproteinase inhibitor).

Marine Lipid Concentrate. (Vitaline) Omega-3 1200 mg, EPA 360 mg, DHA 240 mg, E 5 units/Cap., sodium free. Bot. 90s. *OTC.*
Use: Nutritional supplement.

Marinol. (Unimed) Dronabinol 2.5 mg, 5 mg, 10 mg, in sesame oil. Parabens. Gelatin Cap. Bot. 25s, 60s (except 5 mg), 100s (except 10 mg). *c-III.*
Use: Antiemetic, antivertigo agent.

•**maritime pine.** (mair-ih-time) *NF.*
Use: Pharmaceutic aid.

•**marizomib.** (MAR-i-ZOE-mib) USAN.
Use: Antineoplastic.

Marlissa. (Glenmark Generics) Ethinyl estradiol 30 mcg, levonorgestrel 0.15 mg. Lactose. Tab. 28s (w/7 inert tablets). *Rx.*
Use: Oral monophasic contraceptive.

Marlyn Formula 50. (Marlyn Nutraceuticals) Vitamin B_6 with 18 amino acids. Cap. Bot. 100s, 250s, 1000s. *OTC.*
Use: Nutritional supplement.

Marnatal-F. (Marnel) Folic acid 1 mg, calcium 200 mg, iron 60 mg, vitamins D 400 units, E 30 units, B_1 3 mg, B_2 3.4 mg, B_3 20 mg, B_6 5 mg, B_{12} 12 mcg,

C 100 mg, Cu, Mg. Maltodextrin. Cap. 30s. *Rx.*
Use: Prenatal vitamin with minerals.

•**maropitant citrate.** (mar-oh-PIT-ant) USAN.
Use: Antiemetic.

Marplan. (Validus) Isocarboxazid 10 mg. Lactose. Tab. Bot. 100s. *Rx.*
Use: Antidepressant.

Marqibo. (Talon Therapeutics) Vincristine sulfate liposome 5 mg. Inj. for liposomal Susp. Kit (each kit contains a vial of vincristine sulfate injection [5 mg per 5 mL], a vial containing sphingomyelin/ cholesterol liposome injection [103 mg/ mL], and a vial containing sodium phosphate injection [355 mg per 25 mL]. After preparation, each vial contains mannitol 500 mg, sphingomyelin 73.5 mg, cholesterol 29.5 mg, sodium citrate 36 mg, sodium phosphate 355 mg, and sodium chloride 225 mg). *Rx.*
Use: Antimitotic agent, vinca alkaloid.

Mar-Spas. (Marnel) L-hyoscyamine sulfate 0.25 mg. Aspartame, phenylalanine 3.5 mg. Spearmint flavor. Orally Disintegrating Tab. 100s. *Rx.*
Use: Gastrointestinal anticholinergic/antispasmodic.

Marten-Tab. (Marnel) Butalbital 50 mg, acetaminophen 325 mg. Tab. Bot. 100s. *Rx.*
Use: Analgesic.

MAS-ER. (Teva Pharmaceuticals) Amphetamine mixture 5 mg (dextroamphetamine saccharate 1.25 mg, amphetamine aspartate monohydrate 1.25 mg, dextroamphetamine sulfate 1.25 mg, amphetamine sulfate 1.25 mg), 10 mg (dextroamphetamine saccharate 2.5 mg, amphetamine aspartate monohydrate 2.5 mg, dextroamphetamine sulfate 2.5 mg, amphetamine sulfate 2.5 mg), 15 mg (dextroamphetamine saccharate 3.75 mg, amphetamine aspartate monohydrate 3.75 mg, dextroamphetamine sulfate 3.75 mg, amphetamine sulfate 3.75 mg), 20 mg (dextroamphetamine saccharate 5 mg, amphetamine aspartate monohydrate 5 mg, dextroamphetamine sulfate 5 mg, amphetamine sulfate 5 mg), 25 mg (dextroamphetamine saccharate 6.25 mg, amphetamine aspartate monohydrate 6.25 mg, dextroamphetamine sulfate 6.25 mg, amphetamine sulfate 6.25 mg), 30 mg (dextroamphetamine saccharate 7.5 mg, amphetamine aspartate monohydrate 7.5 mg, dextroamphetamine sulfate 7.5 mg, amphetamine sulfate 7.5 mg). Sugar spheres. ER Cap. 100s. *c-II.*
Use: CNS stimulant, amphetamine.

Masophen. (Mason) Acetaminophen 325 mg, 500 mg. Tab. 100s. *OTC.*
Use: Analgesic.

Masophen Extra Strength. (Mason) Acetaminophen 500 mg. Cap. 100s. *OTC.*
Use: Analgesic.

Masse Breast Cream. (Johnson & Johnson) Glyceryl monostearate, glycerin, cetyl alcohol, lanolin, peanut oil, Span-60, stearic acid, Tween-60, sodium benzoate, propylparaben, methylparaben, potassium hydroxide. Tube 2 oz. *OTC.*
Use: Emollient.

Massengill Baking Soda Freshness. (GlaxoSmithKline) Sanitized water, sodium bicarbonate. Soln. Bot. 180 mL. *OTC.*
Use: Vaginal agent.

Massengill Disposable Douche. (GlaxoSmithKline) Water, SD alcohol 40, lactic acid, sodium lactate, octoxynol-9, cetylpyridinium chloride, propylene glycol, diazolidinyl urea, EDTA, parabens, fragrance, color. Bot. 180 mL. *OTC.*
Use: Vaginal agent.

Massengill Extra Cleansing w/Puraclean. (GlaxoSmithKline) Vinegar, water, cetylpyridinium chloride, diazolidinyl urea, EDTA. Soln. Bot. 180 mL. *OTC.*
Use: Vaginal agent.

Massengill Feminine Cleansing Wash. (GlaxoSmithKline) Sodium laureth sulfate, magnesium oleth sulfate, sodium oleth sulfate, magnesium oleth sulfate, PEG-120 methyl glucose dioleate, parabens. Liq. Bot. 240 mL. *OTC.*
Use: Vaginal agent.

Massengill Feminine Deodorant Spray. (GlaxoSmithKline) Aerosol Bot. 3 oz. *OTC.*
Use: Vaginal agent.

Massengill Liquid. (GlaxoSmithKline) Lactic acid, SD alcohol 40, octoxynol-9, water, sodium bicarbonate. Bot. 120 mL. *OTC.*
Use: Vaginal agent.

Massengill Medicated. (GlaxoSmithKline) Povidone-iodine 0.3% when added to sanitized fluid. Bot. 6 oz. *OTC.*
Use: Vaginal agent.

Massengill Medicated Disposable Douche w/Cepticin. (GlaxoSmithKline) Povidone-iodine 10%. Liq. Vial 5 mL w/180 mL bot. of sanitized water. *OTC.*
Use: Vaginal agent.

Massengill Medicated Douche w/Cepticin. (GlaxoSmithKline) Povidone-iodine

12%. Liq. concentrate. Bot. 120 mL, 240 mL. *OTC.*
Use: Vaginal agent.

Massengill Powder. (GlaxoSmithKline) Ammonium alum, PEG-8, methyl salicylate, eucalyptus oil, menthol, thymol, phenol. Jar 120 g, 240 g, 480 g, 660 g. UD Packette 10s, 12s. *OTC.*
Use: Vaginal agent.

Massengill Soft Cloth. (GlaxoSmithKline) Hydrocortisone 0.5%, diazolidinyl urea, DMDM hydantoin, isopropyl myristate, methylparaben, polysorbate 60, propylene glycol, propylparaben, sorbitan stearate, steareth-2, steareth-21. Towelettes 10s. *OTC.*
Use: Vaginal agent.

Massengill Unscented. (GlaxoSmithKline) Water, SD alcohol 40, lactic acid, sodium lactate, octoxynol-9, cetylpyridinium chloride, propylene glycol, diazolidinyl urea, parabens, EDTA. Soln. Bot. 180 mL. *OTC.*
Use: Vaginal agent.

Massengill Vinegar & Water Extra Cleansing with Puraclean. (GlaxoSmithKline) Vinegar, water, cetylpyridinium chloride, diazolidinyl urea, EDTA. Soln. Bot. 180 mL. *OTC.*
Use: Vaginal agent.

Massengill Vinegar & Water Extra Mild. (GlaxoSmithKline) Vinegar, water, preservative free. Soln. Bot. 180 mL. *OTC.*
Use: Vaginal agent.

Massengill Vinegar-Water Disposable Douche. (GlaxoSmithKline) Water and vinegar solution. Bot. 180 mL. *OTC.*
Use: Vaginal agent.

mast cell stabilizer.
Use: Ophthalmic agent.
See: Bepotastine Besilate.
Cromolyn Sodium.
Pemirolast Potassium.

Master Formula. (Barth's) Vitamins A 10,000 units, D 400 units, C 180 mg, B_1 7 mg, B_2 14 mg, niacin 4.6 mg, B_6 292 mcg, pantothenic acid 210 mcg, B_{12} 25 mcg, biotin 2.9 mcg, E 50 units, Ca 800 mg, P 387 mg, Fe 10 mg, I 0.1 mg, Cl 7.78 mg, inositol 11.6 mg, aminobenzoic acid 35 mcg, rutin 30 mg, citrus bioflavonoid complex 30 mg/4 Tab. Bot. 120s, 600s, 1200s. *OTC.*
Use: Mineral, vitamin supplement.

Mastisol. (Ferndale) Nonirritating medical adhesive. Bot. 4 oz.
Use: Adhesive.

matrix metalloproteinase inhibitor.
Use: Corneal ulcers. [Orphan Drug]

Matulane. (Sigma-Tau) Procarbazine hydrochloride 50 mg. Talc, mannitol, parabens. Cap. Bot. 100s. *Rx.*
Use: Antineoplastic.

Matzim LA. (Watson Pharma) Diltiazem hydrochloride 120 mg, 180 mg, 240 mg, 300 mg, 360 mg, and 420 mg. Lactose, sucrose. ER Tab. 30s, 90s, 1,000s. *Rx.*
Use: Calcium channel blocking agent.

•**mavacoxib.** (MAY-va-KOX-ib) USAN.
Use: Anti-inflammatory; analgesic.

•**mavatrep.** (MAV-a-trep) USAN.
Use: Analgesic.

Mavik. (Abbott) Trandolapril 1 mg, 2 mg, 4 mg, lactose. Tab. Bot. 100s, UD 100s. *Rx.*
Use: Antihypertensive; renin angiotensin system antagonist; angiotensin-converting enzyme inhibitor.

•**mavoglurant.** (MAV-oh-GLOO-rant) USAN.
Use: Treatment of Parkinson disease, fragile X syndrome, obsessive compulsive disorder.

•**mavrilimumab.** (MAV-ri-LIM-ue-mab) USAN.
Use: Antirheumatic agent.

Maxair Autohaler. (Medicis) Pirbuterol acetate 0.2 mg/actuation. Aer. Autohaler 2.8 g (80 inhalations), 14 g (400 inhalations). *Rx.*
Use: Bronchodilator, sympathomimetic.

Maxalt. (Merck) Rizatriptan benzoate 5 mg, 10 mg. Lactose. Tab. UD 18s. *Rx.*
Use: Antimigraine, serotonin 5-HT_1 receptor agonist.

Maxalt-MLT. (Merck) Rizatriptan benzoate 5 mg, 10 mg, lyophilized, mannitol, aspartame, phenylalanine 1.05 mg (5 mg only), 2.1 mg (10 mg only). Tab., orally disintegrating. UD 18s (in 6 unit-of-use carrying case of 3 tablets). *Rx.*
Use: Antimigraine, serotonin, 5-HT_1 receptor agonist.

Max EPA. (Various Mfr.) Omega-3 polyunsaturated fatty acids 1000 mg. Cap. containing EPA 180 mg, DHA 60 mg. Cap. Bot. 50s, 60s, 100s. *OTC.*
Use: Nutritional supplement.

Maxichlor PEH DM. (MCR American) Chlorpheniramine maleate 4 mg, dextromethorphan hydrobromide 20 mg, phenylephrine hydrochloride 10 mg. Tab. 100s. *Rx.*
Use: Upper respiratory combination, antitussive combination.

Maxidex. (Alcon) Dexamethasone 0.1%. Benzalkonium chloride 0.01%, EDTA, hypromellose 0.5%, polysorbate 80, sodium chloride, dibasic sodium phosphate. Ophth. Susp. *Drop-Tainers* 5 mL,

15 mL. *Rx.*
Use: Corticosteroid, ophthalmic.
Maxidone. (Watson) Hydrocodone bitartrate 10 mg, acetaminophen 750 mg, lactose. Tab. Bot. 100s, 500s. *c-III.*
Use: Narcotic analgesic combination.
Maxifed DM. (MCR American) **Liq.:** Dextromethorphan hydrobromide 10 mg, guaifenesin 200 mg, pseudoephedrine hydrochloride 20 mg per 5 mL. Alcohol 0.1%, parabens, sorbitol, sucralose. Sugar free. Orange cream flavor. 473 mL. **Tab.:** Dextromethorphan hydrobromide 20 mg, guaifenesin 400 mg, pseudoephedrine hydrochloride 40 mg. 100s. *Rx.*
Use: Upper respiratory combination, antitussive and expectorant.
Maxifed DMX. (MCR American) Dextromethorphan HBr 20 mg, guaifenesin 400 mg, pseudoephedrine hydrochloride 60 mg. Tab. 100s. *Rx.*
Use: Upper respiratory combination, antitussive and expectorant combination.
Maxiflor. (Allergan) Diflorasone diacetate 0.05%. Cream, Oint. Tubes 15 g, 30 g, 60 g. *Rx.*
Use: Corticosteroid, topical.
Maxiflu DM. (MCR American) Acetaminophen 500 mg, dextromethorphan hydrobromide 20 mg, guaifenesin 400 mg, pseudoephedrine hydrochloride 60 mg. Tab. 100s. *Rx.*
Use: Upper respiratory combination, antitussive and expectorant combination.
Maxilube. (Mission Pharmacal) Water, silicone oil, glycerin, carbomer 934, triethanolamine, sodium lauryl sulfate, parabens. Jelly 90 g, 150 g. *OTC.*
Use: Vaginal agent.
Maximum Bayer Aspirin. (Bayer Consumer Care) Aspirin (Acetylsalicylic Acid; ASA) 500 mg. **Tab.:** 10s, 30s, 60s, 100s. **Capl.:** 60s. *OTC.*
Use: Analgesic.
Maximum Blue Label. (Vitaline) Vitamins A 2500 units, D 16.7 units, E 66.7 mg, B_1 16.7 mg, B_2 8.3 mg, B_3 31.7 mg, B_5 66.7 mg, B_6 16.7 mg, B_{12} 16.7 mcg, C 200 mg, folic acid 0.13 mg, Zn 5 mg, Ca, Cr, Cu, I, K, Mg, Mn, Mo, Se, Si, V, biotin 50 mcg, SOD, l-lysine. Tab. Bot. 180s. *OTC.*
Use: Mineral, vitamin supplement.
Maximum D3. (Pro-Pharma) Cholecalciferol 10,000 IU. Cap. 5s. *OTC.*
Use: Vitamin supplement.
Maximum Green Label. (Vitaline) Vitamins A 2500 units, D 16.7 units, E 66.7 mg, B_1 16.7 mg, B_2 8.3 mg, B_3 31.7 mg, B_5 66.7 mg, B_6 16.7 mg, B_{12} 16.7 mcg, C 200 mg, folic acid 0.13 mg, Zn 5 mg, Ca, Cr, I, K, Mg, Mn, Mo, Se, Si, V, biotin 50 mcg, SOD, l-lysine. Tab. Bot. 180s. *OTC.*
Use: Mineral, vitamin supplement.
Maximum Pain Relief Pamprin. (Chattem) Acetaminophen 250 mg, magnesium salicylate 250 mg, pamabrom 25 mg. Capl. Bot. 16s, 32s. *OTC.*
Use: Analgesic combination.
Maximum Red Label. (Vitaline) Iron 3.3 mg, vitamins A 2500 units, D 67 units, E 66.7 mg, B_1 16.7 mg, B_2 8.3 mg, B_3 31.7 mg, B_5 66.7 mg, B_6 16.7 mg, B_{12} 16.7 mcg, C 200 mg, folic acid 0.13 mg, Zn 5 mg, Ca, Cr, Su, I, K, Mg, Mo, Se, Si, V, biotin 50 mcg, choline, inositol, bioflavonoids, l-lysine, PABA. Tab. Bot. 180s. *OTC.*
Use: Mineral, vitamin supplement.
Maximum Relief ex•lax. (Novartis) Sennosides 25 mg, sucrose. Tab. Bot. 24s, 48s. *OTC.*
Use: Laxative.
Maximum Strength Anbesol. (Whitehall) Benzocaine 20%. Alcohol 50%, saccharin. Liq. Bot. 9 mL. *OTC.*
Use: Topical local anesthetic.
Maximum Strength Aqua-Ban. (Thompson Medical) Pamabrom 50 mg, lactose. Tab. Bot. 30s. *OTC.*
Use: Diuretic.
Maximum Strength Benadryl. (Parke-Davis) **Cream:** Diphenhydramine hydrochloride 2%, parabens in a greaseless base. Jar 15 g. **Spray, nonaerosol:** Diphenhydramine hydrochloride 2%, alcohol 85%. Bot. 60 mL. *OTC.*
Use: Antihistamine, topical.
Maximum Strength Benadryl Itch Relief. (Warner Lambert) Diphenhydramine hydrochloride. **Cream:** 2%, zinc acetate 1%, parabens, aloe vera. 14.2 g. **Stick:** 2%, zinc acetate 1%. Alcohol 73.5%, aloe vera. 14 mL. *OTC.*
Use: Antihistamine.
Maximum Strength Clearasil Clearstick.
See: Clearasil.
Maximum Strength Clearasil Clearstick for Sensitive Skin.
See: Clearasil.
Maximum Strength Cortaid. (Pharmacia) Hydrocortisone 1% in parabens, mineral oil, white petrolatum. Oint. Tube 15 g, 30 g. *OTC.*
Use: Corticosteroid, topical.
Maximum Strength Cortaid Faststick. (Pharmacia) Hydrocortisone 1%,

alcohol 55%, methylparaben. Stick, roll-on. 14 g. *OTC.*
Use: Corticosteroid, topical.

Maximum Strength Dristan. (Whitehall-Robins) Pseudoephedrine hydrochloride 30 mg, acetaminophen 500 mg. Cap. Bot. 24s, 48s, 100s. *OTC.*
Use: Decongestant, analgesic.

Maximum Strength Dristan Cold. (Whitehall-Robins) Pseudoephedrine hydrochloride 30 mg, brompheniramine maleate 2 mg, acetaminophen 500 mg. Capl. Pkg. 16s, Bot. 36s. *OTC.*
Use: Decongestant, analgesic, antihistamine.

Maximum Strength D-2000. (21st Century) Cholecalciferol 2,000 units. Calcium 180 mg. Gluten free. Tab. 110s. *OTC.*
Use: Fat-soluble vitamin.

Maximum Strength Dynafed Plus. (BDi) Acetaminophen 500 mg, pseudoephedrine 30 mg. Tab. Bot. 30s. *OTC.*
Use: Analgesic, decongestant.

Maximum Strength Flexall 454. (Chattem) Menthol 16%, aloe vera gel, eucalyptus oil, methyl salicylate, SD alcohol 38-B, thyme oil. Gel Tube 90 g. *OTC.*
Use: Liniment.

Maximum Strength Halls-Plus. (Warner Lambert) Menthol 10 mg, corn syrup, sucrose. Loz. Pkg. 10s, 20s. *OTC.*
Use: Anesthetic.

Maximum Strength Ivarest. (Blistex) Calamine 14%, diphenhydramine hydrochloride 2%. Lanolin oil, petrolatum, propylene glycol. Cream. 56 g. *OTC.*
Use: Poison ivy treatment.

Maximum Strength KeriCort-10. (Bristol-Myers Squibb) Hydrocortisone 1%, parabens, cetyl alcohol, stearyl alcohol. Cream Tube 56.7 g. *OTC.*
Use: Corticosteroid, topical.

Maximum Strength Meted. (Sirius Labs) Sulfur 5%, salicylic acid 3%. Shampoo. Bot. 118 mL. *OTC.*
Use: Antiseborrheic combination.

Maximum Strength Nasal Decongestant. (Taro) Oxymetazoline hydrochloride 0.05%, 0.002% phenylmercuric acetate, benzalkonium chloride. Spray Bot. 15 mL, 30 mL. *OTC.*
Use: Decongestant.

Maximum Strength No-Aspirin Sinus Medication. (Walgreen) Acetaminophen 500 mg, pseudoephedrine hydrochloride 30 mg. Tab. Bot. 50s. *OTC.*
Use: Analgesic, decongestant.

Maximum Strength NoDoz. (Novartis Consumer Health) Caffeine 200 mg, sucrose. Tab. Pkg. 36s. *OTC.*
Use: CNS stimulant, analeptic.

Maximum Strength Orajel Gel. (Del) Benzocaine 20%, saccharin. Tube 9.45 mL. *OTC.*
Use: Anesthetic, local.

Maximum Strength Orajel Liquid. (Del) Benzocaine 20%, ethyl alcohol 44.2%, phenol, tartrazine, saccharin. Liq. Bot. 13.3 mL. *OTC.*
Use: Anesthetic, local.

Maximum Strength Ornex. (Menley & James Labs, Inc.) Pseudoephedrine hydrochloride 30 mg, acetaminophen 500 mg. Cap. Bot. 24s, 48s. *OTC.*
Use: Analgesic, decongestant.

Maximum Strength Sine-Aid. (McNeil Consumer) Pseudoephedrine hydrochloride 30 mg, acetaminophen 500 mg. Cap., Tab., or Gelcap. **Cap. & Tab.:** Bot. 50s. **Gelcaps:** Bot. 40s. *OTC.*
Use: Analgesic, decongestant.

Maximum Strength Sinutab Nighttime. (Warner Lambert) Pseudoephedrine hydrochloride 10 mg, diphenhydramine hydrochloride 8.33 mg, acetaminophen 167 mg/5 mL. Liq. Alcohol free. 120 mL. *OTC.*
Use: Analgesic, antihistamine, decongestant.

Maximum Strength Sinutab Without Drowsiness. (Warner Lambert) Pseudoephedrine hydrochloride 30 mg, acetaminophen 500 mg. Tab. or Capl. Bot. 24s, 48s (tab. only). *OTC.*
Use: Analgesic, decongestant.

Maximum Strength Sudafed Severe Cold Formula. (McNeil-PPC) Dextromethorphan HBr 15 mg, pseudoephedrine hydrochloride 30 mg, acetaminophen 500 mg. Tab. 10s. *OTC.*
Use: Analgesic, antitussive, decongestant.

Maximum Strength Sudafed Sinus. (McNeil-PPC) Pseudoephedrine hydrochloride 30 mg, acetaminophen 500 mg. Tab. or Capl. Bot. 24s, 48s. *OTC.*
Use: Analgesic, decongestant.

Maximum Strength Wart Remover. (Stiefel) Salicylic acid 17%, alcohol 29%, castor oil, flexible collodion. Liq. 13.3 mL. *OTC.*
Use: Keratolytic.

Maxiphen DM. (MCR American) Dextromethorphan HBr 20 mg, guaifenesin 400 mg, phenylephrine hydrochloride 10 mg. Tab. 100s. *Rx.*
Use: Upper respiratory combination, antitussive and expectorant.

Maxiphen-G DM. (AMBI) Dextromethorphan HBr 30 mg, phenylephrine hydrochloride 20 mg, guaifenesin 1000 mg. ER Tab. 100s. *Rx.*
Use: Upper respiratory combination, antitussive and expectorant combination.

Maxipime. (Hospira) Cefepime hydrochloride 500 mg, 1 g, 2 g. Inj., Pow. for Soln. (contains arginine). Single-dose vial, *ADD-Vantage* single-dose vial (except 500 mg). *Rx.*
Use: Anti-infective, cephalosporin and related antibiotic.

Maxitrol Ointment. (Alcon) Dexamethasone 0.1%, neomycin 0.35%, polymyxin B sulfate 10,000 units/g. Tube 3.5 g. *Rx.*
Use: Anti-infective, ophthalmic.

Maxitrol Ophthalmic Suspension. (Alcon) Dexamethasone 0.1%, neomycin (as sulfate) 0.35%, polymyxin B sulfate 10,000 units/mL, benzalkonium chloride 0.004%, hydroxypropyl methylcellulose 0.5%, hydrochloric acid, sodium chloride, polysorbate 20, sodium hydroxide. *Drop-Tainer* 5 mL. *Rx.*
Use: Anti-infective, ophthalmic; steroid antibiotic combination.

Maxi-Tuss DM. (MCR American) Dextromethorphan HBr 20 mg, guaifenesin 200 mg per 5 mL. Glucose, menthol, parabens, saccharin, black cherry flavor. Liq. Bot. 473 mL. *Rx.*
Use: Upper respiratory combination, antitussive, expectorant.

Maxi-Tuss HC. (MCR American) Hydrocodone bitartrate 2.5 mg, chlorpheniramine maleate 4 mg, phenylephrine hydrochloride 10 mg per 5 mL. Liq. Bot. 473 mL. *c-III.*
Use: Upper respiratory combination, antitussive, antihistamine, decongestant.

Maxivate. (Bristol-Myers Squibb) Betamethasone dipropionate 0.05%. Cream. Oint. Tube 15 g. 45 g. *Rx.*
Use: Corticosteroid, topical.

Maxi-Vite. (Ivax) Vitamins A 10,000 units, D 400 units, E 15 mg, B_1 10 mg, B_2 10 mg, B_3 100 mg, B_5 20 mg, B_6 5 mg, B_{12} 5 mcg, C 200 mg, Ca 53.5 mg, Fe 1.5 mg, folic acid 0.4 mg, biotin 1 mcg, I, P, Cu, Mg, Mn, Zn 1.5 mg, PABA, rutin, glutamic acid, inositol, choline bitartrate, bioflavonoids, l-lysine, betaine, lecithin. Tab. Bot. 60s. *OTC.*
Use: Mineral, vitamin supplement.

Maxovite. (Tyson) Vitamins A 2083 units, D 16.7 units, E 16.7 mg, B_1 5 mg, B_2 4.2 mg, B_3 4.2 mg, B_5 4.2 mg, B_6 54.2 mg, B_{12} 10.8 mcg, C 250 mg, folic acid 0.33 mg, Zn 5 mg, Ca, Cr, Cu, Fe, I, K, Mg, Mn, Se, biotin 11.7 mcg. Tab. Bot. 120s, 240s. *OTC.*
Use: Mineral, vitamin supplement.

Maxzide. (Bertek) Hydrochlorothiazide 50 mg, triamterene 75 mg. Tab. Bot. 100s, 500s, UD 100s. *Rx.*
Use: Antihypertensive; diuretic.

Maxzide-25MG. (Bertek) Triamterene 37.5 mg, hydrochlorothiazide 25 mg. Tab. Bot. 100s, UD 100s. *Rx.*
Use: Diuretic combination.

Mayotic. (Merz) Hydrocortisone 1%, neomycin sulfate 5 mg, polymyxin B sulfate 10,000 units/mL, thimerosal 0.01%. Susp. Bot. 10 mL w/dropper. *Rx.*
Use: Otic.

•**maytansine.** (MAY-tan-SEEN) USAN.
Use: Antineoplastic.

•**mazapertine succinate.** (mazz-ah-PURR-teen) USAN.
Use: Antipsychotic.

Mazicon. (Roche) Flumazenil 0.1 mg/mL. Inj. Vial 5 mL, 10 mL. *Rx.*
Use: Antidote.

•**mazindol.** (MAZE-in-dole) *USP.*
Use: Anorexic; appetite suppressant; Duchenne muscular dystrophy. [Orphan Drug]

M-Caps. (Mill-Mark) Methionine 200 mg. Cap. Bot. 50s, 1000s. *Rx.*
Use: Diaper rash preparation.

M-Clear. (R.A. McNeil) Codeine phosphate 9 mg, guaifenesin 200 mg. Maltodextrin, tartrazine. Cap. 100s. *c-v.*
Use: Upper respiratory combination, antitussive with expectorant.

M-Clear Jr. (R.A. McNeil) Hydrocodone bitartrate 2.5 mg, potassium guaiacolsulfonate 175 mg per 5 mL. Sugar, alcohol, and dye free. Saccharin, sorbitol. Syrup. 473 mL. *c-III.*
Use: Antitussive with expectorant.

M-Clear WC. (R.A. McNeil) Codeine phosphate 6.3 mg, guaifenesin 100 mg per 5 mL. Alcohol and sugar free. PEG, saccharin, sorbitol. Liq. 473 mL. *c-v.*
Use: Upper respiratory combination, antitussive with expectorant.

MCT Oil. (Bristol-Myers Squibb) Triglycerides of medium chain fatty acids. Lipid fraction of coconut oil; fatty acid shorter than C_8 < 6%, C_8 (octanoic) 67%, C_{10} (decanoic) 23%, longer than C_{10} 4%. Bot. Qt. *OTC.*
Use: Nutritional supplement, enteral.

MDP-Squibb. (Bristol-Myers Squibb) Technetium Tc 99 medronate. Reaction vial pkg. 10s.
Use: Radiopaque agent.

MD-76 R. (Mallinckrodt) Diatrizoate meglumine 660 mg, diatrizoate sodium 100 mg, iodine 370 mg/mL. Inj. Vials. 50 mL. Bot. 100 mL, 150 mL, 200 mL. Power injector syringe. 125 mL. *Rx.*
Use: Radiopaque agent, parenteral.

MD-60. (Mallinckrodt) Diatrizoate meglumine 52%, diatrizoate sodium 8% (29.2% iodine). Inj. Vial 30 mL, 50 mL.
Use: Radiopaque agent.

meadinin. Mixture of Amoidin & Amidin alk. of Ammi Majus Linn.

measles, mumps, and rubella virus vaccine live. (MEE-zuhls, mumps, and ru-BELL-uh)
Use: Immunization.
See: M-M-R II.

measles, mumps, rubella, and varicella virus vaccine, live, attenuated.
Use: Immunization.
See: ProQuad.

measles prophylactic serum.
See: Immune Globulin (Intramuscular).

•**measles virus vaccine, live.** (MEE-zuhls) *USP.* Modified live-virus measles vaccine.
Use: Immunization.
W/Mumps virus vaccine, rubella virus vaccine.
See: M-M-R II.

•**mebendazole.** (meh-BEND-uh-zole) *USP.*
Use: Anthelmintic.
See: Vermox.

mebendazole. (Copley) Mebendazole 100 mg. Chew. Tab. Pkg. 12s, 36s. *Rx.*
Use: Anthelmintic.

•**mebeverine hydrochloride.** (MEH-BEH-ver-een) USAN.
Use: Spasmolytic agent; muscle relaxant.

•**mebrofenin.** (MEH-broe-FEN-in) *USP.*
Use: Diagnostic aid (hepatobiliary function determination).

•**mebutamate.** (meh-BYOO-ta-mate) USAN.
Use: Antihypertensive.

•**mecamylamine hydrochloride.** (mek-ah-MILL-ah-meen) *USP.*
Use: Antihypertensive, antiadrenergic.

•**mecasermin.** (mek-a-SER-min) USAN.
Use: Insulin-like growth factor.
See: Increlex.

•**mecetronium ethylsulfate.** (MEH-seh-TROE-nee-uhm ETH-ill-SULL-fate) USAN.
Use: Antiseptic.

mechlorethamine derivative.
Use: Alkylating agent; ethylenimine/methylmelamine.
See: Bendamustine Hydrochloride.

•**mechlorethamine hydrochloride.** (meh-klor-ETH-ah-meen) *USP.*
Use: Antineoplastic, alkylating agent.
See: Mustargen.
Valchlor.

mecholin hydrochloride.
See: Methacholine Chloride.

Mecholyl Ointment. (Gordon Laboratories) Methacholine chloride 0.25%, methyl salicylate 10% in ointment base. Jar 4 oz, 1 lb, 5 lb. *OTC.*
Use: Analgesic, topical.

meclastine. Clemastine.

•**meclizine hydrochloride.** (MEK-lih-zeen) *USP.*
Use: Antinauseant; antiemetic.
See: Antivert.
Antivert/50.
Antivert/25.
Antrizine.
Bonine.
Dizmiss.
Dramamine II.
Dramamine Less Drowsy Formula.
Travel Sickness.

meclizine hydrochloride. (Various Mfr.) Meclizine hydrochloride. **Tab.: 12.5 mg:** Bot. 30s, 60s, 100s, 500s, 1000s, UD 100s. **25 mg:** Bot. 12s, 20s, 30s, 60s, 100s, 500s, 1000s, UD 32s, 100s. **50 mg:** Bot. 100s. **Chew Tab.: 25 mg:** Bot. 20s, 30s, 60s, 100s, 1000s, UD 100s. *Rx-OTC.*
Use: Antiemetic/antivertigo agent.

•**meclocycline.** (meh-kloe-SIGH-kleen) USAN.
Use: Anti-infective.

•**meclofenamate sodium.** (mek-loe-FEN-uh-mate) *USP.*
Use: Nonsteroidal anti-inflammatory agent.

meclofenamate sodium. (Various Mfr.) Meclofenamate sodium 50 mg, 100 mg. Cap. Bot. 100s, 500s, 1000s. *Rx.*
Use: Nonsteroidal anti-inflammatory agent.

•**meclofenamic acid.** (MEH-kloe-fen-AM-ik) USAN.
Use: Anti-inflammatory.

•**mecloqualone.** (MEH-kloe-KWAH-lone) USAN.
Use: Sedative; hypnotic.

•**meclorisone dibutyrate.** (MEH-KLAHR-ih-sone die-BYOO-tih-rate) USAN.
Use: Anti-inflammatory, topical.

•**mecobalamin.** (MEH-koe-BAHL-ah-min) USAN.
Use: Vitamin (hematopoietic).

Mecodrin.
See: Amphetamine.
•**mecrylate.** (MEH-krih-late) USAN.
Use: Surgical aid (tissue adhesive).
mecysteine. Methyl Cysteine.
Medadyne. (Dal-Med Pharmaceuticals) **Liq.:** Methyl benzethonium chloride, benzocaine, tannic acid, camphor, chlorothymol, menthol, benzyl alcohol, alcohol 61%. Bot. 15 mL, 30 mL. **Throat Spray:** Lidocaine, cetyl dimethyl ammonium chloride, ethyl alcohol. Bot. 30 mL. *OTC.*
Use: Mouth and throat preparation.
Meda-Hist Expectorant. (Medwick) Bot. 4 oz, pt, gal.
Use: Decongestant, antitussive.
Medalox Gel. (Davol) Magnesium aluminum hydroxide gel. Bot. 12 oz, pt, gal. *OTC.*
Use: Antacid.
Medamint. (Dal-Med Pharmaceuticals) Benzocaine 10 mg/Loz. Pkg. 12s, 24s. *OTC.*
Use: Mouth and throat preparation.
Medatussin Pediatric. (Dal-Med Pharmaceuticals) Dextromethorphan HBr 5 mg, guaifenesin 50 mg, potassium citrate, citric acid, sorbitol, saccharin. Syr. Bot. 120 mL. *OTC.*
Use: Antitussive, expectorant.
•**medazepam hydrochloride.** (med-AZE-eh-pam) USAN. Under study.
Use: Anxiolytic.
Medebar Plus. (Mallinckrodt) Barium sulfate 100%. Simethicone. Susp. Bot. 1900 mL. 650 mL w/enema tip-tubing assemblies. *Rx.*
Use: Radiopaque agent; GI contrast agent.
Medent. (SJ Pharmaceuticals) Pseudoephedrine hydrochloride 120 mg, guaifenesin 500 mg. Tab. Bot. 100s.
Use: Decongestant, expectorant.
Medent-DMI. (SJ Pharmaceuticals) Dextromethorphan hydrobromide 20 mg, guaifenesin 400 mg, pseudoephedrine hydrochloride 60 mg. Tab. 100s. *OTC.*
Use: Upper respiratory combination, antitussive and expectorant combination.
Mederma. (Merz) PEG-4, onion (allium cepa) extract, xanthan gum, allantoin, fragrance, methylparaben. Gel. Tube. 50 g. *OTC.*
Use: Helps scars appear softer and smoother.
Medescan. (Mallinckrodt) Barium sulfate 2.3%. Sorbitol, saccharin, sodium benzoate. Susp. Bot. 250 mL, 450 mL, 1900 mL. *Rx.*
Use: Radiopaque agent; GI contrast agent.
Medicaine Cream. (Walgreen) Benzocaine 3%, resorcinol 2%. Tube 1.25 oz. *OTC.*
Use: Antipruritic.
Medicated Acne Cleanser. (C & M Pharmacal) Sulfur 4%, resorcinol 2%, SD alcohol 40 11.65%, methylparaben. Lot. Bot. 120 mL. *OTC.*
Use: Dermatologic, acne.
Medicated Body. (Major) Menthol 0.15%, zinc oxide 1%, talc. Pow. 283 g. *OTC.*
Use: Skin protectant.
Medicated Healer. (Walgreen) Strong ammonia soln. 10%, camphor 2.6%. Bot. 6 oz. *OTC.*
Use: Emollient.
Medicated Powder. (Johnson & Johnson) Zinc oxide, talc, fragrance, menthol. Plastic container 3 oz, 6 oz, 11 oz. *OTC.*
Use: Antipruritic.
Medicidin-D. (Medique) Phenylephrine hydrochloride 5 mg, chlorpheniramine maleate 2 mg, acetaminophen 325 mg. Sucrose. Tab. 100s, 200s, 500s. *OTC.*
Use: Upper respiratory combination, decongestant, antihistamine, and analgesic.
Medi-Derm. (Two Hip) Capsaicin 0.035%, menthol 5%, methyl salicylate 20%. Alcohols, cypress oil, glyceryl, propylene glycol, polysorbate 80. Cream 120 g. *OTC.*
Use: Rub and liniment.
Medi-First Extra Strength Pain Relief. (Medique Products) Acetaminophen 110 mg, aspirin 162 mg, caffeine 32.4 mg, salicylamide 152 mg. Tab. 100s, 250s, 500s. *OTC.*
Use: Nonnarcotic analgesic combination.
Medi-First With Lidocaine. (Medique Products) Lidocaine hydrochloride 0.5%, benzalkonium chloride 0.13%. Ethyl alcohol, mineral oil, parabens, paraffin, petrolatum, wax. Cream. Packet. 0.9 g. *OTC.*
Use: Topical local anesthetic combination.
Medihaler-Iso. (3M) Isoproterenol sulfate 80 mcg/actuation. Aer. Inhaler 15 mL (≥ 300 doses) with adapter and 15 mL refill. *Rx.*
Use: Sympathomimetic bronchodilator.
Mediotic-HC. (Dayton) Hydrocortisone 1%, pramoxine hydrochloride 1%, chloroxylenol 0.1%, benzalkonium chloride 0.01%. Drops. Vial. 15 mL with dropper. *Rx.*
Use: Miscellaneous otic preparation.

Medipak. (Armenpharm Ltd.) First-aid kit.

Medi-Phite. (Davol) Vitamins B_1 and B_{12}. Syr. Bot. 4 oz, pt, gal. *OTC.*
Use: Vitamin supplement.

Mediplast. (Beiersdorf) Salicylic acid plaster 40%. Box 25s. *OTC.*
Use: Keratolytic.

Mediplex Plus. (US Pharm) Vitamins E (dl-alpha tocopheryl) 50 units, B_1 25 mg, B_2 10 mg, B_3 100 mg, B_5 25 mg, B_6 10 mg, B_{12} 25 mcg, C 300 mg, folic acid 0.4 mg, Zn 18 mg, Cu, Mg, Mn. Bot. Tab. 100s. *OTC.*
Use: Multivitamin.

Mediplex Tabules. (US Pharm) Vitamins E 60 units, B_1 25 mg, B_2 10 mg, B_3 100 mg, B_5 25 mg, B_6 10 mg, B_{12} 25 mcg, C 300 mg, Zn 4 mg, Cu, Mg, Mn. Bot. 100s. *OTC.*
Use: Mineral, vitamin supplement.

Medi-Quik. (Mentholatum) **Aerosol:** Lidocaine hydrochloride, benzalkonium chloride. 90 mL. **Spray:** Lidocaine 2%, benzalkonium chloride 0.13%, camphor 0.2%, benzyl alcohol. 85 mL. *OTC.*
Use: Antiseptic; anesthetic, local.

•**medorinone.** (MEH-doe-RIH-nohn) USAN.
Use: Cardiovascular agent.

Medotar. (Medco) Coal tar 1%, octoxynol-5, zinc oxide, white petrolatum. Oint. 454 g. *OTC.*
Use: Antipsoriatic; antipruritic.

•**medrogestone.** (MEH-droe-JEST-ohn) USAN.
Use: Hormone, progestin.

Medrol. (Upjohn) Methylprednisolone. Lactose, sucrose. Tab. **2 mg:** 100s. **4 mg:** Bot. 30s, 100s, UD 100s. Dosepack 21s. **8 mg:** 25s. **16 mg:** 50s. ADT Pak 14s. **24 mg:** 25s. **32 mg:** 25s. *Rx.*
Use: Corticosteroid.

•**medronate disodium.** (MEH-droe-nate) USAN. *Formerly Disodium Methylene Diphosphonate; MDP.*
Use: Pharmaceutic aid.

•**medronic acid.** (meh-DRAH-nik) USAN.
Use: Pharmaceutic aid.

Medrosphol Hg-197. Merprane.

Medrox. (Pharmaceutica North America) Capsaicin 0.0375%, menthol 5%, methyl salicylate 20%. **Oint.:** Cetyl alcohol, glycerin, parabens, PEG-150. 60 g. **Patch:** Menthol 5%, glycerin, polysorbate 80, aloe vera, EDTA disodium, urea, parabens. 5s. *OTC.*
Use: Rub and liniment.

•**medroxalol.** (meh-DROX-ah-LAHL) USAN.
Use: Antihypertensive.

•**medroxalol hydrochloride.** (meh-DROX-ah-LAHL) USAN.
Use: Antihypertensive.

Medrox-Rx. (Pharmaceutica North America) Methyl salicylate 20%, menthol 7%, capsaicin 0.05%, aloe, cetyl alcohol, glycerin, PEG, phenoxyethanol, triethanolamine. Oint. 120 g. *Rx.*
Use: Rub and liniment.

•**medroxyprogesterone acetate.** (meh-DROX-ee-pro-JESS-tuh-rone) *USP.*
Tall Man: medroxyPROGESTERone
Use: Hormone, progestin.
See: Depo-Provera.
Depo-Sub Q Provera 104.
Provera.
W/Conjugated Estrogens.
See: Premphase.
Prempro.

medroxyprogesterone acetate. (CMC) Medroxyprogesterone acetate 50 mg, 100 mg/mL. Vial 5 mL.
Use: Hormone, progestin.

medroxyprogesterone acetate. (Sicor) Medroxyprogesterone acetate 150 mg/mL. PEG 28.9 mg, polysorbate 80 2.41 mg, sodium chloride 8.68 mg, methylparaben 1.37 mg, propylparaben 0.15 mg. Inj. Vials. 1 mL. *Rx.*
Use: Contraceptive.

medroxyprogesterone acetate. (Wyeth) Medroxyprogesterone acetate 10 mg. Tab. Bot. 50s, 250s. *Rx.*
Use: Sex hormone, progestin.

medroxyprogesterone acetate. (Various Mfr.) Medroxyprogesterone acetate. **Tab.:** 2.5 mg, 5 mg, 10 mg. 100s, 500s, 1,000s. **Inj., Susp.:** 150 mg/mL. May contain parabens, PEG, polysorbate 80. 1 mL vial and prefilled syringe. *Rx.*
Use: Sex hormone, progestin.

MED-Rx. (Iopharm) Pseudoephedrine hydrochloride 60 mg, guaifenesin 600 mg. CR Tab. Box 28s. Guaifenesin 600 mg. CR Tab. Box 28s. *Rx.*
Use: Decongestant, expectorant.

•**medrysone.** (MEH-drih-sone) USAN.
Use: Ophthalmic, corticosteroid, topical.

•**mefenamic acid.** (MEH-fen-AM-ik) *USP.*
Use: Nonsteroidal anti-inflammatory agent.
See: Ponstel.

mefenamic acid. (Paddock) Mefenamic acid 250 mg. Lactose. Cap. 100s. *Rx.*
Use: Nonsteroidal anti-inflammatory agent.

•**mefenidil.** (meh-FEN-ih-dill) USAN.
Use: Cerebral vasodilator.

•**mefenidil fumarate.** (meh-FEN-ih-dill) USAN.
Use: Cerebral vasodilator.

•**mefenorex hydrochloride.** (meh-FEN-oh-rex) USAN. Under study.
Use: Anorexic.

•**mefexamide.** (meh-FEX-am-IDE) USAN.
Use: Stimulant (central).

•**mefloquine hydrochloride.** (MEH-flow-kwin) USAN.
Use: Antimalarial.

mefloquine hydrochloride. (Geneva) Mefloquine hydrochloride 250 mg (equiv. to mefloquine base 228 mg) May contain lactose. Tab. 25s, UD 25s. *Rx.*
Use: Antimalarial.

•**mefruside.** (MEFF-ruh-side) USAN.
Use: Diuretic.

Mega B. (Arco) Vitamins B_1 100 mg, B_2 100 mg, B_3 100 mg, B_5 100 mg, B_6 100 mg, B_{12} 100 mcg, folic acid 100 mcg, d-biotin 100 mcg, PABA 100 mg. Tab. Bot. 100s. *OTC.*
Use: Vitamin supplement.

Megace. (Bristol-Myers Oncology) Megestrol acetate. **Tab.:** 40 mg. Lactose. Bot. 250s, 500s. **Susp.:** 40 mg/mL. Alcohol ≤ 0.06%, sucrose, lemon-lime flavor. Bot. 240 mL. *Rx.*
Use: Sex hormone, progestin.

Megace ES. (Par Pharmaceutical, Inc.) Megestrol acetate 125 mg/mL. Alcohol ≤ 0.06%, sucrose. Lemon-lime flavor. Susp. 150 mL. *Rx.*
Use: Sex hormone, progestin.

Megadophilus. (Natren) *L. acidophilus.* **Cap.:** 2 billion CFU. Preservative free. 30s, 60s, 90s. **Pow.:** 2 billion CFU/g. Preservative free. 1.25 oz, 1.75 oz, 2.5 oz, 3 oz, 4.5 oz. *OTC.*
Use: Probiotic.

Megadophilus Dairy Free. (Natren) *L. acidophilus* 2 billion CFU/g. Preservative free. Pow. 1.75 oz, 3 oz. *OTC.*
Use: Probiotic.

•**megalomicin potassium phosphate.** (meh-GAL-OH-my-sin) USAN.
Use: Anti-infective.

Mega Vegi-Dophilus. (Natren) *L. acidophilus* 2 billion CFU/g. Preservative free. Pow. 2.5 oz, 4.5 oz. *OTC.*
Use: Probiotic.

Megavite Fruits & Veggies. (Mason Vitamins) Iron 18 mg, calcium 120 mg, vitamins A 15,000 units, D 1,200 units, E 15 units, B_1 4.5 mg, B_2 5.1 mg, B_3 20 mg, B_5 30 mg, B_6 2 mg, B_{12} 18 mcg, C 180 mg, folic acid 0.8 mg, Cu, I, Mg, Mn, P, Zn, biotin, choline, inositol, *Nature Fruit, Veggie and Green Proprietary Blend*, PABA. Maltodextrin, soy. Preservative free. Tab. 60s. *OTC.*
Use: Multivitamin with minerals (including iron).

Mega VM-80. (NBTY) Vitamins A 10,000 units, D 1000 units, E 100 mg, B_1 80 mg, B_2 80 mg, B_3 80 mg, B_5 80 mg, B_6 80 mg, B_{12} 80 mcg, C 250 mg, Fe 1.2 mg, folic acid 0.4 mg, Ca 4.5 mg, Zn 3.58 mg, choline, inositol, biotin 80 mcg, PABA, bioflavonoids, betaine, hesperidin, Cu, I, K, Mg, Mn. Tab. Bot. 60s, 100s. *OTC.*
Use: Mineral, vitamin supplement.

•**megestrol acetate.** (meh-JESS-trole) *USP.*
Use: Sex hormone, progestin.
See: Megace.
Megace ES.

megestrol acetate. (Various Mfr.) Megestrol acetate. **Susp.:** 40 mg/mL. Alcohol, sorbitol, sucrose. 240 mL. **Tab.:** 20 mg, 40 mg. Bot. 100s, 500s (40 mg only), UD 100s. Blister pkg. 25s (40 mg only). *Rx.*
Use: Sex hormone, progestin.

meglitinides.
Use: Antidiabetic.
See: Nateglinide.
Repaglinide.

•**meglumine.** (meh-GLUE-meen) *USP.*
Use: Diagnostic aid (radiopaque medium).

meglumine, diatrizoate injection.
Use: Diagnostic aid (radiopaque medium).
See: Cystografin.
Gastrografin.
Hypaque-M 90%.
Hypaque-M 75%.
Hypaque-76.
Reno-M-Dip.
W/Meglumine iodipamide.
See: Sinografin.
W/Sodium diatrizoate.
See: Gastrografin.
Renografin-60.
Renovist II.

meglumine, iodipamide injection.
Use: Diagnostic aid; radiopaque medium.
See: Cholografin Meglumine.
W/Meglumine diatrizoate.
See: Sinografin.

meglumine, iothalamate injection.
Use: Diagnostic aid; radiopaque medium.

•**meglutol.** (MEH-glue-tahl) USAN.
Use: Antihyperlipoproteinemic.

MEK inhibitors.
See: Trametinib.

Mekinist. (GlaxoSmithKline) Trametinib 0.5 mg (equiv. to trametinib dimethyl sulfoxide 0.5635 mg), 2 mg (equiv. to trametinib dimethyl sulfoxide 2.254 mg). Film coated. Mannitol. Tab. 30s. *Rx.*
Use: Kinase inhibitor, MEK inhibitor.

•**melafocon A.** (MEH-lah-FOE-kahn) USAN.
Use: Contact lens material (hydrophobic).

melanoma cell vaccine.
Use: Invasive melanoma. [Orphan Drug]

melanoma vaccine.
Use: Stage III to IV melanoma. [Orphan Drug]

melarsoprol. (Mel B)
Use: Anti-infective.
See: Arsobal.

melatonin.
Use: Treatment of circadian rhythm sleep disorders in blind patients. [Orphan Drug]

melatonin receptor agonists.
Use: Sedative and hypnotic, nonbarbiturate.
See: Ramelteon.
Tasimelteon.

Mel B.
See: Melarsoprol.

•**melengestrol acetate.** (meh-len-JESS-trole) USAN.
Use: Antineoplastic; hormone, progestin.

Melfiat-105 Unicelles. (Numark) Phendimetrazine tartrate 105 mg, sucrose. SR Cap. Bot. 100s. *c-III.*
Use: CNS stimulant, anorexiant.

Melhoral Child Tablet. (Sanofi-Synthelabo) Acetylsalicylic acid. *OTC.*
Use: Analgesic.

melitoxin.
See: Dicumarol.

•**melitracen hydrochloride.** (meh-lih-TRAY-sen) USAN.
Use: Antidepressant.

•**melizame.** (MEH-lih-zame) USAN.
Use: Sweetener.

mellose. Methylcellulose.

Melonex. Metahexamide.
Use: Oral antidiabetic.

•**meloxicam.** (mell-OX-ih-kam) USAN.
Use: Nonsteroidal anti-inflammatory agent.
See: Mobic.

meloxicam. (Roxane) Meloxicam 7.5 mg/5 mL. Oral Susp. 100 mL. *Rx.*
Use: Nonsteroidal anti-inflammatory agent.

meloxicam. (Various Mfr.) Meloxicam 7.5 mg, 15 mg. Tab. 30s, 60s, 100s, 250s, 500s, 1000s. *Rx.*
Use: Nonsteroidal anti-inflammatory agent.

Melpaque HP. (Stratus) Hydroquinone 4% in a sunblocking base of mineral oil, parabens, talc, EDTA, sodium metabisulfite. Cream. Tinted. Tube 14.2 g, 28.4 g. *Rx.*
Use: Dermatologic.

•**melphalan.** (MELL-fuh-lan) *USP.*
Use: Alkylating agent, nitrogen mustard.
See: Alkeran.

melphalan. (Bioniche Pharma Group) Melphalan hydrochloride 50 mg. Inj., lyophilized Pow. For Soln. Single-use vial (with povidone 20 mg) with 10 mL vial of sterile diluents (with sodium citrate 0.2 g, propylene glycol 6 mL, ethanol (96%) 0.52 mL. *Rx.*
Use: Alkylating agent, nitrogen mustard.

Melquin HP. (Stratus) Hydroquinone 4%, mineral oil, petrolatum, cetostearyl alcohol, glycerin, sodium metabisulfite. Vanishing base. Cream. Tube 14.2 g, 28.4 g. *Rx.*
Use: Dermatologic.

•**memantine hydrochloride.** (me-MAN-teen) USAN.
Use: Alzheimer disease.
See: Namenda.
Namenda XR.

MembraneBlue. (Dutch Ophthalmic) Trypan blue 0.15%. Ophth. Soln. 0.5 mL single-use *Luer Lok* with glass syringe. *Rx.*
Use: Ophthalmic surgical adjunct.

•**memotine hydrochloride.** (MEH-moe-teen) USAN.
Use: Antiviral.

•**menabitan hydrochloride.** (meh-NAB-ih-tan) USAN.
Use: Analgesic.

Menactra A/C/Y/W-135. (Sanofi Pasteur) Each 0.5 mL contains 4 mcg each of groups A, C, Y, and W-135. Inj. Soln. Single-dose syringes and vials (conjugated to approximately 48 mcg of diphtheria toxoid protein carrier). Stopper to the vial contains dry, natural latex rubber. *Rx.*
Use: Agent for active immunization, bacterial vaccine.

•**menadiol sodium diphosphate.** (men-ah-DIE-ole) *USP.*
Use: Vitamin (prothrombogenic).

•**menadione.** (men-ah-DIE-ohn) *USP.*
Use: Oral & IM; Vitamin K therapy; vitamin (prothrombogenic).

menadione diphosphate sodium.
See: Menadiol sodium diphosphate.

menaphthene.
See: Menadione.

menaphthone.
See: Menadione.

menaquinone.
See: Menadione.

M-End DMX. (R.A. McNeil) Dexbrompheniramine maleate 0.667 mg, dextromethorphan hydrobromide 10 mg, pseudoephedrine hydrochloride 20 mg. Glycerin, propylene glycol, saccharin, sorbitol, sucralose. Alcohol free, dye free, gluten free, and sugar free. Tutti-frutti flavor. Syrup. 473 mL. *OTC.*
Use: Upper respiratory combination, antitussive combination.

M-End Max D. (R.A. McNeil) Codeine phosphate 6 mg, dexbrompheniramine maleate 0.667 mg, pseudoephedrine hydrochloride 20 mg. Glycerin, propylene glycol, saccharin, sorbitol. Alcohol free, dye free, gluten free, and sugar free. Tutti-frutti flavor. Liq. 473 mL. *c-v.*
Use: Upper respiratory combination, antitussive combination.

M-End PE. (R.A. McNeil) Brompheniramine maleate 1.33 mg, codeine phosphate 6.33 mg, phenylephrine hydrochloride 3.33 mg per 5 mL. Saccharin, sorbitol. Cotton candy flavor. Liq. 354 mL. *c-v.*
Use: Upper respiratory combination, antitussive combination.

M-End WC. (R.A. McNeil) Brompheniramine maleate 1.3 mg, codeine phosphate 6.3 mg, pseudoephedrine hydrochloride 10 mg per 5 mL. Saccharin, sorbitol. Cherry flavor. Liq. 473 mL. *c-v.*
Use: Upper respiratory combination, antitussive combination.

Menest. (Monarch) Esterified estrogens. 0.3 mg, 0.625 mg, 1.25 mg, 2.5 mg. Lactose. Film-coated. Tab. Bot. 50s. (2.5 mg only), 100s (except 2.5 mg). *Rx.*
Use: Estrogen, hormone.

Menhibrix. (GlaxoSmithKline) *Neisseria meningitidis* C capsular polysaccharide 5 mcg, *N. meningitidis* Y capsular polysaccharide 5 mcg, *Haemophilus* b capsular polysaccharide 2.5 mcg (conjugated to tetanus toxoid 5 mcg, 6.5 mcg, and 6.25 mcg, respectively) per 0.5 mL (after reconstitution) (also contains *Tris* (trometamol)-hydrochloride 96.8 mcg, sucrose 12.6 mcg, and residual formaldehyde 0.72 mcg or less. Preservative free. Inj., lyophilized Pow. for Soln. Single-dose vial w/saline diluent. *Rx.*
Use: Vaccine combination.

meningococcal vaccine.
Use: Agent for active immunization, bacterial vaccine.
See: Menactra A/C/Y/W-135.
Menomune A/C/Y/W-135.

•**menoctone.** (meh-NOCK-tone) USAN. Under study.
Use: Antimalarial.

•**menogaril.** (MEN-oh-gar-ILL) USAN.
Use: Antineoplastic.

Menoject L.A. (Merz) Testosterone cypionate, estradiol cypionate. Vial 10 mL. *Rx.*
Use: Androgen; estrogen combination.

Menolyn. (Arcum) Ethinyl estradiol 0.05 mg. Tab. Bot. 100s, 1000s. *Rx.*
Use: Estrogen.

Menomune A/C/Y/W-135. (Sanofi Pasteur) When reconstituted, each 0.5 mL contains 50 mcg isolated product from each of groups A, C, Y, and W-135. Freeze-dried. Lactose 2.5 to 5 mg per dose. Inj. Lyophilized Pow. for Soln. Single-dose vial w/preservative-free distilled water diluent 0.78 mL. 10-dose vial w/diluent 6 mL w/thimerosal 1:10,000 (stopper to vial contains dry, natural latex rubber). *Rx.*
Use: Immunization.

Menopur. (Ferring) Follicle-stimulating hormone activity 75 units, luteinizing hormone activity 75 units. Pow. or Pellets for Inj., lyophilized. In vials with diluent. *Rx.*
Use: Ovulation stimulant.

Menostar. (Bayer HealthCare) Estradiol 1 mg (0.014 mg/day). Transdermal system. 4s. *Rx.*
Use: Sex hormone, estrogen.

•**menotropins.** (MEN-oh-trope-inz) USAN. *Formerly Human Follicle-Stimulating Hormone.*
Use: Sex hormone; ovulation stimulant; gonadotropin; gonad-stimulating principle.
See: Follistim AQ.
Menopur.
Pergonal.
Repronex.

Men-Phor. (Geritrex) Camphor 0.5%, menthol 0.5%, carbopol, cetearyl alcohol, cetyl alcohol, hydantoin, castor oil, petrolatum. Lot. 222 mL. *OTC.*
Use: Topical combination.

Mentane. (Hoechst) Velnacrine.
Use: Cholinesterase inhibitor for Alzheimer disease.

Mentax. (Mylan) Butenafine hydrochloride 1%. Benzyl and cetyl alcohol, glycerin, white petrolatum. Cream. Tubes.

15 g, 30 g. *Rx.*
Use: Anti-infective, antifungal, topical.
Menthoderm. (Pharmaceutica North America) Methyl salicylate 15%, menthol 10%. Glycerin, parabens, polysorbate 20, propylene glycol, tartrazine, triethanolamine, SD-alcohol, urea. Oint. 60 g, 120 g. *OTC.*
Use: Rub and liniment.
•**menthol.** (MEN-thole) *USP.*
Use: Topical antipruritic; local analgesic; nasal decongestant; antitussive.
See: Absorbine Jr Back Patch.
Bengay Patch.
Biofreeze.
Blue Gel Muscular Pain Reliever.
Blue Ice.
Breathe Right Children's Colds.
Breathe Right Colds.
Cēpacol Menthol Regular Strength.
Cold & Hot Pain Relief Therapy Patch.
Flexall.
Gold Bond Pain Relieving Foot Roll-On.
Icy Hot Back Pain Relief.
Icy Hot Pain Relieving Gel.
Icy Hot PM Medicated.
Icy Hot Pop & Peel.
Icy Hot Pro-Therapy.
Icy Hot Roll.
Menthol Cough Drops.
Mineral Freez.
N'Ice.
Ricola Herb Throat Drops.
Stopain Cold Pain Relieving.
Stopain Cold Roll-On.
Stopain Cold Spray.
Therapy Ice.
Victors.
Zims Max Freeze.
See: Allantoin, Camphor.
Nose Better.
W/Benzethonium Chloride.
See: Gold Bond Antiseptic First Aid Quick Spray.
W/Benzocaine.
See: Cēpacol Maximum Numbing Sore Throat.
Cēpacol Sore Throat Pain Relief Maximum Numbing.
Sting-Kill.
W/Benzocaine, Camphor.
See: Chiggerex.
W/Benzocaine, Cetylpyridinium Chloride.
See: Orasep.
W/Benzocaine, Methyl Salicylate.
See: Dendracin Neurodendtraxcin.
W/Camphor.
See: Mentholatum.
TheraPatch Vapor Patch for Kids Cough Suppressant.
Tiger Balm.
Tom's of Maine Natural Cough & Cold Rub Cough Suppressant.
W/Camphor, Eucalyptus Oil.
See: Vicks VapoRub.
W/Camphor, Methyl Salicylate.
See: Bayer Muscle and Joint.
W/Capsaicin.
See: Capzasin Quick Relief.
Zostrix Hot and Cold Therapy.
W/Capsaicin, Lidocaine, Methyl Salicylate.
See: Terocin.
W/Capsaicin, Methyl Salicylate.
See: Bio-Therm Pain Relieving Lotion.
Medi-Derm.
Medrox.
New Terocin.
Ultracin.
Xoten-C Pain Relief.
Ziks.
W/Combinations.
See: Cēpacol Sore Throat.
Cēpacol Sore Throat From Post Nasal Drip.
Chloraseptic Kids Sore Throat.
Chloraseptic Sore Throat.
Chloraseptic Sore Throat Relief.
Eucalyptamint.
Eucalyptamint Maximum Strength.
Hall's Mentho-Lyptus Sugar Free.
W/Lidocaine Hydrochloride.
See: LenzaGel.
LenzaPatch.
W/Methyl Nicotinate, Methyl Salicylate.
See: Musterole Deep Strength.
W/Methyl Salicylate.
See: Analgesic Balm.
Analgesic Balm-GRX.
Icy Hot Chill Stick.
Menthoderm.
Pain Bust-R II.
Pain Relieving Rub.
W/Zinc Oxide.
See: Calmasyn.
Calmoseptine.
Mentholatum. (Mentholatum Co.) Menthol 1.3%, camphor 9%. Petrolatum. Oint. Tube 28 g, 84 g. *OTC.*
Use: Upper respiratory combination, topical.
Mentholatum Cherry Chest Rub for Kids. (Mentholatum Co.) Camphor 4.7%, menthol 2.6%, eucalyptus oil 1.2%. Petrolatum. Oint. Tube 28 g. *OTC.*
Use: Upper respiratory combination, topical.
Mentholatum Deep Heating Lotion. (Mentholatum Co.) Menthol 6%, methyl salicylate 20%, lanolin derivative in lotion base. Bot. 2 oz, 4 oz. *OTC.*
Use: Analgesic, topical.

Mentholatum Deep Heating Rub. (Mentholatum Co.) Menthol 5.8%, methyl salicylate 12.7%, eucalyptus oil, turpentine oil, anhydrous lanolin, vehicle and fragrance. Tube 1.25 oz, 3.33 oz, 5 oz. *OTC.*
Use: Analgesic, topical.

Menthol Cough Drops. (Major) Menthol 6.5 mg. Eucalyptus oil, glucose syrup, sucrose. Lozenges. 30s. *OTC.*
Use: Mouth and throat product.

Mentholin. (Apco) Methyl salicylate 30%, chloroform 20%, hard soap 3%, camphor gum 2.2%, menthol 0.8%, alcohol 35%. Bot. 2 oz. *OTC.*
Use: Analgesic, topical.

menthyl anthranilate.
See: Meradimate

Menveo. (Novartis) Serogroups A 10 mcg, C 5 mcg, Y 5 mcg, W-135 5 mcg per 0.5 mL. Preservative free. Inj., lyophilized Pow. for Soln. Single-dose vial (supplied as a vial containing group A meningococcal (MenA) lyophilized conjugate component and a vial containing MenCYW-135 liquid. *Rx.*
Use: Agent for active immunization, bacterial vaccine.

•**meobentine sulfate.** (meh-OH-BEN-teen) USAN.
Use: Cardiovascular agent (antiarrhythmic).

mepacrine hydrochloride.
Use: Anthelmintic; antimalarial.

•**mepartricin.** (meh-PAR-trih-sin) USAN.
Use: Antifungal; antiprotozoal.

mepavlon. Meprobamate.

•**mepenzolate bromide.** (meh-PEN-zoe-late) *USP.*
Use: Anticholinergic.
See: Cantil.

mepenzolate methyl bromide. Mepenzolate bromide.
Use: Anticholinergic.

•**meperidine hydrochloride.** (meh-PEHR-ih-deen) *USP.*
Use: Opioid analgesic.
See: Demerol.

meperidine hydrochloride. (Hospira) Meperidine hydrochloride 10 mg/mL. Inj. Single-dose container (this vial only for use with a compatible Hospira *PCA* pump set with injector and a compatible Hospira infusion device). 30 mL. *c-II.*
Use: Opioid analgesic.

meperidine hydrochloride. (Roxane) Meperidine hydrochloride 50 mg/5 mL. Sorbitol. Oral Soln. 500 mL. *c-II.*
Use: Opioid analgesic.

meperidine hydrochloride. (Various Mfr.) Meperidine hydrochloride **Tab.:** 50 mg, 100 mg. Bot. 100s, 500s, 1000s, UD 25s. **Inj.:** 25 mg/mL, 50 mg/mL, 75 mg/mL, 100 mg/mL. Vials. 1 mL. Amps. 1 mL. *c-II.*
Use: Opioid analgesic.

mephenesin.
Use: Muscle relaxant.
See: Myanesin.

mephenesin carbamate. Methoxydone.

•**mephobarbital.** (meh-foe-BAR-bih-tahl) *USP.*
Use: Anticonvulsant; hypnotic; sedative.

mephone. Mephentermine.

Mephyton. (Valeant) Phytonadione (vitamin K) 5 mg. Lactose. Tab. Bot. 100s. *Rx.*
Use: Fat-soluble vitamin.

Mepiben. (Schein) Methylpiperidyl benzhydryl ether.
Use: Antihistamine.

mepiperphenidol bromide.
Use: Anticholinergic.

•**mepivacaine hydrochloride.** (meh-PIHV-ah-cane) *USP.*
Use: Anesthetic, local amide.
See: Carbocaine.
Polocaine.
Polocaine MPF.
Scandonest.
W/Levonordefrin.
See: Carbocaine with Neo-Cobefrin.
Scandonest L.

mepivacaine hydrochloride. (Septodont) Mepivacaine hydrochloride 3%. Inj. Dental Cart. 1.8 mL. *Rx.*
Use: Anesthetic, local amide.

•**meprednisone.** (meh-PRED-nih-sone) *USP.*
Use: Corticosteroid, topical.

•**meprobamate.** (meh-pro-BAM-ate) *USP.*
Use: Anxiolytic; hypnotic; sedative; antianxiety agent.
See: Arcoban.
W/Conjugated Estrogens.
See: PMB 400.
PMB 200.

meprobamate. (Various Mfr.) Meprobamate 200 mg, 400 mg. Tab. Bot. 20s, 100s, 500s (400 mg only), 1000s, UD 100s (400 mg only). *c-IV.*
Use: Antianxiety agent.

meprobamate/aspirin. (Various Mfr.) Aspirin 325 mg, meprobamate 200 mg. Tab. Bot. 100s, 500s. *Rx.*
Use: Analgesic combination.

meprobamate/benactyzine.
Use: Miscellaneous psychotherapeutic agent.

meprobamate, n-isopropyl.
See: Carisoprodol.
Meprogesic Q. (Various Mfr.) Aspirin 325 mg, meprobamate 200 mg. Tab. Bot. 100s, 500s. *Rx.*
Use: Analgesic combination.
Meprolone Tabs. (Major) Methylprednisolone 4 mg. Bot. 25s, 100s. *Rx.*
Use: Corticosteroid.
Mepron. (GlaxoSmithKline) Atovaquone 750 mg/5 mL. Susp. Bot. 210 mL. *Rx.*
Use: Anti-infective.
meprylcaine hydrochloride.
Use: Anesthetic, local.
•**meptazinol hydrochloride.** (mep-TAZE-ih-nahl) USAN.
Use: Analgesic.
mepyrapone.
See: Metopirone.
•**mequidox.** (MEH-kwih-dox) USAN. Under study.
Use: Anti-infective.
•**mequinol.** (MEH-kwih-noll) USAN.
Use: Hyperpigmentation.
mequinolate. Name used for Proquinolate.
•**meradimate.** (mer-ADD-ih-mate) USAN. *Formerly menthyl anthranilate.*
Use: Sunscreen.
•**meralein sodium.** (MER-ah-leen) USAN.
Use: Anti-infective, topical.
merbromin. *OTC.*
Use: Antiseptic, topical.
•**mercaptopurine.** (mer-cap-toe-PURE-een) *USP.*
Use: Antineoplastic.
See: Purinethol.
Purixan.
mercaptopurine. (PAR) Mercaptopurine 50 mg. May contain lactose. Tab. 25s, 30s, 60s, 250s. *Rx.*
Use: Antineoplastic.
mercazole.
See: Methimazole.
•**mercufenol chloride.** (MER-cue-FEEN-ole) USAN.
Use: Anti-infective, topical.
mercuranine.
See: Merbromin.
mercurial, antisyphilitics. Mercuric oleate, mercuric salicylate.
mercuric oleate. Oleate of mercury.
Use: Parasitic and fungal skin diseases.
mercuric oxide ophthalmic ointment, yellow.
Use: Local anti-infective, ophthalmic.
mercuric salicylate. Mercury subsalicylate.
Use: Parasitic and fungal skin diseases.
mercuric succinimide. Bis-Succinimidatomercury.
mercurochrome.
See: Merbromin.
•**mercury, ammoniated.** (mer-cue-REE, ah-MOHN-ee-ated) *USP.*
Use: Anti-infective, topical.
mercury compounds.
See: Antiseptic, Mercurials.
mercury oleate. $Mercury^{++}$ oleate.
Use: Pharmaceutic aid.
mercury-197-203.
See: Chlormerodrin.
Merdex. (Faraday) Docusate sodium 100 mg. Tab. Vial 60 mL. *Rx-OTC.*
Use: Laxative.
•**mericitabine.** (MER-i-SYE-ta-been) USAN.
Use: Treatment of hepatitis C.
•**merimepodib.** (me-ri-ME-poe-dib) USAN.
Use: Inosine monophosphate dehydrogenase inhibitor.
•**merisoprol acetate Hg 197.** (mer-EYE-so-prole) USAN.
Use: Radiopharmaceutical.
•**merisoprol acetate Hg 203.** (mer-EYE-so-prole) USAN.
Use: Radiopharmaceutical.
Meritene Powder. (Novartis) Vanilla flavor: Specially processed nonfat dry milk, corn syrup solids, sucrose, fructose, calcium caseinate, sodium chloride, natural and artificial flavors, lecithin, vitamins and minerals. Can 1 lb, 4.5 lb, 25 lb. Packet 1.14 oz. Vanilla, chocolate, eggnog, milk chocolate, plain flavors. *OTC.*
Use: Nutritional supplement.
merodicein. Sodium meralein.
•**meropenem.** (meh-row-PEN-em) USAN.
Use: Anti-infective.
See: Merrem I.V.
meropenem. (Various Mfr.) Meropenem 500 mg, 1 g. Sodium 45.1 mg (500 mg), 90.2 mg (1 g). Inj., Pow. for Soln. Vial. 20 mL, 30 mL. *Rx.*
Use: Anti-infective agent, carbapenem.
meroxapol 105.
Use: Irrigating solution.
See: Saf-Clens.
merprane.
Use: Diagnostic aid.
Merrem I.V. (AstraZeneca) Meropenem 500 mg, 1 g. Pow. for Inj. Vial 20 mL, 30 mL. *Rx.*
Use: Anti-infective.
Mervan. (Continental Pharma, Belgium) Alclofenac.
Use: Anti-inflammatory.
•**mesalamine.** (me-SAL-uh-MEEN) *USP.*
Use: Anti-inflammatory.
See: Apriso.

Asacol HD.
Canasa.
Delzicol.
Lialda.
Pentasa.
Rowasa.
sfRowasa.

mesalamine. (Various Mfr.) Mesalamine 4 g/60 mL. May contain EDTA, potassium metabisulfite. Enemas. 7s in disposable bot. *Rx.*
Use: Treatment of inflammatory bowel disease.

mescomine.
See: Methscopolamine Bromide.

•**meseclazone.** (meh-SAK-lah-zone) USAN.
Use: Anti-inflammatory.

Mesehist DM. (Trigen Laboratories) Chlorpheniramine maleate 2 mg, dextromethorphan hydrobromide 15 mg, pseudoephedrine hydrochloride 15 mg per 5 mL. Parabens, potassium citrate, potassium sorbate, propylene glycol, sorbitol, sucralose. Alcohol free and sugar free. Orange flavor. Liq. 473 mL. *Rx.*
Use: Upper respiratory combination, antitussive combination.

Mesehist WC. (Trigen Laboratories) Brompheniramine maleate 1.3 mg, codeine phosphate 6.3 mg, pseudoephedrine hydrochloride 10 mg. Cherry flavoring, parabens, potassium citrate, potassium sorbate, propylene glycol, sorbitol, sucralose. Alcohol free and sugar free. Liq. 473 mL. *c-v.*
Use: Upper respiratory combinations, antitussive combination.

•**mesifilcon A.** (MEH-sih-FILL-kahn A) USAN.
Use: Contact lens material; hydrophilic.

•**mesna.** (MESS-nah) USAN.
Use: Cytoprotective agent.
See: Mesnex.

mesna. (Baxter) Mesna 400 mg. Lactose. Film-coated. Tab. 10 blisters. *Rx.*
Use: Cytoprotective agent.

mesna. (Various Mfr.) Mesna 100 mg/mL. Benzyl alcohol 10.4 mg, EDTA 0.25 mg/mL. Inj. Multidose vials. 10 mL. *Rx.*
Use: Cytoprotective agent.

Mesnex. (Baxter) Mesna. **Inj.:** 100 mg/mL. EDTA 0.25 mg/mL, benzyl alcohol 10.4 mg. Multidose vials. 10 mL. **Tab.:** 400 mg. Lactose, simethicone. Film-coated. Blisters. 10. *Rx.*
Use: Antidote; cytoprotective agent.

•**mespiperone C 11.** (meh-SPIH-peh-rone c 11) USAN.
Use: Radiopharmaceutical.

•**mesterolone.** (MESS-TER-oh-lone) USAN.
Use: Androgen.

mestibol. Monomestrol.

Mestinon. (ICN) Pyridostigmine bromide. **ER Tab.:** 180 mg. 30s. **Syrup:** 60 mg/5 mL. Sucrose, sorbitol, alcohol 5%, raspberry flavor. 480 mL. **Tab.:** 60 mg. Lactose. 100s, 500s. *Rx.*
Use: Muscle stimulant.

•**mestranol.** (MESS-trah-nole) *USP.*
Use: Contraceptive; estrogen.
W/Ethynodiol Diacetate.
See: Ovulen-28.
Ovulen-21.
W/Norethindrone.
See: Necon 1/50.
Norinyl.
Norinyl 1 + 50.
W/Norethynodrel.
See: Enovid-E 21.

•**mesuprine hydrochloride.** (MEH-suh-PREEN) USAN.
Use: Vasodilator; muscle relaxant.

Metabolin. (Thurston) Vitamins A 833 units, D 66 units, B_1 833 mcg, B_2 500 mcg, B_6 0.083 mcg, calcium pantothenate 833 mcg, niacinamide 5 mg, folic acid 0.066 mcg, p-aminobenzoic acid 0.416 mcg, inositol 833 mcg, B_{12} 500 mcg, C 5 mg, Ca 33.1 mg, P 14.6 mg, Fe 2.5 mg, I 0.15 mg. Tab. Bot. 100s, 500s, 1000s. *OTC.*
Use: Mineral, vitamin supplement.

•**metabromsalan.** (MET-ah-BROME-sah-lan) USAN.
Use: Antimicrobial; disinfectant.

metabutethamine hydrochloride.
Use: Anesthetic, local.

metabutoxycaine hydrochloride.
Use: Anesthetic, local.

metacaraphen hydrochloride.
See: Netrin.

metacortandracin.
See: Prednisone.

metacortandralone.
See: Prednisolone.

metacortin.
See: Meticorten.

•**metacresol.** (met-ah-KREE-sole) *USP.*
Use: Antiseptic, topical; antifungal.

Metadate CD. (UCB) Methylphenidate hydrochloride 10 mg, 20 mg, 30 mg, 40 mg, 50 mg, 60 mg. PEG, sugar. ER Cap. 100s. *c-II.*
Use: Central nervous system stimulant.

Metadate ER. (Celltech) Methylphenidate hydrochloride 20 mg. Cetyl alcohol, lactose, color-additive free. ER Tab. 100s.

c-II.
Use: Central nervous system stimulant.

meta-delphene. Diethyltoluamide.

Metafolbic. (Breckenridge Pharmaceuticals) Vitamins B_2 5 mg, B_6 50 mg, B_{12} 1,000 mcg, L-methylfolate calcium 6 mg. Gluten free, lactose free. Tab. 90s. *Rx.*
Use: Multivitamin.

Metaglip. (Bristol-Myers Squibb) Glipizide/metformin hydrochloride 2.5 mg/ 250 mg. Film-coated. Tab. 100s. *Rx.*
Use: Antidiabetic combination.

metaglycodol.
Use: Central nervous system depressant.

•**metalol hydrochloride.** (MEH-ta-lahl) USAN. Under study.
Use: Antiadrenergic beta-receptor.

Metamucil. (Procter & Gamble) **Cap.:** Psyllium husk 0.52 g. 100s, 160s. **Pow.:** Psyllium hydrophilic mucilloid, sodium 1 mg, potassium 31 mg/Dose. **Regular Flavor:** w/dextrose. Jar 7 oz, 14 oz, 21 oz. Packette 5.4 g. Box 100s. **Orange and Strawberry Flavors:** w/flavoring, sucrose and coloring. Jar 7 oz, 14 oz, 21 oz. **Wafer:** Psyllium husk 3.4 g, carbohydrates 17 g, sodium 20 mg, fat 5 g, 120 cal/dose, sugar, fructose, molasses, sucrose, cinnamon spice, apple crisp flavors. Ctn. 24s. *OTC.*
Use: Laxative.

Metamucil Instant Mix. (Procter & Gamble) Psyllium hydrophilic mucilloid with citric acid, sucrose, potassium bicarbonate, sodium bicarbonate. Powder when combined with water forms an effervescent, flavored liquid. **Lemon Lime Flavor:** w/calcium carbonate. Cartons of 16, 30, or 100 packets of 3.4 g. **Orange Flavor:** w/flavoring and coloring. Ctn. 16 or 30 packets of 3.4 g. *OTC.*
Use: Laxative.

Metamucil Orange Flavor, Original Texture. (Procter & Gamble) Approximately psyllium husk 3.4 g, carbohydrates 10 g, sodium 5 mg, 40 cal/dose, sucrose. Pow. Can. 210 g, 420 g, 538 g, 630 g. *OTC.*
Use: Laxative.

Metamucil Orange Flavor, Smooth Texture. (Procter & Gamble) Approximately psyllium husk 3.4 g, sodium 5 mg, carbohydrates 12 g, 45 cal/dose, sucrose. Pow. Can. 420 g, 630 g, 1368 g, 100 UD single-dose packs (100s). *OTC.*
Use: Laxative.

Metamucil Original Texture. (Procter & Gamble) Approximately psyllium husk 3.4 g, carbohydrates 6 g, sodium 3 mg, 25 cal/dose, sucrose. Pow. Can. 822 g, Pack. 30. *OTC.*
Use: Laxative.

Metamucil, Sugar Free. (Procter & Gamble) Psyllium hydrophilic mucilloidin sugar-free formula. **Regular Flavor:** Jar 3.7 oz, 7.4 oz, 11.1 oz. Packet 3.4 g. Box 100s. **Orange Flavor:** Jar 3.7 oz, 7.4 oz, 11.1 oz. *OTC.*
Use: Laxative.

Metamucil Sugar Free, Orange Flavor, Smooth Texture. (Procter & Gamble) Approximately psyllium husk 3.4 g, carbohydrates 5 g, sodium 5 mg, 20 cal/ dose, aspartame, phenylalanine 25 mg. Pow. Can. 210 g, 420 g, 630 g, 660 g. *OTC.*
Use: Laxative.

Metamucil, Sugar Free, Smooth Texture. (Procter & Gamble) Approximately psyllium husk 3.4 g, carbohydrates 5 g, sodium 4 mg, 20 cal/dose. Pow. Can. 425 g, Pack. 30s, 100s. *OTC.*
Use: Laxative.

Metandren. (Novartis) Methyltestosterone. **Linguet:** 5 mg, 10 mg Bot. 100s. **Tab.:** 10 mg, 25 mg Bot. 100s. *Rx.*
Use: Androgen.

Metanx. (Pamlab) **Tab.:** Vitamins B_6 35 mg (as pyridoxal-5' phosphate), B_{12} 2,000 mcg (as methylcobalamin), folate 3 mg (as L-methylfolate calcium). 90s, 500s. **Cap.:** Vitamins B_6 35 mg, B_{12} 2,000 mcg, folate 3 mg, algae-S powder 90.314 mg. Glucose free and lactose free. 90s. *OTC.*
Use: Nutritional supplement, multivitamin.

metaphenylbarbituric acid.
See: Mephobarbital.

metaphyllin.
See: Aminophylline.

Metaprel Syrup. (Novartis) Metaproterenol sulfate 10 mg/5 mL. Bot. Pt. *Rx.*
Use: Bronchodilator.

•**metaproterenol polistirex.** (MEH-tuh-pro-TEHR-uh-nahl pahl-ee-STIE-rex) USAN.
Use: Bronchodilator.

•**metaproterenol sulfate.** (MEH-tuh-pro-TEHR-uh-nahl) *USP.*
Use: Bronchodilator, sympathomimetic.

metaproterenol sulfate. (Silarx) Metaproterenol sulfate 10 mg per 5 mL. EDTA, saccharin, sorbitol. Black cherry flavor. Syrup. 473 mL. *Rx.*
Use: Bronchodilator, sympathomimetic.

metaproterenol sulfate. (Various Mfr.) Metaproterenol sulfate 10 mg, 20 mg. Tab. 100s, 1000s. *Rx.*
Use: Bronchodilator, sympathomimetic.

•**metaraminol bitartrate.** (met-uh-RAM-in-ole) *USP.*
Use: Adrenergic; vasopressor.

Metastron. (Medi-Physics, Amersham Healthcare) Strontium-89 chloride 10.9 to 22.6 mg/mL. Preservative free. Inj. Vial 10 mL.
Use: Radiopharmaceutical.

•**metaxalone.** (meh-TAX-ah-lone) USAN.
Use: Muscle relaxant.
See: Skelaxin.

metaxalone. (Various Mfr.) Metaxalone 800 mg. Tab. 100s, 500s, 1,000s. *Rx.*
Use: Skeletal muscle relaxant, centrally acting.

Meted, Maximum Strength. (Medicis) Sulfur 5%, salicylic acid 3%. Shampoo. Bot. 118 mL. *OTC.*
Use: Antiseborrheic combination.

•**meteneprost.** (meh-TEN-eh-PRAHST) USAN.
Use: Oxytocic; prostaglandin.

•**metesind glucuronate.** (MEH-teh-sind glue-CURE-oh-nate) USAN.
Use: Antineoplastic (specific thymidylate synthase inhibitor).

metethoheptazine.
Use: Analgesic.

•**metformin.** (MET-fore-min) USAN.
Tall Man: metFORMIN
Use: Oral hypoglycemic; antidiabetic.
See: Riomet.

•**metformin hydrochloride.** (MET-fore-min) *USP.*
Tall Man: metFORMIN
Use: Antidiabetic agent, biguanide.
See: Fortamet.
Glucophage.
Glucophage XR.
Glumetza.
Riomet.
W/Glipizide.
See: Metaglip.
W/Glyburide.
See: Glucovance.
W/Linagliptin.
See: Jentadueto.
W/Pioglitazone Hydrochloride.
See: ActoPlus Met.
ActoPlus Met XR.
W/Rosiglitazone Maleate.
See: Avandamet.
W/Saxagliptin.
See: Kombiglyze XR.
W/Sitagliptin.
See: Janumet.
Janumet XR.

metformin hydrochloride. (Various Mfr.) Metformin hydrochloride. **ER Tab.:** 500 mg, 750 mg. 100s. **Tab.:** 500 mg, 850 mg, 1,000 mg. Bot. 100s, 500s, 1,000s, 2,000s (500 mg only), UD 100s. *Rx.*
Use: Antidiabetic agent, biguanide.

methacholine bromide. Mecholin bromide.
Use: Cholinergic.

•**methacholine chloride.** (METH-uh-KOH-leen) *USP.*
Use: Cholinergic.
See: Mecholyl Ointment.
Provocholine.

•**methacrylic acid copolymer.** (meth-ah-KRILL-ik ASS-id koe-PAHL-ih-mer) *NF.*
Use: Pharmaceutic aid (tablet coating agent).

•**methacycline.** (meth-ah-SIGH-kleen) USAN.
Use: Anti-infective.

Methadex. (Major) Dexamethasone 0.1%, neomycin 3.5 mg, polymyxin B sulfate 10,000 units. Benzalkonium chloride 0.004%, hypromellose, sodium chloride, polysorbate 20. Ophth. Susp. 5 mL. *Rx.*
Use: Ophthalmic steroid antibiotic combination.

•**methadone hydrochloride.** (METH-uh-dohn) *USP.*
Use: Opioid analgesic; narcotic abstinence syndrome suppressant.
See: Diskets.
Dolophine Hydrochloride.
Methadose.

methadone hydrochloride. (AAI Pharma) Methadone hydrochloride 10 mg/mL. Chlorobutanol 0.5%. Inj. Multidose vial 20 mL. *c-II.*
Use: Opioid analgesic.

methadone hydrochloride. (Roxane) Methadone hydrochloride 5 mg/mL, 10 mg/5 mL. May contain alcohol, sorbitol. Citrus flavor. Oral Soln. 500 mL. *c-II.*
Use: Opioid analgesic.

methadone hydrochloride. (Various Mfr.) Methadone hydrochloride. **Dispersible Tab. for Susp.:** 40 mg. Bot. 100s. **Oral Conc.:** 10 mg/mL. 946 mL, 1 L. **Tab.:** 5 mg, 10 mg. 100s, UD 100s. *c-II.*
Use: Opioid analgesic.

methadone hydrochloride diskets. (Various Mfr.) Methadone hydrochloride 40 mg. Dispersible Tab. Bot. 100s. *c-II.*
Use: Opioid analgesic.

methadone hydrochloride intensol. (Roxane) Methadone hydrochloride 10 mg/mL. Oral Conc. Bot. 30 mg with calibrated dropper. *c-II.*
Use: Opioid analgesic.

Methadose. (Mallinckrodt) Methadone hydrochloride. **Tab.:** 10 mg. 100s. **Disp. Tab.:** 40 mg. 100s. **Oral Conc.:** 10 mg/mL. Sucrose, cherry flavor. Also available sugar free, dye free, unflavored. 1 L. *c-II.*
Use: Opioid analgesic.

•**methadyl acetate.** (METH-ah-dill) USAN.
Use: Analgesic, narcotic.

•**methafilcon B.** (METH-ah-FILL-kahn B) USAN.
Use: Contact lens material (hydrophilic).

Methagual. (Gordon Laboratories) Guaiacol 2%, methyl salicylate 8% in petrolatum. Oint. 2 oz, lb. *OTC.*
Use: Analgesic, topical.

methalamic acid. Name used for lothalamic acid.

•**methalthiazide.** (METH-al-THIGH-ah-zide) USAN.
Use: Antihypertensive; diuretic.

methaminodiazepoxide.
See: Librium.

methamoctol.
Use: Adrenergic.

methamphetamine-dl hydrochloride.
See: dl-Methamphetamine Hydrochloride.

•**methamphetamine hydrochloride.** (meth-am-FET-uh-meen) *USP.*
Use: CNS stimulant, amphetamine.
See: Desoxyn.

methamphetamine hydrochloride. (Mylan) Methamphetamine hydrochloride 5 mg. Lactose. Tab. 100s. *c-II.*
Use: CNS stimulant, amphetamine.

methampyrone.
See: Dipyrone.

methandriol. (Various Mfr.) Methylandrostenediol.

methandriol dipropionate.
See: Arbolic.

Methaphor. (Borden) Protein hydrolysate (l-leucine, l-isoleucine, l-methionine, l-phenylalanine, l-tyrosine); methionine, camphor, benzethonium chloride, in Dermabase vehicle. Oint. Tube 1.5 oz. *OTC.*
Use: Dermatologic, amino acid supplement.

•**methaqualone.** (METH-ah-kwan-lone) USAN.
Use: Hypnotic, sedative.

Methatropic Capsules. (Ivax) Choline 115 mg, inositol 83 mg, methionine 110 mg, vitamins B_1 3 mg, B_2 3 mg, B_3 10 mg, B_5 2 mg, B_6 2 mg, B_{12} 2 mcg, desiccated liver 86 mg. Bot. 100s. *OTC.*
Use: Vitamin supplement.

•**methazolamide.** (meth-ah-ZOLE-ah-mide) *USP.*
Use: Carbonic anhydrase inhibitor.

methazolamide. (Various Mfr.) Methazolamide 25 mg or 50 mg. Tab. Bot. 100s. *Rx.*
Use: Carbonic anhydrase inhibitor.

Methblue 65. (Manne) Methylene blue 65 mg. Tab. Bot. 100s, 1000s. *Rx.*
Use: Antidote, cyanide.

Meth-Choline. (Schein) Choline 115 mg, inositol 83 mg, methionine 110 mg, vitamins B_1 3 mg, B_2 3 mg, B_3 10 mg, B_5 2 mg, B_6 2 mg, B_{12} 2 mcg, desiccated liver 56 mg, liver concentrate 30 mg. Cap. Bot. 100s, 250s, 1000s. *OTC.*
Use: Vitamin supplement.

Meth-Dia-Mer Sulfa. Trisulfapyrimidines. Tab.
Use: Triple sulfonamide therapy.
See: Chemozine.
Triple Sulfa.

Meth-Dia-Mer Sulfonamides Suspension. Trisulfapyrimidines Oral Suspension.
Use: Triple sulfonamide therapy.
See: Chemozine.
Triple Sulfa.

•**methdilazine hydrochloride.** (METH-dill-ah-ZEEN) *USP.*
Use: Antipruritic.

•**methenamine.** (meh-THEN-uh-meen) *USP. Formerly Hexamethylenamine.*
Use: Anti-infective, urinary.
W/Atropine Sulfate, Benzoic Acid, Hyoscyamine Sulfate, Methylene Blue, Phenyl Salicylate.
See: Uritact DS
W/Benzoic Acid, Hyoscyamine Sulfate, Methylene Blue, Phenyl Salicylate.
See: Hyophen.
W/Hyoscyamine Sulfate, Methylene Blue, Phenyl Salicylate, Sodium Biphosphate.
See: Urimax.
W/Hyoscyamine Sulfate, Methylene Blue, Phenyl Salicylate, Sodium Phosphate Monobasic.
See: Phosphasal.
Uticap.
Utrona-C.
W/Hyoscyamine Sulfate, Methylene Blue, Sodium Phosphate Monobasic.
See: Uryl.
W/Combinations.
See: Cystamine.
Cystex.
Cysto.
MHP-A.
Prosed/DS.
Urelle.
Uretron D/S.

Urimar-T.
Urisan-P.
Uriseptic.
Uro Blue.
Urogesic Blue.
Uro Phosphate.

methenamine and monobasic sodium phosphate tablets.
Use: Anti-infective, urinary.

methenamine anhydromethylene citrate. Formanol, uropurgol, urotropin.

•**methenamine hippurate.** (meth-EE-nah-meen HIP-you-rate) *USP.*
Use: Anti-infective, urinary.
See: Hiprex.
Urex.

methenamine hippurate. (CorePharma) Methenamine hippurate 1 g. Saccharin. Tab. 100s. *Rx.*
Use: Anti-infective, methenamine.

methenamine hippurate. (Mylan) Methenamine hippurate 1 g. Saccharin. Tabs. 100s. Rx. Anti-effective, methenamine.

•**methenamine mandelate.** (meth-EE-nah-meen MAN-deh-late) *USP.*
Use: Anti-infective, urinary.
W/Hyoscyamine.
See: Urisedamine.
W/Sodium Acid Phosphate Monobasic Monohydrate.
See: Utac.

methenamine mandelate. (Various Mfr.) **Tab.:** 0.5 g, 1 g. Tab. 100s, 1000s. **Susp.:** 0.5 g/5 mL. Susp. Bot. 480 mL.
Use: Anti-infective, urinary.

•**methenolone acetate.** (meth-EEN-oh-lone) USAN.
Use: Anabolic.

•**methenolone enanthate.** (meth-EEN-oh-lone eh-NAN-thate) USAN.
Use: Anabolic.

Metheponex. (Rawl) Choline 0.54 g, dl-methionine 1.80 g, inositol 0.27 g, whole desiccated liver 8.10 g, vitamins B_1 18 mg, B_2 36 mg, niacinamide 90 mg, B_6 3.6 mg, calcium pantothenate 3.6 mg, biotin 10.8 mcg, B_{12} 5.4 mcg and amino acid/daily therapeutic dose. Cap. Bot. 100s, 500s. *Rx.*
Use: Antidiabetic; nutritional supplement.

metheptazine.
Use: Analgesic.

methestrol.
See: Promethestrol Dipropionate.

methetharimide bemegride. USAN.
Use: Anticonvulsant.

Methibon. (Barrows) Choline dihydrogen citrate 278 mg, dl-methionine 111 mg, inositol 83.3 mg, vitamin B_{12} 2 mcg, liver concentrate, desiccated liver 86.6 mg. Cap. Bot. 100s. *Rx.*
Use: Antidiabetic; nutritional supplement.

•**methicillin sodium.** (meth-ih-SILL-in) USAN.
Use: Anti-infective.

•**methimazole.** (meth-IMM-uh-zole) *USP.*
Use: Antithyroid agent.
See: Northyx.
Tapazole.

methimazole. (Par Pharm) Methimazole 5 mg, 10 mg. Lactose. Tab. Bot. 100s. *Rx.*
Use: Antithyroid agent.

Methiokaps. (Pal-Pak, Inc.) dl-methionine 200 mg. Cap. Bot. 1000s. *Rx.*
Use: Diaper rash product.

methiomeprazine hydrochloride. (GlaxoSmithKline)
Use: Antiemetic.

•**methionine.** (meh-THIGH-oh-NEEN) *USP.*
Note: Also see Racemethionine.
Use: Amino acid.
See: M-Caps.

•**methionine C 11 injection.** (meh-THIGH-oh-NEEN) *USP.*
Use: Radiopharmaceutical.

methionyl brain-derived neurotrophic factor, recombinant.
Use: Amyotrophic lateral sclerosis agent. [Orphan Drug]

Methioplex. (Lincoln Diagnostics) Methionine 25 mg, vitamins B_1 50 mg, niacinamide 100 mg, B_2 2 mg, choline 50 mg, B_6 2 mg, panthenol 2 mg, benzyl alcohol 1%, distilled water q.s./mL. Vial 30 mL. *Rx.*
Use: Nutritional supplement.

•**methisazone.** (METH-eye-SAH-zone) USAN.
Use: Antiviral.

Methitest. (Global) Methyltestosterone 10 mg. Lactose, sugar. Tab. Bot. 100s. *c-III.*
Use: Sex hormone, androgen.

methitural sodium.
Use: Hypnotic, sedative.

•**methixene hydrochloride.** (meh-THIX-een) USAN.
Use: Muscle relaxant.

•**methocarbamol.** (meth-oh-CAR-buh-mahl) *USP.*
Use: Muscle relaxant.
See: Robaxin.
Robaxin-750.

methocarbamol. (Various Mfr.) Methocarbamol. **Tab.:** 500 mg, 750 mg. Bot.

60s (750 mg only), 100s, 500s, UD 100s.
Use: Muscle relaxant.

methocel. Methylcellulose.

•**methohexital.** (meth-oh-HEX-ih-tahl) *USP.*
Use: Pharmaceutic necessity for methohexital sodium for injection.

•**methohexital sodium for injection.** (METH-oh-HEX-ih-tahl) *USP.*
Use: Anesthetic, general; anesthetic (intravenous).
See: Brevital Sodium.

•**methoin.** (METH-eh-toe-in) USAN.
Use: Anticonvulsant.

•**methopholine.** (METH-oh-foe-leen) USAN.
Use: Analgesic.
See: Versidyne.

Methopto Forte 1%. (Professional Pharmacal) Methylcellulose pow. 10 mg (1% soln.), boric acid 12 mg, potassium chloride 7.3 mg, benzalkonium chloride 0.04 mg, glycerin 12 mg/mL w/sodium carbonate to adjust pH and purified water. Bot. 15 mL. *OTC.*
Use: Artificial tears.

Methopto Forte 0.5%. (Professional Pharmacal) Methylcellulose pow. 5 mg (0.5% soln.), boric acid 12 mg, potassium chloride 7.3 mg, benzalkonium chloride 0.4 mg, glycerin 12 mg/mL w/sodium carbonate to adjust pH and purified water. Bot. 15 mL. *OTC.*
Use: Artificial tears.

Methopto 0.25%. (Professional Pharmacal) Methylcellulose pow. 2.5 mg (0.25% soln.), boric acid 12 mg, potassium chloride 7.3 mg, benzalkonium chloride 0.04 mg, glycerin 12 mg/mL w/sodium carbonate to adjust pH and purified water. Bot. 15 mL, 30 mL. *OTC.*
Use: Artificial tears.

methopyraphone.
See: Metopirone.

methorate.
See: Dextromethorphan Hydrobromide.

Methorbate S.C. (Standex) Methenamine 40.8 mg, atropine sulfate 0.03 mg, hyoscyamine sulfate 0.03 mg, salol 18.1 mg, benzoic acid 4.5 mg, methylene blue 5.4 mg. Tab. Bot. 100s. *Rx.*
Use: Anti-infective, urinary.

d-methorphan hydrobromide.
See: Dextromethorphan Hydrobromide.

methorphinan. Racemorphan hydrobromide. Dromoran.

•**methotrexate.** (meth-oh-TREK-sate) *USP. Formerly Amethopterin.*
Use: Leukemia in children; antineoplastic; antipsoriatic; juvenile rheumatoid arthritis; folic acid antagonist.
See: Mexate-AQ.
Otrexup.
Rheumatrex Dose Pack.
Trexall.

methotrexate. (Various Mfr.) Methotrexate 2.5 mg (as sodium). Tab. 36s, 100s, 5,000s, UD 20s. *Rx.*
Use: Antimetabolite, folic acid antagonist.

methotrexate sodium. (Various Mfr.) Methotrexate sodium. **Inj.:** 25 mg/mL (as base). Preservative free. Single-use vials. 2 mL, 4 mL, 8 mL, 10 mL, 20 mL, 40 mL. **Pow. for Inj., lyophilized:** 1 g (as base) (sodium 7 mEq/vial). Preservative free. Single-use vials. *Rx.*
Use: Antimetabolite, folic acid antagonist.

methotrexate sodium. (Various Mfr.) Methotrexate sodium 25 mg/mL (as base). Benzyl alcohol 0.9%. Must not be used for intrathecal or high-dose therapy. Inj. Vials. 2 mL, 10 mL. *Rx.*
Use: Antimetabolite, folic acid antagonist.

methotrexate sodium. (Wyeth) Methotrexate sodium 2.5 mg/mL Vial 2 mL; 25 mg/mL. Vial 2 mL w/preservatives; 20 mg, 50 mg, 100 mg Vial cryodesiccated, preservative free; 50 mg, 100 mg, 200 mg Vial; 25 mg/mL solution preservative free.
Use: Leukemia therapy; psoriasis; osteogenic sarcoma. [Orphan Drug]

methotrexate with laurocapram.
Use: Topical treatment of *Mycosis fungoides.* [Orphan Drug]

•**methoxsalen.** (meth-OX-ah-len) *USP.*
Use: Pigmenting agent.
See: 8-MOP.
Oxsoralen.
Oxsoralen Ultra.
Uvadex.

8-methoxsalen.
Use: Treatment of diffuse systemic sclerosis, rejection of cardiac allografts. [Orphan Drug]
See: Uvadex.

methoxyphenamine hydrochloride. *USP.*
Use: Adrenergic (bronchodilator).

W/Dextromethorphan hydrochloride, orthoxine, sodium citrate.
See: Orthoxicol.

methoxypromazine maleate.
Use: CNS depressant.

methoxypsoralen, oral.
Use: Psoralen.
See: Oxsoralen.

Oxsoralen Ultra.
•**methscopolamine bromide.** (METH-skoe-POL-a-meen) *USP.*
Use: Anticholinergic.
See: Pamine.
Pamine Forte.
Pamine FQ Kit.
W/Butabarbital Sodium, Dried Aluminum Hydroxide Gel and Magnesium Trisilicate.
See: Eulcin.
methscopolamine bromide. (Boca Pharmacal) Methscopolamine bromide 2.5 mg, 5 mg. Tab. 60s (5 mg only), 100s (2.5 mg only), 5 blisters of 12 tablets (5 mg only). *Rx.*
Use: Anticholinergic/antispasmodic.
methscopolamine nitrate. Scopolamine methyl nitrate, preps. Mescomine.
W/Chlorpheniramine Maleate.
See: AeroHist.
AllePak Dose Pack.
Allergy DN.
AlleRx DF Dose Pack.
NoHist EXT.
RelCof CPM.
SymPak PDX.
W/Chlorpheniramine Maleate, Phenylephrine Hydrochloride.
See: AeroHist Plus.
AeroKid.
CPM 8/PE 20/MSC 1.25.
Dehistine.
Denaze.
DriHist SR.
Drysec.
Duradryl.
Duravent.
Duravent-DA.
Extendryl.
NoHist-Plus.
OMNIhist II LA.
PCM.
PE-CPM-MSN 8-2-0.75.
PE-HCL-CPM-MSN 10-2-0.75.
Phenylephrine CM.
QV Allergy.
Ralix.
RelCof PE.
Rescon-MX.
ScopoHist.
ScopoHist-PE.
SymPak PDX.
Triall.
Zinx PCM.
W/Chlorpheniramine Maleate, Pseudoephedrine Hydrochloride.
See: CPM 8/PSE 90/MSC 2.5.
DryMax.
Histatab.
Relcof PSE.
Time-Hist QD.
W/Chlorpheniramine Tannate.
See: Dexodryl.
W/Chlorpheniramine Tannate, Phenylephrine Tannate.
See: AH-chew.
AH-chew Ultra.
Redur-PCM.
W/Dexchlorpheniramine Maleate, Phenylephrine Hydrochloride.
See: Dexphen M.
Extendryl.
Re-Drylex.
W/Dexchlorpheniramine Maleate, Pseudoephedrine Hydrochloride.
See: CoryZa-D.
D-Hist D.
Histatab D.
W/Phenylephrine Hydrochloride.
See: Extendryl PEM.
W/Pseudoephedrine Hydrochloride.
See: AllePak Dose Pack.
Allergy DN.
Amdry-D.
PSE 120/MSC 2.5.
SudaTrate.
•**methsuximide.** (meth-SUCK-sih-mide) *USP.*
Use: Anticonvulsant.
See: Celontin.
•**methyclothiazide.** (METH-ee-kloe-THIGH-ah-zide) *USP.*
Use: Antihypertensive; diuretic.
See: Enduron.
W/Deserpidine.
See: Enduronyl.
methyclothiazide. (Various Mfr.) Methyclothiazide 2.5 mg, 5 mg. Tab. 100s (2.5 mg only), 100s. *Rx.*
Use: Diuretic.
methylacetylcholine.
See: Methacholine.
•**methyl alcohol.** (METH-ill) *NF.*
Use: Pharmaceutic acid (solvent).
methyl aminolevulinate.
Use: Photochemotherapy.
See: Metvixia.
•**methyl aminolevulinate hydrochloride.** (METH-il a-MEE-noe-LEV-ue-LIN-ate) USAN.
Use: Antineoplastic.
methylamphetamine hydrochloride and sulfate.
See: Desoxyephedrine Hydrochloride.
methylandrostenediol. Methandriol.
•**methylatropine nitrate.** (METH-ill-AT-row-peen) USAN.
Use: Anticholinergic.
•**methylbenzethonium chloride.** (meth-ill-benz-eth-OH-nee-uhm) *USP.*

Use: Bactericide, local anti-infective (topical).
See: Diaparene.

methylbenztropine.
See: Ethybenztropine.

methylbromtropin mandelate. Homatropine Methylbromide, USP.

•**methylcellulose.** (METH-ill-SELL-you-lohs) *USP.*
Use: Pharmaceutic aid (suspending agent).
See: Cellothyl.
Citrucel Fiber Shake.
Cologel.
W/Carboxymethylcellulose.
See: Ex-Caloric.

methyl cysteine hydrochloride. Cysteine methyl ester hydrochloride.
Use: Mucolytic agent.

•**methyldopa.** (meth-ill-DOE-puh) *USP. Formerly Alpha-Methyldopa.*
Use: Antihypertensive.
W/Chlorothiazide.
See: Aldoclor.

methyldopa. (Various Mfr.) Methyldopa 250 mg, 500 mg. Tab. Bot. 100s, 500s, 1000s (250 mg only), UD 100s. *Rx.*
Use: Antihypertensive.

methyldopa/hydrochlorothiazide. (Various Mfr.) Methyldopa/hydrochlorothiazide 250 mg/15 mg, 250 mg/25 mg. Tab. Bot. 100s, 500s, 1000s, UD 100s. *Rx.*
Use: Antihypertensive combination.

methyldopa/hydrochlorothiazide. (Various Mfr.) Methyldopa/hydrochlorothiazide 500 mg/30 mg, 500 mg/50 mg. Tab. Bot. 100s, 250s, 500s. *Rx.*
Use: Antihypertensive combination.

•**methyldopate hydrochloride.** (meth-ill-DOE-pate) *USP.*
Use: Antihypertensive.

•**methylene blue.** (METH-ih-leen) *USP.*
Use: Antidote; cyanide.
See: Methblue 65.
W/Atropine Sulfate, Benzoic Acid, Hyoscyamine Sulfate, Methenamine, Phenyl Salicylate.
See: Uritact DS.
W/Benzoic Acid, Hyoscyamine Sulfate, Methenamine, Phenyl Salicylate.
See: Hyophen.
W/Hyoscyamine Sulfate, Methenamine, Phenyl Salicylate, Sodium Biphosphate.
See: Urimax.
W/Hyoscyamine Sulfate, Methenamine, Phenyl Sailcylate, Sodium Phosphate Monobasic.
See: Phosphasal.
Uticap.
Utrona-C.
W/Hyoscyamine Sulfate, Methenamine, Sodium Phosphate Monobasic.
See: Uryl.

methylene blue. (Various Mfr.) Methylene blue 10 mg/mL. Inj. Vial 1 mL, 10 mL. *Rx.*
Use: GU antiseptic; antidote; cyanide.

•**methylene chloride.** (METH-ih-leen) *NF.*
Use: Pharmaceutic aid (solvent).

•**methylergonovine maleate.** (METH-ill-err-go-NO-veen) *USP.*
Use: Uterine-active agent.

methylergonovine maleate. (Gavis Pharmaceuticals) Methylergonovine maleate 0.2 mg. Lactose, parabens. Tab. 28s, 100s. *Rx.*
Use: Uterine-active agent.

methylergonovine maleate. (PharmaForce) Methylergonovine maleate 0.2 mg/mL. Inj., Soln. Vial. 1 mL. *Rx.*
Use: Uterine-active agent.

L-methylfolate.
Use: Water-soluble vitamin.
See: Deplin 15.
Deplin 7.5.
L-Methylfolate Formula 15.
L-Methylfolate Formula 7.5.
L-Methylfolate Forte 7.5.
L-Methyl-MC NAC.
ViloFane-Dp.

L-methylfolate calcium 15. (Zerxis) L-methylfolate 15 mg. Coated. PEG. Gluten free, lactose free. Tab. 90s. *Rx.*
Use: Water-soluble vitamin.

L-methylfolate calcium 7.5. (Zerxis) L-methylfolate 7.5 mg. Coated. PEG. Gluten free, lactose free. Tab. 90s. *Rx.*
Use: Water-soluble vitamin.

L-methylfolate Ca, Me-Cbl, NAC. (Zerxis) Folate 6 mg, N-acetylcysteine 600 mg, B_{12} 2,000 mcg. Coated. Gluten free, lactose free. Tab. 90s. *Rx.*
Use: Multivitamin.

L-methylfolate Ca, P-5-P, Me-Cbl. (Zerxis) Folate 3 mg, B_6 35 mg, B_{12} 2,000 mcg. Coated. Gluten free and lactose free. Tab. 90s. *Rx.*
Use: Multivitamin.

L-methylfolate formula 15. (Zerxis) L-methylfolate 15 mg. Schizochytrium algal oil, glucose, mannitol, soy, sunflower oil. Cap. 90s. *Rx.*
Use: Water-soluble vitamin.

L-methylfolate formula 7.5. (Zerxis) L-methylfolate 7.5 mg. Schizochytrium algal oil, glucose, mannitol, soy, sunflower oil. Cap. 90s. *Rx.*
Use: Water-soluble vitamin.

L-methylfolate forte 7.5. (Breckenridge Pharmaceutical) L-methylfolate 7.5 mg.

Schizochytrium algal oil, glucose, mannitol, soy, sunflower oil. Cap. 90s. *Rx.*
Use: Water-soluble vitamin.
methylglucamine diatrizoate, injection. A water-soluble radiopaque iodine cpd. N-methylglucamine salt of Diatrizoate.
See: Diatrizoate Meglumine.
methylglucamine iodipamide, injection.
See: Meglumine Iodipamide, Injection.
W/Diatrizoate methylglucamine.
See: Sinografin.
methylglyoxal-bis-guanylhydrazone. Methyl GAG.
Methylin. (Shionogi Pharm) Methylphenidate hydrochloride. **Chew. Tab.:** 2.5 mg, phenylalanine 0.42 mg; 5 mg, phenylalanine 0.84 mg; 10 mg, phenylalanine 1.68 mg. Aspartame, grape flavor. 100s. **Oral Soln.:** 5 mg per 5 mL, 10 mg per 5 mL. Glycerin. Grape flavor. 500 mL. *c-II.*
Use: Central nervous system stimulant.
•**methyl isobutyl ketone.** (METH-ill eye-so-BYOO-till KEE-tone) *NF.*
Use: Pharmaceutic aid (alcohol denaturant).
methylmelamines/ethylenimines.
See: Ethylenimines/Methylmelamines.
methylmercadone. Name used for Nifuratel.
•**methylnaltrexone bromide.** (METH-il-nal-TREX-one BROE-mide)
Use: Detoxification agent, antidote.
See: Relistor.
•**methyl nicotinate.** (METH-ill NIK-oh-TIN-ate) USAN.
W/Methyl salicylate, menthol.
See: Musterole Deep Strength.
Methylone. (Paddock) Methylprednisolone acetate 40 mg/mL. Vial 5 mL. *Rx.*
Use: Corticosteroid.
•**methyl palmoxirate.** (METH-ill pal-MOX-ihr-ate) USAN.
Use: Antidiabetic.
•**methylparaben.** (meth-ill-PAR-ah-ben) *NF.*
Use: Pharmaceutic aid (antifungal agent).
•**methylparaben sodium.** (meth-ill-PAR-ah-ben) *NF.*
Use: Pharmaceutic aid (antimicrobial preservative).
methylphenethylamine.
See: Amphetamine Hydrochloride.
•**methylphenidate.** (meth-ill-FEN-ih-date) USAN.
Use: Central nervous system stimulant.
methylphenidate. (Breckenridge) Methylphenidate hydrochloride 5 mg per 5 mL, 10 mg per 5 mL. May contain glycerin, PEG. Grape flavor. Soln. 500 mL. *c-II.*
Use: CNS stimulant.
•**methylphenidate hydrochloride.** (meth-ill-FEN-ih-date) *USP.*
Use: Central nervous system stimulant.
See: Concerta.
Daytrana.
Metadate CD.
Metadate ER.
Methylin.
Quillivant.
Ritalin.
Ritalin LA.
Ritalin-SR.
methylphenidate hydrochloride. (Actavis South Atlantic) Methylphenidate hydrochloride 20 mg, 30 mg, 40 mg. Sugar spheres. ER Cap. 100s, 250s. *c-II.*
Use: Central nervous system stimulant.
methylphenidate hydrochloride. (Kremers Urban Pharmaceuticals) Methylphenidate hydrochloride 10 mg, 50 mg, 60 mg. May contain PEG, sugar spheres. ER Cap. 100s. *c-II.*
Use: Central nervous system stimulant.
methylphenidate hydrochloride. (Various Mfr.) Methylphenidate hydrochloride. **Tab.:** 5 mg, 10 mg, 20 mg. 100s, 1,000s (5 mg only). **ER Tab.:** 10 mg, 18 mg, 20 mg, 27 mg, 36 mg, 54 mg. May contain lactose, PEG. 100s. **ER Cap.:** 10 mg, 20 mg, 30 mg, 40 mg, 50 mg, 60 mg. May contain sugar, PEG. 100s. *c-II.*
Use: Central nervous system stimulant.
methylphenidylacetate hydrochloride.
See: Methylphenidate Hydrochloride.
methylphenobarbital.
See: Mephobarbital.
d-methylphenylamine sulfate.
See: Dextroamphetamine Sulfate.
methylphytyl naphthoquinone.
Use: Vitamin supplement.
See: Phytonadione.
methyl polysiloxane.
See: Mylicon.
Simethicone.
methylpred-40. (Seatrace) Methylprednisolone acetate 40 mg/mL. Vial 5 mL, 10 mL. *Rx.*
Use: Corticosteroid.
•**methylprednisolone.** (METH-ill-pred-NIH-suh-lone) *USP.*
Tall Man: methylPREDNISolone
Use: Adrenocortical steroid, glucocorticoid.
See: Medrol.
methylprednisolone. (Cadista) Methylprednisolone 32 mg. Lactose. Tab. 25s. *Rx.*

Use: Adrenocortical steroid, glucocorticoid.

methylprednisolone. (Various Mfr.) Methylprednisolone 4 mg, 8 mg, 16 mg. May contain lactose (except 4 mg). Tab. **4 mg:** 21s, 100s, unit-of-use 21s. **8 mg:** 25s. **16 mg:** 50s. *Rx.*
Use: Adrenocortical steroid, glucocorticoid.

•**methylprednisolone acetate.** (METH-ill-pred-NIH-suh-lone) *USP.*
Tall Man: methylPREDNISolone
Use: Adrenocortical steroid, glucocorticoid.
See: Depo-Medrol.

methylprednisolone acetate. (Various Mfr.) Methylprednisolone acetate 40 mg/mL, 80 mg/mL. Susp. Inj. Vials. 5 mL, 10 mL (except 80 mg). *Rx.*
Use: Adrenocortical steroids, glucocorticoids.

•**methylprednisolone hemisuccinate.** (METH-ill-pred-NIH-suh-lone hem-ih-SUCK-sih-nate) *USP.*
Tall Man: methylPREDNISolone
Use: Adrenocortical steroid.

•**methylprednisolone sodium phosphate.** (METH-ill-pred-NIH-suh-lone) USAN.
Tall Man: methylPREDNISolone
Use: Corticosteroid, topical.

•**methylprednisolone sodium succinate.** (METH-ill-pred-NIH-suh-lone) *USP.*
Tall Man: methylPREDNISolone
Use: Adrenocorticoid steroid; corticosteroid, topical; glucocorticoid.
See: A-Methapred.
Solu-Medrol.

methylprednisolone sodium succinate. (Various Mfr.) Methylprednisolone sodium succinate 40 mg/vial, 125 mg/vial, 500 mg/vial, 1 g/vial. Inj., Pow. for Soln. Vials. 1 mL (except 125 mg), 2 mL (125 mg only), 3 mL (40 mg only), 4 mL (500 mg only), 5 mL (125 mg only), 8 mL (1 g only), 20 mL (500 mg only), 50 mL (1 g only). *Rx.*
Use: Adrenocortical steroid, glucocorticoid.

•**methylprednisolone suleptanate.** (METH-ill-pred-NIH-suh-lone sull-EPP-tah-NATE) USAN.
Tall Man: methylPREDNISolone
Use: Adrenocortical steroid; anti-inflammatory.

methylpyrimal.
See: Sulfamerazine.

methylrosaniline chloride.
Use: Anthelmintic; anti-infective.
See: Gentian Violet.

•**methyl salicylate.** (METH-ill sal-ISS-ih-late) *NF.*
Use: Rubefacient rub (topical).
W/Benzocaine, Menthol.
See: Dendracin Neurodendtraxcin.
W/Camphor, Menthol.
See: Bayer Muscle and Joint.
W/Capsaicin, Lidocaine, Menthol.
See: Terocin.
W/Capsaicin, Menthol.
See: Bio-Therm Pain Relieving Lotion.
Medi-Derm.
Medrox.
New Terocin.
Ultracin.
Xoten-C Pain Relief.
Ziks.
W/Iodine.
See: Iodex With Methyl Salicylate.
W/Menthol.
See: Analgesic Balm.
Analgesic Balm-GRX.
Icy Hot Chill Stick.
Menthoderm.
Pain Bust-R II.
Pain Relieving Rub.
W/Menthol, Methyl Nicotinate.
See: Musterole Deep Strength.

•**methylsamidorphan.** (METH-il-SAM-i-DOR-fan) USAN.
Use: Gastrointestinal agent.

methyl sulfanil amidoisoxazole. Sulfamethoxazole.

•**methyltestosterone.** (METH-ill-tess-TAHS-ter-ohn) *USP.*
Tall Man: methylTESTOSTERone
Use: Sex hormone, androgen.
See: Methitest.
Testred.
Virilon.
W/Esterified Estrogens.
See: Covaryx.
Covaryx HS.

methyltestosterone. (Various Mfr.) Methyltestosterone. **Tab.:** 10 mg, 25 mg. Bot. 100s. **Tab., buccal:** 10 mg. Bot. 100s. *c-III.*
Use: Sex hormone, androgen.

methyltestosterone and esterified estrogens. (Lannett) Esterified estrogens 1.25 mg, methyltestosterone 2.5 mg. Tartrazine. Film-coated. Tab. 100s, 1000s. *Rx.*
Use: Sex hormone.

methyltestosterone and esterified estrogens H.S. (Lannett) Esterified estrogens 0.625 mg, methyltestosterone 1.25 mg. Lactose. Film-coated. Tab. 100s, 1000s. *Rx.*
Use: Sex hormone.

methylthionine chloride. *Name used for Methylene Blue.*

methylthionine hydrochloride. *Name used for Methylene Blue.*

methylthiouracil. *USP.*
Use: Antithyroid agent.

methyl violet.
See: Gentian Violet, Crystal Violet, Methylrosaniline Chloride.

methyndamine. *Name used for Tetrydamine.*

•**metiamide.** (meh-TIE-aim-ide) USAN. Histamine H_2 antagonist.
Use: Treatment for peptic ulcer; antiulcerative.

•**metiapine.** (meh-TIE-ah-PEEN) USAN.
Use: Antipsychotic.

meticlopindol. *Name used for Clopidol.*

•**metioprim.** (meh-TIE-oh-PRIM) USAN.
Use: Anti-infective.

•**metipranolol.** (meh-tih-PRAN-oh-lahl) USAN.
Use: Antihypertensive (beta-blocker, ophthalmic).

metipranolol. (Falcon Ophthalmics) Metipranolol 0.3%, povidone, hydrochloric acid, NaCl, EDTA, benzalkonium chloride 0.004%. Ophth. Soln. Bot. 5 mL, 10 mL. *Rx.*
Use: Antihypertensive, beta-blocker, ophthalmic.

metipranolol hydrochloride.
Use: Antihypertensive (beta-blocker, ophthalmic).
See: OptiPranolol.

metizoline.
Use: Decongestant.

•**metizoline hydrochloride.** (meh-TIH-zoe-leen) USAN.
Use: Adrenergic vasoconstrictor.

•**metkephamid acetate.** (MET-KEFF-am-id) USAN.
Use: Analgesic.

•**metoclopramide hydrochloride.** (MET-oh-kloe-PRA-mide) *USP.*
Use: Antiemetic; gastrointestinal stimulant.
See: Metozolv.

metoclopramide hydrochloride. (Various Mfr.) Metoclopramide hydrochloride (as monohydrochloride monohydrate). **Inj.:** 5 mg/mL. Vials. 2 mL, 10 mL, 30 mL. Amps. 2 mL. **Syrup:** 5 mg/mL. 480 mL, UD 10 mL. **Tab.:** 5 mg, 10 mg. 100s; 500s; 1000s; 2500s, UD 100s (10 mg only). *Rx.*
Use: Gastrointestinal stimulant.

metofurone. Name used for Nifurmerone.

•**metogest.** (MET-oh-JEST) USAN.
Use: Hormone.

•**metolazone.** (meh-TOLE-uh-ZONE) *USP.*
Use: Antihypertensive; diuretic.
See: Zaroxolyn.

metolazone. (Various Mfr.) Metolazone 2.5 mg, 5 mg, 10 mg. Tab. 100s, 1000s (2.5 mg only). *Rx.*
Use: Diuretic.

•**metopimazine.** (meh-toe-PIH-mazz-EEN) USAN.
Use: Antiemetic.

Metopirone. (Laboratoire HRA Pharma) Metyrapone 250 mg. Softgel Cap. Pkg. 18s. *Rx.*
Use: In vivo diagnostic aid.

•**metoprine.** (MET-oh-preen) USAN.
Use: Antineoplastic.

•**metoprolol.** (meh-TOE-pro-lahl) USAN.
Use: Antiadrenergic/sympatholytic, beta-adrenergic blocker.

•**metoprolol fumarate.** (meh-TOE-pro-lahl) *USP.*
Use: Antihypertensive.

•**metoprolol succinate.** (meh-TOE-pro-lahl) USAN.
Use: Antihypertensive; antianginal; treatment of myocardial infarction.
See: Toprol XL.

metoprolol succinate. (Various Mfr.) Metoprolol 25 mg (metoprolol succinate 23.75 mg equiv. to metoprolol tartrate 25 mg), 50 mg (metoprolol succinate 47.5 mg equiv. to metoprolol tartrate 50 mg), 100 mg (metoprolol succinate 95 mg equiv. to metoprolol tartrate 100 mg), 200 mg (metoprolol succinate 190 mg equiv. to metoprolol tartrate 200 mg). May contain maltodextrin, polydextrose (100 mg, 200 mg only). Film-coated. ER Tab. 100s, 1000s (except 50 mg), UD 100s (100 mg, 200 mg only). *Rx.*
Use: Antiadrenergic/sympatholytic.

•**metoprolol tartrate.** (meh-TOE-pro-lahl) *USP.*
Use: Antiadrenergic (beta-receptor).
W/Hydrochlorothiazide
See: Lopressor.
Lopressor HCT.

metoprolol tartrate. (Hospira) Metoprolol tartrate 1 mg/mL. Inj. Amp. *Carpuject* sterile cartridge units with Interlink System Cannula, *Carpuject* sterile cartridge units with *Luer-Lock. Rx.*
Use: Antiadrenergic/sympatholytic, beta-adrenergic blocker.

metoprolol tartrate. (Purepac) Metoprolol tartrate. **Tab.:** 50 mg, 100 mg, lactose. Bot. 100s, 1000s, UD 100s. **Inj.:** 1 mg/mL. Amp. 5 mL. *Rx.*
Use: Antiadrenergic/sympatholytic; beta-adrenergic blocker.

metoprolol tartrate. (Various Mfr.) Metoprolol tartrate 25 mg, 50 mg, 100 mg. Tab. 30s, 90s, 100s, 1000s. *Rx.*
Use: Antiadrenergic, sympatholytic, beta-adrenergic blocker.

metoprolol tartrate/hydrochlorothiazide. (Mylan) Hydrochlorothiazide/metoprolol tartrate 25 mg/50 mg, 25 mg/100 mg, 50 mg/100 mg. Lactose. Tab. 100s, 500s. *Rx.*
Use: Antihypertensive.

metoquine.
Use: Antimalarial.

•**metoquizine.** (MET-oh-kwih-zeen) USAN.
Use: Anticholinergic; antiulcerative.

Metozolv ODT. (Salix) Metoclopramide 5 mg (equiv. to metoclopramide hydrochloride 5.91 mg), 10 mg (equiv. to metoclopramide hydrochloride 11.82 mg). Acesulfate K, mannitol. Mint flavor. Tab., orally disintegrating. UD 100s. *Rx.*
Use: GI stimulant.

•**metreleptin.** (MET-re-LEP-tin) USAN.
Use: Obesity and related disorders.
See: Myalept.

•**metrifonate.** (meh-TRIH-foe-nate) *USP.*
Formerly trichlorfon.
Use: Cholinesterase inhibitor.

•**metrizamide.** (meh-TRIH-zam-ide) USAN.
Use: Myelography; diagnostic aid (radiopaque medium).
See: Amipaque.

•**metrizoate sodium.** (meh-trih-ZOE-ate) USAN.
Use: Diagnostic aid (radiopaque medium).

MetroCream. (Galderma) Metronidazole 0.75%. Glycerin, benzyl alcohol. Cream. Tube. 45 g. *Rx.*
Use: Topical anti-infective, antibiotic.

MetroGel. (Galderma) Metronidazole 1%. Parabens, EDTA. Gel. Tubes. 45 g. *Rx.*
Use: Dermatologic, acne.

MetroGel-Vaginal. (Medicis) Metronidazole 0.75%, EDTA, parabens. Gel Tube (with 5 applicators) 70 g. *Rx.*
Use: Anti-infective, vaginal.

Metrogesic. (Lexis Laboratories) Salicylamide 325 mg, acetaminophen 162 mg, phenacetin 65 mg. Tab. Bot. 100s.
Use: Analgesic.

metrogestone.
Use: Hormone, progestin.

MetroLotion. (Galderma) Metronidazole 0.75%. Benzyl alcohol, stearyl alcohol, glycerin, mineral oil. Lot. Bot. 59 mL. *Rx.*
Use: Topical anti-infective, antibiotic.

•**metronidazole.** (meh-troe-NID-uh-zole) *USP.*
Tall Man: metroNIDAZOLE
Use: Antiprotozoal (trichomonas); antitrichomonal.
See: Flagyl.
Flagyl ER.
Flagyl 375.
MetroCream.
MetroGel.
MetroGel-Vaginal.
MetroLotion.
Metryl.
Noritate.
Rosadan.
Rosadan Cream Kit.
Rozex.
Vandazole.
W/Bismuth Subcitrate Potassium, Tetracycline Hydrochloride.
See: Pylera.

metronidazole. (Able) Metronidazole 375 mg. Cap. 30s, 50s, 100s, 500s, 1000s. *Rx.*
Use: Anti-infective.

metronidazole. (B. Braun) Metronidazole 5 mg/mL. Inj. Vial 100 mL. *Rx.*
Use: Anti-infective.

metronidazole. (Fougera) Metronidazole. **Cream:** 0.75%. Benzyl alcohol, glycerin, lactic acid. 45 g. **Gel:** 0.75%. EDTA, parabens. 45 g. *Rx.*
Use: Topical anti-infective, antibiotic.

metronidazole. (Prasco) Metronidazole 0.75%. EDTA, parabens. Vaginal Gel. Tubes with vaginal applicators. 70 g. *Rx.*
Use: Vaginal preparation; anti-infective.

metronidazole. (Various Mfr.) Metronidazole. **Gel:** 1%. May contain edetate disodium, parabens, propylene glycol. 60 g tube and 55 g pump. **Gel; vaginal:** 1.3%. May contain benzyl alcohol, PEG, parabens, propylene glycol. 5 g prefilled applicator. **Lot.:** 0.75%. May contain benzyl alcohol. 59 mL. **Tab.:** 250 mg, 500 mg. 4s, 14s, 50s (500 mg only); 100s; 250s (250 mg only); 500s, UD 25s, UD 100s. *Rx.*
Use: Anti-infective.

•**metronidazole benzoate.** (meh-troe-NIH-dah-zole BEN-zoe-ate) *USP.*
Tall Man: metroNIDAZOLE
Use: Anti-infective.

•**metronidazole hydrochloride.** (meh-troe-NIH-dah-zole) USAN.
Tall Man: metroNIDAZOLE
Use: Anti-infective.

metronidazole in sodium chloride. (Various Mfr.) Metronidazole 5 mg/mL.

Sodium chloride. Inj., Soln. Single-dose container. 100 mL. *Rx.*
Use: Anti-infective agent.

•**metronidazole phosphate.** (meh-troe-NIH-dah-zole) USAN.
Tall Man: metroNIDAZOLE
Use: Antibacterial; anti-infective; antiprotozoal.

Metrozole. (Lexis Laboratories) Metronidazole 250 mg, 500 mg. Tab. **250 mg:** Bot. 100s, 250s. **500 mg:** Bot. 100s. *Rx.*
Use: Amebicide; anti-infective.

MET-RX. (Met-Rx USA) **Pow. for Drink:** Fat 2 g, Na 37 mg, K 900 mg, carbohydrate 22 g, protein, < 1 g dietary fiber, sugar, vitamins A, D, C, E, B_1, B_5, B_6, B_{12}, biotin, Mg, Zn, Ca, folate, P, Cu, Fe, riboflavin, iodine. 72 g. **Food Bar:** Fat 4 g, Na 110 mg, K 700 mg, carbohydrate 50 g, protein 27 g, sugar, Ca, vitamins A, D, B_1, B_2, B_3, B_5, B_6, B_{12}, C, E, folate, biotin, P, Mg, Cu, Fe, I, Zn. 100 g. *OTC.*
Use: Nutritional therapy.

Metryl. (Teva) Metronidazole 250 mg. Tab. Bot. 100s, 250s, 500s, UD 100s. *Rx.*
Use: Amebicide, anti-infective.

Metryl 500. (Teva) Metronidazole 500 mg. Tab. Bot. 100s, 500s. *Rx.*
Use: Amebicide; anti-infective.

•**meturedepa.** (meh-TOO-ree-DEH-pah) USAN.
Use: Antineoplastic.

Metussin. (Faraday) Dextromethorphan. Bot. 4 oz. *OTC.*
Use: Antitussive.

Metussin Jr. (Faraday) Dextromethorphan. Bot. 4 oz. *OTC.*
Use: Antitussive.

Metvixia. (PhotoCure ASA) Methyl aminolevulinate 16.8%. Almond oil, EDTA, glycerin, parabens, peanut oil, white petrolatum. Cream. 2 g. *Rx.*
Use: Photochemotherapy.

•**metyrapone.** (meh-TEER-ah-pone) *USP.*
Use: In vivo diagnostic aid (pituitary function determination); adrenocortical enzyme inhibitor.
See: Metopirone.

•**metyrapone tartrate.** (meh-TEER-ah-pone) USAN.
Use: Diagnostic aid (pituitary function determination).

metyrapone tartrate injection.
Use: Diagnostic aid.

•**metyrosine.** (meh-TIE-roe-seen) *USP.*
Use: Antihypertensive.
See: Demser.

Mevacor. (Merck) Lovastatin 20 mg, 40 mg. Lactose. Tab. Bot. 1000s, 10,000s; UD 100s (20 mg only); unit-of-use 60s; unit-of-use 90s. *Rx.*
Use: Antihyperlipidemic; HMG-CoA reductase inhibitor.

mevinolin.
See: Lovastatin.

Mexate-AQ. (Bristol-Myers Squibb Oncology/Virology) Methotrexate 50 mg, 100 mg, 250 mg/preservative-free liquid vial. *Rx.*
Use: Antineoplastic.

•**mexiletine hydrochloride.** (MEX-ih-leh-teen) *USP.*
Use: Antiarrhythmic agent.
See: Mexitil.

mexiletine hydrochloride. (Various Mfr.) Mexiletine hydrochloride 150 mg, 200 mg, 250 mg. Cap. 30s, 60s, 90s (150 mg only); 100s; 120s, 240s (150 mg only). *Rx.*
Use: Antiarrhythmic agent.

Mexitil. (Boehringer Ingelheim) Mexiletine hydrochloride 150 mg, 200 mg, 250 mg. Cap. Bot. 100s, UD 100s. *Rx.*
Use: Antiarrhythmic.

•**mexrenoate potassium.** (mex-REN-oh-ate) USAN.
Use: Aldosterone antagonist.

Mexsana Medicated Powder. (Schering-Plough) Corn starch, kaolin, triclosan, zinc oxide. Can 3 oz, 6.25 oz, 11 oz. *OTC.*
Use: Diaper rash preparation.

Meyenberg Goat Milk. (Jackson-Mitchell) Evaporated and powdered cans of goat milk. Foil pack 4 oz. (makes 1 quart). *OTC.*
Use: Cows' milk allergies.

MG Cold Sore Formula. (Outdoor Recreation) Menthol 1%, lidocaine, propylene glycol in alcohol base. Soln. Bot. 7.5 mL. *OTC.*
Use: Cold sores; fever blisters.

MG400. (Triton) Colloidal sulfur in Guy-Base II 5%, salicylic acid 3%. Shampoo. Bot. 240 mL, pt. *OTC.*
Use: Antiseborrheic.

MG-Oroate. (Miller Pharmacal Group) Magnesium (as magnesium orotate) 33 mg. Tab. Bot. 100s. *OTC.*
Use: Vitamin supplement.

MG-Plus Protein. (Miller Pharmacal Group) Magnesium-protein complex made with specially isolated soy protein 133 mg. Tab. Bot. 100s. *OTC.*
Use: Vitamin supplement.

MG217 Medicated Tar. (Triton) **Shampoo:** Coal tar solution 15%. Bot. 120 mL, 240 mL. **Oint.:** Coal tar solu-

tion 10%, petrolatum, cetyl alcohol. 107 g. **Lot.:** Coal tar solution 5%, moisturizing base, cetyl alcohol, mineral oil. 120 mL. *OTC.*
Use: Antipruritic; antieczematic; keratolytic.

MG217 Medicated Tar-Free. (Triton) Colloidal sulfur 5%, salicylic acid 3%. Shampoo. Bot. 120 mL, 240 mL. *OTC.*
Use: Antiseborrheic; antipruritic.

MG217 Sal-Acid. (Triton) Salicylic acid 3%, vitamin E. Oint. Tube. 60 g. *OTC.*
Use: Keratolytic.

MHP-A. (Cypress) Methenamine 40.8 mg, phenyl salicylate 18.1 mg, atropine sulfate 0.03, hyoscyamine sulfate 0.03 mg, benzoic acid 4.5 mg, methylene blue 5.4 mg. Tab. 100s. *Rx.*
Use: Anti-infective, urinary.

Miacalcin. (Novartis) Calcitonin-salmon. **Inj.:** 200 units/mL. Phenol. Vial 2 mL. **Nasal Spray:** 200 units/activation (0.09 mL/dose). Sodium chloride 8.5 mg. Metered dose glass bot. with pump. 2 mL. *Rx.*
Use: Paget disease; antihypercalcemic; postmenopausal osteoporosis.

Mi-Acid Gelcaps. (Major) Calcium carbonate 311 mg, magnesium carbonate 232 mg, parabens, EDTA. Bot. 50s. *OTC.*
Use: Antacid.

Mi-Acid Liquid. (Major) Aluminum hydroxide 200 mg, magnesium hydroxide 200 mg, simethicone 20 mg/5 mL. Bot. 355 mL, 780 mL. *OTC.*
Use: Antacid; antiflatulent.

Mi-Acid II Liquid. (Major) Aluminum hydroxide 400 mg, magnesium hydroxide 400 mg, simethicone 40 mg/5 mL. Bot. 355 mL. *OTC.*
Use: Antacid; antiflatulent.

Mi-Acid Maximum Strength. (Major) Aluminum hydroxide 400 mg, magnesium hydroxide 400 mg, simethicone 40 mg per 5 mL. Parabens, saccharin, sorbitol. Lemon/mint flavor. Liq. 360 mL.
Use: Antacid combination.

Miaderm Radiation Relief. (Aiden Industries) Caprylic/capric triglyceride, alcohol, PEG, dimethicone, glycerin, aloe, lanolin, sodium hyaluronate, disodium EDTA, sodium benzoate. Lot. 118.3 mL. *OTC.*
Use: Miscellaneous topical combination.

miadone.
See: Methadone Hydrochloride.

•**mianserin hydrochloride.** (my-AN-ser-in) USAN. Under study.
Use: Serotonin inhibitor; antihistamine.

•**mibampator.** (mye-BAM-pa-tor) USAN.
Use: CNS agent.

•**mibolerone.** (my-BOLE-ehr-ohn) USAN.
Use: Anabolic; androgen.

•**micafungin sodium.** (mi-ka-FUN-gin) USAN.
Use: Antifungal.
See: Mycamine.

Micardis. (Boehringer Ingelheim) Telmisartan 20 mg, 40 mg, 80 mg. Sorbitol. Tab. Blister Pack. 28s. *Rx.*
Use: Antihypertensive.

Micardis HCT. (Boehringer Ingelheim) Telmisartan/hydrochlorothiazide 40 mg/12.5 mg, 80 mg/12.5 mg, 80 mg/25 mg. Sorbitol, lactose. Tab. Blister pack 30s. *Rx.*
Use: Antihypertensive.

Micatin. (Ortho) Miconazole nitrate 2%. Mineral oil. Cream. 15 g, 30 g. *OTC.*
Use: Antifungal, topical.

Mi-Cebrin. (Eli Lilly) Vitamins B_1 10 mg, B_2 5 mg, B_6 1.7 mg, pantothenic acid 10 mg, niacinamide 30 mg, B_{12} (activity equivalent) 3 mcg, C 100 mg, E 5.5 units, A 10,000 units, D 400 units, Fe 15 mg, Cu 1 mg, I 0.15 mg, Mn 1 mg, Mg 5 mg, Zn 1.5 mg. Tab. Pkg. 60s, 100s, 1000s, Blister pkg. 10 × 10s. *OTC.*
Use: Mineral, vitamin supplement.

Mi-Cebrin T. (Eli Lilly) Vitamins B_1 15 mg, B_2 10 mg, B_6 2 mg, pantothenic acid 10 mg, niacinamide 100 mg, B_{12} 7.5 mcg, C 150 mg, E 5.5 units, A 10,000 units, D 400 units, Fe 15 mg, Cu 1 mg, I 0.15 mg, Mn 1 mg, Mg 5 mg, Zn 1.5 mg. Tab. Bot. 30s, 100s, 1000s, Blister pkg. 10 × 10s. *OTC.*
Use: Mineral, vitamin supplement.

micofur.
Use: Antifungal; anti-infective, topical.

•**miconazole.** (my-KAHN-uh-zole) *USP.*
Use: Antifungal.

•**miconazole nitrate.** (my-CONE-ah-zole) *USP.*
Use: Antifungal agent, topical anti-infective.
See: Aloe Vesta.
Azolen.
Baza Antifungal.
Critic-Aid Clear AF.
Cruex.
Desenex.
Desenex Jock Itch.
Fungoid Tincture.
Lotrimin AF.
Micatin.
Micro-Guard.
Miranel AF.

Monistat 1 Combination Pack Triple Action.
Monistat 1 Day or Night Combination Pack.
Monistat 7.
Monistat 7 Combination Pack Dual Action.
Monistat 7 Combination Pack Triple Action.
Monistat 3.
Monistat 3 Combination Pack Dual Action.
Monistat 3 Combination Pack Triple Action.
Neosporin AF.
Podactin.
Remedy With Phytoplex Antifungal Clear.
Tetterine.
Triple Paste AF.
Vagistat-3 Combination Pack.
Zeasorb-AF.

miconazole nitrate. (Taro) Miconazole nitrate 2%. Benzoic acid, mineral oil, apricot kernel oil. Cream. Tube 15 g, 30 g. *OTC.*
Use: Antifungal agent, topical anti-infective.

miconazole nitrate. (Various Mfr.) Miconazole nitrate 2%. Vag. Cream. Tube 15 g, 30 g, 45 g. *OTC.*
Use: Antifungal, vaginal.

micoren. (Novartis) A respiratory stimulant; pending release.

MICRhoGAM. (Ortho-Clinical Diagnostics) Rh_0 (D) immune globulin microdose ≈ 5% ± 1% gamma globulin, sodium chloride 2.9 mg/mL, polysorbate 80 0.01%, glycine 15 mg/mL, preservative free. Soln. for Inj. Pkg. containing single-dose prefilled syringes, injection control form, patient ID card 5s, 25s. *Rx.*
Use: Immune globulin.

MICRhoGAM Ultra-Filtered Plus. (Ortho-Clinical Diagnostics) Rh_0(D) immune globulin microdose 50 mcg (250 units/dose). Glycine 15 mg/mL, polysorbate 80 0.01%, sodium chloride 2.9 mg/mL. Preservative free. Inj., Soln. Package w/single-dose syringe, control form, and patient ID card. 1s, 5s, 25s. *Rx.*
Use: Biologic and immunologic agent, immune globulin.

microbubble contrast agent.
Use: Aid in ID of intracranial tumors. [Orphan Drug]

Microcult-GC Test. (Bayer Consumer Care) Miniaturized culture test for the detection of *Neisseria gonorrhoeae.* Test Kit 25s.
Use: Diagnostic aid.

microfibrillar collagen hemostat.
Use: Hemostatic, topical.
See: Hemopad.

Microgestin Fe 1/20. (Watson) Ethinyl estradiol 20 mcg, norethindrone acetate 1 mg. Lactose. Tab. Pack 28s with 7 tabs. with ferrous fumarate 75 mg per tab. *Rx.*
Use: Sex hormone, contraceptive hormone.

Microgestin Fe 1.5/30. (Watson) Ethinyl estradiol 30 mcg, norethindrone acetate 1.5 mg. Lactose. Tab. Pack 28s with 7 tabs with ferrous fumarate 75 mg per tab. *Rx.*
Use: Sex hormone, contraceptive hormone.

Microgestin 1/20. (Watson) Ethinyl estradiol 20 mcg, norethindrone acetate 1 mg. Lactose. Tab. 21s. *Rx.*
Use: Monophasic oral contraceptive.

Micro-Guard. (Coloplast) Miconazole nitrate 2%. Cream. Tube. 57 g. *OTC.*
Use: Topical anti-infective, antifungal.

Micro-K Extencaps. (Wyeth) Potassium chloride (8 mEq) 600 mg. Cap. Bot. 100s, 500s, *Dis-Co* pack 100s. *Rx.*
Use: Electrolyte supplement.

Micro-K 10 Extencaps. (Wyeth) Potassium chloride 750 mg (10 mEq). Cap. Bot. 100s, 500s, *Dis-co* UD 100s. *Rx.*
Use: Electrolyte supplement.

Microlipid. (Nestle Healthcare Nutrition) Fat emulsion 50%, safflower oil, polyglycerol esters of fatty acids, soy lecithin, xanthan gum, ascorbic acid. Cal 4500, fat 500 g/L, 80 mOsm/Kg. H_2O. 120 mL. *Rx.*
Use: Nutritional supplement.

Micronor.
See: Ortho Micronor.

Microsol. (Star) Sulfamethizole 0.5 g, 1 g. Tab. Bot. 100s, 1000s. *Rx.*
Use: Anti-infective; urinary.

Microsol-A. (Star) Phenazopyridine 50 mg, sulfamethizole 0.5 g. Tab. Bot. 100s, 1000s. *Rx.*
Use: Anti-infective; urinary.

Microstix Candida. (Bayer Consumer Care) Test for *Candida* species in vaginal specimens. Box 25s.
Use: Diagnostic aid.

Microstix-3 Reagent Strips. (Bayer Consumer Care) For recognition of nitrite in urine and for semiquantitation of bacterial growth. Bot. 25s with 25 incubation pouches.
Use: Diagnostic aid.

MicroTrak Chlamydia Trachomatis Direct Specimen Test. (Syva) To detect

and identify chlamydia trachomatis. Slide test 60s.
Use: Diagnostic aid.

MicroTrak HSV 1/HSV 2 Culture Confirmation/Typing Test. (Syva) For identification and typing of herpes simplex in tissue culture. Test kit 1s.
Use: Diagnostic aid.

MicroTrak Neisseria Gonorrhea Culture Test. (Syva) For endocervical, urethral, rectal, and pharyngeal cultures. Test kit 85s.
Use: Diagnostic aid.

Microzide. (Watson) Hydrochlorothiazide 12.5 mg. Lactose. Cap. Bot. 100s. *Rx.*
Use: Diuretic.

Micrurus fulvius antivenin. (Wyeth) Inj. Combination package: One vial antivenin, one vial diluent (Bacteriostatic Water for Injection 10 mL).
Use: Antivenin.

Mictrin Plus. (Johnson & Johnson) Water, SD alcohol 38-B, glycerin, poloxamer 407, flavor, sodium saccharin, glutamic acid buffer, cetylpyridinium chloride, FD & C Yellow #5, Blue #1. Bot. 12 oz, 24 oz. *OTC.*
Use: Mouth preparation.

•**midaflur.** (MY-dah-flure) USAN.
Use: Hypnotic; sedative.

midamaline hydrochloride.
Use: Anesthetic, local.

Midamor. (Merck & Co.) Amiloride 5 mg. Tab. Bot. 100s. *Rx.*
Use: Diuretic; antihypertensive.

Midaneed. (Hanlon) Vitamins A 5000 units, D 500 units, B_1 5 mg, B_2 3 mg, B_6 0.5 mcg, B_{12} 5 mcg, C 100 mg, niacinamide 10 mg, calcium pantothenate 5 mg. Cap. Bot. 100s. *OTC.*
Use: Mineral, vitamin supplement.

•**midazolam hydrochloride.** (meh-DAZE-oh-lam) USAN.
Use: Anesthetic (injectable).

midazolam hydrochloride. (Roxane) Midazolam hydrochloride 2 mg/mL. EDTA, saccharin, sorbitol, cherry flavor. Syrup. 118 mL. *c-IV.*
Use: General anesthetic.

midazolam hydrochloride. (Various Mfr.) Midazolam hydrochloride 1 mg/mL, 5 mg/mL. Inj. Vial 1 mL (5 mg only), 2 mL, 5 mL. *Carpuject* Vial 10 mL. Syr. 2 mL (5 mg only). *c-IV.*
Use: Anesthetic.

•**midazolam maleate.** (meh-DAZE-oh-lam) USAN.
Use: Anesthetic, intravenous.

•**midodrine hydrochloride.** (MIH-doe-DREEN) USAN.
Use: Antihypotensive; vasoconstrictor.
See: ProAmatine.

midodrine hydrochloride. (Avkare) Midodrine hydrochloride 10 mg. Tab. 90s. *Rx.*
Use: Vasopressor used in shock.

midodrine hydrochloride. (Global) Midodrine hydrochloride 2.5 mg, 5 mg. Tab. 100s, 500s, 1,000s. *Rx.*
Use: Vasopressor used in shock.

midodrine hydrochloride. (Mylan) Midodrine hydrochloride 10 mg. Tab. 100s. *Rx.*
Use: Vasopressor used in shock.

midodrine hydrochloride. (Various Mfr.) Midodrine hydrochloride 2.5 mg, 5 mg. Tab. 100s, 500s (except 2.5 mg). *Rx.*
Use: Vasopressor used in shock.

Midol Cramp & Body Aches. (Bayer Consumer Care) Ibuprofen 200 mg. Tab. Bot. 24s. *OTC.*
Use: Analgesic; NSAID.

Midol Extended Relief. (Bayer Consumer Care) Naproxen 200 mg (naproxen sodium 220 mg). Sodium 20 mg. Tab. 24s. *OTC.*
Use: Nonsteroidal anti-inflammatory agent.

Midol Maximum Strength Cramp Formula. (Bayer Consumer Care) Ibuprofen 200 mg. Tab. 24s. *OTC.*
Use: Nonsteroidal anti-inflammatory agent.

Midol Menstrual Complete. (Bayer Consumer Care) Acetaminophen 500 mg, caffeine 60 mg, pyrilamine maleate 15 mg. Capl. Pkg. 8s, 16s, 32s. Gelcaps. Pkg. 12s, 24s. *OTC.*
Use: Analgesic combination.

Midol Pre-Menstrual Syndrome. (Bayer Consumer Care) Acetaminophen 500 mg, pamabrom 25 mg, pyrilamine maleate 15 mg. Capl. Bot. 24s. Gelcap: EDTA. Bot. 24s. *OTC.*
Use: Analgesic.

Midol Teen Formula. (Bayer Consumer Care) Acetaminophen 500 mg, pamabrom 25 mg. Capl. Bot. 24s. *OTC.*
Use: Analgesic.

•**midostaurin.** (mi-doe-STOR-in) USAN.
Use: Antineoplastic.

Midrin. (Caraco) Isometheptene mucate 65 mg, acetaminophen 325 mg, dichloralphenazone 100 mg. Cap. 100s. *c-IV.*
Use: Antimigraine.

Midstream Pregnancy Test Kit. (Ivax) Stick for urine test. Kit 1s. *OTC.*
Use: Pregnancy test.

•**mifamurtide.** (mif-AM-ure-tide) USAN.
Use: Investigational treatment for osteosarcoma.

Mifeprex. (Danco Labs) Mifepristone 200 mg. Tab. Single-dose blister pack containing 3 tabs. *Rx.*
Use: Uterine-active agent; abortifacient.

mifepristone.
Use: Uterine-active agent; abortifacient.
See: Korlym.
Mifeprex.

•**mifobate.** (mih-FOE-bate) USAN.
Use: Antiatherosclerotic.

•**migalastat.** (mi-GAL-a-stat) USAN.
Use: Treatment of Fabry disease.

•**migalastat hydrochloride.** (mi-GAL-a-stat) USAN.
Use: Treatment of Fabry disease.

Migergot. (G & W) Caffeine 100 mg, ergotamine tartrate 2 mg. Supp. 12s. *Rx.*
Use: Agent for migraine, migraine combination.

•**miglitol.** (mih-GLIH-tole) USAN.
Use: Antidiabetic.
See: Glyset.

•**miglustat.** (MIG-loo-stat)
Use: Gaucher disease.
See: Zavesca.

migraine agents.
See: Ergotamine Derivatives.
Serotonin 5-HT_1 Receptor Antagonist.

migraine combinations.
See: Isometheptene/Dichloralphenazone/Acetaminophen.

Migranal. (Valeant) Dihydroergotamine mesylate 4 mg/mL, caffeine 10 mg, dextrose 50 mg. Nasal spray. Vial w/nasal sprayer. 3.5 mL. *Rx.*
Use: Antimigraine.

MigraTen. (Pharmelle) Isometheptene mucate 65 mg, caffeine 100 mg, acetaminophen 325 mg. Cap. 100s. *Rx.*
Use: Migraine combination.

Migrazone. (Breckenridge) Acetaminophen 325 mg, dichloralphenazone 100 mg, isometheptene mucate 65 mg. Cap. 100s. *c-IV.*
Use: Agent for migraine, migraine combination.

MIH.
Use: Antineoplastic.
See: Matulane.

•**milacemide hydrochloride.** (mill-ASS-eh-mide) USAN.
Use: Anticonvulsant; antidepressant.

•**milameline hydrochloride.** (mill-AM-eh-leen) USAN.
Use: Antidementia (partial muscarinic agonist).

mild silver protein.
See: Silver Protein, Mild.

•**milenperone.** (mih-LEN-per-OHN) USAN.
Use: Antipsychotic.

•**milipertine.** (MIH-lih-PURR-teen) USAN.
Use: Antipsychotic.

milk of bismuth. (Various Mfr.) Bismuth hydroxide, bismuth subcarbonate.
Use: Orally; intestinal disturbances.

•**milk of magnesia.** (mag-NEE-zhuh) *USP. Formerly Magnesia Magma.*
Use: Antacid; laxative.
See: Magnesium hydroxide.

Milk of Magnesia. (Various Mfr.). Magnesium hydroxide 325 mg, 390 mg. **Tab.:** 250s, 1000s. **Liq.:** 120 mL, 360 mL, 720 mL, pt, qt, gal, UD 10 mL, 15 mL, 20 mL, 30 mL, 100 mL, 180 mL, 400 mL. **Susp.:** 400 mg/5 mL. Bot. 180 mL, 360 mL, 480 mL, UD 30 mL, gal. *OTC.*
Use: Antacid; laxative.

Milk of Magnesia-Concentrated. (Roxane) Equivalent to milk of magnesia 30 mL susp. Bot. 100 mL, 400 mL, UD 10 mL. *OTC.*
Use: Antacid; laxative.

•**milk thistle extract.** *NF.*
Use: Anti-inflammatory.

Millazine. (Major) Thioridazine. **10 mg, 15 mg/Tab.:** Bot. 100s. **25 mg/Tab.:** Bot. 100s, 1000s. **100 mg, 150 mg, 200 mg/Tab.:** Bot. 100s, 500s. *Rx.*
Use: Antipsychotic.

Millipred. (Laser Pharmaceutical) Prednisolone. **Oral Soln.:** 10 mg/5 mL. Dye free. Corn syrup, edetate disodium, methylparaben, saccharin. Grape flavor. 237 mL. **Tab.:** 5 mg. Lactose. 100s, 1,000s. *Rx.*
Use: Adrenocortical steroid, glucocorticoid.

•**milnacipran hydrochloride.** (mil-NA-si-pran) USAN.
Use: Treatment of fibromyalgia.
See: Savella.

•**milodistim.** (my-low-DIH-stim) USAN.
Use: Immunomodulator (antineutropenic).

Milophene. (Milex) Clomiphene citrate 50 mg. Tab. Bot. 30s. *Rx.*
Use: Sex hormone; ovulation stimulant.

Milpar. (Sanofi-Synthelabo) Magnesium hydroxide, mineral oil. *OTC.*
Use: Antacid; laxative.

•**milrinone lactate.** (MILL-rih-nohn) *USP.*
Use: Cardiovascular agent, congestive heart failure.

milrinone lactate. (Bedford) Milrinone lactate (as base) 1 mg/mL, dextrose 47 mg/mL, lactic acid 0.282 mg/mL.

Single-dose vials. 10 mL, 20 mL, 50 mL. *Rx.*
Use: Cardiovascular agent, congestive heart failure.

Milroy Artificial Tears. (Milton Roy) Bot. 22 mL.
Use: Artificial tears.

miltefosine.
Use: Anti-infective agent, antiprotozoal.
See: Impavido.

Miltown. (Wallace) Meprobamate 200 mg, 400 mg. Tab. Bot. 100s; 500s, 1000s (400 mg only). *c-iv.*
Use: Anxiolytic; antianxiety agent.

Miltown 600. (Wallace) Meprobamate 600 mg. Tab. Bot. 100s. *c-iv.*
Use: Anxiolytic.

•**mimbane hydrochloride.** (MIM-bane) USAN.
Use: Analgesic.

Mimvey. (Teva) Estradiol 1 mg/norethindrone acetate 0.5 mg. Film coated. Lactose, PEG. Tab. Blister pack. 28s. *Rx.*
Use: Sex hormone, estrogen/progestin combination.

•**minalrestat.** (min-AL-reh-stat) USAN.
Use: Aldose reductase inhibitor.

•**minaprine.** (MIN-ah-preen) USAN.
Use: Psychotherapeutic agent.

•**minaprine hydrochloride.** (MIN-ah-preen) USAN.
Use: Antidepressant.

Minastrin 24 Fe. (Warner Chilcott) Ethinyl estradiol 20 mcg, norethindrone acetate 1 mg. **Chew. Tab.:** Lactose, sugar. Spearmint flavor. 28s w/4 inert tablets (mannitol, sucralose). **Cap., softgel:** Glycerin, sesame oil, sorbitol. 28s w/4 inert tablets (glycerin, soybean oil, sorbitol). *Rx.*
Use: Monophasic oral contraceptive.

•**minaxolone.** (min-AX-oh-lone) USAN.
Use: Anesthetic.

mincard.
Use: Diuretic.

Mineral Freez. (Geritrex) Menthol 2%. Alcohol. Gel. 226.8 g. *OTC.*
Use: Rub and liniment.

Mineral Ice, Therapeutic. (Bristol-Myers Squibb) Menthol 2%, ammonium hydroxide, carbomer 934, cupric sulfate, isopropyl alcohol, magnesium sulfate, thymol. Gel Tube 105 g, 240 g, 480 g. *OTC.*
Use: Liniment.

mineralocorticoids.
Use: Adrenalocortical steroids.
See: Fludrocortisone Acetate.

•**mineral oil.** (MIN-er-al) *USP.*
Use: Laxative; pharmaceutic aid (solvent, oleaginous vehicle).
See: Kondremul Plain.
Min-O-Ear.
Petrolatum.
Soothe XP.

mineral oil. (Various Mfr.) Mineral oil. Liq. Bot. 180 mL, 473 mL. *OTC.*
Use: Laxative.

•**mineral oil, light.** (MIN-er-al) *NF.*
Use: Pharmaceutic aid (tablet and capsule lubricant, vehicle).
See: Soothe XP.

minerals.
See: Calcium.
Calcium Acetate.
Calcium Carbonate.
Calcium Citrate.
Calcium Glubionate.
Calcium Gluconate.
Calcium Lactate.
Calcium Microcrystalline Hydroxyapatite.
Magnesium.
Magnesium Citrate.
Magnesium Gluconate.
Magnesium Oxide.
Phosphate.
Sodium Phosphates.
Tricalcium Phosphate.

Mineral Zinc. (Mason) Ca 122 mg (calcium content expressed in mg elemental calcium), zinc 10 mg. Gluten free, preservative free, and sugar free. Tab. 100s. *OTC.*
Use: Nutritional supplement, multimineral.

Minerin. (Major) Glyceryl, lanolin alcohol, mineral oil, PEG, propylene glycol. Fragrance free. Lot. 473 mL. *OTC.*
Use: Emollient.

Minibex. (Faraday) Vitamins B_1 6 mg, B_2 3 mg, B_6 0.5 mg, C 50 mg, niacinamide 10 mg, calcium pantothenate 3 mg, B_{12} 2 mcg, folic acid 0.1 mg. Cap. Bot. 100s, 250s, 1000s. *OTC.*
Use: Mineral, vitamin supplement.

MiniCaps Vitamin-D Omega-3. (Sancilio) Omega-3 350 mg (DHA 100 mg, EPA 225 mg, other omega-3s 25 mg), fish oil 400 mg, vitamin D 1,000 units. Glycerin, mineral oil, orange oil. Cap., softgel. 30s, 500s, UD 100s. *OTC.*
Use: Multivitamin.

Minidyne 10%. (Pedinol Pharmacal) Povidone-iodine 10%, citric acid, sodium phosphate dibasic. Soln. Bot. 15 mL. *OTC.*
Use: Antimicrobial; antiseptic.

Minipress. (Pfizer) Prazosin hydrochloride 1 mg, 2 mg, 5 mg. Cap. Bot. 250s.

Rx.
Use: Antihypertensive, antiadrenergic.

Miniprin Low Dose. (Time-Cap Labs) Aspirin 81 mg. Lactose. Tab., enteric coated. 120s. *OTC.*
Use: Salicylate.

Minirin. (Ferring) Desmopressin acetate 0.1 mg, chlorobutanol 5 mg/mL. Nasal spray. 5 mL (50 doses of 10 mcg). *Rx.*
Use: Posterior pituitary hormones.

Minitec. (Bristol-Myers Squibb) Sodium pertechnetate Tc 99 m generator.
Use: Radiopaque agent.

Minitec Generator (Complete with Components). (Bristol-Myers Squibb) Medotopes Kit.
Use: Diagnostic aid.

Minitran. (Medicis) Nitroglycerin 0.1 mg/h (9 mg), 0.2 mg/h (18 mg), 0.4 mg/h (36 mg), 0.6 mg/h (54 mg). Transdermal Patch. 30s. *Rx.*
Use: Antianginal.

Minit-Rub. (Bristol-Myers Squibb) Methyl salicylate 15%, menthol 3.5%, camphor 2.3% in anhydrous base. Tube 1.5 oz, 3 oz. *OTC.*
Use: Analgesic, topical.

Minivelle. (Noven Pharmaceuticals) Estradiol 0.0375 mg (total estradiol 0.62 mg; 2.48 cm^2), 0.05 mg (total estradiol 0.83 mg; 3.3 cm^2), 0.075 mg (total estradiol 1.24 mg; 4.95 cm^2), 0.1 mg (total estradiol 1.65 mg; 6.6 cm^2) per 24 h. Patch; transdermal. Calendar pack (8 and 24 systems). *Rx.*
Use: Sex hormone, estrogen.

Minocin. (Triax) Minocycline hydrochloride. **Cap., pellet filled:** 50 mg, 100 mg. 50s (100 mg), 100s (50 mg), kit w/*T^3 Calming Wipes* (sodium hyaluronate; alcohol free; 30s). **Inj., lyophilized Pow. for Soln.:** 100 mg. Vial. *Rx.*
Use: Anti-infective, tetracycline.

•**minocromil.** (MIH-no-KROE-mill) USAN.
Use: Antiallergic (prophylactic).

•**minocycline.** (mihn-oh-SIGH-kleen) USAN.
Use: Anti-infective.
See: Vectrin.
Ximino.

•**minocycline hydrochloride.** (mihn-oh-SIGH-kleen) *USP.*
Use: Anti-infective, tetracycline.
See: Arestin.
Dynacin.
Minocin.
Solodyn.

minocycline hydrochloride. (Various Mfr.) Minocycline hydrochloride. **Tab.:** 50 mg, 75 mg, 100 mg. May contain lactose. 50s (100 mg only), 60s (100 mg), 100s (except 100 mg). **ER Tab.:** 45 mg, 80 mg, 90 mg, 135 mg. Film coated. May contain lactose. 30s, 100s. **Cap.:** 50 mg, 75 mg, 100 mg. 50s (100 mg only), 60s (except 75 mg), 100s (except 100 mg), 500s (100 mg only), UD 50s (100 mg only). *Rx.*
Use: Tetracycline.

minocycline hydrochloride. *Rx.*
Use: Anti-infective, tetracycline.

Min-O-Ear. (Geritrex) Mineral oil. Otic Soln. 22 mL. *Rx.*
Use: Otic preparation.

•**minoxidil.** (min-OX-ih-dill) *USP.*
Use: Antihypertensive; vasodilator; antialopecia agent.
See: Rogaine.
Rogaine Extra Strength for Men.
Rogaine Men's Extra Strength.

minoxidil. (Rugby) Minoxidil 10 mg. Tab. Bot. 500s. *Rx.*
Use: Antihypertensive.

minoxidil. (Schein) Minoxidil 2.5 mg. Tab. Bot. 100s, 500s, 1000s. *Rx.*
Use: Antihypertensive.

Minoxidil Extra Strength for Men. (Apotex USA) Minoxidil 5%. Alcohol 30%. Top. Soln. Bot. 60 mL (1s and 2s). *OTC.*
Use: Alopecia.

Minoxidil for Men. (Various Mfr.) Minoxidil 2%. Alcohol 60%, propylene glycol. Soln., Top. 60 mL. *OTC.*
Use: Dermatological agent.

Minto-Chlor Syrup. (Pal-Pak, Inc.) Codeine sulfate 10 mg, potassium citrate 219 mg/5 mL, alcohol 2%. Gal. *c-v.*
Use: Antitussive, expectorant.

Mintox. (Major) **Susp.:** Aluminum hydroxide 200 mg, magnesium hydroxide 200 mg, simethicone 20 mg. Benzyl alcohol, parabens, saccharin, sorbitol, sodium 1 mg per 5 mL. Mint creme flavor. 355 mL. **Chew. Tab.:** Aluminum hydroxide/magnesium hydroxide. **200 mg/200 mg:** Saccharin. Mint flavor. 100s. **300 mg/150 mg:** Aspartame, phenylalanine, sorbitol. 24s. *OTC.*
Use: Antacid.

Mintox Plus Extra Strength Liquid. (Major) Aluminum hydroxide 500 mg, magnesium hydroxide 450 mg, simethicone 40 mg/5 mL. Bot. 355 mL. *OTC.*
Use: Antacid, antiflatulent.

Mintox Plus Tablets. (Major) Aluminum hydroxide 200 mg, magnesium hydroxide 200 mg, simethicone 25 mg. Chew. Tab. 100s. *OTC.*
Use: Antacid; antiflatulent.

Mint Sensodyne. (Block Drug) Potassium nitrate 5%, saccharin, sorbitol.

Toothpaste. Tube 28.3 g. *OTC.*
Use: Toothpaste for sensitive teeth.

Mintuss MR. (Breckenridge) Hydrocodone bitartrate 5 mg, pyrilamine maleate 5 mg, phenylephrine hydrochloride 5 mg per 5 mL. Sugar and alcohol free. Menthol, sucrose. Pineapple-orange flavor. Syrup. 473 mL. *c-III.*
Use: Antitussive combination.

Minute-Gel. (Oral-B) Acidulated phosphate fluoride 1.23%. Gel. Bot. 16 oz. *Rx.*
Use: Dental caries agent.

Miochol-E. (Novartis Ophthalmic) Acetylcholine chloride 1:100, mannitol 2.8% when reconstituted. Soln. In 2 mL Univials. *Rx.*
Use: Antiglaucoma agent.

•**mioflazine hydrochloride.** (MY-ah-FLAY-zeen) USAN.
Use: Vasodilator (coronary).

Miostat Intraocular Solution. (Alcon) Carbachol 0.01%. Vial 1.5 mL. Pkg. 12s.
Use: Antiglaucoma agent.

miotics, cholinesterase inhibitors.
Use: Glaucoma agents.
See: Echothiophate Iodide.
Eserine Salicylate.
Eserine Sulfate.
Floropryl.

•**mipafilcon A.** (mih-paff-ILL-kahn A) USAN.
Use: Contact lens material (hydrophilic).

•**mipomersen sodium.** (Mi-poe-MER-sen) USAN.
Use: Antihyperlipidemic agent.
See: Kynamro.

•**mirabegron.** (mye-ra-BE-ron) USAN.
Use: Genitourinary agent.
See: Myrbetriq.

MiraFlow Extra Strength. (Ciba Vision) Isopropyl alcohol 15.7%, poloxamer 407, amphoteric 10. Thimerosal free. Soln. Bot. 12 mL. *OTC.*
Use: Contact lens care.

Miral. (Armenpharm Ltd.) Dexamethasone 0.75 mg. Tab. Bot. 100s, 1000s.
Use: Corticosteroid.

MiraLax. (Schering-Plough) Polyethylene glycol 3350 17 g, 119 g, 238 g, 510 g. Pow. for oral soln. Single-dose packet (17 g only). 12s. 119 g (119 g), 239 g (238 g), 510 g (510 g). *OTC.*
Use: Laxative; bowel evacuant.

Miranel AF. (Humco) Miconazole nitrate 2%. Alcohol, camphor, EDTA, eucalyptus oil, menthol, oregano oil, propylene glycol, tea tree oil, urea. Soln. 28 g. *OTC.*
Use: Topical anti-infective, antifungal.

Mirapex. (Boehringer Ingelheim) Pramipexole dihydrochloride 0.125 mg, 0.25 mg, 0.5 mg, 0.75 mg, 1 mg, 1.5 mg. Mannitol. Tab. Bot. 90s, UD 100s (except 0.125 mg, 0.75 mg). *Rx.*
Use: Antiparkinson agent.

Mirapex ER. (Boehringer Ingelheim) Pramipexole dihydrochloride 0.375 mg, 0.75 mg, 1.5 mg, 2.25 mg, 3 mg, 3.75 mg, 4.5 mg. ER Tab. 30s. *Rx.*
Use: Dopaminergic, dopamine receptor agonist, nonergot.

Miraphen PSE. (Major) Pseudoephedrine hydrochloride 120 mg, guaifenesin 600 mg. ER Tab. Bot. 500s. *Rx.*
Use: Upper respiratory combination, decongestant, expectorant.

Mircette. (Duramed) **Phase 1:** Desogestrel 0.15 mg, ethinyl estradiol 20 mcg. 21 tabs. **Phase 2:** Ethinyl estradiol 10 mcg. 5 tabs. Lactose. Tab. Blister Cards. 28s with 2 inert tabs. *Rx.*
Use: Sex hormone, contraceptive hormone.

Mirena. (Bayer) T-shaped unit containing a reservoir of levonorgestrel 52 mg covered by a silicone membrane. Intrauterine system. Pkg. 1s w/inserter. *Rx.*
Use: Sex hormone; contraceptive.

•**mirfentanil hydrochloride.** (MIHR-FEN-tan-ill) USAN.
Use: Analgesic.

•**mirincamycin hydrochloride.** (mihr-IN-kah-MY-sin) USAN.
Use: Anti-infective; antimalarial.

•**mirisetron maleate.** (my-RIH-seh-trahn) USAN.
Use: Antianxiety.

•**mirtazapine.** (mihr-TAZZ-ah-PEEN) USAN.
Use: Antidepressant, tetracyclic compound.
See: Remeron.
Remeron SolTab.

mirtazapine. (Various Mfr.) Mirtazapine. **Orally Disintegrating Tab.:** 15 mg, 30 mg, 45 mg. May contain aspartame, corn syrup, mannitol, phenylalanine, xylitol. UD 30s. **Tab.:** 7.5 mg, 15 mg, 30 mg, 45 mg. May contain lactose. 30s, 90s (15 mg, 30 mg, 45 mg), 100s (15 mg, 30 mg, 45 mg), 500s, 1000s. Rx.
Use: Antidepressant, tetracyclic compound.

Mirvaso. (Galderma) Brimonidine tartrate 0.33%. Glycerin, methylparaben, propylene glycol, titanium dioxide. Gel. 30 g, 45 g. *Rx.*
Use: Dermatologic alpha-adrenergic agonist.

•**misonidazole.** (MY-so-NIH-dah-zole) USAN.
Use: Antiprotozoal (trichomonas).

•**misoprostol.** (MY-so-PRAHST-ole) USAN.
Use: Antiulcerative.
See: Cytotec.
W/Diclofenac sodium.
See: Arthrotec.

misoprostol. (Various Mfr.) Misoprostol 100 mcg, 200 mcg. Tab. Unit-of-use 60s, 100s (200 mcg only), 120s (120 mcg only). *Rx.*
Use: Antiulcerative.

Mission Prenatal. (Mission Pharmacal) Ferrous gluconate 260 mg (iron 30 mg), vitamins C 100 mg, B_1 5 mg, B_6 3 mg, B_2 2 mg, B_3 10 mg, B_5 1 mg, B_{12} 2 mcg, A 4000 units, D 400 units, Ca, zinc 15 mg. Tab. Bot. 100s. *OTC.*
Use: Mineral, vitamin supplement.

Mission Prenatal F.A. (Mission Pharmacal) Ferrous gluconate 260 mg (iron 30 mg), vitamins C 100 mg, B_1 5 mg, B_6 10 mg, B_2 2 mg, B_3 10 mg, B_{12} 2 mcg, folic acid 0.8 mg, A acetate 4000 units, D 400 units, Ca, B_5 1 mg. Tab. Bot. 100s. *OTC.*
Use: Mineral, vitamin supplement.

Mission Prenatal H.P. (Mission Pharmacal) Ferrous gluconate 260 mg (iron 30 mg), vitamins C 100 mg, B_1 5 mg, B_6 25 mg, B_2 2 mg, B_3 10 mg, B_5 1 mg, B_{12} 2 mcg, folic acid 0.8 mg, A 4000 units, D 400 units, Ca. Tab. Bot. 100s. *OTC.*
Use: Mineral, vitamin supplement.

Mission Prenatal Rx. (Mission Pharmacal) Vitamins A 8000 units, D 400 units, C 240 mg, B_1 4 mg, B_2 2 mg, B_3 20 mg, B_5 10 mg, B_6 20 mg, B_{12} 8 mcg, folic acid 1 mg, Fe 60 mg, Ca 175 mg, I, Zn 15 mg, Cu. Tab. Bot. 100s. *Rx.*
Use: Mineral, vitamin supplement.

Mission Surgical Supplement. (Mission Pharmacal) Vitamins C 500 mg, B_1 2.5 mg, B_2 2.6 mg, B_3 30 mg, B_5 16.3 mg, B_6 3.6 mg, B_{12} 9 mcg, A 5000 units, D 400 units, E 45 units, Fe 27 mg, Zn 22.5 mg. Tab. Bot. 100s. *OTC.*
Use: Mineral, vitamin supplement.

•**mitemcinal fumarate.** (mye-TEM-cin-al) USAN.
Use: GERD.

•**mitindomide.** (my-TIN-doe-MIDE) USAN.
Use: Antineoplastic.

•**mitocarcin.** (MY-toe-CAR-sin) USAN. Antibiotic derived from *Streptomyces* species.
Use: Antineoplastic.

•**mitocromin.** (MY-toe-KROE-min) USAN. Produced by *Streptomyces virdochromogenes.*
Use: Antineoplastic.

•**mitogillin.** (MY-toe-GIH-lin) USAN. An antibiotic obtained from a "unique strain" of *Aspergillus restrictus.*
Use: Antitumorigenic antibiotic; antineoplastic.

mitoguazone. (CTRC Research Foundation)
Use: Treatment of diffuse non-Hodgkin lymphoma. [Orphan Drug]

mitolactol.
Use: Adjuvant therapy in the treatment of primary brain tumors. [Orphan Drug]

•**mitomalcin.** (MY-toe-MAL-sin) USAN. Produced by *Streptomyces malayensis.* Under study.
Use: Antineoplastic.

•**mitomycin.** (MY-toe-MY-sin) *USP.* In literature as Mitomycin C. Antibiotic isolated from *Streptomyces caespitosis.*
Tall Man: mitoMYcin
Use: Anti-infective, antibiotic; antineoplastic.

mitomycin. (Various Mfr.) Mitomycin 5 mg (mannitol 10 mg), 20 mg (mannitol 40 mg), 40 mg (mannitol 80 mg). Pow. for Inj. Vials. *Rx.*
Use: Antibiotic.

mitomycin C.
See: Mitomycin.

Mitosol. (Mobius Therapeutics) Mitomycin 0.2 mg. Mannitol 0.4 mg. Lyophilized Pow. for Soln.; Ophth. Kit (contains 1 vial containing mitomycin 0.2 mg; one 1 mL syringe of sterile water for injection w/connector; 1 plunger rod, one vial adapter w/spike; one 1 mL tuberculin syringe, Luer lock; 1 sponge container; six 3 mm absorbent sponges; six 6 mm absorbent sponges; 6 half-moon sponges; 1 instrument wedge sponge; 1 alcohol prep pad, sterile; 1 chemotherapy waste bag). *Rx.*
Use: Ophthalmic surgical adjunct.

•**mitosper.** (MY-toe-sper) USAN. Substance derived from *Aspergillus* of the glaucus group.
Use: Antineoplastic.

•**mitotane.** (MY-toe-TANE) *USP. Formerly o,p'-DDD.*
Use: Antineoplastic.
See: Lysodren.

•**mitoxantrone hydrochloride.** (MY-toe-ZAN-trone) *USP.*
Tall Man: mitoXANtrone

Use: Antineoplastic; immunologic agent; anthracenedione.

mitoxantrone hydrochloride. (Various Mfr.) Mitoxantrone free base 2 mg/mL. Preservative free. Inj. Multi-dose vials. 10 mL, 12.5 mL, 15 mL. *Rx.*
Use: Anthracenedione; antineoplastic.

•**mitumomab.** (mih-TOO-moe-mab) USAN.
Use: Antitumor monoclonal antibody.

•**mitumprotimut-T.** (MYE-tum-PROE-ti-mut T) USAN.
Use: Treatment of B-cell non-Hodgkin lymphoma.

•**mivacurium chloride.** (MYE-va-KUE-ree-um) *Rx.*
Use: Muscle relaxant–adjunct to anesthesia, nondepolarizing neuromuscular blockers.

•**mivobulin isethionate.** (mih-VOE-byoo-lin eye-seh-THIGH-oh-nate) USAN.
Use: Antineoplastic (microtubule inhibitor).

Mixed E 400 Softgels. (Naturally) Vitamin E 400 IU. Cap. Bot. 60s, 90s, 180s. *OTC.*
Use: Vitamin supplement.

Mixed E 1000 Softgels. (Naturally) Vitamin E 1000 IU. Cap. Bot. 30s, 60s *OTC.*
Use: Vitamin supplement.

Mixed Respiratory Vaccine. Each mL contains *Staphylococcus aureus* 1,200 million organisms, *Streptococcus* (both *viridans* and nonhemolytic) 200 million organisms, *Streptococcus (Diplococcus) pneumoniae* 150 million organisms, *Moraxella (Branhamella, Neisseria) catarrhalis* 150 million organisms, *Klebsiella pneumoniae* 150 million organisms, and *Haemophilus influenzae* types a and b 150 million organisms. Vial. 20 mL.
Use: Bacterial vaccine.
See: MRV.

mixed vespid Hymenoptera venom. *Rx.*
Use: Agent for immunization.
See: Albay.
Pharmalgen.
Venomil.

•**mixidine.** (MIX-ih-deen) USAN.
Use: Vasodilator (coronary).

mixture 612. Dimethyl phthalate solution, compound.

M-M-R II. (Merck) Mixture of 3 viruses: ≥ 1000 measles $TCID_{50}$ (tissue culture infectious doses), ≥ 20,000 mumps $TCID_{50}$, and ≥ 1000 rubella $TCID_{50}$ per 0.5 mL dose. Neomycin 25 mcg. Pow. for Inj. Single dose vial w/diluent. *Rx.*
Use: Agent for immunization.

Mobic. (Boehringer Ingelheim/Abbott) Meloxicam. **Oral Susp.:** 7.5 mg/5 mL. Saccharin, sorbitol. Raspberry flavor. 100 mL. **Tab.:** 7.5 mg, 15 mg. Lactose. Bot. 100s. *Rx.*
Use: Nonsteroidal anti-inflammatory agent.

Mobidin. (B.F. Ascher) Magnesium salicylate, anhydrous 600 mg. Tab. Bot. 100s, 500s. *Rx.*
Use: Antiarthritic.

Mobisyl Creme. (B.F. Ascher) Trolamine salicylate in vanishing creme base. Tube 100 g. *OTC.*
Use: Analgesic, topical.

•**mocetinostat.** (MOE-se-TIN-oh-stat) USAN.
Use: Antineoplastic.

•**mocetinostat dihydrobromide.** (MOE-se-TIN-oh-stat dye-HYE-droe-BROE-mide) USAN.
Use: Antineoplastic.

•**moclobemide.** (moe-KLOE-beh-mide) USAN.
Use: Antidepressant.

•**modafinil.** (moe-DAFF-ih-nill) USAN.
Use: CNS stimulant, analeptic.
See: Provigil.

modafinil. (Various Mfr.) Modafinil 100 mg, 200 mg. Lactose. Tab. 30s, 90s. *c-IV.*
Use: CNS stimulant, analeptic.

•**modaline sulfate.** (MODE-al-een) USAN.
Use: Antidepressant.

Modane. (Savage) Bisacodyl 5 mg. Lactose. Tab., delayed release. 100s. *OTC.*
Use: Laxative.

Modane Mild. (Pharmacia) Phenolphthalein 60 mg. Tab. Bot. 10s, 30s, 100s. *OTC.*
Use: Laxative.

Modane Versabran. (Pharmacia) Psyllium hydrophilic mucilloid in wheat bran base. Dose 3.4 g, Bot. 10 oz. *OTC.*
Use: Laxative.

•**modecainide.** (moe-deh-CANE-ide) USAN.
Use: Cardiovascular (antiarrhythmic).

Moderiba. (AbbVie) Ribavirin 200 mg, 400 mg, 600 mg. Film coated. Lactose. Tab. 168s and *Moderiba* 600 dose packs (200 mg); *Moderiba* 600, 800, and 1,000 dose packs (400 mg); *Moderiba* 1,000 and 1,200 dose packs (600 mg). **Note:** Each *Moderiba* 600 dose pack contains 7 ribavirin 200 mg tablets and 7 ribavirin 400 mg tablets. Each *Moderiba* 800 dose pack contains 14 ribavirin 400 mg tablets. Each *Moderiba* 1,000 dose pack contains

7 ribavirin 400 mg tablets and 7 ribavirin 600 mg tablets. Each *Moderiba* 1,200 dose pack contains 14 ribavirin 600 mg tablets. *Rx.*
Use: Antiviral agent.

Modicon. (Janssen) Norethindrone 0.5 mg, ethinyl estradiol 35 mcg. Lactose. Tab. *Dialpak* and *Veridate* 28s with 7 inert tabs. *Rx.*
Use: Sex hormone, contraceptive hormone.

modinal.
See: Gardinol Type Detergents.

•**modithromycin.** (moe-IDTH-roe-MYE-sin) USAN.
Use: Antibiotic.

Moducal. (Bristol-Myers Squibb) Maltodextrin. Pow. Can 13 oz. *OTC.*
Use: Nutritional supplement.

Moduretic. (Merck & Co.) Hydrochlorothiazide 50 mg, amiloride 5 mg. Tab. Bot. 100s, UD 100s. *Rx.*
Use: Antihypertensive; diuretic.

moenomycin. Phosphorus-containing glycolipide antibiotic. Active against gram-positive organisms. Under study.

•**moexipril hydrochloride.** (moe-EX-ah-prill) USAN.
Use: Renin angiotensin system antagonist, angiotensin-converting enzyme inhibitor.
See: Univasc.
W/Hydrochlorothiazide.
See: Uniretic.

moexipril hydrochloride. (Various Mfr.) Moexipril hydrochloride 7.5 mg, 15 mg. Lactose. Film-coated. Tab. Unit-of-use 90s, 100s, 500s. *Rx.*
Use: Renin angiotensin system antagonist, angiotensin-converting enzyme inhibitor.

moexipril hydrochloride/hydrochlorothiazide. (Teva) Moexipril hydrochloride/hydrochlorothiazide 7.5 mg/12.5 mg, 15 mg/12.5 mg, 15 mg/25 mg. Tartrazine (except 15 mg/12.5 mg). Film-coated. Tab. 100s. *Rx.*
Use: Antihypertensive combination.

•**mofegiline hydrochloride.** (moe-FEH-jih-leen) USAN.
Use: Antiparkinsonian.

•**mogamulizumab.** (moe-GAM-ue-LIZ-oo-mab) USAN.
Use: Antineoplastic.

Moist Again. (Lake Consumer) Aloe vera, EDTA, methylparaben, glycerin. Gel. Tube 70.8 g. *OTC.*
Use: Vaginal agent.

Moi-Stir. (Kingswood) Dibasic sodium phosphate, calcium chloride, sodium chloride, potassium chloride, Mg, sorbitol, sodium carboxymethylcellulose, parabens. Soln. Bot. 120 mL spray. *OTC.*
Use: Saliva substitute.

Moi-Stir Swabsticks. (Kingswood) Dibasic sodium phosphate, Mg, calcium chloride, sodium chloride, potassium chloride, sorbitol, sodium carboxymethylcellulose, parabens. Swabsticks. Pkt. 3s. *OTC.*
Use: Saliva substitute.

Moisture Eyes Preservative Free. (Bausch & Lomb) Propylene glycol 0.95%, boric acid, NaCl, sodium borate, edetate disodium. Preservative free. Soln.; Ophth. 0.6 mL (UD 30s). *OTC.*
Use: Artificial tears.

molar phosphate.
W/Fluoride ion.
See: Coral.

•**molgramostim.** (mahl-GRAH-moe-STIM) USAN.
Use: Hematopoietic stimulant; antineutropenic.

•**molinazone.** (moe-LEEN-ah-zone) USAN.
Use: Analgesic.

•**molindone hydrochloride.** (moe-LIN-dohn) *USP.*
Use: Antipsychotic.

Mollifene Ear Drops. (Pfeiffer) Glycerin, camphor, cajaput oil, eucalyptus oil, thyme oil. Soln. Bot. 24 mL. *OTC.*
Use: Otic.

Mollifene Ear Wax Removing Formula. (Pfeiffer) Carbamide peroxide 6.5%, anhydrous glycerin. Propylene glycol, sodium stannate. Drops. 15 mL with dropper. *OTC.*
Use: Otic preparation.

•**molsidomine.** (mole-SIH-doe-meen) USAN.
Use: Antianginal; vasodilator (coronary).

molybdenum solution. (American Quinine) Molybdenum 25 mcg/mL (as 46 mcg/mL ammonium molybdate tetrahydrate). Inj. Vial 10 mL. *Rx.*
Use: Nutritional supplement, parenteral.

Molycu. (Burns) Meprobamate 400 mg, copper 60 mg/mL. *Rx.*
Use: Antidote.

Moly-Pak. (SoloPak Pharmaceuticals, Inc.) Molybdenum 25 mcg. Inj. Vial 10 mL. *Rx.*
Use: Nutritional supplement, parenteral.

•**momelotinib.** (MOE-me-LOE-ti-nib) USAN.
Use: Antineoplastic.

•**momelotinib dihydrochloride.** (MOE-me-LOE-ti-nib) USAN.
Use: Antineoplastic.

Momentum. (Whitehall-Robins) Aspirin 500 mg, phenyltoloxamine citrate 15 mg. Capl. Bot. 24s, 48s. *OTC.*
Use: Analgesic.

Momentum Muscular Backache Formula. (Whitehall-Robins) Magnesium salicylate tetrahydrate 580 mg (equivalent to 467 mg magnesium salicylate anhydrous). Capl. Box. 48s. *OTC.*
Use: Analgesic compound.

•**mometasone furoate.** (moe-MET-uh-SONE FEW-roh-ate) *USP.*
Use: Corticosteroid, topical; intranasal steroid; oral inhalation.
See: Asmanex Twisthaler.
Elocon.
Propel.
W/Formoterol Fumarate.
See: Dulera.

mometasone furoate. (Clay Park) Mometasone furoate. **Cream:** 0.1%. White petrolatum, stearyl alcohol. 15 g, 45 g. **Top. Soln.:** 0.1%. Isopropyl alcohol 40%, glycerin. 30 mL, 60 mL. *Rx.*
Use: Topical corticosteroid.

mometasone furoate. (Taro) Mometasone furoate 0.1%. Isopropyl alcohol. Lot. Bot. 30 mL, 60 mL. *Rx.*
Use: Anti-inflammatory agent; topical corticosteroid.

mometasone furoate. (Various Mfr.) Mometasone furoate 0.1%. Oint. 15 g, 45 g. *Rx.*
Use: Topical corticosteroid.

mometasone furoate monohydrate.
Use: Respiratory inhalant, intranasal steroid.
See: Nasonex.

monacetyl pyrogallol. Eugallol. Pyrogallol monoacetate.
Use: Keratolytic.

Monafed. (Monarch) Guaifenesin 600 mg, lactose. SR Tab. Bot. 100s. *Rx.*
Use: Expectorant.

monalium hydrate. Hydrated magnesium aluminate. Magaldrate.
See: Riopan.

•**monatepil maleate.** (moe-NAT-eh-pill) USAN.
Use: Antianginal; antihypertensive.

•**monensin.** (mah-NEN-sin) *USP.*
Use: Antifungal; anti-infective; antiprotozoal.

•**monensin sodium.** (mah-NEN-sin) *USP.*
Use: Antifungal; anti-infective; antiprotozoal.

Monistat 1. (Insight Pharmaceuticals) Tioconazole 6.5%. Vag. Oint. Prefilled single-dose applicator 4.6 g. *OTC.*
Use: Antifungal, vaginal.

Monistat 1 Combination Pack Dual Action. (Insight Pharmaceuticals) Miconazole nitrate. **Supp.:** 1200 mg, petrolatum w/parafin. Pkg. 1s w/applicator. **Cream:** 2%, stearyl and cetyl alcohol. Tube 9 g. *Rx.*
Use: Antifungal, vaginal.

Monistat 1 Combination Pack Triple Action. (Insight Pharmaceuticals) Miconazole nitrate. **Supp.; vaginal:** 1,200 mg. Glycerin, mineral oil, petrolatum. 1s w/applicator. **Cream:** 2%. Alcohols, benzoic acid. 9 g. *OTC.*
Use: Antifungal, vaginal.

Monistat 1 Day or Night Combination Pack. (Insight Pharmaceuticals) Miconazole nitrate. **Supp.; vaginal:** 1,200 mg. Glycerin, mineral oil, white petrolatum. 1s w/applicator. **Cream:** 2%. Alcohols, benzoic acid. Tube. 9 g. *OTC.*
Use: Antifungal, vaginal.

Monistat 7. (Insight Pharmaceuticals) Miconazole nitrate. **Vag. Supp.:** 100 mg. Box 7s w/applicator. **Vag. Cream:** 2%. Tube 35 g, 45 g w/1 applicator or 7 *Ultraslim* disp. applicators, or 7 prefilled applicators w/5 g cream. *OTC.*
Use: Antifungal, vaginal.

Monistat 7 Combination Pack Dual Action. (Insight Pharmaceuticals) **Vaginal Supp.:** Miconazole nitrate 100 mg. In 7s with applicator. **Topical Cream:** Miconazole nitrate 2%. Tube. *OTC.*
Use: Antifungal, vaginal.

Monistat 7 Combination Pack Triple Action. (Insight Pharmaceuticals) Miconazole nitrate. **Cream; vaginal:** 100 mg. Alcohols, benzoic acid. 45 g w/7 applicators. **Cream; Top.:** 2%. Alcohol, benzoic acid. 9 g. *OTC.*
Use: Antifungal, vaginal.

Monistat 3. (Insight Pharmaceuticals) Miconazole nitrate 4%. Vag. Cream. Pkg. Prefilled applicator (3). *OTC.*
Use: Antifungal, vaginal.

Monistat 3 Combination Pack Dual Action. (Insight Pharmaceuticals) Miconazole nitrate. **Vag. Supp.:** 200 mg. 3s w/1 reusable applicator or 3 disp. applicators. **Top. Cream:** 2%. Tube. *OTC.*
Use: Antifungal, vaginal.

Monistat 3 Combination Pack Triple Action. (Insight Pharmaceuticals) Miconazole nitrate. **Supp.; vaginal:** 200 mg. Glycerin, vegetable oil. 3s w/applicators. **Cream:** 2%. Alcohols, benzoic acid.

9 g. *OTC.*
Use: Antifungal, vaginal.

monoamine oxidase inhibitors.
Use: Antidepressant.
See: Isocarboxazid.
Phenelzine Sulfate.
Tranylcypromine Sulfate.

•**mono- and di-acetylated monoglycerides.** (mahn-OH and di-ah-SEE-till-ated mahn-OH-GLIH-sir-ides) *NF.* A mixture of glycerin esterified mono- and diesters of edible fatty acids followed by direct acetylation.
Use: Pharmaceutic aid (plasticizer).

•**mono- and di-glycerides.** (mahn-OH and di-GLIH-sir-ides) *NF.* A mixture of mono- and diesters of fatty acids from edible oils.
Use: Fatty acids; pharmaceutic aid (emulsifying agent).

monobactams.
See: Aztreonam.

•**monobenzone.** (MON-oh-BEN-zone) *USP.*
Use: Pigment agent.

Monocal. (Mericon) Fluoride 3 mg, Ca 250 mg. Tab. Bot. 100s. *OTC.*
Use: Mineral supplement.

Monocaps Tablets. (Freeda) Iron 14 mg, vitamins A 10,000 units, D 400 units, E 15 units, B_1 15 mg, B_2 15 mg, B_3 41 mg, B_5 15 mg, B_6 15 mcg, B_{12} 15 mcg, C 125 mg, folic acid 0.1 mg, biotin 15 mg, PABA, L-lysine, Ca, Cu, I, K, Mg, Mn, Se, Zn 12 mg, lecithin. Tab. Bot. 100s, 250s, 500s. *OTC.*
Use: Mineral, vitamin supplement.

Monocete EZ Swabs. (Pedinol) Monochloroacetic acid 80%. PEG 200. Swab. 15s. *Rx.*
Use: Destructive agent, chloroacetic acid.

monochloroacetic acid.
Use: Cauterizing agent.
See: Monocete EZ Swabs.

monochlorophenol-para.
See: Camphorated Para-chlorophenol.

Monoclate-P. (CSL Behring) Human antihemophilic factor 250 units, 500 units, 1,000 units, 1,500 units. Albumin (human) ≈ 1% to 2%, histidine, mannitol 0.8%, ≤ 50 ng murine monoclonal antibody per 100 AHF units, sodium. Heat treated, monoclonal antibody purified. Inj., lyophilized Pow. for Soln. Single-dose vial and diluent. *Rx.*
Use: Antihemophilic agent.

monoclonal antibodies.
See: Alemtuzumab.
Belimumab.
Bevacizumab.
Cetuximab.
Denosumab.
Eculizumab.
Gemtuzumab Ozogamicin.
Ibritumomab Tiuxetan.
Ipilimumab.
Obinutuzumab.
Ofatumumab.
Omalizumab.
Palivizumab.
Panitumumab.
Ramucirumab.
Raxibacumab.
Rituximab.
Siltuximab.
Tositumomab and Iodine I 131 Tositumomab.
Trastuzumab.

monoclonal antibodies (murine) anti-idiotype melanoma associated antigen.
Use: Invasive cutaneous melanoma. [Orphan Drug]

monoclonal antibody for immunization against lupus nephritis. (Medclone, Inc.)
Use: Immunization. [Orphan Drug]

monoclonal antibody (human) against hepatitis B virus.
Use: Prophylaxis in hepatitis B reinfection in liver transplants. [Orphan Drug]

monoclonal antibody to CD4, 5a8. (Biogen)
Use: Postexposure prophylaxis for HIV. [Orphan Drug]

•**monoctanoin.** (MAHN-ahk-tuh-NO-in) USAN.

monocycline hydrochloride.
See: Minocin IV.

Mono-Diff Test. (Wampole)
Use: Diagnostic aid; mononucleosis.

Monodox. (Oclassen) Doxycycline monohydrate 75 mg, 100 mg. Cap. 50s, 250s (100 mg); 100s (75 mg). *Rx.*
Use: Anti-infective; tetracycline.

•**monoethanolamine.** (mahn-oh-eth-an-OLE-ah-meen) *NF.*
Use: Pharmaceutic aid (surfactant).

Monoject PreFill Advanced. (Kendall) Heparin 10 units/mL, 100 units/mL. Preservative free. 3 mL, 5 mL, 10 mL (10 units/mL only) prefilled syringes. *Rx.*
Use: Anticoagulant.

Monojel. (Sherwood Davis & Geck) Glucose 40%. UD 25 g. *OTC.*
Use: Hyperglycemic.

Monoket. (Schwarz Pharma) Isosorbide mononitrate 10 mg, 20 mg. Lactose. Tab. Bot. 100s; 180s, UD 100s (20 mg only). *Rx.*
Use: Vasodilator.

Mono-Latex. (Wampole) Two-minute latex agglutination slide test for the qualitative or semiquantitative detection of infectious mononucleosis heterophile antibodies in serum or plasma. Test kit 20s, 50s, 1000s.
Use: Diagnostic aid.

monolaurin.
Use: Treatment of congenital primary ichthyosis. [Orphan Drug]
See: Glylorin.

MonoNessa. (Watson) Norgestimate 0.25 mg, ethinyl estradiol 35 mcg. Lactose. Tab. Pkg. 28s. *Rx.*
Use: Sex hormone, contraceptive hormone.

Mononine. (CSL Behring) Factor IX (human) ≈ 250 units, ≈ 500 units, ≈ 1,000 units (monoclonal antibody purified). Actual number of units shown on each bottle. Histidine ≈ 10 mM, mannitol 3%, polysorbate 80 0.0075%, sodium chloride 0.066 M, ≤ 50 ng of mouse protein per 100 factor IX activity units (murine monoclonal antibody used in purification). Inj., lyophilized Pow. for Soln. Kit (kits include sterile water for injection 5 mL, double-ended needle for reconstitution, vented filter spike for withdrawal, winged infusion set, and alcohol swabs) w/single-dose vial and diluent. *Rx.*
Use: Antihemophilic agent.

mononucleosis tests.
Use: Diagnostic aid.
See: Mono-Diff Test.
Mono-Latex.
Mono-Plus.
Monospot.
Monosticon Dri-Dot.
Mono-Sure Test.

Monopar. Stilbazium Iodide.
Use: Anthelmintic.

monophen.
Use: Cholecystography.

Mono-Plus. (Wampole) To diagnose infectious mononucleosis from serum, plasma, or fingertip blood. Test kits 24s.
Use: Diagnostic aid.

Monopril. (Bristol-Myers Squibb) Fosinopril sodium 10 mg, 20 mg, 40 mg. Lactose. Tab. Bot. 90s, 1000s (except 40 mg), UD 100s (20 mg only). *Rx.*
Use: Renin angiotensin system antagonist, angiotensin-converting enzyme inhibitor.

Monopril-HCT. (Bristol-Myers Squibb) Fosinopril sodium/hydrochlorothiazide 10 mg/12.5 mg, 20 mg/12.5 mg. Lactose. Tab. Bot. 100s. *Rx.*
Use: Antihypertensive.

•**monosodium glutamate.** (mahn-oh-SO-dee-uhm GLUE-tah-mate) *NF.*
Use: Pharmaceutic aid (flavor, perfume).

monosodium phosphate.
See: Sodium Biphosphate.

Monospot. (Ortho-Clinical Diagnostics) Diagnosis of infectious mononucleosis. Test kit 20s.
Use: Diagnostic aid.

monostearin. (Various Mfr.) Glyceryl monostearate.

Monosticon Dri-Dot. (Organon Teknika) Diagnosis of infectious mononucleosis. Test kit 40s, 100s.
Use: Diagnostic aid.

Mono-Sure Test. (Wampole) One-minute hemagglutination slide test for the differential qualitative detection and quantitative determination of infectious mononucleosis heterophile antibodies in serum or plasma. Kit 20s.
Use: Diagnostic aid.

Monosyl. (Arcum) Secobarbital sodium 1 gr, butabarbital 0.5 gr. Tab. Bot. 100s, 1000s. *c-II.*
Use: Hypnotic; sedative.

Monotard Human Insulin. (Bristol-Myers Squibb; Novo/Nordisk) Human insulin zinc 100 units/mL. Susp. Vial 10 mL. *OTC.*
Use: Antidiabetic.

•**monothioglycerol.** (mahn-oh-thigh-oh-GLIS-er-ole) *NF.*
Use: Pharmaceutic aid (preservative).

Mono-Vacc Test O.T. (Aventis Pasteur) 5 tuberculin units by the Mantoux method. Multiple puncture disposable device. Box 25s (tamper-proof). *Rx.*
Use: Diagnostic aid, tuberculosis.

Monovisc. (Anika Therapeutics) Hyaluronan 22 mg/mL. Sodium chloride. Inj., Soln. Prefilled syringe. 4 mL. *Rx.*
Use: Physical adjunct.

monoxychlorosene. A stabilized, buffered, organichypochlorous acid derivative.
See: Oxychlorosene.

Monsel Solution. (Wade) Bot. 2 oz, 4 oz.
Use: Styptic solution.

•**montelukast sodium.** (mahn-teh-LOO-kast) USAN.
Use: Antiasthmatic, leukotriene receptor antagonist.
See: Singulair.

montelukast sodium. (Dr. Reddy's Laboratories) Montelukast 4 mg/packet (equiv. to montelukast sodium 4.2 mg). Mannitol. Gran. UD 30s. *Rx.*
Use: Leukotriene receptor antagonist.

montelukast sodium. (Various Mfr.) Montelukast. **Tab.:** 10 mg (equiv. to mon-

telukast sodium 10.4 mg). May contain lactose, PEG. 30s, 90s, 1,000s, 10,000s, UD 100s. **Chew. Tab.:** 4 mg (equiv. to montelukast sodium 4.2 mg), 5 mg (equiv. to montelukast sodium 5.2 mg). May contain aspartame, mannitol, phenylalanine, sucralose. 30s, 90s, 500s, 1,000s, UD 30s, UD 100s. *Rx.*
Use: Leukotriene receptor antagonist.

Monurol. (Forest) Fosfomycin tromethamine 3 g/Gran. Single-dose packet. *Rx.*
Use: Anti-infective, urinary.

•**morantel tartrate.** (moe-RAN-tell) USAN.
Use: Anthelmintic.

Moranyl. Suramin.

Morco. (Archer-Taylor) Cod liver oil ointment, zinc oxide, benzethonium chloride, benzocaine 1%. 1.5 oz, lb. *OTC.*
Use: Antiseptic; antipruritic, topical.

More-Dophilus. (Freeda) Lactobacillus acidophilus 12.4 billion units. Pow. 1 oz, 4 oz. *OTC.*
Use: Antidiarrheal; nutritional supplement.

Morgidox. (Medimetriks) Doxycycline hyclate 100 mg. Lactose. Tab. UD 30s and 60s and kits of 30s and 60s with *Acu-Wash* cleanser. *Rx.*
Use: Anti-infective, tetracycline.

•**moricizine hydrochloride.** (MAHR-IH-sizz-een) USAN.
Use: Cardiovascular agent (antiarrhythmic).

•**morniflumate.** (MAR-nih-FLEW-mate) USAN.
Use: Anti-inflammatory.

Moroline. (Schering-Plough) Petrolatum. Jar 1.75 oz, 3.75 oz, 15 oz. *OTC.*
Use: Dermatologic; lubricant; protectant.

Morpen. (Major) Ibuprofen 400 mg, 600 mg. Tab. Bot. 500s. *Rx.*
Use: Analgesic; NSAID.

morphine hydrochloride. (Various Mfr.) Pow. Bot. 1 oz, 5 oz. *c-II.*
Use: Analgesic.

•**morphine sulfate.** (MORE-feen) *USP.*
Use: Opioid analgesic; sedative.
See: Astramorph PF.
Avinza.
DepoDur.
Duramorph.
Infumorph 500.
Infumorph 200.
Kadian.
MS Contin.
MSIR.
Oramorph SR.
RMS.
Roxanol.
Roxanol 100.
Roxanol T.

morphine sulfate. (Abbott, Baxter) Morphine sulfate 0.5 mg/mL. Inj. Amps and vials 10 mL. *c-II.*
Use: Analgesic, narcotic agonist.

morphine sulfate. (Eli Lilly) Morphine sulfate 10 mg, 15 mg, 30 mg, Soln. Tab. Bot. 100s. *c-II.*
Use: Analgesic, narcotic.

morphine sulfate. (Endo) Morphine sulfate 15 mg, 30 mg, 60 mg, 100 mg, lactose. ER Tab. Bot. 100s, 500s. *c-II.*
Use: Analgesic, narcotic agonist.

morphine sulfate. (Ethex) Morphine sulfate 20 mg/mL, alcohol free. Soln. Bot 30 mL, 120 mL, 240 mL. *c-II.*
Use: Analgesic, narcotic agonist.

morphine sulfate. (Paddock) Morphine sulfate. Compounding Pow. Bot. 25 g. *c-II.*
Use: Analgesic, narcotic agonist.

morphine sulfate. (Ranbaxy) Morphine sulfate 10 mg, 15 mg, 30 mg. Lactose, sucrose. Soluble Tab. for Inj. Bot. 100s. *c-II.*
Use: Opioid analgesic.

morphine sulfate. (Roxane) Morphine sulfate 10 mg/5 mL, 20 mg/5 mL. Oral Soln. Bot. 100 mL, 500 mL. UD 5 mL (10 mg only), 10 mL (10 mg only). *c-II.*
Use: Opioid analgesic.

morphine sulfate. (Various Mfr.) Morphine sulfate. **Tab.:** 15 mg, 30 mg. 100s, UD 100s. **ER Tab.:** 15 mg, 30 mg, 60 mg, 100 mg, 200 mg (for use only in opioid-tolerant patients). 50s (30 mg only), 100s, 500s (except 200 mg), UD 100s (except 200 mg). 150 punch cards (15 mg, 30 mg, 60 mg only). **ER Cap.:** 10 mg, 20 mg, 30 mg, 50 mg, 60 mg, 80 mg, 100 mg, 200 mg. May contain PEG, sucrose. 30s, 100s. **Oral Soln., concentrate:** 20 mg/mL. Alcohol free. 15 mL, 30 mL, 120 mL, 240 mL with calibrated dropper or spoon. **Inj.:** 1 mg/mL (Vial 10 mL, 30 mL. Amp. 10 mL), 2 mg/mL (Vial 30 mL, syringe, *Carpuject*, *Tubex* 1 mL); 4 mg/mL (Disp. Syringe 1 mL, 2 mL. *Tubex* and *Carpuject* 1 mL), 5 mg/mL (Vial 1 mL), 8 mg/mL (Vial, Amp., *Carpuject*, 1 mL), 10 mg/mL (1 mL *Carpuject*, Vial, Amp.; Multidose vial 10 mL), 15 mg/mL (Amp., *Carpuject*, Vial 1 mL, Multidose vial 20 mL). **Soln. for Inj.:** 25 mg/mL (Syringe 4 mL, 10 mL, 20 mL, 40 mL; Single-use vials [may contain sulfites]); 50 mg/mL (Syringe 10 mL, 20 mL, 40 mL, 50 mL; Single-use vials [may

contain sulfites]). **Rec. Supp.:** 5 mg, 10 mg, 20 mg, 30 mg. Box 12s. *c-II.*
Use: Opioid analgesic.

morphine sulfate. (Watson) Morphine sulfate 15 mg; 30 mg; 60 mg; 100 mg, 200 mg (for use in opioid-tolerant patients only). Lactose (except 100 mg, 200 mg). Film-coated. CR Tab. 100s. *c-II.*
Use: Opioid analgesic.

morphine sulfate in 5% dextrose. (Hospira) Morphine sulfate 1 mg/mL. Inj. 100 mL, 250 mL. *c-II.*
Use: Opioid analgesic.

•**morrhuate sodium.** (MORE-you-ate) *USP.*
Use: Sclerosing agent.
See: Scleromate.

morrhuate sodium. (Various Mfr.) Morrhuate sodium 50 mg/mL. Inj. Multiple-use vials. 30 mL. *Rx.*
Use: Sclerosing agent.

Morton Salt Substitute. (Morton Grove) Potassium chloride, fumaric acid, tricalcium phosphate, monocalcium phosphate. Na < 0.5 mg/5 g (0.02 mEq/5 g), K 2800 mg/5 g (72 mEq/5 g) 88.6 g. *OTC.*
Use: Salt substitute.

Morton Seasoned Salt Substitute. (Morton Grove) Potassium chloride, spices, sugar, fumaric acid, tricalcium phosphate, monocalcium phosphate. Na < 1 mg/5 g (< 0.04 mEq/5 g), K 2165 mg/5 g (56 mEq/5 g). Bot. 85.1 g. *OTC.*
Use: Salt substitute.

Mosco. (Medtech) Salicylic acid 17.6%. Jar. 10 mL. *OTC.*
Use: Keratolytic.

•**motavizumab.** (moe-ta-VIZ-ue-mab) USAN.
Use: Prevention of respiratory syncytial virus.

•**motesanib.** (moe-TES-a-nib) USAN.
Use: Antiangiogenesis agent.

•**motexafin gadolinium.** (moe-TEX-a-fin gad-OH-lihn-ee-uhm) USAN.
Use: Investigational antineoplastic.

•**motexafin lutetium.** (moe-TEX-a-fin) USAN.
Use: Photoantineoplastic.

Motilium. (Janssen) Domperidone maleate. *Rx.*
Use: Antiemetic.

Motion Aid. (Vangard Labs, Inc.) Dimenhydrinate 50 mg. Tab. Bot. 100s, 1000s, UD 10 × 10s.
Use: Antiemetic; antivertigo.

Motion Cure. (Wisconsin Pharmacal Co.) Meclizine 25 mg. Chew. Tab. 12s.
Use: Antiemetic; antivertigo.

motion sickness agents.
See: Antinauseants.
Bucladin.
Dramamine.
Emetrol.
Marezine.
Scopolamine Hydrobromide.

Motofen. (Valeant) Difenoxin hydrochloride 1 mg, atropine sulfate 0.025 mg. Tab. Bot. 50s, 100s. *c-IV.*
Use: Antidiarrheal.

•**motretinide.** (MOE-TREH-tih-nide) USAN.
Use: Keratolytic.

Motrin, Children's. (McNeil Consumer Healthcare) Ibuprofen 100 mg/5 mL, sucrose. Susp. Bot. 120 mL, 480 mL. *Rx-OTC.*
Use: Analgesic, nonsteroidal anti-inflammatory agent.

Motrin Children's Cold. (McNeil Consumer Healthcare) Pseudoephedrine hydrochloride 15 mg, ibuprofen 100 mg/5 mL. Acesulfame K, sucrose, sucralose. Tropical punch, berry, or grape flavors. Dye free. Susp. Bot. 118 mL. *OTC.*
Use: Upper respiratory combination, decongestant, analgesic.

Motrin IB. (McNeil Consumer Healthcare) Ibuprofen. **Tab.:** 200 mg. Bot. 100s. **Gelcap.:** 200 mg. Pkg. 8s. *OTC.*
Use: Analgesic; nonsteroidal anti-inflammatory agent.

Motrin, Infant's. (McNeil Consumer Healthcare) Ibuprofen 40 mg/mL. Sorbitol, sucrose. Berry flavor. Oral Drops. 30 mL with dropper. *OTC.*
Use: Nonsteroidal anti-inflammatory agent.

Motrin, Junior Strength. (McNeil Consumer Healthcare) Ibuprofen. **Chew. Tab.:** 100 mg. Aspartame, phenylalanine 6 mg, orange flavor. Pkg. 24s **Tab.:** 100 mg. 24s. *OTC.*
Use: Analgesic, nonsteroidal anti-inflammatory agent.

Motrin Migraine Pain. (McNeil Consumer Healthcare) Ibuprofen 200 mg. Capl. Bot. 24s, 50s, 100s. *OTC.*
Use: Analgesic, nonsteroidal anti-inflammatory agent.

mouth and throat products.
See: Amlexanox.
Benzocaine.
Benzyl Alcohol.
Carbamide Peroxide.
Doxycycline.
Menthol.
Minocycline Hydrochloride.

Pilocarpine Hydrochloride.
Saliva Substitutes.
Sulfuric Acid/Sulfonated Phenolics.
Tetracycline Hydrochloride.

MouthKote. (Parnell) Xylitol, sorbitol, yerba santa, citric acid, ascorbic acid, sodium benzoate, saccharin, lemon-lime flavor. Soln. Spray Bot. 60 mL, 240 mL. *OTC.*
Use: Saliva substitute.

MoviPrep. (Salix) PEG 3350 100 g, sodium sulfate 7.5 g, sodium chloride 2.691 g, potassium chloride 1.015 g. Ascorbic acid 4.7 g, sodium ascorbate 5.9 g, phenylalanine 2.33 mg. Lemon flavor. Pow. for Reconstitution. Cartons with disposable container and 4 pouches. *Rx.*
Use: Laxative.

•**moxalactam disodium for injection.** (MOX-ah-LACK-tam) *USP.*
Use: Anti-infective.
See: Moxam.

Moxam. (Eli Lilly) Moxalactam disodium. Vial 1 g/10 mL Traypak 10s; Vial 2 g/20 mL Traypak 10s; Vial 10 g/100 mL Traypak 6s. *Rx.*
Use: Anti-infective; cephalosporin.

Moxatag. (Shionogi Pharma) Amoxicillin 775 mg. Film-coated. ER Tab. 30s, UD 10s. *Rx.*
Use: Penicillin, aminopenicillin.

•**moxazocine.** (MOX-AZE-oh-seen) USAN.
Use: Analgesic; antitussive.

•**moxetumomab pasudotox.** (MOX-e-TOOM-oh-mab pa-SOO-doe-tox) USAN.
Use: Antineoplastic.

Moxeza. (Alcon Vision) Moxifloxacin hydrochloride 0.5%. Boric acid, sodium chloride. Soln., Ophth. 3 mL *Drop-Tainer. Rx.*
Use: Ophthalmic and otic agent, ophthalmic antibiotic.

•**moxifloxacin hydrochloride.** (mox-ih-FLOX-ah-sin) USAN.
Use: Anti-infective; fluoroquinolone; antibiotic, ophthalmic.
See: Avelox.
Avelox IV.
Moxeza.
Vigamox.

moxifloxacin hydrochloride. (Various Mfr.) Moxifloxacin hydrochloride 400 mg. May contain lactose, PEG. Tab. 30s, 100s, 500s, 1,000s, UD 50s. *Rx.*
Use: Anti-infective, fluoroquinolone.

•**moxilubant maleate.** (MOX-ill-yoo-bahnt) USAN.
Use: Treatment of rheumatoid arthritis and psoriasis (leukotriene B_4 receptor antagonist).

•**moxnidazole.** (MOX-NIH-dazz-ole) USAN.
Use: Antiprotozoal (trichomonas).

M-Oxy. (Mallinckrodt) Oxycodone hydrochloride 5 mg. Tab. Bot. 100s. *c-II.*
Use: Opioid analgesic.

Moxy Compound. (Major) Theophylline 130 mg, ephedrine 25 mg, hydroxyzine hydrochloride 10 mg. Tab. Bot. 100s. *Rx.*
Use: Antiasthmatic compound.

Moyco Fluoride Rinse. (Moyco Union Broach Division) Fluoride 2%. Flavor. Bot. 128 oz. with pump. *Rx-OTC.*
Use: Dental caries agent.

Mozobil. (Genzyme) Plerixafor 20 mg/mL. Sodium chloride 5.9 mg. Preservative free. Inj., Soln. Single-use vial. *Rx.*
Use: Hematopoietic agent, stem cell mobilizer.

6-MP.
Use: Antimetabolite.
See: Purinethol.

MRV. (Bayer Consumer Care) 2,000 million organisms/mL from *Staphylococcus aureus* (1200 million), *Streptococcus*, viridans and nonhemolytic (200 million), *Streptococcus pneumoniae* (150 million), *Branhamella catarrhalis* (150 million), *Klebsiella pneumoniae* (150 million), *Haemophilus influenzae* (150 million). Inj. Vial 20 mL. *Rx.*
Use: Immunization.

MS Contin. (Purdue Frederick) Morphine sulfate 15 mg; 30 mg; 60 mg; 100 mg, 200 mg (for use only in opioid-tolerant patients). Lactose (except 100 mg, 200 mg). CR Tab. Bot. 100s, 500s (except 200 mg), UD 25s (except 200 mg). *c-II.*
Use: Opioid analgesic.

MSIR. (Purdue Frederick) Morphine sulfate. **Oral Soln.:** 10 mg/5 mL, 20 mg/5 mL. Sugar, sucrose. EDTA. Bot. 120 mL. **Oral Soln. (concentrate):** 20 mg/mL. EDTA. 30 mL with calibrated dropper. *c-II.*
Use: Opioid analgesic.

MS/L-Concentrate. (Richwood Pharmaceuticals) Morphine sulfate 100 mg/5 mL. Oral Soln. Bot. 120 mL w/calibrated dropper. *c-II.*
Use: Analgesic; narcotic.

MS/S. (Richwood Pharmaceuticals) Morphine sulfate 5 mg, 10 mg, 20 mg, 30 mg. Supp. 12s. *c-II.*
Use: Analgesic; narcotic.

MTC. Mitomycin. *Rx.*
Use: Anti-infective.
See: Mutamycin.

mTOR inhibitor.
Use: Protein-tyrosine kinase inhibitor.
See: Everolimus.
Temsirolimus.

MTP-PE. (Novartis) Muramyl-tripeptide.
Use: Immunomodulator.

MTX. *Rx.*
Use: Antineoplastic; antipsoriatic.
See: Methotrexate.

MTX Support. (Theralogix) Cyanocobalamin 1,000 mcg, folic acid 0.5 mg. Tab. 180s. *OTC.*
Use: Multivitamin.

•**mubritinib.** (mue-bri-TYE-nib) USAN.
Use: Antineoplastic agent.

MucaphEd. (Edwards Pharmaceuticals) Guaifenesin 400 mg, phenylephrine hydrochloride 10 mg. Lactose, maltodextrin, mineral oil. Tab. 100s. *OTC.*
Use: Upper respiratory combination, decongestant and expectorant combination.

mucilloid of psyllium seed.
W/Dextrose.
See: Metamucil.

mucin.
See: Gastric Mucin.

Mucinex. (Reckitt Benckiser) Guaifenesin 600 mg (100 mg immediate-release, 500 mg extended-release). ER Tab. Bot. 20s, 40s, 500s. *OTC.*
Use: Expectorant.

Mucinex Children's. (Reckitt Benckiser) Guaifenesin 100 mg per 5 mL. Alcohol free. Parabens, saccharin. Grape flavor. Liq. 118 mL. *OTC.*
Use: Expectorant.

Mucinex Children's Cold, Cough and Sore Throat. (Reckitt Benckiser) Acetaminophen 162.5 mg, dextromethorphan hydrobromide 5 mg, guaifenesin 100 mg, phenylephrine hydrochloride 2.5 mg per 5 mL. Edetate disodium, glycerin, propylene glycol, sodium 3 mg, sodium benzoate, sorbitol, sucralose. Mixed berry flavor. Liq. 118 mL. *OTC.*
Use: Upper respiratory combination, antitussive and expectorant combination.

Mucinex Children's Stuffy Nose & Cold. (Reckitt Benckiser) Guaifenesin 100 mg, phenylephrine hydrochloride 2.5 mg. Dextrose, parabens, saccharin, sorbitol, sucralose. Alcohol free. Mixed berry flavor. Liq. 118 mL. *OTC.*
Use: Upper respiratory combination, decongestant and expectorant combination.

Mucinex Cough for Kids. (Reckitt Benckiser) Dextromethorphan hydrobromide 5 mg, guaifenesin 100 mg. Dextrose, parabens, saccharin, sucralose. Alcohol free. Cherry flavor. Liq. 118 mL. *OTC.*
Use: Upper respiratory combination, antitussive with expectorant.

Mucinex Cough Mini-Melts for Kids. (Reckitt Benckiser) Dextromethorphan hydrobromide 5 mg, guaifenesin 100 mg. Aspartame, phenylalanine 2 mg, sorbitol. Orange cream flavor. Gran. 12s. *OTC.*
Use: Upper respiratory combination, antitussive with expectorant.

Mucinex D. (Reckitt Benckiser) Pseudoephedrine hydrochloride 60 mg, guaifenesin 600 mg. ER Tab. 18s. *OTC.*
Use: Upper respiratory combination, decongestant and expectorant combination.

Mucinex DM. (Reckitt Benckiser) Dextromethorphan HBr 30 mg, guaifenesin 600 mg. ER Tab. 20s, 40s. *OTC.*
Use: Antitussive with expectorant, upper respiratory combination.

Mucinex DM Maximum Strength. (Reckitt Benckiser) Dextromethorphan hydrobromide 60 mg, guaifenesin 1,200 mg. ER Tab. 14s. *OTC.*
Use: Upper respiratory combination, antitussive with expectorant.

Mucinex Fast-Max Cold and Sinus. (Reckitt Benckiser) Acetaminophen 325 mg, guaifenesin 200 mg, phenylephrine hydrochloride 5 mg. Coated. PEG. Cap. 20s, 30s. *OTC.*
Use: Upper respiratory combination, decongestant and expectorant combination.

Mucinex Fast-Max Cold, Flu and Sore Throat. (Reckitt Benckiser) Acetaminophen 325 mg, dextromethorphan hydrobromide 10 mg, guaifenesin 200 mg, phenylephrine hydrochloride 5 mg. Coated. PEG. Cap. 20s, 30s. *OTC.*
Use: Upper respiratory combination, antitussive and expectorant combination.

Mucinex Fast-Max Severe Congestion and Cold. (Reckitt Benckiser) Acetaminophen 325 mg, dextromethorphan hydrobromide 10 mg, guaifenesin 200 mg, phenylephrine hydrochloride 5 mg. Coated. PEG. Cap. 20s, 30s. *OTC.*
Use: Upper respiratory combination, antitussive and expectorant combination.

Mucinex for Kids. (Reckitt Benckiser) Guaifenesin 100 mg per 5 mL. Parabens, saccharin. Alcohol free. Grape

flavor. Liq. 118 mL. *OTC.*
Use: Expectorant.

Mucinex Maximum Strength. (Reckitt Benckiser) Guaifenesin 1,200 mg. ER Tab. 28s. *OTC.*
Use: Expectorant.

Mucinex Mini-Melts for Kids. (Reckitt Benckiser) Guaifenesin 50 mg, 100 mg per packet. Aspartame, phenylalanine 0.6 mg, 1 mg, sorbitol. Grape, bubble gum flavor. Gran. 12s. *OTC.*
Use: Expectorant.

MUC 9 + 4 Pediatric. (Fujisawa Healthcare) Vitamin A 2300 units, D 400 units, E 7 mg, B_1 1.2 mg, B_2 1.4 mg, B_3 17 mg, B_5 5 mg, B_6 1 mg, B_{12} 1 mcg, C 80 mg, biotin 20 mcg, folic acid 0.14 mg, K 200 mcg/5 mL, mannitol 375 mg. Pow. Vial. 10 mL. *Rx.*
Use: Nutritional supplement, parenteral.

Muco-Fen DM. (Ivax) Guaifenesin 1000 mg, dextromethorphan HBr 60 mg. Dye free. Long-acting Tab. Bot. 100s. *Rx.*
Use: Upper respiratory combination, antitussive, expectorant.

Muco-Fen LA. (Ivax) Guaifenesin 600 mg, dye free. TR Tab. Bot. 100s. *Rx.*
Use: Expectorant.

mucolytics.
Use: Respiratory.

Mucotrol. (Edwards Pharmaceuticals) Sorbitol, *Cyamopsis tetragonolobus*, aloe, acesulfame K, glycyrrhiza, *Centella asiatica, Polygonum cuspidatum, Angelica* spp., *Camella sinensis.* Sugar free. Wafer, concentrated gel. 21s, 45s. *Rx.*
Use: Mouth and throat product.

MucusRelief. (Major) Guaifenesin 400 mg. Maltodextrin. Dye free. Tab. 60s. *OTC.*
Use: Respiratory agent, expectorant.

MucusRelief DM. (Major) Dextromethorphan hydrobromide 20 mg, guaifenesin 400 mg. Maltodextrin, PEG. Tab. 30s. *OTC.*
Use: Upper respiratory combination, antitussive with expectorant.

MucusRelief Sinus. (Major) Phenylephrine hydrochloride 10 mg, guaifenesin 400 mg. Tab. 60s. *OTC.*
Use: Upper respiratory combination, decongestant and expectorant combination.

Mudd. (Chattem) Natural hydrated magnesium aluminum silicate. Topical preparation. *OTC.*
Use: Cleanser.

Mudrane GG Elixir. (ECR) Theophylline 20 mg, ephedrine hydrochloride 4 mg, guaifenesin 26 mg, phenobarbital 2.5 mg/5 mL, alcohol 20%. Bot. pt, 0.5 gal. *Rx.*
Use: Antiasthmatic combination.

Mudrane-2. (ECR) Potassium iodide 195 mg, aminophylline (anhydrous) 130 mg. Tab. Bot. 100s. *Rx.*
Use: Antiasthmatic combination.

MuGard. (Access Pharmaceuticals) Benzyl alcohol, carbomer homopolymer A, citric acid, glycerin, potassium hydroxide, saccharin. Oral Rinse. 237 mL. *Rx.*
Use: Mouth and throat product.

Multa-Gen 12 + E. (Jones Pharma) Vitamin A 5000 units, D 400 units, B_1 2 mg, B_2 2 mg, B_6 0.5 mg, B_{12} 3 mcg, C 37.5 mg, E 15 units, folic acid 0.2 mg, nicotinamide 20 mg. Cap. Bot. 60s, 500s, 1000s. *OTC.*
Use: Vitamin supplement.

Multaq. (Sanofi-Aventis) Dronedarone 400 mg. Film coated. Lactose. Tab. 60s, 180s, 500s, UD 100s. *Rx.*
Use: Cardiovascular agent, antiarrhythmic agent.

Multi-B Complex. (Integrative Therapeutics) Vitamins B_1 50 mg, B_2 60 mg, B_3 75 mg, B_5 50 mg, B_6 55 mg, B_{12} 100 mcg, folic acid 400 mcg, biotin 50 mcg, choline 50 mg, inositol 50 mg, PABA 25 mg. Gluten free, preservative free. 60s. *OTC.*
Use: Multivitamin.

Multi-B-Plex. (Forest) Vitamins B_1 100 mg, B_2 1 mg, nicotinamide 100 mg, pantothenic acid 10 mg, B_6 10 mg/mL. Inj. Vial 10 mL, 30 mL. *Rx.*
Use: Mineral, vitamin supplement.

Multi-B-Plex Capsules. (Forest) Vitamins B_1 50 mg, B_2 5 mg, niacinamide 50 mg, calcium pantothenate 5.4 mg, B_6 0.2 mg, C 150 mg, B_{12} 1 mcg. Cap. Bot. 100s, 1000s. *OTC.*
Use: Mineral, vitamin supplement.

Multi-Day. (NBTY) Vitamins A 5000 units, D 400 units, E 30 mg, B_1 1.5 mg, B_2 1.7 mg, B_3 20 mg, B_5 10 mg, B_6 2 mg, B_{12} 6 mcg, C 60 mg, FA 0.4 mL. Tab. Bot. 100s. *OTC.*
Use: Vitamin supplement.

Multi-Day Plus Iron. (NBTY) Fe 18 mg, A 5000 units, D 400 units, E 15 mg, B_1 1.5 mg, B_2 1.7 mg, B_3 20 mg, B_6 2 mg, B_{12} 6 mcg, C 60 mg, FA 0.4 mg. Tab. Bot. 100s. *OTC.*
Use: Vitamin supplement.

Multi-Day Plus Minerals. (NBTY) Fe 18 mg, A 6500 units, D 400 units, E 30 mg, B_1 1.5 mg, B_2 1.7 mg, B_3 20 mg, B_5 10 mg, B_6 2 mg, B_{12} 6 mcg, C

60 mg, FA 0.4 mg, Ca, Cl, Cr, Cu, I, K, Mg, Mn, Mo, P, Se, Zn 15 mg, biotin 30 mcg. Tab. Bot. 100s. *OTC.*
Use: Vitamin supplement.

Multi-Day with Calcium and Extra Iron Tablets. (NBTY) Fe 27 mg, A 5000 units, D 400 units, E 30 mg, B_1 1.5 mg, B_2 1.7 mg, B_3 20 mg, B_5 10 mg, B_6 2 mg, B_{12} 6 mcg, C 60 mg, FA 0.4 mg, Ca, Zn 15 mg, tartrazine. Tab. Bot. 100s. *OTC.*
Use: Mineral, vitamin supplement.

Multifol. (Breckenridge) Ca 125 mg, iron (as ferrous fumarate) 65 mg, vitamin A 6000 units, D 400 units, E 30 units, B_1 1.1 mg, B_2 1.8 mg, B_3 15 mg, B_6 2.5 mg, B_{12} 5 mcg, C 60 mg, FA 1 mg. Tab. UD 100s. *Rx.*
Use: Multivitamin.

Multigen. (Breckenridge Pharmaceutical) Vitamin B_{12} 10 mcg, desiccated stomach substance 50 mg, Fe 70 mg (from ferrous asparto glycinate), succinic acid 75 mg, vitamin C 152 mg (as calcium ascorbate and calcium threonate). Film coated. Tab. 90s. *Rx.*
Use: Trace element, iron.

Multi-Germ Oil. (Viobin) Corn, sunflower and wheat germ oils. Bot. 4 oz, 8 oz, pt, qt. *OTC.*
Use: Nutritional supplement.

MultiHance. (Bracco Diagnostics) Gadobenate dimeglumine 529 mg/mL. Preservative free. Single-dose vials. 5 mL, 10 mL, 15 mL, 20 mL. *Rx.*
Use: Radiopaque agent.

Multi-Jets. (Kirkman) Vitamins A 10,000 units, D_2 400 units, B_1 20 mg, B_2 8 mg, C 120 mg, niacinamide 10 mg, calcium pantothenate 5 mg, B_6 0.5 mg, E 50 units, desiccated liver 100 mg, dried debittered yeast 100 mg, choline bitartrate 62 mg, inositol 30 mg, dl-methionine 30 mg, B_{12} 7 mcg, Fe 2.6 mg, Ca (dical phosphate) 58 mg, P (dical phosphate) 45 mg, I (potassium iodide) 0.114 mg, Mg sulfate 1 mg, Cu sulfate 1.99 mg, Mn sulfate 1.11 mg, KCl iodide 79 mg. Tab. Bot. 100s. *OTC.*
Use: Mineral, vitamin supplement.

multikinase inhibitors.
Use: Treatment of advanced renal cell carcinoma.
See: Regorafenib.
Sorafenib.

Multilex. (Rugby) Fe 15 mg, vitamins A 10,000 units, D 400 units, E 5.5 mg, B_1 10 mg, B_2 5 mg, B_3 30 mg, B_5 10 mg, B_6 1.7 mg, B_{12} 3 mcg, C 100 mg, Zn 1.5 mg, Cu, I, Mg, Mn. Film coated. Mannitol, PEG, sodium benzoate. Tab. 100s. *OTC.*
Use: Mineral, vitamin supplement.

Multilex T & M Tablets. (Rugby) Fe 15 mg, vitamins A 10,000 units, D 400 units, E 5.5 mg, B_1 15 mg, B_2 10 mg, B_3 100 mg, B_5 10 mg, B_6 2 mg, B_{12} 7.5 mcg, C 150 mg, Cu, I, Mg, Mn, Zn 1.5 mg, sugar. Tab. Bot. 100s. *OTC.*
Use: Mineral, vitamin supplement.

Multilyte. (Fujisawa Healthcare) Vitamins A 5000 units, D 400 units, E 15 mg, B_1 3 mg, B_2 3.4 mg, B_3 36 mg, B_5 14 mg, B_6 4.4 mg, B_{12} 6 mcg, C 120 mg, FA 0.4 mg, Zn 10.5 mg, biotin 100 mcg, Ca, K, Mg, Mn, phenylalanine. Tab. Pkg. 12s. *OTC.*
Use: Mineral, vitamin supplement.

Multilyte-40. (American Pharmaceutical Partners) Na 25 mEq, K ≈ 40 mEq, Ca 5 mEq, Mg 8 mEq, Cl ≈ 33 mEq, acetate ≈ 40 mEq, gluconate 5 mEq/25 mL, osmolarity ≈ 6015 mOsm/L. Single-dose vial 25 mL. *Rx.*
Use: Intravenous nutritional therapy, intravenous replenishment solution.

Multilyte-20. (American Pharmaceutical Partners) Na 25 mEq, K 20 mEq, Ca 5 mEq, Mg 5 mEq, Cl 30 mEq, acetate 25 mEq/25 mL, osmolarity ≈ 4205 mOsm/L. Single-dose vial 25 mL. *Rx.*
Use: Intravenous nutritional therapy, intravenous replenishment solution.

Multi-Mineral Tablets. (NBTY) Ca 166.7 mg, P 75.7 mg, I 25 mcg, Fe 3 mg, Mg 66.7 mg, Cu 0.33 mg, Zn 2.5 mg, K 12.5 mg, Mn 8.3 mg. Tab. Bot. 100s. *OTC.*
Use: Mineral, vitamin supplement.

Multinatal Plus. (Brookstone Pharmaceuticals) Vitamin C 60 mg, E 30 units, B_1 3 mg, B_2 3.4 mg, B_3 20 mg, B_6 50 mg, B_{12} 12 mcg. Folic acid 1 mg, Ca 200 mg, Fe 30 mg, Mg 100 mg, Zn 15 mg, Cu 2 mg. Film coated. Tab. 30s. *Rx.*
Use: Vitamin supplement.

Multipals. (Faraday) Vitamins A 5000 units, D 400 units, C 50 mg, B_1 3 mg, B_6 0.5 mg, B_2 3 mg, calcium pantothenate 5 mg, niacinamide 20 mg, B_{12} 2 mcg. Tab. Bot. 100s, 250s, 1000s. *OTC.*
Use: Mineral, vitamin supplement.

Multipals-M. (Faraday) Vitamins A 6000 units, D 400 units, B_1 3 mg, B_2 3 mg, B_6 0.5 mg, B_{12} 5 mcg, C 60 mg, E 2 units, niacinamide 20 mg, calcium pantothenate 5 mg, Fe 10 mg, I 0.15 mg, Cu 1 mg, Mg 6 mg, Mn 1 mg, K 5 mg. Tab. Bot. 100s, 250s, 1000s. *OTC.*
Use: Mineral, vitamin supplement.

Multiple Electrolytes and 5% Travert. (Baxter Healthcare) Invert sugar 50 g/L, calories 196 cal/L, Na^+ 56 mEq, K^+ 25 mEq, Mg^{++} 6 mEq, Cl^- 56 mEq, phosphate 12.5 mEq, lactate 25 mEq/L, osmolarity 449 mOsm/L, sodium 5 mEq/L sodium bisulfite. Soln. Bot. 1000 mL. *Rx.*
Use: Intravenous nutritional therapy, intravenous replenishment solution.

Multiple Electrolytes and 10% Travert. (Baxter Healthcare) Invert sugar 100 g/L, calories 384 cal/L, Na^+ 56 mEq, K^+ 25 mEq, Mg^{++} 6 mEq, Cl^- 56 mEq, phosphate 12.5 mEq, lactate 25 mEq/L, osmolarity 726 mOsm/L, sodium 5 mEq/L, sodium bisulfite. Soln. Bot. 1000 mL. *Rx.*
Use: Intravenous nutritional therapy, intravenous replenishment solution.

Multiple Vitamin Mineral Formula. (Kirkman) Vitamins A 5000 units, D_2 400 units, C 50 mg, B_1 2.5 mg, B_2 2.5 mg, B_6 0.5 mg, B_{12} 1 mcg, niacinamide 15 mg, calcium pantothenate 5 mg, E 0.1 units, Ca 100 mg, Fe 7.5 mg, Mg 2.5 mg, K 2.5 mg, Zn 0.15 mg, Mn 0.5 mg, I 0.07 mg. Tab. Bot. 100s. *OTC.*
Use: Mineral, vitamin supplement.

Multiple Vitamins Chewable. (Kirkman) Vitamins A 5000 units, D 400 units, C 50 mg, B_1 3 mg, B_2 2.5 mg, B_6 1 mg, B_{12} 1 mcg, niacinamide 20 mg. Tab. Bot. 100s. *OTC.*
Use: Vitamin supplement.

Multiple Vitamins w/Iron. (Kirkman) Vitamins A 5000 units, D 400 units, C 50 mg, B_1 3 mg, B_2 2.5 mg, B_6 1 mg, B_{12} 1 mcg, niacinamide 20 mg, Fe 10 mg. Tab. Bot. 100s. *OTC.*
Use: Mineral, vitamin supplement.

Multi Prenatal. (Nature Made) Folic acid 0.8 mg, calcium 250 mg, iron 27 mg, vitamins A 4,000 units, D 400 units, E 11 units, B_1 1.5 mg, B_2 1.7 mg, B_3 18 mg, B_6 2.6 mg, B_{12} 4 mcg, C 100 mg, Zn. Glycerides of fatty acids, maltodextrin, PEG. Gluten free, preservative free. Tab. 250s. *Rx.*
Use: Prenatal vitamin with minerals.

Multi 75. (Fibertone) Vitamins A 25,000 units, D 500 units, E 150 units, B_1 75 mg, B_2 75 mg, B_3 75 mg, B_5 75 mg, B_6 75 mg, B_{12} 75 mcg, C 250 mg, FA 0.4 mg, Ca 50 mg, Fe 10 mg, biotin, I, Mg, Zn 15 mg, Cu, PABA, K, Mn, Cr, Se, Mo, B, Si, choline bitartrate, inositol, rutin, lemon bioflavonoid complex, hesperidin, betaine, hydrochloride. TR Tab. Bot. 60s, 90s. *OTC.*
Use: Mineral, vitamin supplement.

Multistix 8 Reagent Strips. (Siemans Medical) Urinalysis reagent strip test for detecting glucose, ketone, blood, pH, protein, nitrite, bilirubin, leukocytes. Strip Box. 100s.
Use: Diagnostic aid.

Multistix 8 SG Reagent Strips. (Siemans Medical) Urinalysis reagent strip test for glucose, ketone, specific gravity, blood, pH, protein nitrite, leukocytes. Strip Box 100s.
Use: Diagnostic aid.

Multistix-N. (Bayer Consumer Care) Glucose, protein, pH, blood, ketones, bilirubin, urobilinogen, nitrate, leukocytes. Kit. 100s.
Use: Diagnostic aid.

Multistix 9 Reagent Strips. (Siemans Medical) Urinalysis reagent strip test for glucose, bilirubin, ketone, blood, pH, protein, urobilinogen, nitrite, leukocytes. Strip Box 100s.
Use: Diagnostic aid.

Multistix 9 SG Reagent Strips. (Siemans Medical) Urinalysis reagent strip test for glucose, bilirubin, ketone, specific gravity, blood, pH, protein, nitrite, leukocytes. Strip Box 100s.
Use: Diagnostic aid.

Multistix-N S.G. Reagent Strips. (Bayer Consumer Care) Urinalysis reagent strip test for pH, protein, glucose, ketones, bilirubin, blood nitrite, urobilinogen, specific gravity. Strip Bot. 100s.
Use: Diagnostic aid.

Multistix Reagent Strips. (Siemans Medical) Urinalysis reagent strip test for pH, protein, glucose, ketone, bilirubin, blood. Strip Box 100s.
Use: Diagnostic aid.

Multistix 7. (Siemans Medical) Urinalysis reagent strip test for glucose ketone, blood, pH, protein, nitrite, leukocytes. Strip Box 100s.
Use: Diagnostic aid.

Multistix 10 SG Reagent Strips. (Siemans Medical) Reagent strip test for glucose, bilirubin, ketone, specific gravity, blood, pH, protein, urobilinogen, nitrite, leukocytes in urine. Strip Box 100s.
Use: Diagnostic aid.

Multistix 2 Reagent Strips. (Siemans Medical) Urinalysis reagent strip test for nitrite and leukocytes. Strip Bot. 100s.
Use: Diagnostic aid.

Multi-Symptom Tylenol Cold. (McNeil Consumer) Pseudoephedrine hydrochloride 30 mg, chlorpheniramine maleate 2 mg, dextromethorphan HBr

15 mg, acetaminophen 325 mg. Capl. or Tab. Bot. 24s, 50s. *OTC.*
Use: Analgesic, antihistamine, antitussive, decongestant.

Multi-Thera-M. (NBTY) Iron 27 mg, vitamins A 5500 units, D 400 units, E 30 mg, B_1 3 mg, B_2 3.4 mg, B_3 30 mg, B_5 10 mg, B_6 3 mg, B_{12} 9 mcg, C 120 mg, folic acid 0.4 mg, biotin 15 mcg, Zn 15 mg, Ca, Cl, Cr, Cu, I, K, Mg, Mn, Mo, Se. Tab. Bot. 130s. *OTC.*
Use: Mineral, vitamin supplement.

Multi-Thera Tablets. (NBTY) Vitamins A 5500 units, D 400 units, E 30 mg, B_1 3 mg, B_2 3.4 mg, B_3 30 mg, B_5 10 mg, B_6 3 mg, B_{12} 9 mcg, C 120 mg, folic acid 0.4 mg, biotin 15 mcg. Tab. Bot. 100s. *OTC.*
Use: Vitamin supplement.

Multitrace-5. (American Regent) Chromium (as chloride) 4 mcg, copper (as sulfate) 0.4 mg, manganese (as sulfate) 0.1 mg, selenium (as selenious acid) 20 mcg, zinc (as sulfate) 1 mg. Benzyl alcohol 0.9%. Inj. Multidose vial. 10 mL. *Rx.*
Use: Trace metal combination.

Multitrace-5 Concentrate. (American Regent) Zinc sulfate 5 mg, copper sulfate 1 mg, manganese sulfate 0.5 mg, chromium chloride 10 mcg, selenium 60 mcg, benzyl alcohol 0.9%. Inj. Soln. Vial 1 mL, 10 mL. *Rx.*
Use: Mineral supplement.

Multitrace-4. (American Regent) Chromium (as chloride) 4 mcg, copper (as sulfate) 0.4 mg, manganese (as sulfate) 0.1 mg, zinc (as sulfate) 1 mg. Benzyl alcohol 0.9%. Inj. Multidose vial. 10 mL. *Rx.*
Use: Trace metal combination.

Multitrace-4 Concentrate. (American Regent) Chromium (as chloride) 10 mcg, copper (as sulfate) 1 mg, manganese (as sulfate) 0.5 mg, zinc (as sulfate) 5 mg. Benzyl alcohol 0.9%. Inj. 1 mL single-dose vial, 10 mL multidose vial. *Rx.*
Use: Trace metal combination.

Multitrace-4 Neonatal. (American Regent) Chromium (as chloride) 0.85 mcg, copper (as sulfate) 0.1 mg, manganese (as sulfate) 0.025 mg, zinc (as sulfate) 1.5 mg. Inj. Single-dose vial. 2 mL. *Rx.*
Use: Trace metal combination.

Multitrace-4 Pediatric. (American Regent) Chromium (as chloride) 1 mcg, copper (as sulfate) 0.1 mg, manganese (as sulfate) 0.025 mg, zinc (as sulfate) 1 mg. Preservative free. Inj. Single-dose vial. 3 mL. *Rx.*
Use: Trace metal combination.

Multi-Vita. (Rosemont) Vitamins A 1500 units, D 400 units, E 5 mg, B_1 0.5 mg, B_2 0.6 mg, B_3 8 mg, B_6 0.4 mg, B_{12} 2 mcg, C 35 mg/mL. Alcohol free. Drop. Bot. 50 mL. *OTC.*
Use: Vitamin supplement.

Multi-Vita Drops. (Rosemont) Vitamins A 1500 units, D 400 units, E 5 mg, B_1 0.5 mg, B_2 0.6 mg, B_3 8 mg, B_6 0.4 mg, B_{12} 2 mcg, C 35 mg/mL. Alcohol free. Drop. Bot. 50 mL. *OTC.*
Use: Mineral, vitamin supplement.

Multi-Vita Drops w/Fluoride. (Rosemont) Fluoride 0.5 mg, vitamins A 1500 units, D 400 units, E 5 mg, B_1 0.5 mg, B_2 0.6 mg, B_3 8 mg, B_6 0.4 mg, B_{12} 2 mcg, C 35 mg/mL. Alcohol free. Drop. Bot. 50 mL. *Rx.*
Use: Vitamin supplement; dental caries agent.

Multi-Vita Drops w/Iron. (Rosemont) Iron 10 mg, vitamins A 1500 units, D 400 units, E 5 mg, B_1 0.5 mg, B_2 0.6 mg, B_3 8 mg, B_6 0.4 mg, C 35 mg/mL. Alcohol free. Drop. Bot. 50 mL. *OTC.*
Use: Mineral, vitamin supplement.

multivitamin concentrate injection. (Fujisawa Healthcare) Vitamins A 10,000 units, D 1000 units, E 5 units, B_1 50 mg, B_2 10 mg, B_3 100 mg, B_5 25 mg, B_6 15 mg, C 500 mg/Inj. Vial 5 mL. *Rx.*
Use: Vitamin supplement.

multivitamin infusion (neonatal formula).
Use: Nutritional supplement for low birth weight infants. [Orphan Drug]

Multi-Vitamin Mineral w/Beta Carotene. (Mission Pharmacal) Iron 27 mg, A 5000 units, D 400 units, E 30 units, B_1 2.25 mg, B_2 2.6 mg, B_3 20 mg, B_5 10 mg, B_6 3 mg, B_{12} 9 mcg, C 90 mg, folic acid 0.4 mg, biotin 0.45 mg, Ca, Cl, Cr, Cu, I, K, Mg, Mn, Mo, P, Se, Zn 15 mg, Vitamin K. Tab. Bot. 130s. *OTC.*
Use: Mineral, vitamin supplement.

Multi-Vitamins Capsules. (Forest) Vitamins A 5000 units, D 400 units, B_1 1.5 mg, B_2 2 mg, B_6 0.1 mg, C 37.5 mg, calcium pantothenate 1 mg, niacinamide 20 mg. Cap. Bot. 100s, 1000s, 5000s. *OTC.*
Use: Mineral, vitamin supplement.

Multivitamins Capsules. (Solvay) Vitamins A 5000 units, D 400 units, B_1 2.5 mg, B_2 2.5 mg, C 50 mg, B_3 20 mg, B_5 5 mg, B_6 0.5 mg, B_{12} 2 mcg, E 10 units. Cap. Bot. 100s, UD 100s. *OTC.*
Use: Mineral, vitamin supplement.

Multivitamins with A, B, D, E and K Plus Zinc. (SourceCF) **Tab., Chew.:** Vitamins A 16,000 units, D 1,000 units, E 200 units, B_1 1.5 mg, B_2 1.7 mg, B_3 10 mg, B_5 12 mg, B_6 1.9 mg, B_{12} 6 mcg, C 100 mg, K 800 mcg, folic acid 200 mcg, Zn, biotin 100 mcg. Sucralose, sucrose. Bubble gum flavor. 90s. **Cap. softgels:** Vitamins A 16,000 units, D 1,000 units, E 200 units, B_1 1.5 mg, B_2 1.7 mg, B_3 20 mg, B_5 12 mg, B_6 1.9 mg, B_{12} 6 mcg, C 100 mg, K 800 mcg, folic acid 200 mcg, Zn, biotin 100 mcg. Hydrogenated vegetable oil, soybean oil, sucralose. 60s. **Pediatric Drops:** Vitamins A 4,627 units, D 500 units, E 50 units, B_1 0.5 mg, B_2 0.6 mg, B_3 6 mg, B_5 3 mg, B_6 0.6 mg, B_{12} 4 mcg, C 45 mg, K 400 mcg, Zn, biotin 15 mcg per mL. EDTA, sucralose, sucrose. 60 mL w/dropper.
Use: Nutritional supplement, multivitamin.

multivitamins with iron.
Use: Nutritional combination products.
See: BiferaRx.
Tandem DHA.

multivitamins with iron and other minerals.
Use: Nutritional combination products.
See: Biotect Plus.
Tandem OB.
Tandem Plus.
TotalDay.

multivitamins with minerals.
Use: Nutritional combination products.
See: Advanced Ear Health Formula.
Calcium-Folic Acid Plus D.
Corvite Free.
Daily Betic.
D1000 Plus.
Invites Rx.
K-PAX Immune Support.
Multivitamin with A, B, D, E, and K Plus Zinc.
Nutravance.
One-Daily.
PreserVision Lutein.
Prosteon.
Strovite One.
Udamin.
Udamin SP.
UpCal D.

Multi-Vitamin With Fluoride & Iron. (Boca) Fluoride 0.25 mg, vitamins A 1,500 units, D 400 units, E 5 units, B_1 0.5 mg, B_2 0.6 mg, B_3 8 mg, B_6 0.4 mg, C 35 mg. Ferrous sulfate, glycerin, methylparaben, polysorbate 80, sodium benzoate. Liq. 50 mL. *Rx.*
Use: Multivitamin with minerals.

Multivitamin with Fluoride Drops. (Hi-Tech) Fluoride 0.5 mg, vitamins A 1500 units, D 400 units, E 5 units, B_1 0.5 mg, B_2 0.6 mg, B_3 8 mg, B_6 0.4 mg, B_{12} 2 mcg, C 35 mg, F 0.25 mg. Drop. Bot. 50 mL. *Rx.*
Use: Vitamin supplement; dental caries agent.

Multivitamin with Fluoride Drops. (Major) Fluoride 0.5 mg, vitamins A 1500 units, D 400 units, E 4.1 units, B_1 0.5 mg, B_2 0.6 mg, B_3 8 mg, B_6 0.4 mg, B_{12} 2 mg, C 35 mg. Drop. Bot. 50 mL. *OTC.*
Use: Vitamin supplement; dental caries agent.

Multi-Vit Drops. (Alra) Vitamins A 500 units, D 400 units, E 5 mg, B_1 0.5 mg, B_2 0.6 mg, B_3 8 mg, B_6 0.4 mg, B_{12} 2 mcg, C 35 mg/mL. Bot. 50 mL. *OTC.*
Use: Vitamin supplement.

Multi-Vit Drops w/Iron. (Alra) Iron 10 mg, vitamins A 1500 units, D 400 units, E 5 units, B_1 0.5 mg, B_2 0.6 mg, B_3 8 mg, B_6 0.4 mg, C 35 mg/mL. Methylparaben. Drop. Bot. 50 mL. *OTC.*
Use: Mineral, vitamin supplement.

Multi-Vit with Fluoride. (Qualitest) Fluoride 0.25 mg, vitamins A 1,500 units (as vitamin A palmitate), D_3 400 units (as cholecalciferol), E 5 units (as d-alpha-tocopheryl acid succinate), B_1 0.5 mg, B_2 0.6 mg, B_3 8 mg, B_6 0.4 mg, B_{12} 2 mcg, C 35 mg. Glycerin. Drops. 50 mL. *Rx.*
Use: Multivitamin.

Multorex. (Health for Life Brands) Vitamins A 6000 units, D 1250 units, C 50 mg, E 5 units, B_1 3 mg, B_2 3 mg, B_6 0.5 mg, niacinamide 20 mg, calcium pantothenate 5 mg, B_{12} 5 mcg, Ca 59 mg, P 45 mg. Cap. Bot. 100s, 250s, 1000s.
Use: Mineral, vitamin supplement.

Mulvidren-F Softabs. (Wyeth) Fluoride 1 mg, vitamins A 4000 units, D 400 units, B_1 1.6 mg, B_2 2 mg, B_3 10 mg, B_5 2.8 mg, B_6 1 mg, B_{12} 3 mcg, C 75 mg, saccharin. Tab. Bot. 100s. *Rx.*
Use: Mineral, vitamin supplement; dental caries agent.

•**mumps skin test antigen.** *USP.*
Use: Diagnostic aid (dermal reactivity indicator).

•**mumps virus vaccine live.** *USP.*
Use: Immunization.

mumps virus vaccine, live attenuated. Jeryl Lynn (B level) strain.
W/Measles virus vaccine, rubella virus vaccine.
See: M-M-R.

•**muparfostat.** (mue-PAR-foe-stat) USAN.
Use: Antineoplastic.

•**muparfostat sodium.** (mue-PAR-foe-stat) USAN.
Use: Antineoplastic.

•**mupirocin.** (myoo-PIHR-oh-sin) *USP.*
Use: Anti-infective (topical and nasal).
See: Bactroban.
Centany.

mupirocin. (Various Mfr.) Mupirocin 2%. Polyethylene glycol base. Oint. 15 g, 22 g, 30 g. *Rx.*
Use: Topical anti-infective, antibiotic.

•**mupirocin calcium.** (myoo-PIHR-oh-sin) USAN.
Use: Anti-infective, topical.
See: Bactroban.

mupirocin calcium. (Prasco Laboratories) Mupirocin 2%. Alcohols, benzyl alcohol, mineral oil. Cream. 15 g, 30 g. *Rx.*
Use: Topical anti-infective, antibiotic agent.

•**muplestim.** (myoo-PLEH-stim) USAN.
Use: Hematopoietic stimulant; antineutropenic.

•**muraglitazar.** (myoo-ra-GLI-ta-zar) USAN.
Use: Investigational antidiabetic.

muriatic acid.
See: Hydrochloric Acid.

Muri-Lube. (Fujisawa Healthcare) Mineral Oil "Light." Vial 2 mL, 10 mL. *Rx.*
Use: Lubricant.

Murine Ear Drops. (Ross) Carbamide peroxide 6.5%, alcohol 6.3%, glycerin, polysorbate 20. Drops. 15 mL. *OTC.*
Use: Otic preparation.

Murine Ear Wax Removal System. (Ross) Carbamide peroxide 6.5% in anhydrous glycerin w/ear washing syringe. Bot. 0.5 oz. and ear washer 1 oz. *OTC.*
Use: Otic.

Murine Plus. (MedTech) Tetrahydrozoline hydrochloride 0.05%. Polyvinyl alcohol 0.5%, povidone 0.6%, benzalkonium chloride, dextrose, EDTA, sodium bicarbonate, sodium chloride, sodium citrate, sodium phosphate mono- and dibasic. Ophth. Soln. Bot. 15 mL. *OTC.*
Use: Vasoconstrictor; ophthalmic decongestant.

Murine Regular Formula. (Ross) Sodium chloride, potassium chloride, sodium phosphate, glycerin, benzalkonium chloride 0.01%, EDTA 0.05%. Drop. Bot. 15, 30 mL. *OTC.*
Use: Artificial tears.

Murine Tears for Dry Eyes. (MedTech) PVP 0.6%, PVA 0.5%, benzalkonium chloride, dextrose, EDTA, KCl, NaCl, sodium bicarbonate, sodium citrate, sodium phosphate. Soln.; Ophth. 15 mL, 30 mL. *OTC.*
Use: Artificial tears.

•**muromonab-CD3.** (MYOO-row-MOE-nab) USAN.
Use: Monoclonal antibody (immunosuppressant).

Muro 128 Ointment. (Bausch & Lomb) Sodium chloride 5% in sterile ointment base. Tube 3.5 g. *OTC.*
Use: Hyperosmolar.

Muro 128 Solution. (Bausch & Lomb) Sodium chloride 2%, 5%. Soln. Bot. 15 mL, 30 mL (5% only). *OTC.*
Use: Hyperosmolar.

Muro's Opcon A Solution. (Bausch & Lomb) Naphazoline hydrochloride 0.025%, pheniramine maleate 0.3%. Bot. 15 mL. *OTC.*
Use: Antihistamine (ophthalmic), decongestant.

Muro's Opcon Solution. (Bausch & Lomb) Naphazoline hydrochloride 0.1%. Bot. 15 mL. *OTC.*
Use: Decongestant; ophthalmic.

Muro Tears Solution. (Bausch & Lomb) Hydroxypropyl methylcellulose, dextran 40. Soln. Bot. 15 mL. *OTC.*
Use: Artificial tears.

muscle adenylic acid. (Various Mfr.) Active form of adenosine 5-monophosphate.

muscle relaxants.
See: Curare.
Flexeril.
Lioresal.
Mephenesin.
Meprobamate.
Neuromuscular Blockers, Nondepolarizing.
Norflex.
Pancuronium Bromide.
Parafon Forte DSC.
Robaxin.
Rocuronium Bromide.
Soma.
Succinylcholine Chloride.

Muse. (Meda Pharmaceuticals) Alprostadil 125 mcg, 250 mcg, 500 mcg, 1000 mcg. Pellet. Individual foil pouches. *Rx.*
Use: Anti-impotence agent.

mustaral oil.
See: Allyl Isothiocyanate.

Mustargen. (Recordati Rare Diseases) Mechlorethamine hydrochloride 10 mg. Pow. for Inj. Vial. Set of 4s. *Rx.*
Use: Antineoplastic, alkylating agent.

Musterole Deep Strength. (Schering-

Plough) Methyl salicylate 30%, menthol 3%, methyl nicotinate 0.5%. Rub. 37 g, 90 g. *OTC.*
Use: Analgesic, topical.

Musterole Extra Strength. (Schering-Plough) Camphor 5%, menthol 3%, methyl salicylate, lanolin, oil of mustard, petrolatum. 27 g, 30 g, 67.5 g. *OTC.*
Use: Liniment.

mustin.
See: Mechlorethamine Hydrochloride.

mutalin. (Spanner) Protein and iodine. Vial 30 mL.

•**muzolimine.** (MYOO-ZOLE-ih-meen) USAN.
Use: Antihypertensive; diuretic.

M.V.I. Pediatric. (Hospira) Vitamin A 2300 units, D 400 units, E 7 units, B_1 1.2 mg, B_2 1.4 mg, B_3 17 mg, B_5 5 mg, B_6 1 mg, B_{12} 1 mcg, C 80 mg, biotin 20 mcg, FA 0.14 mg, vitamin K 200 mcg, mannitol 375 mg. Inj. Vial. *Rx.*
Use: Nutritional supplement, parenteral.

M-Vit. (R.A. McNeil) Folic acid 1 mg, iron 27 mg, vitamins A 2,000 units, E 30 units, B_1 20 mg, B_2 20 mg, B_3 100 mg, B_5 25 mg, B_6 25 mg, B_{12} 50 mcg, C 500 mg, Cr, Cu, Mg, Mn, Se, Zn, biotin 150 mcg, lemon bioflavonoids 50 mg. Coated. Tab. 100s. *Rx.*
Use: Prenatal vitamin with minerals.

M.V.I.-12. (Hospira) Vitamins A 3300 units, D 200 units, E 10 units, B_1 3 mg, B_2 3.6 mg, B_3 40 mg, B_5 15 mg, B_6 4 mg, B_{12} 5 mcg, C 100 mg, biotin 60 mcg, FA 0.4 mg. Inj. Vials. 5 mL single-dose, 50 mL multiple-dose; Unit vial: 10 mL two-chambered vials. *Rx.*
Use: Nutritional supplement, parenteral.

M.V.M. (Tyson) Iron 3.6 mg, vitamins A 400 units, E 60 units, B_1 20 mg, B_2 10 mg, B_3 10 mg, B_5 100 mg, B_6 31 mg, B_{12} 160 mcg, C 50 mg, folic acid 0.08 mg, Ca, Cr, Cu, I, K, Mg, Mo, Zn 6 mg, biotin 160 mcg, PABA, Mn, Se, tryptophan. Cap. Bot. 150s. *OTC.*
Use: Mineral, vitamin supplement.

Myadec. (Parke-Davis) Iron 18 mg, A 5000 units, D 400 units, E 30 units, B_1 1.7 mg, B_2 2 mg, B_3 20 mg, B_5 10 mg, B_6 3 mg, B_{12} 6 mcg, C 60 mg, folic acid 0.4 mg, biotin 30 mcg, vitamin K, Ca, P, I, Mg, Cu, Zn 15 mg, Mn, K, Cl, Cr, Mo, Se, Ni, Si, V, B, Sn. Tab. Bot. 130s. *OTC.*
Use: Mineral, vitamin supplement.

myagen. Bolasterone.
Use: Anabolic agent.

Myalept. (Bristol-Myers Squibb) Metreleptin 11.3 mg. Sucrose, glycine. Preservative free. Inj., lyophilized Pow. for Soln. Vial. *Rx.*
Use: Lipodystrophy agent.

Myambutol. (X-Gen) Ethambutol hydrochloride. Tab. **100 mg:** Bot. 100s. **400 mg:** Bot. 100s, 1000s, UD 10s. *Rx.*
Use: Antituberculous.

myanesin.
See: Mephenesin.

Myapap Drops. (Rosemont) Acetaminophen 80 mg/0.8 mL. Bot. 15 mL w/dropper. *OTC.*
Use: Analgesic.

Myapap Elixir. (Rosemont) Acetaminophen 160 mg/5 mL. Bot. 4 oz, pt, gal. *OTC.*
Use: Analgesic.

Myapap with Codeine Elixir. (Rosemont) Acetaminophen 120 mg, codeine phosphate 12 mg/5 mL. Bot. 4 oz, pt, gal. *c-v.*
Use: Analgesic, antitussive.

Mybanil. (Rosemont) Codeine phosphate 10 mg, bromodiphenhydramine hydrochloride 12.5 mg/5 mL, alcohol 5%. Bot. 4 oz, pt, gal. *c-v.*
Use: Antihistamine, antitussive.

Mycadec DM Drops. (Rosemont) Pseudoephedrine 25 mg, carbinoxamine maleate 2 mg, dextromethorphan HBr 4 mg/mL. Bot. 30 mL. *Rx.*
Use: Antihistamine, antitussive, decongestant.

Mycadec DM Syrup. (Rosemont) Carbinoxamine maleate 4 mg, pseudoephedrine hydrochloride 60 mg, dextromethorphan HBr 15 mg/5 mL, alcohol 0.6%. Bot. 4 oz, pt, gal. *Rx.*
Use: Antihistamine, antitussive, decongestant.

Mycadec Drops. (Rosemont) Pseudoephedrine hydrochloride 25 mg, dextromethorphan HBr 4 mg, carbinoxamine maleate 2 mg/mL. Bot. 30 mL. *Rx.*
Use: Antihistamine, antitussive, decongestant.

Mycamine. (Astellas Pharma, Inc.) Micafungin sodium 50 mg, 100 mg. Lactose. Pow. for Inj., lyophilized. Single-use vials. *Rx.*
Use: Antifungal agent.

Mycartal. (Sanofi-Synthelabo) Pentaerythritol tetranitrate. *Rx.*
Use: Coronary vasodilator.

Mycelex. (Ortho McNeil) Clotrimazole. **Cream:** 1%. Tube 15 g, 30 g, 90 g (2 × 45 g). **Topical Soln.:** 1%. Bot. 10 mL, 30 mL. *Rx-OTC.*
Use: Antifungal, topical.

Mycelex-7. (Ortho-McNeil) Clotrimazole 1%, benzyl alcohol, cetostearyl alco-

hol. Vag. Cream. Tube 45 g w/1 applicator or 7 disp. applicators. *OTC.*
Use: Antifungal, vaginal.

Mycelex-7 Combination Pack. (Ortho-McNeil) Clotrimazole. **Cream:** 1%, benzyl alcohol, cetostearyl alcohol, polysorbate 80. Tube 7 g. **Supp.:** 100 mg, lactose, povidone. Pkg. 7s w/applicator. *OTC.*
Use: Antifungal, vaginal.

Mycelex Troches. (Bayer Consumer Care) Clotrimazole 10 mg. Troche 70s, 140s. *Rx.*
Use: Antifungal.

Mychel-S. (Houba) Sterile chloramphenicol sodium succinate. Vial 1 g/15 mL. Box 5s. *Rx.*
Use: Anti-infective.

Mycifradin. (Pharmacia) Neomycin sulfate 125 mg/5 mL (equivalent to 87.5 mg neomycin). Oral soln. Bot. Pt. *Rx.*
Use: Anti-infective.

Mycinaire Saline Mist. (Pfeiffer) Sodium chloride 0.65%, benzalkonium chloride. Soln. Spray Bot. 45 mL. *OTC.*
Use: Nasal decongestant.

Mycinette. (Pfeiffer) Benzocaine 15 mg, sorbitol, saccharin, menthol. Loz. 12s. *OTC.*
Use: Anesthetic, local; antiseptic; expectorant.

Mycinette Sore Throat. (Pfeiffer) Phenol 1.4%, alum 0.3%, alcohol free, sugar free. Spray 180 mL. *OTC.*
Use: Mouth and throat preparation.

Myci-Spray. (Edwards) Phenylephrine hydrochloride 0.25%, pyrilamine maleate 0.15%/mL. Bot. 20 mL. *OTC.*
Use: Antihistamine, decongestant.

Mycitracin. (Pharmacia) Bacitracin 500 units, neomycin sulfate 5 mg, polymyxin B sulfate 5000 units/g. Oint. Tube 0.5 oz. Box 36s; 1 oz; UD 1/32 oz. Box 144s. *OTC.*
Use: Anti-infective, topical.

Mycitracin Triple Antibiotic, Maximum Strength. (Pharmacia) Polymyxin B sulfate 5000 units/g, neomycin 3.5 mg/g, bacitracin 500 units/g, parabens, mineral oil, white petrolatum. Oint. Tube 30 g, UD 0.94 g. *OTC.*
Use: Anti-infective, topical.

Mycobutin. (Pharmacia) Rifabutin 150 mg. Cap. Bot. 100s. *Rx.*
Use: Antituberculosal.

Mycocide NS. (Woodward) Tolnaftate 1%. Propylene glycol. Soln. 30 mL. *Rx.*
Use: Topical anti-infective, antifungal.

Mycodone Syrup. (Rosemont) Hydrocodone bitartrate 5 mg, homatropine HBr 1.5 mg/5 mL. Bot. 4 oz, pt, gal. *c-III.*
Use: Antitussive.

Mycogen-II. (Bristol-Myers Squibb) Nystatin 100,000 units/g, triamcinolone acetonide 0.1%. **Cream:** Vanishing base. White petrolatum. 15 g, 30 g, 60 g, 120 g. **Oint.:** Mineral oil, gel base. 15 g, 30 g, 60 g, 120 g. *Rx.*
Use: Antifungal, topical corticosteroid.

Mycomist. (Gordon Laboratories) Chlorophyll, formalin, benzalkonium chloride. Bot. 4 oz, plastic bot. 1 oz. *OTC.*
Use: Antifungal for clothing.

mycophenolate. (Various Mfr.) Mycophenolate mofetil 250 mg. Cap. 30s, 100s, 120s, 500s, 1,000s, 3,500s. *Rx.*
Use: Immunologic agent, immunosuppressive.

•**mycophenolate mofetil.** (my-koe-FEN-oh-late MOE-fe-till) USAN.
Use: Transplantation (immunosuppressant).
See: CellCept.

•**mycophenolate sodium.** (mye-koe-FEN-oh-late) USAN.
Use: Immunosuppressant (transplantation).
See: Myfortic.

•**mycophenolic acid.** (MY-koe-fen-AHL-ik) USAN.
Use: Antineoplastic.
See: Myfortic.

mycophenolic acid. (Various Mfr.) Mycophenolic acid (as mycophenolate sodium) 180 mg, 360 mg. May contain maltodextrin, PEG. Tab., delayed release. 120s, 240s. *Rx.*
Use: Immunologic agent, immunosuppressive.

Mycoplasma Pneumonia IFA IgM Test. (Wampole) Indirect fluorescent assay for IgM antibodies to *Mycoplasma pneumoniae*. Box test 100s.
Use: Diagnostic aid.

Mycoplasma Pneumonia IFA Test. (Wampole) Indirect fluorescent assay for antibodies to *Mycoplasma pneumoniae* Box test 100s.
Use: Diagnostic aid.

Mycostatin. (Bristol-Myers Squibb) Nystatin. **Tab.:** 500,000 units, lactose. Bot. 100s. **Cream:** 100,000 units/g in aqueous base. Tube 15 g, 30 g. **Oint.:** 100,000 units/g in Plastibase (polyethylene and mineral oil). Tube 15 g, 30 g. **Troche:** 200,000 units. 30s. **Vaginal Tab:** 100,000 units, lactose 0.95 g, ethyl cellulose, stearic acid, starch. Pkg. 15s, 30s. **Pow.:** (topical) 100,000 units/g in talc. Shaker bot. 15 g. *Rx.*
Use: Antifungal.

Mycostatin Pastilles. (Bristol-Myers Squibb Oncology/Virology) Nystatin, 200,000 units. Troche. 30s. *Rx.*
Use: Antifungal.

Myco-Triacet. (Various Mfr.) Triamcinolone acetonide 0.1%, neomycin sulfate 0.25%, gramicidin 0.25 mg, nystatin 100,000 units/g. **Cream:** 15 g, 30 g, 60 g, 480 g. **Oint.:** 15 g, 30 g, 60 g. *Rx.*
Use: Antifungal; corticosteroid, topical.

Myco-Triacet II. (Teva) Nystatin 100,000 units, triamcinolone acetonide 1 mg/g. **Cream:** White petrolatum and mineral oil. Tube 15 g, 30 g, 60g. **Oint.:** Tube 15 g, 30 g, 60 g. *Rx.*
Use: Antifungal; corticosteroid, topical.

Mycotussin Expectorant. (Rosemont) Pseudoephedrine hydrochloride 60 mg, hydrocodone bitartrate 5 mg, guaifenesin 200 mg/5 mL, alcohol 12.5%. Liq. Bot. 4 oz, pt, gal. *c-III.*
Use: Antitussive, decongestant, expectorant.

Mycotussin Liquid. (Rosemont) Pseudoephedrine hydrochloride 60 mg, hydrocodone bitartrate 5 mg/5 mL, alcohol 5%. Bot. 4 oz, pt, gal. *c-III.*
Use: Antitussive, decongestant.

Mydacol. (Rosemont) Vitamins B_1 5 mg, B_2 2.5 mg, niacinamide 50 mg, B_6 1 mg, B_{12} 1 mcg, pantothenic acid 10 mg, I 100 mcg, Fe 15 mg, Mg 2 mg, Zn 2 mg, choline 100 mg, Mn 2 mg/30 mL. Liq. Bot. Pt, gal. *OTC.*
Use: Mineral, vitamin supplement.

Mydfrin 2.5%. (Alcon) Phenylephrine hydrochloride 2.5%. Benzalkonium chloride 0.01%, EDTA, sodium bisulfite, boric acid. Ophth. Soln. *Drop-Tainers.* 3 mL, 5 mL. *Rx.*
Use: Mydriatic; ophthalmic decongestant.

Mydral. (OcuSoft) Tropicamide 0.5%, 1%. Benzalkonium chloride 0.01%, EDTA. Soln. 2 mL (1% only), 15 mL. *Rx.*
Use: Ophthalmic and otic agent, cycloplegic mydriatic.

Mydriacyl. (Alcon) Tropicamide 1%. Soln. 3 mL, 15 mL *Drop-Tainer. Rx.*
Use: Cycloplegic; mydriatic.

mydriatics, parasympatholytic types.
See: Homatropine Hydrobromide.
Scopolamine Salts.

mydriatics, sympathomimetic types.
See: Amphetamine Sulfate.
Ephedrine Sulfate.
Epinephrine Hydrochloride.
Neo-Synephrine Hydrochloride.
Phenylephrine Hydrochloride.

Myelo-Kit. (Sanofi-Synthelabo) Omnipaque 180, 240 in various sizes and one sterile myelogram tray.
Use: Radiopaque agent.

•**myeloperoxidase.** (MY-el-oh-per OX-i-dase) USAN.
Use: Anti-infective.

Myfed. (Rosemont) Triprolidine hydrochloride 1.25 mg, pseudoephedrine hydrochloride 30 mg/5 mL. Syr. Bot. 4 oz, pt, gal. *OTC.*
Use: Antihistamine, decongestant.

Myfedrine. (Rosemont) Pseudoephedrine 30 mg/5 mL. Liq. Bot. 473 mL. *OTC.*
Use: Decongestant.

Myfedrine Plus. (Rosemont) Pseudoephedrine hydrochloride 30 mg, chlorpheniramine maleate 2 mg/5 mL. Syr. Bot. 4 oz, pt, gal. *OTC.*
Use: Antitussive, decongestant.

Myferon 150. (M.E. Pharmaceuticals) Polysaccharide iron complex 150 mg. Cap. UD 100s. *OTC.*
Use: Trace element.

Myfortic. (Novartis) Mycophenolate (as sodium) 180 mg, 360 mg. Lactose. Film-coated. DR Tab. 120s. *Rx.*
Use: Immunosuppressant.

Mygel Liquid. (Geneva) Aluminum hydroxide 200 mg, magnesium hydroxide 200 mg, simethicone 20 mg, Na 1.38 mg/5 mL. Liq. Bot. 360 mL. *OTC.*
Use: Antacid; antiflatulent.

Mygel Suspension. (Geneva) Aluminum hydroxide 200 mg, magnesium hydroxide 200 mg, simethicone 20 mg/5 mL. Bot. 360 mL. *OTC.*
Use: Antacid; antiflatulent.

Mygel II Suspension. (Geneva) Aluminum hydroxide 400 mg, magnesium hydroxide 400 mg, simethicone 40 mg/5 mL. Bot. 360 mL. *OTC.*
Use: Antacid; antiflatulent.

MyHist-DM. (Larken) Dextromethorphan HBr 15 mg, pyrilamine maleate 12.5 mg, phenylephrine hydrochloride 7.5 mg per 5 mL. Alcohol, dye, and sugar free. EDTA, parabens, saccharin, sorbitol. Grape flavor. Liq. 473 mL. *Rx.*
Use: Upper respiratory combination, antitussive combination.

Myhistine DH. (Rosemont) Codeine phosphate 10 mg, chlorpheniramine maleate 2 mg, pseudoephedrine hydrochloride 30 mg/5 mL. Liq. Bot. 4 oz, pt, gal. *c-V.*
Use: Antihistamine, antitussive, decongestant.

Myhistine Elixir. (Rosemont) Chlorpheniramine maleate 2 mg, phenylephrine hydrochloride 5 mg/5 mL, alcohol 5%. Liq. Bot. 4 oz, pt, gal. *OTC.*
Use: Antihistamine, decongestant.

Myhistine Expectorant. (Rosemont) Codeine phosphate 10 mg, guaifenesin 100 mg, pseudoephedrine hydrochloride 30 mg/5 mL, alcohol 7.5%. Liq. Bot. 4 oz, pt, gal. *c-v.*
Use: Antitussive, decongestant, expectorant.

Myidone Tabs. (Major) Primidone 250 mg. Tab. Bot. 100s, 1000s. *Rx.*
Use: Anticonvulsant.

Mykacet Cream. (Alra) Nystatin 100,000 units, triamcinolone acetonide 0.1%/g. Tube 15 g, 30 g, 60 g. *Rx.*
Use: Antifungal; corticosteroid, topical.

My-K Elixir. (Rosemont) Potassium 20 mEq/15 mL, alcohol 5%, saccharin. Bot. Pt, gal. *Rx.*
Use: Electrolyte supplement.

My-K Formula 77 Liquid. (Rosemont) Doxylamine succinate 3.75 mg, dextromethorphan HBr 7.5 mg/5 mL, alcohol 10%. Liq. Bot. 180 mL. *OTC.*
Use: Antihistamine, antitussive.

Mykinac. (Alra) Nystatin 100,000 units/g in cream base. Cream Tube 15 g, 30 g. *OTC.*
Use: Antifungal, topical.

My-K Nasal Spray. (Rosemont) Oxymetazoline hydrochloride 0.05%. Soln. Bot. 0.5 oz. *OTC.*
Use: Decongestant.

Mykrox. (Medeva) Metolazone 0.5 mg. Tab. Bot. 100s. *OTC.*
Use: Diuretic.

Mylagen Gelcaps. (Ivax) Calcium carbonate 311 mg, magnesium carbonate 232 mg. Pkg. 24s. *OTC.*
Use: Antacid.

Mylagen Liquid. (Ivax) Magnesium hydroxide 200 mg, aluminum hydroxide 200 mg, simethicone 20 mg/5 mL. Bot. 355 mL. *OTC.*
Use: Antacid; antiflatulent.

Mylagen II Liquid. (Ivax) Aluminum hydroxide 400 mg, magnesium hydroxide 400 mg, simethicone 40 mg/5 mL. Bot. 355 mL. *OTC.*
Use: Antacid; antiflatulent.

Mylase 100. Alpha-amylase.
See: Diastase.

Myleran. (GlaxoSmithKline) Busulfan 2 mg. Lactose. Film-coated. Tab. Bot. 25s. *Rx.*
Use: Alkylating agent.

Mylicon. (AstraZeneca) Simethicone 40 mg. **Chew. Tab.:** Bot. 100s, 500s, UD 100s. **Drops:** 40 mg/0.6 mL. Bot. 30 mL. *OTC.*
Use: Antiflatulent.

Mylicon-80. (AstraZeneca) Simethicone 80 mg. Chew. Tab. Bot. 100s, Box 12s, 48s, UD 100s. *OTC.*
Use: Antiflatulent.

Mylicon-125. (AstraZeneca) Simethicone 125 mg. Chew. Tab. In 12s, 50s. *OTC.*
Use: Antiflatulent.

Mylocaine 4% Solution. (Rosemont) Lidocaine hydrochloride 4%. Bot. 50 mL, 100 mL. *Rx.*
Use: Anesthetic, local.

Mylocaine 2% Viscous Solution. (Rosemont) Lidocaine hydrochloride 2%. Bot. 100 mL. *Rx.*
Use: Anesthetic, local.

Mymethasone. (Rosemont) Dexamethasone 0.5 mg/5 mL, alcohol 5%. Elix. Bot. 100 mL, 240 mL. *Rx.*
Use: Corticosteroid.

Mynatal. (ME Pharmaceuticals) Ca 300 mg, Fe 65 mg, vitamins A 5000 units, D 400 units, E 30 mg, B_1 3 mg, B_2 3.4 mg, B_3 20 mg, B_5 10 mg, B_6 10 mg, B_{12} 12 mcg, C 120 mg, folic acid 1 mg, biotin 30 mcg, Cr, Cu, I, Mg, Mn, Mo, Zn 25 mg. Cap. Bot. 100s, 500s. *Rx.*
Use: Mineral, vitamin supplement.

Mynatal FC. (ME Pharmaceuticals) Ca 250 mg, Fe 60 mg, vitamin A 5000 units, D 400 units, E 30 units, B_1 3 mg, B_2 3.4 mg, B_3 20 mg, B_5 10 mg, B_6 10 mg, B_{12} 12 mcg, C 100 mg, folic acid 1 mg, biotin 30 mcg, Zn 25 mg, I, Mg, Cr, Cu, Mo, Mn. Capl. Bot. 100s. *Rx.*
Use: Mineral, vitamin supplement.

Mynatal P.N. Captabs. (ME Pharmaceuticals) Ca 125 mg, Fe 60 mg, vitamins A 4000 units, D 400 units, B_1 3 mg, B_2 3 mg, B_3 10 mg, B_6 2 mg, B_{12} 3 mcg, C 50 mg, folic acid 1 mg, Zn 18 mg. Tab. Bot. 100s. *Rx.*
Use: Mineral, vitamin supplement.

Mynatal P.N. Forte. (ME Pharmaceuticals) Fe 60 mg, vitamin A 5000 units, D 400 units, E 30 units, C 80 mg, B_1 3 mg, B_2 3.4 mg, B_3 20 mg, B_6 4 mg, B_{12} 12 mcg, folic acid 1 mg, Ca 250 mg, Zn 25 mg, I, Mg, Cu. Capl. Bot. 100s. *Rx.*
Use: Mineral, vitamin supplement.

Mynatal Rx. (ME Pharmaceuticals) Ca 200 mg, Fe 60 mg, vitamin A 4000 units, D 400 units, E 15 mg, B_1 1.5 mg, B_2 1.6 mg, B_3 17 mg, B_5 7 mg, B_6 4 mg, B_{12} 2.5 mcg, C 80 mg, folic acid 1 mg, biotin 0.03 mg, Zn 25 mg, Mg, Cu. Capl. Bot. 100s. *Rx.*
Use: Mineral, vitamin supplement.

Mynate 90 Plus. (ME Pharmaceuticals) Ca 250 mg, Fe 90 mg, vitamin A 4000 units, D 400 units, E 30 units, B_1 3 mg, B_2 3.4 mg, B_3 20 mg, B_6 20 mg,

B_{12} 12 mcg, C 120 mg, folic acid 1 mg, Zn 25 mg, DSS, I, Cu. Capl. Bot. 100s. *Rx.*
Use: Mineral, vitamin supplement.

Myo-B. (Sigma-Tau) Adenosine-5-monophosphoric acid, vitamin B_{12}. Inj. Vial 10 mL. *Rx.*

Myobloc. (Solstice Neurosciences) RimabotulinumtoxinB 5,000 units/mL, human serum albumin 0.05%, sodium succinate 0.01 M, sodium chloride 0.1 M. Preservative free. (One unit corresponds to the calculated median lethal intraperitoneal dose (LD_{50}) in mice.) Inj. Soln. Single-use vial. 0.5 mL, 1 mL, 2 mL. *Rx.*
Use: Botulinum toxin.

Myocide NS. (Woodward) Benzalkonium chloride, propylene glycol, methylparaben. Soln. 30 mL. *OTC.*
Use: Antiseptic.

Myodil.
See: Iophendylate Injection.

Myoflex Creme. (Novartis Consumer) Trolamine salicylate 10% in a vanishing cream base. Tube 2 oz, 4 oz, Jar 8 oz, lb, Pump dispenser 3 oz. *OTC.*
Use: Analgesic, topical.

Myolin. (Roberts) Orphenadrine citrate 30 mg/mL. Inj. Vial 10 mL. *Rx.*
Use: Muscle relaxant.

Myorgal. (Mysuran) Ambenonium Chloride.
Use: Cholinergic.

Myorisan. (Versapharm) Isotretinoin 10 mg, 20 mg, 40 mg. Edetate disodium, vegetable oil, soybean oil. Cap., softgel. UD 30s, UD 100s. *Rx.*
Use: First-generation retinoid.

Myoscint. (Centocor) Imciromab pentetate 0.5 mg for conjugation with indium-111. Kit.
Use: Radioimmunoscintigraphy agent. [Orphan Drug]

Myotalis. (Vita Elixir) Digitalis 1.5 gr. EC Tab. *Rx.*
Use: Cardiovascular agent.

Myotonachol. (Glenwood) Bethanechol chloride 10 mg, 25 mg. Tab. Bot. 100s. *Rx.*
Use: Urinary tract product.

Myotoxin. (Vita Elixir) **#1:** Digitoxin 0.1 mg. Tab. **#2:** Digitoxin 0.2 mg. Tab. *Rx.*
Use: Cardiovascular agent.

Myozyme. (Genzyme Corporation) Alglucosidase alfa 50 mg. Preservative free. Pow. for Inj., lyophilized. Single-use vials. 20 mL. *Rx.*
Use: Enzyme replacement therapy.

Myphentol Elixir. (Rosemont) Phenobarbital 16.2 mg, hyoscyamine SO_4 or HBr 0.1037 mg, atropine sulfate 0.0194 mg, scopolamine HBr 0.0065 mg/5 mL, alcohol 23%. Bot. 4 oz, pt, gal. *Rx.*
Use: Anticholinergic; antispasmodic; hypnotic; sedative.

Myphetane DX Cough. (Morton Grove) Brompheniramine maleate 2 mg, pseudoephedrine hydrochloride 30 mg, dextromethorphan HBr 10 mg/5 mL. Alcohol 0.95%, methylparaben, sugar. Butterscotch flavor. Syrup. 473 mL. *Rx.*
Use: Upper respiratory combination, antitussive combination.

Myproic Acid. (Rosemont) Valproic acid 250 mg (as sodium valproate)/5 mL. Syrup. Bot. Pt. *Rx.*
Use: Anticonvulsant.

Myrbetriq. (Astellas) Mirabegron 25 mg, 50 mg. Film coated. Butylated hydroxytoluene, PEG. ER Tab. 30s, 90s, UD 100s. *Rx.*
Use: Urinary acidifier, acid phosphate.

Myriatin Drops. (Sanofi-Synthelabo) Atropine methonitrate BP. *Rx.*
Use: Antispasmodic.

myristica oil.
Use: Flavor.

•**myristyl alcohol.** (mih-RIST-ill) *NF.*
Use: Pharmaceutic aid (stiffening agent).

Myrj 53. (AstraZeneca) Polyoxyl 50 stearate.
Use: Surface active agent.

Myrj 52 and M2s. (AstraZeneca) Polyoxyethylene 40 stearate. Mixture of free polyoxyethylene glycol and its mono- and di-stearates.
Use: Surface active agent.

Myrj 45. (AstraZeneca) Mixture of free polyoxyethylene glycol and its mono- and di-stearates. Polyoxyl 8 stearate.
Use: Surface active agent.

Mysoline. (Valeant) Primidone 50 mg, 250 mg. Lactose. Tab. 100s. *Rx.*
Use: Anticonvulsant.

Mysuran. Ambenonium Chloride.
Use: Muscle stimulant.
See: Mytelase.

Mytussin. (Morton Grove Pharmaceuticals) Guaifenesin 100 mg/5 mL, alcohol 3.5%. Syrup. Bot. 4 oz, pt, gal. *OTC.*
Use: Expectorant.

Mytussin DM. (Morton Grove Pharmaceuticals) Guaifenesin 100 mg, dextromethorphan HBr 10 mg per 5 mL. Alcohol free, sugar, menthol, saccharin, cherry flavor. Syrup. Bot. 118 mL, 3.8 L. *OTC.*
Use: Upper respiratory combination, antitussive, expectorant.

Myverol. (Eastman Kodak) Glyceryl monostearate.

My-Vitalife. (ME Pharmaceuticals) Ca 130 mg, Fe 27 mg, vitamins A 6500 units, D 400 units, E 30 mg, B_1 1.5 mg, B_2 1.7 mg, B_3 20 mg, B_5 10 mg, B_6 2 mg, B_{12} 6 mcg, C 60 mg, folic acid 0.4 mg, Cr, Cu, K, I, Mg, Mn, Mo, P, Se, Zn 15 mg, vitamin K, biotin 30 mcg. Cap. Bot. 60s. *OTC.*
Use: Mineral, vitamin supplement.

My Way. (Gavis Pharmaceuticals) Levonorgestrel 1.5 mg. Lactose. Tab. UD 1s. *OTC.*
Use: Emergency contraceptive.

Myzilra. (Qualitest) **Phase 1:** Ethinyl estradiol 30 mcg, levonorgestrel 0.05 mg. Film coated. Lactose, PEG. 6s. **Phase 2:** Ethinyl estradiol 40 mcg, levonorgestrel 0.075 mg. Film coated. 5s. **Phase 3:** Ethinyl estradiol 30 mcg, levonorgestrel 0.125 mg. Film coated. 10s.Tab. 28s w/7 inert tablets. *Rx.*
Use: Oral triphasic contraceptive.

N

Na-Ana-Tal. (Churchill) Phenobarbital 0.25 g, phenacetin 2 g, aspirin 3 g, nicotinic acid 50 mg. Tab. Bot. 100s, Liq. Bot. 16 oz. *c-IV.*
Use: Analgesic; hypnotic; sedative.

•**nabazenil.** (nab-AZE-eh-nill) USAN.
Use: Anticonvulsant.

Nabi-HB. (Biotest Pharmaceuticals) Hepatitis B immune globulin (human) 5% ± 1% protein. Glycine 0.15 M, solvent/detergent treated. Preservative free. Soln. for Inj. Single-dose vial 1 mL, 5 mL. *Rx.*
Use: Immune globulin.

•**nabilone.** (NAB-ih-lone) USAN.
Use: Anxiolytic; antiemetic/antivertigo agent.
See: Cesamet.

•**nabitan hydrochloride.** (NAB-ih-tan) USAN. *Formerly Nabutan Hydrochloride.*
Use: Analgesic.

•**nabiximols.** (nab-IX-i-mols) USAN.
Use: Analgesic.

•**naboctate hydrochloride.** (NAB-ock-tate) USAN.
Use: Antiglaucoma agent; antinauseant.

•**nabumetone.** (nab-YOU-meh-TONE) *USP.*
Use: Nonsteroidal anti-inflammatory agent.

nabumetone. (Various Mfr.) Nabumetone 500 mg, 750 mg. Tab. 100s, 500s, 1000s. *Rx.*
Use: Nonsteroidal anti-inflammatory agent.

n-acetylcysteine.
See: Acetylcysteine.

n-acetyl-p-aminophenol. Acetaminophen.

•**nadide.** (NAD-ide) USAN. *Formerly Diphosphopyridine Nucleotide, Nicotinamide Adenine Dinucleotide.*
Use: Antagonist to alcohol and narcotics.

Nadinola (Deluxe) for Oily Skin. (Strickland) Hydroquinone 2%. Bot. 1.25 oz, 2.25 oz. *Rx.*
Use: Dermatologic.

Nadinola for Dry Skin. (Strickland) Hydroquinone 2%. Bot. 1.25 oz, 2.25 oz. *Rx.*
Use: Dermatologic.

Nadinola (Ultra) for Normal Skin. (Strickland) Hydroquinone 2%. Bot. 1.25 oz, 3.75 oz, Tube 1.85 oz. *Rx.*
Use: Dermatologic.

•**nadolol.** (nay-DOE-lahl) *USP.*
Use: Antihypertensive; antianginal; beta-adrenergic blocker.
See: Corgard.

nadolol. (Various Mfr.) Nadolol 20 mg, 40 mg, 80 mg, 120 mg, 160 mg. Tab. Bot. 30s (80 mg only), 100s; 500s (80 mg, 120 mg, 160 mg only); 1000s (except 20 mg); UD 100s (20 mg, 40 mg, 80 mg only). *Rx.*
Use: Antiadrenergic/sympatholytic, beta-adrenergic blocker.

nadolol and bendroflumethiazide.
Use: Antihypertensive; antianginal beta blocker.
See: Corzide.

nadolol/bendroflumethiazide. (IMPAX Laboratories) Nadolol/bendroflumethiazide 40 mg/5 mg, 80 mg/5 mg. Lactose, mannitol. Tab. 100s, 500s. *Rx.*
Use: Antihypertensive combination.

naepaine hydrochloride.
Use: Anesthetic, local.

•**nafamostat mesylate.** (naff-AM-oh-stat) USAN.
Use: Anticoagulant; antifibrinolytic.

•**nafarelin acetate.** (NAFF-uh-RELL-in) USAN.
Use: LHRH agonist; agonist; hormone. [Orphan Drug]
See: Synarel.

Nafazair A. (Bausch & Lomb) Naphazoline hydrochloride 0.025%, pheniramine maleate 0.3%, benzalkonium chloride 0.01%, EDTA, boric acid, sodium borate. Bot. 15 mL. *Rx.*
Use: Decongestant combination, ophthalmic.

nafcillin. (Baxter) Inj., Soln. Nafcillin. **1 g:** Dextrose 1.8 g. Premixed, frozen 50 mL single-dose *Galaxy* container. **2 g:** Dextrose 3.6 g. Premixed, frozen 100 mL single-dose *Galaxy* container. *Rx.*
Use: Penicillin, penicillin-resistant penicillin.

Nafcillin Injection. (Baxter) Nafcillin sodium 1 g, 2 g (as base). Premixed, frozen, single-dose *Galaxy* containers. 50 mL (1 g only), 100 mL (2 g only). *Rx.*
Use: Anti-infective, penicillin.

•**nafcillin sodium.** (naff-SILL-in) *USP.*
Use: Anti-infective.
See: Nafcillin Injection.

nafcillin sodium. (Sandoz) Nafcillin sodium (as base) 1 g, 2 g. Pow. for Inj. *Add-Vantage* vials. *Rx.*
Use: Penicillin, anti-infective.

Na-Feen. (Pacemaker) Fluoride 1 mg/Dose. Tab. Bot. 100s, 500s, 1000s; Liq. 2 oz. *Rx.*
Use: Dental caries agent.

• **nafenopin.** (naff-EN-oh-pin) USAN.
Use: Antihyperlipoproteinemic.

• **nafimidone hydrochloride.** (naff-IH-mih-DOHN) USAN.
Use: Anticonvulsant.

• **naflocort.** (NAFF-lah-cort) USAN.
Use: Adrenocortical steroid (topical).

• **nafoxidine hydrochloride.** (naff-OX-ih-deen) USAN.
Use: Antiestrogen.

• **nafronyl oxalate.** (NAFF-row-NILL OX-ah-late) USAN.
Use: Vasodilator.

• **naftifine hydrochloride.** (NAFF-tih-FEEN) USAN.
Use: Antifungal agent, topical anti-infective.
See: Naftin.

Naftin. (Merz Pharmaceutical) Naftifine hydrochloride. **Cream:** 1%, 2%. 30 g, 45 g (2% only), 60 g, 90 g (1% only). **Gel: 1%:** Alcohol, edetate disodium, polysorbate 80. 40 g, 60 g, 90 g. **2%:** Alcohol, benzyl alcohol, edetate disodium, propylene glycol. 45 g. *Rx.*
Use: Antifungal agent, topical anti-infective.

Naganol.
See: Suramin.
Naphuride Sodium.

Naglazyme. (BioMarin) Galsulfase 1 mg/mL (expressed as protein content). Preservative free. Soln. for Inj. Single-use vial (contains sodium chloride 43.8 mg, sodium phosphate monobasic monohydrate 6.2 mg, sodium phosphate dibasic heptahydrate 1.34 mg, polysorbate 80 0.25 mg) 5 mL. *Rx.*
Use: Mucopolysaccharidosis VI.

• **nagrestipen.** (na-GRES-ti-pen) USAN.
Use: Stem cell inhibitory protein.

Nailicure. (Purepac) Denatonium benzoate in a clear nail polish base. Liq. Bot. 0.33 oz. *OTC.*
Use: Nail-biting deterrent.

Nail Plus. (Faraday) Gelatin Cap. Bot. 100s, 200s.

• **nalbuphine hydrochloride.** (NAL-byoo-FEEN) USAN.
Use: Narcotic agonist-antagonist analgesic.
See: Nubain.

nalbuphine hydrochloride. (Various Mfr.) Nalbuphine hydrochloride 10 mg/mL, 20 mg/mL. Inj. Vials. 1 mL, 10 mL. *Rx.*
Use: Narcotic agonist-antagonist analgesic.

Naldecon Senior EX. (Sandoz) Guaifenesin 200 mg/5 mL, saccharin, sorbitol. Alcohol free. Liq. Bot. 120 mL. *OTC.*
Use: Expectorant.

• **naldemedine.** (nal-DEM-e-deen) USAN.
Use: Gastrointestinal agent.

• **naldemedine tosylate.** (nal-DEM-e-deen) USAN.
Use: Gastrointestinal agent.

Nalfon. (Xspire Pharma) Fenoprofen calcium 200 mg, 400 mg. Cap. 90s (400 mg only), 100s (200 mg only), 500s (400 mg only). *Rx.*
Use: Analgesic; NSAID.

• **nalidixate sodium.** (nal-ih-DIK-sate) USAN. Under study.
Use: Anti-infective.

• **nalidixic acid.** (nal-ih-DIK-sik) *USP.*
Use: Anti-infective.

• **nalmefene hydrochloride.** (NAL-meh-FEEN) USAN. *Formerly Naletrene.*
Use: Antagonist to narcotics.

nalmetrene.
Use: Antagonist to narcotics.

• **nalmexone hydrochloride.** (NAL-mex-ohn) USAN.
Use: Analgesic; narcotic.

• **nalorphine hydrochloride.** (nal-OR-feen) *USP.*

• **naloxegol.** (nal-OX-ee-gol) USAN.
Use: Treatment of opioid-induced constipation.

• **naloxegol oxalate.** (nal-OX-ee-gol) USAN.
Use: Treatment of opioid-induced constipation.

• **naloxone hydrochloride.** (nal-OX-one) *USP.*
Use: Detoxification agent, antidote.
W/Buprenorphine Hydrochloride.
See: Zubsolv.

naloxone hydrochloride. (Amphastar) Naloxone hydrochloride 1 mg/mL. Inj., Soln. Single-dose, prefilled syringe. 2 mL. *Rx.*
Use: Detoxification agent, antidote.

naloxone hydrochloride. (Various Mfr.) Naloxone hydrochloride. **Inj.:** 0.4 mg/mL. Amps. 1 mL. Syringes. 1 mL. Vials. 1 mL, 2 mL, 10 mL. **Neonatal Inj.:** 0.02 mg/mL. Vial. 2 mL. *Rx.*
Use: Detoxification agent, antidote.

• **naltrexone hydrochloride.** (nal-TREX-ohn) USAN.
Use: Antidote, antagonist to narcotics.
See: ReVia.
Vivitrol.

naltrexone hydrochloride. (Various Mfr.) Naltrexone hydrochloride 50 mg. Tab. Bot. 30s, 100s, 500s. *Rx.*
Use: Narcotic antagonist; antidote.

•**naluzotan.** (na-lue-ZOE-tan) USAN.
Use: CNS agent.

•**naluzotan hydrochloride.** (na-lue-ZOE-tan) USAN.
Use: CNS agent.

Namenda. (Forest Laboratories) Memantine hydrochloride. **Oral Soln.:** 2 mg/mL. Sorbitol, parabens. Alcohol free. Peppermint flavor. 360 mL. **Tab.:** 5 mg, 10 mg. Lactose. Film-coated. 60s, 200s, 2000s, UD 100s, titration paks (blister pack containing 49 tabs [28 × 5 mg and 21 × 10 mg]). *Rx.*
Use: Alzheimer disease.

Namenda XR. (Forest Laboratories) Memantine hydrochloride 7 mg, 14 mg, 21 mg, 28 mg. PEG, sugar. ER Cap. 30s, 90s (14 mg, 28 mg), UD 100s (14 mg, 28 mg), titration pack (contains 28 capsules [7 × 7 mg, 7 × 14 mg, 7 × 21 mg, 7 × 28 mg]). *Rx.*
Use: NMDA receptor antagonist.

•**naminidil.** (nam-IN-i-dil) USAN.
Use: Alopecia.

namol xenyrate.
See: Namoxyrate.

•**namoxyrate.** (nam-OX-ee-rate) USAN.
Use: Analgesic.
See: Namol Xenyrate.

namuron.
See: Cyclobarbital Calcium.

•**nandrolone cyclotate.** (NAN-drole-ohn SIH-kloe-tate) USAN.
Use: Anabolic.

•**nandrolone decanoate.** (NAN-drole-ohn deh-KAN-oh-ate) *USP.*
Use: Anabolic steroid.

•**nandrolone phenpropionate.** (NAN-drole-ohn PROE-pee-oh-nate) *USP.*
Use: Androgen.

NanoVM 4-8 Years. (Solace) Iron 10 mg, calcium 800 mg, vitamins A 1,332 units, D 400 units, E 10 units, B_1 0.6 mg, B_2 0.6 mg, B_3 8 mg, B_5 3 mg, B_6 0.6 mg, B_{12} 1.2 mcg, C 25 mg, K 55 mcg, folic acid 0.2 mg, Cr, Cu, I, K, Mg, Mn, Mo, P, Se, Zn, biotin. Pow. 200 g. *OTC.*
Use: Multivitamin with mineral.

NanoVM 1-3 Years. (Solace) Iron 7 mg, calcium 500 mg, vitamins A 1,000 units, D 400 units, E 9 units, B_1 0.5 mg, B_2 0.5 mg, B_3 6 mg, B_5 2 mg, B_6 0.5 mg, B_{12} 0.9 mcg, C 15 mg, K 30 mcg, folic acid 150 mcg, Cr, Cu, I, K, Mg, Mn, Mo, P, Se, Zn, biotin. Pow. 200 g. *OTC.*
Use: Multivitamin with minerals.

•**nantradol hydrochloride.** (NAN-trah-DAHL) USAN.
Use: Analgesic.

Naotin. (Drug Products) Sodium nicotinate. Amp. (equivalent to 10 mg nicotinic acid/mL) 10 mL, Box 25s, 100s. *Rx.*
Use: Vitamin B_3 supplement.

NAPA. (Medco Research; Parke-Davis) Acecainide hydrochloride.
Use: Cardiovascular agent.

•**napactadine hydrochloride.** (nap-ACK-tah-deen) USAN.
Use: Antidepressant.

•**napamezole hydrochloride.** (nap-am-EH-zole) USAN.
Use: Antidepressant.

NAPAmide Caps. (Major) Disopyramide phosphate 100 mg or 150 mg. Bot. 100s, 500s, UD 100s. *Rx.*
Use: Antiarrhythmic.

naphazoline. (Various Mfr.) Naphazoline hydrochloride. 0.1%. Ophth. Soln. Bot. 15 mL. *Rx.*
Use: Adrenergic, vasoconstrictor; ophthalmic decongestant.

•**naphazoline hydrochloride.** (naff-AZZ-oh-leen) *USP.*
Use: Adrenergic, vasoconstrictor; nasal decongestant, arylalkylamine; ophthalmic decongestant.
See: Advanced Eye Relief, Redness Instant Relief.
Advanced Eye Relief, Redness Maximum Relief.
AK-Con.
Clear Eyes ACR Seasonal Relief.
Clear Eyes for Redness Relief.
Clear Eyes Tears Plus Redness Relief.
Muro's Opcon.
Naphcon.
Privine.
20/20 Eye Drops.
W/Pheniramine Maleate.
See: Naphcon-A.
Opcon-A.
Visine-A.

naphazoline hydrochloride and antazoline phosphate. (Various Mfr.) Naphazoline hydrochloride 0.05%, antazoline phosphate 0.5%. Soln. 5 mL, 15 mL. *OTC.*
Use: Antihistamine; decongestant, ophthalmic.

naphazoline hydrochloride and pheniramine maleate. (Various Mfr.) Naphazoline hydrochloride 0.025%, pheniramine maleate 0.3%. Soln. Bot. 15 mL. *OTC.*
Use: Antihistamine; decongestant, ophthalmic.

naphazoline hydrochloride/pheniramine maleate. (Altaire Pharmaceuticals) Naphazoline hydrochloride

0.027%/pheniramine maleate 0.315%. Benzalkonium chloride 0.01%, disodium edetate 0.1%, boric acid, hydroxypropyl methylcellulose, sodium borate, sodium chloride. Soln. 15 mL, 30 mL. *OTC.*
Use: Ophthalmic decongestant/antihistamine combination.

Naphcon. (Alcon) Naphazoline hydrochloride 0.012%. Benzalkonium chloride 0.01%, EDTA. Ophth. Soln. Bot. 15 mL. *OTC.*
Use: Mydriatic; vasoconstrictor; ophthalmic decongestant.

Naphcon-A. (Alcon) Naphazoline hydrochloride 0.025%, pheniramine maleate 0.3%. Soln. Bot. 15 mL. *OTC.*
Use: Decongestant combination, ophthalmic.

Napholine. (Horizon) Naphazoline hydrochloride 0.1%. Soln. Bot. 15 mL. *Rx.*
Use: Mydriatic; vasoconstrictor.

Naphthyl-B Salicylate. Betol, Naphthosalol, Salinaphthol.
Use: GI & GU, antiseptic.

naphuride sodium. Suramin Sodium.

•**napitane mesylate.** (NAP-ih-tane) USAN.
Use: Antidepressant.

Naprelan. (Victory Pharma) Naproxen 375 mg (naproxen sodium 412.5 mg), 500 mg (naproxen sodium 550 mg), 750 mg (naproxen sodium 825 mg). CR Tab. 30s (750 mg), 100s (375 mg), 60s (750 mg), 75s (500 mg). *Rx.*
Use: Nonsteroidal anti-inflammatory agent.

Naprosyn. (Roche) Naproxen. **Tab.:** 250 mg, 375 mg, 500 mg. Bot. 100s, 500s. **Susp.:** 125 mg/5 mL. Sorbitol, sucrose, parabens, orange-pineapple flavor. Bot. 473 mL. *Rx.*
Use: Analgesic; nonsteroidal anti-inflammatory agent.

•**naproxcinod.** (na-PROKS-sin-od) USAN.
Use: Osteoarthritis.

•**naproxen.** (nah-PROX-ehn) *USP.*
Use: Analgesic; nonsteroidal anti-inflammatory agent; antipyretic.
See: EC-Naprosyn.
Naprosyn.

naproxen. (Various Mfr.) Naproxen. **Tab.:** 250 mg, 375 mg, 500 mg. Bot. 30s, 100s, 500s, 1000s, UD 100s, UD 300s (500 mg only); unit-of-use 30s, 60s, 90s, 120s; *Robot ready* 25s (except 375 mg). **DR Tab.:** 375 mg, 500 mg. Bot. 100s, 500s. **Susp.:** 125 mg/5 mL. Methylparaben, sorbitol, sucrose, pineapple-orange flavor. Bot. 15 mL, 20 mL, 500 mL. *Rx.*
Use: Analgesic; nonsteroidal anti-inflammatory agent; antipyretic.

•**naproxen etemesil.** (na-PROX-en et-e-ME-sil) USAN.
Use: CNS agent.

•**naproxen sodium.** (nah-PROX-ehn) *USP.*
Use: Analgesic; nonsteroidal anti-inflammatory agent; antipyretic.
See: Aleve.
All Day Relief.
Anaprox.
Anaprox DS.
Midol Extended Relief.
Naprelan.
W/Diphenhydramine Hydrochloride.
See: Aleve PM.
W/Pseudoephedrine Hydrochloride.
See: Aleve-D Sinus & Cold.

naproxen sodium. (Ivax) Naproxen sodium 200 mg (220 mg naproxen sodium). Tab. Bot. 24s. *OTC.*
Use: Anti-inflammatory.

naproxen sodium. (Various Mfr.) Naproxen 200 mg (naproxen sodium 220 mg), 250 mg (naproxen sodium 275 mg), 500 mg (naproxen sodium 550 mg). Tab. Bot. 24s, 50s (200 mg only); 100s, 500s, 1000s, UD 100s (except 200 mg). *Rx-OTC.*
Use: Analgesic; nonsteroidal anti-inflammatory agent.

naproxen sodium and pseudoephedrine hydrochloride.
Use: Upper respiratory combination, decongestant, analgesic.
See: Aleve Cold & Sinus.
Aleve Sinus & Headache.

•**naproxol.** (nay-PROX-ole) USAN.
Use: Analgesic; anti-inflammatory; antipyretic.

•**napsagatran.** (nap-sah-GAT-ran) USAN.
Use: Antithrombotic.

•**narafilcon B.** (NAR-a-FIL-kon) USAN.
Use: Contact lens material (hydrophilic).

•**naranol hydrochloride.** (NARE-ah-nahl) USAN.
Use: Antipsychotic.

•**naratriptan hydrochloride.** (NAHR-ah-trip-tan) *USP.*
Use: Antimigraine, serotonin 5-HT_1 receptor antagonist.
See: Amerge.

naratriptan hydrochloride. (Various Mfr.) Naratriptan hydrochloride 1 mg, 2.5 mg. Film coated. May contain lactose, PEG, polyvinyl alcohol. Tab. Blister pack. 9s. *Rx.*
Use: Agent for migraine, serotonin 5-HT_1 receptor agonist.

narcotic agonist-antagonist analgesics.
See: Buprenorphine Hydrochloride.

Butorphanol Tartrate.
Nalbuphine Hydrochloride.
Pentazocine.

narcotic antitussive.
See: Codeine Sulfate.

Nardil. (Parke-Davis) Phenelzine sulfate 15 mg. Mannitol. Film-coated. Tab. Bot. 60s. *Rx.*
Use: Antidepressant, monoamine oxidase inhibitor.

•**narlaprevir.** (nar-la-PRE-vir) USAN.
Use: Antiviral.

•**narnatumab.** (nar-NAT-ue-mab) USAN.
Use: Antineoplastic.

•**naronapride.** (nar-ON-a-pride) USAN.
Use: Gastrointestinal agent.

•**naronapride dihydrochloride.** (nar-ON-a-pride) USAN.
Use: Gastrointestinal agent.

Naropin. (AAP Pharmaceuticals) Ropivacaine hydrochloride 2 mg/mL (0.2%), 5 mg/mL (0.5%), 7.5 mg/mL (0.75%), 10 mg/mL (1%). Preservative free. Inj. *PolyAmp DuoFit Sterile Paks* 10 mL (0.2%, 1% only), 20 mL. Single-dose vial 30 mL (0.5% only). Single-dose infusion bot. 100 mL, 200 mL (0.2% only). *Rx.*
Use: Anesthetic, local injectable.

Nasabid. (Jones Pharma) Pseudoephedrine hydrochloride 90 mg, guaifenesin 250 mg, sucrose. Cap., prolonged-action. Bot. 100s. *Rx.*
Use: Decongestant; expectorant.

Nasabid SR. (Jones Medical) Pseudoephedrine hydrochloride 90 mg, guaifenesin 600 mg. SR Tab. Bot. 100s. *Rx.*
Use: Decongestant; expectorant.

Nasacort Allergy 24 HR. (Sanofi-Aventis) Triamcinolone acetonide 55 mcg/actuation. Benzalkonium chloride, dextrose, edetate disodium, polysorbate 80. Spray, Susp.; intranasal. 10.5 g (providing 60 sprays) or 16.5 g (providing 120 sprays) with metered-dose pump unit and nasal adapter. *OTC.*
Use: Respiratory inhalant product, intranasal steroid.

Nasadent. (Scherer) Sodium metaphosphate, glycerin, dicalcium phosphate dihydrate, sodium carboxymethylcellulose, oil of spearmint, sodium benzoate, saccharin. *OTC.*
Use: Ingestible dentifrice.

NaSal. (Bayer Consumer Care) Sodium chloride 0.65%, benzalkonium chloride. Alcohol free. Soln. Drop bot. 15 mL. Spray bot. 30 mL. *OTC.*
Use: Nasal decongestant.

NasalCrom. (Medtech) Cromolyn sodium 40 mg/mL, benzalkonium Cl, EDTA. Nasal Soln. Delivers 5.2 mg/spray. Metered spray device 13 mL or 26 mL. *OTC.*
Use: Antiasthmatic.

Nasal Decongestant, Children's Non-Drowsy. (Various Mfr.) Pseudoephedrine hydrochloride 15 mg/5 mL. Liq. Bot. 118 mL. *OTC.*
Use: Nasal decongestant, arylalkylamine.

Nasal Decongestant, Maximum Strength. (Taro) Oxymetazoline hydrochloride 0.05%. Soln. Spray bot. 15 mL, 30 mL. *OTC.*
Use: Nasal decongestant, imidazoline.

Nasal Decongestant Oral. (Various Mfr.) Pseudoephedrine hydrochloride 7.5 mg/0.8 mL. Drops. Bot. 15 mL, 30 mL w/dropper. *OTC.*
Use: Nasal decongestant, arylalkylamine.

nasal decongestants.
See: Arylalkylamines.
Ephedrine Hydrochloride.
Imidazolines.
Naphazoline Hydrochloride.
Oxymetazoline Hydrochloride.
Phenylephrine Hydrochloride.
Pseudoephedrine Hydrochloride.
Pseudoephedrine Sulfate.
Tetrahydrozoline Hydrochloride.
Xylometazoline Hydrochloride.

Nasal Decongestant Sinus Non-Drowsy. (Topco) Pseudoephedrine hydrochloride 30 mg, acetaminophen 500 mg. Tab. Pkg. 24s. *OTC.*
Use: Upper respiratory combination, decongestant, analgesic.

Nasal•Ease with Zinc. (Health Care Products) Zinc acetate, aloe vera, calendula extract, parabens, tocopherol acetate, EDTA, glycerin. Soln. Gel. Tube 14.1 g. *OTC.*
Use: Nasal decongestant.

Nasal•Ease with Zinc Gluconate. (Health Care Products) Zinc gluconate, sodium chloride, benzalkonium chloride, glycerin. Soln. Spray. Bot. 30 mL. *OTC.*
Use: Nasal decongestant.

Nasal Jelly. (Kondon) Phenol, camphor, menthol, eucalyptus oil, lavender oil. Oint. Tube. 20 g. *OTC.*
Use: Decongestant.

Nasal Moist. (Blairex) Sodium chloride 0.65%, alcohol and dye free. Soln. Spray bot. 45 mL. Mist pump bot. 15 mL. Gel bot. 28.5 g, unit-of-use 2 mL, aloe vera. *OTC.*
Use: Nasal decongestant.

Nasal Relief. (Rugby) Oxymetazoline hydrochloride 0.05%, EDTA, phenylmercuric acetate, sodium chloride. Soln. Spray bot. 15 mL. *OTC.*
Use: Nasal decongestant, imidazoline.

NaSal Saline. (Sanofi-Synthelabo) Nasal spray and drops. Sodium Cl 0.65% buffered w/phosphates. Benzalkonium chloride, sodium chloride. Alcohol free. Bot. 15 mL. Spray Bot. 15 mL. *OTC.*
Use: Moisturizer, nasal.

Nasal Spray. (Various Mfr.) Sodium chloride. Soln. Spray bot. 45 mL. *OTC.*
Use: Nasal decongestant.

•**nasaruplase beta.** (na-SA-rue-plase) USAN.
Use: Ischemic stroke, acute.

Nascobal. (Par Pharmaceuticals) Cyanocobalamin 500 mcg per 0.1 mL (500 mcg/actuation). Benzalkonium chloride. Intranasal spray. 2.3 mL (≈ 8 doses/bottle). *Rx.*
Use: Water-soluble vitamin.

Nashville Rabbit Antithymocyte. (Applied Medical Research) Antithymocyte serum. *Rx.*
Use: Immunosuppressant.

Nasohist. (Hawthorn) Chlorpheniramine maleate 1 mg, phenylephrine hydrochloride 2 mg per mL. Saccharin, sorbitol. Orange-vanilla flavor. Soln., Conc. 30 mL. *Rx.*
Use: Upper respiratory combination, decongestant and antihistamine.

Nasohist DM. (Hawthorn) Chlorpheniramine maleate 1 mg, phenylephrine hydrochloride 2 mg, dextromethorphan HBr 3 mg per mL. Saccharin, sorbitol. Orange-vanilla flavor. Soln., Conc. 30 mL. *Rx.*
Use: Upper respiratory combination, antitussive combination.

Nasonex. (Schering) Mometasone furoate monohydrate 0.05% (50 mcg/actuation). Glycerin, 0.25% w/w phenylethyl alcohol, citric acid, benzalkonium chloride, polysorbate 80. Spray Susp. Intranasal. Bot. 17 g (120 sprays) w/metered-dose manual pump spray unit. *Rx.*
Use: Respiratory inhalant, intranasal steroid.

NasOpen. (GM Pharmaceuticals) Chlorcyclizine hydrochloride 9.375 mg, pseudoephedrine hydrochloride 30 mg per 5 mL. Glycerin, propylene glycol, sorbitol, sucralose. Alcohol free, dye free, gluten free, and sugar free. Cotton candy flavor. Liq. 473 mL. *Rx.*
Use: Upper respiratory combination, decongestant and antihistamine.

NasOpen PE. (GM Pharmaceuticals) Phenylephrine hydrochloride 3.3 mg, thonzylamine hydrochloride 16.7 mg. Glycerin, maltitol, propylene glycol, saccharin, sodium 2.3 mg per 5 mL, sorbitol, sucralose. Alcohol free, gluten free, and sugar free. Cotton candy flavor. Liq. 118 mL. *OTC.*
Use: Upper respiratory combination, decongestant and antihistamine.

Nasophen. (Premo) Phenylephrine hydrochloride 0.25%, 1%. Bot. Pt. *OTC.*
Use: Decongestant.

Nasotuss. (Hawthorn Pharmaceuticals) Chlorcyclizine hydrochloride 25 mg, codeine phosphate 10 mg, phenylephrine hydrochloride 10 mg. Glycerin, propylene glycol, sorbitol, sucralose. Alcohol free, dye free, and sugar free. Raspberry flavor. Liq. 473 mL. *c-v.*
Use: Upper respiratory combination, antitussive combination.

Natabec. (Parke-Davis) Vitamins A 4000 units, D 400 units, B_1 3 mg, B_2 2 mg, B_6 3 mg, C 50 mg, B_{12} 5 mcg, B_3 10 mg, elemental calcium 240 mg, elemental iron 30 mg. Kapseal. Bot. 100s. *OTC.*
Use: Mineral, vitamin supplement.

Natabec-F.A. (Parke-Davis) Vitamins A 4000 units, D 400 units, B_1 3 mg, B_2 2 mg, B_6 3 mg, C 50 mg, B_{12} 5 mcg, B_3 10 mg, elemental calcium 240 mg, elemental iron 30 mg, folic acid 0.1 mg. Kapseal, magnesium, bisulfites. Bot. 100s. *OTC.*
Use: Mineral, vitamin supplement.

Natabec with Fluoride. (Parke-Davis) Vitamins A 4000 units, D 400 units, B_1 3 mg, B_2 2 mg, B_6 3 mg, C 50 mg, B_{12} 5 mcg, B_3 10 mg, elemental calcium 240 mg, elemental iron 30 mg, elemental fluoride 1 mg. Kapseal. Bot. 100s. *Rx.*
Use: Vitamin supplement, dental caries agent.

NataChew. (Eckson) Folic acid 1 mg, Fe 28 mg, vitamins A 2,700 units, D 400 units, E 20 units, B_1 2 mg, B_2 3 mg, B_3 20 mg, B_6 10 mg, B_{12} 12 mcg, C 120 mg. PEG, sucralose, sugar. Tab. 90s. *Rx.*
Use: Prenatal vitamin with minerals.

Natacyn. (Alcon) Natamycin 5%. Bot. 15 mL. *Rx.*
Use: Antifungal agent, ophthalmic.

NatalCare Plus. (Ethex) Vitamin A 4000 units, C 120 mg, calcium sulfate

200 mg, Fe 27 mg, D 400 units, E 22 units, B_1 1.84 mg, B_2 3 mg, niacinamide 20 mg, B_6 10 mg, folic acid 1 mg, B_{12} 12 mcg, Zn 25 mg, Cu 2 mg. Tab. Bot. 100s. *Rx.*
Use: Mineral, vitamin supplement.

NatalCare Three. (Ethex) Ca 200 mg, Fe (as ferrous fumarate) 27 mg, vitamin A (as beta carotene) 3000 units, D 400 units, E (as dl-alpha tocopheryl acetate) 30 units, B_1 1.8 mg, B_2 4 mg, B_3 20 mg, B_6 25 mg, B_{12} 12 mcg, C 120 mg, folic acid 1 mg, Zn 25 mg, Cu, Mg. Tab. Bot. 100s. *Rx.*
Use: Vitamin, mineral supplement.

Natalins. (Bristol-Myers Squibb) Ca 200 mg, Fe 30 mg, vitamins A 4000 units, D 400 units, E 15 units, B_1 1.5 mg, B_2 1.6 mg, B_3 17 mg, B_6 2.6 mg, B_{12} 2.5 mcg, C 70 mg, folic acid 0.5 mg, Mg, Cu, Zn 15 mg. Tab. Bot. 100s. *OTC.*
Use: Mineral, vitamin supplement.

•**natalizumab.** (nay-tal-IZ-oo-mab) USAN.
Use: Immunomodulator, immunologic agent.
See: Tysabri.

Natalvirt CA. (Virtus Pharmaceuticals) **Tab.:** Folic acid 1 mg, calcium 125 mg, iron 35 mg, vitamins D 400 units, E 30 units, B_1 3 mg, B_2 3.4 mg, B_3 20 mg, B_6 25 mg, C 120 mg, Cu, I, Zn, docusate sodium 50 mg. UD 30s. **Cap., softgel:** DHA 300 mg. Glycerin, vitamin E. UD 30s. *Rx.*
Use: Prenatal vitamin with minerals.

Natalvirt 90 DHA. (Virtus Pharmaceuticals) **Tab.:** Folic acid 1 mg, calcium 160 mg, iron 90 mg, vitamins D 400 units, E 30 units, B_1 3 mg, B_2 3.4 mg, B_3 20 mg, B_6 20 mg, C 120 mg, Cu, I, Zn, docusate sodium 50 mg. UD 30s. **Cap., softgel:** DHA 300 mg. Glycerin, vitamin E. UD 30s. *Rx.*
Use: Prenatal vitamin with minerals.

•**natamycin.** (NAT-uh-MY-sin) *USP.*
Use: Anti-infective, ophthalmic.
See: Natacyn.

Natarex Prenatal. (Major) Ca 200 mg, iron 60 mg, vitamins A 4000 units, D 400 units, E 15 mg, B_1 1.5 mg, B_2 1.6 mg, B_3 17 mg, B_5 7 mg, B_6 4 mg, B_{12} 2.5 mcg, C 80 mg, folic acid 1 mg, Cu, Mg, Zn 25 mg, biotin 30 mcg. Tab. Bot 100s. *Rx.*
Use: Mineral, vitamin supplement.

Nata-San. (Sandia) Vitamins A 4000 units, D 400 units, B_1 5 mg, B_2 4 mg, B_6 10 mg, nicotinic acid 10 mg, C 100 mg, B_{12} activity 5 mcg, ferrous fumarate 200 mg (elemental iron 65 mg), calcium carbonate 500 mg (Ca 196 mg), Cu (sulfate) 0.5 mg, Mg (sulfate) 0.1 mg, Mn (sulfate) 0.1 mg, K (sulfate) 0.1 mg, Zn (sulfate) 0.5 mg. Tab. Bot. 100s, 1000s. *OTC.*
Use: Mineral, vitamin supplement.

Nata-San F.A. (Sandia) Vitamins A 4000 units, D 400 units, B_1 5 mg, B_2 4 mg, B_6 10 mg, nicotinic acid 10 mg, C 100 mg, B_{12} activity 5 mcg, folic acid 1 mg, Fe 65 mg, Ca 200 mg, Cu (sulfate) 0.5 mg, Mg (sulfate) 0.1 mg, Mn (sulfate) 0.1 mg, K (sulfate) 0.1 mg, Zn (sulfate) 0.5 mg. Tab. Bot. 100s, 1000s. *Rx.*
Use: Mineral, vitamin supplement.

NataTab FA. (Ethex) Vitamin A 4000 units, C 120 mg, Ca 200 mg, Fe 29 mg, D 400 units, E 30 units, B_1 3 mg, B_2 3 mg, niacin 20 mg, B_6 3 mg, folic acid 1 mg, B_{12} 8 mcg, iodine, zinc 15 mg, lactose. Tab. Bot. 100s. *Rx.*
Use: Vitamin, mineral supplement.

Natazia. (Bayer HealthCare Pharmaceuticals) **Phase 1:** Estradiol valerate 3 mg. **Phase 2:** Dienogest 2 mg, estradiol valerate 2 mg. **Phase 3:** Dienogest 3 mg, estradiol valerate 2 mg. **Phase 4:** Estradiol valerate 1 mg.Film coated. Lactose. Tab. 28s w/2 inert tablets. *Rx.*
Use: 4-Phasic oral contraceptive.

•**nateglinide.** (na-te-GLYE-nide) USAN.
Use: Antidiabetic; meglitinide.
See: Starlix.

nateglinide. (Dr Reddy's Labs) Nateglinide 60 mg, 120 mg. Mannitol. Tab. 30s, 90s, 100s, 500s, UD 100s. *Rx.*
Use: Antidiabetic agent, meglitinide.

nateglinide. (Par Pharmaceutical) Nateglinide 60 mg, 120 mg. Lactose. Tab. UD 30s. *Rx.*
Use: Antidiabetic agent, meglitinide.

Natelle-EZ. (Tiber Labs) Ca 100 mg, Fe 25 mg, vitamin A 2700 units, D_3 400 units, E 20 units, B_1 3 mg, B_2 3.5 mg, B_3 20 mg, B_5 8 mg, B_6 30 mg, B_{12} 12 mcg, C 120 mg, folic acid 800 mcg, biotin 30 mcg, Cu, Mg, Se, Zn, choline bitartrate. PEG, polyvinyl alcohol. Tab. 30s. *Rx.*
Use: Multivitamin with calcium and iron.

Natodine. (Faraday) Iodine in organic form as found in kelp 1 mg. Tab. Bot. 100s, 250s. *OTC.*

Natrapel. (Tender) Citronella 10% in 15% Aloe vera base. *OTC.*
Use: Insect repellent.

Natrecor. (Scios Nova) Nesiritide 1.58 mg, mannitol. Pow. for Inj., lyophilized. Single-use vial 1.5 mg. *Rx.*
Use: Vasodilator, human B-type natriuretic peptide.

Natrico. (Drug Products) Potassium nitrate 2 g, sodium nitrite 1 g, nitroglycerin 0.25 g, *Crataegus oxyacantha* 0.25 g. Pulvoid. Bot. 100s, 1000s. *Rx.*
Use: Antihypertensive.

Natroba. (ParaPRO/Pernix Therapeutics) Spinosad 0.9%. Alcohols, butylated hydroxytoluene, propylene glycol. Susp. 120 mL. *Rx.*
Use: Scabicide/Pediculicide.

Naturacil. (Bristol-Myers Squibb) Psyllium seed husks 3.4 g, carbohydrate 9.6 g, Na 11 mg, 54 cal/2 pieces. Ctn. 24s, 40s. *OTC.*
Use: Laxative.

Natur-Aid. (Scot-Tussin) Lactose, pectin, and carob-lemon juice. Pow. 90%. Bot. 8 oz. *OTC.*
Use: Increase in normal intestinal flora.

Natural Balance Tears. (Major Pharmaceuticals) Hypromellose 0.4%, benzalkonium chloride 0.01%, edetate disodium, potassium chloride, sodium chloride, sodium phosphate. Soln.; Ophth. 15 mL. *OTC.*
Use: Artificial tear solution.

Natural Diuretic Water Tablet. (AmLab) Buchu leaves 1 g, uva ursi 1 g, trilicum 1 g, parsley 1 g, juniper berries 1 g, asparagus 1 g, alfalfa powder 1 gr. Tab. Bot. 100s. *OTC.*
Use: Diuretic.

Natural E 400. (Mason) Vitamin E 400 units (as d-alpha tocopheryl acetate). Glycerin, soybean oil. Cap., softgels. 90s. *OTC.*
Use: Fat-soluble vitamin.

Natural E 200. (Mason) Vitamin E 200 units. Preservative free and sugar free. Cap., softgels. 100s. *OTC.*
Use: Fat-soluble vitamin.

Natural Fiber Laxative. (Apothecary Prods.) Approx. psyllium hydrophilic mucilloid 3.4 g/7 g dose, 14 cal/dose, sodium free. Pow. Can. 390 g. *OTC.*
Use: Laxative.

natural lung surfactant.
See: Survanta.

natural penicillins.
Use: Anti-infective.
See: Penicillin G (Aqueous).
Penicillin G Potassium.
Pfizerpen.

Natural Psyllium Fiber. (Plus Pharma) Psyllium hydrophilic mucilloid fiber 3.4 g, sodium 3 mg, 25 calories per dose. Dextrose. Pow. 368 g. *OTC.*
Use: Laxative.

Natural Psyllium Fiber, Orange. (Plus Pharma) Psyllium hydrophilic mucilloid fiber 3.4 g, sodium 3 mg, 25 calories per dose. Sucrose. Orange flavor. Pow. 368 g. *OTC.*
Use: Laxative.

natural vitamin A in oil.
See: Oleovitamin A.

Natural Vitamin E. (Freeda Vitamins) Vitamin E 1,150 units (as d-alpha tocopherol) per 1.25 mL. Gluten, lactose, and sugar free. Liq. 114 mL. *OTC.*
Use: Fat-soluble vitamin.

Naturalyte. (Unico Holdings) Na 45 mEq, K 20 mEq, Cl 35 mEq, citrate 48 mEq, dextrose 25 g/L. Soln. Bot. 240 mL, 1 liter. *OTC.*
Use: Electrolyte, mineral supplement.

Nature's Aid Laxative Tabs. (Walgreen) Docusate sodium 100 mg, yellow phenolphthalein 65 mg. Tab. Bot. 60s. *OTC.*
Use: Laxative.

Nature's Remedy. (Block Drug) Aloe 100 mg, cascara sagrada 150 mg, lactose. Tab. Bot. 15s, 30s, 60s. *OTC.*
Use: Laxative.

Nature's Wash Plus. (Geritrex) Aloe vera, parabens, propylene glycol, urea, vitamin E, wheat germ oil. Soap. 3,785 mL. *OTC.*
Use: Emollient bath preparation.

Nature-Throid. (RLC Labs) Thyroid desiccated 16.25 mg (1/4 gr) (lactose, PEG 400), 32.4 mg (1/2 gr), 48.75 mg (3/4 gr) (lactose), 64.8 mg (1 gr), 81.25 mg (1 1/4 gr) (lactose), 97.5 mg (1 1/2 gr) (lactose), 113.75 mg (1 3/4 gr) (lactose), 129.6 mg (2 gr), 146.25 mg (2 1/4 gr) (lactose), 162.5 mg (2 1/2 gr) (lactose), 194.4 mg (3 gr), 260 mg (4 gr) (lactose), 325 mg (5 gr) (lactose). Note: 1 grain (gr) = 64.8 mg. Tab. 100s; 30s, 60s, 90s, 990s, 1,000s, 1,008s (48.75 mg, 81.25 mg, 97.5 mg, 113.75 mg, 146.25 mg, 162.5 mg, 260 mg, 325 mg). *Rx.*
Use: Thyroid hormone.

Natur-Lax Tablets. (Faraday) Rhubarb root, cape aloes, cascara sagrada extract, mandrake root, parsley, carrot. Protein-coated tab. Bot. 100s. *OTC.*
Use: Laxative.

Naus-A-Tories. (Table Rock) Pyrilamine maleate 25 mg, secobarbital 30 mg. Supp. Box 12s. *c-II.*
Use: Antiemetic.

Nausatrol. (Medique Products) Dextrose 1.87 g, fructose 1.87 g, phosphoric acid 21.5 mg per 5 mL. Cherry flavoring, glycerin, methylparaben, potassium sorbate. Soln. 15 mL packet (20s). *OTC.*
Use: Miscellaneous antiemetic, phosphorated carbohydrate solution.

Nausea Relief. (Ivax) Dextrose 1.87 g, fructose 1.87 g, phosphoric acid 21.5 mg. Methylparaben. Soln. 118 mL. *OTC.*
Use: Antiemetic; antivertigo.

Nausetrol. (Walsh Dohmen) Dextrose 1.87 g, fructose 1.87 g, phosphoric acid 21.5 mg per 5 mL. Glycerin, methylparaben. Cherry flavor. Soln. 118 mL. *OTC.*
Use: Antiemetic; antivertigo.

Navane. (Roerig) Thiothixene 2 mg, 10 mg, 20 mg. Lactose. Cap. 100s. *Rx.*
Use: Antipsychotic.

•**navarixin.** (NAV-a-RIX-in) USAN.
Use: Treatment of asthma and chronic obstructive pulmonary disease.

•**naveglitazar.** (nav-e-GLI-ta-zar) USAN.
Use: Diabetes.

Navelbine. (Pierre Fabre Pharmaceuticals) Vinorelbine tartrate 10 mg/mL, preservative free. Inj. Single-use Vial 1 mL, 5 mL. *Rx.*
Use: Antineoplastic; vinca alkaloid.

•**navitoclax.** (na-VIT-oh-klax) USAN.
Use: Antineoplastic.

•**navitoclax dihydrochloride.** (na-VIT-oh-klax) USAN.
Use: Antineoplastic.

•**naxagolide hydrochloride.** (nax-A-go-LIDE) USAN.
Use: Antiparkinsonian; dopamine agonist.

•**naxifylline.** (na-xee-FYE-leen) USAN.
Use: Edema.

Nazafair. (Various Mfr.) Naphazoline hydrochloride 0.1%. Soln. Bot. 15 mL. *Rx.*
Use: Mydriatic; vasoconstrictor.

ND-Gesic. (Hyrex) Acetaminophen 300 mg, pyrilamine maleate 12.5 mg, chlorpheniramine maleate 2 mg, phenylephrine hydrochloride 5 mg. Tab. Bot. 100s, 1000s. *OTC.*
Use: Analgesic; antihistamine; decongestant.

n-diethylvanillamide.
See: Ethamivan.

NDNA. (Wampole) Anti-native DNA test by IFA. Confirmatory test for active SLE. Test 48s. *Rx.*
Use: Diagnostic aid.

•**nebacumab.** (neh-BACK-you-mab) USAN. *Formerly Septomonab.*
Use: Monoclonal antibody, antiendotoxin.

•**nebivolol.** (neh-BIV-oh-lole) USAN.
Use: Antiadrenergic/sympatholytic, beta-adrenergic blocking agents.
See: Bystolic.

•**nebivolol hydrochloride.** (neh-BIV-oh-lole) USAN.
Use: Antihypertensive, beta blocker.

•**nebramycin.** (neh-brah-MY-sin) USAN. A complex of antibiotic substances produced by *Streptomyces tenebrarius.*
Use: Anti-infective.

NebuPent. (American Pharmaceutical Partners) Pentamidine isethionate 300 mg. Aer. single-dose vial. *Rx.*
Use: Anti-infective.

Nebu-Prel. (Mahon) Isoproterenol sulfate 0.4%, phenylephrine hydrochloride 2%, propylene glycol 10%. Liq. Vial 10 mL. *Rx.*
Use: Bronchodilator.

•**neceprevir.** (nes-E-pre-vir) USAN.
Use: Treatment of hepatitis C.

•**neceprevir sodium.** (nes-E-pre-vir) USAN.
Use: Treatment of hepatitis C.

•**necitumumab.** (NE-si-TOOM-oo-mab) USAN.
Use: Antineoplastic.

Necon 1/50. (Watson) Mestranol 50 mcg, norethindrone 1 mg. Lactose. Tab. Pkt. 21s, 28s (7 inert tabs.). *Rx.*
Use: Sex hormone, contraceptive hormone.

Necon 1/35. (Watson) Ethinyl estradiol 35 mcg, norethindrone 1 mg. Lactose. Tab. Pkt. 21s, 28s (7 inert tabs.). *Rx.*
Use: Sex hormone, contraceptive hormone.

Necon 7/7/7. (Watson) **Phase 1:** Norethindrone 0.5 mg, ethinyl estradiol 35 mcg. 7 tabs. **Phase 2:** Norethindrone 0.75 mg, ethinyl estradiol 35 mcg. 7 tabs. **Phase 3:** Norethindrone 1 mg, ethinyl estradiol 35 mcg. 7 tabs. Tab. 28s (7 inert tabs.). *Rx.*
Use: Sex hormone, contraceptive hormone.

Necon 10/11. (Watson) **Phase 1:** Norethindrone 0.5 mg, ethinyl estradiol 35 mcg. 10 tabs. **Phase 2:** Norethindrone 1 mg, ethinyl estradiol 35 mcg. 11 tabs. Lactose. Tab. Pkt. 28s (7 inert tabs.). *Rx.*
Use: Sex hormone, contraceptive hormone.

Necon 0.5/35. (Watson) Ethinyl estradiol 35 mcg, norethindrone 0.5 mg. Lactose. Tab. Pkt. 21s, 28s (7 inert tabs). *Rx.*
Use: Sex hormone, contraceptive hormone.

•**nedocromil.** (NEH-doe-KROE-mill) USAN.
Use: Antiallergic, prophylactic.

•**nedocromil calcium.** (NEH-doe-KROE-mill) USAN.
Use: Antiallergic, prophylactic.

•**nedocromil sodium.** (NEH-doe-KROE-mill) USAN.
Use: Mast cell stabilizer, ophthalmic agent.
See: Alocril.

N.E.E. (Lexis Laboratories) Ethinyl estradiol 35 mcg, norethindrone 1 mg. Tab. 6 pcks. 21s, 28s. *Rx.*
Use: Contraceptive.

NeevoDHA. (Pamlab) L-methylfolate calcium 1.13 mg, calcium 110 mg, iron 27 mg, vitamins D 200 units, E 23 units, B_1 1.4 mg, B_2 1.4 mg, B_3 18 mg, B_6 25 mg, B_{12} 1,000 mcg, C 85 mg, I, Mg, Se, algal oil, soy lecithin. Glycerin, sorbitol. Cap. 90s. *Rx.*
Use: Prenatal vitamin with minerals.

•**nefazodone hydrochloride.** (neff-AZE-oh-dohn) USAN.
Use: Antidepressant.

nefazodone hydrochloride. (Various Mfr.) Nefazodone hydrochloride 50 mg, 100 mg, 150 mg, 200 mg, 250 mg. Tab. 60s, 100s (50 mg only). *Rx.*
Use: Antidepressant.

•**neflumozide hydrochloride.** (neh-FLEW-moe-ZIDE) USAN.
Use: Antipsychotic.

•**nefocon A.** (NEE-FOE-kahn A) USAN.
Use: Contact lens material, hydrophilic.

•**nefopam hydrochloride.** (NEFF-oh-pam) USAN.
Use: Muscle relaxant; analgesic.

Negacide. (Sanofi-Synthelabo) Nalidixic acid. *Rx.*
Use: Anti-infective, urinary.

•**nelarabine.** (neh-LAY-rah-bean) USAN.
Use: Antineoplastic; DNA demethylation agent.
See: Arranon.

•**nelezaprine maleate.** (neh-LEH-zah-PREEN) USAN.
Use: Muscle relaxant.

•**nelfilcon A.** (nell-FILL-kahn A) USAN.
Use: Contact lens material, hydrophilic.

•**nelfinavir mesylate.** (nell-FIN-ah-veer) USAN.
Use: Antiviral.
See: Viracept.

•**nelipepimut-S.** (NEL-i-PEP-i-mut) USAN.
Use: Cancer immunotherapy for prevention and delay of cancer recurrence.

•**nelotanserin.** (NEL-oh-tan-SER-in) USAN.
Use: CNS agent.

Nelulen. (Watson) **1/35 E:** Ethynodiol diacetate 1 mg, ethinyl estradiol 35 mcg. Tab. Pack 21s, 28s. **1/50 E:** Ethynodiol diacetate 1 mg, ethinyl estradiol 50 mcg. Tab. Pack 21s, 28s. *Rx.*
Use: Contraceptive.

•**nelzarabine.** (nell-ZARE-ah-bean) USAN.
Use: Antineoplastic.

nemazine. Under study.
Use: Anti-inflammatory.

•**nemazoline hydrochloride.** (neh-MAZZ-oh-leen) USAN.
Use: Decongestant, nasal.

Nembutal Sodium. (Ovation) Pentobarbital sodium 50 mg/mL. Alcohol 10%, propylene glycol. Inj. 2 mL amp; 20 mL and 50 mL vial. *c-II.*
Use: Hypnotic; sedative.

•**nemifitide ditriflutate.** (ne-MI-fi-tide dye-trye-FLOO-tate) USAN.
Use: Antidepressant.

Neoasma. (Tarmac Products) Theophylline 125 mg, guaifenesin 100 mg. Tab. UD 30s. *Rx.*
Use: Antiasthmatic combination.

Neo-Benz-All. (Xttrium) Benzalkonium Cl 20.1%. Packet 25 mL 15s. To make gal of 1:750 soln. Also Aqueous Neo-Benz-All 1:750 soln. Packet 20 mL, 50s. *OTC.*
Use: Antiseptic; antimicrobial.

NeoBenz Micro SD. (SkinMedica) Benzoyl peroxide 3.5%, 5.5%, 8.5%. Cetyl alcohol, stearyl alcohol, parabens. Cream. 0.5 g applicators. 30s. *Rx.*
Use: Topical anti-infective.

NeoBenz Micro Wash. (SkinMedical) Benzoyl peroxide 7%. Castor oil, edetate disodium, methylparaben, PEG-6, PEG-15, PEG-40. Top. Wash. 180 g. *Rx.*
Use: Anti-infective, topical; antibiotic agent.

Neo Beserol. (Sanofi-Synthelabo) Aspirin, methocarbamol. *Rx.*
Use: Analgesic; muscle relaxant.

Neocalamine. (Various Mfr.) Red ferric oxide 30 g, yellow ferric oxide 40 g, zinc oxide 930 g. *OTC.*
Use: Astringent; antiseptic.

Neocate One +. (Scientific Hospital Supplies, Inc.) Protein 2.5 g (amino acids 3 g), carbohydrates 14.6 g, fat 3.5 g, vitamins A, D, E, K, B_1, B_2, B_3, B_5, B_6, B_{12}, folic acid, biotin, C, choline, inositol, Ca, P, Mg, Fe, Zn, Mn, Cu, I, Mo, Cr, Se, Cl, Na 20 mg (0.9 mEq), K 93 mg (2.4 mEq) per 100 mL, 100 cal/mL. Liq. Bot. 237 mL. *OTC.*
Use: Nutritional supplement, enteral.

Neo-Cholex. (Lafayette) Fat emulsion containing 40% w/v pure vegetable oil. Bot. 60 mL. *Rx.*
Use: Cholecystokinetic.

Neocidin. (Major) Polymyxin B sulfate 10,000 units, neomycin sulfate 1.75 mg, gramicidin 0.025 mg/mL. Soln. Bot.

10 mL. *Rx.*
Use: Anti-infective, ophthalmic.

Neo-Cobefrin.
Use: Vasoconstrictor.

Neocurb. (Taylor Pharmaceuticals) Phendimetrazine tartrate 35 mg. Tab. Bot. 100s, 1000s. *c-III.*
Use: Anorexiant.

Neocylate. (Schwarz Pharma) Potassium salicylate 280 mg, aminobenzoic acid 250 mg. Tab. Bot. 100s, 1000s. *OTC.*
Use: Analgesic.

Neocyten. (Schwarz Pharma) Orphenadrine citrate 30 mg/mL. Vial 10 mL. *Rx.*
Use: Muscle relaxant.

Neo-Dexair. (Bausch & Lomb) Dexamethasone sodium phosphate 0.1%, neomycin sulfate 0.35%, polysorbate 80, EDTA, benzalkonium Cl 0.02%, sodium bisulfite 0.1%. Soln. Bot. 5 mL. *Rx.*
Use: Anti-infective; corticosteroid, ophthalmic.

Neo-Diaral. (Roberts) Loperamide 2 mg. Cap. Bot. UD 8s, 250s. *OTC.*
Use: Antidiarrheal.

Neo DM. (Laser) **Drops:** Dextromethorphan HBr 2.75 mg, chlorpheniramine maleate 0.75 mg, phenylephrine hydrochloride 1.75 mg per 1 mL. Alcohol and sugar free. Saccharin, sorbitol. Black cherry flavor. 30 mL with dropper. **Syrup:** Dextromethorphan HBr 30 mg, pseudoephedrine hydrochloride 50 mg, brompheniramine maleate 3 mg per 5 mL. Saccharin, sorbitol. Berry vanilla flavor. 30 mL, 470 mL. **Susp.:** Dextromethorphan tannate 30 mg, brompheniramine tannate 10 mg, phenylephrine tannate 25 mg per 5 mL. Alcohol and sugar free. Aspartame, parabens, phenylalanine 7 mg/5 mL. Cherry flavor. 473 mL. **Elix:** Brompheniramine maleate 3 mg, dextromethorphan hydrobromide 30 mg, pseudoephedrine hydrochloride 15 mg per 5 mL saccharin, sorbitol. Berry vanilla flavor. 473 mL. *Rx-OTC.*
Use: Upper respiratory combination, antitussive combination.

neodrenal.
See: Isoproterenol.

Neo-Durabolic. (Roberts) Nandrolone decanoate injection. **50 mg/mL, 100 mg/mL:** Vial 2 mL. **200 mg/mL:** Vial 1 mL. *c-III.*
Use: Anabolic steroid.

Neo-fradin. (Pharma-Tek) Neomycin sulfate 125 mg/5 mL, parabens. Oral Soln. Bot. 480 mL. *Rx.*
Use: Amebicide.

Neofrin. (Ocusoft) Phenylephrine hydrochloride 2.5% (benzalkonium chloride 0.01%, boric acid, EDTA, sodium borate, sodium bisulfite), 10% (benzalkonium chloride, sodium phosphate mono- and dibasic). Ophth. Soln. 15 mL. *Rx.*
Use: Ophthalmic decongestant.

Neogesic. (Pal-Pak, Inc.) Aspirin 194.4 mg, acetaminophen 129.6 mg, caffeine 32.4 mg. Tab. Bot. 1000s. *OTC.*
Use: Analgesic combination.

Neo HC. (Laser) Chlorpheniramine maleate 3 mg, hydrocodone bitartrate 5 mg, phenylephrine hydrochloride 7.5 mg. Glycerin, saccharin, sorbitol. Alcohol free and sugar free. Orange cream flavor. Syr. 473 mL. *c-III.*
Use: Upper respiratory combination, antitussive combination.

Neo-Mist Nasal Spray. (A.P.C.) Phenylephrine hydrochloride 0.5%, cetalkonium Cl 0.02%. Spray Bot. 20 mL. *OTC.*
Use: Antiseptic; decongestant.

Neo-Mist Pediatric 0.25% Nasal Spray. (A.P.C.) Phenylephrine hydrochloride 0.25%, cetalkonium Cl 0.02%. Squeeze Bot. 20 mL. *OTC.*
Use: Antiseptic; decongestant.

neomycin.
W/Bacitracin Zinc, Lidocaine, Polymyxin B Sulfate.
See: Lanabiotic.
W/Bacitracin Zinc, Polymyxin B Sulfate.
See: Neosporin Original.
Triple Antibiotic.
W/Bacitracin Zinc, Polymyxin B Sulfate, Pramoxine Hydrochloride.
See: Neosporin Plus Pain Relief.
Tri-Biozene.
W/Dexamethasone, Polymyxin B Sulfate.
See: Methadex.
Poly-Dex.
W/Polymyxin B Sulfate, Pramoxine Hydrochloride.
See: Neosporin Plus Pain Relief.

neomycin and polymyxin B sulfate. (Watson Pharma) Neomycin 40 mg, polymyxin B sulfate 200,000 units/mL. Soln., intravesical. Amp. 1 mL. *Rx.*
Use: Anti-infective.

•**neomycin and polymyxin B sulfates and bacitracin.** *USP.* Ointment; ophthalmic ointment.
Use: Anti-infective, antibiotic, topical.

•**neomycin and polymyxin B sulfates and bacitracin zinc.** *USP.* Ointment; ophthalmic ointment.
Use: Anti-infective, topical.

neomycin and polymyxin B sulfates and bacitracin zinc ophthalmic ointment. (Various Mfr.) Polymyxin B sul-

fate 10,000 units, neomycin 3.5 mg, bacitracin zinc 400 units/g, white petrolatum, mineral oil. Tube. 3.5 g. *Rx.*
Use: Anti-infective; corticosteroid, ophthalmic.

•**neomycin and polymyxin B sulfates and dexamethasone.** *USP.* Ophthalmic ointment; ophthalmic suspension.

neomycin and polymyxin B sulfates and dexamethasone ophthalmic ointment. (Various Mfr.) Dexamethasone 0.1%, neomycin sulfate 0.35%, polymyxin B sulfate 10,000 units. Tube 3.5 g.

neomycin and polymyxin B sulfates and dexamethasone ophthalmic suspension. (Various Mfr.) Dexamethasone 0.1%, neomycin sulfate 0.35%, polymyxin B sulfate 10,000 units/mL, benzalkonium chloride 0.004%, hydroxypropyl methylcellulose 0.5%, hydrochloric acid, sodium chloride, polysorbate 20, sodium hydroxide. 5 mL. *Rx.*

•**neomycin and polymyxin B sulfates and gramicidin.** *USP.* Cream; ophthalmic solution.
Use: Anti-infective, topical.

•**neomycin and polymyxin B sulfates and hydrocortisone.** *USP.* Otic solution; ophthalmic suspension; otic suspension.
Use: Anti-infective; corticosteroid, otic.

neomycin and polymyxin B sulfates and hydrocortisone. (Falcon) Hydrocortisone 1%, neomycin sulfate equiv. to 0.35% neomycin as base, polymyxin B sulfate 10,000 units/mL. Thimerosal 0.001%, cetyl alcohol, glyceryl monostearate, mineral oil, propylene glycol. Susp. 7.5 mL *Drop-Tainers. Rx.*
Use: Otic preparations.

•**neomycin and polymyxin B sulfates and hydrocortisone acetate cream.** *USP.*
Use: Anti-infective; corticosteroid, topical.

•**neomycin and polymyxin B sulfates and hydrocortisone acetate ophthalmic suspension.** *USP.*
Use: Anti-infective; corticosteroid, ophthalmic.

neomycin and polymyxin B sulfates and hydrocortisone acetate ophthalmic suspension. (Various Mfr.) Hydrocortisone 1%, neomycin sulfate 0.35%, polymyxin B sulfate 10,000 units. Bot. 7.5 mL, 10 mL.
Use: Anti-infective; corticosteroid, ophthalmic.

neomycin and polymyxin B sulfates and hydrocortisone otic suspension. (Steris) Polymyxin B sulfate equiv. to 10,000 polymyxin B units, neomycin sulfate equiv. to 3.5 mg neomycin base/mL. Hydrocortisone 1%, thimerosal 0.01%, cetyl alcohol, propylene glycol, polysorbate 80. Susp. 10 mL.

•**neomycin and polymyxin B sulfates and pramoxine hydrochloride cream.** *USP.*
Use: Anti-infective, topical anesthetic.

•**neomycin and polymyxin B sulfates and prednisolone acetate ophthalmic suspension.** *USP.*
Use: Anti-infective; corticosteroid, ophthalmic.

•**neomycin and polymyxin B sulfates, bacitracin, and hydrocortisone acetate.** *USP.* Ointment; ophthalmic ointment.
Use: Anti-infective; corticosteroid, topical.

•**neomycin and polymyxin B sulfates, bacitracin, and lidocaine ointment.** *USP.*
Use: Anti-infective; anesthetic, topical.

•**neomycin and polymyxin B sulfates, bacitracin zinc, and hydrocortisone.** *USP.* Ointment; ophthalmic ointment.
Use: Anti-infective; corticosteroid.

•**neomycin and polymyxin B sulfates, bacitracin zinc, and hydrocortisone acetate ophthalmic ointment.** *USP.*
Use: Anti-infective; antifungal; anti-inflammatory, topical.

•**neomycin and polymyxin B sulfates, bacitracin zinc, and lidocaine ointment.** *USP.*
Use: Anti-infective, anesthetic.

•**neomycin and polymyxin B sulfates, gramicidin, and hydrocortisone acetate cream.** *USP.*
Use: Anti-infective; corticosteroid.

neomycin and polymyxin B sulfates solution for irrigation.
Use: Irrigant, ophthalmic; anti-infective, topical.
See: Neosporin G.U. Irrigant.

neomycin base.
Use: Anti-infective.
W/Combinations.
See: Maxitrol.
Neosporin Plus.
Neotal.

•**neomycin boluses.** *USP.*
Use: Anti-infective.

•**neomycin palmitate.** (NEE-oh-MY-sin PAL-mih-tate) USAN.
Use: Anti-infective.

neomycin/polymyxin B sulfates/hydrocortisone otic. (Various Mfr.) Hydrocortisone 1%, neomycin 3.5 mg, polymyxin B sulfate 10,000 units. Cetyl alcohol, glyceryl monostearate, mineral oil, polyoxyl 40 stearate, propylene glycol, thimerosal 0.001%. Ophth. Susp. *Drop-Tainer.* 7.5 mL *Rx.*
Use: Steroid antibiotic combination.

•**neomycin sulfate.** (NEE-oh-MY-sin) *USP.* Cream; Ointment; Ophthalmic Ointment, Oral Solution; Tablets.
Use: Anti-infective.
See: Mycifradin.
Neo-fradin.
Neo-Tabs.
W/Bacitracin Zinc, Hydrocortisone Acetate, Polymyxin B Sulfate.
See: Coracin.
W/Bacitracin Zinc, Polymyxin B Sulfate.
See: Mycitracin.
Neosporin Maximum Strength.
Neotal.
Neo-Thrycex.
Ocutricin.
Tigo.
Trimixin.
Triple Antibiotic.
W/Colistin Sulfate, Hydrocortisone Acetate, Thonzonium.
See: Coly-Mycin S Otic.
Cortisporin-TC.
W/Dexamethasone, Polymyxin B Sulfate.
See: Maxitrol.
W/Hydrocortisone Acetate, Polymyxin B Sulfate.
See: Cortisporin.
W/Polymyxin B Sulfate.
See: Neosporin G.U. Irrigant.

neomycin sulfate. (Pharmacia) Neomycin sulfate. Pow. micronized for compounding. Bot. 100 g.
Use: Anti-infective.

•**neomycin sulfate and bacitracin ointment.** *USP.*
Use: Anti-infective, topical.

•**neomycin sulfate and bacitracin zinc ointment.** *USP.*
Use: Anti-infective, topical.

•**neomycin sulfate and dexamethasone sodium phosphate cream.** *USP.*
Use: Anti-infective; corticosteroid, topical.

•**neomycin sulfate and dexamethasone sodium phosphate ophthalmic ointment.** *USP.*
Use: Anti-infective; corticosteroid, ophthalmic.

•**neomycin sulfate and dexamethasone sodium phosphate ophthalmic solution.** *USP.* (Various Mfr.) Dexamethasone sodium phosphate 0.1%, neomycin sulfate 0.35%. Bot. 5 mL.
Use: Anti-infective; corticosteroid, ophthalmic.

•**neomycin sulfate and fluocinolone acetonide cream.** *USP.*
Use: Anti-infective; corticosteroid, topical.

•**neomycin sulfate and fluorometholone ointment.** *USP.*
Use: Anti-infective; corticosteroid, topical.

•**neomycin sulfate and flurandrenolide.** *USP.* Cream; Lotion; Ointment.
Use: Anti-infective; corticosteroid, topical.

•**neomycin sulfate and gramicidin ointment.** *USP.*
Use: Anti-infective, topical.

•**neomycin sulfate and hydrocortisone.** *USP.* Cream; Ointment; Otic Suspension, USP.
Use: Anti-infective; corticosteroid, topical.

•**neomycin sulfate and hydrocortisone acetate.** *USP.* Cream; Lotion; Ointment; Ophthalmic Ointment; Ophthalmic Suspension.
Use: Anti-infective; corticosteroid.

•**neomycin sulfate and methylprednisolone acetate cream.** *USP.*
Use: Anti-infective; corticosteroid, topical.

•**neomycin sulfate and prednisolone acetate ointment.** *USP.*
Use: Anti-infective; corticosteroid, topical.

•**neomycin sulfate and prednisolone acetate ophthalmic ointment.** *USP.*
Use: Anti-infective; corticosteroid, topical.

•**neomycin sulfate and prednisolone acetate ophthalmic suspension.** *USP.*
Use: Anti-infective; corticosteroid, topical.

•**neomycin sulfate and prednisolone sodium phosphate ophthalmic ointment.** *USP.*
Use: Anti-infective; corticosteroid, topical.

•**neomycin sulfate and triamcinolone acetonide cream.** *USP.*
Use: Anti-infective; corticosteroid, topical.

•**neomycin sulfate and triamcinolone acetonide ophthalmic ointment.** *USP.*

Use: Anti-infective; corticosteroid, ophthalmic.

neomycin sulfate, polymyxin B sulfate, and gramicidin solution. (Various Mfr.) Polymyxin B sulfate 10,000 units/mL, neomycin sulfate 1.75 mg/mL, gramicidin 0.025 mg/mL, sodium chloride, alcohol 0.5%, propylene glycol, hydrochloric acid, thimerosal 0.001%, poloxamer 188, ammonium hydroxide. Bot. 10 mL. *Rx.*
Use: Anti-infective, ophthalmic.

neomycin sulfate, polymyxin B sulfate, and lidocaine.
Use: Anti-infective; anesthetic, local.

•**neomycin sulfate, sulfacetamide sodium, and prednisolone acetate ophthalmic ointment.** *USP.*
Use: Anti-infective; corticosteroid, topical.

•**neomycin undecylenate.** (NEE-oh-MY-sin UHN-de-sih-LEN-ate) USAN.
Use: Anti-infective; antifungal.

Neopham 6.4%. (Pharmacia) Essential and nonessential amino acids 6.4%. Inj. 250 mL, 500 mL. *Rx.*
Use: Nutritional supplement, parenteral.

Neo Picatyl. (Sanofi-Synthelabo) Glycobiarsoln. *Rx.*
Use: Amebicide.

NeoProfen. (Recordati Rare Diseases) Ibuprofen lysine 17.1 mg (equiv. to ibuprofen 10 mg/mL [±]). Preservative free. Soln. for Inj. Single-use vials. *Rx.*
Use: Agent for patent ductus arteriosus.

Neo Quipenyl. (Sanofi-Synthelabo) Primaquine phosphate. *Rx.*
Use: Antimalarial.

Neoral. (Novartis) Cyclosporine. **Soft Gelatin Cap.:** 25 mg, 100 mg, dehydrated alcohol 11.9%. UD 30s. **Oral Soln.:** 100 mg/mL, dehydrated alcohol 11.9%. Bot. 50 mL. *Rx.*
Use: Immunosuppressant.

Neosalus. (Quinnova) **Aer., Foam.:** Dimethicone, glycerin, parabens. 70 g, 200 g. **Cream:** Dimethicone, glycerin, parabens, trolamine. 60 g, 100 g. *Rx.*
Use: Emollient.

neo-skiodan. Iodopyracet, Diodrast.

Neosporin AF. (Johnson & Johnson) Miconazole nitrate 2%. Mineral oil. Cream. 14 g. *OTC.*
Use: Anti-infective, topical; antifungal agent.

Neosporin G.U. Irrigant. (Monarch) Neomycin sulfate 40 mg, polymyxin B sulfate 200,000 units/mL. Amp. 1 mL. Box 10s, 50s, Multiple-dose vial 20 mL. *Rx.*
Use: Irrigant, genitourinary.

Neosporin Maximum Strength. (Johnson & Johnson) Polymyxin B sulfate 10,000 units, neomycin 3.5 mg, bacitracin 500 units/g, white petrolatum. Oint. Tube 15 g. *OTC.*
Use: Anti-infective, topical.

Neosporin Ophthalmic Solution. (Monarch) Polymyxin B sulfate 10,000 units, neomycin 1.75 mg, gramicidin 0.025 mg/mL, alcohol 0.5%, thimerosal 0.001%, propylene glycol, sodium chloride. Bot. 10 mL. *Drop-dose. Rx.*
Use: Anti-infective, ophthalmic.

Neosporin Original. (Johnson & Johnson) Polymyxin B sulfate 5000 units, neomycin 3.5 mg, bacitracin zinc 400 units per g. Cocoa butter, cottonseed oil, olive oil, white petrolatum. Oint. Tubes. 14 g, 28 g, UD 0.9 g (10s). *OTC.*
Use: Anti-infective, antibiotic, topical.

Neosporin Plus Pain Relief. (Johnson & Johnson) **Oint.:** Polymyxin B sulfate 10,000 units, neomycin 3.5 mg, bacitracin zinc 500 units, pramoxine hydrochloride 10 mg per g. White petrolatum. Tubes. 15 g, 30 g. **Cream:** Polymyxin B sulfate 10,000 units, neomycin 3.5 mg, pramoxine hydrochloride 10 mg per g. Methylparaben, mineral oil, white petrolatum. Tubes. 15 g. *OTC.*
Use: Anti-infective, antibiotic, topical.

neostibosan. Ethylstibamine.

neostigmine.
Use: Cholinergic.
See: Neostigmine Bromide.
Neostigmine Methylsulfate.

neostigmine and atropine sulfate.
Use: Muscle stimulant.
See: Neostigmine Min-I-Mix.

•**neostigmine bromide.** (nee-oh-STIGG-meen) *USP.*
Use: Cholinergic.
See: Prostigmin Bromide.

neostigmine bromide. (Lannett) Neostigmine bromide. 15 mg. Tab. 100s and 1000s.
Use: Cholinergic.

•**neostigmine methylsulfate.** (nee-oh-STIGG-meen METH-ill-SULL-fate) *USP.*
Use: Cholinergic.
See: Bloxiverz.
Prostigmin.

neostigmine methylsulfate. (Various Mfr.) Neostigmine methylsulfate 1:2000 (0.5 mg/mL), 1:1000 (1 mg/mL). Inj. Vials. 1 mL, 2 mL, 10 mL (1:2000 only). Multidose vials. 10 mL. *Rx.*
Use: Cholinergic; urinary cholinergic.

Neostigmine Min-I-Mix. (I.M.S., Ltd.) Atropine sulfate 1.2 mg, neostigmine

methylsulfate 2.5 mg. Inj. Vial. *Rx.*
Use: Cholinergic muscle stimulant.

Neo-Strepsan.
See: Sulfathiazole.

Neo-Synephrine. (Hospira) Phenylephrine hydrochloride 1% (10 mg/mL). Sodium bisulfite. Inj. Uni-Nest amps. 1 mL. *Rx.*
Use: Mydriatic; vasopressor.

Neo-Synephrine Extra Strength. (Bayer Consumer Care) Phenylephrine hydrochloride 1%, benzalkonium chloride. Drop. bot., Spray bot. 15 mL. *Formerly Neo-Synephrine 4-Hour Extra Strength. OTC.*
Use: Nasal decongestant, arylalkylamine.

Neo-Synephrine Mild Strength. (Bayer Consumer Care) Phenylephrine hydrochloride 0.25%, benzalkonium chloride. Soln. Spray bot. 15 mL. *Formerly Neo-Synephrine 4-Hour Mild Formula. OTC.*
Use: Nasal decongestant, arylalkylamine.

Neo-Synephrine Regular Strength. (Bayer Consumer Care) Phenylephrine hydrochloride 0.5%, benzalkonium chloride. Soln. Spray bot., Drop. bot. 15 mL. *Formerly Neo-Synephrine 4-Hour Regular Formula. OTC.*
Use: Nasal decongestant, arylalkylamine.

Neo-Synephrine Hydrochloride. (Sanofi-Synthelabo) Phenylephrine hydrochloride. **Spray:** 0.25% children and adult, 0.5% adult. **Regular:** Squeeze bot. 0.5 oz. **0.5% mentholated:** Squeeze bot. 0.5 oz. **Drops:** 0.125% infant; 0.25% children and adult; 0.5% adult; 1% adult extra strength. Bot. 1 oz; 0.25% and 1%, also bot. 16 oz. **Jelly:** 0.5%. Tube. 18.75 g. *OTC.*
Use: Decongestant.

Neo-Synephrine 12-Hour Extra Moisturizing. (Bayer Consumer Care) Oxymetazoline hydrochloride 0.05%, benzalkonium chloride, edetate sodium, sodium chloride. Soln. Spray Bot. 15 mL. *OTC.*
Use: Nasal decongestant, imidazoline.

Neo-Tabs. (Pharma-Tek) Neomycin sulfate 500 mg (equivalent to 350 mg neomycin base). Tab. Bot. 100s. *Rx.*
Use: Amebicide.

Neotal. (Roberts) Zinc bacitracin 400 units, polymyxin B sulfate 5000 units, neomycin sulfate 5 mg, petrolatum and mineral oil base/g. Tube 3.5 g. *Rx.*
Use: Anti-infective, ophthalmic.

Neo-Thrycex. (Del) Bacitracin, neomycin sulfate, polymyxin B sulfate. Oint. Tube 0.5 oz. *Rx.*
Use: Anti-infective, topical.

Neotricin Ophthalmic Ointment. (Bausch & Lomb) Polymyxin B sulfate 10,000 units, neomycin sulfate 3.5 mg, bacitracin 400 units/g. In 3.5 g. *Rx.*
Use: Anti-infective, ophthalmic.

Neotricin Ophthalmic Solution. (Bausch & Lomb) Polymyxin B sulfate 10,000 units, neomycin sulfate 1.75 mg, gramicidin 0.025 mg/mL. Dropper bot. 10 mL. *Rx.*
Use: Anti-infective, ophthalmic.

Neo-Trobex Injection. (Forest) Vitamins B_1 150 mg, B_6 10 mg, riboflavin 5-phosphate sodium 2 mg, niacinamide 150 mg, panthenol 10 mg, choline Cl 20 mg, inositol 20 mg/mL. Vial 30 mL. *Rx.*
Use: Vitamin supplement.

Neotrol. (Horizon) Phenylephrine hydrochloride 0.25%, pyrilamine maleate 0.2%, cetalkonium Cl 0.05%, tyrothricin 0.03%, phenylmercuric acetate 1:50,000. Soln. Squeeze Bot. 20 mL. *OTC.*
Use: Antihistamine; decongestant.

NeoTuss. (A.G. Marin Pharmaceuticals) Dextromethorphan hydrobromide 30 mg, guaifenesin 200 mg. Glycerin, menthol, parabens, propylene glycol, sorbitol, sucralose. Alcohol free, dye free, and sugar free. Grape menthol flavor. Liq. 473 mL. *OTC.*
Use: Upper respiratory combination, antitussive with expectorant.

NeoTuss-D. (A.G. Marin Pharmaceuticals) Dextromethorphan hydrobromide 30 mg, guaifenesin 200 mg, phenylephrine hydrochloride 7.5 mg. Glycerin, parabens, propylene glycol, sucralose. Alcohol free, dye free, and sugar free. Raspberry flavor. Liq. 474 mL. *Rx.*
Use: Upper respiratory combination, antitussive and expectorant combination.

Neoval. (Halsey Drug) Vitamins A 10,000 units, D 400 units, B_1 10 mg, B_2 5 mg, B_6 2 mg, B_{12} 3 mcg, C 100 mg, E 5 mg, pantothenic acid 10 mg, niacinamide 30 mg, Fe 15 mg, Cu 1 mg, Mg 5 mg, Mn 1 mg, Zn 1.5 mg, I 0.15 mg. Tab. Bot. 100s. *OTC.*
Use: Mineral, vitamin supplement.

Neoval T. (Halsey Drug) Vitamins A 10,000 units, D 400 units, B_1 15 mg, B_2 10 mg, B_6 2 mg, C 150 mg, B_{12} 7.5 mcg, E 5 mg, pantothenic acid 10 mg, E 5 mg, niacinamide 100 mg,

Fe 15 mg, Mg 5 mg, Mn 1 mg, Zn 1.5 mg, Cu 1 mg. Tab. Bot. 1000s. *OTC.*
Use: Mineral, vitamin supplement.

•**nepafenac.** (neh-pah-FEN-ack) USAN.
Use: Ophthalmic nonsteroidal anti-inflammatory agent.
See: Ilevro.
Nevanac.

nepafenac. (Alcon) Nepafenac 0.3%. Benzalkonium chloride 0.005%, boric acid, carboxymethylcellulose, edetate disodium, propylene glycol, sodium chloride, sodium hydroxide and/or hydrochloric acid. Susp.; Ophth. 1.7 mL dropper bottle. *Rx.*
Use: Ophthalmic nonsteroidal anti-inflammatory drug.

NephPlex Rx. (Nephro-Tech) B_1 1.5 mg, B_2 1.7 mg, B_3 20 mg, B_5 10 mg, B_6 10 mg, B_{12} 6 mcg, C 60 mg, folic acid 1 mg, biotin 300 mcg, Zn 12.5 mg. Tab. Bot. 100s. *Rx.*
Use: Mineral, vitamin supplement.

5.4% NephrAmine. (McGaw) Amino acid concentration 5.4%, nitrogen 0.65 g/100 mL. **Essential amino acids:** Isoleucine 560 mg, leucine 880 mg, lysine 640 mg, methionine 880 mg, phenylalanine 880 mg, threonine 400 mg, tryptophan 200 mg, valine 640 mg, histidine 250 mg/100 mL. **Nonessential amino acids:** Cysteine < 20 mg/100 mL, sodium 5 mEq, acetate 44 mEq, chloride 3 mEq/L, sodium bisulfite. Inj. 250 mL. *Rx.*
Use: Nutritional supplement, parenteral.

nephridine.
See: Epinephrine.

Nephro-Calci. (Watson) Calcium carbonate 1500 mg (elemental calcium 600 mg). Tab. Bot. 100s. *OTC.*
Use: Mineral supplement, calcium.

Nephrocaps. (Fleming) Vitamins B_1 1.5 mg, B_2 1.7 mg, B_3 20 mg, B_5 5 mg, B_6 10 mg, B_{12} 6 mcg, C 100 mg, folate 1 mg, biotin 150 mcg. Glycerin, lecithin, soybean oil, wax. Cap., softgel. 30s, 90s. *Rx.*
Use: Multivitamin.

Nephrocaps QT. (Fleming) Vitamins D 1,750 units, B_1 1.5 mg, B_2 1.7 mg, B_3 20 mg, B_5 5 mg, B_6 10 mg, B_{12} 6 mcg, C 100 mg, folic acid 1 mg, biotin. Mannitol, sucralose. Fruit punch flavor. Tab., quick-dissolve. 30s, 90s. *Rx.*
Use: Multivitamin.

Nephronex. (Llorens) Biotin 300 mcg, folic acid 0.9 mg, vitamins B_1 1.5 mg, B_2 1.7 mg, B_3 20 mg, B_5 10 mg, B_6 10 mg, B_{12} 10 mcg, C 60 mg per 5 mL. Aspartame, parabens, phenylalanine. Alcohol free, dye free, and sugar free. Liq. 236.5 mL. *OTC.*
Use: Nutritional supplement, multivitamin.

Nephron FA. (Nephro-Tech) Fe 66.6 mg, C 40 mg, B_1 1.5 mg, B_2 1.7 mg, B_3 20 mg, B_5 10 mg, B_6 10 mg, B_{12} 6 mcg, biotin 300 mcg, FA 1 mg, docusate sodium 75 mg. Tab. Bot. 100s. *Rx.*
Use: Mineral, vitamin supplement.

Nephro-Vite Rx. (R & D Laboratories, Inc.) Vitamins B_1 1.5 mg, B_2 1.7 mg, B_3 20 mg, B_5 10 mg, B_6 10 mg, B_{12} 6 mcg, C 60 mg, folic acid 1 mg, d-biotin 300 mcg. Tab. Bot. 100s. *Rx.*
Use: Mineral, vitamin supplement.

Nephro-Vite Vitamin B Complex & C Supplement. (R & D Laboratories, Inc.) Vitamins B_1 1.5 mg, B_2 1.7 mg, B_3 20 mg, B_5 10 mg, B_6 10 mg, B_{12} 6 mcg, C 60 mg, folic acid 800 mcg, biotin 300 mcg. Tab. Bot. 100s. *OTC.*
Use: Mineral, vitamin supplement.

Nephrox. (Fleming & Co.) Aluminum hydroxide 320 mg, mineral oil 10%/5 mL. Bot. Pt. *OTC.*
Use: Antacid.

Nepro. (Ross) Protein 6.6 g (as Ca, Mg, and Na caseinates), fat 22.7 g (as 90% high-oleic safflower oil, 10% soy oil), carbohydrate 51.1 g (as sucrose, hydrolyzed corn starch), vitamins A, D, E, K, C, B_1, B_2, B_5, B_6, B_{12}, biotin, FA, Na, K, Cl, Ca, P, Mg, I, Mn, Cu, Zn, Fe, Se/240 mL. 59.4 calories. Liq. Can. 240 mL. *OTC.*
Use: Nutritional supplement, enteral.

•**neramexane mesylate.** (ner-a-MEX-ane) USAN.
Use: Depression; Alzheimer disease; pain.

neraval.
Use: Anesthetic, general.

•**nerelimomab.** (neh-reh-LI-moe-mab) USAN.
Use: Monoclonal antibody.

Nervine Nighttime Sleep-Aid. (Bayer Consumer Care) Diphenhydramine hydrochloride 25 mg. Tab. Bot. 12s, 30s, 50s. *OTC.*
Use: Sleep aid.

Nesacaine. (AAP Pharmaceuticals) Chloroprocaine hydrochloride 1% (10 mg/mL), 2% (20 mg/mL). Methylparaben, EDTA. Inj. Multidose vial. 30 mL. *Rx.*
Use: Anesthetic, local injectable.

Nesacaine-MPF. (AAP Pharmaceuticals) Chloroprocaine hydrochloride 2% (20 mg/mL), 3% (30 mg/mL). Preservative free. Inj. Single-dose vials. 20 mL.

Rx.
Use: Anesthetic, local injectable.
Nesa Nine Cap. (Standex) Vitamins A 5000 units, D 400 units, C 37.5 mg, B_1 1.5 mg, B_2 2 mg, niacinamide 20 mg, B_6 0.1 mg, calcium pantothenate 1 mg, E 2 units. Cap. Bot. 100s. *OTC.*
Use: Mineral, vitamin supplement.
nesdonal sodium.
See: Pentothal.
Thiopental Sodium.
Nesina. (Takeda) Alogliptin 6.25 mg (equiv. to alogliptin benzoate 8.5 mg), 12.5 mg (equiv. to alogliptin benzoate 17 mg), 25 mg (equiv. to alogliptin benzoate 34 mg). Film coated. Mannitol. Tab. 30s, 90s, 500s (except 6.25 mg). *Rx.*
Use: Antidiabetic agent, dipeptidyl peptidase-4 inhibitor.
•**nesiritide.** (ni-SIR-i-tide) USAN.
Use: Vasodilator, human B-type natriuretic peptide.
See: Natrecor.
•**nesiritide citrate.** (ni-SIR-i-tide) USAN.
Use: Treatment of congestive heart failure.
•**nesofilcon A.** (nes-oh-FIL-kon) USAN.
Use: Contact lens material.
Nestabs. (Women's Choice Pharmaceuticals) Folic acid 1 mg, Ca 220 mg, Fe 32 mg, vitamins D 450 units, E 30 units, B_1 3 mg, B_2 3 mg, B_3 20 mg, B_6 50 mg, B_{12} 10 mcg, C 120 mg, I, Zn, choline 55 mg. PEG, saccharin. Film coated. Tab. 90s. *Rx.*
Use: Prenatal vitamin with minerals.
Nestabs ABC Tablets and Softgel Capsules. (Women's Choice Pharmaceuticals) Folic acid 1 mg, calcium 200 mg, iron 32 mg, vitamins D 450 units, E 30 units, B_1 3 mg, B_2 3 mg, B_3 20 mg, B_6 50 mg, B_{12} 10 mcg, C 120 mg, I, Zn, choline 55 mg. **Tab.:** Film coated. Maltodextrin. UD 30s. **Cap., softgel:** EPA 180 mg, DHA 120 mg. Glycerin. UD 30s. *Rx.*
Use: Prenatal vitamin with minerals.
Nestabs CBF. (Fielding) Vitamins A 4000 units, D 400 units, E 30 units, C 120 mg, folic acid 1 mg, B_1 3 mg, B_2 3 mg, niacinamide 20 mg, B_6 3 mg, B_{12} 8 mcg, Ca 200 mg, I, Zn 15 mg, Fe 50 mg. Tab. Bot. 100s. *Rx.*
Use: Mineral, vitamin supplement.
Nestabs DHA Tablets and Capsules. (Women's Choice Pharmaceuticals) Folic acid 1 mg, Ca 200 mg, Fe 32 mg, vitamins D 450 units, E 30 units, B_1 3 mg, B_2 3 mg, B_3 20 mg, B_6 50 mg, B_{12} 10 mcg, C 120 mg, I, Zn, choline 55 mg. **Tab.:** Film coated. PEG, saccharin. UD 30s. **Cap., softgel:** DHA 230 mg, EPA 30 mg, vitamin E 2 units, glycerin. UD 30s. *Rx.*
Use: Prenatal vitamin with minerals.
Nestabs FA. (Fielding) Vitamins A 4000 units, D 400 units, E 30 units, C 120 mg, B_1 3 mg, B_2 3 mg, B_3 20 mg, B_6 3 mg, B_{12} 8 mcg, Ca 200 mg, Fe 29 mg, folic acid 1 mg, Zn 15 mg, I. Tab. Bot. 100s. *Rx.*
Use: Mineral, vitamin supplement.
Nestle VHC 2.25. (Nestle Clinical Nutrition) Protein 90 g, carbohydrate 196 g, fat 120 g, vitamins A, B_1, B_2, B_3, B_5, B_6, B_{12}, C, D, E, K, folic acid, biotin, chloride, choline, Ca, Cr, Cu, Fe, I, Mg, Mn, Mo, P, Se, Zn, Na 1200 mg, K 1732 mg/L. Liq. Can. 250 mL. *OTC.*
Use: Enteral nutrition.
•**nesvacumab.** (nes-VAK-ue-mab) USAN.
Use: Antineoplastic.
•**netilmicin sulfate.** (ne-til-MYE-sin) USAN.
•**netoglitazone.** (net-oh-GLIT-a-zone) USAN.
Use: Antidiabetic.
•**netrafilcon A.** (NET-rah-FILL-kahn A) USAN.
Use: Contact lens material, hydrophilic.
netrin. Under Study.
Use: Anticholinergic.
See: Metacaraphen Hydrochloride.
•**netupitant.** (net-UE-pi-tant) USAN.
Use: Antiemetic.
Neulasta. (Amgen) Pegfilgrastim 10 mg/mL, preservative free. Soln. for Inj. Dispensing pack containing single-dose syr. w/needle. *Rx.*
Use: Hematopoietic, colony stimulating factor.
Neumega. (Wyeth) Oprelvekin 5 mg. Dibasic sodium phosphate heptahydrate 1.6 mg, monobasic sodium phosphate monohydrate 0.55 mg. Preservative free. Pow. for Inj. Soln., lyophilized. Single-dose vial with diluent. *Rx.*
Use: Hematopoietic, interleukin.
Neupogen. (Amgen) Filgrastim (G-CSF). Inj. Polysorbate 80. Preservative free. **300 mcg/0.5 mL:** Prefilled syringe. 0.5 mL. **300 mcg/mL:** Single-dose vial. 1 mL. **480 mcg/0.8 mL:** Single-use prefilled syringe. 0.8 mL. **480 mcg/1.6 mL:** Single-use vial. 1.6 mL. *Rx.*
Use: Immunomodulator.
Neupro. (UCB Inc) Rotigotine 1 mg/24 hours (2.25 mg per 5 cm^2), 2 mg/24 hours (4.5 mg per 10 cm^2), 3 mg/

24 hours (6.75 mg per 15 cm^2), 4 mg/ 24 hours (9 mg per 20 cm^2), 6 mg/ 24 hours (13.5 mg per 30 cm^2), 8 mg/ 24 hours (18 mg per 40 cm^2). Patch; transdermal. Carton. 30s. *Rx.*
Use: Dopaminergic; dopamine receptor agonist, nonergot.

NeuRecover-DA. (NeuroGenesis) DL-phenylalanine 460 mg, L-glutamine 25 mg, vitamin A 333.3 units, B_1 1.65 mg, B_2 0.85 mg, B_3 33 mg, B_5 15 mg, B_6 3 mg, B_{12} 5 mcg, FA 0.065 mg, C 100 mg, E 5 units, biotin 0.05 mg, Ca 25 mg, Cr 0.01 mg, Fe 1.5 mg, Mg 25 mg, Zn 2.5 mg. Cap. Bot. 180s. *OTC.*
Use: Amino acid.

NeuRecover-SA. (NeuroGenesis) DL-phenylalanine 250 mg, L-tyrosine 150 mg, L-glutamine 50 mg, vitamins B_1 1.65 mg, B_2 2.5 mg, B_3 16.6 mg, B_5 15 mg, B_6 3.36 mg, B_{12} 5 mcg, FA 0.067 mg, C 100 mg, Ca 25 mg, Fe 1.5 mg, Mg 25 mg, Zn 5 mg. Cap. Bot. 180s. *OTC.*
Use: Amino acid.

Neurodep Injection. (Medical Products Panamericana) Vitamins B_1 50 mg, B_2 5 mg, B_3 125 mg, B_5 6 mg, B_6 5 mg, B_{12} 1000 mcg, C 50 mg/mL. Inj. Vial 10 mL. *Rx.*
Use: Vitamin supplement, parenteral.

neuromuscular blockers, nondepolarizing.
Use: Muscle relaxants; adjuncts to anesthesia.
See: Cisatracurium Besylate.
Mivacurium Chloride.
Pancuronium Bromide.
Rocuronium Bromide.

Neurontin. (Pfizer) Gabapentin. **Cap.:** 100 mg, 300 mg, 400 mg, lactose, talc. Bot. 100s, UD 50s. **Tab.:** 600 mg, 800 mg, talc. Bot. 100s, 500s, UD 50s. **Oral Soln.:** 250 mg/5 mL, xylitol, cool strawberry anise flavor. Bot. 480 mL. *Rx.*
Use: Anticonvulsant.

neurosin.
See: Calcium Glycerophosphate.

NeuroSlim. (NeuroGenesis) DL-phenylalanine 500 mg, L-glutamine 15 mg, L-tyrosine 25 mg, L-carnitine 10 mg, L-arginine pyroglutamate 10 mg, ornithine aspartate 10 mg, Cr 0.033 mg, Se 0.012 mg, vitamins B_1 0.33 mg, B_2 0.5 mg, B_3 3.3 mg, B_5 0.012 mg, B_6 0.333 mg, B_{12} 1 mcg, E 5 units, biotin 0.05 mg, FA 0.066 mg, Fe 1 mg, Zn 2.5 mg, Ca 35 mg, I 0.025 mg, Cu 0.33 mg, Mg 25 mg. Cap. Bot. 180s. *OTC.*
Use: Amino acid.

neurotrophin-1.
Use: Motor neuron disease/amyotrophic lateral sclerosis. [Orphan Drug]

Neut. (Abbott) Sodium bicarbonate 4%. Vial (2.4 mEq each of sodium and bicarbonate), disodium edetate anhydrous 0.05% as stabilizer. Pintop Vial 5 mL, 10 mL. Box 25s, 100s. *Rx.*
Use: Nutritional supplement, parenteral.

NeutraGuard Advanced. (Pascal) Fluoride sodium 1.1%, wintermint flavor. Dental Gel. 60 g. *Rx.*
Use: Prevention of dental caries.

Neutrahist. (Cypress Pharmaceuticals) Chlorpheniramine maleate 0.8 mg, pseudoephedrine hydrochloride 9 mg per 5 mL. Saccharin, sorbitol. Cherry flavor. Drops. 30 mL w/dropper. *Rx.*
Use: Upper respiratory combination, decongestant and antihistamine.

Neutrahist PDX. (Cypress) Dextromethorphan hydrobromide 3 mg, chlorpheniramine maleate 0.8 mg, pseudoephedrine hydrochloride 9 mg. Glycerin, propylene glycol, saccharin, sorbitol. Alcohol free and sugar free. Grape flavor. Drops. 30 mL w/dropper. *OTC.*
Use: Upper respiratory combination, antitussive combination.

neutral acriflavine.
See: Acriflavine.

Neutralin. (Dover Pharmaceuticals) Calcium carbonate, magnesium oxide. Tab. Sugar, lactose, and salt free. UD Box 500s. *OTC.*
Use: Antacid.

neutral protamine hagedorn-insulin.
See: Insulin.
N.P.H. Iletin II.

•**neutramycin.** (NEW-trah-MY-sin) USAN. A neutral macrolide antibiotic produced by a variant strain of *Streptomyces rimosus.*
Use: Anti-infective.

NeutrapHor Skin Protectant. (pH R&D) Dimethicone 1%, mineral oil, white petrolatum, lanolin alcohol, phenoxyethanol. Cream. 57 g, 10 mL packet. *OTC.*
Use: Miscellaneous skin protectant.

NeutraSal. (Invado Pharmaceuticals) Calcium chloride 50 mg, dibasic sodium phosphate 10 mg, monobasic sodium phosphate 10 mg, silicon dioxide 2 mg, sodium chloride 450 mg, sodium bicarbonate 16 mg. Pow. 30s, 120s. *OTC.*
Use: Saliva substitute.

neutroflavin.
See: Acriflavine.

Neutrogena Antiseptic Cleanser for Acne-Prone Skin. (Neutrogena)

Benzethonium Cl, butylene glycol, methylparaben, menthol, peppermint oil, eucalyptus, mint, rosemary oils, witch hazel extract, camphor. Liq. Bot. 135 mL. *OTC.*
Use: Dermatologic, acne.

Neutrogena Body Lotion. (Neutrogena) Glyceryl stearate, isopropyl myristate, PEG-100 stearate, butylene glycol, imidazolidinyl urea, carbomer 934, parabens, sodium lauryl sulfate, triethanolamine, cetyl alcohol. Lot. Bot. 240 mL. *OTC.*
Use: Emollient.

Neutrogena Body Oil. (Neutrogena) Isopropyl myristate, sesame oil, PEG-40 sorbitan peroleate, parabens. Bot. 240 mL. *OTC.*
Use: Emollient.

Neutrogena Chemical-Free Sunblocker. (Neutrogena) Titanium dioxide, parabens, diazolidinyl urea, shea butter. SPF 17. Lot. Bot. 120 mL. *OTC.*
Use: Sunscreen.

Neutrogena Cleansing for Acne-Prone Skin. (Neutrogena) TEA-stearate, triethanolamine, glycerin, sodium tallowate, sodium cocoate, TEA-oleate, sodium ricinoleate, acetylated lanolin alcohol, cocamide DEA, TEA lauryl sulfate, tocopherol. Bar 105 g. *OTC.*
Use: Dermatologic, cleanser.

Neutrogena Clear Pore. (Neutrogena) Benzoyl peroxide 3.5%, glycerin, titanium dioxide, EDTA, menthol. Cleanser/mask. 125 mL. *OTC.*
Use: Dermatologic, acne.

Neutrogena Drying. (Neutrogena) Witch hazel, isopropyl alcohol, EDTA, parabens, tartrazine. Gel. Tube 22.5 mL. *OTC.*
Use: Dermatologic, acne.

Neutrogena Dry Skin Soap. (Neutrogena) Triethanolamine, stearic acid, tallow, glycerin, coconut oil, castor oil, sodium hydroxide, oleic acid, laneth-10 acetate, cocamide DEA, nonoxynol-14, PEG-14 octoate, BHT, O-tolyl biguanide. Bar 105 g, 165 g. Scented or unscented. *OTC.*
Use: Dermatologic, cleanser.

Neutrogena Glow Sunless Tanning. (Neutrogena) Octyl methoxycinnamate, cetyl alcohol, diazolidinyl urea, parabens, EDTA. SPF 8. Lot. Bot. 120 mL. *OTC.*
Use: Sunscreen.

Neutrogena Intensified Day Moisture. (Neutrogena) Octyl methoxycinnamate, 2-phenylbenzimidazole sulfonic acid, titanium dioxide, cetyl alcohol, diazolidinyl urea, parabens, EDTA. SPF 15. Cream 67.5 g. *OTC.*
Use: Dermatologic, moisturizer.

Neutrogena Lip Moisturizer. (Neutrogena) Octyl methoxycinnamate, benzophenone-3, corn oil, castor oil, mineral oil, lanolin oil, petrolatum, lanolin, stearyl alcohol. SPF 15. Lip balm 4.5 g. *OTC.*
Use: Lip protectant.

Neutrogena Moisture SPF 15. (Neutrogena) Octyl methoxycinnamate, benzophenone-3, glycerin, PEG-100 stearate, dimethicone, PEG-6000 monostearate, triethanolamine, parabens, imidazolidinyl urea, carbomer 954, PABA free. Lot. Bot. 120 mL. *OTC.*
Use: Sunscreen.

Neutrogena Moisture SPF 5. (Neutrogena) Octyl methoxycinnamate, petrolatum, cetyl alcohol, parabens, diazolidinyl urea, EDTA, cetyl alcohol. Lot. Bot 60 mL, 120 mL. *OTC.*
Use: Dermatologic, moisturizer.

Neutrogena Non-Drying Cleansing. (Neutrogena) Glycerin, caprylic/capric triglyceride, PEG-20 almond glycerides, cetyl ricinoleate, isohexadecane, TEA-cocoyl glutamate, PEG-20 methyl glucose sesquistearate, stearyl alcohol, cetyl alcohol, EDTA, dipotassium glycyrrhizate, stearyl glycyrrhetinate, bisabolol, parabens, acrylates/C 10-30 alkyl acrylate crosspolymer, triethanolamine, diazolidinyl urea. Lot. Bot. 165 mL. *OTC.*
Use: Dermatologic, cleanser.

Neutrogena Norwegian Formula Emulsion. (Neutrogena) Glycerin base 2%. Pump dispenser 5.25 oz. *OTC.*
Use: Emollient.

Neutrogena Norwegian Formula Hand Cream. (Neutrogena) Glycerin base 41%. Tube 2 oz. *OTC.*
Use: Emollient.

Neutrogena No-Stick Sunscreen. (Neutrogena) SPF 30. Homosalate 15%, octyl methoxycinnamate 7.5%, benzophenone-36%, octyl salicylate 5%, EDTA, parabens, diazolidinyl urea/Cream. Waterproof 118 g. *OTC.*
Use: Sunscreen.

Neutrogena Oil-Free Acne Wash. (Neutrogena) Salicylic acid 2%, EDTA, propylene glycol, tartrazine, aloe extract. Liq. Bot. 180 mL. *OTC.*
Use: Dermatologic, acne.

Neutrogena Oily Skin Formula Soap. (Neutrogena) Triethanolamine, glycerin, fatty acids. Bar 3.5 oz. *OTC.*
Use: Dermatologic, cleanser.

Neutrogena Original Formula Soap. (Neutrogena) Triethanolamine, glycerin,

fatty acids. Bar 3.5 oz, 5.5 oz. *OTC.*
Use: Dermatologic, cleanser.

Neutrogena Soap. (Neutrogena) TEA-stearate, triethanolamine, glycerin, sodium tallowate, sodium cocoate, sodium ricinoleate, TEA-oleate, cocamide DEA, tocopherol. Bar 105 g, 165 g. *OTC.*
Use: Dermatologic, cleanser.

Neutrogena Sunblock. (Neutrogena) **SPF 8:** Octyl methoxycinnamate, menthyl anthranilate, titanium dioxide, mineral oil. Cream 67.5 g. **SPF 15:** Octyl methoxycinnamate, octyl salicylate, menthyl anthranilate, mineral oil, titanium dioxide, propylparaben. Cream 67.5 g. **SPF 25:** Octyl methoxycinnamate, benzophenone-3, octyl salicylate, castor oil, cetearyl alcohol, propylparaben, shea butter. Stick 12.6 g. **SPF 30:** Octocrylene, octyl methoxycinnamate, menthyl anthranilate, zinc oxide, mineral oil, vitamin E. Cream 67.5 g. *OTC.*
Use: Sunscreen.

Neutrogena Sunscreen. (Neutrogena) Ethylhexyl p-methoxycinnamate 7%, oxybenzone 4%, titanium dioxide 2%. Tube 3 oz. *OTC.*
Use: Sunscreen.

Neutrogena T/Gel Original. (Neutrogena Corp) Coal tar extract 2%. Shampoo. Bot. 132 mL, 255 mL, 480 mL. *OTC.*
Use: Dermatologic.

Neutrogena T/Sal. (Neutrogena) Salicylic acid 2%, solubilized coal tar extract 2%. Shampoo. Bot. 135 mL. *OTC.*
Use: Antiseborrheic.

Neutrogena Ultra Sheer Dry-Touch Sunblock. (Neutrogena) Avobenzone 3%, homosalate 15%, octisalate 5%, octocrylene 2.8%, oxybenzone 6%. EDTA, glyceryl, PEG 100. SPF 70. Lot. 88 mL. *OTC.*
Use: Sunscreen.

Nevanac. (Alcon) Nepafenac 0.1%. Benzalkonium chloride 0.005%, EDTA, sodium chloride, tyloxapol, sodium hydroxide, hydrochloric acid. Ophth. Susp. Bot. 3 mL with dropper. *Rx.*
Use: Ophthalmic nonsteroidal anti-inflammatory drug.

•**nevirapine.** (neh-VIE-rah-peen) *USP.*
Use: Antiviral.
See: Viramune.
Viramune XR.

nevirapine. (Various Mfr.) Nevirapine. **Tab.:** 200 mg. May contain lactose. 30s, 60s, UD 10s. **Susp.:** 50 mg per 5 mL. Parabens, polysorbate 80, sorbitol, sucrose. 240 mL. *Rx.*
Use: Antiretroviral agent, non-nucleoside reverse transcriptase inhibitor.

New Terocin. (Alexso) Capsaicin 0.025%, menthol 10%, methyl salicylate 25%. Aloe, borago seed oil, cetyl alcohol, glyceryl, lavender oil, lidocaine, parabens, PEG, propylene glycol, triethanolamine. Lot. 120 mL. *OTC.*
Use: Rub and liniment.

Nexa Plus. (Upsher-Smith) Folic acid 1.25 mg, calcium 160 mg, Fe 29 mg, vitamins D 800 units, E 30 units, B_6 25 mg, C 28 mg, DHA 350 mg, biotin 250 mcg, docusate calcium 55 mg. Beeswax, corn oil, glycerin, lecithin, soybean oil, sunflower oil. Cap., softgel. 30s. *Rx.*
Use: Prenatal vitamin with minerals.

Nexa Select. (Upsher-Smith) Folic acid 1.25 mg, Ca 160 mg, Fe 29 mg, vitamins D 800 units, E 30 units, B_6 25 mg, B_{12} 25 mcg, C 28 mg, DHA 325 mg, docusate sodium 55 mg. Beeswax, glycerin, soybean oil. Cap. 30s. *Rx.*
Use: Prenatal vitamin with minerals.

Nexavar. (Bayer) Sorafenib 200 mg (equiv. to sorafenib tosylate 274 mg). Film coated. PEG. Tab. 120s. *Rx.*
Tall Man: NexAVAR
Use: Multikinase inhibitor.

•**nexeridine hydrochloride.** (NEX-eh-RIH-deen) USAN.
Use: Analgesic.

Nexium. (AstraZeneca) Esomeprazole. **DR Cap.:** 20 mg, 40 mg. Sugar spheres. Enteric-coated Gran. Bot. 90s, 1000s, unit-of-use 30s, UD 100s. **DR Pow. for Susp.:** 2.5 mg, 5 mg, 10 mg, 20 mg, 40 mg. Dextrose. Contains enteric-coated granules. Unit-dose packets. 30s. *Rx.*
Tall Man: NexIUM
Use: Proton pump inhibitor.

Nexium I.V. (AstraZeneca) Esomeprazole 20 mg, 40 mg. EDTA. Inj., Pow. or Cake for Soln. Single-use vials. 10s. *Rx.*
Tall Man: NexIUM
Use: Proton pump inhibitor.

Nexplanon. (Schering) Etonogestrel 68 mg. Implant; subdermal. Preloaded needle with disposable applicator (each etonogestrel implant rod consists of an EVA copolymer core containing 68 mg of synthetic progestin etonogestrel and barium sulfate surrounded by an EVA copolymer skin). *Rx.*
Use: Sex hormone, contraceptive hormone.

Next Choice One Dose. (Watson Laboratories) Levonorgestrel 1.5 mg. Lactose. Tab. UD 1s. *OTC.*
Use: Emergency contraceptive.

Nexterone. (Prism Pharmaceuticals)

Amiodarone hydrochloride. **Inj., Soln.: 50 mg/mL:** 3 mL, 10 mL, 30 mL single-dose vials; 3 mL prefilled syringe. **1.5 mg/mL and 1.8 mg/mL:** Premixed in dextrose. Single-dose *Galaxy* containers. 100 mL, 200 mL. *OTC.*
Use: Cardiovascular agent, antiarrhythmic agent.

NF Formulas Children's. (Integrative Therapeutics) Iron 2.5 mg, calcium 100 mg, vitamins A 500 units, D 100 units, E 7.5 units, B_1 0.5 mg, B_2 0.5 mg, B_3 2.5 mg, B_5 2.5 mg, B_6 0.5 mg, B_{12} 1.5 mcg, C 30 mg, K 20 mcg, folate 0.1 mg, Cr, Cu, I, K, Mg, Mn, Mo, P, Se, Zn, biotin, cranberry fruit extract, elder fruit extract, grape seed extract, inositol, Stevia leaf extract. Fructose, maltodextrin, peppermint leaves, sorbitol, soybean oil. Gluten free, preservative free. Cherry flavor. Chew. Tab. 120s. *OTC.*
Use: Multivitamin with minerals.

NF Formulas Spectra Probiotic With Cofactors Caplets. (Integrative Therapeutics) 1 billion live organisms blend of *L. acidophilus*, *B. bifidum*, *B. infantis*, *B. longum*, *L. helveticus*, *L. casei*, *L. salivarius*, *S. thermophilus*. Maltodextrin. Gluten free, preservative free, and sugar free. Tab. 90s. *OTC.*
Use: Probiotic

NF Formulas Spectra Probiotic With Cofactors UltraCaps. (Integrative Therapeutics) 1 billion live organisms blend of *L. acidophilus*, *B. bifidum*, *B. infantis*, *B. longum*, *L. helveticus*, *L. casei*, *L. salivarius*, *S. thermophilus*. Gluten free, preservative free, and sugar free. Tab. 90s. *OTC.*
Use: Probiotic.

N.G.T. (Geneva) Triamcinolone acetonide 0.1%, nystatin 100,000 units/g. Cream. Tube 15 g. *Rx.*
Use: Antifungal; corticosteroid, topical.

NG-29.
Use: Diagnostic aid. [Orphan Drug]

Niacal. (Jones Pharma) Calcium lactate 324 mg, niacin 25 mg. Tab. Peppermint flavor. Bot. 100s, 1000s. *OTC.*
Use: Vasodilator; vitamin supplement.

•**niacin.** (NYE-uh-sin) *USP.*
Use: Antihyperlipidemic; vitamin, enzyme co-factor.
See: Flush-Free Niacin.
Lipo-Nicin.
Niacal.
Niacin Extended Release.
Niacin Flush-Free.
Niacin No Flush.
Niacor.
Niaspan.
Ni Cord XL.
Nicotinic Acid.
Slo-Niacin.
W/Lovastatin.
See: Advicor.
W/Simvastatin.
See: Simcor.

•**niacinamide.** (nye-ah-SIN-ah-mide) *USP.*
Use: Vitamin, enzyme co-factor.

niacinamide (nicotinamide). (Various Mfr.) Niacinamide (nicotinamide) 100 mg, 500 mg. Tab. Bot. 100s, 250s. *Rx-OTC.*
Use: Water-soluble vitamin.

niacin ER. (Various Mfr.) Niacin 250 mg, 500 mg, 750 mg, 1,000 mg. ER Tab. 30s (500 mg only), 60s (500 mg only), 100s, 200s (500 mg only), 250s (250 mg and 500 mg only), 300s (500 mg only). *Rx.*
Use: Water-soluble vitamin.

Niacin Flush-Free. (Mason) Niacin. **Cap.:** 750 mg. Inositol 211.5 mg. Preservative free and sugar free. 50s. **Tab.:** 400 mg. Gluten free, preservative free, and sugar free. 110s. *OTC.*
Use: Water-soluble vitamin.

Niacin No Flush. (Windmill) Niacin 100 mg, 250 mg. Preservative free and sugar free. Tab. 60s. *OTC.*
Use: Water-soluble vitamin.

Niacor. (Upsher-Smith) Niacin 500 mg. Lactose. Tab. Bot. 100s. *Rx.*
Use: Water-soluble vitamin.

Nialexo-C. (Roberts) Niacin 50 mg, vitamin C 30 mg. Tab. Bot. 100s. *OTC.*
Use: Vitamin supplement.

Niarb Super. (Miller Pharmacal Group) Magnesium 100 mg, vitamin C 200 mg, niacinamide 200 mg (as ascorbate). Tab. Bot. 100s. *OTC.*
Use: Mineral, vitamin supplement.

Niaspan. (Abbott) Niacin 500 mg, 750 mg, 1000 mg. ER Tab. Bot. 100s. *Rx.*
Use: Water-soluble vitamin.

Niazide. (Major) Trichlormethiazide 4 mg. Tab. Bot. 100s, 1000s. *Rx.*
Use: Diuretic.

niazo. Neotropin.
Use: Antiseptic, urinary.

•**nibroxane.** (nye-BROX-ane) USAN.
Use: Antimicrobial, topical.

nicamindon.
See: Nicotinamide.

•**nicardipine hydrochloride.** (NYE-CAR-dih-peen) USAN.
Tall Man: niCARdipine
Use: Calcium channel blocker.

See: Cardene IV.
Cardene SR.

nicardipine hydrochloride. (Teva) Nicardipine hydrochloride 2.5 mg/mL. Inj., Soln. Single-use vial. 10 mL. *Rx.*
Use: Cardiovascular agent, calcium channel blocking agent.

nicardipine hydrochloride. (Various Mfr.) Nicardipine hydrochloride 20 mg, 30 mg. Cap. Bot. 90s, 500s. *Rx.*
Use: Calcium channel blocker.

NicAzel Forte. (Elorac) Vitamin B_6 8 mg, folic acid 500 mcg, Cu, Zn, *Azerizin* (blend of nicotinamide, azelaic acid, quercetin, and curcumin) 700 mg. Tab. 60s. *Rx.*
Use: Multivitamin with minerals (except iron).

N'Ice. (Insight Pharmaceuticals) Ascorbic acid 60 mg. Acesulfame potassium, menthol. Sugar free. Tangerine flavor. Loz. 24s. *OTC.*
Use: Water-soluble vitamin.

N'Ice. (Insight Pharmaceuticals) Menthol 5 mg. Sugar free. Assorted, cherry, menthol, orange, citrus, and honey lemon flavors. Loz. 24s. *OTC.*
Use: Anesthetic, local; cough suppressant.

N'ice 'n Clear. (GlaxoSmithKline) Menthol 5 mg, sorbitol. Loz. Pkg. 16s. *OTC.*
Use: Anesthetic, local.

•**nicergoline.** (nice-ERR-go-leen) USAN.
Use: Vasodilator.

Nichols Syphon Powder. (Last) Sodium bicarbonate, sodium Cl, sodium borate. Pouch 12.2 g (add to 32 oz. water to yield isotonic soln.).

•**niclosamide.** (nye-CLOSE-ah-mide) USAN.
Use: Anthelmintic.

nicobion.
See: Nicotinamide.

NicoDerm CQ. (GlaxoSmithKline Consumer) Nicotine 7 mg, 14 mg, 21 mg/day (dose absorbed in 24 hours). Transdermal system. Box 7s (21 mg only), 14s, original and clear patches. *OTC.*
Use: Smoking deterrent.

nicoduozide. A mixture of nicothazone and isoniazid.

•**nicorandil.** (NIH-CAR-an-dill) USAN.
Use: Coronary vasodilator.

Ni Cord XL Caps. (Scot-Tussin) Nicotinic acid 400 mg. Cap. Bot. 100s, 500s. *OTC.*
Use: Vitamin supplement.

NicoRelief. (Major Pharmaceuticals) Nicotine polacrilex 2 mg, 4 mg. **Loz.:** Aspartame, mannitol, phenylalanine 5.1 mg, sodium 16 mg. Mint flavor. 72s. **Gum:** Acesulfame potassium, calcium 100 mg, sodium 11 mg, sorbitol. Original flavor. 50s, 110s. *OTC.*
Use: Smoking deterrent.

Nicorette. (GlaxoSmithKline Consumer) Nicotine polacrilex. **Chewing gum:** 2 mg, 4 mg/square; orange, mint, and original flavors. Chewing gum. Box 48, 108, 168 pieces. **Lozenge:** 2 mg, 4 mg. Aspartame, mannitol, phenylalanine 3.4 mg. 72s. *OTC.*
Use: Smoking deterrent.

Nicorette Mini. (GlaxoSmithKline Consumer) Nicotine polacrilex 2 mg, 4 mg. Acesulfame potassium, mannitol, sodium 5 mg. Mint flavor. Loz. 20s, 81s. *OTC.*
Use: Smoking deterrent.

nicotamide.
See: Nicotinamide.

nicothazone. Nicotinal dehydethiose micarbazone.

nicotilamide.
See: Nicotinamide.

nicotinamide. Niacinamide, USP. Vitamin B_3, aminicotin, dipegyl, nicamindon, nicotamide, nicotilamide, nicotinic acid amide.

nicotinamide adenine dinucleotide.
Name used for Nadide.

nicotinamide with zinc-copper and folic acid. (Brookstone Pharmaceuticals) Nicotinamide 750 mg, zinc oxide 25 mg, cupric oxide 1.5 mg, folic acid 500 mcg. Tab. 60s. *Rx.*
Use: Multivitamin, mineral combination.

•**nicotine.** (NIK-oh-teen) *USP.*
Use: Smoking cessation adjunct.
See: Nicotine Inhalation System.
Nicotine Nasal Spray.
Nicotine Polacrilex.
Nicotine Transdermal System.

nicotine gum. (Various Mfr.) Nicotine polacrilex 2 mg, 4 mg/square. Chewing gum. Box 48, 108 pieces. *OTC.*
Use: Smoking deterrent.

nicotine inhalation system.
Use: Smoking deterrent.
See: Nicotrol Inhaler.

nicotine nasal spray.
Use: Smoking deterrent.
See: Nicotrol NS.

•**nicotine polacrilex.** (NIK-oh-teen PAHL-ah-KRILL-ex) *USP.*
Use: Smoking cessation adjunct.
See: Commit.
NicoRelief.
Nicorette.
Nicorette Mini.
Nicotine Gum.
Thrive.

nicotine polacrilex. (Perrigo) Nicotine (as polacrilex) 2 mg. Phenylalanine 3.4 mg, aspartame, mannitol. Mint flavor. Loz. 48s. *OTC.*
Use: Smoking deterrent.

nicotine resin complex.
See: Nicotine Polacrilex.

•**nicotine transdermal system.** (NIK-oh-teen) *USP.*
Use: Smoking cessation adjunct.

nicotine transdermal system.
Use: Smoking deterrent.
See: Habitrol.
NicoDerm CQ.
Prostep.

nicotine transdermal system. (Various Mfr.) Nicotine 7 mg, 14 mg, 21 mg/day (dose absorbed in 24 hours). Transdermal system. Box 7s, 30s. *OTC.*
Use: Smoking deterrent.

nicotinic acid. Niacin, USP.

nicotinic acid. (Rugby) Nicotinic acid 1,000 mg. Gluten free, preservative free, sugar free. Tab., controlled release. 100s. *OTC.*
Use: Water-soluble vitamin.

nicotinic acid. (Various Mfr.) Nicotinic acid. **Tab.:** 50 mg, 100 mg, 250 mg, 500 mg. Bot. 100s, 250s (50 mg, 100 mg only), 1000s (500 mg only). **TR Tab.:** 250 mg, 500 mg. Bot. 100s, 250s (250 mg only), 1000s (500 mg only). **SR Tab.:** 500 mg. Bot. 100s. **ER Cap.:** 250 mg, 400 mg. Bot. 100s, 1000s (250 mg only). **SR Cap.:** 125 mg, 500 mg. Bot. 100s. **TR Cap.:** 250 mg, 500 mg. Bot. 100s, 1000s (500 mg only). *Rx-OTC.*
Use: Water-soluble vitamin.

nicotinic acid amide. Niacinamide, USP.
See: Niacinamide.

nicotinic acid with combinations.
See: Niacin w/Combinations.

•**nicotinyl alcohol.** (NIK-oh-TIN-ill AL-koe-hahl) USAN.
Use: Vasodilator, peripheral.

nicotinyl tartrate. 3-Pyridinemethanol tartrate.

Nicotrol Inhaler. (Pfizer) Nicotine 4 mg delivered (10 mg/cartridge). Inhaler Kit contains mouthpiece, storage trays each containing 6 cartridges, 1 plastic storage case, patient information leaflet. Box 42s, 168s. *Rx.*
Use: Smoking deterrent.

Nicotrol NS. (Pfizer) Nicotine 0.5 mg per actuation (10 mg/mL). Parabens, EDTA. Spray pump. Bot. 10 mL. (≈ 200 applications). Each unit has a glass container mounted with metered spray pump. *Rx.*
Use: Smoking deterrent.

nieraline.
See: Epinephrine.

Nifedical XL. (Teva) Nifedipine 30 mg, 60 mg. Lactose. Film-coated. ER Tab. Bot. 100s, 300s. *Rx.*
Use: Calcium channel blocker.

•**nifedipine.** (nye-FED-ih-peen) *USP.*
Tall Man: NIFEdipine
Use: Calcium channel blocker; urinary tract agent. [Orphan Drug]
See: Adalat CC.
Afeditab CR.
Nifediac CC.
Nifedical XL.
Procardia.
Procardia XL.

nifedipine. (Mylan) Nifedipine 30 mg, 60 mg, 90 mg. ER Tab. Bot. 100s, 300s (except 90 mg). *Rx.*
Use: Calcium channel blocker.

nifedipine. (Teva) Nifedipine 30 mg, 60 mg, 90 mg. Lactose (except 30 mg). Film-coated. ER Tab. 100s, 300s (except 90 mg), 1000s (except 90 mg). *Rx.*
Use: Calcium channel blocker.

nifedipine. (Various Mfr.) Nifedipine 10 mg, 20 mg. May be liquid filled. Cap. 100s, 300s. *Rx.*
Use: Calcium channel blocker.

Niferex-150. (Ther-Rx) Elemental iron (from ferrous asparto glycinate and polysaccharide iron complex) 150 mg, vitamin C (calcium ascorbate and calcium threonate) 50 mg, succinic acid 50 mg. Cap. 90s. *OTC.*
Use: Mineral supplement.

Niferex-150 Forte. (Ther-Rx) Elemental iron (from ferrous asparto glycinate and polysaccharide-iron complex) 150 mg, vitamin C (as calcium ascorbate and calcium threonate) 60.8 mg, folic acid 1 mg, vitamin B_{12} 25 mcg. Cap. 90s. *Rx.*
Use: Mineral, vitamin supplement.

Niferex-PN Forte. (Ther-Rx) Calcium 250 mg, iron 60 mg, vitamins A 5000 units, D 400 units, E 30 mg, B_1 3 mg, B_2 3.4 mg, B_3 20 mg, B_6 4 mg, B_{12} 12 mcg, C 80 mg, folic acid 1 mg, Cu, I, Mg, Zn 25 mg. Bot. 100s. *Rx.*
Use: Mineral, vitamin supplement.

•**nifluridide.** (nye-FLURE-ih-DIDE) USAN.
Use: Ectoparasiticide.

•**nifungin.** (nih-FUN-jin) USAN. Substance derived from *Aspergillus giganteus.*

•**nifuradene.** (NYE-fyoor-ad-EEN) USAN.
Use: Anti-infective.

•**nifuraldezone.** (NYE-fer-AL-dee-zone) USAN. (Eaton Medical)
Use: Anti-infective.

•**nifuratel.** (NYE-fyoor-at-ell) USAN.

Use: Anti-infective; antifungal; antiprotozoal, trichomonas.

•**nifuratrone.** (nye-FYOOR-ah-trone) USAN.
Use: Anti-infective.

•**nifurdazil.** (NYE-fyoor-dazz-ill) USAN.
Use: Anti-infective.

nifurethazone.
Use: Anti-infective.

•**nifurimide.** (nye-FYOOR-ih-MIDE) USAN.
Use: Anti-infective.

•**nifurmerone.** (NYE-fyoor-MER-ohn) USAN.
Use: Antifungal.

nifuroxime.
Use: Antifungal; anti-infective, topical; antiprotozoal.
See: Micofur.

•**nifurpirinol.** (nye-fer-PIHR-ih-nole) USAN.
Use: Anti-infective.

•**nifurquinazol.** (NYE-fyoor-KWIN-azz-ole) USAN.
Use: Anti-infective.

•**nifurthiazole.** (NYE-fyoor-THIGH-ah-zole) USAN.
Use: Anti-infective.

nifurtimox.
Use: CDC anti-infective agent.
See: Lampit.

Nighttime Cold Softgels. (Goldline) Dextromethorphan HBr 10 mg, doxylamine succinate 6.25 mg, pseudoephedrine hydrochloride 30 mg, acetaminophen 250 mg. Alcohol free. Sorbitol. Softgels. 12s. *OTC.*
Use: Antitussive combination.

Nighttime Pamprin. (Chattem) Diphenhydramine hydrochloride 50 mg, acetaminophen 650 mg. Pow. Pkg. 4s. *OTC.*
Use: Sleep aid.

Nighttime Sleep Aid. (Rugby) Diphenhydramine hydrochloride 50 mg. Tab. Bot. 50s. *OTC.*
Use: Antihistamine, nonselective ethanolamine.

nigrin. Streptonigrin.
Use: Antineoplastic.

Niko-Mag. (Scruggs) Magnesium oxide 500 mg. Cap. Bot. 100s, 1000s. *OTC.*
Use: Antacid.

Nikotime TD Caps. (Major) Niacin 125 mg, 250 mg. TD Cap. Bot. 100s, 1000s. *OTC.*
Use: Vitamin supplement.

Nilandron. (Covis) Nilutamide 50 mg, 150 mg, lactose. Tab. Bot. 90s (50 mg only), 30s (150 mg only). *Rx.*
Use: Antineoplastic; hormone, antiandrogen.

•**nilotinib.** (nye-LOE-ti-nib) USAN.
Use: Protein-tyrosine kinase inhibitor.
See: Tasigna.

Nil Tuss. (Minnesota Pharm) Dextromethorphan HBr 10 mg, chlorpheniramine maleate 1.25 mg, phenylephrine hydrochloride 5 mg, ammonium Cl 83 mg/5 mL. Syr. Bot. Pt. *OTC.*
Use: Antihistamine; antitussive; decongestant; expectorant.

•**nilutamide.** (nye-LOO-tah-mide) USAN.
Use: Antineoplastic; hormone, antiandrogen.
See: Nilandron.

•**nilvadipine.** (NILL-vah-DIH-peen) USAN.
Use: Antagonist, calcium channel.

Nil Vaginal Cream. (Century) Sulfanilamide 15%, 9-aminoacridine hydrochloride 0.2%, allantoin 1.5%. Bot. 4 oz. w/applicator. *OTC.*
Use: Anti-infective, vaginal.

•**nimazone.** (nih-mah-ZONE) USAN.
Use: Anti-inflammatory.

Nimbex. (Abbott) Cisatracurium besylate 2 mg/mL, Vial 5 mL, 10 mL; 10 mg/mL, Vial 20 mL. Inj. *Rx.*
Use: Nondepolarizing neuromuscular blocker; muscle relaxant.

Nimbus. (Biomerica) Monoclonal antibody-based enzyme immunoassay. Screens for urinary chorionic gonadotropin. Pkg. 10s, 25s, 50s. *Rx.*
Use: Diagnostic aid.

•**nimodipine.** (NYE-MOE-dih-peen) *USP.*
Tall Man: niMODipine
Use: Vasodilator, calcium channel blocker.
See: Nymalize.

nimodipine. (Various Mfr.) Nimodipine 30 mg. Liquid filled. Cap. UD 30s, 100s. *Rx.*
Use: Calcium channel blocking agent.

•**nintedanib.** (nin-TED-a-nib) USAN.
Use: Antineoplastic.

•**nintedanib esylate.** (nin-TED-a-nib) USAN.
Use: Antineoplastic.

Nion B Plus C. (Nion Corp.) Vitamins B_1 15 mg, B_2 10.2 mg, B_3 50 mg, B_5 10 mg, C 300 mg. Capl. Bot 100s. *OTC.*
Use: Vitamin supplement.

Niong. (US Ethicals) Nitroglycerin 2.6 mg, 6.5 mg. CR Tab. Bot. 100s. *Rx.*
Use: Antianginal.

Nipent. (Hospira) Pentostatin 10 mg/vial. Mannitol 50 mg/vial. Pow. for Inj. Vial. Single-dose. *Rx.*
Use: Antineoplastic.

•**niraparib.** (nye-RAP-a-rib) USAN.
Use: Antineoplastic.

Niratron. (Progress) Chlorpheniramine maleate 4 mg/5 mL. Bot. pt. *Rx.*
Use: Antihistamine.

Niravam. (Azur Pharma) Alprazolam 0.25 mg, 0.5 mg, 1 mg, 2 mg. Sucralose, sucrose. Orange flavor. Orally Disintegrating Tab. 100s. *Rx.*
Use: Antianxiety agent.

•**niridazole.** (nye-RIH-dah-ZOLE) USAN.
Use: Antischistosomal.

Niron Komplete. (Eckson) Iron 30 mg, vitamins B_{12} 12 mcg, C 120 mg, E 20 units, folic acid 1 mg. PEG. Tab. 30s. *Rx.*
Use: Multivitamin with iron.

•**nisbuterol mesylate.** (NISS-BYOO-teh-role) USAN.
Use: Bronchodilator.

•**nisobamate.** (NYE-so-BAM-ate) USAN.
Use: Anxiolytic; hypnotic; sedative.

•**nisoldipine.** (nye-SOLE-dih-peen) USAN.
Use: Calcium channel blocker.
See: Sular.

nisoldipine. (Mylan) Nisoldipine 20 mg, 30 mg, 40 mg. Polydextrose. Film-coated ER Tab. 100s, 500s. *Rx.*
Use: Cardiovascular agent, calcium channel blocking agent.

nisoldipine. (Prasco Laboratories) Nisoldipine 8.5 mg, 17 mg, 34 mg. Film coated. Glyceryl, lactose. ER Tab. 100s. *Rx.*
Use: Calcium channel blocking agent.

•**nisoxetine.** (NISS-OX-eh-teen) USAN.
Use: Antidepressant.

•**nisterime acetate.** (nye-STEER-eem) USAN.
Use: Androgen.

•**nitarsone.** (NITE-AHR-sone) USAN.
Use: Antiprotozoal, histomonas.

•**nitazoxanide.** (nye-tah-ZOX-ah-nide)
Use: Antiprotozoals.
See: Alinia.

Nite Time Children's. (Topco) Pseudoephedrine hydrochloride 10 mg, chlorpheniramine maleate 0.67 mg, dextromethorphan HBr 5 mg per 5 mL. Sucrose, cherry flavor, alcohol free. Liq. Bot. 118 mL. *OTC.*
Use: Upper respiratory combination, decongestant, antihistamine, antitussive.

Nite Time Cold Formula. (Alra) Pseudoephedrine hydrochloride 10 mg, doxylamine succinate 1.25 mg, dextromethorphan HBr 5 mg, acetaminophen 167 mg, alcohol 25%. Liq. Bot. 180 mL, 300 mL. *OTC.*
Use: Analgesic; antihistamine; antitussive; decongestant.

Nite Time Cold Formula for Adults. (Alpharma) Dextromethorphan HBr 5 mg, doxylamine succinate 2.1 mg, pseudoephedrine hydrochloride 10 mg, acetaminophen 167 mg per 5 mL. Alcohol 10%, saccharin, sucrose. Liq. Bot. 296 mL. *OTC.*
Use: Upper respiratory combination, antitussive, antihistamine, decongestant, analgesic.

Nithiodote. (Hope Pharmaceuticals) Sodium nitrite 30 mg/mL, sodium thiosulfate 250 mg/mL (administration of 1 vial of each medication constitutes a single dose). Potassium chloride 4.4 mg. Inj., Soln. Kit w/one 10 mL sodium nitrite vial and one 50 mL sodium thiosulfate vial. *Rx.*
Use: Detoxification agent, antidote.

•**nitisinone.** (nit-IS-i-none) USAN.
Use: Tyrosinemia.
See: Orfadin.

•**nitralamine hydrochloride.** (nye-TRAL-ah-meen) USAN.
Use: Antifungal.

•**nitramisole hydrochloride.** (nye-TRAM-ih-sole) USAN.
Use: Anthelmintic.

nitrates.
Use: Vasodilator.
See: Amyl Nitrate.
Isosorbide Dinitrate.
Isosorbide Mononitrate.
Nitroglycerin.

•**nitrazepam.** (nye-TRAY-zeh-pam) USAN.
Use: Anticonvulsant; hypnotic; sedative.

Nitrek. (Bertek) Nitroglycerin 0.2 mg/h (22.4 mg), 0.4 mg/h (44.8 mg), 0.6 mg/h (67.2 mg). Transdermal Patch. Box 30s. *Rx.*
Use: Vasodilator.

•**nitrendipine.** (NIGH-TREN-dih-peen) USAN.
Use: Antihypertensive.

•**nitric acid.** (NYE-trick) *NF.*
Use: Pharmaceutic aid, acidifying agent.
See: Nitric Oxide.

nitric acid silver. Silver Nitrate.

nitric oxide.
Use: Respiratory inhalant; primary pulmonary hypertension agent. [Orphan Drug]
See: INOmax.

Nitro-Bid. (Savage) Nitroglycerin 2% in lanolin-white petrolatum base. Lactose. Oint. Tube 30 g, 60 g, UD 1 g. *Rx.*
Use: Vasodilator.

Nitrocap. (Freeport) Nitroglycerin 2.5 mg. TR Cap. Bot. 100s. *Rx.*
Use: Antianginal.

•**nitrocycline.** (NYE-troe-SIGH-kleen) USAN.
Use: Anti-infective.

•**nitrodan.** (NYE-troe-dan) USAN.
Use: Anthelmintic.

Nitrodisc. (Roberts) Nitroglycerin. Transdermal nitroglycerin discs releasing 16 mg, 24 mg, 32 mg. Patch. Ctn. 30s, 100s. *Rx.*
Use: Antianginal.

Nitro-Dur. (Key) Nitroglycerin 0.1 mg/h (20 mg), 0.2 mg/h (40 mg), 0.3 mg/h (60 mg), 0.4 mg/h (80 mg), 0.6 mg/h (120 mg), 0.8 mg/h (160 mg). Transdermal Patch. 30s, UD 30s. *Rx.*
Use: Vasodilator.

Nitrofan Caps. (Major) Nitrofurantoin 50 mg, 100 mg. Cap. Bot. 100s, 500s. *Rx.*
Use: Anti-infective, urinary.

nitrofurans.
See: Nitrofurantoin.

•**nitrofurantoin.** (nye-troe-FYOOR-an-toyn) *USP.*
Use: Anti-infective, urinary.
See: Furadantin.
Macrobid.
Macrodantin.

nitrofurantoin. (Amneal Pharmaceuticals) Nitrofurantoin 25 mg per 5 mL. Glycerin, parabens, saccharin, sorbitol. Tutti-frutti flavor. Susp. 230 mL. *Rx.*
Use: Anti-infective, nitrofuran.

nitrofurantoin. (Various Mfr.) Nitrofurantoin as macrocrystals 50 mg, 100 mg. Cap. Bot. 100s, 500s, 1000s. *Rx.*
Use: Anti-infective, urinary.

nitrofurantoin. (Various Mfr.) Nitrofurantoin (as monohydrate/macrocrystals) 100 mg. Cap. 100s, 500s. *Rx.*
Use: Anti-infective, urinary.

•**nitrofurazone.** (nye-troe-FYOOR-a-zone) *USP.*
Use: Anti-infective, topical.

Nitrogard. (Forest) Transmucosal nitroglycerin 2 mg, 3 mg. Buccal CR Tab. Bot. 100s, UD 100s. *Rx.*
Use: Vasodilator.

•**nitrogen.** (NYE-troe-jen) *NF.*
Use: Pharmaceutic aid, air displacement.

nitrogen monoxide. Laughing Gas, Nitrous Oxide.
Use: Anesthetic, general; analgesic.

nitrogen mustard.
See: Mustargen.

nitrogen mustard derivatives.
See: Leukeran.
Mustargen.
Triethylenemelamine.

nitrogen mustards.
Use: Alkylating agents.
See: Chlorambucil.
Cyclophosphamide.
Ifosfamide.
Mechlorethamine Hydrochloride.
Melphalan.

•**nitroglycerin.** (nye-troe-GLH-suh-rin) *USP.*
Use: Vasodilator.
See: Minitran.
Niong.
Nitrek.
Nitro-Bid.
Nitrodisk.
Nitro-Dur.
Nitrogard.
Nitrolingual.
Nitro-Lyn.
NitroMist.
Nitrostat.
Nitro-Time.
Rectiv.
Transderm-Nitro.

nitroglycerin. (Wilshire Pharmaceuticals) Nitroglycerin 0.4 mg per metered spray. Alcohol 20%, peppermint oil. Spray, lingual. 4.9 g and 12 g (60 and 200 metered doses). *Rx.*
Use: Vasodilator, nitrate.

nitroglycerin. (Various Mfr.) Nitroglycerin. **ER Cap.:** 2.5 mg, 6.5 mg, 9 mg. Bot. 30s (9 mg only), 60s, 100s, UD 60s (2.5 mg only), UD 100s. **Oint.:** 2%. Tube 30 g, 60 g. **Soln. for Inj.:** 5 mg/mL. Single-dose vials. 5 mL, 10 mL. **Sublingual Tab.:** 0.3 mg (1/200 gr), 0.4 mg (1/150 gr), 0.6 mg (1/100 gr). May contain lactose. 25s (0.4 mg only), 100s. *Rx.*
Use: Vasodilator.

•**nitroglycerin, diluted.** (nye-troe-GLIH-suh-rin) *USP. Formerly Glyceryl Trinitrate.*
Use: Vasodilator, coronary.

nitroglycerin in 5% dextrose. (Various Mfr.) Nitroglycerin 100 mcg/mL, 200 mcg/mL, 400 mcg/mL. Inj. Glass containers. 250 mL, 500 mL. *Rx.*
Use: Vasodilator.

nitroglycerin injection. (Abbott) Nitroglycerin 25 mg/mL. Vial 5 mL, 10 mL.
Use: Antianginal; vasodilator.
See: Tridil.

nitroglycerin, intravenous.
Use: Vasodilator.

nitroglycerin patch.
Use: Antianginal.
See: Nitrek.

nitroglycerin transdermal. (Mylan) Nitroglycerin 0.1 mg/h. Transdermal Patch.

30s. *Rx.*
Use: Vasodilator.

nitroglycerin transdermal. (Various Mfr.) Nitroglycerin 0.2 mg/h (16 mg to 62.5 mg), 0.4 mg/h (32 mg to 125 mg), or 0.6 mg/h (75 mg to 187.5 mg). Transdermal Patch. Box 30s. *Rx.*
Use: Vasodilator.

nitroglycerin transdermal system. (Hercon Laboratories, Inc.) Nitroglycerin 37.3 mg, 74.6 mg, 111.9 mg. Patch Pkg. 30s. *Rx.*
Use: Vasodilator.

nitroglycerol.
See: Nitroglycerin.

Nitrolan. (Elan) Protein 60 g, fat 40 g, carbohydrates 160 g, Na 690 mg, K 1.17 g/L, lactose free. With appropriate vitamins and minerals. Liq. In 237 mL *Tetra Pak* containers and 1000 mL *New Pak* closed systems with and without *Color Check. OTC.*
Use: Nutritional supplement.

Nitrolin. (Schein) Nitroglycerin 2.5 mg, 9 mg. SR Cap. **2.5 mg:** Bot. 100s. **9 mg:** Bot. 60s. *Rx.*
Use: Antianginal.

Nitrolingual. (Sciele Pharma) Nitroglycerin 0.4 mg/metered dose. Alcohol 20%, peppermint oil. Aerosol Spray, lingual. 4.9 g and 12 g (60 and 200 metered doses). *Rx.*
Use: Vasodilator.

Nitro-Lyn. (Lynwood) Nitroglycerin 2.5 mg. Cap. Bot. 100s. *Rx.*
Use: Antianginal.

nitromannite.
See: Mannitol Hexanitrate.

nitromannitol.
See: Mannitol Hexanitrate.

Nitromed. (US Ethicals) Nitroglycerin 2.6 mg, 6.5 mg. CR Tab. Bot. 100s. *Rx.*
Use: Antianginal.

•**nitromersol.** (nye-troe-MER-sole) *USP.*
Use: Anti-infective, topical.

•**nitromide.** (NYE-troe-mide) USAN.
Use: Anti-infective.

•**nitromifene citrate.** (nye-TROE-mih-feen) USAN.
Use: Antiestrogen.

NitroMist. (Akrimax Pharmaceuticals) Nitroglycerin 0.4 mg per spray. Aerosol spray, lingual. 8.5 g (230 metered doses). *Rx.*
Use: Vasodilator.

Nitronet. (US Ethicals) Nitroglycerin 2.6 mg, 6.5 mg. CR Tab. Bot. 100s. *Rx.*
Use: Antianginal.

Nitropress. (Marathon) Sodium nitroprusside 50 mg/2 mL. Vial. *Rx.*
Use: Antihypertensive.

nitroprusside sodium.
Use: Antihypertensive.
See: Nitropress (Abbott).
Sodium Nitroprusside.

nitrosoureas.
Use: Alkylating agent; antineoplastic.
See: Carmustine.
Lomustine.
Streptozocin.

Nitrostat. (Parke-Davis) Nitroglycerin 0.3 mg (1/200 g), 0.4 mg (1/150 g), 0.6 mg (1/100 g). Lactose. Sublingual Tab. Bot. 25s (0.4 mg only), 100s. *Rx.*
Use: Vasodilator.

Nitrostat IV. (Parke-Davis) Nitroglycerin for infusion. **0.8 mg/mL:** Amp. 10 mL. **5 mg/mL:** Amp. 10 mL, Vial 10 mL. **10 mg/mL:** Vial 10 mL. *Rx.*
Use: Antianginal.

Nitro-Time. (Time-Cap Labs) Nitroglycerin 2.5 mg, 6.5 mg, 9 mg, lactose, sucrose. ER Cap. Bot. 60s, 90s, 100s. *Rx.*
Use: Vasodilator.

nitrous acid, sodium salt. Sodium Nitrite.

•**nitrous oxide.** (NYE-trus OX-ide) *USP.* Laughing Gas. Nitrogen Monoxide.
Use: Anesthesia, inhalation.

nitrous oxide. (Airgas) Nitrous oxide 100% (provided as a liquefied compressed gas). Gas, Inhal. Cylinder.
Use: General anesthetic, gas.

•**nivazol.** (NIH-vah-ZOLE) USAN.
Use: Corticosteroid, topical.

Nivea Creme. (Beiersdorf) Glycerin, lanolin alcohol, mineral oil, petrolatum, wax, paraffin. Cream. 192 g. *OTC.*
Use: Emollient.

Nivea Moisturizing. (Beiersdorf) **Cream:** Mineral oil, petrolatum, lanolin alcohol, glycerin, microcrystalline wax, paraffin, magnesium sulfate, decyloleate, octyl dodecanol, aluminum stearate, citric acid, magnesium stearate. 120 g, 180 g, 300 g, 480 g. **Lot.:** Mineral oil, lanolin, isopropyl myristate, cetearyl alcohol, glyceryl stearate, acrylamide/sodium acrylate copolymer, simethicone, methychloroisothiazolinone, methylisothiazolinone. In 180 mL, 300 mL, 450 mL. *OTC.*
Use: Emollient.

Nivea Moisturizing Creme Soap. (Beiersdorf) Sodium tallowate, sodium cocoate, glycerin, petrolatum, titanium dioxide, NaCl, octyldodecanol, macadamia nut oil, aloe, sodium thiosulfate, lanolin alcohol, pentasodium pentetate, EDTA, BHT, beeswax. Bar 90 g, 150 g. *OTC.*
Use: Dermatologic, cleanser.

Nivea Oil. (Beiersdorf) Emulsion of neutral aliphatic hydrocarbons. **Liq.:** Bot. 2 oz, 4 fl oz, pt, qt. **Cream:** Tube 1 oz, 2⅓ oz, Jar 4 oz, 6 oz, 1 lb, 5 lb. tin. **Soap:** Bath or toilet size. *OTC.*
Use: Emollient.

Nivea Original Moisture. (Beiersdorf) Cetearyl alcohol, glycerin, glyceryl, lanolin alcohol, mineral oil. Lot. 400 mL. *OTC.*
Use: Emollient.

Nivea Soft. (Beiersdorf) Glycerin, glyceryl, lanolin alcohol, mineral oil, petrolatum, alcohols, dimethicone, jojoba seed oil. Cream. 192 g. *OTC.*
Use: Emollient.

Nivea Sun. (Beiersdorf) Octyl methoxycinnamate, octyl salicylate, benzophenone-3, 2-phenylbenzimidazole-5-sulfonic acid. Lot. Bot. 120 mL. *OTC.*
Use: Sunscreen.

•**nivimedone sodium.** (nih-VIH-meh-dohn) USAN.
Use: Antiallergic.

•**nivocasan.** (nye-VOE-ka-san) USAN.
Use: Apoptosis prevention during cell stress.

•**nivolumab.** (nye-VOL-ue-mab) USAN.
Use: Antineoplastic.

Nix Complete Lice Treatment System. (Insight) Permethrin 1%. Cetyl alcohol, isopropyl alcohol 20%, parabens. Liq., Top. 59 mL w/comb, gloves, cape, and drop cloth. *OTC.*
Use: Scabicide/pediculicide.

Nix Creme Rinse. (Insight) Permethrin 1%. Isopropyl alcohol 20%, cetyl alcohol, parabens. Liq. (cream rinse). 60 mL with comb. *OTC.*
Use: Pediculicide.

•**nizatidine.** (nye-ZAT-ih-deen) *USP.*
Use: Histamine H_2 antagonist.
See: Axid.
Axid AR.
Axid Pulvules.

nizatidine. (Various Mfr.) Nizatidine. **Cap.:** 150 mg, 300 mg. 30s (300 mg only), 60s (150 mg only), 100s, 500s, 1000s (150 mg only), UD 100s (150 mg only). **Soln.:** 15 mg/mL. Glycerin, parabens, saccharin, sucrose. Bubble gum flavor. 480 mL. *Rx.*
Use: Histamine H_2 antagonist.

Nizoral. (McNeil Consumer) Ketoconazole 2%. Shampoo. 120 mL. *Rx.*
Use: Antifungal agent; topical anti-infective.

Nizoral A-D. (McNeil Consumer) Ketoconazole 1%. Tetrasodium EDTA. Shampoo. Bot. 207 mL. *OTC.*
Use: Antifungal agent; topical anti-infective.

N-methyl-D-aspartate receptor antagonists.
Use: Treatment of Alzheimer dementia.
See: Memantine hydrochloride.

n-methylhydrazine.
Use: Antineoplastic.
See: Procarbazine Hydrochloride.

n-methylisatin beta-thiosemicarbazone. Under study.
Use: Smallpox protection.

n, n-diethylvanillamide.
See: Ethamivan.

No-Aspirin. (Walgreen) Acetaminophen 325 mg. Tab. Bot. 100s. *OTC.*
Use: Analgesic.

No-Aspirin Extra Strength. (Walgreen) Acetaminophen 500 mg. Tab. **Tab.:** Bot. 60s, 100s. **Cap.:** Bot. 50s, 100s. *OTC.*
Use: Analgesic.

•**noberastine.** (no-BER-ast-een) USAN.
Use: Antihistamine.

Noble Formula. (Ontos) Pyrithione zinc 0.25%. **Cream:** Alcohol, almond oil, rose hip oil, vitamin E. 120 mL. **Spray:** Alcohol. 120 mL. *OTC.*
Use: Dermatological agent.

Noble Formula HC. (Ontos) Hydrocortisone 1%. Alcohols, almond oil pyrithione zinc, rose hip oil. Cream. 120 g. *OTC.*
Use: Anti-inflammatory agent, topical corticosteroid.

•**nocodazole.** (no-KOE-DAH-zole) USAN.
Use: Antineoplastic.

Nodolor. (Macoven Pharmaceuticals) Acetaminophen 325 mg, dichloralphenazone 100 mg, isometheptene mucate 65 mg. Lactose. Cap. 100s. *c-IV.*
Use: Migraine combination.

No Drowsiness Allerest. (Novartis) Pseudoephedrine hydrochloride 30 mg, acetaminophen 500 mg. Tab. Bot. 20s. *OTC.*
Use: Analgesic; decongestant.

No Drowsiness Sinarest. (Medeva) Pseudoephedrine hydrochloride 30 mg, acetaminophen 500 mg. Tab. Bot. 24s. *OTC.*
Use: Analgesic; decongestant.

nofetumomab merpentan.
See: Verluma.

•**nogalamycin.** (no-GAL-ah-MY-sin) USAN.
Use: Antineoplastic.

NoHist EXT. (Larken) Chlorpheniramine maleate 8 mg, methscopolamine nitrate 2.5 mg. ER Tab. 100s. *Rx.*

Use: Upper respiratory combination, decongestant, antihistamine, and anticholinergic.

NoHist LQ. (Larken) Chlorpheniramine maleate 4 mg, phenylephrine hydrochloride 10 mg. Edetate disodium, glycerin, parabens, propylene glycol, saccharin. Alcohol free and sugar free. Bubble gum flavor. Liq. 473 mL. *OTC.*
Use: Upper respiratory combination, decongestant and antihistamine.

NoHist-Plus. (Larken) Chlorpheniramine maleate 2 mg, methscopolamine nitrate 1.25 mg, phenylephrine hydrochloride 10 mg. Mannitol, saccharin, sugar. Chew. Tab. 100s. *Rx.*
Use: Upper respiratory combination, decongestant, antihistamine, anticholinergic combination.

Nokane. (Wren) Salicylamide 4 g, n-acetyl-p-aminophenol 4 g, caffeine 0.5 gr. Tab. Bot. 40s. *OTC.*
Use: Analgesic combination.

•**nolinium bromide.** (no-LIN-ee-uhm) USAN.
Use: Antisecretory; antiulcerative.

•**nomegestrol.** (NOE-me-JES-trol) USAN.
Use: Hormonal contraceptive.

•**nomegestrol acetate.** (NOE-me-JES-trol) USAN.
Use: Hormonal contraceptive.

Nometic. Diphenidol.
Use: Antiemetic.

•**nomifensine maleate.** (NO-mih-FEN-seen) USAN.
Use: Antidepressant.

Nonamin. (Western Research) Ca 100 mg, Cl 90 mg, Mg 50 mg, Zn 3.75 mg, Fe 4.5 mg, Cu 0.5 mg, I 37.5 mcg, K 49 mg, P 100 mg. Tab. Bot. 1000s. *OTC.*
Use: Mineral supplement.

Non-Aspirin Extra Strength. (Mason) Acetaminophen 500 mg. Tab. 100s. *OTC.*
Use: Analgesic.

nonbarbiturate sedative/hypnotic agents.
See: Sedative/Hypnotic Agents (Nonbarbiturate).

Non-Drowsy Allergy. (Major) Loratadine 10 mg. Lactose. Tab. 30s. *OTC.*
Use: Antihistamine, peripherally selective piperidine.

Non-Drowsy Allergy Relief. (Major) Loratadine 10 mg. Phenylalanine 0.9 mg, aspartame, lactose, mannitol. Cherry flavor. Orally Disintegrating Tab. 10s. *OTC.*
Use: Antihistamine, peripherally selective piperidine.

Non-Drowsy Allergy Relief for Kids. (Major) Loratadine 5 mg per 5 mL. Glycerin, sucrose. Fruit flavor. Syrup. 120 mL. *OTC.*
Use: Antihistamine, peripherally selective piperidine.

Non-Drowsy Contac Sinus. (GlaxoSmithKline) Pseudoephedrine hydrochloride 30 mg, acetaminophen 500 mg. Cap. Bot. 24s. *OTC.*
Use: Analgesic; decongestant.

None. (Forest) Heparin sodium 1000 units/mL. No preservatives. Amps 5 mL. Box 25s. *Rx.*
Use: Anticoagulant.

Non-Habit Forming Stool Softener. (Rugby) Docusate sodium 100 mg, sorbitol, parabens. Cap. Bot. 100s, 1000s. *OTC.*
Use: Laxative.

nonnarcotic analgesic combinations.
See: Acetaminophen/Aspirin/Caffeine.
Acetaminophen/Butalbital.
Acetaminophen/Butalbital/Caffeine.
Acetaminophen/Caffeine/Magnesium Salicylate.
Acetaminophen/Magnesium Salicylate.
Acetaminophen/Phenyltoloxamine Citrate.
Diclofenac Sodium/Misoprostol.
Naproxen/Lansoprazole.

nonnarcotic antitussives.
See: Benzonatate.
Carbetapentane Tannate.
Dextromethorphan Hydrobromide.
Dextromethorphan Hydrobromide/Benzocaine.
Diphenhydramine Hydrochloride.

non-nucleoside reverse transcriptase inhibitors. *Rx.*
Use: Antiretroviral.
See: Delavirdine Mesylate.
Efavirenz.
Efavirenz/Emtricitabine/Tenofovir Disoproxil Fumarate.
Etravirine.
Nevirapine.
Rescriptor.
Rilpivirine.

nonoxynol. (Ortho-McNeil) *OTC.*
Use: Contraceptive, spermicide.

•**nonoxynol-15.** (NAHN-ox-sih-nahl) USAN.
Use: Pharmaceutic aid, surfactant.

•**nonoxynol-4.** (NAHN-ox-sih-nahl) USAN.
Use: Pharmaceutic aid, surfactant.

•**nonoxynol-9.** (NAHN-ox-sih-nahl) *USP.*
Use: Spermicide; pharmaceutic aid, wetting and solubilizing agent.
See: Today Sponge.

•**nonoxynol-10.** (nahn-OCK-sih-nahl) *NF.*
Use: Pharmaceutic aid, surfactant.
•**nonoxynol-30.** (NAHN-ox-sih-nahl) USAN. Under study.
Use: Pharmaceutic aid, surfactant.
nonselective alkylamines.
Use: Antihistamine.
See: Alkylamines, nonselective.
nonselective ethanolamines.
Use: Antihistamine.
See: Ethanolamines, nonselective.
nonselective piperazines.
Use: Antihistamine.
See: Piperazines, nonselective.
nonselective piperidines.
Use: Antihistamine.
See: Piperidines, nonselective.
nonsteroidal anti-inflammatory agents.
See: Celecoxib.
Diclofenac Potassium.
Diclofenac Sodium.
Etodolac.
Fenoprofen Calcium.
Flurbiprofen.
Ibuprofen.
Indomethacin.
Ketoprofen.
Ketorolac Tromethamine.
Meclofenamate Sodium.
Mefenamic Acid.
Meloxicam.
Nabumetone.
Naproxen.
Oxaprozin.
Piroxicam.
Selective COX-2 Inhibitors.
Sulindac.
Tolmetin Sodium.
nonsteroidal anti-inflammatory agents, ophthalmic.
See: Bromfenac.
Diclofenac Sodium.
Flurbiprofen Sodium.
Ketorolac Tromethamine.
Nepafenac.
Suprofen.
nonsteroidal anti-inflammatory agents, topical.
See: Diclofenac.
nonylphenoxypolyethoxy ethanol. Nonoxynol.
Use: Contraceptive, spermicide.
See: Delfen.
No Pain-HP. (Young Again Products) Capsaicin 0.075%. Roll-on. 60 mL. *OTC.*
Use: Analgesic, topical.
Nora-BE. (Watson) Norethindrone 0.35 mg. Lactose. Tab. 28s. *Rx.*
Use: Sex hormone, contraceptive hormone.
•**noracymethadol hydrochloride.** (nahr-ASS-ih-METH-ah-dole) USAN.
Use: Analgesic.
•**norbolethone.** (nahr-BOLE-eth-ohn) USAN.
Use: Anabolic.
Norcet Tablets. (Holloway) Hydrocodone bitartrate 5 mg, acetaminophen 500 mg. Tab. Bot. 100s. *c-III.*
Use: Analgesic combination; narcotic.
Norco. (Watson) Hydrocodone bitartrate 10 mg, acetaminophen 325 mg. Tab. Bot. 100s, 500s. *c-III.*
Use: Analgesic; narcotic.
Norco 5/325. (Watson) Hydrocodone bitartrate 5 mg, acetaminophen 325 mg, sucrose. Tab. Bot. 100s, 500s. *c-III.*
Use: Narcotic analgesic combination.
Norcuron. (Organon Teknika) Vecuronium bromide 10 mg/5 mL. **With diluent:** Vial 5 mL lyophilized powder and 5 mL Amp. of sterile water for injection. Box 10s. **Without diluent:** Vial 5 mL lyophilized powder. Box 10s. **Prefilled syringe:** Vial 10 mL lyophilized powder and 10 mL syringe w/bacteriostatic water for injection. Box 10s. *Rx.*
Use: Muscle relaxant.
norcycline.
Use: Anti-infective.
Norditropin. (Novo Nordisk) Somatropin. 5 mg/1.5 mL, 10 mg/1.5 mL, 15 mg/1.5 mL, 30 mg/3 mL. Histidine 1 mg (5 mg, 10 mg only), 1.7 mg (15 mg only), 3.3 mg (30 mg only); poloxamer 188; phenol 4.5 mg, 9 mg (30 mg only); mannitol 60 mg (5 mg, 10 mg only), 58 mg (15 mg only), 117 mg (30 mg only). Inj. *Nordiflex* prefilled pens and cartridges (5 mg, 15 mg only). *Rx.*
Use: Hormone, growth.
Norel AD. (US Pharm) Acetaminophen 325 mg, chlorpheniramine maleate 4 mg, phenylephrine hydrochloride 10 mg. Tab. 20s. *OTC.*
Use: Upper respiratory combination; decongestant, antihistamine, and analgesic combination.
norelgestromin/ethinyl estradiol.
Use: Sex hormone, contraceptive hormone.
See: Ortho Evra.
Xulane.
Norel LA. (US Pharm) Phenylephrine hydrochloride 40 mg, carbinoxamine maleate 8 mg. ER Tab. 100s. *Rx.*
Use: Decongestant and antihistamine.
Norel SR. (US Pharm) Phenylephrine hydrochloride 40 mg, chlorpheniramine maleate 8 mg, phenyltoloxamine citrate 50 mg, acetaminophen 325 mg. ER

Tab. 100s. *Rx.*
Use: Upper respiratory combination, decongestant, antihistamine, and analgesic.

•**norepinephrine bitartrate.** (NOR-eh-pih-NEFF-reen bye-TAR-trate) *USP. Formerly levarterenol bitartrate.*
Use: Adrenergic, vasoconstrictor, vasopressor.
See: Levophed.

norepinephrine bitartrate. (Abbott) Norepinephrine bitartrate (as base) 1 mg/mL. Sodium metabisulfite 0.46 mg, sodium chloride 8.2 mg. Inj. Amps. 4 mL. *Rx.*
Use: Vasopressor.

•**norethindrone.** (nor-ETH-in-drone) *USP.*
Use: Progestin.
See: Jolivette.
Micronor.
Nor-Q.D.
Ortho Micronor.
W/Ethinyl Estradiol.
See: Alyacen 1/35.
Alyacen 7/7/7.
Aranelle.
Balziva.
Brevicon.
Briellyn.
Cyclafem 1/35.
Cyclafem 7/7/7.
Dasetta 1/35.
Dasetta 7/7/7.
Femcon Fe.
GenCept.
Generess Fe.
Gildagia.
Heather.
Jencycla.
Jenest-28.
Junel Fe 1/20.
Junel Fe 1.5/30.
Leena.
Loestrin Fe 1/20.
Loestrin Fe 1.5/30.
Loestrin 21 1/20.
Loestrin 21 1.5/30.
Lo Loestrin Fe.
Microgestin Fe 1/20.
Microgestin Fe 1.5/30.
Modicon.
Norinyl 1 + 35.
Nortrel 1/35.
Nortrel 7/7/7.
Nortrel 0.5/35.
Ortho-Novum 1/35.
Ortho-Novum 7/7/7.
Ovcon-35.
Philith.
Pirmella 1/35.
Pirmella 7/7/7.
Tri-Legest Fe.
Tri-Norinyl.
Wera.
Wymzya Fe.
Zenchent.
W/Mestranol.
See: Necon 1/50.
Norinyl.
Norinyl 1 + 50.

norethindrone. (Barr) Norethindrone acetate 5 mg. Tab. Bot. 50s. *Rx.*
Use: Sex hormone, progestin.

norethindrone. (Glenmark Pharmaceuticals) Norethindrone 0.35 mg. Lactose. Tab. 28s. *Rx.*
Use: Oral contraceptive, progestin-only product.

•**norethindrone acetate.** (nor-ETH-in-drone) *USP.*
Use: Sex hormone, progestin.
See: Aygestin.
W/Ethinyl Estradiol.
See: Estrostep Fe.
Femhrt.
Gildess Fe 1.5/30.
Gildess 1.5/30.
Gildess 1/20.
Gildess 1/20 Fe.
Jinteli.
Junel 21 Day 1/20.
Junel 21 Day 1.5/30.
Larin Fe 1.5/30.
Larin Fe 1/20.
Loestrin 24 Fe.
Lomedia 24 Fe.
Microgestin 1/20.
Minastrin 24 Fe.
Tilia Fe.
Tri-Legest Fe.
W/Estradiol.
See: CombiPatch.
Mimvey.
W/Leuprolide Acetate.
See: Lupaneta Pack 1-Month.
Lupaneta Pack 3-Month.

norethindrone acetate/ethinyl estradiol and ferrous fumarate. (Warner Chilcott) Ethinyl estradiol 20 mcg, norethindrone acetate 1 mg. Lactose, sugar. Chew. Tab. 28s w/4 inert tablets (ferrous fumarate 75 mg, mannitol, sucralose; spearmint flavor). *Rx.*
Use: Monophasic oral contraceptive.

•**norethynodrel.** (nor-eh-THIGH-no-drell) *USP.*
Use: Hormone, progestin.
See: Enovid.

Norflex. (Graceway Pharmaceuticals) Orphenadrine citrate 30 mg/mL. Sodium bisulfite. Inj. Amp. 2 mL. *Rx.*
Use: Muscle relaxant.

•**norfloxacin.** (nor-FLOX-uh-SIN) *USP.*
Use: Anti-infective.
See: Noroxin.

•**norflurane.** (nor-FLUR-ane) USAN. Under study.
Use: Anesthetic, general.

•**norgestimate.** (nore-JEST-ih-mate) USAN. *Formerly Dexnorgestrel Acetime.*
Use: Hormone, progestin.
W/Estradiol.
See: Prefest.
W/Ethinyl Estradiol.
See: Estarylla.
MonoNessa.
Ortho-Cyclen.
Ortho Tri-Cyclen.
Previfem.
Tri-Linyah.
Tri-Previfem.

norgestimate and ethinyl estradiol. (Glenmark Pharmaceuticals) Ethinyl estradiol 35 mcg, norgestimate 0.25 mg. Lactose. Tab. 28s w/7 inert tablets (lactose). *Rx.*
Use: Monophasic oral contraceptive.

norgestimate and ethinyl estradiol. (Glenmark Pharmaceuticals) **Phase 1:** Ethinyl estradiol 35 mcg, norgestimate 0.18 mg. **Phase 2:** Ethinyl estradiol 35 mcg, norgestimate 0.215 mg. **Phase 3:** Ethinyl estradiol 35 mcg, norgestimate 0.25 mg.Lactose. Tab. 21s w/7 inert tablets. *Rx.*
Use: Triphasic oral contraceptive.

•**norgestomet.** (nore-JESS-toe-met) USAN.
Use: Hormone, progestin.

•**norgestrel.** (nor-JESS-trell) *USP.*
Use: Contraceptive; hormone, progestin.
W/Ethinyl Estradiol.
See: Elinest.
Low-Ogestrel.
Ogestrel.

•**norgestrel and ethinyl estradiol tablets.** *USP.*
Use: Contraceptive.
See: Norinyl 1 + 35.

Norinyl. (Roche) Norethindrone 2 mg, mestranol 0.1 mg. Tab. *Memorette* Disp. of 20s. Refill folders of 20s. *Rx.*
Use: Contraceptive.

Norinyl 1 + 50. (Watson) Norethindrone 1 mg, mestranol 50 mcg. Lactose. Tab. *Wallette* 28s with 7 inert tabs. *Rx.*
Use: Sex hormone, contraceptive hormone.

Norinyl 1 + 35. (Watson) Norethindrone 1 mg, ethinyl estradiol 35 mcg. Lactose. Tab. *Wallette* 28s with 7 inert tabs. *Rx.*
Use: Sex hormone, contraceptive hormone.

Norisodrine Aerosol. (Abbott) Norisodrine hydrochloride (isoproterenol hydrochloride) 0.25% (2.8 mg/mL) in inert chlorofluorohydrocarbon propellants, alcohol 33%, ascorbic acid 0.1% as preservative. Aerosol 15 mL. Box 12s. *Rx.*
Use: Bronchodilator.

Norisodrine/Calcium Iodide Syrup. (Abbott) Isoproterenol sulfate 3 mg, calcium iodide, anhydrous 150 mg/5 mL, alcohol 6%. Bot. Pt. *Rx.*
Use: Bronchodilator.

Noritate. (Valeant) Metronidazole 1%. Parabens, glycerin. Cream. Tubes. 30 g. *Rx.*
Use: Topical anti-infective; antibiotic.

Norlestrin Fe 1/50 Tablets. (Parke-Davis) Norethindrone acetate 1 mg, ethinyl estradiol 50 mcg. Compact 21 yellow Tab., 7 brown 75 mg ferrous fumarate Tab. Pkg. 5 compacts. Pkg. 5 refills; Ctn. 10 × 5 refills. *Rx.*
Use: Contraceptive.

Norlestrin Fe 2.5/50 Tablets. (Parke-Davis) Norethindrone acetate 2.5 mg, ethinyl estradiol 50 mcg. Compact 21 Tab., 7 brown 75 mg ferrous fumarate Tab. Pkg. 5 compacts. Pkg. 5 refills; Ctn. 10 × 5 refills. *Rx.*
Use: Contraceptive.

Norlestrin-28 1/50 Tablet. (Parke-Davis) Norethindrone acetate 1 mg, ethinyl estradiol 50 mcg. Compact 21 yellow, 7 white (inert) tablets. Pkg. 5 compacts. Pkg. 5 refills; Ctn. 10 × 5 refills. *Rx.*
Use: Contraceptive.

Norlestrin-21 1/50 Tablets. (Parke-Davis) Norethindrone acetate 1 mg, ethinyl estradiol 50 mcg. Compact 21s. Pkg. 5 compacts. Pkg. 5 refills; Ctn. 10 × 5 refills. *Rx.*
Use: Contraceptive.

Norlestrin-21 2.5/50 Tablets. (Parke-Davis) Norethindrone acetate 2.5 mg, ethinyl estradiol 50 mcg. Tab. Compact 21s. Pkg. 5 compacts. Pkg. 5 refills; Ctn. 10 × 5 refills. *Rx.*
Use: Contraceptive.

Normaderm Cream & Lotion. (Doak Dermatologics) Buffered lactic acid in vanishing bases. **Cream:** Jar 3 ¾ oz, 16 oz. **Lot.:** Bot. 4 oz, 16 oz, 128 oz. *OTC.*
Use: Dermatologic, emollient.

normal human serum albumin. Albumin Human.

normal human serum albumin. (Baxter Healthcare) Normal human serum albumin. **5% Inj.:** 50 mL, 250 mL, 500 mL **25% Inj.:** 20 mL, 50 mL, 100 mL. *Rx.*
Use: Blood volume supporter.

Normaline. (Apothecary Prods.) Sodium chloride 250 mg. Tab. Bot. 200s, 500s. *OTC.*
Use: Ophthalmic.

normal saline.
See: Sodium Chloride 0.9%.

Normocarb HF 35. (Apotex) Sodium 140 mEq/L, magnesium 1.5 mEq/L, chloride 106.5 mEq/L. Osmolarity 283 mOsm/L. Vial. 240 mL. *Rx.*
Use: Electrolyte.

Normocarb HF 25. (Apotex) Sodium 140 mEq/L, magnesium 1.5 mEq/L, chloride 116.5 mEq/L, bicarbonate 25 mEq/L. Osmolarity 283 mOsm/L. Vial. 240 mL. *Rx.*
Use: Electrolyte.

Normol. (Alcon) Sterile, isotonic solution of thimerosal 0.004%, chlorhexidine gluconate 0.005%, edetate disodium 0.1%. Bot. 8 oz. *OTC.*
Use: Contact lens care.

Normosol-M. (Abbott) Na^+ 40 mEq, K^+ 13 mEq, Mg^{++} 3 mEq, Cl^- 40 mEq, acetate 16 mEq, osmolarity 10% mOsm/L, pH ≈ 6. Soln. Single-dose container 1000 mL. *Rx.*
Use: Intravenous nutritional therapy, intravenous replenishment solution.

Normosol-M and 5% Dextrose. (Hospira) Dextrose 50 g, calories 170, Na^+ 40 mEq, K^+ 13 mEq, Mg^{++} 3 mEq, Cl^- 40 mEq, acetate 16 mEq, osmolarity 363 mOsm/L. Soln. Bot. 500 mL, 1000 mL. *Rx.*
Use: Intravenous nutritional therapy, intravenous replenishment solution.

Normosol-R. (Hospira) Na^+ 140 mEq, K^+ 5 mEq, Mg^{++} 3 mEq, Cl^- 98 mEq, acetate 27 mEq, gluconate 23 mEq, osmolarity 294 mOsm/L, preservative free, ph ≈ 6. Soln. Single-dose container 500 mL, 1000 mL. *Rx.*
Use: Intravenous nutritional therapy, intravenous replenishment solution.

Normosol-R and 5% Dextrose. (Abbott) Dextrose 50 g, calories 185, Na^+ 140 mEq, K^+ 5 mEq, Mg^{++} 3 mEq, Cl^- 98 mEq, acetate 27 mEq, gluconate 23 mEq, osmolarity 547 mOsm/L. Soln. Bot. 500 mL, 1000 mL. *Rx.*
Use: Intravenous nutritional therapy, intravenous replenishment solution.

Normosol-R pH 7.4. (Abbott) Na^+ 140 mEq, K^+ 5 mEq, Mg^{++} 3 mEq, Cl^- 98 mEq, acetate 27 mEq, gluconate 23 mEq, osmolarity 295 mOsm/L, preservative free. Soln. Single-dose container 500 mL, 1000 mL. *Rx.*
Use: Intravenous nutritional therapy, intravenous replenishment solution.

Normotensin. (Marcen) Mucopolysaccharide 20 mg, sodium nucleate 25 mg, epinephrine-neutralizing factor 25 units, sodium citrate 10 mg, inositol 5 mg, phenol 0.5%/mL. IM Soln. for Inj. Multidose vial 10 mL, 30 mL. *Rx.*
Use: Antihypertensive.

Norolon. (Sanofi-Synthelabo) Chloroquine phosphate. *Rx.*
Use: Antimalarial.

Noroxin. (Merck & Co.) Norfloxacin 400 mg. Tab. 100s, UD 20s. *Rx.*
Use: Urinary anti-infective, fluoroquinolone.

Norpace. (Pharmacia) Disopyramide phosphate 100 mg, 150 mg, lactose. Cap. Bot. 100s, 1000s. *Rx.*
Use: Antiarrhythmic.

Norpace CR. (Pharmacia) Disopyramide phosphate 100 mg, 150 mg, sucrose. ER Cap. Bot. 100s, 500s, UD 100s. *Rx.*
Use: Antiarrhythmic.

Norphyl. (Vita Elixir) Aminophylline 100 mg. Tab. *Rx.*
Use: Bronchodilator.

Norpramin. (Sanofi Aventis) Desipramine hydrochloride 10 mg, 25 mg, 50 mg, 75 mg, 100 mg, 150 mg. Mannitol, sucrose. Film-coated. Tab. 50s (150 mg only), 100s (except 150 mg). *Rx.*
Use: Antidepressant.

Nor-QD. (Watson) Norethindrone 0.35 mg. Lactose. Tab. 28s. *Rx.*
Use: Sex hormone, contraceptive hormone.

Nortemp Children's. (Ballay) Acetaminophen 160 mg/5 mL. Alcohol free. Butylparaben, corn syrup, sorbitol. Cotton candy flavor. Oral Susp. 118 mL. *OTC.*
Use: Analgesic.

Nortemp Infants' Drops. (Ballay) Acetaminophen 100 mg/mL. Methylparaben, propylene glycol, saccharin, sodium benzoate. Alcohol free and sugar free. Cherry flavor. Soln., concentrate. 30 mL w/dropper. *OTC.*
Use: Analgesic.

Northera. (Chelsea Therapeutics) Droxidopa 100 mg, 200 mg, 300 mg. Mannitol. Cap. 90s. *Rx.*
Use: Vasopressor.

Northyx. (Centrix) Methimazole 5 mg, 10 mg, 15 mg, 20 mg. Lactose. Tab. 100s. *Rx.*
Use: Thyroid drug, antithyroid agent.

Nortrel 1/35. (Barr) Ethinyl estradiol 35 mcg, norethindrone 1 mg. Lactose. Tab. Pkt. 21s, 28s (7 inert tabs.). *Rx.*
Use: Sex hormone, contraceptive hormone.

Nortrel 7/7/7. (Barr) **Phase 1:** Norethindrone 0.5 mg, ethinyl estradiol 35 mcg. **Phase 2:** Norethindrone 0.75 mg, ethinyl estradiol 35 mcg. **Phase 3:** Norethindrone 1 mg, ethinyl estradiol 35 mcg.Lactose. Tab. 21s w/7 white inert tablets. *Rx.*
Use: Oral contraceptive.

Nortrel 0.5/35. (Barr) Ethinyl estradiol 35 mcg, norethindrone 0.5 mg. Lactose. Tab. Pkt. 21s, 28s (7 inert tabs.). *Rx.*
Use: Sex hormone, contraceptive hormone.

nortriptyline. (Various Mfr.) Nortriptyline 10 mg, 25 mg, 50 mg, 75 mg. Cap. 100s, 500s. *Rx.*
Use: Antidepressant.

•**nortriptyline hydrochloride.** (nor-TRIP-tih-leen) *USP.*
Use: Antidepressant.
See: Pamelor.

nortriptyline hydrochloride. (Various Mfr.). **Soln.:** Nortriptyline base 10 mg/5 mL. Alcohol 4%, sorbitol. Bot. 480 mL. **Cap.:** Nortriptyline hydrochloride 10 mg, 25 mg, 50 mg, 75 mg. Bot. 100s, 500s, 1,000s; blister pack 25s (except 75 mg), 100s, 600s; UD 100s (except 75 mg). *Rx.*
Use: Antidepressant.

Norval. Docusate sodium.
Use: Laxative.

Norvasc. (Pfizer) Amlodipine. **2.5 mg:** Bot. 90s, 100s; **5 mg:** Bot. 90s, 100s, 300s, UD 100s; **10 mg:** Bot. 90s, 100s, UD 100s. *Rx.*
Use: Calcium channel blocker.

Norvir. (AbbVie) Ritonavir. **Soft Gel Cap.:** 100 mg. Bot. 30s, 120s. **Oral Soln.:** 80 mg/mL. Saccharin, ethanol, peppermint and caramel flavors. Bot. 240 mL. **Tab.:** 100 mg. Film coated. Sorbitan. 30s. *Rx.*
Use: Antiretroviral, protease inhibitor.

Norwich Extra Strength. (Lee) Aspirin 500 mg. Tab. Bot. 150s. *OTC.*
Use: Analgesic.

Norwich Regular Strength. (Lee) Aspirin 325 mg. Coated. Tab. 100s. *OTC.*
Use: Analgesic.

Nosalt. (GlaxoSmithKline) Potassium Cl, potassium bitartrate, adipic acid, mineral oil, fumaric acid. Na < 10 mg/5 g (0.43 mEq/5 g), K 2502 mg/5 g (64 mEq/5 g). Pkg. 330 g. *OTC.*
Use: Salt substitute.

Nosalt Seasoned. (GlaxoSmithKline) Potassium Cl, dextrose, onion, and garlic, spices, lactose, cream of tartar, paprika, silica, disodium inosinate, disodium guanylate, turmeric. Na < 5 mg/5 g (0.2 mEq/5 g), K 1328 mg/5 g (34 mEq/5 g). Pkg. 240 g. *OTC.*
Use: Salt substitute.

•**noscapine.** (NAHS-kah-peen) *USP.*
Use: Antitussive.

noscapine hydrochloride. l-Narcotine-hydrochloride.
Use: Antitussive.
See: Noscaps.

Noscaps. (Table Rock) Noscapine 7.5 mg, chlorpheniramine maleate 1 mg, phenylephrine hydrochloride 5 mg, N-acetyl-p-aminophenol 150 mg, salicylamide 150 mg, vitamin C 20 mg. Cap. Bot. 100s, 500s. *OTC.*
Use: Analgesic; antihistamine; decongestant; vitamin C.

Nose Better. (Oakhurst) Allantoin 0.5%, camphor 0.75%, menthol 0.5%. Lanolin, methylparaben. Gel. Tube 12.9 g. *OTC.*
Use: Upper respiratory combination, topical.

Noskote. (Schering-Plough) Oxybenzone 3%, homosalate 8%. SPF 8. Cream 13.2 g, 30 g. *OTC.*
Use: Sunscreen.

Noskote Sunblock. (Schering-Plough) Padimate O 8%, oxybenzone 3%, benzyl alcohol. SPF 15. Cream. Tube 30 g. *OTC.*
Use: Sunscreen.

Nostril. (Boehringer Ingelheim) Phenylephrine hydrochloride 0.25%, 0.5%, benzalkonium Cl 0.004% in buffered aqueous soln. Bot. 15 mL, pump spray. *OTC.*
Use: Decongestant.

Nōstrilla Complete Congestion Relief 12-Hour. (Insight) Oxymetazoline hydrochloride 0.05%. Benzalkonium chloride, camphor, edetate disodium, eucalyptol, menthol. Soln., Intranasal Spray. 15 mL. *OTC.*
Use: Nasal decongestant, imidazoline.

Nōstrilla Conditioning Double Moisture. (Insight) Oxymetazoline hydrochloride 0.05%. Benzalkonium chloride, eucalyptol, sodium chloride, spearmint oil, winter green oil. Soln., Intranasal Spray. 15 mL. *OTC.*
Use: Nasal decongestant, imidazoline.

Nōstrilla 12-Hour. (Insight) Oxymetazoline hydrochloride 0.05%, benzalkonium chloride, glycine, sorbitol. Soln. Spray bot. 15 mL. *OTC.*
Use: Nasal decongestant, imidazoline.

Notuss-Forte. (SJ Pharmaceutical) Chlorpheniramine maleate 4 mg, hydrocodone bitartrate 5 mg, pseudoephedrine hydrochloride 40 mg. Saccharin,

sorbitol. Alcohol free, dye free, gluten free, and sugar free. Vanilla flavor. Syr. 473 mL. *c-III.*
Use: Upper respiratory combination, antitussive combination.

Nouriva Repair. (Ferndale) Petrolatum, paraffin, mineral oil, sorbitan oleate, carnauba wax, ceramide 3, cholesterol, glycerin, oleic acid, palmitic acid, acrylates/C 10–30 albyl acrylate crosspolymer, tromethamine. Cream. 30 g. *OTC.*
Use: Emollient.

Novacort. (Primus) Hydrocortisone acetate 2%, pramoxine 1%. Alcohols, aloe, glycerin. Gel. Tubes. 29 g. *Rx.*
Use: Anti-inflammatory agent.

Nova-Dec. (Rugby) Iron 18 mg, vitamins A 5000 units, D 400 units, E 30 units, B_1 1.7 mg, B_2 2 mg, B_3 20 mg, B_5 10 mg, B_6 3 mg, B_{12} 6 mcg, C 60 mg, folic acid 0.4 mg, Ca, Cr, Cu, I, Mg, Mo, Mn, P, Se, K, Zn 15 mg, vitamin K, Cl, Ni, Sn, V, B, biotin 30 mcg. Tab. Bot. 130s. *OTC.*
Use: Mineral, vitamin supplement.

Novadyne Expectorant. (Various Mfr.) Pseudoephedrine 30 mg, codeine phosphate 10 mg, guaifenesin 100 mg/5 mL, alcohol 7.5%. Bot. 120 mL, pt, gal. *c-III.*
Use: Antitussive; decongestant; expectorant.

NovaFerrum 50. (Gensavis) Polysaccharide iron complex 50 mg. Cap. 90s. *OTC.*
Use: Trace element.

NovaFerrum Liquid Pediatric. (Gensavis) Polysaccharide iron complex 15 mg per mL. Benzoate, glycerin, potassium sorbate. Raspberry grape flavor. Soln., concentrate. 120 mL. *OTC.*
Use: Trace element.

NovaFerrum 125. (Gensavis) Polysaccharide iron complex 125 mg, vitamin D_3 100 units per 5 mL. Glycerin, potassium sorbate, sodium benzoate. Alcohol free and sugar free. Raspberry grape flavor. Liq. 180 mL. *OTC.*
Use: Trace element.

Novagest Expectorant with Codeine. (Major) Pseudoephedrine hydrochloride 30 mg, codeine phosphate 10 mg, guaifenesin 100 mg per 5 mL. Alcohol 8.2%, sugar, menthol, parabens. Liq. Bot. 118 mL, 473 mL. *c-v.*
Use: Upper respiratory combination, antitussive, decongestant, expectorant.

Novahistine DH. (Deston Therapeutics) Dihydrocodeine bitartrate 7.25 mg, chlorpheniramine maleate 2 mg, phenylephrine hydrochloride 5 mg per 5 mL. Alcohol and sugar free. EDTA, parabens, saccharin, sorbitol. Strawberry flavor. Liq. 473 mL. *c-III.*
Use: Antitussive combination.

novamidon.
See: Aminopyrine.

Novamine. (Clintec Nutrition) Amino acid concentration 11.4%, for infusion. Nitrogen 1.8 g/100 mL. Essential amino acids (mg/100 mL): Isoleucine 570, leucine 790, lysine 900, methionine 570, phenylalanine 790, threonine 570, tryptophan 190, valine 730. Nonessential amino acids (mg/100 mL): Alanine 1650, arginine 1120, histidine 680, proline 680, serine 450, tyrosine 30, glycine 790, glutamic acid 570, aspartic acid 330, acetate 114 mEq/L, sodium metabisulfite 30 mg/100 mL. In 250 mL, 500 mL, 1 liter. *Rx.*
Use: Parenteral nutritional supplement.

Novamine Without Electrolytes. (Clintec Nutrition) Amino acid concentration 8.5%, for infusion. Nitrogen 1.35 g/100 mL. Essential amino acids (mg/100 mL): Isoleucine 420, leucine 590, lysine 673, methionine 420, phenylalanine 590, threonine 420, tryptophan 140, valine 550. Nonessential amino acids (mg/100 mL): Alanine 1240, arginine 840, histidine 500, proline 500, serine 340, tyrosine 20, glycine 590, glutamic acid 420, aspartic acid 250, acetate 88 mEq/L, sodium bisulfite 30 mg/100 mL. In 500 mL, 1 liter. *Rx.*
Use: Nutritional supplement, parenteral.

Novarel. (Ferring) Chorionic gonadotropin 10,000 units per vial with 10 mL diluent (1,000 units per mL), mannitol, benzyl alcohol 0.9%. Pow. for Inj. Vials. 10 mL. *Rx.*
Use: Ovulation stimulant.

NovaSource Renal. (Novartis Nutrition) Protein (sodium and calcium caseinates, arginine, taurine, carnitine) 74 g, carbohydrates (corn syrup, fructose, hydrolyzed corn starch) 200 g, fat (high oleic sunflower oil, corn oil, medium chain triglycerides, soy lecithin) 100 g/L, vitamins A, B_1, B_2, B_3, B_5, B_6, B_{12}, C, D, E, K, folic acid, biotin, choline, Ca chloride, Cu, Fe, I, Mg, Mn, P, Se, Zn, Na 1000 mg (43.5 mEq)/L, Na 1600 mg/complete feeding *Brik* Paks) (70 mEq)/L (closed system), K 810 mg (20.8 mEq)/L, K 1100 mg/complete feeding *Brik* Paks (28.2 mEq)/L (closed system), H_2O 700 mOsm/kg (complete feeding *Brik* Paks), H_20 960 mOsm/kg (closed system), 2 cal/mL, vanilla flavor. Liq. *Tetra Brik* Paks 237 mL (27s),

closed system containers 1000 mL (6s). *OTC.*
Use: Enteral nutritional therapy.

novatropine.
See: Homatropine Methylbromide.

Novocain. (Abbott) Procaine hydrochloride 1%, 10%. Inj. *Uni-Amp* 2 mL. Single-dose amp. 6 mL w/acetone sodium bisulfite (1% only). Multidose vial 30 mL w/acetone sodium bisulfite, chlorobutanol (1% only). *Rx.*
Use: Anesthetic, local ester.

Novocain for Spinal Anesthesia. (Sanofi-Synthelabo) Procaine hydrochloride 10% soln. Amp. 2 mL. Box 25s. *Rx.*
Use: Anesthetic, spinal.

Novoeight. (Novo Nordisk) Antihemophilic factor (recombinant) 250 units, 500 units, 1,000 units, 1,500 units, 2,000 units, 3,000 units. Polysorbate 80, sucrose, sodium chloride. Preservative free. Inj., lyophilized Pow. for Soln. Single-use vial w/diluent and adapter. *Rx.*
Use: Antihemophilic factor.

Novolin N. (Novo Nordisk) Human insulin (rDNA) 100 units/mL. Inj. Vials. 10 mL. *OTC.*
Tall Man: NovoLIN
Use: Antidiabetic, insulin.

Novolin N PenFill. (Novo Nordisk) Human insulin (rDNA) 100 units/mL. Cartridges. 5 × 1.5. Use with *NovoPen* and *Novolin Pen. OTC.*
Tall Man: NovoLIN
Use: Antidiabetic, insulin.

Novolin N Prefilled. (Novo Nordisk) Human insulin (rDNA) 100 units/mL. Inj. Prefilled syringes. 5 × 1.5 mL. *OTC.*
Tall Man: NovoLIN
Use: Antidiabetic, insulin.

Novolin R. (Novo Nordisk) Human insulin (rDNA) 100 units/mL. Inj. Vials. 10 mL. *OTC.*
Tall Man: NovoLIN
Use: Antidiabetic, insulin.

Novolin R PenFill. (Novo Nordisk) Human insulin (rDNA) 100 units/mL. Cartridges. 5 × 1.5. Use with *NovoPen* and *Novolin Pen. OTC.*
Tall Man: NovoLIN
Use: Antidiabetic, insulin.

Novolin R Prefilled. (Novo Nordisk) Human insulin (rDNA) 100 units/mL. Inj. Prefilled syringes. 5 × 1.5 mL. *OTC.*
Tall Man: NovoLIN
Use: Antidiabetic, insulin.

Novolin 70/30. (Novo Nordisk) Human insulin (rDNA) 100 units/mL. Inj. Vials. 10 mL. *OTC.*
Tall Man: NovoLIN
Use: Antidiabetic, insulin.

Novolin 70/30 PenFill. (Novo Nordisk) Human insulin (rDNA) 100 units/mL. Cartridges. 5 × 1.5 mL. Use with *NovoPen* and *Novolin Pen. OTC.*
Tall Man: NovoLIN
Use: Antidiabetic, insulin.

Novolin 70/30 Prefilled. (Novo Nordisk) Human insulin (rDNA) 100 units/mL. Inj. Prefilled syringes. 5 × 1.5 mL. *OTC.*
Tall Man: NovoLIN
Use: Antidiabetic, insulin.

NovoLog. (Novo Nordisk) Human insulin aspart 100 units/mL. Metacresol 1.72 mg/mL. Inj. *PenFill* cartridges. 3 mL. Vials. 10 mL. *FlexPen* prefilled syringes. 3 mL. *Rx.*
Tall Man: NovoLOG
Use: Antidiabetic, insulin.

NovoSeven RT. (Novo Nordisk) Coagulation factor VIIa, recombinant 1 mg, 2 mg, 5 mg, 8 mg. Preservative free. Inj., lyophilized Pow. for Soln. Single-use vial w/histidine diluent. *Rx.*
Use: Hematological agent, antihemophilic agent.

Noxafil. (Schering Corporation) Posaconazole. **Susp.:** 40 mg/mL. Polysorbate 80, sodium benzoate, glucose, glycerin. Cherry flavored. 105 mL with calibrated dosing spoon. **Tab., delayed release:** 100 mg. Film coated. Alcohol, PEG. 60s. *Rx.*
Use: Antifungal agent, triazole antifungal.

Noxzema Antiseptic Cleanser Sensitive Skin Formula. (Noxell Corp.) Benzalkonium Cl 0.13%. Bot. 4 oz, 8 oz. *OTC.*
Use: Dermatologic, cleanser.

Noxzema Antiseptic Skin Cleanser. (Noxell Corp.) SD 40 alcohol 63%. Bot. 4 oz, 8 oz. *OTC.*
Use: Dermatologic, cleanser.

Noxzema Antiseptic Skin Cleanser Extra Strength Formula. (Noxell Corp.) SD 40 alcohol 36%, isopropyl alcohol 34%. Bot. 4 oz, 8 oz. *OTC.*
Use: Dermatologic, cleanser.

Noxzema Clear Ups. (Noxell Corp.) Salicylic acid 0.5% on pads. Jar 50s. *OTC.*
Use: Dermatologic, acne.

Noxzema Clear Ups Acne Medicine Maximum Strength Lotion. (Noxell Corp.) Benzoyl peroxide 10%. Bot. 1 oz. Vanishing formula. *OTC.*
Use: Dermatologic, acne.

Noxzema Clear Ups Maximum Strength. (Noxell Corp.) Salicylic acid 2% on pads. Jar. 50s. *OTC.*
Use: Dermatologic, acne.

Noxzema Medicated Skin Cream. (Noxell Corp.) Menthol, camphor, clove oil, eucalyptus oil, phenol. Jar 2.5 oz, 4 oz, 6 oz, 10 oz. Tube 4.5 oz. Bot. 6 oz., 14 oz. Pump Bottle 10.5 oz. *OTC.*
Use: Counterirritant.

Noxzema On-The-Spot. (Noxell Corp.) Benzoyl peroxide 10% in vanishing and tinted lotion. Bot. 0.25 oz. *OTC.*
Use: Dermatologic, acne.

Nplate. (Amgen) Romiplostim 250 mcg, 500 mcg. Mannitol, sucrose, L-histidine, polysorbate 20. Preservative free. Inj., lyophilized Pow. for Soln. Single-use vial. 250 mcg, 500 mcg. *Rx.*
Use: Hematopoietic agent, thrombopoietin mimetic agent.

NP Thyroid. (Acella Pharmaceuticals) Thyroid dessicated (porcine derived) 30 mg (½ gr), 60 mg (1 gr), 90 mg (1½ gr). Dextrose, maltodextrin, mineral oil. Tab. 100s. *Rx.*
Use: Thyroid hormone.

NRS Nasal Relief. (Rugby) Oxymetazoline hydrochloride 0.05%. Benzalkonium chloride, EDTA, sodium chloride. Spray. 15 mL. *OTC.*
Use: Nasal decongestant, imidazoline.

NTS Transdermal System. (Circa) Nitroglycerin transdermal system 5 mg/24 hours or 15 mg/24 hours. Box 30s. *Rx.*
Use: Antianginal.

NTZ Long-Acting. (Sanofi-Synthelabo) Oxymetazoline hydrochloride 0.05%, benzalkonium Cl, phenylmercuric acetate 0.002% as preservatives. Drops. Bot. 1 oz. Spray Bot. 1 oz. *OTC.*
Use: Decongestant.

Nubain. (Endo) Nalbuphine hydrochloride 10 mg/mL, 20 mg/mL. Parabens. Amp (available as sulfite/paraben free) 1 mL. Vial 10 mL. *Rx.*
Use: Narcotic agonist-antagonist analgesic.

Nu-Bolic. (Seatrace) Nandrolone phenpropionate 25 mg/mL. Vial 5 mL. *c-III.*
Use: Anabolic steroid.

nucite.
See: Inositol.

nucleoside analog reverse transcriptase inhibitor combinations.
Use: Antiretroviral.
See: Abacavir/Lamivudine.
Emtricitabine/Tenofovir/Disoproxil Fumarate.
Lamivudine And Zidovudine.

nucleoside reverse transcriptase inhibitors.
Use: Antiretroviral.
See: Abacavir Sulfate.
Didanosine.
Emtricitabine.
Lamivudine.
Stavudine.
Telbivudine.
Zalcitabine.
Zidovudine.

nucleotide analog reverse transcriptase inhibitor.
Use: Antiretroviral.
See: Tenofovir Disoproxil Fumarate.

Nu-COPD. (CarWin Associates) Guaifenesin 400 mg, phenylephrine hydrochloride 10 mg. Tab. 100s. *OTC.*
Use: Upper respiratory combination, decongestant and expectorant combination.

NuCort. (WraSer) Hydrocortisone acetate 2%. Aloe, benzyl alcohol, camphor, cetyl alcohol, glycerin, glyceryl stearate, PEG-7. Lot. 60 mL. *Rx.*
Use: Anti-inflammatory agent; corticosteroid, topical.

Nucotuss Expectorant. (Alpharma) Pseudoephedrine hydrochloride 60 mg, codeine phosphate 20 mg, guaifenesin 200 mg per 5 mL. Alcohol 12.5%. Syrup. Bot. 473 mL. *c-III.*
Use: Upper respiratory combination, antitussive, decongestant, expectorant.

Nucotuss Pediatric Expectorant. (Alpharma) Pseudoephedrine hydrochloride 30 mg, codeine phosphate 10 mg, guaifenesin 100 mg per 5 mL. Alcohol 6%, strawberry flavor. Syrup. Bot. 473 mL. *c-V.*
Use: Upper respiratory combination, antitussive, decongestant, expectorant.

Nucynta. (Janssen Pharmaceuticals) Tapentadol hydrochloride. **Tab.:** 50 mg, 75 mg, 100 mg. Film coated. Lactose. 100s, UD 10s. **Soln.:** 20 mg/mL (equiv. to tapentadol hydrochloride 23 mg/mL). Sucralose, raspberry flavoring. 100 mL and 200 mL w/calibrated dosing syringe. *c-II.*
Use: CNS agent, opioid analgesic.

Nucynta ER. (Janssen Pharmaceuticals) Tapentadol 50 mg (equiv. to tapentadol hydrochloride 58.24 mg), 100 mg (equiv. to tapentadol hydrochloride 116.48 mg), 150 mg (equiv. to tapentadol hydrochloride 174.72 mg), 200 mg (equiv. to tapentadol hydrochloride 232.96 mg), 250 mg (equiv. to tapentadol hydrochloride 291.2 mg). Film coated. PEG. ER Tab. 60s, UD 10s. *c-II.*
Use: Opioid analgesic.

Nuedexta. (Avanir) Dextromethorphan hydrobromide 20 mg/quinidine sulfate

10 mg. Lactose. Cap. 60s. *Rx.*
Use: Psychotherapeutic combination.

•**nufenoxole.** (NEW-fen-OX-ole) USAN.
Use: Antiperistaltic.

Nuhist. (Dayton) Phenylephrine tannate 5 mg, chlorpheniramine tannate 4.5 mg per 5 mL. Methylparaben, saccharin, sucrose. Susp. 473 mL. *Rx.*
Use: Decongestant and antihistamine.

Nu-Iron 150. (Merz) Polysaccharide-iron complex equivalent to 150 mg iron. Parabens, EDTA, castor oil, sucrose. Cap. Bot. 100s. *OTC.*
Use: Mineral supplement.

Nu-Iron Plus Elixir. (Merz) Polysaccharide iron complex 300 mg, folic acid 3 mg, vitamin B_{12} 75 mcg/15 mL. Bot. 237 mL. *Rx.*
Use: Mineral, vitamin supplement.

Nu-Iron-V. (Merz) Polysaccharide iron 60 mg, folic acid 1 mg, vitamins A 4000 units, C 50 mg, D 400 units, B_1 3 mg, B_2 3 mg, B_3 10 mg, B_6 2 mg, B_{12} 3 mcg, Ca. Tab. Bot. 100s. *Rx.*
Use: Mineral, vitamin supplement.

Nulecit. (Watson Labs) Elemental iron 12.5 mg/mL (as sodium ferric gluconate complex). Benzyl alcohol 9 mg/mL, sucrose 20%. Inj., Soln. Vial. 5 mL. *Rx.*
Use: Trace element.

NuLev. (Meda Pharmaceuticals) Hyoscyamine sulfate 0.125 mg. Lactose, mannitol. Peppermint flavor. Chew. Tab., dispersible. 100s. *Rx.*
Use: Anticholinergic/antispasmodic, belladonna alkaloid.

Nullo. (Monticello) Chlorophyllin copper complex 100 mg. Coated. Tab. 60s, 135s. *OTC.*
Use: Gastrointestinal agent, systemic deodorizer.

Nulojix. (Bristol-Myers Squibb) Belatacept 250 mg. Sucrose. Inj., lyophilized Pow. for Soln. Single-use vial w/silicone-free disposable syringe. *Rx.*
Use: Immunologic agent, immunosuppressive.

Nul-Tach. (Davis & Sly) Potassium 16 mg, magnesium 13 mg, ascorbic acid 250 mg. Tab. Bot. 100s. *Rx.*
Use: Antiarrythmic.

NuLYTELY. (Braintree) PEG 3350 420 g, sodium bicarbonate 5.72 g, sodium chloride 11.2 g, potassium chloride 1.48 g, cherry, lemon-lime, orange flavors. Pow. for Recon. Disp. Jugs 4 L. *Rx.*
Use: Laxative.

Numby Stuff. (Iomed) Lidocaine hydrochloride 2% for iontophoretic dermal delivery. Epinephrine 1:100,000 per 30 mL multiple-unit fliptop vial. *Rx.*
Use: Topical local anesthetic, amide local anesthetic.

Numoisyn. (Align) **Loz.:** Sorbitol 0.3 g, polyethylene glycol, malic acid, sodium citrate, calcium phosphate dibasic, hydrogenated cottonseed oil, citric acid, magnesium stearate, silicon dioxide. 100s. **Soln.:** Sorbitol, linseed (flaxseed) extract, *Chondrus crispus*, parabens, sodium benzoate, potassium sorbate, dipotassium phosphate. 30 mL, 300 mL. *Rx.*
Use: Saliva substitute.

Numotizine Cataplasm. (Hobart) Guaiacol 0.26 g, beechwood creosote 1.302 g, methyl salicylate 0.26 g/100 g. Jar 4 oz. *OTC.*
Use: Analgesic, topical.

Numotizine Cough Syrup. (Hobart) Guaifenesin 5 g, ammonium Cl 5 g, sodium citrate 20 g, menthol 0.04 g/fl oz. Bot. 3 oz, pt, gal. *OTC.*
Use: Expectorant.

Nu-Natal Advanced. (Rising) Ca 200 mg, Fe (as carbonyl iron) 90 mg, vitamin D 400 units, E 30 units, B_1 3 mg, B_2 3.4 mg, B_3 20 mg, B_6 20 mg, B_{12}12 mcg, C 120 mg, FA 1 mg, CU 2 mg, Mg, dioctyl sodium sulfosuccinate 50 mg, Zn 25 mg. Mineral oil. Film-coated. Tab. UD 90s. *Rx.*
Use: Multivitamin.

Nunol.
See: Phenobarbital.

NuOx. (Gentex) Benzoyl peroxide 6%, sulfur 3%. Benzyl alcohol, disodium EDTA, glycerin. Gel. 43 g. *Rx.*
Use: Acne product combination.

Nupercainal. (Ciba Consumer) Dibucaine 1%. Acetone, sodium bisulfite, lanolin, mineral oil, white petrolatum. Oint. 30 g, 60 g. *OTC.*
Use: Topical local anesthetic.

Nuquin HP. (Stratus) **Cream:** 4% hydroquinone, octyl methoxycinnamate, glycerin, cetyl alcohol, cetostearyl alcohol, stearyl alcohol, sodium metabisulfite. Tube 14.2 g, 28.4 g, 56.7 g. **Gel:** 4% hydroquinone, 30 mg dioxybenzone per g. Alcohol, sodium metabisulfite, EDTA. Tube 14.2 g, 28.4 g. *Rx.*
Use: Dermatologic.

Nu-Salt. (Cumberland Packing Corp.) Potassium Cl, potassium bitartrate, calcium silicate, natural flavor derived from yeast. Sodium 0.85 mg/5 g (< 0.04 mEq/5 g), potassium 2640 mg/5 g (68 mEq/5 g). Pkg. 90 g. *OTC.*
Use: Salt substitute.

Nu-Tears. (Optopics) Polyvinyl alcohol

1.4%, EDTA, NaCl, benzalkonium chloride, potassium chloride. Soln. Bot. 15 mL. *OTC.*
Use: Artificial tears.

Nu-Tears II. (Optopics) Polyvinyl alcohol 1%, PEG-400 1%, EDTA, benzalkonium chloride. Soln. Bot. 15 mL. *OTC.*
Use: Artificial tears.

Nu-Thera. (Kirkman) Vitamins A 10,000 units, D 400 units, B_1 10 mg, B_2 5 mg, niacinamide 100 mg, B_6 1 mg, B_{12} 5 mcg, C 150 mg, Ca 103 mg, P 80 mg, Fe 10 mg, Mg 5.5 mg, Mn 1 mg, K 5 mg, Zn 1.4 mg. Cap. Bot. 100s. *OTC.*
Use: Mineral, vitamin supplement.

nutmeg oil.
Use: Pharmaceutic aid, flavor.

Nutracort. (Galderma) Hydrocortisone 1%. Cream Jar 4 oz. Tube 30 g, 60 g. *Rx.*
Use: Corticosteroid, topical.

Nutraderm. (Galderma) Oil-in-water emulsion. **Lot.:** Plastic bot. 8 oz, 16 oz. **Cream:** Tube 1.5 oz, 3 oz, Jar lb. *OTC.*
Use: Emollient.

Nutraderm Advanced Formula. (Valeant Pharmaceuticals) Glycerin, white petrolatum, alcohols, cholesterol, urea, parabens. Lot. 473 mL. *OTC.*
Use: Emollient.

Nutraderm Bath Oil. (Galderma) Mineral oil, PEG-4 dilaurate, lanolin oil, butylparaben, benzophenone-3, fragrance, D & C Green No. 6. Bot. 8 oz. *OTC.*
Use: Emollient.

Nutraloric. (Nutraloric) A chocolate, vanilla, or strawberry flavored liquid containing, when mixed with whole milk to make 1 L, 91.7 g protein, 175 g carbohydrates, 125 g fat, 875 mg Na, 3166.7 mg, K 2.2 calories/mL. Pow. Can 480 g. *OTC.*
Use: Nutritional supplement.

Nutrament Drink Box. (Drackett) Protein 10 g, fat 7 g, carbohydrate 35 g, vitamins, minerals/240 calories/8 oz. Liq. Drink Box. *OTC.*
Use: Nutritional supplement.

Nutrament Liquid. (Mead Johnson Nutritionals) Protein (calcium and sodium caseinates, skim milk, soy protein isolates [in all flavors except chocolate]) 44.5 g, carbohydrate (sugar, corn syrup) 144.6 g, fat (canola oil, high oleic sunflower oil, corn oil, soy lecithin) 27.8 g/L, vitamins A, B_1, B_2, B_3, B_5, B_6, B_{12}, C, D, E, K, biotin, folate, Ca, Cr, Cu, Fe, I, Mg, Mn, Mo, P, Se, Zn, Na 695 mg, K 1390 mg/L, 1 cal/mL, vanilla, strawberry, chocolate, banana, coconut, and eggnog flavors. Liq. Can. 12 oz. *OTC.*
Use: Nutritional supplement.

Nutramigen. (Bristol-Myers Squibb) Hypoallergenic formula that supplies 640 calories/qt. Protein 18 g, fat 25 g, carbohydrates 86 g, vitamins A 2000 units, D 400 units, E 20 units, C 52 mg, folic acid 100 mcg, B_1 0.5 mg, B_2 0.6 mg, niacin 8 mg, B_6 0.4 mg, B_{12} 2 mcg, biotin 50 mcg, pantothenic acid 3 mg, K-1 100 mcg, Cl 85 mg, inositol 30 mg, Ca 600 mg, P 400 mg, I 45 mcg, Fe 12 mg, Mg 70 mg, Cu 0.6 mg, Zn 5 mg, Mn 200 mcg, Cl 550 mg, K 700 mg, Na 300 mg/qt of formula (4.9 oz pow.). Liq. Can 16 oz, 390 mL concentrate, 1 qt ready-to-use. *OTC.*
Use: Nutritional supplement.

Nutramin. (Thurston) Vitamins A 666 units, D 66 units, B_1 666 mcg, B_2 333 mcg, niacinamide 2 mg, folic acid 0.0444 mcg, Ca 16.6 mg, P 8.33 mg, Fe 1.33 mg, I 0.15 mg. Tab. Bot. 200s, 500s, 1000s. *OTC.*
Use: Mineral, vitamin supplement.

Nutramin Granular. (Thurston) Vitamins A 333 units, D 333 units, B_1 3.3 mg, B_2 1.6 mg, niacinamide 10 mg, folic acid 0.133 mg, Ca 250 mg, P 115 mg, Fe 6.6 mg, I 0.15 mg/5 g. Bot. 10 oz, 32 oz. *OTC.*
Use: Mineral, vitamin supplement.

Nutraplus. (Valeant) Urea 10% in emollient cream base or lotion base with preservatives. **Cream:** Tube 3 oz, Jar lb. **Lot.:** Glyceryl, lanolin alcohol, parabens, PEG, wax, white petrolatum. 236 mL. *OTC.*
Use: Emollient.

Nutra-Soothe. (Pertussin) Colloidal oatmeal, light mineral oil. Emollient bath preparation. Pow. Pkts. 9s. *OTC.*
Use: Dermatologic.

Nutravance. (Breckenridge) Vitamins A 3,000 units, B_1 20 mg, B_2 5 mg, B_3 25 mg, B_5 15 mg, B_6 25 mg, B_{12} 50 mcg, C 300 mg, D_3 400 units, E 100 units, Cr, Cu, Mg, Mn, Se, Zn, alpha-lipoic acid 15 mg, biotin 100 mcg, lutein 5 mg. Film coated. PEG. Tab. 100s. *Rx.*
Use: Multivitamin with minerals (except iron).

Nutravims. (Health for Life Brands) Vitamins A 6000 units, D 1250 units, C 50 mg, E 5 units, B_{12} 5 mcg, B_1 3 mg, B_2 3 mg, B_6 0.5 mg, niacinamide 20 mg, calcium pantothenate 5 mg, Zn 1.5 mg, Mn 1 mg, I 0.15 mg, K 5 mg, Mg 4 mg, Fe 15 mg, Ca 59 mg, P 45 mg. Cap. Bot. 100s, 250s, 1000s. *OTC.*
Use: Mineral, vitamin supplement.

Nutren 1.5 Liquid. (Clintec Nutrition) Casein, maltodextrin, corn syrup, sucrose, MCT, corn oil, vitamins A, B_1, B_2, B_3, B_5, B_6, B_{12}, C, D, E, K, folic acid, biotin, choline, Ca, Cl, Cu, Fe, I, Mg, Mn, P, Zn. 250 mL. *OTC.*
Use: Nutritional supplement.

Nutren 1.0 Liquid. (Clintec Nutrition) Potassium and sodium caseinate, maltodextrin, sucrose, MCT, corn oil, lecithin, vitamins A, B_1, B_2, B_3, B_5, B_6, B_{12}, C, D, E, K, folic acid, biotin, choline, Ca, Cl, Cu, Fe, I, Mg, Mn, P, Zn. Can 250 mL. *OTC.*
Use: Nutritional supplement.

Nutren 2.0 Liquid. (Nestle Nutrition) Biotin 800 mcg, calcium 1,340 mg, calories 2,000 kcal/L, carbohydrate 196 g, chloride 1,876 mg, choline 900 mg, chromium 80 mcg, copper 2.8 mg, fat 104 g, golic acid 1,080 mcg, iodine 200 mcg, iron 24 mg, L-carnitine 160 mg, magnesium 536 mg, manganese 5.2 mg, molybdenum 240 mcg, pantothenic acid 28 mg, phosphorus 1,340, potassium 1,920 mg, protein 80 g/L, selenium 80 mcg, sodium 1,300 mg, taurine 160 mg, vitamin A 6,400 units, vitamin B_1 4 mg, vitamin B_2 4.8 mg, vitamin B_3 56 mg, vitamin B_6 8 mg, vitamin B_{12} 16 mcg, vitamin C 280 mg, vitamin D 532 units, vitamin E 56 units, vitamin K 100 mcg, zinc 28 mg per L. Gluten and lactose free. Corn syrup, maltodextrin, sucrose. Liq. 1,000 mL. *OTC.*
Use: Nutritional supplement.

Nutr-E-Sol. (Advanced Nutritional Therapy) Vitamin E 798 IU per 30 mL. Sugar and dye free. Liq. 473 mL. *OTC.*
Use: Vitamin supplement.

NutreStore. (Emmaus Medical) Glutamine 5 g/packet. Pow. for Soln. 84s. *Rx.*
Use: Gastrointestinal agent.

Nutrex. (Holloway) Ca 162 mg, Fe 27 mg, vitamins A 5000 units, D 400 units, E 30 mg, B_1 2.25 mg, B_2 2.6 mg, B_3 20 mg, B_5 10 mg, B_6 3 mg, B_{12} 9 mcg, C 90 mg, folic acid 0.4 mg, Cu, I, K, Mg, Mn, P, Zn 22.5 mg, biotin 45 mcg. Tab. Bot. 100s. *OTC.*
Use: Mineral, vitamin supplement.

Nutricon Tablets. (Taylor Pharmaceuticals) Ca 200 mg, Fe 20 mg, vitamins A 2500 units, D 200 units, E 15 mg, B_1 1.5 mg, B_2 1.5 mg, B_3 10 mg, B_5 5 mg, B_6 2 mg, B_{12} 5 mcg, C 50 mg, folic acid 0.4 mg, Cu, I, Mg, Zn 3.75 mg, biotin 150 mcg. Bot. 120s. *OTC.*
Use: Mineral, vitamin supplement.

Nutri-E. (Nutri Vention) Vitamin E.
Cream: 200 units/g. Jar 1 oz, 2 oz.
Oil: 1 oz. **Oint.:** 200 units/g. Tube 1 oz, 1.5 oz. **Cap.:** 200 units. Bot. 80s; 400 units. Bot. 60s, 100s; 800 units. Bot. 55s. *OTC.*
Use: Vitamin supplement.

Nutrifac ZX. (Rising Pharmaceuticals) Vitamin A 5000 units, D_3 400 units, E (succinate) 50 units, B_1 20 mg, B_2 20 mg, B_3 100 mg, B_5 25 mg, B_6 25 mg, B_{12} 50 mcg, C 500 mg, folic acid 1 mg, Zn 20 mg, Ca, Cr, Cu, Mg, Mn, Se, biotin 200 mcg, tartrazine, mineral oil. Tab. 60s. *Rx.*
Use: Multivitamin.

NutriFocus. (Ross) Protein (Na caseinate, milk protein isolate, soy protein isolate, arginine) 61.7 g, carbohydrate (corn syrup, sugar, fructooligosaccharides) 212.3 g, fat (canola oil, high-oleic safflower oil, corn oil, lecithin) 48.8 g/L, vitamins A, B_1, B_2, B_3, B_5, B_6, B_{12}, C, D, E, K, folic acid 417 mcg/L, beta carotene, biotin, choline, Ca, chloride, Cr, Cu, Fe, I, Mg, Mn, Mo, P, Se, Zn, Na 917 mg, K 1668 mg/L, fiber 20.85 g/L, 1.5 cal/mL, lactose and gluten free, chocolate and vanilla flavors. Liq. Can. 240 mL. *OTC.*
Use: Enteral nutritional therapy.

NutriHeal. (Nestle) Protein 62.4 g, carbohydrate 112.8 g, fat 33.2 g, Na 876 mg/L, K 1248 mg/L, cal 1/mL. Vitamins A, B_1, B_2, B_3, B_5, B_6, B_{12}, C, D, E, K, beta carotene, biotin, chloride, choline, folic acid, Ca, Cr, Cu, Fe, I, Mg, Mn, Mo, P, Se, Zn. Vanilla flavor. Liq. Can. 250 mL. *OTC.*
Use: Nutritional supplement.

Nutrilan. (Elan) A vanilla, chocolate, or strawberry flavored liquid containing 38 g protein, 37 g fat, 143 g carbohydrates, 632.5 mg Na, 1.073 g K/L. With appropriate vitamins and minerals. In 237 mL *Tetra Pak* containers. *OTC.*
Use: Nutritional supplement.

Nutrilipid. (McGaw) Soybean oil intravenous fat emulsion. **10%:** Calories 1.1/mL. Bot. 250 mL, 500 mL. **20%:** Calories 2/mL. Bot. 250 mL, 500 mL. *Rx.*
Use: Nutritional supplement, parenteral.

Nutrilyte. (American Regent) Na^+ 25 mEq, $K^+ \approx$ 40 mEq, Ca^{++} 5 mEq, Mg^{++} 8 mEq, $Cl^- \approx$ 33 mEq, acetate $\approx$ 41 mEq, gluconate 5 mEq/20 mL, osmolarity $\approx$ 7562 mOsm/L. Conc. Soln. Single-dose vial 20 mL, pharmacy bulk pkg. 100 mL. *Rx.*
Use: Intravenous nutritional therapy, intravenous replenishment solution.

Nutrilyte II. (American Regent) Na^+ 35 mEq, K^+ 20 mEq, Ca^{++} 4.5 mEq,

Mg^{++} 5 mEq, Cl^- 35 mEq, acetate 29.5 mEq/20 mL, osmolarity ≈ 6,212 mOsm/L. Conc. Soln. Single-dose vial 20 mL, pharmacy bulk pkg. Vial 100 mL. *Rx.*
Use: Intravenous nutritional therapy, intravenous replenishment solution.

Nutri-Plex Tablets. (Faraday) Vitamins B_1 5 mg, B_2 5 mg, B_6 5 mg, pantothenic acid 25 mg, B_{12} 12.5 mcg, niacinamide 50 mg, iron gluconate 30 mg, choline bitartrate 50 mg, inositol 50 mg, PABA 15 mg, C 150 mg/2 Tab. Bot. 100s, 250s. *OTC.*
Use: Mineral, vitamin supplement.

Nutrisource Modular System. (Novartis) Individual Nutrisource modules available: protein, amino acids, amino acids (high branched chain), carbohydrate, lipid (medium chain triglycerides), lipid (long branched chain triglycerides), vitamins, minerals. Cans of liquid. Packets of powder. *OTC.*
Use: Nutritional supplement.

Nutri-Tab OB. (WH Nutritionals) Folic acid 1 mg, Ca 200 mg, Fe 32 mg, vitamins D 450 units, E 30 units, B_1 3 mg, B_2 3 mg, B_3 20 mg, B_6 50 mg, B_{12} 10 mcg, C 120 mg, choline 55 mg. I, Zn. PEG. Tab. 90s. *Rx.*
Use: Prenatal vitamin with minerals.

Nutri-Val. (Marcen) Vitamins A 5000 units, D 500 units, B_1 10 mg, B_2 5 mg, B_{12} activity 5 mcg, B_6 5 mcg, C 50 mg, hesperidin 5 mg, niacinamide 15 mg, folic acid 0.2 mg, calcium pantothenate 50 mg, choline bitartrate 50 mg, betaine hydrochloride 25 mg, lipo-K 0.4 mg, duodenum substance 50 mg, pancreas substance 50 mg, inositol 25 mg, Cy-yeast hydrolysates 50 mg, rutin 5 mg, l-lysine hydrochloride 5 mg, E 5 units, Ossonate (glucuronic complex) 8 mg, glutamic acid 30 mg, lecithin 5 mg, Fe 20 mg, I 0.15 mg, Ca 50 mg, P 40 mg, B 0.1 mg, Cu 1 mg, Mn 1 mg, Mg 1 mg, K 5 mg, Zn 0.5 mg, biotin 0.02 mg. Cap. Bot. 100s, 500s, 1000s. *OTC.*
Use: Mineral, vitamin supplement.

Nutri-Vite Natural Multiple Vitamin and Minerals. (Faraday) Vitamins A 15,000 units, D 400 units, B_1 1.5 mg, B_2 3 mg, B_{12} 15 mcg, niacin 500 mcg, B_6 20 mcg, choline 1.75 mg, folic acid 13 mcg, pantothenic acid 50 mcg, p-aminobenzoic acid 12 mcg, inositol 1.72 mg, C 60 mg, citrus bioflavonoids 15 mg, E 50 units, iron gluconate 15 mg, Ca 192 mg, P 85 mg, I 0.15 mg, red bone marrow 30 mg/3 Tab. Protein-coated Tab. Bot. 100s, 250s. *OTC.*
Use: Mineral, vitamin supplement.

Nutrizyme. (Enzyme Process) Vitamins A 5000 units, D 400 units, C 60 mg, B_1 1.5 mg, B_2 1.7 mg, niacinamide 20 mg, B_6 2 mg, pantothenate 10 mg, B_{12} 6 mcg, E 30 units, Fe 10 mg, Cu 1 mg, Zn 1 mg, Folac in 0.025 mg. Tab. Bot. 90s, 250s. *OTC.*
Use: Mineral, vitamin supplement.

Nutropin. (Genentech) Somatropin 10 mg. Mannitol 90 mg, glycine 3.4 mg. Pow. for Inj. (lyophilized). w/multiple-dose vials of diluent (bacteriostatic water for injection w/benzyl alcohol 0.9%). *Rx.*
Use: Hormone, growth.

Nutropin AQ. (Genentech) Somatropin 5 mg per 2 mL, 10 mg per 2 mL, 20 mg per 2 mL. Sodium chloride, sodium citrate. Inj. 2 mL vials (10 mg per 2 mL), 2 mL pen cartridges (except 5 mg per 2 mL), 2 mL multidose prefilled *Nuspin* injection device. *Rx.*
Use: Hormone, growth.

Nutrox Capsules. (Tyson) Vitamins A 10,000 units, E 150 units, B_1 25 mg, B_2 25 mg, B_3 50 mg, B_5 22 mg, C 80 mg, l-cysteine, taurine, glutathione, zinc oxide 15 mg, Se. Cap. Bot. 90s. *OTC.*
Use: Mineral, vitamin supplement.

Nuvail. (Innocutis) Poly-ureaurethane 16%. Soln.; topical. 15 mL w/applicator. *Rx.*
Use: Management of nail dystrophy.

NuvaRing. (Organon) Etonogestrel 0.12 mg, ethinyl estradiol 2.7 mg/sachet. Box 1s, 3s. *Rx.*
Use: Sex hormone, contraceptive hormone.

Nuvigil. (Cephalon) Armodafinil 50 mg, 150 mg, 200 mg, 250 mg. Lactose. Tab. 30s (200 mg only), 60s (except 200 mg). *c-IV.*
Use: Central nervous system stimulant, analeptic.

Nuzine Ointment. (Hobart) Guaiacol 1.66 g, oxyquinoline sulfate 0.42 g, zinc oxide 2.5 g, glycerine 1.66 g, lanum (anhydrous) 43.76 g, petrolatum 50 g/100 g. Tube 1 oz. *OTC.*
Use: Anorectal preparation.

NXY-059.
Use: Investigational neuroprotectant.

Nycoff. (Dover Pharmaceuticals) Dextromethorphan HBr. Tab. UD Box 500s. Sugar, lactose, and salt free. *OTC.*
Use: Antitussive.

Nyco-White. (Whiteworth Towne) Nystatin, neomycin, gramicidin, triamcinolone. Cream. Tube 15 g, 30 g, 60 g. *Rx.*
Use: Anti-infective, topical.

Nyco-Worth. (Whiteworth Towne) Nystatin. Cream. Tube 15 g. *Rx.*
Use: Antifungal, topical.

Nydrazid. (Apothecon) Isoniazid 100 mg/mL, chlorobutanol 0.25%. Inj. Vial 10 mL. *Rx.*
Use: Antituberculosal.

•**nylestriol.** (NYE-less-TRY-ole) USAN.
Use: Estrogen.

Nymalize. (Arbor) Nimodipine 3 mg/mL. Ethanol, glycerin, methylparaben, polyethylene glycol. Soln. 473 mL; UD 20 mL cups. *Rx.*
Use: Calcium channel blocker.

NyQuil.
See: Vicks NyQuil.

Nyral. (Pal-Pak, Inc.) Cetylpyridinium Cl 0.5 mg, benzocaine 5 mg/Loz. w/parabens. Pkg. 100s, 1000s. *OTC.*
Use: Antiseptic.

•**nystatin.** (nye-STAT-in) *USP.*
Use: Antifungal.
See: Mycostatin.
Nystop.
Pedi-Dri.
W/Diphenhydramine Hydrochloride, Hydrocortisone.
See: First Duke's Mouthwash.
W/Diphenhydramine Hydrochloride, Hydrocortisone, Tetracycline Hydrochloride.
See: First Mary's Mouthwash.

nystatin. (Paddock) Nystatin 50 million units, 150 million units, 500 million units, 1 billion units, 2 billion units, 5 billion units. *Rx.*
Use: Antifungal.

nystatin. (Various Mfr.) Nystatin. **Pow.:** 100,000 units/g. Dispensed in talc. 15 g, 60 g. **Susp.:** 100,000 units/mL. 5 mL, 60 mL, 480 mL. **Tab.:** 500,000 units. 100s. *Rx.*
Use: Antifungal.

nystatin and triamcinolone acetonide.
Use: Antifungal; anti-infective; corticosteroid, topical.
See: Mycolog.

nystatin and triamcinolone acetonide cream.
Use: Antifungal; corticosteroid, topical.

nystatin and triamcinolone acetonide ointment.
Use: Antifungal; corticosteroid, topical.

Nystop. (Paddock) Nystatin 100,000 units/g. Dispersed in talc. Pow. 15 g, 30 g. *Rx.*
Use: Antifungal.

Nytcold Medicine. (Rugby) Pseudoephedrine hydrochloride 10 mg, doxylamine succinate 1.25 mg, dextromethorphan HBr 5 mg, acetaminophen 167 mg, alcohol 25%, glucose, saccharin, sucrose, cherry flavor. Liq. Bot. 177 mL. *OTC.*
Use: Analgesic; antihistamine; antitussive; decongestant.

Nytime Cold Medicine. (Rugby) Acetaminophen 1000 mg, doxylamine succinate 7.5 mg, pseudoephedrine hydrochloride 60 mg, dextromethorphan HBr 30 mg/30 mL, alcohol 25%. Bot. 6 oz, 10 oz. *OTC.*
Use: Analgesic; antihistamine; antitussive; decongestant.

Nytol. (Block Drug) Diphenhydramine hydrochloride 25 mg. Tab. Bot. 16s, 32s, 72s. *OTC.*
Use: Sleep aid.

Nytol Maximum Strength. (Glaxo Consumer Healthcare) Diphenhydramine hydrochloride 50 mg. Lactose. Tab. 8s, 16s. *OTC.*
Use: Antihistamine, nonselective ethanolamine.

O

O.A.D. (Sween) Ostomy. Bot. 1.25 oz, 4 oz, 8 oz. *OTC.*
Use: Deodorant; ostomy.

Oasis. (Zitar) Artificial saliva. Bot. 6 oz. *OTC.*
Use: Antixerostomia agent.

•**oatmeal, colloidal.** *USP.*
Use: Antipruritic, topical.
See: Aveeno.

•**obatoclax mesylate.** (oh-BAT-oh-klax) USAN.
Use: Antineoplastic.

OB Complete. (Vertical) **Tab:** Vitamins A 2,100 units, B_1 2 mg, B_2 3.4 mg, B_3 10 mg, B_6 10 mg, B_{12} 15 mcg, C 120 mg, D_3 315 units, E 20 units, folic acid 1.25 mg, Cu, Mg, Zn, Fe 50 mg. UD 100s. **Chew. Tab.:** Vitamins B_1 2 mg, B_2 3 mg, B_3 10 mg, B_6 10 mg, B_{12} 15 mcg, C 120 mg, D 800 units, E 30 units, folic acid 1 mg, Mg, Zn, Ca 20 mg, Fe 20 mg, DHA 100 mg. Sucralose, wild berry flavoring. UD 30s. *Rx.*
Use: Prenatal vitamin with minerals.

OB Complete 400. (Vertical) Folic acid 1 mg, Fe 50 mg, vitamins D 1,000 units, E 30 units, B_1 2 mg, B_2 3.4 mg, B_3 10 mg, B_6 40 mg, B_{12} 20 mcg, C 110 mg, Cu, Zn, purified fish oil 400 mg (DHA 320 mg; EPA, ALA, and linoleic acid 40 mg). Beeswax. Softgels. UD 30s. *Rx.*
Use: Prenatal vitamin with minerals.

OB Complete One. (Vertical) Folic acid 1 mg, Ca 55 mg, Fe 50 mg, vitamins D 1,200 units, E 30 units, B_1 2 mg, B_2 4mg, B_3 10 mg, B_6 30 mg, B_{12} 50 mcg, C 70 mg, purified fish oil 476 mg (DHA 300 mg, EPA 40 mg), biotin 200 mcg, Cu, I, Mg, Zn. Beeswax, glycerin, orange flavoring, soybean oil. Softgels. UD 30s. *Rx.*
Use: Prenatal vitamin with minerals.

OB Complete Petite. (Vertical) Folic acid 1 mg, iron 40 mg, vitamins D 1,000 units, E 30 units, B_1 2 mg, B_2 3.4 mg, B_6 30 mg, B_{12} 15 mcg, C 125 mg, Cu, Zn, DHA 200 mg. Beeswax, lecithin, soybean oil. Cap., softgel. 30s. *Rx.*
Use: Prenatal vitamin with minerals.

OB Complete Premier. (Vertical) Folic acid 1 mg, Ca 100 mg, Fe 50 mg, vitamins A 2,100 units, D 800 units, E 20 units, B_1 2 mg, B_2 3.4 mg, B_3 10 mg, B_6 10 mg, B_{12} 15 mcg, C 120 mg, Cu, Mg, Zn. Tab. UD 30s. *Rx.*
Use: Prenatal vitamin with minerals.

OB Complete with DHA. (Vertical) Vitamin D_3 400 units, vitamin E 30 units, vitamin B_1 2 mg, vitamin B_2 3.4 mg, vitamin B_6 10 mg, vitamin B_{12} 15 mcg, vitamin C 120 mg, folic acid 1.25 mg, DHA 200 mg, zinc 25 mg, copper 1 mg, iron 28 mg. Softgel Cap. 60s. *Rx.*
Use: Multivitamin with minerals.

Obepar. (Tyler) Vitamins A 3000 units, D 300 units, B_1 3 mg, B_2 2 mg, nicotinamide 10 mg, B_6 3 mg, calcium pantothenate 2 mg, B_{12} 3 mcg, C 37.5 mg, Ca 150 mg, Fe 5 mg, Mg 1 mg, Mn 0.1 mg, K 1 mg, Zn 0.15 mg. Cap. Bot. 100s. *OTC.*
Use: Mineral, vitamin supplement.

•**obeticholic acid.** (oh-BET-i-KOL-ik) USAN.
Use: Treatment of primary biliary cirrhosis.

Obe-Tite. (Scot-Tussin) Phendimetrazine tartrate 35 mg. Tab. Bot. 100s, 500s. *c-III.*
Use: Anorexiant.

Obezine. (Western Research) Phendimetrazine tartrate 35 mg. Tab. *Handi count* 28 (36 bags of 28s). *c-III.*
Use: Anorexiant.

•**obidoxime chloride.** (OH-bih-DOX-eem) USAN.
Use: Cholinesterase reactivator.

•**obinutuzumab.** (OH-bi-nue-TOOZ-ue-mab) USAN.
Use: Antineoplastic.
See: Gazyva.

•**oblimersen sodium.** (ob-li-MER-sen) USAN.
Use: Anticancer therapy.

Obrical. (Canright) Calcium lactate 500 mg, vitamins D 400 units, ferrous sulfate exsiccated 35 mg, B_1 1 mg, B_2 1 mg, C 10 mg. Tab. Bot. 100s, 1000s. *OTC.*
Use: Mineral, vitamin supplement.

Obrical-F. (Canright) Ferrous sulfate 50 mg, calcium lactate 500 mg, vitamins D 400 units, B_1 1 mg, B_2 1 mg, C 10 mg, folic acid 0.67 mg. Tab. Bot. 100s, 1000s. *OTC.*
Use: Mineral, vitamin supplement.

Obrite. (Milton Roy) Contact lens and eye glass cleaner. Plastic spray Bot. 30 mL, 55 mL. *OTC.*
Use: Contact lens and eye glass care.

Obstetrix-100. (Seyer) Ca 250 mg, Fe 100 mg, vitamin A 2700 units, D_3 400 units, E (as dl-alpha tocopheryl) 30 units, B_1 3 mg, B_2 3.4 mg, B_3 20 mg, B_6 20 mg, B_{12} 12 mcg, C 250 mg, folic acid 1 mg, Zn 25 mg, sodium docusate 50 mg. Tab. UD 30s. *Rx.*
Use: Vitamin, mineral supplement.

OB-Tinic. (Roberts) Fe 65 mg, vitamins A 6000 units, D 400 units, E 30 units, B_1 1.1 mg, B_2 1.8 mg, B_3 15 mg, B_6 2.5 mg, B_{12} 5 mcg, C 60 mg, folic acid 1 mg, Ca Tab. Bot. 100s. *Rx.*
Use: Mineral, vitamin supplement.

Obtrex. (Pronova) Vitamin A 2700 units, E 18 mg, C 120 mg, selenium 65 mcg, D_3 400 units, folic acid 1 mg, zinc 25 mg, B_1 3 mg, B_2 3.4 mg, B_3 20 mg, B_6 40 mg, B_{12} 2 mcg, magnesium 30 mg, sodium docusate 50 mg. Tab. 60s. *Rx.*
Use: Vitamin, mineral supplement.

O-Cal f.a. (bPharmics) **Tab.:** Ca 200 mg, Fe 66 mg, vitamins A 5000 units, D 400 units, E 30 mg, B_1 3 mg, B_2 3 mg, B_3 20 mg, B_6 4 mg, B_{12} 12 mcg, C 90 mg, folic acid 1 mg, fluoride 1.1 mg, Mg, I, Cu, Zn 15 mg. Bot. 100s. *Rx.*
Use: Mineral, vitamin supplement.

O-Cal Prenatal. (Pharmics) Ca 200 mg, Fe 15 mg, vitamin A 2500 units, D 400 units, E 30 units, B_1 1.5 mg, B_2 1.6 mg, B_3 17 mg, B_6 12 mg, B_{12} 12 mcg, C 70 mg, folic acid 1 mg, Zn 15 mg, Cu, I, Mg. Tab. Bot. 100s. *Rx.*
Use: Multivitamin.

•**ocaperidone.** (oke-ah-PURR-ih-dohn) USAN.
Use: Antipsychotic.

•**ocaratuzumab.** (oh-KAR-a-TOOZ-ue-mab) USAN.
Use: Antineoplastic.

Occlusal HP. (Medicis) Salicylic acid 17%. Soln. Bot. 10 mL. *OTC.*
Use: Keratolytic.

Occucoat. (Bausch & Lomb) Hydroxypropyl methylcellulose 2%. Soln. Syringe 1 mL with cannula. *Rx.*
Use: Ophthalmic.

Ocean. (Valeant) Sodium Cl 0.65%, benzalkonium chloride. Soln. Spray Bot. 45 mL, 473 mL. *OTC.*
Use: Nasal decongestant.

Ocean Complete. (Valeant) Sodium chloride. Glycerin. Soln., spray; intranasal. 177 mL. *OTC.*
Use: Nasal decongestant.

Ocean for Kids. (Valeant) Sodium chloride 0.65%. Alcohol free. Benzalkonium chloride, EDTA, glycerin. Nasal spray. 37.5 mL. *OTC.*
Use: Nasal decongestant.

Ocean Nasal Moisturizer. (Valeant) Hyaluronan. Glycerin, parabens, trolamine. Gel; intranasal. 14 g. *OTC.*
Use: Nasal decongestant.

Ocean Plus. (Fleming & Co.) Caffeine 2.5%, benzyl alcohol. Soln. Bot. 15 mL. *OTC.*
Use: Moisturizer, nasal.

OC8. (Sebela) Benzoyl peroxide 7%. Edetate disodium, PEG, propylene glycol. Gel. 45 g. *OTC.*
Use: Topical anti-infective, antibiotic.

Ocella. (Barr Laboratories) Drospirenone 3 mg, ethinyl estradiol 30 mcg. Lactose. Film coated. Tab. Blister packs 28s, w/7 inert tablets. *Rx.*
Use: Oral contraceptive, monophasic contraceptive.

•**ocfentanil hydrochloride.** (ock-FEN-tah-NILL) USAN.
Use: Analgesic, narcotic.

•**ocinaplon.** (oh-SIN-ah-plahn) USAN.
Use: Anxiolytic.

•**oclacitinib.** (OK-la-SI-ti-nib) USAN.
Use: Dermatological agent.

•**oclacitinib maleate.** (OK-la-SI-ti-nib) USAN.
Use: Dermatological agent.

•**ocrelizumab.** (oh-kre-LIZ-oo-mab) USAN.
Use: Rheumatoid arthritis.

•**ocriplasmin.** (OK-ri-PLAS-min) USAN.
Use: Cardiovascular agent.
See: Jetrea.

•**ocrylate.** (AH-krih-late) USAN.
Use: Surgical aid, tissue adhesive.

•**octabenzone.** (OCK-tah-BEN-zone) USAN.
Use: Ultraviolet screen.

octadecanoic acid.
See: Stearic Acid.

octadecanoic acid, sodium salt.
See: Sodium Stearate.

octadecanoic acid, zinc salt.
See: Zinc Stearate.

octadecanol-l.
See: Stearyl Alcohol.

octafluoropropane.
Use: Radiopaque agent.
See: Definity.

•**octanoic acid.** (OCK-tah-NO-ik) USAN.
Use: Antifungal.

octapeptide sequence.
Use: Antiviral.
See: Flumadine.

Octaplas. (Octapharma USA) Human plasma protein 45 to 70 mg/mL (available for blood groups A, B, AB, and O). Inj., Soln. 200 mL. *Rx.*
Use: Hematological agent.

Octarex. (Health for Life Brands) Vitamins A 5000 units, D 1000 units, B_1 1.5 mg, B_2 2 mg, B_6 0.1 mg, calcium pantothenate 1 mg, niacinamide 20 mg, C 37.5 mg, E 1 unit, B_{12} 1 mcg. Cap. Bot. 100s, 1000s. *OTC.*
Use: Mineral, vitamin supplement.

Octavims. (Health for Life Brands) Vitamins A 6000 units, D 1250 units, C 50 mg, E 5 units, B_1 3 mg, B_2 3 mg, B_6 0.5 mg, niacinamide 20 mg, calcium pantothenate 5 mg, B_{12} 5 mcg, Ca 59 mg, P 45 mg. Cap. Bot. 100s, 250s, 1000s. *OTC.*
Use: Mineral, vitamin supplement.

•**octazamide.** (OCK-TAY-zah-mide) USAN.
Use: Analgesic.

•**octenidine hydrochloride.** (OCK-TEN-ih-deen) USAN.
Use: Anti-infective, topical.

•**octenidine saccharin.** (OCK-TEN-ih-deen SACK-ah-rin) USAN.
Use: Dental plaque inhibitor.

•**octicizer.** (OCK-tih-SIGH-zer) USAN. Santicizer 141.
Use: Pharmaceutic aid, plasticizer.

•**octinoxate.** (ok-TIN-ox-ate) *USP. Formerly octylmethoxycinnamate.*
Use: Sunscreen.
W/Combinations.
See: Keri Age Defy & Protect.
Lubriderm Daily Moisture with SPF 15.
TI-Screen Sports.

•**octisalate.** (ok-ti-SAL-ate) *USP. Formerly octyl salicylate.*
Use: Sunscreen.
W/Avobenzone, Homosalate, Octocrylene, Oxybenzone.
See: Neutrogena Ultra Sheer Dry-Touch Sunblock.
W/Octinoxate, Oxybenzone.
See: Lubriderm Daily Moisture with SPF 15.
TI-Screen Sports.
W/Octyl Methoxycinnamate.
See: Scar Cream Maximum Strength.

Octocaine. (Septodont) Lidocaine hydrochloride 2%, epinephrine 1:50,000, sodium bisulfite. Inj. Cartridge 1.8 mL. *Rx.*
Use: Anesthetic, local.

•**octocrylene.** (OCK-toe-KRIH-leen) *USP.*
Use: Ultraviolet screen.
W/Avobenzone, Ecamsule.
See: Anthelios SX.
UV Protective.
W/Avobenzone, Ecamsule, Titanium Dioxide.
See: Capital Soleil 20.
W/Avobenzone, Homosalate, Oxybenzone, Octisalate.
See: Neutrogena Ultra Sheer Dry-Touch Sunblock.

•**octodrine.** (OCK-toe-DREEN) USAN. Under study.
Use: Adrenergic, vasoconstrictor; anesthetic, local.

•**octoxynol 9.** (ock-TOXE-ih-nahl 9) *NF.*
Use: Pharmaceutic aid, surfactant.

OctreoScan. (Mallinckrodt) Pentetreotide 10 mcg, indium In 111 chloride sterile solution. Kit. Vials. 10 mL. *Rx.*
Use: Radiopaque agent.

•**octreotide.** (ock-TREE-oh-tide) USAN.
Use: Antisecretory, gastric.

•**octreotide acetate.** (ock-TREE-oh-tide) USAN.
Use: Somatostatin analog.
See: Sandostatin.
Sandostatin LAR Depot.

octreotide acetate. (Various Mfr.) Octreotide acetate 0.05 mg/mL, 0.1 mg/mL, 0.2 mg/mL, 0.5 mg/mL, 1 mg/mL. Inj. Single-dose vials. 1 mL (except 0.2 mg/mL and 1 mg/mL). Multi-dose vials. 5 mL (0.2 mg/mL and 1 mg/mL only). *Rx.*
Use: Somatostatin analog.

•**octreotide pamoate.** (ock-TREE-oh-tide PAM-oh-ate) USAN.
Use: Antineoplastic.

•**octriptyline phosphate.** (ock-TRIP-tih-leen) USAN.
Use: Antidepressant.

•**octrizole.** (OCK-TRY-zole) USAN.
Use: Ultraviolet screen.

•**octyldodecanol.** (OK-til-doe-DEK-a-nole) *NF.*
Use: Pharmaceutic aid, oleaginous vehicle.

octyl methoxycinnamate.
See: Octinoxate.

octylphenoxy polyethoxyethanol. (Antara) A mono-ether of a polyethylene glycol. Igepal CA 630.

octyl salicylate.
See: Octisalate.

Ocudox Convenience Kit. (OcuSOFT Inc) Doxycycline hyclate 50 mg. Lactose, PEG. Cap. 60s in kit w/30 *OcuSOFT Lid Scrub* pads and *Tears Again Liposome Spray* (15 mL). *Rx.*
Use: Anti-infective, tetracycline.

Ocufen. (Allergan) Flurbiprofen sodium 0.03%. Polyvinyl alcohol 1.4%, thimerosal 0.005%, EDTA. Ophth. Soln. Bot. 2.5 mL w/dropper. *Rx.*
Use: NSAID, ophthalmic.

•**ocufilcon A.** (OCK-you-FILL-kahn A) USAN.
Use: Contact lens material, hydrophilic.

•**ocufilcon B.** (OCK-you-FILL-kahn B) USAN.
Use: Contact lens material, hydrophilic.

•**ocufilcon C.** (OCK-you-FILL-kahn C) USAN.
Use: Contact lens material, hydrophilic.

•**ocufilcon D.** (OCK-you-FILL-kahn D) USAN.
Use: Contact lens material, hydrophilic.

•**ocufilcon E.** (OCK-you-FILL-kahn E) USAN.
Use: Contact lens material, hydrophilic.

•**ocufilcon F.** (OCK-you-FILL-kahn F) USAN.
Use: contact lens material, hydrophilic.

Ocuflox. (Allergan) Ofloxacin 3 mg/mL, benzalkonium chloride 0.005%. Soln. Bot. 1 mL, 5 mL, 10 mL. *Rx.*
Use: Anti-infective, ophthalmic.

ocular lubricants.
Use: Ophthalmic.
See: Akwa Tears.
Artificial Tears.
Dry Eyes.
Duolube.
Duratears Naturale.
GenTeal PM.
GenTeal Severe Eye Relief.
Hypotears.
Lacri-Lube NP.
Lacri-Lube S.O.P.
Lipo-Tears.
LubriTears.
OcuCoat PF.
Puralube.
Refresh PM.
Systane Nighttime.
Tears Again.
Tears Again Advanced.
Tears Again Night & Day.
Tears Naturale P.M.
Tears Renewed.
Vit-A-Drops.

Ocu-Lube. (Bausch & Lomb) Petrolatum sterile, preservative and lanolin free. Oint. Tube 3.5 g. *OTC.*
Use: Lubricant, ophthalmic.

Ocumeter.
See: Decadron Phosphate.

OCuSOFT VMS. (OCuSOFT) Vitamins A 5000 units, E 30 units, C 60 mg, Cu, Se, Zn 40 mg. Tab. Bot. 60s. *OTC.*
Use: Mineral, vitamin supplement.

Ocutricin. (Bausch & Lomb) Polymyxin B sulfate 10,000 units, bacitracin zinc 400 units, neomycin sulfate 3.5 mg. Oint. Tube 3.5 g. *Rx.*
Use: Antibiotic, ophthalmic.

Ocuvite. (Bausch & Lomb) Vitamins A 5000 units, E 30 units, C 60 mg, Zn 40 mg, Cu, Se 40 mcg. Tab. Bot. 120s. *OTC.*
Use: Mineral, vitamin supplement.

Ocuvite Extra. (Bausch & Lomb) Vitamin A 1000 units, C 300 mg, E 100 units, Zn 40 mg, B_3 40 mg, B_2 3 mg, Cu, Se, Mn, l-glutathione, lutein 2 mg. Tab. Bot. 50s. *OTC.*
Use: Vitamin supplement.

Ocuvite Eye + Multi. (Bausch & Lomb) Vitamins A 500 units, D 200 units, E 25 units, B_1 0.75 mg, B_2 0.85 mg, B_3 10 mg, B_5 5 mg, B_6 1 mg, B_{12} 3 mcg, C 75 mg, K 15 mcg, folic acid 0.2 mg, Ca, Cr, Cu, I, Mg, Mn, Mo, P, Se, Zn, biotin 15 mcg, lutein 5 mg, lycopene 150 mcg, zeaxanthin 1 mg. PEG. Tab. 60s. *OTC.*
Use: Multivitamin with minerals (except iron).

Ocuvite Lutein. (Bausch & Lomb) Vitamin E 30 units, C 60 mg, Zn 15 mg, Cu, lutein 6 mg. Lactose. Cap. 36s. *OTC.*
Use: Mineral, vitamin supplement.

•**odelepran.** (oh-DEL-e-pran) USAN.
Use: Treatment of alcohol dependence.

•**odelepran hydrochloride.** (oh-DEL-e-pran) USAN.
Use: Treatment of alcohol dependence.

oestergon.
See: Estradiol.

Oesto-Mins. (Tyson) Ascorbic acid 500 mg, Ca 250 mg, Mg 250 mg, K 45 mg, vitamin D 100 units/4.5 g. Pow. Bot. 200 g. *OTC.*
Use: Vitamin supplement.

oestradiol.
See: Estradiol.

oestrasid.
See: Dienestrol.

oestrin.
See: Estrone.

oestroform.
See: Estrone.

•**ofatumumab.** (OH-fa-TUE-mue-mab) USAN.
Use: Antineoplastic.

OFF-Ezy Corn & Callous Remover. (Del) Salicylic acid 17% in a collodion-like vehicle of 65% ether and 21% alcohol. Kit. 13.5 mL with callous smoother and 3 corn cushions. *OTC.*
Use: Keratolytic.

OFF-Ezy Corn Remover. (Del) Salicylic acid 13.57%, inflexible collodion base, ether 65%, alcohol 21%. Liq. Bot. 0.45 oz. *OTC.*
Use: Keratolytic.

OFF-Ezy Wart Remover. (Del) Salicylic acid 17% in flexible collodion base, ether 65%, alcohol 21%. Liq. Bot. 13.5 mL. *OTC.*
Use: Keratolytic.

Ofirmev. (Cadence Pharmaceuticals) Acetaminophen 10 mg/mL. Mannitol. Inj., Soln. Single-use vial. 100 mL. *Rx.*
Use: Analgesic.

•**ofloxacin.** (oh-FLOX-uh-SIN) *USP.*
Use: Anti-infective.
See: Floxin.
Ocuflox.

ofloxacin. (Pacific Pharma) Ofloxacin 0.3% (3 mg/mL). Benzalkonium chloride 0.005%. Ophth. Soln. 5 mL, 10 mL. *Rx.*
Use: Otic antibiotic.

ofloxacin. (Various Mfr.) Ofloxacin. **Soln.:** 0.3% (3 mg/mL). Benzalkonium chloride 0.005%. Dropper bot. 5 mL, 10 mL. **Tab.:** 200 mg, 300 mg, 400 mg. 50s (except 400 mg), 100s. *Rx.*
Use: Otic preparation; anti-infective.

•**ofornine.** (ah-FAR-neen) USAN.
Use: Antihypertensive.

Ogestrel 0.5/50. (Watson) Norgestrel 0.5 mg, ethinyl estradiol 50 mcg. Lactose. Tab. Pack 28s with 7 inert tabs. *Rx.*
Use: Sex hormone, contraceptive hormone.

•**oglufanide disodium.** (oh-GLOO-fa-nide) USAN. Previously Glufanide disodium.
Use: Immunomodulator; angiogenesis inhibitor (Kaposi sarcoma).

Oilatum Soap. (GlaxoSmithKline) Polyunsaturated vegetable oil 7.5%. Bar 120 g, 240 g. *OTC.*
Use: Dermatologic, cleanser.

oil of camphor with combinations.
See: Sloan's Liniment.

Oil of Olay Daily UV Protectant. (Procter & Gamble) SPF 15. **Cream:** Titanium dioxide, ethylhexyl p-methoxycinnamate, 2-phenylbenzimidazole-5-sulfonic acid, glycerin, triethanolamine, imidazolidinyl urea, parabens, carbomer, PEG-10, EDTA, castor oil, tartrazine. Scented and unscented. 51 g. **Lot.:** Ethylhexyl p-methoxycinnamate, 2-phenylbenzimidazole-5-sulfonic acid, titanium dioxide, cetyl alcohol, imidazolidinyl urea, parabens, EDTA, castor oil, tartrazine. Bot. 105 g, 157.7 g. *OTC.*
Use: Sunscreen.

Oil of Olay Foaming Face Wash. (Procter & Gamble) Potassium cocoyl hydrolyzed collagen, glycerin, EDTA. Liq. Bot. 90 mL, 210 mL. *OTC.*
Use: Dermatologic, acne.

oil of pine with combinations.
See: Sloan's Liniment.

ointment and lotion base.
See: Hydrocerin.

ointment base, washable.
See: Cetaphil.
Velvachol.

•**ointment, bland lubricating ophthalmic.** *USP.*
Use: Lubricant, ophthalmic.

•**ointment, hydrophilic.** *USP.*
Use: Pharmaceutic aid, oil-in-water emulsion ointment base.

•**ointment, rose water.** *USP.*
Use: Pharmaceutic aid, emollient, ointment base.

•**ointment, white.** *USP.*
Use: Pharmaceutical aid, oleaginous ointment base.

•**ointment, yellow.** *USP.*
Use: Pharmaceutic aid, ointment base.

•**olaflur.** (OH-lah-flure) USAN.
Use: Dental caries agent.

olamine.
See: Ethanolamine.

•**olanexidine hydrochloride.** (OH-lan-EX-i-deen) USAN.
Use: Antimicrobial.

•**olanzapine.** (oh-LAN-zah-PEEN) USAN.
Tall Man: OLANZapine
Use: Antipsychotic, dibenzapine derivative.
See: Zyprexa.
Zyprexa Relprevv.
Zyprexa Zydis.
W/Fluoxetine Hydrochloride.
See: Symbyax.

olanzapine. (Prasco) Olanzapine 10 mg. Lactose 50 mg, tartaric acid 3.5 mg. Inj., Pow. for Soln. 10 mg vial. *Rx.*
Use: Antipsychotic agent, dibenzapine derivative.

olanzapine. (Various Mfr.) Olanzapine. **Tab.:** 2.5 mg, 5 mg, 7.5 mg, 10 mg, 15 mg, 20 mg. May contain lactose, PEG. 30s, 60s, 100s, 500s, 1,000s, UD 50s (15 mg and 20 mg only), UD 100s. **Tab., orally disintegrating:** 5 mg, 10 mg, 15 mg, 20 mg. May contain aspartame, mannitol, parabens, phenylalanine. 30s, UD 30s, UD 100s. *Rx.*
Use: Antipsychotic agent, dibenzapine derivative.

olanzapine/fluoxetine. (Teva Pharmaceuticals) Olanzapine/fluoxetine hydrochloride 3 mg/25 mg, 6 mg/25 mg, 6 mg/50 mg, 12 mg/25 mg, 12 mg/50 mg Cap. 30s. *Rx.*
Use: Psychotherapeutic combination.

•**olaratumab.** (oh-LAR-a-TUE-mab) USAN.
Use: Antineoplastic.

•**olcorolimus.** (OL-kor-OH-li-mus) USAN.
Use: Inhibition of smooth muscle cell proliferation.

old tuberculin.
See: Mono-Vacc Test O.T.
Tuberculin, Old, Tine Test.

oleandomycin phosphate. Phosphate of

an antibacterial substance produced by *Streptomyces antibioticus*.
Use: Anti-infective.

oleandomycin, triacetyl. Troleandomycin, USP.

•**oleic acid.** (oh-LAY-ik) *NF.*
Use: Pharmaceutic aid, emulsion adjunct.

•**oleic acid I 131.** (oh-LAY-ik) USAN.
Use: Radiopharmaceutical.

•**oleic acid I 125.** (oh-LAY-ik) USAN.
Use: Radiopharmaceutical.

oleovitamin A.
See: Vitamin A.

•**oleovitamin A and D.** (OH-lee-oh-VYE-ta-min) *USP.*
Use: Vitamin supplement.
See: Super D Perles.

oleovitamin D, synthetic.
Use: Vitamin supplement.

Oleptro. (Labopharm) Trazodone hydrochloride 150 mg, 300 mg. Film coated. PEG. ER Tab. 30s, 90s, 500s, UD 30s. *Rx.*
Use: Antidepressant.

•**oleyl alcohol.** (oh-LAY-il) *NF.*
Use: Pharmaceutic aid, emulsifying agent, emollient.
See: Pataday.
Patanol.

•**olive oil.** *NF.*
Use: Emollient, pharmaceutic aid, setting retardant for dental cements.

•**olmesartan.** (ole-mih-SAR-tan) USAN.
Use: Antihypertensive.

•**olmesartan medoxomil.** (ole-mih-SAR-tan meh-DOX-oh-mill) USAN.
Use: Antihypertensive.
See: Benicar.
W/Amlodipine Besylate.
See: Azor.
W/Hydrochlorothiazide.
See: Benicar HCT.

•**olodaterol.** (OH-loe-DA-ter-ol) USAN.
Use: Treatment of chronic obstructive pulmonary disorder.

•**olodaterol hydrochloride.** (OH-loe-DA-ter-ol) USAN.
Use: Treatment of chronic obstructive pulmonary disorder.

•**olopatadine hydrochloride.** (oh-low-pat-AD-een) USAN.
Use: Antiallergic, allergic rhinitis, urticaria, allergic conjunctivitis, asthma.
See: Pataday.
Patanase.
Patanol.

olopatadine hydrochloride. (Alcon) Olopatadine hydrochloride 0.2%. Benzalkonium chloride 0.01%, EDTA, povidone, dibasic sodium phosphate, sodium chloride, hydrochloric acid/sodium hydroxide. Soln., Ophth. 2.5 mL fill in 4 mL bottle. *Rx.*
Use: Ophthalmic antihistamine.

•**olsalazine sodium.** (OLE-SAL-uh-zeen) USAN. *Formerly Sodium azodisalicylate, azodisal sodium.*
Use: Maintenance of remission of ulcerative colitis in patients intolerant of sulfasalazine; anti-inflammatory, gastrointestinal.
See: Dipentum.

Olux. (GlaxoSmithKline) Clobetasol propionate 0.05%, ethanol 60%, cetyl alcohol, stearyl alcohol. Foam. Can. 50 g, 100 g. *Rx.*
Use: Anti-inflammatory.

Olux-E. (GlaxoSmithKline) Clobetasol propionate 0.5 mg. Cetyl alcohol, light mineral oil, white petrolatum. Foam. 100 g. *Rx.*
Use: Anti-inflammatory.

•**olvanil.** (OLE-van-ill) USAN.
Use: Analgesic.

Olysio. (Janssen Therapeutics) Simeprevir 150 mg (equiv. to simeprevir sodium 154.4 mg). Lactose. Cap. 7s, 28s. *Rx.*
Use: Antiviral agent.

•**omacetaxine mepesuccinate.** (OH-ma-set-AX-een MEP-i-SUX-in-ate) USAN.
Use: Antineoplastic, protein synthesis inhibitor.
See: Synribo.

Omacor. (Ross) Eicosapentanaenoic acid (EPA) 465 mg, docosahexaenoic acid (DHA) 375 mg, α-tocopherol 4 mg. Cap. 120s. *Rx.*
Use: Dietary supplement.

•**omadacycline.** (oh-MAD-a-SYE-kleen) USAN.
Use: Antibiotic.

•**omadacycline tosylate.** (oh-MAD-a-SYE-kleen) USAN.
Use: Antibiotic.

•**omafilcon B.** (OH-ma-FIL-kon) USAN.
Use: Contact lens polymer (hydrophilic).

•**omalizumab.** (oh-mah-lie-ZOO-mab) USAN.
Use: Monoclonal antibody.
See: Xolair.

omapatrilat.
Use: Vasopeptidase inhibitor.

•**omarigliptin.** (oh-MAR-i-GLIP-tin) USAN.
Use: Antidiabetic agent.

•**omecamtiv mecarbil.** (OM-e-KAM-tiv me-KAR-bil) USAN.
Use: Cardiovascular agent.

Omeclamox-Pak. (Pernix Therapeutics) Consists of 10 daily administration cards. **Cap., delayed release:** Omeprazole 20 mg. Lactose, mannitol. 2s. **Cap.:** Amoxicillin 500 mg. 4s. **Tab.:** Clarithromycin 500 mg. Film coated. Lactose. 2s. *Rx.*
Use: Gastrointestinal agent, *H. pylori* agent.

Omega Essentials With Vitamin D-3. (Physician Recommended Nutriceuticals) Omega-3. **Cap., softgel:** 667 mg (DHA 140 mg, EPA 420 mg, other omega-3s 107 mg), vitamin D 250 units. Soy. Dairy free, gluten free. 60s. **Liq.:** 1,150 mg (DHA 450 mg, EPA 650 mg, other omega-3 fatty acids 50 mg), vitamin D 1,000 units. Orange oil, rosemary oil. Dairy free, gluten free. 240 mL. *OTC.*
Use: Multivitamin and mineral with omega-3 polyunsaturated fatty acids.

Omega Oil. (Block Drug) Methyl nicotinate, methyl salicylate, capsicum oleoresin, histamine dihydrochloride, isopropyl alcohol 44%. Bot. 2.5 oz, 4.85 oz. *OTC.*
Use: Analgesic, topical.

•**omega-3-acid ethyl esters.** USAN.
Use: Hypolipidemic.
See: Omtryg.

Omega 3 Complex. (ChronoHealth) DHA 192 mg, EPA 251 mg, vitamin E 11 units (as mixed tocopherols) Cap., softgels. Unit of use 1s. *OTC.*
Use: Fish oil.

omega-3 (n-3) polyunsaturated fatty acids. From cold water fish oils.
Use: Dietary supplement to reduce risk of coronary artery disease.
See: Animi-3.
Cardi-Omega 3.
Lovaza.
Max EPA.
Omacor.
Promega.
Sea-Omega 50.
SuperEPA.

•**omeprazole.** (oh-MEH-pray-ZAHL) *USP.*
Use: Proton pump inhibitor.
See: Prilosec.
Prilosec OTC.
W/Sodium Bicarbonate.
See: Zegerid.
Zegerid OTC.

omeprazole. (Various Mfr.) Omeprazole. **Tab., delayed release:** 20 mg. May contain lactose. 14s. **Cap., delayed release:** 10 mg, 20 mg, 40 mg. May contain lactose, sucrose (40 mg). Enteric-coated granules. 30s (except 40 mg), 100s, 1,000s (40 mg), UD 30s (40 mg). *Rx-OTC.*
Use: Proton pump inhibitor.

omeprazole/amoxicillin/clarithromycin.
Use: Helicobacter pylori agent.
See: Omeclamox-Pak.

•**omeprazole sodium.** (oh-MEH-pray-ZOLE) USAN.
Use: Antisecretory, gastric.

omeprazole/sodium bicarbonate. (Various Mfr.) Omeprazole/sodium bicarbonate. **Cap.:** 20 mg/1,100 mg, 40 mg/1,100 mg. 30s, 500s. **Pow. for Susp.:** 20 mg/1,680 mg, 40 mg/1,680 mg. Sucrose, sucralose, xylitol. UD 30s. *Rx.*
Use: Proton pump inhibitor combination.

omeprazole/sodium bicarbonate/magnesium hydroxide. (Various Mfr.) Omeprazole/sodium bicarbonate/magnesium hydroxide 20 mg/750 mg/343 mg, 40 mg/750 mg/343 mg. Sodium 209 mg. Tab. 30s. *Rx.*
Use: Proton pump inhibitor combination.

OM 401.
Use: Sickle cell disease. [Orphan Drug]

•**omiganan pentahydrochloride.** (oh-me-GAN-an PEN-ta-HYE-droe-KLOR-ide) USAN.
Use: Antimicrobial.

Omnaris. (Nycomed) Ciclesonide 50 mcg/actuation. Edetate sodium. Spray Susp. Intranasal. 125 g glass bot. (120 actuations) with metered-dose pump with oxygen absorber sachet. *Rx.*
Use: Respiratory inhalant, intranasal steroid.

Omnicol. (Delta Pharmaceutical Group) Dextromethorphan HBr 15 mg, chlorpheniramine maleate 4 mg, phenylephrine hydrochloride 5 mg, phenindamine tartrate 4 mg, salicylamide 227 mg, acetaminophen 100 mg, caffeine alkaloid 10 mg, ascorbic acid 25 mg. Tab. Bot. 100s. *OTC.*
Use: Antitussive, antihistamine, decongestant, analgesic.

Omnihemin. (Delta Pharmaceutical Group) Fe 110 mg, vitamins C 150 mg, B_{12} 7.5 mcg, folic acid 1 mg, Zn 1 mg, Cu 1 mg, Mn 1 mg, Mg 1 mg. Tab. or Soln. 5 mL. **Tab.:** Bot. 100s. **Soln.:** Bot. Pt. *Rx.*
Use: Mineral, vitamin supplement.

OmniHIB. (GlaxoSmithKline) Purified *Haemophilus influenzae* type b capsular polysaccharide 10 mcg, tetanus toxoid 24 mcg/0.5 mL, sucrose 8.5%. Pow. for Inj. (lyophilized). Vial w/0.6 mL

syringe of diluent. *Rx.*
Use: Immunization.

OMNIhist II L.A. (Dexo Pharma) Phenylephrine hydrochloride 25 mg, chlorpheniramine maleate 8 mg, methscopolamine nitrate 2.5 mg. Dye free. Tab. Bot. 100s. *Rx.*
Use: Upper respiratory combination, anticholinergic, antihistamine, decongestant combination.

Omninatal. (Delta Pharmaceutical Group) Fe 60 mg, Cu 2 mg, Zn 15 mg, vitamins A 8000 units, D 400 units, C 90 mg, Ca 200 mg, folic acid 1.5 mg, B_1 2.5 mg, B_2 3 mg, niacinamide 20 mg, pyridoxine hydrochloride 10 mg, pantothenic acid 15 mg, B_{12} 8 mcg. Tab. Bot. 100s. *Rx.*
Use: Mineral, vitamin supplement.

Omnipaque 140. (Nycomed) Iohexol 302 mg equivalent to iodine 140 mg/mL. EDTA. Inj. Vials. 50 mL, Bot. *Rx.*
Use: Radiopaque agent, parenteral.

Omnipaque 300. (Nycomed) Iohexol 647 mg equivalent to iodine 300 mg/mL. EDTA. Inj. Vials. 10 mL, 30 mL, 50 mL. Bot. 50 mL. Flex. Cont. 100 mL, 150 mL. Prefilled Syringes. 50 mL. 75 mL fill in 100 mL Bot. 100 mL fill in 100 mL Bot. 125 mL fill in 200 mL Bot. 150 mL fill in 200 mL Bot. 125 mL fill in 150 mL Flex. Cont. *Rx.*
Use: Radiopaque agent, parenteral.

Omnipaque 350. (Nycomed) Iohexol 755 mg equivalent to iodine 350 mg/mL. EDTA. Inj. Vials. 50 mL. Bot. 50 mL. Flex. Cont. 100 mL, 150 mL, 200 mL. Prefilled Syringes. 50 mL. 75 mL fill in 100 mL Bot., 100 mL fill in 100 mL Bot., 125 mL fill in 200 mL Bot., 150 mL fill in 200 mL Bot., 200 mL fill in 200 mL Bot., 250 mL fill in 300 mL Bot., 125 mL fill in 150 mL Flex. Cont. *Rx.*
Use: Radiopaque agent, parenteral.

Omnipaque 240. (Nycomed) Iohexol 518 mg equivalent to iodine 240 mg/mL. EDTA. Inj. Vials. 10 mL, 20 mL, 50 mL. Bot. 50 mL. Flex. Cont. 100 mL, 150 mL, 200 mL. Prefilled Syringes. 50 mL. 100 mL fill in 100 mL Bot. 150 mL fill in 200 mL Bot. 200 mL fill in 200 mL Bot. *Rx.*
Use: Radiopaque agent, parenteral.

Omnipen. (Wyeth) **Cap.:** Ampicillin anhydrous 250 mg, 500 mg. Bot. 100s, 500s. **Pow. for Oral Susp.:** Ampicillin trihydrate 125 mg, 250 mg/5 mL when reconstituted. Pow. for Oral Susp. Bot. 100 mL, 150 mL, 200 mL. *Rx.*
Use: Anti-infective, penicillin.

Omnipen-N. (Wyeth) Ampicillin sodium 125 mg, 250 mg, 500 mg, 1 g, 2 g, 10 g. Pow. for Inj. Vial, Piggyback and *ADD-Vantage* vials (only 500 mg, 1 g, 2 g). *Rx.*
Use: Anti-infective, penicillin.

Omnipred. (Alcon) Prednisolone 1% (as acetate). Susp., Ophth. *Drop-Tainer* (with benzalkonium chloride 0.01%, EDTA, polysorbate 80, glycerin, hydroxypropyl methylcellulose). 5 mL, 10 mL. *Rx.*
Use: Ophthalmic and otic agent, corticosteroid.

Omniscan. (GE Healthcare) Gadodiamide 287 mg/mL. Preservative free. Inj. Soln. Vials. 5 mL, 10 mL, 20 mL, 50 mL. Prefilled Syringes. 10 mL, 15 mL, 20 mL. *Rx.*
Use: Radiopaque agent, parenteral.

Omnitabs. (Halsey Drug) Vitamins A 5000 units, D 400 units, C 50 mg, B_1 3 mg, B_2 2.5 mg, niacin 20 mg, B_6 1 mg, B_{12} 1 mcg, pantothenic acid 0.9 mg Tab. Bot. 100s. *OTC.*
Use: Vitamin supplement.

Omnitabs with Iron. (Halsey Drug) Vitamins A 5000 units, D 400 units, B_1 3 mg, B_2 2.5 mg, B_6 1 mg, B_{12} 1 mcg, C 50 mg, niacinamide 20 mg, calcium pantothenate 1 mg, Fe 15 mg. Tab. Bot. 100s. *OTC.*
Use: Mineral, vitamin supplement.

Omnitrope. (Sandoz) Somatropin. **Pow. for Inj., lyophilized:** 5.8 mg ($\approx$ 17.4 units). Glycine 27.6 mg. Vials with diluent (bacteriostatic water for injection containing benzyl alcohol 1.5% as a preservative). **Inj., Soln.:** 5 mg/mL. Benzyl alcohol, mannitol 52.5 mg, poloxamer 188 3 mg. Cartridges. *Rx.*
Use: Growth hormone.

•**omoconazole nitrate.** (oh-moe-KAHN-ah-zole) USAN.
Use: Antifungal.

•**omtriptolide sodium.** (ohm-TRIP-toe-lide) USAN.
Use: Antineoplastic.

Omtryg. (Trygg Pharma) Omega-3-acid ethyl esters A $\geq$ 900 mg (EPA $\approx$ 465 mg and DHA $\approx$ 375 mg). Alpha tocopherol, sunflower oil. Cap., liquid filled. 120s. *Rx.*
Use: Multivitamin with minerals and omega-3 polyunsaturated fatty acids.

•**onabotulinumtoxinA.** (ON-a-bot-u-lin-um-tox-in-a) USAN.
Use: Botulinum toxin.
See: Botox.
Botox Cosmetic.

•**onamelatucel-L.** (ON-a-MEL-a-TOO-sel) USAN.
Use: Antineoplastic.

•**onartuzumab.** (ON-ar-TOOZ-oo-mab) USAN.
Use: Treatment of cancer.

Oncaspar. (Sigma Tau) Pegaspargase 750 units/mL. Preservative free. Inj. Single-use vials. *Rx.*
Use: Antineoplastic agent.

Oncet. (Wakefield) Hydrocodone bitartrate 5 mg, acetaminophen 500 mg. Cap. Bot. 100s. *c-III.*
Use: Analgesic; antitussive.

OncoRad ov103.
Use: Antineoplastic. [Orphan Drug]

Oncovite. (Mission Pharmacal) Vitamin A 10,000 units, C 500 mg, D_3 400 units, E 200 units, B_1 0.37 mg, B_2 0.5 mg, B_6 25 mg, B_{12} 1.5 mcg, folate 0.4 mg, Zn 7.5 mg, sugar. Tab. Bot. 120s. *OTC.*
Use: Vitamin supplement.

•**ondansetron.** (ahn-DAN-SEH-trahn) *USP.*
Use: Antiemetic/antivertigo agent, 5-HT_3 receptor antagonist.
See: Zofran ODT.
Zuplenz.

ondansetron. (Sandoz) Ondansetron 4 mg, 8 mg. Aspartame, mannitol, parabens, phenylalanine < 0.3 mg. Strawberry flavor. Tab., orally disintegrating. UD 10s (8 mg), UD 30s. *Rx.*
Use: Antiemetic/antivertigo agent, 5-HT_3 receptor antagonist.

•**ondansetron hydrochloride.** (ahn-DAN-SEH-trahn) USAN.
Use: Anxiolytic; antiemetic; antischizophrenic.
See: Zofran.

ondansetron hydrochloride. (Sandoz) Ondansetron hydrochloride 4 mg, 8 mg. Phenylalanine < 0.3 mg, aspartame, mannitol, parabens. Strawberry flavor. Orally Disintegrating Tab. UD 10s (8 mg only), UD 30s. *Rx.*
Use: Antiemetic/antivertigo agent.

ondansetron hydrochloride. (Various Mfr.) Ondansetron hydrochloride. **Inj.:** 2 mg/mL. May contain parabens. Sodium chloride. Single-dose and multidose vials. 32 mg/50 mL. Preservative free. Citric acid 26 mg, dextrose 2,500 mg, sodium citrate 11.5 mg. Single-dose containers. 50 mL. **Soln.:** 4 mg/5 mL. May contain saccharin, sorbitol. Strawberry flavor. 50 mL. **Tab.:** 4 mg, 8 mg, 16 mg, 24 mg. Polydextrose (16 mg only), lactose. Film-coated. 30s, 100s (8 mg, 16 mg only), 500s, UD 1s (24 mg only), UD 3s (except 16 mg, 24 mg), UD 100s (except 16 mg), blister card 1s (16 mg only). *Rx.*
Use: Antiemetic/antivertigo agent.

ondansetron hydrochloride and dextrose. (Hospira) Ondansetron hydrochloride (as hydrochloride dihydrate) 32 mg per 50 mL. Preservative free. Dextrose 2500 mg, citric acid 26 mg, sodium citrate 11.5 mg. Inj. Single-dose flexible plastic containers. *Rx.*
Use: Antiemetic/antivertigo agent.

Ondrox. (LSI) Ca 50 mg, vitamins A 6000 units, D 300 units, E 50 units, B_1 0.75 mg, B_2 0.75 mg, B_3 10 mg, B_5 5 mg, B_6 1 mg, B_{12} 3 mcg, C 125 mg, folic acid 200 mcg, biotin 15 mcg, I, Mg, Cu, P, vitamin K, Cr, Mn, Mo, Se, V, B, Si, Zn 7.5 mg, inositol, citrus bioflavonoids, N-acetylcysteine, l-methionine, l-glutamine, taurine. Tab. Bot. 60s, 180s. *OTC.*
Use: Mineral, vitamins supplements.

One-A-Day Essential. (Bayer Consumer Care) Vitamins A 5000 units, E 30 units, C 60 mg, folic acid 0.4 mg, B_1 1.5 mg, B_2 1.7 mg, B_3 20 mg, B_6 2 mg, B_{12} 6 mcg, B_5 10 mg, D 400 units. Tab. Sodium free. Bot. 75s, 130s. *OTC.*
Use: Vitamin supplement.

One-A-Day Extras Antioxidant. (Bayer Consumer Care) Vitamin E 200 units, C 250 mg, A 5000 units, Zn 7.5 mg, Cu, Se, Mn, tartrazine. Softgel Cap. Bot. 50s. *OTC.*
Use: Vitamin supplement.

One-A-Day Extras Vitamin E. (Bayer Consumer Care) Vitamin E 400 units. Softgel Cap. Bot. 60s. *OTC.*
Use: Vitamin supplement.

One-A-Day 55 Plus. (Bayer Consumer Care) Vitamin A 6000 units, C 120 mg, B_1 4.5 mg, B_2 3.4 mg, B_3 20 mg, D 400 units, E 60 units, B_6 6 mg, folic acid 0.4 mg, biotin 30 mcg, B_5 20 mg, K 25 mcg, Ca 220 mg, I, Mg, Cu, Zn 15 mg, Cr, Se, Mo, Mn, K, Cl. Tab. Bot. 50s, 80s. *OTC.*
Use: Mineral, vitamin supplement.

One-A-Day Kids. (Bayer Consumer Care) Vitamin A 5000 units, C 60 mg, D 400 units, E 30 units, B_1 1.5 mg, B_2 1.7 mg, B_3 20 mg, B_5 10 mg, B_6 2 mg, B_{12} 6 mcg, folic acid 400 mcg, biotin 40 mcg, calcium 100 mg, iron 18 mg, phosphorus 100 mg, iodine 150 mcg, magnesium 20 mg, zinc 15 mg, copper 2 mg, sorbitol, aspartame, phenylalanine. Chew. Tab. 50s. *OTC.*
Use: Vitamin, mineral supplement.

One-A-Day Kids Scooby-Doo! Fizzy Vites. (Bayer Consumer Care) Ca 50 mg, Fe (as ferrous fumarate) 9 mg, vitamin A 1500 units, D 200 units, E 15 units, B_1 0.75 mg, B_2 0.85 mg, B_3

7.5 mg, B_5 5 mg, B_6 1 mg, B_{12} 3 mcg, C 170 mg, FA 200 mcg, biotin 20 mcg, P, I, Mg, Zn, Cu, Na. Aspartame, phenylalanine, sucrose, vegetable oil. Chew. Tab. 60s. *OTC.*
Use: Multivitamin.

One-A-Day Maximum Formula. (Bayer Consumer Care) Fe 18 mg, vitamins A 5000 units, D 400 units, E 30 units, B_1 1.5 mg, B_2 1.7 mg, B_3 20 mg, B_5 10 mg, B_6 2 mg, B_{12} 6 mcg, C 60 mg, folic acid 0.4 mg, Ca, Cl, Cr, Cu, I, K, Mg, Mn, Mo, P, Se, Zn 15 mg, biotin 30 mcg. Tab. Bot. 60s, 100s. *OTC.*
Use: Mineral, vitamin supplement.

One-A-Day Men's Health Formula. (Bayer Consumer Care) Vitamins A 3,500 units, D 700 units, E 22.5 units, B_1 1.35 mg, B_2 1.7 mg, B_3 18 mg, B_5 16 mg, B_6 3 mg, B_{12} 18 mcg, C 60 mg, K 20 mcg, folic acid 400 mcg, Ca, Cr, Cu, Mg, Mn, Se, Zn, biotin 75 mcg, lycopene 300 mcg. Film coated. Tab. 60s. *OTC.*
Use: Multivitamin.

One-A-Day Men's Vitamins. (Bayer Consumer Care) Vitamin A 5000 units, C 200 mg, B_1 2.25 mg, B_2 2.55 mg, B_3 20 mg, D 400 units, E 45 units, B_6 3 mg, folic acid 0.4 mg, B_{12} 9 mcg, B_5 10 mg. Tab. Bot. 60s, 100s. *OTC.*
Use: Mineral, vitamin supplement.

One-A-Day Vitacraves Adults Multivitamin Gummies. (Bayer Consumer Care) Vitamins A 2,000 units, D 200 units, E 20 units, B_5 5 mg, B_6 1 mg, B_{12} 5 mcg, C 30 mg, folic acid 0.2 mg, I, Zn, biotin 75 mcg, choline 30 mcg, inositol 20 mcg. Glucose, sucrose, vegetable oil. Chew. Tab. 50s. *OTC.*
Use: Multivitamin with minerals (except iron).

One-A-Day Weight Smart. (Bayer Consumer Care) Ca 300 mg, Fe (as ferrous fumarate) 18 mg, vitamin A 2500 units, D 400 units, E 30 units, B_1 1.9 mg, B_2 2.125 mg, B_3 25 mg, B_5 12.5 mg, B_6 2.5 mg, B_{12} 7.5 mcg, FA 400 mcg, vitamin K, Mg, Zn, Se, Cu, Mn, Cr, EGCG, dextrose, glucose. Tab. 50s, 100s. *OTC.*
Use: Multivitamin.

One-A-Day Women's Formula. (Bayer Consumer Care) Ca 450 mg, Fe 27 mg, vitamins A 5000 units, D 400 units, E 30 mg, B_1 1.5 mg, B_2 1.7 mg, B_3 20 mg, B_5 10 mg, B_6 2 mg, B_{12} 6 mcg, C 60 mg, folic acid 0.4 mg, Zn 15 mg, tartrazine. Tab. Bot. 60s, 100s. *Rx.*
Use: Mineral, vitamin supplement.

One-A-Day Women's Plus Healthy Skin Support. (Bayer Consumer Care) Iron 18 mg, calcium 300 mg, vitamins A 2,500 units, D 1,000 units, E 30 units, B_1 1.5 mg, B_2 1.7 mg, B_3 5 mg, B_5 5 mg, B_6 2 mg, B_{12} 6 mcg, C 90 mg, folic acid 0.4 mg, Cr, Cu, Mg, Se, Zn, biotin, lutein. Tab. 80s. *OTC.*
Use: Multivitamin with minerals (including iron).

One-Daily. (Geri-Care) Fe 18 mg, vitamin A 5,000 units, D 400 units, B_1 2 mg, B_2 2.5 mg, B_3 20 mg, B_5 1 mg, B_6 1 mg, B_{12} 1 mcg, C 50 mg. PEG. Tab. 100s, 1,000s. *OTC.*
Use: Multivitamin with minerals.

One Daily Adults 50+. (21st Century HealthCare) Vitamins A 2,500 units, D 400 units, E 33 units, B_1 4.5 mg, B_2 3.4 mg, B_3 20 mg, B_5 15 mg, B_6 6 mg, B_{12} 25 mcg, C 120 mg, folate 400 mcg, Ca, Cr, Cu, I, K, Mg, Mn, Mo, Se, Zn. Biotin 30 mcg, chloride 34 mg, potassium 40 mg. Tab. 100s. *OTC.*
Use: Nutritional supplement.

One-Daily Multi-Vitamin with Minerals. (Geri-Care) Vitamins A 5,000 units, C 50 mg, D 400 units, B_1 2 mg, B_2 2.5 mg, B_3 20 mg, B_5 1 mg, B_6 1 mg, B_{12} 1 mcg, Ca 19 mg, Fe 4.5 mg, P, I, Zn, Cr, Mn, Mg, Se. Mineral oil, sucrose. Tab. 100s. *OTC.*
Use: Multivitamin.

1+1-F Creme. (Oxypure) Clioquinol 3%, hydrocortisone 1%, pramoxine hydrochloride 1%. Tube 30 g. *Rx.*
Use: Corticosteroid; anesthetic, local; antifungal, topical.

•**onercept.** (O-ner-sept) USAN.
Use: Anti-tumor-necrosis factor activity.

One-Tablet-Daily. (Various Mfr.) Vitamins A 5000 units, D 400 units, E 30 mg, B_1 1.5 mg, B_2 1.7 mg, B_3 20 mg, B_5 10 mg, B_6 2 mg, B_{12} 6 mcg, C 60 mg, folic acid 0.4 mg. Tab. Bot. 30s, 100s, 250s, 365s, 1000s. *OTC.*
Use: Vitamin supplement.

One-Tablet-Daily Plus Iron. (Various Mfr.) Iron 18 mg, vitamins A 5000 units, D 400 units, E 15 mg, B_1 1.5 mg, B_2 1.7 mg, B_3 20 mg, B_6 2 mg, B_{12} 6 mcg, C 60 mg, folic acid 0.4 mg. Tab. Bot. 100s, 250s, 365s. *OTC.*
Use: Mineral, vitamin supplement.

One-Tablet-Daily with Iron. (Ivax) Fe 18 mg, A 5000 units, D 400 units, E 30 mg, B_1 1.5 mg, B_2 1.7 mg, B_3 20 mg, B_5 10 mg, B_6 2 mg, B_{12} 6 mcg, C 60 mg, folic acid 0.4 mg. Tab. Bot. 100s. *OTC.*
Use: Mineral, vitamin supplement.

One-Tablet-Daily with Minerals. (Ivax) Fe 18 mg, vitamins A 5000 units, D 400 units, E 30 units, B_1 1.5 mg, B_2 1.7 mg, B_3 20 mg, B_5 10 mg, B_6 2 mg, B_{12} 6 mcg, C 60 mg, folic acid 0.4 mg, Ca, Cl, Cr, Cu, I, K, Mg, Mn, Mo, P, Se, Zn 15 mg, biotin 30 mcg. Tab. Bot. 100s, 1000s. *OTC.*
Use: Mineral, vitamin supplement.

1000-BC, IM, or IV. (Solvay) Vitamins B_1 25 mg, B_2 2.5 mg, B_6 5 mg, panthenol 5 mg, B_{12} 500 mcg, niacinamide 75 mg, C 100 mg/mL. Vial 10 mL. *Rx.*
Use: Vitamin supplement.

1-2-3 Ointment No. 20. (Durel) Burow's solution, lanolin, zinc oxide (Lassar's paste). Jar oz, 1 lb, 6 lb. *OTC.*
Use: Anti-inflammatory, topical.

1-2-3 Ointment No. 21. (Durel) Burow's solution 1 part, lanolin 2, zinc oxide (Lassar's paste) 1.5 oz, cold cream 1.5 oz. Jar oz, 1 lb, 6 lb. *OTC.*
Use: Anti-inflammatory, topical.

Onfi. (Lundbeck Inc) Clobazam. **Susp.:** 2.5 mg/mL. Maltitol, parabens, polysorbate 80, propylene glycol, sucralose. Berry flavor. 120 mL. **Tab.:** 10 mg, 20 mg. Lactose. 100s. *c-IV.*
Use: Anticonvulsant, benzodiazepine.

Onglyza. (Bristol-Myers Squibb) Saxagliptin 2.5 mg (equiv. to saxagliptin hydrochloride 2.79 mg), 5 mg (equiv. to saxagliptin hydrochloride 5.58 mg). Film coated. Lactose. Tab. 30s, 90s, 500s (5 mg only), UD 100s (5 mg only). *Rx.*
Use: Antidiabetic agent, dipeptidyl peptidase-4 inhibitor.

Onmel. (Merz Pharmaceuticals) Itraconazole 200 mg. Lactose, vegetable oil. Tab. UD 28s. *Rx.*
Use: Antifungal, triazole antifungal.

•**onobotulinumtoxinA.** USAN.
Use: Botulinum Toxin.
See: Botox.
Botox Cosmetic.

Onoton Tablets. (Sanofi-Synthelabo) Pancreatin, hemicellulose, ox bile extracts. *OTC.*
Use: Digestive aid.

Onset Forte Micro-Coated. (Medique) Phenylephrine hydrochloride 5 mg, chlorpheniramine maleate 2 mg, acetaminophen 162.5 mg. Tab. 100s, 500s. *OTC.*
Use: Upper respiratory combination, decongestant, antihistamine, and analgesic.

•**onsifocon A.** (on-si-FOE-kon A) USAN.
Use: Hydrophobic.

Onsolis. (Meda Pharmaceuticals) Fentanyl citrate 200 mcg, 400 mcg, 600 mcg, 800 mcg, 1,200 mcg per film. Saccharin, parabens, peppermint oil. Film, soluble; buccal. Foil package. 30s. *c-II.*
Use: CNS agent, opioid analgesic.

•**ontazolast.** (ahn-TAH-zoe-last) USAN.
Use: Antiasthmatic, leukotriene antagonist.

On-the-Spot Acne Treatment. (Neutrogena) Benzoyl peroxide 2.5%. Disodium EDTA, glycerin, glyceryl, parabens, wax. Oil free. Gel. 21.26 mL. *OTC.*
Use: Topical anti-infective, antibiotic agent.

Ontosein.
See: Orgotein.

•**ontuxizumab.** (ON-tux-IZ-ue-mab) USAN.
Use: Antineoplastic.

Opana. (Endo Pharmaceuticals) Oxymorphone hydrochloride. **Inj., Soln.:** 1 mg/mL. Amps. 1 mL. **Tab.:** 5 mg, 10 mg. Lactose. Tab. 100s, UD 100s. *c-II.*
Use: Opioid analgesic.

Opana ER. (Endo Pharmaceuticals) Oxymorphone hydrochloride 5 mg, 10 mg, 20 mg, 30 mg, 40 mg. Lactose (40 mg only), methylparaben. Film-coated. ER Tab. 100s, UD 100s. *c-II.*
Use: Opioid analgesic.

Opcon. (Bausch & Lomb) Naphazoline hydrochloride 0.1%. Soln. Bot. 15 mL. *OTC.*
Use: Mydriatic; vasoconstrictor.

Opcon-A. (Bausch & Lomb) 0.027% naphazoline hydrochloride, 0.315% pheniramine maleate, 0.5% hydroxypropyl methylcellulose, 0.01% benzalkonium chloride, 0.1% EDTA, NaCl, boric acid, sodium buffers. Soln. Bot. 15 mL. *OTC.*
Use: Mydriatic; vasoconstrictor; antihistamine.

o,p'-DDD.
Use: Miscellaneous antineoplastic.
See: Lysodren

•**opebacan.** (oh-PE-bay-kan) USAN.
Use: Antimicrobial

Operand. (Aplicare) **Aerosol:** Iodine 0.5%. 90 mL. **Skin cleanser:** Iodine 1%. 90 mL. **Oint.:** Iodine 1%. 30 g, lb, packette 1.2 g, 2.7 g. **Perineal wash conc.:** Iodine 1%. 240 mL. **Prep soln.:** Iodine 1%. 60 mL, 120 mL, 240 mL, pt, qt. **Soln:** Prep pad 100s, swab stick 25s. **Surgical scrub:** Povidone-iodine 7.5%. 60 mL, 120 mL, 240 mL, pt, qt, gal, packette 22.5 mL. **Whirlpool conc.:** Iodine 1%. Gal. *OTC.*
Use: Antiseptic; antimicrobial.

Operand Douche. (Aplicare) Povidone-iodine. Soln. Bot. 60 mL, 240 mL, UD 15 mL. *OTC.*
Use: Vaginal agent.
o-phenylphenol.
W/Amyl complex, phenylmercuric nitrate.
See: Lubraseptic Jelly.
Ophthacet. (Vortech Pharmaceuticals) Sodium sulfacetamide 10%. Soln. 15 mL. *Rx.*
Use: Anti-infective, ophthalmic.
ophthalmic agents.
See: Alocril.
Nedocromil Sodium.
Pemirolast Potassium.
ophthalmic alpha adrenergic agonists.
See: Brimonidine Tartrate.
ophthalmic antibiotics.
See: Erythromycin.
Gatifloxacin.
Gentamicin.
Levofloxacin.
Moxifloxacin Hydrochloride.
ophthalmic antihistamines.
See: Alcaftadine.
Azelastine.
Emedastine Difumarate.
Epinastine Hydrochloride.
Ketotifen Fumarate.
Olopatadine Hydrochloride.
ophthalmic decongestant agents.
See: Naphazoline Hydrochloride.
Oxymetazoline Hydrochloride.
Phenylephrine Hydrochloride.
Tetrahydrozoline Hydrochloride.
ophthalmic diagnostic products.
See: Fluorexon.
Indocyanine Green.
Lissamine Green.
Rose Bengal.
Tear Test Strips.
ophthalmic hyperosmolar preparations.
See: Sodium Chloride, Hypertonic.
ophthalmic nonsurgical adjuncts.
See: SteriLid.
ophthalmic phototherapy.
See: Verteporfin.
ophthalmic proteolytic enzymes.
See: Ocriplasmin.
ophthalmic surgical adjuncts.
See: Botox.
Botulinum Toxin Type A.
Hydroxypropyl Methylcellulose.
Sodium Hyaluronate.
Trypan Blue.
Ophtha P/S. (Edwards) Prednisolone acetate 0.5%, sodium sulfacetamide 10%, hydroxyethyl cellulose, EDTA, polysorbate 80, sodium thiosulfate, benzalkonium chloride 0.025%. Susp. Bot. 5 mL. *Rx.*
Use: Corticosteroid; anti-infective, ophthalmic.
Ophtha P/S Ophthalmic Suspension. (Edwards) Sodium sulfacetamide 10%, prednisolone acetate 0.5%. Bot. 5 mL w/dropper. *Rx.*
Use: Corticosteroid; anti-infective, ophthalmic.
Ophthetic. (Allergan) Proparacaine hydrochloride 0.5%. Benzalkonium chloride 0.01%, glycerin, sodium chloride, hydrochloride acid and/or sodium hydroxide. Bot. 15 mL. *Rx.*
Use: Anesthetic, ophthalmic.
opioid agonists-antagonist analgesics.
See: Buprenorphine.
opioid analgesic combinations.
See: Acetaminophen, Caffeine, Dihydrocodeine Bitartrate.
Acetaminophen, Hydrocodone Bitartrate.
Acetaminophen, Oxycodone Hydrochloride.
Butalbital, Aspirin, Caffeine with Codeine Phosphate.
Hydrocodone Bitartrate, Ibuprofen.
Meperidine Hydrochloride, Promethazine Hydrochloride.
opioid analgesics.
See: Alfentanil Hydrochloride.
Codeine.
Fentanyl Citrate.
Fentanyl Transdermal System.
Hydromorphone Hydrochloride.
Levomethadyl Acetate Hydrochloride.
Levorphanol Tartrate.
Meperidine Hydrochloride.
Methadone Hydrochloride.
Morphine Sulfate.
Opium.
Oxycodone Hydrochloride.
Oxymorphone Hydrochloride.
Propoxyphene Hydrochloride.
Propoxyphene Napsylate.
Remifentanil Hydrochloride.
Sufentanil Citrate.
Tapentadol Hydrochloride.
Tramadol Hydrochloride.
•**opipramol hydrochloride.** (oh-PIH-prah-mole) USAN.
Use: Antipsychotic; antidepressant; tranquilizer.
•**opium.** (OH-pee-uhm) *USP.*
Use: Opioid analgesic; pharmaceutic necessity for powdered opium.
See: Opium Tincture, Deodorized.
Paregoric.
opium and belladonna. (Wyeth) Powdered opium/belladonna extract 30 mg/16.2 mg, 60 mg/15 mg, 60 mg/16.2 mg.

May have a cocoa butter or polyethylene glycol/polysorbate 60 base. Supp. 12s (except 60 mg/15 mg), 20s (except 30 mg/16.2 mg). *c-II.*
Use: Analgesic, narcotic; anticholinergic; antispasmodic.

•**opium powdered.** (OH-pee-uhm) *USP.*
Use: Pharmaceutical necessity for Paregoric.

opium tincture, camphorated.
Use: Antidiarrheal.
See: Paregoric

opium tincture, deodorized. (Ranbaxy) Anhydrous morphine equivalent to 10 mg/mL. Alcohol 19%. Liq. Bot. 120 mL, 473 mL. *c-II.*
Use: Opioid analgesic.

•**oprelvekin.** (oh-PRELL-veh-kin) USAN.
Use: Hematopoietic, interleukin.
See: Neumega.

•**oprozomib.** (oh-PROZ-oh-mib) USAN.
Use: Antineoplastic.

Opsumit. (Actelion) Macitentan 10 mg. Film coated. Lactose. Tab. 30s, UD 15s. *Rx.*
Use: Vasodilator, endothelin receptor antagonist.

Optase. (Onset Therapeutics) Balsam peru 87 mg, castor oil 788 mg, trypsin 0.12 mg. Oleth 10, safflower oil. Gel. 6 g, 95 g. *Rx.*
Use: Topical enzyme combination.

Opti-Bon Eye Drops. (Barrows) Phenylephrine hydrochloride, berberine sulfate, boric acid, sodium Cl, sodium bisulfite, glycerin, camphor, water, peppermint water, thimerosal 0.004%. Bot. 1 oz. *OTC.*
Use: Ophthalmic.

Opticaps. (Health for Life Brands) Vitamins A 32,500 units, D 3250 units, B_1 15 mg, B_2 5 mg, B_6 0.5 mg, C 150 mg, E 5 units, calcium pantothenate 3 mg, niacinamide 150 mg, B_{12} 20 mcg, Fe 11.26 mg, choline bitartrate 30 mg, inositol 30 mg, pepsin 32.5 mg, diastase 32.5 mg, Ca 30 mg, P 25 mg, Mg 0.7 mg, Fr. dicalcium phosphate 110 mg, Mn 1.3 mg, K 0.68 mg, Zn 0.45 mg, hesperidin compound 25 mg, biotin 20 mcg, brewer's yeast 50 mg, wheat germ oil 20 mg, hydrolyzed yeast 81.25 mg, protein digest 47.04 mg, amino acids 34.21 mg. Cap. Bot. 30s, 60s, 90s, 1000s. *OTC.*
Use: Mineral, vitamin supplement.

Opticare PMS. (Standard Drug Co.) Fe 2.5 mg, vitamins 2083 units, D 17 units, E 14 units, B_1 4.2 mg, B_2 4.2 mg, B_3 4.2 mg, B_5 4.2 mg, B_6 50 mg, B_{12} 10.4 mcg, C 250 mg, folic acid 0.03 mg, Cr, Cu, I, K, Mg, Mn, Se, Zn 4.2 mg, biotin 10.4 mcg, choline bitartrate, bioflavonoids, inositol, PABA, rutin, Ca, amylase activity, protease activity, lipase activity, betaine, tartrazine. Bot. 150s. *OTC.*
Use: Mineral, vitamin supplement.

Opti-Clean II Especially For Sensitive Eyes. (Alcon) EDTA 0.1%, polyquaternium 1 0.001%, polymeric cleaners, Tween 21. Thimerosal free. Bot. 12 mL, 20 mL. *OTC.*
Use: Contact lens care.

Opti-Clear. (Major) Tetrahydrozoline hydrochloride 0.05%. Benzalkonium chloride 0.01%, boric acid, EDTA, sodium borate, sodium chloride. Ophth. Soln. 15 mL. *OTC.*
Use: Ophthalmic decongestant.

Opti-Free. (Alcon) Citrate buffer, sodium chloride, EDTA 0.05%, polyquaternium 1 0.001%. Soln. Bot. 10 mL, 20 mL. *OTC.*
Use: Contact lens rewetting solution.

Opti-Free Express Multi-Purpose. (Alcon) Isotonic. Myristamidopropyl dimethylamine 0.0005%, polyquaternium-1 0.001%, citrate, sodium chloride, boric acid, sorbitol, EDTA. Soln. 118 mL. *OTC.*
Use: Soft contact lens disinfection system.

Opti-Free Non-Hydrogen Peroxide-Containing System. (Alcon) Isotonic. Citrate buffer, NaCl, EDTA 0.05%, polyquaternium-1 0.001%. Thimerosal free. Soln. 118 mL, 237 mL, 355 mL. *OTC.*
Use: Contact lens disinfection system.

Opti-Free Surfactant Cleaning Solution. (Alcon) EDTA 0.01%, polyquaternium 1 0.001%, microclens polymeric cleaners, Tween 21. Thimerosal free. Soln. Bot. 12 mL, 20 mL. *OTC.*
Use: Contact lens care.

Optigene 3. (Pfeiffer) Tetrahydrozoline hydrochloride 0.05%. Benzalkonium chloride 0.01%, boric acid, EDTA 0.1%, sodium borate. Ophth. Soln. Bot. 15 mL. *OTC.*
Use: Mydriatic, vasoconstrictor; ophthalmic decongestant.

Optilets-500. (Abbott) Vitamins B_1 15 mg, B_2 10 mg, B_3 100 mg, B_5 20 mg, B_6 5 mg, C 500 mg, A 10,000 units, D 400 units, E 30 units, B_{12} 12 mcg. Filmtab. Bot. 120s. *OTC.*
Use: Mineral, vitamin supplement.

Optilets-M-500. (Abbott) Vitamins C 500 mg, B_3 100 mg, B_5 20 mg, $B_1$15 mg,

A 5000 units, B_2 10 mg, B_6 5 mg, D 400 units, B_{12} 12 mcg, E 30 units, Fe 20 mg, Mg, Zn 1.5 mg, Cu, Mn, I. Filmtab. Bot. 120s. *OTC.*
Use: Mineral, vitamin supplement.

OptiMARK. (Mallinckrodt) Gadoversetamide 330.9 mg/mL. Calcium versetamide sodium 28.4 mg, calcium chloride dihydrate 0.7 mg per mL. Preservative free. Inj., Soln. Vials. 5 mL, 10 mL, 15 mL, 20 mL. Syringes. 10 mL, 15 mL, 20 mL, 30 mL. *Rx.*
Use: Radiopaque agent, parenteral.

Optimental. (Ross) Protein 12.2 g, fat 6.7 g, carbohydrate 32.9 g, vitamin A 1950 units, D 67 units, E 50 units, K 20 mcg, C 50 mg, folic acid 135 mcg, B_1 0.5 mg, B_2 0.57 mg, B_6 0.67 mg, B_{12} 2 mcg, B_3 6.7 mg, choline 100 mg, biotin 100 mcg, B_5 3.4 mg, Na 250 mg, K 420 mg, chloride 320 mg, Ca 250 mg, P 250 mg, Mg 100 mg, I 38 mcg, Mn 0.84 mg, Cu 0.34 mg, Zn 3.8 mg, Fe 3 mg, Se 12 mcg, Cr 20 mcg, Mo 25 mcg, sucrose, canola oil, soy oil. Liq. Bot. 237 mL. *OTC.*
Use: Nutritional therapy, enteral.

Optimine. (Key) Azatadine maleate 1 mg, lactose. Tab. Bot. 100s. *Rx.*
Use: Antihistamine, nonselective piperidine.

Optimox Prenatal. (Optimox) Ca 100 mg, iron 5 mg, vitamins A 833 units, D 67 units, E 2 mg, B_1 0.5 mg, B_2 0.6 mg, B_3 6.7 mg, B_5 3.3 mg, B_6 0.73 mg, B_{12} 0.87 mcg, C 30 mg, folic acid 0.13 mg, Cr, Cu, I, K, Mg, Mn, Se, Zn 3.17 mg. Tab. Bot. 360s. *OTC.*
Use: Mineral, vitamin supplement.

Optimyd. (Schering-Plough) Prednisolone phosphate 0.5%, sodium sulfacetamide 10%, sodium thiosulfate. Sterile Soln. Drop Bot. 5 mL. *Rx.*
Use: Anti-infective; corticosteroid; ophthalmic.

Optinate Omega-3 L-Vcaps. (First Horizon) **Cap.:** Docosahexaenoic acid 250 mg. Blister packs of 5s. **Tab.:** Calcium 200 mg, iron 90 mg, vitamin D_3 400 units, E 10 units, B_1 3 mg, B_2 3.4 mg, niacinamide 20 mg, B_6 20 mg, B_{12} 12 mcg, C 120 mg, folate 1 mg, biotin 30 mcg, pantothenic acid 6 mg, copper 2 mg, zinc 15 mg, magnesium 30 mg, docusate sodium 50 mg. Lactose, sucrose. Film-coated. Blister packs of 5s. *Rx.*
Use: Multivitamin.

Opti-One. (Alcon) EDTA 0.05%, polyquaternium-1 0.001%, sodium chloride, citrate buffer. Soln. 10 mL. *OTC.*
Use: Contact lens rewetting solution.

Opti-One Multi-Purpose. (Alcon) EDTA 0.05%, polyquaternium-1 0.001%, sodium chloride. Buffered, isotonic. Soln. Bot. 118 mL, 237 mL, 355 mL, 473 mL. *OTC.*
Use: Contact lens care.

Opti-One Rewetting. (Alcon) EDTA 0.05%, polyquaternium 1 0.001%, sodium chloride, citrate buffer, isotonic. Drops. Bot. 10 mL. *OTC.*
Use: Contact lens care.

OptiPranolol. (Bausch & Lomb) Metipranolol hydrochloride 0.3%, benzalkonium chloride 0.004%, glycerin, EDTA, povidone, hydrochloric acid, sodium chloride, sodium hydroxide and/or hydrochloric acid. Soln. Bot. 5 mL, 10 mL w/dropper. *Rx.*
Use: Antiglaucoma agent; beta-adrenergic blocker.

Optiray 160. (Mallinckrodt) Ioversol 339 mg, iodine 160 mg/mL. EDTA. Inj. Bot. 50 mL, 100 mL. *Rx.*
Use: Radiopaque agent, parenteral.

Optiray 300. (Mallinckrodt) Ioversol 636 mg, iodine 300 mg/mL. EDTA. Inj. Bot. 50 mL, 100 mL, 150 mL. 200 mL fill in 250 mL Bot. Hand-held syringe. 50 mL. Power injector syringe. 100 mL fill in 125 mL. *Rx.*
Use: Radiopaque agent, parenteral.

Optiray 350. (Mallinckrodt) Ioversol 741 mg, iodine 350 mg/mL. EDTA. Inj. Bot. 50 mL, 100 mL, 150 mL. 75 mL fill in 100 mL Bot., 200 mL fill in 250 mL Bot. Hand-held syringes. 30 mL, 50 mL. Power injector syringes. 50 mL fill in 125 mL, 75 mL fill in 125 mL, 100 mL fill in 125 mL. Power Injector Syringes. 125 mL. *Rx.*
Use: Radiopaque agent, parenteral.

Optiray 320. (Mallinckrodt) Ioversol 678 mg, iodine 320 mg/mL. EDTA. Inj. Vials. 20 mL, 30 mL. Bot. 50 mL, 100 mL, 150 mL. 75 mL fill in 150 mL Bot. 200 mL fill in 250 mL Bot. Hand-held syringes. 30 mL, 50 mL. Power injector syringes. 50 mL fill in 125 mL, 75 mL fill in 125 mL, 100 mL fill in 125 mL Power injector syringes. 125 mL. *Rx.*
Use: Radiopaque agent, parenteral.

Optiray 240. (Mallinckrodt) Ioversol 509 mg, iodine 240 mg/mL. EDTA. Inj. Bot. 50 mL, 100 mL, 150 mL, 200 mL fill in 250 mL Bot. Hand-held syringes. 50 mL. Power injector syringes. 125 mL. *Rx.*
Use: Radiopaque agent, parenteral.

Opti-Soft Especially for Sensitive Eyes. (Alcon) Buffered, isotonic. EDTA 0.1%, polyquaternium 1 0.001%, NaCl, borate buffer. For lenses w/≤ 45% water content. Soln. Bot. 118 mL, 237 mL, 355 mL. *OTC.*
Use: Contact lens care.

Optison. (GE Healthcare) Perflutren 0.22 ± 0.11 mg/mL. Protein type A microspheres 5 to 8 × 10^8, albumin human 10 mg, N-acetyltryptophan 0.2 mg, caprylic acid 0.12 mg. Preservative free. Inj., Susp. Single-use vials. 3 mL. *Rx.*
Use: Radiopaque agent, parenteral agent.

Optivar. (MedPointe Healthcare) Azelastine hydrochloride 0.05%. Benzalkonium chloride 0.125 mg, EDTA, dihydrate, hydroxypropylmethylcellulose, sodium hydroxide. Soln., Ophth. 6 mL w/dropper. *Rx.*
Use: Ophthalmic antihistamine.

Optive. (Allergan) Carboxymethylcellulose sodium 0.5%, glycerin 0.9%. Ophth. Soln. 15 mL. *OTC.*
Use: Artificial tear solution.

Optivite for Women. (Optimox) Vitamins A 2083 units, D 16.7 units, E 14 mg, B_1 4.2 mg, B_2 4.2 mg, B_3 4.2 mg, B_5 4.2 mg, B_6 50 mg, B_{12} 10.4 mcg, C 250 mg, Fe 2.5 mg, folic acid 0.03 mg, Zn 4.2 mg, choline 52 mg, inositol 10 mg, Cr, Cu, I, K, Mg, Mn, Se, citrus bioflavonoids, PABA, rutin, pancreatin, biotin. Tab. Bot. 180s. *OTC.*
Use: Mineral, vitamin supplement.

Optivite P.M.T. (Optimox) Vitamins A 2083 units, D, E 16.7 mg, B_1 4.2 mg, B_2 4.2 mg, B_3 4.2 mg, B_5 4.2 mg, B_6 50 mg, B_{12} 10.4 mcg, C 250 mg, Fe 2.5 mg, FA 0.03 mg, Zn 4.2 mg, choline, Ca, Cr, Cu, I, K, Mg, Mn, Se, bioflavonoids, betaine, PABA, rutin, pancreatin, biotin, inositol. Tab. Bot. 180s. *OTC.*
Use: Mineral, vitamin supplement.

OptiZen. (InnoZen) Polysorbate 80 0.5%. EDTA, NaCl, sodium phosphate, sorbic acid. Drops. 10 mL. *OTC.*
Use: Artificial tears.

Orabase. (Colgate) Benzocaine 20%. Paste, Dental. 5 g. *OTC.*
Use: Local anesthetic, topical; ester local anesthetic.

Orabase-B. (Colgate) Benzocaine 20%, mineral oil. Paste; dental. 5 g, 15 g. *OTC.*
Use: Mouth and throat preparation.

Orabase Baby. (Colgate) Benzocaine 7.5%, alcohol free, fruit flavor. Gel. Tube 7.2 mL. *OTC.*
Use: Anesthetic, local.

Orabase HCA. (Colgate) Hydrocortisone acetate 0.5%, polyethylene 5%, mineral oil. Gel. Tube 5 mL. *Rx.*
Use: Corticosteroid, dental.

Orabase Lip. (Colgate) Benzocaine 5%, allantoin 1.5%, menthol 0.5%, petrolatum, lanolin, parabens, camphor, phenol/g. Cream. Tube 10 g. *OTC.*
Use: Anesthetic, local.

Orabase Plain. (Colgate) Gelatin, pectin & sodium carboxymethyl cellulose in polyethylene and mineral gel. Paste. Tube 5 g, 15 g. *OTC.*
Use: Mouth and throat preparation.

Orabloc. (Pierrel) Articaine hydrochloride 4%. With epinephrine bitartrate 1:100,000 (0.018 mg/mL), 1:200,000 (0.009 mg/mL). Sodium metabisulfite. Inj., Soln. Single-use cartridge. 1.8 mL. *Rx.*
Use: Injectable local anesthetic, amide local anesthetic.

Oracea. (Galderma) Doxycycline 40 mg (30 mg immediate release and 10 mg delayed release). PEG, sugar. Cap. 30s. *Rx.*
Use: Anti-infective, tetracycline.

Oracit. (Carolina Medical Products) Sodium citrate 490 mg, citric acid 640 mg/5 mL. Parabens. Each mL contains sodium ion 1 mEq and is equiv. to bicarbonate 1 mEq. Soln. 500 mL, UD 15 mL, UD 30 mL. *Rx.*
Use: Alkalinizer, systemic.

Oraderm Lip Balm. (Schattner) Sodium phenolate, sodium tetraborate, phenol, base containing an anionic emulsifier. ⅛ oz. *OTC.*
Use: Anesthetic; antiseptic, local.

Orafate. (McCullough Mueller Enterprises) Sucralfate 10%. Parabens, saccharin. Paste; oral. 30 mL. *Rx.*
Use: Gastrointestinal agent.

ORA5. (McHenry Laboratories, Inc.) Copper sulfate, iodine, potassium iodide, alcohol 1.5%. Liq. Bot. 3.75 mL, 30 mL. *OTC.*
Use: Mouth preparation.

ORAfix Special. (Hogil) Tube 1.4 oz, 2.4 oz. *OTC.*
Use: Denture adhesive.

ORAfix Ultra. (Hogil) Tube 3.2 oz. *OTC.*
Use: Denture adhesive.

Oragrafin Calcium Granules. (Bristol-Myers Squibb) Ipodate calcium (61.7% iodine) 3 g/8 g Pkg. 25 × 1 dose pkg.
Use: Radiopaque agent.

Orahesive. (Colgate Oral) Gelatin, pectin, sodium carboxymethylcellulose. Pow. Bot. 25 g. *OTC.*
Use: Denture adhesive.

Orajel. (Del) Benzocaine 10% in a special base. Gel. Tube 0.2 oz, 0.5 oz. *OTC.*
Use: Anesthetic, local.

Orajel Baby. (Del) Benzocaine 7.5%. **Gel; dental:** Saccharin, sorbitol. Alcohol free. 9.45 g. **Liq.; dental:** Parabens, saccharin, sorbitol. Very berry flavor. 13.3 mL. *OTC.*
Use: Topical local anesthetic, ester local anesthetic.

Orajel Baby Nighttime. (Del) Benzocaine 10%. Saccharin, sorbitol. Alcohol free. Cherry flavor. Gel; dental. 6 g. *OTC.*
Use: Topical local anesthetic, ester local anesthetic.

Orajel Brace-Aid. (Del) Benzocaine 20%. Saccharin. Gel; dental. 14.1 g. *OTC.*
Use: Topical local anesthetic, ester local anesthetic.

Orajel D. (Del) Benzocaine 10%, saccharin. Gel. Tube 9.45 mL. *OTC.*
Use: Topical local anesthetic, ester local anesthetic.

Orajel Maximum Strength. (Del) Benzocaine 20%. **Gel; dental:** Saccharin. 9.45 g. **Liq.; dental:** Ethyl alcohol 44.2%, phenol, saccharin. 13.3 mL. *OTC.*
Use: Topical local anesthetic, ester local anesthetic.

Orajel Mouth-Aid. (Del) Benzocaine 20%. **Liq.:** Cetylpyridinium chloride 0.1%, ethyl alcohol 70%, saccharin. 13.5 mL. **Gel; dental:** Benzalkonium chloride 0.02%, zinc chloride 0.1%, saccharin. Sugar free. 5.6 g, 10 g. *OTC.*
Use: Topical local anesthetic, ester local anesthetic.

Orajel Perioseptic. (Del) Carbamide peroxide 15%, saccharin, methylparaben, EDTA, sorbitol, ethyl alcohol. Liq. Bot. 240 mL. *OTC.*
Use: Mouth and throat product.

Orajel P.M. Nighttime Formula Toothache Pain Relief. (Del) Benzocaine 20%. Menthol, methyl salicylate, saccharin. Cream; dental. 5.4 g. *OTC.*
Use: Topical local anesthetic, ester local anesthetic.

Orajel Regular Strength. (Church Dwight) Benzocaine 10%. PEG, saccharin. Gel; dental. 5.1 g, 7.1 g, 9.4 g. *OTC.*
Use: Topical local anesthetic, ester local anesthetic.

Oral-B Muppets Fluoride Toothpaste. (Oral-B) Fluoride 0.22%. Pump 4.3 oz. *OTC.*
Use: Dental caries agent.

oral contraceptives.
See: Alesse.
Altavera.
Apri.
Aviane.
Beyaz.
Brevicon.
Briellyn.
Caziant.
Chateal.
Dasetta 1/35.
Daysee.
Desogen.
Enovid-E 21.
Estarylla.
Estrostep Fe.
Falmina.
GenCept.
Generess Fe.
Gianvi.
Heather.
Jencycla.
Jenest-28.
Kurvelo.
Levlen.
Levlite.
Levora.
Loestrin 21 1/20.
Loestrin 21 1.5/30.
Loestrin Fe 1/20.
Loestrin Fe 1.5/30.
Lo Loestrin Fe.
Lo/Ovral.
Loryna.
Low-Ogestrel.
Microgestin Fe 1/20.
Microgestin Fe 1.5/30.
Micronor.
Mircette.
Modicon.
MonoNessa.
Necon 0.5/35.
Necon 1/35.
Necon 1/50.
Necon 10/11.
Nelulen.
Nordette.
Norinyl 1+35.
Norinyl 1+50.
Nor-QD.
Nortrel 0.5/35.
Nortrel 1/35.
Ocella.
Ogestrel 0.5/50.
Ortho Cept.
Ortho-Cyclen.
Ortho-Novum 1/35.
Ortho-Novum 1/50.
Ortho-Novum 7/7/7.
Ortho-Novum 10/11.
Ortho Tri-Cyclen.
Ovcon-35.
Ovcon-50.

Ovral.
Ovulen-21.
Ovulen-28.
Plan B.
Preven.
Seasonale.
Seasonique.
Syeda.
Tri-Estarylla.
Tri-Levlen.
Tri-Norinyl.
Triphasil.
Trivora.
Viorele.
Yasmin.
Zarah.
Zeosa.
Zovia 1/35E.
Zovia 1/50E.

Oral Drops/Canker Sore Relief. (Weeks & Leo) Carbamide peroxide 10% in anhydrous glycerin base. Bot. 30 mL. *OTC.*
Use: Mouth preparation.

Oral Pain Relief Maximum Strength. (Major) Benzocaine 20%. PEG, saccharin. Gel, dental. 14.2 g. *OTC.*
Use: Ester local anesthetic.

oral rehydration salts.
Use: Electrolyte combination.

Oral Wound Rinse. (Carrington) Acemannan hydrogel. Fructose. Mouthwash. 7.4 g. *OTC.*
Use: Mouth and throat product.

Oralyte. (Rugby) Sodium 45 mEq/L, potassium 20 mEq/L, chloride 35 mEq/L, dextrose 25 g/L, zinc 7.8 mg/L. Acesulfame K, sucralose (flavored solutions only). Unflavored, bubble gum, fruit, and grape flavors. Soln. 1 L ready-to-use. *OTC.*
Use: Electrolyte mixture.

Oralyte Freeze Pops. (Rugby) Sodium 45 mEq/L, potassium 20 mEq/L, chloride 35 mEq/L. Acesulfame potassium, benzoic acid, dextrose 25 g/L, potassium citrate, sucralose. Wild berry, grape, orange, and cherry flavors. 62.5 mL ready-to-freeze pops (16s). *OTC.*
Use: Electrolyte mixture.

OraMagic Plus. (MPM Medical) Benzocaine 10%. Aloe vera extract, maltodextrin, xylitol. Liq.; dental. 60 mL. *OTC.*
Use: Mouth and throat product.

OraMagicRx. (MPM Medical) *Aloemannon-Plus* (high molecular weight complex carbohydrates, mannons, and low molecular weight constituents extracted from aloe vera), citric acid, lemon/lime flavor, maltodextrin, potassium benzoate, potassium sorbate, xanthan, xylitol. Alcohol free. Pow. for Oral Rinse. 25 g, 37.5 g. *Rx.*
Use: Mouth and throat product.

Oramide. (Major) Tolbutamide 0.5 g. Tab. Bot. 100s, 1000s. *Rx.*
Use: Antidiabetic.

Oraminic II. (Vortech Pharmaceuticals) Brompheniramine maleate 10 mg/mL. Inj. Vial. 10 mL multidose. *Rx.*
Use: Antihistamine.

Oramorph SR. (AAIPharma) Morphine sulfate 15 mg, 30 mg, 60 mg, 100 mg (for use only in opioid-tolerant patients). Lactose. CR Tab. Bot. 50s (30 mg only), 100s, 250s (30 mg only), 500s (15 mg only), UD 25s (60 mg and 100 mg only), UD 100s (15 mg and 30 mg only). *c-II.*
Use: Opioid analgesic.

orange flower oil.
Use: Flavor; perfume; vehicle.

orange flower water.
Use: Flavor; perfume.

•**orange oil.** *NF.*
Use: Flavor.

•**orange peel tincture, sweet.** *NF.*
Use: Flavor.

•**orange spirit, compound.** *NF.*
Use: Flavor.

•**orange syrup.** *NF.*
Use: Flavored vehicle.

Orap. (Teva) Pimozide 1 mg, 2 mg, lactose. Tab. Bot. 100s. *Rx.*
Use: Antipsychotic.

Orapred. (Sciele) Prednisolone 15 mg (equiv. to prednisolone sodium phosphate 20.2 mg)/5 mL. Alcohol 2%, fructose, monammonium glycyrrhizinate, sorbitol. Dye free. Grape flavor. Oral Soln. 20 mL, 237 mL. *Rx.*
Use: Adrenocortical steroid, glucocorticoid.

Orapred ODT. (Concordia) Prednisolone 10 mg (equiv. to prednisolone sodium phosphate 13.4 mg), 15 mg (equiv. to prednisolone sodium phosphate 20.2 mg), 30 mg (equiv. to prednisolone sodium phosphate 40.3 mg). Mannitol, sucralose, sucrose. Grape flavor. Orally Disintegrating Tab. UD 48s. *Rx.*
Use: Andrenocortical steroid, glucocorticoid.

Oraqix. (Dentsply Pharmaceutical) Lidocaine 2.5%, prilocaine 2.5%. Gel. Single-use cartridge w/applicator 20s. 1.7 g. *Rx.*
Use: Topical local anesthetic combination.

OraQuick Advance Rapid HIV-1/2 Antibody Test. (OraSure Technologies) Collection kit: Test device, absorbent packet, developer solution vial, test stands, and specimen collection loops for 25 or 100 tests. Device for in vitro immunoassay. For professional use only.
Use: Diagnostic aid.

Orasep. (Llorens) Benzocaine 2%, cetylpyridinium chloride 0.1%, menthol 0.5%. Castor oil, parabens, propylene glycol, saccharin. Alcohol free. Soln. 30 mL. *OTC.*
Use: Mouth and throat product.

Orasept. (Pharmakon) Tannic acid 12.16%, methyl benzethonium hydrochloride 1.53%, ethyl alcohol 53.31%, camphor, menthol, benzyl alcohol, spearmint oil, cassia oil. Liq. Bot. 15 mL. *OTC.*
Use: Mouth and throat preparation.

Orasept, Throat. (Pharmakon) Benzocaine 0.996%, methyl benzethonium Cl 1.037%, sorbitol 70%, menthol, peppermint, saccharin. Throat spray. 45 mL. *OTC.*
Use: Mouth and throat preparation.

Orasol. (Ivax) Benzocaine 6.3%. Alcohol 70%, camphor, menthol, phenol 0.5%, povidone-iodine. Liq.; dental. 14.79 mL. *OTC.*
Use: Anesthetic, local.

OraSure HIV-1. (Epitope) Collection kit: Cotton fiber on a stick with collection vial. Device for oral specimen collection. For professional use only.
Use: Diagnostic aid.

OraVerse. (Septodont) Phentolamine mesylate 0.4 mg per 1.7 mL. D-mannitol, edetate disodium. Preservative free. Inj., Soln. Dental cartridge. *Rx.*
Use: Agent for pheochromocytoma.

Orazinc. (Mericon Industries) Zinc sulfate 220 mg. Cap. Bot. 100s, 1000s. *OTC.*
Use: Mineral supplement.

orbenin. Sodium cloxacillin.
Use: Anti-infective.
See: Cloxapen.

Orbiferrous. (Orbit) Ferrous fumarate 300 mg, vitamins B_{12} 12 mcg, C 50 mg, B_1 3 mg, defatted desiccated liver 50 mg. Tab. Bot. 60s, 500s. *OTC.*
Use: Mineral, vitamin supplement.

Orbit. (Spanner) Vitamins A 6250 units, D 400 units, B_1 3 mg, B_2 3 mg, B_6 2 mg, B_{12} 5 mcg, C 75 mg, niacinamide 20 mg, calcium pantothenate 10 mg, E 15 units, biotin 15 mcg, Fe 20 mg. Tab. Bot. 100s. *OTC.*
Use: Mineral, vitamin supplement.

Orbivan. (ECR Pharmaceuticals) Acetaminophen 300 mg, butalbital 50 mg, caffeine 40 mg. Cap. 100s. *Rx.*
Use: Nonnarcotic analgesic combination, nonnarcotic analgesic with barbiturates.

Orbivan CF. (ECR Pharmaceuticals) Acetaminophen 300 mg, butalbital 50 mg. Tab. 100s. *Rx.*
Use: Nonnarcotic analgesic with barbiturate.

•**orbofiban acetate.** (ore-boe-FIE-ban) USAN.
Use: Fibrinogen receptor antagonist; platelet aggregation inhibitor, antithrombotic.

•**orconazole nitrate.** (ahr-KOE-nah-zole) USAN.
Use: Antifungal.

•**oregovomab.** (oh-re-GOE-voe-mab) USAN.
Use: Monoclonal antibody (ovarian cancer).

Orencia. (Bristol-Myers Squibb) Abatacept. **Inj., lyophilized Pow. for Soln.:** 250 mg. Maltose 500 mg. Preservative free. Single-use vials w/syringe. **Inj., Soln.:** 125 mg/mL. Sucrose 170 mg. Preservative free. Single-use vial w/syringe. *Rx.*
Use: Immunomodulator, immunologic agent.

Orenitram. (United Therapeutics Corp.) Treprostinil 0.125 mg (equiv. to treprostinil diolamine 0.159 mg), 0.25 mg (equiv. to treprostinil diolamine 0.317 mg), 1 mg (equiv. to treprostinil diolamine 1.27 mg), 2.5 mg (equiv. to treprostinil diolamine 3.17 mg). Maltodextrin, PEG, xylitol. ER Tab. 100s. *Rx.*
Use: Vasodilator, peripheral vasodilator.

Orexin. (Roberts) Vitamins B_1 8.1 mg, B_6 4.1 mg, B_{12} 25 mcg. Chew. Tab. Bot. 100s. *OTC.*
Use: Vitamin supplement.

Orfadin. (Sobi) Nitisinone 2 mg, 5 mg, 10 mg. Cap. 60s. *Rx.*
Use: Tyrosinemia.

Organidin. (Wallace) **Tab.:** 30 mg. Bot. 100s. **Elix.:** 60 mg/5 mL. 21.75% alcohol, glucose, saccharin. Bot. Pt., gal. **Soln.:** 50 mg/mL. Bot. 30 mL w/dropper.
Use: Expectorant.

Organ-I NR. (Qualitest) Guaifenesin 200 mg. Maltodextrin. Tab. 100s. *OTC.*
Use: Expectorant.

Orglagen. (Ivax) Orphenadrine citrate 100 mg. Tab. Bot. 100s, 1000s. *Rx.*
Use: Muscle relaxant.

•**orgotein.** (OR-goe-teen) USAN. A group of soluble metalloproteins isolated from

liver, red blood cells, and other mammalian tissues.
Use: Anti-inflammatory; antirheumatic.

orgotein. (Diagnostic Data) Pure water-soluble protein with a compact conformation maintained by 4 g atoms of chelated divalent metals, produced from bovine liver as a Cu-Zn mixed chelate having superoxide dismutase activity. Ontosein, Palosein.

oriental ginseng.
See: Ginseng, Asian.

Original Alka-Seltzer Effervescent. (Bayer Consumer Care) 1700 mg sodium bicarbonate, 325 mg aspirin, 1000 mg citric acid, 9 mg phenylalanine, 506 mg Na, aspartame. Tab. Pkg. 24s. *OTC.*
Use: Antacid.

Original Eclipse Sunscreen. (Tri Tec) Padimate O, glyceryl PABA, SPF 10. Lot. Bot. 120 mL. *OTC.*
Use: Sunscreen.

Original Sensodyne. (Block Drug) Strontium chloride hexahydrate 10%, saccharin, sorbitol. Toothpaste. Tube 59.5 g. *OTC.*
Use: Mouth and throat preparation.

•**oritavancin diphosphate.** (or-IT-a-VAN-sin) USAN.
Use: Antibacterial.

•**orlistat.** (ORE-lih-stat) USAN.
Use: Inhibitor, pancreatic lipase.
See: Alli.
Xenical.

•**ormaplatin.** (ORE-mah-PLAT-in) USAN.
Use: Antineoplastic.

•**ormetoprim.** (ore-MEH-toe-PRIM) USAN.
Use: Anti-infective.

Ornex No Drowsiness. (B.F. Ascher) Pseudoephedrine hydrochloride 30 mg, acetaminophen 325 mg. Lactose, PEG. Tab. Bot. 24s, 48s. *OTC.*
Use: Upper respiratory combination, analgesic, decongestant.

•**ornidazole.** (ahr-NIH-DAH-zole) USAN.
Use: Anti-infective.

•**ornithine phenylacetate.** (OR-ni-theen) USAN.
Use: Ammonia detoxifying agent.

•**orpanoxin.** (AHR-pan-OX-in) USAN.
Use: Anti-inflammatory.

Orpeneed VK. (Hanlon) Penicillin, buffered, 400,000 units. Tab. Bot. 100s. *Rx.*
Use: Anti-infective, penicillin.

•**orphenadrine citrate.** (ore-FEN-uh-dreen) *USP.*
Use: Antihistamine, muscle relaxant.
See: Banflex.
Flexon.
Myolin.
Norflex.
W/Aspirin, Caffeine.
See: Orphenadrine Compound.
Orphenadrine Compound-DS.

orphenadrine citrate. (Apothecon) Orphenadrine citrate 100 mg. Lactose. SR Tab. 100s, 500s. *Rx.*
Use: Muscle relaxant.

orphenadrine citrate. (Various Mfr.) Orphenadrine citrate. **Inj:** 30 mg/mL. Amps. 2 mL. Vials. 10 mL. **Tab.:** 100 mg. Bot. 30s, 100s, 500s, 1000s. *Rx.*
Use: Antihistamine; muscle relaxant.

Orphenadrine Compound. (Sandoz) Aspirin 385 mg, caffeine 30 mg, orphenadrine citrate 25 mg. Lactose. Tab. 100s. *Rx.*
Use: Skeletal muscle relaxant.

Orphenadrine Compound-DS. (Sandoz) Aspirin 770 mg, caffeine 60 mg, orphenadrine citrate 50 mg. Lactose. Tab. 100s. *Rx.*
Use: Skeletal muscle relaxant.

Orphengesic Forte. (Various Mfr.) Orphenadrine citrate 50 mg, aspirin 770 mg, caffeine 60 mg, lactose. Tab. Bot. 100s, 500s. *Rx.*
Use: Analgesic, muscle relaxant.

Orsythia. (Qualitest) Ethinyl estradiol 20 mcg, levonorgestrel 0.1 g. Film coated. Lactose, PEG. Tab. 28s w/7 film-coated inert tablets (lactose, PEG). *Rx.*
Use: Monophasic oral contraceptive.

Ortac-DM. (ION Laboratories, Inc.) Dextromethorphan 10 mg, phenylephrine hydrochloride 5 mg, guaifenesin 100 mg/5 mL. Liq. Bot. 4 oz. *OTC.*
Use: Antitussive, decongestant, expectorant.

ortal sodium. Sodium 5-ethyl-5-hexylbarbiturate. Hexethal sodium.

ortedrine.
See: Amphetamines.

•**orteronel.** (or-TER-oh-nel) USAN.
Use: Antineoplastic.

orthesin.
See: Benzocaine.

Ortho All-Flex Diaphragm. (Ortho-McNeil) Diaphragm kit (all flex arcing spring) in plastic compact, sizes 55, 60, 65, 70, 75, 80, 85, 90, 95 mm. *Rx.*
Use: Contraceptive.

orthocaine.
See: Orthoform.

Ortho-Cept. (Janssen) Desogestrel 0.15 mg, ethinyl estradiol 30 mcg. Lactose. Tab. *Dialpak* and *Veridate* 28s

with 7 inert tabs. *Rx.*
Use: Sex hormone, contraceptive hormone.

Ortho-Cyclen. (Janssen) Norgestimate 0.25 mg, ethinyl estradiol 35 mcg. Lactose. Tab. *Dialpak* and *Veridate* 28s with 7 inert tabs. *Rx.*
Use: Sex hormone, contraceptive hormone.

Ortho Diaphragm. (Ortho-McNeil) Diaphragm kit, coil spring sizes 50, 55, 60, 65, 70, 75, 80, 85, 90, 95, 100, 105 mm. *Rx.*
Use: Contraceptive.

Ortho Diaphragm-White. (Ortho-McNeil) Diaphragm kit, flat spring sizes 55, 60, 65, 70, 75, 80, 85, 90, 95 mm. *Rx.*
Use: Contraceptive.

Ortho Dienestrol Vaginal Cream. (Ortho-McNeil) Dienestrol 0.01%. Cream. Tube 78 g with or without applicator. *Rx.*
Use: Estrogen.

Ortho Evra. (Janssen) Norelgestromin 150 mcg, ethinyl estradiol 35 mcg per 24 h. Patch; transdermal. 1s, 3s. *Rx.*
Use: Sex hormone, contraceptive hormone.

Orthoflavin. (Enzyme Process) Vitamins C 150 mg, E 25 mg. Tab. Bot. 100s, 250s. *OTC.*
Use: Vitamin supplement.

Orthoform. (Columbus) Tyrothricin 0.5 mg, tetracaine hydrochloride 0.5%, epinephrine 1/1000 Soln. 2%/g. Oint. Tube oz. *Rx.*
Use: Anti-infective, ophthalmic.

ortho-hydroxybenzoic acid. Salicylic Acid, USP.

orthohydroxyphenylmercuric chloride.
Use: Antiseptic.
W/Benzocaine, Parachlorometaxylenol, Benzalkonium Chloride, Phenol.
See: Unguentine.

Ortho Micronor. (Ortho-McNeil) Norethindrone 0.35 mg. Lactose. Tab. *Dialpak* 28s. *Rx.*
Use: Sex hormone, contraceptive hormone.

Ortho-Novum 1/35. (Janssen) Norethindrone 1 mg, ethinyl estradiol 35 mcg. Lactose. Tab. *Dialpak* and *Veridate* 28s with 7 inert tabs. *Rx.*
Use: Sex hormone, contraceptive hormone.

Ortho-Novum 7/7/7. (Janssen) **Phase 1:** Norethindrone 0.5 mg, ethinyl estradiol 35 mcg. 7 tabs. **Phase 2:** Norethindrone 0.75 mg, ethinyl estradiol 35 mcg. 7 tabs. **Phase 3:** Norethindrone 1 mg, ethinyl estradiol 35 mcg. 7 tabs. Lactose. Tab. *Dialpak* and *Veridate* 28s with 7 inert tabs. *Rx.*
Use: Sex hormone, contraceptive hormone.

Ortho Personal Lubricant. (Johnson & Johnson) Greaseless, water-soluble, and non-staining aqueous hydrocolloid gel. Acid buffered to vaginal pH. Tube 2 oz, 4 oz. *OTC.*
Use: Lubricant.

Ortho Tri-Cyclen. (Janssen) **Phase 1:** Norgestimate 0.18 mg, ethinyl estradiol 35 mcg. 7 tabs. **Phase 2:** Norgestimate 0.215 mg, ethinyl estradiol 35 mcg. 7 tabs. **Phase 3:** Norgestimate 0.25 mg, ethinyl estradiol 35 mcg. 7 tabs. Lactose. Tab. *Dialpak* and *Veridate* 28s with 7 inert tabs. *Rx.*
Use: Sex hormone, contraceptive hormone.

Ortho Tri-Cyclen Lo. (Janssen) **Phase 1:** Norgestimate 0.18 mg, ethinyl estradiol 25 mcg. 7 tabs. **Phase 2:** Norgestimate 0.215 mg, ethinyl estradiol 25 mcg. 7 tabs. **Phase 3:** Norgestimate 0.25 mg, ethinyl estradiol 25 mcg. 7 tabs. Talc, lactose. Tab. *Dialpak* and *Veridate* 28s with 7 inert tabs. *Rx.*
Use: Sex hormone, contraceptive hormone.

Orthovisc. (Anika) Hyaluronan 15 mg. Sodium chloride 9 mg/mL. Inj. Prefilled syringe. 2 mL. *Rx.*
Use: Physical adjunct.

OrthoWash. (Omnil Oral) Sodium fluoride (as acidulated phosphate solution) 0.044%. Grape flavor. Rinse. 480 mL. *Rx.*
Use: Prevention of dental caries.

orthoxine. Methoxyphenamine.

orticalm.
Use: Hypotensive; tranquilizer.

•**orvepitant.** (or-VEE-pi-tant) USAN.
Use: CNS agent.

•**orvepitant maleate.** (or-VEE-pi-tant) USAN.
Use: CNS agent.

orvus.
See: Gardinol Type Detergents.

Os-Cal Extra D. (GlaxoSmithKline) Vitamin D_3 500 units (as cholecalciferol), calcium 500 mg (as calcium carbonate). Alcohol, corn syrup, parabens, PEG, sucrose. Gluten free. Tab. 60s, 120s. *OTC.*
Use: Nutritional combination product.

Os-Cal 500. (GlaxoSmithKline Consumer) Calcium carbonate 1250 mg (elemental calcium 500 mg). **Tab.:** Oyster shell powder, corn syrup, parabens. Bot. 75s. **Chew. Tab.:** Dextrose. Bot. 60s. *OTC.*
Use: Mineral supplement.

Os-Cal 500 + D. (GlaxoSmithKline Consumer) **Chew. Tab.:** Calcium 500 mg, vitamin D 400 units. Aspartame, phenylalanine, sorbitol, sucrose. Lemon chiffon flavor. 60s. **Tab.:** Calcium 500 mg, vitamin D 200 units, corn syrup, parabens, polydextrose. Bot. 75s, 160s. *OTC.*
Use: Mineral, vitamin supplement.

Os-Cal Fortified. (GlaxoSmithKline Consumer) Ca 250 mg, Fe (as ferrous fumarate) 5 mg, Mg, Mn, zinc 0.5 mg, D 125 units, B_1 1.7 mg, B_2 1.7 mg, B_3 15 mg, B_6 2 mg, C 50 mg, E 0.8 units, parabens, corn syrup solids, EDTA. Tab. Bot. 100s. *OTC.*
Use: Mineral, vitamin supplement.

Os-Cal Fortified Multivitamin & Minerals. (GlaxoSmithKline Consumer) Vitamins A 1668 units, D 125 units, E 0.8 units, B_1 1.7 mg, B_2 1.7 mg, B_3 15 mg, B_6 2 mg, C 50 mg, Fe 5 mg, Ca 250 mg, Zn 0.5 mg, Mn, Mg, EDTA, parabens. Tab. Bot. 100s. *OTC.*
Use: Mineral, vitamin supplement.

Os-Cal Plus. (GlaxoSmithKline Consumer) Ca 250 mg, vitamins D 125 units, A 1666 units, C 33 mg, B_2 0.66 mg, B_1 0.5 mg, B_6 0.5 mg, niacinamide 3.33 mg, Zn 0.75 mg, Mn 0.75 mg, Fe 16.6 mg. Tab. Bot. 100s. *OTC.*
Use: Mineral, vitamin supplement.

Os-Cal 250. (GlaxoSmithKline Consumer) Oyster shell powder as calcium 250 mg, vitamin D 125 units, and trace minerals (Cu, Fe, Mg, Mn, Zn, silica). Tab. Bot. 100s, 240s, 500s, 1000s. *OTC.*
Use: Mineral, vitamin supplement.

Os-Cal 250 + D. (GlaxoSmithKline Consumer) Calcium carbonate 625 mg, vitamin D 125 units. Tab. Bot. 100s. *OTC.*
Use: Mineral, vitamin supplement.

Os-Cal Ultra. (GlaxoSmithKline Consumer) Ca 600 mg, vitamin D 200 units, C 60 mg, E 15 units, Mg 20 mg, Zn 7.5 mg, Cu, Mn, boron 250 mcg. Lactose, sucrose. Tab. 120s. *OTC.*
Use: Nutritional supplement.

Oscimin. (Larken Labs) Hyoscyamine sulfate. **Tab.:** 0.125 mg. Lactose, mannitol. Peppermint flavor. 100s. **Tab., sublingual:** 0.125 mg. Lactose, mannitol. Peppermint flavor. 100s. **Tab., disintegrating:** 0.125 mg. Lactose, mannitol. Peppermint flavor. 100s. *Rx.*
Use: Gastrointestinal anticholinergic/antispasmodic, belladonna alkaloid.

Oscimin SR. (Larken Labs) Hyoscyamine sulfate 0.375 mg. Lactose. ER Tab. 100s. *Rx.*
Use: Gastrointestinal anticholinergic/antispasmodic, belladonna alkaloid.

•**oseltamivir phosphate.** (oh-sel-TAM-i-vir) USAN.
Use: Antiviral.
See: Tamiflu.

Oseni. (Takeda Pharmaceuticals America) Alogliptin benzoate/pioglitazone hydrochloride 12.5 mg/15 mg, 12.5 mg/30 mg, 12.5 mg/45 mg, 25 mg/15 mg, 25 mg/30 mg, 25 mg/45 mg. Film coated. Lactose. Tab. 30s, 90s, 500s. *Rx.*
Use: Antidiabetic combination product.

Osmitrol. (Baxter PPI) Mannitol in water. **5%:** 1000 mL. **10%:** 500 mL, 1000 mL. **15%:** 150 mL, 500 mL. **20%:** 250 mL, 500 mL. Mannitol in 0.3% Na. **5%:** 1000 mL. Mannitol in 0.45% Na. **20%:** 500 mL. *Rx.*
Use: Diuretic.
See: Mannitol.

Osmolite. (Ross) Isotonic liquid food containing 1.06 calories/mL. Two quarts (2000 calories) provides 100% US RDA vitamins and minerals for adults and children. Osmolality: 300 mOsm/kg water. Ready-to-Use: Bot. Can 8 fl oz, 32 fl oz. *OTC.*
Use: Nutritional supplement.

Osmolite HN. (Ross) High nitrogen isotonic liquid food containing 1.06 calories/mL; 1400 calories provides 100% USRDA vitamins and minerals for adults and children. Osmolality: 300 mOsm/kg water. Ready-to-Use: Bot. 8 fl oz. Can 8 fl oz, 32 fl oz. *OTC.*
Use: Nutritional supplement.

OsmoPrep. (Salix Pharmaceuticals) Sodium phosphate 1.5 g (sodium phosphate monobasic monohydrate 1.102 g, sodium phosphate dibasic 0.398 g). Gluten free. 100s. *Rx.*
Use: Laxative.

osmotic diuretics.
See: Ismotic.
Mannitol.
Osmitrol.
Osmoglyn.
Ureaphil.

•**ospemifene.** (os-PEM-i-feen) USAN.
Use: Selective estrogen receptor modulator; post-menopausal vaginal atrophy.
See: Osphena.

Osphena. (Shionogi) Ospemifene 60 mg. Film coated. Lactose, mannitol, PEG. Tab. 100s, UD 30s. *Rx.*
Use: Sex hormone, selective estrogen receptor modulator.

ospolot.
Use: Anticonvulsant drug; pending release.

Ossonate. (Marcen) Cartilage mucopolysaccharide extract, chondroitin sulfate 50 mg. Cap. Bot. 100s, 500s, 1000s.

Ossonate-Plus. (Marcen) Ossonate mucopolysaccharide extract 50 mg, acetaminophen 300 mg, salicylamide 200 mg. Cap. Bot. 100s, 500s, 1000s. *OTC.*
Use: Antiarthritic.

Ossonate-Plus, Inj. (Marcen) Ossonate cartilage mucopolysaccharide extract 12.5 mg, case in hydrolysates 80 mg, sulfur 20 mg, sodium citrate 5 mg, benzyl alcohol 0.5%, phenol 0.5%/mL. Multidose 10 mL vial. *Rx.*
Use: Muscle relaxant, pain reliever.

Ossonate-75. (Marcen) Chondroitin sulfate 37.5 mg, benzyl alcohol 0.5%, phenol 0.5%, sodium citrate 5 mg/mL. Vial 10 mL. *Rx.*
Use: Infantile and atopic eczemas; drug allergies; dermatoses associated with intestinal toxemias.

Osteo-D. (Teva)
See: Secalciferol.

Osteolate. (Fellows) Sodium thiosalicylate 50 mg, benzyl alcohol 2%/mL. Inj. Vial 30 mL. *Rx.*
Use: Analgesic.

Osteo-Mins. (Tyson) **Pow.:** Vitamin C 500 mg, Ca 250 mg, Mg 250 mg, K 45 mg, 100 units D/4.5 g, sugar free. 200 g. *OTC.*
Use: Vitamin supplement.

Osteon/D. (Taylor Pharmaceuticals) Ca 600 mg, P 400 mg, Mg 240 mg, vitamin D 400 units. Tab. Bot. 180s. *Rx.*
Use: Mineral, vitamin supplement.

Ostiderm Roll-On. (Pedinol Pharmacal) Aluminum chlorohydrate, camphor, alcohol, EDTA, diazolidinyl urea. Bot. 88.7 mL. *OTC.*
Use: Antipruritic; astringent, topical.

OstiGen Melts. (US Food & Pharmaceuticals) Vitamin D 150 units, Ca 350 mg, vitamin K, P, Mg, Cu, Na, K. Chocolate, chocolate mint, and caramel flavors. Sugar free. Orally Disintegrating Tab. 90s. *OTC.*
Use: Multivitamin.

Osto-K. (Parthenon) Potassium 1 mEq (39 mg from gluconate, Cl, and citrate), vitamin C 25 mg, sodium 0.52 mg. Tab. Bot. 60s. *OTC.*
Use: Mineral, vitamin supplement.

Otezla. (Celgene Corporation) Apremilast 10 mg, 20 mg, 30 mg. Film coated. Alcohol, lactose, PEG. Tab. Starter pack (for 2 weeks and includes a 13 tablet blister titration pack containing 10, 20, and 30 mg tablets w/an additional fourteen 30 mg tablets), 60s (30 mg only), UD 28s (30 mg only). *Rx.*
Use: Immunomodulator.

Otic Care. (Pure Tek) Antipyrine 5.4%, benzocaine 1.4%, U-polycosanol alcohol 0.0097%. Soln.; Otic. 14 mL w/dropper. *Rx.*
Use: Otic preparation.

Otic Domeboro. (Bayer) Acetic acid 2%, aluminum acetate solution. Soln. 60 mL with dropper. *Rx.*
Use: Otic.

Otic Edge. (River's Edge) Antipyrine 5.4%, benzocaine 1.4%, policosanol 0.0097%. Acetic acid, glycerin. Soln., Otic. 14 mL w/dropper. *Rx.*
Use: Otic preparation.

Otic-HC. (Roberts) Chloroxylenol 1 mg, pramoxine hydrochloride 10 mg, hydrocortisone alcohol 10 mg, benzalkonium Cl 0.2 mg/mL. Bot. 12 mL. *Rx.*
Use: Otic.

Oticin. (Teral) Parachlorometaxylenol 0.01 g, proxazocain hydrochloride 0.1 g. Drops, otic. 10 mL w/dropper. *Rx.*
Use: Miscellaneous otic preparation.

Oticin HC. (Teral) Hydrocortisone 1 g, parachlormetaxylenol 0.01 g, proxazocaine hydrochloride 0.1 g. Edetate disodium. Drops, otic. 10 mL w/dropper. *Rx.*
Use: Miscellaneous otic preparation.

Otic-Neo-Cort Dome.
See: Neo-Cort Dome.

Otic-Plain. (Roberts) Chloroxylenol 1 mg, pramoxine hydrochloride 10 mg, benzalkonium Cl 0.2 mg/mL. Bot. 12 mL. *Rx.*
Use: Otic.

Otic Solution No. 1. (Foy Laboratories) Hydrocortisone alcohol 10 mg, pramoxine hydrochloride 10 mg, benzalkonium Cl 0.2 mg, acetic acid glacial 20 mg/mL w/propylene glycol q.s. Bot. *Rx.*
Use: Otic.

•**otlertuzumab.** (OT-ler-TOOZ-ue-mab) USAN.
Use: Antineoplastic.

Otocain. (Abana) Benzocaine 20%, benzethonium chloride 0.1%, glycerin 1%, polyethylene glycol 300. Soln. Bot. 15 mL. *Rx.*
Use: Otic preparation.

Oto-End 10. (Larken Laboratories) Chloroxylenol 0.1%, hydrocortisone 1%, pramoxine hydrochloride 1%. Edetate disodium. Soln., Otic. 10 mL w/dropper. *Rx.*
Use: Ophthalmic and otic agent, otic preparation.

Otogesic HC Solution. (Lexis Laboratories) Polymyxin B sulfate 10,000 units, neomycin sulfate 3.5 mg, hydrocortisone 10 mg/mL, potassium metabisulfite 0.1%. Bot. 10 mL. *Rx.*
Use: Otic.

Otogesic HC Suspension. (Lexis Laboratories) Polymyxin B sulfate 10,000 units, neomycin sulfate 3.5 mg, hydrocortisone 10 mg/mL, benzalkonium Cl 0.01%. Bot. 10 mL. *Rx.*
Use: Otic.

Otomar-HC. (Marnel) Chloroxylenol 1 mg, hydrocortisone 10 mg, pramoxine hydrochloride 10 mg/mL. Otic Soln. Plastic dropper vials 10 mL. *Rx.*
Use: Otic preparation.

Otosporin. (Calmic) Hydrocortisone 1%, neomycin sulfate 5 mg, polymyxin B 10,000 units. Soln. 10 mL with dropper. *Rx.*
Use: Steroid and antibiotic combination.

Otozin. (Allegis Pharmaceuticals) Antipyrine 5.4%, benzocaine 1%, glycerin 2%, zinc acetate dihydrate 1%. Soln., otic. 10 mL w/dropper. *Rx.*
Use: Miscellaneous otic preparation.

Otrexup. (Antares Pharma) Methotrexate 10 mg per 0.4 mL, 15 mg per 0.4 mL, 20 mg per 0.4 mL, 25 mg per 0.4 mL. Sodium chloride. Preservative free. Inj., Soln. Single-use auto injector. *Rx.*
Use: Antimetabolite, folic acid antagonist.

Otrivin. (Novartis) Xylometazoline hydrochloride 0.1%, benzalkonium chloride, sodium chloride, EDTA. Soln. Dropper Bot. 25 mL. Spray Bot. 20 mL. *OTC.*
Use: Nasal decongestant, imidazoline.

Otrivin Pediatric Nasal. (Novartis) Xylometazoline hydrochloride 0.05%, benzalkonium chloride, EDTA. Soln. Dropper Bot. 25 mL. *OTC.*
Use: Nasal decongestant, imidazoline.

Ovace. (Mission Pharmacal) Sulfacetamide sodium 10%. Disodium EDTA, methylparaben, PEG. Soap. 355 mL. *Rx.*
Use: Topical anti-infective, antibiotic agent.

Ovace Plus. (Mission Pharmacal) Sulfacetamide sodium 10%. **Cream:** Benzyl alcohol, caprylic/capric triglyceride, cetyl alcohol, dimethicone, disodium EDTA, glycerin, glyceryl stearate, parabens, paraffin, PEG, zinc oxide. 57 g. **Soap:** Alcohol, disodium EDTA, glyceryl, methylparaben, PEG, wax. 355 mL. **Shampoo:** Parabens, PEG. 237 mL. *Rx.*
Use: Topical anti-infective, antibiotic agent.

ovarian extract. Aqueous extract of whole ovaries of cattle.
Use: Estrogen.

ovarian substance. (Various Mfr.) Whole ovarian substance from cattle, sheep, or swine. *Rx.*
Use: Estrogen.

Ovastat. (Medac GmbH c/o Princeton Regulatory Assoc.)
See: Treosulfan.

Ovcon-35. (Warner Chilcott) Norethindrone 0.4 mg, ethinyl estradiol 35 mcg. Lactose. Tab. Pack 28s with 7 inert tabs. *Rx.*
Use: Sex hormone, contraceptive hormone.

•**ovemotide.** (oh-VEM-oh-tide) USAN.
Use: Melanoma peptide vaccine.

Overtime. (BDI) Caffeine 200 mg. Tab. Bot. 100s, 500s. *OTC.*
Use: CNS stimulant, analeptic.

Ovide. (Taro) Malathion 0.5%. In a vehicle of isopropyl alcohol 78%, terpineol, dipentene, and pine needle oil. Lot. Bot. 59 mL. *Rx.*
Use: Pediculicide, scabicide.

Ovidrel. (Serono) Choriogonadotropin alfa 250 mcg/0.5 mL, mannitol 28.1 mg, 85% O-phosphoric acid 505 mcg. Inj. Single-dose prefilled syringes. *Rx.*
Use: Sex hormone, ovulation stimulant.

ovifollin.
See: Estrone.

Ovlin. (Sigma-Tau) **Tab.:** Ethinyl estradiol 0.02 mg, conjugated estrogens 0.2 mg. Bot. 100s, 1000s. **Inj.:** Estrone 2 mg, ethinyl estradiol 0.05 mg, vitamin B_{12} 1000 mcg/mL. Vial 30 mL. *Rx.*
Use: Estrogen.

Ovocylin Dipropionate. (Novartis) Estradiol dipropionate. *Rx.*
Use: Estrogen.

ovulation stimulants.
See: Choriogonadotropin Alfa.
Chorionic Gonadotropin.
Clomiphene Citrate.
Gonadotropins.
Lutropin Alfa.
Menotropins.

ovulation tests.
See: Clearblue Easy Ovulation Test.
First Response Ovulation Predictor Test Kit.
Fortel Ovulation.

Ovulen-28. (Pharmacia) Ethynodiol diacetate 1 mg, mestranol 0.1 mg. Tab. w/7 inert Tab. *Compack* 28s: 21 active tab., 7 placebo tab. *Compack* dispenser 28s. Box 6 × 28. Refill 28s, Box 12 × 28. *Rx.*
Use: Contraceptive.

Ovulen-21. (Pharmacia) Ethynodiol diacetate 1 mg, mestranol 0.1 mg. Tab. *Compack* Disp. 21s, 6 × 21, 24 × 21. Refill 21s, 12 × 21. *Rx.*
Use: Contraceptive.

Ovustick Self-Test. (Monoclonal Antibodies) Home test for ovulation. Test kit 10s.
Use: Diagnostic aid.

Oxabid. (Jamieson-McKames) Magnesium oxide 140 mg or magnesium oxide heavy 400 mg. Cap. Bot. 100s. *OTC.*
Use: Antacid.

•**oxacillin sodium.** (ox-uh-SILL-in) *USP.*
Use: Anti-infective.

oxacillin sodium. (Various Mfr.) Oxacillin sodium 500 mg, 1 g, 2 g, 10 g. Pow. for Inj. Vial (except 10 g), piggyback vial (1 g, 2 g only), *ADD-Vantage* vials (1 g, 2 g only), Bulk Vial (10 g only). *Rx.*
Use: Anti-infective, penicillin.

oxadimedine hydrochloride.
Use: Antiarrhythmic.

oxafuradene. (OX-ah-FYOOR-ah-deen) Name used for Nifuradene.
Use: Platelet aggregation agent.

•**oxagrelate.** (OX-ah-greh-LATE) USAN.
Use: Platelet aggregation inhibitor.

•**oxaliplatin.** (ox-AL-ih-PLA-tin) *USP.*
Use: Antineoplastic.
See: Eloxatin.

oxaliplatin. (Various Mfr.) Oxaliplatin. **Inj.; Soln, Conc.:** 5 mg/mL. Preservative free. Single-use vial. 10 mL, 20 mL. **Inj., lyophilized Pow. for Soln.:** 50 mg, 100 mg. May contain lactose. Preservative free. Single-use vial. *Rx.*
Use: Antineoplastic agent, platinum coordination complex.

oxalodinones.
Use: Anti-infective.
See: Linezolid.

•**oxamarin hydrochloride.** (OX-ah-mah-rin) USAN.
Use: Hemostatic.

•**oxamisole hydrochloride.** (ox-AM-ih-sole) USAN.
Use: Immunoregulator.

•**oxamniquine.** (ox-AM-nih-kwin) *USP.*
Use: Antischistosomal, treatment of schistosomiasis.

oxanamide.
Use: Anxiolytic.

Oxandrin. (Savient) Oxandrolone 2.5 mg, 10 mg, lactose. Tab. Bot. 100s (2.5 mg only), 60s (10 mg only). *c-III.*
Use: Anabolic steroid.

•**oxandrolone.** (ox-AN-droe-lone) *USP.*
Use: Anabolic steroid.
See: Oxandrin.

oxandrolone. (Sandoz) Oxandrolone 2.5 mg, 10 mg. Lactose. Tab. 100s, 1000s. *c-III.*
Use: Anabolic steroid.

•**oxantel pamoate.** (OX-an-tell PAM-oh-ate) USAN.
Use: Anthelmintic.

•**oxaprotiline hydrochloride.** (OX-ah-PRO-tih-leen) USAN.
Use: Antidepressant.

•**oxaprozin.** (OX-ah-pro-zin) *USP.*
Use: Nonsteroidal anti-inflammatory agent.
See: Daypro.
Daypro ALTA.

oxaprozin. (Eon Labs) Oxaprozin 600 mg. Film-coated. Tab. Bot. 100s, 500s, 1000s, blister 100s. *Rx.*
Use: Nonsteroidal anti-inflammatory agent.

•**oxarbazole.** (ox-AHR-bah-zole) USAN.
Use: Antiasthmatic.

•**oxatomide.** (ox-AT-ah-mid) USAN.
Use: Antiallergic, antiasthmatic.

•**oxazepam.** (ox-AZ-e-pam) *USP.*
Use: Anxiolytic, sedative.

oxazepam. (Various Mfr.) Oxazepam 10 mg, 15 mg, 30 mg. Cap. 100s, 500s, UD 100s. *c-IV.*
Use: Anxiolytic.

ox bile extract. Purified ox gall.
See: Bile Extract.

•**oxcarbazepine.** (OC-kar-BAZ-e-peen) USAN.
Tall Man: OXcarbazepine
Use: Anticonvulsant; antiepileptic.
See: Oxtellar XR.
Trileptal.

oxcarbazepine. (Sandoz) Oxcarbazepine 60 mg/mL. Ethanol, saccharin, sorbitol. Susp. 250 mL w/dosing syringe and adapter. *Rx.*
Use: Anticonvulsant.

oxcarbazepine. (Various Mfr.) Oxcarbazepine 150 mg, 300 mg, 600 mg. Tab. 30s, 100s, 500s, 1000s, UD 100s. *Rx.*
Use: Anticonvulsant.

•**oxelumab.** (ox-EL-ue-mab) USAN.
Use: Treatment of asthma.

•**oxendolone.** (ox-EN-doe-lone) USAN.
Use: Antiandrogen (benign prostatic hypertrophy).

•**oxethazaine.** (ox-ETH-a-zane) USAN.
Use: Anesthetic, local.

•**oxetorone fumarate.** (ox-EH-toe-rone) USAN.
Use: Antimigraine.

•**oxfendazole.** (ox-FEN-da-zole) USAN.
Use: Anthelmintic.

•**oxfenicine.** (ox-FEN-ih-seen) USAN.
Use: Vasodilator.

ox gall.
See: Ox Bile Extract.

•**oxibendazole.** (ox-ee-BEND-ah-zole) USAN.
Use: Anthelmintic.

•**oxiconazole nitrate.** (ox-ee-KAHN-ah-zole) USAN.
Use: Antifungal.
See: Oxistat.

oxidized bile acids.
See: Bile Acids, Oxidized.

oxidized cellulose. Absorbable cellulose. Cellulosic acid.
Use: Hemostatic.
See: Oxycel.
Surgicel.

•**oxidopamine.** (OX-ih-DOE-pah-meen) USAN.
Use: Adrenergic (ophthalmic).

•**oxidronic acid.** (OX-ih-DRAHN-ik) USAN.
Use: Regulator (calcium).

Oxi-Freeda. (Freeda) Vitamin A 5000 units, E 150 mg, B_3 40 mg, C 100 mg, B_1 20 mg, B_2 20 mg, B_5 20 mg, B_6 20 mg, B_{12} 10 mcg, Zn 15 mg, Se, glutathione, L-cysteine. Tab. Bot. 100s, 250s. *OTC.*
Use: Mineral, vitamin supplement.

•**oxifungin hydrochloride.** (OX-ih-FUN-jin) USAN.
Use: Antifungal.

•**oxilorphan.** (ox-ih-LORE-fan) USAN.
Use: Narcotic antagonist.

•**oximonam.** (OX-ih-MOE-nam) USAN.
Use: Anti-infective.

•**oximonam sodium.** (OX-ih-MOE-nam) USAN.
Use: Anti-infective.

oxine.
See: Oxyquinoline Sulfate.

•**oxiperomide.** (ox-ih-PURR-oh-mide) USAN.
Use: Antipsychotic.

Oxipor VHC. (Medtech) Coal tar soln. 25% (equiv. to 5% coal tar), alcohol 79%. Lot. Bot. 56 mL. *OTC.*
Use: Antipsoriatic.

•**oxiramide.** (ox-EER-am-ide) USAN.
Use: Cardiovascular agent.

Oxistat. (Pharmaderm) Oxiconazole nitrate 1%. Cream. Tube 15 g, 30 g, 60 g; Lot. Bot. 30 mL. *Rx.*
Use: Antifungal, topical.

•**oxisuran.** (OX-ih-SUH-ran) USAN.
Use: Antineoplastic.

•**oxmetidine hydrochloride.** (ox-MEH-tih-DEEN) USAN.
Use: Antiulcerative.

•**oxmetidine mesylate.** (ox-MEH-tih-DEEN) USAN.
Use: Antiulcerative.

•**oxogestone phenpropionate.** (ox-oh-JESS-tone fen-PRO-pih-oh-nate) USAN.
Use: Hormone, progestin.

Oxolamine. (Arcum) Crystalline hydroxycobalamin 1000 mcg/mL. Vial 10 mL. *Rx.*
Use: Vitamin supplement.

•**oxolinic acid.** (ox-oh-LIH-nik acid) USAN.
Use: Anti-infective.

Oxothiazolidine Carboxylate. (Clintec Nutrition) Phase I restoration of glutathione depletion in HIV, ARC, AIDS; prevention of inflammation-induced HIV replication. *Rx.*
Use: Immunomodulator.

l-2-oxothiazolidine-4-carboxylic acid.
Use: Treatment of adult respiratory distress syndrome. [Orphan Drug]
See: Procysteine.

•**oxprenolol hydrochloride.** (ox-PREH-no-lole) *USP.* Under study.
Use: Beta-adrenergic receptor blocker, vasodilator (coronary).

Oxsoralen. (ICN Pharmaceuticals) Methoxsalen 1% (10 mg/mL), acetone, alcohol 71%. Lot. Bot. 30 mL. *Rx.*
Use: Dermatologic.

Oxsoralen-Ultra. (ICN Pharmaceuticals) Methoxsalen 10 mg. Soft Gelatin Cap. Bot. 50s. *Rx.*
Use: Dermatologic.

Oxtellar XR. (Supernus Pharmaceuticals) Oxcarbazepine 150 mg, 300 mg, 600 mg. PEG. ER Tab. 100s. *Rx.*
Use: Anticonvulsant.

•**oxtriphylline.** (ox-TRY-fih-lin) *USP.*
Use: Bronchodilator.
W/Guaifenesin.
See: Brondecon.

•**oxybenzone.** (ox-ee-BEN-zone) *USP.*
Use: Ultraviolet screen.
W/Avobenzone, Homosalate, Octisalate, Octocrylene.
See: Neutrogena Ultra Sheer Dry-Touch Sunblock.
W/Dioxybenzone, Benzophenone.
See: Solbar.
W/Combinations.
See: Coppertone.
Keri Age Defy & Protect.
Lubriderm Daily Moisture with SPF 15.
Noskote.
Shade.

Super Shade.
TI-Screen Sports.

•**oxybutynin chloride.** (OX-ee-BYOO-tih-nin) *USP.*
Use: Anticholinergic.
See: Ditropan XL.
Gelnique 10%.
Gelnique 3%.
Oxytrol.
Oxytrol for Women.

oxybutynin chloride. (Various Mfr.) Oxybutynin chloride. **ER Tab.:** 5 mg, 10 mg, 15 mg. May contain lactose (15 mg). 100s, 500s (5 mg, 10 mg only). **Tab.:** 5 mg. Bot. 100s, 500s, 1000s, blister pack 25s, UD 100s. **Syr.:** 5 mg/5 mL. Bot. 473 mL. *Rx.*
Use: Antispasmodic; anticholinergic.

Oxycel. (Becton Dickinson & Co.) Cellulosic acid in absorbable hemostatic agent prepared from cellulose. Resembles ordinary surgical gauze or cotton. Pledget 2 × 1 × 1 inch. 10s. Pad 3 × 3 inch. 8 ply. 10s. Strip 5 × 0.5 inch. 4 ply. 18 × 2 inch. 4 ply. 10s. 36 × 0.5 inch. 4 ply. *Rx.*
Use: Hemostatic, topical.

Oxycet. (Halsey Drug) Oxycodone hydrochloride 5 mg, acetaminophen 325 mg. Tab. Bot. 100s, 500s, Hospital pack 250s. *c-II.*
Use: Narcotic analgesic combination.

Oxy-Chinol. (Ferndale) Potassium oxyquinoline sulfate 1 g. Tab. Bot. 100s, 1000s. *OTC.*
Use: Antimicrobial, deodorant.

•**oxychlorosene.** (OCK-sih-KLOR-ah-seen) USAN. Monoxychlorosene. Hydrocarbon derivative containing 14 carbons and hypochlorous acid. The hydrocarbon chain also has a phenyl substituent which in turn holds a sulfonic acid group.
Use: Anti-infective, topical.
See: Clorpactin WCS-90.

•**oxychlorosene sodium.** (OCK-sih-KLOR-ah-seen) USAN. Sodium salt of the complex derived from hypochlorous acid and tetradecylbenzene sulfonic acid. Action of active chlorine.
Use: Anti-infective, topical.

•**oxycodone.** (OX-ee-KOE-dohn) USAN.
Tall Man: oxyCODONE
Use: Analgesic, narcotic w/combinations.
See: Endocet.
W/Acetaminophen.
See: Primlev.

oxycodone and acetaminophen. (Mallinckrodt) Oxycodone hydrochloride/acetaminophen 7.5 mg/325 mg, 7.5 mg/500 mg, 10 mg/325 mg, 10 mg, 650 mg. Tab. 20s, 100s, 500s, 1,000s, UD 100s. *c-II.*
Use: Narcotic analgesic.

oxycodone and acetaminophen. (Various Mfr.) Oxycodone hydrochloride/acetaminophen. **Cap.:** 5 mg/500 mg. 100s, 500s, 1,000s, UD 25s. **Tab.:** 2.5 mg/325 mg, 5 mg/325 mg, 7.5 mg/325 mg, 10 mg/325 mg, 5 mg/500 mg, 7.5 mg/500 mg, 10 mg/650 mg. 100s, 500s (except 2.5 mg/325 mg, 7.5 mg/500 mg, 10 mg/650 mg), UD 100s (except 2.5 mg/325 mg, 5 mg/500 mg). *c-II.*
Use: Analgesic combination, narcotic.

oxycodone and aspirin. (Various Mfr.) Oxycodone hydrochloride 4.5 mg, oxycodone terephthalate 0.38 mg, aspirin 325 mg. Tab. Bot. 100s, 500s, 1000s, UD 25s. *c-II.*
Use: Analgesic combination, narcotic.

•**oxycodone hydrochloride.** (OX-ee-KOE-dohn) *USP.*
Tall Man: oxyCODONE
Use: Opioid analgesic.
See: M-oxy.
OxyContin.
OxyFAST.
OxyIR.
Roxicodone.
Roxicodone Intensol.
W/Acetaminophen
See: Primalev.
Xolox.
W/Combinations.
See: Endocet.
Percocet.
Percodan.
Perloxx.

oxycodone hydrochloride. (Amide) Oxycodone hydrochloride 15 mg, 30 mg. Lactose. IR Tab. 100s, UD 100s. *c-II.*
Use: Opioid analgesic.

oxycodone hydrochloride. (Endo) Oxycodone hydrochloride 10 mg, 20 mg, 40 mg. CR Tab. 30s, 500s. *c-II.*
Use: Opioid analgesic.

oxycodone hydrochloride. (Ethex) Oxycodone hydrochloride. **Cap.:** 5 mg. Lactose. 100s, UD 100s. **Tab.:** 10 mg, 20 mg. 100s, UD 100s. *c-II.*
Use: Opioid analgesic.

oxycodone hydrochloride. (Teva) Oxycodone hydrochloride 80 mg. Lactose. Film-coated. ER Tab. 100s. *c-II.*
Use: Opioid analgesic.

oxycodone hydrochloride. (Various Mfr.) Oxycodone hydrochloride. **CR Tab.:** 80 mg. Lactose. 100s, 500s, 1,000s.

Oral Soln.: 5 mg/5 mL. 500 mL. **Soln. Concentrate:** 20 mg/mL. 30 mL. **Tab.:** 5 mg, 15 mg, 30 mg. Bot. 100s, 500s (except 15 mg, 30 mg), UD 100s. *c-II.*
Use: Opioid analgesic, narcotic agonist.

oxycodone hydrochloride/acetaminophen. (Various Mfr.) Acetaminophen 325 mg, oxycodone hydrochloride 2.5 mg. Tab. 30s, 100s, 500s, 1,000s. *c-II.*
Use: Opioid analgesic combination.

oxycodone hydrochloride and ibuprofen. (Various Mfr.) Oxycodone hydrochloride 5 mg, ibuprofen 400 mg. May contain lactose, polydextrose. Film-coated. Tab. 30s, 100s, 500s. *c-II.*
Use: Narcotic analgesic.

•**oxycodone terephthalate.** (OX-ee-KOE-dohn teh-REFF-thah-late) *USP.*
Tall Man: oxyCODONE
Use: Analgesic, narcotic.

OxyContin. (Purdue) Oxycodone hydrochloride 10 mg, 15 mg, 20 mg, 30 mg, 40 mg, 60 mg, 80 mg. Lactose. CR Tab. Bot. 100s, UD 25s (except 15 mg, 30 mg, 60 mg). *c-II.*
Tall Man: OxyCONTIN
Use: Opioid analgesic.

Oxy Cover. (GlaxoSmithKline) Benzoyl peroxide 10%. Cream. 30 g. *OTC.*
Use: Dermatologic, acne.

oxyethylene oxypropylene polymer.
See: Poloxalkol.

W/Danthron, vitamin B_1, carboxymethyl cellulose.
See: Evactol.

OxyFAST. (Purdue Pharma LP) Oxycodone hydrochloride 20 mg/mL. Saccharin. Conc. Soln. Dropper Bot. 30 mL. *c-II.*
Use: Opioid analgesic.

•**oxyfilcon A.** (OX-ee-FILL-kahn A) USAN.
Use: Contact lens material (hydrophilic).

OXY 5 Acne-Pimple Medication. (GlaxoSmithKline) Benzoyl peroxide 5% in lotion base. Lot. Bot. oz. *OTC.*
Use: Dermatologic, acne.

•**oxygen.** (OX-i-jen) *USP.*
Use: Gas, medicinal.

•**oxygen 93 percent.** (OX-i-jen) *USP.*
Use: Gas, medicinal.

OxyIR. (Purdue Pharma) Oxycodone hydrochloride 5 mg. Sucrose. Cap. Bot. 100s. *c-II.*
Use: Opioid analgesic.

OXY Medicated Cleanser and Maximum Strength Pads. (Mentholatum) Salicylic acid 2%, SD alcohol 44%, citric acid, menthol, propylene glycol. Cleanser. Bot. 120 mL. Pads 50s, 90s. *OTC.*
Use: Dermatologic, acne.

OXY Medicated Cleanser and Regular Strength Pads. (Mentholatum) Salicylic acid 0.5%, SD alcohol 28%, citric acid, menthol, propylene glycol. Cleanser. Bot. 120 mL. Pads 50s, 90s. *OTC.*
Use: Dermatologic, acne.

OXY Medicated Cleanser and Sensitive Skin Pads. (Mentholatum) Salicylic acid 0.5%, alcohol 22%, disodium lauryl sulfosuccinate, menthol, trisodium EDTA. Cleanser. Bot. 120 mL. Pads 50s, 90s. *OTC.*
Use: Dermatologic, acne.

OXY Medicated Soap. (Mentholatum) Triclosan 1%, bentonite, cocoamphodipropionate, iron oxides, glycerin, magnesium silicate, sodium borohydride, sodium cocoate, sodium tallowate, talc, EDTA, titanium dioxide. Bar. 97.5 g. *OTC.*
Use: Dermatologic, acne.

•**oxymetazoline hydrochloride.** (OX-ee-MET-azz-oh-leen) *USP.*
Use: Nasal decongestant, imidazoline; adrenergic (vasoconstrictor); mydriatic.
See: Afrin All Night No Drip.
Afrin Extra Moisturizing.
Afrin No-Drip 12-Hour.
Afrin No-Drip 12-Hour Extra Moisturizing.
Afrin Severe Congestion with Menthol.
Afrin Sinus 12 Hour Relief.
Afrin 12-Hour Original.
Dristan 12-Hr Nasal.
Duramist Plus 12-Hr Decongestant.
Duration.
Genasal.
Nasal Decongestant, Maximum Strength.
Nasal Relief.
Neo-Synephrine 12-Hour Extra Moisturizing.
Nōstrilla Complete Congestion Relief 12-Hour.
Nōstrilla Conditioning Double Moisture.
Nōstrilla 12-Hour.
NRS Nasal Relief.
12 Hour Nasal.
Twice-A-Day 12-Hour Nasal.
Vicks Sinex 12 Hour.
Vicks Sinex 12-Hour Decongestant Ultrafine Mist Moisturizing Nasal Spray.
Vicks Sinex 12 Hour UltraFine Mist for Sinus Relief.
Visine LR.

oxymetazoline hydrochloride. (Various Mfr.) Oxymetazoline hydrochloride 0.05%. Soln. Spray Bot. 15 mL, 30 mL. *OTC.*
Use: Nasal decongestant, imidazoline.

•**oxymetholone.** (OCK-sih-METH-oh-lone) *USP.*
Use: Anabolic steroid.
See: Anadrol-50.

•**oxymorphone hydrochloride.** (ox-ee-MORE-fone) *USP.*
Use: Opioid analgesic.
See: Opana.
Opana ER.

oxymorphone hydrochloride. (Actavis Elizabeth) Oxymorphone hydrochloride 7.5 mg, 15 mg. ER Tab. 100s, 500s. *c-II.*
Use: Opioid analgesic.

oxymorphone hydrochloride. (Endo Pharmaceuticals) Oxymorphone hydrochloride 5 mg, 10 mg. Lactose. Tab. 100s, UD 100s. *c-II.*
Use: Opioid analgesic.

oxymorphone hydrochloride. (Global Pharmaceuticals) Oxymorphone hydrochloride 5 mg, 10 mg, 20 mg, 30 mg, 40 mg. Lactose. ER Tab. 30s, 100s, 1,000s. *c-II.*
Use: Opioid analgesic.

OXY Night Watch. (Mentholatum) Salicylic acid 1%, cetyl alcohol, silica, propylene glycol, stearyl alcohol, sodium laureth sulfate, parabens, EDTA. Lot. Bot. 60 mL. *OTC.*
Use: Dermatologic, acne.

OXY Night Watch Maximum Strength. (Mentholatum) Salicylic acid 2%, cetyl alcohol, EDTA, parabens, stearyl alcohol. Lot. Bot. 60 mL. *OTC.*
Use: Dermatologic, acne.

OXY Night Watch Sensitive Skin. (Mentholatum) Salicylic acid 1%, cetyl alcohol, EDTA, stearyl alcohol, parabens. Lot. Bot. 60 mL. *OTC.*
Use: Dermatologic, acne.

OXY Oil-Free Maximum Strength Acne Wash. (Mentholatum) Benzoyl peroxide 10%, parabens, diazolidinyl urea. Liq. 237 mL. *OTC.*
Use: Dermatologic, acne.

•**oxypertine.** (OX-ee-PURR-teen) USAN. Integrin hydrochloride.
Use: Psychotherapeutic agent, antidepressant.

•**oxyphenbutazone.** (ox-ee-fen-BYOO-tah-zone) *USP.*
Use: Analgesic, antiarthritic, anti-inflammatory, antipyretic, antirheumatic.

•**oxyphenisatin acetate.** (OX-ee-fen-EYE-sah-tin) USAN.
Use: Laxative.
See: Endophenolphthalein.
Isacen.
Prulet.

•**oxypurinol sodium.** (OX-ee-PYOO-ree-nahl) USAN.
Use: Investigational xanthine oxidase inhibitor.

•**oxyquinoline.** (OX-ih-KWIN-oh-lin) USAN.
Use: Disinfectant.

oxyquinoline benzoate. (Merck & Co.) Pkg. lb.
Use: Disinfectant.

•**oxyquinoline sulfate.** (OX-ih-KWIN-oh-lin) *NF.*
Use: Disinfectant, pharmaceutic aid (complexing agent).
See: Chinositol.
W/Combinations.
See: Acid Jelly.
Fem ph.
Oxyzal Wet Dressing.
Rectal Medicone Unguent.

OXY-Scrub. (Mentholatum) Abradant cleanser containing dissolving abradant particles of sodium tetraborate decahydrate. Tube 2.65 oz. *OTC.*
Use: Dermatologic, acne.

Oxysept 1. (Allergan) Microfiltered hydrogen peroxide 3% w/sodium tannate and sodium nitrate, preservative free, buffered. Soln. Bot. 355 mL. *OTC.*
Use: Contact lens care.

•**oxytetracycline.** (OX-i-TET-ra-SYE-kleen) *USP.*
Use: Anti-infective.
See: Terramycin.

•**oxytetracycline and nystatin capsules.** *USP.*
Use: Anti-infective, antifungal.

•**oxytetracycline and nystatin for oral suspension.** *USP.*
Use: Anti-infective, antifungal.

•**oxytetracycline calcium.** (OX-i-TET-ra-SYE-kleen) *USP.*
Use: Anti-infective.

•**oxytetracycline hydrochloride.** (OX-i-TET-ra-SYE-kleen) *USP.* An antibiotic from *Streptomyces rimosus.*
Use: Anti-infective; antirickettsial.
W/Hydrocortisone.
See: Terra-Cortril.

•**oxytetracycline hydrochloride and hydrocortisone acetate ophthalmic suspension.** *USP.*
Use: Anti-infective, anti-inflammatory.

•**oxytetracycline hydrochloride and hydrocortisone ointment.** *USP.*
Use: Anti-infective; anti-inflammatory.

•**oxytetracycline hydrochloride and polymyxin B sulfate ointment.** *USP.*
Use: Anti-infective.

•**oxytetracycline hydrochloride and polymyxin B sulfate ophthalmic ointment.** *USP.*
Use: Anti-infective.

•**oxytetracycline hydrochloride and polymyxin B sulfate topical powder.** *USP.*
Use: Anti-infective.

•**oxytetracycline hydrochloride and polymyxin B sulfate vaginal inserts.** *USP.*
Use: Anti-infective.

oxytetracycline-polymyxin B. Mix of oxytetracycline hydrochloride and polymyxin B sulfate.
Use: Anti-infective.

•**oxytocin.** (ox-ih-TOE-sin) *USP.*
Use: Oxytocic.
See: Pitocin.

oxytocin. (Various Mfr.) Oxytocin 10 units/mL. Inj. Vials. 3 mL, 10 mL. *Rx.*
Use: Uterine active agent.

oxytocin nasal solution.
Use: Oxytocic.

oxytocin, synthetic.
See: Pitocin.

Oxytrol. (Watson) Oxybutynin 36 mg (delivers 3.9 mg/day over 3 to 4 days). Transdermal Patch. 8s. *Rx.*
Use: Anticholinergic.

Oxytrol for Women. (Schering-Plough Healthcare) Oxybutynin chloride 3.9 mg per 24 hours (36 mg total oxybutynin). 39 cm^2 system. Patch; transdermal. Boxes of 4 and 8 systems. *OTC.*
Use: Urinary anticholinergic.

OXY Wash. (Mentholatum) Benzoyl peroxide 10%. Liq. Bot. 120 mL. *OTC.*
Use: Dermatologic, acne.

Oxyzal Wet Dressing. (Gordon Laboratories) Benzalkonium Cl 1:2000, oxyquinoline sulfate, distilled water. Dropper bot. 1 oz, 4 oz. *OTC.*
Use: Dermatologic, counterirritant.

Oysco D. (Rugby) Ca 250 mg, D 125 units. Tab. Bot. 100s, 250s, 1000s. *OTC.*
Use: Mineral, vitamin supplement.

Oysco 500. (Rugby) Calcium carbonate 1250 mg (elemental calcium 500 mg), as oyster shell calcium. Tab. Bot. 60s, 250s. *OTC.*
Use: Mineral supplement.

Oyst-Cal-D. (Ivax) Calcium 250 mg, vitamin D 125 units. Tab. Bot. 100s, 1000s. *OTC.*
Use: Mineral, vitamin supplement.

Oyst-Cal 500. (Goldline) Calcium carbonate 1250 mg (elemental calcium 500 mg), as oyster shell calcium. Preservative free. Tartrazine. Tab. Bot. 60s, 120s. *OTC.*
Use: Mineral supplement.

Oyster Calcium. (NBTY) Ca 275 mg, D 200 units, A 800 units. Tab. Bot. 100s. *OTC.*
Use: Mineral, vitamin supplement.

Oystercal-D. (NBTY) Calcium 250 mg, vitamin D 125 units. Tab. Bot. 100s, 250s. *OTC.*
Use: Mineral, vitamin supplement.

Oyster Shell Calcium. (Various Mfr.) Calcium carbonate 1250 mg (elemental calcium 500 mg). Tab. Bot. 60s, 150s, 300s, 1000s, UD 100s. *OTC.*
Use: Mineral supplement.

Oyster Shell Calcium 500 mg + D. (Major) Calcium 500 mg, vitamin D 200 units. Tab. **60s, 150s, 300s, 1,000s:** Tartrazine. **100s:** Coconut oil, maltodextrin, PEG, propylene glycol. *OTC.*
Use: Nutritional supplement.

Oyster Shell Calcium With Vitamin D. (Major) Calcium 250 mg, vitamin D 125 units. Maltodextrin. Tab. 100s, 300s, 1,000s, UD 100s. *OTC.*
Use: Nutritional supplement.

oyster shells.
See: Os-Cal.
Oysco 500.
Oyst-Cal 500.

•**ozanezumab.** (OH-za-NEZ-ue-mab) USAN.
Use: Treatment of ALS and multiple sclerosis.

•**ozolinone.** (oh-ZOE-lih-NOHN) USAN.
Use: Diuretic.

•**ozoralizumab.** (oh-ZOR-a-LIZ-oo-mab) USAN.
Use: Immunomodulator.

Ozurdex. (Allergan) Dexamethasone 0.7 mg. Implant, intravitreal. Pouch w/single-use applicator. *Rx.*
Use: Ophthalmic and otic agent, corticosteroid.

P

Pabalate-SF. (Wyeth) Potassium salicylate 300 mg, potassium aminobenzoate 300 mg. Tab. Bot. 100s, 500s. *OTC.*
Use: Antirheumatic.

PABA-Salicylate. (Various Mfr.) Sodium salicylate, p-aminobenzoate, vitamin C. Tab. Bot. 100s, 500s. *OTC.*
Use: Analgesic; vitamin combination.

PABA sodium. (Various Mfr.) Sodium p-aminobenzoate. *OTC.*
Use: Vitamin supplement.

Pabasone. (Pinex) Sodium salicylate 5 g, para-aminobenzoic acid 5 g, ascorbic acid 20 mg. Tab. Bot. 100s. *OTC.*
Use: Analgesic; vitamin supplement.

P-A-C. Preparations of phenacetin, aspirin, caffeine.
See: A.P.C. preparations.
Empirin preparations.

P-A-C Analgesic. (Lee) Aspirin 400 mg, caffeine 32 mg. Tab. Bot. 100s, 1000s. *OTC.*
Use: Analgesic combination.

Pacemaker Prophylaxis Pastes with Fluoride. (Pacemaker) Silicone dioxide and diatomaceous earth, sodium fluoride 4.4%. Light abrasive, cinnamon/cherry. Medium abrasive, orange. Heavy abrasive, mint. Paste. Bot. 8 oz.
Use: Dental caries agent.

Pacerone. (Upsher Smith) Amiodarone hydrochloride 100 mg, 200 mg, 400 mg. Lactose. Tab. Bot. 30s (100 mg, 400 mg only), 60s (200 mg only), 90s (200 mg only), 100s (400 mg only), 500s (except 100 mg), UD 100s. *Rx.*
Use: Antiarrhythmic.

Paclin VK. (Armenpharm Ltd.) Penicillin phenoxymethyl 125 mg, 250 mg. Tab. Bot. 100s, 1000s. *Rx.*
Use: Anti-infective, penicillin.

•**paclitaxel.** (pak-lih-TAX-uhl) *USP.*
Tall Man: PACLitaxel
Use: Antineoplastic; antimitotic agent.
See: Abraxane.

paclitaxel. (SuperGen) Paclitaxel 6 mg/mL. May contain dehydrated alcohol, polyoxyethylated castor oil. Inj., Soln., concentrate. Multidose vial. 5 mL, 16.7 mL, 25 mL, 50 mL. *Rx.*
Use: Antimitotic agent.

•**paclitaxel poliglumex.** (pak-lih-TAX-uhl pol-ee-GLOO-mex) USAN.
Tall Man: PACLitaxel
Use: Antineoplastic.

Pacnex HP. (Medimetriks Pharmaceuticals) Benzoyl peroxide 7%. Alcohol, aloe, edetate disodium, glycerin, glyceryl, green tea, PEG, propylene glycol. Pad. UD 60s. *Rx.*
Use: Topical anti-infective, antibiotic.

Pacnex LP. (Medimetriks Pharmaceuticals) Benzoyl peroxide 4.25%. Alcohol, aloe, edetate disodium, glycerin, glyceryl, green tea, PEG, propylene glycol. Pad. UD 60s. *Rx.*
Use: Topical anti-infective, antibiotic.

P-A-C Revised Formula Analgesic. (Pharmacia) Aspirin 400 mg, caffeine 32 mg. Tab. Bot. 100s, 1000s. *OTC.*
Use: Analgesic.

•**padimate A.** (PAD-ih-mate A) USAN.
Use: Ultraviolet screen.

•**padimate O.** (PAD-ih-mate O) *USP.*
Use: Ultraviolet screen.
See: Coppertone.
Eclipse.
Shade.
Super Shade.
Tropical Blend.
W/Combinations.
See: Glyquin.

•**paflufocon A.** (PA-floo-FOE-kon A) USAN.
Use: Contact lens material, hydrophobic.

•**paflufocon B.** (PA-flo-FOE-kon B) USAN.
Use: Contact lens material, hydrophobic.

•**paflufocon C.** (PA-flo-FOE-kon C) USAN.
Use: Contact lens material, hydrophobic.

•**paflufocon D.** (PA-flo-FOE-kon D) USAN.
Use: Contact lens material, hydrophobic.

•**paflufocon D-HEM-iberfilcon A.** (pafloo-FOE-kon eye-ber-FIL-kon A) USAN.
Use: Contact lens material, hybrid.

•**paflufocon E.** (PA-flo-FOE-kon E) USAN.
Use: Contact lens material, hydrophobic.

•**pafuramidine maleate.** (PA-fur-AM-i-deen) USAN.
Use: Anti-infective.

•**pagoclone.** (PAG-oh-klone) USAN.
Use: Anxiolytic.

PAH.
See: Sodium aminohippurate.

Painaid. (Zee Medical) Aspirin 162 mg, salicylamide 152 mg, acetaminophen 110 mg, caffeine 32.4 mg. Tab. 24s. *OTC.*
Use: Nonnarcotic analgesic.

Painaid Back Relief Formula. (Zee Medical) Acetaminophen 250 mg, magnesium salicylate 250 mg. Castor oil, magnesium 17 mg. Tab. UD 2s (100s, 250s). *OTC.*
Use: Nonnarcotic analgesic combination.

Painaid BRF Back Relief Formula. (Zee Medical) Magnesium salicylate tetrahydrate 250 mg, acetaminophen 250 mg. Tab. 24s. *OTC.*
Use: Nonnarcotic analgesic.

Painaid ESF Extra-Strength Formula. (Zee Medical) Acetaminophen 250 mg, aspirin 250 mg, caffeine 65 mg. Tab. 24s. *OTC.*
Use: Nonnarcotic analgesic.

Painaid PMF Premenstrual Formula. (Zee Medical) Acetaminophen 500 mg, pamabrom 25 mg. Tab. 24s. *OTC.*
Use: Nonnarcotic analgesic.

Pain and Fever. (Rugby) Acetaminophen. **Tab.:** 325 mg. Bot. 100s. **Tab. and Capl.:** 500 mg. Bot. 100s, 1000s. *OTC.*
Use: Analgesic.

Pain and Fever Children's. (Rugby) Acetaminophen 80 mg. Aspartame, dextrose, phenylalanine, sugar. Fruit flavor. Chew. Tab. 30s *OTC.*
Use: Analgesic.

Pain and Fever Reliever Children's. (Rugby) Acetaminophen. **Soln., Conc., Oral:** 100 mg/mL. Alcohol free. Butylparaben, corn syr., sorbitol. Cherry flavor. 15 mL. **Soln., Oral:** 160 mg/5 mL. Sorbitol, sucrose. Cherry flavor. 118 mL. *OTC.*
Use: Analgesic.

Pain Bust-R II. (Continental Consumer Products) Methyl salicylate 17%, menthol 12%. Cream. Jar 90 g. *OTC.*
Use: Liniment.

Pain Doctor. (E. Fougera) Capsaicin 0.025%, methyl salicylate 25%, menthol 10%, parabens, propylene glycol. Cream. Tube 60 g. *OTC.*
Use: Anesthetic, local.

Pain Gel Plus. (Mentholatum Co.) Menthol 4%, aloe, vitamin E. Gel. Tube 57 g. *OTC.*
Use: Liniment.

Pain-gesic. (Mason Remedies) Phenyltoloxamine citrate 30 mg, acetaminophen 325 mg. Lactose. Tab. 100s. *OTC.*
Use: Upper respiratory combination, decongestant, antihistamine, and analgesic.

Pain Relief. (Walgreen) Methyl salicylate 15%, menthol 10%. Oint. Tube 1.5 oz, 3 oz. *OTC.*
Use: Analgesic, topical.

Pain Relief Extra Strength. (Basic) Acetaminophen 500 mg. Tab. Bot. 100s. *OTC.*
Use: Analgesic, local.

Pain Reliever. (Magno-Humphries) Acetaminophen 325 mg. Tab. 100s, 250s, 1000s. *OTC.*
Use: Analgesic.

Pain Reliever Extra Strength. (Magno-Humphries) Acetaminophen 500 mg. Tab. 100s, 250s, 1000. *OTC.*
Use: Analgesic.

Pain Reliever PM Extra Strength. (Magno-Humphries) Diphenhydramine hydrochloride 25 mg, acetaminophen 500 mg. Tab. 100s. *OTC.*
Use: Nonprescription sleep aid.

Pain Relievers-Tension Headache Relievers. (Weeks & Leo) Acetaminophen 325 mg, phenyltoloxamine citrate 30 mg. Tab. Bot. 40s, 100s. *OTC.*
Use: Analgesic combination.

Pain Relieving Rub. (G & W Labs) Menthol 10%, methyl salicylate 15%. Cetyl alcohol, glycerin, glyceryl, triethanolamine. Cream. 114 g. *OTC.*
Use: Rub and liniment.

Paire OB Plus DHA Tablets and Softgel Capsules. (Centrix) Folic acid 1 mg, iron 28 mg, vitamins D 400 units, E 10 units, B_1 1.5 mg, B_2 1.6 mg, B_3 17 mg, B_5 10 mg, B_6 50 mg, B_{12} 12 mcg, Cu, I, Se, Zn, biotin 30 mcg. **Tab.:** Maltodextrin, polydextrose. UD 30s. **Cap., softgel:** DHA 200 mg. Glycerin. UD 30s. *Rx.*
Use: Prenatal vitamin with minerals.

Paladin. (Pal Midwest Ltd.) Petrolatum, starch, lanolin, zinc oxide, mineral oil, boric acid, beeswax, vitamin A and D concentrate. Oint. 2 oz. *OTC.*
Use: Diaper rash products.

Palbar No. 2. (Roberts) Atropine sulfate 0.012 mg, scopolamine HBr 0.005 mg, hyoscyamine HBr 0.018 mg, phenobarbital 32.4 mg. Tab. Bot. 100s. *Rx.*
Use: Anticholinergic; antispasmodic; sedative; hypnotic.

•**palbociclib.** (PAL-boe-SYE-klib) USAN.
Use: Antineoplastic.

•**palbociclib isethionate.** (PAL-boe-SYE-klib) USAN.
Use: Antineoplastic.

Palcaps 10. (Breckenridge) Lipase 10,000 units, protease 37,500 units, amylase (porcine-derived enzymes) 33,200 units. Sucrose. Enteric-coated microspheres. DR Cap. 100s, 250s. *Rx.*
Use: Digestive enzyme.

•**paldimycin.** (pal-dih-MY-sin) USAN.
Use: Anti-infective.

palestrol.
See: Diethylstilbestrol.

Palgic. (Pamlab) Carbinoxamine maleate 4 mg/5 mL. Parabens. Sugar free. Bubble gum flavor. Liq. 118 mL, 473 mL.

Rx.
Use: Antihistamine.

Palgic-D. (Pamlab) Pseudoephedrine hydrochloride 80 mg, carbinoxamine maleate 8 mg. Dye free. ER Tab. Bot. 100s. *Rx.*
Use: Upper respiratory combination, antihistamine, decongestant.

Palgic DS. (Pamlab) Carbinoxamine maleate 2 mg, pseudoephedrine hydrochloride 25 mg per 5 mL. Strawberry/pineapple flavor. Syr. Bot. 15 mL, 473 mL. *Rx.*
Use: Upper respiratory combination, antihistamine, decongestant.

•**palifermin.** (pal-ee-FER-min) USAN.
Use: Keratinocyte growth factor; mucositis.
See: Kepivance.

•**palifosfamide.** (PAL-i-FOS-fa-mide) USAN.
Use: Antineoplastic.

•**palifosfamide tromethamine.** (PAL-i-FOS-fa-mide) USAN.
Use: Antineoplastic.

•**palinavir.** (pal-LIH-nah-veer) USAN.
Use: Antiviral.

palinum.
Use: Hypnotic; sedative.
See: Cyclobarbital calcium.

•**paliperidone.** (pal-ee-PER-i-done) USAN.
Use: Antipsychotic, schizophrenia.
See: Invega.
Invega Sustenna.

•**paliperidone palmitate.** (pal-ee-PER-i-done PAL-mih-tate) USAN.
Use: Antipsychotic, schizophrenia.

palivizumab.
Use: Antibody.
See: Synagis.

•**palmoxirate sodium.** (pal-MOX-ihr-ate) USAN.
Use: Antidiabetic.

Palomar "E". (Pal Midwest) Vitamin E, boric acid, beeswax, lanolin, mineral oil, petroleum, starch, zinc oxide. Oint. 2 oz. *OTC.*
Use: Emollient.

•**palonosetron hydrochloride.** (pal-oh-NO-seh-trahn) USAN.
Use: 5-HT_3 receptor antagonist; antiemetic/antivertigo agent.
See: Aloxi.

•**palovarotene.** (PA-loe-VAR-oh-teen) USAN.
Use: Treatment of emphysema.

PALS. (Palisades Pharmaceuticals) Chlorophyllin copper complex 100 mg. Tab. Bot. 30s, 100s, 1000s, UD 30s. *OTC.*
Use: Deodorant, systemic.

•**pamabrom.** (PAM-a-brom) USAN.
See: Maximum Strength Aqua-Ban.
W/Acetaminophen, Pyridoxine Hydrochloride.
See: Vitelle Lurline PMS.
W/Acetaminophen.
See: Midol Teen Formula.
Painaid PMF Premenstrual Formula.
Women's Tylenol Multi-Symptom Menstrual Relief.
W/Acetaminophen, Magnesium Salicylate.
See: Pamprin Maximum Pain Relief.
W/Acetaminophen, Pyrilamine Maleate.
See: Midol Pre-Menstrual Syndrome.
Pamprin Multi-Symptom Maximum Strength.
Vitelle Lurline PMS.

•**pamapimod.** (pa-MAP-i-mod) USAN.
Use: Treatment of rheumatoid arthritis.

•**pamaqueside.** (pam-ah-KWEH-side) USAN.
Use: Antiatherosclerotic; hypocholesterolemic.

•**pamatolol sulfate.** (PAM-ah-TOE-lole) USAN.
Use: Anti-adrenergic, β-receptor.

Pamelor. (Mallinckrodt) Nortriptyline hydrochloride 10 mg, 25 mg, 50 mg, 75 mg. Benzyl alcohol, EDTA, parabens. Cap. 100s, 500s (25 mg only), UD 100s (except 75 mg). *Rx.*
Use: Antidepressant.

•**pamidronate disodium.** (pam-IH-DROE-nate) USAN.
Use: Bisphosphonate.

pamidronate disodium. (Faulding) Pamidronate disodium 6 mg/mL. Mannitol 400 mg. Inj. Vials. 10 mL. *Rx.*
Use: Bisphosphonate.

pamidronate disodium. (Sandoz) Pamidronate disodium 30 mg (mannitol 470 mg), 90 mg (mannitol 375 mg). Pow. for Inj., lyophilized. Vials. *Rx.*
Use: Bisphosphonate.

pamidronate disodium. (Various Mfr.) Pamidronate disodium 3 mg/mL, 9 mg/mL. May contain mannitol. Inj. Vials. 10 mL. *Rx.*
Use: Bisphosphonate.

Pamine. (Kenwood/Bradley) Methscopolamine bromide 2.5 mg. Tab. Bot. 100s, 500s. *Rx.*
Use: Anticholinergic/antispasmodic.

Pamine Forte. (Kenwood Therapeutics) Methscopolamine bromide 5 mg. Tab. 60s. *Rx.*
Use: Anticholinergic/antispasmodic.

Pamine FQ Kit. (Kenwood Therapeutics) Methscopolamine bromide 5 mg with *Flora-Q* capsules containing 8 million CFUs of *Lactobacillus acidophilus, L. paracasei, Bifidobacteriura*, and *Streptococcus thermophilus*. Gluten free. Tab. Packs of 60 methscopolamine bromide tablets and 30 *Flor-Q* capsules. *Rx.*
Use: GI anticholinergic/antispasmodic, quaternary anticholinergic.

p-aminosalicylic acid salts.
See: Aminosalicylic acid salts.

Pamprin Extra Strength Multi-Symptom Relief Formula. (Chattem) Acetaminophen 400 mg, pamabrom 25 mg, pyrilamine maleate 15 mg. Tab. Bot. 12s, 24s, 48s. *OTC.*
Use: Analgesic combination.

Pamprin Maximum Cramp Relief Formula Caplets. (Chattem) Acetaminophen 500 mg, pamabrom 25 mg, pyrilamine maleate 15 mg. Tab. Bot. 8s, 16s, 32s. *OTC.*
Use: Analgesic combination.

Pamprin Maximum Pain Relief Caplets. (Chattem) Acetaminophen 250 mg, magnesium salicylate 250 mg, pamabrom 25 mg. Tab. Bot. 16s, 32s. *OTC.*
Use: Analgesic combination.

Pamprin Multi-Symptom Maximum Strength. (Chattem) Acetaminophen 500 mg, pamabrom 25 mg, pyrilamine maleate 15 mg. **Cap.:** Bot. 24s, 48s. **Tab.:** Bot. 12s, 24s, 48s. *OTC.*
Use: Analgesic combination.

•**panadiplon.** (pan-ad-IH-plone) USAN.
Use: Anxiolytic.

Panadol Extra Strength. (GlaxoSmithKline) Acetaminophen 500 mg. Tab. 30s, 60s. *OTC.*
Use: Analgesic.

Panadol, Infants'. (GlaxoSmithKline) Acetaminophen 100 mg/mL. Drops. Bot. 15 mL with 0.8 mL dropper. *OTC.*
Use: Analgesic.

Panadol, Jr. (GlaxoSmithKline) Acetaminophen 160 mg. Cap. Box. 30s. *OTC.*
Use: Analgesic.

Panafil White. (Rystan) Papain 10,000 units enzyme activity, hydrophilic base/g, urea 10%. Oint. Tube oz. *Rx.*
Use: Enzyme, topical.

Panalgesic. (ECR) Methyl salicylate 55.01%, menthol 1.25%, camphor 3.1%, in alcohol 22%, emollients, color. Liq. 4 oz, pt, 0.5 gal. *OTC.*
Use: Analgesic, topical.

Panasol. (Seatrace) Prednisone 5 mg. Tab. Bot. 100s. *Rx.*
Use: Corticosteroid.

Panatuss DXP. (Seyer) Dexbrompheniramine maleate 2 mg, dextromethorphan hydrobromide 20 mg, phenylephrine hydrochloride 10 mg. Aspartame, parabens, PEG, phenylalanine 15 mg per 5 mL, propylene glycol, sucrose. Alcohol free. Raspberry flavor. Syrup. 118 mL. *Rx.*
Use: Upper respiratory combination, antitussive combination.

Pan C-500. (Freeda) Hesperidin 100 mg, citrus bioflavonoids 100 mg, vitamin C 500 mg. Sodium and sugar free. Tab. Bot. 100s, 250s, 500s. *OTC.*
Use: Water-soluble vitamin.

Pancof. (Pan American) Dihydrocodeine bitartrate 7.5 mg, chlorpheniramine maleate 2 mg, pseudoephedrine hydrochloride 15 mg per 5 mL. Saccharin, sorbitol, alcohol free, dye free, sugar free. Syr. 473 mL. *c-III.*
Use: Antitussive combination.

Pancof-EXP. (Pan American) Dihydrocodeine bitartrate 7.5 mg, guaifenesin 100 mg, pseudoephedrine 15 mg per 5 mL. Saccharin, sorbitol, menthol. Alcohol and dye free. Syr. Bot. 25 mL, 473 mL. *Rx.*
Use: Upper respiratory combination, antitussive, expectorant, decongestant.

Pancof XP. (Pan American) Hydrocodone bitartrate 3 mg, guaifenesin 90 mg per 5 mL. Menthol, saccharin, sorbitol. Syr. 3700 mL. *c-III.*
Use: Antitussive with expectorant.

•**pancopride.** (PAN-koe-pride) USAN.
Use: Antiemetic, anxiolytic, peristaltic stimulant.

pancreatic enzyme.
See: Ox bile extract.
Pepsin.

pancreatic substance. Substance from fresh pancreas of hog or ox, containing the enzymes amylopsin, trypsin, steapsin.

•**pancreatin.** (PAN-kree-ah-tin) *USP.* Pancreatic enzymes obtained from hog or cattle pancreatic tissue.
Use: Enzyme (digestant adjunct).

Pancreatin Quadruple Strength. (Twinlab) Amylase 50,000 units, lipase 4,000 units, protease 50,000 units. Medium chain triglycerides. Cap. 50s. *OTC.*
Use: Digestive enzyme.

Pancreaze. (Janssen Pharmaceuticals) Amylase/lipase/protease 17,500 units/4,200 units/10,000 units; 43,750 units/10,500 units/25,000 units; 70,000 units/16,800 units/40,000 units; 61,000 units/21,000 units/37,000 units. Enteric-coated microtablets. Cap., delayed

release (porcine-derived enzymes). 100s. *Rx.*
Use: Digestive enzyme.

•**pancrelipase.** (pan-KREE-lih-pace) *USP.* Preparation of hog pancreas with high content of steapsin and adequate amounts of pancreatic enzymes.
Use: Enzyme (digestant adjunct).

pancrelipase. (X-Gen Pharmaceuticals) Amylase 27,000 units, lipase 5000 units, protease 17,000 units. Enteric-coated beads. Cap., delayed release. 100s. *Rx.*
Use: Digestive enzyme.

Pancretide. (Baxter PPI) Pancreatic polypeptide in normal saline.
Use: Fibrinolytic conditions.

pancuronium.
See: Pancuronium bromide.

•**pancuronium bromide.** (PAN-cue-ROW-nee-uhm) USAN.
Use: Neuromuscular blocker, muscle relaxant.

pancuronium bromide. (Various Mfr.) Pancuronium bromide. **1 mg/mL:** Vials 10 mL with benzyl alcohol. **2 mg/mL:** Benzyl alcohol. Vials 2 mL, 5 mL. Amps with benzyl alcohol. *Rx.*
Use: Neuromuscular blocker, muscle relaxant.

Pandel. (Collagenex) Hydrocortisone probutate 0.1%, white petrolatum, light mineral oil, stearyl alcohol, parabens. Cream. Tube 15 g, 45 g, 80 g. *Rx.*
Use: Corticosteroid, topical.

P & S. (Ivax) Mineral oil, water, glycerin, fragrance, phenol, sodium chloride. Liq. 4 oz, 8 oz. *OTC.*
Use: Antiseborrheic.

P & S Shampoo. (Aero Pharmaceuticals) Salicylic acid 2%. Lactic acid, parabens, tetrasodium EDTA, triethanolamine, urea. Shampoo. 236 mL. *OTC.*
Use: Keratolytic agent.

Panfil G. (Pan American) **Cap.:** Dyphylline 200 mg, guaifenesin 100 mg, lactose. Bot. 100s. **Syr.:** Dyphylline 100 mg, guaifenesin 50 mg/5 mL, parabens, sorbitol, sucrose, vanilla flavor. Bot. 473 mL. *Rx.*
Use: Antiasthmatic; expectorant.

Panhematin. (Recordati Rare Diseases) Hematin 313 mg (when mixed with sterile water for injection, each 43 mL provides the equivalent of approximately 301 mg of hemin [7 mg/mL]). Sorbitol 300 mg. Preservative free. Single-dose vial. *Rx.*
Use: Hematinic.

Panitol. (Wesley) Allylisobutyl barbituric acid 15 mg, acetaminophen 300 mg. Tab. Bot. 100s, 1000s. *Rx.*
Use: Analgesic; hypnotic; sedative.

•**panitumumab.** (pan-i-TUE-moo-mab) USAN.
Use: Antineoplastic; monoclonal antibody.
See: Vectibix.

Panlor DC. (Pan American) Acetaminophen 356.4 mg, caffeine 30 mg, dihydrocodeine bitartrate 16 mg. Cap. Bot. 100s. *c-III.*
Use: Analgesic.

PanMist-DM. (Pan American) **Syr.:** Dextromethorphan HBr 15 mg, guaifenesin 100 mg, pseudoephedrine hydrochloride 40 mg per 5 mL. Strawberry flavor. Alcohol, sugar, and dye free. Bot. 15 mL, 473 mL. **ER Tab.:** Dextromethorphan HBr 32 mg, guaifenesin 595 mg, pseudoephedrine hydrochloride 48 mg. Bot. 100s. *Rx.*
Use: Upper respiratory combination, antitussive, expectorant, decongestant.

PanMist JR. (Pan American) Pseudoephedrine hydrochloride 48 mg, guaifenesin 595 mg, dye free. ER Tab. Bot. 100s. *Rx.*
Use: Upper respiratory combination, decongestant, expectorant.

PanMist LA. (Pan American) Pseudoephedrine hydrochloride 85 mg, guaifenesin 795 mg. ER Tab. Bot. 100s. *Rx.*
Use: Upper respiratory combination, decongestant, expectorant.

PanMist S. (Pan American) Pseudoephedrine hydrochloride 40 mg, guaifenesin 200 mg. Alcohol free, grape flavor. Syr. Bot. 15 mL, 473 mL. *Rx.*
Use: Upper respiratory combination, decongestant, expectorant.

Panmycin. (Pharmacia) Tetracycline hydrochloride 250 mg. Cap. Bot. 100s, 1000s. *Rx.*
Use: Anti-infective, tetracycline.

•**panobinostat.** (PAN-oh-BIN-oh-stat) USAN.
Use: Antineoplastic.

PanOxyl. (GlaxoSmithKline) Benzoyl peroxide. **Bar:** 10%. Cetostearyl alcohol, glycerin, castor oil, mineral oil in a rich lathering, mild surfactant cleansing base. Soap free. 113 g. **Liq.:** 2.5%. Cetearyl alcohol. Soap free. 156 g. **Wash:** 10%. Alcohol, methylparaben. 156 g. *OTC.*
Use: Dermatologic, acne.

PanOxyl AQ 2½, 5, 10. (GlaxoSmithKline) Benzoyl peroxide 2.5%, 5%, 10%, methylparaben, EDTA, glycerin. Gel. Tube 57 g, 113 g. *Rx.*
Use: Dermatologic, acne.

panparnit hydrochloride. Caramiphen hydrochloride.
Use: Antiparkinsonian.
Panretin. (Ligand) Alitretinoin 0.1%. Dehydrated alcohol. Gel. Tube 60 g. *Rx.*
Use: Second-generation retinoid.
Panscol. (Ivax) Salicylic acid 3%, lactic acid 2%, phenol (< 1%). **Oint.:** Jar 3 oz. **Lot.:** Bot. 4 oz. *OTC.*
Use: Emollient.
•**panthenol.** (PAN-theh-nahl) *USP.* Alcohol corresponding to pantothenic acid.
Use: Vitamin; emollient.
W/Combinations.
See: Lifer-B.
Panthoderm. (Aventis) Dexpanthenol 2% in water-miscible cream. Cream. Tube 1 oz. Jar 2 oz, lb. *OTC.*
Use: Emollient.
pantocaine.
See: Tetracaine hydrochloride.
Pantocrin-F. (Spanner) Plurigland, ovarian, anterior and posterior pituitary, adrenal, thyroid extracts. Vial 30 mL. *Rx.*
Use: Hormone.
•**pantoprazole.** (pan-TOE-pra-zole) USAN.
Use: Antiulcerative.
•**pantoprazole sodium.** (pahn-TOE-prazz-ole) USAN.
Use: Proton pump inhibitor.
See: Protonix.
Protonix I.V.
pantoprazole sodium. (Akorn) Pantoprazole sodium 40 mg. May contain edetate disodium. Inj., lyophilized Pow. for Soln. Single-dose vial. *Rx.*
Use: Proton pump inhibitor.
pantoprazole sodium. (Teva) Pantoprazole 20 mg (as pantoprazole sodium 22.6 mg), 40 mg (as pantoprazole sodium 45.1 mg). May contain lactose. DR Tab. 90s. *Rx.*
Use: Proton pump inhibitor.
pantothenic acid.
Use: Vitamin B_5 supplement.
See: Calcium Pantothenate.
pantothenic acid salts.
See: Calcium pantothenate.
Sodium pantothenate.
pantothenol.
See: Dexpanthenol.
pantothenyl alcohol.
See: Dexpanthenol.
pantothenylol.
See: Panthenol.
Panvitex Geriatric. (Forest) Safflower oil 340 mg, vitamins A 10,000 units, D 400 units, B_1 5 mg, B_6 1 mg, B_2 2.5 mg, B_{12} activity 2 mcg, C 75 mg, niacinamide 40 mg, calcium pantothenate 4 mg, E 2 units, inositol 15 mg, choline bitartrate 31.4 mg, Ca 75 mg, P 58 mg, Fe 30 mg, Mn 0.5 mg, K 2 mg, Zn 0.5 mg, Mg 3 mg. Cap. Bot. 100s, 1000s. *OTC.*
Use: Mineral, vitamin supplement.
Panvitex Plus Minerals. (Forest) Vitamins A 5000 units, D 400 units, B_1 3 mg, B_2 2.5 mg, niacinamide 20 mg, B_6 1.5 mg, calcium pantothenate 5 mg, B_{12} 2.5 mcg, C 50 mg, E 3 units, Ca 215 mg, P 166 mg, Fe 13.4 mg, Mg 7.5 mg, Mn 1.5 mg, K 5 mg, Zn 1.4 mg. Cap. Bot. 100s, 1000s. *OTC.*
Use: Mineral, vitamin supplement.
Panvitex Prenatal. (Forest) Ferrous fumarate 150 mg, cobalamin concentration 2 mcg, vitamins A 6000 units, D 400 units, B_1 1.5 mg, B_2 2.5 mg, niacinamide 15 mg, B_6 3 mg, C 100 mg, Ca 250 mg, calcium pantothenate 5 mg, folic acid 0.2 mg. Cap. Bot. 100s, 1000s. *OTC.*
Use: Mineral, vitamin supplement.
Panvitex T-M. (Forest) Vitamins A 10,000 units, D 400 units, B_1 10 mg, B_6 1 mg, B_2 5 mg, B_{12} 5 mcg, C 150 mg, niacinamide 100 mg, Ca 103 mg, P 80 mg, Fe 10 mg, Mn 1 mg, K 5 mg, Zn 1.4 mg, Mg 5.56 mg. Cap. Bot. 100s, 1000s. *OTC.*
Use: Mineral, vitamin supplement.
PAP. (Abbott Diagnostics) Enzyme immunoassay for measurement of prostatic acid phosphatase. Test kit 100s.
Use: Diagnostic aid.
Papadeine #3. (Vangard Labs, Inc.) Codeine phosphate 30 mg, acetaminophen 300 mg. Tab. Bot. 100s, 1000s. *c-III.*
Use: Analgesic combination; narcotic.
•**papain.** (pap-ANE) *USP.* A proteolytic substance derived from *Carica papaya.*
Use: Proteolytic enzyme.
W/Combinations.
See: Ziox 405.
Pap-a-Lix. (Freeport) n-acetyl-aminophenol 120 mg, alcohol 10%/5 mL. Bot. 4 oz, gal. *OTC.*
Use: Analgesic.
•**papaverine hydrochloride.** (pap-PAV-uhr-een) *USP.*
Use: Vasodilator.
See: Pavagen TD.
papaverine hydrochloride. (Various Mfr.) Papaverine hydrochloride. **Inj.:** 30 mg/mL. Vial 2 mL, multiple-dose vial 10 mL. **TR Cap.:** 150 mg. 100s, 1000s. *Rx.*
Use: Vasodilator.

papillomavirus vaccine, quadrivalent, human.
Use: Active immunization agent, viral vaccine.
See: Gardasil.

Paplex Ultra. (Medicis) Salicylic acid 26% in flexible collodion. Bot. 15 mL. *OTC.*
Use: Keratolytic.

para-aminobenzoic acid. (Various Mfr.) para-aminobenzoic acid. **Tab.:** 100 mg. Bot. 100s, 250s. **SR Tab.:** 100 mg. Bot. 100s. *OTC.*
Use: Sunscreen; agent for scleroderma.

para-aminobenzoic acid (PABA).
Use: Sunscreen; agent for scleroderma.
See: Potaba.

•**para-aminosalicylic acid.** *USP.* Aminosalicylic acid. *Rx.*
Use: Antituberculosis.

Parabaxin. (Parmed Pharmaceuticals, Inc.) Methocarbamol 500 mg, 750 mg. Tab. Bot. 100s. *Rx.*
Use: Muscle relaxant.

parabrom.
See: Pyrabrom.

parabromidylamine.
See: Brompheniramine.
Dimetane Decongestant.

Paracaine. (Ocusoft) Proparacaine hydrochloride 0.5%. Soln. 15 mL. *Rx.*
Use: Ophthalmic local anesthetic.

paracarbinoxamine maleate. Carbinoxamine.

paracetaldehyde.
See: Parldehyde.

Paracet Forte. (Major) Chlorzoxazone, acetaminophen. Tab. Bot. 100s, 1000s. *Rx.*
Use: Muscle relaxant.

parachloramine hydrochloride. Meclizine hydrochloride.
See: Bonine.

parachlorometaxylenol.
Use: Phenolic antiseptic.
W/Pramoxine hydrochloride, hydrocortisone, benzalkonium Cl, acetic acid.
See: Rezamid.

•**parachlorophenol.** (PAR-a-KLOR-oh-FEE-nole) *USP.*
Use: Anti-infective, topical.

•**parachlorophenol, camphorated.** (PAR-a-KLOR-oh-FEE-nole) *USP.*
Use: Anti-infective, topical.

paracodin.
See: Dihydrocodeine.

Paraeusal Liquid. (Paraeusal) Liq. Bot. 2 oz, 6 oz, 12 oz.
Use: Minor skin irritations.

Paraeusal Solid. (Paraeusal) Oint. Jar 1 oz, 2 oz, 16 oz.
Use: Dermatologic, counterirritant.

•**paraffin.** (PAR-ah-fin) *NF.*
Use: Pharmaceutic aid (stiffening agent).

•**paraffin, synthetic.** (PAR-ah-fin) *NF.*
Use: Pharmaceutic aid (stiffening agent).

Paraflex. (McNeil Pharm.) Chlorzoxazone 250 mg. Tab. Bot. 100s. *Rx.*
Use: Muscle relaxant.

Parafon Forte DSC. (Janssen) Chlorzoxazone 500 mg. Cap. Bot. 100s, 500s, UD 100s. *Rx.*
Use: Muscle relaxant.

paraform. Paraformaldehyde (No Manufacturer Available).

paraformaldehyde.
Use: Essentially the same as formaldehyde.
See: Formaldehyde.
Trioxymethylene (an incorrect term for paraformaldehyde).

paraglycylarsanilic acid. N-carbamylmethyl-p-aminobenzenearsonic acid, the free acid of tryparsamide.

Parahist HD. (Pharmics) Phenylephrine hydrochloride 5 mg, chlorpheniramine maleate 2 mg, hydrocodone bitartrate 1.67 mg, alcohol free. Liq. Bot. 473 mL. *c-III.*
Use: Antihistamine; antitussive; decongestant.

Para-Jel. (Health for Life Brands) Benzocaine 5%, cetyl dimethyl benzyl ammonium Cl. Tube 0.25 oz. *OTC.*
Use: Anesthetic, local.

•**paraldehyde.** (par-AL-deh-hide) *USP.*
Use: Hypnotic; sedative.

paramephrin.
See: Epinephrine.

•**paramethasone acetate.** (PAR-ah-meth-ah-zone) *USP.*
Use: Corticosteroid, topical.
See: Haldrone.

para-monochlorophenol.
See: Camphorated para-chlorophenol.

•**paranyline hydrochloride.** (PAR-ah-NYE-leen) USAN.
Use: Anti-inflammatory.

•**parapenzolate bromide.** (pa-rah-PEN-zoe-late) USAN.
Use: Anticholinergic.

Paraplatin. (Bristol-Myers Squibb) Carboplatin 50 mg, 150 mg, 450 mg. Mannitol. Inj., lyophilized Pow. for Soln. Single-use vial. *Rx.*
Use: Antineoplastic agent, platinum coordination complex.

pararosaniline embonate. Pararosaniline pamoate.

•**pararosaniline pamoate.** (par-ah-row-ZAN-ih-lin PAM-oh-ate) USAN.
Use: Antischistosomal.

parasympatholytic agents. Cholinergic blocking agents.
See: Anticholinergic agents.
Antispasmodics.
Mydriatics.
Parkinsonism agents.

parasympathomimetic agents.
See: Cholinergic agents.

•**parathyroid hormone.** (par-a-THYE-roid) USAN.
Use: Anti-osteoporotic.

Paratrol. (Walgreen) Pyrethrins 0.2%, piperonyl butoxide technical 2%, deodorized kerosene 0.8%. Liq. Bot. 2 oz. *OTC.*
Use: Pediculicide.

Parazone. (Henry Schein) Chlorzoxazone 250 mg, acetaminophen 300 mg. Tab. Bot. 100s, 1000s. *Rx.*
Use: Muscle relaxant; analgesic.

•**parbendazole.** (par-BEN-dah-ZOLE) USAN. Under study.
Use: Anthelmintic.

Parcillin. (Parmed Pharmaceuticals, Inc.) Crystalline potassium penicillin G 240 mg, 400,000 units. Tab. Bot. 100s, 1000s. Pow. for Syr. 400,000 units/5 mL. 80 mL. *Rx.*
Use: Anti-infective, penicillin.

•**parconazole hydrochloride.** (par-KOE-nah-zole) USAN.
Use: Antifungal.

Parcopa. (Azur Pharma) Carbidopa/levodopa 10 mg/100 mg (phenylalanine 3.4 mg), 25 mg/100 mg (phenylalanine 3.4 mg), 25 mg/250 mg (phenylalanine 8.4 mg). Aspartame, mannitol. Mint flavor. Orally Disintegrating Tab. 100s. *Rx.*
Use: Antiparkinson agent.

•**pardoprunox.** (par-doe-PRUE-nox) USAN.
Use: Parkinson disease; restless legs syndrome.

•**pardoprunox hydrochloride.** (par-doe-PRUE-nox) USAN.
Use: Parkinson disease; restless legs syndrome.

•**parecoxib.** (pa-re-KOX-ib) USAN.
Use: Anti-inflammatory; analgesic.

•**paregoric.** (par-eh-GORE-ik) *USP.*
Use: Antiperistaltic.

paregoric. (Various Mfr.) Morphine anhydrous equivalent 2 mg/5 mL. Alcohol 45%, may contain benzoic acid. Liq. Bot. 473 mL. *c-III.*
Use: Antiperistaltic; opioid analgesic.

Paremyd. (Akorn) Hydroxyamphetamine HBr 1%, tropicamide 0.25%. Soln. Bot. 5 mL, 15 mL. *Rx.*
Use: Cycloplegic, mydriatic.

parenabol. Boldenone undecylenate.

•**pareptide sulfate.** (PAR-epp-tide) USAN.
Use: Antiparkinsonian.

Par Estro. (Parmed Pharmaceuticals, Inc.) Conjugated estrogens 1.25 mg. Tab. Bot. 100s. *Rx.*
Use: Estrogen.

Par-F. (Pharmics) Fe 60 mg, Ca 250 mg, vitamins C 120 mg, A 5000 units, D 400 units, B_1 3 mg, B_2 3.4 mg, B_{12} 12 mcg, B_6 12 mg, B_3 20 mg, Cu, I, Mg, Zn 15 mg, E 30 units, folic acid 1 mg. Tab. Bot. 100s. *Rx.*
Use: Mineral, vitamin supplement.

•**pargyline hydrochloride.** (PAR-jih-leen) *USP.*
Use: Antihypertensive.

•**paricalcitol.** (pah-ri-KAL-si-tole) *USP.*
Use: Hyperparathyroidism.
See: Zemplar.

paricalcitol. (Various Mfr.) Paricalcitol 1 mcg, 2 mcg, 4 mcg. May contain BHT, glycerin, soya lecithin. Cap., softgel. 30s. *Rx.*
Use: Fat-soluble vitamin.

Parkelp. (Phillip R. Park) Pacific sea kelp.
Tab.: Bot. 100s, 200s, 500s, 800s.
Gran.: Bot. 2 oz, 7 oz, 1 lb, 3 lb. *OTC.*
Use: Nutritional supplement.

parkinsonism, agents for. Parasympatholytic agents.
See: Akineton.
Benztropine Mesylate.
Caramiphen Hydrochloride.
Cogentin.
Dopar.
Eldepryl.
Kemadrin.
Larodopa.
Lodosyn.
Parlodel.
Permax.
Sinemet.
Symmetrel.
Trihexyphenidyl Hydrochloride.
Trihexy-2.

Parlodel. (Novartis) Bromocriptine mesylate. Lactose. **Tab.:** 2.5 mg. Bot. 30s, 100s. **Cap.:** 5 mg. Bot. 30s, 100s. *Rx.*
Use: Antiparkinsonian.

Parmeth. (Parmed Pharmaceuticals, Inc.) Promethazine hydrochloride 50 mg. Cap. Bot. 100s, 1000s. *Rx.*
Use: Antiemetic; antihistamine; antivertigo.

parminyl. Salicylamide, phenacetin, caffeine, acetaminophen.

Par-Natal-FA. (Parmed Pharmaceuticals, Inc.) Vitamins A 4000 units, D 400 units, thiamine hydrochloride 2 mg, riboflavin 2 mg, pyridoxine hydrochloride 0.8 mg, ascorbic acid 50 mg, niacinamide 10 mg, I 0.15 mg, folic acid 0.1 mg, cobalamin concentrate 2 mcg, Fe 50 mg, Ca 240 mg. Cap. Bot. 100s, 1000s. *OTC.*
Use: Mineral, vitamin supplement.

Par-Natal Plus 1 Improved. (Parmed Pharmaceuticals, Inc.) Elemental calcium 200 mg, elemental iron 65 mg, vitamins A 4000 units, D 400 units, E 11 mg, B_1 1.5 mg, B_2 3 mg, B_3 20 mg, B_6 10 mg, B_{12} 12 mcg, C 120 mg, folic acid 1 mg, Zn 25 mg, Cu. Tab. Bot. 500s. *Rx.*
Use: Mineral, vitamin supplement.

Parnate. (Covis) Tranylcypromine sulfate 10 mg. Lactose. Film-coated. Tab. Bot. 100s. *Rx.*
Use: Antidepressant, monoamine oxidase inhibitor.

parodyne.
See: Antipyrine.

paroleine.
See: Petrolatum Liquid.

•**paromomycin sulfate.** (par-oh-moe-MY-sin) *USP.* An antibiotic substance obtained from cultures of certain *Streptomyces* species, one of which is *Streptomyces rimosus.*
Use: Antiamebic.
See: Humatin.

paromomycin sulfate. (Caraco Pharmaceutical Laboratories) Paromomycin 250 mg. Cap. 100s. *Rx.*
Use: Oral aminoglycoside.

parothyl. (Henry Schein) Meprobamate 400 mg, tridihexethyl Cl 25 mg. Tab. Bot. 100s. *c-IV.*
Use: Anticholinergic; anxiolytic; antispasmodic.

•**paroxetine.** (pa-ROX-e-teen) USAN.
Use: Antidepressant, selective serotonin reuptake inhibitor.
See: Brisdelle.

paroxetine. (Various Mfr.) Paroxetine hydrochloride 10 mg, 20 mg, 30 mg, 40 mg. Tab. 30s, 100s, 1000s, UD 100s. *Rx.*
Use: Antidepressant, selective serotonin reuptake inhibitor.

•**paroxetine hydrochloride.** (pa-ROX-e-teen) *USP.*
Tall Man: PARoxetine
Use: Antidepressant, selective serotonin reuptake inhibitor.
See: Paxil.
Paxil CR.

paroxetine hydrochloride. (Apotex USA) Paroxetine hydrochloride 10 mg/5 mL. Oral Susp. 250 mL. *Rx.*
Use: Antidepressant, selective serotonin reuptake inhibitor.

paroxetine hydrochloride. (Mylan) Paroxetine 12.5 mg, 25 mg, 37.5 mg. Lactose, PEG, polydextrose. Film-coated. CR Tab. 30s, 100s (12.5 and 25 mg only), 500s (12.5 and 25 mg only). *Rx.*
Use: Antidepressant, selective serotonin reuptake inhibitor.

•**paroxetine mesylate.** (pa-ROX-e-teen) USAN.
Tall Man: PARoxetine
Use: Antidepressant, selective serotonin reuptake inhibitor.
See: Pexeva.

parpanit.
See: Caramiphen hydrochloride.

•**parsatuzumab.** (PAR-sa-TUE-zue-mab) USAN.
Use: Antineoplastic.

parsley concentrate. Garlic concentrate. *Rx.*

Par-Supp. (Parmed Pharmaceuticals, Inc.) Estrone 0.2 mg, lactose 50 mg. Vaginal Supp. Pkg. 12s.
Use: Estrogen.

•**partricin.** (PAR-trih-sin) USAN. Antibiotic produced by *Streptomyces aureofaciens.*
Use: Antifungal; antiprotozoal.

Partuss A.C. (Parmed Pharmaceuticals, Inc.) Guaifenesin 100 mg, pheniramine maleate 7.5 mg, codeine phosphate 10 mg, alcohol 3.5%/5 mL. Bot. 4 oz. *c-v.*
Use: Antihistamine; antitussive; expectorant.

Parvlex. (Freeda) Iron 100 mg, vitamins B_1 20 mg, B_2 20 mg, B_3 20 mg, B_5 1 mg, B_6 10 mg, B_{12} 50 mcg, C 50 mg, folic acid 0.1 mg, Cu, Mn. Tab. Bot. 100s, 250s. *OTC.*
Use: Mineral, vitamin supplement.

Pas-C. (Hellwig) Pascorbic. p-aminosalicylic acid 0.5 g with vitamin C. Tab. Bot. 1000s. *Rx.*
Use: Antituberculosal.

•**pascolizumab.** (pas-co-LIZ-oo-mab) USAN.
Use: Asthma.

Paser. (Jacobus Pharm) Aminosalicylic acid 4 g. Oral DR Gran. Pkt. *Rx.*
Use: Antituberculosis agent.

•**pasireotide.** (PAS-i-REE-oh-tide) USAN.
Use: Endocrine and metabolic agent.
See: Signifor.

passiflora. Dried flowering and fruiting

tops of *Passiflora incarnata*. Phenobarbital, valerian, hyoscyamus.

Pataday. (Alcon) Olopatadine hydrochloride 0.2%. Benzalkonium chloride. Ophth. Soln. 2.5 mL. *Rx.*
Use: Ophthalmic antihistamine.

Patanase. (Alcon Labs) Olopatadine 0.6% (equiv. to olopatadine hydrochloride 665 mcg). Benzalkonium chloride 0.01%, edetate disodium. Spray, Soln., Intranasal. Metered-dose manual spray pump and applicator. 30.5 g (240 actuations). *Rx.*
Use: Respiratory inhalant, intranasal antihistamine.

Patanol. (Alcon) Olopatadine hydrochloride 0.1%. Soln. *Drop-Tainer* 5 mL. *Rx.*
Use: Antihistamine, ophthalmic.

•**pateclizumab.** (PA-tek-LIZ-ue-mab) USAN.
Use: Immunomodulator.

patent ductus arteriosus, agents for.
See: Alprostadil.
Ibuprofen Lysine.
Indomethacin Sodium.
Indomethacin Sodium Trihydrate.

Path. (Parker) Buffered neutral formalin soln. 10%. Bot. 1 gal, 5 gal. Jar 4 oz.
Use: Tissue specimen fixative.

Pathocil. (Wyeth) Dicloxacillin sodium. **Cap.:** 250 mg, 500 mg. Bot. 50s (500 mg only), 100s (250 mg only). **Pow. for Oral Susp.:** 62.5 mg/5 mL. Bot. to make 100 mL. *Rx.*
Use: Anti-infective, penicillin.

•**patiromer.** (pa-TIR-oh-mer) USAN.
Use: Treatment of hyperkalemia.

•**patiromer calcium.** (pa-TIR-oh-mer) USAN.
Use: Treatment of hyperkalemia.

•**paulomycin.** (PAW-low-MY-sin) USAN.
Use: Anti-infective.

Pavagen TD. (Rugby) Papaverine hydrochloride 150 mg. TR Cap. Bot. 100s, 500s, 1000s. *Rx.*
Use: Vasodilator.

Paxil. (Apotex) Paroxetine hydrochloride. **Tab.:** 10 mg, 20 mg, 30 mg, 40 mg. Film-coated. Bot. 30s; 90s (20 mg only), SUP 100s (20 mg only). **Oral Susp.:** 10 mg/5 mL. Parabens, saccharin, sorbitol, orange flavor. Bot. 250 mL. *Rx.*
Use: Antidepressant, selective serotonin reuptake inhibitor.

Paxil CR. (Apotex) Paroxetine hydrochloride 25 mg, 37.5 mg. Lactose. Enteric coated. CR Tab. 30s. *Rx.*
Use: Antidepressant, selective serotonin reuptake inhibitor.

•**pazinaclone.** (pah-ZIN-ah-klone) USAN.
Use: Anxiolytic.

Pazo Hemorrhoid. (Bristol-Myers Squibb) Zinc oxide 5%, ephedrine sulfate 0.2%, camphor 2% in lanolin-petrolatum base. Oint. Tube 28 g. *OTC.*
Use: Anorectal preparation.

Pazol XS. (Stratus) Coal tar 1%, salicylic acid 2%, sulfur 2%. Shampoo. 118 mL. *OTC.*
Use: Antiseborrheic combination.

•**pazopanib hydrochloride.** (paz-OH-pa-nib) USAN.
Use: Antineoplastic.
See: Votrient.

•**pazoxide.** (pay-ZOX-ide) USAN.
Use: Antihypertensive.

PB-Hyos. (Kylemore) Atropine sulfate 0.0194 mg, hyoscyamine hydrobromide or sulfate 0.1037 mg, phenobarbital 16.2 mg, scopolamine hydrobromide 0.0065 mg. Alcohol 23%, glycerin, saccharin, sorbitol, sucrose. Grape flavor. Elix. 473 mL. *c-IV.*
Use: Gastrointestinal anticholinergic/antispasmodic, gastrointestinal anticholinergic combination.

PB 100. (Schlicksup) Phenobarbital 1.5 g. Tab. Bot. 1000s. *c-IV.*
Use: Hypnotic; sedative.

PBZ. (Novartis) Tripelennamine hydrochloride 25 mg, 50 mg. Tab. Bot. 100s. *Rx.*
Use: Antihistamine.

PBZ-SR. (Novartis) Tripelennamine hydrochloride 100 mg. SR Tab. Bot. 100s. *Rx.*
Use: Antihistamine.

PCE Dispertab. (Abbott) Erythromycin 333 mg (lactose), 500 mg. Polymer-coated particles. Tab. Bot. 60s (333 mg only), 100s (500 mg only). *Rx.*
Use: Anti-infective, erythromycin.

p-chlorometaxylenol. Benzocaine, benzyl alcohol, propylene glycol.
W/Hydrocortisone, pramoxine hydrochloride.
See: 20-Caine Burn Relief.

p-chlorophenol.
See: Parachlorophenol.

PCM. (Boca Pharmacal) Phenylephrine hydrochloride 10 mg, chlorpheniramine maleate 2 mg, methscopolamine nitrate 1.25 mg. Lactose, mannitol, sugar. Chew. Tab. 100s. *Rx.*
Use: Upper respiratory combination, decongestant, antihistamine, and anticholinergic.

PCMX.
See: Parachlorometaxylenol.

PC-Tar. (Geritrex) Coal tar 1%. EDTA. Shampoo. 180 mL. *OTC.*
Use: Photochemotherapy.

PDP Liquid Protein. (Wesley) Protein 15 g (from protein hydrolysates), cal 60/30 mL. Bot. Pt, qt, gal. *OTC.*
Use: Protein supplement.

Peacock's Bromides. (Natcon) **Liq.:** Potassium bromide 6 g, sodium bromide 6 g, ammonium bromide 3 g/5 mL. Bot. 8 oz. **Tab.:** Potassium bromide 3 g, sodium bromide 3 g, ammonium bromide 1.5 g. Bot. 100s. *Rx.*
Use: Hypnotic; sedative.

•**peanut oil.** (PEE-nut) *NF.*
Use: Pharmaceutic aid (solvent).

Pearls IC. (Enzymatic Therapy) 1 billion CFU blend of *L. acidophilus, L. rhamnosus, B. bifidum, B. lactic, B. longum, B. breve.* Coconut oil, glycerin, palm oil, soy lecithin. Preservative free. Cap. 30s, UD 90s. *OTC.*
Use: Probiotic.

PE-CPM-MSN 8-2-0.75. (Kylemore) Chlorpheniramine maleate 2 mg, methscopolamine nitrate 0.75 mg, phenylephrine hydrochloride 8 mg. Glycerin, parabens, PEG, potassium, *Prosweet,* sorbate, sucrose, saccharin, sorbitol, sucralose. Grape flavor. Syrup. 473 mL. *Rx.*
Use: Upper respiratory combination; decongestant, antihistamine, and anticholinergic combination.

Pectamol. (British Drug House) Diethylaminoethoxyethyl-a,a-diethylphenylacetate citrate. Bot. 4 fl oz, 16 fl oz, 80 fl oz, 160 fl oz.
Use: Antitussive.

•**pectin.** (PECK-tin) *USP.*
Use: Protectant; pharmaceutic aid, suspending agent.
W/Benzocaine.
See: Cēpacol Sore Throat + Coating Relief Maximum Numbing.
W/Combinations.
See: Furoxone.
Kaopectate.

Pedenex. (Health for Life Brands) Caprylic acid, zinc undecylenate, sodium propionate. Tube 1.5 oz. Foot pow. spray 5 oz. *OTC.*
Use: Antifungal, topical.

PediaCare Children's Cough & Congestion. (Medtech) Dextromethorphan hydrobromide 5 mg, guaifenesin 100 mg. Dextrose, glycerin, potassium sorbate, parabens, propylene glycol, saccharin, sodium 3 mg per 5 mL, sucrose. Cherry flavor. Liq. 118 mL. *OTC.*
Use: Upper respiratory combination, antitussive with expectorant.

PediaCare Children's Cough & Sore Throat. (Medtech) Acetaminophen 160 mg, dextromethorphan hydrobromide 5 mg. Acesulfame K, corn syrup, glycerin, sodium benzoate, sorbitol. Cherry flavor. Liq. 118 mL. *OTC.*
Use: Upper respiratory combination, antitussive combination.

PediaCare Children's Long-Acting Cough. (McNeil) Dextromethorphan HBr 7.5 mg per 5 mL. Alcohol and sugar free. Saccharin, sorbitol. Grape flavor. Oral Soln. 120 mL. *OTC.*
Use: Nonnarcotic antitussive.

PediaCare Children's Multi-Symptom Cold. (McNeil) Phenylephrine hydrochloride 5 mg, dextromethorphan HBr 5 mg per 5 mL. Sorbitol, sodium 10 mg/5 mL. Grape flavor. Liq. Bot. 118 mL. *OTC.*
Use: Upper respiratory combination, decongestant, antihistamine, antitussive.

PediaCare Children's NightTime Cough. (McNeil) Diphenhydramine 12.5 mg per 5 mL. Sucrose. Cherry flavor. Liq. Bot. 120 mL. *OTC.*
Use: Antitussive.

PediaCare Children's Pain Reliever Fever Reducer IB. (Medtech) Ibuprofen 100 mg per 5 mL. Glycerin, sodium benzoate, sucrose. Dye free. Berry flavor. Susp. 118 mL. *OTC.*
Use: Nonsteroidal anti-inflammatory agent.

PediaCare Cold & Flu Hydration. (Medtech) Potassium 180 mg, sodium 240 mg, vitamin C 9 mg. Dextrose, sucralose. Grape flavor. Pow. for Soln. Packet 8 g. *OTC.*
Use: Electrolyte.

PediaCare Infants' Pain Reliever Fever Reducer IB. (Medtech) Ibuprofen 40 mg/mL. Glycerin, sodium benzoate, sorbitol, sucrose. Dye free. Berry flavor. Susp., Conc. 15 mL, 30 mL w/dropper. *OTC.*
Use: Nonsteroidal anti-inflammatory agent.

Pediacof. (Sanofi-Synthelabo) Codeine phosphate 5 mg, phenylephrine hydrochloride 2.5 mg, chlorpheniramine maleate 0.75 mg, potassium iodide 75 mg/5 mL, sodium benzoate 0.2%, alcohol 5%. Syr. Bot. 16 fl oz. *c-v.*
Use: Antihistamine; antitussive; decongestant; expectorant.

Pediaderm AF. (Arbor Pharmaceuticals) Nystatin 100,000 units/g. Aluminum hydroxide gel, medical antifoam AF emulsion, parabens, PEG 400, propylene glycol, titanium dioxide, white petro-

latum. Cream. 30 g w/diaper defense cream (beeswax, light mineral oil, parabens, paraffin, PEG-30, vitamin E, white petrolatum, zinc oxide. *Rx.*
Use: Topical anti-infective, antifungal agent.

Pediaderm TA. (Arbor Pharmaceuticals) Triamcinolone acetonide 0.1%. Cetyl alcohol, glyceryl, cetyl esters wax, polysorbate 80, propylene glycol. Cream. 30 g w/protective emollient (petrolatum, glycerin, mineral oil, cetyl alcohol, parabens). *Rx.*
Use: Anti-inflammatory agent, topical corticosteroid.

Pediahist DM. (Boca Pharmacal) Pseudoephedrine hydrochloride 30 mg, brompheniramine maleate 2 mg, dextromethorphan hydrobromide 5 mg, guaifenesin 50 mg per 5 mL. Alcohol free. Corn syrup. Grape flavor. Syrup. 473 mL. *Rx.*
Use: Antitussive combination, antitussive and expectorant combination, upper respiratory combination.

Pedia-Lax. (Fleet) Magnesium hydroxide 400 mg. Watermelon flavor. Chew. Tab. 30s. *OTC.*
Use: Laxative.

Pedialyte. (Abbott) **Soln.:** Sodium 45 mEq/L, potassium 20 mEq/L, chloride 35 mEq/L. Dextrose 25 g/L, zinc 7.8 mg/L, sucralose (except unflavored), acesulfame K (except unflavored), potassium citrate. Strawberry, fruit, grape, and bubble gum flavor, and unflavored. Ready-to-use. 1 L. **Singles Soln.:** Sodium 9 mEq/8.5 g, potassium 4 mEq/8.5 g, chloride 7 mEq/8.5 g. Zinc 1.6 mg/L, dextrose 5.3 g/L, sucralose, acesulfame K, potassium citrate. Fruit, cherry, and apple flavors. 200 mL. **Pow. Packs:** Sodium 10.6 mEq/8.5 g, 4.7 mEq/8.5 g, 8.3 mEq/8.5 g. Dextrose 22.8 g/L, sucralose, acesulfame K, potassium citrate. Fruit punch, grape, apple, and strawberry flavor. Packet. 8.5 g. *OTC.*
Use: Electrolyte.

Pedialyte Freezer Pops. (Abbott) Sodium 45 mEq/L, potassium 20 mEq/L, chloride 35 mEq/L. Dextrose 25 g/L, potassium citrate, potassium sorbate, sodium benzoate, sucralose, acesulfame K. Grape, cherry, orange, and blue raspberry flavors. Liq. ready-to-freeze pops (16s). 62.5 mL. *OTC.*
Use: Electrolyte.

Pediamycin. (Ross) Erythromycin ethylsuccinate for oral suspension 100 mg/2.5 mL. Drops. Bot. 50 mL (Dropper enclosed). *Rx.*
Use: Anti-infective, erythromycin.

Pediapred. (Celltech Pharmaceuticals) Prednisolone 5 mg/5 mL (equiv. to prednisolone sodium phosphate 6.7 mg/5 mL). Methylparaben, EDTA, sorbitol. Raspberry flavor. Oral Soln. Bot. 120 mL. *Rx.*
Use: Adrenocortical steroid, glucocorticoid.

Pedia Relief Cough-Cold. (Major) Chlorpheniramine maleate 1 mg, dextromethorphan hydrobromide 5 mg, pseudoephedrine hydrochloride 15 mg per 5 mL. Alcohol free. Cherry flavor. Liq. 118 mL. *OTC.*
Use: Upper respiratory combination, antitussive combination.

Pedia Relief Decongestant Plus Cough Infants'. (Major) Pseudoephedrine hydrochloride 9.375 mg, dextromethorphan HBr 3.125 mg per 1 mL. Sorbitol, cherry flavor, alcohol free. Drops. Bot. 15 mL w/dropper. *OTC.*
Use: Upper respiratory combination, decongestant, antitussive.

Pediarix. (GlaxoSmithKline) Diphtheria toxoid 25 Lf, tetanus toxoid 10 Lf, inactivated pertussis toxin 25 mcg, filamentous hemagglutinin 25 mcg, pertactin 8 mcg, hepatitis B surface antigen 10 mcg, D-antigen units type 1 poliovirus 40, DU type 2 poliovirus 8, DU type 3 poliovirus 32, sodium chloride 4.5 mg, aluminum adjuvant ($\leq$ 0.85 mg aluminum by assay). Preservative free. Vial. Single-dose, prefilled syringes. *Rx.*
Use: Vaccine.

PediaSure. (Abbott Nutrition) Protein 30 g (L-carnitine, milk protein concentrate, whey protein concentrate, taurine), carbohydrate 131 g (corn maltodextrin, sucrose), fat 38 g (high-oleic safflower oil, soy oil, medium chain triglycerides)/L. Na 380 mg/L, K 1310 mg/L, 480 (vanilla, strawberry, and banana cream), 540 (chocolate), 560 (orange cream) mOsm/kg H_2O, 1 cal/mL. Vitamins A, B_1, B_2, B_3, B_5, B_6, B_7, B_{12}, C, D, E, K, inositol, Cl^-, Cr, Ca, P, Mg, I, Mn, Cu, Se, Zn, Fe, folic acid. Gluten and lactose free. Vanilla, chocolate, strawberry, banana cream, orange cream flavors. Ready-to-use cans and bots. 240 mL. *OTC.*
Use: Infant food, enteral nutritional therapy.

PediaSure with Fiber. (Ross) Protein 30 g (sodium caseinate, low-lactose whey, carnitine, taurine), carbohydrate 113.5 g (maltodextrin, sucrose, soy fiber [total dietary fiber 5 g]), fat 49.7 g (high-

oleic safflower oil, soy oil, medium chain triglyceride oil, lecithin)/L, vitamins A, B_1, B_2, B_3, B_6, B_{12}, C, D, E, K, folic acid, Ca, Fe, I, Mg, P, Se, Zn, Na 380 mg (16.5 mEq), K 1310 mg (33.5 mEq), cal 1/L, vanilla flavor, lactose and gluten free. Liq. Bot. 8 oz. *OTC.*
Use: Enteral nutritional therapy, defined formula diet.

PediaTan. (ProEthic) Chlorpheniramine (as tannate) 8 mg. Methylparaben, sodium saccharin, sorbitol. Sugar free. Bubble gum flavor. Oral Susp. 473 mL. *Rx.*
Use: Antihistamine.

Pediatex. (Zyber) Carbinoxamine maleate 1.67 mg/5 mL. Alcohol and dye free. Saccharin, sorbitol. Cotton candy flavor. Liq. 15 mL, 473 mL. *Rx.*
Use: Antihistamine, nonselective ethanolamine.

Pediatex-D. (Zyber) Pseudoephedrine hydrochloride 12.5 mg, carbinoxamine maleate 1.67 mg per 5 mL. Sugar, alcohol, and dye free. Cotton candy flavor. Liq. Bot. 20 mL, 473 mL. *Rx.*
Use: Upper respiratory combination, decongestant, antihistamine.

Pediatex-DM. (Zyber) Pseudoephedrine hydrochloride 15 mg, carbinoxamine maleate 2 mg, dextromethorphan HBr 15 mg per 1 mL. Saccharin, sorbitol, cotton candy flavor. Liq. Bot. 20 mL, 473 mL. *Rx.*
Use: Upper respiratory combination, decongestant, antihistamine, antitussive.

Pediatex HC. (Zyber) Pseudoephedrine hydrochloride 17.5 mg, chlorpheniramine maleate 2.5 mg, hydrocodone bitartrate 1.67 mg per 5 mL. Sugar free. Saccharin, sorbitol. Cotton candy flavor. Syr. 20 mL, 480 mL. *c-III.*
Use: Pediatric antitussive combination.

Pediatex 12. (Zyber) Carbinoxamine tannate 3.2 mg/5 mL. Methylparaben, saccharin, sucrose. Candy apple flavor. Oral Susp. 20 mL, 473 mL. *Rx.*
Use: Antihistamine.

Pediatex 12 D. (Zyber) Pseudoephedrine tannate 45.2 mg, carbinoxamine tannate 3.6 mg per 5 mL. Magnasweet, methylparaben, saccharin, sucrose. Candy apple flavor. Susp. Bot. 20 mL, 473 mL. *Rx.*
Use: Pediatric decongestant and antihistamine.

Pediatric Advil Drops. (Wyeth Consumer Healthcare) Ibuprofen 100 mg/2.5 mL. EDTA, glycerin, sorbitol, sucrose, grape flavor. Susp. Bot. 7.5 mL. *OTC.*
Use: Anti-inflammatory.

Pediatric Cough. (Weeks & Leo) Ammonium Cl 300 mg, sodium citrate 600 mg/oz. Syr. Bot. 4 oz. *OTC.*
Use: Expectorant.

Pediatric Cough & Cold. (Ivax) Dextromethorphan HBr 5 mg, chlorpheniramine maleate 1 mg, pseudoephedrine hydrochloride 15 mg per 5 mL. Alcohol free. Liq. 120 mL. *OTC.*
Use: Upper respiratory combination, antitussive combination.

Pediatric Cough & Cold Medicine. (Silarx) Dextromethorphan HBr 5 mg, chlorpheniramine maleate 1 mg, pseudoephedrine hydrochloride 15 mg per 5 mL. Alcohol free. Sorbitol. Liq. 120 mL. *OTC.*
Use: Upper respiratory combination, antitussive combination.

Pediatric Electrolyte. (Major) Sodium 45 mEq/L, potassium 20 mEq/L, chloride 35 mEq/L, zinc 7.8 mg/L, dextrose 25 g/L, acesulfame potassium, potassium citrate, sucralose. Bubble gum flavor. Soln. 1 L ready-to-use. *OTC.*
Use: Electrolyte.

Pediatric Maintenance Solution. (Abbott) IV solution w/dose calculated according to age, weight, clinical condition. Bot. 250 mL. *Rx.*
Use: Electrolytes, nutrient replacement.

Pediatric Multiple Trace Element. (American Regent) Zn (as sulfate) 0.5 mg, Cu (as sulfate) 0.1 mg, Mn (as sulfate) 0.03 mg, Cr (as chloride) 1 mcg/mL. Soln. Vial 10 mL. *Rx.*
Use: Nutritional supplement, parenteral.

Pedi-Boot Mist Kit. (Pedinol Pharmacal) Cetylpyridinium Cl, triacetin, chloroxylenol. Bot. 2 oz. *OTC.*
Use: Antifungal; antiseptic; deodorant.

Pedicran with Iron. (Scherer) Vitamin B_{12} (crystallized) 25 mcg, ferric pyrophosphate, soluble (elemental iron 30 mg) 250 mg, thiamine mononitrate 10 mg, nicotinamide 10 mg, alcohol 1%/5 mL. Bot. 4 oz, pt. *OTC.*
Use: Mineral, vitamin supplement.

pediculicides/scabicides.
See: Lindane.
Malathion.
Permethrin.

Pedi-Dri. (Pedinol Pharmacal) Nystatin 100,000 units/g, talc. Pow. Plastic Bot. w/shaker cap. 56.7 g. *Rx.*
Use: Antifungal; antiperspirant; deodorant; foot powder.

Pediox. (Atley) Pseudoephedrine hydrochloride 15 mg, chlorpheniramine maleate 2 mg. Aspartame, phenylalanine, mannitol, sorbitol, xylitol, grape fla-

vor. Chew. Tab. 100s. *Rx.*
Use: Decongestant and antihistamine.

Pediox-S. (Atley) Chlorpheniramine maleate 4 mg/5 mL. Aspartame, methylparaben, phenylalanine 8.419 mg/5 mL, sucralose. Cotton candy flavor. Susp. 118 mL. *Rx.*
Use: Antihistamine, nonselective alkylamine.

Pedipirox Nail Lacquer. (Pedinol) Ciclopirox 8%. Isopropyl alcohol. Soln., Top. 3.3 mL, 6.6 mL w/brushes. *Rx.*
Use: Topical anti-infective, antifungal agent.

Pedi-Pro. (Pedinol) Benzalkonium chloride, menthol. Pow. 56.7 g. *OTC.*
Use: Antifungal; antiperspirant; deodorant.

Pedituss Cough. (Major) Phenylephrine hydrochloride 2.5 mg, chlorpheniramine maleate 0.75 mg, codeine phosphate 5 mg, potassium iodide 75 mg/5 mL, alcohol 5%, saccharin, sorbitol, sucrose. Syr. Bot. Pt., gal. *c-v.*
Use: Antihistamine; antitussive; decongestant; expectorant.

Pedolatum. (King) Salicylic acid, sodium salicylate. Oint. Pkg. 0.5 oz. *OTC.*
Use: Analgesic, topical.

Pedric Senior. (Pal-Pak, Inc.) Acetaminophen 320 mg. *OTC.*
Use: Analgesic.

PedvaxHIB. (Merck & Co.) Purified capsular polysaccharide of *Haemophilus influenzae* type b, *Neisseria meningitidis* OMPC 250 mcg/dose when reconstituted, sodium chloride 0.9%, lactose 2 mg, thimerosal 1:20,000. Pow. for Inj. or Soln. Single-dose vial with vial of aluminum hydroxide diluent or single-dose vial. *Rx.*
Use: Immunization.

•**pefcalcitol.** (pef-KAL-si-tol) USAN.
Use: Treatment of plaque psoriasis.

•**pefloxacin.** (PEH-FLOX-ah-sin) USAN.
Use: Anti-infective.

•**pefloxacin mesylate.** (pe-FLOX-a-sin) USAN.
Use: Anti-infective.

PEG. (Medco Lab) Polyethylene glycol. Oint. Jar 16 oz. *OTC.*
Use: Pharmaceutical aid, ointment base.

•**pegademase bovine.** (peg-AD-ah-MASE BOE-vine) USAN.
Use: Replacement therapy (adenosine deaminase deficiency); modified enzyme for use in ADA deficiency. [Orphan Drug]
See: Adagen.

•**pegadricase.** (peg-AD-ri-kase) USAN.
Use: Treatment of hyperuricemia.

•**pegamotecan.** (peg-am-oh-TEE-kan) USAN.
Use: Gastrointestinal.

Peganone. (Recordati Rare Diseases) Ethotoin 250 mg. Lactose. Tab. 100s. *Rx.*
Use: Anticonvulsant.

•**pegaptanib octasodium.** (pag-AP-ta-nib) USAN.
Use: Age-related macular degeneration disease.

•**pegaptanib sodium.** (pag-AP-ta-nib) USAN.
Use: Age-related macular degeneration disease.
See: Macugen.

•**pegaspargase.** (peh-ASS-par-jase) USAN.
Use: Antineoplastic.
See: Oncaspar.

Pegasys. (Roche) Peginterferon alfa-2a 180 mcg. Inj. Single-use vials (sodium chloride 8 mg, polysorbate 80 0.05 mg, benzyl alcohol 10 mg) 1 mL; prefilled syringes (sodium chloride 4 mg, polysorbate 80 0.025 mg, benzyl alcohol 5 mg) 0.5 mL; available in vial (4 single-use vials, 4 1-mL syringes with needles, 8 alcohol swabs) and prefilled syringe (4 single-use prefilled syringes, 4 needles, and 4 alcohol swabs) monthly convenience packs. *Rx.*
Use: Immunologic agent, immunomodulator.

•**pegbovigrastim.** (peg-BOE-vi-GRA-stim) USAN.
Use: Reducing clinical mastitis in dairy cows.

•**pegdinetanib.** (PEG-dye-NET-a-nib) USAN.
Use: Antineoplastic.

pegfilgrastim.
Use: Hematopoietic, colony stimulating factor.
See: Neulasta.

PEG-glucocerebrosidase. (Enzon)
Use: Treatment of Gaucher disease. [Orphan Drug]

•**peginesatide.** (PEG-in-ES-a-tide) USAN.
Use: Treatment of anemia associated with chronic kidney disease.

•**peginesatide acetate.** (PEG-in-ES-a-tide) USAN.
Use: Treatment of anemia associated with chronic kidney disease.

•**peginterferon alfa-2a.** (peg-IN-ter-FEER-ahn AL-fuh-2a) USAN.
Use: Immunologic agent, immunomodulator.
See: Pegasys.

•**peginterferon alfa-2b.** (peg-IN-ter-FEER-ahn AL-fuh-2b) USAN.
Use: Immunologic agent, immunomodulator.
See: PEG-Intron.
Sylatron.

•**peginterferon beta-1a.** (peg-IN-ter-FEER-on) USAN.
Use: Treatment of multiple sclerosis.

•**peginterferon lambda-1a.** (PEG-in-ter-FEER-on LAM-da) USAN.
Use: Treatment of chronic hepatitis C infection.

PEG-interleukin-2. (Cetus)
Use: Immunomodulator. [Orphan Drug]

PEG-Intron. (Schering) Peginterferon alfa-2b 50 mcg/0.5 mL, 80 mcg/0.5 mL, 120 mcg/0.5 mL, 150 mcg/0.5 mL when reconstituted. Pow. for Inj., lyophilized. Vial 2 mL (contains dibasic and monobasic sodium phosphate 1.11 mg, polysorbate 80 0.074 mg, and sucrose 59.2 mg) with 1.25 mL diluent vial, 2 syringes, and 2 alcohol swabs and *Redipen* (contains dibasic and monobasic sodium phosphate 1.013 mg, polysorbate 80 0.0675 mg, and sucrose 54 mg) with 1 B-D needle and 2 alcohol swabs. *Rx.*
Use: Immunologic agent, immunomodulator.

PEG-L-asparaginase. (Enzon) *Rx.*
Use: Antineoplastic.

•**peglicol 5 oleate.** (PEG-lih-kahl 5 OH-lee-ate) USAN.
Use: Pharmaceutic aid, emulsifying agent.

•**pegloticase.** (peg-LOE-ti-kase) USAN.
Use: Gout.
See: Krystexxa.

•**pegnivacogin.** (peg-NYE-va-KOG-in) USAN.
Use: Anticoagulant.

•**pegnivacogin sodium.** (peg-NYE-va-KOG-in) USAN.
Use: Anticoagulant.

•**pegorgotein.** (peg-AHR-gah-teen) USAN.
Use: Free oxygen radical scavenger.

•**pegoterate.** (PEG-oh-TEER-ate) USAN.
Use: Pharmaceutic aid, suspending agent.

•**pegoxol 7 stearate.** (peg-OX-ole 7 STEE-ah-rate) USAN.
Use: Pharmaceutic aid, emulsifying agent.

•**pegsunercept.** (peg-SOO-ner-sept) USAN.
Use: TNF-inhibitor; anti-inflammatory (Crohn disease, RA).

PEG 3350.
Use: Laxative.
See: Dulcolax Balance.
GlycoLax.
MoviPrep.
TriLyte.
W/Sodium Bicarbonate, Sodium Chloride, Potassium Chloride.
See: TriLyte.
W/Sodium Bicarbonate, Sodium Chloride, Sodium Sulfate, Potassium Chloride.
See: GaviLyte-C.
GaviLyte-G.

PEG-3350 & electrolytes. (Kremers Urban Pharmaceuticals) 240 g of PEG 3350, 22.72 g of sodium sulfate, 6.72 g of sodium bicarbonate, 5.84 g of sodium chloride, 2.98 g of potassium chloride. Pow. for Soln. 4 L. *Rx.*
Use: Laxative, bowel evacuant.

PEG-3350, sodium chloride, sodium bicarbonate, potassium chloride. (Mylan) PEG 3350 420 g, sodium bicarbonate 5.72 g, sodium chloride 11.2 g, potassium chloride 1.48 g. Pow. for Soln. Disposable jug w/cherry, lemon lime, orange, and pineapple flavor packs. 4 L. *Rx.*
Use: Laxative, bowel evacuant.

•**pegvisomant.** (peg-VI-soe-mant) USAN.
Use: Acromegaly; proliferative diabetic retinopathy.

PE HCL-CPM-MSN 10-2-0.75. (Kylemore) Chlorpheniramine maleate 2 mg, methscopolamine nitrate 0.75 mg, phenylephrine hydrochloride 10 mg. Glycerin, parabens, propylene glycol, sodium benzoate, sucrose. Grape flavor. Syrup. 473 mL. *Rx.*
Use: Upper respiratory combination; decongestant, antihistamine, and anticholinergic combination.

PE-Hist DM. (Larkin) Chlorpheniramine maleate 2 mg, dextromethorphan hydrobromide 15 mg, phenylephrine hydrochloride 5 mg. Methylparaben, saccharin, sucrose. Alcohol free. Syrup. 473 mL. *Rx.*
Use: Upper respiratory combination, antitussive combination.

•**pelanserin hydrochloride.** (peh-LAN-ser-in) USAN.
Use: Antihypertensive; vasodilator (serotonin S_2 and α_1 adrenergic receptor blocker).

•**pelareorep.** (PEL-a-REE-oh-rep) USAN.
Use: Antineoplastic.

•**peldesine.** (PELL-deh-seen) USAN.
Use: Antineoplastic; antipsoriatic.

pelentan. Ethyl Biscoumacetate. (No Manufacturer Available).

PeleVerus Clear. (LTC Products) Zinc acetate 0.9%, beeswax, panthenol, petrolatum, vitamin E. Oint. 100 g. *OTC.*
Use: Miscellaneous skin protectant.

•**peliglitazar.** (pel-ee-GLI-ta-zar) USAN.
Use: Antidiabetic.

•**peliomycin.** (PEE-lee-oh-MY-sin) USAN. An antibiotic derived from *Streptomycin luteogriseus.*
Use: Antineoplastic.

•**pelitinib.** (pel-i-TYE-nib) USAN.
Use: Antineoplastic.

•**pelitrexol.** (PEL-i-trex-ol) USAN.
Use: Antineoplastic.

•**pelretin.** (PELL-REH-tin) USAN.
Use: Antikeratinizer.

•**pelrinone hydrochloride.** (PELL-rih-nohn) USAN.
Use: Cardiovascular agent.

•**pemedolac.** (peh-MEH-doe-LACK) USAN.
Use: Analgesic.

•**pemerid nitrate.** (PEM-eh-rid) USAN.
Use: Antitussive.

pemetrexed. (pem-eh-TREX-ehd)
Use: Antimetabolite.
See: Alimta.

•**pemetrexed disodium.** (pem-eh-TREX-ehd) USAN.
Tall Man: PEMEtrexed
Use: Antineoplastic.

•**pemirolast potassium.** (peh-mihr-OH-last) USAN.
Use: Antiallergic; inhibitor (mediator release).

Penagen-VK. (Grafton) Penicillin V. **Tab.:** 250 mg. Bot. 100s. **Pow.:** 250 mg/100 mL. *Rx.*
Use: Anti-infective, penicillin.

•**penamecillin.** (PEN-ah-meh-SILL-in) USAN.
Use: Anti-infective.

•**penbutolol sulfate.** (pen-BYOO-toe-lole) *USP.*
Use: Antiadrenergic/sympatholytic, beta-adrenergic blocking agent.
See: Levatol.

•**penciclovir.** (pen-SIGH-kloe-VEER) USAN.
Use: Antiviral.
See: Denavir.

PENcream. (Humco) Caprylic/capric triglyceride, cetearyl alcohol, ceteareth 20, glyceryl stearate, isopropyl palmitate, PEG 100, propylene glycol, octyldodecanol, lecithin, ethylhextlglycerin, phenoxyethanol. Cream. 45 g. *OTC.*
Use: Ointment and lotion base.

Penecare. (Schwarz Pharma) **Cream:** Lactic acid, mineral oil, imidurea. Tube 120 g. **Lot.:** Lactic acid, imidurea. Bot. 240 mL. *OTC.*
Use: Emollient.

Penecort. (Allergan) Hydrocortisone 1%, 2.5%, benzyl alcohol, petrolatum, stearyl alcohol, propylene glycol, isopropyl myristate, polyoxyl 40 stearate, carbomer 934, sodium lauryl sulfate, edetate disodium w/sodium hydroxide to adjust pH, purified water. Cream. **1%:** Tube 30 g, 60 g. **2.5%:** Tube 30 g. *Rx.*
Use: Corticosteroid, topical.

•**penfluridol.** (pen-FLEW-rih-dahl) USAN.
Use: Antipsychotic.

•**penicillamine.** (PEN-ih-SILL-ah-meen) *USP.*
Use: Chelating agent; metal complexing agent, cystinuria, rheumatoid arthritis.
See: Cuprimine.
Depen.

penicillin. (pen-ih-SILL-in) Unless clarified, it means an antibiotic substance or substances produced by growth of the molds *Penicillium notatum* or *P. chrysogenum.*
Use: Anti-infective.

penicillin aluminum. *Rx.*
Use: Anti-infective, penicillin.

penicillinase-resistant penicillins.
Use: Anti-infective.
See: Dicloxacillin Sodium.
Nafcillin Sodium.
Oxacillin Sodium.

•**penicillin calcium.** (pen-ih-SILL-in) *USP. Rx.*
Use: Anti-infective, penicillin.

penicillin, dimethoxy-phenyl. Methicillin sodium.
Use: Anti-infective, penicillin.

penicillin G, aqueous.
Use: Anti-infective.
See: Penicillin G potassium.
Pfizerpen.

•**penicillin G benzathine.** (pen-ih-SILL-in G BENZ-ah-theen) *USP.*
Use: Anti-infective.
See: Bicillin L-A.
Permapen.

penicillin G benzathine/penicillin G procaine.
Use: Anti-infective.
See: Bicillin C-R.
Bicillin C-R 900/300.

•**penicillin G potassium.** (pen-ih-SILL-in) *USP.*
Use: Anti-infective.
See: Pfizerpen.

penicillin G potassium. (Various Mfr.) Penicillin G potassium. **Inj., Soln.:** 1 million units, 2 million units, 3 million units. Premixed, frozen 50 mL single-use *Galaxy* container. **Inj., Pow. for Soln.:** 1 million units (≈6.8 mg of sodium [0.3 mEq] and 65 mg of potassium [1.68 mEq] per million units), 5 million units (≈6.8 mg of sodium [0.3 mEq] and 65.6 mg of potassium [1.68 mEq] per million units), 20 million units (≈6.8 mg of sodium [0.3 mEq] and 65.6 mg of potassium [1.68 mEq] per million units). Vial. *Rx.*
Use: Anti-infective, penicillin.

•**penicillin G procaine.** (pen-ih-SILL-in G PRO-cane) *USP.*
Use: Anti-infective.

penicillin G procaine. (Monarch) Penicillin G procaine 600,000 units/vial. Inj. 1 mL *Tubex*; 1,200,000 units/vial. Inj. 2 mL *Tubex*. Parabens, povidone. *Rx.*
Use: Anti-infective, penicillin.

•**penicillin G procaine and dihydrostreptomycin sulfate intramammary infusion.** *USP.*
Use: Anti-infective.

•**penicillin G procaine and dihydrostreptomycin sulfate injectable suspension.** *USP.*
Use: Anti-infective.

•**penicillin G procaine and novobiocin sodium intramammary infusion.** *USP.*
Use: Anti-infective.

penicillin G procaine combinations.
See: Bicillin C-R.

•**penicillin G procaine, dihydrostreptomycin sulfate, and prednisolone injectable suspension.** *USP.*
Use: Anti-infective; anti-inflammatory.

•**penicillin G procaine, dihydrostreptomycin sulfate, chlorpheniramine maleate, and dexamethasone injectable suspension.** *USP.*
Use: Anti-infective; antihistamine; anti-inflammatory.

•**penicillin G procaine, neomycin and polymyxin B sulfates, and hydrocortisone acetate topical suspension.** *USP.*
Use: Anti-infective; anti-inflammatory.

penicillin G procaine/penicillin G benzathine.
Use: Anti-infective.
See: Bicillin C-R.
Bicillin C-R 900/300.

penicillin G procaine, sterile. Sterile Susp., Intramammary infusion, Procaine Penicillin.
Use: Anti-infective.

penicillin G procaine w/aluminum stearate suspension, sterile.
Use: Anti-infective.

•**penicillin G sodium.** (PEN-ih-SILL-in G) *USP.*
Use: Anti-infective.

penicillin G sodium. (Marsam) Penicillin G sodium 5,000,000 units/Vial. Pow. for Inj. Vial. *Rx.*
Use: Anti-infective, penicillin.

penicillin G sodium. (Sandoz) Penicillin G sodium 5,000,000 units. Sodium 1.68 mEq/million vials. Pow. for Inj. Vials. *Rx.*
Use: Anti-infective, penicillin.

•**penicillin G sodium for injection.** *USP.*
Use: Anti-infective.

penicillin hydrabamine phenoxymethyl.
Use: Anti-infective.

penicillin O chloroprocaine.
Use: Anti-infective, penicillin.

penicillin O, sodium. Allylmercaptomethyl penicillin.
Use: Anti-infective.

penicillin, phenoxyethyl.
Use: Anti-infective, penicillin.

penicillin phenoxymethyl benzathine.
Use: Anti-infective, penicillin.
See: Penicillin V benzathine.

penicillin phenoxymethyl hydrabamine.
Use: Anti-infective, penicillin.
See: Penicillin V hydrabamine.

penicillins.
Use: Anti-infective.
See: Aminopenicillins.
Extended-Spectrum Penicillins.
Natural Penicillins.
Penicillinase-Resistant Penicillins.

penicillin S benzathine and penicillin G procaine suspension, sterile.
Use: Anti-infective.

penicillins, extended spectrum.
Use: Anti-infective.
See: Piperacillin Sodium.
Piperacillin Sodium/Tazobactam Sodium.
Ticarcillin/Clavulanate.
Ticarcillin Disodium.

penicillins, natural.
Use: Anti-infective.
See: Penicillin G (Aqueous).
Penicillin G Benzathine and Procaine Combined, Intramuscular.
Penicillin G Benzathine, Intramuscular.
Penicillin G Procaine, Injectable.
Penicillin V (Phenoxymethyl Penicillin).

•**penicillin V.** (pen-ih-SILL-in V) *USP. Formerly Penicillin Phenoxymethyl.*

A biosynthetic penicillin formed by fermentation, with suitable precursors of *Penicillin notatum*.
Use: Anti-infective.
See: Penicillin VK.
Veetids.

•**penicillin V benzathine.** (pen-ih-SILL-in V BEN-zah-theen) *USP. Formerly Penicillin Benzathine Phenoxymethyl.*
Use: Anti-infective.

•**penicillin V hydrabamine.** (pen-ih-SILL-in V HIGH-drah-BAM-een) *USP. Formerly Penicillin Hydrabamine Phenoxymethyl.*
Use: Anti-infective.

Penicillin VK. (Various Mfr.) Penicillin v. **Tab.:** 250 mg, 500 mg. Bot. 100s, 500s (500 mg only), 1000s (250 mg only). **Pow. for Oral Soln.:** 125 mg/5 mL, 250 mg/5 mL when reconstituted. Bot. 100 mL, 200 mL. *Rx.*
Use: Anti-infective, penicillin.

•**penicillin V potassium.** (pen-ih-SILL-in) *USP. Formerly Penicillin Potassium Phenoxymethyl.*
Use: Anti-infective.
See: Beepen VK.
Betapen VK.
Bopen-VK.
Pen-Vee K.
Pfizerpen VK.
Suspen.
V-Cillin K.

penidural.
Use: Anti-infective.

Pen-Kera Creme with Keratin Binding Factor. (B.F. Ascher) Bot. 8 oz. *OTC.*
Use: Emollient.

Penlac Nail Lacquer. (Valeant) Ciclopirox 8%. Isopropyl alcohol. Top. Soln. Bot. 3.3 mL, 6.6 mL w/brushes. *Rx.*
Use: Anti-infective, topical; antifungal.

Pennsaid. (Nuvo) Diclofenac 1.5% (1 mL contains diclofenac sodium 16.05 mg), 2% (1 g contains diclofenac sodium 20 mg). Alcohol, glycerin, propylene glycol (1.5%); ethanol, propylene glycol (2%). Soln.; topical. 150 mL (1.5%), 112 g (2%). *Rx.*
Use: Anti-inflammatory agent; nonsteroidal anti-inflammatory drug, topical.

Penntuss. (Medeva) Codeine (as polistirex) 10 mg, chlorpheniramine maleate 4 mg/5 mL. Bot. Pt. *c-v.*
Use: Antitussive; antihistamine.

•**pentabamate.** (PEN-tah-BAM-ate) USAN.
Use: Anxiolytic.

Pentacarinat. (Aventis) Pentamidine isethionate 300 mg. Inj. Single-dose vial. *Rx.*
Use: Anti-infective.

Pentacel. (Sanofi Pasteur) Diphtheria toxoid 15 Lf, tetanus toxoid 5 Lf, pertussis toxin detoxified 20 mcg, filamentous hemagglutinin 20 mcg, pertactin 3 mcg, fimbriae types 2 and 3 five mcg, type 1 inactivated poliovirus (Mahoney) 40 D-antigen units, type 2 inactivated poliovirus (MEF-1) 8 D-antigen units, type 3 inactivated poliovirus (Saukett) 32 D-antigen units, lyophilized polyribosyl-ribilol-phosphate of *Haemophilus influenzae* type B 10 mcg bound to tetanus toxoid 24 mcg per 0.5 mL. Aluminum phosphate 1.5 mg (aluminum 0.33 mg), residual formaldehyde ≤ 5 mcg, residual glutaraldehyde < 50 ng, residual bovine serum albumin ≤ 50 ng, 2-phenoxyethanol 3.3 mg (0.6% v/v), neomycin < 4 pg, polymyxin B sulfate < 4 pg. Preservative free. Inj., Susp. Single-dose vial for reconstitution. *Rx.*
Use: Vaccine combination, diphtheria and tetanus toxoids and acellular pertussis adsorbed, inactivated poliovirus and *haemophilus influenzae* type B conjugate vaccine combined.

pentacosactride.
Use: Corticotrophic peptide.

•**pentaerythritol tetranitrate diluted.** (pen-tuh-eh-Rith-rih-tole teh-truh-NYE-trate) *USP.*
Use: Vasodilator.
See: Arcotrate No. 1.
Arcotrate No. 2.
Duotrate 45.
Pentetra Paracote.
Peritrate.
Petro-20 mg.
Tetratab.
Tetratab No. 1.
Vasolate.
Vasolate-80.
W/Combinations.
See: Arcotrate No. 3.
Bitrate.
Dimycor.

•**pentafilcon A.** (PEN-tah-FILL-kahn A) USAN.
Use: Contact lens material, hydrophilic.

pentafluoropropane.
W/Tetrafluoroethane.
See: Gebauer's Spray and Stretch.

•**pentalyte.** (PEN-tah-lite) USAN.
Use: Electrolyte combination.

•**pentamidine isethionate.** (pen-TAM-i-deen EYE-se-THYE-oh-nate) USAN.
Use: Anti-infective.
See: NebuPent.

Pentam 300.
Pentacarinat.

pentamidine isethionate. (Abbott) Pentamidine isethionate 300 mg. Pow. for Inj., lyophilized. Single-dose fliptop vials. *Rx.*
Use: Anti-infective.

•**pentamorphone.** (PEN-tah-MORE-fone) USAN.
Use: Analgesic; narcotic.

pentamoxane hydrochloride.
Use: Anxiolytic.

Pentam 300. (American Pharmaceutical Partners) Pentamidine isethionate 300 mg. Single-dose vials. *Rx.*
Use: Anti-infective.

•**pentamustine.** (PEN-tah-MUSS-teen) USAN.
Use: Antineoplastic.

pentaphonate. Dodecyltriphenylphosphonium pentachlorophenolate.
Use: Anti-infective.

•**pentapiperium methylsulfate.** (PEN-tah-PIP-ehr-ee-uhm METH-ill-SULL-fate) USAN.
Use: Anticholinergic.

pentapyrrolidinium bitartrate.
See: Pentolinium tartrate.

Pentasa. (Shire US) Mesalamine 250 mg, 500 mg. Sugar. CR Cap. Bot. 120s (500 mg only), 240s (250 mg only), UD 80s. *Rx.*
Use: Anti-inflammatory.

pentasodium colistinmethanesulfonate. Sterile Colistimethate Sodium.

•**pentastarch.** (PEN-tah-starch) USAN.
Use: Leukophoresis adjunct, red cell sedimenting agent. [Orphan Drug]

Penta-Stress. (Penta) Vitamins A 10,000 units, D 500 units, B_1 10 mg, B_2 10 mg, B_6 1 mg, calcium pantothenate 5 mg, niacinamide 50 mg, C 100 mg, E 2 units, B_{12} 3.3 mcg. Cap. Bot. 90s, 1000s, Jar 250s. *OTC.*
Use: Mineral, vitamin supplement.

Penta-Viron. (Penta) Calcium carbonate 500 mg, ferrous fumarate 100 mg, vitamins C 50 mg, D 167 units, A 3.333 units, B_1 3.3 mg, B_2 3.3 mg, B_6 2 mg, calcium pantothenate 1.6 mg, niacinamide 16.7 mg, E 2 units. Cap. Bot. 100s, 1000s, Jar 250s. *OTC.*
Use: Mineral, vitamin supplement.

Pentazine. (Century) Promethazine 50 mg/mL. Inj. Vial 10 mL. *Rx.*
Use: Antihistamine.

Pentazine VC w/Codeine. (Century) Promethazine hydrochloride 6.25 mg, codeine phosphate 10 mg. Liq. Bot. 118 mL, pt, gal. *c-v.*
Use: Antihistamine; antitussive.

Pentazine w/Codeine. (Century) Promethazine expectorant. Bot. 4 oz, 16 oz, gal.
Use: Antihistamine.

•**pentazocine.** (pen-TAZ-oh-seen) *USP.*
Use: Narcotic agonist-antagonist analgesic.
See: Talwin.

•**pentazocine and aspirin.** (pen-TAZ-oh-seen and AS-pir-in) *USP. Formerly pentazocine hydrochloride and aspirin.*
Use: Analgesic.

•**pentazocine and naloxone.** (pen-TAZ-oh-seen and NAL-ox-one) *USP. Formerly pentazocine and naloxone hydrochloride.*
Use: Analgesic.

pentazocine and naloxone. (Royce) Pentazocine 50 mg, naloxone hydrochloride 0.5 mg. Tab. Box. 100s, 500s, 1000s. *Rx.*
Use: Analgesic.

•**pentazocine hydrochloride.** (pen-TAZ-oh-seen) *USP.*
Use: Analgesic.

pentazocine hydrochloride and acetaminophen. (Watson) Pentazocine hydrochloride 25 mg, acetaminophen 650 mg. Tab. Bot. 100s, 500s, 1000s. *c-iv.*
Use: Analgesic combination.

•**pentazocine injection.** (pen-TAZ-oh-seen) *USP. Formerly pentazocine lactate injection.*
Use: Analgesic.
See: Talwin.

•**pentetate calcium trisodium.** (PEN-teh-tate KAL-see-uhm try-SO-dee-uhm) USAN.
Use: Chelating agent, plutonium.

pentetate calcium trisodium. (Akorn) Pentetate calcium trisodium 200 mg/mL. Inj. 5 mL single-use ampules. *Rx.*
Use: Chelating agent, plutonium, americium, or curium.

•**pentetate calcium trisodium Yb 169.** (PEN-teh-tate) USAN.
Use: Radiopharmaceutical.

•**pentetate indium disodium In 111.** (PEN-teh-tate IN-dee-uhm) USAN.
Use: In vivo diagnostic aid, radiopharmaceutical.
See: Indium DTPA In 111.

pentetate zinc trisodium. (Akorn) Pentetate zinc trisodium 200 mg/mL. Inj. 5 mL single-use ampules. *Rx.*
Use: Detoxification agent, chelating agent.

•**pentetic acid.** (PEN-teh-tick) *USP.*
Use: Diagnostic aid.
Pentetra-Paracote. (Paddock) Pentaerythritol tetranitrate 30 mg, 80 mg. Cap. Bot. 100s, 500s, 1000s. *Rx.*
Use: Antianginal.
pentetreotide.
Use: Radiopaque agent, parenteral.
See: OctreoScan.
•**pentiapine maleate.** (pen-TIE-ah-PEEN) USAN.
Use: Antipsychotic.
•**pentigetide.** (pent-EYE-jeh-TIDE) USAN.
Use: Antiallergic.
Pentina. (Freeport) *Rauwolfia serpentina,* 100 mg. Tab. Bot. 1000s. *Rx.*
Use: Antihypertensive.
•**pentisomicin.** (pent-IH-so-MY-sin) USAN.
Use: Anti-infective.
•**pentizidone sodium.** (pen-TIH-ZIH-dohn) USAN.
Use: Anti-infective.
•**pentobarbital.** (pen-toe-BAR-bih-tahl) *USP.*
Tall Man: PENTobarbital
Use: Hypnotic; sedative.
See: Nembutal.
W/Combinations
See: Cafergot PB.
•**pentobarbital sodium.** (pen-toe-BAR-bih-tahl) *USP.*
Tall Man: PENTobarbital
Use: Hypnotic; sedative.
See: Nembutal Sodium.
W/Ergotamine tartrate, caffeine alkaloid, bellafoline.
See: Cafergot PB.
pentobarbital sodium. (Wyeth) Pentobarbital sodium 50 mg/mL. Inj. *Tubex* 2 mL. *c-II.*
Use: Hypnotic; sedative.
pentobarbital, soluble.
See: Pentobarbital Sodium.
pentolinium tartrate. Pentamethylene-1:5-bis (1′-methylpyrrolidinium bitartrate).
Use: Antihypertensive.
Pentol Tabs. (Major) Pentaerythritol tetranitrate. **Tab.: 10 mg:** Bot. 1000s. **20 mg:** Bot. 100s, 1000s. **SA Tab.: 80 mg:** Bot. 250s, 1000s. *Rx.*
Use: Antianginal.
•**pentomone.** (PEN-toe-MONE) USAN.
Use: Prostate growth inhibitor.
•**pentopril.** (PEN-toe-prill) USAN.
Use: Enzyme inhibitor, angiotensin-converting.
•**pentosan polysulfate sodium.** (PEN-toe-san PAHL-in-SULL-fate) USAN.
Use: Anti-inflammatory, interstitial cystitis.
See: Elmiron.
•**pentostatin.** (PEN-toe-STAT-in) USAN.
Use: Potentiator; leukemia; antineoplastic. [Orphan Drug]
See: Nipent.
pentostatin. (Bedford) Pentostatin 10 mg. Mannitol 50 mg. Inj., Lyophilized Pow. for Soln., Conc. Single-dose vials. *Rx.*
Use: Antimetabolite, purine analogs and related agent.
•**pentoxifylline.** (pen-TOX-IH-fill-in) *USP.*
Use: Hemorrheologic agent.
See: Trental.
pentoxifylline. (Copley) Pentoxifylline 400 mg. Film-coated. CR Tab. Bot. 100s, 500s, bulk pack 5000s. *Rx.*
Use: Hemorrheologic agent.
pentoxifylline extended-release. (Purepac) Pentoxifylline 400 mg. ER Tab. Bot. 100s, 500s, 1000s. *Rx.*
Use: Hemorrheologic agent.
Pentrax. (Medicis) Coal tar extract 5%. Shampoo. Bot. 236 mL. *OTC.*
Use: Antiseborrheic.
•**pentrinitrol.** (pen-TRY-nye-TROLE) USAN.
Use: Vasodilator, coronary.
Pent-T-80. (Mericon Industries) Pentaerythritol tetranitrate 80 mg. TD Cap. Bot. 100s, 1000s. *Rx.*
Use: Antianginal.
Pen-V. (Ivax) Penicillin 250 mg, 500 mg. Tab. Bot. 100s, 1000s. *Rx.*
Use: Anti-infective, penicillin.
Pen-Vee K. (Wyeth) Penicillin V 250 mg, 500 mg Tab. Bot. 100s, 500s, UD 100s. *Rx.*
Use: Anti-infective, penicillin.
Pen-Vee K for Oral Solution. (Wyeth) Penicillin V 125 mg/5 mL, 250 mg/5 mL. Bot. 100 mL, 150 mL (250 mg/5 mL only), 200 mL. *Rx.*
Use: Anti-infective, penicillin.
Pepcid. (Marathon Pharmaceuticals) Famotidine. **Tab.:** 20 mg, 40 mg. Film-coated. Bot. 1000s, 10,000. Unit-of-use 30s, 90s, 100s. UD 100s. *Uniblister* 31s. **Pow. for Oral Susp.:** 40 mg/5 mL when reconstituted. Parabens, sucrose. Cherry, banana, mint flavors. Bot. 400 mg. *Rx.*
Use: Histamine H_2 antagonist.
Pepcid AC. (Marathon Pharmaceuticals) Famotidine. **Chew. Tab.:** 10 mg. Phenylalanine 1.4 mg, lactose, aspartame, mannitol. Pkg. 6s, 18s, 30s, 50s, 60s, 68s. **Gelcap:** 10 mg. Bot. 30s, 50s, 60s, 90s. **Tab.:** 10 mg. Pkg. 2s, 6s, 18s, 30s, 60s, 90s. *OTC.*
Use: Histamine H_2 antagonist.

Pepcid AC Maximum Strength. (Marathon Pharmaceuticals) Famotidine 20 mg. Tab. 25s. *OTC.*
Use: Histamine H_2 antagonist.

Pepcid AC Maximum Strength EZ Chews. (Marathon Pharmaceuticals) Famotidine 20 mg. Dextrose, lactose, sucralose. Cool mint, berry, and cream flavors. Tab. 25s, 50s. *OTC.*
Use: Gastrointestinal agent, histamine H_2 antagonist.

Pepcid Complete Dual Action. (McNeil Consumer) Famotidine 10 mg, calcium carbonate 800 mg, magnesium hydroxide 165 mg. Lactose, sugar. Mint flavor. Chew. Tab. 5s, 15s, 25s, 50s. *OTC.*
Use: Histamine H_2 antagonist combination.

Pepcid RPD. (Marathon Pharmaceuticals) Famotidine 20 mg, 40 mg. Aspartame, mint flavor, mannitol, phenylalanine 1.05 mg (20 mg only), 2.1 mg (40 mg only). Orally disintegrating Tab. UD 30s, 100s. *Rx.*
Use: Histamine H_2 antagonist.

•**peplomycin sulfate.** (PEP-low-MY-sin) USAN.
Use: Antineoplastic.

•**peppermint.** *NF.*
Use: Pharmaceutic aid, flavor, perfume; antitussive; expectorant; nasal decongestant.

•**peppermint oil.** *NF.*
Use: Pharmaceutic aid, flavor.

•**peppermint spirit.** *USP.*
Use: Pharmaceutic aid, flavor, perfume.

•**peppermint water.** *NF.*
Use: Pharmaceutic aid, vehicle, flavored.

Pepsicone. (Sanofi-Synthelabo) **Gel:** Aluminum hydroxide, magnesium hydroxide, simethicone. **Tab.:** Aluminum hydroxide, magnesium hydroxide, simethicone. *OTC.*
Use: Antacid; antiflatulent.

pepsin.
Use: Digestive aid.
W/Combinations
See: Biloric.

•**pepstatin.** (pep-STAT-in) USAN.
Use: Enzyme inhibitor, pepsin.

Peptamen. (Clintec Nutrition) Enzymatically hydrolyzed whey proteins, maltodextrin, starch, MCT, sunflower oil, lecithin, vitamins A, B_1, B_2, B_3, B_5, B_6, B_{12}, C, D, E, K, folic acid, biotin, choline, Ca, Cl, Cu, Fe, I, Mg, Mn, P, Zn. Liq. Can 500 mL. *OTC.*
Use: Nutritional supplement.

Peptenzyme. (Schwarz Pharma) Alcohol 16%. Pleasantly aromatic. Bot. Pt.
Use: Pharmaceutic aid.

Peptic Relief. (Rugby) Bismuth subsalicylate. **Chew. Tab.:** 262 mg. Cherry flavoring, dextrose, sorbitol. 30s. **Liq. Susp.:** 262 mg per 15 mL. Benzoic acid, saccharin. Sugar free. 237 mL. *OTC.*
Use: Antidiarrheal.

Peptinex. (Novartis Nutrition) Protein (whey protein hydrolysate, taurine, L-carnitine) 50 g, carbohydrate (hydrolyzed cornstarch) 160 g, fat (soybean oil, medium chain triglycerides, soy lecithin) 17 g/L, vitamins A, B_1, B_2, B_3, B_5, B_6, B_{12}, C, D, E, K, biotin, choline, folic acid, Ca, Cl, Cr, Cu, Fe, I, Mg, Mn, Mo, P, Se, Zn, Na 1010 mg (44 mEq), K 1490 mg (38 mEq)/L, H_2O 320 mOsm/kg, 1 cal/mL, vanilla flavor. Liq. *Tetra Brik* Paks 8 oz. *OTC.*
Use: Enteral nutritional therapy.

Peptinex DT. (Novartis Nutrition) Protein (casein hydrolysate, amino acids) 50 g, carbohydrate (maltodextrin, modified cornstarch) 164 g, fat (medium chain triglycerides, soybean oil) 17.4 g/L, vitamins A, B_1, B_2, B_3, B_5, B_6, B_{12}, C, D, E, K, biotin, choline, folic acid, Ca, Cl, Cr, Cu, Fe, I, Mg, Mn, Mo, P, Se, Zn, Na 1700 mg (74 mEq), K 800 mg (21 mEq)/L, H_2O 460 mOsm/kg, 1 cal/mL, lactose and gluten free. Liq. Can 250 mL; closed system containers 1 L, 1.5 L. *OTC.*
Use: Enteral nutritional therapy.

Pepto-Bismol. (Procter & Gamble) **Chew. Tab.:** Bismuth subsalicylate 262.5 mg. Pkg. 24s, 42s. **Liq.:** Bismuth subsalicylate 262 mg/15 mL. Bot. 4 oz, 8 oz, 12 oz, 16 oz. **Tab.:** Bismuth subsalicylate 262 mg, < 2 mg sodium. Capl. Sugar free. Bot. 24s, 40s. *OTC.*
Use: Antidiarrheal.

Pepto-Bismol InstaCool. (Procter & Gamble) Bismuth subsalicylate 262 mg. Mannitol, saccharin, sodium < 1 mg/tablet. Sugar free. Peppermint flavor. Chew. Tab. 30s. *OTC.*
Use: Antidiarrheal.

Pepto-Bismol Maximum Strength. (Procter & Gamble) 524 mg/15 mL. Liq. Bot. 120 mL, 240 mL, 360 mL. *OTC.*
Use: Antidiarrheal.

Pepto Children's. (Procter & Gamble) Calcium carbonate 400 mg (elemental calcium 160 mg). Mannitol, sorbitol, sugar. Sodium free. Bubble gum and watermelon flavors. Chew. Tab. 24s. *OTC.*
Use: Mineral.

•**perakizumab.** (PER-a-KIZ-ue-mab) USAN.
Use: Immunologic agent.
•**peramivir.** (per-AM-i-vir) USAN.
Use: Neuraminidase inhibitor.
•**perampanel.** (per-AM-pa-nel) USAN.
Use: Anticonvulsant.
See: Fycompa.
Perandren Phenylacetate. (Novartis) Testosterone phenylacetate. *c-III.*
Use: Androgen.
percaine.
Use: Local anesthetic.
See: Dibucaine hydrochloride.
perchloroethylene.
See: Tetrachloroethylene.
Percocet. (Endo) Oxycodone hydrochloride/acetaminophen 2.5 mg/325 mg, 5 mg/325 mg, 7.5 mg/325 mg, 7.5 mg/500 mg, 10 mg/325 mg, 10 mg/650 mg. Tab. Bot. 100s, 500s (except 7.5 mg/325 mg), UD 100s (except 7.5 mg/325 mg). *c-II.*
Use: Analgesic combination; narcotic.
Percodan. (Endo Pharmaceuticals) Oxycodone hydrochloride 4.5 mg, oxycodone terephthalate 0.38 mg, aspirin 325 mg. Tab. Bot. 100s, 500s, 1000s, UD 250s. *c-II.*
Use: Analgesic combination; narcotic.
Percogesic. (Medtech) Acetaminophen 325 mg, diphenhydramine hydrochloride 12.5 mg. Mineral oil, PEG. Tab. 90s. *OTC.*
Use: Upper respiratory combination, analgesic, antihistamine.
Percogesic Extra Strength. (Medtech) Diphenhydramine hydrochloride 12.5 mg, acetaminophen 500 mg. Tab. Bot. 60s. *OTC.*
Use: Upper respiratory combination, antihistamine, analgesic.
Percomorph Liver Oil. May be blended with 50% other fish liver oils; each g contains vitamins A 60,000 units, D 8500 units.
Percy Medicine. (Merrick Medicine) Bismuth subnitrate 959 mg, calcium hydroxide 21.9 mg/10 mL, alcohol 5%. *OTC.*
Use: Antidiarrheal.
Perdiem. (Novartis) Blend of psyllium 82%, senna 18% as active ingredients in granular form. Sodium content (0.08 mEq) 1.8 mg/rounded tsp. (6 g). Can. 100 g, 250 g, UD 6 g. *OTC.*
Use: Laxative.
Perdiem Fiber Therapy. (Novartis) Psyllium 4.03 g, sodium 1.8 mg, potassium 36.1 mg, 4 cal/6 g, sucrose, dye free, mint flavor. Gran. Can. 100 g, 250 g. *OTC.*
Use: Laxative.
Pere-Diosate. (Towne) Docusate sodium 100 mg, casanthranol 30 mg. Cap. Bot. 100s. *OTC.*
Use: Laxative.
Perestan. (Henry Schein) Docusate sodium 100 mg, casanthranol 30 mg. Cap. Bot. 100s, 1000s. *OTC.*
Use: Laxative.
•**perfilcon A.** (per-FILL-kahn A) USAN.
Use: Contact lens material, hydrophilic.
•**perflenapent.** (per-FLEN-ah-pent) USAN.
Use: Diagnostic aid, ultrasound contrast agent.
•**perflexane.** (per-FLEKS-ane) USAN.
Use: Diagnostic aid, ultrasound contrast agent.
•**perflisopent.** (per-FLYE-soh-pent) USAN.
Use: Diagnostic aid, ultrasound contrast agent.
•**perflubrodec.** (per-FLOO-broe-deck) USAN.
Use: Anemia.
•**perflubron.** (per-FLEW-brahn) *USP.*
Use: Contrast agent; blood substitute.
•**perflubutane.** (per-FLOO-bue-tane) USAN.
Use: Ultrasound contrast agent.
•**perflutren.** (per-FLOO-tren) *USP.*
Use: Radiopaque agent, parenteral.
See: Definity.
•**perflutren protein-type A microspheres injectable suspension.** (per-FLOO-tren PROE-teen) *USP. Formerly perflutren protein-type A microspheres for injection.*
Use: Diagnostic aid.
See: Optison.
Perforomist. (Dey) Formoterol fumarate 20 mcg/2 mL. Inh. Soln. Unit-dose vials. Cartons of 60s. *Rx.*
Use: Bronchodilator.
•**perfosfamide.** (per-FOSS-fam-ide) USAN.
Use: Antineoplastic. [Orphan Drug]
•**pergolide mesylate.** (PURR-go-lide) *USP.*
Use: Antiparkinson agent.
Pergrava. (Arcum) Vitamins A 2000 units, D 300 units, B_1 2 mg, B_2 2 mg, nicotinamide 10 mg, B_6 2 mg, B_{12} 5 mcg, C 60 mg, Ca 40 mg. Cap. Bot. 100s, 1000s. *OTC.*
Use: Mineral, vitamin supplement.
Pergrava No. 2. (Arcum) Vitamins A 2000 units, D 300 units, B_1 2 mg, B_2 2 mg, nicotinamide 10 mg, B_6 2 mg, C

60 mg, calcium lactate monohydrate 200 mg, ferrous gluconate 31 mg, folic acid 0.1 mg. Cap. Bot. 100s, 1000s. *OTC.*
Use: Mineral, vitamin supplement.

perhexiline. (per-HEX-ih-leen)
Use: Antianginal.

•**perhexiline maleate.** (per-HEX-ih-leen) USAN.
Use: Vasodilator, coronary.

perhydrol.
See: Hydrogen Peroxide 30%.

Peri-Care. (Sween) Vitamins A and D in petroleum ointment base. Tube 0.5 oz, 1.75 oz. Jar 2 oz, 5 oz, 8 oz. *OTC.*
Use: Emollient.

Peri-Colace. (Purdue) Docusate sodium 50 mg, sennosides 8.6 mg. Tab. 10s, 30s, 60s. *OTC.*
Use: Laxative.

Peridex. (Procter & Gamble) Chlorhexidine gluconate 0.12%, alcohol 11.6%, glycerin, PEG-40 sorbitan diisostearate, flavor, sodium saccharin, FD&C blue No. 1, water. Bot. 480 mL. *Rx.*
Use: Mouth preparation.

Peridin-C. (Beutlich) Hesperidin methyl cholcone (bioflavonoids) 50 mg, hesperidin complex 150 mg, ascorbic acid 200 mg. Tab. Bot. 100s, 500s. *OTC.*
Use: Water-soluble vitamin.

Peries. (Xttrium) Medicated pads w/witch hazel, glycerin. Jar pad 40s. *OTC.*
Use: Hygienic wipe and local compress.

Periguard. (DermaRite) Aloe vera, lanolin, mineral oil, parabens, vitamin A, vitamin D, vitamin E. Oint. 100 g. *OTC.*
Use: Dermatological agent, protectant.

•**perindopril.** (per-IN-doe-prill) USAN.
Use: ACE inhibitor.

•**perindopril erbumine.** (per-IN-doe-prill ehr-BYOO-meen) USAN.
Use: Angiotensin-converting enzyme inhibitor.
See: Aceon.

perindopril erbumine. (Roxane) Perindopril erbumine 2 mg, 4 mg, 8 mg. May contain lactose. Tab. 30s, 100s, 500s (except 2 mg). *Rx.*
Use: Renin angiotensin antagonist, angiotensin-converting enzyme inhibitor.

PerioChip. (Adria) Chlorhexidine gluconate 2.5 mg. Chip Blister pack 10s. *Rx.*
Use: Anesthetic.

Perio-Eze 20. (Moyco Union Broach Division) Oral paste.
Use: Analgesic, topical.

PerioGard. (Colgate Oral) Chlorhexidine gluconate 0.12%, alcohol 11.6%, glycerin, PEG-40, sorbitol diisostearnate, saccharin. Rinse. Bot. 473 mL w/15 mL dose cup. *Rx.*
Use: Anesthetic.

PerioMed. (Omnii Oral) Stannous fluoride concentrate 0.64%. Alcohol-free. Tropical fruit, mint, and cinnamon flavor. Rinse. 283.5 g. *Rx.*
Use: Prevention of dental caries.

PeriShield. (Ameriderm Laboratories) White petrolatum, lanolin, mineral oil, paraffin, corn oil, aloe, retinyl palmitate, chloroxylenol, sodium borate, zinc oxide. Oint. 452 g. *OTC.*
Use: Skin protectant.

Peri Sofcap. (Alton) Docusate sodium with peristim. Bot. 100s, 1000s. *OTC.*
Use: Laxative.

Peritrate. (Parke-Davis) Pentaerythritol tetranitrate. **Tab.: 10 mg:** Bot. 100s, 1000s. **20 mg:** Bot. 100s, 1000s, UD 100s. **40 mg:** Bot. 100s. *Rx.*
Use: Antianginal.

Peritrate S.A. (Parke-Davis) Pentaerythritol tetranitrate 80 mg (20 mg in immediate-release layer, 60 mg in sustained-release base). Tab. Bot. 100s, 1000s, UD 100s. *Rx.*
Use: Antianginal.

Peri-Wash. (Sween) Bot. 4 oz, 8 oz, 1 gal., 5 gal., 30 gal., 55 gal.
Use: Anorectal preparation.

Peri-Wash II. (Sween) Bot. 4 oz, 8 oz, 1 gal., 5 gal., 30 gal., 55 gal.
Use: Anorectal preparation.

Perjeta. (Genentech Inc) Pertuzumab 30 mg/mL. Sucrose. Preservative free. Inj., Soln. Single-use vial. 14 mL. *Rx.*
Use: Antineoplastic agent, monoclonal antibody.

Perlane. (Medicis) Hyaluronic acid 20 mg/mL. Inj., Gel. Single-use, prefilled syringes. *Rx.*
Use: Physical adjunct.

Perlane-L. (Medicis Aesthetics) Hyaluronic acid 20 mg/mL. Lidocaine 0.3%. Inj., gel. Single-use, prefilled syringe. *Rx.*
Use: Physical adjunct.

•**perlapine.** (PURR-lah-peen) USAN.
Use: Hypnotic; sedative.

Perlatan.
See: Estrone.

Perloxx. (Athlon Pharmaceuticals) Oxycodone hydrochloride/acetaminophen 2.5 mg/300 mg, 5 mg/300 mg, 7.5 mg/300 mg. Tab. 100s. *c-II.*
Use: Narcotic analgesic.

•**permanganic acid, potassium salt.**
USP. Potassium permanganate.

Permapen. (Roerig) Penicillin G

benzathine 1,200,000 units/dose with polyvinylpyrrolidone, parabens. Inj. *Isoject* 2 mL. *Rx.*
Use: Anti-infective, penicillin.

•**permethrin.** (per-METH-rin) USAN. Synthetic pyrethrin.
Use: Pediculicide for treatment of head lice, ectoparasiticide.
See: Acticin.
Elimite.
Nix.
Nix Complete Lice Treatment System.

permethrin. (Various Mfr.) Permethrin. **Cream:** 5%. 60 g. **Lot.:** 1%. 60 mL with comb. *OTC.*
Use: Scabicide, pediculicide.

Permitil. (Schering) Fluphenazine hydrochloride. **Concentrate:** 5 mg/mL, alcohol 1%, parabens. Dropper Bot. 118 mL. **Tab.:** 2.5 mg, 5 mg, 10 mg, lactose. Bot. 100s (except 10 mg), 1000s (10 mg only). *Rx.*
Use: Antipsychotic.

Pernox. (Bristol-Myers Squibb) Microfine granules of polyethylene 20%, sulfur 2%, salicylic acid 2% in a combination of soapless cleansers and wetting agents. Lot. Bot. 6 oz. *OTC.*
Use: Dermatologic, acne.

Pernox Lathering Abradant Scrub. (Ranbaxy) Sulfur, salicylic acid. Lot. Bot. 141 g. *OTC.*
Use: Dermatologic, acne.

Pernox Medicated Lathering Scrub Cleanser. (Bristol-Myers Squibb) Polyethylene granules 26%, sulfur 2%, salicylic acid 1.5% w/soapless surface-active cleansers and wetting agents. Regular or lemon. Tube 2 oz, 4 oz. *OTC.*
Use: Dermatologic, acne.

Pernox Scrub for Oily Skin. (Ranbaxy) Sulfur, salicylic acid, EDTA. Cleanser. 56 g, 113 g. *OTC.*
Use: Dermatologic, acne.

Pernox Shampoo. (Bristol-Myers Squibb) Sodium laureth sulfate, water, lauramide DEA, quaternium 22, PEG-75 lanolin/hydrolyzed animal protein, fragrance, sodium Cl, lactic acid, sorbic acid, disodium EDTA, FD&C yellow No. 6 and blue No. 1. Bot. 8 oz. *OTC.*
Use: Cleanser; conditioner.

peroxidase.
W/Glucose oxidase, potassium, iodide.
See: Diastix Reagent Strips.

peroxide, dibenzoyl. Benzoyl Peroxide, Hydrous.

peroxides.
See: Carbamide Peroxide.
Hydrogen Peroxide.
Urea Peroxide.

Peroxyl. (Colgate Oral) Hydrogen peroxide 1.5% in a mint-flavored base. Gel. Tube 15 mL. *OTC.*
Use: Mouth preparation.

Peroxyl Dental Rinse. (Colgate Oral) Hydrogen peroxide 1.5% in mint-flavored base, alcohol 6%. Bot. 240 mL, pt. *OTC.*
Use: Mouth preparation.

•**perphenazine.** (per-FEN-uh-ZEEN) *USP.*
Use: Antiemetic; antipsychotic; anxiolytic.

perphenazine. (Various Mfr.) Perphenazine 2 mg, 4 mg, 8 mg, 16 mg. Tab. Bot. 100s, 500s (4 mg, 8 mg only), 1000s, UD 100s. *Rx.*
Use: Antipsychotic.

perphenazine/amitriptyline.
See: Etrafon-A.
Etrafon Forte.
Etrafon 2-25.

perphenazine/amitriptyline. (Various Mfr.) Perphenazine/amitriptyline 2 mg/10 mg, 2 mg/25 mg, 4 mg/10 mg, 4 mg/25 mg, 4 mg/50 mg. Tab. Bot. 21s (2 mg/10 mg only), 100s, 250s (4 mg/10 mg and 4 mg/50 mg only), 500s (except 4 mg/50 mg), 800s (4 mg/25 mg only), 1000s (except 4 mg/50 mg).
Use: Miscellaneous psychotherapeutic.

Perry Medical Prenatal. (Kirkman) Folic acid 0.4 mg, Ca 100 mg, Fe 13.5 mg, vitamins A 3,000 units, D 200 units, E 15 mg, B_1 1.5 mg, B_2 1 mg, B_3 10 mg, B_5 5 mg, B_6 2 mg, B_{12} 4 mcg, C 50 mg. Cu, I, Mg, Zn. Gluten free. Cap. 200s. *OTC.*
Use: Prenatal vitamin with minerals.

Persangue. (Arcum) Ferrous gluconate 192 mg, vitamins C 150 mg, B_1 3 mg, B_2 3 mg, B_{12} 50 mcg. Cap. Bot. 100s, 500s. *OTC.*
Use: Mineral, vitamin supplement.

Persantine. (Boehringer Ingelheim) Dipyridamole 25 mg, 50 mg, 75 mg. Tab. **25 mg, 50 mg:** Bot. 100s, 1000s, UD 100s. **75 mg:** Bot. 100s, 500s, UD 100s. *Rx.*
Use: Antiplatelet.

•**persic oil.** (PER-sik) *NF.*
Use: Vehicle.

pertechnetic acid, sodium salt.
Sodium Pertechnetate Tc-99m Solution.

Pertscan-99m. (Abbott Diagnostics) Radiodiagnostic. Inj. Tc-99m.
Use: Diagnostic aid.

Pertussin. (Pertussin) Dextromethorphan HBr 15 mg/5 mL, alcohol 9.5%. Syr. Bot. 3 oz, 6 oz. *OTC.*
Use: Antitussive.

Pertussin All-Night PM. (Pertussin) Acetaminophen 167 mg, doxylamine

succinate 1.25 mg, pseudoephedrine hydrochloride 10 mg, dextromethorphan HBr 5 mg/5 mL, alcohol 25%. Liq. Bot. 240 mL. *OTC.*
Use: Analgesic; antihistamine; antitussive; decongestant.

Pertussin CS. (Pertussin) Dextromethorphan HBr 3.5 mg, guaifenesin 25 mg/5 mL, 8.5% alcohol. Bot. 90 mL. *OTC.*
Use: Antitussive; expectorant.

Pertussin ES. (Pertussin) Dextromethorphan HBr 15 mg/5 mL, alcohol 9.5%, sugar, sorbitol. Liq. Bot. 120 mL. *OTC.*
Use: Antitussive.

•**pertussis immune globulin.** (per-TUSS-iss) *USP. Formerly Pertussis Immune Human Globulin.*
Use: Immunization.

pertussis vaccine. (Michigan Department of Health) Vial 5 mL.
Use: Immunization.

•**pertussis vaccine acellular.** *USP.*
Use: Immunization.
W/Diphtheria and tetanus toxoids.
See: Adacel.
Boostrix.
Daptacel.
Infanrix.

pertussis vaccine, acellular, and diphtheria and tetanus toxoids, adsorbed.
Use: Immunization.
See: Adacel.
Boostrix.
Daptacel.
Infanrix.

•**pertussis vaccine adsorbed.** *USP.*
Use: Immunization.

•**pertuzumab.** (per-TUE-zue-mab) USAN.
Use: Antineoplastic.
See: Perjeta.

Pertzye. (Digestive Care) Lipase/protease/amylase 8,000 USP units/28,750 USP units/30,250 USP units, 16,000 USP units/57,500 USP units/60,500 USP units. Enteric-coated microspheres. Sodium. Cap., delayed release. 100s. *Rx.*
Use: Digestive enzyme.

Peruvian balsam.
Use: Local protectant, rubefacient.
W/Benzocaine, Zinc Oxide Bismuth Subgallate, Boric Acid.
See: Hemorrhoidal Ointment.
W/Lidocaine, Bismuth Subgallate, Zinc Oxide, Aluminum Subacetate.
See: Xylocaine.

•**perzinfotel.** (per-zin-FOE-tel) USAN.
Use: NMDA receptor antagonist.

peson. Sodium Lyapolate. Polyethylene sulfonate sodium.
Use: Anticoagulant.

Peterson's Ointment. (Peterson) Carbolic acid, camphor, tannic acid, zinc oxide. Tube w/pipe 1 oz. Jar 16 oz. Can 1.4 oz, 3 oz. *OTC.*
Use: Anorectal preparation.

Pethadol. (Halsey Drug) Meperidine hydrochloride 50 mg, 100 mg. Tab. Bot. 100s, 1000s. *c-II.*
Use: Analgesic; narcotic.

pethidine hydrochloride.
See: Meperidine Hydrochloride.

PETN.
See: Pentaerythritol Tetranitrate.

petrichloral. Pentaerythritol chloral.
Use: Sedative.

•**petrolatum.** (pe-troe-LAY-tum) *USP.*
Use: Pharmaceutic aid (ointment base).
See: Aloe Vesta.

petrolatum gauze.
Use: Surgical aid.

•**petrolatum, hydrophilic.** (pe-troe-LAY-tum hye-droe-FIL-ik) *USP.*
Use: Pharmaceutic aid, absorbent, ointment base; topical protectant.

•**petrolatum, liquid.** (pe-troe-LAY-tum) *USP.* Mineral Oil, Light Mineral Oil, Adepsine Oil, Glymol, Liquid Paraffin, Parolein, White Mineral Oil, Heavy Liquid Petrolatum.
Use: Laxative.
See: Fleet Mineral Oil.
Mineral Oil.
Saxol.

petrolatum, liquid, emulsion.
Use: Lubricant, laxative.
W/Irish Moss, Casanthranol.
See: Haley's M. O.

petrolatum, red veterinarian. (AstraZeneca) Also known as RVP.
W/Zinc Oxide, 2-ethoxyethyl p-methoxy-cinnamate.
See: RVPaque.

•**petrolatum, white.** (pe-troe-LAY-tum) *USP.*
Use: Pharmaceutic aid, oleaginous ointment base; topical protectant.
See: Moroline.

Petro-Phylic Soap. (Doak Dermatologics) Hydrophilic Petrolatum. Cake 4 oz.
Use: Emollient; anti-infective, topical.

Petro-20. (Foy Laboratories) Pentaerythritol tetranitrate 20 mg. Tab. Bot. 100s, 1000s. *Rx.*
Use: Antianginal.

•**pevonedistat.** (PE-voe-NED-i-stat) USAN.
Use: Antineoplastic.

•**pevonedistat hydrochloride.** (PE-voe-NED-i-stat) USAN.
Use: Antineoplastic.

•**pexastimogene devacirepvec.** (PEX-a-STIM-oh-jeen DEE-vas-i-REP-vek) USAN.
Use: Antineoplastic.

•**pexelizumab.** (peks-e-li-ZOO-mab) USAN.
Use: Monoclonal antibody.

Pexeva. (Noven Therapeutics) Paroxetine mesylate 10 mg, 20 mg, 30 mg, 40 mg. Tab. 30s, 100s (20 mg only), 500s (20 mg only). *Rx.*
Use: Antidepressant, selective serotonin reuptake inhibitor.

Pfeiffer's Cold Sore. (Pfeiffer) Gum benzoin 7%, camphor, menthol, thymol, eucalyptol, alcohol 85%. Lot. Bot. 15 mL. *OTC.*
Use: Cold sores; fever blisters; moisturizer.

PF4RIA. (Abbott Diagnostics) Platelet factor 4 radioimmunoassay for the quantitative measurement of total PF4 levels in plasma.
Use: Diagnostic aid.

Pfizerpen. (Pfizer) Penicillin G potassium 5,000,000 units, 20,000,000 units/vial, sodium ≈ 6.8 mg (0.3 mEq), potassium 65.6 mg (1.68 mEq)/million units. Pow. for Inj. Vial. *Rx.*
Use: Anti-infective, penicillin.

Pfizerpen VK. (Pfizer) Penicillin V potassium. Tab. **250 mg:** Bot. 1000s. **500 mg:** Bot. 100s. *Rx.*
Use: Anti-infective, penicillin.

PGA.
See: Folic Acid.

PGE.
Use: Prostaglandin.
See: Alprostadil.

pH acid. (Ivax) Bot. 8 oz.
Use: Dermatologic.

Phadiatop RIA Test. (Pharmacia) Determination of IgE antibodies specific to inhalant allergens in human serum. Kit 60s.
Use: Diagnostic aid.

Phanatuss Cough. (Pharmakon) Dextromethorphan HBr 10 mg, guaifenesin 85 mg, potassium citrate 75 mg, citric acid 35 mg/5 mL, sorbitol, menthol. Syr. Bot. 118 mL. *OTC.*
Use: Antitussive; expectorant.

Phanatuss DM. (Pharmakon) Dextromethorphan HBr 10 mg, guaifenesin 100 mg per 5 mL. Parabens, saccharin, menthol, alcohol free, sugar free. Syr. Bot. 118 mL. *OTC.*
Use: Upper respiratory combination, antitussive, expectorant.

pH Antiseptic Skin Cleanser. (Walgreen) Alcohol 63%. Bot. 16 oz. *OTC.*
Use: Astringent; cleanser.

Pharazine. (Halsey Drug) Bot. 4 oz, pt, gal.
Use: A series of cough and cold products.

Pharbechlor. (Pharbest Pharmaceuticals) Chlorpheniramine maleate 4 mg. Tab. 100s, 1,000s. *OTC.*
Use: Antihistamine, nonselective alkylamine.

Pharbetol. (Pharbest Pharmaceuticals) Acetaminophen 325 mg. Tab. 100s. *OTC.*
Use: CNS agent.

Pharbetol Extra Strength. (Pharbest Pharmaceuticals) Acetaminophen 500 mg. Tab. 1,000s. *OTC.*
Use: CNS agent.

Pharmadine. (Sherwood Davis & Geck) Povidone-iodine. **Oint.:** Pkt. 1 g, 1.5 g, 2 g, 30 g, 1 lb. **Perineal wash:** 240 mL. **Skin cleanser:** 240 mL. **Soln.:** 15 mL, 120 mL, 240 mL, pt, qt. **Soln., swabs:** 100s. **Soln., swabsticks:** 1 or 3/packet in 250s. **Spray:** 120 g. **Surgical scrub:** 30 mL, pt, qt, gal, foil-pack 15 mL. **Surgical scrub sponge/brush:** 25s. **Swabsticks, lemon glycerin:** 100s. **Whirlpool soln.:** Gal. *OTC.*
Use: Antiseptic.

Pharmaflur. (Pharmics) Sodium fluoride 2.21 mg. Tab. Bot. 1000s. *Rx.*
Use: Dental caries agent.

Pharmalgen Hymenoptera Venoms. (ALK) Freeze-dried venom or venom protein. Vials of 120 mcg, 1100 mcg for each of honey bee, white-faced hornet, yellow hornet, yellow jacket, or wasp. Vials of 360 mcg, 3300 mcg for mixed vespids (white-faced hornet, yellow hornet, yellow jacket). Diagnostic kit: 5 × 1 mL vial. Treatment kit: 6 × 1 mL vial or 1 × 1.1 mg multiple-dose vial. Starter Kit: 6 × 1 mL, prediluted 0.01 mcg to 100 mcg/mL.
Use: Antivenom.

Pharmalgen Standardized Allergenic Extracts. (ALK) 100,000 allergenic units. Vial. Box 5 × 1 mL.
Use: Diagnostic aid.

Phazyme. (GlaxoSmithKline) Simethicone. **Cap.:** 180 mg. 12s. **Drops:** 40 mg/0.6 mL, saccharin. Bot. 30 mL w/dropper. **Tab.:** 60 mg. Bot. 50s, 100s, 1000s. *OTC.*
Use: Antiflatulent.

Phazyme 95. (GlaxoSmithKline) Simethicone 95 mg. Tab. Bot. 100s. *OTC.*
Use: Antiflatulent.

Phazyme 125. (GlaxoSmithKline) Simethicone 125 mL. Cap. Bot. 50s. *OTC.*
Use: Antiflatulent.

Phazyme Quick Dissolve. (GlaxoSmithKline) Simethicone 125 mg. Phenylalanine 0.4 mg, aspartame, mannitol, sorbitol. Mint flavor. Chew. Tab. 18s, 48s. *OTC.*
Use: Antiflatulent.

•**phemfilcon A.** (FEM-fill-kahn A) USAN.
Use: Contact lens material, hydrophilic.

phenacaine hydrochloride.
Use: Anesthetic, local.

Phenacal. (NeuroGenesis/Matrix Tech.) D,l-phenylalanine 500 mg, l-glutamine 15 mg, l-tyrosine 25 mg, l-carnitine 10 mg, l-arginine pyroglutamate 10 mg, l-ornithine/l-aspartate 10 mg, Cr 0.033 mg, Se 0.012 mg, vitamin B_1 0.33 mg, B_2 5 mg, B_3 3.3 mg, B_5 0.33 mg, B_6 0.33 mg, B_{12} 1 mcg, E 5 units, biotin 0.05 mg, folic acid 0.066 mg, Fe 1 mg, Zn 2.5 mg, Ca 35 mg, I 0.25 mg, Cu 0.33 mg, Mg 25 mg. Cap. Bot. 42s, 180s. *OTC.*
Use: Nutritional supplement.

phenacetin. Acetophenetidin. Ethoxyacetanilide.
Note: This drug has been withdrawn from the market because of liver and kidney toxicity. This drug is no longer official in the USP.
Use: Antipyretic; analgesic.

Phenadex Senior. (Alra) Dextromethorphan HBr 10 mg, guaifenesin 200 mg/5 mL. Liq. Bot. 118 mL. *OTC.*
Use: Antitussive; expectorant.

Phenadoz. (Watson Pharma) Promethazine hydrochloride 12.5 mg, 25 mg. Cocoa butter. Supp. 12s. *Rx.*
Use: Antihistamine, nonselective phenothiazine.

phenamazoline hydrochloride.
Use: Vasoconstrictor.

Phenameth. (Major) Promethazine 25 mg. Tab. Bot. 1000s. *Rx.*
Use: Antiemetic; antihistamine.

Phenameth DM. (Major) Promethazine hydrochloride 6.25 mg, dextromethorphan HBr 15 mg/5 mL, alcohol. Syr. Bot. 120 mL. *Rx.*
Use: Antihistamine; antitussive.

Phenameth VC w/Codeine. (Major) Phenylephrine hydrochloride 5 mg, promethazine hydrochloride 6.25 mg, codeine phosphate 10 mg/5 mL, alcohol 7%. Syr. Bot. Pt, gal. *c-v.*
Use: Antihistamine; antitussive; decongestant.

Phenameth w/Codeine. (Major) Promethazine hydrochloride 6.25 mg, codeine phosphate 10 mg/5 mL, alcohol 7%. Syr. Bot. 4 oz, pt, gal. *c-v.*
Use: Antihistamine; antitussive.

phenantoin. Mephenytoin.

Phenapap. (Rugby) Pseudoephedrine hydrochloride 30 mg, acetaminophen 325 mg. Tab. Bot. 100s. *OTC.*
Use: Upper respiratory combination, decongestant, analgesic.

Phenapap Sinus Headache & Congestion. (Rugby) Pseudoephedrine hydrochloride 30 mg, chlorpheniramine 2 mg, acetaminophen 325 mg. Tab. Bot. 30s, 100s, 1000s. *OTC.*
Use: Analgesic; antihistamine; decongestant.

phenaphthazine. Sodium dinitro phenylazonaphthol disulfonate.

phenarsone sulfoxylate. Methanesulfinic acid disodium salt.
Use: Antiamebic.

Phenaseptic. (Rugby) Phenol 1.4%, saccharin, cherry flavor. Throat spray. Bot. 177 mL. *OTC.*
Use: Mouth and throat product.

Phenaspirin Compound. (Davis & Sly) Phenobarbital 0.25 g, aspirin 3.5 g. Cap. Bot. 1000s. *Rx.*
Use: Analgesic; hypnotic; sedative.

PhenaVent LA. (Ethex) Phenylephrine hydrochloride 30 mg, guaifenesin 600 mg. Film-coated. Tab. 100s. *Rx.*
Use: Decongestant, expectorant.

phenazocine hydrobromide.
Use: Analgesic.

PhenazoForte Plus. (Creekwood Pharmaceutical) Butalbital 15 mg, hyoscyamine hydrobromide 300 mcg, phenazopyridine hydrochloride 150 mg. Lactose, mineral oil, PEG. Tab. 30s. *Rx.*
Use: Renal and genitourinary agent, interstitial cystitis combination.

phenazone.
See: Antipyrine.

•**phenazopyridine hydrochloride.** (fen-AZZ-oh-PIH-rih-deen) *USP.*
Use: Analgesic, urinary.
See: AZO Standard.
AZO Standard Maximum Strength.
Baridium.
Geridium.
Prodium.
Pyridium.
Urogesic.
UTI Relief.

W/Butabarbital, Hyoscyamine Hydrobromide.
See: Phenazopyridine Plus.

W/Butalbital, Hyoscyamine Hydrobromide.
See: PhenazoForte Plus.
W/Combinations.
See: Urisan-P.

phenazopyridine hydrochloride. (Various Mfr.) Phenazopyridine hydrochloride 100 mg, 200 mg. Tab. 100s, 1000s, UD 100s. *Rx.*
Use: Interstitial cystitis agent.

Phenazopyridine Plus. (Breckenridge) Phenazopyridine hydrochloride 150 mg, hyoscyamine hydrobromide 0.3 mg, butabarbital 15 mg. Tab. 30s. *Rx.*
Use: Interstitial cystitis agent.

•**phenbutazone sodium glycerate.** (fen-BYOO-tah-zone so-dee-uhm GLIH-seh-rate) USAN.
Use: Anti-inflammatory.

•**phencarbamide.** (FEN-car-BAM-id) USAN.
Use: Anticholinergic; spasmolytic.

Phencarb GG. (Boca Pharmacal) Carbetapentane citrate 20 mg, guaifenesin 100 mg, phenylephrine hydrochloride 10 mg per 5 mL. EDTA, sorbitol, sugar. Spearmint flavor. Syr. 473 mL. *Rx.*
Use: Antitussive and expectorant combination, upper respiratory combination.

Phenchlor-Eight. (Freeport) Chlorpheniramine maleate 8 mg. TR Cap. Bot. 1000s. *Rx.*
Use: Antihistamine.

Phenchlor-Twelve. (Freeport) Chlorpheniramine maleate 12 mg. TR Cap. Bot. 1000s. *Rx.*
Use: Antihistamine.

•**phencyclidine hydrochloride.** (fen-SIGH-klih-deen) USAN.
Use: Anesthetic.

phendimetrazine. (Various Mfr.) Phendimetrazine tartrate 35 mg. Tab. Bot. 100s, 1000s, 5000s. *c-III.*
Use: CNS stimulant, anorexiant.

•**phendimetrazine tartrate.** (fen-die-MEH-trah-zeen) *USP.*
Use: CNS stimulant, anorexiant.
See: Anorex.
Bontril PDM.
Bontril Slow Release.
Delcozine.
Di-Ap-Trol.
Elphemet.
Melfiat-105 Unicelles.
Obe-Tite.
Phendimetrazine.
Phen-70.
Prelu-2.
Reducto, Improved.
Rexigen Forte.
Slim-Tabs.

phendimetrazine tartrate. (Sandoz) Phendimetrazine tartrate 105 mg. Sucrose. ER Cap. 100s, 1000s. *c-III.*
Use: Anorexiant.

Phendry. (LuChem Pharmaceuticals, Inc.) Diphenhydramine hydrochloride 12.5 mg/5 mL, alcohol 14%. Elix. Bot. Pt, gal. *OTC.*
Use: Antihistamine.

Phendry Children's Allergy Medicine. (LuChem Pharmaceuticals, Inc.) Diphenhydramine hydrochloride 12.5 mg/5 mL, alcohol 14%. Elix. Bot. 120 mL. *OTC.*
Use: Antihistamine.

phenelzine dihydrogen sulfate.
See: Nardil.

•**phenelzine sulfate.** (FEN-uhl-zeen) *USP.*
Use: Antidepressant.
See: Nardil.

phenelzine sulfate. (Gavis Pharmaceuticals) Phenelzine sulfate 15 mg. Film coated. Edetate disodium, mannitol, PEG. Tab. 60s. *Rx.*
Use: Antidepressant, monoamine oxidase inhibitor.

Phenergan. (West-Ward) Promethazine hydrochloride 25 mg/mL, 50 mg/mL. EDTA, sodium metabisulfite 0.25 mg/mL. Inj. Amp. 1 mL. *Rx.*
Use: Antihistamine, nonselective phenothiazine.

Phenergan with Codeine. (Wyeth) Promethazine hydrochloride 6.25 mg, codeine phosphate 10 mg/5 mL. Bot. 4 oz, 6 oz, 8 oz, pt, gal. *c-V.*
Use: Antihistamine; antitussive.

Phenergan with Dextromethorphan. (Wyeth) Promethazine hydrochloride 6.25 mg, dextromethorphan HBr 15 mg/5 mL, alcohol 7%. Bot. 4 oz, 6 oz, pt, gal. *Rx.*
Use: Antihistamine; antitussive.

pheneridine.
Use: Analgesic.

i-phenethylbiguanide monohydrochloride. Phenformin hydrochloride.

Phenex-1. (Ross) Protein 15 g, fat 23.9 g, carbohydrates 46.3 g, linoleic acid 1800 mg, Fe 9 mg, Na 190 mg, K 675 mg, Cal 480/100 g. With appropriate vitamins and minerals. Phenylalanine free. Pow. Can 350 g. *OTC.*
Use: Nutritional supplement.

Phenex-2. (Ross) Protein 30 g, fat 15.5 g, carbohydrates 30 g, Na 880 mg, K 1370 mg, Cal 410/mL. With appropriate vitamins and minerals. Phenylalanine free. Pow. Can 325 g. *OTC.*
Use: Nutritional supplement.

Phenflu G. (AMBI) Dextromethorphan HBr 30 mg, guaifenesin 600 mg, phenylephrine hydrochloride 15 mg, acetaminophen 500 mg. Dye free. Tab. 100s. *Rx.*
Use: Upper respiratory combination, antitussive and expectorant combination.
phenformin hydrochloride.
Note: Withdrawn from market in 1977. Available under IND exemption.
Use: Hypoglycemic.
Phenhist DH w/Codeine. (Rugby) Pseudoephedrine hydrochloride 30 mg, chlorpheniramine maleate 2 mg, codeine phosphate 10 mg/5 mL, alcohol 5%. Liq. Bot. 120 mL, 480 mL. *c-v.*
Use: Antihistamine; antitussive; decongestant.
Phenhist Expectorant. (Rugby) Pseudoephedrine hydrochloride 30 mg, codeine phosphate 10 mg, guaifenesin 100 mg/5 mL, alcohol 7.5%. Liq. Bot. 118 mL, pt, gal. *c-v.*
Use: Antihistamine; antitussive; decongestant.
•**phenindamine tartrate.** (fen-IN-dah-meen) USAN.
Use: Antihistamine, nonselective piperidine.
W/Phenylephrine Hydrochloride, Aspirin, Caffeine, Aluminum Hydroxide, Magnesium Carbonate.
See: Dristan.
W/Phenylephrine Hydrochloride, Caramiphen Ethanedisulfonate.
See: Dondril.
W/Phenylephrine Hydrochloride, Chlorpheniramine Maleate, Belladonna Alkaloids.
See: Comhist LA.
W/Phenylephrine Hydrochloride, Chlorpheniramine Maleate, Drytane.
See: Comhist.
W/Phenylephrine Hydrochloride, Pyrilamine Maleate, Chlorpheniramine Maleate, Dextromethorphan HBr.
See: Histalet.
pheniodol.
See: Iodoalphionic acid.
pheniprazine hydrochloride.
Use: Antihypertensive.
•**pheniramine maleate.** (fen-IR-a-meen) *USP.*
Use: Antihistamine.
See: Citra Forte.
Partuss AC.
Tritussin.
W/Acetaminophen, Phenylephrine Hydrochloride.
See: Theraflu Cold & Sore Throat.
Theraflu Flu & Sore Throat.
Theraflu Nighttime Severe Cold.
W/Caffeine Citrate, Phenylephrine Hydrochloride, Sodium Salicylate.
See: Scot-Tussin Original Multi-Action Cold and Allergy.
W/Dextromethorphan Hydrobromide, Phenylephrine Hydrochloride.
See: Theraflu Cold & Cough.
W/Naphazoline Hydrochloride.
See: Naphcon-A.
Opcon-A.
Visine-A.
•**phenmetrazine hydrochloride.** (fen-MEH-trah-zeen) *USP.*
Use: Anorexic.
•**phenobarbital.** (fee-no-BAR-bih-tahl) *USP.*
Tall Man: PHENobarbital
Use: Anticonvulsant; hypnotic; sedative.
See: Luminal Sodium.
Solfoton.
W/Atropine Sulfate.
See: Antrocol.
W/Atropine Sulfate, Hyoscyamine Hydrobromide or Sulfate, Scopolamine Hydrobromide.
See: Antispasmodic.
Donnatal.
Donnatal Extentabs.
PB-Hyos.
Quadrapax.
Se-Donna PB Hyos.
phenobarbital. (Pharmaceutical Associates) Phenobarbital 15 mg/5 mL. Elix. Bot. Pt, UD 5 mL, 10 mL, 20 mL. *c-IV.*
Use: Anticonvulsant; hypnotic; sedative.
phenobarbital. (Various Mfr.) Phenobarbital. **Tab.: 15 mg, 30 mg:** Bot. 100s, 1000s, 5000s, UD 100s. **60 mg:** Bot. 100s, 1000s, UD 100s. **100 mg:** 100s, 1000s. **Elix.:** 20 mg/5 mL. Bot. Pt, gal, UD 5 mL, UD 7.5 mL.
Use: Anticonvulsant; hypnotic; sedative.
phenobarbital and theobromine combinations.
See: Theobromine w/phenobarbital combinations.
•**phenobarbital sodium.** (fee-no-BAR-bih-tahl) *USP.*
Tall Man: PHENobarbital
Use: Anticonvulsant; hypnotic; sedative.
See: Luminal Injection.
phenobarbital sodium. (Wyeth) Phenobarbital sodium Inj. **30 mg/mL, 60 mg/mL:** *Tubex* 1 mL. **65 mg/mL:** Vial 1 mL. *c-IV.*
Use: Anticonvulsant; hypnotic; sedative.
phenobarbital sodium in propylene glycol. (Vitarine) Amp. 0.13 g: 1 mL, Box

25s, 100s. *c-IV.*
Use: Anticonvulsant; hypnotic; sedative.

phenobarbital with aminophylline.
See: Aminophylline.

phenobarbital with central nervous system stimulants.
See: Arcotrate No. 3.
Spabelin.

phenobarbital with homatropine methylbromide.
See: Homatropine methylbromide and phenobarbital combinations.

phenobarbital with hyoscyamus.
See: Hyoscyamus products and phenobarbital combinations.

phenobarbital with mannitol hexanitrate.
Use: Anticonvulsant; sedative; hypnotic.
See: Mannitol hexanitrate with phenobarbital combinations.

phenobarbital with theophylline.
See: Theophylline with phenobarbital combinations.

Pheno-Bella. (Ferndale) Belladonna extract 10.8 mg, phenobarbital 16.2 mg. Tab. Bot. 100s, 1000s. *Rx.*
Use: Anticholinergic; antispasmodic; hypnotic; sedative.

•**phenol.** (FEE-nole) *USP.*
Use: Pharmaceutic aid, preservative; topical antipruritic; mouth and throat product.
See: Chloraseptic Kids Sore Throat.
Chloraseptic Sore Throat.
Green Throat Spray.
Phenaseptic.
Red Throat Spray.
Triaminic Sore Throat Spray.
W/Benzocaine.
See: Anbesol.
W/Lidocaine.
See: Skeeter Stik.
W/Resorcinol, Boric Acid, Basic Fuchsin, Acetone.
See: Castellani's Paint.

•**phenolate sodium.** (FEEN-oh-late) USAN.
Use: Disinfectant.

Phenolax. (Pharmacia) Phenolphthalein 64.8 mg. Wafer. Bot. 100s. *OTC.*
Use: Laxative.

•**phenol, camphorated topical gel.** (FEE-nole) *USP.*
Use: Topical antipruritic.

•**phenol, liquefied.** (FEE-nole) *USP.*
Use: Topical antipruritic.

•**phenolphthalein.** (fee-nahl-THAY-leen) *USP.*
Use: Indicator.

phenolsulfonates.
See: Sulfocarbolates.

phenolsulfonic acid. Sulfocarbolic acid. Used in Sulphodine. (Strasenburgh).

phenoltetrabromophthalein. Disulfonate Disodium.
See: Sulfobromophthalein Sodium.

Pheno Nux. (Pal-Pak, Inc.) Phenobarbital 16.2 mg, nux vomica extract 8.1 mg, calcium carbonate 194.4 mg. Tab. Bot. 1000s. *c-IV.*
Use: Sedative; hypnotic; antacid.

phenothiazine. Thiodiphenylamine.

phenothiazine derivatives.
See: Chlorpromazine Hydrochloride.
Fluphenazine.
Mesoridazine.
Perphenazine.
Prochlorperazine.
Thioridazine Hydrochloride.
Trifluoperazine Hydrochloride.

phenothiazines, nonselective.
See: Promethazine Hydrochloride.

Phenoturic. (Truett) Phenobarbital 40 mg/5 mL. Elix. Bot. Pt, gal. *c-IV.*
Use: Hypnotic; sedative.

•**phenoxybenzamine hydrochloride.** (fen-ox-ee-BEN-zuh-meen) *USP.*
Use: Antihypertensive.
See: Dibenzyline.

phenoxymethyl penicillin.
See: Penicillin V.

phenoxymethyl penicillin potassium.
See: Penicillin V potassium.

phenoxynate. Mixture of phenylphenols 17% to 18%, octyl and related alkylphenols 2% to 3%.

•**phenprocoumon.** (fen-PRO-koo-mahn) USAN.
Use: Anticoagulant.

Phen-70. (Parmed Pharmaceuticals, Inc.) Phendimetrazine tartrate 70 mg. Tab. Bot. 100s, 1000s. *c-III.*
Use: Anorexiant.

Phental. (Armenpharm Ltd.) Belladonna alkaloids, phenobarbital 0.25 g. Tab. Bot. 1000s. *c-IV.*
Use: Anticholinergic; antispasmodic; hypnotic; sedative.

Phentamine. (Major) Phentermine hydrochloride 30 mg. Cap. (equivalent to 24 mg base). Bot. 100s. *c-IV.*
Use: Anorexiant.

•**phentermine.** (FEN-ter-meen) USAN.
Use: Anorexic.
See: Adipex-P.
Wilpowr.

•**phentermine hydrochloride.** (FEN-ter-meen) *USP.*
Use: CNS stimulant, anorexiant.
See: Adipex-P.
Suprenza.

W/Topiramate.
See: Qsymia.
phentermine hydrochloride. (Various Mfr.) Phentermine hydrochloride. **Tab.:** 37.5 mg (equiv. to 30 mg phentermine base). 30s, 60s, 100s, 250s, 500s, 1,000s. **Cap.:** 15 mg (equiv. to 12 mg phentermine base), 30 mg (equiv. to 24 mg phentermine base), 37.5 mg (equiv. to 30 mg phentermine base). May contain lactose. 100s, 1,000s. *c-IV.*
Use: CNS stimulant, anorexiant.
phentetiothalein sodium. Iso-Iodeikon.
Use: Radiopaque agent.
phentolamine hydrochloride.
Use: Antihypertensive.
•**phentolamine mesylate.** (fen-TOLE-uh-meen) *USP. Formerly Phentolamine Methanesulfonate.*
Use: Agent for Pheochromocytoma.
See: OraVerse.
phentolamine mesylate for injection. (Bedford) Phentolamine mesylate 5 mg. Mannitol. Pow. for Inj. Vial 2 mL. *Rx.*
Use: Antiadrenergic.
phentolamine methanesulfonate. Phentolamine mesylate.
Phentolox w/APAP. (Global Source) Phenyltoloxamine citrate 30 mg, acetaminophen 325 mg. Tab. Bot. 1000s. *Rx.*
Use: Antihistamine; analgesic.
phentydrone.
Use: Systemic fungicide.
Phenydex. (Roxmar) Dextromethorphan HBr 20 mg, guaifenesin 200 mg, phenylephrine hydrochloride 10 mg, pyrilamine maleate 25 mg per 5 mL. Sugar, alcohol, and dye free. Phenylalanine. Cherry menthol flavor. Liq. 118 mL. *Rx.*
Use: Antitussive and expectorant.
Phenydex Pediatric. (Roxmar) Phenylephrine hydrochloride 2.5 mg, dextromethorphan HBr 5 mg, guaifenesin 50 mg per 5 mL. Phenylalanine, tutti frutti flavor. Liq. 118 mL. *Rx.*
Use: Pediatric antitussive and expectorant.
n-phenylacetamide.
See: Acetanilid.
•**phenylalanine.** (fen-ill-AL-ah-NEEN) *USP.*
Use: Amino acid.
W/Combinations.
See: Amoxicillin.
Amoxil.
Benadryl Children's Allergy Fastmelt.
Pepcid AC.
phenylalanine ammonia-lyase.
Use: Hyperphenylalaninemia. [Orphan Drug]
phenylalanine mustard.
See: Melphalan.
•**phenyl aminosalicylate.** (FEN-ill ah-MEE-no-sah-LIH-sih-late) USAN.
Use: Anti-infective.
phenylazo. (A.P.C.) Phenylazodiaminopyridine hydrochloride 1.5 g. Tab. Bot. 1000s. *Rx.*
Use: Analgesic, urinary.
phenylazodiaminopyridine.
See: Phenazopyridine.
phenylazodiaminopyridine hydrobromide.
See: Phenazopyridine Hydrobromide.
phenylazodiaminopyridine hydrochloride.
See: Phenazopyridine Hydrochloride.
phenylazo sulfisoxazole. (A.P.C.) Sulfisoxazole 0.5 g, phenylazopyridine 50 mg. Tab. Bot. 1000s. *Rx.*
Use: Anti-infective, sulfonamide.
phenylbenzimidazole sulfonic acid.
See: Ensulizole.
•**phenylbutazone.** (fen-ill-BYOO-tah-zone) *USP.*
Use: Antirheumatic.
phenylbutylpiperadine derivatives.
Use: Antipsychotic.
See: Haloperidol.
Pimozide.
phenylcarbinol.
See: Benzyl Alcohol, NF.
Phenyl Chlor-Tan Pediatric. (Hi-Tech) Phenylephrine tannate 5 mg, chlorpheniramine tannate 4.5 mg per 5 mL. Methylparaben, saccharin, sucrose. Susp. 473 mL. *Rx.*
Use: Decongestant and antihistamine, upper respiratory combination.
phenylcinchoninic acid. Name used for cinchophen.
•**phenylephrine bitartrate.** *USP.*
W/Aspirin, Chlorpheniramine Maleate.
See: Alka-Seltzer Plus Cold.
Alka-Seltzer Plus Sparkling Original Cold Formula.
W/Aspirin, Dextromethorphan Hydrobromide.
See: Alka-Seltzer Plus Day & Night Cold.
W/Aspirin, Dextromethorphan Hydrobromide, Doxylamine Succinate.
See: Alka-Seltzer Plus Day & Night Cold.
Alka-Seltzer Plus Night Cold.
phenylephrine CM. (Boca Pharmacal) Phenylephrine hydrochloride 40 mg, chlorpheniramine maleate 8 mg, methscopolamine nitrate 2.5 mg. ER Tab. 30s, 100s. *Rx.*

Use: Decongestant, antihistamine, and anticholinergic, upper respiratory combination.

phenylephrine-guaifenesin. (Acella) Phenylephrine hydrochloride 1.5 mg, guaifenesin 20 mg. Drops. 30 mL. *Rx.*
Use: Upper respiratory combination/decongestant and expectorant combination.

•**phenylephrine hydrochloride.** (fen-ill-EFF-rin) *USP.*
Use: Adrenergic; mydriatic; sympathomimetic; vasoconstrictor; nasal decongestant, arylalkylamine.
See: AH-Chew.
AK-Dilate.
Altafrin.
Anu-Med.
Formulation R.
4-Way Fast Acting.
4-Way Menthol.
Isopto Frin.
Little Colds for Infants and Children.
Mydfrin 2.5%.
Neofrin.
Neo-Synephrine.
Neo-Synephrine Extra Strength.
Neo-Synephrine Mild Strength.
Neo-Synephrine Regular Strength.
Refresh Redness Relief.
Relief.
Rhinall.
Sudafed PE.
Sudafed PE Maximum Strength Nasal Decongestant.
Super-Anahist Nasal Spray.
Triaminic Thin Strips Cold.
Zincfrin.

W/Acetaminophen.
See: Alka-Seltzer Plus Sinus.
Comtrex Maximum Strength Day & Night Flu Therapy.
Comtrex Maximum Strength Day & Night Severe Cold & Sinus.
Contac Cold + Flu Day.
Dilotab II.
Excedrin Sinus Headache.
Mapap Sinus Congestion and Pain Maximum Strength.
Robitussin Adult Peak Cold Nasal Relief.
Sine-Off Non-Drowsy Maximum Strength.
Sinutab Sinus.
Sudafed PE Sinus Headache.
Vicks DayQuil Sinex.

W/Acetaminophen, Chlorpheniramine Maleate.
See: Alka-Seltzer Multi-Symptom Cold Relief.
Alka-Seltzer Plus Fast Crystal Packs.
Comtrex Maximum Strength Day & Night Flu Therapy.
Comtrex Maximum Strength Day & Night Severe Cold & Sinus.
Contac Cold + Flu.
Contac Cold + Flu Maximum Strength.
Contac Cold + Flu Night.
Dristan Cold Multi-Symptom Formula.
Dryphen Multi-Symptom Formula.
Medicidin-D.
Norel AD.
Onset Forte Micro-Coated.
Pyrroxate Extra Strength.
Robitussin Adult Peak Cold Nighttime Nasal Relief.
Sine Off Sinus/Cold.
Tylenol Allergy Multi-Symptom.
Tylenol Allergy Multi-Symptom Convenience Pack.
Tylenol Plus Children's Cold.
Tylenol Sinus Congestion & Pain Daytime.
Tylenol Sinus Congestion & Pain Nighttime.

W/Acetaminophen, Chlorpheniramine Maleate, Dextromethorphan Hydrobromide.
See: Alka-Seltzer Plus Cold & Cough.
Comtrex Maximum Strength Day & Night Cold & Cough.
Dimetapp Children's Multi-Symptom Cold & Flu.
Robitussin Cough, Cold & Flu Nighttime.
Theraflu Nighttime Severe Cold.
Tylenol Cold Head Congestion Nighttime.
Tylenol Cold Multi-Symptom Nighttime.
Tylenol Plus Children's Flu.
Tylenol Plus Children's Multi-Symptom Cold.

W/Acetaminophen, Chlorpheniramine Maleate, Phenyltoloxamine Citrate.
See: Trital SR.

W/Acetaminophen, Dexbrompheniramine.
See: Sinadrin PE.

W/Acetaminophen, Dextromethorphan Hydrobromide.
See: Alka-Seltzer Plus Day & Night Cold.
Alka-Seltzer Plus Day Cold.
Alka-Seltzer Plus Day Non-Drowsy Cold.
Comtrex Maximum Strength Day & Night Cold & Cough.
Mapap Cold Formula Multi-Symptom.
Theraflu Daytime Severe Cold & Cough.
Theraflu Severe Cold & Cough Daytime/Nighttime.

Theraflu Warming Relief Daytime Multi-Symptom Cold.
Tylenol Cold Head Congestion Daytime.
Tylenol Cold Multi-Symptom Daytime.
Vicks DayQuil Multi-Symptom Cold/Flu Relief.
Vicks Nature Fusion Cold & Flu Relief.

W/Acetaminophen, Dextromethorphan Hydrobromide, Diphenhydramine Hydrochloride.
See: Respa C & C.

W/Acetaminophen, Dextromethorphan Hydrobromide, Doxylamine Succinate.
See: Alka-Seltzer Plus Day & Night Cold.
Alka-Seltzer Plus Night Cold Formula.
Alka-Seltzer Plus Severe Sinus Congestion Allergy & Cough.
Tylenol Cold Multi-Symptom Nighttime.

W/Acetaminophen, Dextromethorphan Hydrobromide, Guaifenesin.
See: Mucinex Children's Cold, Cough and Sore Throat.
Mucinex Fast-Max Cold, Flu and Sore Throat.
Mucinex Fast-Max Severe Congestion and Cold.
Phenflu G.
Sine-Off Cough/Cold.
Sudafed PE Multi-Symptom Cold and Cough.

W/Acetaminophen, Diphenhydramine Hydrochloride.
See: Benadryl Allergy & Cold.
Benadryl Allergy & Sinus Headache.
Benadryl Severe Allergy & Sinus Headache Maximum Strength.
Sudafed PE Multi-Symptom Severe Cold.
Sudafed PE Nighttime Cold Maximum Strength.
Theraflu Nighttime Severe Cough & Cold.
Theraflu Severe Cold & Cough Daytime/Nighttime.
Theraflu Sugar-Free Nighttime Severe Cough & Cold.
Theraflu Warming Relief Flu & Sore Throat.
Tylenol Allergy Multi-Symptom Convenience Pack.
Tylenol Allergy Multi-Symptom Nighttime.
Tylenol Plus Children's Cold & Allergy.

W/Acetaminophen, Guaifenesin.
See: Mucinex Fast-Max Cold and Sinus.
Sine-Off Multi Symptom Relief.
Tylenol Sinus Congestion & Pain Severe Daytime.

W/Acetaminophen, Pheniramine Maleate.
See: Theraflu Cold & Sore Throat.
Theraflu Flu & Sore Throat.
Theraflu Nighttime Severe Cold.

W/Antipyrine, Benzocaine.
See: Ear-Gesic.

W/Benzalkonium Chloride.
See: Mydfrin Ophthalmic.
Rhinall.

W/Brompheniramine Maleate.
See: Brohist D.
BrōveX PEB.
Cenhist.
Dimetapp Children's Cold & Allergy.
Entre-B.
LoHist PEB.
Ru-Hist D.
Rynex PE.
Vazobid-PD.

W/Brompheniramine Maleate, Carbetapentane Citrate.
See: V-Cof.

W/Brompheniramine Maleate, Codeine Phosphate.
See: M-End PE.
Poly-Tussin AC.

W/Brompheniramine Maleate, Dextromethorphan Hydrobromide.
See: Alahist DM.
BPM-DM-PHEN.
BrōveX PEB DM.
BROM/PE/DM.
Children's Dimaphen DM.
Dimetapp Children's Cold & Cough.
LoHist-DM.
LoHist PEB DM.
TGQ 7.5PEH/4BRM/15DM.
TL-Hist DM.

W/Brompheniramine Maleate, Dextromethorphan Hydrobromide, Guaifenesin.
See: Bromhist-PDX.

W/Brompheniramine Maleate, Dihydrocodeine Bitartrate.
See: Poly-Tussin DHC.

W/Caffeine Citrate, Pheniramine Maleate, Sodium Salicylate.
See: Scot-Tussin Original Multi-Action Cold and Allergy.

W/Carbetapentane Citrate, Dexchlorpheniramine Maleate.
See: Corzall-PE.

W/Carbetapentane Citrate, Diphenhydramine Tannate.
See: D-Tann CD.

W/Carbetapentane Citrate, Guaifenesin.
See: Albatussin.
Carbatab-12.
Carbatuss.

Extendryl GCP.
Gentex 30.
Levall.
Phencarb GG.
Zinx GCP.
W/Chlophedianol Hydrochloride, Guaifenesin.
See: Vanacof GPE.
W/Chlophedianol Hydrochloride, Thonzylamine Hydrochloride.
See: Vanacof APE.
W/Chlorcyclizine Hydrochloride.
See: Dallergy.
W/Chlorcyclizine Hydrochloride, Codeine Phosphate.
See: Nasotuss.
W/Chlorpheniramine Maleate.
See: AccuHist.
AMBI 10PEH/4CPM.
Actifed Cold & Allergy.
Cardec.
Dallergy.
Ed A-Hist.
Ed ChlorPed D.
Extendryl PEM.
LoHist.
Nasohist.
NoHist LQ.
Rescon-Jr.
Virdec.
W/Chlorpheniramine Maleate, Dextromethorphan Hydrobromide.
See: AMBI 10PEH/4CPM/20DM.
Balamine DM.
Cardec DM.
Corfen-DM.
CP DEC-DM.
DM/PE/CPM.
Donatussin DM.
Ed-A-Hist DM.
Father John's Medicine Plus.
Maxichlor PEH DM.
Nasohist DM.
Neo DM.
PE-Hist DM.
Relahist-DM.
Rondec-DM.
Rondex-DM.
Sonahist DM.
TGQ 15DM/5PEH/2CPM.
Trigofen DM.
Virdec DM.
Z-Dex 12D.
ZoDen DM.
W/Chlorpheniramine Maleate, Dextromethorphan Hydrobromide, Guaifenesin.
See: Chlordex GP.
DM/CPM/PE/GG.
Donatussin.
W/Chlorpheniramine Maleate, Hydrocodone Bitartrate.
See: Neo HC.
Notuss-Forte.
Relacon-HC.
W/Chlorpheniramine Maleate, Methscopolamine Nitrate.
See: AeroHist Plus.
AeroKid.
Ah-Chew Ultra.
CPM 8/PE 20/MSC 1.25.
Dehistine.
Denaze.
DriHist SR.
Drysec.
Duradryl.
Duravent.
Duravent-DA.
Extendryl.
NoHist-Plus.
OMNIhist II LA.
PCM.
PE-CPM-MSN 8-2-0.75.
PE HCL-CPM-MSN 10-2-0.75.
Phenylephrine CM.
QV Allergy.
Ralix.
RelCof PE.
Rescon-MX.
ScopoHist.
ScopoHist-PE.
SymPak PDX.
Triall.
Zinx PCM.
W/Chlorpheniramine Maleate, Pyrilamine Maleate.
See: Polyhist PD.
Pyrichlor PE.
Triplex AD.
W/Codeine Phosphate, Diphenhydramine Hydrochloride.
See: Airacof.
W/Codeine Phosphate, Guaifenesin.
See: Giltuss Ped-C.
W/Codeine Phosphate, Promethazine Hydrochloride.
See: Promethazine VC w/Codeine.
W/Codeine Phosphate, Pyrilamine Maleate.
See: Pro-Red AC.
W/Dexbrompheniramine Maleate, Dextromethorphan Hydrobromide.
See: Panatuss DXP.
W/Dexchlorpheniramine Maleate.
See: Ala-Hist PE.
W/Dexchlorpheniramine Maleate, Methscopolamine Nitrate.
See: Extendryl.
Dexphen M.
Re-Drylex.

W/Dextromethorphan Hydrobromide.
See: Little Colds Decongestant Plus Cough.
PediaCare Children's Multi-Symptom Cold.
Theraflu Thin Strips Daytime Cough & Cold.
Triaminic Children's Thin Strips Day Time Cold & Cough.
Triaminic Daytime Cold & Cough.
W/Dextromethorphan Hydrobromide, Guaifenesin.
See: AMBI 10PEH/400GFN/20DM.
Biobron SF.
Biogil.
BioGtuss.
Bio T Pres.
Bio T Pres Pediatric.
Biotuss.
Bio-Tussi.
Bio-Tussi Pediatric.
Broncotron-D.
Brontuss DX.
Dacex PE.
Deconex DM.
Deconex DMX.
Despec NR.
Dynatuss EX.
Endacon.
ExeCof.
ExeTuss-DM.
GFN 1200/DM 20/PE 40.
Giltuss.
Giltuss Pediatric.
Giltuss TR.
Guaifen.
Maxiphen DM.
NeoTuss-D.
Phlemex Forte.
Phlemex-PE.
Robitussin Children's Cough & Cold CF.
SINUtuss DM.
TriTuss.
TriTuss ER.
Tussi-Pres.
Tussi-Pres Pediatric.
Tusso DM.
Tusso DMR.
Tusso XR.
Vanacof DM.
Z-Dex.
Z-Dex Pediatric.
Zotex.
Zotex Pediatric.
W/Dextromethorphan Hydrobromide, Pheniramine Maleate.
See: Theraflu Cold & Cough.
W/Dextromethorphan Hydrobromide, Pyrilamine Maleate.
See: MyHist-DM.
Poly Hist DM.
Pyril DM.
Theraflu Cold & Cough.
W/Dihydrocodeine Bitartrate.
See: Alahist DHC.
W/Dihydrocodeine Bitartrate, Guaifenesin.
See: Donatuss DC.
Poly-Tussin EX.
W/Dihydrocodeine Bitartrate, Pyrilamine Maleate.
See: Poly Hist DHC.
W/Diphenhydramine Hydrochloride.
See: Aldex-CT.
Benadryl-D Children's Allergy & Sinus.
Delsym Children's Night Time Cough & Cold.
Delsym Night Time Cough & Cold.
Dimetapp Children's Nighttime Cold & Congestion.
PediaCare Children's NightRest Multi-Symptom Cold.
Robitussin Pediatric Cough & Cold Nighttime.
Sudafed PE Day & Night.
Sudafed PE Nighttime Nasal Decongestant.
Theraflu Thin Strips Nighttime Cold & Cough.
Triaminic Children's Thin Strips Night Time Cold & Cough.
Triaminic Night Time Cold & Cough.
ZoDen PD.
W/Guaifenesin.
See: Donatussin.
ED Bron GP.
Entex LQ.
ExeTuss GP.
J-Max.
Liquibid D-R.
Liquibid PD-R.
Lusair.
MucaphEd.
Mucinex Children's Stuffy Nose & Cold.
MucusRelief Sinus.
Nu-COPD.
PhenaVent LA.
Reese's OneTab Congestion & Cough.
Refenesen PE.
Rescon 66.
SINUtab PE.
Sudafed PE Non-Drying Sinus.
TG 10PEH/380GFN.
Triaminic Chest & Nasal Congestion.
ZoDen.
W/Hydrocodone Bitartrate, Pyrilamine Maleate.
See: Tussplex.

W/Methscopolamine Nitrate.
See: Extendryl PEM.
W/Thonzylamine Hydrochloride.
See: NasOpen PE.
phenylephrine hydrochloride. (Various Mfr.) Phenylephrine hydrochloride. **Soln.:** 1%. 480 mL. **Ophth. Soln.:** 2.5%, 10%. 2.5 mL, 5 mL (10% only), 15 mL (2.5% only). **Inj.:** 1% (10 mg/mL). Vials. 1 mL, 5 mL. *Rx-OTC.*
Use: Nasal decongestant, arylalkylamine; ophthalmic decongestant; vasopressor used in shock.
phenylephrine tannate.
W/Brompheniramine Tannate.
See: BrōveX ADT.
Relhist.
W/Brompheniramine Tannate, Carbetapentane Tannate.
See: Vazotan Tannate.
W/Brompheniramine Tannate, Dextromethorphan Tannate.
See: Neo DM.
W/Carbetapentane Tannate, Pyrilamine Tannate.
See: Tussi-12D S.
W/Chlorpheniramine Tannate.
See: Phenyl Chlor-Tan Pediatric.
Ry-Tann.
TanalHist-D Pediatric.
Tannate Pediatric.
W/Chlorpheniramine Tannate, Methscopolamine Nitrate.
See: AH-Chew.
AH-Chew Ultra.
Redur-PCM.
W/Pyrilamine Maleate.
See: Poly Hist Forte.
Pyril D.
•**phenylethyl alcohol.** (fen-ill-ETH-ill) *USP.*
Use: Pharmaceutic aid, antimicrobial.
phenyl-ethyl-hydrazine, beta. Phenelzine dihydrogen sulfate.
See: Nardil.
phenylethylmalonylurea.
See: Phenobarbital.
Phenyl-Free 1. (Mead Johnson Nutritionals) Corn syr. solids 49.2%, casein hydrolysate 18.7% (enzymic digest of casein containing amino acids and small peptides), corn oil 18%, modified tapioca starch 9.57%, protein equivalent 15%, fat 18%, carbohydrate 60%, minerals (ash) 3.6%, phenylalanine 75 mg/100 g pow., vitamins A 1600 units, D 400 units, E 10 units, C 52 mg, folic acid 100 mcg, B_1 0.5 mg, B_2 0.6 mg, niacin 8 mg, B_6 0.4 mg, B_{12} 2 mcg, biotin 0.05 mg, pantothenic acid 3 mg, vitamin K-1 100 mcg, choline 85 mg, inositol 30 mg, Ca 600 mg, P 450 mg, I 45 mcg, Fe 12 mg, Mg 70 mg, Cu 0.6 mg, Zn 4 mg, Mn 1 mg, C 450 mg, K 650 mg, Na 300 mg/qt. at normal dilution of 20 k cal/fl oz, Can 2 1/2 lb. *OTC.*
Use: Nutritional supplement.
Phenylhistine DH. (Qualitest) Chlorpheniramine maleate 2 mg, codeine phosphate 10 mg, pseudoephedrine hydrochloride 30 mg. Alcohol 5%, saccharin, sorbitol, sucrose. Liq. 118 mL, 473 mL. *c-v.*
Use: Upper respiratory combination, antitussive combination.
phenylic acid.
See: Phenol.
phenylketonuria agents.
See: Dihydrochloride.
Sapropterin.
•**phenylmercuric acetate.** (fen-ill-mer-CURE-ik ASS-eh-tate) *NF.*
Use: Pharmaceutic aid, antimicrobial; preservative, bacteriostatic.
W/Benzocaine, chlorothymol, resorcin.
See: Lanacane.
phenylmercuric acetate. (Various Mfr.) Phenylmercuric acetate. Bot. 1 lb, 5 lb, 10 lb.
Use: Pharmaceutic aid, antimicrobial; preservative, bacteriostatic.
phenylmercuric borate. (F. W. Berk) Pkg. Custom packed.
W/Benzyl alcohol, benzocaine, butyl p-aminobenzoate.
See: Dermathyn.
phenylmercuric chloride. Chlorophenylmercury.
•**phenylmercuric nitrate.** (fen-ill-mer-CURE-ik) *NF.*
Use: Pharmaceutic aid, antimicrobial; preservative, bacteriostatic.
W/Amyl, phenylphenol complex.
See: Lubraseptic Jelly.
phenylmercuric nitrate. (A.P.L.) Phenylmercuric nitrate. **Oint. 1:1500:** 1 oz, 4 oz, lb. (Chicago Pharm) Loz. w/benzocaine. Bot. 100s, 1000s. **Ophth. Oint., 1:3000:** Tube ⅛ oz. **Soln. 1:20,000:** Bot. pt, gal. **Vaginal supp., 1:5000:** Box 12s.
Use: Pharmaceutic aid, antimicrobial; preservative, bacteriostatic.
phenylmercuric picrate.
Use: Antimicrobial.
phenylphenol-o.
W/Amyl complex, phenylmercuric nitrate.
See: Lubraseptic.
phenylpropylmethylamine hydrochloride. Vonedrine hydrochloride.
phenyl salicylate.
See: Salol.

W/Atropine Sulfate, Benzoic Acid, Hyoscyamine Sulfate, Methenamine, Methylene Blue.
See: Uritact DS.
W/Benzoic Acid, Hyoscyamine Sulfate, Methenamine, Methylene Blue.
See: Hyophen.
W/Hyoscyamine Sulfate, Methenamine, Methylene Blue, Sodium Biphosphate.
See: Urimax.
W/Hyoscyamine Sulfate, Methenamine, Methylene Blue, Sodium Phosphate Monobasic.
See: Phosphasal.
Uticap.
Utrona-C.
phenyl-tert-butylamine.
See: Phentermine.
phenylthilone.
Use: Anticonvulsant.
•**phenyltoloxamine citrate.** *USP.*
Use: Antihistamine.
W/Acetaminophen.
See: Biphenox.
Pain-gesic.
Relagesic.
Zflex.
W/Acetaminophen, Aspirin, Caffeine, Salicylamide.
See: Levacet.
W/Acetaminophen, Caffeine, Magnesium Salicylate.
See: Durabac Forte.
W/Acetaminophen, Caffeine, Salicylamide.
See: Durabac.
W/Acetaminophen, Chlorpheniramine Maleate, Phenylephrine Hydrochloride.
See: Trital SR.
W/Acetaminophen, Salicylamide.
See: Duraxin.
Ed-Flex.
W/Hyoscyamine Sulfate.
See: Digex NF.
Phenylzin. (Ciba Vision) Zinc sulfate 0.25%, phenylephrine hydrochloride 0.12%. Bot. 15 mL. *Rx.*
Use: Decongestant, ophthalmic.
•**phenyramidol hydrochloride.** (FEN-ih-RAM-ih-dole) USAN.
Use: Analgesic; muscle relaxant.
Phenytek. (Mylan) Phenytoin extended 200 mg, 300 mg. Cap. 30s, 100s. *Rx.*
Use: Anticonvulsant, hydantoin.
•**phenytoin.** (FEN-ih-toe-in) *USP. Formerly Diphenylhydantoin.*
Use: Anticonvulsant.
See: Dilantin.
Dilantin-125.
Phenytek.
Phenytoin Infatabs.
phenytoin. (Mylan) Phenytoin 50 mg. May contain sugar. Chew. Tab. 100s, 500s. *Rx.*
Use: Anticonvulsant, hydantoin.
phenytoin. (Various Mfr.) Phenytoin 125 mg per 5 mL. May contain alcohol, sucrose, sodium benzoate, glycerin. Susp. 240 mL. *Rx.*
Use: Anticonvulsant, hydantoin.
Phenytoin Infatabs. (Greenstone) Phenytoin 50 mg. May contain saccharin, sucrose. Chew. Tab. 100s. *Rx.*
Use: Anticonvulsant, hydantoin.
•**phenytoin sodium.** (FEN-ih-toe-in) *USP. Formerly Diphenylhydantoin Sodium.*
Use: Anticonvulsant; cardiac depressant, antiarrhythmic.
See: Dilantin.
W/Phenobarbital.
See: Dilantin with Phenobarbital Kapseals.
phenytoin sodium. (Caraco) Phenytoin sodium 200 mg, 300 mg. ER Cap. 30s, 100s, 500s. *Rx.*
Use: Anticonvulsant, hydantoin.
phenytoin sodium. (Wockhardt USA) Phenytoin sodium 30 mg. ER Cap. 100s, 1,000s. *Rx.*
Use: Anticonvulsant, hydantoin.
phenytoin sodium. (Various Mfr.) Phenytoin sodium. **ER Cap.:** 30 mg, 100 mg. May contain lactose, mannitol, sugar (100 mg). 100s, 1,000s (30 mg); 30s, 100s, 500s, 1,000s, UD 100s (100 mg). **Inj., Soln.:** 50 mg/mL. May contain alcohol, propylene glycol. 2 mL, 5 mL. *Rx.*
Use: Anticonvulsant, hydantoin.
pheochromocytoma, agents for.
See: Metyrosine.
Phenoxybenzamine Hydrochloride.
Phentolamine Mesylate.
Pherazine DM. (Halsey Drug) Promethazine 6.25 mg, dextromethorphan HBr 15 mg, alcohol 7%/5 mL. Bot. 4 oz, 6 oz, pt, gal. *Rx.*
Use: Antihistamine; antitussive.
Pherazine VC. (Halsey Drug) Phenylephrine hydrochloride 5 mg, promethazine hydrochloride 6.25 mg, alcohol 7%/5 mL. Syr. Bot. Pt, gal. *Rx.*
Use: Antihistamine; decongestant.
Pherazine VC with Codeine. (Halsey Drug) Phenylephrine hydrochloride 5 mg, promethazine hydrochloride 6.25 mg, codeine phosphate 10 mg, alcohol 7%/5 mL. Syr. Bot. Pt, gal. *c-v.*
Use: Antihistamine; antitussive; decongestant.
Pherazine w/Codeine. (Halsey Drug) Promethazine hydrochloride 6.25 mg, codeine phosphate 10 mg/5 mL, alcohol

7%, sorbitol, sucrose. Syr. Bot. 120 mL, pt, gal. *c-v.*
Use: Antihistamine; antitussive.

phethenylate. Also sodium salt.

Phicon. (T.E. Williams Pharmaceuticals) Pramoxine hydrochloride 0.5%, vitamin A 7500 units, E 2000 units/30 g. Cream. Tube 60 g. *OTC.*
Use: Emollient.

Phicon F. (T.E. Williams Pharmaceuticals) Undecylenic acid 8%, pramoxine hydrochloride 0.05%. Cream. 60 g. *OTC.*
Use: Anesthetic, local; antifungal.

Philith. (Northstar) Ethinyl estradiol 35 mcg, norethindrone 0.4 mg. Lactose, PEG. Tab. 28s w/7 inert tablets (lactose, PEG). *Rx.*
Use: Monophasic oral contraceptive.

Phillips'. (Bayer Consumer Care) Magnesium (as magnesium oxide) 500 mg. Polyvinyl alcohol. Tab. 24s. *OTC.*
Use: Laxative.

Phillips' Chewable. (Bayer Consumer Care) Magnesium hydroxide 311 mg. Tab. 100s, 200s.
Use: Laxative, antacid.

Phillips' Colon Health. (Bayer Consumer Care) 1.5 billion cell blend of *L. acidophilus, B. bifidum, B. longum.* Cap. 30s. *OTC.*
Use: Probiotic.

Phillips' Colon Health Probiotic Fiber. (Bayer Consumer Care) 1 billion cell blend of *L. acidophilus, B. bifidum, B. longum* per 3.3 g. Pow. 3.5 oz. *OTC.*
Use: Probiotic.

Phillips' LaxCaps. (Bayer Consumer Care) Docusate sodium 83 mg, phenolphthalein 90 mg. Cap. Bot. 8s, 24s, 48s. *OTC.*
Use: Laxative.

Phillips' Liqui-Gels. (Bayer Consumer Care) Docusate sodium 100 mg, parabens, sorbitol. Softgel Cap. Bot. 10s, 30s, 50s. *OTC.*
Use: Laxative.

Phillips' Milk of Magnesia. (Bayer Consumer Care) Magnesium hydroxide 400 mg/5 mL, saccharin (mint), sorbitol, sugar (cherry), mint, cherry, regular flavors. Susp. Bot. 120 mL, 360 mL, 780 mL. *OTC.*
Use: Laxative; antacid.

Phillips' Milk of Magnesia Concentrated. (Bayer Consumer Care) Magnesium hydroxide 800 mg/5 mL, sorbitol, sugar, strawberry creme flavor. Susp. Bot. 240 mL. *OTC.*
Use: Laxative; antacid.

Phish Omega. (Pharmics) Natural salmon oil concentrate containing EPA 120 mg, DHA 100 mg. Cap. Bot. 60s. *OTC.*
Use: Vitamin supplement.

Phish Omega Plus. (Pharmics) Natural fish oil concentrate containing EPA 300 mg, DHA 200 mg. Cap. Bot. 60s. *OTC.*
Use: Vitamin supplement.

pHisoDerm. (Chattem) Sodium octoxynol-2 ethane sulfonate, white petrolatum, water, mineral oil (with lanolin alcohol and oleyl alcohol), sodium benzoate, octoxynol-3, tetrasodium EDTA, methylcellulose, cocamide MEA, imidazolidinyl urea. **Regular:** 150 mL, 270 mL, 480 mL, gal. **Oily skin:** 150 mL, 480. *OTC.*
Use: Dermatologic, cleanser.

pHisoDerm for Baby. (Chattem) Sodium octoxynol-2 ethane sulfonate, petrolatum, octoxynol-3, mineral oil (with lanolin alcohol and oleyl alcohol), cocamide MEA, imidazolidinyl urea, sodium benzoate, tetrasodium EDTA, methylcellulose, hydrochloric acid. Liq. Bot. 150 mL, 270 mL. *OTC.*
Use: Dermatologic, cleanser.

pHisoHex. (Sanofi-Synthelabo) Entsufon sodium, hexachlorophene 3%, petrolatum, lanolin cholesterols, methylcellulose, polyethylene glycol, polyethylene glycol monostearate, lauryl myristyl diethanolamide, sodium benzoate, water, pH adjusted with hydrochloric acid. Emulsion, Bot. 5 oz, pt, gal. Wall dispensers pt. Unit packets 0.25 oz. Box 50s, Pedal operated dispenser 30 oz. *OTC.*
Use: Antimicrobial, antiseptic.

pHisoMed. (Sanofi-Synthelabo) Hexachlorophene. *OTC.*
Use: Antimicrobial; antiseptic.

pHisoPuff. (Sanofi-Synthelabo) Nonmedicated cleansing sponge. Box sponge 1s. *OTC.*
Use: Dermatologic, cleanser.

P-Hist DM. (Midlothian Laboratories) Dextromethorphan HBr 5 mg, brompheniramine maleate 1 mg, pseudoephedrine hydrochloride 12 mg per 1 mL. Alcohol and dye free. Magnasweet, menthol, sucrose. Grape flavor. Concentrate Soln. 30 mL with dropper. *Rx.*
Use: Pediatric antitussive combination.

Phlemex Forte. (Cypress) Dextromethorphan HBr 30 mg, guaifenesin 1200 mg, phenylephrine hydrochloride 30 mg. Dye free. ER Tab. 100s. *Rx.*
Use: Upper respiratory combination, antitussive and expectorant combination.

Phlemex-PE. (Cypress) Phenylephrine hydrochloride 20 mg, dextromethorphan HBr 20 mg, guaifenesin 800 mg. ER Tab. 100s. *Rx.*
Use: Antitussive and expectorant combination, upper respiratory combination.

PhosChol. (American Lecithin) Phosphatidylcholine (highly purified lecithin). **Softgel:** 565 mg, 900 mg. Bot. 100s, 300s. **Liq. Conc.:** 3000 mg/5 mL. Bot. 240 mL, 480 mL. *OTC.*
Use: Nutritional supplement.

phoscolic acid.
Use: Adjuvant.

Phos-Flur Oral Rinse Supplement. (Colgate Oral Pharmaceuticals) Acidulated phosphate sodium fluoride 0.05%, fluoride 1 mL/5 mL. Bot. 250 mL, 500 mL, gal. *Rx.*
Use: Dental caries preventative.

PhosLo. (Fresenius) Calcium acetate. **Cap.:** 667 mg (elemental calcium 169 mg). Polyethylene glycol 8000. 200s. **Gelcap:** 667 mg (elemental calcium 169 mg). Polyethylene glycol 8000. 200s. *Rx.*
Use: Mineral supplement.

PHOS-NaK. (Cypress) Potassium 280 mg, phosphorus 250 mg, sodium 160 mg/packet, fruit flavor. Pow. Packets. 1.5 g (100s). *OTC.*
Use: Phosphorus replacement.

Phosphasal. (BioComp Pharma) Hyoscyamine sulfate 0.12 mg, methenamine 81.6 mg, methylene blue 10.8 mg, phenyl salicylate 36.2 mg, sodium phosphate monobasic 40.8 mg. PEG. Tab. 100s. *Rx.*
Use: Anti-infective, methenamine combination.

phosphate.
See: Potassium Phosphate.
Sodium Phosphate.

phosphate binders.
Use: Phosphate reduction.
See: Lanthanum Carbonate.
Sevelamer Carbonate.
Sevelamer Hydrochloride.

Phospha 250 Neutral. (Rising Pharmaceuticals) Dibasic sodium phosphate 852 mg, monobasic potassium phosphate 155 mg, monobasic sodium phosphate 130 mg (contains potassium 1.1 mEq, sodium 13 mEq). Film-coated. Tab. 100s. *Rx.*
Use: Urinary acidifier, acid phosphate.

phosphentaside. Adenosine-5-monophosphate. Adenylic acid.

phosphocysteamine.
Use: Cystinosis. [Orphan Drug]

phosphodiesterase type 5 inhibitors.
Use: Impotence agents.
See: Avanafil.
Sildenafil Citrate.
Tadalafil.
Vardenafil Hydrochloride.

phosphonoformic acid.
See: Foscarnet sodium.

phosphorated carbohydrate solution.
See: Emetrol.
Nausea Relief.
Nausatrol.
Nausetrol.

•**phosphoric acid.** (fos-FORE-ik) *NF.*
Use: Pharmaceutic aid, solvent.
W/Dextrose, Fructose.
See: Emetrol.
Nausatrol.
Nausea Relief.
Nausetrol.

phosphoric acid, diluted.
Use: Pharmaceutic aid, solvent.

phosphorus.
Use: Phosphorus replacement.
See: K-Phos Neutral.
PHOS-NaK.
Uro-KP-Neutral.
W/Calcium Glycerophosphate.
See: Prelief.

Phospho-Soda. (C.B. Fleet) Sodium biphosphate 48 g, sodium phosphate 18 g/100 mL. Bot. 1.5 oz, 3 oz, 8 oz. Flavored, unflavored. *OTC.*
Use: Laxative.

Phosphotec. (Bristol-Myers Squibb) Technetium Tc-99m pyrophosphate kit. 10 vials/kit.
Use: Radiodiagnostic.

photochemotherapy.
See: Aminolevulinic acid hydrochloride.
Methoxasalen.
Methyl Aminolevulinate.
Psoralens.
Tar-containing preparations.

photochemotherapy, ophthalmic.
See: Verteporfin.
Visudyne.

Photofrin. (Pinnacle Biologics) Porfimer sodium 75 mg. Preservative free. Freeze-dried cake or Pow. for Inj. Vial. *Rx.*
Use: Antineoplastic.

Photoplex Sunscreen. (Allergan) Butyl methoxydibenzoylmethane 3%, padimate O 7%. Lot. 120 mL. *OTC.*
Use: Sunscreen.

Phrenilin Forte. (Valeant) Acetaminophen 650 mg, butalbital 50 mg, benzyl alcohol, parabens, EDTA. Cap. Bot. 100s, 500s. *Rx.*
Use: Analgesic; hypnotic; sedative.

Phrenilin w/Caffeine and Codeine. (Valeant) Codeine phosphate 30 mg, acetaminophen 325 mg, caffeine 40 mg, butalbital 50 mg. Cap. 100s. *c-III.*
Use: Narcotic analgesic.

Phresh 3.5 Finnish Cleansing Liquid. (3M) Water, cocamidopropyl betaine, lactic acid, polyoxyethylene distearate, polyoxyethylene monostearate, hydroxyethyl cellulose, sodium phosphate, methylparaben. Bot. 6 oz. *OTC.*
Use: Soapless cleansing agent.

pH-Stabil. (Healthpoint Medical) Skin protection cream. Bot. 8 oz. Cream. Tube 2 oz. *OTC.*
Use: Dermatologic.

Phthalamaquin. (Penick) Quinetolate.
Use: Antiasthmatic.

phthalazine, i-hydrazino-, monohydrochloride. Hydralazine hydrochloride.

phthalazinones, peripherally selective.
Use: Antihistamine.
See: Azelastine Hydrochloride.

phylcardin.
See: Aminophylline.

phyllindon.
See: Aminophylline.

Phylorinol. (Schaffer) Phenol 0.6%, boric acid, strong iodine solution, sorbitol 70% solution, sodium copper chlorophyll. Liq. Bot. 240 mL. *OTC.*
Use: Mouth and throat preparation.

Phylorinol Mouthwash. (Schaffer) Phenol 0.6%, methyl salicylate, sorbitol. Bot. 240 mL. *OTC.*
Use: Mouth and throat preparation.

physical adjuncts.
See: Calcium Hydroxylapatite.
Hyaluronan.
Hyaluronic Acid.
Hyaluronidase.
Poly-l-lactic Acid.

physiological irrigating solution.
See: Physiolyte.
Physiosol.
TIS-U-SOL.

Physiolyte. (McGaw) Sodium Cl 530 mg, sodium acetate 370 mg, sodium gluconate 500 mg, potassium Cl 37 mg, magnesium Cl 30 mg/100 mL. Soln. Bot. 500 mL, 2 L, 4 L. *Rx.*
Use: Irrigant, ophthalmic.

Physiosol Irrigation. (Hospira) Bot. 250 mL, 500 mL, 1000 mL glass or Aqualite (semirigid) containers. *Rx.*
Use: Irrigant, ophthalmic.

•**physostigmine salicylate.** (FYE-soe-STIG-meen) *USP.*
Use: Anticholinergic.
See: Antilirium.

physostigmine salicylate. (Akorn) Physostigmine salicylate 1 mg/mL. Benzyl alcohol 2%, sodium metabisulfite 0.1%. Inj. Amp. 2 mL. *Rx.*
Use: Cholinergic, antidote.

•**physostigmine sulfate.** (FYE-soe-STIG-meen) *USP.*
Use: Cholinergic, ophthalmic.

•**phytate persodium.** (FIE-tate per-SO-dee-uhm) USAN.
Use: Pharmaceutic aid.

•**phytate sodium.** (FYE-tate) USAN. Sodium salt of inositol hexaphosphoric acid.
Use: Chelating agent, calcium.

phytic acid. Inositol hexophosphoric acid.

•**phytonadione.** (fye-toe-nuh-DIE-ohn) *USP.*
Use: Fat-soluble vitamin.
See: Vitamin K.

phytonadione. (Hospira) Vitamin K 2 mg/mL, 10 mg/mL. Dextrose, benzyl alcohol 9 mg. Inj. Emulsion. Ampuls. 0.5 mL (2 mg/mL only), 1 mL (10 mg/mL only). *Rx.*
Use: Fat-soluble vitamin.

•**piboserod hydrochloride.** (pi-BOE-ser-od) USAN.
Use: Irritable bowel syndrome.

Picato. (LEO Pharma Inc) Ingenol mebutate 0.015%, 0.05%. Benzyl alcohol, isopropyl alcohol. Gel. Single-use tube. *Rx.*
Use: Topical immunomodulator.

•**picenadol hydrochloride.** (pih-SEN-AID-ole) USAN.
Use: Analgesic.

•**piclamilast.** (pih-KLAM-ill-ast) USAN.
Use: Antiasthmatic, type IV phosphodiesterase inhibitor.

•**picoplatin.** (PI-koe-PLA-tin) USAN.
Use: Antineoplastic.

•**picotrin diolamine.** (PIH-koe-trin die-OH-lah-meen) USAN.
Use: Keratolytic.

picrotoxin. Cocculin.
Use: Respiratory.

•**pictilisib.** (pik-TIL-i-sib) USAN.
Use: Antineoplastic.

•**picumeterol fumarate.** (PIKE-you-MEH-teh-role) USAN.
Use: Bronchodilator.

•**pidilizumab.** (PI-di-LIZ-ue-mab) USAN.
Use: Antineoplastic.

•**pifarnine.** (pih-FAR-neen) USAN.
Use: Antiulcerative, gastric.

pigment agent combinations.
See: Solage.
Tri-Luma.

pigment agents.
See: Dihydroxyacetone.
Hydroquinone.
Monobenzone.

•**pilocarpine.** (PYE-loe-KAR-peen) *USP.*
Use: Antiglaucoma; ophthalmic cholinergic; miotic.

•**pilocarpine hydrochloride.** (PYE-loe-KAR-peen) *USP.*
Use: Cholinergic, ophthalmic; topically as a miotic, xerostomia and keratoconjunctivitis sicca; mouth and throat product. [Orphan Drug]
See: Isopto Carpine.
Piloptic.
Salagen.

pilocarpine hydrochloride. (Actavis Elizabeth) Pilocarpine hydrochloride 5 mg, 7.5 mg. Film-coated. Tab. 100s. *Rx.*
Use: Mouth and throat products.

pilocarpine hydrochloride. (Sandoz) Pilocarpine hydrochloride 5 mg. Tab. 100s. *Rx.*
Use: Treatment of dry mouth.

pilocarpine hydrochloride. (Various Mfr.) Pilocarpine hydrochloride. **0.5%:** 15 mL, 30 mL. **1%:** 2 mL, 15 mL, 30 mL, UD 1 mL. **2%, 4%:** 2 mL, 15 mL, 30 mL. **6%:** 15 mL.
Use: Cholinergic, ophthalmic; topically as a miotic, xerostomia and keratoconjunctivitis sicca. [Orphan Drug]

•**pilocarpine nitrate.** (PYE-loe-KAR-peen) *USP.*
Use: Cholinergic, ophthalmic.

Piloptic. (Optopics) Pilocarpine hydrochloride 0.5%, 1%, 2%, 3%, 4%, 6%. Soln. Bot. 15 mL. *Rx.*
Use: Antiglaucoma.

Pilostat. (Bausch & Lomb) Pilocarpine hydrochloride 0.5%, 1%, 2%, 3%, 4%, 6%. Soln. Bot. 15 mL, twinpack 2 × 15 mL. *Rx.*
Use: Antiglaucoma.

Pima. (Fleming & Co.) Potassium iodide 325 mg/5 mL. Sugar. Black-raspberry flavor. Syrup. Pt., gal. *Rx.*
Use: Thyroid drug.

•**pimagedine hydrochloride.** (pih-MAH-jeh-deen) USAN.
Use: Inhibitor (advanced glycosylation end-product formation inhibitors).

•**pimasertib.** (PIM-a-SER-tib) USAN.
Use: Antineoplastic.

•**pimecrolimus.** (PIM-e-KROE-li-mus) USAN.
Use: Immunomodulator, topical.
See: Elidel.

•**pimetine hydrochloride.** (PIM-eh-teen) USAN.
Use: Antihyperlipoproteinemic.

piminodine esylate.
Use: Analgesic.

piminodine ethanesulfonate.
Use: Analgesic; narcotic.

•**pimobendan.** (pie-MOE-ben-dan) USAN.
Use: Cardiovascular agent.

•**pimozide.** (pih-moe-ZIDE) *USP.*
Use: Antipsychotic.
See: Orap.

•**pinacidil.** (pie-NASS-ih-DILL) USAN.
Use: Antihypertensive.

•**pinadoline.** (pih-nah-DOE-leen) USAN.
Use: Analgesic.

•**pindolol.** (PIN-doe-lahl) *USP.*
Use: Antiadrenergic/sympatholytic, beta-adrenergic blocking agent, vasodilator.
See: Visken.

pindolol. (Various Mfr.) Pindolol 5 mg, 10 mg. Tab. Bot. 100s, 500s, 1000s. *Rx.*
Use: Antiadrenergic/sympatholytic, beta-adrenergic blocker.

pine needle oil.
Use: Perfume; flavor.

pine tar.
Use: Local antieczematic; rubefacient.

pine tar oil.
See: Grandpa's Wonder Pine Tar Conditioner.

Pinex Concentrate Cough. (Last) Dextromethorphan HBr 7.5 mg/5 mL (after diluting 3 oz. concentrate to make 16 oz. solution). Syr. Bot. 3 oz. *OTC.*
Use: Antitussive.

Pinex Cough. (Last) Dextromethorphan HBr 7.5 mg/5 mL. Syr. Bot. 3 oz, 6 oz. *OTC.*
Use: Antitussive.

Pinex Regular. (Last) Potassium guaiacolsulfonate, oil of pine and eucalyptus, extract of grindelia, alcohol 3%/30 mL. Syr. Bot. 3 oz, 8 oz. Also cherry flavored 3 oz. Super and concentrated 3 oz. *OTC.*
Use: Expectorant.

Pink Bismuth. (Ivax) Pink bismuth 130 mg/15 mL. Liq. Bot. 240 mL. *OTC.*
Use: Antidiarrheal.

Pinnacaine. (Sircle Labs) Benzocaine 20%, benzethonium chloride, glycerin, PEG. Soln.; Otic. 15 mL w/dropper. *Rx.*
Use: Miscellaneous otic preparation.

•**pinoxepin hydrochloride.** (pih-NOX-eh-PIN) USAN.
Use: Antipsychotic.

Pin-Rid. (Apothecary Prods.) Pyrantel pamoate 180 mg (equivalent to 62.5 mg

pyrantel base). Cap., soft gel. 24s. *OTC.*
Use: Anthelmintic.

Pin-X. (Effcon) **Chew. Tab.:** Pyrantel pamoate 720.5 mg (equiv. to pyrantel base 250 mg). Dextrose, maltodextrin, sorbitol. Orange flavor. 12s. **Susp.:** Pyrantel pamoate 50 mg/mL. Parabens, sorbitol. Caramel flavor. 30 mL. *OTC.*
Use: Anthelmintic.

•**pioglitazone hydrochloride.** (PIE-oh-GLIH-tah-zone) USAN.
Use: Antidiabetic.
See: Actos.
W/Alogliptin Benzoate.
See: Oseni.
W/Glimepiride.
See: Duetact.
W/Metformin Hydrochloride.
See: ActoPlus Met.
ActoPlus Met XR.

pioglitazone hydrochloride. (Mylan) Pioglitazone hydrochloride 15 mg, 30 mg, 45 mg. Lactose. Tab. 30s, 90s, 500s. *Rx.*
Use: Antidiabetic agent, thiazolidinedione.

pioglitazone hydrochloride/glimepiride. (Sandoz) Pioglitazone hydrochloride/glimepiride 30 mg/2 mg, 30 mg/4 mg. Lactose. Tab. 30s, 1,000s, UD 28s. *Rx.*
Use: Antidiabetic combination product.

pioglitazone hydrochloride/metformin hydrochloride. (Mylan) Pioglitazone hydrochloride/metformin hydrochloride 15 mg/500 mg, 15 mg/850 mg. PEG, polydextrose. Tab. 60s, 180s, 500s (15 mg/850 mg only), 1,000s (15 mg/500 mg only). *Rx.*
Use: Antidiabetic combination.

•**pipamperone.** (pih-PAM-peer-OHN) USAN. *Formerly Floropipamide.*
Use: Antipsychotic.

•**pipazethate.** (pip-AZZ-eh-thate) USAN.
Use: Cough suppressant; antitussive.

pipazethate hydrochloride.
Use: Antitussive.

•**piperacetazine.** (pih-PURR-ah-SET-ah-zeen) USAN.
Use: Antipsychotic.

•**piperacillin.** (PI-per-a-SIL-in) *USP.*
Use: Anti-infective.

•**piperacillin sodium.** (PI-per-a-SIL-in) *USP.*
Use: Anti-infective.

piperacillin sodium and tazobactam sodium.
Use: Anti-infective.
See: Zosyn.

piperacillin sodium/tazobactam sodium. (WG Critical Care) Piperacillin/tazobactam 40.5 g (as piperacillin sodium 36 g/tazobactam sodium 4.5 g). Preservative free. Inj., Pow. for Soln. Bulk vial (contains sodium 2.35 mEq (54 mg) per gram of piperacillin. *Rx.*
Use: Penicillin, extended-spectrum penicillin.

piperacillin sodium/tazobactam sodium. (Various Mfr.) Piperacillin/tazobactam 2 g/0.25 g, 3 g/0.375 g, 4 g/0.5 g. Sodium 108 mg (2 g/0.25 g), 162 mg (3 g/0.375 g), 216 mg (4 g/0.5 g). Preservative free. Inj., Pow. for Soln., concentrate. Single-dose vial. *Rx.*
Use: Penicillin, extended-spectrum penicillin.

•**piperamide maleate.** (PIH-per-ah-mid) USAN.
Use: Anthelmintic.

•**piperazine.** (pi-PER-a-zeen) *USP.*
Use: Anthelmintic.

•**piperazine citrate.** (pi-PER-a-zeen) *USP.* Piperazine Citrate Telra Hydrous Tripiperazine Dicitrate.
Use: Anthelmintic.
See: Bryrel.
Ta-Verm.

•**piperazine edetate calcium.** (pi-PER-a-zeen) USAN.
Use: Anthelmintic.

piperazine estrone sulfate.
See: Estropipate.

piperazine hexahydrate. Tivazine.

piperazine phosphate.
Use: Anthelmintic.

piperazines, nonselective.
Use: Antihistamine.
See: Chlorcyclizine Hydrochloride.
Hydroxyzine.

piperazines, peripherally selective.
Use: Antihistamine.
See: Cetirizine Hydrochloride.
Dihydrochloride.
Levocetirizine Dihydrochloride.

piperidine phosphate.
Use: Psychiatric drug.

piperidines, nonselective.
Use: Antihistamine.
See: Cyproheptadine.
Phenindamine Tartrate.

piperidines, peripherally selective.
Use: Antihistamine.
See: Desloratadine.
Fexofenadine Hydrochloride.
Loratadine.

piperidolate hydrochloride.
Use: Anticholinergic.

piperonyl butoxide.
Use: Pediculicide.
W/Pyrethrins.
See: RID.

piperoxan hydrochloride. Fourneau 933. Benzodioxane. Diagnosis of hypertension.
Use: Diagnostic aid.

pipethanate hydrochloride.
Use: Anxiolytic.

•**piposulfan.** (PIP-oh-SULL-fan) USAN.
Use: Antineoplastic.

•**pipotiazine palmitate.** (PIP-oh-TIE-ah-zeen PAL-mih-tate) USAN.
Use: Antipsychotic.

•**pipoxolan hydrochloride.** (pih-POX-oh-lan) USAN.
Use: Muscle relaxant.

•**piprozolin.** (PIP-row-ZOE-lin) USAN.
Use: Choleretic.

•**piquindone hydrochloride.** (PIH-kwin-dohn) USAN.
Use: Antipsychotic.

•**piquizil hydrochloride.** (PIH-kwih-zill) USAN.
Use: Bronchodilator.

•**piracetam.** (pir-A-se-tam) USAN.
Use: Cognition adjuvant; cerebral stimulant, myoclonus. [Orphan Drug]

•**pirandamine hydrochloride.** (pih-RAN-dah-meen) USAN.
Use: Antidepressant.

•**pirazmonam sodium.** (pihr-AZZ-moe-nam) USAN.
Use: Antimicrobial.

•**pirazolac.** (PIHR-AZE-oh-lack) USAN.
Use: Antirheumatic.

•**pirbenicillin sodium.** (pihr-ben-IH-SILL-in) USAN.
Use: Anti-infective.

•**pirbuterol acetate.** (pihr-BUE-ter-ol) USAN.
Use: Bronchodilator, sympathomimetic.
See: Maxair Autohaler.

•**pirbuterol hydrochloride.** (pihr-BUE-ter-ol) USAN.
Use: Bronchodilator.

•**pirenperone.** (PIHR-en-PURR-ohn) USAN.
Use: Anxiolytic.

•**pirenzepine hydrochloride.** (PIHR-en-zeh-PEEN) USAN.
Use: Antiulcerative.

•**piretanide.** (pihr-ETT-ah-nide) USAN.
Use: Diuretic.

•**pirfenidone.** (PEER-FEN-ih-dohn) USAN.
Use: Analgesic; anti-inflammatory; antipyretic.

Piridazol.
See: Sulfapyridine.

•**piridicillin sodium.** (pihr-RIH-dih-SILL-in) USAN.
Use: Anti-infective.

•**piridronate sodium.** (pihr-IH-DROE-nate) USAN.
Use: Regulator, calcium.

•**piriprost.** (PIR-i-prost) USAN.
Use: Antiasthmatic.

•**piriprost potassium.** (PIR-i-prost) USAN.
Use: Antiasthmatic.

piriton.
See: Chlorpheniramine.

•**piritrexim isethionate.** (pih-rih-TREX-im eye-seh-THIGH-oh-nate) USAN.
Use: Antiproliferative. [Orphan Drug]

•**pirlimycin hydrochloride.** (PIHR-lih-MY-sin) USAN.
Use: Anti-infective.

•**pirmagrel.** (PIHR-mah-GRELL) USAN.
Use: Inhibitor, thromboxane synthetase.

Pirmella 1/35. (Lupin) Ethinyl estradiol 35 mcg, norethindrone 1 mg. Lactose. Tab. 28s w/7 inert tablets (lactose). *Rx.*
Use: Monophasic oral contraceptive.

Pirmella 7/7/7. (Lupin) **Phase 1:** Ethinyl estradiol 35 mcg, norethindrone 0.5 mg. 7s. **Phase 2:** Ethinyl estradiol 35 mcg, norethindrone 0.75 mg. 7s. **Phase 3:** Ethinyl estradiol 35 mcg, norethindrone 1 mg. 7s. Lactose. 7 inert tablets (lactose). *Rx.*
Use: Triphasic oral contraceptive.

•**pirmenol hydrochloride.** (PIHR-MEH-nahl) USAN.
Use: Cardiovascular agent, antiarrhythmic.

•**pirnabine.** (PIHR-NAH-bean) USAN.
Use: Antiglaucoma agent.

•**piroctone.** (pir-OK-tone) USAN.
Use: Antiseborrheic.

•**piroctone olamine.** (pir-OK-tone OLE-a-meen) USAN.
Use: Antiseborrheic.

•**pirodavir.** (pih-ROW-dav-ihr) USAN.
Use: Antiviral.

•**piroglide tartrate.** (PIHR-oh-GLIE-ride) USAN.
Use: Antidiabetic.

•**pirolate.** (PIHR-oh-late) USAN.
Use: Antiasthmatic.

•**pirolazamide.** (PIHR-ole-aze-ah-mide) USAN.
Use: Cardiovascular agent, antiarrhythmic.

•**piroxantrone hydrochloride.** (PIH-row-ZAN-trone) USAN.
Use: Antineoplastic.

•**piroxicam.** (phr-OX-i-kam) *USP.*
Use: Anti-inflammatory.
See: Feldene.

piroxicam. (Various Mfr.) Piroxicam

10 mg, 20 mg. Cap. Bot. 100s; 500s, 1000s, UD 100s (10 mg only). *Rx.*
Use: Nonsteroidal anti-inflammatory agent.

•**piroxicam betadex.** (phr-OX-i-kam BAY-ta-dex) USAN.
Use: Analgesic; anti-inflammatory; antirheumatic.

•**piroxicam cinnamate.** (phr-OX-i-kam SIN-a-mate) USAN.
Use: Anti-inflammatory.

•**piroxicam olamine.** (phr-OX-i-kam OLE-a-meen) USAN.
Use: Anti-inflammatory; analgesic.

•**piroximone.** (PIHR-ox-ih-MONE) USAN.
Use: Cardiovascular agent.

•**pirprofen.** (pihr-PRO-fen) USAN.
Use: Anti-inflammatory.

•**pirquinozol.** (PIHR-KWIN-oh-zole) USAN.
Use: Antiallergic.

•**pirsidomine.** (pihr-SIH-doe-meen) USAN.
Use: Vasodilator.

pitavastatin.
Use: HMG-CoA Reductase Inhibitor.
See: Livalo.

Pitayine.
See: Quinidine.

Pitocin. (JHP Pharmaceuticals) Oxytocin. Inj. 1 mL amps (chlorobutanol 0.5%), 1 mL *Steri-Dose* disposable syringes, 1 mL *Steri-Vials.* 10 units/mL. *Rx.*
Use: Oxytocic.

Pitressin Synthetic. (JHP Pharm) Vasopressin 20 pressor units/mL. Chlorobutanol 0.5%. Inj., Soln. 1 mL vial. *Rx.*
Use: Posterior pituitary hormone, vasopressin.

Pitts Carminative. (Del) Bot. 2 oz.
Use: Antiflatulent.

pituitary, anterior. The anterior lobe of the pituitary gland supplies protein hormones classified under following headings.
See: Corticotropin.
Gonadotropin.
Growth hormone.
Thyrotropic Principle.

Pituitary Function Test.
See: Metopirone.

pituitary, posterior, hormones.
See: DDAVP.
Desmopressin Acetate.
Pitressin.
Stimate.
Vasopressin.

•**pituitary, posterior, injection.** *USP.*
Use: Hormone, antidiuretic.

•**pivampicillin hydrochloride.** (piv-AM-pi-SIL-in) USAN.
Use: Anti-infective.

•**pivampicillin pamoate.** (piv-AM-pi-SIL-in PAM-oh-ate) USAN.
Use: Anti-infective.

•**pivampicillin probenate.** (piv-AM-pi-SIL-in PROE-be-nate) USAN.
Use: Anti-infective.

•**pivopril.** (PIH-voe-PRILL) USAN.
Use: Antihypertensive.

•**pixantrone.** (PIX-an-trone) USAN.
Use: Antineoplastic.

•**pixantrone dimaleate.** (PIX-an-trone) USAN.
Use: Treatment of non-Hodgkin lymphoma.

pix carbonis.
See: Coal tar.

Pix Juniperi.
Use: Sunscreen; moisturizer.
See: Juniper tar.

•**pizotyline.** (pih-ZOE-tih-leen) USAN.
Use: Anabolic; antidepressant; serotonin inhibitor, migraine.

placebo capsules. (Cowley) No. 3 orange red; No. 4 yellow. Bot. 1000s.
Use: Placebo.

placebo tablets. (Cowley) 1 g white; 2 g white; 3 g white, red or yellow, pink, orange; 4 g white; 5 g white. Bot. 1000s.
Use: Placebo.

•**placulumab.** (pla-KUL-ue-mab) USAN.
Use: Monoclonal antibody.

Plan B. (Teva Women's Health) Levonorgestrel 0.75 mg. Lactose. Tab. Blister pack 2s. *OTC.*
Use: Sex hormone, contraceptive hormone.

Plan B One-Step. (Teva Women's Health) Levonorgestrel 1.5 mg. Lactose. Tab. 1s. *OTC.*
Use: Emergency contraceptive.

Planocaine.
See: Procaine hydrochloride.

planochrome.
See: Merbromin.

plantago, ovata coating.
See: Konsyl.
Metamucil.

•**plantago seed.** (PLAN-tah-go seed) *USP.*
Use: Laxative.

Plaquenil. (Covis) Hydroxychloroquine sulfate 200 mg. Film coated. PEG. Tab. 100s. *Rx.*
Use: Antirheumatic agent.

Plasbumin-5. (Talecris) Normal serum albumin (human) 5% USP fractionated from normal serum plasma, heat treated against hepatitis virus. Albumin

12.5 g/250 mL. Inj. Vial 50 mL. Bot. with IV set 250 mL, 500 mL. *Rx.*
Use: Plasma protein fraction.

Plasbumin-20. (Talecris) Normal serum albumin (human) 20%. Inj. Vial. 50 mL, 100 mL. *Rx.*
Use: Plasma protein fraction.

Plasbumin-25. (Talecris) Normal serum albumin (human) 25% USP fractionated from normal serum plasma, heat treated against hepatitis virus. Albumin 12.5 g/50 mL. Inj. Vial 20 mL. Bot. with IV set 50 mL, 100 mL. *Rx.*
Use: Plasma protein fraction.

plasma expanders.
See: Hetastarch.
Plasma Protein Fraction.
Tetrastarch.

plasma expanders or substitutes.
See: Dextran 6% and LMD 10%.
Macrodex.

Plasma-Lyte A ph 7.4. (Baxter PPI) Na 140 mEq, K 5 mEq, Mg 3 mEq, Cl 98 mEq, acetate 27 mEq, gluconate 23 mEq, osmolarity 294 mOsm/L, pH 7.4. Soln. Plastic Bot. 500 mL, 1000 mL. *Rx.*
Use: Intravenous nutritional therapy, intravenous replenishment solution.

Plasma-Lyte 56 and 5% Dextrose. (Baxter PPI) Na 40 mEq, K 13 mEq, Mg 3 mEq, Cl 40 mEq, acetate 16 mEq, dextrose 50 g, calories 170, osmolarity 363 mOsm/L. Soln. Plastic Bot. 500 mL, 1000 mL. *Rx.*
Use: Intravenous nutritional therapy, intravenous replenishment solution.

Plasma-Lyte 56 in Water. (Baxter PPI) Na 40 mEq, K 13 mEq, Mg 3 mEq, Cl 40 mEq, acetate 16 mEq/L. Plastic Bot. 500 mL, 1000 mL. *Rx.*
Use: Nutritional supplement, parenteral.

Plasma-Lyte M and 5% Dextrose. (Baxter PPI) Na 40 mEq, K 16 mEq, Ca 5 mEq, Mg 3 mEq, Cl 40 mEq, acetate 12 mEq, lactate 12 mEq, dextrose 50 g, calories 180, osmolarity 377 mOsm/L. Soln. Plastic Bot. 500 mL, 1000 mL. *Rx.*
Use: Intravenous nutritional therapy, intravenous replenishment solution.

Plasma-Lyte 148. (Baxter PPI) Na 140 mEq, K 5 mEq, Mg 3 mEq, Cl 98 mEq, acetate 27 mEq, gluconate 23 mEq, osmolarity 294 mOsm/L, ph ≈ 5.5. Soln. Bot. 500 mL, 1000 mL. *Rx.*
Use: Intravenous nutritional therapy, intravenous replenishment solution.

Plasma-Lyte 148 and 5% Dextrose. (Baxter PPI) Dextrose 50 g, calories 190, Na 140 mEq, K 5 mEq, Mg 3 mEq, Cl 98 mEq, acetate 27 mEq, osmolarity 547 mOsm, gluconate 23 mEq/L. Soln. Bot. 500 mL, 1000 mL. *Rx.*
Use: Intravenous nutritional therapy, intravenous replenishment solution.

Plasma-Lyte R. (Baxter PPI) Na 140 mEq, K 10 mEq, Ca 5 mEq, Mg 3 mEq, Cl 103 mEq, acetate 47 mEq, lactate 8 mEq, osmolarity 312 mOsm/L, ph ≈ 5.5. Soln. Bot. 1000 mL. *Rx.*
Use: Intravenous nutritional therapy, intravenous replenishment solution.

Plasma-Lyte R and 5% Dextrose. (Baxter PPI) Dextrose 50 g, calories 180, Na^+ 140 mEq, K^+ 10 mEq, Ca^{++} 5 mEq, Mg^{++} 3 mEq, Cl^- 103 mEq, lactate 8 mEq, acetate 47 mEq, osmolarity 564 mOsm/L, sodium bisulfite. Soln. Bot. 1000 mL. *Rx.*
Use: Intravenous nutritional therapy, intravenous replenishment solution.

Plasma-Lyte R Injection. (Baxter PPI) Na 140 mEq, K 10 mEq, Ca 5 mEq, Mg 3 mEq, Cl 103 mEq, acetate 47 mEq, lactate 8 mEq/L. Bot. 1000 mL. *Rx.*
Use: Nutritional supplement, parenteral.

Plasmanate. (Talecris) Plasma protein fraction (human) 5%. USP Vial 50 mL. Bot. 250 mL, 500 mL with set. *Rx.*
Use: Plasma protein fraction.

Plasma-Plex. (Centeon) Plasma protein fraction 5%. Inj. Vial 250 mL, 500 mL. *Rx.*
Use: Plasma protein fraction.

•**plasma protein fraction.** *USP. Formerly Plasma Protein Fraction, Human.*
Use: Blood-volume supporter.
See: Albumin.
Plasmanate.
Plasma-Plex.
Protenate.

plasma protein fraction. (Baxter PPI) For the plasma protein preparation obtained from human plasma using the Cohn fractionation technique. Bot. 250 mL.
Use: Blood volume supporter.

plasma protein (human).
Use: Hematological agent.
See: Octaplas.

plasmochin naphthoate. Pamaquine naphthoate.
Use: Antimalarial.

•**platelet concentrate.** *USP.*
Use: Platelet replenisher.

Platelet Factor 4. (Abbott Diagnostics) Radioimmunoassay for quantitative measurement of total PF4 levels in plasma. Test kit 100s.
Use: Diagnostic aid.

platinum coordination complex.
Use: Antineoplastic.

See: Carboplatin.
Oxaliplatin.

Plavix. (Bristol-Myers Squibb) Clopidogrel 75 mg (equiv. to clopidogrel bisulfate 97.875 mg), 300 mg (equiv to clopidogrel bisulfate 391.5 mg). Castor oil, lactose, mannitol. Film-coated. Tab. Bot. 30s, 90s, 500s (75 mg only), UD 4s (300 mg only), UD 30s (300 mg only), UD 100s. *Rx.*
Use: Antiplatelet, aggregation inhibitor.

Plax. (McNeil-PPC) Sorbitol solution, alcohol 8.7%, tetrasodium pyrophosphate, benzoic acid, poloxamer 407, sodium benzoate, sodium lauryl sulfate, sodium saccharin, xanthan gum. Original, mint, sensation, and softmint flavors. Mouthwash. 118 mL, 237 mL, 473 mL, 710 mL. *OTC.*
Use: Anti-infective.

•**plazomicin.** (PLA-zoe-MYE-sin) USAN.
Use: Treatment of gram-negative bacterial infections.

•**plecanatide.** (ple-KAN-a-tide) USAN.
Use: Gastrointestinal agent.

•**pleconaril.** (pleh-KOE-nah-rill) USAN.
Use: Antiviral.

PledgaClin. (JSJ Pharmaceuticals) Clindamycin phosphate 1%. Isopropyl alcohol 50%, propylene glycol. Pledget. 69s. *Rx.*
Use: Topical anti-infective, antibiotic agent.

Plegisol. (Hospira) Calcium Cl dihydrate 17.6 mg, magnesium Cl hexahydrate 325.3 mg, potassium Cl 119.3 mg, sodium Cl 643 mg/100 mL. Approximately 260 mOsm/L. Single-dose container 1000 mL without sodium bicarbonate. *Rx.*
Use: Cardiovascular agent.

•**plerixafor.** (pler-IX-a-fore) USAN.
Use: Stem cell mobilizer.
See: Mozobil.

Pletal. (Otsuka America Pharmaceutical) Cilostazol 50 mg. Tab. Bot. 60s. *Rx.*
Use: Antiplatelet.

Plewin. (Sanofi-Synthelabo) Glycobiarsol, chloroquine phosphate. Tab. *Rx.*
Use: Amebicide.

Plexion. (Medicis) Sulfur 5%, sodium sulfacetamide 10%, cetyl alcohol, stearyl alcohol, EDTA, parabens. Cleanser. Bot. 170 g, 340 g. *Rx.*
Use: Keratolytic.

Plexion Cleansing Cloths. (Medicis) Sulfur 5%, sodium sulfacetamide 10%. Glycerine, glyceryl stearate, propylene glycol, propylene glycol oleate, alcohols, EDTA, parabens. Cloths. 30s. *Rx.*
Use: Keratolytic agent.

Plexion SCT. (Medicis) Sulfur 5%, sodium sulfacetamide 10%, witch hazel, benzyl alcohol. Cream. Tube 120 g. *Rx.*
Use: Keratolytic.

Plexion TS. (Medicis) Sulfur 5%, sodium sulfacetamide 10%. Mineral oil, glyceryl stearate, propylene glycol, propylene glycol oleate, alcohols, EDTA, sodium thiosulfate, coco-glycerides. Susp. Topical. 30 g. *Rx.*
Use: Keratolytic agent.

Plexolan. (Last) Zinc oxide, lanolin. Cream. Tube 1.25 oz, 3 oz. Jar 16 oz. *OTC.*
Use: Dermatologic.

Plexon. (Sigma-Tau) Testosterone 10 mg, estrone 1 mg, liver 2 mcg, pyridoxine hydrochloride 10 mg, panthenol 10 mg, inositol 20 mg, choline Cl 20 mg, vitamin B_2 2 mg, B_{12} 100 mcg, procaine hydrochloride 1%, niacinamide 100 mg/mL. Vial 10 mL.
Use: Hormone; mineral, vitamin supplement.

Pliagel. (Alcon) NaCl, KCl, poloxamer 407, sorbic acid 0.25%, EDTA 0.5%. Soln. Bot. 25 mL. *OTC.*
Use: Contact lens care.

Pliaglis. (Galderma) Lidocaine 7%, tetracaine 7%. Parabens, petrolatum, polyvinyl alcohol. Cream 30 g. *Rx.*
Use: Topical local anesthetic.

•**plicamycin.** (PLYE-ka-MYE-sin) *USP.*
Use: Antineoplastic.

•**plinabulin.** (PLIN-a-BUE-lin) USAN.
Use: Antineoplastic.

•**plomestane.** (PLOE-mess-TANE) USAN.
Use: Antineoplastic, aromatase inhibitor.

•**plovamer.** (PLOE-va-mer) USAN.
Use: Treatment of multiple sclerosis.

•**plovamer acetate.** (PLOE-va-mer) USAN.
Use: Treatment of multiple sclerosis.

Pluravit. (Sanofi-Synthelabo) Multivitamin. Drops.
Use: Vitamin supplement.

Ply Hist Forte. (Poly) Phenylephrine hydrochloride 10 mg, pyrilamine maleate 25 mg. Tab. 100s. *OTC.*
Use: Upper respiratory combination, decongestant and antihistamine.

PMB 400. (Wyeth) Conjugated estrogens 0.45 mg, meprobamate 400 mg, lactose, sucrose. Tab. Bot. 100s. *Rx.*
Use: Anxiolytic, estrogen.

PMB 200. (Wyeth) Conjugated estrogens

0.45 mg, meprobamate 200 mg, lactose, sucrose. Tab. Bot. 60s. *Rx.*
Use: Anxiolytic, estrogen.

P.M.P. Compound. (Mericon Industries) Chlorpheniramine maleate 4 mg, phenylephrine hydrochloride 15 mg, salicylamide 300 mg, scopolamine methylnitrate 0.8 mg. Tab. Bot. 100s, 1000s. *Rx.*
Use: Analgesic; antihistamine; decongestant.

P.M.P. Expectorant. (Mericon Industries) Codeine phosphate 10 mg, phenylephrine hydrochloride 10 mg, guaifenesin 40 mg, chlorpheniramine maleate 2 mg/5 mL. Bot. Gal. *c-v.*
Use: Antihistamine; antitussive; decongestant; expectorant.

pneumococcal vaccine, polyvalent.
Use: Agent for active immunization, bacterial vaccine.
See: Pneumovax 23.

Pneumomist. (ECR) Guaifenesin 600 mg. SR Tab. Bot. 100s. *Rx.*
Use: Expectorant.

Pneumotussin. (ECR) Hydrocodone bitartrate 2.5 mg, guaifenesin 300 mg. Dye free. Tab. Bot. 100s. *c-III.*
Use: Upper respiratory combination, antitussive, expectorant.

Pneumotussin HC. (ECR) Hydrocodone bitartrate 5 mg, guaifenesin 100 mg/5 mL. Syr. Bot. 120 mL, 480 mL. *c-III.*
Use: Antitussive; expectorant.

Pneumovax 23. (Merck) 23 polysaccharide isolates 25 mcg each/0.5 mL dose. Phenol 0.25%. Inj. Vials. 1-dose, 5-dose. *Rx.*
Use: Agent for active immunization, bacterial vaccine.

PNS Unna Boot. (Pedinol Pharmacal) Nonsterile gauze bandage 10 yds × 3". Box 12s.
Use: Ambulatory procedure in treatment of leg ulcers and varicosities.

PNV Ferrous Fumarate/Docusate/Folic Acid. (Virtus) Folic acid 1 mg, calcium 200 mg, iron 29 mg, vitamins A 1,000 units, D 400 units, E 30 units, B_1 3 mg, B_2 3 mg, B_3 15 mg, B_5 7 mg, B_6 20 mg, B_{12} 12 mcg, C 100 mg, Zn, docusate sodium 25 mg. PEG. Tab. 100s. *Rx.*
Use: Prenatal vitamin with minerals.

PNV-First. (Acella) Folic acid 1 mg, iron 29 mg, vitamins A 1,100 units, D 1,000 units, E 20 units, B_1 1.6 mg, B_2 1.8 mg, B_3 15 mg, B_6 2.5 mg, B_{12} 12 mcg, C 30 mg, Cu, I, Mg, Zn, DHA 200 mg. Beeswax, glycerin, lecithin. Cap., softgel. 30s. *Rx.*
Use: Prenatal vitamin with minerals.

PNV OB + DHA. (PharmaPure Rx) Vitamins C 120 mg, D_3 400 units, E 30 units, B_1 3 mg, B_2 3.4 mg, B_3 20 mg, B_6 20 mg, folic acid 1 mg, Fe 27 mg, Ca 125 mg, Zn, Cu, I. **Caplets:** Docusate sodium 50 mg. PEG, polydextrose, soybean oil, sucrose. Preservative free and gluten free. UD 30s. **Cap., softgels:** DHA 250 mg, EPA, and other omega-3 fatty acids. Glycerin. Preservative free and gluten free. UD 30s. *Rx.*
Use: Prenatal vitamin with minerals.

•**pobilukast edamine.** (poe-BIH-loo-kast EH-dah-meen) USAN.
Use: Antiasthmatic, leukotriene antagonist.

pochlorin. Prophyrinic and chlorophyllic compound.
Use: Antihypercholesterolemic agent.

Podactin. (Reese) Miconazole nitrate 2%. Benzoic acid, glyceryl, mineral oil. Cream. 28.35 g. *OTC.*
Use: Topical anti-infective, antifungal.

Pod-Ben-25. (C & M Pharmacal) Podophyllin 25% in benzoin tincture. Bot. 1 oz. *Rx.*
Use: Keratolytic.

Podoben. (American Pharmaceutical) Podophyllum resin extract 25%. Bot. 5 mL. *Rx.*
Use: Keratolytic.

Podocon-25. (Paddock) Podophyllum resin 25% in benzoin tincture. Soln. 15 mL. *Rx.*
Use: Keratolytic.

•**podofilox.** (pah-dah-FILL-ox) USAN.
Use: Antimitotic.
See: Condylox.

podofilox. (Various Mfr.) Podofilox 0.5%. Alcohol 95%. Top. Soln. 3.5 mL. *Rx.*
Use: Antimitotic.

Podofin. (Syosset) Podophyllum resin (podophyllin) 25% in tincture of benzoin. Liq. 15 mL. *Rx.*
Use: Keratolytic.

podophyllin.
See: Podophyllum resin.

podophyllotoxin derivatives.
See: Teniposide.

•**podophyllum.** (pode-oh-FIL-um) *USP.*
Use: Pharmaceutic necessity.

•**podophyllum resin.** (pode-oh-FIL-um REZ-in) *USP.*
Use: Caustic.
See: Podoben.
Podofin.

podophyllum resin. (Various Mfr.) Podophyllin. Pkg. 1 oz, 0.25 lb, 1 lb.
Use: Caustic.

Point-Two Mouthrinse. (Colgate Oral Pharmaceuticals) Sodium fluoride 0.2% in a flavored neutral liquid. Bot. 120 mL. *Rx.*
Use: Dental caries agent.

•**poison ivy extract, alum precipitated.** (poy-zuhn EYE-vee EX-tract, AL-uhm pree-SIP-ih-tay-tehd) USAN.
Use: Ivy poisoning counteractant.

•**polacrilin.** (POL-a-KRILL-in) USAN. Methacrylic acid with divinylbenzene. A synthetic ion-exchange resin, supplied in the hydrogen or free acid form. Amberlite IRP-64.
Use: Pharmaceutic aid.

•**polacrilin potassium.** (POL-a-KRILL-in) *NF.* A synthetic ion-exchange resin, prepared through the polymerization of methacrylic acid and divinylbenzene, further neutralized with potassium hydroxide to form the potassium salt of methacrylic acid and divinylbenzene. Supplied as a pharmaceutical-grade ion-exchange resin in a particle size of 100- to 500-mesh.
Use: Pharmaceutic aid, tablet disintegrant.
See: Amberlite IRP-88.

Poladex Tabs. (Major) Dexchlorpheniramine maleate. Tab. **4 mg:** Bot. 100s, 250s, 1000s. **6 mg:** Bot. 100s, 1000s. *Rx.*
Use: Antihistamine.

polamethene resin caprylate. The physiochemical complex of the acid-binding ion exchange resin, polyamine-methylene resin and caprylic acid.

Polaramine. (Schering-Plough) Dexchlorpheniramine maleate, lactose. **Tab.:** 2 mg, lactose. Bot. 100s. **Syr.:** 2 mg/5 mL alcohol 6%, sorbitol, menthol, parabens, sugar, orange-like flavor. Bot. 473 mL. *Rx.*
Use: Antihistamine, nonselective alkylamine.

Polaramine Expectorant. (Schering-Plough) Dexchlorpheniramine maleate 2 mg, pseudoephedrine sulfate 20 mg, guaifenesin 100 mg/5 mL, alcohol 7.2%, menthol, sorbitol, sugar. Liq. Bot. 473 mL. *Rx.*
Use: Upper respiratory combination, antihistamine, decongestant, expectorant.

Polaramine Repetabs. (Schering-Plough) Dexchlorpheniramine maleate 4 mg, 6 mg, parabens, lactose, sugar. TR Tab. Bot. 100s. *Rx.*
Use: Antihistamine, nonselective alkylamine.

Poldeman. (Sanofi-Synthelabo) Kaolin. Susp. *OTC.*
Use: Antidiarrheal.

Poldeman AD. (Sanofi-Synthelabo) Kaolin. Susp. *OTC.*
Use: Antidiarrheal.

Poldemicina. (Sanofi-Synthelabo) Kaolin. Susp. *OTC.*
Use: Antidiarrheal.

•**poldine methylsulfate.** (POLE-deen METH-ill-SULL-fate) *USP.*
Use: Anticholinergic.

•**policapram.** (PAH-lee-CAP-ram) USAN.
Use: Pharmaceutic aid, tablet binder.

Polident Dentu-Grip. (Block Drug) Carboxymethylcellulose gum, ethylene oxide polymer. Pkg. 0.675 oz, 1.75 oz, 3.55 oz. *OTC.*
Use: Denture adhesive.

polidocanol.
Use: Sclerosing agent.
See: Asclera.
Varithena.

•**polifeprosan 20.** (pahl-ee-FEH-pro-SAHN 20) USAN.
Use: Pharmaceutic aid, biodegradable polymer for controlled drug delivery.

•**poligeenan.** (PAHL-ih-JEE-nan) USAN. Polysaccharide produced by extensive hydrolysis of carragheen from red algae.
Use: Pharmaceutic aid, dispersing agent.

•**poliglecaprone 90.** (POL-ee-GLEK-a-prone 90) USAN.
Use: Surgical aid, surgical suture coating (absorbable).

•**poliglecaprone 25.** (POL-ee-GLEK-a-prone 25) USAN.
Use: Surgical aid, surgical suture material (absorbable).

•**poliglusam.** (pahl-ee-GLUE-sam) USAN.
Use: Antihemorrhagic, hemostatic; dermatologic, wound therapy.

•**polignate sodium.** (poe-LIG-nate) USAN.
Use: Enzyme inhibitor, pepsin.

Poli-Grip. (Block Drug) Karaya gum, magnesium oxide in petrolatum mineral oil base, peppermint and spearmint flavor. Tube 0.75 oz, 1.5 oz, 2.5 oz. *OTC.*
Use: Denture adhesive.

poliomyelitis vaccine, inactivated. (Aventis Pasteur) (Purified, Salk Type IPV) Poliovirus vaccine, inactivated. Amp. 5 × 1 mL. Vial 10 dose. *Rx.*
Use: Immunization.
See: IPOL.
Poliovirus Vaccine, Inactivated

•**poliovirus vaccine, inactivated.** (POE-lee-oh-VYE-russ) *USP. Formerly Poliomyelitis Vaccine.*

Use: Immunization.
See: IPOL.

poliovirus vaccine, inactivated. (Aventis Pasteur) Amp. 1 mL. Box 5s. Vial 10 dose. Subcutaneous administration.
Use: Agent for immunization, active.

poliovirus vaccine, inactivated, diphtheria and tetanus toxoids and acellular pertussis adsorbed, hepatitis B (recombinant), combined.
Use: Active immunization, toxoid.
See: Diphtheria and Tetanus Toxoids and Acellular Pertussis Adsorbed, Hepatitis B (Recombinant), Inactivated Poliovirus Vaccine Combined.

•**polipropene 25.** (pahl-ee-PRO-peen 25) USAN.
Use: Pharmaceutic aid, tablet excipient.

•**polixetonium chloride.** (pahl-ix-eh-TOE-nee-uhm) USAN.
Use: Pharmaceutic aid, preservative.

Polocaine. (APP Pharmaceutical) Mepivacaine hydrochloride. **1%, 2%:** Mannitol. Inj. Multidose vial 50 mL. **3%:** Sodium bisulfite. Inj. Dental cartridge 1.8 mL. *Rx.*
Use: Anesthetic, local amide.

Polocaine MPF. (APP Pharmaceutical) Mepivacaine hydrochloride. **1%, 1.5%:** Inj. Methylparaben. Single-dose vial 30 mL. **2%:** Inj. Single-dose vial 20 mL. *Rx.*
Use: Anesthetic, local amide.

Poloris Poultices. (Block Drug) Benzocaine 7.5 mg, capsicum 4.6 mg in poultice base. Pkg. 5 unit, 12 unit. *Rx.*
Use: Anesthetic, local.

•**poloxalene.** (PAHL-OX-ah-leen) *USP.* Liquid nonionic surfactant polymer of polyoxypropylene polyoxyethylene type.
Use: Pharmaceutic aid, surfactant.

poloxalkol. Polyoxyethylene polyoxypropylene polymer.

•**poloxamer.** (pahl-OX-ah-mer) *NF.*
Use: Pharmaceutic aid (ointment and suppository base, surfactant, tablet binder and coating agent, emulsifying agent).

poloxamer-iodine.
See: Prepodyne.

poloxamer 188.
Use: Cathartic; sickle cell crisis; severe burns. [Orphan Drug]

poloxamer 188 lf.
Use: Pharmaceutic aid, surfactant.

poloxamer 182 d.
Use: Pharmaceutic aid, surfactant.

poloxamer 182 lf.
Use: Food additive; pharmaceutic aid.

poloxamer 331.
Use: Food additive, surfactant; AIDS-related toxoplasmosis. [Orphan Drug]

polyamine resin.
See: Polyamine-Methylene Resin.

polyanhydroglucose. Polyanhydroglucuronic acid.

Polybase. (Paddock) Preblended polyethylene glycol suppository base for incorporation of medications where a water-soluble base is indicated. Jar 1 lb, 5 lb.
Use: Pharmaceutical aid, suppository base.

polybenzarsol. Benzocal.

Poly-Bon Drops. (Barrows) Vitamins A 3000 units, D 400 units, C 60 mg, B_1 1 mg, B_2 1.2 mg, niacinamide 8 mg/0.6 mL. Bot. 50 mL. *OTC.*
Use: Vitamin supplement.

•**polybutester.** (PAHL-ee-byoot-ESS-ter) USAN.
Use: Surgical aid, surgical suture material.

•**polybutilate.** (PAHL-ee-BYOO-tih-late) USAN.
Use: Surgical aid, surgical suture coating.

•**polycarbophil.** (POL-ee-KAR-boe-fil) *USP.*
Use: Laxative.
See: Bulk Forming Fiber Laxative.
Equalactin.
FiberCon.
Fiber-Lax.
FiberNorm.
Konsyl Fiber.

Polycillin. (Bristol-Myers Squibb) Ampicillin trihydrate. **Cap.: 250 mg:** Bot. 100s, 500s, 1000s, UD 100s. **Cap.: 500 mg:** Bot. 100s, 500s, UD 100s. **Pediatric Drops:** 100 mg/mL. Dropper bot. 20 mL. **Susp.: 125 mg/5 mL:** Bot. 80 mL, 100 mL, 150 mL, 200 mL, UD 5 mL. **Susp.: 250 mg/5 mL:** Bot. 80 mL, 100 mL, 150 mL, 200 mL, UD 5 mL. **Susp.: 500 mg/5 mL:** Bot. 100 mL, UD 5 mL. *Rx.*
Use: Anti-infective, penicillin.

polycosanol.
W/Acetic Acid, Antipyrine, Benzocaine.
See: AABP.
Auralgan.

Polycose. (Ross) Glucose polymers derived from controlled hydrolysis of corn starch. Calories 380, carbohydrate 94 g, water 6 g, Na 110 mg, K 10 mg, Cl 223 mg, Ca 30 mg, P 5 mg/100 g. Pow. Can 12.3 oz. Case 6s. *OTC.*
Use: Nutritional supplement.

Poly-Dex. (OcuSoft) Dexamethasone

0.1%, neomycin 3.5 mg, polymyxin B sulfate 10,000 units. Benzalkonium chloride 0.004%, sodium chloride, hypromellose, polysorbate 80. Susp.; Ophth. 5 mL. *Rx.*
Use: Ophthalmic steroid antibiotic combination.

•**polydextrose.** (PAH-lee-DEX-trose) USAN.
Use: Food additive.

polydimethylsiloxane (silicone oil).
Use: Ophthalmic.
See: AdatoSil 5000.

Polydine. (Century) **Oint.:** Povidone-iodine 10%. 24 g, lb. **Soln.:** Povidone-iodine solution 10%. pt, gal. **Surgical scrub:** Povidone-iodine in scrub solution 5.5. pt, gal. *OTC.*
Use: Antiseptic.

•**polydioxanone.** (PAHL-ee-die-OX-ah-nohn) USAN.
Use: Surgical aid, surgical suture material (absorbable).

Poly ENA Test System for RNP and SM. (Wampole) Qualitative identification of auto antibodies to extractable nuclear antigens in human serum by gel precipitation technique. Aid in the diagnosis of SLE, MCTD, PSS, SS. Box test 48s.
Use: Diagnostic aid.

Poly ENA Test System for RNP, SM, SSA, and SSB. (Wampole) Qualitative identification of auto antibodies to extractable nuclear antigens in human serum by gel precipitation techniques. Aid in the diagnosis of SLE, MCTD, PSS, SS. Box test 96s.
Use: Diagnostic aid.

Poly ENA Test System for SSA and SSB. (Wampole) Qualitative identification of auto antibodies to extractable nuclear antigens in human serum by gel precipitation techniques. Aid in the diagnosis of SLE, MCTD, PSS, SS. Box test 48s.
Use: Diagnostic aid.

polyene antifungals.
See: Amphotericin B Desoxycholate.
Amphotericin B, Lipid-Based.
Nystatin.

•**polyethadene.** (PAHL-ee-ETH-ah-DEEN) USAN.
Use: Antacid.

•**polyethylene excipient.** (POL-ee-ETH-i-leen) *NF.*
Use: Pharmaceutic aid, stiffening agent.

•**polyethylene glycol.** (POL-ee-ETH-i-leen GLYE-kol) *NF.*
Use: Pharmaceutic aid (ointment and suppository base, tablet excipient, solvent, tablet and capsule lubricant).
See: Dulcolax Balance.
GaviLAX.
GlycoLax.
MiraLax.
Zanfel.

polyethylene glycol. (Braintree) PEG 3350 255 g, 527 g. Pow. for Oral Soln. 16 oz (255 g only), 32 oz (527 g only). *Rx.*
Use: Laxative.

polyethylene glycol and electrolytes.
Use: Rehydration; bowel evacuant.
See: Colyte.
GoLYTELY.
NuLYTELY.

•**polyethylene glycol monomethyl ether.** (POL-ee-ETH-i-leen GLYE-kol) *NF.*
Use: Pharmaceutic aid, excipient.

polyethylene glycol 3350 and electrolytes. (Mylan) PEG 3350 236 g, sodium sulfate 22.74 g, sodium bicarbonate 6.74 g, NaCl 5.86 g, KCl 2.97 g. Pow. for Soln. Disposable jug. *Rx.*
Use: Laxative, bowel evacuant.

•**polyethylene granules.** (POL-ee-ETH-i-leen)
Use: Poison ivy treatment.
See: Zanfel.
Zanfel Wash.

•**polyethylene oxide.** (POL-ee-ETH-i-leen OX-ide) *NF.*
Use: Pharmaceutic aid, suspending and viscosity agent, tablet binder.

•**polyferose.** (PAHL-ee-feh-rohs) USAN. An iron carbohydrate chelate containing approximately 45% of iron in which the metallic (Fe) ion is sequestered within a polymerized carbohydrate derived from sucrose.
Use: Hematinic.

Poly-F Fluoride. (Major) Fluoride 0.5 mg, vitamins A 1500 units, D 400 units, E 5 mg, B_1 0.5 mg, B_2 0.6 mg, B_3 8 mg, B_6 0.4 mg, B_{12} 2 mcg, C 35 mg/mL. Drops. Bot. 50 mL. *Rx.*
Use: Mineral, vitamin supplement.

•**polyglactin 910.** (POL-ee-GLAK-tin 910) USAN.
Use: Surgical aid, surgical suture coating (absorbable).

•**polyglactin 370.** (POL-ee-GLAK-tin 370) USAN. Lactic acid polyester with glycolic acid.
Use: Surgical aid, surgical suture coating (absorbable).

•**polyglycolic acid.** (PAHL-ee-glie-KAHL-ik) USAN.
Use: Surgical aid, surgical suture material.

•**polyglyconate.** (PAHL-ee-GLIE-koe-nate) USAN.
Use: Surgical aid, surgical suture material (absorbable).

Poly Hist DHC. (Poly Pharmaceuticals) Dihydrocodeine bitartrate 7.5 mg, phenylephrine hydrochloride 5 mg, pyrilamine maleate 7.5 mg. Glycerin, propylene glycol, saccharin, sorbitol. Alcohol free, dye free, gluten free, and sugar free. Fruit gum flavor. Liq. 473 mL. *c-III.*
Use: Upper respiratory combination, antitussive combination.

Poly Hist DM. (Poly Pharmaceuticals) Dextromethorphan HBr 15 mg, pyrilamine maleate 12.5 mg, phenylephrine hydrochloride 7.5 mg per 5 mL. Sugar, alcohol, and dye free. Glycerin, propylene glycol, saccharin, sorbitol. Grape flavor. Liq. 20 mL, 480 mL. *Rx.*
Use: Antitussive combination, upper respiratory combination.

Poly Hist NC. (Poly Pharmaceuticals) Codeine phosphate 10 mg, pseudoephedrine hydrochloride 15 mg, triprolidine hydrochloride 1.25 mg. Glycerin, propylene glycol, saccharin, sorbitol. Alcohol free, dye free, and sugar free. Cotton candy flavor. Liq. 473 mL. *c-v.*
Use: Upper respiratory combination, antitussive combination.

poly I; poly C12U.
Use: AIDS; antineoplastic. [Orphan Drug]

Poly-Iron 150. (Cypress) Polysaccharide iron complex 150 mg. PEG, tartrazine. Cap. 100s. *OTC.*
Use: Trace element.

poly-l-lactic acid.
Use: Restoration/correction of facial fat loss in individuals with HIV.
See: Sculptra.

•**polyisobutylene.** (POL-ee-EYE-soe-BUE-ti-leen). *NF.*
Use: Synthetic polymer.

•**polymacon.** (PAHL-ee-MAY-kahn) USAN.
Use: Contact lens material, hydrophilic.

polymeric oxygen.
Use: Sickle cell disease. [Orphan Drug]

polymeric phosphate binders.
Use: Treatment of hyperphosphatemia.
See: Sevelamer hydrochloride.

•**polymetaphosphate P 32.** (pahl-ee-met-ah-FOSS-fate) USAN.
Use: Radiopharmaceutical.

Polymox. (Bristol-Myers Squibb) Amoxicillin trihydrate. **Cap.:** 250 mg. Bot. 100s, 500s, UD 100s; 500 mg. Bot. 50s, 100s, 500s, UD 100s. **Oral Susp.:** 125 mg, 250 mg/5 mL. Bot. 80 mL, 100 mL, 150 mL. **Ped. Drops:** 50 mg/mL. Bot. 15 mL. *Rx.*
Use: Anti-infective, penicillin.

polymyxin B. (Various Mfr.) Antimicrobial substances produced by *Bacillus polymyxa.*

•**polymyxin B sulfate.** (POL-ee-MIX-in) *USP.*
Use: Anti-infective.
W/Bacitracin Zinc.
See: AK-Poly-Bac.
Betadine First Aid Antibiotics Plus Moisturizer.
Double Antibiotic.
Polysporin.
W/Bacitracin Zinc, Hydrocortisone Acetate, Neomycin Sulfate.
See: Coracin.
W/Bacitracin Zinc, Lidocaine, Neomycin.
See: Lanabiotic.
W/Bacitracin Zinc, Neomycin, Polymyxin B Sulfate.
See: Mycitracin.
Neosporin Maximum Strength.
Neosporin Original Triple Antibiotic.
Neotal.
Neo-Thrycex.
Ocutricin.
Tigo.
Trimixin.
Triple Antibiotic.
W/Bacitracin Zinc, Neomycin, Polymyxin B Sulfate, Pramoxine Hydrochloride.
See: Neosporin Plus Pain Relief.
Tri-Biozene.
W/Dexamethasone, Neomycin.
See: Maxitrol.
Methadex.
Poly-Dex.
W/Hydrocortisone Acetate, Neomycin Sulfate.
See: Cortisporin.
W/Neomycin Sulfate.
See: Neosporin G.U. Irrigant.
W/Trimethoprim.
See: Polytrim.

polymyxin B sulfate and hydrocortisone.
Use: Anti-infective; anti-inflammatory, otic.

•**polymyxin B sulfate and trimethoprim ophthalmic solution.** (POL-ee-MIX-in) *USP.*
Use: Anti-infective, ophthalmic.

polymyxin-neomycin-bacitracin. (Various Mfr.) Oint. *OTC.*
Use: Anti-infective, topical.

polynoxylin. Anaflex.

polyoxyethylene 8 stearate.
See: Polyoxyl 8 Stearate.
polyoxyethylene 50 stearate.
See: Polyoxyl 50 stearate.
polyoxyethylene 40 monostearate.
See: Polyoxyl 40 stearate.
Myrj 52 & M2S.
polyoxyethylene lauryl ether.
W/Benzoyl Peroxide, Ethyl Alcohol.
See: Benzagel.
Desquam-X.
polyoxyethylene nonyl phenol.
W/Sodium Edetate, Docusate Sodium, 9-Aminoacridine Hydrochloride.
See: Vagisec Plus.
polyoxyethylene sorbitan monolaurate. Polysorbate 20.
W/Ferrous Gluconate, Vitamins.
See: Simron Plus.
polyoxyethylene 20 sorbitan monoleate.
See: Polysorbate 80.
polyoxyethylene 20 sorbitan trioleate. Tween 85. (Zeneca Pharmaceuticals), Polysorbate 85.
polyoxyethylene 20 sorbitan tristearate. Tween 65. (Zeneca Pharmaceuticals), Polysorbate 65.
•**polyoxyl 8 stearate.** (POL-ee-OX-il 8 STEER-ate) USAN.
Use: Pharmaceutic aid, surfactant.
See: Myrj 45.
polyoxyl 50 stearate. *Formerly Polyoxyethylene 50 stearate.*
Use: Pharmaceutic aid, surfactant, emulsifying agent.
•**polyoxyl 40 hydrogenated castor oil.** (POL-ee-OX-il 40 hye-DROJ-en-AY-ted KAS-tor) *NF.*
Use: Pharmaceutic aid, surfactant, emulsifying agent.
•**polyoxyl 40 stearate.** (POL-ee-OX-il 40 STEER-ate) *NF.* Macrogic Stearate 2000 (I.N.N.) Polyoxyethylene 40 monostearate.
Use: Pharmaceutic aid; hydrophilic oint., surfactant; surface-active agent.
See: Myrj 52 & M2S.
•**polyoxyl 10 oleyl ether.** (POL-ee-OX-il 10 oh-LAY-il EE-ther) *NF.*
Use: Pharmaceutic aid, surfactant.
•**polyoxyl 35 castor oil.** (POL-ee-OX-il 35 KAS-tor) *NF.*
Use: Pharmaceutic aid, surfactant, emulsifying agent.
•**polyoxyl 20 cetostearyl ether.** (POL-ee-OX-il 20 SEE-toe-STEER-il EE-ther) *NF.*
Use: Pharmaceutic aid, surfactant.
•**polyoxypropylene 15 stearyl ether.** (POL-ee-OX-ee-PROE-pi-leen 15 STEER-il EE-ther) USAN. *Formerly PPG-15 Stearyl Ether.*
Use: Pharmaceutic aid, solvent.
polypropylene glycol. An addition polymer of propylene oxide and water.
Use: Pharmaceutic aid, suspending agent.
polysaccharide-iron complex.
Use: Mineral supplement.
See: EZFE 200.
Ferrex 150.
iFerex 150.
Myferon.
NovaFerrum 50.
NovaFerrum Liquid Pediatric.
NovaFerrum 125.
Nu-Iron 150.
Poly-Iron 150.
ProFe.
W/Ferrous Fumarate.
See: Tandem.
polysaccharide iron complex. (Various Mfr.) Iron (as polysaccharide iron complex) 150 mg. Cap. Bot. 100s. *OTC.*
Use: Mineral supplement.
polysonic lotion. (Parker) Multipurpose ultrasound lotion with high coupling efficiency. Bot. 8.5 oz, gal.
Use: Diagnostic aid, therapeutic aid.
•**polysorbate 80.** (POL-ee-SOR-bate 80) *NF.*
Use: Pharmaceutic aid, surfactant; artificial tears.
See: OptiZen.
W/Glycerin.
See: Refresh Dry Eye Therapy.
•**polysorbate 85.** (POL-ee-SOR-bate 85) USAN.
Use: Pharmaceutic aid, surfactant.
•**polysorbate 40.** (POL-ee-SOR-bate 40) *NF.*
Use: Pharmaceutic aid, surfactant.
•**polysorbate 60.** (POL-ee-SOR-bate 60) *NF.*
Use: Pharmaceutic aid, surfactant.
•**polysorbate 65.** (POL-ee-SOR-bate 65) USAN.
Use: Pharmaceutic aid, surfactant.
•**polysorbate 20.** (POL-ee-SOR-bate 20) *NF.*
Use: Pharmaceutic aid, surfactant.
Polysporin. (Pfizer) Polymyxin B sulfate 10,000 units, bacitracin zinc 500 units per g. White petrolatum base. Oint. Tubes. ≈ 15 g, ≈ 30 g. *OTC.*
Use: Anti-infective, antibiotic, topical.
polysulfides. Polythionate.
Polytabs-F Chewable Vitamin. (Major) Fluoride 1 mg, vitamins A 2500 units, D 400 units, E 15 mg, B_1 1.05 mg, B_2 1.2 mg, B_3 13.5 mg, B_6 1.05 mg, B_{12}

4.5 mcg, C 60 mg, folic acid 0.3 mg. Chew. Tab. Bot. 100s, 1000s. *Rx.*
Use: Mineral, vitamin supplement.

Poly Tan DM. (Poly) Dextromethorphan tannate 30 mg, dexbrompheniramine tannate 4 mg, pyrilamine maleate 3.5 mg, phenylephrine tannate 25 mg per 5 mL. Alcohol and sugar free. Aspartame, parabens, phenylalanine 7 mg per 5 mL. Candy apple flavor. Susp. 15 mL, 473 mL. *Rx.*
Use: Upper respiratory combination, antitussive combination.

Polytar Shampoo. (GlaxoSmithKline) Polytar 4.5% (coal tar soln., solubilized crude coal tar equiv. to 0.5% coal tar). Lanolin. 177 mL, 355 mL. *OTC.*
Use: Antiseborrheic.

Polytar Soap. (GlaxoSmithKline) Coal tar soln. 2.5% (equiv. to coal tar 0.5%). Glycerin, ethyl alcohol, peanut oil. 113 g. *OTC.*
Use: Dermatologic.

•**polytef.** (PAHL-ee-teff) USAN.
Use: Prosthetic aid.

Polytinic. (Pharmics) Elemental iron 100 mg, vitamin C 300 mg, folic acid 1 mg. tab. Bot. 100s. *Rx.*
Use: Mineral, vitamin supplement.

Polytrim. (Allergan) Polymyxin B sulfate 10,000 units, trimethoprim 1 mg/mL, benzalkonium chloride 0.04 mg/mL, sodium chloride, sodium hydroxide. Bot. 5 mL, 10 mL. *Rx.*
Use: Anti-infective, ophthalmic.

Polytuss-DM. (Rhode) Dextromethorphan HBr 15 mg, chlorpheniramine maleate 1 mg, guaifenesin 25 mg/5 mL. Bot. 4 oz, 8 oz. *OTC.*
Use: Antihistamine; antitussive; expectorant.

Poly-Tussin. (Poly Pharmaceuticals) Chlorcyclizine hydrochloride 9.375 mg, codeine phosphate 10 mg. Glycerin, propylene glycol, saccharin, sorbitol. Alcohol free, dye free, gluten free, and sugar free. Cherry flavor. Liq. 473 mL. *c-v.*
Use: Upper respiratory combination, antitussive combination.

Poly-Tussin AC. (Poly Pharmaceuticals) Brompheniramine maleate 2 mg, codeine phosphate 10 mg, phenylephrine hydrochloride 7.5 mg per 5 mL. Saccharin, sorbitol. Alcohol free. Raspberry-bubblegum flavor. Liq. 473 mL. *c-v.*
Use: Upper respiratory combination, antitussive combination.

Poly-Tussin D. (Poly Pharmaceuticals) Chlorcyclizine hydrochloride 9.375 mg, codeine phosphate 10 mg, pseudoephedrine hydrochloride 30 mg. Glycerin, propylene glycol, saccharin, sorbitol. Alcohol free, dye free, gluten free, and sugar free. Berry vanilla flavor. Liq. 473 mL. *c-v.*
Use: Upper respiratory combination, antitussive combination.

Poly-Tussin DHC. (Poly Pharmaceuticals) Brompheniramine maleate 4 mg, dihydrocodeine bitartrate 3 mg, phenylephrine hydrochloride 7.5 mg per 5 mL. PEG, saccharin. Grape flavor. Liq. 473 mL. *c-v.*
Use: Upper respiratory combination, antitussive combination.

Poly-Tussin EX. (Poly Pharmaceuticals) Dihydrocodeine bitartrate 7.5 mg, guaifenesin 50 mg, phenylephrine hydrochloride 7.5 mg. Glycerin, propylene glycol, saccharin, sorbitol. Alcohol free, dye free, gluten free, and sugar free. Grape flavor. Liq. 473 mL. *c-III.*
Use: Upper respiratory combination, antitussive and expectorant combination.

poly-ureaurethane.
Use: Management of nail dystrophy.
See: Nuvail.

•**polyurethane foam.** (PAHL-ih-you-ree-thane foam) USAN.
Use: Prosthetic aid, internal bone splint.

Poly-Vent DM. (Poly Pharmaceuticals) Dextromethorphan hydrobromide 15 mg, guaifenesin 400 mg, pseudoephedrine hydrochloride 45 mg. Tab. 60s. *OTC.*
Use: Upper respiratory combination, antitussive and expectorant combination.

Poly-Vent IR. (Poly Pharmaceuticals) Guaifenesin 380 mg, pseudoephedrine hydrochloride 60 mg. Gluten free. Tab. 100s. *OTC.*
Use: Upper respiratory combination, decongestant and expectorant combination.

polyvidone. *Name previously used for Povidone.*

Poly-Vi-Flor. (Zylera) **Chew. Tab.:** Fluoride 0.25 mg, 0.5 mg, 1 mg. L-methylfolate calcium 0.2 mg, *Lipidomin* (blend of vitamins A, D, E) 2,415 units, *Drotamin* (blend of vitamins C, B_1, B_2, B_3, B_6) 73.65 mg. Biphasic. Fructose, sorbitol, sucralose, sucrose. Berry flavor. 30s. **Susp., concentrate:** Fluoride 0.25 mg, L-methylfolate calcium 0.2 mg, ferrous bisglycinate hydrochloride 7 mg, *Lipidomin* (blend of vitamins A, D, E) 1,905 units, *Drotamin* (blend of vitamins C, B_1, B_2, B_3, B_6) 46.5 mg. Biphasic,

enteric-coated microbead suspension. 50 mL w/dropper. *Rx.*
Use: Multivitamin with fluoride.

Poly-Vi-Flor With Iron. (Zylera) **Chew. Tab.:** Fluoride 0.5 mg, L-methylfolate calcium 0.2 mg, Fe 10 mg, *Lipidomin* (blend of vitamins A, D, E) 2,415 units, *Drotamin* (blend of vitamins C, B_1, B_2, B_3, B_6) 73.65 mg. Biphasic. Fructose, sorbitol, sucralose, sucrose. Berry flavor. 30s. **Susp., concentrate:** Fluoride 0.25 mg, L-methylfolate calcium 0.2 mg, ferrous bisglycinate hydrochloride 7 mg, *Lipidomin* (blend of vitamins A, D, E) 1,905 units, *Drotamin* (blend of vitamins C, B_1, B_2, B_3, B_6) 46.5 mg. Biphasic enteric-coated microbead suspension. 50 mL w/dropper. *Rx.*
Use: Multivitamin with fluoride.

•**polyvinyl acetate phthalate.** (POL-ee-VYE-nil ASS-e-tate THAL-ate) *NF.*
Use: Pharmaceutic aid, coating agent.

•**polyvinyl alcohol.** (POL-ee-VYE-nil) *USP.* Ethanol, homopolymer.
Use: Pharmaceutic aid, viscosity-increasing agent.
See: Liquifilm Forte.
Puralube Tears.
W/Hydroxypropyl Methylcellulose.
See: Liquifilm Wetting.

polyvinylpyrrolidone. *Name previously used for Povidone.*

Poly-Vi-Sol. (Bristol-Myers Squibb) **Drops:** Vitamins A 1500 units, D 400 units, C 35 mg, B_1 0.5 mg, B_2 0.6 mg, E 5 units, B_6 0.4 mg, B_3 8 mg, B_{12} 2 mcg/mL. Bot. 50 mL. **Chew. Tab.:** Vitamins A 2500 units, E 15 units, D 400 units, C 60 mg, B_1 1.05 mg, B_2 1.2 mg, B_3 13.5 mg, B_6 1.05 mg, B_{12} 4.5 mcg, folic acid 0.3 mg. Bot. 100s. **Chew. Tab. With Iron:** Above formula plus Fe 12 mg, Zn 8 mg. Tab. Bot. 100s. Circus shape Tab. Bot. 100s. *OTC.*
Use: Vitamin supplement.

Poly-Vi-Sol w/Iron. (Bristol-Myers Squibb) **Chew. Tab.:** Fe 12 mg, vitamins A 2500 units, D 400 units, E 15 mg, B_1 1.05 mg, B_2 1.2 mg, B_3 13.5 mg, B_6 1.05 mg, B_{12} 4.5 mcg, C 60 mg, folic acid 0.3 mg, Cu, Zn 8 mg, sugar. Bot. 100s. **Drops:** Vitamins A 1500 units, D 400 units, E 5 units, C 35 mg, B_1 0.5 mg, B_2 0.6 mg, B_3 8 mg, B_6 0.4 mg, Fe 10 mg/mL. Bot. 50 mL. *OTC.*
Use: Mineral, vitamin supplement.

Poly-Vi-Sol w/Minerals. (Bristol-Myers Squibb) Fe 12 mg, vitamins A 2500 units, D 400 units, E 15 mg, B_1 1.05 mg, B_2 1.2 mg, B_3 13.5 mg, B_6 1.06 mg, B_{12} 4.5 mcg, C 60 mg, folic acid 0.3 mg, Cu, Zn 8 mg. Chew. Tab. Bot. 60s, 100s. *OTC.*
Use: Mineral, vitamin supplement.

Poly-Vita. (Major) Vitamins A 1,500 units, D 400 units, E 5 units, B_1 0.5 mg, B_2 0.6 mg, B_3 8 mg, B_6 0.4 mg, B_{12} 2 mcg, C 35 mg per mL. Glycerin, polysorbate 80, potassium sorbate, propylene glycol, sodium benzoate. Alcohol free, sugar free. Fruit flavor. Drops. 50 mL w/dropper. *OTC.*
Use: Multivitamin.

Poly Vitamin. (Rugby) Vitamins A 2,500 units, D 400 units, E 15 units, B_1 1.05 mg, B_2 1.2 mg, B_3 13.5 mg, B_6 1.05 mg, B_{12} 4.5 mcg, C 60 mg, folic acid 0.3 mg. Sucralose, sucrose. Fruit flavor. Chew. Tab. 100s. *Rx.*
Use: Multivitamin.

Poly-Vitamin Drops. (Schein) Vitamins A 1500 units, D 400 units, E 5 units, B_1 0.5 mg, B_2 0.6 mg, B_3 8 mg, B_6 0.4 mg, B_{12} 1.5 mcg, C 35 mg/mL. Dropper. Bot. 50 mL. *OTC.*
Use: Vitamin supplement.

Polyvitamin Drops with Iron. (Various Mfr.) Fe 10 mg, vitamins A 1500 units, D 400 units, E 5 mg, B_1 0.5 mg, B_2 0.6 mg, B_3 8 mg, B_6 0.4 mg, C 35 mg/mL. Bot. 50 mL. *OTC.*
Use: Mineral, vitamin supplement.

Polyvitamin Drops w/Iron and Fluoride. (Various Mfr.) Fluoride 0.25 mg, Vitamins A 1500 units, D 400 units, E 5 units, B_1 0.5 mg, B_2 0.6 mg, B_3 8 mg, B_6 0.4 mg, C 35 mg, Fe 10 mg. Bot. 50 mL. *Rx.*
Use: Mineral, vitamin supplement; dental caries agent.

Polyvitamin Fluoride. (Various Mfr.) Fluoride 0.25 mg, vitamins A 1500 units, D 400 units, E 5 units, B_1 0.5 mg, B_2 0.6 mg, B_3 8 mg, B_6 0.4 mg, B_{12} 2 mcg, C 35 mg/mL. Dropper. Bot. 50 mL. *Rx.*
Use: Mineral, vitamin supplement; dental caries agent.

Polyvitamin Fluoride w/Iron. (Various Mfr.) Fluoride 1 mg, vitamins A 2500 units, D 400 units, E 15 mg, B_1 1.05 mg, B_2 1.2 mg, B_3 13.5 mg, B_6 1.05 mg, B_{12} 4.5 mcg, C 60 mg, folic acid 0.3 mg, Fe 12 mg, Cu, Zn 10 mg. Tab. Bot. 100s, 1000s. *Rx.*
Use: Mineral, vitamin supplement; dental caries agent.

Poly-Vitamins w/Fluoride. (Various Mfr.) Fluoride 1 mg, vitamins A 2500 units, D 400 units, E 15 mg, B_1 1.05 mg, B_2 1.2 mg, B_3 13.5 mg, B_6 1.05 mg, B_{12} 4.5 mcg, C 60 mg, folic acid 0.3 mg. Chew. Tab. Bot. 100s, 1000s. *Rx.*

Use: Mineral, vitamin supplement; dental caries agent.

Poly-Vitamins w/Fluoride 0.5 mg. (Various Mfr.) **Drops:** Fluoride 0.5 mg, vitamins A 1500 units, D 400 units, E 5 units, B_1 0.5 mg, B_2 0.6 mg, B_3 8 mg, B_6 0.4 mg, B_{12} 2 mcg, C 35 mg/mL. Bot. 50 mL. **Tab.:** Fluoride 0.5 mg, vitamins A 2500 units, D 400 units, E 15 mg, B_1 1 mg, B_2 1.2 mg, B_3 13.5 mg, B_6 1 mg, B_{12} 4.5 mcg, C 60 mg, folic acid 0.3 mg. Bot. 100s, 1000s. *Rx.*
Use: Mineral, vitamin supplement; dental caries agent.

Polyvitamin w/Fluoride. (Rugby) Fluoride 0.5 mg, vitamins A 1500 units, D 400 units, E 5 mg, B_1 0.5 mg, B_2 0.6 mg, B_3 8 mg, B_6 0.4 mg, B_{12} 2 mcg, C 35 mg/mL. Dropper Bot. 50 mL. *Rx.*
Use: Mineral, vitamin supplement; dental caries agent.

Poly-Vitamin w/Iron. (Hi-Tech) Iron 10 mg, vitamins A 1,500 units, D 400 units, E 5 units, B_1 0.5 mg, B_2 0.6 mg, B_3 8 mg, B_6 0.4 mg, C 35 mg per mL. Cherry flavoring, glycerin, methylparaben, orange oil, polysorbate 80, sodium benzoate. Soln. concentrate. 50 mL with dropper. *OTC.*
Use: Multivitamin with iron.

Poly-Vita With Iron Drops. (Major) Iron 10 mg, vitamins A 1,500 units, D 400 units, E 5 units, B_1 0.5 mg, B_2 0.6 mg, B_3 8 mg, B_6 0.4 mg, C 35 mg per mL. Glycerin, polysorbate 80, potassium sorbate, propylene glycol, sodium benzoate. Alcohol free, sugar free. Fruit flavor. Soln., concentrate. 50 mL w/dropper. *OTC.*
Use: Multivitamin with iron.

Polyvite with Fluoride. (Geneva) Fluoride 0.25 mg, vitamins A 1500 units, D 400 units, E 5 mg, B_1 0.5 mg, B_2 0.6 mg, B_3 8 mg, B_6 0.4 mg, B_{12} 2 mcg, C 35 mg/mL. Dropper Bot. 50 mL. *Rx.*
Use: Mineral, vitamin supplement; dental caries agent.

•**pomaglumetad methionil.** (POE-ma-GLOO-me-tad) USAN.
Use: CNS agent.

•**pomalidomide.** (POE-ma-LID-oh-mide) USAN.
Use: Immunomodulator.
See: Pomalyst.

Pomalyst. (Celgene Corporation) Pomalidomide 1 mg, 2 mg, 3 mg, 4 mg. Mannitol. Cap. 21s, 100s. *Rx.*
Use: Immunomodulator.

•**ponalrestat.** (poe-NAHL-ress-TAT) USAN.
Use: Antidiabetic.

Ponaris. (Jamol Lab Inc.) Nasal emollient of mucosal lubricating and moisturizing botanical oils. Cajeput, eucalyptus, peppermint in iodized cottonseed oil. Bot. 1 oz w/dropper. *OTC.*
Use: Moisturizer, nasal.

•**ponatinib.** (poe-NA-ti-nib) USAN.
Use: Antineoplastic.

•**ponatinib hydrochloride.** (poe-NA-ti-nib) USAN.
Use: Antineoplastic.
See: Iclusig.

•**ponezumab.** (poe-NEZ-oo-mab) USAN.
Use: CNS agent.

Ponstel. (Sciele Pharma) Mefenamic acid 250 mg. Lactose. Cap. Bot. 100s. *Rx.*
Use: Nonsteroidal anti-inflammatory agent.

Pontocaine. (Sanofi-Synthelabo) **Cream:** Tetracaine hydrochloride 1%, glycerin, light mineral oil, methylparaben, sodium metabisulfite. Tube 28.35 g. **Oint.:** Tetracaine 0.5%, menthol, white petrolatum. Tube 28.35 g. *OTC.*
Use: Anesthetic, topical.

Pontocaine Hydrochloride. (Hospira) Tetracaine hydrochloride. **Inj. 0.2%:** Dextrose 6%. Amp 2 mL. **0.3%:** Dextrose 6%. Amp 5 mL. **1%:** Acetone sodium bisulfite. Amp 2 mL. **Pow. for reconstitution:** *Niphanoid* (instantly soluble). Amp. *Rx.*
Use: Anesthetic, injectable local.

Pontocaine 2% Aqueous Solution. (Sanofi-Synthelabo) Tetracaine hydrochloride 20 mg, chlorobutanol 4 mg/mL of 2% soln. Bot. 30 mL, Box 12s. Bot. 118 mL, Box 6s. *Rx.*
Use: Anesthetic, local.

Po-Pon-S. (Shire US) Vitamins A 2000 units, D 100 units, E 5 mg, B_1 5 mg, B_2 3 mg, B_3 35 mg, B_5 15 mg, B_6 4 mg, B_{12} 6 mcg, C 100 mg, Ca, P. Tab. Bot. 60s, 240s. *OTC.*
Use: Vitamin, mineral supplement.

poppy-seed oil. The ethyl ester of the fatty acids of the poppy w/iodine.

poractant alfa.
Use: Lung surfactant.
See: Curosurf.

porcine islet preparation, encapsulated.
Use: For type I diabetes patients already on immunosuppression. [Orphan Drug]

•**porfimer sodium.** (PORE-fih-muhr) USAN.
Use: Antineoplastic.
See: Photofrin.

•**porfiromycin.** (par-FIH-row-MY-sin) USAN.
Use: Anti-infective; antineoplastic.

Pork NPH Iletin II. (Eli Lilly) Purified pork insulin 100 units/mL in isophane insulin suspension (insulin w/protamine and zinc). Inj. Bot. 10 mL.
Use: Antidiabetic.

Pork Regular Iletin II. (Eli Lilly) Insulin 100 units/mL. Purified pork. Inj. Vial 10 mL.
Use: Antidiabetic.

•**porofocon A.** (POR-oh-FOE-kon A) USAN.
Use: Contact lens material, hydrophobic.

•**porofocon B.** (POR-oh-FOE-kon B) USAN.
Use: Contact lens material, hydrophobic.

Portabiday. (Washington Ethical) Concentrated soln. of alkylamine lauryl sulfate, a mild detergent with pH approx. 6 for use with *Portabiday* Vaginal Cleansing Kit. Bot. 3 oz. *OTC.*
Use: Vaginal agent.

Portagen. (Bristol-Myers Squibb) A nutritionally complete dietary powder containing as a % of the calories protein 14% as caseinate, fat 41% (medium chain triglycerides 86%, corn oil 14%), carbohydrate 45% as corn syr. solids and sucrose, vitamins A 5000 units, D 500 units, E 20 units, C 52 mg, B_1 1 mg, B_2 1.2 mg, B_6 1.4 mg, B_{12} 4 mcg, niacin 13 mg, folic acid 0.1 mg, choline 83 mg, biotin 0.05 mg, Ca 600 mg, P 450 mg, Mg 133 mg, Fe 12 mg, I 47 mcg, Cu 1 mg, Zn 6 mg, Mn 0.8 mg, Cl 550 mg, Na 300 mg, K 800 mg, pantothenic acid 6.7 mg, K-1 0.1 mg/qt. 20 Kcal/fl oz. Can 1 lb. *OTC.*
Use: Nutritional supplement, enteral.

Portia. (Barr) Levonorgestrel 0.15 mg, ethinyl estradiol 30 mcg. Lactose. Film-coated. Tab. Packs. 21s, 28s (with 7 inert tabs. [lactose]. *Rx.*
Use: Sex hormone, contraceptive hormone.

porton asparaginase.
See: Erwinia L-asparaginase.

•**posaconazole.** (poe-sa-KONE-a-zole) USAN.
Use: Antifungal.
See: Noxafil.

positive and negative hCG urine controls. (Wampole) Positive and negative human urine controls for urine pregnancy tests. 1 set, 1 vial each.
Use: Diagnostic aid.

Poslam Psoriasis Ointment. (Last) Sulfur 5%, salicylic acid 2%. Jar 1 oz.
Use: Antipsoriatic.

posterior pituitary hormones.
See: DDAVP.
Desmopressin Acetate.
Pitressin.
Stimate.
Vasopressin.

•**posterior pituitary injection.** *USP.*
Use: Hormone, antidiuretic.

postlobin-O.
See: Pituitary, Posterior, Hormones.

postlobin-V.
See: Pituitary, Posterior, Hormones.

Posture. (Iverness Medical) Elemental calcium 600 mg. Preservative free. Tab. Bot. 90s. *OTC.*
Use: Mineral supplement, calcium.

Posture D 600. (Wyeth) Calcium phosphate 600 mg, vitamin D 125 units. Tab. Bot. 60s. *OTC.*
Use: Mineral supplement.

Potaba. (Glenwood) Aminobenzoate potassium. **Cap.:** 500 mg. Bot. 250s, 1000s. **Tab.:** 500 mg. Bot. 100s, 1000s. **Envule (Pow.):** 2 g. Box 50s. *Rx.*
Use: Water-soluble vitamin.

Potachlor 10%. (Rosemont) Potassium and chloride 20 mEq/15 mL. Alcohol 5%. Bot. Pt, gal. Alcohol 3.8%. Bot. Pt, gal, UD 15 mL, 30 mL. *Rx.*
Use: Electrolyte supplement.

Potachlor 20%. (Rosemont) Potassium and chloride 40 mEq/15 mL. Alcohol free. Liq. Bot. pt, gal. *Rx.*
Use: Electrolyte supplement.

•**potash, sulfurated.** (PTO-ash SUL-fur-AY-ted) *USP.*
Use: Source of sulfide.

potassic saline lactated injection.
Use: Electrolyte replacement.

potassium.
Use: Electrolyte.
W/Sodium, Vitamin C.
See: PediaCare Cold & Flu Hydration.

•**potassium acetate.** (poe-TASS-ee-um) *USP.* Acetic acid, potassium salt.
Use: Electrolyte replacement; to avoid Cl when high concentration of potassium is needed.

potassium acetate. (Various Mfr.) Potassium acetate 40 mEq. Inj. 20 mL in 50 mL Vial.
Use: Electrolyte replacement; to avoid Cl when high concentration of potassium is needed.

potassium acid phosphate.
See: K-Phos.

potassium acid phosphate/sodium acid phosphate.
Use: Genitourinary.
See: K-Phos No. 2.

•**potassium aspartate and magnesium aspartate.** (poe-TASS-ee-um a-SPAR-tate and mag-NEE-zee-um a-SPAR-tate) USAN.
Use: Nutrient.

•**potassium benzoate.** (poe-TASS-ee-um BEN-zoe-ate) *NF.*
Use: Pharmaceutic aid, preservative.

•**potassium bicarbonate.** (poe-TASS-ee-um bye-KAR-bo-nate) *USP.*
Use: Pharmaceutic necessity; electrolyte replacement.
See: K-Bicarb.
W/Citric Acid, Sodium Bicarbonate.
See: Alka-Seltzer Gold.

•**potassium bicarbonate and potassium chloride effervescent tablets for oral solution.** *USP.*
Use: Electrolyte supplement.

•**potassium bicarbonate and potassium chloride for effervescent oral solution.** *USP.*
Use: Electrolyte supplement.

•**potassium bicarbonate and sodium bicarbonates and citric acid effervescent tablets for oral solution.** *USP.*
Use: Electrolyte supplement.

•**potassium bicarbonate effervescent tablets for oral solution.** *USP.*
Use: Electrolyte supplement.

•**potassium bitartrate.** *USP.*
Use: Cathartic.

•**potassium carbonate.** *USP.*
Use: Potassium therapy; pharmaceutic aid, alkalizing agent.

potassium channel blockers.
See: Dalfampridine.

potassium channel openers.
See: Ezogabine.

•**potassium chloride.** *USP.*
Use: Electrolyte replacement; potassium deficiency, hypopotassemia.
See: Cena-K.
Choice 10.
Choice 20.
Kaochlor.
Kaochlor-Eff.
Kaon Cl.
Kaon Cl-10.
Kaon Cl 20%.
K-Lor.
Klor-Con.
Klorvess.
Klotrix.
K-Lyte/Cl.
K-Lyte/Cl 50.
K-Tab.
Micro-K Extencaps.
Ten-K.
W/PEG 3350, Sodium Bicarbonate, Sodium Chloride.
See: Suclear.
W/PEG 3350, Sodium Bicarbonate, Sodium Chloride, Sodium Sulfate.
See: GaviLyte-C.
GaviLyte-G.

potassium chloride. (Abbott) Potassium chloride. **Ampules:** 20 mEq, 10 mL; 40 mEq, 20 mL. **Pintop Vials:** 10 mEq, 5 mL in 10 mL; 20 mEq, 10 mL in 20 mL; 30 mEq, 12.5 mL in 30 mL; 40 mEq, 12.5 mL in 30 mL. **Fliptop Vials:** 20 mEq, 10 mL in 20 mL; 40 mEq, 20 mL in 50 mL. **Univ. Add. Syr.:** 5 mEq/5 mL, 20 mEq/10 mL, 30 mEq/20 mL, 40 mEq/20 mL (Eli Lilly and Co.) Amp. (40 mEq) 20 mL, 6s, 25s. *Rx.*
Use: Nutritional therapy.

potassium chloride. (KV Pharmaceutical Co.) Microencapsulated potassium chloride 600 mg equivalent to 8 mEq. ER Cap. 100s, 500s. *Rx.*
Use: Electrolyte.

potassium chloride. (Major) Potassium 20 mEq/15 mL. Glycerin, saccharin, sodium benzoate, sorbitol. Sugar free. Cherry flavor. Soln. 473 mL. *Rx.*
Use: Electrolyte.

potassium chloride. (Roxane) Potassium chloride. **Oral soln.:** Sugar free. 40 mEq/30 mL. Bot. 6 oz, 500 mL, 1 L, 5 L 20%. 80 mEq/30 mL. Bot. 500 mL, 1 L, 5 L. **Pow.:** 20 mEq/4 g. Pkt. 30s, 100s. *Rx.*
Use: Electrolyte supplement.

potassium chloride. (Wyeth) Potassium chloride 10%, 20%. Sugar free. Soln. 16 oz, gal. *Rx.*
Use: Electrolyte supplement.

potassium chloride. (Various Mfr.) Potassium chloride. **ER Tab.:** 20 mEq. 30s, 90s, 100s, 500s. **Inj., Soln., concentrate: 2 mEq/mL:** Equiv. to 149 mg/mL of potassium chloride. 250 mL and 500 mL pharmacy bulk packages. **10 mEq:** Equiv. to 149 mg/mL of potassium chloride. 5 mL and 10 mL single-dose vials and 50 mL and 100 mL flexible plastic containers. **20 mEq:** Equiv. to 149 mg/mL of potassium chloride. 10 mL single-dose vials and 50 mL and 100 mL flexible plastic containers. **30 mEq:** Equiv. to 149 mg/mL of potassium chloride. 15 mL single-dose vials and 100 mL flexible plastic containers. **40 mEq:** Equiv. to 149 mg/mL of potassium chloride. 20 mL and 30 mL

single-dose vials and 100 mL flexible plastic containers. **60 mEq:** Equiv. to 149 mg/mL of potassium chloride. Parabens. 30 mL multiple-use vials. *Rx.*
Use: Electrolyte.

•**potassium chloride in dextrose and sodium chloride injection.** *USP.*
Use: Electrolyte supplement.

potassium chloride in 5% dextrose. (Various Mfr.) Dextrose 50 g; calories 170; K^+ 10, 20, 30, or 40 mEq; Cl^- 10, 20, 30, or 40 mEq, osmolarity ≈ 272, 292 to 295, 310 to 312, or 330 to 333 mOsm/L. Soln. Bot. 500 mL (330 to 333 mOsm only), 1000 mL. *Rx.*
Use: Intravenous nutritional therapy, intravenous replenishment solution.

potassium chloride in 5% dextrose and lactated Ringer's. (Baxter Healthcare) Dextrose 50 g, calories 170, Na^+ 130 mEq, K^+ 24 or 44 mEq, Ca^{++} 2.7 mEq, Cl^- 129 or 149 mEq, lactate 28 mEq, osmolarity 565 or 604 mOsm/L. Soln. 1,000 mL. *Rx.*
Use: Intravenous nutritional therapy, intravenous replenishment solution.

potassium chloride in 5% dextrose and lactated Ringer's. (Hospira) Dextrose 50 g, kcal 179, Na+ 130 mEq, K+ 24 mEq, Ca++ 2.7 mEq, Cl– 129 mEq, lactate 28 mEq, 563 mOsm per liter. Inj. 1,000 mL. *Rx.*
Use: Intravenous nutritional therapy.

potassium chloride in 5% dextrose and 0.45% sodium chloride. (Various Mfr.) Dextrose 50 g; calories 170; Na^+ 77 mEq; K^+ 10, 20, 30, or 40 mEq, Cl^- 87, 97, 107, or 117 mEq; osmolarity ≈ 425, 445 to 447, ≈ 465, or 487 to 490 mOsm/L. Soln. Bot. 500 mL (445 to 447 mOsm only); 1000 mL. *Rx.*
Use: Intravenous nutritional therapy, intravenous replenishment solution.

potassium chloride in 5% dextrose and 0.9% sodium chloride. (Various Mfr.) Dextrose 50 g; calories 170; Na^+ 154 mEq; K^+ 20 or 40 mEq, Cl^- 174 or 194 mEq; osmolarity ≈ 600 or 640 mOsm/L. Soln. Bot. 1000 mL. *Rx.*
Use: Intravenous nutritional therapy, intravenous replenishment solution.

potassium chloride in 5% dextrose and 0.33% sodium chloride. (Various Mfr.) Dextrose 50 g; calories 170; Na^+ 56 mEq; K^+ 20, 30, or 40 mEq, Cl^- 76, 86, or 96 mEq; osmolarity 405, 425, or 446 mOsm/L. Soln. Bot. 500 mL (405 mOsm only); 1000 mL. *Rx.*
Use: Intravenous nutritional therapy, intravenous replenishment solution.

potassium chloride in 5% dextrose and 0.2% sodium chloride. (Various Mfr.) Dextrose 50 g; calories 170; Na^+ 34 mEq; K^+ 10, 20, 30, or 40 mEq, Cl^- 44, 54, 64, or 74 mEq; osmolarity ≈ 340, 360, 380, or 400 mOsm/L. Soln. Bot. 250 mL, 500 mL (≈ 360 mOsm only); 1000 mL. *Rx.*
Use: Intravenous nutritional therapy, intravenous replenishment solution.

•**potassium chloride in lactated Ringer's and dextrose injection.** *USP.*
Use: Electrolyte supplement.

•**potassium chloride in sodium chloride injection.** *USP.*
Use: Electrolyte supplement.

potassium chloride in 10% dextrose and 0.2% sodium chloride. (B. Braun) Dextrose 100 g, calories 340, Na^+ 34 mEq; K^+ 20 mEq, Cl^- 54 mEq; osmolarity 615 mOsm/L. Soln. Bot. 250 mL. *Rx.*
Use: Intravenous nutritional therapy, intravenous replenishment solution.

potassium chloride in 3.3% dextrose and 0.3% sodium chloride. (B. Braun) Dextrose 33 g, calories 110, Na^+ 51 mEq, K^+ 20 mEq, Cl^- 71 mEq, osmolarity 310 mOsm/L. Soln. Bot. 1000 mL. *Rx.*
Use: Intravenous nutritional therapy, intravenous replenishment solution.

potassium chloride in 0.9% sodium chloride. (Various Mfr.) Na^+ 154 mEq, K^+ 20 or 40 mEq, Cl^- 174 or 194 mEq, osmolarity ≈ 350 or 390 mOsm/L. Soln. Bot. 1000 mL. *Rx.*
Use: Intravenous nutritional therapy, intravenous replenishment solution.

•**potassium chloride K 42.** (poe-TASS-ee-um K 42) USAN.
Use: Radiopharmaceutical.

potassium chloride, sodium chloride, and calcium carbonate.
Use: Salt replacement.
See: Sustain.

potassium chloride with potassium gluconate.
Use: Electrolyte supplement.

•**potassium citrate.** (poe-TASS-ee-um SIT-rate) *USP.* Tripotassium citrate.
Use: Alkalizer. [Orphan Drug]
See: Urocit-K.
W/Citric Acid, Sodium Citrate.
See: Cytra.
Polycitra K Crystals.
W/Dextromethorphan Hydrobromide, Guaifenesin.
See: Sorbutuss NR.

W/Sodium citrate.
See: Bicitra.
potassium citrate. (Upsher-Smith) Potassium citrate 5 mEq, 10 mEq. Wax matrix. ER Tab. 100s. *Rx.*
Use: Urinary alkalinizer.
potassium citrate. (Various Mfr.) Potassium citrate 5 mEq (540 mg), 10 mEq (1,080 mg), 15 mEq (1,620 mg). ER Tab. 100s. *Rx.*
Use: Urinary alkalinizer.
potassium citrate monohydrate.
W/Citric Acid Monohydrate.
See: Taron-Crystals.
potassium clavulanate/amoxicillin.
Use: Anti-infective, penicillin.
See: Amoclan.
Amoxicillin and potassium clavulanate.
Augmentin.
potassium clavulanate/ticarcillin.
Use: Anti-infective, penicillin.
See: Ticarcillin and clavulanate potassium.
•**potassium glucaldrate.** (poe-TASS-ee-um gloo-KAL-drate) USAN.
Use: Antacid.
•**potassium gluconate.** (poe-TASS-ee-um GLOO-koe-nate) *USP.*
Use: Electrolyte replacement.
See: Kaon.
potassium gluconate. (Various Mfr.) Potassium 40 mEq provided by potassium gluconate 9.36 g/30 mL, alcohol 5%. Elix. Bot. Pt, Patient-Cup 15 mL. *Rx.*
Use: Electrolyte supplement.
•**potassium gluconate and potassium chloride for oral solution.** *USP.*
Use: Replacement therapy.
•**potassium gluconate and potassium chloride solution.** *USP.*
Use: Replacement therapy.
•**potassium gluconate and potassium citrate oral solution.** *USP.*
Use: Electrolyte supplement.
•**potassium gluconate, potassium citrate, and ammonium chloride oral solution.** *USP.*
Use: Electrolyte supplement.
potassium glutamate. The monopotassium salt of l-glutamic acid.
potassium G penicillin.
See: Penicillin G potassium.
•**potassium guaiacolsulfonate.** (poe-TASS-ee-um GWYE-a-kol-SUL-foe-nate) *USP.* Sulfoguaiacol. Potassium Hydroxymethoxybenzene sulfonate. Used in many cough preps.
Use: Expectorant.
See: Pinex Regular.
•**potassium hydroxide.** (poe-TASS-ee-um hye-DROX-ide) *NF.*
Use: Pharmaceutic aid, alkalinizing agent.
potassium in sodium chloride. (Various Mfr.) Potassium Cl 0.15%, 0.22%, 0.3% in sodium Cl 0.9%. Soln. for Inj. 1000 mL. *Rx.*
Use: Intravenous replenishment solution, nutritional supplement.
•**potassium iodide.** (poe-TASS-ee-um EYE-oh-dide) *USP.*
Use: Expectorant; antifungal; supplement, iodine; thyroid drug.
See: Iosat.
ThyroSafe.
ThyroShield.
W/Combinations.
See: Diastix Reagent Strips.
Elixophyllin-KI.
KIE.
Mudrane.
Mudrane-2.
W/Iodine.
See: Strong Iodine Solution (Lugol's Solution).
potassium iodide. (Roxane) Potassium iodide 1 g/mL. Soln. 30 mL, 240 mL. *Rx.*
Use: Thyroid drug.
potassium iodide. (Various Mfr.) Potassium iodide 1 g/mL. Soln. 30 mL, 240 mL, pt. *Rx.*
Use: Thyroid drug.
•**potassium metabisulfite.** (poe-TASS-ee-um MET-a-bye-SUL-fite) *NF.*
Use: Pharmaceutic aid, antioxidant.
•**potassium metaphosphate.** (poe-TASS-ee-um MET-a-FOS-fate) *NF.*
Use: Pharmaceutic aid, buffering agent.
•**potassium nitrate.** (poe-TASS-ee-um NYE-trate) *USP.*
W/Silver Nitrate.
See: Grafco.
W/Sodium Fluoride.
See: Sensodyne Iso-Active Multi Action.
Sensodyne Iso-Active Whitening.
potassium p-aminobenzoate.
See: Potaba.
W/Potassium salicylate.
See: Pabalate-SF.
potassium penicillin G.
Use: Anti-infective, penicillin.
See: Penicillin G, Potassium.
potassium penicillin V.
Use: Anti-infective, penicillin.
See: Phenoxymethyl penicillin potassium.
•**potassium perchlorate.** (poe-TASS-ee-um per-KLOR-ate) *USP.*
Use: Hyperthyroidism.

•**potassium permanganate.** (poe-TASS-ee-um per-MAN-ga-nate) *USP.* Permanganic acid, potassium salt.
Use: Anti-infective, topical.
potassium phenethicillin. Phenethicillin potassium.
Use: Anti-infective.
potassium phenoxymethyl penicillin.
Use: Anti-infective.
See: Penicillin V potassium.
potassium phosphate. (Various Mfr.) Phosphate 3 mM, potassium 4.4 mEq per mL. Inj. Vials. 5 mL, 10 mL, 15 mL, 30 mL, 50 mL. *Rx.*
Use: Intravenous nutritional therapy, mineral.
•**potassium phosphate, dibasic.** (poe-TASS-ee-um FOS-fate) *USP.*
Use: Calcium regulator.
•**potassium phosphate, monobasic.** (poe-TASS-ee-um FOS-fate) *NF.* Dipotassium hydrogen phosphate.
Use: Pharmaceutic aid, buffering agent; source of potassium.
W/Dibasic Sodium Phosphate, Monobasic Sodium Phosphate.
See: Phospha 250 Neutral.
potassium phosphate, monobasic. (Abbott) Potassium phosphate monobasic 15 mM, 5 mL in 10 mL vial; 45 mM, 15 mL in 20 mL/Inj. vial.
Use: Pharmaceutic aid, buffering agent; source of potassium.
potassium reagent strips. (Bayer Consumer Care) Quantitative dry reagent strip test for potassium in serum or plasma. Bot. 50s.
Use: Diagnostic aid.
potassium-removing resins.
See: Sodium Polystyrene Sulfonate.
potassium rhodanate.
See: Potassium Thiocyanate.
potassium salicylate.
See: Neocylate.
W/Potassium P-Aminobenzoate.
See: Pabalate-SF.
potassium salt.
See: Potassium sorbate.
•**potassium sodium tartrate.** (poe-TASS-ee-um SOE-dee-um TAR-trate) *USP.*
Use: Laxative.
•**potassium sorbate.** (poe-TASS-ee-um SOR-bate) *NF.*
Use: Pharmaceutic aid, antimicrobial.
•**potassium sulfate.** (poe-TAS-ee-um) USAN.
Use: Bowel evacuant.
W/Magnesium Sulfate, Sodium Sulfate.
See: Suclear.
Suprep Bowel Prep.
potassium sulfocyanate. Potassium Rhodanate.
See: Potassium thiocyanate.
potassium thiocyanate. Potassium sulfocyanate, potassium rhodanate.
potassium thiphencillin.
Use: Anti-infective.
potassium troclosene. (Monsanto) Potassium dichloroisocyanurate.
Use: Anti-infective.
Potiga. (GlaxoSmithKline) Ezogabine 50 mg, 200 mg, 300 mg, 400 mg. Film coated. PEG. Tab. 90s. *Rx.*
Use: Anticonvulsant, calcium channel opener.
•**povidone.** (POE-vi-done) *USP. Formerly Polyvidone, Polyvinylpyrrolidone.*
Use: Pharmaceutic aid, dispersing and suspending agent.
•**povidone-iodine.** *USP.*
Use: Anti-infective, topical.
See: Betadine.
Betadine PrepStick.
Betadine PrepStick Plus.
GRX Dyne.
GRX Dyne Scrub.
Massengill Medicated.
W/Lidocaine Hydrochloride.
See: ProTech First-Aid Stik.
povidone-iodine complex.
See: Betadine.
•**povidone I 131.** (POE-vi-done) USAN.
Use: Radiopharmaceutical.
•**povidone I 125.** (POE-vi-done) USAN.
Use: Radiopharmaceutical.
PowerMate. (Green Turtle Bay Vitamin Co.) Vitamins A 5000 units, E 100 units, B_3 12.5 mg, C 250 mg, Zn 2.5 mg, Se 7.5 mcg, n-acetyl-L-cysteine 25 mg, glutathione 5 mg, gingko biloba 5 mg, green tea extract 100 mg, pine bark extract 5 mg, echinacea 50 mg, golden seal root 20 mg, coenzyme Q10 2 mg, yeast free. Tab. Bot. 50s. *OTC.*
Use: Amino acid
PowerSleep. (Green Turtle Bay Vitamin Co.) L-glutamine 250 mg, 5-HTP 25 mg, melatonin 0.25 mg, vitamin B_3 25 mg, B_6 5 mg, inositol 100 mg, Ca 25 mg, passion flower extract 100 mg, valerian powder 75 mg. Tab. Bot. 60s. *OTC.*
Use: Amino acid.
PowerVites. (Green Turtle Bay Vitamin Co.) Vitamin A 2500 units, D 150 units, E 12.5 units, C 125 mg, B_1 6.3 mg, B_2 6.3 mg, B_3 25 mg, B_5 25 mg, B_6 12.5 mg, B_{12} 6.3 mcg, biotin, folic acid 0.15 mg, B, Ca, Mg, Cu, Zn 2.5 mg, Cr, Mn, K, Se, betaine, hesperidin. Tab.

Bot. 40s, 100s, 200s. *OTC.*
Use: Mineral, vitamin supplement.

Poyaliver Stronger. (Forest) Liver inj. (equivalent to 10 mcg B_{12}), vitamin B_{12} 100 mcg, folic acid 10 mcg, niacinamide 1%/mL. Vial 10 mL. *Rx.*
Use: Nutritional supplement, parenteral.

Poyamin Jel Injection. (Forest) Cyanocobalamin 1000 mcg/mL. Vial 10 mL.
Use: Nutritional supplement, parenteral.

Poyaplex. (Forest) Vitamins B_1 100 mg, niacinamide 100 mg, B_6 10 mg, B_2 1 mg, panthenol 10 mg, B_{12} 5 mcg/mL. Vial 10 mL, 30 mL. *Rx.*
Use: Nutritional supplement, parenteral.

•**pozanicline.** (poe-ZAN-i-kleen) USAN.
Use: CNS agent.

•**pozanicline tartrate.** (poe-ZAN-i-kleen) USAN.
Use: CNS agent.

P.P.D. tuberculin.
See: Tuberculin Purified Protein Derivative.

P.P. factor. Pellagra preventive factor.
See: Nicotinic Acid.

ppg-15 stearyl ether.
Use: Pharmaceutic aid, surfactant.

PR. (PruGen) Cyclomethicone, dimethicone, hexyl laurate, polyglyceryl-4-isostearate, propylparaben. Dye free. Cream. 56.7 g kit w/*PruDrate* moisturizing cream. *Rx.*
Use: Emollient.

•**practolol.** (PRAK-toe-lole) USAN.
Use: Antiadrenergic, β-receptor.

Pradaxa. (Boehringer Ingelheim Pharmaceuticals) Dabigatran etexilate 75 mg (equiv. to dabigatran etexilate mesylate 86.48 mg), 150 mg (equiv. to dabigatran etexilate mesylate 172.95 mg). Cap. 60s, UD 60s. *Rx.*
Use: Anticoagulant, thrombin inhibitor.

•**pradefovir mesylate.** (prad-e-FOE-veer) USAN.
Use: Antiviral.

•**pralatrexate.** (PRAL-a-TREX-ate) USAN.
Tall Man: PRALAtrexate
Use: Folic acid antagonist.
See: Folotyn.

•**pralidoxime chloride.** (PRAL-i-DOX-eem) *USP.*
Use: Cholinesterase reactivator; antidote.
See: Protopam Chloride.

pralidoxime chloride. (Survival Technical) Pralidoxime chloride 600 mg, benzyl alcohol, aminocaproic acid. Inj. Vial 2 mL. *Rx.*
Use: Antidote.

pralidoxime chloride/atropine.
Use: Detoxification agent, antidote.
See: DuoDote.

•**pralidoxime iodide.** (PRAL-i-DOX-eem EYE-oh-dide) USAN.
Use: Cholinesterase reactivator.

•**pralidoxime mesylate.** (PRAL-i-DOX-eem) USAN.
Use: Cholinesterase reactivator.

pralidoxime methiodide.
See: Pralidoxime Iodide.

•**pralmorelin dihydrochloride.** (pral-more-ELL-in die-HIGH-droe-KLOR-ide) USAN.
Use: Growth hormone-releasing factor.

•**pralnacasan.** (PRAL-na-ka-san) USAN.
Use: Rheumatoid arthritis.

PramCort. (Rochester Pharmaceuticals) Hydrocortisone acetate 1%, pramoxine hydrochloride 1%. Alcohol, ceresin wax, lanolin alcohol, mineral oil, propylene glycol, triethanolamine, white petrolatum. Cream. 30 g. *Rx.*
Use: Topical corticosteroid combination.

PrameGel. (Bioglan) Pramoxine hydrochloride 1%. Emollient base with menthol 0.5%, benzyl alcohol, SD alcohol 40. Gel. 118 mL. *OTC.*
Use: Topical local anesthetic.

Pram-HCA. (Acella) Hydrocortisone acetate 2.35%, pramoxine hydrochloride 1%. Aloe, disodium EDTA, mineral oil, parabens, PEG, petrolatum, propylene glycol, triethanolamine, vitamin E, wax. Cream; rectal. 30 g w/2 wipes and 1 applicator. *Rx.*
Use: Anorectal preparation, steroid-containing product.

•**pramiconazole.** (PRAM-i-KON-a-zole) USAN.
Use: Antifungal.

Pramilet FA. (Ross) Vitamins A 4000 units, B_1 3 mg, B_2 2 mg, B_6 3 mg, B_{12} 3 mcg, C 60 mg, D 400 units, B_5 1 mg, B_3 10 mg, Ca 250 mg, Cu, I, Fe 40 mg, Mg, Zn, folic acid 1 mg. Filmtab. Bot. 100s. *Rx.*
Use: Mineral, vitamin supplement.

•**pramipexole dihydrochloride.** (pram-ih-PEX-ole) USAN.
Use: Antiparkinsonian; antischizophrenic; antidepressant.
See: Mirapex.
Mirapex XR.

pramipexole dihydrochloride. (Various Mfr.) Pramipexole dihydrochloride. **Tab.:** 0.125 mg, 0.25 mg, 0.5 mg, 0.75 mg, 1 mg, 1.5 mg. May contain mannitol. 90s, 500s, 1,000s (except 0.75 mg), UD 100s (except 0.75 mg, 1.5 mg).

ER Tab.: 0.375, 0.75 mg, 1.5 mg, 2.25 mg, 3 mg, 3.75 mg, 4.5 mg. May contain mannitol, soy lecithin. 30s. *Rx.*
Use: Antiparkinson agent, dopaminergic, nonergot dopamine receptor agonist.

•**pramiracetam hydrochloride.** (PRAM-i-RA-se-tam) USAN. *Formerly Amacetam Hydrochloride.*
Use: Cognition adjuvant.

•**pramiracetam sulfate.** (PRAM-i-RA-se-tam) USAN. *Formerly Amacetam Sulfate.*
Use: Cognition adjuvant.

•**pramlintide acetate.** (PRAM-lin-tide) USAN.
Use: Antidiabetic agent, amylin analog.
See: Symlin.

Pramosone. (Sebela) Hydrocortisone acetate/pramoxine hydrochloride 1%/1%, 2.5%/1%. **Cream:** Hydrophilic base. Potassium sorbate 0.1%, sorbic acid 0.1%. 30 g, 60 g (1%/1% only), 120 g. **Lot.:** Hydrophilic base. Glycerin, potassium sorbate 0.1%, sorbic acid 0.1%. 60 mL, 120 mL, 240 mL (1%/1% only). **Oint.:** Emollient base. White petrolatum. 30 g, 120 g. *Rx.*
Use: Anti-inflammatory agent, topical corticosteroid combination.

Pramosone E. (Sebela) Hydrocortisone acetate 2.5%, pramoxine 1%. *Hydrolipid* base. Cetostearyl alcohol, mineral oil, propylparaben, triethanolamine, white petrolatum. Cream. 28.4 g, 57 g. *Rx.*
Use: Topical corticosteroid combination.

Pramoxine-HC. (Ascend Laboratories) Chloroxylenol 1 mg, hydrocortisone 10 mg, pramoxine hydrochloride 10 mg. Isopropyl alcohol, propylene glycol. Drops; Otic. 10 mL. *Rx.*
Use: Miscellaneous otic preparation.

•**pramoxine hydrochloride.** (pram-OX-een) *USP.*
Use: Anesthetic, topical.
See: Campho-Phenique Cold Sore Treatment and Scab Relief.
Itch-X.
Ivy Wash.
PrameGel.
Prax.
ProctoFoam NS.
Sarna Sensitive Anti-Itch.
Tronothane Hydrochloride.
Tucks.
Vagisil Maximum Strength.
W/Bacitracin Zinc.
See: Bacitraycin Plus.
W/Bacitracin Zinc, Neomycin, Polymyxin B Sulfate.
See: Neosporin Plus Pain Relief.
Tri-Biozene.
W/Benzalkonium Chloride.
See: Bactine Pain Relieving Cleansers.
W/Benzalkonium Chloride, Chloroxylenol, Hydrocortisone.
See: Cortic-ND.
Mediotic-HC.
W/Calamine.
See: Aveeno Anti-Itch.
Caladryl.
Calagesic.
W/Chloroxylenol, Hydrocortisone.
See: Oto-End 10.
Otomar-HC.
Pramoxine-HC.
Zoto-HC.
W/Chloroxylenol, Zinc Acetate Dihydrate.
See: ZinOtic ES.
W/Clioquinol, Hydrocortisone.
See: 1 + 1-F Creme.
W/Dimethicone.
See: Gold Bond Intensive Healing.
W/Hydrocortisone.
See: Cortane-B.
W/Hydrocortisone Acetate.
See: Analpram-E.
EndaRoid.
Epifoam.
HC Pram 1%.
HC Pramoxine.
HC Pram 2.5%.
PramCort.
Pram-HCA.
Pramosone.
Pramosone E.
ProCort.
Proctofoam-HC.
ZyPram.
W/Neomycin, Polymyxin B Sulfate.
See: Neosporin Plus Pain Relief.
W/Zinc Acetate.
See: Calaclear.
Callergy Clear.

pramoxine hydrochloride. (Libertas Pharma) Pramoxine hydrochloride 1%. Cetyl alcohol, parabens, propylene glycol, trolamine, wax. Aer., foam. 15 g. *OTC.*
Use: Topical local anesthetic.

PrandiMet. (Novo Nordisk) Repaglinide 1 mg/metformin hydrochloride 500 mg, repaglinide 2 mg/metformin hydrochloride 500 mg. PEG, sorbitol. Tab. 20s, 100s. *Rx.*
Use: Antidiabetic agent, antidiabetic combination product.

Prandin. (Novo Nordisk) Repaglinide 0.5 mg, 1 mg, 2 mg. Tab. Bot. 100s, 500s, 1000s. *Rx.*
Use: Antidiabetic, meglitinide.

•**pranolium chloride.** (pray-NO-lee-uhm) USAN.
Use: Cardiovascular agent, antiarrhythmic.

•**prasugrel hydrochloride.** (pra-SOO-grel) USAN.
Use: Platelet antagonist.
See: Effient.

Pravachol. (Bristol-Myers Squibb) Pravastatin sodium 20 mg, 40 mg, 80 mg. Lactose. Tab. 90s, 500s (80 mg only), 1,000s (20 mg only), UD 100s. *Rx.*
Use: Antihyperlipidemic, HMG-CoA reductase inhibitor.

•**pravadoline maleate.** (pray-AH-doe-leen) USAN.
Use: Analgesic.

•**pravastatin sodium.** (PRUH-vuh-stuh-tin) USAN.
Use: Antihyperlipidemic, HMG-CoA reductase inhibitor.
See: Pravachol.

pravastatin sodium. (Various Mfr.) Pravastatin sodium 10 mg, 20 mg, 40 mg, 80 mg. May contain lactose. Tab. 30s (except 80 mg), 90s, 100s, 500s, 1000s. *Rx.*
Use: Antihyperlipidemic agent, HMG-CoA reductase inhibitor.

Prax. (Sebela) Pramoxine hydrochloride 1%. **Lot.:** Hydrophilic base with potassium sorbate 0.1%, sorbic acid 0.1%, mineral oil, cetyl alcohol, glycerin, lanolin. 120 mL, 240 mL. **Wipes:** Glycerin. 12s. *OTC.*
Use: Topical local anesthetic.

praziquantel.
Use: Anthelmintic.
See: Biltricide.

•**prazosin hydrochloride.** (PRAY-zoe-sin) *USP.*
Use: Antihypertensive, antiadrenergic.
See: Minipress.

prazosin hydrochloride. (Various Mfr.) Prazosin hydrochloride 1 mg, 2 mg, 5 mg. Cap. Bot. 100s, 250s, 500s, 1000s (except 5 mg).
Use: Antihypertensive, antiadrenergic.

Pre-Attain. (Sherwood Davis & Geck) Sodium caseinate, maltodextrin, corn oil, soy lecithin, vitamins A, B_1, B_2, B_3, B_5, B_6, B_{12}, C, D, E, K, folic acid, Ca, Cl, Cu, Fe, I, Mg, Mn, P, Zn. Liq. Can 250 mL, closed system 1000 mL. *OTC.*
Use: Nutritional supplement.

PreCare. (Ther-Rx) Vitamin C 50 mg, Ca 250 mg, Fe 40 mg, D_3 6 mcg, E 3.5 mg, B_6 2 mg, folic acid 1 mg, Mg, Zn 15 mg, Cu, mannitol, sucrose, vanilla flavor. Chew. Tab. UD 100s. *Rx.*
Use: Vitamin, mineral supplement.

PreCare Conceive. (Ther-Rx) Vitamin C 60 mg, Ca 200 mg, Fe 30 mg, E 30 units, thiamin 3 mg, riboflavin 3.4 mg, niacin 20 mg, pyridoxine 50 mg, folic acid 1 mg, Mg, cyanocobalamin 12 mcg, Zn 15 mg, Cu, lactose. Tab. UD 100s. *Rx.*
Use: Vitamin, mineral supplement.

PreCare Premier. (Thera-Rx) Vitamin C 50 mg, D_3 240 units, E 3.5 units, B_1 3 mg, B_2 3.4 mg, B_3 20 mg, B_6 50 mg, folic acid 1 mg, B_{12} 12 mcg, calcium 250 mg, sumalate iron 30 mg, magnesium 25 mg, zinc 15 mg, copper 2 mg, docusate sodium 50 mg, succinic acid 35 mg. Lactose, PEG, polydextrose, sucrose, vegetable oil. Tab. 30s. *Rx.*
Use: Nutritional supplement.

PreCare Prenatal. (Ther-Rx) Ca 250 mg, Fe (as ferrous fumarate) 40 mg, E (dl-alpha tocopheryl acetate) 3.5 mg, D_3 6 mcg, B_1 3 mg, B_2 3.4 mg, B_3 20 mg, B_6 12 mcg, C 50 mg, folic acid 1 mg, Mg, Zn 15 mg, Cu. Dye free. Tab. UD 100s. *Rx.*
Use: Vitamin, mineral supplement.

Precedex. (Hospira) Dexmedetomidine hydrochloride. **Inj., Soln.:** 4 mcg/mL. Sodium chloride. Preservative free. Single-use bottle. 50 mL, 100 mL. **Inj., Soln., concentrate:** 100 mcg/mL. Sodium chloride. Preservative free. Single-use vial. 2 mL. *Rx.*
Use: Sedative; hypnotic (nonbarbiturate).

Precef for Injection. (Bristol-Myers Squibb) Ceforanide 500 mg, 1 g/Vial or piggyback. *Rx.*
Use: Anti-infective, cephalosporin.

Precision High Nitrogen Diet. (Novartis) Vanilla flavor: Maltodextrin, pasteurized egg white solids, sucrose, natural and artificial flavors, medium chain triglycerides, partially hydrogenated soybean oil, polysorbate 80, mono- and diglycerides, vitamins, minerals. Pow. Packet 2.93 oz. *OTC.*
Use: Nutritional supplement.

Precision LR Diet. (Novartis) Orange flavor: Maltodextrin, pasteurized egg white solids, sucrose, medium chain triglycerides, partially hydrogenated soybean oil with BHA, citric acid, natural and artificial flavors, mono- and diglycerides, polysorbate 80, FD&C Yellow No. 5 and No. 6, vitamins, minerals. Pow. Packet 3 oz. *OTC.*
Use: Nutritional supplement.

Precose. (Bayer) Acarbose 25 mg, 50 mg, 100 mg. Tab. Bot. 100s, UD

100s (except 25 mg). *Rx.*
Use: Antidiabetic.

Predamide Ophthalmic. (Maurry) Sodium sulfacetamide 10%, prednisolone acetate 0.5%, hydroxyethyl cellulose, polysorbate 80, sodium thiosulfate, benzalkonium Cl 0.025%. Bot. 5 mL, 15 mL. *Rx.*
Use: Anti-infective; corticosteroid, ophthalmic.

Pred Forte. (Allergan) Prednisolone acetate 1%. Benzalkonium chloride, EDTA, polysorbate 80, hydroxypropyl methylcellulose, sodium bisulfite, boric acid, sodium chloride, sodium citrate. Ophth. Susp. Bot. 1 mL, 5 mL, 10 mL, 15 mL. *Rx.*
Use: Corticosteroid, ophthalmic.

Pred-G. (Allergan) **Oint.:** Prednisolone acetate 0.6%, gentamicin sulfate 0.3%, chlorobutanol 0.5%. Oint. Tube 3.5 g. **Ophth. Susp.:** Prednisolone acetate 1%, gentamicin sulfate 0.3%, benzalkonium chloride 0.005%, polyvinyl alcohol 1.4%, EDTA, hydrochloric acid, hydroxypropyl methylcellulose, sodium chloride, polysorbate 80, sodium citrate dihydrate, sodium hydroxide. Bot. 2 mL, 5 mL, 10 mL. *Rx.*
Use: Corticosteroid; anti-infective, ophthalmic.

Predicort-AP. (Oxypure) Prednisolone sodium phosphate 20 mg, prednisolone acetate 80 mg/mL. Vial 10 mL. *Rx.*
Use: Corticosteroid.

Predicort-RP. (Oxypure) Prednisolone sodium phosphate equivalent to prednisolone phosphate 20 mg, niacinamide 25 mg/mL. Vial 10 mL. *Rx.*
Use: Corticosteroid.

Pred Mild. (Allergan) Prednisolone acetate 0.12%. Benzalkonium chloride, EDTA, polysorbate 80, hydroxypropyl methylcellulose, sodium bisulfite, boric acid, sodium chloride, sodium citrate. Ophth. Susp. Bot. 5 mL, 10 mL. *Rx.*
Use: Corticosteroid, ophthalmic.

•**prednazate.** (PRED-nah-zate) USAN.
Use: Anti-inflammatory.

•**prednicarbate.** (PRED-nih-CAR-bate) USAN.
Use: Corticosteroid, topical.
See: Dermatop.

prednicarbate. (Fougera) Prednicarbate 0.1%. Cetostearyl alcohol, EDTA, lanolin alcohols, mineral oil, white petrolatum. Cream. 15 g, 60 g. *Rx.*
Use: Anti-inflammatory agent, topical corticosteroid.

prednicarbate. (Fougera) Prednicarbate 0.1%. Glyceryl, white petrolatum. Oint. 15 g, 60 g. *Rx.*
Use: Anti-inflammatory agent; corticosteroid, topical.

•**prednimustine.** (PRED-nih-MUSS-teen) USAN.
Use: Antineoplastic. [Orphan Drug]

•**prednisolone.** (pred-NIS-oh-lone) *USP.* Metacortandralone.
Tall Man: prednisoLONE
Use: Corticosteroid; adrenocortical steroid, glucocorticoid.
See: AsmalPred Plus.
Cordrol.
Millipred.
Orapred.
Orapred ODT.
Prelone.
Veripred 20.

prednisolone. (Halsey Drug) Prednisolone 15 mg/5 mL, alcohol 5%. Syr. Bot. 236 mL, 473 mL. *Rx.*
Use: Corticosteroid.

prednisolone. (Various Mfr.) Prednisolone. **Syr.:** 15 mg/mL. Sucrose. 240 mL, 480 mL. **Tab.:** 5 mg. 100s, 1000s, 5000s. *Rx.*
Use: Adrenocortical steroid, glucocorticoid.

•**prednisolone acetate.** (pred-NIS-oh-lone) *USP.*
Tall Man: prednisoLONE
Use: Corticosteroid, topical; adrenocortical steroid, glucocorticoid.
See: Flo-Pred.
Omnipred.
Pred.
Pred Forte.
Pred Mild.
Predicort-AP.
Sigpred.
Steraject.
W/Combinations.
See: Blephamide.
Blephamide Ophthalmic Ointment.
Pred-G.
Pred-G S.O.P.

prednisolone acetate. (Various Mfr.) Prednisolone acetate 1%. Benzalkonium chloride 0.01%, EDTA, polysorbate 80, glycerin, hypromellose, dibasic sodium phosphate. Ophth. Susp. Bot. 5 mL, 10 mL, 15 mL. *Rx.*
Use: Corticosteroid, ophthalmic.

prednisolone acetate and prednisolone sodium phosphate. (Various Mfr.) Prednisolone acetate 80 mg, prednisolone sodium phosphate 20 mg/mL. Inj. Vial 10 mL. *Rx.*
Use: Corticosteroid.

prednisolone butylacetate.
Use: Corticosteroid.

prednisolone cyclopentylpropionate. *Use:* Corticosteroid.

•**prednisolone hemisuccinate.** (pred-NIS-oh-lone HEM-ee-SUX-i-nate) *USP.*
Tall Man: prednisoLONE
Use: Corticosteroid, topical.

•**prednisolone sodium metazoate.** (pred-NIS-oh-lone) USAN.
Use: Gastrointestinal agent.

•**prednisolone sodium phosphate.** (pred-NIS-oh-lone) *USP.*
Tall Man: prednisoLONE
Use: Corticosteroid, topical; adrenocortical steroid, glucocorticoid.
See: AsmalPred Plus.
Orapred.
Orapred ODT.
Pediapred.
Prednisol.
W/Prednisolone acetate.
See: Optimyd.
Vasocidin Ophthalmic Solution.

prednisolone sodium phosphate. (Bausch & Lomb) Prednisolone sodium phosphate 1%. Hypromellose, monobasic and dibasic sodium phosphate, sodium chloride, EDTA, benzalkonium chloride 0.01%. Ophth. Soln. 5 mL, 10 mL, 15 mL. *Rx.*
Use: Ophthalmic corticosteroid.

prednisolone sodium phosphate. (Mission Pharmacal) Prednisolone 25 mg per 5 mL (equiv. to prednisolone sodium phosphate 33.6 mg per 5 mL). Corn syrup, edetate disodium, glycerin, methylparaben, saccharin. Dye free. Grape flavor. Soln. 237 mL. *Rx.*
Use: Adrenocortical steroid, glucocorticoid.

prednisolone sodium phosphate. (Upstate Pharma) Prednisolone sodium phosphate 6.75 mg (prednisolone 5 mg) per 5 mL. Oral Soln. 120 mL. *Rx.*
Use: Adrenocortical steroid, glucocorticoid.

prednisolone sodium phosphate. (Various Mfr.) Prednisolone 5 mg per 5 mL (equiv. to prednisolone sodium phosphate 6.7 mg per 5 mL), 15 mg per 5 mL (equiv. to prednisolone sodium phosphate 20.2 mg per 5 mL). Soln. 120 mL (5 mg per 5 mL), 237 mL (15 mg per 5 mL). *Rx.*
Use: Adrenocortical steroid, glucocorticoid.

prednisolone sodium phosphate. (Various Mfr.) Prednisolone sodium phosphate 20.2 mg (prednisolone 15 mg) per 5 mL. Oral Soln. 237 mL. *Rx.*
Use: Adrenocortical steroid, glucocorticoid.

•**prednisolone sodium succinate for injection.** *USP.*
Tall Man: prednisoLONE
Use: Corticosteroid, topical.

•**prednisolone tebutate.** (pred-NIS-oh-lone TEB-ue-tate) *USP.*
Tall Man: prednisoLONE
Use: Corticosteroid, topical.
See: Metalone.

prednisolone tertiary-butylacetate.
See: Prednisolone Tebutate.

•**prednisone.** (PRED-nih-sone) *USP.*
Tall Man: predniSONE
Use: Corticosteroid; adrenocortical steroid, glucocorticoid.
See: Rayos.

prednisone. (Roxane) Prednisone. **Oral Soln.:** 5 mg/5 mL. Alcohol 5%, EDTA, fructose, saccharin. 120 mL, 500 mL, UD 5 mL. **Tab.:** 1 mg, 2.5 mg. Lactose. 100s, 1000s (1 mg only), UD 100s. *Rx.*
Use: Glucocorticoid, adrenocortical steroid.

prednisone. (Various Mfr.) Prednisone 5 mg, 10 mg, 20 mg, 50 mg. Tab. Bot. 100s, 500s (except 50 mg), 1000s, 5000s (5 mg only), UD 100s. *Rx.*
Use: Adrenocortical steroid, glucocorticoid.

Prednisone Intensol. (Roxane) Prednisone 5 mg/mL. Alcohol 30%. Oral Soln. Bot. 30 mL w/calibrated dropper. *Rx.*
Use: Adrenocortical steroid, glucocorticoid.

•**prednival.** (PRED-nih-val) USAN.
Use: Corticosteroid.

Predsulfair. (Bausch & Lomb) **Drops:** Prednisolone acetate 0.5%, sodium sulfacetamide 10%, hydroxypropyl methylcellulose, polysorbate 80 0.5%, sodium thiosulfate, benzalkonium Cl 0.01%. Bot. 5 mL, 15 mL. **Oint.:** Prednisolone acetate 0.5%, sodium sulfacetamide 10%, mineral oil, white petrolatum, lanolin, parabens. 3.5 g. *Rx.*
Use: Anti-infective; corticosteroid, ophthalmic.

Prefest. (Teva Women's Health) Estradiol 1 mg; estradiol 1 mg/norgestimate 0.09 mg. Lactose. Tab. Blister card 30s (15 each tablet). *Rx.*
Use: Sex hormone, estrogen and progestin combination.

Preflex Daily Cleaning Especially for Sensitive Eyes. (Alcon) Isotonic, aqueous solution of sorbic acid, sodium phosphates, sodium Cl, tyloxapol, hydroxyethyl cellulose, polyvinyl alco-

hol, EDTA. Bot. 30 mL. *OTC.*
Use: Contact lens care.

PreFol-DHA. (Method Pharmaceuticals) Folic acid 1.2 mg, calcium 160 mg, iron 26 mg, vitamins D 400 units, E 30 units, B_6 25 mg, C 28 mg, DHA 300 mg, docusate sodium 55 mg. Beeswax, lecithin, soybean oil. Cap., softgel. 30s. *Rx.*
Use: Prenatal vitamin with minerals.

•**pregabalin.** (preh-GAB-ah-lin) USAN.
Use: Anticonvulsant.
See: Lyrica.

Pregestimil. (Bristol-Myers Squibb) Protein hydrolysate formula supplies 640 calories/qt. protein 18 g, fat 26 g, carbohydrate 86 g, vitamins A 2000 units, D 400 units, E 15 units, C 52 mg, folic acid 100 mcg, thiamine hydrochloride 0.5 mg, riboflavin 0.6 mg, niacin 8 mg, B_6 0.4 mg, B_{12} 2 mcg, biotin 0.05 mg, pantothenic acid 3 mg, K-1 100 mcg, choline 85 mg, inositol 30 mg, Ca 600 mg, P 400 mg, I 45 mcg, Fe 12 mg, Mg 70 mg, Cu 0.6 mg, Zn 4 mg, Mn 0.2 mg, Cl 550 mg, K 700 mg, Na 300 mg/qt. (20 Kcal/fl oz.). Pow. Can lb. *OTC.*
Use: Nutritional supplement, enteral.

Pregnaslide Latex hCG Test with Fast Trak Slides. (Wampole) Latex agglutination slide test for the qualitative detection of hCG in urine. Test 24s. Test kit 96s.
Use: Diagnostic aid.

pregneninolone.
See: Ethisterone.

pregnenolone.
Use: Treatment of rheumatoid arthritis.

•**pregnenolone succinate.** (preg-NEN-oh-lone) USAN.
Use: Nonhormonal sterol derivative.

Pregnosis Slide Test. (Roche) Latex agglutination inhibition slide test. 50s, 200s.
Use: Diagnostic aid.

Pregnyl. (Organon) Chorionic gonadotropin 10,000 units/vial with diluent 10 mL (1000 units per mL), benzyl alcohol 0.9%. Vial 10 mL. *Rx.*
Use: Ovulation stimulant.

Preject Preinjection Topical Anesthetic. (Colgate Oral) Benzocaine 20% in polyethylene glycol base. Jar 2 oz. *OTC.*
Use: Anesthetic, local.

Prelestrin. (Taylor Pharmaceuticals) Conjugated estrogens 0.625 mg, 1.25 mg. Tab. Bot. 100s, 1000s. *Rx.*
Use: Estrogen.

Prelief. (AKPharma) Calcium glycerophosphate 65 mg, phosphorus 50 mg. Tab. 120s. *OTC.*
Use: Antacid.

Prelone. (Aero) Prednisolone 15 mg/5 mL. Alcohol 5%, saccharin, sucrose. Cherry flavor. Syr. 240 mL. *Rx.*
Use: Adrenocortical steroid, glucocorticoid.

Prelu-2. (Roxane) Phendimetrazine tartrate 105 mg, sucrose. Cap. Bot. 100s. *c-III.*
Use: CNS stimulant, anorexiant.

Premarin. (Wyeth-Ayerst) Conjugated estrogens. 0.3 mg, 0.45 mg, 0.625 mg, 0.9 mg, 1.25 mg. Lactose, sucrose. Tab. Bot. 100s (except 0.625 mg), 1000s (except 0.45 mg, 0.9 mg), UD 100s (0.45 mg, 0.625 mg only). *Rx.*
Use: Estrogen, sex hormone.

Premarin Intravenous. (Wyeth-Ayerst) Conjugated estrogens 25 mg. Inj. *Secules* each with 5 mL sterile diluent. Lactose 200 mg, simethicone 0.2 mg, sodium citrate 12.2 mg, benzyl alcohol 2%. *Rx.*
Use: Estrogen.

Premarin Vaginal. (Wyeth-Ayerst) Conjugated estrogens 0.625 mg/g in a nonliquefying base. Benzyl alcohol, cetyl alcohol, mineral oil. Cream. Tube with or without calibrated applicator 42.5 g. *Rx.*
Use: Estrogen, sex hormone.

Premarin w/Meprobamate.
See: PMB 400.
PMB 200.

Premphase. (Wyeth-Ayerst) Conjugated estrogens 0.625 mg. Medroxyprogesterone acetate 5 mg/conjugated estrogens 0.625 mg. Lactose, PEG, sucrose. Tab. UD 28s (14 of each tablet). *Rx.*
Use: Sex hormone, estrogen, progestin combination.

Prempro. (Wyeth-Ayerst) Conjugated estrogens/medroxyprogesterone acetate 0.3 mg/1.5 mg, 0.45 mg/1.5 mg, 0.625 mg/2.5 mg, 0.625 mg/5 mg. Lactose, PEG, sucrose. Tab. UD 28s. *Rx.*
Use: Sex hormone, estrogen, progestin combination.

Prēmsyn PMS. (Chattem) Acetaminophen 500 mg, pamabrom 25 mg, pyrilamine maleate 15 mg. Cap. Bot. 20s, 40s. *OTC.*
Use: Analgesic; antihistamine; diuretic.

Prenaissance. (Acella) Vitamins B_6 25 mg, C 28 mg, D 800 units, E 30 units, folic acid 1.25 mg, Ca 160 mg, Fe 29 mg, DHA 325 mg, docusate sodium 55 mg. Glycerin, orange flavoring, soybean oil. Cap., softgel. 30s. *Rx.*
Use: Prenatal vitamin with minerals.

Prenaissance DHA. (Acella) Folic acid 1 mg, calcium 125 mg, iron 27 mg, vitamins D 400 units, E 30 units, B_1 3 mg, B_2 3.4 mg, B_3 20 mg, B_6 20 mg, C 120 mg, Cu, I, Zn, docusate sodium 50 mg. **Tab.:** UD 30s. **Cap., softgel:** DHA 250 mg, EPA ≤ 2 mg. Glycerin. UD 30s. *Rx.*
Use: Prenatal vitamin with minerals.

Prenaissance Harmony DHA. (Acella) Folic acid 1 mg, Ca 219 mg, Fe 27 mg, vitamins A 2,850 mg, D 840 units, E 3 units, B_1 1.8 mg, B_2 4 mg, B_3 20 mg, B_6 50 mg, B_{12} 12 mcg, C 120 mg. Cu, Mg, Zn. Gluten free. **Cap., softgel:** Enteric coated. Omega-3 fatty acids ≥ 380 mg (as DHA ≥ 268 mg, other omega-3 ≥ 112 mg), glycerin, vitamin E oil. UD 30s. **Tab.:** UD 30s. *Rx.*
Use: Prenatal vitamin with minerals.

Prenaissance Next-B. (Acella) Folic acid 1.22 mg, calcium 124.23 mg, B_6 42 mg, ginger root extract 100 mg. Tartrazine. Tab. 60s. *Rx.*
Use: Prenatal vitamin with minerals.

Prenaissance 90 DHA. (Acella) Folic acid 1 mg, calcium 160 mg, iron 90 mg, vitamins D 400 units, E 30 units, B_1 3 mg, B_2 3.4 mg, B_3 20 mg, B_6 20 mg, C 120 mg, Cu, I, Zn, docusate sodium 50 mg. **Tab.:** UD 30s. **Cap., softgel:** DHA 300 mg, EPA ≤ 2 mg. Glycerin. UD 30s. *Rx.*
Use: Prenatal vitamin with minerals.

Prenaissance Plus. (Acella) Folate 1 mg, Ca 100 mg, Fe 28 mg, vitamins D 400 units, E 30 units, B_6 25 mg, DHA 250 mg, docusate sodium 50 mg. Beeswax, glycerin, soybean oil. Cap., softgels. 30s. *Rx.*
Use: Prenatal vitamin with minerals.

Prenaissance Promise. (Acella) Folic acid 1 mg, calcium 125 mg, iron 35 mg, vitamins D 400 units, E 30 units, B_1 3 mg, B_2 3.4 mg, B_3 20 mg, B_6 25 mg, C 120 mg, Cu, I, Zn, docusate sodium 50 mg. **Tab.:** UD 30s. **Cap., softgel:** DHA 300 mg, EPA ≤ 2 mg. Glycerin. UD 30s. *Rx.*
Use: Prenatal vitamin with minerals.

•**prenalterol hydrochloride.** (PREE-NAL-teh-role) USAN.
Use: Adrenergic.

Prena1 Chew With Quatrefolic. (BocaGreenMD) Folate 1 mg, vitamins D 400 units, B_2 1.7 mg, B_6 2 mg, B_{12} 8 mcg. Mannitol. Gluten free, lactose free, sugar free. Vanilla flavor. Chew. Tab. 30s. *Rx.*
Use: Prenatal vitamin with minerals.

Prena1 Pearl. (BocaGreenMD) Folic acid 1.4 mg, iron 30 mg, vitamins D 400 units, E 30 units, B_1 1.7 mg, B_2 2 mg, B_3 20 mg, B_5 10 mg, B_6 25 mg, B_{12} 8 mcg, C 30 mg, I, Zn. Biotin 300 mcg, DHA 200 mg. Beeswax, glycerin, sunflower lecithin. Cap., softgel. UD 30s. *Rx.*
Use: Prenatal vitamin with minerals.

Prena1 Plus With Quatrefolic. (BocaGreenMD) **Tab.:** Folate 1 mg, calcium 150 mg, Fe 30 mg, vitamins D 600 units, E 30 units, B_1 3 mg, B_2 3.4 mg, B_3 20 mg, B_5 10 mg, B_6 25 mg, B_{12} 12 mcg, C 60 mg, biotin 300 mg, Cu, I, Zn. Inulin, medium chain triglycerides. 30s. **Cap., softgel:** DHA 300 mg. Lecithin, rosemary extract, sunflower oil. 30s. *Rx.*
Use: Prenatal vitamin with minerals.

Prena1 With Quatrefolic. (BocaGreenMD) Folic acid 1 mg, iron 30 mg, vitamins D 400 units, E 21 units, B_1 1.5 mg, B_2 1.7 mg, B_3 20 mg, B_5 10 mg, B_6 25 mg, B_{12} 8 mcg, C 60 mg, Zn. Biotin 300 mcg, DHA 200 mg. Beeswax, glycerol, orange oil, rosemary extract, soybean lecithin, sunflower oil. Gluten free, lactose free, and sugar free. Cap., softgel. UD 30s. *Rx.*
Use: Prenatal vitamin with minerals.

PréNata. (Sancillo) Folic acid 1 mg, Fe 29 mg, vitamins D 400 units, E 11 units, B_1 2 mg, B_2 3 mg, B_3 20 mg, B_6 10 mg, B_{12} 12 mcg, C 120 mg. Sucralose, xylitol. Gluten free, sugar free. Fruit flavor. Chew. Tab. 90s. *Rx.*
Use: Prenatal vitamin with minerals.

Prenatabs RX. (Cypress) Ca 200 mg, Fe (as carbonyl iron) 29 mg, vitamin A 4000 units, D 400 units, E (dl-alpha tocopheryl acetate) 30 units, B_1 3 mg, B_2 3 mg, B_3 20 mg, B_5 7 mg, B_6 3 mg, B_{12} 8 mcg, C 120 mg, folic acid 1 mg, biotin 30 mcg, Zn 15 mg, Cu, I, Mg. Tab. Bot. 90s. *Rx.*
Use: Mineral, vitamin supplement.

Prenatal. (Major) Folic acid 0.8 mg, calcium 263 mg, iron 27 mg, vitamins A 4,000 units, D 400 units, E 11 units, B_1 1.5 mg, B_2 1.7 mg, B_3 18 mg, B_6 2.6 mg, B_{12} 4 mcg, C 100 mg, Zn. BHT, maltodextrin, sodium benzoate, sucrose. Tab. 30s, 100s. *OTC.*
Use: Prenatal vitamin with minerals.

Prenatal. (PlusPHARMA) Vitamins A 4,000 units, C 120 mg, D_3 400 units, E 30 units, B_1 1.8 mg, B_2 1.7 mg, B_3 20 mg, B_6 2.6 mg, B_{12} 8 mcg, Ca 200 mg, Fe 28 mg, folic acid 800 mcg, Zn. Maltodextrin, propylene glycol, sucrose, sodium benzoate, sunflower oil.

Tab. 100s. *Rx.*
Use: Prenatal vitamin.

PreNatal. (21st Century HealthCare) Folic acid 0.8 mg, calcium 200 mg, iron 28 mg, vitamins A 4,000 units, D 400 units, E 30 units, B_1 1.8 mg, B_2 1.7 mg, B_3 20 mg, B_6 2.6 mg, B_{12} 8 mcg, C 120 mg, Zn. **Tab.:** 60s. **Cap., softgel:** DHA 200 mg. Glycerin, rosemary extract, soy lecithin, sunflower oil. 60s. *OTC.*
Use: Prenatal vitamin with minerals.

Prenatal AD. (Cypress) Ca 200 mg, Fe (carbonyl iron) 90 mg, vitamin A 2700 units, D_3 400 units, E (dl-alpha tocopheryl acetate) 30 units, B_1 3 mg, B_2 3.4 mg, B_3 20 mg, B_6 20 mg, B_{12} 12 mcg, C 120 mg, folic acid 1 mg, Zn 25 mg, Cu, Mg, docusate sodium 50 mg. Tab. Bot. 90s. *Rx.*
Use: Mineral, vitamin supplement.

Prenatal Folic Acid + Iron. (Everett) Vitamins, minerals, folic acid 1 mg. Tab. Bot. 100s. *Rx.*
Use: Mineral, vitamin supplement.

Prenatal Hematinic With Folic Acid. (Cypress Pharmaceuticals) Folic acid 1 mg, Fe 324 mg. Film coated. Tab. 100s. *Rx.*
Use: Prenatal vitamin with minerals.

Prenatal H.P. (Mission Pharmacal) Vitamins A 4000 units, C 100 mg, D_3 400 units, B_1 4 mg, B_2 2 mg, B_3 10 mg, B_5 1 mg, B_6 20 mg, B_{12} 2 mcg, folate 0.8 mg, Ca 50 mg, Fe 30 mg, sugar. Tab. Bot. 100s. *OTC.*
Use: Mineral, vitamin supplement.

Prenatal Maternal. (Ethex) Ca 250 mg, Fe 4 mg, B_2 60 mg, vitamins A 5000 units, D 400 units, E 30 mg, B_1 2.9 mg, B_2 3.4 mg, B_3 20 mg, B_5 10 mg, B_6 12.2 mg, B_{12} 12 mcg, C 100 mg, folic acid 1 mg, Cr, Cu, I, Mg, Mn, Mo, Zn 25 mg, biotin 30 mcg. Tab. Bot. 100s. *Rx.*
Use: Mineral, vitamin supplement.

Prenatal Multi + DHA. (Nature Made) Folic acid 0.8 mg, calcium 150 mg, iron 27 mg, vitamins A 4,000 units, D 400 units, E 11 units, B_1 1.5 mg, B_2 1.7 mg, B_3 18 mg, B_6 2.6 mg, B_{12} 4 mcg, C 100 mg, Zn, omega-3 fatty acids 228 mg (DHA 200 mg and EPA 28 mg). Beeswax, glycerin, soy lecithin, soybean oil. Gluten free, preservative free. Cap., softgel. 90s. *Rx.*
Use: Prenatal vitamin with minerals.

Prenatal 19. (Cypress) Ca 200 mg, Fe 29 mg, vitamin A 1000 units, D 400 units, E (dl-alpha tocopheryl acetate) 30 units, B_1 3 mg, B_2 3 mg, B_3 15 mg, B_5 7 mg, B_6 20 mg, B_{12} 12 mcg, C 100 mg, folic acid 1 mg, Zn 20 mg, docusate sodium 25 mg. Tab. Bot. 100s. *Rx.*
Use: Mineral, vitamin supplement.

Prenatal 19 Chewable. (Cypress) Ca 200 mg, Fe 29 mg, vitamin A 1000 units, D 400 units, E (dl-alpha tocopheryl acetate) 30 units, B_1 3 mg, B_2 3 mg, B_3 15 mg, B_5 7 mg, B_6 20 mg, B_{12} 12 mcg, C 100 mg, folic acid 1 mg, Zn 20 mg, docusate sodium 25 mg, orange flavor. Tab. Bot. 100s. *Rx.*
Use: Mineral, vitamin supplement.

Prenatal 1. (VitaMed MD) Vitamin C 60 mg, D_3 400 units, E 21 units, B_1 1.5 mg, B_2 1.7 mg, B_3 20 mg, B_5 10 mg, B_6 25 mg, B_{12} 8 mcg, Fe 30 mg, folic acid 975 mcg, biotin 300 mcg, DHA 200 mg, Zn. Sunflower oil. Cap., softgels. 30s. *Rx.*
Use: Prenatal vitamin.

Prenatal PC 40. (Integrity) Ca 250 mg, Fe (as ferrous fumarate and carbonyl iron) 40 mg, vitamin D_3 6 mcg, E (dl-alpha tocopheryl acetate) 3.5 mg, B_1 3 mg, B_2 3.4 mg, B_3 20 mg, B_6 20 mg, B_{12} 12 mcg, C 50 mg, folic acid 1 mg, Zn 15 mc, CU, Mg, polydextrose. Tab. UD 100s. *Rx.*
Use: Multivitamin.

Prenatal Plus. (Ivax) Vitamins A (as acetate and carotene) 4000 units, D 400 units, E 22 mg, C 120 mg, folic acid 1 mg, B_1 1.84 mg, B_2 3 mg, B_3 20 mg, B_6 10 mg, B_{12} 12 mcg, Ca 200 mg, Fe 65 mg, Cu 2 mg, Zn 25 mg. Tab. Bot. 100s. *Rx.*
Use: Mineral, vitamin supplement.

Prenatal Plus Iron. (Major) Vitamins A 4000 units, D 400 units, E 22 mg, C 120 mg, folic acid 1 mg, B_1 1.84 mg, B_2 3 mg, niacinamide 20 mg, B_6 10 mg, B_{12} 12 mcg, Ca 200 mg, Cu 2 mg, Fe 27 mg, Zn 25 mg. Tab. Bot. 100s. *Rx.*
Use: Vitamin, mineral supplement.

Prenatal Rx with Beta Carotene. (Various Mfr.) Ca 200 mg, Fe 60 mg, vitamins A 4000 units, D 400 units, E 15 mg, B_1 1.5 mg, B_2 1.6 mg, B_3 17 mg, B_5 7 mg, B_6 4 mg, B_{12} 2.5 mcg, C 80 mg, folic acid 1 mg, biotin 30 mcg, Cu, Mg, Zn 25 mg. Tab. 100s, 500s. *Rx.*
Use: Mineral, vitamin supplement.

Prenatal Vitamins. (Basic Vitamins) Folic acid 0.8 mg, calcium 200 mg, iron 28 mg, vitamins A 4,000 units, D 400 units, E 30 units, B_1 1.8 mg, B_2 1.7 mg, B_3 20 mg, B_6 2.6 mg, B_{12} 8 mcg, C 120 mg, Zn. Mannitol. Preservative

free. Tab. 90s. *OTC.*
Use: Prenatal vitamin with minerals.

Prenatal Vitamins. (Rugby) Folic acid 0.8 mg, calcium 200 mg, iron 28 mg, vitamins A 4,000 units, D 400 units, E 30 units, B_1 1.8 mg, B_2 1.7 mg, B_3 20 mg, B_6 2.6 mg, B_{12} 8 mcg, C 120 mg, Zn. Maltodextrin, PEG. Tab. 100s. *Rx.*
Use: Prenatal vitamin with minerals.

PreNatal Vitamins Plus. (Boca Pharmacal) Folic acid 1 mg, calcium 200 mg, iron 27 mg, vitamins A 4,000 units, D 400 units, E 22 units, B_1 1.84 mg, B_2 3 mg, B_3 20 mg, B_6 10 mg, B_{12} 12 mcg, C 120 mg, Cu, Zn. Glucose, maltodextrin, PEG, soy, sucrose. Tab. 100s, 500s. *Rx.*
Use: Prenatal vitamin with minerals.

Prenatal with Folic Acid. (Eon Labs) Vitamins A 6000 units, D 400 units, E 30 units, folic acid 1 mg, C 60 mg, B_1 1.1 mg, B_2 1.8 mg, B_6 2.5 mg, B_{12} 5 mcg, niacin 15 mg, Ca 125 mg, Fe 65 mg. Tab. Bot. 100s, 1000s. *Rx.*
Use: Mineral, vitamin supplement.

Prenatal with Folic Acid. (Geneva) Ca 200 mg, Fe 60 mg, vitamins A 4000 units, D 400 units, E 11 mg, B_1 1.5 mg, B_2 1.7 mg, B_3 18 mg, B_6 2.6 mg, B_{12} 4 mcg, C 100 mg, folic acid 0.8 mg, Zn 25 mg. Tab. Bot. 100s. *OTC.*
Use: Mineral, vitamin supplement.

Prenatal Z. (Ethex) Ca 300 mg, Fe 65 mg, vitamins A 5000 units, D 400 units, E 30 mg, B_1 3 mg, B_2 3 mg, B_3 20 mg, B_6 12.2 mg, B_{12} 12 mcg, C 80 mg, folic acid 1 mg, Zn 20 mg, I, Mg. Tab. Bot. 100s. *Rx.*
Use: Mineral, vitamin supplement.

Prenate AM With Quatrefolic. (Avion Pharmaceuticals) Folate 1 mg, calcium 200 mg, vitamins B_6 75 mg, B_{12} 12 mcg, ginger extract, lingonberry. Film coated. Tab. 30s. *Rx.*
Use: Prenatal vitamin with minerals.

Prenate Chewable with Quatrefolic. (Avion Pharmaceuticals) Folate 1 mg, calcium 500 mg, vitamins D 300 units, B_6 10 mg, B_{12} 125 mcg, B, Mg, biotin 280 mcg, blueberry extract 25 mg. Fructose. Chocolate flavor. Chew. Tab. 30s. *Rx.*
Use: Prenatal vitamin with minerals.

Prenate Elite. (Sciele) Vitamins A 2500 units, C 80 mg, D_3 400 units, E 10 units, B_1 3 mg, B_2 3.4 mg, B_5 6 mg, B_6 20 mg, B_{12} 12 mcg, folate 1 mg, biotin 300 mcg, Ca 120 mg, Fe 27 mg, I, Cu, Mg, Zn. Hydrogenated soybean oil, hydrogenated vegetable oil, polyvinyl alcohol, povidone, sucrose. Tab. 90s. *Rx.*
Use: Nutritional combination product, prenatal vitamin with minerals.

Prenate Elite with Quatrefolic. (Avion Pharmaceuticals) Folate 1 mg, calcium 100 mg, iron 26 mg, vitamins A 2,600 units, D 450 units, E 10 units, B_1 3 mg, B_2 3.5 mg, B_3 21 mg, B_5 6 mg, B_6 21 mg, B_{12} 13 mcg, C 75 mg, Cu, I, Mg, Zn, biotin 330 mcg. Film coated. Tab. 90s. *Rx.*
Use: Prenatal vitamin with minerals.

Prenate Enhance With Quatrefolic. (Avion Pharmaceuticals) Folate 1 mg, calcium 155 mg, iron 28 mg, vitamins D 1,000 units, E 10 units, B_6 25 mg, B_{12} 12 mcg, C 85 mg, I, Mg, biotin 500 mcg, DHA 400 mg. Beeswax, glycerin, soy lecithin, vegetable shortening. Cap., softgel. 30s. *Rx.*
Use: Prenatal vitamin with minerals.

Prenate Essential. (Shionogi Pharma) Folate 1 mg, vitamin C 85 mg, D_3 200 units, E 10 units, B_6 25 mg, B_{12} 12 mcg, Ca 140 mg, Fe 28 mg, biotin 250 mcg, DHA 300 mg, EPA 40 mg, I, Mg. Glycerin, propylene glycol, sorbitol, vegetable oil. Cap., softgels. UD 30s. *Rx.*
Use: Prenatal vitamin with minerals.

Prenate Essential With Quatrefolic. (Avion Pharmaceuticals) Folate 1 mg, calcium 145 mg, iron 29 mg, vitamins D 220 units, E 10 units, B_6 26 mg, B_{12} 13 mcg, C 90 mg, I, Mg, biotin 280 mcg, DHA 300 mg, EPA 40 mg. Beeswax, glycerin, soy lecithin, tartrazine, vegetable oil. Cap., softgel. 30s. *Rx.*
Use: Prenatal vitamin with minerals.

Prenate Mini. (Avion Pharmaceuticals) Folic acid 1 mg (as *Quatrefolic* 600 mcg, folic acid 400 mcg), Ca 100 mg, Fe 29 mg, vitamins D 220 units, E 10 units, B_6 26 mg, B_{12} 13 mcg, C 60 mg, DHA 350 mg, blueberry extract 25 mg, biotin 280 mcg, I, Mg. Beeswax, corn oil, fish oil, glycerin, soy, vegetable oil. Cap., softgel. 30s. *Rx.*
Use: Prenatal vitamin with minerals.

Prenate 90. (Sanofi-Synthelabo) Vitamins A 4000 units, D 400 units, E 30 mg, C 120 mg, folic acid 1 mg, B_1 3 mg, B_2 3.4 mg, B_6 20 mg, B_{12} 12 mcg, B_3 20 mg, DSS, Ca 250 mg, I, Fe 90 mg, Cu, Zn 20 mg. FC Tab. Bot. 100s, 1000s. *Rx.*
Use: Mineral, vitamin supplement.

PreNate Plus. (Boca) Vitamins A 4,000 units, D 400 units, E 22 units, B_1 1.84 mg, B_2 3 mg, B_3 20 mg, B_6 10 mg, B_{12} 12 mcg, C 120 mg, Cu, Zn, folate

1 mg, Ca 200 mg, Fe 27 mg. Maltodextrin, mineral oil, sucrose. Tab. 100s. *Rx.*
Use: Prenatal vitamin with minerals.

PreNexa. (Upsher-Smith) Vitamins B_6 25 mg, C 28 mg, D_3 400 units, E (as d-alpha tocopherol acetate) 30 units, folic acid 1.25 mg, Ca 160 mg, Fe 27 mg, DHA 300 mg, docusate sodium 55 mg. Glycerin, palm kernel oil, sodium benzoate, soybean oil, sunflower oil. Cap. 30s. *Rx.*
Use: Prenatal vitamin with minerals.

•**prenylamine.** (PREH-nill-ah-meen) USAN. Segontin; synadrin lactate.
Use: Coronary vasodilator.

Preorbotic. (MedChem Manufacturing) *L. acidophilus* 250 million CFU, *B. bifidum* 250 million CFU, *L. casei* 124 million CFU, *L. rhamnosus* 120 million CFU, inulin juice complex 150 mg, mannan oligosaccharide complex 50 mg. Cap. 60s. *OTC.*
Use: Probiotic.

Preparation H. (Wyeth Consumer Health) **Cream:** Glycerin 14.4%, phenylephrine hydrochloride 0.25%, pramoxine hydrochloride 1%, white petrolatum 15%. Aloe, cetyl alcohol, EDTA, mineral oil, parabens, stearyl alcohol. 15 g, 26 g. **Oint.:** Petrolatum 71.9%, mineral oil 14%, shark liver oil 3%, phenylephrine hydrochloride 0.25%, corn oil, glycerin, lanolin, lanolin alcohol, parabens, tocopherol. 30 g, 60 g. **Supp.:** Shark liver oil 3%, cocoa butter 79%, corn oil, EDTA, parabens, tocopherol. 12s, 24s, 36s, 48s. *OTC.*
Use: Anorectal preparation.

Preparation H Cooling. (Wyeth Consumer Health) Witch hazel 50%, phenylephrine hydrochloride 0.25%, alcohol 7.5%, EDTA, parabens. Gel. Tube 51 g. *OTC.*
Use: Anorectal preparation.

Prepcat. (Mallinckrodt) Barium sulfate 1.5%. Simethicone, sorbitol, strawberry flavor. Susp. Bot. 450 mL. *Rx.*
Use: Radiopaque agent, GI contrast agent.

Prepcat 2000. (Lafayette) Barium sulfate 1.2% w/w suspension. Bot. 2000 mL, Case Bot. 4s.
Use: Radiopaque agent.

Prepcort. (Whitehall-Robins) Hydrocortisone 0.5%. Cream. Tube 0.5 oz, 1 oz.
Use: Corticosteroid.

Pre-Pen. (ALK-Abelló) Benzylpenicilloyl polylysine 6×10^{-5} per 25 mL. Inj., Soln. Single-dose amp. *Rx.*
Use: In vivo diagnostic aid.

Prepidil. (Pharmacia) Dinoprostone 0.5 mg. Gel. Syringes (with 2 shielded catheters 10 and 20 mm tip) 3 g. *Rx.*
Use: Cervical ripening.

Prepodyne. (West) Titratable iodine. **Soln.:** 1%. Bot. Pt, gal. **Scrub:** 0.75%. Bot. 6 oz, gal. **Swabs:** Saturated with soln. Pkt. 1s, Box 100s. **Swabsticks:** Saturated with soln. Pkt. 1s, Box 50s. Pkt. 3s, Box 75s.
Use: Antiseptic, topical.

Prepopik. (Ferring Pharmaceuticals) Sodium picosulfate 10 mg/magnesium oxide 3.5 mg/citric acid 12 g per packet. Lactose, saccharin. Orange flavor. Pow. for Soln. 16.1 g packet (2s). *Rx.*
Use: Laxative, bowel evacuant.

PreQue 10. (Watson) Folic acid 0.5 mg, Fe 15 mg, vitamins A 1,250 units, D 120 units, E 15 units, B_1 1 mg, B_2 1.7 mg, B_{12} 1 mcg, C 30 mg, Cu, Mg, Se, Zn, CoQ10 50 mg, docusate sodium 25 mg, DHA 50 mg, lycopene 5 mg. Coated. Alga oil, glucose, mannitol, PEG, sodium benzoate, sodium caseinate, soy, sucrose, sunflower oil. Tab. 60s. *Rx.*
Use: Prenatal vitamin with minerals.

Presalin. (Roberts) Aspirin 260 mg, salicylamide 120 mg, acetaminophen 120 mg, aluminum hydroxide 100 mg. Tab. Bot. 50s. *OTC.*
Use: Analgesic combination; antacid.

Presera. (Quinnova Pharmaceuticals) Dimethicone, glycerin, propylene glycol, trolamine. Fragrance free, preservative free. Aer., Foam. 200 g. *Rx.*
Use: Emollient.

PreserVision Eye Vitamin AREDS 2 Formula. (Bausch & Lomb) **Tab.:** Vitamin A 7,160 units, E 100 units, C 113 mg, Zn 17.4 mg, Cu. Lactose. 120s. **Cap., softgel:** Vitamin C 113 mg, vitamin E 100 units, omega-3 250 mg, lutein 2.5 mg, zeaxanthin 0.5 mg, EPA 81.25 mg, DHA 43.75 mg, Zn, Cu. Fish oil, glycerin, soy. 120s. *OTC.*
Use: Mineral, vitamin supplement.

PreserVision Lutein. (Bausch & Lomb) Vitamin C 226 mg, E 200 units, Cu 0.8 mg, lutein 5 mg, Zn 34.75 mg. Softgel Cap. 50s. *OTC.*
Use: Nutritional combination product, multivitamin with minerals.

pressor agents.
See: Sympathomimetic agents.

Pressorol. (Baxter PPI) Metaraminol bitartrate 10 mg/mL. Inj. Vial 10 mL. *Rx.*
Use: Vasoconstrictor.

PreSun Active. (Bristol-Myers Squibb) Octyl methoxycinnamate, oxybenzone,

octyl salicylate, 69% SD alcohol 40. PABA free. Waterproof. SPF 15, 30. Gel. 120 g. *OTC.*
Use: Sunscreen.

PreSun 8 Creamy. (Bristol-Myers Squibb) Padimate O 5%, oxybenzone 2%. Waterproof. SPF 8. Bot. 4 oz. *OTC.*
Use: Sunscreen.

PreSun 8 Lotion. (Bristol-Myers Squibb) Padimate O 7.3%, oxybenzone 2.3%, SD alcohol 40 60%. SPF 8. Bot. 4 oz. *OTC.*
Use: Sunscreen.

PreSun 15 Creamy. (Bristol-Myers Squibb) Padimate O 8%, oxybenzone 3%, benzyl alcohol. Waterproof. SPF 15. Bot. 4 oz. *OTC.*
Use: Sunscreen.

PreSun 15 Facial Sunscreen. (Bristol-Myers Squibb) Padimate O (octyl dimethyl PABA) 8%, oxybenzone 3%. SPF 15. Bot. 2 oz. *OTC.*
Use: Sunscreen.

PreSun 15 Facial Sunscreen Stick. (Bristol-Myers Squibb) Octyl dimethyl PABA 8%, oxybenzone 3%. SPF 15. Stick 0.42 oz. *OTC.*
Use: Sunscreen.

PreSun 15 Lip Protector. (Bristol-Myers Squibb) Padimate O 8%, oxybenzone 3%. SPF 15. Stick 4.5 g. *OTC.*
Use: Sunscreen.

PreSun 15 Lotion. (Bristol-Myers Squibb) Padimate O 5%, PABA 5%, oxybenzone 3%, SD alcohol 40 58%. SPF 15. Bot. 4 oz. *OTC.*
Use: Sunscreen.

PreSun 15 Sensitive Skin Sunscreen. (Bristol-Myers Squibb) Octyl methoxycinnamate, oxybenzone, octyl salicylate, cetyl alcohol, PABA free, waterproof, SPF 15. Cream. Bot. 120 mL. *OTC.*
Use: Sunscreen.

PreSun for Kids. (Bristol-Myers Squibb) **Cream:** Octyl methoxycinnamate, oxybenzone, octyl salicylate, cetyl alcohol, PABA free. Waterproof. SPF 29. Bot. 120 mL. **Liq.:** Padimate O, octyl methoxycinnamate, oxybenzone, octyl salicylate, SD alcohol 40 19%. Waterproof. SPF 23. Spray Bot. 105 mL. *OTC.*
Use: Sunscreen.

PreSun 4 Creamy. (Bristol-Myers Squibb) Padimate O 1.4%, alcohol, titanium dioxide. Waterproof. Lot. SPF 4. Bot. 4 oz. *OTC.*
Use: Sunscreen.

PreSun Moisturizing. (Bristol-Myers Squibb) Octyl dimethyl PABA, oxybenzone, cetyl alcohol, diazolidinyl urea. SPF 46. Lot. Bot. 120 mL. *OTC.*
Use: Sunscreen.

PreSun Moisturizing Sunscreen with Keri, SPF 15. (Bristol-Myers Squibb) Octyl dimethyl PABA, oxybenzone, cetyl alcohol, diazolidinyl urea. Waterproof. Lot. Bot. 120 mL. *OTC.*
Use: Sunscreen.

PreSun Moisturizing Sunscreen with Keri, SPF 25. (Bristol-Myers Squibb) Octyl methoxycinnamate, oxybenzone, octyl salicylate, petrolatum, cetyl alcohol, diazolidinyl urea. Waterproof. Lot. Bot. 120 mL. *OTC.*
Use: Sunscreen.

PreSun Spray Mist. (Bristol-Myers Squibb) Octyl dimethyl PABA, octyl methoxycinnamate, oxybenzone, octyl salicylate, 19% SD alcohol 40, C12-15 alcohols benzoate. Waterproof. SPF 23. Liq. Bot. 120 mL. *OTC.*
Use: Sunscreen.

PreSun 39 Creamy Sunscreen. (Bristol-Myers Squibb) Padimate O, oxybenzone, cetyl alcohol. Waterproof. SPF 39. Cream Bot. 120 mL. *OTC.*
Use: Sunscreen.

PreSun 29 Sensitive Skin Sunscreen. (Bristol-Myers Squibb) Octyl methoxycinnamate, oxybenzone, octyl salicylate. Waterproof. SPF 29. Bot. 4 oz. *OTC.*
Use: Sunscreen.

PreSun 23. (Bristol-Myers Squibb) Padimate O, octyl methoxycinnamate, oxybenzone, octyl salicylate, SD alcohol 40 19%. Waterproof. SPF 23. Spray mist. Bot. 105 mL. *OTC.*
Use: Sunscreen.

PreSun Ultra. (Bristol-Myers Squibb) Avobenzone 3%, octyl methoxycinnamate 7.5%, octyl salicylate 5%, oxybenzone 6%. SPF 30. SD alcohol 65.5%. Gel. 120 mL. *OTC.*
Use: Sunscreen.

Pretend-U-Ate. (Vitalax) Enriched candy-appetite pacifier. Pkg. 20s. *OTC.*
Use: Dietary aid.

prethcamide. Mixture of crotethamide and cropropamide.
See: Micoren.

Pretts Diet Aid. (Milance Laboratories, Inc.) Alginic acid 200 mg, sodium carboxymethylcellulose 100 mg, sodium bicarbonate 70 mg. Chew. Tab. Bot. 60s. *OTC.*
Use: Dietary aid.

Pretty Feet & Hands. (B.F. Ascher) Paraffin, triethanolamine, parabens. Cream 90 g. *OTC.*
Use: Emollient.

Pretz Irrigation. (Parnell) Sodium chloride, yerba santa. Soln. Spray bot.

273 mL. *OTC.*
Use: Nasal decongestant.

Pretz Moisturizing. (Parnell) Sodium chloride, glycerin, yerba santa. Soln. Spray bot. 50 mL. *OTC.*
Use: Nasal decongestant.

Prevacid. (Takeda Pharmaceuticals) Lansoprazole. **DR Cap.:** 15 mg, 30 mg. Enteric-coated granules. PEG, sugar spheres, sucrose. 100s (30 mg only), 30s (15 mg only). **Orally Disintegrating DR Tab.:** 15 mg, 30 mg. Aspartame, lactose, mannitol, PEG, phenylalanine 2.5 mg (15 mg), 5.1 mg (30 mg). Strawberry flavor. Enteric-coated granules. UD 100s. *Rx.*
Use: Proton pump inhibitor.

Prevacid SoluTab. (TAP) Lansoprazole 15 mg (phenylalanine 2.5 mg), 30 mg (phenylalanine 5.1 mg). Mannitol, lactose, aspartame, strawberry flavor. DR Orally Disintegrating Tab. UD 30s. *Rx.*
Use: Proton pump inhibitor.

Prevacid 24 Hour. (Novartis) Lansoprazole 15 mg (contains enteric-coated granules). PEG, sugar spheres, sucrose. Cap., delayed release. 14s, 28s, 42s. *OTC.*
Use: Proton pump inhibitor.

Prevalite. (Upsher Smith) Cholestyramine 4 g (as anhydrous cholestyramine resin)/5.5 g powder. Aspartame, phenylalanine 14.1 mg/5.5 g, orange flavor. Pow. for Oral Susp. 5.5 g packets. 42s, 60s. Cans. 231 g (42 doses). *Rx.*
Use: Antihyperlipidemic; bile acid sequestrant.

PreviDent 5000 Plus. (Colgate Oral) Sodium fluoride 1.1%, sorbitol, saccharin, spearmint and fruit flavors. Dental Cream. Tube 51 g (1s, 2s). *Rx.*
Use: Caries prevention.

PreviDent Rinse. (Colgate Oral) Neutral sodium fluoride 0.2%, alcohol 6%, mint flavor. Sol. Bot. 250 mL, gal (w/pump dispenser). *Rx.*
Use: Dental caries agent.

Preview. (Lafayette) Barium sulfate 60% w/v suspension. Bot. 355 mL, Case 24 bot.
Use: Radiopaque agent.

Preview 2000. Barium sulfate 60% w/v suspension. Bot. 2000 mL, Case 4 Bot.
Use: Radiopaque agent.

Previfem. (Qualitest) Ethinyl estradiol 35 mcg, norgestimate 0.25 mg. Lactose. Tab. 28s w/7 white inert tablets. *Rx.*
Use: Oral contraceptive, monophasic contraceptive.

Prevision. Mestranol, USP.

Prevnar 13. (Pfizer) Total saccharides 30.8 mcg (each 0.5 mL dose contains ≈ 2.2 mcg of each of *Streptococcus pneumonia* serotypes 1, 3, 4, 5, 6A, 7F, 9V, 14, 18C, 19A, 19F, and 23F saccharides; and 4.4 mcg of serotype 6B saccharides) per 0.5 mL dose. Inj., Susp. Single-dose, prefilled syringe (also contains CRM_{197} carrier protein 34 mcg, 100 mcg of polysorbate 80, succinate buffer 295 mcg, aluminum 125 mcg as aluminum phosphate adjuvant per dose). 0.5 mL. *Rx.*
Use: Agent for active immunization, bacterial vaccine.

Prevpac. (Takeda Pharmaceuticals) Two *Prevacid* (lansoprazole) 30 mg delayed-release Cap. (PEG, sucrose, sugar spheres). Four *Trimox* (amoxicillin) 500 mg Cap. Two *Biaxin* (clarithromycin) 500 mg (film coated) Tab. Daily administration pack.
Use: H. pylori eradication.

Prexonate. (Tennessee Pharmaceutic) Vitamins A acetate 5000 units, D 500 units, B_6 2 mg, B_1 5 mg, B_2 2 mg, C 100 mg, B_{12} 2.5 mcg, calcium pantothenate 1 mg, niacinamide 15 mg, folic acid 1 mg, Fe 45 mg, Ca 500 mg, intrinsic factor 3 mg. Tab. Bot. 100s, 1000s. *Rx.*
Use: Mineral, vitamin supplement.

•**prezatide copper acetate.** (PREH-zat-IDE KAH-per) USAN.
Use: Immunomodulator.

Prezista. (Tibotec Therapeutics) Darunavir ethanolate. **Tab.:** 75 mg, 150 mg, 400 mg, 600 mg. Film coated. 60s (400 mg and 600 mg), 240s (150 mg), 480s (75 mg). **Susp.:** 100 mg/mL. Methylparaben, sucralose, strawberry cream flavoring. 200 mL. *Rx.*
Use: Antiretroviral, protease inhibitor.

Prialt. (Azur Pharma) Ziconotide 25 mcg/mL (used only for ziconotide-naive pump priming), 100 mcg/mL. Preservative free. L-methionine. Inj. Single-use vials. 1 mL, 2 mL, 5 mL (100 mcg/mL only); 20 mL (25 mcg/mL only). *Rx.*
Use: Management of severe chronic pain.

•**pridefine hydrochloride.** (PRIH-deh-FEEN) USAN.
Use: Antidepressant.

•**pridopidine.** (pri-DOE-pi-deen) USAN.
Use: CNS agent.

•**pridopidine hydrochloride.** (pri-DOE-pi-deen) USAN.
Use: CNS agent.

Prid Salve. (Walker) Ichthammol, Phenol, Lead Oleate, Rosin, Beeswax,

Lard. Tin 20 g. *OTC.*
Use: Drawing salve.

•**prifelone.** (PRIH-feh-LONE) USAN.
Use: Anti-inflammatory, dermatologic.

Priftin. (Aventis) Rifapentine 150 mg. EDTA, polyethylene glycol. Tab. Bot. 32s. *Rx.*
Use: Antituberculosal.

•**priliximab.** (prih-LICK-sih-mab) USAN.
Use: Monoclonal antibody (autoimmune lymphoproliferative diseases, organ transplantation).

•**prilocaine.** (PRIL-oh-kane) USAN.
Use: Anesthetic, local.
W/Lidocaine.
See: EMLA.
EMLA Anesthetic.
Oraqix.

•**prilocaine and epinephrine injection.** *USP.*
Use: Anesthetic, local.

•**prilocaine hydrochloride.** (PRIL-oh-kane) *USP.*
Use: Anesthetic, local amide.
See: Citanest Forte.
Citanest Plain.

prilocaine hydrochloride. (Septodont) Prilocaine hydrochloride 4%. Epinephrine 0.005 mg/mL, sodium metabisulfite 0.5 mg. Inj., Soln. 1.8 mL cartridge. *Rx.*
Use: Injectable local anesthetic, amide local anesthetic.

Prilosec. (AstraZeneca) Omeprazole. **DR Cap.:** 10 mg, 20 mg, 40 mg. Lactose, mannitol. Enteric-coated granules. 100s (40 mg only), 1000s, unit-of-use 30s. **DR Susp.:** 2.5 mg, 10 mg. Dextrose, sugar spheres. UD 30s. *Rx.*
Tall Man: PriLOSEC
Use: Proton pump inhibitor.

Prilosec OTC. (Proctor and Gamble) Omeprazole magnesium 20 mg. Sucrose, talc. DR Tab. 14s, 28s, 42s. *OTC.*
Tall Man: PriLOSEC
Use: Proton pump inhibitor.

primacaine.
Use: Anesthetic, local.

•**primaquine phosphate.** (PRIM-uh-kween) *USP.*
Use: Antimalarial.

primaquine phosphate. (Sanofi-Synthelabo) Primaquine phosphate 26.3 mg. Film coated. Tab. 100s.
Use: Antimalarial.

primaquine phosphate. (Sanofi-Synthelabo)
Use: Treatment of AIDS-associated PCP. [Orphan Drug]

Primatene. (Wyeth Consumer Healthcare) Ephedrine hydrochloride 12.5 mg, guaifenesin 200 mg. Tab. 24s, 60s. *OTC.*
Use: Upper respiratory combination, decongestant and expectorant combination.

Primatene M. (Wyeth Consumer Healthcare) Theophylline 118 mg, ephedrine hydrochloride 24 mg, pyrilamine maleate 16.6 mg. Tab. Bot. 24s, 60s. *OTC.*
Use: Antihistamine, bronchodilator.

Primatene Mist. (Wyeth Consumer Healthcare) Epinephrine bitartrate 0.3 mg. Bot. 10 mL w/mouthpiece. Spray. *OTC.*
Use: Bronchodilator.

Primatene P. (Wyeth Consumer Healthcare) Theophylline 118 mg, ephedrine hydrochloride 24 mg, phenobarbital 8 mg. Tab. Bot. 24s, 60s. *OTC.*
Use: Bronchodilator; hypnotic; sedative.

Primatuss Cough Mixture 4. (Rugby) Doxylamine succinate 3.75 mg, dextromethorphan HBr 7.5 mg/5 mL, alcohol 10%. Liq. Bot. 180 mL. *OTC.*
Use: Antihistamine; antitussive.

Primatuss Cough Mixture 4D. (Rugby) Pseudoephedrine hydrochloride 20 mg, dextromethorphan HBr 10 mg, guaifenesin 67 mg/5 mL, alcohol 10%. Liq. Bot. 120 mL. *OTC.*
Use: Antitussive; decongestant; expectorant.

Primaxin I.V. (Merck) Imipenem 250 mg, cilastatin 250 mg, sodium 0.8 mEq. Imipenem 500 mg, cilastatin 500 mg, sodium 1.6 mEq. Pow. for Inj. Vials, infusion bottles, *ADD-Vantage* vials. *Rx.*
Use: Anti-infective.

•**primidolol.** (prih-MID-oh-lahl) USAN.
Use: Antianginal; antihypertensive; cardiovascular agent, antiarrhythmic.

•**primidone.** (PRIM-ih-dohn) *USP.*
Use: Anticonvulsant.
See: Mysoline.

primidone. (Various Mfr.) Primidone 50 mg, 250 mg. May contain lactose. Tab. 100s, 500s, 1,000s, UD 100s. *Rx.*
Use: Anticonvulsant.

Primlev. (Akrimax Pharmaceutical) Acetaminophen/oxycodone hydrochloride 300 mg/5 mg, 300 mg/7.5 mg, 300 mg/10 mg. Tab. 100s. *c-II.*
Use: Opioid analgesic combination.

primostrum. A prep. of primiparous colostrum.

Primsol. (Ascent Pediatrics) Trimethoprim 50 mg/5 mL, parabens, sorbitol, alcohol free, bubble gum flavor. Oral Soln. Bot. 473 mL. *Rx.*
Use: Anti-infective.

•**prinaberel.** (prin-a BER-el) USAN.
Use: Anti-inflammatory.

Principen with Probenecid. (Bristol-Myers Squibb) Ampicillin (as trihydrate) 3.5 g, probenecid 1 g/regimen. Single-dose Bot. 9s. *Rx.*
Use: Anti-infective, penicillin.

Prinivil. (Merck) Lisinopril 5 mg, 10 mg, 20 mg. Mannitol. Tab. Unit-of-use 90s. *Rx.*
Use: Renin angiotensin antagonist, angiotensin-converting enzyme inhibitor.

•**prinomastat.** (pri-NOE-ma-stat) USAN.
Use: Antineoplastic; antiangiogenic; retinal and subfoveal choroidal neovascularization.

•**prinomide tromethamine.** (PRIH-no-MIDE troe-METH-ah-meen) USAN.
Use: Antirheumatic.

•**prinoxodan.** (prin-OX-oh-dan) USAN.
Use: Cardiovascular agent.

Prinzide. (Merck) Lisinopril/hydrochlorothiazide 10 mg/12.5 mg, 20 mg/12.5 mg, 20 mg/25 mg. Tab. Unit-of-use 30s (20 mg/25 mg only), unit-of-use 100s. *Rx.*
Use: Antihypertensive.

Pristiq. (Wyeth) Desvenlafaxine 50 mg (equiv. to desvenlafaxine succinate 76 mg), 100 mg (equiv. to desvenlafaxine succinate 152 mg). Dextrose. ER Tab. 14s, 30s, 90s, 10 blisters of 10s. *Rx.*
Use: Antidepressant, serotonin and norepinephrine reuptake inhibitor.

Privigen. (CSL Behring) Immune globulin (human) 10% (100 mg/mL). Preservative free. Inj., Soln. Single-use vials. 5 g, 10 g, 20 g. *Rx.*
Use: Immune globulin.

Privine. (Insight) Naphazoline hydrochloride, benzalkonium chloride, EDTA. Soln. Dropper bot. 25 mL. Spray bot. 20 mL. *OTC.*
Use: Nasal decongestant, imidazoline.

•**prizidilol hydrochloride.** (PRIH-zie-DILL-ole) USAN.
Use: Antihypertensive.

PR Natal 400. (PruGen) Vitamins A 3,000 units, B_1 1.8 mg, B_2 4 mg, B_3 20 mg, B_6 25 mg, B_{12} 12 mcg, C 120 mg, D 400 units, E 30 units, folic acid 1 mg, Ca 200 mg, Mg, Zn, Cu, Fe 29 mg. **Tab.:** Film coated. Maltodextrin, polydextrose. 30s. **Cap., softgels:** Omega-3 fatty acids 400 mg (DHA ≥ 275 mg, EPA, other omega-3 fatty acids), glycerin. 30s. *Rx.*
Use: Prenatal vitamin with minerals.

PR Natal 400 ec. (PruGen) Vitamins A 3,000 units, B_1 1.8 mg, B_2 4 mg, B_3 20 mg, B_6 25 mg, B_{12} 12 mcg, C 120 mg, D 400 units, E 3 units, folic acid 1 mg, Ca 200 mg, Mg, Zn, Cu, Fe 29 mg. **Tab.:** Film coated. Maltodextrin, polydextrose. 30s. **Cap., softgels:** Enteric coated. Omega-3 fatty acids 400 mg (DHA ≥ 275 mg, EPA, other omega-3 fatty acids). 30s. *Rx.*
Use: Prenatal vitamin with minerals.

PR Natal 430. (PruGen) Vitamins A 3,000 units, B_1 1.8 mg, B_2 4 mg, B_3 20 mg, B_6 25 mg, B_{12} 12 mcg, C 120 mg, D 400 units, E 30 units, folic acid 1 mg, Ca 200 mg, Mg, Zn, Cu, Fe 29 mg. **Tab.:** Film coated. Maltodextrin, polydextrose. 30s. **Cap., softgel:** Omega-3 fatty acids 430 mg (DHA ≥ 295 mg, EPA, other omega-3 fatty acids). 30s. *Rx.*
Use: Prenatal vitamin with minerals.

PR Natal 430 ec. (PruGen) Vitamins A 3,000 units, B_1 1.8 mg, B_2 4 mg, B_3 20 mg, B_6 25 mg, B_{12} 12 mcg, C 120 mg, D 400 units, E 3 units, folic acid 1 mg, Ca 200 mg, Mg, Zn, Cu, Fe 29 mg. **Tab.:** Film coated. Maltodextrin, polydextrose. 30s. **Cap., softgel:** Enteric coated. Omega-3 fatty acids 430 mg (DHA ≥ 295 mg, EPA, other omega-3 fatty acids). 30s. *Rx.*
Use: Prenatal vitamin with minerals.

Pro-Acet Douche Concentrate. (Pro-Acet) Lactic, citric, and acetic acids, sodium lauryl sulfate, lactose, dextrose, sodium acetate. Pkg. polyethylene envelope 10 mL. Contents of 1 envelope to be diluted with 2 quarts of water. Douche 6 oz, 12 oz. Travel Packet 10 mL. *OTC.*
Use: Vaginal agent.

•**proadifen hydrochloride.** (pro-AD-ih-fen) USAN.
Use: Synergist, nonspecific.

ProAir HFA. (Ivax) Albuterol (as sulfate) 90 mcg/actuation. Contains no chlorofluorocarbons. Aerosol. 8.5 g (200 inhalations). *Rx.*
Use: Bronchodilator; sympathomimetics.

ProAmatine. (Shire) Midodrine hydrochloride 2.5 mg, 5 mg, 10 mg. Tab. Bot. 100s. *Rx.*
Use: Orthostatic hypotension; vasopressor.

Probarbital Sodium. 5-Ethyl-5-isopropylbarbiturate sodium.

Probax. (Fischer) Propolis 2%, petrolatum, mineral oil, lanolin. Gel. Tube 3.5 g. *OTC.*
Use: Mouth and throat preparation.

Probec-T. (Roberts) Vitamins B_1 12.2 mg,

B_2 10 mg, B_3 100 mg, B_5 18.4, B_6 4.1 mg, B_{12} 5 mcg, C 600 mg. Tab. Bot. 60s. *OTC.*
Use: Mineral, vitamin supplement.

Proben-C. (Rugby) Probenecid 500 mg, colchicine 0.5 mg. Tab. Bot. 100s, 1000s. *Rx.*
Use: Antigout agent.

•**probenecid.** (pro-BEN-uh-sid) *USP.*
Use: Uricosuric.
W/Ampicillin.
See: Principen w/Probenecid.

probenecid and colchicine. (Various Mfr.) Probenecid 500 mg, colchicine 0.5 mg. Tab. Bot. 100s, 1000s. *Rx.*
Use: Agent for gout.

•**probenecid and colchicine tablets.** (pro-BEN-uh-sid and KOHL-chih-seen) *USP.*
Use: Agent for gout.

•**probicromil calcium.** (pro-BYE-KROE-mill) USAN.
Use: Antiallergic, prophylactic.

Pro-Bionate. (NaTREN) *Lactobacillus acidophilus* strain NAS 2 billion units/g. **Pow.:** 52.5 g, 90 g. **Cap.:** Bot. 30s, 60s. *OTC.*
Use: Antidiarrheal; nutritional supplement.

Probiotic Acidophilus. (Nature's Bounty) *L. acidophilus* > 100 million colonies. Maltodextrin. Gluten free, lactose free, preservative free, and sugar free. Cap. 100s. *OTC.*
Use: Probiotic.

Probiotic & Acidophilus Extra-Strength Formula. (Windmill) 300 million organism blend of *L. acidophilus, B. coagulans, L. plantarum, B. bifidum, L. casei.* Cap. 60s. *OTC.*
Use: Probiotic.

Pro-biotic Blend. (Nature's Blend) 2 billion bacteria blend of *L. acidophilus, L. casei, B. bifidum, B. longum.* Gluten free, preservative free, and sugar free. Cap. 100s. *OTC.*
Use: Probiotic.

Probiotic Complex Acidophilus. (Nature's Bounty) 2 billion CFU blend of *L. acidophilus, B. bifidum, L. bulgaricus, L. brevis, B. lactis.* Sugar free. Cap. 60s. *OTC.*
Use: Probiotic.

Probiotic Formula. (Rugby) *L. acidophilus* 2 billion CFU, *L. salivarius* 2 billion CFU, *L. plantarum* 2 billion CFU, *L. casei* 2 billion CFU, *B. lactis* 2 billion CFU. Preservative free. Cap. 30s. *OTC.*
Use: Probiotic.

Probiotic Gold Extra Strength Acidophilus. (Nature's Bounty) *L. acidophilus* 500 million CFU. Gluten free, lactose free, preservative free, and sugar free. Cap. 60s. *OTC.*
Use: Probiotic.

Probiotic Pearls. (Integrative Therapeutics) 1 billion CFU blend of *L. acidophilus* and *B. longum.* Palm oil, vegetable glycerin. Gluten free, preservative free, and sugar free. Cap. 30s, UD 90s. *OTC.*
Use: Probiotic.

Probiotic Pearls Advantage. (Integrative Therapeutics) 5 billion CFU blend of *L. plantarum, B. lactis, L. acidophilus, B. longum.* Vegetable glycerin, vegetable oil. Preservative free and sugar free. Cap. 60s. *OTC.*
Use: Probiotic.

Probiotic With Prebiotic. (Mason) *B. coagulans* spores 1 billion CFU. Sugar free. Cap. 40s. *OTC.*
Use: Probiotic.

•**probucol.** (PRO-byoo-kahl) *USP.*
Use: Antihyperlipidemic.
See: Lorelco.

•**probutate.** (pro-BYOO-tate) USAN. Formerly buteprate.
Use: Radical.

•**procainamide hydrochloride.** (pro-CANE-uh-mide) *USP.*
Use: Cardiovascular agent, antiarrhythmic.

procainamide hydrochloride. (Hospira) Procainamide hydrochloride 100 mg/mL. Methylparaben. Inj. Soln. Vials. 10 mL. *Rx.*
Use: Antiarrhythmic agent.

procainamide hydrochloride. (Various Mfr.) Procainamide hydrochloride 500 mg/mL. Inj. Vial. 2 mL. *Rx.*
Use: Antiarrhythmic.

•**procaine and tetracaine hydrochlorides and levonordefrin injection.** *USP.*
Use: Anesthetic, local.

procaine base.
Use: Anesthetic, local.
See: Anucaine.

•**procaine hydrochloride.** (pro-CANE) *USP.* Bernocaine, Chlorocaine, Ethocaine, Irocaine, Kerocaine, Syncaine.
Use: Anesthetic, injectable local.
See: Novocain.

procaine hydrochloride. (Various Mfr.) Procaine hydrochloride 2%. May contain sodium metabisulfite. Inj. Multiple-dose vials. 30 mL.
Use: Anesthetic, injectable local.

•**procaine hydrochloride and epinephrine injection.** *USP.*
Use: Anesthetic, local.

procaine hydrochloride and levonordefrin injection.
Use: Anesthetic, local.

procaine, penicillin G suspension, sterile.
Use: Anti-infective, penicillin.
See: Penicillin G Procaine.
Pfizerpen.

procaine, penicillin G w/aluminum stearate suspension, sterile.
Use: Anti-infective, penicillin.
See: Penicillin G Procaine with Aluminum Stearate Suspension, Sterile.

procaine, tetracaine and nordefrin hydrochlorides injection.
Use: Anesthetic, local.

procaine, tetracaine and phenylephrine hydrochlorides injection.
Use: Anesthetic.

Pro-Cal. (Pro-Biotiks) Ca 750 mg, Mg 160 mg, P 580 mg, vitamin D 400 units, C 30 mg. Levulose. Tab. 120s, 240s. *OTC.*
Use: Nutritional supplement, vitamin.

ProcalAmine Injection. (McGaw) Injection of amino acid 3%, glycerin 3%, electrolytes. Bot. 1000 mL. *Rx.*
Use: Nutritional supplement, parenteral.

•**procarbazine hydrochloride.** (pro-CAR-buh-ZEEN) *USP.* (Roche) Natulan.
Use: Cytostatic; antineoplastic.
See: Matulane.

Procardia. (Pfizer) Nifedipine 10 mg. Saccharin. Cap., liquid filled. 100s, 300s. *Rx.*
Use: Calcium channel blocker.

Procardia XL. (Pfizer) Nifedipine. Film-coated. ER Tab. **30 mg, 60 mg:** Bot. 100s, 300s, 5000s, UD 100s. **90 mg:** Bot 100s, UD 100s. *Rx.*
Use: Calcium channel blocker.

•**procaterol hydrochloride.** (PRO-CAT-ehr-ole) USAN.
Use: Bronchodilator.

ProCentra. (FSC Laboratories) Dextroamphetamine sulfate 5 mg per 5 mL. Benzoic acid, saccharin, sorbitol. Bubble gum flavor. Soln. 473 mL. *c-II.*
Use: Amphetamine.

Proception Sperm Nutrient Douche. (Milex) Ringer type glucose douche. Bot. sufficient for 10 douches. *OTC.*
Use: Vaginal agent.

•**prochlorperazine.** (PROE-klor-PER-a-zeen) *USP.*
Use: Antipsychotic, phenothiazine derivative.
See: Compro.

prochlorperazine. (Various Mfr.) Prochlorperazine 25 mg. Supp. 12s. *Rx.*
Use: Antipsychotic, phenothiazine derivative.

•**prochlorperazine edisylate.** (PROE-klor-PER-a-zeen e-DIS-i-late) *USP.*
Use: Antipsychotic, phenothiazine derivative.
See: Compazine.

prochlorperazine edisylate. (Various Mfr.) Prochlorperazine edisylate 5 mg/mL. May contain benzyl alcohol, sodium saccharin. Inj., Soln. Vials. 2 mL, 10 mL. *Rx.*
Use: Antipsychotic, phenothiazine derivative.

prochlorperazine ethanedisulfonate. Prochlorperazine Edisylate, USP.
Use: Anxiolytic.

prochlorperazine/isopropamide. (Various Mfr.) Isopropamide iodide 5 mg, prochlorperazine maleate 10 mg. Cap. Bot. 100s, 500s, 1000s, UD 100s. *Rx.*
Use: Anticholinergic; antispasmodic; antiemetic; antivertigo.

•**prochlorperazine maleate.** (PROE-klor-PER-a-zeen) *USP.*
Use: Antipsychotic, phenothiazine derivative.
See: Compazine.

prochlorperazine maleate. (Various Mfr.) Prochlorperazine maleate 5 mg, 10 mg. May contain lactose, PEG. Tab. 100s, 1,000s (10 mg only). *Rx.*
Use: Antipsychotic, phenothiazine derivative.

•**procinonide.** (pro-SIN-oh-nide) USAN.
Use: Adrenocortical steroid.

•**proclonol.** (PRO-klah-nole) USAN. Under study.
Use: Anthelmintic; antifungal.

Pro Comfort Athlete's Foot Spray. (Scholl) Tolnaftate 1%. Aer. Can 4 oz. *OTC.*
Use: Antifungal, topical.

Pro Comfort Jock Itch Spray Powder. (Scholl) Tolnaftate 1%. Aer. Can 3.5 oz. *OTC.*
Use: Antifungal, topical.

ProCoMycin. (Physicians Science and Nature) Polymyxin B sulfate 10,000 units/g, neomycin 3.5 mg/g, bacitracin zinc 500 units/g, lidocaine 40 mg. Aloe, avocado oil, cetearyl alcohol, parabens. Oint. 15 g. *OTC.*
Use: Topical anti-infective, antibiotic combination.

Procort. (Roberts) Hydrocortisone 1%. **Cream:** Tube 30 g. **Spray:** Can. 45 mL. *OTC.*
Use: Corticosteroid, topical.

ProCort. (Women's Choice Pharmaceuticals) Hydrocortisone acetate 1.85%, pramoxine hydrochloride 1.15% (in a hydrophilic/hydrophobic base). Cream; rectal. 60 g w/15 single-use applicators. *OTC.*
Use: Anorectal preparation, steroid-containing product.

Procrit. (Janssen Products) Epoetin alfa, recombinant 2000 units/mL, 3000 units/mL, 4000 units/mL, 10,000 units/mL, 20,000 units/mL, 40,000 units/mL. Inj. Soln. Single-dose vials. 1 mL, preservative free with albumin (human) 2.5 mg/mL (except 20,000 units/mL). Multidose vials. 1 mL (20,000 units/mL only) and 2 mL (10,000 units only), preserved with benzyl alcohol 1% and with albumin (human) 2.5 mg/mL. *Rx.*
Use: Hematopoietic.

Proctocort. (Salix) **Cream; rectal:** Hydrocortisone 1%. Stearyl and cetyl alcohols. 28.35 g. **Supp.; rectal:** Hydrocortisone acetate 30 mg. In hydrogenated vegetable oil base. 12s, 24s. *Rx.*
Use: Anorectal preparation, steroid-containing product.

ProctoFoam. (Alaven Pharmaceutical) Pramoxine hydrochloride 1%. Cetyl alcohol, glyceryl, parabens, PEG-100, propylene glycol, trolamine. Aer. Foam. 15 g w/applicator. *OTC.*
Use: Topical local anesthetic.

ProctoFoam-HC. (Meda Pharmaceuticals) Hydrocortisone acetate 1%, pramoxine hydrochloride 1% in hydrophilic foam base. Bot. aerosol container, Aerosol foam 10 g w/applicator. *Rx.*
Use: Corticosteroid; anesthetic, local.

Pro-Cute. (Ferndale) Silicone, hexachlorophene, lanolin. Cream. 2 oz, lb. *OTC.*
Use: Emollient.

ProCycle Gold. (Cyclin) Vitamins A 833.3 units, D 66.7 units, E 66.7 units, C 30 mg, B_1 1.7 mg, B_2 1.7 mg, B_3 3.3 mg, B_5 1.7 mg, B_6 3.3 mg, B_{12} 21 mcg, folic acid 66.7 mg, Ca 166.7 mg, Fe 3 mg, Zn 2.5 mg, B, Cu, Cr, I, Mg, Mn, Se, PABA, inositol, rutin, biotin, hesperidin, pancreatin, betaine. Tab. Sugar free. Bot. 100s. *OTC.*
Use: Mineral, vitamin supplement.

•**procyclidine hydrochloride.** (pro-SI-klih-deen) *USP.*
Use: Muscle relaxant; antiparkinsonian.

Procysbi. (Raptor Pharmaceuticals) Cysteamine 25 mg (equiv. to cysteamine bitartrate 74 mg), 75 mg (equiv. to cysteamine bitartrate 221 mg). Cap., delayed release. 60s (25 mg), 250s (75 mg). *Rx.*
Use: Endocrine and metabolic agent.

Procysteine. (Free Radical Sciences)
See: L_2-Oxothiazolidine$_4$-carboxylic acid.

Proderm Topical Dressing. (Dow Hickam) Castor oil 650 mg, Peruvian balsam 72.5 mg/0.82 mL. Aer. 4 oz. *OTC.*
Use: Dermatologic, wound therapy.

•**prodilidine hydrochloride.** (pro-DIH-lih-deen) USAN.
Use: Analgesic.

Prodium. (Breckenridge) Phenazopyramide hydrochloride 95 mg. Tab. 12s, 30s. *OTC.*
Use: Analgesic.

•**prodolic acid.** (PRO-dole-ik acid) USAN.
Use: Anti-inflammatory.

Prodrin. (Gentex Pharma) Acetaminophen/caffeine/isometheptene mucate 500 mg/20 mg/130 mg, 325 mg/20 mg/65 mg. Tab. 50s. *Rx.*
Use: Agent for migraine, migraine combination.

Pro-Est. (Burgin-Arden) Progesterone 25 mg, estrogenic substance 25,000 units, sodium carboxymethylcellulose 1 mg, sodium Cl 0.9%, benzalkonium Cl 1:10,000, sodium phosphate dibasic 0.1% in water. *Rx.*
Use: Estrogen, progestin combination.

•**profadol hydrochloride.** (PRO-fah-dahl) USAN.
Use: Analgesic.

Profamina.
See: Amphetamine.

ProFe. (Pro-Pharma) Polysaccharide iron complex 180 mg. Cap. 30s. *OTC.*
Use: Trace element.

ProFe Forte. (Pro-Pharma) Folic acid 1 mg, Fe 155 mg, vitamins B_1 1.5 mg, B_2 1.7 mg, B_3 20 mg, B_5 10 mg, B_6 25 mg, B_{12} 1,000 mcg, C 45 mg, biotin 150 mcg. Cap. 90s. *OTC.*
Use: Prenatal vitamin with minerals.

Profen Forte. (Ivax) Pseudoephedrine hydrochloride 90 mg, guaifenesin 800 mg. ER Tab. Bot. 100s. *Rx.*
Use: Upper respiratory combination; decongestant, expectorant.

Profen Forte DM. (Ivax) Pseudoephedrine hydrochloride 90 mg, dextromethorphan HBr 60 mg, guaifenesin 800 mg. SR Tab. Bot. 100s. *Rx.*
Use: Upper respiratory combination, antitussive, decongestant, expectorant.

Profen II. (Ivax) Pseudoephedrine hydrochloride 45 mg, guaifenesin 800 mg. ER Tab. Bot. 100s. *Rx.*

Use: Upper respiratory combination, decongestant, expectorant.

Profen II DM. (Ivax) Pseudoephedrine hydrochloride 45 mg, guaifenesin 800 mg, dextromethorphan HBr 30 mg. ER Tab. Bot. 100s. *Rx.*
Use: Upper respiratory combination, antitussive, decongestant, expectorant.

Professional Care Lotion, Extra Strength. (Walgreen) Zinc oxide 0.25% in a lotion base. Lot. Bot. 16 oz. *OTC.*
Use: Astringent; antiseptic, dermatologic.

Profiber. (Sherwood Davis & Geck) Sodium caseinate, dietary fiber from soy, calcium caseinate, hydrolyzed cornstarch, corn oil, soy lecithin, vitamins A, B_1, B_2, B_3, B_5, B_6, B_{12}, C, D, E, K, folic acid, biotin, choline, Ca, Cl, Cr, Cu, Fe, I, Mg, Mn, Mo, P, Se, Zn. Liq. Can 250 mL, closed system 1000 mL. *OTC.*
Use: Nutritional supplement.

Profilnine SD. (Grifols) Factor IX, II, X, and low amounts of VII (human). Preservative free. Solvent/detergent treated. Inj., lyophilized Pow. for Soln. Inj. Kit w/single-dose vials and sterile water for injection. *Rx.*
Use: Antihemophilic agent.

proflavine dihydrochloride. 3,6-Diaminoacridine dihydrochloride.

proflavine sulfate. 3,6-Diaminoacridine sulfate.

Pro-Flora Concentrate. (Integrative Therapeutics) 1 billion CFU blend of *L. rhamnosus, B. lactis, L. acidophilus, B. longum, B. breve, B. bifidum.* Palm oil, vegetable glycerin. Gluten free, preservative free, and sugar free. Cap. 30s. *OTC.*
Use: Probiotic.

Pro-Flora Immune. (Integrative Therapeutics) 1 billion CFU blend of *L. plantarum, B. lactis, L. acidophilus, B. longum.* Palm oil, vegetable glycerin. Gluten free, preservative free, and sugar free. Cap. 30s. *OTC.*
Use: Probiotic.

•**progabide.** (pro-GAB-ide) USAN.
Use: Anticonvulsant, muscle relaxant.

Progens. (Major) Conjugated estrogens. Tab. **0.625 mg:** Bot. 100s, 1000s. **1.25 mg:** Bot. 1000s. **2.5 mg:** Bot. 100s, 1000s. *Rx.*
Use: Estrogen.

Pro-Gesic. (Nastech) Trolamine salicylate 10%, propylene glycol, methylparahydroxybenzoic acid, propyl parahydroxybenzoic acid, EDTA. Liq. Bot. 75 mL. *OTC.*
Use: Liniment.

•**progesterone.** (pro-JESS-ter-ohn) *USP.* Flavolutan, Luteogan, Luteosan, Lutren.
Use: Hormone, progestin.
W/Oil.
See: Crinone.
Endometrin.
Prochieve.
Prometrium.

progesterone. (Teva) Progesterone 100 mg, 200 mg. Peanut oil. Cap., micronized softgel. 100s. *Rx.*
Use: Sex hormone, progestin.

progesterone. (Various Mfr.) Progesterone Pow. 1 g, 10 g, 25 g, 100 g, 1000 g.
Use: Hormone, progestin.

progesterone in oil. (Various Mfr.) Progesterone 50 mg/mL. May contain sesame oil, benzyl alcohol. Inj. Multidose vials. 10 mL. *Rx.*
Use: Sex hormone, progestin.

progestins. Progesterone.
Use: Sex hormone.
See: Estrogens and Progestins Combined.
Hydroxyprogesterone Caproate.
Leuprolide Acetate.
Medroxyprogesterone Acetate.
Megestrol Acetate.
Micronor.
Norethindrone.
Norethindrone Acetate.
Nor-QD.
Progesterone.

•**proglumide.** (pro-GLUE-mid) USAN. (Wallace)
Use: Anticholinergic.

Proglycem. (Baker Norton) **Cap.:** Diazoxide 50 mg. Bot. 100s. **Oral Susp.:** Diazoxide 50 mg/mL. Alcohol 7.25%, parabens, sorbitol. Chocolate-mint flavor. 30 mL w/calibrated dropper. *Rx.*
Use: Hyperglycemic.

Prograf. (Astellas) Tacrolimus. **Cap.:** 0.5 mg, 1 mg, 5 mg. Lactose. 100s, blister cards of 10s. **Inj.:** 5 mg/mL. Polyoxyl 60 hydrogenated castor oil (HCO-60) 200 mg/mL, dehydrated alcohol 80%. Amp. 1 mL. *Rx.*
Use: Immunosuppressant.

proguanil hydrochloride.
See: Chloroguanide hydrochloride.
W/Atovaquone.
See: Malarone.
Malarone Pediatric.

ProHance. (Bracco Diagnostics) Gadoteridol 279.3 mg/mL. Preservative free. Inj. Soln. Single-dose vials. 5 mL fill in 15 mL; 10 mL, 15 mL, 20 mL fill in 30 mL. Prefilled syringes. 10 mL and

17 mL fill in 20 mL. *Rx.*
Use: Radiopaque agent, parenteral.

ProHIBiT. (Aventis Pasteur) Purified capsular polysaccharide of *Haemophilus influenzae* type b 25 mcg, conjugated diphtheria toxoid protein 18 mcg/0.5 mL dose. Also called PRP-D. Inj. Vial 0.5 mL, 2.5 mL, 5 mL. Syr. 0.5 mL. *Rx.*
Use: Immunization.

Prohist CF. (Poly Pharmaceuticals) Chlophedianol hydrochloride 25 mg, triprolidine hydrochloride 2.5 mg. Glycerin, propylene glycol, saccharin, sorbitol. Grape flavor. Liq. 473 mL. *Rx.*
Use: Upper respiratory combination, antitussive combination.

Prohist DM. (ProEthic) Dextromethorphan HBr 5 mg, brompheniramine maleate 1 mg, pseudoephedrine hydrochloride 12 mg per 1 mL. Alcohol and dye free. Magnasweet, menthol, saccharin, sucrose. Grape flavor. Drops. 30 mL with dropper. *Rx.*
Use: Upper respiratory combination, antitussive combination.

•**proinsulin human.** (PRO-in-suh-LIN HYOO-muhn) USAN.
Use: Antidiabetic.

Prolactin RIA. (Abbott Diagnostics) Quantitative measurement of total circulating human prolactin. Test unit 50s, 100s.
Use: Diagnostic aid.

Prolactin RIAbead. (Abbott Diagnostics) Radioimmunoassay for the quantitative measurement of prolactin in human serum and plasma.
Use: Diagnostic aid.

proladyl. Pyrrobutamine.
Use: Antihistamine.

prolase. Proteolytic enzyme from *Carica papaya.*
See: Papain.

Prolastin-C. (Talecris) Alpha-1 proteinase inhibitor (human) 1,000 mg. Preservative free. Inj., lyophilized Pow. for Soln. Single-use vial (with sodium; specific activity is ≥ 0.7 mg of functional alpha-1 proteinase inhibitor per mg of total protein; total alpha-1 proteinase inhibitor functional activity in mg is stated on label of each vial) w/20 mL of diluent (sterile water for inj.), transfer needle, and filter needle. *Rx.*
Use: Respiratory enzyme.

Prolensa. (Bausch & Lomb) Bromfenac sodium 0.07%. Soln.; Ophth. Dropper bottle (w/benzalkonium chloride, boric acid, edetate disodium, povidone, sodium borate, sodium sulfite, tyloxapol). 1.6 mL, 3 mL. *Rx.*
Use: Ophthalmic nonsteroidal anti-inflammatory drug.

Proleukin. (Prometheus) Aldesleukin (interleukin-2) 22 × 10^6 IU/vial (18 million IU [1.1 mg] per mL when reconstituted). Mannitol 50 mg, sodium dodecyl sulfate 0.18 mg, monobasic 0.17 mg and dibasic 0.89 mg sodium phosphate. Preservative free. Pow. for Inj., lyophilized. Single-use vials. *Rx.*
Use: Biological response modifiers.

Prolia. (Amgen) Denosumab 60 mg/mL. Sorbitol 4.7%. Preservative free. Inj., Soln. Single-use, prefilled syringe and vial. *Rx.*
Use: Monoclonal antibody.

•**proline.** (PRO-leen) *USP.*
Use: Amino acid.

•**prolintane hydrochloride.** (pro-LIN-tane) USAN.
Use: Antidepressant.

Proloprim. (GlaxoSmithKline) Trimethoprim 100 mg. Tab. Bot. 100s, UD 100s (in sesame oil with benzyl alcohol). *Rx.*
Use: Anti-infective, urinary.

Promacet. (MCR American) Acetaminophen 650 mg, butalbital 50 mg. Tab. 100s. *Rx.*
Use: Nonnarcotic analgesic.

Promachlor. (Geneva) Chlorpromazine hydrochloride 10 mg, 25 mg, 50 mg, 100 mg, 200 mg. Tab. Bot. 100s, 1000s. *Rx.*
Use: Antiemetic; antivertigo; antipsychotic.

Promacta. (GlaxoSmithKline) Eltrombopag 12.5 mg, 25 mg, 50 mg, 75 mg, 100 mg. Mannitol. Film-coated. Tab. 30s. *Rx.*
Use: Hematopoietic agent, thrombopoietin receptor agonist.

Promega. (Parke-Davis) Omega-3 (N-3) polyunsaturated fatty acids 1000 mg, containing EPA 350 mg, DHA 150 mg, vitamins E (3% RDA), A, B_1, B_2, B_3, Ca, Fe (< 2% RDA). Cap., cholesterol and sodium free. Bot. 30s. *OTC.*
Use: Mineral, vitamin supplement.

Promega Pearls. (Parke-Davis) EPA 168 mg, DHA 72 mg, cholesterol < 2 mg, E 1 units, < 2% RDA of A, B_1, B_2, B_3, Fe, Ca. Cap. Bot. 60s, 90s. *OTC.*
Use: Vitamin supplement.

Prometa. (Muro) Metaproterenol sulfate 10 mg/5 mL, with saccharin and sorbitol, strawberry flavor. Syr. Bot. 480 mL. *Rx.*
Use: Bronchodilator.

promethazine. (Alpharma) Promethazine 25 mg, hard fat. Supp. 12s. *Rx.*
Use: Antihistamine, nonselective phenothiazine.

•**promethazine hydrochloride.** (pro-METH-uh-zeen) *USP.*
Use: Antiemetic; antihistamine, nonselective phenothiazine.
See: Pentazine.
Phenadoz.
Phenergan.
Promethegan.
Sigazine.
W/Codeine Phosphate, Phenylephrine Hydrochloride.
See: Promethazine VC w/Codeine.
W/Dextromethorphan Hydrobromide.
See: Promethazine w/Dextromethorphan Cough.
W/Phenylephrine Hydrochloride.
See: Promethazine VC.

promethazine hydrochloride. (Able Labs) Promethazine hydrochloride 12.5 mg. May contain lactose. Tab. 30s, 100s, 500s, 1000s. *Rx.*
Use: Antihistamine.

promethazine hydrochloride. (Ivax) Promethazine hydrochloride 12.5 mg. May contain hard fat. Supp. 12s. *Rx.*
Use: Antihistamine.

promethazine hydrochloride. (Various Mfr.) Promethazine hydrochloride. **Tab.:** 25 mg, 50 mg. May contain lactose. Bot. 30s, 100s, 500s, 1000s. **Supp.:** 25 mg, 50 mg. May contain hard fat (25 mg only). Pkg. 12s. **Inj.:** 25 mg/mL, 50 mg/mL. May contain EDTA. Amp. 1 mL. *Rx.*
Use: Antiemetic; antihistamine, nonselective phenothiazine; sedative.

promethazine hydrochloride and phenylephrine hydrochloride. (Various Mfr.) Phenylephrine hydrochloride 5 mg, promethazine hydrochloride 6.25 mg/5 mL. Alcohol 7%, may contain sorbitol, sugar, parabens. Syr. Bot. 118 mL, 473 mL, 3.8 L. *Rx.*
Use: Upper respiratory combination, decongestant, antihistamine.

promethazine hydrochloride, phenylephrine hydrochloride, and codeine phosphate. (Alpharma) Codeine phosphate 10 mg, promethazine hydrochloride 6.25 mg, phenylephrine hydrochloride 5 mg per 5 mL. Alcohol 7%, parabens, sucrose, saccharin, sugar. Strawberry flavor. Syr. 118 mL, 237 mL, 473 mL. *c-v.*
Use: Antitussive combination, upper respiratory combination.

promethazine hydrochloride w/codeine. (Various Mfr.) Codeine phosphate 10 mg, promethazine hydrochloride 6.25 mg per 5 mL. May contain corn syr., parabens, saccharin. Syr. Bot. 118 mL, 473 mL. *c-v.*
Use: Upper respiratory combination, antitussive combination.

Promethazine VC. (Various Mfr.) Phenylephrine hydrochloride 5 mg, promethazine hydrochloride 6.25 mg per 5 mL. May contain alcohol 7%, menthol, parabens, saccharin sucrose. Syr. Bot. 118 mL, 237 mL, 473 mL. *Rx.*
Use: Antihistamine and decongestant, upper respiratory combination.

Promethazine VC w/Codeine. (Qualitest) Promethazine hydrochloride 6.25 mg, phenylephrine hydrochloride 5 mg, codeine phosphate 10 mg per 5 mL. Alcohol 7%, menthol, parabens, saccharin, sucrose. Strawberry flavor. Syr. Bot. 118 mL. *c-v.*
Use: Upper respiratory combination, antitussive combination.

promethazine w/dextromethorphan cough. (Morton Grove) Dextromethorphan HBr 15 mg, promethazine hydrochloride 6.25 mg per 5 mL. Alcohol 7.1%, EDTA, methylparaben, sugar. Syr. Bot. 118 mL, 473 mL. *Rx.*
Use: Upper respiratory combination, antitussive combination.

Promethegan. (G & W) Promethazine hydrochloride 12.5 mg, 25 mg, 50 mg. Supp., Rectal. 12s, 1000s. *Rx.*
Use: Antihistamine, nonselective phenothiazine.

promethestrol dipropionate.
Use: Estrogen.

Prometh VC w/Codeine Cough. (Alpharma) Codeine phosphate 10 mg, promethazine hydrochloride 6.25 mg, phenylephrine hydrochloride 5 mg per 5 mL. Alcohol 7%, parabens, sugar, saccharin. Syr. Bot. 118 mL, 237 mL, 473 mL, 3.8 L. *c-v.*
Use: Upper respiratory combination, antitussive, antihistamine, decongestant.

Prometh w/Codeine Cough. (Alpharma) Codeine phosphate 10 mg, promethazine hydrochloride 6.25 mg per 5 mL. Alcohol 7%, corn syr., parabens, saccharin. Syr. Bot. 118 mL. *c-v.*
Use: Upper respiratory combination, antitussive, antihistamine.

Prometh w/Dextromethorphan. (Alpharma) Dextromethorphan HBr 15 mg, promethazine hydrochloride 6.25 mg per 5 mL. Alcohol 7%, parabens, saccharin, lemon/mint flavor. Syr. Bot. 118 mL, 237 mL, 473 mL, 3.8 L. *Rx.*
Use: Upper respiratory combination, antitussive, antihistamine.

Prometol. (Viobin) Concentrated wheat germ oil. **3 min/Cap.:** Bot. 100s, 250s.

10 min/Cap.: Bot. 100s. *OTC.*
Use: Supplement.

Prometrium. (AbbVie) Progesterone 100 mg, 200 mg. Peanut oil. Cap. Micronized Soft Gel. Bot. 100s. *Rx.*
Use: Progestin, sex hormone.

prominal.
See: Mephobarbital.

Promine. (Major) Procainamide 250 mg, 375 mg, 500 mg. Cap. Bot. 100s, 250s, 1000s, UD 100s (375 mg/Cap. w/500s instead of 250s). *Rx.*
Use: Antiarrhythmic.

Promine S.R. (Major) Procainamide. **SR Tab.:** 250 mg. Bot. 100s, 250s; 500 mg. Bot. 100s, 250s, 1000s; 750 mg. **SR Cap.:** 250 mg, 375 mg, 500 mg. Bot. 100s, 250s. *Rx.*
Use: Antiarrhythmic.

Promiseb. (Promius Pharma) Castor oil, disodium EDTA, PEG-30. Cream. 30 g. *Rx.*
Use: Emollient.

Promist HD. (UCB) Hydrocodone bitartrate 2.5 mg, pseudoephedrine hydrochloride 30 mg, chlorpheniramine maleate 2 mg/5 mL, alcohol 5%, menthol, saccharin, sorbitol. Bot. Pt. *c-III.*
Use: Antihistamine; antitussive; decongestant.

Promist LA. (UCB) Pseudoephedrine hydrochloride 120 mg, guaifenesin 500 mg. Tab. Bot. 100s. *Rx.*
Use: Decongestant; expectorant.

Pro-Mix R.D.P. (Navaco) Protein 15 g (from whey protein), fat 0.8 g, carbohydrate 1 g, Na 46 mg, K 165 mg, Cl 46 mg, Ca 73.6 mg, P 64.4 mg, Fe 0.3 mg, Cr, Cu, Mg, Mn, Mo, Se, Zn, 72 Cal./5 Tbsp. (20 g). Pow. Packet 20 g, can 300 g. *OTC.*
Use: Nutritional supplement.

Promylin Enteric Coated Microzymes. (Shear/Kershman) Enteric-coated pancrelipase. Lipase 4000 units, amylase 20,000 units, protease 25,000 units. *Rx.*
Use: Digestive enzymes.

Pro-Nasyl. (Progonasyl) o-Iodobenzoic acid 0.5%, triethanolamine 5.5% in a special neutral hydrophilic base compounded from oleic acid, mineral oil, vegetable oil. Bot. 15 mL, 60 mL.
Use: Treatment of sinusitis.

Pronemia Hematinic. (Wyeth) Iron 115 mg, B_{12} 15 mcg, IFC 75 mg, C 150 mg, folic acid 1 mcg. Cap. Bot. 30s. *Rx.*
Use: Iron w/B_{12} and intrinsic factor.

Pronto. (Del) Pyrethrins 0.33%, piperonyl butoxide 4%, benzyl alcohol, decyl alcohol, isopropyl alcohol. Shampoo. 60 mL, 120 mL with comb. *OTC.*
Use: Pediculicide.

Propac. (Biosearch Medical Products) Protein 3 g (from whey protein), carbohydrate 0.2 g, fat 0.3 g, Cl 3 mg, K 20 mg, Na 9 mg, Ca 24 mg, P 12 mg, 16 Cal/Tbsp. (4 g). Pow. Packet 19.5 g, Can 350 g. *OTC.*
Use: Nutritional supplement.

propaesin. (Various Mfr.) Propyl p-Aminobenzoate.

•**propafenone hydrochloride.** (pro-pah-FEN-ohn) *USP.*
Use: Antiarrhythmic agent.
See: Rythmol.
Rythmol SR.

propafenone hydrochloride. (Par Pharmaceuticals) Propafenone hydrochloride 225 mg, 325 mg, 425 mg. Lactose. ER Cap. 60s, 90s, 100s, 500s, 1,000s. *Rx.*
Use: Antiarrhythmic agent.

propafenone hydrochloride. (Various Mfr.) Propafenone 150 mg, 225 mg, 300 mg. Tab. Bot. 100s, 500s (except 300 mg). *Rx.*
Use: Antiarrhythmic agent.

Propagon-S. (Spanner) Estrone 2 mg, 5 mg/mL. Vial 10 mL. *Rx.*
Use: Estrogen.

Propain HC. (Springbok) Acetaminophen 500 mg, hydrocodone bitartrate 5 mg. Cap. Bot. 100s, 500s. *c-III.*
Use: Analgesic combination; narcotic.

•**propane.** (PROE-pane) *NF.*
Use: Aerosol propellant.

propanediol diacetate, 1,2.
See: VoSoL.

1,2,3-propanetriol, trinitrate. Nitroglycerin Tab., USP.

•**propanidid.** (pro-PAN-ih-did) USAN.
Use: Anesthetic, intravenous.

propanolol. Propranolol.

•**propantheline bromide.** (pro-PAN-thuh-leen) *USP.*
Use: Anticholinergic.

propantheline bromide. (Various Mfr.) Propantheline bromide 15 mg. Tab. 100s, 500s, 1000, UD 100s. *Rx.*
Use: Anticholinergic.

PROPApH Astringent Cleanser Maximum Strength. (Del) Salicylic acid 2%, aloe vera gel, SD alcohol 40-2 55.1%. Liq. Bot. 355 mL. *OTC.*
Use: Dermatologic, acne.

PROPApH Cleansing for Oily Skin. (Del) Salicylic acid 0.6%, SD alcohol 40, EDTA, menthol. Lot. Bot. 180 mL. *OTC.*
Use: Dermatologic, acne.

PROPApH Cleansing for Sensitive Skin. (Del) Salicylic acid 0.5%, SD alcohol 40, aloe vera gel, EDTA, menthol. Pads. In 45s. *OTC.*
Use: Dermatologic, acne.

PROPApH Cleansing Lotion for Normal/Combination Skin. (Del) Salicylic acid 0.5%, SD alcohol 40, EDTA. Lot. Bot. 180 mL. Pads. 45s. *OTC.*
Use: Antiacne.

PROPApH Cleansing Maximum Strength. (Del) Salicylic acid 2%, SD alcohol 40, aloe vera gel, EDTA, propylene glycol, menthol. Pads. In 45s. *OTC.*
Use: Dermatologic, acne.

PROPApH Cleansing Pads. (Del) Salicylic acid 0.5%, SD alcohol 40, EDTA, menthol. Pads. 45s. *OTC.*
Use: Dermatologic, acne.

PROPApH Foaming Face Wash. (Del) Salicylic acid 2%, aloe vera gel, EDTA, menthol. Alcohol, oil and soap free. Liq. Bot. 180 mL. *OTC.*
Use: Dermatologic, acne.

PROPApH Maximum Strength Acne Cream. (Del) Salicylic acid 2%, acetylated lanolin alcohol, cetearyl alcohol, stearyl alcohol, EDTA, menthol. Tube 19.5 g. *OTC.*
Use: Dermatologic, acne.

PROPApH Medicated Acne Cream with Aloe. (Del) Salicylic acid 2%. Tube 1 oz. *OTC.*
Use: Dermatologic, acne.

PROPApH Medicated Acne Stick with Aloe. (Del) Salicylic acid 2%. Stick 0.05 oz. *OTC.*
Use: Dermatologic, acne.

PROPApH Medicated Cleansing Pads with Aloe. (Del) Salicylic acid 0.5%, SD alcohol 40 25%, aloe. Jar containing 45 pads. *OTC.*
Use: Dermatologic, acne.

PROPApH Peel-Off Acne Mask. (Del) Salicylic acid 2%, tartrazine, parabens, polyvinyl alcohol, vitamin E acetate, SD alcohol 40. Mask. 60 mL. *OTC.*
Use: Dermatologic, acne.

PROPApH Skin Cleanser with Aloe. (Del) Salicylic acid USP 0.5%, SD alcohol 40 25%. Liq. Bot. 6 oz, 10 oz. *OTC.*
Use: Dermatologic, acne.

•**proparacaine hydrochloride.** (pro-PAR-ah-cane) *USP.*
Use: Anesthetic local, ophthalmic.
See: Alcaine.
Ophthetic.
Paracaine.
W/Fluorescein Sodium.
See: Flucaine.
Fluoracaine.

proparacaine hydrochloride. (Various Mfr.) Proparacaine hydrochloride 0.5%. Soln. 15 mL. *Rx.*
Use: Anesthetic local, ophthalmic.

proparacaine hydrochloride and fluorescein sodium. (Various Mfr.) Proparacaine hydrochloride 0.5%, fluorescein sodium 0.25%. Povidone, glycerin, EDTA, thimerosal 0.01%. Soln. Bot. 5 mL with dropper. *Rx.*
Use: Anesthetic local, ophthalmic.

proparacaine hydrochloride/procaine hydrochloride.
Use: Anesthetic.

•**propatyl nitrate.** (PRO-pah-till) USAN. Investigational drug in US but available in England.
Use: Coronary vasodilator.

Propecia. (Merck) Finasteride 1 mg, lactose. Film-coated. Tab. Unit-of-use 30s, *ProPak* carton of 3 unit-of-use bottles of 30. *Rx.*
Use: Androgen hormone inhibitor; hair growth.

Propel. (Intersect ENT) Mometasone furoate 370 mcg (mometasone furoate is embedded in a bioabsorbable polymer matrix containing poly-[DL-lactide-co-glycolide] and polyethylene glycol, which provides for the gradual release of the drug). PEG. Implant, intranasal. Single use w/delivery system. *Rx.*
Use: Respiratory agent.

•**propenzolate hydrochloride.** (pro-PEN-zoe-late) USAN.
Use: Anticholinergic.

propesin. Name used for *Risocaine.*

Prophene 65. (Halsey Drug) Propoxyphene hydrochloride 65 mg. Cap. Bot. 100s, 500s, 1000s. *c-iv.*
Use: Analgesic; narcotic.

prophenpyridamine maleate.
See: Pheniramine maleate.
W/Combinations
See: Trimahist.
Vasotus.

Pro-Phree. (Ross) Fat 31 g, carbohydrate 60 g, linoleic acid 2250 mg, Fe 11.9 mg, Na 250 mg, K 875 mg, with appropriate vitamins and minerals, 520 Cal/100 g. Protein free. Pow. Can 350 g. *OTC.*
Use: Nutritional supplement.

•**propikacin.** (PRO-pih-KAY-sin) USAN.
Use: Anti-infective.

Propimex-1. (Ross) Protein 15 g, fat 23.9 g, carbohydrate 46.3 g, linoleic acid 1800 mg, Fe 9 mg, Na 190 mg, K 675 mg, with appropriate vitamins and minerals, 480 Cal/100 g. Methionine and

valine free. Pow. Can 350 g. *OTC.*
Use: Nutritional supplement.

Propimex-2. (Ross) Protein 30 g, fat 15.5 g, carbohydrate 30 g, Na 880 mg, K 1370 mg, with appropriate vitamins and minerals, 410 Cal/mL. Methionine and valine free. Pow. Can 325 g. *OTC.*
Use: Nutritional supplement for propionic or methylmalonic acidemia.

•**propiolactone.** (PRO-pee-oh-LACK-tone) USAN.
Use: Disinfectant, sterilizing agent of vaccines and tissue grafts.

•**propionic acid.** (pro-pee-AHN-ik) *NF.*
Use: Antimicrobial; pharmaceutic aid, acidifying agent.

propionyl erythromycin lauryl sulfate.
See: Erythromycin Propionate Lauryl Sulfate.

•**propiram fumarate.** (PRO-pih-ram) USAN.
Use: Analgesic.

Propisamine.
See: Amphetamine.

propitocaine. Prilocaine.

•**propofol.** (PRO-puh-FOLE) *USP.*
Use: Anesthetic, intravenous.
See: Diprivan.
Fresenius Propoven.

propofol. (Baxter Healthcare) Propofol 10 mg/mL, soybean oil 100 mg/mL, glycerol 22.5 mg/mL, egg yolk phospholipid 12 mg/mL, sodium metabisulfite 0.25 mg/mL, ph = 4.5 to 6.4. Inj. Emulsion. Single-use vial 20 mL; Single-use infusion vial 50 mL, 100 mL. *Rx.*
Use: Anesthetic.

Propoquin. Amopyroquin hydrochloride.
Use: Antimalarial.

•**propoxycaine and procaine hydrochlorides and levonordefrin injection.** *USP.*
Use: Anesthetic, local.

•**propoxycaine and procaine hydrochlorides and norepinephrine bitartrate injection.** *USP.*
Use: Anesthetic, local.

•**propoxycaine hydrochloride.** (pro-POX-ih-cane) *USP.*
Use: Anesthetic, local.

propoxychlorinol. Toloxychlorinol.

•**propoxyphene hydrochloride.** (proe-POX-i-feen) *USP.*
Use: Analgesic.
See: Darvon Pulvules.
Dolene Plain.
Pro-Gesic.
W/Combinations.
See: Dolene, AP-65.
Dolene Compound-65.

propoxyphene hydrochloride. (Various Mfr.) Propoxyphene hydrochloride 65 mg. Cap. Bot. 100s. *c-IV.*
Use: Opioid analgesic.

•**propoxyphene hydrochloride, aspirin, and caffeine capsules.** *USP.*
Use: Analgesic.

•**propoxyphene napsylate.** (proe-POX-i-feen NAP-si-late) *USP.*
Use: Analgesic.

•**propoxyphene napsylate and aspirin tablets.** *USP.*
Use: Analgesic.

•**propranolol hydrochloride.** (pro-PRAN-oh-lahl) *USP.*
Use: Antiadrenergic/sympatholytic, beta-adrenergic blocker.
See: Hemangeol.
Inderal LA.
Inderal XL.
InnoPran XL.
Propranolol Intensol.

propranolol hydrochloride. (Various Mfr.) Propranolol hydrochloride. **Tab.:** 10 mg, 20 mg, 40 mg, 60 mg, 80 mg. May contain lactose. 90s (20 mg only), 100s, 500s (80 mg only), 1,000s (except 60 mg and 80 mg), UD 100s (except 60 mg and 80 mg). **ER Cap.:** 60 mg, 80 mg, 120 mg, 160 mg. 100s, 500s, 1,000s, UD 100s. **Inj.:** 1 mg/mL. Vial 1 mL. *Rx.*
Use: Antiadrenergic/sympatholytic, beta-adrenergic blocker.

propranolol hydrochloride solution. (Roxane) Propranolol hydrochloride 4 mg/mL, 8 mg/mL, parabens, saccharin, sorbitol, dye free, strawberry-mint flavor. Oral Soln. 500 mL. *Rx.*
Use: Antiadrenergic/sympatholytic, beta-adrenergic blocker.

propranolol/hydrochlorothiazide. (Various Mfr.) Propranolol hydrochloride/hydrochlorothiazide 40 mg/25 mg, 80 mg/25 mg. Bot. 100s, 1000s (80 mg/25 mg only). *Rx.*
Use: Antihypertensive.

propranolol intensol. (Roxane) Propranolol hydrochloride 80 mg/mL, alcohol and dye free. Concentrated Oral Soln. Bot. 30 mL with dropper. *Rx.*
Use: Antiadrenergic/sympatholytic, beta-adrenergic blocker.

•**propylene carbonate.** (PRO-pi-leen CAR-boe-nate) *NF.*
Use: Pharmaceutic aid, gelling agent.

•**propylene glycol.** (PRO-pi-leen GLYE-kol) *USP.*
Use: Pharmaceutic aid, humectant, solvent, suspending agent.

•**propylene glycol alginate.** (PRO-pi-leen GLYE-kol AL-ji-nate) *NF.*
Use: Pharmaceutic aid, suspending, viscosity-increasing agent.

propylene glycol diacetate.
Use: Pharmaceutic aid, solvent.

•**propylene glycol monostearate.** (PRO-pi-leen GLYE-kol mon-oh-STEER-ate) *NF.*
Use: Pharmaceutic aid, emulsifying agent.

•**propyl gallate.** (PRO-pill GAL-ate) *NF.*
Use: Pharmaceutic aid; antioxidant.

•**propylhexedrine.** (pro-pill-HEX-ih-dreen) *USP.*
Use: Adrenergic, vasoconstrictor; appetite suppressant; antihistamine.

•**propyliodone.** (pro-pill-EYE-oh-dohn) *USP.*
Use: Diagnostic aid, radiopaque medium.
See: Dionosil Oily.

propylnoradrenaline-iso.
See: Isoproterenol.

propyl p-aminobenzoate. (Various Mfr.) Propaesin.
Use: Anesthetic, local.

•**propylparaben.** (PROE-pil-PAR-a-ben) *NF.* Propyl Chemosept (Chemo Puro).
Use: Pharmaceutic aid, antifungal agent.

•**propylparaben sodium.** (PROE-pil-PAR-a-ben) *NF.*
Use: Pharmaceutic aid, antimicrobial preservative.

•**propylthiouracil.** (pro-puhl-thigh-oh-YOU-rah-sill) *USP.*
Use: Antithyroid agent.

propylthiouracil. (Various Mfr.) Propylthiouracil 50 mg. Tab. Bot. 100s, 1000s. *Rx.*
Use: Antithyroid agent.

Pro-Q. (CollaGenex) Dimethicone, glycerin, parabens. Foam. 76 mL, 161 mL. *OTC.*
Use: Protectant.

ProQuad. (Merck & Co.) Mixture of 4 viruses: ≥ 3.00 log_{10} $TCID_{50}$ (50% tissue culture infectious dose) of measles virus; 4.3 log_{10} $TCID_{50}$ of mumps virus; 3.00 log_{10} $TCID_{50}$ of rubella virus; and ≥ 3.99 log_{10} plaque-forming units of varicella virus per 0.5 mL. Also contains sucrose, hydrolyzed gelatin, sodium chloride, sorbitol, monosodium L-glutamate, sodium phosphate dibasic, human albumin, sodium bicarbonate, potassium phosphate monobasic, potassium chloride, potassium phosphate dibasic, residual components of MRC-5 cells including DNA and protein, neomycin, bovine calf serum. Preservative free. Pow. for Inj., lyophilized. Single-dose vials. 1s with diluent. *Rx.*
Use: Agent for immunization.

•**proquazone.** (PRO-kwah-zone) USAN.
Use: Anti-inflammatory.

Pro-Red AC. (Pro-Pharma) Codeine phosphate 9 mg, pyrilamine maleate 8.33 mg, phenylephrine hydrochloride 5 mg. Alcohol free and sugar free. Glycerin, saccharin, sorbitol. Cotton candy flavor. Syr. 473 mL. *c-v.*
Use: Upper respiratory combination, antitussive combination.

•**prorenoate potassium.** (pro-REN-oh-ate) USAN.
Use: Aldosterone antagonist.

Prorone. (Sigma-Tau) Progesterone 25 mg/mL. Aqueous or oil susp. Vial 10 mL. *Rx.*
Use: Hormone, progestin.

•**proroxan hydrochloride.** (pro-ROCK-san) USAN. *Formerly Pyrroxane, Pirrousan.*
Use: Antiadrenergic, α-receptor.

Proscar. (Merck) Finasteride 5 mg, lactose. Tab. 1000s, Unit-of-use 30s, 100s, UD 100s. *Rx.*
Use: Androgen hormone inhibitor.

•**proscillaridin.** (pro-sih-LARE-ih-din) USAN. Talusin, Tradenal.
Use: Cardiovascular agent.

Prosed/DS. (Ferring) Methenamine 81.6 mg, phenyl salicylate 36.2 mg, methylene blue 10.8 mg, benzoic acid 9 mg, hyoscyamine sulfate 0.12 mg. Sugar. Sugar coated. Tab. 100s. *Rx.*
Use: Anti-infective, urinary.

ProSight Lutein. (Major) Ca 22 mg, vitamin E 30 units, C 60 mg, Zn 15 mg, Cu 2 mg. Cap. Bot. 36s. *OTC.*
Use: Nutritional combination product.

Pro Skin. (Marlyn Nutraceuticals) Vitamins A 6250 units, E 100 units, C 100 mg, B_5 10 mg, Zn 10 mg, Se. Cap., Bot. 60s. *OTC.*
Use: Mineral, vitamin supplement.

ProSobee. (Bristol-Myers Squibb) Milk free formula supplies 640 cal/qt, protein 19.2 g, fat 34 g, carbohydrate 64 g, vitamins A 2000 units, D 400 units, E 20 units, C 52 mg, folic acid 100 mcg, B_1 0.5 mg, B_2 0.6 mg, niacin 8 mg, B_6 0.4 mg, B_{12} 2 mcg, biotin 50 mg, pantothenic acid 3 mg, K-1 100 mcg, choline 50 mg, inositol 30 mg, Ca 600 mg, P 475 mg, I 65 mcg, Fe 12 mg, Mg 70 mg, Cu 0.6 mg, Zn 5 mg, Mn 1.6 mg, Cl 530 mg, K 780 mg, Na 230 mg/Qt. (20 Kcal/fl oz). Concentrated liq. can

13 fl oz; Ready-to-Use Liq. Can 8 fl oz, 32 fl oz. Pow., Can 14 oz. *OTC.*
Use: Nutritional supplement.

ProSobee Concentrate. (Bristol-Myers Squibb) P-soy protein isolate, l-methionine. CHO. Corn syr. solids, soy and coconut oil, lecithin, mono- and diglycerides. Protein 20.3 g, CHO 65.4 g, fat 33.6 g, Fe 12 mg, 640 cal/serving. Concentrate 390 mL. *OTC.*
Use: Nutritional supplement.

Pro-Sof w/Casanthranol SG. (Vangard Labs, Inc.) Casanthranol 30 mg, docusate sodium 100 mg. Cap. Bot. 100s, 1000s.
Use: Laxative.

prostacyclin analog.
Use: Vasodilator.
See: Iloprost.

prostaglandin agonist.
Use: Antiglaucoma agent.
See: Bimatoprost.
Latanoprost.
Lumigan.
Tafluprost.
Travatan.
Travoprost.

prostaglandin E_2.
See: Dinoprostone.

prostaglandins.
Use: Abortifacient; agent for impotence; agent for cervical ripening; patent ductus arteriosus; antiulcerative.
See: Carboprost Tromethamine.
Dinoprostone.
Misoprostol.

•**prostalene.** (PRAHST-ah-leen) USAN.
Use: Prostaglandin.

ProstaScint. (Cytogen) Each kit contains capromab pendetide 0.5 mg/mL of sodium phosphate buffered saline and 1 vial of sodium acetate 82 mg in 2 mL sterile water for inj. Preservative free. Includes 1 sterile 0.22 mcm *Millex GV filter*, prescribing information, and 2 identification labels. *Rx.*
Use: In vivo diagnostic aid.

Pro-Stat AWC. (Medical Nutrition) Protein 17 g/30 mL (amino acids including histidine, isoleucine, leucine, lysine, methionine, phenylalanine, threonine, tryptophan, valine, alanine, arginine, aspartic acid, cystine, glutamic acid, glycine, proline, serine, tyrosine, hydroxylysine, hydroxyproline), carbohydrates 10.2 g/30 mL (sugar, xylitol), sodium 13 mg/30 mL, potassium 17 mg/30 mL, 3.6 Kcal/mL. Fructose, phosphorus, potassium citrate, potassium sorbate, sodium benzoate, sucralose, vitamin C, zinc. Lactose free, gluten free, and soy free. Wild cherry punch flavor. Liq. 887 mL. *OTC.*
Use: Nutritional supplement.

Pro-Stat 101. (Medical Nutrition) Protein 15 g/30 mL (collagen hydrolysate, amino acids [including histidine, isoleucine, leucine, lysine, methionine, phenylalanine, threonine, tryptophan, valine, alanine, arginine, aspartic acid, cystine, glutamic acid, glycine, proline, serine, tyrosine, hydroxylysine, hydroxyproline]). Fructose, potassium sorbate, sodium 14.5 mg/30 mL, sucralose, xylitol. Gluten free and lactose free. Natural, butter pecan, and wild cherry flavors. Liq. 887 mL. *OTC.*
Use: Nutritional supplement.

Pro-Stat Profile. (Medical Nutrition) Protein 11.3 g/30 mL (amino acids including histidine, isoleucine, leucine, lysine, methionine, phenylalanine, threonine, tryptophan, valine, alanine, arginine, aspartic acid, cystine, glutamic acid, glycine, proline, serine, tyrosine, hydroxylysine, hydroxyproline), carbohydrates 10.2 g/30 mL (sugar), sodium 15 mg/30 mL, potassium 16 mg/30 mL, 2.8 Kcal/mL. Acesulfame K, fructose, phosphorus, potassium sorbate, sodium benzoate, sucralose. Lactose free, gluten free, soy free. Fruit flavor. Liq. 887 mL. *OTC.*
Use: Nutritional supplement.

Pro-Stat Renal Care. (Medical Nutrition) Protein 15 g/30 mL (amino acids including histidine, isoleucine, leucine, lysine, methionine, phenylalanine, threonine, tryptophan, valine, alanine, arginine, aspartic acid, cystine, glutamic acid, glycine, proline, serine, tyrosine, hydroxylysine, hydroxyproline), carbohydrates 8 g/30 mL (glycerin), sodium 15 mg/30 mL, potassium 18 mg/30 mL, 2.4 Kcal/mL. Neotame, phosphorus, polydextrose, potassium sorbate, sodium benzoate, sucralose. Sugar free, lactose free, gluten free, soy free. Tangerine flavor. Liq. 887 mL. *OTC.*
Use: Nutritional supplement.

Pro-Stat 64. (Medical Nutrition) Protein 15 g/30 mL (collagen hydrolysate, amino acids [including histidine, isoleucine, leucine, lysine, methionine, phenylalanine, threonine, tryptophan, valine, alanine, arginine, aspartic acid, cystine, glutamic acid, glycine, proline, serine, tyrosine, hydroxylysine, hydroxyproline]). Acesulfame-K, glycerin, potassium sorbate, sodium 14.5 mg/30 mL, sucralose, xylitol. Gluten free, lactose free, and sugar free. Natural, grape, and

wild cherry punch flavors. Liq. 887 mL. *OTC.*
Use: Nutritional supplement.

Prosteon. (Theralogix) Vitamin D_3 500 units, K 25 mcg, B, Ca, Mg, Sr. Tab. 240s. *OTC.*
Use: Multivitamin with minerals.

ProStep. (Wyeth) Transdermal nicotine 11 mg, 22 mg/day. Patch 7s. *Rx.*
Use: Smoking deterrent.

Prostigmin Bromide. (AstraZeneca) Neostigmine bromide 15 mg. Tab. Bot. 100s, 1000s. *Rx.*
Use: Muscle stimulant.

Prostin E2. (Pfizer) Dinoprost 20 mg. Supp. Containers of 1 each. *Rx.*
Use: Abortifacient.

Prostin VR Pediatric. (Pfizer) Alprostadil 500 mcg/mL. Amp. 1 mL. *Rx.*
Use: Arterial patency agent.

Prostonic. (Seatrace) Thiamine hydrochloride 10 mg, alanine 130 mg, glutamic acid 130 mg, amino-acetic acid 130 mg. Cap. Bot. 100s. *Rx.*
Use: Palliative relief of benign prostatic hypertrophy.

Protabolin. (Taylor Pharmaceuticals) Methandriol dipropionate 50 mg/mL. Vial 10 mL. *Rx.*
Use: Hormone.

•**protamine sulfate.** (PRO-tuh-meen) *USP.*
Use: Coagulant, heparin antagonist.
W/Insulin Lispro.
See: Humalog Mix 50/50.
Humalog Mix 75/25.

protamine sulfate. (Various Mfr.) Protamine sulfate 10 mg/mL. Preservative free. Inj. Vials 5 mL, 25 mL.
Use: Coagulant, heparin antagonist.

protargin mild.
See: Silver Protein, Mild.

Protargol. (Sterwin) Strong silver protein. Pow. Bot. 25 g. *Rx.*
Use: Antiseptic.

protease.
W/Amylase, Lipase.
See: Bio-Zyme.
Creon.
Palcaps 10.
Pancreatin Quadruple Strength.
Pancreaze.
Pancrelipase.
Pertzye.
Tri-Pase 8.
Tri-Pase 16.
Tyler Panplex 2-Phase.
Tyler Similase Jr.
Ultresa.
Viokace.
Zenpep.

protease inhibitors.
Use: Antiretroviral.
See: Atazanavir Sulfate.
Darunavir Ethanolate.
Fosamprenavir Calcium.
Indinavir Sulfate.
Lopinavir/Ritonavir.
Nelfinavir Mesylate.
Ritonavir.
Saquinavir Mesylate.
Tipranavir.

proteasome inhibitors.
See: Bortezomib.
Carfilzomib.

ProTech First-Aid Stik. (Triton) Lidocaine hydrochloride 2.5%, povidone iodine 10%. Liq. 14 mL dab-on applicator. *OTC.*
Use: Topical local anesthetic combination.

ProtectNatal. (Gil Pharmaceutical) Vitamins A 1,250 units, C 125 mg, D_3 200 units, E 25 units, B_1 5 mg, B_2 5 mg, B_3 10 mg, B_5 12.5 mg, B_6 5 mg, B_{12} 100 mcg, Fe 13.5 mg, folic acid 0.5 mg, biotin 25 mcg, Ca 75 mg, I, Mg, Zn, Cu, Se, Mn, Cr, Mo, coenzyme Q10 15 mg, EPA 112 mg, DHA 75 mg, omega-3 fish oil 700 mg, papaya, whey, bromelain. Enteric coated. Glucose, mineral oil, PEG, parabens, sucrose. Gluten free and sugar free. Tab. 60s. *Rx.*
Use: Prenatal vitamin.

Protegra Softgels. (Wyeth) Vitamins E 200 units, C 250 mg, beta-carotene 3 mg, Zn 7.5 mg, Cu, Se, Mn. Cap. Bot. 50s. *OTC.*
Use: Vitamin supplement.

proteinase inhibitor, alpha 1.
See: Prolastin.

protein C concentrate (human).
Use: Thrombolytic agent, human protein C.
See: Ceprotin.

protein C1 inhibitors.
See: C1 Inhibitor (Human).

•**protein hydrolysate injection.** (PROE-teen hye-DROL-i-sate) *USP.*
Use: Fluid, nutrient replacement.
See: Amigen.
Aminogen.
Lacotein.

protein hydrolysates oral.
Use: Enteral nutritional supplement.
See: Nutramigen.
Pregestimil.
W/Vitamin B_{12}.
See: Stuart Amino Acids and B_{12}.

protein substrates.
See: Cysteine Hydrochloride.

protein synthesis inhibitors.
See: Omacetaxine Mepesuccinate.

protein-tyrosine kinase inhibitors.
See: Dasatinib.
Imatinib.
mTOR Inhibitor.
Nilotinib.
Sunitinib Malate.

Protenate. (Baxter PPI) Plasma protein fraction (Human) 5%. Inj. Vial 250 mL, 500 mL w/administration set. *Rx.*
Use: Plasma protein fraction.

ProThelial. (McCullough Mueller Enterprises) Sucralfate 10%. Parabens, saccharin. Paste; oral. 125 mL, 250 mL. *Rx.*
Use: Gastrointestinal agent.

Prothers. (ICN) Soap free. White petrolatum, disodium cocamido MIPA-sulfosuccinate, pentane, ammonium laureth sulfate, PEG-150 distearate, hydroxypropyl methylcellulose, imidazolidinyl urea, parabens, propylene glycol stearate, hydrogenated soy glyceride, sodium stearyl lactylate. Liq. Bot. 180 mL. *OTC.*
Use: Dermatologic, cleanser.

prothipendyl hydrochloride.
Use: Sedative.

prothrombin complex concentrate (human).
Use: Systemic hemostatic.

Proticuleen. (Spanner) Vitamin B_{12} activity 10 mcg, folic acid 10 mg, B_{12} crystalline 50 mcg, niacinamide 75 mg/mL. Multiple-dose vial 10 mL. IM Inj. *Rx.*
Use: Nutritional supplement, parenteral.

Protonix. (Wyeth-Ayerst) Pantoprazole sodium. **DR Susp.:** 40 mg (as pantoprazole sodium sesquihydrate 45.1 mg). Enteric-coated gran. UD 30s. **DR Tab.:** 20 mg (as pantoprazole sodium sesquihydrate 22.6 mg), 40 mg (as pantoprazole sodium sesquihydrate 45.1 mg). Mannitol. Tab. Bot. 90s, UD 100s (40 mg only). *Rx.*
Use: Proton pump inhibitor.

Protonix I.V. (Wyeth-Ayerst) Pantoprazole sodium 40 mg. EDTA. Inj., freeze-dried, Pow. for Soln. Vials. *Rx.*
Use: Proton pump inhibitor.

proton pump inhibitors.
See: Esomeprazole Magnesium.
Esomeprazole Strontium.
Lansoprazole.
Omeprazole.
Omeprazole/Sodium Bicarbonate.
Omeprazole/Sodium Bicarbonate/ Magnesium Hydroxide.
Pantoprazole Sodium.
Rabeprazole Sodium.

Protopam Chloride. (Wyeth-Ayerst) Pralidoxime chloride 1 g. Pow. for Inj. Single-use vial. 20 mL. *Rx.*
Use: Antidote.

Protopic. (Astellas Pharma) Tacrolimus 0.03%, 0.1%. Mineral oil, white petrolatum. Oint. Tube 30 g, 60 g, 100 g. *Rx.*
Use: Immunomodulator, topical.

Protosan. (Recsei) Protein 87.5%, lactose 0.5%, fat 1.3%, ash 3.5%, Na 0.02%. Jar 1 lb, 5 lb. *OTC.*
Use: Nutritional supplement.

Prot-O-Sea. (Barth's) Protein 90%, containing amino acids and minerals. Bot. 100s, 500s. *OTC.*
Use: Nutritional supplement.

Protran Plus. (Vangard Labs, Inc.) Meprobamate 150 mg, ethoheptazine citrate 75 mg, aspirin 250 mg. Tab. Bot. 100s. 500s. *Rx.*
Use: Analgesic, anxiolytic combination.

•**protriptyline hydrochloride.** (pro-TRIP-tih-leen) *USP.*
Use: Antidepressant.
See: Vivactil.

protriptyline hydrochloride. (Various Mfr.) Protriptyline hydrochloride 5 mg, 10 mg. Tab. Bot. 100s, 1000s. *Rx.*
Use: Antidepressant.

Provella. (Upsher-Smith) *L. acidophilus* 2 billion CFU, *L. fermentum*, *L. plantarum*, *L. reuteri*, *L. rhamnosus*, *B. bifidum*. Sodium 20 mg. Gluten free and preservative free. Tab. 30s. *OTC.*
Use: Probiotic.

Provenge. (Dendreon Corporation) Sipuleucel-T 50 million autologous $CD54^{+}$ cells (activated with prostatic acid phosphatase linked to granulocyte-macrophage colony-stimulating factor). Inj., Susp. Patient-specific infusion bags. 250 mL. *Rx.*
Use: Miscellaneous antineoplastic.

Proventil HFA. (Key) Albuterol sulfate 90 mcg/actuation. Aer. Can. 6.7 g/ (200 inhalations). Contains no chlorofluorocarbons (CFCs). *Rx.*
Use: Bronchodilator, sympathomimetic.

Provera. (Pfizer) Medroxyprogesterone acetate 2.5 mg, 5 mg, 10 mg. Lactose, sucrose. Tab. 100s, 500s (10 mg only). *Rx.*
Use: Sex hormone, progestin.

Provida OB. (US Pharmaceutical Corporation) Folic acid 1.25 mg, iron 40 mg, vitamins D 400 units, B_1 2.5 mg, B_2 3.5 mg, B_3 10 mg, B_5 6 mg, B_6 25 mg, B_{12} 12 mcg, C 60 mg, Cu, Mg, Zn, biotin 300 mcg, *Lactobacillus casei* KE-99 200 billion CFU/g 30 mg. Cap. 30s. *Rx.*
Use: Prenatal vitamin with minerals.

Provigil. (Cephalon) Modafinil 100 mg, 200 mg. Lactose. Tab. 100s. *c-IV.*
Use: CNS stimulant, analeptic.

ProVisc. (Alcon) Sodium hyaluronate 10 mg/mL. Sodium chloride 8.4 mg/mL. Inj. Disposable syringe. 0.4 mL, 0.55 mL, 0.85 mL. *Rx.*
Use: Ophthalmic surgical adjunct.

Provocholine. (Methapharm) Methacholine chloride 100 mg/5 mL. Soln. for Inhalation. Vial 5 mL. *Rx.*
Use: Diagnostic aid.

Prox/APAP. (Forest) Propoxyphene hydrochloride 65 mg, acetaminophen 650 mg. Tab. Bot. 100s, 500s. *c-IV.*
Use: Analgesic combination; narcotic.

•**proxazole.** (PROX-a-zole) USAN.
Use: Analgesic; anti-inflammatory; muscle relaxant.

•**proxazole citrate.** (PROX-a-zole) USAN.
Use: Relaxant, smooth muscle; analgesic; anti-inflammatory.

•**proxicromil.** (prox-ih-KROE-mill) USAN.
Use: Antiallergic.

Proxigel. (Schwarz Pharma) Carbamide peroxide 10% in a water-free gel base. Tube 34 g w/applicator. *OTC.*
Use: Antiseptic, cleanser.

•**proxorphan tartrate.** (PROX-ahr-fan TAR-trate) USAN.
Use: Analgesic; antitussive.

Proxy 65. (Parmed Pharmaceuticals, Inc.) Propoxyphene hydrochloride 65 mg, acetaminophen 650 mg. Tab. Bot. 100s, 500s. *c-IV.*
Use: Analgesic combination; narcotic.

Prozac. (Eli Lilly/Dista) Fluoxetine hydrochloride. **Cap.:** 10 mg, 20 mg, 40 mg. 30s (except 10 mg); 100s (except 40 mg); 2,000s (20 mg only). **Oral Soln.:** 20 mg/5 mL. Alcohol 0.23%, sucrose, mint flavor. 120 mL. *Rx.*
Tall Man: PROzac
Use: Antidepressant, selective serotonin reuptake inhibitor.

Prozac Weekly. (Eli Lilly/Dista) Fluoxetine hydrochloride 90 mg. Sucrose, sugar. Enteric-coated pellets. Cap., delayed release. UD 4s. *Rx.*
Tall Man: PROzac
Use: Antidepressant, selective serotonin reuptake inhibitor.

•**prucalopride.** (proo-KAL-oh-pride) USAN.
Use: Constipation.

prucalopride hydrochloride.
Use: Constipation.

•**prucalopride succinate.** (proo-KAL-oh-pride) USAN.
Use: Constipation.

PruClair. (PruGen) *Butyrospermum parkii*, glyceryl stearate, glycyrrhetinic acid, PEG-100 stearate, alcohols, allantoin, DMDM hydantoin, disodium EDTA, ethylhexylglycerin, sodium hyaluronate, tocopheryl acetate. Cream. 100 g. *Rx.*
Use: Miscellaneous topical combination.

Prudents. (Bariatric) Acetylphenylisatin 5 mg. Chewable protein and amino acid. Tab. Bot. 30s, 100s. *OTC.*
Use: Laxative.

Prudoxin. (Healthpoint Medical) Doxepin hydrochloride 5%. Cream, Top. 45 g. *Rx.*
Use: Topical antihistamine preparation.

Prulet. (Mission Pharmacal) White phenolphthalein 60 mg. Tab. Strips 12s, 40s. *OTC.*
Use: Laxative.

PruMyx. (PruGen) Olive oil, glycerin, palm glycerides, vegetable oil, lecithin, squalane, betaine, palmitamide MEA, sarcosine, acetamide MEA, hydroxyethyl cellulose, sodium carbomer, carbomer, xanthan gum. Preservative free and fragrance free. Cream. 140 g. *Rx.*
Use: Miscellaneous topical combination.

prune powder concentrated dehydrated.
See: Diacetyl-dihydroxyphenylisatin.

Prurilo. (Whorton Pharmaceuticals, Inc.) Menthol 0.25%, phenol 0.25%, calamine lotion in special lubricating base. Bot. 4 oz, 8 oz. *OTC.*
Use: Dermatologic, counterirritant.

•**prussian blue insoluble.** (PRUSH-un) USAN.
Use: Antidote.

prussian blue oral.
Use: Chelating agents; detoxification agent.
See: Radiogardase.

•**pruvanserin.** (prue-VAN-ser-in) USAN.
Use: 5-HT_2 receptor antagonist; insomnia.

•**pruvanserin hydrochloride.** (prue-VAN-ser-in) USAN.
Use: 5-HT_2 receptor antagonist; insomnia.

PSE 120/MSC 2.5. (Cypress) Pseudoephedrine hydrochloride 120 mg, methscopolamine nitrate 2.5 mg. Dye free. ER Tab. Bot. 60s. *Rx.*
Use: Upper respiratory combination, decongestant, antihistamine, and anticholinergic.

Pseudo-Car DM. (Geneva) Pseudoephedrine hydrochloride 60 mg, carbinoxamine maleate 4 mg, dextromethorphan HBr 15 mg/5 mL, alcohol < 0.6%. Bot. Pt, gal. *Rx.*
Use: Antihistamine; antitussive; decongestant.

Pseudo-Chlor. (Various Mfr.) Pseudoephedrine hydrochloride 120 mg, chlorpheniramine maleate 8 mg. Cap. Bot. 100s, 250s. *Rx.*
Use: Antihistamine; decongestant.

Pseudo Cough. (Boca Pharmacal) Dextromethorphan HBr 15 mg, guaifenesin 175 mg, pseudoephedrine hydrochloride 32 mg per 5 mL. Alcohol free. Acesulfame K, saccharin, sorbitol. Grape flavor. Liq. 118 mL, 473 mL. *Rx.*
Use: Upper respiratory combination, antitussive and expectorant combination.

•**pseudoephedrine hydrochloride.** (SOO-doe-e-FED-rin) *USP.*
Use: Adrenergic, vasoconstrictor.
See: Congestaid.
ElixSure Children's Congestion.
Genaphed.
Kid Kare.
Nasal Decongestant, Children's Non-Drowsy.
Nasal Decongestant Oral.
Simply Stuffy.
Sinustop.
Sudafed.
Sudafed Children's Non-Drowsy.
Sudafed Non-Drowsy, Maximum Strength.
Sudafed Non-Drowsy 12 Hour Long-Acting.
Sudafed Non-Drowsy 24 Hour Long-Acting.
SudoGest Non-Drowsy.
Triaminic AM Decongestant Formula.
Unifed.
Zephrex-D.
W/Acetaminophen.
See: Dilotab II.
Mapap Sinus Maximum Strength.
Ornex No Drowsiness.
W/Acetaminophen, Chlorpheniramine Maleate.
See: Advil Allergy Sinus.
BC Allergy, Sinus, Headache.
W/Acetaminophen, Dextromethorphan Hydrobromide, Guaifenesin.
See: Duraflu.
Flutabs.
Maxiflu DM.
Maxiflu G.
Tylenol Cold Severe Congestion.
W/Acetaminophen, Guaifenesin.
See: Tylenol Sinus Severe Congestion.
W/Belladonna Alkaloids, Chlorpheniramine Maleate.
See: Respa A.R.
W/Brompheniramine Maleate.
See: BPM Pseudo 6/45 mg.
Brotapp.
BrōveX PSB.
BrōveX PSE.
J-Tan D PD.
Lodrane D.
Lodrane LD.
LoHist PSB.
Rynex PSE.
SymPak II.
ULTRAbrom PD.
W/Brompheniramine Maleate, Chlophedianol Hydrochloride.
See: Dicel CD.
W/Brompheniramine Maleate, Codeine Phosphate.
See: CPB WC.
Mar-Cof BP.
M-End WC.
Mesehist WC.
W/Brompheniramine Maleate, Dextromethorphan Hydrobromide.
See: Brometane-DX Cough.
Bromfed DM.
Bromhist-DM.
Bromhist PDX.
Brotapp DM.
BrōveX PSE DM.
Dimaphen DM Cough, Cold & Allergy.
DM/PSE/BPM.
Myphetane DX Cough.
Neo DM.
Pediahist DM.
Prohist DM.
Q-Tapp DM Cold and Cough.
Rondec DM.
TGQ 50PSE/3BRM/30DM.
TGQ 40PSE/4BRM/20DM.
TGQ 30PSE/3BRM/15DM.
W/Brompheniramine Maleate, Dextromethorphan Hydrobromide, Guaifenesin.
See: Bromhist DM Pediatric.
Histacol DM Pediatric.
Pediahist DM.
W/Brompheniramine Maleate, Dihydrocodeine Bitartrate.
See: J-COF DHC.
W/Carbetapentane Citrate, Guaifenesin.
See: Exall-D.
W/Carbinoxamine Maleate.
See: Palgic-DS.
Rondec TR.
W/Cetirizine Hydrochloride.
See: All Day Allergy-D.
Zyrtec-D.
W/Chlophedianol Hydrochloride.
See: Clofera.
W/Chlophedianol Hydrochloride, Chlorcyclizine Hydrochloride.
See: Biclora-D.
W/Chlophedianol Hydrochloride, Chlorpheniramine Maleate.
See: Biclora.

W/Chlophedianol Hydrochloride, Guaifenesin.
  See: Certuss-D.
    Vanacof Dx.
W/Chlophedianol Hydrochloride, Pseudoephedrine Hydrochloride.
  See: Chlo Tuss.
W/Chlorcyclizine Hydrochloride.
  See: NasOpen.
    Stahist AD.
W/Chlorcyclizine Hydrochloride, Codeine Phosphate.
  See: Poly-Tussin D.
W/Chlorpheniramine Maleate.
  See: AMBI 60PSE/4CPM.
    Colfed-A.
    Deconamine.
    Duratuss DA.
    LoHist-D.
    Neutrahist.
    Sudafed Sinus & Allergy.
    SudaHist.
    SudoGest Sinus & Allergy Maximum Strength.
    Zinx Chlor-D.
W/Chlorpheniramine Maleate, Codeine Phosphate.
  See: Phenylhistine DH.
W/Chlorpheniramine Maleate, Dextromethorphan Hydrobromide.
  See: Allres DS.
    AMBI 60PSE/4CPM/20DM.
    CPM/PSE DM.
    Dicel DM.
    Esocor P.
    KidKare Children's Cough/Cold.
    Mesehist DM.
    Neutrahist PDX.
    Pedia Relief Cough-Cold.
    Pediatric Cough & Cold.
    Pediatric Cough & Cold Medicine.
    Rescon DM.
    Triaminic-D Children's.
W/Chlorpheniramine Maleate, Dihydrocodeine Bitartrate.
  See: Pancof.
    Tricof.
W/Chlorpheniramine Maleate, Guaifenesin, Hydrocodone Bitartrate.
  See: ZTuss Expectorant.
W/Chlorpheniramine Maleate, Hydrocodone Bitartrate.
  See: Notuss-Forte.
    Pediatex HC.
    Tussend.
W/Chlorpheniramine Maleate, Methscopolamine Nitrate.
  See: CPM 8/PSE 90/MSC 2.5.
    DryMax.
    Histatab.
    Relcof PSE.
    ScopoHist.
    Time-Hist QD.
W/Codeine Phosphate.
  See: EndaCof-DC.
W/Codeine Phosphate, Dexbrompheniramine Maleate.
  See: M-End Max D.
W/Codeine Phosphate, Guaifenesin.
  See: Ambifed CD.
    Ambifed CDX.
    Cheratussin DAC.
    Guiatuss DAC.
    Lortuss EX.
    Tusnel C.
    Zodryl DEC 80.
    Zodryl DEC 50.
    Zodryl DEC 40.
    Zodryl DEC 60.
    Zodryl DEC 30.
    Zodryl DEC 35.
    Zodryl DEC 25.
    Z-Tuss E.
W/Codeine Phosphate, Triprolidine Hydrochloride.
  See: Poly Hist NC.
W/Dexbrompheniramine Maleate, Dextromethorphan Hydrobromide.
  See: M-End DMX.
W/Dexchlorpheniramine Maleate.
  See: HexaFed.
    Rescon.
W/Dexchlorpheniramine Maleate, Dextromethorphan Hydrobromide.
  See: TanaCof-DM.
    Tanafed DMX.
    Tannate DMP-DEX.
W/Dexchlorpheniramine Maleate, Methscopolamine Nitrate.
  See: CoryZa-D.
    D-Hist D.
    Histatab D.
W/Dextromethorphan Hydrobromide.
  See: Robitussin Pediatric Cough & Cold Formula.
W/Dextromethorphan Hydrobromide, Acetaminophen.
  See: 666 Cold Preparation Maximum Strength.
W/Dextromethorphan Hydrobromide, Doxylamine Succinate.
  See: Lortuss DM.
W/Dextromethorphan Hydrobromide, Guaifenesin.
  See: Aldex GS DM.
    Ambifed-G DM.
    AMBI 60/580/30.
    AMBI 60PSE/400GFN/20DM.
    AMBI 40PSE/400GFN/20DM.
    Bionel.
    Bionel Pediatric.
    Capmist DM.

Despec.
Donatussin DM.
Entex PAC.
Entre-Cough.
GFN 600/PSE 60/DM 30.
Liquicough DM.
Maxifed DM.
Maxifed DMX.
Medent DMI.
PanMist-DM.
Poly-Vent DM.
Pseudo Cough.
Q-Tussin CF.
Relacon DM NR.
Relasin DM.
Robaben CF.
Robitussin Cough & Cold D.
Sudafed Multi-Symptom Cold & Cough.
TGQ 30PSE/150GFN/15DM.
Tidafen DM.
TL-DEX DM.
Touro CC-LD.
Trispec PSE.
Tusnel.
Tusnel-DM Pediatric.
Tusnel Pediatric.
Z-Cof DMX.
Z-Cof 8DM.
Z-Cof I.

W/Dihydrocodeine, Guaifenesin.
See: Despec-EXP.
Pancof-EXP.

W/Diphenhydramine Hydrochloride.
See: Respa-SA.
Tekral.

W/Doxylamine Succinate.
See: Lortuss LQ.

W/Guaifenesin.
See: Aldex GS.
Altarussin-PE.
Congestac.
Entex T.
ExeFen-IR.
Mucinex D.
Poly-Vent IR.
Respaire-30.
Rydex G.
Sudafed Maximum Strength Non-Drowsy Non-Drying Sinus.
Tenar PSE.
TG 45PSE/400GFN.

W/Guaifenesin, Theophylline.
See: Broncomar.

W/Ibuprofen.
See: Advil Children's Cold.
Advil Cold & Sinus.
Children's Motrin Cold.

W/Methscopolamine Nitrate.
See: AllePak Dose Pack.
Allergy DN.
Amdry-D.
PSE 120/MSC 2.5.
SudaTrate.

W/Naproxen Sodium.
See: Aleve-D Sinus & Cold.

W/Triprolidine Hydrochloride.
See: Altafed.
Aprodine.
Ed A-Hist PSE.
Entre-Hist PSE.
Genac.
Hist PSE.
Silafed.

pseudoephedrine hydrochloride. (Ohm) Pseudoephedrine hydrochloride 120 mg. Castor oil. ER Tab. 10s. *OTC.*
Use: Nasal decongestant, arylalkylamine.

pseudoephedrine hydrochloride. (Various Mfr.) Pseudoephedrine hydrochloride. **Tab.:** 30 mg, 60 mg. Bot. 24s (30 mg only), 100s, 1000s, blister pack 100s. **Liq.:** 30 mg/5 mL. Bot. 120 mL, 473 mL. *OTC.*
Use: Nasal decongestant, arylalylamine.

pseudoephedrine hydrochloride and triprolidine hydrochloride. (Various Mfr.) Pseudoephedrine hydrochloride 60 mg, triprolidine hydrochloride 2.5 mg. Tab. Bot. 100s, 1000s, UD 100s. *Rx.*
Use: Antihistamine; decongestant.

•**pseudoephedrine hydrochloride, carbinoxamine maleate, and dextromethorphan hydrobromide oral solution.** *USP.*
Use: Decongestant, antihistamine, antitussive.

•**pseudoephedrine polistirex.** (SOO-doe-e-FED-rin POL-ee-SYE-rex) USAN.
Use: Decongestant, nasal.
W/Combinations.
See: Atuss-12 DM.

•**pseudoephedrine sulfate.** (SOO-doe-e-FED-rin) *USP.*
Use: Bronchodilator.
See: Afrinol Repetabs.
W/Desloratadine.
See: Clarinex-D 24 Hour.
W/Dexbrompheniramine Maleate.
See: Drixoral Cold & Allergy.
Drixoral Cold & Allergy Maximum Strength.
W/Loratadine.
See: Alavert Allergy & Sinus D-12 Hour.
Allergy Relief & Nasal Decongestant.
Claritin-D 12 Hour.
Claritin-D 24 Hour.
Clear-Atadine D.
Loratadine D.

pseudoephedrine tannate.
W/Brompheniramine Tannate.
See: B-Vex PD.
Lodrane D.
W/Carbinoxamine Tannate, Dextromethorphan Tannate.
See: Carb PSE 12 DM.
Pseudo-Gest. (Major) Pseudoephedrine hydrochloride 30 mg, 60 mg. Tab. Bot. 24s, 100s. *OTC.*
Use: Decongestant.
Pseudo-Gest Plus. (Major) Pseudoephedrine hydrochloride 60 mg, chlorpheniramine maleate 4 mg. Tab. Bot. 24s, 100s, 200s. *OTC.*
Use: Antihistamine; decongestant.
Pseudo-Hist. (Holloway) Pseudoephedrine hydrochloride 30 mg, chlorpheniramine maleate 10 mg. Cap. Bot. 100s. *OTC.*
Use: Antihistamine; decongestant.
Pseudo-Hist Expectorant. (Holloway) Pseudoephedrine 15 mg, hydrocodone bitartrate 2.5 mg, guaifenesin 100 mg, alcohol 5%. Bot. 480 mL. *c-III.*
Use: Antitussive; decongestant; expectorant.
pseudomonas test.
Use: Urine test.
pseudomonic acid A.
Use: Anti-infective, topical.
See: Bactroban.
Pseudo Plus. (Weeks & Leo) Pseudoephedrine hydrochloride 60 mg, chlorpheniramine maleate 4 mg. Tab. Bot. 40s. *OTC.*
Use: Antihistamine; decongestant.
Pseudo Syrup. (Major) Pseudoephedrine 30 mg/5 mL. Liq. Bot. 120 mL, pt, gal. *OTC.*
Use: Decongestant.
psoralens.
See: Methoxsalen.
Psor-a-set. (Hogil) Salicylic acid 2%. Soap. Bar 97.5 g. *OTC.*
Use: Keratolytic.
Psorcon E. (Dermik) Diflorasone diacetate 0.05%. **Oint.:** Emollient, occlusive base, lanolin alcohol, white petrolatum. Tube 15 g, 30 g, 60 g. **Cream:** Hydrophilic base, stearyl alcohol, cetyl alcohol, mineral oil. Tube 15 g, 30 g, 60 g. *Rx.*
Use: Corticosteroid, topical.
Psorent. (NeoStrata) Coal tar solution 15% (equiv. to coal tar 2.3%). Soln. 100 mL. *OTC.*
Use: Miscellaneous tar-containing product.
Psoriasin Medicated. (Alva-Amco Pharmacal) Salicylic acid 3%. Dye free and fragrance free. Soap. 177 mL. *OTC.*
Use: Keratolytic agent.
Psorinail. (Summers) Coal tar solution w/isopropyl alcohol 2.5%, 3-butylene glycol I, acetyl mandelic acid. Liq. Bot. 30 mL. *OTC.*
Use: Antipsoriatic, topical.
Psorion. (ICN) Betamethasone dipropionate 0.05%, mineral oil, white petrolatum, propylene glycol. Cream. Tube 15 g, 45 g. *Rx.*
Use: Corticosteroid, topical.
psychotherapeutic agents.
See: Atomoxetine Hydrochloride.
Fluoxetine Hydrochloride.
Olanzapine.
Sodium Oxybate.
Tranquilizers.
psychotherapeutic combinations.
See: Dextromethorphan Hydrobromide/Quinidine Sulfate.
Olanzapine/Fluoxetine Hydrochloride.
psyllium.
Use: Laxative.
See: Fiberall Natural Flavor
Fiberall Orange Flavor.
Fiberall Tropical Fruit Flavor.
Fiber Therapy Original Texture.
Genfiber.
Genfiber, Orange Flavor.
Geri-Mucil.
Hydrocil Instant.
Konsyl.
Konsyl-D.
Konsyl Easy Mix Formula.
Konsyl Orange Sugar Free.
Metamucil.
Metamucil Orange Flavor, Original Texture.
Metamucil Orange Flavor, Smooth Texture.
Metamucil Original Texture.
Metamucil, Sugar Free, Orange Flavor, Smooth Texture.
Metamucil, Sugar Free, Smooth Texture.
Natural Fiber Laxative.
Natural Psyllium Fiber.
Perdiem Fiber Therapy.
Reguloid.
Reguloid, Orange.
Reguloid, Sugar Free Orange.
Reguloid, Sugar Free Regular.
Serutan.
Syllact.
W/Sennosides.
See: Senna Prompt.
•**psyllium hemicellulose.** (SIL-ee-um HEM-ee-SEL-ue-lose) *USP.*
Use: Laxative.
•**psyllium husk.** (SIL-ee-um) *USP.*
Use: Laxative, cathartic.

psyllium hydrocolloid.
Use: Laxative.
psyllium seed gel.
Use: Laxative.
pteroic acid. The compound formed by the linkage of carbon 6 of 2-amine-4-hydroxypteridine by means of a methylene group with the nitrogen of p-aminobenzoic acid.
pteroylglutamic acid.
See: Folic acid.
pteroylmonoglutamic acid. Pteroylglutamic acid.
See: Folic acid.
P-Tex. (Poly Pharmaceuticals) Brompheniramine tannate 10 mg/5 mL. Alcohol and sugar free. Peach flavor. Oral Susp. 480 mL. *Rx.*
Use: Antihistamine.
PTFE. (Ethicon) Polytef.
PTU.
See: Propylthiouracil.
Pulexn DM. (Ballay Pharmaceuticals) Dextromethorphan HBr 10 mg, guaifenesin 100 mg per 5 mL. Saccharin, sorbitol. Syr. 473 mL. *Rx.*
Use: Antitussive with expectorant.
Pulmicort Flexhaler. (AstraZeneca) Budesonide 90 mcg (each actuation delivers ≈ 80 mcg/metered dose), 180 mcg (each actuation delivers ≈ 160 mcg/metered dose). Lactose. Inh. Pow. 60 dose *Flexhaler* (90 mcg only), 120 dose *Flexhaler* (180 mcg only). *Rx.*
Use: Corticosteroid.
Pulmicort Respules. (AstraZeneca) Budesonide 0.25 mg/2 mL, 0.5 mg/2 mL, 1 mg/2 mL. EDTA. Inh. Susp. Single-dose envelopes. 30s. *Rx.*
Use: Respiratory inhalant, corticosteroid.
Pulmocare. (Abbott Nutrition) Protein 62.6 g (L-carnitine, taurine), carbohydrate 105.7 g (corn maltodextrin, sucrose), fat 93.3 g (canola oil, corn oil, high oleic safflower oil, medium chain triglycerides, soy lecithin)/L. Sodium 1310 mg/L, potassium 1960 mg/L, 475 mOsm/kg H_2O, 1.5 cal/mL. Vitamins A, B_1, B_2, B_3, B_5, B_6, B_7, B_{12}, C, D, E, K, Ca, choline, Cl^-, Cr, Cu, Fe, folic acid, I, Mg, Mn, Mo, P, Se, Zn. Gluten and lactose free. Vanilla and strawberry flavors and unflavored. Liq. 240 mL, 1 L. *OTC.*
Use: Enteral nutritional therapy, defined formula diet.
pulmonary surfactant replacement. (Scios Nova)
Use: Diagnostic aid, thyroid. [Orphan Drug]
pulmonary surfactant replacement, porcine.
Use: Diagnostic aid, thyroid. [Orphan Drug]
See: Curosurf.
Pulmosin. (Spanner) Guaiacol 0.1 g, eucalyptol 0.08 g, camphor 0.05 g, iodoform 0.02 g/2 mL. Multiple-dose vial 30 mL. IM. Inj. *Rx.*
Pulmozyme. (Genentech) Dornase alfa 1 mg, calcium chloride dihydrate 0.15 mg, NaCl 8.77 mg/mL. Soln. for Inh. Amps. Single-use 2.5 mL. *Rx.*
Use: Anti-infective.
•**pumice.** (PUM-iss) *USP.*
Use: Abrasive, dental.
punctum plug. (Eagle Vision) Silicone plug. 0.5 mm, 0.6 mm, 0.7 mm, 0.8 mm. Pkg. 2 plugs, 1 inserter tool. *Rx.*
Use: Punctal plug.
Puralube. (Fera Pharmaceuticals) White petrolatum 85%, mineral oil 15%. Oint., Ophth. 3.5 g, UD 1 g (20s). *OTC.*
Use: Ocular lubricant.
Puralube Tears. (E. Fougera) Polyvinyl alcohol 1%, polyethylene glycol 400 1%, EDTA, benzalkonium Cl. Soln. Bot. 15 mL. *OTC.*
Use: Lubricant, ophthalmic.
Pure C 500. (Mason) Ascorbic acid 500 mg. Tab. 100s. *OTC.*
Use: Water-soluble vitamin.
PureFe OB Plus. (PharmaPure Rx) Folic acid 1 mg, vitamin C 200 mg, B_1 10 mg, B_2 6 mg, B_3 30 mg, B_5 10 mg, B_6 5 mg, B_{12} 15 mcg, Fe 277.2 mg, Mg, Zn, Cu, Mn. Gluten free and preservative free. Cap. 90s. *Rx.*
Use: Prenatal vitamin with minerals.
PureFe Plus. (PharmaPure Rx) Vitamins C 200 mg, B_1 10 mg, B_2 6 mg, B_3 30 mg, B_5 10 mg, B_6 5 mg, B_{12} 15 mcg, Fe 106 mg, folic acid 1 mg, Zn, Cu, Mn, Mg. Preservative free, gluten free, soy free. Cap. 100s. *Rx.*
Use: Multivitamin with minerals.
Puresept Murine Saline. (Ross) **Disinfecting soln.:** Sterile hydrogen peroxide solution 3%, sodium stannate, sodium nitrate, phosphate buffers, thimerosal free. 237 mL. **Murine Saline Soln.:** Buffered isotonic solution w/borate buffers, NaCl, sorbic acid 0.1%, EDTA 0.1%. 60, 237, 355 mL. Includes cups and lens holder. *OTC.*
Use: Contact lens care.
PureVit DualFe Plus. (PharmaPure Rx) Vitamins C 200 mg, B_1 10 mg, B_2 6 mg, B_3 30 mg, B_5 10 mg, B_6 5 mg, B_{12} 15 mcg, folic acid 1 mg, Fe 277.2 mg,

Zn, Cu, Mn. Preservative free, gluten free, and soy free. Cap. 90s. *Rx.*
Use: Multivitamin with minerals.

Puri-Clens. (Sween) UD 2 oz. Bot. 8 oz.
Use: Dermatologic, wound therapy.

purified oxgall.
See: Bile Extract, Ox.

purified protein derivative of tuberculin.
Use: Mantoux TB test.
See: Aplisol.
Aplitest.
Tubersol.

purified type II collagen.
Use: Juvenile rheumatoid arthritis. [Orphan Drug]

purine analogs and related agents.
Use: Antimetabolite.
See: Allopurinol.
Cladribine.
Clofarabine.
Fludarabine Phosphate.
Mercaptopurine.
Pentostatin.
Rasburicase.
Thioguanine.

Purinethol. (Gate Pharmaceuticals) Mercaptopurine 50 mg. Tab. 60s. *Rx.*
Use: Antineoplastic.

Purixan. (AnovoRx Distribution) Mercaptopurine 20 mg/mL. Aspartame, parabens, phenylalanine, raspberry juice, sucrose. Susp. 100 mL. *Rx.*
Use: Antimetabolite, purine analog and related agent.

•**puromycin.** (PURE-oh-MY-sin) USAN.
Use: Antineoplastic; antiprotozoal, trypanosoma.

•**puromycin hydrochloride.** USAN.
Use: Antineoplastic; antiprotozoal, trypanosoma.

purple foxglove.
See: Digitalis.

Purpose Shampoo. (Johnson & Johnson) Water, amphoteric-19, PEG-44 sorbitan laurate, PEG-150 distearate, sorbitan laurate, boric acid, fragrance, benzyl alcohol. Bot. 8 oz. *OTC.*
Use: Dermatologic.

Purpose Soap. (Johnson & Johnson) Sodium tallowate, sodium cocoate, glycerin, NaCl, BHT, EDTA. Bar 108 g, 180 g. *OTC.*
Use: Dermatologic, cleanser.

Pursettes Premenstrual. (DEP Corp.) Acetaminophen 500 mg, pamabrom 25 mg, pyrilamine maleate 15 mg. Tab. Bot. 24s. *OTC.*
Use: Analgesic; antihistamine; diuretic.

PVP-I. (Day-Baldwin) Povidone-iodine. Oint. Tube 1 oz, Jar lb, Foilpac 1.5 g. *OTC.*
Use: Antiseborrheic; antiseptic.

Py-Co-Pay Tooth Powder. (Block Drug) Sodium Cl, sodium bicarbonate, calcium carbonate, magnesium carbonate, tricalcium phosphate, eugenol, methyl salicylate. Can 7 oz. *OTC.*
Use: Dentifrice.

Pylera. (Aptalis) Bismuth subcitrate potassium 140 mg/metronidazole 125 mg/tetracycline hydrochloride 125 mg. Cap. 120s. *Rx.*
Use: Helicobacter pylori agent.

•**pyrabrom.** (PEER-ah-brahm) USAN.
Use: Antihistamine.

Pyracol. (Davis & Sly) Pyrathyn hydrochloride 0.08 g, ammonium Cl 0.778 g, citric acid 0.52 g, menthol 0.006 g/fl oz. Bot. pt.

pyraminyl maleate.
See: Pyrilamine Maleate.

pyranilamine maleate.
See: Pyrilamine Maleate.

pyranisamine bromotheophyllinate.
See: Pyrabrom.

pyranisamine maleate.
See: Pyrilamine Maleate.

•**pyrantel pamoate.** (pi-RAN-tel PAM-oh-ate) *USP.*
Use: Anthelmintic.
See: Pin-Rid.
Pin-X.

•**pyrantel tartrate.** (pi-RAN-tel) USAN.
Use: Anthelmintic.

•**pyrazinamide.** (peer-uh-ZIN-uh-mide) *USP.* Aldinamide, Zinamide.
Use: Antituberculosis agent.

pyrazinamide. (Various Mfr.) Pyrazinamide 500 mg. Tab. 60s, 90s, 100s, 500s, UD 100s.
Use: Anti-tuberculosis agent.

pyrazinecarboxamide.
See: Pyrazinamide.

•**pyrazofurin.** (pihr-AZZ-oh-FYOO-rin) USAN.
Use: Antineoplastic.

pyrazoline.
See: Antipyrine.

pyrbenzindole.
See: Benzindopyrine Hydrochloride.

pyrethrins.
Use: Pediculicide.
W/Piperonyl Butoxide.
See: RID.

•**pyrethrum extract.** (pye-REE-thrum) *USP.*
Use: Pediculicide.

Pyribenzamine.
See: PBZ.

Pyrichlor PE. (Breckenridge) Chlorpheniramine maleate 2 mg, phenylephrine hydrochloride 10 mg, pyrilamine maleate 10 mg per 5 mL. Glycerin, saccharin, sodium benzoate, sorbitol. Alcohol free and sugar free. Grape flavor. Liq. 473 mL. *Rx.*
Use: Upper respiratory combination, decongestant and antihistamine.

Pyridamole. (Major) Dipyridamole. Tab. **25 mg:** Bot. 1000s, 2500s. **50 mg, 75 mg:** 100s, 1000s. *Rx.*
Use: Antianginal; antiplatelet.

Pyridene. (Health for Life Brands) Phenylazo Diamino Pyridine hydrochloride 100 mg. Tab. Bot. 24s, 100s, 1000s. *Rx.*
Use: Analgesic, urinary.

Pyridium. (Gemini) Phenazopyridine hydrochloride 100 mg, 200 mg. Sucrose, lactose. Tab. Bot. 100s, 1000s, UD 100s. *Rx.*
Use: Interstitial cystitis agent.

•**pyridostigmine bromide.** (pihr-id-oh-STIG-meen) *USP.*
Use: Cholinergic.
See: Mestinon.

pyridostigmine bromide. (Various Mfr.) Pyridostigmine bromide 60 mg. Tab. 100s, 500s. *Rx.*
Use: Cholinergic.

Pyridox. (Oxford Pharmaceutical Services) **No. 1:** Pyridoxine hydrochloride 100 mg. Tab. **No. 2:** Pyridoxine hydrochloride 200 mg. Tab. Bot. 100s. *OTC.*
Use: Vitamin supplement.

pyridoxal. Vitamin B_6. *OTC.*
Use: Vitamin supplement.

pyridoxamine. Vitamin B_6. *OTC.*
Use: Vitamin supplement.
See: Pyridoxine Hydrochloride.

•**pyridoxine hydrochloride.** (peer-ih-DOX-een) *USP.*
Use: Enzyme co-factor vitamin, water-soluble vitamin.
See: Aminoxin.
Vitamin B_6.
W/Acetaminophen, Pamabrom.
See: Vitelle Lurline PMS.
W/Doxylamine Succinate.
See: Diclegis.

pyridoxine hydrochloride. (Various Mfr.) Pyridoxine hydrochloride 100 mg/mL. Chorobutanol anhydrous 5 mg. Inj. Vials. 1 mL. *Rx.*
Use: Enzyme co-factor vitamin, water-soluble vitamin.

pyridoxol.
See: Pyridoxine Hydrochloride.
Vitamin B_6.

pyrilamine bromotheophyllinate.
See: Bromaleate.
Pyrabrom.

•**pyrilamine maleate.** (peer-IL-a-meen) *USP.*
Use: Antihistamine.
W/Acetaminophen, Caffeine.
See: Midol Menstrual Complete.
W/Acetaminophen, Pamabrom.
See: Pamprin Multi-Symptom Maximum Strength.
W/Chlophedianol Hydrochloride.
See: Vanacof-8.
W/Chlorpheniramine Maleate, Phenylephrine Hydrochloride.
See: Pyrichlor PE.
W/Codeine Phosphate, Phenylephrine Hydrochloride.
See: Pro-Red AC.
W/Dextromethorphan Hydrobromide.
See: Capron DM.
W/Dextromethorphan Hydrobromide, Phenylephrine Hydrochloride.
See: MyHist-DM.
Poly Hist DM.
Pyril DM.
W/Dihydrocodeine Bitartrate, Phenylephrine Hydrochloride.
See: Poly Hist DHC.
W/Hydrocodone Bitartrate, Phenylephrine Hydrochloride.
See: Tussplex.
W/Phenylephrine Hydrochloride.
See: Poly Hist Forte.
Pyril D.
W/Zinc Oxide.
See: Z-Xtra.

pyrilamine tannate.
Use: Antihistamine.
W/Carbetapentane Tannate, Phenylephrine Tannate.
See: Tussi-12D S.
W/Dextromethorphan Hydrobromide, Pseudoephedrine Hydrochloride.
See: Viravan-T.
W/Pseudoephedrine Hydrochloride.
See: Viravan-P.

Pyril D. (Macoven) Phenylephrine hydrochloride 5 mg, pyrilamine maleate 16 mg. Glycerin, methylparaben, saccharin, sodium benzoate, sucrose. Grape flavor. Susp. 473 mL. *OTC.*
Use: Upper respiratory combination, decongestant and antihistamine.

Pyril DM. (Macoven) Dextromethorphan hydrobromide 15 mg, phenylephrine hydrochloride 5 mg, pyrilamine maleate 16 mg. Glycerin, glycyrrhizinate, methylparaben, sodium benzoate, sucrose, sucralose. Grape flavor. Susp. 473 mL. *Rx.*
Use: Upper respiratory combination, antitussive combination.

•**pyrimethamine.** (pihr-ih-METH-ah-meen) *USP.*
Use: Antimalarial.
See: Daraprim.
pyrimidine analogs.
Use: Antimetabolite.
See: Capecitabine.
Cytarabine.
Floxuridine.
Fluorouracil.
Gemcitabine Hydrochloride.
pyrimidine antagonist, topical.
Use: Dermatologic agent.
See: Fluorouracil.
•**pyrinoline.** (PIHR-ih-NO-leen) USAN.
Use: Cardiovascular agent, antiarrhythmic.
Pyrinyl Plus. (Rugby) Pyrethrins 0.33%, piperonyl butoxide 4%, benzyl alcohol. Shampoo. 59 mL. *OTC.*
Use: Pediculicide.
pyrithen.
See: Chlorothen Citrate.
•**pyrithione sodium.** (PEER-ih-THIGH-ohn) USAN.
Use: Antimicrobial, topical.
•**pyrithione zinc.** (PEER-ih-THIGH-ohn zingk) USAN. Zinc Omadine.
Use: Antifungal; anti-infective; antiseborrheic.
See: Denorex Everyday Dandruff.
Dermazine.
DHS Zinc.
Head & Shoulders.
Noble Formula.
Zincon.
ZNP Bar.
W/Ketoconazole.
See: Xolegel Duo Convenience Pack.
Pyrogallic Acid. (Gordon Laboratories) Pyrogallic acid 25%, chlorobutanol. Oint. Jar 1 oz, 1 lb.
Use: Dermatologic, wart therapy.
pyrogallol. Pyrogallic acid.
Pyrohep. (Major) Cyproheptadine hydrochloride 4 mg. Tab. Bot. 250s, 500s. *Rx.*
Use: Antihistamine.
•**pyrovalerone hydrochloride.** (PIE-row-val-EH-rone) USAN.
Use: Central stimulant.
•**pyroxamine maleate.** (pihr-OX-ah-meen) USAN.
Use: Antihistamine.
•**pyroxylin.** (pihr-OX-ih-lin) *USP.* Soluble gun cotton. Cellulose nitrate.
Use: Pharmaceutic necessity for collodion.
pyrrobutamine phosphate.
Use: Antihistamine.
•**pyrrocaine.** (PIHR-oh-cane) USAN.
Use: Anesthetic, local.
pyrrocaine hydrochloride.
Use: Anesthetic, local.
pyrrocaine hydrochloride and epinephrine injection.
Use: Anesthetic, local.
•**pyrroliphene hydrochloride.** (pihr-OLE-ih-feen) USAN.
Use: Analgesic.
•**pyrrolnitrin.** (pihr-OLE-nye-trin) USAN. Under study.
Use: Antifungal.
Pyrroxate Extra-Strength. (Lee) Phenylephrine hydrochloride 10 mg, chlorpheniramine maleate 4 mg, acetaminophen 650 mg. PEG. Tab. 24s. *OTC.*
Use: Decongestant, antihistamine, and analgesic, upper respiratory combination.
•**pyrvinium pamoate.** (pihr-VIN-ee-uhm PAM-oh-ate) *USP.*
Use: Anthelmintic.
PYtest. (Tri-Med) 1 mCi ^{14}-C-urea. Cap. UD 1s, 10s, 100s. *Rx.*
Use: Diagnostic aid.
PYtest Kit. (Tri-Med) Breath test for detecting *H. pylori.* Kit. 1 PYtest Cap. and breath collection equipment. *Rx.*
Use: Diagnostic aid.

Q

QB. (Major) Theophylline 150 mg, guaifenesin 90 mg. Liq. Bot. Pt, gal. *Rx.*
Use: Bronchodilator, expectorant.

QDALL. (Atley) Pseudoephedrine hydrochloride 100 mg, chlorpheniramine maleate 12 mg. Sucrose. Cap. 100s. *Rx.*
Use: Decongestant and antihistamine.

Q-dryl. (Qualitest Pharmaceuticals) Diphenhydramine hydrochloride 12.5 mg per 5 mL. Glycerin, saccharin, sodium 5 mg, sucrose. Alcohol free. Cherry flavor. Liq. 237 mL. *OTC.*
Use: Antihistamine, nonselective ethanolamine.

QNASL. (Teva) Beclomethasone dipropionate 80 mcg/actuation. Spray; intranasal. 8.7 g canister (120 metered doses per canister) with nasal actuator. *Rx.*
Use: Respiratory inhalant, intranasal steroid.

Q-Pap. (Qualitest) Acetaminophen 325 mg. Tab. 100s. *OTC.*
Use: Analgesic.

Q-Pap Children's. (Qualitest) Acetaminophen. **Elix.:** 160 mg/5 mL. Alcohol free. Sorbitol, sucrose. Grape flavor. 118 mL, 3785 mL. **Liq.:** 160 mg/5 mL. Alcohol free. Sorbitol, sucrose. Cherry and grape flavors. 118 mL, 473 mL, 3785 mL. **Oral Susp.:** 160 mg/5 mL. Alcohol free. Butylparaben, corn syrup, sorbitol. Grape and bubble gum flavors. 118 mL. *Rx.*
Use: Analgesic.

Q-Pap Extra Strength. (Qualitest) Acetaminophen 500 mg. Tab. 100s. *OTC.*
Use: Analgesic.

Q-Pap Infants. (Qualitest) Acetaminophen 100 mg/mL. Alcohol free. Butylparaben, saccharin. Fruit flavor. Soln., Conc., Oral. 15 mL. *OTC.*
Use: Analgesic.

Qsymia. (Vivus) Phentermine hydrochloride/ER topiramate 3.75 mg/23 mg, 7.5 mg/46 mg, 11.25 mg/69 mg, 15 mg/92 mg. Sucrose, tartrazine. ER Cap. 14s (3.75 mg/23 mg only), 30s. *c-IV.*
Use: CNS stimulant, anorexiant combination product.

Q-Tapp DM Cold & Cough. (Qualitest) Dextromethorphan HBr 5 mg, brompheniramine maleate 1 mg, pseudoephedrine hydrochloride 15 mg per 5 mL. Alcohol free. Corn syrup, saccharin, sorbitol. Grape flavor. Elixir. 118 mL. *OTC.*
Use: Upper respiratory combination, antitussive combination.

Q.T. Quick Tanning Suntan by Coppertone. (Schering-Plough) Ethylhexyl p-methoxycinnamate, dihydroxyacetone. SPF 2. Lot. Bot. 120 mL. *OTC.*
Use: Sunscreen.

Qua-Bid. (Quaker City Pharmacal) Papaverine hydrochloride 150 mg. TR Cap. Bot. 100s, 1000s. *OTC.*
Use: Vasodilator.

•**quadazocine mesylate.** (kwad-AZE-oh-SEEN) USAN.
Use: Opioid antagonist.

Quadramet. (DuPont) Samarium SM 153 lexidronam 1850 MBq/mL (50 mCi/mL) at calibration. Inj. Frozen, single-dose vial. 10 mL. In 2 mL fill (3700 MBq), 3 mL fill (5550 MBq). *Rx.*
Use: Treatment for bone lesions.

Quadrapax. (Acella Pharmaceuticals) Atropine sulfate 0.0194 mg, scopolamine hydrobromide 0.0065 mg, hyoscyamine hydrobromide or sulfate 0.1037 mg. Alcohol 23%, glycerin, saccharin, sorbitol, sucrose. Grape flavor. Elix. 473 mL. *c-IV.*
Use: Gastrointestinal anticholinergic combination.

quadruple sulfonamides.
See: Sulfonamides.

Qualaquin. (AR Scientific) Quinine sulfate 324 mg. Cap. 30s, 100s, 500s, 1,000s. *Rx.*
Use: Antimalarial.

Qual-Tussin. (Pharmaceutical Associates) Dextromethorphan HBr 7.5 mg, guaifenesin 100 mg, phenylephrine hydrochloride 10 mg, chlorpheniramine maleate 2 mg per 5 mL. Parabens, saccharin, sucrose. Fruit flavor. Syrup. 473 mL. *Rx.*
Use: Antitussive and expectorant.

Quartette. (Teva Women's Health) **Phase 1:** Ethinyl estradiol 0.02 mg, levonorgestrel 0.15 mg. 42s. **Phase 2:** Ethinyl estradiol 0.025 mg, levonorgestrel 0.15 mg. 21s. **Phase 3:** Ethinyl estradiol 0.03 mg, levonorgestrel 0.15 mg. 21s. **Phase 4:** Ethinyl estradiol 0.01 mg. 7s. Film coated. Lactose, PEG. *Rx.*
Use: 4-phasic oral contraceptive.

Quasense. (Watson Pharma) Ethinyl estradiol 30 mcg, levonorgestrel 0.15 mg. Lactose. Tab. 91s with 7 inert tablets (lactose). *Rx.*
Use: Contraceptive hormone, sex hormone.

quaternary anticholinergics.
See: Glycopyrrolate.

•**quazepam.** (KWAZ-e-pam) *USP.*
Use: Sedative/hypnotic, nonbarbiturate.
See: Doral.

•**quazinone.** (KWAZ-i-none) USAN.
Use: Cardiovascular agent.

•**quazodine.** (KWAZ-oh-deen) USAN.
Use: Cardiovascular agent.

•**quazolast.** (KWAZ-oh-last) USAN.
Use: Antiasthmatic mediator release inhibitor.

Qudexy XR. (Upsher-Smith) Topiramate 25 mg, 50 mg, 100 mg, 150 mg, 200 mg. ER Cap. 30s, 90s, 500s. *Rx.*
Use: Anticonvulsant.

Quelicin. (Hospira) Succinylcholine Cl. **Inj. 20 mg/mL:** Fliptop vial 10 mL, *Abboject* Syringe 5 mL. **100 mg/mL:** Amp. 10 mL. **Quelicin-500:** 5 mL in Pintop vial 10 mL. **Quelicin-1000:** 100 mg/mL. Parabens. Preservative free, single-use vial. 5 mL, 10 mL. Multidose vial. 20 mL. *Rx.*
Use: Muscle relaxant.

Quelidrine Cough. (Abbott) Dextromethorphan HBr 10 mg, chlorpheniramine maleate 2 mg, ephedrine hydrochloride 5 mg, phenylephrine hydrochloride 5 mg, ammonium Cl 40 mg, ipecac fluid extract 0.005 mL, ethyl alcohol 2%/ 5 mL. Syrup. Bot. 4 oz. *Rx.*
Use: Antihistamine; antitussive; bronchodilator; decongestant; expectorant.

Quercetin. (Freeda) Quercetin (from eucalyptus) 50 mg, 250 mg. Sugar and sodium free. Tab. Bot. 100s, 250s. *OTC.*
Use: Water-soluble vitamin.

Quertine.
Use: Bioflavonoid supplement.

Questran. (Par) Anhydrous cholestyramine resin 4 g per 9 g powder. Sucrose. Pow. for Oral Susp. Packets. 9 g (60s). Cans. 378 g. *Rx.*
Use: Antihyperlipidemic; bile acid sequestrant.

Questran Light. (Par) Anhydrous cholestyramine resin 4 g per 6.4 g powder. Maltodextrin, aspartame, phenylalanine 28.1 mg per 6.4 g, orange vanilla flavor. Pow. for Oral Susp. Packets. 6.4 g (60s). Cans. 268 g. *Rx.*
Use: Antihyperlipidemic; bile acid sequestrant.

•**quetiapine fumarate.** (cue-TIE-ah-peen) USAN.
Tall Man: QUEtiapine
Use: Antipsychotic, dibenzapine derivative.
See: Seroquel.
Seroquel XR.

quetiapine fumarate. (Various Mfr.) Quetiapine fumarate 25 mg, 50 mg, 100 mg, 150 mg, 200 mg, 300 mg, 400 mg. May contain lactose. Tab. 30s, 60s, 100s, 500s, UD 100s. *Rx.*
Use: Antipsychotic agent, dibenzapine derivative.

Quiagel. (Rugby) Kaolin 6 g, pectin 142.8 mg, hyoscyamine sulfate 0.1037 mg, atropine sulfate 0.0194 mg, scopolamine HBr 0.0065 mg/30 mL. Susp. Bot. Pt, gal. *Rx.*
Use: Antidiarrheal.

Quibron Plus. (Bristol-Myers Squibb) Ephedrine hydrochloride 25 mg, theophylline (anhydrous) 150 mg, butabarbital 20 mg, guaifenesin 100 mg. Cap. Bot. 100s. *Rx.*
Use: Antiasthmatic combination.

Quibron Plus Elixir. (Bristol-Myers Squibb) Theophylline 150 mg, ephedrine hydrochloride 25 mg, guaifenesin 100 mg, butabarbital 20 mg, alcohol 15%. Elix. Bot. Pt. *Rx.*
Use: Antiasthmatic combination.

Quick-K. (Western Research) Potassium bicarbonate 650 mg (potassium 6.5 mEq). Tab. Bot. 30s, 100s. *Rx.*
Use: Electrolyte supplement.

Quick Melts Children's Non-Aspirin. (Marlex) Acetaminophen 80 mg. Bubble gum flavor (gluten free, mannitol, sorbitol, sucralose, sugar), grape flavor (gluten and sugar free, corn syrup, mannitol, sorbitol, sucralose), watermelon flavor (gluten and sugar free, mannitol, sorbitol, sucralose). Tab., disintegrating. 30s. *OTC.*
Use: Analgesic.

Quick Melts Jr. Strength Non-Aspirin. (Marlex) Acetaminophen 160 mg. Bubble gum flavor (gluten free, mannitol, sorbitol, sucralose, sugar), grape flavor (gluten and sugar free, corn syrup, mannitol, sorbitol, sucralose). Tab., disintegrating. 30s. *OTC.*
Use: Analgesic.

Quiebar. (Nevin) Butabarbital sodium. **Spantab:** 1.5 gr. TR Spantab. Bot. 50s, 500s. **Elix.:** 30 mg/5 mL. Bot. Pt, gal. **Tab.:** 15 mg. Bot. 100s, 1000s; 30 mg. Bot. 1000s. **A.C. Cap.:** Bot. 100s, 500s. *c-III.*
Use: Hypnotic; sedative.

Quiebel. (Nevin) Butabarbital sodium 15 mg, belladonna extract 15 mg. Cap. Bot. 100s, 1000s. Elix. Pt, gal. *c-III.*
Use: Anticholinergic; antispasmodic; hypnotic; sedative.

Quiecof. (Nevin) Dextromethorphan HBr 7.5 mg, chlorpheniramine maleate

0.75 mg, guaiacol glyceryl ether 25 mg/5 mL. Bot. 4 oz, pt, gal. *OTC.*
Use: Antitussive; antihistamine; expectorant.

Quiet Night. (Rosemont) Pseudoephedrine hydrochloride 10 mg, doxylamine succinate 1.25 mg, dextromethorphan HBr 5 mg, acetaminophen 167 mg/5 mL. Liq. Bot. 180 mL, 300 mL. *OTC.*
Use: Analgesic; antihistamine; antitussive; decongestant.

Quiet Time. (Whiteworth Towne) Acetaminophen 600 mg, ephedrine sulfate 8 mg, dextromethorphan HBr 15 mg, doxylamine succinate 7.5 mg, alcohol 25 mg/30 mL. Bot. 180 mL. *OTC.*
Use: Analgesic; antihistamine; antitussive; decongestant.

•**quiflapon sodium.** (KWIH-flap-ahn) USAN.
Use: Antiasthmatic; inflammatory bowel disease suppressant.

Quik-Cept. (Laboratory Diagnostics) Slide test for pregnancy, rapid latex inhibition test. Kit 25s, 50s, 100s.
Use: Diagnostic aid.

Quik-Cult. (Laboratory Diagnostics) Slide test for fecal occult blood. Kit 150s, 200s, 300s, and tape test.
Use: Diagnostic aid.

•**quilizumab.** (kwi-LIZ-ue-mab) USAN.
Use: Treatment of asthma.

Quillivant XR. (NextWave Pharmaceuticals) Methylphenidate hydrochloride 25 mg per 5 mL (≈20% immediate-release and 80% extended-release methylphenidate). Banana flavoring, sodium benzoate, sucralose, sucrose. Pow. for Susp., extended release. 60 mL, 120 mL, 180 mL. *c-II.*
Use: CNS stimulant.

•**quilostigmine.** (Kwill-oh-STIG-meen) USAN.
Use: Cholinergic, cholinesterase inhibitor; treatment of Alzheimer disease.

Quinaglute Dura-Tabs. (Berlex) Quinidine gluconate 324 mg. Tab. Bot. 100s, 250s, 500s, UD 100s. Unit-of-use 90s, 120s. *Rx.*
Use: Antiarrhythmic.

•**quinaldine blue.** (kwin-AL-deen) USAN.
Use: Diagnostic agent, obstetrics.

•**quinaprilat.** (KWIN-ah-PRILL-at) *USP.*
Use: Antihypertensive; enzyme inhibitor, angiotensin-converting.

•**quinapril hydrochloride.** (KWIN-uh-PRILL) USAN.
Use: Antihypertensive; enzyme inhibitor, angiotensin-converting.
See: Accupril.
W/Hydrochlorothiazide.
See: Accuretic.
Quinaretic.

quinapril hydrochloride. (Various Mfr.) Quinapril hydrochloride 5 mg, 10 mg, 20 mg, 40 mg. May contain lactose. Tab. 90s, 1,000s (except 5 mg). *Rx.*
Use: Angiotensin-converting enzyme inhibitor.

quinapril hydrochloride/hydrochlorothiazide. (Greenstone) Hydrochlorothiazide/quinapril hydrochloride 12.5 mg/10 mg, 12.5 mg/20 mg, 25 mg/20 mg. Lactose. Film-coated. Tab. 90s. *Rx.*
Use: Antihypertensive combination.

Quinaretic. (Amide) Hydrochlorothiazide/quinapril hydrochloride 12.5 mg/20 mg, 25 mg/20 mg. Film-coated. Tab. 30s, 100s, 500s. *Rx.*
Use: Antihypertensive combination.

•**quinazosin hydrochloride.** (kwin-AZZ-oh-sin) USAN.
Use: Antihypertensive.

•**quinbolone.** (KWIN-bole-ohn) USAN.
Use: Anabolic.

•**quindecamine acetate.** (kwin-DECK-ah-meen) USAN.
Use: Anti-infective.

•**quindonium bromide.** (kwin-DOE-nee-um) USAN.
Use: Cardiovascular agent, antiarrhythmic.

•**quinelorane hydrochloride.** (kwih-NELL-oh-RANE) USAN.
Use: Antihypertensive; antiparkinsonian.

•**quinetolate.** (Kwin-EH-toe-late) USAN.
Use: Muscle relaxant.

•**quinfamide.** (KWIN-fah-mide) USAN.
Use: Antiamebic.

•**quingestanol acetate.** (kwin-JESS-tan-ahl) USAN.
Use: Hormone, progestin.

•**quingestrone.** (kwin-JESS-trone) USAN.
Use: Hormone, progestin.

quinidine.
Tall Man: quiNIDine
Use: Antiarrhythmic.
See: Quinidine Gluconate.
Quinidine Sulfate.

•**quinidine gluconate.** (KWIN-ih-deen) *USP.*
Tall Man: quiNIDine
Use: Cardiovascular agent, antiarrhythmic.

quinidine gluconate. (Lilly) Quinidine gluconate 80 mg/mL (50 mg/mL quinidine), EDTA 0.005%, phenol 25%. Inj. Vials. 10 mL multidose. *Rx.*
Use: Antiarrhythmic.

quinidine gluconate. (Various Mfr.)

Quinidine gluconate 324 mg. SR Tab. Bot. 100s, 250s, 500s. *Rx.*
Use: Antiarrhythmic.

•**quinidine sulfate.** (KWIN-ih-deen) *USP.*
Tall Man: quiNIDine
Use: Cardiovascular agent, antiarrhythmic.

quinidine sulfate. (Mutual) Quinidine sulfate 100 mg (equiv. to 83 mg base). Tab. 50s, 100s, 250s, 500s, 1000s. *Rx.*
Use: Antiarrhythmic agent, quinidine.

quinidine sulfate. (Various Mfr.) Quinidine sulfate. **Tab.:** 200 mg, 300 mg. Bot. 100s, 1000s. **SR Tab.:** 300 mg. 100s, 250s. *Rx.*
Use: Cardiovascular agent, antiarrhythmic.

quinine and urea hydrochloride.
Use: Sclerosing agent.

•**quinine ascorbate.** (KWIE-nine ass-CORE-bate) USAN. *Formerly quinine biascorbate.*
Tall Man: quiNINE
Use: Smoking deterrent.

quinine bisulfate.
Use: Analgesic; antimalarial; antipyretic.

quinine dihydrochloride.
Use: Antimalarial.

quinine ethylcarbonate.
See: Euquinine.

quinine glycerophosphate. Quinine compound with glycerol phosphate.

•**quinine sulfate.** (KWIE-nine) *USP.*
Tall Man: quiNINE
Use: Antimalarial.
W/Dextromethorphan Hydrobromide.
See: Nuedexta.

quinine sulfate. (Mutual Pharmaceutical) Quinine sulfate 324 mg (equiv. to quinine 269 mg). Cap. 30s, 100s. *Rx.*
Use: Antimalarial preparation, cinchona alkaloid.

quinisocaine.
See: Dimethisoquin Hydrochloride.

quinolinone derivatives.
Use: Antipsychotic.
See: Aripiprazole.

quinophan.
See: Cinchophen.

Quinora. (Key) Quinidine sulfate 300 mg. Tab. Bot. 100s, 1000s, UD 100s. *Rx.*
Use: Antiarrhythmic.

quinoxyl.
See: Chiniofon.

•**quinpirole hydrochloride.** (KWIN-pihr-ole) USAN.
Use: Antihypertensive.

quinprenaline. Quinterenol sulfate.

Quin-Release. (Major) Quinidine gluconate 324 mg. SR Tab. Bot. 100s, 250s, 500s, UD 100s. *Rx.*
Use: Antiarrhythmic.

Quinsana Plus. (Stephan) Tolnafate 1%, cornstarch, talc. Pow. In 90 g. *OTC.*
Use: Antifungal, topical.

Quintabs. (Freeda) Vitamins A 10,000 units, D 400 units, E 29 mg, B_1 25 mg, B_2 25 mg, B_3 100 mg, B_5 25 mg, B_6 25 mg, B_{12} 25 mcg, C 300 mg, folic acid 0.1 mg, inositol, PABA. Tab. Bot. 100s, 250s. *OTC.*
Use: Vitamin supplement.

Quintabs-M. (Freeda) Iron 15 mg, Vitamins A 10,000 units, D 400 units, E 50 mg, B_1 30 mg, B_2 30 mg, B_3 150 mg, B_5 30 mg, B_6 30 mg, B_{12} 30 mcg, C 300 mg, folic acid 0.4 mg, Ca, Cu, K, Mg, Mn, Se, Zn 30 mg, PABA. Tab. Bot. 100s, 250s, 500s. *OTC.*
Use: Mineral, vitamin supplement.

•**quinterenol sulfate.** (kwin-TER-en-ahl) USAN.
Use: Bronchodilator.

•**quinuclium bromide.** (kwih-NEW-klee-uhm) USAN.
Use: Antihypertensive.

•**quinupristin.** (kwih-NEW-priss-tin) USAN.
Use: Anti-infective.
W/Dalfopristin
See: Synercid.

•**quipazine maleate.** (KWIP-ah-zeen) USAN.
Use: Antidepressant; oxytocic.

quipenyl naphthoate.
See: Plasmochin Naphthoate.

•**quisinostat.** (kwi-SIN-oh-stat) USAN.
Use: Antineoplastic.

•**quisinostat hydrochloride.** (kwi-SIN-oh-stat) USAN.
Use: Antineoplastic.

Quixin. (Santen) Levofloxacin 0.5% (5 mg/mL), benzalkonium chloride 0.005%. Soln. Bot. 2.5 mL, 5 mL. *Rx.*
Use: Antibiotic.

•**quizartinib.** (kwiz-AR-ti-nib) USAN.
Use: Antineoplastic.

•**quizartinib dihydrochloride.** (kwiz-AR-ti-nib) USAN.
Use: Antineoplastic.

Qutenza. (NeurogesX) Capsaicin 8%. Patch. Single-use patch w/cleansing gel. *Rx.*
Use: Dermatological agent, counterirritant.

QV-Allergy. (Pharmaceutical Associates) Phenylephrine hydrochloride 10 mg, chlorpheniramine maleate 2 mg, methscopolamine nitrate 0.625 mg per 5 mL. Sucrose. Grape flavor. Syrup. 473 mL. *Rx.*

Use: Upper respiratory combination, decongestant, antihistamine, and anticholinergic combination.

QVAR. (Ivax) Beclomethasone dipropionate 40 mcg, 80 mcg per actuation. Aer. Can. 7.3 g (100 actuations w/actuator). *Rx.*

Use: Respiratory inhalant, corticosteroid.

R

RabAvert. (Chiron) Rabies antigen ≥ 2.5 IU/mL. Freeze-dried, fixed virus strain Flury LEP grown in cultures of chicken fibroblasts. With human albumin < 0.3 mg, processed bovine gelatin < 12 mg, potassium glutamate 1 mg, sodium EDTA 0.3 mg, neomycin < 1 mcg, chlortetracycline < 20 ng, amphotericin B < 2 ng, ovalbumin < 3 ng per dose. Inj., Lyophilized Pow. for Reconstitution. Single-dose vial with 1 vial diluent, 1 disposable syringe, 1 longer needle for reconstitution, and 1 smaller needle for injection. *Rx.*
Use: Active immunization, viral vaccine.

•**rabeprazole sodium.** (rab-EH-pray-zahl) USAN.
Tall Man: RABEprazole
Use: Proton pump inhibitor.
See: AcipHex.
AcipHex Sprinkle.

rabeprazole sodium. (Various Mfr.) Rabeprazole sodium 20 mg. Enteric coated. May contain lactose, mannitol, PEG. Tab., delayed release. 30s, 90s. *Rx.*
Use: Proton pump inhibitor.

rabies antigen.
Use: Immunization.

•**rabies immune globulin.** (RAY-beez ih-MYOON GLAB-byoo-lin) *USP.*
Use: Immunization.
See: HyperRab S/D.
Imogam Rabies-HT.

rabies immune globulin (RIG), human.
See: Rabies immune globulin.

•**rabies vaccine.** (RAY-beez vaccine) *USP.*
Use: Active immunization agent, viral vaccine.
See: Imovax Rabies.
RabAvert.

•**rabusertib.** (RA-bue-SER-tib) USAN.
Use: Antineoplastic.

•**racemethionine.** (RAY-see-meh-THIGH-oh-neen) *USP. Formerly Methionine.*
Use: Acidifier, urinary.

racemic calcium pantothenate.
See: Calcium Pantothenate, Racemic.

racemic desoxynorephedrine. Amphetamine.

racemic ephedrine hydrochloride. Racephedrine hydrochloride.

racemic pantothenic acid.
See: Calcium Pantothenate.

•**racephedrine hydrochloride.** (RAYSE-e-FED-rin) USAN.
Use: Vasoconstrictor; decongestant, nasal.

racephedrine hydrochloride. (Pharmacia) Racephedrine hydrochloride **Cap.:** 3/8 gr. Bot. 40s, 250s, 1000s. **Soln.:** 1%. Bot. 1 fl oz, pt, gal.
Use: Vasoconstrictor; decongestant, nasal.

•**racephenicol.** (race-FEN-ih-KAHL) *USP.*
Use: Anti-infective.

•**racepinephrine hydrochloride.** (race-epp-ih-NEFF-rin) *USP.*
Use: Bronchodilator; vasopressor.
See: Asthmanephrin.
MicroNefrin.
Nephron.
S2.

•**raclopride C11.** (RACK-low-pride) *USP.*
Use: Radiopharmaceutical.

•**radafaxine hydrochloride.** (rad-a-FAX-een) USAN.
Use: Antidepressant, antianxiety.

•**radavirsen.** (RAD-a-VIR-sen) USAN.
Use: Treatment of influenza.

•**radezolid.** (ra-DEZ-oh-lid) USAN.
Use: Antibacterial agent.

•**radezolid hydrochloride.** (ra-DEZ-oh-lid) USAN.
Use: Antibacterial agent.

RadiaPlexRx. (MPM Medical) Aloe vera, diazolidinyl urea and iodopropynyl butylcarbamate, EDTA, glycerin, glyceryl stearate, isopropyl palmitate, lipowax, mineral oil, myritol, phenoxyethanol, polydimethylsiloxane fluid, sodium hyaluronate, triethanolamine. Top. Gel. 170 g. *Rx.*
Use: Flexible hydroactive dressing.

Radiesse. (Bioform Medical) Calcium hydroxylapatite (particle size range is 25 to 45 microns). Implant, Subcutaneous. Single-use prefilled syringes. 0.3 mL, 1.3 mL. *Rx.*
Use: Physical adjunct.

radioactive isotopes.
See: Albumin, Aggregated Iodinated.
Chlormerodrin Hg 197.
Chlormerodrin Hg 203.
Cyanocobalamin Co 57.
Cyanocobalamin Co 60.
Radio-Iodinated Serum Albumin.
Selenomethionine Se 75.
Sodium Chromate Cr 51.
Sodium Iodide I 131.
Sodium Iodide I 125.
Sodium Phosphate P 32.
Sodium Radio Chromate.
Sodium Radio Iodide.
Sodium Radio Phosphate.
Strontium Nitrate Sr 85.
Technetium Tc 99m.
Triolein I 131.
Xenon Xe 133.

Radiogardase. (HEYL Chemisch-pharmazeutische Fabrik GmbH & Co.) Prussian blue oral 0.5 g (blue powder in gelatin capsules). Cap. 30s. *Rx.*
Use: Chelating agent; detoxification agent.

radiogold (^{198}Au) solution. Gold Au-198 injection.
Use: Irradiation therapy.

radio-iodide (^{131}I), sodium.
Use: Radiopharmaceutical.
See: Iodotope.

radio-iodinated (^{131}I) serum albumin. (Human) Iodinated I-131 albumin.

radio-iodinated (^{125}I) serum albumin. *See:* (Human) Iodinated I-125 albumin.

radiopaque agents.
See: Gastrointestinal Contrast Agents (Iodinated).
Gastrointestinal Contrast Agents (Miscellaneous).
Radiopaque Agents, Miscellaneous.

radiopaque agents, miscellaneous.
See: Diatrizoate Meglumine.
Diatrizoate Meglumine 52% and Diatrizoate Sodium 8%.
Diatrizoate Meglumine 52.7% and Iodipamide Meglumine 26.8%.
Diatrizoate Meglumine 66% and Diatrizoate Sodium 10%.
Ethiodized Oil.
Ferumoxides.
Gadobenate Dimeglumine.
Gadodiamide.
Gadopentetate Dimeglumine.
Gadoterate Meglumine.
Gadoteridol.
Gadoversetamide.
Iodipamide Meglumine 52%.
Iodixanal.
Iohexol.
Iopamidol.
Iopromide.
Iosulfan Blue.
Iothalamate Meglumine.
Ioversol.
Mangafodipir Trisodium.
Pentetreotide.
Perflutren.
Perflutren, Protein Based.
Technetium Tc-99m Mebrofenin.

radiopaque polyvinyl chloride.
Use: Radiopaque agent, GI contrast agent.
See: Sitzmarks.

radiopharmaceuticals.
See: Radium Ra 223 Dichloride.

radio-phosphate (^{32}P), sodium.
Use: Radiopharmaceutical.

radioselenomethionine 75 Se. Selenomethionine Se 75.

radiotolpovidone I-131. Tolpovidone I-131.

•**radium Ra 223 dichloride.** (RAY-dee-um) USAN.
Use: Antineoplastic.
See: Xofigo.

•**rafoxanide.** (ray-FOX-ah-nide) USAN.
Use: Anthelmintic.

Ragus. (Miller Pharmacal Group) Mg 27 mg, vitamins C 100 mg, Ca 580 mg, P 450 mg, l-lysine 25 mg, dl-methionine 50 mg, A 5000 units, D 400 units, E 10 mg, B_1 20 mg, B_2 3 mg, B_6 5 mg, B_{12} 9 mcg, niacinamide 80 mg, pantothenic acid 5 mg, Fe 20 mg, Cu 1 mg, Mn 2 mg, K 10 mg, Zn 2 mg, I 0.1 mg/3 Tab. Bot. 100s. *OTC.*
Use: Mineral, vitamin supplement.

Ragwitek. (Merck Sharp & Dohme) Short ragweed pollen allergen extract 12 Amb a 1-unit. Mannitol. Tab., disintegrating; sublingual. UD 30s, UD 90s. *Rx.*
Use: Allergenic extract.

•**ralimetinib.** (RAL-i-ME-ti-nib) USAN.
Use: Antineoplastic.

•**ralimetinib mesylate.** (RAL-i-ME-ti-nib) USAN.
Use: Antineoplastic.

•**ralitoline.** (rah-LIT-oh-leen) USAN.
Use: Anticonvulsant.

Ralix. (Cypress) Phenylephrine hydrochloride 40 mg, chlorpheniramine maleate 8 mg, methscopolamine nitrate 2.5 mg. ER Tab. 100s. *Rx.*
Use: Decongestant, antihistamine, and anticholinergic, upper respiratory combination.

R A Lotion. (Medco Lab) Resorcinol 3%, alcohol 43%. Lot. Plastic Bot. 120 mL, 240 mL, 480 mL. *OTC.*
Use: Dermatologic, acne.

•**raloxifene hydrochloride.** (ral-OX-ih-FEEN) USAN. *Formerly Keoxifene Hydrochloride.*
Use: Antiestrogen.
See: Evista.

raloxifene hydrochloride. (Various Mfr.) Raloxifene hydrochloride 60 mg (equiv. to 55.71 mg free base). May contain polydextrose, PEG. Tab. 30s, 100s, 1,000s. *Rx.*
Use: Sex hormone, selective estrogen receptor modulator.

•**ralpancizumab.** (RAL-pan-SIZ-ue-mab) USAN.
Use: Treatment of dyslipidemia.

•**raltegravir.** (ral-TEG-ra-vir) USAN.
Use: Antiretroviral agent, integrase inhibitor.
See: Isentress.

•**raltegravir potassium.** (ral-TEG-ra-vir) USAN.
Use: Antiviral.
•**raltitrexed.** (ral-tih-TREX-ehd) USAN.
Use: Advanced colorectal cancer treatment (thymidylate synthase inhibitor), antineoplastic.
•**raluridine.** (ral-YOUR-ih-deen) USAN.
Use: Antiviral.
•**ramatercept.** (ra-MAT-er-sept) USAN.
Use: Musculoskeletal agent.
•**ramelteon.** (ram-EL-tee-on) USAN.
Use: Sleep disorders.
See: Rozerem.
•**ramipril.** (ruh-MIH-prill) USAN.
Use: Antihypertensive, enzyme inhibitor (angiotensin-converting), congestive heart failure.
See: Altace.
ramipril. (Various Mfr.) Ramipril 1.25 mg, 2.5 mg, 5 mg, 10 mg. Cap. 30s, 90s, 100s, 500s, 1,000s (except 1.25 mg), UD 30s (1.25 mg only), UD 100s (except 1.25 mg). *Rx.*
Use: Renin angiotensin system antagonist, angiotensin-converting enzyme inhibitor.
•**ramoplanin.** (ram-oh-PLAN-in) USAN.
Use: Investigational anti-infective.
•**ramucirumab.** (RA-mue-SIR-ue-mab) USAN.
Use: Antineoplastic.
See: Cyramza.
ranestol. Triclofenol piperazine.
Use: Anthelmintic.
Ranexa. (Gilead Sciences) Ranolazine 500 mg, 1,000 mg. Lactose (1,000 mg only), PEG (500 mg only). Film-coated. ER Tab. 60s, 500s. *Rx.*
Use: Miscellaneous antianginal agent.
•**ranibizumab.** (ra-NIB-i-ZUE-mab) USAN.
Use: Age-related macular degeneration.
See: Lucentis.
•**ranimycin.** (ran-ih-MY-sin) USAN.
Use: Anti-infective.
•**ranitidine.** (ra-NI-ti-deen) USAN.
Use: Histamine H_2 antagonist.
See: Zantac.
Zantac Efferdose.
Zantac 150 Maximum Strength.
Zantac 75.
ranitidine. (Various Mfr.) Ranitidine (as base). **Cap.:** 150 mg, 300 mg. 30s (300 mg only), 60s (150 mg only), 100s (300 mg only), 500s (150 mg only). **Inj.:** 25 mg/mL. Single-dose vials. 2 mL. Multidose vials. 6 mL with phenol 5 mg/mL. **Tab.:** 75 mg, 150 mg, 300 mg. Bot. 10s (75 mg only); 20s (75 mg only); 30s (except 150 mg); 60s (except 300 mg); 100s (except 75 mg); 250s (300 mg only); 500s (150 mg only); 1000s, 5000s, UD 100s (150 mg only). *Rx-OTC.*
Use: Histamine H_2 antagonist.
•**ranitidine hydrochloride.** (ra-NI-ti-deen) *USP.*
Use: Histamine H_2 antagonist.
ranitidine hydrochloride. (Various Mfr.) Ranitidine 15 mg/mL. May contain alcohol, parabens, saccharin, sorbitol. Peppermint flavor. Soln. 473 mL. *Rx.*
Use: Histamine H_2 antagonist.
•**ranolazine.** (RAY-no-lah-ZEEN) USAN.
Use: Antianginal agent, miscellaneous.
See: Ranexa.
Rapaflo. (Watson Pharma) Silodosin 4 mg, 8 mg. Cap. 30s, 100s (4 mg); 30s, 90s, 1,000s (8 mg). *Rx.*
Use: Antiadrenergic agent—peripherally acting, alpha-1-adrenergic blocker.
Rapamune. (Wyeth Laboratories) Sirolimus. **Oral Soln.:** 1 mg/mL. Ethanol. 60 mL glass bot. with oral syringe adaptor. **Tab.:** 0.5 mg, 1 mg, 2 mg. Lactose, PEG, sucrose. 100s, *Redipak* UD 100s. *Rx.*
Use: Immunologic, immunosuppressive.
Rapid B-12 Energy. (Mason) Cyanocobalamin 200 mcg per spray. Glycerin, potassium sorbate. Peppermint flavor. Spray, Soln.; sublingual. 30 mL. *OTC.*
Use: Water-soluble vitamin.
Rapid Test Strep. (SmithKline Diagnostics) Latex slide agglutination test for identification of group A streptococci. Box. 25s, 100s.
Use: Diagnostic aid.
•**rasagiline.** (ra-SA-ji-leen) USAN.
Use: Antiparkinson agent.
See: Azilect.
•**rasagiline mesylate.** (ra-SA-ji-leen) USAN.
Use: Antiparkinson agent.
•**rasburicase.** (raz-BYORR-ih-kays) USAN.
Use: Antimetabolite.
See: Elitek.
rastinon. Tolbutamide.
Use: Antidiabetic.
rattlesnake bite therapy.
See: Antivenin (Crotalidae).
Rauneed. (Hanlon) Rauwolfia 50 mg, 100 mg. Tab. Bot. 100s. *Rx.*
Use: Antihypertensive.
Raunescine. (Penick) An alkaloid of *Rauwolfia serpentina.* Under study.
Use: Antihypertensive.
Raunormine. (Penick) 11-Desmethoxy reserpine. *Rx.*

Raurine. (Westerfield) Reserpine. **Tab.:** 0.1 mg. Bot. 100s. **Delayed-Action Cap.:** 0.5 mg. Bot. 100s. *Rx.*
Use: Antihypertensive.

Rauserfia. (New Eng. Phr. Co.) *Rauwolfia serpentina* 50 mg, 100 mg. Tab. Bot. 100s. *Rx.*
Use: Antihypertensive.

Rautina. (Fellows) *Rauwolfia serpentina* whole root 50 mg, 100 mg. Tab. Bot. 1000s. *Rx.*
Use: Antihypertensive.

Rauval. (Pal-Pak, Inc.) *Rauwolfia* whole root 50 mg, 100 mg. Tab. Bot. 100s, 500s, 1000s. *Rx.*
Use: Antihypertensive.

•**rauwolfia serpentina.** (rah-WOOL-fee-ah ser-pen-TEE-nah) *USP.*
Use: Antihypertensive.
See: Rauneed.
Rauval.
Rawfola.
T-Rau.

rauwolfia serpentina active principles (alkaloids). Deserpidine, rescinnamone.
See: Reserpine.

rauwolscine. An alkaloid of *Rauwolfia canescens.* Under study.
Use: Antihypertensive.

Ravicti. (Hyperion Therapeutics) Glycerol phenylbutyrate 1.1 g/mL. Liq. Multi-use bottle. 25 mL. *Rx.*
Use: Endocrine and metabolic agent.

Ravocaine. (Cook-Waite Laboratories, Inc.) Propoxycaine hydrochloride 4 mg, procaine 20 mg, norepinephrine bitartrate equivalent to 0.033 mg levophed base, sodium Cl 3 mg, acetone sodium bisulfite not more than 2 mg. Cartridge 1.8 mL. *Rx.*
Use: Anesthetic, local.

ravuconazole.
Use: Antifungal.

Rawfola. (Foy Laboratories) *Rauwolfia serpentina* 50 mg. Tab. Bot. 1000s. *Rx.*
Use: Antihypertensive.

Rawl Vite. (Rawl) Vitamins A 10,000 units, D 500 units, B_1 10 mg, B_2 5 mg, B_6 1 mg, calcium pantothenate 5 mg, nicotinamide 50 mg, C 125 mg, E 2.5 units. Tab. Bot. 100s. *OTC.*
Use: Mineral, vitamin supplement.

Rawl Whole Liver Vitamin B Complex. (Rawl) Whole liver 500 mg, amino acids found in the whole liver, vitamins B_1 1 mg, B_2 2 mg, niacinamide 5 mg, choline Cl 12 mg, B_6 0.2 mg, calcium pantothenate 0.2 mg, inositol 5 mg, biotin 0.6 mcg, B_{12} 0.3 mcg. Cap. Bot. 100s, 500s. *OTC.*
Use: Mineral, vitamin supplement.

•**raxibacumab.** (RAX-ee-BAK-ue-mab) USAN.
Use: Anthrax infection.

raxibacumab. (Glaxosmithkline) Raxibacumab 50 mg/mL. Glycine, polysorbate 80, sucrose. Preservative free. Inj., Soln. Single-use vial. 34 mL. *Rx.*
Use: Monoclonal antibody.

Ray Block. (Del-Ray) Octyl dimethyl PABA 5%, benzophenone-3 3%, SD alcohol. Lot. Bot. 118.3 mL. *OTC.*
Use: Sunscreen.

Ray-D. (Nion Corp.) Vitamin D 400 units, thiamine mononitrate 1 mg, riboflavin 2 mg, niacin 10 mg, I 0.1 mg, Ca 375 mg, P 300 mg/6 Tab. In base of brewer's yeast. Bot. 100s, 500s. *OTC.*
Use: Mineral, vitamin supplement.

•**rayon, purified.** (RAY-ahn) *USP.*
Use: Surgical aid.

Rayos. (Horizon Pharma) Prednisone 1 mg, 2 mg, 5 mg. Lactose. Tab., delayed release. 30s, 100s. *Rx.*
Use: Adrenocortical steroid, glucocorticoid.

raythesin. (Raymer)
See: Propyl p-Aminobenzoate.

Razadyne. (Janssen) Galantamine hydrobromide. **Tab.:** 4 mg, 8 mg, 12 mg. Lactose. Film-coated. Bot. 60s. **Oral Soln.:** 4 mg/mL. Saccharin. Bot. 100 mL with calibrated pipette. *Rx.*
Use: Cholinesterase inhibitor.

Razadyne ER. (Janssen) Galantamine hydrobromide (as base) 8 mg, 16 mg, 24 mg. Sucrose. ER Cap. 30s. *Rx.*
Use: Cholinesterase inhibitor.

•**razaxaban hydrochloride.** (ra-ZAX-a-ban) USAN.
Use: Anticoagulant.

Razepam. (Major) Temazepam 15 mg, 30 mg. Cap. Bot. 100s. *c-IV.*
Use: Hypnotic; sedative.

•**razupenem.** (RAZ-u-PEN-em) USAN.
Use: Antibiotic.

RCF. (Ross) Carbohydrate free low iron soy protein formula base. Carbohydrate and water must be added. For infants unable to tolerate the amount or type of carbohydrate in conventional formulas. Can 14 fl oz. (Concentrated liq.). *OTC.*
Use: Nutritional supplement.

Reabilan. (Elan) Protein 31.5 g, fat 39 g, carbohydrates 131.5 g, Na 702 mg, K 1.252 g/L, lactose free. With appropriate vitamins and minerals. Liq. Bot. 375 mL. *OTC.*
Use: Nutritional supplement.

Reabilan HN. (Elan) Protein 58.2 g, fat

52 g, carbohydrates 158 g, Na 1000 mg, K 1661 mg/L, lactose free. With appropriate vitamins and minerals. Liq. Bot. 375 mL. *OTC.*
Use: Nutritional supplement.

Readi-Cat. (EZ EM) Barium sulfate 1.3%, 2.1%. Saccharin, sorbitol. Orange flavor and vanilla flavor. Susp. 450 mL, 900 mL, 1,900 mL. *Rx.*
Use: Radiopaque agent, miscellaneous gastrointestinal contrast agent.

Readi-Cat 2. (EZ EM) Barium sulfate 2%. Saccharin, sorbitol. Apple flavor, banana flavor, berry flavor, vanilla flavor. Susp. 250 mL, 450 mL, 900 mL, 1,900 mL. *Rx.*
Use: Radiopaque agent, miscellaneous gastrointestinal contrast agent.

Rea-Lo. (Whorton Pharmaceuticals, Inc.) Urea in water-soluble moisturizing oil base. **Lot.:** 15%. Bot. 4 oz, pt. **Cream:** 30%. Jar 2 oz, 16 oz. *OTC.*
Use: Emollient.

Reaphirm Plant Source DHA. (Everett) Vitamin A 1,100 units, C 30 mg, D_3 1,000 units, E 20 units, B_1 1.6 mg, B_2 1.8 mg, B_3 15 mg, B_6 2.5 mg, B_{12} 12 mcg, folic acid 1 mg, Fe 29 mg, I, Mg, Zn, Cu, DHA 200 mg. Beeswax, glycerin, sorbitol, soy lecithin, soybean oil, sunflower oil, vegetable oil. Cap., softgel. UD 30s. *Rx.*
Use: Prenatal vitamin with minerals.

•**rebastinib.** (re-BAS-ti-nib) USAN.
Use: Antineoplastic.

•**rebastinib tosylate.** (re-BAS-ti-nib) USAN.
Use: Antineoplastic.

RE Benzoyl Peroxide. (River's Edge) Benzoyl peroxide 3.5%, 5.5%, 8.5%. Cetearyl alcohol, cetyl alcohol, glycerin, glyceryl, parabens, PEG-3, stearyl alcohol. Cream. In 45 g. *Rx.*
Use: Anti-infective, antibiotic.

Rebetol. (Schering) Ribavirin. **Cap.:** 200 mg. Lactose. Bot 42s, 56s, 70s, 84s. **Oral Soln.:** 40 mg/mL. Glycerin, propylene glycol, sodium benzoate, sorbitol, sucrose. Bubble gum flavor. 100 mL. *Rx.*
Use: Antiviral.

Rebif. (Serono) Interferon beta-1a 8.8 mcg/0.2 mL (2.4 million units) (human albumin 0.8 mg, mannitol 10.9 mg, sodium acetate 0.16 mg in water for injection), 22 mcg/0.5 mL (6 million units) (human albumin 2 mg, mannitol 27.3 mg, sodium acetate 0.4 mg), 44 mcg/0.5 mL (12 million units) (human albumin 4 mg, mannitol 27.3 mg, sodium acetate 0.4 mg). Preservative free. Inj. Prefilled single-use syringe (0.2 mL [8.8 mcg only], 0.5 mL [22 mcg and 44 mcg only]), *Rebidose* autoinjectors, 12s, and titration pack 6s (except 44 mcg). *Rx.*
Use: Immunologic, immunomodulator.

•**rebimastat.** (re-BIM-a-stat) USAN.
Use: Antineoplastic.

reboxetine mesylate.
Use: Antidepressant.

•**recainam hydrochloride.** (reh-CANE-am) USAN.
Use: Cardiovascular agent, antiarrhythmic.

•**recainam tosylate.** (reh-CANE-am TAH-sill-ate) USAN.
Use: Cardiovascular agent, antiarrhythmic.

Recal D. (River's Edge) Vitamin B 250 mcg, Ca citrate 1,342 mg, folic acid 1 mcg, Mg 50 mg, B_6 10 mg, B_{12} 125 mcg, D_3 300 units. Maltodextrin, sugar. Chocolate flavor. Wafer, Chew. 60s. *Rx.*
Use: Multivitamin.

RE Chlordiazepoxide/Clidinium. (River's Edge) Chlordiazepoxide hydrochloride 5 mg, clidinium bromide 2.5 mg. Lactose. Cap. 100s. *Rx.*
Use: GI anticholinergic combination.

•**recilisib.** (RE-si-LIS-ib) USAN.
Use: Radiation protection agent.

•**recilisib sodium.** (RE-si-LIS-ib) USAN.
Use: Radiation protection agent.

Reclast. (Novartis) Zoledronic acid 5 mg/100 mL (as zoledronic acid monohydrate 5.33 mg). Mannitol 4,950 mg. Inj., Soln. 100 mL. *Rx.*
Use: Bisphosphonate.

•**reclazepam.** (reh-CLAY-zeh-pam) USAN.
Use: Hypnotic; sedative.

Reclipsen. (Watson) Ethinyl estradiol 30 mcg, desogestrel 0.15 mg. Lactose. Tab. 28s with 7 inert tablets. *Rx.*
Use: Contraceptive hormone, sex hormone.

Reclomide. (Major) Metoclopramide hydrochloride 10 mg. Tab. Bot. 100s, 500s, 1000s, UD 100s. *Rx.*
Use: Antiemetic, gastrointestinal stimulant.

recombinant human activated protein C.
Use: Thrombolytic agent.
See: Protein C Concentrate (Human).

recombinant human erythropoietin.
Use: Hematopoietic.
See: Darbepoetin Alfa.
Epoetin Alfa, Recombinant.

recombinant human insulin-like growth factor I.
Use: Antibody-mediated growth hormone resistance. [Orphan Drug]

recombinant soluble human CD4. rCD4.
Use: Antiviral, HIV. [Orphan Drug]

recombinant tissue plasminogen activator. *Rx.*
See: Activase.

Recombinate. (Baxter) Recombinant antihemophilic factor 250 units, 500 units, 1,000 units. Albumin (human) ≤ 12.5 mg/mL, histidine, PEG 3350, sodium, von Willebrand Factor ≤ 2 mg per AHF unit. Preservative free. Monoclonal antibody purified. Inj., lyophilized Pow. for Soln. Single-dose Bot. and diluent (sterile water for injection 10 mL). *Rx.*
Use: Antihemophilic agent.

Recombivax HB. (Merck) Hepatitis B vaccine recombinant. Hepatitis B surface antigen. **Pediatric/Adolescent:** 5 mcg/0.5 mL, preservative free. Inj. Single-dose vial 0.5 mL. **Adult:** 10 mcg/mL, thimerosal 50 mcg/mL. Inj. Single-dose vial 1 mL, multi-dose vial 3 mL, prefilled, single-dose syringe 1 mL. **Dialysis:** 40 mcg/mL, thimerosal 50 mcg/mL. Inj. Single-dose vial 1 mL. *Rx.*
Use: Immunization, viral vaccine.

Recortex 10X in Oil. (Forest) 1000 mcg/mL. Vial 10 mL. *Rx.*

Recort Plus. (Reese Pharmaceutical) Hydrocortisone 1%. Benzyl alcohol, glycerin, lactic acid, wax. Cream. 30 g. *OTC.*
Use: Anti-inflammatory agent, topical corticosteroid.

Recothrom. (Zymo Genetics) Thrombin (recombinant) 1,000 units/mL. PEG. Preservative free. Pow. for Soln., lyophilized, Top. 5,000 and 20,000 unit single-use vials; 20,000 unit spray applicator kit. *Rx.*
Use: Hemostatic.

Recover. (Dermik) Bot. 2.25 oz. *OTC.*
Use: Dermatologic.

Rectacort-HC. (Acino Products) Hydrocortisone acetate 25 mg. Vegetable oil. Supp., rectal. 12s, 24s, 50s, 100s. *Rx.*
Use: Anorectal preparation, steroid-containing product.

Rectagene. (Pfeiffer) Live yeast cell derivative supplying 2000 units Skin Respiratory Factor/oz, shark liver oil in a cocoa butter base. Supp. 12s. *OTC.*
Use: Anorectal preparation.

Rectagene Medicated Rectal Balm. (Pfeiffer) Live yeast cell derivative that supplies 2000 units Skin Respiratory Factor/30 g, refined shark liver oil 3%, white petrolatum, lanolin, thyme oil, 1:10,000 phenylmercuric nitrate. Oint. Tube. 56.7 g. *OTC.*
Use: Anorectal preparation.

Rectal Medicone. (Medicore) Benzocaine 2 g, balsam peru 1 g, hydroxyquinoline sulfate 0.25 g, menthol 1/7 g, zinc oxide 3 g. Supp. Box 12s, 24s. *OTC.*
Use: Anesthetic; antiseptic, topical.

Rectal Medicone Unguent. (Medicore) Benzocaine 20 mg, oxyquinoline sulfate 5 mg, menthol 4 mg, zinc oxide 100 mg, balsam peru 12.5 mg, petrolatum 625 mg, lanolin 210 mg/g. Tube 1.5 oz. *OTC.*
Use: Anorectal preparation.

RectiCare. (Ferndale Healthcare) Lidocaine 5%. Benzyl alcohol, cholesterol, polysorbate 80, propylene glycol, trolamine. Cream; rectal. 30 g. *OTC.*
Use: Topical local anesthetic, amide local anesthetic.

Rectiv. (Aptalis Pharma US) Nitroglycerin 0.4%. Lanolin, propylene glycol, white petrolatum. Oint. 30 g tube. *Rx.*
Use: Anorectal preparation.

red blood cells. Human red blood cells given by IV infusion.
Use: Blood replenisher.

red cell tagging solution.
See: A-C-D.

Red Cross Toothache Kit. (Mentholatum Co.) Eugenol 85%, sesame oil. Drops. Bot. 3.7 mL w/cotton pellets and tweezers. *OTC.*
Use: Anesthetic, local.

red ferric oxide.
Use: Pharmaceutic aid (color).

Reditemp-C. (Wyeth) Ammonium nitrate, water, and special additives. Pkg. Large and small sizes. 4 × 10s. *OTC.*
Use: Cold compress.

Re-Drylex. (River's Edge) Dexchlorpheniramine maleate 1 mg, methscopolamine nitrate 1.25 mg, phenylephrine hydrochloride 10 mg. Sorbitol, sugar. Root beer flavor. Syrup. 473 mL. *Rx.*
Use: Upper respiratory combination; decongestant, antihistamine, and anticholinergic combination.

Red Throat Spray. (Clay-Park Labs) Phenol 1.4%. Glycerin, saccharin. Alcohol free. Throat spray. 177 mL. *OTC.*
Use: Mouth and throat product.

Reducto, Improved. (Arcum) Phendimetrazine bitartrate 35 mg. Tab. Bot. 100s, 1000s. *c-III.*
Use: Anorexiant.

Reese's OneTab Congestion and Cough. (Reese) Guaifenesin 400 mg, phenylephrine hydrochloride 10 mg. Lactose, maltodextrin, mineral oil. Dye free. Tab. 30s. *OTC.*
Use: Upper respiratory combination, decongestant and expectorant combination.

Reese's Pinworm. (Reese) Pyrantel pamoate. **Cap., soft gel:** 180 mg (equiv. to pyrantel base 62.5 mg). 24s. **Oral Susp.: 50 mg/mL:** 30 mL. **144 mg/mL:** Equiv. to 50 mg/mL of pyrantel base. Glycerin, saccharin, sodium 4 mg per 5 mL, sorbitol. Banana flavor. 30 mL w/measuring cup. **Tab.:** 180 mg (equiv. to pyrantel base 62.5 mg). 24s. *OTC.*
Use: Anthelmintic.

ReFacto. (Wyeth) Recombinant antihemophilic factor 250 units, 500 units, 1,000 units, 2,000 units. L-histidine, sodium, sucrose. Preservative free and albumin free. Inj., lyophilized Pow. for Soln. Single-use vials and diluent (sodium chloride 0.9% 4 mL). *Rx.*
Use: Antihemophilic agent.

Refenesen PE. (Reese) Guaifenesin 400 mg, phenylephrine hydrochloride 10 mg. Lactose, maltodextrin, mineral oil. Cap. 50s. *OTC.*
Use: Upper respiratory combination, decongestant and expectorant combination.

Refenesen Plus Severe Strength Cough & Cold Medicine. (Reese) Pseudoephedrine hydrochloride 60 mg, guaifenesin 400 mg. Tab. Pkg. 16s. *OTC.*
Use: Upper respiratory combination, decongestant, expectorant.

Refissa. (Suneva Medical) Tretinoin 0.05%. Emollient base. BHT, dimethicone, edetate disodium, lt. mineral oil, parabens, PEG, stearyl alcohol. Cream. 20 g, 40 g. *Rx.*
Use: First-generation retinoid.

Refresh Classic. (Allergan) Polyvinyl alcohol 1.4%, povidone 0.6%, sodium Cl. UD 30s, 50s (0.3 mL single-dose container). *OTC.*
Use: Artificial tears.

Refresh Dry Eye Therapy. (Allergan) Glycerin 1%, polysorbate 80 1%. Preservative free. Castor oil. Ophth. Drops. Single-use containers. 0.4 mL. *OTC.*
Use: Artificial tear solution.

Refresh Lacri-Lube. (Allergan) White petrolatum 56.8%, mineral oil 42.5%, chlorobutanol, lanolin alcohols. Oint.; Ophth. 3.5 g, 7 g. *OTC.*
Use: Ocular lubricant.

Refresh Liquigel. (Allergan) Carboxymethylcellulose sodium 1%, boric acid, calcium chloride, magnesium chloride, potassium chloride, sodium borate, sodium chloride. Soln.; Ophth. 15 mL, 30 mL. *OTC.*
Use: Ophthalmic agent, artificial tear solution.

Refresh Optive Advanced. (Allergan) Carboxymethylcellulose sodium 0.5%, glycerin 1%, polysorbate 80 0.5%, boric acid, castor oil. Soln.; Ophth. 10 mL. *OTC.*
Use: Artificial tears.

Refresh Plus. (Allergan) Carboxymethylcellulose sodium 0.5%, sodium chloride. Preservative free. Soln. 0.3 mL/single-use container 4s, 30s. *OTC.*
Use: Artificial tears.

Refresh PM. (Allergan) White petrolatum 56.8%, mineral oil 41.5%, lanolin alcohol, sodium Cl. Tube 3.5 g. *OTC.*
Use: Lubricant, ophthalmic.

Refresh Redness Relief. (Allergan) Phenylephrine hydrochloride 0.12%. Benzalkonium chloride, edetate disodium, polyvinyl alcohol 1.4%. Soln., Ophth. 15 mL. *OTC.*
Use: Ophthalmic decongestant.

Refresh Tears. (Allergan) Carboxymethylcellulose 0.5%. Drops. Bot. 15 mL w/dropper. *OTC.*
Use: Artificial tears.

•**regadenoson.** (re-ga-DEN-oh-son) USAN.
Use: In vivo diagnostic aid.
See: Lexiscan.

Regain. (NCI Medical Foods) Protein 15 g, carbohydrates 52 g, fat 7 g, Na 45 mg, K 75 mg, Ca 200 mg, P 100 mg, Ca, Fe, vitamin B_{12}, Mg, folic acid, fructose. With dietary fiber. 300 calories. Lactose free. Vanilla, strawberry, and malt flavors. Bar 85 g. *OTC.*
Use: Nutritional supplement.

Regenecare HA. (MPM Medical) Lidocaine hydrochloride 2%. **Gel:** Glycerin, parabens. 85 g. **Spray:** Aloe vera, benzethonium chloride, glycerin, sodium hyaluronate, triethanolamine. 120 mL. *OTC.*
Use: Topical local anesthetic, amide local anesthetic.

Regenecare Wound. (MPM Medical) Lidocaine hydrochloride 2%. Aloe, collagen. Gel. 14 g. *Rx.*
Use: Local anesthetic, topical; amide local anesthetic.

Regimex. (WraSer) Benzphetamine hydrochloride 25 mg. Sorbitol. Tab. 100s. *c-III.*
Use: Sympathomimetic anorexiant.

Reglan. (ANI Pharmaceuticals) Metoclopramide (as monohydrochloride monohydrate) 5 mg, 10 mg. Lactose (5 mg only). Tab. Bot. 100s, 500s, (10 mg only), *Dis-Co* UD 100s. *Rx.*
Use: Antiemetic, gastrointestinal stimulant.

•**regorafenib.** (RE-goe-RAF-e-nib) USAN.
Use: Antineoplastic.
See: Stivarga.

•**regramostim.** (reh-GRAH-moe-STIM) USAN.
Use: Biological response modifier; antineoplastic adjunct; antineutropenic; hematopoietic stimulant.

Regranex. (Smith & Nephew Biotherapeutics) Becaplermin 0.01%. Parabens. Gel. Tube. 2 g, 15 g. *Rx.*
Use: Diabetic neuropathic ulcers.

Regular Strength Bayer Enteric Coated Caplets. (Bayer Consumer Care) Aspirin 325 mg. Bot. 50s, 100s. EC Tab. *OTC.*
Use: Analgesic.

Reguloid. (Rugby) Psyllium husk fiber 95% pure 3.4 g/5 mL, dextrose, 14 cal/tsp. Pow. Can. 369 g, 540 g. *OTC.*
Use: Laxative.

Reguloid, Orange. (Rugby) Psyllium mucilloid 3.4 g, sucrose, orange flavor/tbsp. Pow. Can. 369 g, 540 g. *OTC.*
Use: Laxative.

Reguloid, Sugar Free Orange. (Rugby) Psyllium hydrophilic mucilloid 3.4 g, aspartame, phenylalanine 30 mg/rounded tsp. Pow. Can. 284 g, 426 g. *OTC.*
Use: Laxative.

Reguloid, Sugar Free Regular. (Rugby) Psyllium hydrophilic mucilloid 3.4 g, aspartame, phenylalanine 6 mg/dose. Pow. Can. 284 g, 426 g. *OTC.*
Use: Laxative.

Rehydralyte. (Ross) Sodium 75 mEq, potassium 20 mEq, chloride 65 mEq, citrate 30 mEq, dextrose 25 g/L, 100 calories/L. Ready-to-use Bot. 8 oz. *Rx.*
Use: Fluid, electrolyte replacement.

Rehyla. (Medimetriks) Alcohol, chamomile, edetate disodium, glycerin, glyceryl, PEG, propylene glycol, sodium hyaluronate, wax. Dye free, fragrance free, paraben free. Soap. 473 mL. *OTC.*
Use: Emollient.

•**relacatib.** (REL-a-ka-tib) USAN.
Use: Osteoporosis.

Relacon-DM NR. (Cypress) Dextromethorphan HBr 15 mg, guaifenesin 200 mg, pseudoephedrine hydrochloride 32 mg per 5 mL. Alcohol free. Saccharin, sorbitol. Grape flavor. Liq. 473 mL. *Rx.*
Use: Upper respiratory combination, antitussive and expectorant combination.

Relacon-HC. (Cypress) Hydrocodone bitartrate 3.5 mg, chlorpheniramine maleate 2.5 mg, phenylephrine hydrochloride 10 mg per 5 mL. Alcohol, sugar, and dye free. Raspberry flavor. Liq. 473 mL. *c-III.*
Use: Upper respiratory combination, antitussive combination.

Relagesic. (International Ethical) Phenyltoloxamine citrate 50 mg, acetaminophen 650 mg. Tab. 100s. *Rx.*
Use: Antihistamine and analgesic.

Relahist-DM. (Cypress) Chlorpheniramine maleate 1 mg, dextromethorphan HBr 3 mg, phenylephrine hydrochloride 2 mg per 1 mL. Saccharin, sorbitol. Orange vanilla flavor. Conc. Soln. 30 mL. *Rx.*
Use: Upper respiratory combination; antitussive, decongestant, antihistamine.

Relasin DM. (Cypress) Dextromethorphan HBr 15 mg, guaifenesin 175 mg, pseudoephedrine hydrochloride 32 mg per 5 mL. Alcohol free. Menthol, saccharin, sorbitol. Grape flavor. Liq. 473 mL. *Rx.*
Use: Upper respiratory combination, antitussive and expectorant combination.

relaxin. A purified ovarian hormone of pregnancy (obtained from sows) responsible for pubic relaxation or separation of the symphysis pubis in mammals.

RelCof CPM. (Burel) Chlorpheniramine maleate 8 mg, methscopolamine nitrate 2.5 mg. ER Tab. 100s. *Rx.*
Use: Upper respiratory combination; decongestant, antihistamine, and anticholinergic combination.

RelCof DN PE. (Burel) *RelCof PE*: Chlorpheniramine maleate 8 mg, methscopolamine nitrate 2.5 mg, phenylephrine hydrochloride 20 mg. CR Tab. 10s. *RelCof CPM*: Chlorpheniramine maleate 8 mg, methscopolamine nitrate 2.5 mg. CR Tab. 10s. *Rx.*
Use: Upper respiratory combination; decongestant, antihistamine, and anticholinergic combination.

RelCof DN PSE. (Burel) *RelCof PSE*: Chlorpheniramine maleate 8 mg, methscopolamine nitrate 2.5 mg, pseudoephedrine hydrochloride 120 mg. Lactose. CR Tab. 10s. *RelCof CPM*: Chlorpheniramine maleate 8 mg, methscopolamine nitrate 2.5 mg. CR Tab. 10s. *Rx.*
Use: Upper respiratory combination;

decongestant, antihistamine, and anticholinergic combination.

RelCof PE. (Burel Pharmaceuticals) Chlorpheniramine maleate 8 mg, methscopolamine nitrate 2.5 mg, phenylephrine hydrochloride 20 mg. Tab. 10s, 100s. *Rx.*
Use: Upper respiratory combination; decongestant, antihistamine, and anticholinergic combination.

RelCof PSE. (Burel) Pseudoephedrine hydrochloride 120 mg, chlorpheniramine maleate 8 mg, methscopolamine nitrate 2.5 mg. lactose. ER Tab. 100s. *Rx.*
Use: Upper respiratory combination, decongestant, antihistamine, and anticholinergic combination.

Relenza. (GlaxoSmithKline) Zanamivir 5 mg. Lactose 20 mg. Pow. for Inh. Blister. Box 4 blisters w/ 5 *Rotadisks* and 1 *Disk-haler. Rx.*
Use: Antiviral.

Relhist. (Burel Pharmaceuticals) Brompheniramine tannate 6 mg/phenylephrine tannate 15 mg. Orange flavor. Chew. Tab. 60s. *Rx.*
Use: Upper respiratory combination, decongestant and antihistamine.

Relief Solution. (Allergan) Phenylephrine hydrochloride 0.12%, antipyrine 0.1%. Soln. Bot. 20 mL. *OTC.*
Use: Decongestant combination, ophthalmic.

Reli on Ketone Test Strips. (Bayer) Reagent strips for urine tests. 50s. *OTC.*
Use: Diagnostic aid.

Relistor. (Salix Pharmaceuticals) Methylnaltrexone bromide. Inj., Soln. **12 mg per 0.6 mL:** Edetate calcium disodium 0.24 mg, glycine 0.18 mg. Single-use vial. **8 mg per 0.4 mL:** Edetate calcium disodium 0.16 mg, glycine 0.12 mg. Single-use, prefilled syringe. *Rx.*
Use: Detoxification agent, antidote.

•**relomycin.** (REE-low-MY-sin) USAN. A macrolide antibiotic produced by a variant strain of *Streptomyces hygroscopicus.*
Use: Anti-infective.

Relpax. (Pfizer) Eletriptan 20 mg (equiv. to eletriptan hydrobromide 24.2 mg), 40 mg (equiv. to eletriptan hydrobromide 48.5 mg). Film coated. Lactose. Tab. UD 6s, UD 12s (40 mg only). *Rx.*
Use: Agent for migraine, serotonin 5-HT_1 receptor agonist.

•**remacemide hydrochloride.** (rem-ASS-eh-MIDE) USAN.
Use: Anticonvulsant (neuroprotective).

Rem Cough Medicine. (Last) Dextromethorphan HBr 5 mg/5 mL. Bot. 3 oz, 6 oz. *OTC.*
Use: Antitussive.

Remedy. (Medline) Benzalkonium chloride 0.12%. *Aloe barbadensis,* citrus oils, glycerin, parabens, tetrasodium EDTA, urea. Cleanser. 236 mL. *OTC.*
Use: Anti-infective, topical; antiseptic and germicide.

Remedy Calazime. (Medlline) Menthol 0.2%, zinc oxide 20%. Beeswax, *Carthamus tinctorius* seed oil, citrus oils, glycerin, glycine, methylparaben, olea europaea fruit oil, PEG-8, white petrolatum, zea mays oil. Oint. 113 g. *OTC.*
Use: Miscellaneous protectant.

Remedy With Phytoplex Antifungal Clear. (Medline) Miconazole nitrate 2%. Corn oil, dimethicone, olive oil, petrolatum, safflower seed oil, soybean oil. Oint. 71 g. *OTC.*
Use: Topical anti-infective, antifungal.

Remegel Soft Chewable Antacid. (Warner Lambert) Aluminum hydroxide-magnesium carbonate 476.4 mg. Chew. Tab. Pkg. 8s, 24s. *OTC.*
Use: Antacid.

Remeron. (Organon) Mirtazapine 15 mg, 30 mg, 45 mg. Lactose. Film coated. Tab. 30s. *Rx.*
Use: Antidepressant, tetracyclic compound.

Remeron SolTab. (Organon) Mirtazapine 15 mg, 30 mg, 45 mg. Aspartame, mannitol, sucrose, phenylalanine 2.6 mg (15 mg), 5.2 mg (30 mg), and 7.8 mg (45 mg). Orange flavor. Orally Disintegrating Tab. UD 30s. *Rx.*
Use: Antidepressant, tetracyclic compound.

•**remestemcel-L.** (REM-e-STEM-sel-l) USAN.
Use: Immunomodulator.

Remicade. (Centocor) Infliximab 100 mg. 0.5 mg of polysorbate 80, sucrose 500 mg. Preservative free. Inj., lyophilized, Pow. for Soln. Single-dose vial. *Rx.*
Use: Immunologic agent; immunomodulator.

•**remifentanil hydrochloride.** (reh-mih-FEN-tah-nill) USAN.
Use: Opioid analgesic.
See: Ultiva.

•**remiprostol.** (reh-mih-PROSTE-ole) USAN.
Use: Antiulcerative.

Remivox. (Janssen) Lorcainide hydrochloride. *Rx.*
Use: Antiarrhythmic.

Remodulin. (United Therapeutics)

Treprostinil sodium 1 mg/mL, 2.5 mg/mL, 5 mg/mL (sodium chloride 5.3 mg), 10 mg/mL (sodium chloride 4 mg). Inj. Multi-use vials. 20 mL. *Rx.*
Use: Vasodilator.

•**remogliflozin etabonate.** (re-MOE-gli-FLOE-zin) USAN.
Use: Antidiabetic agent.

•**remoxipride.** (reh-MOX-ih-PRIDE) USAN.
Use: Antipsychotic.

•**remoxipride hydrochloride.** (reh-MOX-ih-PRIDE) USAN.
Use: Antipsychotic.

Remular-S. (Inter. Ethical) Chlorzoxazone 250 mg. Tab. Bot. 100s. *Rx.*
Use: Muscle relaxant.

RE MultiVit with Fluoride. (River's Edge) **1 mg:** Fluoride 1 mg, folate 0.3 mg (as folic acid), vitamins A 2,500 units, B_1 1.05 mg, B_2 1.2 mg, B_3 13.5 mg, B_6 1.05 mg, B_{12} 4.5 mcg, C 60 mg, D 400 units, E 15 units. **0.5 mg:** Fluoride 0.5 mg, folate 0.3 mg, vitamins A 2,500 units, B_1 1.05 mg, B_2 1.2 mg, B_3 13.5 mg, B_6 1.05 mg, B_{12} 4.5 mcg, C 60 mg, D 400 units, E 15 units. **0.25 mg:** Fluoride 0.25 mg, folate 0.3 mg, vitamins A 2,500 units, $B_1$1.05 mg, $B_2$1.2 mg, $B_3$13.5 mg, $B_6$1.05 mg, B_{12}4.5 mcg, C 60 mg, D 400 units, E 15 units. PEG, sugar (0.25 mg only). Chew. Tab. 100s.
Use: Nutritional supplement, multivitamin with fluoride.

Renacidin. (Guardian) Citric acid (anhydrous) 6.602 g, glucono-delta-lactone 0.198 g, magnesium carbonate 3.177 g, benzoic acid 0.023 g per 100 mL. Soln. 500 mL. *Rx.*
Use: Genitourinary irrigant.

ReNaf. (River's Edge) Fluoride 0.25 mg, 0.5 mg, 1 mg. Sugar free. Vanilla, grape, and cherry flavors. Chew. Tab. 120s, 1,000s. *Rx.*
Use: Trace element.

Renagel. (Genzyme) Sevelamer hydrochloride 400 mg, 800 mg. Film-coated. Tab. Bot. 180s (800 mg only), 360s (400 mg only). *Rx.*
Use: Phosphate binder.

renanolone. *Rx.*
Use: Steroid anesthetic.

Renax. (Everett) Vitamin E (as d-alpha tocopheryl succinate) 35 units, B_1 3 mg, B_2 2 mg, B_3 20 mg, B_5 10 mg, B_6 15 mg, B_{12} 12 mg, C 50 mg, folic acid 2.5 mg, Zn 20 mg, biotin 300 mcg, Cr, Se. Capl. Bot. 90s. *Rx.*
Use: Vitamin, mineral supplement.

Renbu. (Wren) Butabarbital sodium 32.4 mg. Tab. Bot. 100s, 1000s. *c-III.*
Use: Hypnotic; sedative.

renin angiotensin system antagonists.
See: Angiotensin-Converting Enzyme Inhibitors.
Angiotensin II Receptor Antagonists.
Direct Renin Inhibitors.
Selective Aldosterone Receptor Antagonists.

renin inhibitors, direct.
See: Aliskirin.

RenoCal-76. (Bracco Diagnostics) Diatrizoate meglumine 660 mg, diatrizoate sodium 100 mg, iodine 370 mg/mL. EDTA. Inj. Vials. 50 mL. Bot. 100 mL, 150 mL, 200 mL. *Rx.*
Use: Radiopaque agent.

renoform.
See: Epinephrine.

Reno-M Dip. (Bracco Diagnostics) Diatrizoate meglumine 300 mg, iodine 141 mg/mL. Inj. Bot. 300 mL. *Formerly Renografin-Dip. Rx.*
Use: Radiopaque agent.

Renormax. (Novartis) Spirapril 3 mg, 6 mg, 12 mg, 24 mg. Tab. *Rx.*
Use: ACE inhibitor.

Reno-Sed. (Vita Elixir) Methenamine 2 g, salol 0.5 g, methylene blue $\frac{1}{10}$ g, benzoic acid $\frac{1}{8}$ g, atropine sulfate $\frac{1}{1000}$ g, hyoscyamine sulfate $\frac{1}{2000}$ g. Tab. *Rx.*
Use: Anti-infective, urinary.

Renova. (Valeant) Tretinoin 0.02%, 0.05%, stearyl alcohol, EDTA; parabens, benzyl alcohol, cetyl alcohol (0.02% only); methylparabens (0.05% only). Cream. Tube. 20 g (0.05% only), 40 g, 60 g (0.05% only). *Rx.*
Use: Retinoid.

Renovist. (Bracco Diagnostics) Diatrizoate methylglucamine 34.3%, diatrizoate sodium 35%, iodine 37%. Inj. Vial 50 mL, Box 25s.
Use: Radiopaque agent.

Renovist II. (Bracco Diagnostics) Diatrizoate sodium 29.1%, meglumine diatrizoate 28.5%, iodine 31%. Inj. Vial 30 mL, 60 mL, Box 25s.
Use: Radiopaque agent.

Renovue-Dip. (Bracco Diagnostics) Iodamide meglumide 24%, iodine 11.1%. Infusion Bot. 300 mL.
Use: Radiopaque agent.

Renovue-65. (Bracco Diagnostics) Iodamide meglumide 65%, organically bound iodine 30%, edetate disodium. Vial 50 mL.
Use: Radiopaque agent.

Rentamine Pediatric. (Major) Phenylephrine tannate 5 mg, chlorpheniramine

tannate 4 mg, carbetapentane tannate/ 5 mL, saccharin, sucrose. Syr. Bot. Pt. *Rx.*
Use: Antihistamine, antitussive, decongestant.

ReNu Multi-Purpose. (Bausch & Lomb) Isotonic. Sodium chloride, sodium borate, boric acid, poloxamine, polyaminopropyl biguanide 0.00005%, EDTA 0.01%. Soln. Bot. 118 mL, 237 mL, 355 mL. *OTC.*
Use: Contact lens disinfection system.

ReNu Saline. (Bausch & Lomb) Isotonic buffered soln. of sodium Cl, boric acid, polyaminopropyl biguanide 0.00003%, EDTA. Soln. Bot. 355 mL. *OTC.*
Use: Contact lens care.

Renvela. (Genzyme) Sevelamer (as sevelamer carbonate). **Tab.:** 800 mg. Film-coated. 30s, 270s. **Pow. for Susp.:** 0.8 g, 2.4 g per packet. Sucralose. Citrus cream flavor. 90s. *Rx.*
Use: Phosphate binder.

ReoPro. (Lilly) Abciximab 2 mg/mL in buffered solution of sodium phosphate 0.01 M, sodium chloride 0.15 M. Preservative free. Inj. Single-use vials. 5 mL. *Rx.*
Use: Antiplatelet, glycoprotein IIb/IIIa inhibitor.

•**repaglinide.** (re-PAG-li-nide) *USP.*
Use: Antidiabetic, meglitinide.
See: Prandin.

repaglinide. (Various Mfr.) Repaglinide 0.5 mg, 1 mg, 2 mg. Tab. 100s, 500s. *Rx.*
Use: Antidiabetic agent, meglitinide.

Repan. (Everett) Butalbital 50 mg, caffeine 40 mg, acetaminophen 325 mg. Tab. Bot. 100s. *Rx.*
Use: Analgesic; hypnotic; sedative.

•**reparixin.** (RE-pa-RIX-in) USAN.
Use: Immunosuppressive.

RepHresh Pro-B. (Lil' Drug Store Products) 2.5 billion CFU of *L. rhamnosus* GR-1, 2.5 billion CFU of *L. reuteri* RC 14. Dextrose. Cap. 30s. *OTC.*
Use: Probiotic.

•**repifermin.** (re-pi-FER-min) USAN.
Use: Mucositis; wound healing.

•**repirinast.** (reh-PIRE-ih-nast) USAN.
Use: Antiallergic; antiasthmatic.

Replesta Children's. (Everidis) Cholecalciferol (D_3) 14,000 units. Dextrose. Orange flavor. Wafer, Chew. 6s. *OTC.*
Use: Fat-soluble vitamin.

Replesta NX. (Everidis) Cholecalciferol (D_3) 14,000 units, vitamin E 34 units. Dextrose. Orange flavor. Wafer, Chew. 8s. *OTC.*
Use: Fat-soluble vitamin.

Replete. (Clintec Nutrition) K caseinate, Ca caseinate, maltodextrin, sucrose, corn oil, lecithin, vitamins A, B_1, B_2, B_3, B_5, B_6, B_{12}, C, D, E, K, folic acid, biotin, choline, Ca, Cl, Cu, Fe, I, Mg, Mn, P, Zn. Liq. Bot. 250 mL. *OTC.*
Use: Nutritional supplement.

Reprexain. (Hawthorn) Hydrocodone bitartrate/ibuprofen 2.5 mg/200 mg, 5 mg/ 200 mg, 10 mg/200 mg. Film coated. PEG, polydextrose (2.5 mg/200 mg only). Tab. 100s. *c-III.*
Use: Opioid analgesic combination.

Reprieve. (Mayer Lab) Caffeine 32 mg, salicylamide 225 mg, vitamin B_1 50 mg, homatropine methylbromide 0.5 mg. Tab. Bot. 8s, 16s. *Rx.*
Use: Analgesic combination.

•**repromicin.** (rep-ROW-MY-sin) USAN.
Use: Anti-infective.

Repronex. (Ferring) Follicle-stimulating hormone and luteinizing hormone 75 units or 150 units. Pow. or pellet for inj., lyophilized. Vial with diluent. *Rx.*
Use: Sex hormone, ovulation stimulant.

•**reproterol hydrochloride.** (re-PROE-ter-ol) USAN.
Use: Bronchodilator.

Reptilase-R. (Abbott Diagnostics) Diagnostic for the investigation of fibrin formation and disturbances in fibrin formation due to causes other than thrombin inhibition.
Use: Diagnostic aid.

Requa's Charcoal. (Requa, Inc.) Wood charcoal 10 g. Tab. Pkg. 50s. Can 125s. *OTC.*
Use: Antiflatulent.

Requip. (GlaxoSmithKline) Ropinirole hydrochloride 0.25 mg, 0.5 mg, 1 mg, 2 mg, 3 mg, 4 mg, 5 mg. Lactose, PEG. Film-coated. Tab. Bot. 100s. *Rx.*
Use: Antiparkinson agent.

Requip XL. (GlaxoSmithKline) Ropinirole 2 mg, 4 mg, 6 mg, 8 mg, 12 mg. Lactose, maltodextrin, mannitol, PEG. Film coated. ER Tab. 30s, 90s (except 12 mg). *Rx.*
Use: Antiparkinson agent.

Resa. (Vita Elixir) Reserpine 0.25 mg. Tab. Bot. *Rx.*
Use: Antihypertensive.

Resaid. (Geneva) Phenylpropanolamine hydrochloride 75 mg, chlorpheniramine maleate 12 mg. Cap. Bot. 100s, 1000s. *Rx.*
Use: Antihistamine, decongestant.

Resaid S.R. (Geneva) Phenylpropanolamine hydrochloride 75 mg, chlorpheniramine maleate 12 mg. SR Cap.

Bot. 100s, 1000s. *Rx.*
Use: Antihistamine, decongestant.

Rescaps-D S.R. (Geneva) Phenylpropanolamine hydrochloride 75 mg, caramiphen edisylate 40 mg. Cap. Bot. 100s. *Rx.*
Use: Antitussive, decongestant.

Rescon. (Capellon) Dexchlorpheniramine maleate 2 mg, pseudoephedrine hydrochloride 60 mg. Lactose. Tab. 90s. *OTC.*
Use: Upper respiratory combination; decongestant, antihistamine, and anticholinergic combination.

Rescon-DM. (Capellon) Dextromethorphan HBr 10 mg, pseudoephedrine hydrochloride 30 mg, chlorpheniramine maleate 2 mg per 5 mL. Alcohol, sugar, and dye free. Parabens, saccharin, sorbitol, fruit punch flavor. Liq. Bot. 118 mL, 473 mL. *OTC.*
Use: Upper respiratory combination, antitussive combination.

Rescon-GG. (Capellon) Phenylephrine hydrochloride 5 mg, guaifenesin 100 mg/5 mL. Alcohol and dye free. Parabens, sorbitol, sugar. Cherry flavor. Liq. Bot 118 mL, 473 mL. *OTC.*
Use: Upper respiratory combination, decongestant, expectorant.

Rescon-JR. (Capellon) Chlorpheniramine maleate 4 mg, phenylephrine hydrochloride 20 mg. ER Tab. 100s. *Rx.*
Use: Upper respiratory combination, decongestant and antihistamine.

Rescon-MX. (Capellon) Dexchlorpheniramine maleate 6 mg, phenylephrine hydrochloride 40 mg. Tab. 90s. *Rx.*
Use: Upper respiratory combination; decongestant, antihistamine, anticholinergic.

Rescriptor. (Agouron) Delavirdine mesylate 100 mg, 200 mg, lactose. Tab. Bot. 180s (200 mg only), 360s (100 mg only). *Rx.*
Use: Antiretroviral, non-nucleoside reverse transcriptase inhibitor.

Rescula. (Sucampo Pharma Americas) Unoprostone isopropyl 0.15%. Benzalkonium chloride 0.015%, edetate disodium, polysorbate 80. Soln.; Ophth. 5 mL bottle w/dropper tip. *Rx.*
Use: Agent for glaucoma.

Reserpaneed. (Hanlon) Reserpine 0.25 mg. Tab. Bot. 100s, 1000s. *Rx.*
Use: Antihypertensive.

•**reserpine.** (reh-SER-peen) *USP.*
Use: Antihypertensive.
See: Broserpine.
De Serpa.
Elserpine.
Raurine.
Reserpaneed.
Sertabs.
Zepine.

•**reserpine, hydralazine hydrochloride, and hydrochlorothiazide tablets.** *USP.*
Use: Antihypertensive.

resiquimod.
Use: Antiviral; antitumor.

•**reslizumab.** (res-li-ZOO-mab) USAN.
Use: Bronchial asthma.

•**resocortol butyrate.** (reh-so-CORE-tole BYOO-tih-rate) USAN.
Use: Corticosteroid; anti-inflammatory, topical.

Resol. (Wyeth) Na 50 mEq, K 20 mEq, Cl 50 mEq, citrate 34 mEq, Ca 4 mEq, Mg 4 mEq, phosphate 5 mEq, glucose 20 g/L. Contains 80 calories/L. Ctn. 32 fl oz. *Rx.*
Use: Fluid, electrolyte replacement.

Resolve/GP Daily Cleaner. (Allergan) Buffered solution with cocoamphocarboxyglycinate, sodium lauryl sulfate, hexylene glycol, alkyl ether sulfate, fatty acid amide surfactant cleaning agents, preservative free. Soln. Bot. 30 mL. *OTC.*
Use: Contact lens care.

Resonium-A. (Sanofi-Synthelabo) Sodium polystyrene sulfonate. *Rx.*
Use: Potassium removing resin.

resorcin.
See: Resorcinol.
W/Benzocaine.
See: Vagisil.

•**resorcinol.** (reh-SORE-sih-nole) *USP.*
Use: Keratolytic.
W/Benzocaine.
See: Unguentine Maximum Strength.
Vagisil.
Vagisil Maximum Strength.
W/Combinations.
See: Adult Acnomel.
Bicozene.
Black and White.
Clearasil Adult Care.
Rezamid.

•**resorcinol and sulfur lotion.** (reh-SORE-sih-nole) *USP.*
Use: Antifungal; parasiticide; scabicide.

•**resorcinol and sulfur topical suspension.** (reh-SORE-sih-nole) *USP.*
Use: Antifungal; parasiticide; scabicide.

•**resorcinol monoacetate.** (re-SORE-sih-nole) *USP.*
Use: Antiseborrheic; keratolytic.

resorcinolphthalein sodium.
Use: Antiseborrheic, topical.
See: Fluorescein Sodium.

Resource. (Novartis Nutrition) Ca and Na

caseinates, soy protein isolate 37 g, sugar, hydrolyzed cornstarch 140 g, corn oil, soy lecithin 37 g, Na 890 mg, K 1600 mg, A, B_1, B_2, B_3, B_5, B_6, B_{12}, C, D, E, K, Ca, P, I, Fe, Mg, Cu, Zn, Mn, Cl, gluten free, vanilla, chocolate, strawberry flavor. Liq. Bot. 237 mL. *OTC.*
Use: Nutritional supplement.

Resource Diabetic. (Novartis Nutrition) Protein (sodium and calcium caseinates, soy protein isolates, carnitine, taurine) 63 g, carbohydrate (hydrolyzed cornstarch, fructose) 99 g, fat (high oleic sunflower oil, soybean oil) 47 g/L, vitamins A, B_1, B_2, B_3, B_5, B_6, B_{12}, C, D, E, K, biotin, choline, folic acid, m-inositol, Ca, chloride, Cr, Cu, Fe, I, Mg, Mn, Mo, P, Se, Zn, Na 970 mg (42 mEq), K 1100 mg (29 mEq), H_2O 450 mOsm/Kg, 1.06 cal/mL, fiber 13 g/L, lactose free, french vanilla, chocolate, strawberry, flavors. Liq. *Tetra Brik* Paks 237 mL (27s), closed system containers 1000 mL, 1500 mL (6s). *OTC.*
Use: Enteral nutritional therapy.

Resource Fruit Beverage. (Novartis Nutrition) Protein (whey protein concentrates) 38 g, carbohydrates (sugar, hydrolyzed cornstarch) 150 g/L, vitamins A, B_1, B_2, B_3, B_5, B_6, B_{12}, C, D, E, K, biotin, choline, folic acid, Ca, chloride, Cu, Fe, I, Mg, Mn, P, Zn, Na < 295 mg (< 13 mEq), K < 93 mg (< 2.4 mEq), H_2O 700 mOsm/Kg, 0.76 cal/mL, lactose free, orange, peach and wild berry flavors. Liq. *Tetra Brik* Paks 237 mL (27s). *OTC.*
Use: Enteral nutritional therapy.

Resource Instant Crystals. (Novartis Nutrition) Maltodextrin, sucrose, hydrogenated soy oil, sodium caseinate, calcium caseinate, soy protein isolate, potassium citrate, polyglycerol esters of fatty acids, vanilla and artificial flavors, vitamins and minerals. Instant Crystals. Pkt. 1.5 oz., 2 oz. *OTC.*
Use: Nutritional supplement.

Resource Just for Kids. (Novartis Nutrition) Protein (sodium and calcium caseinates, whey protein concentrate, carnitine, taurine) 30 g, carbohydrate (hydrolyzed cornstarch, sucrose) 110 g, fat (high oleic sunflower oil, soybean oil, medium chain triglycerides oil) 50 g, vitamins A, B_1, B_2, B_3, B_5, B_6, B_{12}, C, D, E, K, biotin, choline, folic acid, m-inositol, Ca, chloride, Cr, Cu, Fe, I, Mg, Mn, Mo, P, Se, Zn, Na 380 mg (17 mEq)/L, K 1300 mg (33 mEq)/L, H_2O 390 mOsm/Kg, 1 cal/mL, lactose free, french vanilla, chocolate, strawberry flavors. Liq. *Tetra Brik* Paks 237 mL (27s). *OTC.*
Use: Enteral nutritional therapy.

Resource Plus. (Novartis Nutrition) Ca and Na caseinates, soy protein isolate 54.9 g, maltodextrin, sucrose 200 g, corn oil, lecithin 53.3 g, Na 899 mg, K 1740 mg, A, B_1, B_2, B_3, B_5, B_6, B_{12}, C, D, E, K, biotin, choline, Ca, P, I, Fe, Mg, Cu, Zn, Cl, Mn, gluten free, vanilla, chocolate, strawberry flavors. Liq. Bot. 8 oz. *OTC.*
Use: Nutritional supplement.

Respa A.R. (Respa) Pseudoephedrine hydrochloride 90 mg, chlorpheniramine maleate 8 mg, belladonna alkaloids (atropine, hyoscyamine, scopolamine) 0.24 mg. Dye and sugar free. ER Tab. 100s. *Rx.*
Use: Upper respiratory combination, decongestant, antihistamine, and anticholinergic.

Respa C & C. (Respa) Acetaminophen 575 mg, dextromethorphan hydrobromide 30 mg, diphenhydramine hydrochloride 37.5 mg, phenylephrine hydrochloride 18 mg. Tab. 100s. *Rx.*
Use: Upper respiratory combination, antitussive combination.

Respaire-30. (Laser) Guaifenesin 150 mg, pseudoephedrine hydrochloride 30 mg. Sugar. Cap. 100s. *Rx.*
Use: Upper respiratory combination, decongestant and expectorant combination.

Respalor. (Bristol-Myers Squibb) Protein 75 g, carbohydrate 146 g, fat 70 g, Na 1248 mg, K 1456 mg, Fe 12.5 mg, cal/L 1498. Lactose free. Vanilla flavor. With appropriate vitamins and minerals. Liq. Bot. 237 mL. *OTC.*
Use: Nutritional supplement.

Respa-SA. (Respa Pharmaceuticals) Diphenhydramine hydrochloride 37.5 mg, pseudoephedrine hydrochloride 58 mg. Tab. 100s. *Rx.*
Use: Upper respiratory combination, decongestant and antihistamine.

Respihaler Decadron Phosphate. (Merck & Co.)
See: Decadron Phosphate.

Respiracult. (Orion) Culture test for group A beta-hemolytic streptococci. In 10s.
Use: Diagnostic aid.

Respiralex. (Orion) Latex agglutination test to detect group A streptococci in throat and nasopharynx. Kit 1s.
Use: Diagnostic aid.

respiratory enzymes.
See: $Alpha_1$-Proteinase Inhibitor.

respiratory gases.
See: Nitric Oxide.
respiratory inhalant combinations.
See: Budesonide/Formoterol.
Fluticasone Furoate/Vilanterol.
Fluticasone Propionate/Salmeterol.
respiratory inhalants.
See: Corticosteroids.
Intranasal Antihistamines.
Intranasal Steroids.
Mast Cell Stabilizers.
Mucolytics.
Respiratory Gases.
respiratory syncytial virus immune globulin (human) (RSV-IG).
Use: Prophylaxis against respiratory tract infection.
Restasis. (Allergan) Cyclosporine emulsion 0.05%, glycerin, castor oil, polysorbate 80, preservative free. Single-use vials. 0.4 mL. *Rx.*
Use: Immunologic agent.
Rest Easy. (Walgreen) Acetaminophen 1000 mg, pseudoephedrine hydrochloride 60 mg, dextromethorphan HBr 30 mg, doxylamine succinate 7.5 mg/30 mL. Bot. 6 oz, 16 oz. *OTC.*
Use: Analgesic; antihistamine; antitussive; decongestant.
Restora. (US Pharm) *L. casei* 4 billion CFU. Omega-3 oil. Cap. 30s. *OTC.*
Use: Probiotic.
Restoril. (Mallinckrodt) Temazepam 7.5 mg, 15 mg, 22.5 mg, 30 mg. Lactose. Cap. Bot. 30s (7.5 mg and 22.5 mg only), 100s, 500s (15 mg and 30 mg only). *c-IV.*
Use: Sedative/hypnotic, nonbarbiturate.
Restylane. (Medicis Aesthetics) Hyaluronic acid 20 mg/mL. Gel for Inj. Single-use prefilled syringes. *Rx.*
Use: Physical adjunct.
Restylane-L. (Medicis Aesthetics) Hyaluronic acid 20 mg/mL. Lidocaine 0.3%. Inj., gel. Single-use, prefilled syringe. *Rx.*
Use: Physical adjunct.
Re-Tann. (Midlothian Labs) Carbetapentane tannate 25 mg, pseudoephedrine tannate 75 mg per 5 mL. Aspartame, parabens, phenylalanine. Cherry flavor. Susp. 473 mL. *Rx.*
Use: Antitussive combination.
•**retapamulin.** (re-TAP-a-MUE-lin) USAN.
Use: Antibiotic.
See: Altabax.
•**retaspimycin.** (RET-asp-i-MY-sin) USAN.
Use: Antineoplastic agent.
•**retaspimycin hydrochloride.** (RET-asp-i-MY-sin) USAN.
Use: Antineoplastic agent.
Retavase. (Centocor) Reteplase 10.4 units (18.1 mg). Pow. for Inj., lyophilized. Preservative-free. Kits with package insert, 2 single-use reteplase vials of 10.4 U (18.1 mg), 2 single-use diluent vials for reconstitution (10 mL sterile water for injection), 2 sterile 10 mL syringes, 2 sterile dispensing pins, 4 sterile needles, and 2 alcohol swabs. Half kits with package insert, 1 single-use reteplase vial 10.4 U (18.1 mg), 1 single-use diluent vial for reconstitution (10 mL sterile water for injection), and a sterile dispensing pin. *Rx.*
Use: Management of acute myocardial infarction.
•**reteplase, recombinant.** (RE-te-plase) USAN.
Use: Management of acute myocardial infarction; plasminogen activator.
See: Retavase.
•**retigabine.** (re-TIG-a-been) USAN.
Use: Antiepileptic.
Retin-A. (Valeant) **Cream:** Tretinoin 0.1%, 0.05%, 0.025%, stearyl alcohol (0.1% only). Cream. Tube 20 g, 45 g. **Gel:** Tretinoin 0.01%, 0.025%, alcohol 90%. Gel. Tube 15 g, 45 g. *Rx.*
Use: Dermatologic, acne; retinoid.
Retin-A Micro. (Valeant) Tretinoin 0.04%, 0.08%, 0.1%. Glycerin, propylene glycol, benzyl alcohol, EDTA. Gel. 20 g, 45 g (except 0.08%); 50 g pump. *Rx.*
Use: Dermatologic, acne; retinoid.
retinoic acid. Tretinoin.
Use: Keratolytic.
See: Retin A.
9-cis-retinoic acid.
Use: Acute promyelocytic leukemia. [Orphan Drug]
retinoids.
See: Adapalene.
Retinoids, First Generation.
Retinoids, Second Generation.
Tazarotene.
retinoids, first generation.
See: Isotretinoin.
Tretinoin.
retinoids, second generation.
See: Acitretin.
Alitretinoin.
Retinol. (NBTY) Vitamin A 100,000 units, glycol stearate, mineral oil, propylene glycol, lanolin oil, propylene glycol stearate SE, lanolin alcohol, retinol, parabens, EDTA. Cream. Tube 60 g. *OTC.*
Use: Emollient.
Retinol-A. (Young Again Products) Vitamin A palmitate 300,000 units/30 g.

Cream. Tube 60 g. *OTC.*
Use: Emollient.

Retisert. (Bausch & Lomb) Fluocinolone acetonide 0.59 mg. Ophth. Implant. Individual cartons. *Rx.*
Use: Corticosteroid, ophthalmic.

Retrovir. (GlaxoSmithKline) Zidovudine. **Tab.:** 300 mg. Bot. 60s. **Cap:** 100 mg. Bot. 100s. UD 100s. **Syrup:** 50 mg/5 mL, sodium benzoate 0.2%, sucrose, strawberry flavor. Bot. 240 mL. **Inj:** 10 mg/mL. Single-use Vial 20 mL. *Rx.*
Use: Antiretroviral, nucleoside reverse transcriptase inhibitor.

RE Urea 50. (River's Edge) Urea 50%. Cetyl alcohol, disodium EDTA, glycerin, lactic acid, mineral oil PEG-6, titanium dioxide. Soln., Top. Prefilled applicator. 4 mL.
Use: Emollient.

•**revaprazan hydrochloride.** (re-VA-pra-zan) USAN.
Use: Agent for GERD.

Revatio. (Pfizer) Sildenafil citrate. **Tab.:** 20 mg. Lactose. Film-coated. 90s. **Inj., Soln.:** 10 mg per 12.5 mL. Dextrose 50.5 mg/mL. Single-use vial. 12.5 mL. **Pow. for Susp.:** 10 mg/mL (after reconstitution). Grape flavoring, sodium benzoate, sorbitol, sucralose. 112 mL w/oral dosing syringe and bottle adaptor. *Rx.*
Use: Treatment of pulmonary arterial hypertension to improve exercise ability.

Reversol. (Organon Teknika) Edrophonium chloride 10 mg/mL. Inj. Vial. 10 mL. *Rx.*
Use: Muscle stimulant.

ReVia. (Teva Women's Health) Naltrexone hydrochloride 50 mg. Film-coated. Tab. Bot. 30s, 100s. *Rx.*
Use: Antidote.

RevitaDERM Wound Care. (Blaine Labs) Colloidal silver 1%. Alcohol, aloe oil extract, aloe vera, collagen, elastin, glycerin, hyaluronic acid, phenonip, triethanolamine. Gel. 90 g. *OTC.*
Use: Would healing agent.

Revlimid. (Celgene) Lenalidomide 2.5 mg, 5 mg, 10 mg, 15 mg, 20 mg, 25 mg. Lactose. Cap. 28s (except 15 mg, 25 mg), 21s (15 mg, 20 mg, 25 mg only), 100s. *Rx.*
Use: Immunomodulator.

Revonto. (US Worldmeds) Dantrolene sodium 20 mg/vial. Mannitol 3 g/vial. Inj., lyophilized Pow. for Soln. Vial. 65 mL. *Rx.*
Use: Skeletal muscle relaxants, direct acting.

Revs Caffeine T.D. (Eon Labs) Caffeine 250 mg. Cap. Bot. 100s, 1000s. *OTC.*
Use: CNS stimulant.

Rexahistine. (Econo Med Pharmaceuticals) Phenylephrine hydrochloride 5 mg, chlorpheniramine maleate 1 mg, menthol 1 mg, sodium bisulfite 0.1%, alcohol 5%/5 mL. Bot. Gal. *OTC.*
Use: Antihistamine, decongestant.

Rexahistine DH. (Econo-Rx) Codeine phosphate 10 mg, phenylephrine hydrochloride 10 mg, chlorpheniramine maleate 2 mg, menthol 1 mg, alcohol 5%/5 mL. Bot. Gal. *c-v.*
Use: Antihistamine, antitussive, decongestant.

Rexahistine Expectorant. (Econo-Rx) Codeine phosphate 10 mg, phenylephrine hydrochloride 10 mg, chlorpheniramine maleate 2 mg, guaifenesin 100 mg, menthol 1 mg, alcohol 5%/5 mL. Bot. Gal. *c-v.*
Use: Antihistamine, antitussive, decongestant, expectorant.

Rexigen Forte. (ION Laboratories, Inc.) Phendimetrazine tartrate 105 mg. SR Cap. Bot. 100s. *c-III.*
Use: Anorexiant.

rexinoids.
See: Bexarotene.

Reyataz. (Bristol-Myers Squibb) Atazanavir sulfate (as base) 150 mg, 200 mg, 300 mg. Lactose, alcohols, simethicone. Cap. 30s (300 mg only), 60s (except 300 mg). *Rx.*
Use: Antiretroviral, protease inhibitor.

Rezamid. (Summers) Sulfur 5%, resorcinol 2%, SD alcohol 40 28%. Lot. Bot. 56.7 mL. *OTC.*
Use: Dermatologic; acne.

•**rezatomidine.** (RE-za-TOE-mi-deen) USAN.
Use: Treatment of chronic pain.

Rezine. (Marnel) Hydroxyzine hydrochloride 10 mg, 25 mg. Tab. Bot. 100s. *Rx.*
Use: Anxiolytic.

ReZyst IM. (Zyber) 3 billion viable cells blend of *Lactobacillus* and *Bifidobacterium.* Sorbitol, sucralose, xylitol. Berry flavor. Chew. Tab. 60s. *OTC.*
Use: Oral nutritional supplement, probiotic.

RF Latex Test. (Laboratory Diagnostics) Rapid latex agglutination test for the qualitative screening and semi-quantitative determination of rheumatoid factor. Kit 100s.
Use: Diagnostic aid.

R-Frone. (Serono)
See: Interferon Beta.

R-Gene 10. (Pharmacia & Upjohn) Arginine hydrochloride 1 g per 10 mL.

Chloride ion 47.5 mEq per 100 mL. Preservative free. Inj., Soln. 300 mL. *Rx.*
Use: In vivo diagnostic aid.

R-HCTZ-H. (Wyeth) Reserpine 0.1 mg, hydrochlorothiazide 15 mg, hydralazine hydrochloride 25 mg. Tab. Bot. 100s, 500s. *Rx.*
Use: Antihypertensive.

Rheomacrodex. (Medisan) Dextran 40 10% in sodium Cl 0.9% or in dextrose 5%. Soln. Bot. 500 mL. *Rx.*
Use: Plasma expander.

Rheumatex. (Wampole) Latex agglutination test for the qualitative detection and quantitative determination of rheumatoid factor in serum. Kit 100s.
Use: Diagnostic aid.

Rheumaton. (Wampole) Two-minute hemagglutination slide test for the qualitative and quantitative determination of rheumatoid factor in serum or synovial fluid. Test kit 20s, 50s, 150s.
Use: Diagnostic aid.

Rheumatrex Dose Pack. (STADA Pharm) Methotrexate 2.5 mg. Tab. Pkg. 5 mg, 7.5 mg, 10 mg, 12.5 mg, 15 mg/week dose packs. *Rx.*
Use: Antipsoriatic; antirheumatic; antimetabolite.

Rhinabid. (Breckenridge) Phenylephrine hydrochloride 15 mg, brompheniramine maleate 12 mg. Sugar. ER Cap. 100s. *Rx.*
Use: Decongestant and antihistamine.

Rhinabid PD. (Breckenridge) Phenylephrine hydrochloride 7.5 mg, brompheniramine maleate 6 mg. Sugar. ER Cap. 100s. *Rx.*
Use: Pediatric decongestant and antihistamine.

Rhinall. (Scherer) Phenylephrine hydrochloride 0.25%, sodium bisulfite, chlorobutanol, benzalkonium chloride. Soln. Spray Bot. 40 mL. Dropper Bot. 30 mL. *OTC.*
Use: Nasal decongestant, arylalkylamine.

Rhinall 10. (Scherer) Phenylephrine hydrochloride 0.2%. Drop. Bot. oz. *OTC.*
Use: Decongestant.

Rhinaris. (Arbor Pharmaceuticals) Sodium chloride. **Gel, intranasal:** 0.2%. Benzalkonium chloride, PEG, propylene glycol. 28.4 g. **Soln., intranasal:** 0.2%. Benzalkonium chloride, PEG, propylene glycol. Spray. 30 mL. *OTC.*
Use: Nasal decongestant.

Rhinaris Lubricating Mist. (Pharmascience) Polyethylene glycol 15%, propylene glycol 5% (spray only) 20% (gel only), benzalkonium chloride, sodium chloride. Soln. Spray Bot. 30 mL. Gel Tube. 28.35 g. *OTC.*
Use: Nasal decongestant.

Rhinatate. (Major) Phenylephrine tannate 25 mg, chlorpheniramine tannate 8 mg, pyrilamine tannate 25 mg. Tab. Bot. 100s, 250s. *Rx.*
Use: Antihistamine, decongestant.

Rhinatate-NF Pediatric. (Major) Phenylephrine tannate 5 mg, chlorpheniramine tannate 4.5 mg per 5 mL. Methylparaben, saccharin, sucrose. Susp. Bot. 473 mL. *Rx.*
Use: Upper respiratory combination, decongestant, antihistamine.

Rhinatate Pediatric. (Major) Phenylephrine tannate 5 mg, chlorpheniramine tannate 2 mg, pyrilamine tannate 12.5 mg/5 mL, methylparaben, saccharin, sucrose, strawberry-blackberry-currant flavor. Susp. Bot. 473 mL *Rx.*
Use: Upper respiratory combination, decongestant, antihistamine.

Rhinocort Aqua. (AstraZeneca) Budesonide 32 mcg/actuation. Dextrose, polysorbate 80, EDTA. Spray, Intranasal. Bot. 8.6 g (120 metered sprays) with metered-dose pump. *Rx.*
Use: Respiratory inhalant, intranasal steroid.

Rhinolar-EX. (McGregor Pharmaceuticals, Inc.) Phenylpropanolamine hydrochloride 75 mg, chlorpheniramine maleate 8 mg. SR Cap. Dye free. Bot. 60s. *Rx.*
Use: Antihistamine, decongestant.

Rhinolar-EX 12. (McGregor Pharmaceuticals, Inc.) Phenylpropanolamine hydrochloride 75 mg, chlorpheniramine maleate 12 mg. SR Cap. Dye free. Bot. 60s. *Rx.*
Use: Antihistamine; decongestant.

Rhinosyn. (Great Southern) Pseudoephedrine hydrochloride 60 mg, chlorpheniramine maleate 4 mg/5 mL, alcohol 0.45%, sucrose. Liq. Bot. 120 mL, 473 mL. *OTC.*
Use: Antihistamine, decongestant.

Rhinosyn DM. (Great Southern) Pseudoephedrine hydrochloride 30 mg, chlorpheniramine maleate 2 mg, dextromethorphan HBr 15 mg/5 mL, alcohol 1.4%, sucrose. Liq. Bot. 120 mL. *OTC.*
Use: Antihistamine, antitussive, decongestant.

Rhinosyn DMX. (Great Southern) Dextromethorphan HBr 15 mg, guaifenesin 100 mg/5 mL, alcohol 1.4%. Syr. Bot. 120 mL. *OTC.*
Use: Antitussive, expectorant.

Rhinosyn-PD. (Great Southern) Pseudoephedrine hydrochloride 30 mg,

chlorpheniramine maleate 2 mg/5 mL. Liq. Bot. 120 mL. *OTC.*
Use: Antihistamine, decongestant.

Rhinosyn-X. (Great Southern) Pseudoephedrine hydrochloride 30 mg, dextromethorphan HBr 10 mg, guaifenesin 100 mg/5 mL, alcohol 7.5%. Liq. Bot. 120 mL. *OTC.*
Use: Antitussive, decongestant, expectorant.

rhodanate.
See: Potassium Thiocyanate.

rhodanide. More commonly Rhodanate, same as thiocyanate.
See: Potassium Thiocyanate.

•**RH_o(D) immune globulin.** (RH_oD ih-MYOON GLAB-byoo-lin) *USP.*
Use: Immunization.
See: BayRho-D Full Dose.
Gamulin Rh.
$MICRh_o$GAM.
HyperRHO S/D Mini-Dose.
RhoGAM.
Rhophylac.
WinRho SD.
WinRho SDF.

RH_o(D) immune globulin intravenous (human). (RH_oD ih-MYOON GLAB-byoo-lin) *Formerly RH_o Immune Human Globulin.*
Use: Immune thrombocytopenic purpura, immunizing agent (passive). [Orphan Drug]
See: WinRho SDF.

RhoGAM. (Ortho-Clinical Diagnostics) Rh_o(D) immune globulin 5% ± 1% gamma globulin. Sodium chloride 2.9 mg, polysorbate 80 0.01%, glycine 15 mg/mL. Preservative free. Filtrated. Soln. for Inj. Pkg. Prefilled single-dose syringe, package insert, control form, patient ID card. 5s, 25s, 100s. *Rx.*
Use: Immunization.

RhoGAM Ultra Filtered Plus. (Ortho-Clinical Diagnostics) Rh_o(D) immune globulin 300 mcg (1,500 units). Glycine 15 mg/mL, polysorbate 80 0.01%, sodium chloride 2.9 mg/mL. Preservative free. Inj., Soln. Package w/single-dose syringe, control form, and patient ID card. 1s, 5s, 25s. *Rx.*
Use: Biologic and immunological agent, immune globulin.

Rhophylac. (CSL Behring) Rh_o(D) immune globulin IV (human) 1,500 units (300 mcg). Glycine, sodium chloride. Preservative free. Inj. Soln. Prefilled syringes. 2 mL. *Rx.*
Use: Immunization.

Rhythmin. (Sidmak) Procainamide 250 mg, 500 mg. SR Tab. Bot. 100s, 500s, 1000s. *Rx.*
Use: Antiarrhythmic.

RiaSTAP. (CSL Behring) Fibrinogen concentrate (human) ≈ 1 g (900 to 1,300 mg). Albumin 400 to 700 mg. Preservative free. Inj., Lyophilized Pow. for Soln. Single-use vial. *Rx.*
Use: Hemostatic, systemic.

Riax. (Artesa Labs) Benzoyl peroxide 5.5%, 9.5%. Parabens, wax. Foam; topical. 100 g. *Rx.*
Use: Topical anti-infective, antibiotic agent.

•**ribaminol.** (rye-BAM-ih-nahl) USAN.
Use: Memory adjuvant.

RibaPak. (Par) Ribavirin 400 mg, 600 mg. Lactose, PEG 3350. Film-coated. Tab. UD 14s. Also available in a 400 mg and 600 mg combination package (1000 mg/day). *Rx.*
Use: Antiviral agent.

Ribasphere. (Kadmon Pharmaceuticals) Ribavirin. **Cap.:** 200 mg. Lactose. Pellet filled. 42s, 56s, 70s, 84s, 140s, 168s, 180s. **Tab.:** 200 mg, 400 mg, 600 mg. Lactose, PEG 3350. Film-coated. 56s (except 200 mg), 168s (200 mg only), 250s (600 mg only), 500s (except 600 mg); *RibaPak* 800 and 1,000 dose packs (400 mg only), *RibaPak* 1,000 and 1,200 dose packs (600 mg only) (Each *RibaPak* 800 dose pack contains 14 ribavirin 400 mg tablets. Each *RibaPak* 1,000 dose pack contains 7 ribavirin 400 mg tablets and 7 ribavirin 600 mg tablets. Each *RibaPak* 1,200 dose pack contains 14 ribavirin 600 mg tablets.). *Rx.*
Use: Antiviral agents.

Ribatab. (PRX Pharmaceuticals) Ribavirin 400 mg, 600 mg. Lactose, PEG 3350. Film-coated. Tab. UD 14s. Also available in a 400 mg and 600 mg combination package (1000 mg/day). *Rx.*
Use: Antiviral agent.

•**ribavirin.** (rye-buh-VIE-rin) *USP.*
Use: Antiviral.
See: Copegus.
Moderiba.
Rebetol.
Ribasphere.
RibPak.
Ribatab.
Virazole.

ribavirin. (Various Mfr.) Ribavirin. **Cap.:** 200 mg. 42s, 56s, 70s, 84s, 180s, 1,000s, UD 100s. **Tab.:** 200 mg. 168s 180s, 1,000s, UD 50s. *Rx.*
Use: Antiviral agent.

ribavirin. (Zydus) Ribavirin 400 mg, 500 mg. PEG. Film-coated. Tab. 28s,

56s, 60s. *Rx.*
Use: Antiviral agent.

ribavirin and interferon alfa-2b, recombinant.
Use: Antineoplastic.

•**riboflavin.** (RYE-boh-FLAY-vin) *USP.*
Use: Vitamin (enzyme co-factor), water-soluble vitamin.
See: B_2-400.
Cyto B2.
Vitamin B_2.

riboflavin. (Various Mfr.) Riboflavin 50 mg, 100 mg. Tab. Bot. 100s, 250s. *OTC.*
Use: Water-soluble vitamin.

•**riboflavin 5′-phosphate sodium.** (RYE-boh-FLAY-vin) *USP.*
Use: Vitamin.

•**riboprine.** (RYE-boe-PREEN) USAN.
Use: Antineoplastic.

Ribozyme. (Fellows) Riboflavin-5-phosphate sodium 50 mg/mL Inj. Vial 10 mL. *Rx.*

ricin (blocked) conjugated murine MCA. (ImmunoGen)
Use: Antineoplastic. [Orphan Drug]

Ricola Herb Throat Drops. (Ricola USA) Menthol. **1.1 mg:** Aspartame, phenylalanine 1 mg. Sugar free. Lemon mint flavor. 19s. **1.5 mg:** Peppermint, sugar. Lemon mint flavor. 24s. **2 mg:** Honey, natural cherry concentrate, peppermint, sugar. Cherry honey flavor. 24s. Loz. *OTC.*
Use: Mouth and throat product.

•**ricolinostat.** (RI-koe-LIN-oh-stat) USAN.
Use: Antineoplastic.

Ricolon Solution. (Sanofi-Synthelabo) Ricolon concentrate. Soln. *Rx.*
Use: Leucocytotic preparation.

RID. (Bayer) Pyrethrins 0.33%, piperonyl butoxide 4%. **Mousse:** Cetearyl alcohol, SD alcohol, isobutene. 165 mL w/comb. **Shampoo:** SD alcohol. 60 mL, 120 mL, 240 mL, and 120 mL kits containing gel, comb, and lice control spray. *OTC.*
Use: Scabicide/pediculicide.

•**ridaforolimus.** (rid-a-for-OH-li-mus) USAN.
Use: Antineoplastic.

Rid•a•Pain•HP. (Pfeiffer) Capsaicin 0.075%, alcohols, parabens. Cream. Tube. 45 g. *OTC.*
Use: Analgesic.

Ridaura. (GlaxoSmithKline) Auranofin 3 mg. Cap. Bot. 60s. *Rx.*
Use: Antirheumatic.

Rid Lice Control Spray. (Pfizer) Synthetic pyrethroids 0.5%, related compounds 0.065%, aromatic petroleum hydrocarbons 0.664%. Spray. Can 5 oz. *OTC.*
Use: Pediculicide.

Rid Lice Elimination System. (Pfizer) Rid lice killing shampoo, nit removal comb, Rid lice control spray and instruction booklet/unit. *OTC.*
Use: Pediculicide.

•**ridogrel.** (RYE-doe-grell) USAN.
Use: Thromboxane synthetase inhibitor.

•**rifabutin.** (RIFF-uh-BYOO-tin) *USP.*
Use: Anti-infective (antimycobacterial), MAC disease; antituberculosal.
See: Mycobutin.

rifabutin. (Various Mfr.) Rifabutin 150 mg. Cap. 60s, 100s. *Rx.*
Use: Anti-infective, antituberculosis agent.

Rifadin. (Aventis) Rifampin. **150 mg/Cap.:** Bot. 30s. **300 mg/Cap.:** Bot. 30s, 60s, 100s. **Pow. for Inj.:** 600 mg. Vials. *Rx.*
Use: Antituberculous.

•**rifalazil.** (RIFF-ah-lah-zill) USAN.
Use: Antibacterial.

Rifamate. (Aventis) Rifampin 300 mg, isoniazid 150 mg. Cap. Bot. 60s. *Rx.*
Use: Antituberculosal.

•**rifametane.** (RIFF-ah-met-ane) USAN.
Use: Anti-infective.

•**rifamexil.** (riff-ah-MEX-ill) USAN.
Use: Anti-infective.

•**rifamide.** (RIFF-am-ide) USAN.
Use: Anti-infective.

•**rifampin.** (RIFF-am-pin) *USP.* Rifampin, isoniazid, and pyrazinamide. Tablets.
Use: Anti-infective, antituberculostatic.
See: Rifadin.
Rifater.
Rimactane.

rifampin. (Akorn-Strides) Rifampin 600 mg. Lyophilized Pow. for Inj. Vial. *Rx.*
Use: Anti-infective agent, antituberculosis agent.

rifampin. (Various Mfr.) Rifampin 150 mg, 300 mg. Cap. Bot. 30s, 60s (300 mg only), 100s, 500s (300 mg only). *Rx.*
Use: Antituberculosal.

•**rifampin and isoniazid.** *USP.*
Use: Anti-infective (tuberculostatic).
See: IsonaRif.
Rifamate.

•**rifampin, isoniazid, and pyrazinamide.** *USP.*
Use: Anti-infective (tuberculostatic).
See: Rifater.

•**rifampin, isoniazid, pyrazinamide, and ethambutol hydrochloride.** *USP.*
Use: Anti-infective (tuberculostatic).

•**rifamycin.** (RIF-a-MYE-sin) USAN.
Use: Treatment of traveler's diarrhea.

•**rifamycin sodium.** (RIF-a-MYE-sin) USAN.
Use: Treatment of traveler's diarrhea.

•**rifapentine.** (RIFF-ah-pen-teen) USAN.
Use: Anti-infective, antituberculosal.
See: Priftin.

rifapentine.
Use: Pulmonary tuberculosis; *mycobacterium avium* complex in AIDS patients. [Orphan Drug]

Rifater. (Aventis) Rifampin 120 mg, isoniazid 50 mg, pyrazinamide 300 mg. Tab. Bot. 60s. *Rx.*
Use: Antituberculosal.

•**rifaximin.** (riff-AX-ih-min) USAN.
Use: Anti-infective.
See: Xifaxan.

r-IFN-beta. Recombinant interferon beta.

RIG. *Acronym for rabies immune globulin.*
Use: Immunization, rabies.
See: Imogam.

•**rigosertib.** (RIG-oh-SER-tib) USAN.
Use: Antineoplastic.

•**rigosertib sodium.** (RIG-oh-SER-tib) USAN.
Use: Antineoplastic.

•**rilapladib.** (ri-LAP-la-dib) USAN.
Use: Atherosclerosis.

•**rilimogene galvacirepvec.** (ri-LIM-oh-jeen GAL-vas-i-REP-vek) USAN.
Use: Antineoplastic.

•**rilimogene glafolivec.** (ri-LIM-oh-jeen gla-FOL-i-vek) USAN.
Use: Antineoplastic.

•**rilonacept.** (ri-LON-a-sept) USAN.
Use: Immunomodulator.
See: Arcalyst.

•**rilotumumab.** (ril-oh-TOOM-ue-mab) USAN.
Use: Antineoplastic.

•**rilpivirine.** (RIL-pi-VIR-een) USAN.
Use: Treatment of HIV infection.
See: Edurant.
W/Emtricitabine, Tenofovir Disoproxil Fumarate.
See: Complera.

•**rilpivirine hydrochloride.** (RIL-pi-VIR-een) USAN.
Use: Treatment of HIV infection.

Rilutek. (Covis) Riluzole 50 mg. Tab. *Rx.*
Use: Amyotrophic lateral sclerosis agent.

•**riluzole.** (RILL-you-zole) USAN.
Use: Amyotrophic lateral sclerosis agent. [Orphan Drug]
See: Rilutek.

riluzole. (Various Mfr.) Riluzole 50 mg. May contain PEG. Tab. 30s, 60s, 100s, 500s, 1,000s. *Rx.*
Use: Amyotrophic lateral sclerosis agent.

•**rimabotulinumtoxinB.** (RIM-a-BOT-ue-LYE-num-TOX-in-BEE) USAN.
Use: Botulinum toxin.

Rimactane. (Novartis) Rifampin 300 mg. Cap. Bot. 30s, 60s, 100s. *Rx.*
Use: Antituberculous.

Rimadyl. (Roche) *Rx.*
Use: Analgesic, NSAID.
See: Carprofen.

•**rimantadine hydrochloride.** (rih-MAN-tuh-deen) *USP.*
Use: Antiviral.
See: Flumadine.

rimantadine hydrochloride. (Various Mfr.) Rimantadine hydrochloride 100 mg. Tab. 100s, 1,000s. *Rx.*
Use: Antiviral agent.

•**rimcazole hydrochloride.** (RIM-kazz-OLE) USAN.
Use: Antipsychotic.

•**rimegepant.** (ri-ME-je-pant) USAN.
Use: Agent for migraine.

•**rimegepant sulfate.** (ri-ME-je-pant) USAN.
Use: Agent for migraine.

•**rimexolone.** (rih-MEX-oh-lone) USAN.
Use: Ophthalmic corticosteroid.
See: Vexol.

•**rimiterol hydrobromide.** (RIH-mih-TER-ole) USAN.
Use: Bronchodilator.

•**rimonabant.** (RIM-oh-nab-ant) USAN.
Use: Investigational selective cannabinoid type 1 receptor blocker; weight loss.

Rimso-50. (Research Industries) Dimethyl sulfoxide in a 50% aqueous soln. Bot. 50 mL. *Rx.*
Use: Interstitial cystitis agent.

Rinade. (Econo Med Pharmaceuticals) Chlorpheniramine maleate 8 mg, phenylephrine hydrochloride 20 mg, methscopolamine nitrate 2.5 mg. Cap. Bot. 120s. *Rx.*
Use: Anticholinergic; antihistamine, decongestant.

•**rindopepimut.** (RIN-doe-PEP-i-mut) USAN.
Use: Immunotherapeutic agent.

Ringer's in 5% dextrose. (Various Mfr.) Dextrose 50 g, calories 170, Na^+ ≈ 147 mEq, K^+ 4 mEq, Ca^{++} ≈ 4.5 mEq, Ca^- ≈ 4.5 mEq, Cl^- ≈ 156 mEq, osmolarity ≈ 560 mOsm/L. Soln. Bot. 500 mL. 1000 mL. *Rx.*

Use: Intravenous nutritional therapy, intravenous replenishment solution.

•**Ringer's injection.** *USP.*
Use: Fluid, electrolyte replacement; irrigant, ophthalmic.

Ringer's injection. (Various Mfr.) Na^+ ≈ 147 mEq, K^+ 4 mEq, Ca^{++} ≈ 4 mEq, Cl^- ≈ 156 mEq, osmolarity ≈ 310 mOsm/L. Soln. Bot. 500 mL. 1000 mL. *Rx.*
Use: Intravenous nutritional therapy, intravenous replenishment solution.

•**Ringer's injection, lactated.** *USP.*
Use: Fluid, electrolyte replacement.

Ringer's irrigation. (Various Mfr.) Sodium chloride 0.86 g, potassium chloride 0.03 g, calcium chloride 0.033 g/ 100 mL. Bot. 1 liter. *Rx.*
Use: Irrigant, ophthalmic.

•**rintatolimod.** (RIN-ta-TOL-i-mod) USAN.
Use: Antiviral.

•**riociguat.** (RYE-oh-SIG-ue-at) USAN.
Use: Vasodilator, soluble guanylate cyclase stimulator.
See: Adempas.

Riomet. (Ranbaxy) Metformin hydrochloride 500 mg/5 mL. Saccharin, cherry flavor. Oral Soln. Bot. 120 mL, 480 mL. *Rx.*
Use: Antidiabetic agent, biguanide.

Riopan Plus Double Strength Suspension. (Wyeth) Magaldrate 1080 mg, simethicone 40 mg/5 mL. Bot. 360 mL. *OTC.*
Use: Antacid; antiflatulent.

Riopan Plus Double Strength Tablets. (Wyeth) Magaldrate 1080 mg, simethicone 20 mg. Chew. Tab. Bot. 60s. *OTC.*
Use: Antacid; antiflatulent.

Riopan Plus Tablets. (Wyeth) Magaldrate 480 mg, simethicone 20 mg. Chew. Tab. Bot. 50s, 100s. *OTC.*
Use: Antacid; antiflatulent.

•**rioprostil.** (RYE-oh-PRAHS-till) USAN.
Use: Gastric antisecretory.

•**ripazepam.** (rip-AZE-eh-pam) USAN.
Use: Anxiolytic.

Risa-Bid. (Rising) 1 billion CFU blend of *L. acidophilus, L. bulgaricus, B. bifidum, S. thermophilus.* Tab. 100s. *OTC.*
Use: Probiotic.

RisaQuad. (Rising) 8 billion CFU blend of *L. acidophilus, Bifidobacterium, L. paracasei, S. thermophilus.* Gluten free and lactose free. Cap. 30s. *OTC.*
Use: Probiotic.

RisaQuad-2 Double Strength. (Rising) 16 billion CFU blend of *L. acidophilus, Bifidobacterium, L. paracasei, S. thermophilus.* Gluten free, lactose free, and preservative free. Cap. 30s. *OTC.*
Use: Probiotic.

•**risedronate sodium.** (riss-ED-row-nate) USAN.
Use: Bisphosphonate.
See: Actonel.
Atelvia.

•**rismorelin porcine.** (riss-more-ELL-in PORE-sine) USAN.
Use: Hormone, growth hormone-releasing.

•**risocaine.** (RIZZ-oh-cane) USAN.
Use: Anesthetic, local.

•**risotilide hydrochloride.** (rih-SO-tih-LIDE) USAN.
Use: Cardiovascular agent (antiarrhythmic).

Risperdal. (Janssen) Risperidone. **Tab.:** 0.25 mg, 0.5 mg, 1 mg, 2 mg, 3 mg, 4 mg. Lactose. Bot. 60s, 500s (except 4 mg), UD 100s. **Oral Soln.:** 1 mg/mL. Bot. 30 mL w/calibrated pipette. *Rx.*
Tall Man: RisperDAL
Use: Antipsychotic, benzisoxazole derivative.

Risperdal Consta. (Janssen) Risperidone 12.5 mg, 25 mg, 37.5 mg, 50 mg. Inj., Pow. for Soln., ER. Vials/Kits. Dose pack contains prefilled syringe and 2 mL of diluent. *Rx.*
Tall Man: RisperDAL
Use: Antipsychotic, benzisoxazole derivatives.

Risperdal M-Tab. (Janssen) Risperidone 0.5 mg (phenylalanine 0.14 mg), 1 mg (phenylalanine 0.28 mg), 2 mg (phenylalanine 0.42 mg), 3 mg (phenylalanine 0.63 mg), 4 mg (phenylalanine 0.84 mg). Aspartame, mannitol, peppermint oil. Orally disintegrating tab. UD 28s, UD 30s (0.5 mg, 1 mg only). *Rx.*
Tall Man: RisperDAL
Use: Antipsychotic, benzisoxazole derivative.

•**risperidone.** (RISS-PURR-ih-dohn) USAN.
Tall Man: risperiDONE
Use: Antipsychotic, neuroleptic, benzisoxazole derivative.
See: Risperdal.
Risperdal Consta.
Risperdal M-Tab.

risperidone. (Dr. Reddy's Laboratories) Risperidone 0.5 mg, 1 mg, 2 mg, 3 mg, 4 mg. Aspartame, mannitol, phenylalanine 2.1 mg (0.5 mg), 4.21 mg (1 mg), 8.4 mg (2, 3, and 4 mg). Orally disintegrating Tab. UD 30s and 100s. *Rx.*
Use: Antipsychotic agent, benzisoxazole derivative.

risperidone. (Teva) Risperidone. **Tab.:** 0.25 mg, 0.5 mg, 1 mg, 2 mg, 3 mg, 4 mg. Lactose, PEG. Film coated. 60s, 500s (except 4 mg). **Soln.:** 1 mg/mL. Sorbitol. 30 mL w/calibrate pipette. *Rx.*
Use: Antipsychotic agent, benzisoxazole derivative.

risperidone. (Various Mfr.) Risperidone 1 mg/mL. Soln. Bot. w/calibrated pipette. 30 mL. *Rx.*
Use: Antipsychotic agent, benzisoxazole derivative.

•**ristianol phosphate.** (riss-TIE-ah-NOLE) USAN.
Use: Immunoregulator.

Ritalin. (Novartis) Methylphenidate hydrochloride 5 mg, 10 mg, 20 mg. Lactose (except 20 mg), sucrose (20 mg only), talc (20 mg only). Tab. Bot. 100s. *c-II.*
Use: Central nervous system stimulant.

Ritalin LA. (Novartis) Methylphenidate hydrochloride 10 mg, 20 mg, 30 mg, 40 mg. Sugar spheres, talc. ER Cap. Bot. 100s. *c-II.*
Use: Central nervous system stimulant.

Ritalin-SR. (Novartis) Methylphenidate hydrochloride 20 mg, lactose, cetostearyl alcohol, mineral oil, color-additive free. SR Tab. Bot. 100s. *c-II.*
Use: Central nervous system stimulant.

•**ritanserin.** (rih-TAN-ser-in) USAN.
Use: Serotonin antagonist.

•**ritodrine.** (RIH-toe-DREEN) USAN.
Use: Muscle relaxant.

•**ritolukast.** (rih-tah-LOO-kast) USAN.
Use: Antiasthmatic (leukotriene antagonist).

•**ritonavir.** (rih-TON-a-veer) USAN.
Use: Antiretroviral, protease inhibitor.
See: Norvir.

ritonavir/lopinavir.
Use: Antiretroviral, protease inhibitor.
See: Kaletra.

Rituxan. (Biogen Idec/Genentech) Rituximab 10 mg/mL. Polysorbate 80 0.7 mg/mL. Preservative free. Inj. Single-use vial. 10 mL, 50 mL. *Rx.*
Use: Antineoplastic; monoclonal antibody.

•**rituximab.** (rih-TUCK-sih-mab) USAN.
Tall Man: riTUXimab
Use: Antineoplastic (microtubule inhibitor); monoclonal antibody.
See: Rituxan.

•**rivanicline galactarate.** (rye-VAN-i-kleen gal-AK-tar-ate) USAN.
Use: Ulcerative colitis; nicotinic receptor agonist.

•**rivaroxaban.** (RIV-a-ROX-a-ban) USAN.
Use: Selective factor Xa inhibitor.
See: Xarelto.

rivastigmine tartrate.
Use: Cholinesterase inhibitor.
See: Exelon.

rivastigmine tartrate. (Dr. Reddy's Laboratories) Rivastigmine 1.5 mg, 3 mg, 4.5 mg, 6 mg. Cap. 60s, 500s, UD 100s. *Rx.*
Use: Cholinesterase inhibitor.

•**rivipansel.** (RIV-i-PAN-sel) USAN.
Use: Treatment of sickle cell vaso-occlusive crisis.

•**rivipansel sodium.** (RIV-i-PAN-sel) USAN.
Use: Treatment of sickle cell vaso-occlusive crisis.

Rixubis. (Baxter Bioscience) Factor IX (recombinant) 250 units, 500 units, 1,000 units, 2,000 units, 3,000 units. Preservative free. Inj., lyophilized Pow. for Soln. Kit (w/5 mL sterile water for injection and a transfer device) w/single-dose vial (contains calcium chloride 4 mM, L-histidine 20 mM, mannitol 110 mM, 0.005% polysorbate 80, sodium chloride 60 mM, and sucrose 35 mM when reconstituted). *Rx.*
Use: Antihemophilic agent.

•**rizatriptan benzoate.** (rye-zah-TRIP-tan BENZ-oh-ate) USAN.
Use: Antimigraine, serotonin 5-HT_1 receptor agonist.
See: Maxalt.
Maxalt-MLT.

rizatriptan benzoate. (Mylan) Rizatriptan benzoate 5 mg (equiv. to rizatriptan benzoate 7.265 mg), 10 mg (equiv. to rizatriptan benzoate 14.53 mg). May contain aspartame, mannitol, phenylalanine 1.68 mg (5 mg) and 3.36 mg (10 mg), sorbitol. Tab., disintegrating. 6s, 9s, 1,000s. *Rx.*
Use: Agent for migraine, serotonin 5-HT_1 receptor agonist.

rizatriptan benzoate. (Various Mfr.) Rizatriptan 5 mg (equiv. to rizatriptan benzoate 7.265 mg), 10 mg (equiv. to rizatriptan benzoate 14.53 mg). May contain lactose. Tab. 12s, 100s, 500s, UD 6s, UD 12s, UD 18s, UD 30s. *Rx.*
Use: Agent for migraine, serotonin 5-HT_1 receptor agonist.

•**rizatriptan sulfate.** (rye-zah-TRIP-tan) USAN.
Use: Antimigraine.

RMS. (Upsher-Smith) Morphine sulfate 5 mg, 10 mg, 20 mg, 30 mg. Rectal. Supp. Box 12s. *c-II.*
Use: Opioid analgesic.

R-Natal OB. (R3 Pharmaceuticals) Folic

acid 1 mg, iron 20 mg, vitamins D 400 units, E 30 units, B_1 2 mg, B_2 4 mg, B_6 20 mg, B_{12} 30 mcg, C 100 mg, Cu, Zn, DHA 320 mg. Gluten free, lactose free, sugar free. Beeswax, glycerin, soy lecithin. Cap., softgel. 30s. *Rx.*
Use: Prenatal vitamin with minerals.

Robafen. (Major) Guaifenesin 100 mg/5 mL, alcohol 3.5%. Syr. Bot. 118 mL, 240 mL, pt, gal. *OTC.*
Use: Expectorant.

Robafen AC Cough. (Major) Guaifenesin 100 mg, codeine phosphate 10 mg/5 mL, alcohol 3.5%, parabens. Syrup. Bot. 473 mL. *c-v.*
Use: Antitussive; expectorant, narcotic.

Robafen CF. (Major) Pseudoephedrine hydrochloride 30 mg, dextromethorphan HBr 10 mg, guaifenesin 100 mg per 5 mL. Saccharin, sorbitol, alcohol free. Liq. Bot. 237 mL. *OTC.*
Use: Upper respiratory combination, antitussive and expectorant combination.

Robafen DAC. (Major) Pseudoephedrine 30 mg, codeine phosphate 10 mg, guaifenesin 100 mg/5 mL, alcohol 1.4%. Liq. Bot. Pt. *c-v.*
Use: Antitussive, decongestant, expectorant.

Robafen DM. (Major) Dextromethorphan HBr 10 mg, guaifenesin 100 mg/5 mL. **Liq.:** Corn syrup, glucose, glycerin, menthol, saccharin, sodium benzoate. 237 mL. **Syrup:** Alcohol 1.4%. 473 mL. *OTC.*
Use: Antitussive; expectorant.

Robafen PE. (Major) Pseudoephedrine hydrochloride 30 mg, guaifenesin 100 mg/5 mL, glucose, corn syrup, saccharin, alcohol free. Liq. Bot. 118 mL. *OTC.*
Use: Upper respiratory combination, decongestant, expectorant.

robanul.
See: Robinul.

RoBathol Bath Oil. (Pharmaceutical Specialties) Cottonseed oil, alkyl aryl polyether alcohol. Lanolin free. Oil. Bot. 240 mL, 480 mL, gal. *OTC.*
Use: Dermatologic.

•**robatumumab.** (ROE-ba-TOOM-ue-mab) USAN.
Use: Antineoplastic.

Robaxin. (Actient Pharmaceuticals) Methocarbamol 500 mg. Saccharin. Tab. 100s, 500s, *Disco-Pak* 100s. *Rx.*
Use: Muscle relaxant.

Robaxin. (West-Ward) Methocarbamol 100 mg/mL in a soln. of polyethylene glycol 300. Inj. Vial 10 mL. *Rx.*
Use: Muscle relaxant.

Robaxin-750. (Actient Pharmaceuticals) Methocarbamol 750 mg. Saccharin. Tab. Bot. 100s, 500s, *Disco-Pak* 100s. *Rx.*
Use: Muscle relaxant.

Robimycin. (Wyeth) Erythromycin 250 mg. Tab. Bot. 100s, 500s. *Rx.*
Use: Anti-infective, erythromycin.

Robinul. (Shionogi) Glycopyrrolate 1 mg, lactose. Tab. 100s. *Rx.*
Use: Anticholinergic.

Robinul Forte. (Shionogi) Glycopyrrolate 2 mg, lactose. Tab. 100s. *Rx.*
Use: Anticholinergic.

Robinul Injectable. (West-Ward) Glycopyrrolate 0.2 mg/mL, benzyl alcohol 0.9%. Vial 1 mL, 2 mL, 5 mL, 20 mL. *Rx.*
Use: Anticholinergic.

Robitussin Adult Peak Cold Nasal Relief. (Pfizer Consumer Healthcare) Acetaminophen 325 mg, phenylephrine hydrochloride 5 mg. Film coated. PEG. Tab. 20s. *OTC.*
Use: Upper respiratory combination; decongestant and analgesic combination.

Robitussin Adult Peak Cold Nighttime Nasal Relief. (Pfizer Consumer Healthcare) Acetaminophen 325 mg, chlorpheniramine maleate 2 mg, phenylephrine hydrochloride 5 mg. Film coated. PEG. Tab. 20s. *OTC.*
Use: Upper respiratory combination; decongestant, antihistamine, and analgesic combination.

Robitussin Children's Cough & Cold CF. (Pfizer Consumer Healthcare) Dextromethorphan hydrobromide 5 mg, guaifenesin 50 mg, phenylephrine hydrochloride 2.5 mg. Glycerin, propylene glycol, sodium 3 mg, sodium benzoate, sorbitol, sucralose. Liq. 118 mL. *Rx.*
Use: Upper respiratory combination, antitussive and expectorant combination.

Robitussin Children's Cough & Cold Long-Acting. (Pfizer Consumer Healthcare) Chlorpheniramine maleate 1 mg, dextromethorphan hydrobromide 7.5 mg. Glycerin, propylene glycol, sodium 3 mg per 5 mL, sodium benzoate, sorbitol, sucralose. Alcohol free. Fruit punch flavor. Liq. 118 mL. *OTC.*
Use: Upper respiratory combination, antitussive combination.

Robitussin Children's Cough Long-Acting. (Pfizer Consumer Healthcare) Dextromethorphan hydrobromide 7.5 mg per 5 mL. Corn syrup, glycerin,

propylene glycol, saccharin, sodium benzoate. Alcohol free. Fruit punch flavor. Syrup. 118 mL. *OTC.*
Use: Nonnarcotic antitussive.

Robitussin Cough & Cold D. (Wyeth Consumer) Dextromethorphan hydrobromide 15 mg, guaifenesin 200 mg, pseudoephedrine hydrochloride 30 mg per 5 mL. Menthol, PEG, sodium 4 mg, sorbitol, sucralose. Liq. 118 mL. *OTC.*
Use: Upper respiratory combination, antitussive and expectorant combination.

Robitussin Cough & Congestion. (Wyeth Consumer) Dextromethorphan 10 mg, guaifenesin 200 mg per 5 mL. Alcohol free. Corn syrup, menthol, PEG, saccharin, sorbitol. Liq. 118 mL. *OTC.*
Use: Upper respiratory combination, antitussive with expectorant.

Robitussin Cough, Cold & Flu Nighttime. (Wyeth Consumer) Dextromethorphan HBr 5 mg, chlorpheniramine maleate 1 mg, phenylephrine hydrochloride 2.5 mg, acetaminophen 160 mg per 5 mL. Alcohol free. Menthol, sodium 2 mg/5 mL, sorbitol, sucralose. Syrup. 118 mL. *OTC.*
Use: Upper respiratory combination, antitussive combination.

Robitussin Cough DM. (Wyeth Consumer) Dextromethorphan HBr 10 mg, guaifenesin 100 mg per 5 mL. Alcohol free. Glycerin, corn syrup, menthol, saccharin sodium. Liq. 118 mL. *OTC.*
Use: Upper respiratory combination, antitussive with expectorant.

Robitussin Cough Drops. (Wyeth Consumer) Menthol 7.4 mg, 10 mg, eucalyptus oil, sucrose, corn syrup. Loz. Pkg. 9s, 25s, menthol 10 mg, eucalyptus oil, sucrose, corn syrup, honey-lemon flavor. Loz. Pkg. 9s, 25s. *OTC.*
Use: Antitussive.

Robitussin Cough Long-Acting. (Wyeth Consumer) Dextromethorphan HBr 15 mg/5 mL. Alcohol, glucose, corn syrup, saccharin, cherry flavor. Liq. Bot. 118 mL, 237 mL. *OTC.*
Use: Nonnarcotic antitussive.

Robitussin Cough Sugar-Free DM. (Wyeth Consumer) Dextromethorphan HBr 10 mg, guaifenesin 100 mg per 5 mL. Sugar and alcohol free. Acesulfame K, methylparaben, PEG, saccharin. Liq. Bot. 118 mL. *OTC.*
Use: Upper respiratory combination, antitussive with expectorant.

Robitussin Lingering Cold Long-Acting Cough. (Pfizer Consumer Healthcare) Dextromethorphan hydrobromide 15 mg per 5 mL. Alcohol, corn syrup, glucose, glycerin, menthol, saccharin, sodium benzoate. Liq. 118 mL. *OTC.*
Use: Nonnarcotic antitussive.

Robitussin Lingering Cold Long-Acting CoughGels. (Pfizer Consumer Healthcare) Dextromethorphan hydrobromide 15 mg. Coconut oil, glycerin, mannitol, PEG, sorbitol. Liquid-filled. Cap. 20s. *OTC.*
Use: Nonnarcotic antitussive.

Robitussin Mucus + Chest Congestion. (Pfizer Consumer Health) Guaifenesin 100 mg per 5 mL. Corn syrup, glucose, glycerin, menthol, propylene glycol, saccharin, sodium 2 mg, sodium benzoate. Alcohol free. Liq. 118 mL. *OTC.*
Use: Respiratory agent, expectorant.

Robitussin Night Time Pediatric Cough & Cold. (Wyeth Consumer) Diphenhydramine hydrochloride 6.25 mg, phenylephrine hydrochloride 2.5 mg per 5 mL. Alcohol free. Sodium 3 mg/5 mL, sorbitol, sucralose. Liq. 118 mL. *OTC.*
Use: Upper respiratory combination, antitussive combination.

Robitussin Pediatric Cough. (Pfizer Consumer Healthcare) Dextromethorphan hydrobromide 7.5 mg/5 mL. Alcohol and sugar free. Saccharin, sorbitol, cherry flavor. Syrup. 118 mL. *OTC.*
Use: Nonnarcotic antitussive.

Robitussin Pediatric Cough & Cold CF. (Wyeth Consumer) Dextromethorphan HBr 2 mg, guaifenesin 40 mg, phenylephrine hydrochloride 1 mg per 1 mL. Alcohol free. PEG, sorbitol, sucralose. Drops. 30 mL with oral dosing device. *OTC.*
Use: Upper respiratory combination, antitussive and expectorant combination.

Robomol/ASA. (Major) Methocarbamol w/ASA. Tab. Bot. 100s, 500s. *Rx.*
Use: Muscle relaxant; analgesic.

Rocaltrol. (Validus) Calcitriol. **Cap.:** 0.25 mcg, 0.5 mcg, sorbitol, parabens. Bot. 30s (0.25 mcg only), 100s. **Oral Soln.:** 1 mcg/mL. Bot. with dispensers. 15 mL. *Rx.*
Use: Antihypocalcemic; vitamin.

•**rocastine hydrochloride.** (row-KASS-teen) USAN.
Use: Antihistamine.

Rocephin. (Genentech) Ceftriaxone sodium (as base). **Pow. for Inj.:** 500 mg, 1 g, 2 g. **500 mg:** Vials. **1 g, 2 g:** Vials, piggyback vials, *ADD-Vantage* vials. **Inj.:** 1 g, 2 g. Dextrose. Frozen Pre-

mixed. 50 mL plastic containers. *Rx.*
Use: Anti-infective; cephalosporin.

•**rocuronium bromide.** (row-kuhr-OH-nee-uhm) USAN.
Use: Neuromuscular blocker, muscle relaxant.
See: Zemuron.

rocuronium bromide. (Various Mfr.) Rocuronium bromide 10 mg/mL. Inj., Soln. Multidose vial 5 mL, 10 mL. *Rx.*
Use: Muscle relaxant—adjunct to anesthesia, nondepolarizing neuromuscular blocker.

•**rodocaine.** (ROW-doe-cane) USAN.
Use: Anesthetic, local.

roentgenography.
See: Iodine Products, Diagnostic.

•**roflumilast.** (roe-FLUE-mi-last) USAN.
Use: Bronchial asthma; chronic obstructive pulmonary disease.
See: Daliresp.

•**roflurane.** (row-FLEW-rane) USAN.
Use: Anesthetic, general.

Rogaine. (Pfizer Consumer Health) Minoxidil 2%. Topical Soln. Bot. 60 mL w/multiple applicators. *OTC.*
Use: Antialopecia agent.

Rogaine Extra Strength for Men. (Pfizer Consumer Health) Minoxidil 5%. Alcohol. Soln. Bot. 60 mL w/dropper and sprayer applicators. 2s. *OTC.*
Use: Antialopecia agent.

Rogaine Men's Extra Strength. (Pfizer Consumer Health) Minoxidil 5%. Cetyl alcohol, SD alcohol, stearyl alcohol. Aer. Foam, Top. 60 g. *OTC.*
Use: Antialopecia agent.

•**rogletimide.** (row-GLETT-ih-MIDE) USAN.
Use: Antineoplastic (aromatase inhibitor).

Rolaids. (Pfizer Consumer Healthcare) Magnesium hydroxide 110 mg, calcium carbonate 550 mg. Dextrose, sucrose. Peppermint, spearmint, and cherry flavors. Chew. Tab. 12s, 36s, 150s, 250s, 300s. *OTC.*
Use: Antacid.

Rolaids Calcium Rich. (Pfizer Consumer Healthcare) Calcium carbonate 412 mg, magnesium hydroxide 80 mg. Chew. Tab. Bot. 12s, 36s, 75s, 150s. *OTC.*
Use: Antacid.

Rolaids Extra Strength. (Pfizer Consumer Healthcare) Magnesium hydroxide 135 mg, calcium carbonate 675 mg. Dextrose, sucrose. Cool strawberry, freshmint, fruit, tropical punch flavors. Chew. Tab. 10s, 30s, 100s. *OTC.*
Use: Antacid.

Rolaids Extra Strength Plus Gas Relief. (Pfizer Consumer Healthcare) Calcium carbonate 1177 mg, simethicone 80 mg. Corn syrup, maltodextrin, sodium 2 mg, sorbitol, sucrose. Chew. Tab. 6s, 12s, 36s. *OTC.*
Use: Antacid.

Rolaids Extra Strength Softchews. (Pfizer Consumer Healthcare) Calcium carbonate 1,177 mg (elemental calcium 470.8 mg). Corn syrup, corn syrup solids, nonfat dry milk, sucrose. Vanilla creme and wild cherry flavors. Chew. Tab. 18s. *OTC.*
Use: Mineral supplement; antacid.

Rolaids Multi-Symptom. (Pfizer Consumer Healthcare) Magnesium hydroxide 135 mg, calcium carbonate 675 mg, simethicone 60 mg, dextrose, sucrose. Cool mint and berry flavors. Chew. Tab. 10s, 30s, 100s. *OTC.*
Use: Antacid.

Rolatuss Expectorant. (Huckaby Pharmacal) Phenylephrine hydrochloride 5 mg, chlorpheniramine maleate 2 mg, codeine phosphate 9.85 mg, ammonium Cl 33.3 mg/5 mL, alcohol 5%. Bot. 480 mL. *c-v.*
Use: Antihistamine, antitussive, decongestant, expectorant.

Rolatuss Plain. (Major) Phenylephrine hydrochloride 5 mg, chlorpheniramine maleate 2 mg/5 mL. Liq. Bot. 473 mL. *OTC.*
Use: Antihistamine, decongestant.

Rolatuss w/Hydrocodone. (Major) Phenylpropanolamine hydrochloride 3.3 mg, phenylephrine hydrochloride 5 mg, pyrilamine maleate 3.3 mg, pheniramine maleate 3.3 mg, hydrocodone bitartrate 1.67 mg/5 mL. Liq. Bot. 480 mL. *c-III.*
Use: Antihistamine, antitussive, decongestant.

•**roletamide.** (row-LET-am-ide) USAN.
Use: Hypnotic; sedative.

•**rolgamidine.** (role-GAM-ih-deen) USAN.
Use: Antidiarrheal.

Rolicap. (Arcum) Vitamins A acetate 5000 units, D_2 400 units, B_1 3 mg, B_2 2.5 mg, B_6 10 mg, C 50 mg, niacinamide 20 mg, B_{12} 1 mcg. Chew. Tab. Bot. 100s, 1000s. *OTC.*
Use: Vitamin supplement.

•**rolicyprine.** (ROW-lih-SIGH-preen) USAN.
Use: Antidepressant.

•**rolipram.** (ROLE-ih-pram) USAN.
Use: Anxiolytic.

•**rolitetracycline.** (ROW-li-tet-rah-SIGH-kleen) USAN.
Use: Anti-infective.

•**rolitetracycline nitrate.** (ROW-li-tet-rah-SIGH-kleen) USAN. Tetrim.
Use: Anti-infective.

•**rolodine.** (ROW-low-deen) USAN.
Use: Muscle relaxant.

Romach Antacid. (Last) Magnesium carbonate 400 mg, sodium bicarbonate 250 mg. Tab. Strip pack 60s, 500s. *OTC.*
Use: Antacid.

•**romazarit.** (row-MAZZ-ah-rit) USAN.
Use: Anti-inflammatory; antirheumatic.

Romazicon. (Hoffman-La Roche) Flumazenil 0.1 mg/mL, parabens, EDTA. Inj. Vials 5 mL, 10 mL. *Rx.*
Use: Antidote.

Romex. (A.P.C.) **Troche:** Polymyxin B sulfate 1000 units, benzocaine 5 mg, cetalkonium Cl 2.5 mg, gramicidin 100 mcg, chlorpheniramine maleate 0.5 mg, tyrothricin 2 mg. Pkg. 10s. **Liq.:** Guaifenesin 200 mg, dextromethorphan HBr 60 mg, chlorpheniramine maleate 12 mg, phenylephrine hydrochloride 30 mg/fl oz. Bot. 4 oz. *Rx.*
Use: Antihistamine, antitussive, decongestant, expectorant; anti-infective.

Romex Cough & Cold Capsules. (A.P.C.) Guaifenesin 65 mg, dextromethorphan HBr 10 mg, chlorpheniramine maleate 1.5 mg, pyrilamine maleate 12.5 mg, phenylephrine hydrochloride 5 mg, acetaminophen 160 mg. Cap. Bot. 21s. *OTC.*
Use: Antihistamine, antitussive, decongestant, expectorant.

Romex Cough & Cold Tablets. (A.P.C.) Dextromethorphan HBr 7.5 mg, phenylephrine hydrochloride 2.5 mg, ascorbic acid 30 mg. Tab. Box 15s. *OTC.*
Use: Antitussive, decongestant.

•**romidepsin.** (ROE-mi-DEP-sin) USAN.
Tall Man: romiDEPsin
Use: Cutaneous T-cell lymphoma.
See: Istodax.

•**romiplostim.** (roe-MIP-loe-stim) USAN.
Tall Man: romiPLOStim
Use: Hematopoietic agent, thrombopoietin mimetic agent.
See: Nplate.

•**romosozumab.** (ROE-moe-SOZ-ue-mab) USAN.
Use: Treatment of osteoporosis.

•**romyelocel-L.** (ROE-mye-EL-oh-sel el) USAN.
Use: Treatment of myelosuppression.

•**ronacaleret hydrochloride.** (ROE-na-KAL-er-et) USAN.
Use: Antiviral.

Rondamine-DM. (Major) **Drops:** Pseudoephedrine 25 mg, carbinoxamine maleate 2 mg, dextromethorphan HBr 4 mg/mL. Bot. 30 mL. **Syrup:** Dextromethorphan HBr 15 mg, brompheniramine maleate 4 mg, pseudoephedrine hydrochloride 60 mg per 5 mL. Alcohol < 0.2%, grape flavor. Bot. 120 mL. 473 mL, 3.8 L. *Rx.*
Use: Upper respiratory combination, antihistamine, antitussive, decongestant.

Rondec-DM. (Alliant) Dextromethorphan HBr 15 mg, chlorpheniramine maleate 4 mg, phenylephrine hydrochloride 12.5 mg per 5 mL. Alcohol and sugar free. Saccharin, sorbitol. Grape flavor. Syr. Bot. 20 mL, 118 mL, 473 mL. *Rx.*
Use: Upper respiratory combination; antitussive combination.

Rondex DM. (Pack) Dextromethorphan HBr 3 mg, chlorpheniramine maleate 1 mg, phenylephrine hydrochloride 3.5 mg per 1 mL. Alcohol and sugar free. Saccharin, sorbitol. Grape flavor. Oral Drops. 30 mL with dropper. *Rx.*
Use: Upper respiratory combination, antitussive combination.

•**ronidazole.** (row-NYE-dazz-OLE) USAN.
Use: Antiprotozoal.

•**ronnel.** (RAHN-ell) USAN. Fenchlorphos.
Use: Insecticide (systemic).

•**rontalizumab.** (RON-ta-LIZ-ue-mab) USAN.
Use: Treatment of systemic lupus erythematosus.

•**ropidoxuridine.** (roe-PYE-dox-URE-i-deen) USAN.
Use: Treatment of cancer.

ropinirole. (Various Mfr.) Ropinirole hydrochloride. **Tab.:** 0.25 mg, 0.5 mg, 1 mg, 2 mg, 3 mg, 4 mg, 5 mg. May contain lactose, PEG. 100s, 1,000s. **ER Tab.:** 2 mg, 3 mg, 4 mg, 6 mg, 8 mg, 12 mg. May contain glyceryl, lactose, PEG. 30s, 90s, 500s, 1,800s (except 6 mg), UD 100s (3 mg, 6 mg, and 12 mg only). *Rx.*
Use: Antiparkinson agent, dopaminergic.

•**ropinirole hydrochloride.** (row-PIN-ih-role) USAN.
Tall Man: rOPINIRole
Use: Antiparkinsonian (D_2 receptor agonist).
See: Requip.
Requip XL.

•**ropitoin hydrochloride.** (ROW-pih-toe-in) USAN.
Use: Cardiovascular agent (antiarrhythmic).

ropivacaine hydrochloride.
Use: Anesthetic, local injectable.
See: Naropin.

•**ropizine.** (row-PIH-zeen) USAN.
Use: Anticonvulsant.

•**roquinimex.** (row-KWIH-nih-mex) USAN.
Use: Biological response modifier; immunomodulator; antineoplastic.

•**rosabulin.** (ROE-za-BUE-lin) USAN.
Use: Antineoplastic.

Rosadan. (Medimetriks Pharmaceuticals) Metronidazole 0.75%. Glycerin, wax. Cream. 45 g. *Rx.*
Use: Topical anti-infective, antibiotic agent.

Rosadan Cream Kit. (Medimetriks Pharmaceuticals) Metronidazole 0.75%. Glycerin, wax. Cream. 45 g w/*Rehyla* soap (473 mL). *Rx.*
Use: Topical anti-infective, antibiotic agent.

Rosaderm Kit. (River's Edge) Sodium sulfacetamide 10%, sulfur 5%. Disodium EDTA, mineral oil, parabens. Soap. 170 g, 340 g, kits w/*RE Cleansing Lotion. Rx.*
Use: Acne product, combination.

Rosanil. (Galderma) Sulfur 5%, sodium sulfacetamide 10%, EDTA, light mineral oil, parabens. Cleanser. 170 g. *Rx.*
Use: Keratolytic agent.

rosaniline dyes.
See: Fuchsin, Basic.
Methylrosaniline Cl.

•**rosaramicin.** (row-ZAR-ah-MY-sin) USAN. *Formerly Rosamicin.*
Use: Anti-infective.

•**rosaramicin butyrate.** (row-ZAR-ah-MY-sin BYOO-tih-rate) USAN. *Formerly Rosamicin Butyrate.*
Use: Anti-infective.

•**rosaramicin propionate.** (row-ZAR-ah-MY-sin PRO-pee-oh-nate) USAN. *Formerly Rosamicin Propionate.*
Use: Anti-infective.

•**rosaramicin sodium phosphate.** (row-ZAR-ah-MY-sin) USAN. *Formerly Rosamicin Sodium Phosphate.*
Use: Anti-infective.

•**rosaramicin stearate.** (row-ZAR-ah-MY-sin STEE-ah-rate) USAN. *Formerly Rosamicin Stearate.*
Use: Anti-infective.

rose bengal.
Use: Ophthalmic diagnostic product.

rose bengal. (Akorn) Rose bengal 1%. Bot. 5 mL.
Use: Diagnostic, tissue staining.

rose bengal. (Barnes-Hind) Rose bengal 1.3 mg. Strip. Box 100s. *OTC.*
Use: Diagnostic aid.

•**rose bengal sodium I 131 injection.** (rose BEN-gal) *USP.*
Use: Diagnostic aid (hepatic function), radiopharmaceutical.

•**rose bengal sodium I 125.** (rose BEN-gal) USAN.
Use: Radiopharmaceutical.

Rose-C. (Barth's) Vitamin C 300 mg, rose hip extract/5 mL. Liq. Dropper Bot. 2 oz, 8 oz. *OTC.*
Use: Vitamin supplement.

rose hips. (Burgin-Arden) Vitamin C 300 mg, in base of sorbitol. Bot. 4 oz, 8 oz. *OTC.*
Use: Vitamin supplement.

rose hips vitamin C. (Kirkman) Vitamin C 100 mg, 250 mg, 500 mg. Tab. Bot. 100s, 250s, 500s (except 100 mg). *OTC.*
Use: Vitamin supplement.

•**rose oil.** (rose) *NF.*
Use: Pharmaceutic aid; perfume.

rose water ointment.
Use: Emollient, ointment base.

•**rose water, stronger.** (rose) *NF.*
Use: Pharmaceutic aid; perfume.

•**rosiglitazone maleate.** (roe-sih-GLIH-tah-sone) USAN.
Use: Antidiabetic, thiazolidinedione.
See: Avandia.
W/Glimepiride.
See: Avandaryl.
W/Metformin.
See: Avandamet.

•**rosin.** (ROZZ-in) *USP.*
Use: Stiffening agent, pharmaceutical necessity.

•**rosoxacin.** (row-SOX-ah-sin) USAN.
Use: Anti-infective.

Ross SLD. (Ross) Low-residue nutritional supplement for patients restricted to a clear liquid feeding or with fat malabsorption disorders. Packet 1.35 oz. Ctn. 6s. Case 4 ctn. Can 13.5 oz. Case 6s. *OTC.*
Use: Nutritional supplement.

•**rostaporfin.** (roe-sta-POR-fin) USAN.
Use: Cutaneous carcinomas; Kaposi sarcomas; choroidal neovascularization.

•**rosuvastatin calcium.** (roe-SOO-va-sta-tin) USAN.
Use: Antihyperlipidemic agent, HMG-CoA reductase inhibitor.
See: Crestor.

Rotalex Test. (Orion) Latex slide

agglutination test for detection of rotavirus in feces. Kit 1s.
Use: Diagnostic aid.

Rotarix. (GlaxoSmithKline) Rotavirus human 89-12 strain (G1P[8] type); at least 10^6 cell culture infective dose per 1 mL (after reconstitution). Preservative free. Dextran, glucose, sorbitol, sucrose. Pow. for Susp., Lyophilized, Oral. Vials with 1 mL prefilled liquid diluent and transfer adapter for reconstitution. *Rx.*
Use: Agent for active immunization.

RotaTeq. (Merck) Rotavirus outer capsid protein (2.2×10^6 infectious units of G1, 2.8×10^6 infectious units of G2, 2.2×10^6 infectious units of G3, 2×10^6 infectious units of G4, 2.3×10^6 infectious units of rotavirus attachment protein P1A[8]) per 2 mL. Preservative free. Sucrose. Oral Susp. Single-dose tubes. 2 mL (10s). *Rx.*
Use: Immunization.

rotavirus vaccine live.
Use: Immunization.
See: Rotarix.
RotaTeq.

Rotazyme II. (Abbott Diagnostics) Enzyme immunoassay for detection of rotavirus antigen in feces. Test kit 50s.
Use: Diagnostic aid.

•**rotigaptide.** (roe-ti-GAP-tide) USAN.
Use: Antiarrhythmic agent.

•**rotigotine.** (ROE-ti-goe-tine) USAN.
Use: Antiparkinson agent, dopaminergic.
See: Neupro.

•**rotoxamine.** (row-TOX-ah-meen) USAN.
Use: Antihistamine.

•**rovelizumab.** (roe-ve-LYE-zue-mab) USAN.
Use: Immunomodulator.

Rowasa. (Alaven) Mesalamine 4 g/60 mL. EDTA, potassium metabisulfite, white petrolatum. Enema. 7s and 28s with lubricated applicator tip in disposable bots. *Rx.*
Use: Anti-inflammatory.

•**roxadimate.** (rox-AD-ih-mate) USAN.
Use: Sunscreen.

•**roxadustat.** (ROX-a-DOO-stat) USAN.
Use: Hematological agent.

Roxanol. (aaiPharma) Morphine sulfate 20 mg/mL. Oral Soln., concentrate. Bot. 30 mL, 120 mL w/calibrated dropper. *c-II.*
Use: Opioid analgesic.

Roxanol 100. (aaiPharma) Morphine sulfate 100 mg/5 mL. Oral Soln., concentrate. Bot. 240 mL with calibrated spoon. *c-II.*
Use: Opioid analgesic.

Roxanol T. (aaiPharma) Morphine sulfate 20 mg/mL. Flavored. Oral Soln., concentrate. Bot. 30 mL, 120 mL with calibrated dropper. *c-II.*
Use: Opioid analgesic.

•**roxarsone.** (ROX-AHR-sone) USAN.
Use: Anti-infective.

•**roxatidine acetate.** (ROX-ah-tih-DEEN) USAN.
Use: Antiulcer.

Roxicet. (Roxane) **Oral Soln.:** Oxycodone hydrochloride 5 mg, acetaminophen 325 mg/5 mL. Bot. UD 5 mL, 500 mL. **Tab.:** Oxycodone hydrochloride 5 mg, acetaminophen 325 mg, 0.4% alcohol. Bot. 100s, 500s, UD 100s. *c-II.*
Use: Analgesic combination, narcotic.

Roxicodone. (aaiPharma) **Oral Soln.:** Oxycodone hydrochloride 5 mg/5 mL. Sorbitol. Bot. 500 mL, UD 5 mL. **Tab.:** Oxycodone hydrochloride 15 mg, 30 mg. Lactose (15 mg, 30 mg only). Bot. 100s, UD 100s. *c-II.*
Use: Opioid analgesic.

Roxicodone Intensol. (aaiPharma) Oxycodone hydrochloride 20 mg/mL. Conc. Soln. Bot. 30 mL with calibrated dropper. *c-II.*
Use: Opioid analgesic.

•**roxifiban acetate.** (rox-ih-FIE-ban) USAN.
Use: Antithrombotic, fibrinogen receptor antagonist.

Roxiprin. (Roxane) Oxycodone hydrochloride 4.5 mg, oxycodone terephthalate 0.38 mg, aspirin 325 mg. Tab. Bot. 100s, 1000s, UD 100s. *c-II.*
Use: Analgesic combination, narcotic.

•**roxithromycin.** (ROX-ith-row-MY-sin) USAN.
Use: Anti-infective.

Rozerem. (Takeda Pharmaceutical) Ramelteon 8 mg. Lactose. Tab. Bot. 30s, 100s, 500s. *Rx.*
Use: Insomnia.

Rozex. (Galderma) Metronidazole 0.75%. Top. Emulsion. Tube. 60 g. *Rx.*
Use: Anti-inflammatory, dermatologic.

•**rozrolimupab.** (ROZ-roe-LIM-ue-pab) USAN.
Use: Recombinant polyclonal antibody.

R/S. (Summers) Sulfur 5%, resorcinol 2%, alcohol 28%. Lot. Bot. 56.7 mL. *OTC.*
Use: Dermatologic; acne.

R-Tannamine. (Qualitest) Phenylephrine tannate 25 mg, chlorpheniramine tannate 8 mg, pyrilamine tannate 25 mg. Tab. Bot. 100s. *Rx.*
Use: Antihistamine; decongestant.

R-Tannamine Pediatric. (Qualitest) Phenylephrine tannate 5 mg, chlorpheniramine tannate 2 mg, pyrilamine tannate 12.5 mg/5 mL, 120 mL, 473 mL. *Rx.*
Use: Antihistamine; decongestant.

R-Tanna S Pediatric. (Prasco) Phenylephrine tannate 5 mg, chlorpheniramine tannate 4.5 mg per 5 mL. Methylparaben, saccharin, sucrose, grape flavor. Susp. 118 mL. *Rx.*
Use: Decongestant and antihistamine.

R-Tannate. (Various Mfr.) Phenylephrine tannate 25 mg, chlorpheniramine tannate 8 mg, pyrilamine tannate 25 mg. Tab. Bot. 100s. *Rx.*
Use: Antihistamine; decongestant.

R-Tannate Pediatric. (Various Mfr.) Phenylephrine tannate 5 mg, chlorpheniramine tannate 2 mg, pyrilamine tannate 12.5 mg/5 mL, saccharin. Susp. Bot. 473 mL. *Rx.*
Use: Antihistamine; decongestant.

R-3 Screen Test. (Wampole) A three-minute latex-eosin slide test for the qualitative detection of rheumatoid factor activity in serum. Kit 100s.
Use: Diagnostic aid.

rt-PA.
Use: Tissue plasminogen.
See: Activase.

RII retinamide.
Use: Myelodysplastic syndromes. [Orphan Drug]

Rubacell. (Abbott Diagnostics) Passive hemagglutination (PHA) test for the detection of antibody to rubella virus in serum or recalcified plasma.
Use: Diagnostic aid.

Rubacell II. (Abbott Diagnostics) Passive hemagglutination (PHA) test to detect antibody to rubella in serum or recalcified plasma. In 100s, 1000s.
Use: Diagnostic aid.

Rubaquick Diagnostic Kit. (Abbott Diagnostics) Rapid passive hemagglutination (PHA) for the detection of antibodies to rubella virus in serum specimens.
Use: Diagnostic aid.

Ruba-Tect. (Abbott Diagnostics) Hemagglutination inhibition test for the detection and quantitation of rubella antibody in serum. In 100s.
Use: Diagnostic aid.

Rubatrope-57. (Bracco Diagnostics) Cyanocobalamin Co 57 18.5 to 37 kBq. Cap. Bot. 5s and 10s.
Use: Diagnostic aid.

Rubazyme. (Abbott Diagnostics) Enzyme immunoassay for 1 gG antibody to rubella virus. Test kit 100s, 1000s.
Use: Diagnostic aid.

Rubazyme-M. (Abbott Diagnostics) Enzyme immunoassay for IgM antibody to rubella virus in serum. Test kit 50s.
Use: Diagnostic aid.

•**rubella virus vaccine, live.** (roo-BELL-ah) *USP.*
Use: Immunization.

Rubex. (Bristol-Myers Squibb Oncology/Virology) Doxorubicin hydrochloride 100 mg, lactose 500 mg, preservative free. Pow. for Inj. lyophilized. Vial. *Rx.*
Use: Antibiotic.

•**rubidium chloride Rb 86.** (roo-BIH-dee-uhm) USAN.
Use: Radiopharmaceutical.

•**rubidium chloride Rb 82 injection.** (roo-BIH-dee-uhm) *USP.*
Use: Diagnostic aid (radioactive, cardiac disease), radiopharmaceutical.

•**rubitecan.** USAN.
Use: Antineoplastic.

ruboxistaurin.
Use: Investigational protein kinase C beta inhibitor.

•**rucaparib.** (roo-KAP-a-rib) USAN.
Use: Antineoplastic.

•**rucaparib phosphate.** (roo-KAP-a-rib) USAN.
Use: Antineoplastic.

•**rufinamide.** (roo-FIN-a-mide) USAN.
Use: Antiepileptic.
See: Banzel.

RU 486.
Use: Antiprogesterone.

Ru-Hist D. (Allegis Pharmaceuticals) Brompheniramine maleate 4 mg, phenylephrine hydrochloride 10 mg. Tab. 60s. *OTC.*
Use: Upper respiratory combination, decongestant and antihistamine.

Ru-lets M 500. (Rugby) Vitamin C 500 mg, B_3 100 mg, B_5 20 mg, B_1 15 mg, B_2 10 mg, B_6 5 mg, A 10,000 units, B_{12} 12 mcg, D 400 units, E 30 mg, Mg, Fe 20 mg, Cu, Zn 1.5 mg, Mn, I. Tab. Bot. 100s. *OTC.*
Use: Mineral, vitamin supplement.

RuLox Plus. (Rugby) **Susp.:** Aluminum hydroxide 500 mg, magnesium hydroxide 450 mg, simethicone 40 mg/5 mL. Bot. 355 mL. **Tab.:** Aluminum hydroxide 200 mg, magnesium hydroxide 200 mg, simethicone 25 mg. Chew. Bot. 50s. *OTC.*
Use: Antacid; antiflatulent.

RuLox Suspension. (Rugby) Aluminum hydroxide 225 mg, magnesium hydroxide 200 mg/5 mL. Parabens, saccharin, sorbitol. Susp. 360 mL, 769 mL, gal.

OTC.
Use: Antacid.

•**rupintrivir.** (roo-PIN-tri-veer) USAN.
Use: Antiviral.

•**ruplizumab.** (rue-PLYE-zue-mab) USAN.
Use: Immune thrombocytopenic purpura; systemic lupus erythematosus.

•**rusalatide acetate.** (roo-SAL-a-tide) USAN.
Use: Tissue and bone repair.

rust inhibitor.
See: Sodium Nitrite.

•**rutamycin.** (ROO-tah-MY-sin) USAN. From strain of *Streptomyces rutgersensis.* Under study.
Use: Antifungal.

rutgers 612.
See: Ethohexadiol.

rutin. (Various Mfr.) 3-Rhamnoglucoside of 5,7,3′,4-tetrahydroxyflavonol. Eldrin, globulariacitrin, myrticalorin, oxyritin, phytomelin, rutoside, sophorin. Tab. 20 mg, 50 mg, 60 mg, 100 mg. *Rx.*
Use: Vascular disorders.

rutoside.
See: Rutin.

Ru-Tuss II. (Knoll) Phenylpropanolamine hydrochloride 75 mg, chlorpheniramine maleate 12 mg. Cap. Bot. 100s. *Rx.*
Use: Antihistamine, decongestant.

•**ruxolitinib.** (RUX-oh-LI-ti-nib) USAN.
Use: Antineoplastic.

•**ruxolitinib phosphate.** (RUX-oh-LI-ti-nib) USAN.
Use: Antineoplastic.
See: Jakafi.

RVPaque. (ICN) Red petrolatum, zinc oxide, cinoxate, in water-resistant base. Tube 15 g, 37.5 g. *OTC.*
Use: Sunscreen.

Rx Support Heartburn & Acid Reflux. (Mason Vitamins) Ca, folic acid 400 mcg, vitamins B_6 10 mg, B_{12} 200 mcg, D 1,000 units (as cholecalciferol). PEG. Tab. 60s. *OTC.*
Use: Multivitamin with minerals (except iron).

Rx Support Heartburn & Acid Reflux Plus Aloe. (Mason Vitamins) Aloe vera powder 100 mg, Ca, folic acid 400 mcg, vitamins D 1,000 units (as cholecalciferol), B_6 10 mg, B_{12} 200 mcg. PEG. Tab. 60s. *OTC.*
Use: Multivitamin with minerals (except iron).

Rybix ODT. (Victory Pharma) Tramadol hydrochloride 50 mg. Aspartame, mannitol. Mint flavor. Tab., orally disintegrating. UD 30s. *Rx.*
Use: Opioid analgesic.

Rydex G. (Centurion Labs) Guaifenesin 398 mg, pseudoephedrine hydrochloride 38.5 mg. Tab. 100s. *OTC.*
Use: Upper respiratory combination, decongestant and expectorant combination.

Rymed. (Edwards) **Cap.:** Pseudoephedrine hydrochloride 30 mg, guaifenesin 250 mg. Cap. Bot. 100s. **Liq.:** Pseudoephedrine hydrochloride 30 mg, guaifenesin 100 mg/5 mL, alcohol 1.4%. Bot. Pt. *OTC.*
Use: Decongestant, expectorant.

Rymed-TR. (Edwards) Phenylpropanolamine hydrochloride 75 mg, guaifenesin 400 mg. Tab. Bot. 100s. *OTC.*
Use: Decongestant, expectorant.

Ryna-CX. (Wallace) Guaifenesin 100 mg, pseudoephedrine hydrochloride 30 mg, codeine phosphate 10 mg, alcohol 7.5%, saccharin, sorbitol/5 mL. Bot. 4 oz, pt. *c-v.*
Use: Antitussive, decongestant, expectorant.

Rynatan-S Pediatric. (Wallace) Phenylephrine tannate 5 mg, chlorpheniramine tannate 2 mg, pyrilamine tannate 12.5 mg/5 mL. Susp. Bot. 120 mL w/syringe. *Rx.*
Use: Antihistamine, decongestant.

Rynex PE. (Edwards Pharmaceuticals) Brompheniramine maleate 1 mg, phenylephrine hydrochloride 2.5 mg. Parabens, potassium sorbate, propylene glycol, sorbitol, sucralose. Alcohol free, gluten free, and sugar free. Bubble gum flavor. Liq. 473 mL. *Rx.*
Use: Upper respiratory combination, decongestant and antihistamine.

Rynex PSE. (Edwards Pharmaceuticals) Brompheniramine maleate 1 mg, pseudoephedrine hydrochloride 15 mg. Parabens, propylene glycol, sorbitol, sucralose. Alcohol free, gluten free. Orange flavor. Liq. 473 mL. *OTC.*
Use: Upper respiratory combination, decongestant and antihistamine.

Ryneze. (SJ Pharmaceuticals) Chlorpheniramine maleate 4 mg, scopolamine 1.25 mg per 5 mL. Saccharin, sorbitol. Alcohol free, dye free, gluten free, and sugar free. Grape flavor. Liq. 473 mL. *Rx.*
Use: Upper respiratory combination; decongestant, antihistamine, and anticholinergic combination.

Ry-Tann. (Midlothian) Chlorpheniramine tannate 9 mg, phenylephrine tannate 25 mg. Lactose. Tab. 100s. *Rx.*
Use: Upper respiratory combination, decongestant and antihistamine.

Rythmol. (GlaxoSmithKline) Propafenone hydrochloride 150 mg, 225 mg. Film-coated. Tab. 100s, UD 100s. *Rx.*
Use: Antiarrhythmic agent.

Rythmol SR. (GlaxoSmithKline) Propafenone hydrochloride 225 mg, 325 mg, 425 mg. ER Cap. 100s. *Rx.*
Use: Antiarrhythmic agent.

S

Saave+. (NeuroGenesis/Matrix Tech.) Vitamin D 40 mg, L-phenylalanine, L-glutamine 25 mg, vitamins A 333.3 units, B_1 2.417 mg, B_2 0.85 mg, B_3 33 mg, B_5 15 mg, B_6 3 mg, B_{12} 5 mcg, folic acid 0.067 mg, C 100 mg, E 5 units, biotin 0.05 mg, Ca 25 mg, Cr 0.01 mg, Fe 1.5 mg, Mg 25 mg, Zn 2.5 mg. Cap. Yeast and preservative free. Bot. 42s, 180s. *OTC.*
Use: Mineral, vitamin supplement.

•**sabcomeline hydrochloride.** (sab-KOE-meh-leen) USAN.
Use: Treatment of Alzheimer disease.

•**sabeluzole.** (sah-BELL-you-zole) USAN.
Use: Anticonvulsant; antihypoxic.

Sabril. (Lundbeck) Vigabatrin. **Pow. for Soln.:** 500 mg. Packet. **Tab.:** 500 mg. Film coated. PEG. 100s. *Rx.*
Use: Anticonvulsant.

•**saccharin.** (SACK-ah-rin) *NF.*
Use: Pharmaceutic aid (flavor).

saccharin. (Merck & Co.) Saccharin. Pow. Pkg. 1 oz, 0.25 lb, 1 lb. (Bristol-Myers Squibb) Tab. 0.25 g, 0.5 g. Bot. 500s, 1000s; 1 g. Bot. 1000s.
Use: Pharmaceutic aid (flavor).

•**saccharin calcium.** (SACK-ah-rin) *USP.*
Use: Non-nutritive sweetener.

•**saccharin sodium.** (SACK-ah-rin) *USP.*
Use: Sweetener (non-nutritive).
See: Sweeta.

saccharin sodium. (Various Mfr.) Saccharin sodium. Pow., Bot. 1 oz, 0.25 lb, 1 lb. Tab.
Use: Sweetener (non-nutritive).

saccharin soluble.
See: Saccharin Sodium.

Sac-500. (Western Research) Vitamin C 500 mg. TR Cap. Bot. 1000s. *OTC.*
Use: Vitamin supplement.

sacrosidase.
Use: Nutritional therapy.
See: Sucraid.

Saf-Clens. (Calgon Vestal Laboratories) Meroxapol 105, NaCl, potassium sorbate NF, DMDM hydantoin. Spray. Bot. 177 mL. *OTC.*
Use: Dermatologic, wound therapy.

Safeskin. (C & M Pharmacal) A dermatologically acceptable detergent for patients who are sensitive to ordinary detergents. No whiteners, brighteners, or other irritants. Bot. qt.
Use: Laundry detergent for sensitive skin.

Safe Suds. (Ar-Ex) Hypoallergenic, all-purpose detergent for patients whose hands or respiratory membranes are irritated by soaps or detergents. pH 6.8. No enzymes, phosphates, lanolin, fillers, bleaches. Bot. 22 oz.
Use: Detergent.

Safetussin DM. (Kramer) Guaifenesin 100 mg, dextromethorphan HBr 15 mg per 5 mL. Aspartame, menthol, parabens, phenylalanine 4.2 mg/5 mL. Mint flavor. Liq. Bot. 120 mL. *OTC.*
Use: Upper respiratory combination, antitussive, expectorant.

Safety-Coated Arthritis Pain Formula. (Whitehall-Robins) Enteric coated aspirin 500 mg. Tab. Bot. 24s, 60s. *OTC.*
Use: Analgesic.

•**safflower oil.** (SAF-low-er) *USP.*
Use: Pharmaceutic aid (vehicle, oleaginous).

safflower oil.
Use: Nutritional supplement.
See: Microlipid.

•**safinamide.** (saf-IN-a-mide) USAN.
Use: Antiparkinson agent.

•**safinamide mesylate.** (saf-IN-a-mide) USAN.
Use: Antiparkinson agent.

•**safingol.** (saff-IN-gole) USAN.
Use: Antineoplastic (adjunct); antipsoriatic.

•**safingol hydrochloride.** (saff-IN-gole) USAN.
Use: Antineoplastic (adjunct); antipsoriatic.

Safyral. (Bayer) Drospirenone 3 mg, ethinyl estradiol (as betadex clathrate) 30 mcg. Film coated. Lactose, levomefolate calcium 0.451 mg, PEG. Tab. 21s w/7 tablets (levomefolate calcium 0.451 mg). *Rx.*
Use: Oral monophasic contraceptive.

•**sagopilone.** (sa-GOP-i-lone) USAN.
Use: Antineoplastic.

Saizen. (Serono) Somatropin 5 mg (≈ 15 units)/vial, 8.8 mg (≈ 26.4 units)/vial. Sucrose. Pow. for Inj., lyophilized. Vial w/diluent (bacteriostatic water for injection w/benzyl alcohol 0.9%). *Click-easy* cartridge w/diluent (bacteriostatic water for injection and metacresol 0.3%) (8.8 mg only). *Rx.*
Use: Hormone, growth.

SalAc Cleanser. (Medicis) Salicylic acid 2%, benzyl alcohol, glyceryl cocoate. Liq. Bot. 177 mL. *OTC.*
Use: Dermatologic, acne.

salacetin.
See: Acetylsalicylic Acid.

Salacid 60%. (Gordon Laboratories) Salicylic acid 60% in ointment base. Jar

2 oz. *OTC.*
Use: Keratolytic.
Salacid 25%. (Gordon Laboratories) Salicylic acid 25% in ointment base. Jar 2 oz, lb. *OTC.*
Use: Keratolytic.
Salactic Film. (Pedinol Pharmacal) Salicylic acid 16.7% in flexible collodion w/color. Liq. Applicator Bot. 15 mL. *OTC.*
Use: Keratolytic.
Salacyn. (Stratus) Salicylic acid 6%. Cetearyl alcohol, cetyl alcohol, disodium EDTA, glycerin, mineral oil, parabens, PEG-3, PEG-100. **Cream:** 400 g. **Lot.:** 414 mL. *Rx.*
Use: Keratolytic agent.
Salagen. (Eisai) Pilocarpine hydrochloride 5 mg, 7.5 mg. Tab. Bot. 100s. *Rx.*
Use: Mouth and throat product.
Salazide. (Major) Hydroflumethiazide 50 mg, reserpine 0.125 mg. Tab. Bot. 100s, 500s, 1000s. *Rx.*
Use: Antihypertensive combination.
Salazide-Demi. (Major) Hydroflumethiazide 25 mg, reserpine 0.125 mg. Tab. Bot. 100s. *Rx.*
Use: Antihypertensive combination.
salbutamol.
See: Albuterol.
•**salcaprozate sodium.** (sal-KAP-roe-zate) USAN.
Use: Oral absorption promoter.
Salcegel. (Apco) Sodium salicylate 5 g, calcium ascorbate 25 mg, calcium carbonate 1 g, dried aluminum hydroxide gel 2 g. Tab. Bot. 100s. *OTC.*
Use: Analgesic.
Sal-Clens Acne Cleanser. (C & M Pharmacal) Salicylic acid 2%. Gel. Tube 240 g. *OTC.*
Use: Dermatologic, acne.
•**salcolex.** (SAL-koe-lex) USAN.
Use: Analgesic; anti-inflammatory; antipyretic.
Salese With Xylitol. (Nuvora) Eucalyptus oil, glyceryl, sucralose, lemon oil, peppermint oil, wintergreen oil, xylitol, zinc. Alcohol free and sugar free. Peppermint, wintergreen, and mild lemon flavors. Loz. 12s. *OTC.*
Use: Mouth and throat product.
•**salethamide maleate.** (sal-ETH-ah-MIDE) USAN. Under study.
Use: Analgesic.
saletin.
See: Acetylsalicylic Acid.
Saleto. (Mallard) Aspirin 210 mg, acetaminophen 115 mg, salicylamide 65 mg, caffeine 16 mg. Tab. Bot. 100s, 1000s, *Sani-Pak* 1000s. *OTC.*
Use: Analgesic.
Saleto-200. (Roberts) Ibuprofen 200 mg. Tab. Bot. 1000s, UD 50s. *OTC.*
Use: Analgesic; NSAID.
Salex. (Coria) Salicylic acid. **Cream.:** 6%. Alcohols, glycerin, parabens. Bot. 400 g. **Lot.:** 6%. Alcohols, EDTA, glycerin, mineral oil, parabens, PEG 100. 414 mL. **Shampoo:** 6%. Cetearyl alcohol, EDTA, glycerin, parabens. 177 mL. *Rx.*
Use: Keratolytic agent.
•**salicyl alcohol.** (SAL-ih-sill AL-koe-hahl) USAN. *Formerly Saligenin, Saligenol, Salicain.*
Use: Anesthetic, local.
•**salicylamide.** (SAL-i-SIL-a-mide) *USP.*
Use: Analgesic.
W/Acetaminophen, Aspirin, Caffeine.
See: Medi-First Extra Strength Pain Relief.
W/Acetaminophen, Caffeine, Phenyltoloxamine Citrate.
See: Durabac.
W/Aspirin, Caffeine.
See: BC Powder Arthritis Strength.
Stanback Headache Powders.
W/Combinations.
See: Anodynos.
Dapco.
Duraxin.
Ed-Flex.
Levacet.
Nokane.
Painaid.
P.M.P. Compound.
Presalin.
Saleto.
Salipap.
Salocol.
Sinulin.
Sleep Tablets.
salicylanilide.
Use: Antifungal.
salicylated bile extract. Chologestin.
•**salicylate meglumine.** (suh-LIH-sih-late) USAN.
Use: Antirheumatic; analgesic.
salicylates.
See: Aspirin
Aspirin, Buffered.
Diflunisal.
Magnesium Salicylate.
Salsalate.
Sodium Thiosalicylate
salicylazosulfapyridine.
See: Sulfasalazine.
•**salicylic acid.** (sal-ih-SILL-ik) *USP.*
Use: Keratolytic.
See: Ala Seb.

Calicylic.
Compound W for Kids.
Compount W One Step Invisible.
Compound W One Step Wart Remover for Kids.
Hydrisalic.
Keralyt.
Maximum Strength Wart Remover.
MG217 Sal-Acid.
OFF-Ezy Corn & Callous Remover.
P & S.
PROPApH Astringent Cleanser Maximum Strength.
Psor-a-set.
Psoriasin Medicated.
Salactic Film.
Salacyn.
Salex.
Sal-Plant.
Salvax.
SA 6%.
Scalpicin.
Sebulex with Conditioners.
UltraSal-ER.
Virasal.
Wart-Off.

W/Benzoyl Peroxide/Tocopherol.
See: Inova 8/2 Acne Control Therapy.
Inova 4/1 Acne Control Therapy.

W/Combinations.
See: Aveenobar Medicated.
Akne Drying Lotion.
Bensal HP.
Clearasil Clearstick for Sensitive Skin, Maximum Strength.
Clearasil Clearstick, Maximum Strength.
Clearasil Clearstick, Regular Strength.
Clearasil Double Clear.
Clearasil Double Textured Pads.
Clearasil Medicated Deep Cleanser.
Duofilm.
Duo-WR.
Ionax Astringent Cleanser.
Ionil.
Ionil T.
MG217 Medicated Tar Free.
MG217 Sal-Acid.
Neutrogena T/Sal.
Occlusal HP.
Oxy Clean Medicated Pads for Sensitive Skin.
Oxy Night Watch.
Pernox.
PROPApH.
Salicylic Acid Cleansing Bar.
Salicylic Acid & Sulfur Soap.
Salicylic Acid Wart Remover.
Sebulex with Conditioners.

W/Sulfur.
See: Exoderm.

salicylic acid. (Brookstone) Salicylic acid 6%. Glycerin, parabens, polysorbate 20, polysorbate 80, propylene glycol, tolamine. Aer., Foam. 70 g. *Rx.*
Use: Keratolytic agent.

salicylic acid. (Exact-Rx) Salicylic acid 6%. **Cream:** Alcohols, disodium EDTA, glycerin, glyceryl, mineral oil, parabens, PEG, trolamine. 400 g and 454 g kits w/355 mL hydrating cleanser. **Lot.:** Alcohols, disodium EDTA, glycerin, glyceryl, mineral oil, parabens, PEG, trolamine. 400 g and 227 g kits w/355 mL hydrating cleanser. *Rx.*
Use: Keratolytic agent.

salicylic acid. (Kylemore Pharmaceuticals) Salicylic acid 6%. EDTA, SD alcohol. Gel. 40 g. *Rx.*
Use: Keratolytic agent.

salicylic acid. (River's Edge) Salicylic acid 6%. EDTA, SD alcohol 40-2. Gel. 40 g. *Rx.*
Use: Keratolytic agent.

salicylic acid. (Rochester Pharmaceuticals) Salicylic acid 26%. Isopropyl alcohol. Liq. 10 mL w/brush applicator. *Rx.*
Use: Keratolytic agent.

salicylic acid & sulfur soap. (GlaxoSmithKline) Salicylic acid 3%, sulfur 10%, EDTA. Cake 116 g. *OTC.*
Use: Antiseborrheic; keratolytic.

salicylic acid cleansing bar. (GlaxoSmithKline) Salicylic acid 2%, EDTA. Cake 113 g. *OTC.*
Use: Antiseborrheic; keratolytic.

salicylic acid shampoo. (Hi Tech Pharmacal) Salicylic acid 6%. Edetate disodium, glycerin, parabens. Shampoo. 177 mL. *Rx.*
Use: Keratolytic agent.

salicylic acid topical foam.
Use: Keratolytic.

Salicylic Acid Wart Remover. (Acella Pharmaceuticals) Salicylic acid 27.5%. Isopropyl alcohol. Liq. 10 mL w/brush applicator. *Rx.*
Use: Keratolytic agent.

salicylsalicylic acid. Salsalate.
Use: Analgesic.
See: Disalcid.

salicylsulphonic acid. Sulfosalicylic acid.

Saligenin. (City Chemical Corp.) Salicyl alcohol. Bot. 25 g, 100 g. *OTC.*

Saline. (Bausch & Lomb) Buffered isotonic. Thimerosal 0.001%, boric acid, NaCl, EDTA. Soln. Bot. 355 mL. *OTC.*
Use: Contact lens care.

saline laxatives.
See: Epsom Salt.
Fleet Phospho-soda.
Magnesium Citrate.

Milk of Magnesia.
Milk of Magnesia-Concentrated.
Phillips' Milk of Magnesia.
Phillips' Milk of Magnesia, Concentrated.

Saline Solution. (Akorn) Saline solution, isotonic, preserved. Bot. 12 oz. *OTC.*
Use: Contact lens care, soaking.

Saline Spray. (Akorn) Isotonic nonpreserved saline aerosol soln. Bot. 2 oz, 8 oz, 12 oz. *OTC.*
Use: Contact lens care.

SalineX. (Muro) Sodium chloride 0.4%, benzalkonium chloride, propylene glycol, polyethylene glycol, EDTA. Soln. Dropper bot. 15 mL. Mist bot. 50 mL. *OTC.*
Use: Nasal decongestant.

Salipap. (Freeport) Salicylamide 5 g, acetaminophen 5 g. Tab. Bot. 1000s. *OTC.*
Use: Analgesic.

Salithol. (Madland) Balm of methyl salicylate, menthol, camphor. Liq. Bot. pt, gal. Oint. Jar 1 lb, 5 lb. *OTC.*
Use: Analgesic, topical.

Salivart. (Gebauer) Sodium carboxymethylcellulose, sorbitol, sodium chloride, potassium chloride, calcium chloride, magnesium chloride, dibasic potassium phosphate, and nitrogen (as propellant). Preservative free. Soln. Aerosol spray can 75 mL. *OTC.*
Use: Saliva substitute.

Saliva Substitute. (Roxane) Sorbitol, sodium carboxymethylcellulose, methylparaben. Soln. Bot. 120 mL. *OTC.*
Use: Saliva substitute.

saliva substitutes.
Use: Mouth and throat product.
See: Aquoral.
Caphosol.
Entertainer's Secret.
Moi-Stir.
Moi-Stir Swabsticks.
MouthKote.
NeutraSal.
Numoisyn.
Salese.
Salivart.
Saliva Substitute.
Saliva Sure.
XyliMelts.

SalivaSure. (Scandinavian Formulas) Apple acid, citric acid, dibasic calcium phosphate, xylitol. Citrus flavor. Loz. 90s. *OTC.*
Use: Mouth and throat product, saliva substitute.

Salkera. (Onset Therapeutics) Salicylic acid 6%. Aloe, cetostearyl alcohol, edetate disodium, parabens, white petrolatum. Top. Foam. 60 g. *Rx.*
Use: Keratolytic agent.

Salk vaccine.
See: IPOL.
Poliovirus Vaccine, Inactivated.

•**salmeterol xinafoate.** (sal-MEH-teh-role zin-AF-oh-ate) USAN.
Use: Bronchodilator, sympathomimetic.
See: Serevent Diskus.

salmeterol xinafoate/fluticasone propionate.
Use: Bronchodilator, sympathomimetic.
See: Advair Diskus.
Advair HFA.

•**salnacedin.** (sal-NAH-seh-din) USAN.
Use: Anti-inflammatory, topical.

Salocol. (Roberts) Acetaminophen 115 mg, aspirin 210 mg, salicylamide 65 mg, caffeine 16 mg. Tab. Bot. 1000s. *Rx.*
Use: Analgesic combination.

Salonpas. (Hisamitsu America) **Aer., Foam:** Menthol 3%, methyl salicylate 10%. Alcohol, castor oil, PEG. 118 mL. **Spray:** Menthol 3%, methyl salicylate 10%. Alcohol. 118 mL. *OTC.*
Use: Rub and liniment.

Salonpas Arthritis Pain. (Hisamitsu America) Menthol 3%, methyl salicylate 10%. Mineral oil. Patch. 5s. *OTC.*
Use: Rub and liniment.

Salpaba w/Colchicine. (Madland) Sodium salicylate 0.25 g, para-aminobenzoic acid 0.25 g, vitamin C 20 mg, colchicine 0.25 mg. Tab. Bot. 100s, 1000s. *Rx.*
Use: Antigout.

Sal-Plant. (Pedinol Pharmacal) Salicylic acid 17% in flexible collodion vehicle. Gel. Tube 14 g. *OTC.*
Use: Keratolytic.

•**salsalate.** (SAL-sah-late) *USP.*
Use: Analgesic; anti-inflammatory.

salsalate. (Various Mfr.) Salsalate 500 mg, 750 mg. Tab. 100s, 250s, 500s, 1,000s, UD 100s. *Rx.*
Use: Salicylate.

Salten. (Wren) Salicylamide 10 g. Tab. Bot. 100s, 1000s. *OTC.*
Use: Analgesic.

salt replacement products.
See: Slo-Salt-K.
Sodium Chloride.

salts, rehydration, oral.
Use: Electrolyte combination.

SaltStable LO. (Humco) Isopropyl palmitate, lecithin. Cream. 454 g, 4,536 g. *OTC.*
Use: Ointment and lotion base.

salt substitutes.
Use: Sodium-free seasoning agent.
See: Adolph's Salt Substitute.
Adolph's Seasoned Salt Substitute.
Morton Salt Substitute.
Morton Seasoned Salt Substitute.
NoSalt.
Nu-Salt.

salt tablets. (Cross) Sodium Cl 650 mg. Tab. Dispenser 500s. *OTC.*
Use: Salt replenisher.

Salvarsan.
Use: Antisyphilitic.

Salvax. (Quinnova) Salicylic acid 6%. Dimethicone, glycerin, parabens, polysorbate 80, povidone, propylene glycol, trolamine. Aer. Foam. Kit w/150 g *Hydro 35* foam. 70 g, 200 g. *Rx.*
Use: Keratolytic agent.

Salvax Duo. (Quinnova) Salicylic acid 6%, urea 40%, glycerin, parabens. Foam. 70 g. *Rx.*
Use: Miscellaneous topical combination.

Salvite-B. (Faraday) Sodium chloride 7 g, dextrose 3 g, vitamin B_1 1 mg. Tab. Bot. 100s, 1000s. *OTC.*

•**samalizumab.** (SA-ma-LIZ-oo-mab) USAN.
Use: Antineoplastic.

•**samarium Sm 153 lexidronam injection.** (sah-MARE-ee-uhm Sm 153 lex-IH-drah-nam) *USP.*
Use: Antineoplastic; radiopharmaceutical.

•**samarium Sm 153 lexidronam pentasodium.** (sah-MARE-ee-uhm Sm 153 lex-IH-drah-nam) USAN.
Use: Antineoplastic; radiopharmaceutical.
See: Quadramet.

•**samatasvir.** (sa-MAT-as-vir) USAN.
Use: Antiviral.

•**samfilcon A.** (sam-FIL-con) USAN.
Use: Contact lens polymer.

•**samidorphan.** (SAM-i-DOR-fan) USAN.
Use: Treatment of addictive disorders.

•**samidorphan l-malate.** (SAM-i-DOR-fan) USAN.
Use: Treatment of addictive disorders.

Samsca. (Otsuka America) Tolvaptan 15 mg, 30 mg. Lactose. Tab. UD 10s. *Rx.*
Use: Vasopressin receptor antagonist.

Sanctura. (Various Mfr.) Trospium chloride 20 mg. Lactose, sucrose. Tab. 60s, 500s. Blister 14s. *Rx.*
Use: Anticholinergic.

Sancura. (Thompson Medical) Benzocaine, chlorobutanol, chlorothymol, benzoic acid, salicylic acid, benzyl alcohol, cod liver oil, lanolin in a washable petrolatum base. Oint. 30 g, 90 g.
Use: Anesthetic, local.

Sancuso. (ProStrakan) Granisetron 3.1 mg per 24 hours (34.3 mg per 52 cm^2). Patch, Transdermal. 1s. *Rx.*
Use: Antiemetic/antivertigo agent, 5-HT_3 receptor antagonist.

•**sancycline.** (SAN-SIGH-kleen) USAN.
Use: Anti-infective.

Sandimmune. (Novartis) Cyclosporine. **Oral soln.:** 100 mg/mL. Alcohol 12.5%. Bot. 50 mL with syringe. **Inj.:** 50 mg/mL. Polyoxyethylated castor oil 650 mg/mL, alcohol 32.9%. Amp. 5 mL. **Soft Gelatin Cap.:** 25 mg, 100 mg. Sorbitol, dehydrated alcohol ≤ 12.7%. UD 30s. *Rx.*
Tall Man: SandIMMUNE
Use: Immunosuppressant.

sandoptal. Isobutyl allylbarbituric acid.
See: Butalbital.
W/Caffeine, Aspirin, Phenacetin.
See: Fiorinal.
W/Caffeine, Aspirin, Phenacetin, Codeine Phosphate.
See: Fiorinal w/Codeine.

Sandostatin. (Novartis) Octreotide acetate. **0.05 mg/mL, 0.1 mg/mL, 0.5 mg/mL:** Inj. Amp 1 mL. **0.2 mg/mL, 1 mg/mL:** Inj. 5 mL multidose vials. *Rx.*
Tall Man: SandoSTATIN
Use: Somatostatin analog.

Sandostatin LAR Depot. (Novartis) Octreotide acetate 10 mg per 5 mL, 20 mg per 5 mL, 30 mg per 5 mL. Pow. for Inj. Susp. Kits with 2 mL diluent, 1½" 20-gauge needles and instruction booklet. *Rx.*
Tall Man: SandoSTATIN
Use: Somatostatin analog.

Sanestro. (Sandia) Estrone 0.7 mg, estradiol 0.35 mg, estriol 0.14 mg. Tab. Bot. 100s, 1000s. *Rx.*
Use: Estrogen.

•**sanfetrinem cilexetil.** (san-FEH-trih-nem sigh-LEX-eh-till) USAN.
Use: Anti-infective.

•**sanfetrinem sodium.** (san-FEH-trih-nem) USAN.
Use: Anti-infective.

SangCya. (SangStat) Cyclosporine 100 mg/mL, alcohol 10.5%. Oral Soln. Bot. 50 mL. *Rx.*
Use: Immunosuppressive.

•**sanguinarium chloride.** (san-gwih-NARE-ee-uhm) USAN. *Formerly Sanguinarine Chloride.*
Use: Antimicrobial; anti-inflammatory; antifungal.

Sanguis. (Sigma-Tau) Liver 10 mcg, vitamin B_{12} 100 mcg, folic acid 1 mcg/mL. Vial 10 mL. *Rx.*
Use: Nutritional supplement.

Sani-Supp. (G & W) Glycerin. Supp. **Adults:** Box 10s, 25s, 50s. **Pediatric:** Box 10s, 25s. *OTC.*
Use: Laxative.

sanluol.
See: Arsphenamine.

Sanstress. (Sandia) Vitamins A 25,000 units, D 400 units, B_1 10 mg, B_2 5 mg, niacinamide 100 mg, B_6 1 mg, B_{12} 5 mcg, C 150 mg, Ca 103 mg, P 80 mg, Fe 10 mg, Cu 1 mg, I 0.1 mg, Mg 5.5 mg, Mn 1 mg, K 5 mg, Zn 1.4 mg. Cap. Bot. 100s, 1000s. *OTC.*
Use: Mineral, vitamin supplement.

Santiseptic. (Santiseptic) Menthol, phenol, benzocaine, zinc oxide, calamine. Lot. Bot. 4 oz. *OTC.*
Use: Dermatologic, counterirritant.

Santyl. (Knoll) Proteolytic enzyme derived from *Clostridium histolyticum* 250 units/g. Oint. Tube. 15 g, 30 g. *Rx.*
Use: Enzyme, topical.

•**sapacitabine.** (SAP-a-SYE-ta-been) USAN.
Use: Antineoplastic.

•**saperconazole.** (SAP-ehr-KOE-nah-zole) USAN.
Use: Antifungal.

Saphris. (Organon) Asenapine 5 mg, 10 mg. Mannitol, sucralose (black cherry flavor only). Unflavored or black cherry flavor. Tab., sublingual. 60s, UD 100s. *Rx.*
Use: Antipsychotic agent, dibenzapine derivative.

saponated cresol solution.
See: Cresol.

•**saprisartan potassium.** (sap-rih-SAHR-tan) USAN.
Use: Antihypertensive.

•**sapropterin dihydrochloride.** (SAP-roe-TER-in) USAN.
Use: Phenylketonuria (PKU).
See: Kuvan.

•**saquinavir mesylate.** (sack-KWIN-uh-vihr) *USP.*
Use: Antiviral.
See: Invirase.

•**saracatinib.** (SAR-a-KA-ti-nib) USAN.
Use: Antineoplastic.

•**saracatinib difumarate.** (SAR-a-KA-ti-nib) USAN.
Use: Antineoplastic.

Sarafem. (Warner Chilcott) Fluoxetine hydrochloride 10 mg, 15 mg, 20 mg. Tab. UD 28s. *Rx.*
Use: Antidepressant, selective serotonin reuptake inhibitor.

•**sarafloxacin hydrochloride.** (sa-rah-FLOX-ah-SIN) USAN.
Use: Anti-infective (DNA gyrase inhibitor).

•**saralasin acetate.** (sare-AL-ah-sin) USAN.
Use: Antihypertensive.

Saratoga. (Blair) Boric acid, zinc oxide, eucalyptol, white petrolatum. Oint. Tube 1 oz, 2 oz. *OTC.*
Use: Dermatologic, counterirritant.

l-sarcolysin. Melphalan.
Use: Antineoplastic.

Sardo Bath & Shower. (Schering-Plough) Mineral oil, tocopherol. Oil. Bot. 112.5 mL. *OTC.*
Use: Emollient.

Sardo Bath Oil Concentrate. (Schering-Plough) Mineral oil, isopropyl palmitate. Bot. 3.75 oz, 7.75 oz. *OTC.*
Use: Emollient.

Sardoettes. (Schering-Plough) Mineral oil, tocopherol, beta-carotene. Towelettes. Box 25s. *OTC.*
Use: Emollient.

Sardoettes Moisturizing Towelettes. (Schering-Plough) Mineral oil, isopropyl palmitate, impregnated towelling material. Individual packets. Box 25s. *OTC.*
Use: Emollient.

•**sarecycline.** (SAR-e-SYE-kleen) USAN.
Use: Acne product.

•**sarecycline hydrochloride.** (SAR-e-SYE-kleen) USAN.
Use: Acne product.

•**sargramostim.** (sar-GRUH-moe-STIM) USAN.
Use: Antineutropenic; hematopoietic stimulant; leukopoietic (granulocyte macrophage colony-stimulating factor).
See: Leukine.

•**saridegib.** (SAR-i-DEG-ib) USAN.
Use: Antineoplastic.

•**saridegib hydrochloride.** (SAR-i-DEG-ib) USAN.
Use: Antineoplastic.

•**sarilumab.** (sar-IL-ue-mab) USAN.
Use: Monoclonal antibody.

Sarisol No. 2. (Halsey Drug) Butabarbital sodium 30 mg. Tab. Bot. 100s, 1000s. *c-III.*
Use: Hypnotic; sedative.

•**sarizotan hydrochloride.** (sar-i-ZOE-tan) USAN.
Use: Antiparkinson agent.

•**sarmoxicillin.** (sar-MOX-ih-SILL-in) USAN.
Use: Anti-infective.

Sarna. (GlaxoSmithKline) Triclosan 0.2%. Benzyl alcohol, parabens, PEG-75, stearyl alcohol. Fragrance free. Wash. 237 mL. *OTC.*
Use: Anti-infective, topical; antiseptic and germicide.

Sarna Anti-Itch. (GlaxoSmithKline) Camphor 5%, menthol 5%, carbomer 940, cetyl alcohol, DMDM hydantoin. Foam. Bot. 105 mL. *OTC.*
Use: Emollient.

Sarna Sensitive Anti-Itch. (GlaxoSmithKline) Pramoxine hydrochloride 1%. Benzyl alcohol, cetyl alcohol, petrolatum. Fragrance free. Lot. 222 mL. *OTC.*
Use: Topical local anesthetic.

•**sarpicillin.** (sahr-PIH-SILL-in) USAN.
Use: Anti-infective.

SA 6%. (River's Edge) Salicylic acid 6%. **Cream:** Alcohol, ammonium lactate, cetyl alcohol, dimethicone, disodium EDTA, glycerin, glyceryl, mineral oil, parabens, PEG-3, PEG-100, trolamine. 454 g in kit w/cleanser. **Lotion:** Alcohol, disodium EDTA, glycerin, glyceryl, mineral oil, parabens, PEG-100, trolamine. 237 mL in kit w/cleanser. *Rx.*
Use: Keratolytic agent.

SAStid soap. (GlaxoSmithKline) Salicylic acid 3%, sulfur 5%. EDTA, HEDTA. Soap. 100 g. *OTC.*
Use: Dermatologic, acne.

Savella. (Forest) Milnacipran hydrochloride 12.5 mg, 25 mg, 50 mg, 100 mg. Film coated. PEG. Tab. 60s. *Rx.*
Use: Antidepressant, serotonin and norepinephrine reuptake inhibitor.

•**saxagliptin.** (SAX-a-GLIP-tin) USAN.
Use: Antidiabetic.
See: Onglyza.
W/Metformin Hydrochloride.
See: Kombiglyze XR.

saxol.
See: Petrolatum.

saw palmetto.
Use: Dietary supplement.

scabicides/pediculicides.
See: Benzyl Alcohol.
Crotamiton.
Lindane.
Malathion.
Permethrin.
Spinosad.

Scalacort DK. (Avidas Pharmaceuticals) Hydrocortisone 2%. Benzalkonium chloride, isopropyl alcohol. Lot. 29.6 mL and shampoo. *Rx.*
Use: Anti-inflammatory agent, topical corticosteroid.

Scalpicin. (Combe) Salicylic acid 3%, menthol, SD alcohol 40. Shampoo. Bot. 45 mL, 75 mL, 120 mL. *OTC.*
Use: Corticosteroid, topical.

Scan. (Parker) Water-soluble gel. Bot. 8 oz, gal.
Use: Ultrasound aid.

Scandonest. (Septodont) Mepivacaine hydrochloride 3%. Sodium chloride 6 mg. Inj., Soln. Dental cartridge. 1.7 mL. *Rx.*
Use: Injectable local anesthetic, amide local anesthetic.

Scandonest L. (Septodont) Mepivacaine hydrochloride 2% w/levonordefrin 1:20,000. Edetate disodium, sodium chloride 4 mg. Inj., Soln. Dental cartridge. 1.7 mL. *Rx.*
Use: Injectable local anesthetic, amide local anesthetic.

Scar Cream Maximum Strength. (Clay-Park Labs) Octyl methoxycinnamate 7.5%, octyl salicylate 5%. Alcohols, mineral oil, parabens, urea. Cream. 28 g. *OTC.*
Use: Sunscreen.

Scarlet Red Ointment Dressings. (Sherwood Davis & Geck) 5% scarlet red, lanolin, olive oil, petrolatum. Gauze. 5" × 9" strips. *Rx.*
Use: Dermatologic, wound therapy.

Schamberg's. (C & M Pharmacal) Menthol 0.15%, phenol 1%, zinc oxide, peanut oil, lime water. Bot. Pt, gal. *OTC.*
Use: Antipruritic; counterirritant.

•**Schick test control.** *USP. Formerly Diphtheria Toxin, Inactivated Diagnostic.*
Use: Diagnostic aid (dermal reactivity indicator).

Schirmer Tear Test. (Various Mfr.) Sterile tear flow test strips. 250s. *Rx.*
Use: Diagnostic aid, ophthalmic.

Schlesinger's Solution.
See: Morphine Hydrochloride.

Sclerex. (Miller Pharmacal Group) Inositol 2 g, magnesium complex 34 mg, vitamins C 100 mg, calcium succinate 25 mg, A 2500 units, D 200 units, E 100 units, B_1 5 mg, B_2 5 mg, B_6 5 mg, B_{12} 5 mcg, niacin 10 mg, niacinamide 30 mg, pantothenic acid 7.5 mg, folic acid 0.1 mg, Fe 10 mg, Cu 1 mg, Mn 2 mg, Zn 9 mg, I 0.10 mg/3 Tab. Bot. 60s. *OTC.*
Use: Mineral, vitamin supplement.

Scleromate. (Glenwood) Morrhuate sodium 50 mg/mL. Inj. Multiple-use vial. 30 mL. *Rx.*
Use: Sclerosing agent.

sclerosing agents.
Use: Treatment of varicose veins.
See: Ethanolamine Oleate.
Morrhuate Sodium.

Polidocanol.
Sodium Tetradecyl Sulfate.

Sclerosol. (Bryan) Talc 4 g. Aerosol. Single-use aluminum canister with 2 delivery tubes of 15 cm and 25 cm. *Rx.*
Use: Antineoplastic.

•**scopafungin.** (SKOE-pah-FUN-jin) USAN.
Use: Antifungal; anti-infective.

Scope. (Procter & Gamble) Cetylpyridinium Cl, tartrazine, saccharin, SD alcohol 38F 67.9%. Liq. Bot. 90 mL, 180 mL, 360 mL, 720 mL, 1080 mL, 1440 mL. *OTC.*
Use: Mouthwash.

ScopoHist. (Larken) **ER Tab.:** Chlorpheniramine maleate 8 mg, methscopolamine nitrate 1.25 mg, pseudoephedrine hydrochloride 60 mg. 100s. **Syrup:** Chlorpheniramine maleate 2 mg, methscopolamine nitrate 0.75 mg, phenylephrine hydrochloride 8 mg. Sorbitol, sugar. Grape flavor. 473 mL. *Rx.*
Use: Upper respiratory combination; decongestant, antihistamine, and anticholinergic combination.

ScopoHist-PE. (Larken) Chlorpheniramine maleate 8 mg, methscopolamine nitrate 1.25 mg, phenylephrine hydrochloride 20 mg. Lactose. ER Tab. 100s. *Rx.*
Use: Upper respiratory combination; decongestant, antihistamine, and anticholinergic combination.

•**scopolamine hydrobromide.** (skoe-PAHL-uh-meen) *USP. Formerly Hyoscine Hydrobromide.* Hyoscine, l-Scopolamine, Epoxytropine tropate.
Use: Anticholinergic (ophthalmic); cycloplegic; hypnotic; mydriatic; sedative; GI anticholinergic/antispasmodic.
See: Transderm-Scōp.
W/Atropine Sulfate, Hyoscyamine Hydrobromide or Sulfate, Phenobarbital.
See: Antispasmodic.
Donnatal.
Donnatal Extentabs.
PB-Hyos.
Quadrapax.
Se-Donna PB Hyos.
W/Combinations.
See: Belladonna.
Belladonna Alkaloids.
Respa A.R.
Stahist.

scopolamine hydrobromide. (GlaxoSmithKline) Scopolamine HBr 0.86 mg/mL. Inj. Vials. 1 mL. *Rx.*
Use: Amnestic; anxiolytic; sedative; GI anticholinergic/antispasmodic.

scopolamine hydrobromide. (Invenex) Scopolamine HBr 0.3 mg/mL. Inj. Vial 1 mL. *Rx.*
Use: Amnestic; anxiolytic; sedative.

scopolamine hydrobromide. (Various Mfr.) Scopolamine HBr 0.3 mg/mL, 0.4 mg/mL, 1 mg/mL. Inj. Amps. 0.5 mL (0.4 mg/mL only). Vials. 1 mL. *Rx.*
Use: GI anticholinergic/antispasmodic.

scopolamine methobromide.
See: Methscopolamine Bromide.

scopolamine methyl nitrate.
See: Methscopolamine Nitrate.

scopolamine salts.
See: Belladonna.

Scotavite. (Scot-Tussin) Vitamins A 25,000 units, D 400 units, B_1 10 mg, B_2 10 mg, B_6 5 mg, B_{12} 5 mcg, niacinamide 100 mg, calcium pantothenate 20 mg, C 200 mg, d-alpha tocopheryl 15 units, acid succinate iodine 0.15 mg. Tab. Bot. 100s, 500s. *OTC.*
Use: Mineral, vitamin supplement.

Scotcil. (Scot-Tussin) **Tab.:** Potassium penicillin 400,000 units w/calcium carbonate. Bot. 100s, 500s. **Pow.:** 80 mL, 150 mL. *Rx.*
Use: Anti-infective, penicillin.

Scotonic. (Scot-Tussin) Vitamins B_1 10 mg, B_2 5 mg, B_6 1 mg, niacinamide 50 mg, choline Cl 100 mg, inositol 100 mg, B_{12} 25 mcg, Ca 19 mg, Fe 50 mg, folic acid 0.15 mg, alcohol 15%, sodium benzoate 0.1%/45 mL. Bot. Pt, gal. *OTC.*
Use: Mineral, vitamin supplement.

Scott's Emulsion. (GlaxoSmithKline) Vitamins A 1,250 units, D 1,400 units/4 tsp. Bot. 6.25 oz, 12.5 oz. *OTC.*
Use: Vitamin supplement.

Scot-Tussin Allergy Relief Formula Clear. (Scot-Tussin) Diphenhydramine hydrochloride 12.5 mg/5 mL. Alcohol and dye free. Parabens, menthol. Cherry-strawberry flavor. Liq. Bot. 118 mL. *OTC.*
Use: Antihistamine, nonselective ethanolamine.

Scot-Tussin Diabetes. (Scot-Tussin) Dextromethorphan hydrobromide 10 mg per 5 mL. Glycerin, *Magnasweet*, menthol, parabens, propylene glycol. Alcohol free, gluten free, and sugar free. Cherry-strawberry flavor. Liq. 118 mL. *OTC.*
Use: Nonnarcotic antitussive.

Scot-Tussin DM. (Scot-Tussin) Dextromethorphan HBr 15 mg, chlorpheniramine maleate 2 mg per 5 mL. Sugar

and alcohol free. Magnasweet, menthol, parabens. Liq. Bot. 118 mL. *OTC.*
Use: Upper respiratory combination, antitussive combination.

Scot-Tussin DM Cough Chasers. (Scot-Tussin) Dextromethorphan HBr 5 mg. Peppermint oil, sorbitol. Sugar and dye free. Loz. Box 20s. *OTC.*
Use: Nonnarcotic antitussive.

Scot-Tussin Expectorant. (Scot-Tussin) Guaifenesin 100 mg/5 mL. Parabens, phenylalanine, menthol, aspartame. Alcohol and dye free. Grape flavor. Liq. Bot. 118 mL. *OTC.*
Use: Expectorant.

Scot-Tussin Hayfebrol. (Scot-Tussin) Pseudoephedrine hydrochloride 30 mg, chlorpheniramine maleate 2 mg/5 mL. Parabens, menthol, alcohol and dye free. Liq. Bot. 120 mL. *OTC.*
Use: Upper respiratory combination, decongestant, antihistamine.

Scot-Tussin Original Multi-Action Cold and Allergy. (Scot-Tussin) Phenylephrine hydrochloride 4 mg, pheniramine maleate 13 mg, sodium salicylate 83 mg, caffeine citrate 25 mg/5 mL. Saccharin, parabens, cherry-strawberry flavor. Sugar, alcohol, and dye free. Syrup. Liq. Bot. 118 mL, 473 mL, 3.8 L. *OTC.*
Use: Upper respiratory combination, decongestant, antihistamine, analgesic.

Scot-Tussin Pharmacal Allergy. (Scot-Tussin) Diphenhydramine hydrochloride 12.5 mg/5 mL, parabens, menthol. Liq. Dye free, sugar free. Bot. 120 mL. *OTC.*
Use: Antihistamine.

Scot-Tussin Pharmacal DM. (Scot-Tussin) Dextromethorphan HBr 15 mg, chlorpheniramine maleate 2 mg/5 mL, alcohol 10%, sugar free. Liq. Bot. 4 oz, 8 oz. *OTC.*
Use: Antihistamine.

Scot-Tussin Pharmacal DM Cough Chasers. (Scot-Tussin) Dextromethorphan HBr 2.5 mg, dye free, sorbitol. Loz. Pkg. 20s. *OTC.*
Use: Antitussive.

Scot-Tussin Pharmacal DM2. (Scot-Tussin) Dextromethorphan HBr 15 mg, guaifenesin 100 mg, alcohol 1.4%/5 mL. Syrup. Bot. 120 mL, 240 mL. *OTC.*
Use: Antitussive; expectorant.

Scot-Tussin Pharmacal Expectorant. (Scot-Tussin) Guaifenesin 100 mg/5 mL, menthol, aspartame, phenylalanine, parabens, alcohol and dye free. Liq. Bot. 30 mL, 118.3 mL, 240 mL. *OTC.*
Use: Expectorant.

Scot-Tussin Pharmacal Sugar-Free. (Scot-Tussin) Dextromethorphan HBr 15 mg, chlorpheniramine maleate 2 mg/5 mL. Bot. 4 oz, 8 oz, 16 oz, gal. *OTC.*
Use: Antitussive; antihistamine.

Scot-Tussin Pharmacal Sugar-Free Expectorant. (Scot-Tussin) Guaifenesin 100 mg/5 mL w/alcohol 3.5%. Dye, sodium free, and sugar free. *OTC.*
Use: Expectorant.

Scot-Tussin Pharmacal with Sugar. (Scot-Tussin) Phenylephrine hydrochloride 4.17 mg, pheniramine maleate 13.3 mg, sodium citrate 83.33 mg, sodium salicylate 83.33 mg, caffeine citrate 25 mg/5 mL. Bot. 4 oz, 8 oz, 16 oz, gal. *OTC.*
Use: Analgesic combination; antihistamine; decongestant.

Scot-Tussin Senior Clear. (Scot-Tussin) Guaifenesin 200 mg, dextromethorphan HBr 15 mg per 5 mL. Parabens, phenylalanine, aspartame, menthol, alcohol free, sugar free. Liq. Bot. 118 mL. *OTC.*
Use: Upper respiratory combination, antitussive, expectorant.

Sculptra. (Dermik Laboratories) Poly-l-lactic acid (freeze dried). Pow. for Inj. Single-use vials. *Rx.*
Use: Restoration/correction of facial fat loss in individuals with HIV.

Scurenaline.
See: Epinephrine.

Scuroforme.
See: Butyl Aminobenzoate.

S.D.M. #50. (AstraZeneca) Isosorbide dinitrate 50% in lactose. *Rx.*
Use: Vasodilator.

S.D.M. #5. (AstraZeneca) Mannitol hexanitrate 7% in lactose. *Rx.*
Use: Vasodilator.

S.D.M. #40. (AstraZeneca) Isosorbide dinitrate 25% in lactose. *Rx.*
Use: Vasodilator.

S.D.M. #17. (AstraZeneca) Nitroglycerin 10% in lactose. *Rx.*
Use: Vasodilator.

S.D.M. #35. (AstraZeneca) Pentaerythritol tetranitrate 35% in mannitol. *Rx.*
Use: Vasodilator.

S.D.M. #37. (AstraZeneca) Nitroglycerin 10% in ethanol. *Rx.*
Use: Vasodilator.

S.D.M. #27. (AstraZeneca) Nitroglycerin 10% in propylene glycol. *Rx.*
Use: Vasodilator.

S.D.M. #23. (AstraZeneca) Pentaerythritol tetranitrate 20% in lactose. *Rx.*
Use: Vasodilator.

Sea & Ski Baby Lotion Formula. (Carter-Wallace) Octyl-dimethyl PABA. SPF 2. Lot. Bot. 120 mL. *OTC.*
Use: Sunscreen.

Sea & Ski Golden Tan. (Carter-Wallace) Padimate O. SPF 4. Lot. Bot. 120 mL. *OTC.*
Use: Sunscreen.

Sea Greens. (Modern Aids Inc.) Iodine 0.25 mg. Tab. Bot. 220s, 460s. *OTC.*

Sea Master. (Barth's) Vitamins A 10,000 units, D 400 units. Cap. Bot. 100s, 500s. *OTC.*
Use: Vitamin supplement.

Sea-Omega 50. (Rugby) Omega-3 polyunsaturated fatty acid 1000 mg. Cap. containing EPA 300 mg, DHA 200 mg, vitamin E 1 unit. Bot. 30s, 50s. *OTC.*
Use: Nutritional supplement.

Sea-Omega 30. (Rugby) N-3 fat content (mg) EPA 180, DHA 140. 100s. *OTC.*
Use: Nutritional supplement.

Seasonique. (Duramed) **Phase 1:** Levonorgestrel 0.15 mg, ethinyl estradiol 10 mcg. Lactose. Film-coated. Tab. 84s. **Phase 2:** Ethinyl estradiol 10 mcg. Lactose. Film-coated. Tab. 7s. *Rx.*
Use: Contraceptive hormone, sex hormone.

Seba-Lo. (Whorton Pharmaceuticals, Inc.) Acetone-alcohol cleanser. Bot. 4 oz. *OTC.*
Use: Skin cleanser.

Sebana. (Bristol-Myers Squibb) Salicylic acid 2%. Shampoo. Bot. 4 oz, 8 oz, pt, qt, 0.5 gal. *OTC.*
Use: Antiseborrheic.

Sebanatar. (Bristol-Myers Squibb) Salicylic acid 2%, liquor carbonis detergens 3%. Shampoo. Bot. 4 oz, 8 oz, pt, qt, 0.5 gal, gal. *OTC.*
Use: Antiseborrheic.

Seba-Nil Cleansing Mask. (Galderma) Astringent face mask containing SD alcohol 40, sulfated castor oil, methylparaben. Tube 105 g. *OTC.*
Use: Dermatologic, acne.

Seba-Nil Liquid. (Galderma) Alcohol 49.7%, acetone, polysorbate 20. Liq. Bot. 240 mL, pt. *OTC.*
Use: Dermatologic, acne.

Seba-Nil Oily Skin Cleanser. (Galderma) SD alcohol, acetone. Liq. Bot. 240 mL, 473 mL. *OTC.*
Use: Dermatologic, acne.

Sebasorb. (Summers) Activated attapulgite 10%, salicylic acid 2%. Lot. Bot. 45 mL. *OTC.*
Use: Dermatologic, acne.

•**sebelipase alfa.** (SE-be-LYE-pase) USAN.
Use: Enzyme replacement therapy.

SE BPO. (Seton Pharmaceuticals) Benzoyl peroxide 3%, 6%, 9%. Cetyl alcohol, glycerin, sodium hyaluronate, zinc. Cloths, topical. UD 60s. *Rx.*
Use: Topical anti-infective, antibiotic agent.

SE BPO 7%. (Seton Pharmaceuticals) Benzoyl peroxide 7%. Castor oil, dimethicone, edetate disodium, glycerin, methylparaben, PEG-15, PEG-40. Soap. 180 g. *Rx.*
Use: Topical anti-infective, antibiotic agent.

Seb-Prev. (Perrigo) Sulfacetamide sodium 10%. EDTA, methylparaben. Gel. 30 g, 60 g. *Rx.*
Use: Topical anti-infective.

Seb-Prev. (Glades) Sodium sulfacetamide 10%. Propylene glycol, EDTA, methylparaben. Lot. 118 mL. *Rx.*
Use: Dermatologic agent, acne product.

Seb-Prev Wash. (Perrigo) Sulfacetamide sodium 10%. Edetate disodium, PEG, methylparaben. Soap. 340 mL. *Rx.*
Use: Topical anti-infective.

Sebulex with Conditioners. (Bristol-Myers Squibb) Sulfur 2%, salicylic acid 2%. Bot. 4 oz, 8 oz. *OTC.*
Use: Antiseborrheic.

•**secalciferol.** (seh-kal-SIFF-eh-ROLE) USAN.
Use: Regulator (calcium); treatment of familial hypophosphatemic rickets. [Orphan Drug]
See: Osteo-D.

•**seclazone.** (SEK-lah-zone) USAN.
Use: Anti-inflammatory; uricosuric.

•**secobarbital.** (see-koe-BAR-bih-tahl) *USP.*
Use: Hypnotic; sedative.
W/Combinations.
See: Monosyl.

secobarbital elixir.
See: Seconal.

•**secobarbital sodium.** (see-koe-BAR-bih-tahl) *USP.*
Use: Hypnotic; sedative.

secobarbital sodium. (Wyeth) Secobarbital sodium 50 mg/mL. Inj. *Tubex* 2 mL. *c-II.*
Use: Hypnotic; sedative.

secobarbital sodium and amobarbital sodium capsules.
Use: Hypnotic; sedative.
See: Tuinal.

Seconal Sodium Pulvules. (Marathon) Secobarbital sodium 100 mg. Cap. Bot. 100s, UD 100s. *c-II.*
Use: Hypnotic; sedative.

Secran. (Scherer) Vitamins B_1 10 mg, B_3 10 mg, B_{12} 25 mcg, alcohol 17%. Liq. Bot. 480 mL. *OTC.*
Use: Vitamin supplement.

secretin.
Use: Diagnostic aid, gastrointestinal function test.
See: ChiRhoStim.

Sectral. (Reddy Pharmaceuticals) Acebutolol hydrochloride 200 mg, 400 mg. Cap. Bot. 100s, *Redipak* 100s (200 mg only). *Rx.*
Use: Antiadrenergic/sympatholytic, beta-adrenergic blocker.

•**secukinumab.** (SEK-ue-KIN-ue-mab) USAN.
Use: Uveitis, rheumatoid arthritis, psoriasis.

sedaform.
See: Chlorobutanol.

Sedamine. (Health for Life Brands) Phosphorated carbohydrate soln. Bot. 4 oz. *OTC.*
Use: Antinauseant.

Sedamine. (Oxypure) Hyoscyamine sulfate 0.1037 mg, atropine sulfate 0.0194 mg, hyoscine HBr 0.0065 mg, phenobarbital 16.2 mg. Tab. Bot. 100s, 1000s. *Rx.*
Use: Antispasmodic; sedative.

Sedapap. (Merz) Acetaminophen 650 mg, butalbital 50 mg. Tab. Bot. 100s. *Rx.*
Use: Analgesic.

Sedapar. (Parmed Pharmaceuticals, Inc.) Atropine sulfate 0.0195 mg, hyoscine HBr 0.0065 mg, hyoscyamine sulfate 0.104 mg, phenobarbital 0.25 g. Tab. Bot. 1000s. *Rx.*
Use: Antispasmodic; sedative.

sedative/hypnotic agents.
See: Barbiturates.
Bromides.
Butisol Sodium.
Carbamide Compounds.
Chloral Hydrate.
Chlorobutanol.
Paraldehyde.
Phenergan.
Triazolam.

sedative/hypnotic agents, nonbarbiturate.
See: Benzodiazepines.
Chloral Hydrate.
Dexmedetomidine Hydrochloride.
Eszopiclone.
Imidazopyridines.
Melatonin Receptor Agonists.
Paraldehyde.
Propiomazine Hydrochloride.
Pyrazolopyrimidine.

sedeval.
See: Barbital.

Se-Donna PB Hyos. (Seton Pharmaceuticals) Atropine sulfate 0.0194 mg, hyoscyamine hydrobromide or sulfate 0.1037 mg, phenobarbital 16.2 mg, scopolamine hydrobromide 0.0065 mg. Alcohol 23%, glycerin, saccharin, sorbitol, sucrose. Grape flavor. Elix. 473 mL. *c-iv.*
Use: Gastrointestinal anticholinergic/antispasmodic.

•**sedoxantrone trihydrochloride.** (sed-OX-an-trone try-HIGH-droe-KLOR-ide) USAN.
Use: Antineoplastic (DNA topoisomerase II inhibitor).

Sedral. (Vita Elixir) Phenobarbital ⅛ g, theophylline 2 g, ephedrine g. Tab. *Rx.*
Use: Bronchodilator; sedative.

•**seglitide acetate.** (SEH-glih-TIDE) USAN.
Use: Antidiabetic.

selective aldosterone receptor antagonists.
See: Eplerenone.

selective COX-2 inhibitors.
Use: Anti-inflammatory; nonsteroidal anti-inflammatory agent.
See: Celecoxib.

selective estrogen receptor modulator.
Use: Sex hormone.
See: Ospemifene.
Raloxifene Hydrochloride.

selective factor Xa inhibitor.
Use: Anticoagulant.
See: Fondaparinux Sodium.
Rivaroxaban.

selective phosphodiesterase 4 inhibitors.
See: Roflumilast.

selective serotonin reuptake inhibitors.
Use: Antidepressant.
See: Citalopram Hydrobromide.
Escitalopram Oxalate.
$5\text{-}HT_{1A}$ Receptor Agonists.
Fluoxetine Hydrochloride.
Fluvoxamine Maleate.
Paroxetine Hydrochloride.
Sertraline Hydrochloride.

selective vascular endothelial growth factor antagonists.
See: Aflibercept.
Pegaptanib Sodium.
Ranibizumab.

Select-OB + DHA Chewable Tablets and Softgel Capsules. (Everett) Folic acid 1 mg, iron 29 mg, vitamins A 1,700 units, D 400 units, E 30 units, B_1 1.6 mg, B_2 1.8 mg, B_3 15 mg, B_6 2.5 mg, B_{12} 5 mcg,

C 60 mg, Mg, Zn. **Chew. Tab.:** BHT, fructose, mixed berry flavoring, sodium benzoate, sucrose. UD 30s. **Cap., softgel:** DHA 250 mg, lauric acid 20 mg. Glycerin. UD 30s. *Rx.*
Use: Prenatal vitamin with minerals.

•**selegiline hydrochloride.** (se-LE-ji-leen) USAN.
Use: Antiparkinson agent.
See: Carbex.
Eldepryl.
Emsam.
Zelapar.

selegiline hydrochloride. (Various Mfr.) Selegiline 5 mg. May contain lactose. **Cap.:** 60s, 500s, 1,000s. **Tab.:** 60s, 500s. *Rx.*
Use: Antiparkinson agent.

Selenicaps-200. (Key Co) Selenium 200 mcg. Sugar free and wheat free. Cap. 100s. *OTC.*
Use: Trace element.

Selenicel. (Taylor Pharmaceuticals) Selenium yeast complex 200 mcg, vitamins C 100 mg, E 100 mg. Cap. Bot. 90s. *OTC.*
Use: Vitamin supplement.

Selenimin. (Key Co) Selenium 125 mcg. Film coated. Sugar free and wheat free. Tab. 100s. *OTC.*
Use: Trace element.

Selenimin-50. (Key Co) Selenium 50 mcg. Film coated. Sugar free and wheat free. Tab. 100s. *OTC.*
Use: Trace element.

Selenimin-200. (Key Co) Selenium 200 mcg. Film coated. Sugar free and wheat free. Tab. 100s. *OTC.*
Use: Trace element.

•**selenious acid.** (seh-LEE-nee-us) *USP.*
Use: Supplement (trace mineral).

selenium.
Use: Trace element.
See: Selenicaps-200.
Selenimin.
Selenimin-50.
Selenimin-200.
Se-100.
W/Calcium.
See: Vitaline Selenium.

selenium. (Major) Selenium 200 mcg. Contains wheat ingredients. Lactose free, preservative free, and sugar free. ER Tab. 60s. *OTC.*
Use: Trace element.

selenium. (Mason) Selenium 100 mcg. Sugar free. Tab. 100s. *OTC.*
Use: Trace element.

selenium. (McGuff) Selenium 100 mcg. Gluten free, preservative free, and sugar free. Cap. 100s. *OTC.*
Use: Trace element.

selenium. (Nion Corp.) Selenium 50 mcg. Tab. Bot. 100s. *Rx.*
Use: Nutritional supplement, parenteral.

selenium. (Various Mfr.) Selenium. **Cap.:** 200 mcg. 60s, 100s. **Tab.:** 50 mcg, 200 mcg. 50s (200 mg only), 60s (200 mg only), 100s. *OTC.*
Use: Trace element.

selenium disulfide.
See: Selenium Sulfide.

•**selenium sulfide.** (seh-LEE-nee-uhm SULL-fide) *USP.*
Use: Antidandruff; antifungal; antiseborrheic.
See: Head & Shoulders Intensive Treatment.
Selenos.
SelRx.
Selsun.

selenium sulfide. (Kylemore) Selenium sulfide 2.25%. Caprylic/capric triglyceride, edetate disodium, parabens, propylene glycol, urea, zinc. Shampoo, Susp. 180 mL. *Rx.*
Use: Antipsoriatic agent.

selenium sulfide. (Various Mfr.) Selenium sulfide. **Lot./Shampoo:** 1%. 210 mL. **Lot.:** 2.5%. 120 mL. *Rx-OTC.*
Use: Antidandruff; antiseborrheic.

•**selenomethionine Se 75.** (seh-LEE-no-meh-THIGH-oh-neen Se 75) USAN.
Use: Diagnostic aid (pancreas function determination), radiopharmaceutical.
See: Sethotope.

Selenos. (Breckenridge Pharmaceutical) Selenium sulfide 2.25%. Caprylic/capric triglyceride, edetate disodium, parabens, propylene glycol, urea, zinc. Shampoo, Susp. 180 mL. *Rx.*
Use: Anti-psoriatic agent.

•**seletracetam.** (SEL-e-TRA-se-tam) USAN.
Use: Antiepileptic.

•**selexipag.** (se-LEX-i-pag) USAN.
Use: Antihypertensive agent.

Selfemra. (Teva) Fluoxetine hydrochloride 10 mg, 20 mg. Cap. UD 28s. *Rx.*
Use: Antidepressant, selective serotonin reuptake inhibitor.

•**selfotel.** (SELL-fah-tell) USAN.
Use: NMDA antagonist.

•**selodenoson.** (sel-oh-DEN-oh-son) USAN.
Use: Cardiovascular agent.

Selora. (Sanofi-Synthelabo) Potassium Cl. Pow. *OTC.*
Use: Salt substitute.

SelRx. (Artesa Labs) Selenium sulfide 2.3%. Caprylic/capric triglyceride,

disodium EDTA, parabens, propylene glycol, titanium dioxide, urea, zinc. Shampoo. 180 mL. *Rx.*
Use: Antipsoriatic agent.

Selsun. (Abbott) Selenium sulfide 2.5%. Lot. 120 mL. *Rx.*
Use: Antiseborrheic.

Selsun Blue Medicated Treatment. (Chattern) Selenium sulfide 1%. Menthol. Lot./Shampoo. 325 mL. *OTC.*
Use: Antiseborrheic.

•**selumetinib.** (SEL-ue-ME-ti-nib) USAN.
Use: Antineoplastic.

•**selumetinib sulfate.** (SEL-ue-ME-ti-nib) USAN.
Use: Antineoplastic.

Selzentry. (ViiV Healthcare) Maraviroc 150 mg, 300 mg. Film-coated. Tab. Bot. 60s. *Rx.*
Use: Antiretroviral, cellular chemokine receptor antagonist.

•**semaglutide.** (SEM-a-GLOO-tide) USAN.
Use: Treatment of type 2 diabetes.

•**sematilide hydrochloride.** (SEH-may-tih-LIDE) USAN.
Use: Cardiovascular agent (antiarrhythmic).

•**semaxanib.** (sem-AX-an-ib) USAN.
Use: Antineoplastic.

•**semduramicin.** (sem-DER-ah-MY-sin) USAN.
Use: Coccidiostat.

•**semduramicin sodium.** (sem-DER-ah-MY-sin) USAN.
Use: Coccidiostat.

Semprex-D. (Actient Pharmaceuticals) Acrivastine 8 mg, pseudoephedrine hydrochloride 60 mg. Lactose. Cap. Bot. 100s. *Rx.*
Use: Upper respiratory combination, decongestant, antihistamine.

•**semuloparin.** (SEM-ue-loe-PAR-in) USAN.
Use: Antithrombotic.

•**semuloparin sodium.** (SEM-ue-loe-PAR-in) USAN.
Use: Antithrombotic.

•**semustine.** (SEH-muss-teen) USAN.
Use: Antineoplastic.

Se-Natal 19. (Seton) Folic acid 1 mg, calcium 200 mg, iron 29 mg, vitamins A 1,000 units, D 400 units, E 30 units, B_1 3 mg, B_2 3 mg, B_3 15 mg, B_5 7 mg, B_6 20 mg, B_{12} 12 mcg, C 100 mg, Zn. **Tab.:** Docusate sodium 25 mg. 100s. **Chew. Tab.:** Orange juice powder, stevia, sucrose. Orange flavor. 100s. *Rx.*
Use: Prenatal vitamin with minerals.

Senexon. (Rugby) Sennosides. **Liq.:** 8.8 mg/mL. Parabens, sucrose. 237 mL. **Tab.:** 8.6 mg. Lactose. Bot. 100s, 1000s. *OTC.*
Use: Laxative.

•**senicapoc.** (SEN-i-KAY-pok) USAN.
Use: Sickle cell disease.

Senilavite. (Defco) Vitamins A 5,000 units, C 100 mg, B_1 2.5 mg, B_2 2 mg, nicotinamide 10 mg, B_6 1 mg, calcium pantothenate 5 mg, B_{12} w/intrinsic factor concentrate 0.133 units, ferrous fumarate 150 mg, glutamic acid hydrochloride 150 mg, docusate sodium 50 mg. Cap. Bot. 100s. *OTC.*
Use: Nutritional supplement.

Senilezol. (Edwards) Vitamins B_1 0.42 mg, B_2 0.42 mg, $B_3$1.67 mg, B_5 0.83 mg, B_6 0.17 mg, B_{12} 0.83 mcg, ferric pyrophosphate 3.3 mg/15 mL, alcohol 15%. Liq. Bot. 473 mL. *OTC.*
Use: Mineral, vitamin supplement.

•**senna.** (SEN-ah) *USP.*
Use: Laxative.
W/Docusate Sodium.
See: Dok Plus.
Senna Plus.
Senna-S.

senna. (Pharmaceutical Associates) Senna leaf extract 176 mg per 5 mL. Glycerin, parabens, sucrose. Syrup. 237 mL. *OTC.*
Use: Laxative.

senna. (SDA Labs) Sennosides 8.8 mg/5 mL. Parabens, sucrose. Syrup. 236 mL. *OTC.*
Use: Laxative, irritant or stimulant laxative.

senna concentrate, standardized.
Use: Cathartic.
See: Senexon.
Senokot.
W/Docusate Sodium.
See: Senokot-S.
W/Psyllium.
See: Perdiem.

senna fruit extract, standardized.
Use: Cathartic.
See: Dosaflex.
Senokot.

Senna-Gen. (Ivax) Sennosides 8.6 mg, lactose. Tab. Bot. 100s, 1000s. *OTC.*
Use: Laxative.

Senna Plus. (Contract Pharmacal) Docusate sodium 50 mg, senna concentrate (as sennosides) 8.6 mg. Tartrazine. Tab. 100s. *OTC.*
Use: Laxative.

Senna Prompt. (Konsyl) Sennosides 9 mg, psyllium 500 mg. Cap. 90s. *OTC.*
Use: Laxative.

Senna-S. (Akyma) Docusate sodium 50 mg, sennosides 8.6 mg. Tab. 1000s.

OTC.
Use: Laxative.
Senna Smooth. (Novartis Consumer Health) Sennosides 15 mg. Sucrose. Tab. 24s. *OTC.*
Use: Laxative.
•**sennosides.** (SEN-oh-sides) *USP.*
Use: Laxative.
See: Agoral.
Black Draught.
Dr. Edwards' Olive.
Evac-U-Gen.
ex-lax.
ex-lax chocolated.
Fletcher's Castoria.
Gentle Nature Natural Vegetable Laxative.
Lax-Pills.
Little Tummys Laxative.
Maximum Relief ex-lax.
Senexon.
Senna.
Senna-Gen.
Senna Smooth.
Senokot.
SenokotXTRA.
W/Docusate Sodium.
See: Dok Plus.
ex-lax Gentle Strength.
Laxacin.
PeriColace.
Senna Plus.
Senna-S.
W/Psyllium.
See: Senna Prompt.
Senokot. (Purdue) **Gran.:** Sennosides 15 mg/5 mL, sucrose. Can. 56 g, 170 g, 340 g. **Tab.:** Sennosides 8.6 mg, lactose. Bot. 10s, 20s, 50s, 100s, 1000s. UD 100s. *OTC.*
Use: Laxative.
Senokot-S. (Purdue) Docusate sodium 50 mg, senna concentrate 8.6 mg, lactose. Tab. Bot. 10s, 30s, 60s, 1000s, UD 100s. *OTC.*
Use: Laxative.
Senokot Suppositories. (Purdue) Standardized senna concentrate. Supp. Pkg. 6s. *OTC.*
Use: Laxative.
SenokotXTRA. (Purdue) Sennosides 17 mg, lactose. Tab. Bot. 12s, 36s. *OTC.*
Use: Laxative.
Sensi-Care Moisturizing Body. (ConvaTec) Dimethicone 1%, petrolatum 30%, cetyl alcohol, glycerin, urea. Cream. 85 g. *OTC.*
Use: Emollient.
Sensipar. (Amgen) Cinacalcet hydrochloride (as base) 30 mg, 60 mg, 90 mg. Film-coated. Tab. 30s. *Rx.*
Use: Calcium receptor agonist.
Sensitive Eyes. (Bausch & Lomb) Sorbic acid 0.1%, EDTA 0.025%, NaCl, boric acid, sodium borate. Soln. Bot. 118 mL, 237 mL, 355 mL. *OTC.*
Use: Contact lens care.
Sensitive Eyes Daily Cleaner. (Bausch & Lomb) Sorbic acid 0.25%, EDTA 0.5%, NaCl, hydroxypropyl methylcellulose, poloxamine, sodium borate. Soln. Bot. 20 mL. *OTC.*
Use: Contact lens care.
Sensitive Eyes Drops. (Bausch & Lomb) Buffered. Sorbic acid 0.1%, EDTA 0.025%, sodium chloride, boric acid, sodium borate. Soln. Bot. 30 mL. *OTC.*
Use: Contact lens rewetting solution.
Sensitive Eyes Plus. (Bausch & Lomb) Boric acid, sodium borate, KCl, NaCl, polyaminopropyl biguanide 0.00003%, EDTA 0.025%. Soln. Bot. 118 mL, 355 mL. *OTC.*
Use: Contact lens care.
Sensitive Eyes Saline. (Bausch & Lomb) NaCl, borate buffer, sorbic acid 0.1%, EDTA. Soln. Bot. 118 mL, 237 mL, 355 mL. *OTC.*
Use: Contact lens care.
Sensitive Eyes Saline/Cleaning Solution. (Bausch & Lomb) Isotonic solution w/borate buffer, NaCl, poloxamine, sorbic acid 0.15%, sodium borate, boric acid, EDTA 0.1%. Soln. Bot. 237 mL. *OTC.*
Use: Contact lens care.
Sensodyne Fresh Mint Toothpaste. (Block Drug) Potassium nitrate 5%, sodium monofluorophosphate 0.76%, saccharin, sorbitol. Mint flavor. Tube 2.4 oz, 4.6 oz. *OTC.*
Use: Dentrifice.
Sensodyne Iso-Active Multi Action. (Glaxo Consumer Healthcare) Potassium nitrate 5%, sodium fluoride 0.15%. Glycerin, PEG, saccharin, sorbitol, sucralose. Gel, dental. 121.6 g. *OTC.*
Use: Mouth and throat product, preparation for sensitive teeth.
Sensodyne Iso-Active Whitening. (Glaxo Consumer Healthcare) Potassium nitrate 5%, sodium fluoride 0.15%. Glycerin, PEG, saccharin, sorbitol, sucralose. Gel, dental. 121.6 g. *OTC.*
Use: Mouth and throat product, preparation for sensitive teeth.
Sensodyne-SC Toothpaste. (Block Drug) Glycerin, sorbitol, sodium methylcocoyl taurate, PEG-40 stearate, strontium Cl hexahydrate 10%, methyl- and propylparabens. Tinted. Tube 2.1 oz,

4 oz. *OTC.*
Use: Dentrifice.

SensoGARD. (Block Drug) Benzocaine 20%. Parabens. Gel; dental. 0.5 g. *OTC.*
Use: Anesthetic, local.

Sensorcaine. (APP Pharmaceuticals) Bupivacaine hydrochloride 0.25% or 0.5%. Bupivacaine hydrochloride 0.25% or 0.5%, epinephrine 1:200,000, methylparaben 1 mg/mL. Inj. Multidose vial 50 mL. *Rx.*
Use: Anesthetic, local amide.

Sensorcaine MPF. (APP Pharmaceuticals) Bupivacaine hydrochloride 0.25%, 0.5%, 0.75%. Inj. Single-dose amp. 30 mL (except 0.5%). Single-dose vials 10 mL, 30 mL. Bupivacaine hydrochloride 0.25%, 0.5%, or 0.75% with epinephrine 1:200,000. Inj. Single-dose amp. 5 mL (0.5% only), 30 mL (except 0.5%). Single-dose vials 10 mL, 30 mL. *Rx.*
Use: Anesthetic, local amide.

Sensorcaine-MPF Spinal. (APP Pharmaceuticals) Bupivacaine hydrochloride 0.75%, dextrose 8.25%. Inj. Amp. 2 mL. *Rx.*
Use: Anesthetic, local amide.

Se-100. (Bio-Tech Pharmacal) Selenium 100 mcg. Dye free, preservative free, and sugar free. Cap. 100s. *OTC.*
Use: Trace element.

•**sepantronium bromide.** (SEP-an-TROE-nee-um) USAN.
Use: Antineoplastic.

•**sepazonium chloride.** (SEP-ah-ZOE-nee-uhm) USAN.
Use: Anti-infective, topical.

•**seperidol hydrochloride.** (seh-PURR-ih-dahl) USAN.
Use: Neuroleptic; antipsychotic.

•**seprilose.** (SEH-prih-LOHS) USAN.
Use: Antirheumatic.

•**seproxetine hydrochloride.** (sep-ROX-eh-teen) USAN.
Use: Antidepressant.

Septi-Chek. (Roche) Blood culture and simultaneous sub-culture system with three media to support clinically significant pathogens. Quick and easy assembly forms a closed system to protect sub-cultures from contamination.
Use: Diagnostic aid.

Septiphene. (SEP-tih-feen) (Monsanto)
Use: Disinfectant.

Septo. (Vita Elixir) Methylbenzethonium Cl, ethanol 2%, menthol. *OTC.*
Use: Antimicrobial; antiseptic.

•**seractide acetate.** (seer-ACK-tide) USAN.
Use: Corticotrophic peptide, hormone (adrenocorticotrophic).

Ser-A-Gen. (Ivax) Hydrochlorothiazide 15 mg, reserpine 0.1 mg, hydralazine hydrochloride 25 mg. Tab. Bot. 100s, 1000s. *Rx.*
Use: Antihypertensive combination.

Seralyzer. (Bayer Consumer Care) A system for the measurement of enzymes, potassium levels, blood chemistries, and therapeutic drug assays consisting of a reflectance photometer and a series of solid-phase reagent strips.
Use: Diagnostic aid.

•**seratrodast.** (seh-RAH-troe-dast) USAN.
Use: Anti-inflammatory (non-antihistaminic); antiasthmatic (thromboxane receptor antagonist).

•**serazapine hydrochloride.** (ser-AZE-ah-PEEN) USAN.
Use: Anxiolytic.

Sereen. (Foy Laboratories) Chlordiazepoxide hydrochloride 10 mg. Cap. Bot. 500s, 1000s. *c-iv.*
Use: Anxiolytic.

Sereine Cleaning Solution. (Optikem) Cocoamphodiacetate and glycols, EDTA 0.1%, benzalkonium Cl 0.01%. Soln. Bot. 60 mL. *OTC.*
Use: Contact lens care.

Sereine Wetting/Soaking Solution. (Optikem) EDTA 0.1%, benzalkonium Cl 0.01%. Soln. Bot. 120 mL. *OTC.*
Use: Contact lens care, soaking, wetting.

Sereine Wetting Solution. (Optikem) EDTA 0.1%, benzalkonium chloride 0.01%. Soln. Bot. 60 mL, 120 mL. *OTC.*
Use: Contact lens care.

•**serelaxin.** (SER-e-LAX-in) USAN.
Use: Treatment of acute heart failure.

Serene. (Health for Life Brands) Salicylamide 2 g, scopolamine aminoxide HBr 0.2 mg. Cap. Bot. 24s, 60s. *Rx.*
Use: Analgesic; sedative.

Serevent Diskus. (GlaxoSmithKline) Salmeterol xinafoate 50 mcg, lactose. Pow. for Inh. Blisters 28s, 60s. *Rx.*
Use: Bronchodilator, sympathomimetic.

•**sergliflozin.** (SER-gli-FLOE-zin) USAN.
Use: Antidiabetic.

•**sergolexole maleate.** (SER-go-LEX-ole) USAN.
Use: Antimigraine.

sericinase. A proteolytic enzyme.

•**serine.** (SER-een) *USP.*
Use: Amino acid.

•**serlopitant.** (ser-LOE-pi-tant) USAN.
Use: Genitourinary agent.

• **sermetacin.** (ser-MET-ah-sin) USAN.
Use: Anti-inflammatory.

• **sermorelin acetate.** (SER-moe-REH-lin) USAN.
Use: Growth hormone-releasing factor, diagnostic aid. [Orphan Drug]

Serophene. (Serono) Clomiphene citrate 50 mg. Tab. Bot. 10s, 30s. *Rx.*
Use: Ovulation inducer; sex hormone.

Seroquel. (AstraZeneca) Quetiapine (as quetiapine fumarate) 25 mg, 50 mg, 100 mg, 200 mg, 300 mg, 400 mg. Lactose. Film-coated. Tab. Bot. 60s (300 mg only), 100s (except 300 mg), 1000s (25 mg and 50 mg only), UD 100s. *Rx.*
Tall Man: SEROquel
Use: Antipsychotic, dibenzapine derivative.

Seroquel XR. (AstraZeneca) Quetiapine 50 mg (equiv. to quetiapine fumarate 58 mg), 150 mg (equiv. to quetiapine fumarate 173 mg), 200 mg (equiv. to quetiapine fumarate 230 mg), 300 mg (equiv. to quetiapine fumarate 345 mg), 400 mg (equiv. to quetiapine fumarate 461 mg). Lactose. Film-coated. 60s, 500s (50 mg and 150 mg only), UD 100s. *Rx.*
Tall Man: SEROquel
Use: Antipsychotic, dibenzapine derivative.

Serostim. (EMD Serono) Somatropin 4 mg/vial (≈ 12 units), 5 mg/vial (≈ 15 units), 6 mg/vial (≈ 18 units). Sucrose. Inj. lyophilized Pow. for Soln. Single-use vial w/diluent. *Rx.*
Use: Hormone, growth.

serotonin and norepinephrine reuptake inhibitors.
Use: Antidepressant.
See: Desvenlafaxine Succinate.
Duloxetine Hydrochloride.
Levomilnacipran.
Venlafaxine Hydrochloride.

serotonin 5-HT$_1$ receptor agonists.
Use: Antimigraine agents.
See: Almotriptan Malate.
Eletriptan Hydrobromide.
Frovatriptan Succinate.
Naratriptan Hydrochloride.
Rizatriptan Benzoate.
Sumatriptan Succinate.
Zolmitriptan.

serotonin reuptake inhibitors, selective.
Use: Antidepressant.
See: Citalopram Hydrochloride.
Escitalopram.
Fluoxetine Hydrochloride.
Fluvoxamine Maleate.
Paroxetine Hydrochloride.
Sertraline Hydrochloride.

serotonin 2C receptor agonists.
See: Lorcaserin.

Serpasil-Apresoline. (Novartis) **#1:** Reserpine 0.1 mg, hydralazine hydrochloride 25 mg. Tab. Bot. 100s. **#2:** Reserpine 0.2 mg, hydralazine hydrochloride 50 mg. Tab. Bot. 100s. *Rx.*
Use: Antihypertensive combination.

Serpasil-Esidrix. (Novartis) **#1:** Reserpine 0.1 mg, hydrochlorothiazide 25 mg. Tab. **#2:** Reserpine 0.1 mg, hydrochlorothiazide 50 mg. Tab. Bot. 100s, 1000s. *Rx.*
Use: Antihypertensive combination.

Serpazide. (Major) Reserpine 0.1 mg, hydralazine hydrochloride 25 mg, hydrochlorothiazide 15 mg. Tab. Bot. 100s, 1000s. *Rx.*
Use: Antihypertensive combination.

Serratia marcescens extract (polyribosomes).
Use: Primary brain malignancies. [Orphan Drug]

Sertabs. (Table Rock) Reserpine 0.25 mg, 0.5 mg. Tab. Bot. 100s, 500s. *Rx.*
Use: Antihypertensive.

sertaconazole nitrate. (SIR-tah-KAHN-uh-zole)
Use: Antifungal agent, topical anti-infective.
See: Ertaczo.

Sertina. (Fellows) Reserpine 0.25 mg. Tab. Bot. 1000s, 5000s. *Rx.*
Use: Antihypertensive.

• **sertindole.** (ser-TIN-dole) USAN.
Use: Antipsychotic.

• **sertraline hydrochloride.** (SIR-truh-leen) USAN.
Use: Antidepressant, selective serotonin reuptake inhibitor.
See: Zoloft.

sertraline hydrochloride. (Ranbaxy Pharmaceuticals) Sertraline 20 mg/mL (as base). Alcohol 15.8%, menthol. Mint flavor. Oral Concentrate. Soln. Bot. 60 mL with calibrated droppers. *Rx.*
Use: Antidepressant, selective serotonin reuptake inhibitor.

sertraline hydrochloride. (Various Mfr.) Sertraline hydrochloride (as base) 25 mg, 50 mg, 100 mg. May contain lactose, polydextrose. Tab. 30s, 50s, 60s, 90s, 100s, 180s, 480s (except 25 mg), 500s, 1000s, 3000s (50 mg only), 5000s, UD 100s (except 25 mg). *Rx.*
Use: Antidepressant, selective serotonin reuptake inhibitor.

serum, albumin, human, radioiodinated.
See: Albumin Injection.
serum, albumin, normal human.
See: Albumin Human.
serum, globulin (human), immune.
Use: Immunization.
Serutan. (GlaxoSmithKline) Psyllium 2.5 g, sodium < 0.03 g/heaping tsp, saccharin, sugar. Gran. Can. 170 g, 540 g. *OTC.*
Use: Laxative.
•**sesame oil.** (SES-a-me) *NF.*
Use: Pharmaceutic aid (solvent; vehicle, oleaginous).
Sesame Street Complete. (McNeil Consumer) Ca 80 mg, Fe 10 mg, vitamins A 2750 units, D 200 units, E 10 mg, B_1 0.75 mg, B_2 0.85 mg, B_3 10 mg, B_5 5 mg, B_6 0.7 mg, B_{12} 3 mcg, C 40 mg, folic acid 0.2 mg, biotin 15 mg, Cu, I, Mg, Zn 8 mg. Lactose. Tab. Bot. 50s. *OTC.*
Use: Mineral, vitamin supplement.
Sesame Street Plus Iron. (McNeil Consumer) Fe 10 mg, vitamins A 2750 units, D 200 units, E 10 units, B_1 0.75 mg, B_2 0.85 mg, B_3 10 mg, B_5 5 mg, B_6 0.7 mg, B_{12} 3 mcg, C 40 mg, folic acid 0.2 mg. Chew. Tab. Bot. 50s. *OTC.*
Use: Mineral, vitamin supplement.
Sesame Street Vitamins. (McNeil Consumer) **For ages 4 and older:** Vitamins A 5,000 units, B_1 1.5 mg, B_{12} 6 mcg, C 60 mg, D 400 units, E 30 units, folic acid 400 mcg, biotin 300 mcg. Chew. Tab. Bot. 60s. **For ages 2 to 3:** Vitamins A 2,500 units, B_1 0.7 mg, B_2 0.8 mg, B_3 9 mg, B_5 5 mg, B_6 0.7 mg, B_{12} 3 mcg, C 40 mg, D 400 units, E 10 units, folic acid 200 mcg, biotin 150 mcg. Chew. Tab. Bot. 60s. *OTC.*
Use: Vitamin supplement.
Sesame Street Vitamins and Minerals. (McNeil Consumer) **For ages 4 and older:** Vitamins A 5,000 units, B_1 1.5 mg, B_2 1.7 mg, B_3 20 mg, B_5 10 mg, B_6 2 mg, B_{12} 6 mcg, C 60 mg, D 400 units, E 30 units, folic acid 400 mcg, biotin 300 mcg, Ca 100 mg, Fe 18 mg, I 150 mcg, Zn 15 mg, Cu 2 mg. Chew. Tab. Bot. 60s. **For ages 2 to 3:** Vitamins A 2,500 units, B_1 0.7 mg, B_{12} 3 mcg, C 40 mg, D 400 units, E 10 units, folic acid 200 mcg, biotin 150 mcg, Ca 80 mg, Fe 10 mg, I 70 mcg, Zn 8 mg, Cu 1 mg. Chew. Tab. Bot. 60s. *OTC.*
Use: Mineral, vitamin supplement.
SE 10-5 SS. (Seton Pharmaceuticals) Sodium sulfacetamide 10%, sulfur 5%. Benzyl alcohol, witch hazel. Cream. 120 g. *Rx.*
Use: Acne product combination.
Sethotope. (Bristol-Myers Squibb) Selenomethionine selenium 75; available as 0.25, 1 mCi.
Use: Diagnostic imaging.
•**setileuton.** (set-i-LOO-ton) USAN.
Use: Treatment of asthma.
•**setipiprant.** (set-I-pi-prant) USAN.
Use: Treatment of asthma, allergic rhinitis, atopic dermatitis.
•**setoperone.** (SEE-toe-per-OHN) USAN.
Use: Antipsychotic.
•**setrobuvir.** (SET-roe-BUE-vir) USAN.
Use: Treatment of hepatitis C.
•**sevelamer carbonate.** (se-VEL-a-mer) USAN.
Use: Phosphate binder.
See: Renvela.
•**sevelamer hydrochloride.** (se-VEL-a-mer) USAN.
Use: Phosphate binder.
See: Renagel.
•**sevirumab.** (seh-VIE-roo-mab) USAN.
Use: Monoclonal antibody (antiviral).
•**sevoflurane.** (SEE-voe-FLEW-rane) USAN.
Use: Anesthetic, general, volatile liquid.
See: Sojourn.
Ultane.
sex hormones.
See: Anabolic Steroids.
Androgen Hormone Inhibitor.
Androgens.
Contraceptive Hormones.
Danazol.
Esterified Estrogens.
Estradiol.
Estradiol Cypionate.
Estradiol Topical Emulsion.
Estradiol Transdermal System.
Estradiol Valerate.
Estrogen and Androgen Combinations.
Estrogens.
Estrogens and Progestins Combined.
Estrogens, Conjugated.
Estrogens, Miscellaneous Topical.
Estrogens, Miscellaneous Vaginal.
Estrogens, Synthetic.
Estropipate.
Gonadotropin-Releasing Hormone Antagonists.
Gonadotropin-Releasing Hormones.
Ovulation Stimulants.
Progestins.
Raloxifene Hydrochloride.
Selective Estrogen Receptor Modulator.

•**sezolamide hydrochloride.** (seh-ZOLE-ah-MIDE) USAN.
Use: Carbonic anhydrase inhibitor.

SF 5000 Plus. (Cypress Pharmaceutical) Fluoride 1.1%. Glycerin, saccharin, sorbitol. Cream, dental. 51 g. *Rx.*
Use: Trace element.

SF 1.1%. (Cypress) Fluoride 0.5% Parabens, saccharin, sorbitol. Mint flavor. Gel, dental. 56 g. *Rx.*
Use: Trace element.

sfRowasa. (Alaven) Mesalamine 4 g per 60 mL. Edetate disodium. Sulfite free. Susp. 7s, 14s, 28s. *Rx.*
Use: Gastrointestinal agent.

Shade. (Schering-Plough) SPF 15. Contains one or more of the following ingredients: Padimate O, oxybenzone, ethylhexyl-p-methoxycinnamate. Bot. 118 mL, 120 mL, 240 mL. *OTC.*
Use: Sunscreen.

Shade Cream. (O'Leary) Jar 0.25 oz. *OTC.*
Use: Contouring cream.

Shade Sunblock Gel, 15 SPF. (Schering-Plough) Ethylhexyl p-methoxycinnamate, octyl salicylate, oxybenzone, SD alcohol 40. PABA free. SPF 15. Waterproof. Gel. Bot. 120 mL. *OTC.*
Use: Sunscreen.

Shade Sunblock Gel, 30 SPF. (Schering-Plough) Ethylhexyl p-methoxycinnamate, homosalate, oxybenzone, 73% SD alcohol 40. Bot. 120 mL. *OTC.*
Use: Sunscreen.

Shade Sunblock Gel, 25 SPF. (Schering-Plough) Ethylhexyl p-methoxycinnamate, octyl salicylate, homosalate, oxybenzone, SD alcohol 40. PABA free. Gel. Bot. 120 mL. *OTC.*
Use: Sunscreen.

Shade Sunblock Lotion, 15 SPF. (Schering-Plough) Ethylhexyl p-methoxycinnamate, oxybenzone, benzyl alcohol, phenethyl alcohol. PABA free. Waterproof. Lot. Bot. 120 mL. *OTC.*
Use: Sunscreen.

Shade Sunblock Lotion, 45 SPF. (Schering-Plough) Ethylhexyl p-methoxycinnamate, oxybenzone, 2-ethylhexyl salicylate, benzyl alcohol, phenethyl alcohol. PABA free. Waterproof. Lot. Bot. 120 mL. *OTC.*
Use: Sunscreen.

Shade Sunblock Lotion, 30 SPF. Schering-Plough) Ethylhexyl p-methoxycinnamate, 2-ethylhexyl salicylate, homosalate, oxybenzone, benzyl alcohol, phenethyl alcohol. PABA free. Waterproof. Lot. Bot. 120 mL. *OTC.*
Use: Sunscreen.

Shade Sunblock Stick, 30 SPF. (Schering-Plough) Ethylhexyl p-methoxycinnamate, oxybenzone, 2-ethylhexyl salicylate, homosalate. PABA free. Waterproof. Stick. 18 g. *OTC.*
Use: Sunscreen.

Shade UVA Guard. (Schering-Plough) Octyl methoxycinnamate 7.5%, avobenzone 3%, oxybenzone 3%. Waterproof. SPF 15. Lot. 120 mL. *OTC.*
Use: Sunscreen.

Sheik Elite. (Durex) Condom with nonoxynol-9 15%. 3s, 12s, 24s, 36s. *OTC.*
Use: Contraceptive.

•**shellac.** (she-LAK) *NF.*
Use: Pharmaceutic aid (tablet coating agent).

Shellgel. (Cytosol Ophthalmics) Sodium hyaluronate 12 mg/mL, sodium chloride 9 mg/mL. Inj. Disposable syringes. 0.8 mL. *Rx.*
Use: Ophthalmic surgical adjunct.

Shepard's Cream Lotion. (Dermik) Creamy lotion with no lanolin or mineral oil, for entire body. Scented or unscented. Bot. 8 oz, 16 oz. *OTC.*
Use: Emollient.

Sherhist. (Sheryl) Phenylephrine hydrochloride, pyrilamine maleate. Tab. Bot. 100s. Liq. Bot. Pt.
Use: Decongestant; antihistamine.

Shernatal. (Sheryl) Phosphorus free calcium, non-irritating iron, trace minerals and essential vitamins. Tab. Bot. 100s. *OTC.*
Use: Mineral, vitamin supplement.

Shohl's Modified. (Humco) Sodium citrate 500 mg, citric acid 300 mg per 5 mL. Alcohol 0.25%, parabens. Each mL contains sodium ion 1 mEq and is equiv. to bicarbonate 1 mEq. Soln. 473 mL. *Rx.*
Use: Alkalizer, systemic.

short chain fatty acid solution.
Use: Ulcerative colitis. [Orphan Drug]

short ragweed pollen allergen extract.
Use: Allergenic extract.
See: Ragwitek.

Shur-Clens. (GlaxoSmithKline) Poloxamer 188 20%. Soln. Bot. UD 100 mL, 200 mL. *OTC.*
Use: Dermatologic.

Sibelium. (Janssen) Flunarizine hydrochloride. *Rx.*
Use: Vasodilator.

•**sibenadet hydrochloride.** (si-BEN-a-det) USAN.
Use: Chronic obstructive pulmonary disease.

•**sibopirdine.** (sih-BOE-pihr-deen) USAN.
Use: Nootropic; cognition enhancer (Alzheimer disease).

•**sibrafran.** (sib-rah-FIE-ban) USAN.
Use: Antithrombotic; fibrinogen receptor antagonist; platelet aggregation inhibitor.

•**sibutramine hydrochloride.** (sih-BYOO-trah-meen) USAN.
Use: Antidepressant, CNS stimulant, anorexic.

sickle cell test.
Use: Diagnostic aid.
See: Sickledex.

Sickledex. (Ortho-Clinical Diagnostics) Test kit 12s, 100s.
Use: Diagnostic aid to detect hemoglobin S.

•**sifalimumab.** (SYE-fa-LIM-ue-mab) USAN.
Use: Monoclonal antibody.

Sigamine. (Sigma-Tau) Cyanocobalamin injection 1000 mcg/mL. Vial 10 mL, 30 mL. Also Sigamine L.A. Vial 10 mL. *Rx.*
Use: Vitamin supplement.

Sigazine. (Sigma-Tau) Promethazine hydrochloride 50 mg/mL. Vial 10 mL. *Rx.*
Use: Antihistamine.

Signa Creme. (Parker) Conductive cosmetic quality electrolyte cream. Bot. 5 oz, 2 L, 4 L. *OTC.*
Use: Diagnostic aid.

Signa Gel. (Parker) Conductive saline electrode gel. Tube 250 g.
Use: Diagnostic aid, gel.

Signa Pad. (Parker) Premoistened electrode pads.
Use: Diagnostic aid, pad.

Signatal C. (Sigma-Tau) Ca 230 mg, Fe 49.3 mg, vitamins A 4,000 units, D 400 units, B_1 2 mg, B_2 2 mg, B_6 1 mg, B_{12} 2 mcg, folic acid 0.1 mg, niacinamide 10 mg, C 50 mg, I 0.15 mg. SC Tab. Bot. 100s, 1000s. *OTC.*
Use: Mineral, vitamin supplement.

Signate. (Sigma-Tau) Dimenhydrinate 50 mg, propylene glycol 50%, benzyl alcohol 5%/mL. Vial 10 mL. *Rx.*
Use: Antiemetic; antivertigo.

Signifor. (Novartis) Pasireotide diaspartate 0.3 mg/mL, 0.6 mg/mL, 0.9 mg/mL. Mannitol. Inj., Soln. Single-dose ampule. 1 mL. *Rx.*
Use: Somatostatin analog.

Sigpred. (Sigma-Tau) Prednisolone acetate. Vial 10 mL. *Rx.*
Use: Corticosteroid.

Sigtab. (Roberts) Vitamins A 5,000 units, D 400 units, B_1 10.3 mg, B_2 10 mg, C 333 mg, B_3 100 mg, B_6 6 mg, B_5 20 mg, folic acid 0.4 mg, B_{12} 18 mcg, E 15 mg. Tab. Bot. 90s, 500s. *OTC.*
Use: Vitamin supplement.

Sigtab-M. (Roberts) Vitamins A 6000 units, D_3 400 units, E 45 mg, C 100 mg, B_3 25 mg, B_1 5 mg, B_2 5 mg, B_6 3 mg, folic acid 400 mcg, B_5 0.015 mg, biotin 45 mcg, Ca 200 mg, P, Fe 18 mg, Mg, Cu, Zn 15 mg, Mn, K, Cl, Mo, Se, Cr, Ni, Sn, V, Si, B, vitamin K, I. Tab. Bot. 100s. *OTC.*
Use: Mineral, vitamin supplement.

Silace. (Silarx) Docusate sodium. **Liq.:** 10 mg/mL. Parabens. 473 mL. **Syrup:** 60 mg/15 mL. Alcohol ≤ 1%. Bot. 473 mL. *OTC.*
Use: Laxative.

Siladryl. (Silarx) Diphenhydramine hydrochloride 12.5 mg/5 mL. Black cherry flavoring, parabens, propylene glycol, saccharin, sorbitol. Alcohol free and sugar free. Liq. 118 mL, 237 mL. *OTC.*
Use: Antihistamine, nonselective ethanolamine.

Silafed. (Silarx) Pseudoephedrine hydrochloride 30 mg, triprolidine hydrochloride 1.25 mg/5 mL. Methylparaben, sucrose, saccharin. Syrup. Bot. 118 mL. *OTC.*
Use: Upper respiratory combination, antihistamine and decongestant combination.

•**silafilcon A.** (SIH-lah-FILL-kahn A) USAN.
Use: Contact lens material (hydrophilic).

•**silafocon A.** (SIH-lah-FOH-kahn A) USAN.
Use: Contact lens material (hydrophobic).

•**silandrone.** (sil-AN-drone) USAN.
Use: Androgen.

Silapap Children's. (Silarx) Acetaminophen. **Elix.:** 160 mg/5 mL. Alcohol free. Bot. 237 mL. **Liq.:** 160 mg/5 mL. Alcohol and sugar free. Methylparaben, saccharin. 118 mL, 237 mL, 473 mL. *OTC.*
Use: Analgesic.

Silapap Infant's. (Silarx) Acetaminophen 100 mg/mL. Alcohol free. Soln., Conc., Oral. 15 mL, 30 mL. *OTC.*
Use: Analgesic.

•**sildenafil citrate.** (sill-DEN-ah-fil SIH-trate) USAN.
Use: Anti-impotence agent.
See: Revatio.
Viagra.

sildenafil citrate. (Greenstone) Sildenafil

citrate 20 mg. Lactose. Tab. 90s. *Rx.*
Use: Impotence agent, phosphodiesterase type 5 inhibitor.

Silenor. (Somaxon Pharmaceuticals) Doxepin 3 mg (equiv. to doxepin hydrochloride 3.39 mg), 6 mg (equiv. to doxepin hydrochloride 6.78 mg). Tab. 30s, 100s, 500s, UD 30s. *Rx.*
Use: Antidepressant, tricyclic compound.

•**silica, dental-type.** (SILL-ih-kah) *NF.*
Use: Pharmaceutic aid.

•**siliceous earth, purified.** (sih-LIH-shus) *NF.*
Use: Pharmaceutic aid (filtering medium).

•**silicon dioxide.** (SILL-ih-kahn die-OX-ide) *NF. Formerly Silica Gel.*
Use: Pharmaceutic aid (dispersing and suspending agent).
W/Calcium Chloride, Dibasic Sodium Phosphate, Monobasic Sodium Phosphate, Sodium Chloride, Sodium Bicarbonate.
See: NeutraSal.

•**silicon dioxide, colloidal.** (SILL-ih-kahn die-OX-ide) *NF.*
Use: Pharmaceutic aid (tablet/capsule diluent, suspending and thickening agent).

Silicone. (Dow Hickam) Dimethicone. Liq., Bot. oz. Bulk Pkg. Oint.

silicone oil.
See: Polydimethylsiloxane (Silicone Oil).

silicone ointment. Dimethicone Dimethyl Polysiloxane.

silicone powder. (Gordon Laboratories) Talc with silicone. Pkg. 4 oz, 1 lb, 5 lb. *OTC.*
Use: Dusting powder.

silodosin. (sil-OH-doe-sin)
Use: Antiadrenergic agent, peripherally acting; alpha-1–adrenergic blocker.
See: Rapaflo.

•**silodrate.** (SILL-oh-drate) USAN.
Use: Antacid.

Silphen Cough. (Silarx) Diphenhydramine hydrochloride 12.5 mg/5 mL, alcohol 5%, menthol, sucrose, parabens, strawberry flavor. Syr. Bot. 118 mL. *OTC.*
Use: Antihistamine.

Silphen DM. (Silarx) Dextromethorphan HBr 10 mg/5 mL. Alcohol 5%, menthol, methylparaben, sucrose. Syrup. Bot. 118 mL. *OTC.*
Use: Nonnarcotic antitussive.

Siltussin DAS. (Silarx) Guaifenesin 100 mg/5 mL. Strawberry flavor. Liq. 118 mL. *OTC.*
Use: Expectorant.

Siltussin DM. (Silarx) Dextromethorphan HBr 10 mg, guaifenesin 100 mg/5 mL. Saccharin, sucrose, methylparaben, menthol. Alcohol free. Liq. Bot. 118 mL, 237 mL, 473 mL. *OTC.*
Use: Upper respiratory combination, antitussive, expectorant.

Siltussin DM Cough. (Silarx) Dextromethorphan HBr 10 mg, guaifenesin 100 mg per 5 mL. Alcohol free. Sucrose, saccharin, methylparaben. Syrup. 118 mL. *OTC.*
Use: Antitussive with expectorant.

Siltussin SA. (Silarx) Guaifenesin 100 mg/5 mL, strawberry flavor. Liq. 118 mL, 237 mL, 473 mL. *OTC.*
Use: Expectorant.

•**siltuximab.** (sil-TUX-i-mab) USAN.
Use: Monoclonal antibody.
See: Sylvant.

Silvadene. (Monarch) Silver sulfadiazine 10 mg/g in a water–miscible base. Contains white petrolatum, stearyl alcohol, methylparaben 0.3%. Cream. 20 g, 50 g, 85 g, 400 g, 1000 g. *Rx.*
Use: Anti-infective, topical.

silver.
See: Elta SilverGel.
SilvrSTAT.

silver compounds.
See: Silver Nitrate.
Silver Protein, Mild.
Silver Protein, Strong.
Silverseal.

•**silver nitrate.** (SILL-ver NYE-trate) *USP.*
Use: Anti-infective, topical.
W/Potassium Nitrate.
See: Grafco.

•**silver nitrate, toughened.** (SILL-ver NYE-trate) *USP.*
Use: Caustic.

silver protein, mild. Argentum Vitellinum, Cargentos, Mucleinate Mild, Protargin Mild.

silver protein, strong.
See: Protargol.

Silverseal. (Alliqua Biomedical) Silver 99.9%. Dressing; topical. 2" × 3" and 4" × 5". 10s. *Rx.*
Use: Wound healing agent.

silver sulfadiazine. (SILL-ver SULL-fah-DIE-ah-zeen)
Use: Anti-infective, topical.
See: Silvadene.
SSD.
SSD AF.
Thermazene.

silver sulfadiazine. (Various Mfr.) Silver sulfadiazine 1%. May contain alcohols,

methylparaben, petrolatum, propylene glycol. Cream. 20 g, 25 g, 50 g, 85 g, 400 g. *Rx.*
Use: Topical anti-infective, burn preparation.

SilvrSTAT. (ABL Medical) Silver 32 parts per million. Propylene glycol, triethanolamine. Gel. 28.35 g, 85.05 g. *Rx.*
Use: Wound healing agent.

Simbrinza. (Alcon) Brinzolamide 1%/brimonidine tartrate 0.2%. Benzalkonium chloride, boric acid, propylene glycol, tyloxapol. Susp.; Ophth. 8 mL. *Rx.*
Use: Agent for glaucoma.

Simcor. (Abbott) Niacin (extended release)/simvastatin 500 mg/20 mg, 500 mg/40 mg, 750 mg/20 mg, 1,000 mg/40 mg. Lactose, PEG. ER Tab. 90s. *Rx.*
Use: Antihyperlipidemic.

•**simenepag.** (sye-MEN-e-pag) USAN.
Use: Ophthalmic agent.

•**simenepag isopropyl.** (sye-MEN-e-pag) USAN.
Use: Ophthalmic agent.

•**simeprevir.** (sim-E-pre-vir) USAN.
Use: Treatment of hepatitis C.
See: Olysio.

•**simethicone.** (sih-METH-ih-cone) *USP.* Mixture of liquid dimethyl polysiloxanes with silica aerogel.
Use: Antiflatulent.
See: Baby Gas-X Infant.
Bicarsim.
Bicarsim Forte.
Gas Relief.
Gas-X Extra Strength.
Gas-X Thin Strips.
Mylicon.
Mylicon-80.
Phazyme.
Phazyme Quick Dissolve.
W/Aluminum Hydroxide, Magnesium Hydroxide.
See: Di-Gel.
Gas Ban DS.
Maalox Advanced Maximum Strength.
Maalox Advanced Regular Strength.
Mi-Acid Maximum Strength.
Mintox.
Trial AG.
W/Calcium Carbonate.
See: Gas Ban.
Gas-X With Maalox Extra Strength.
Maalox Junior.
Rolaids Extra Strength Plus Gas Relief.
Titralac Plus.
Tums Plus.
W/Calcium Carbonate, Magnesium Hydroxide.
See: Rolaids Multi-Symptom.
W/Citric Acid, Sodium Bicarbonate.
See: E-Z Gas II.
W/Loperadmide Hydrochloride.
See: Imodium Multi-Symptom Relief.

simethicone. (Rugby) Simethicone 180 mg. Glycerin. Cap., softgel. 60s. *OTC.*
Use: Antiflatulent.

Similac Human Milk Fortifier. (Ross) Protein (nonfat milk, whey protein concentrate) 1 g, carbohydrate (corn syrup solids) 1.8 g, fat (fractionated coconut oil [medium chain triglycerides], soy lecithin) 0.36 g per 4 packets (3.6 g), with vitamins A, B_1, B_2, B_3, B_5, B_6, B_{12}, C, D, E, K, folic acid (folacin), biotin, Ca, chloride, Cu, Fe, Mg, Mn, P, Zn, Na 15 mg, K 63 mg, 14 cal/3.6 g. Add to breast milk. Pow. Pkt. 0.9 g (50s). *OTC.*
Use: Enteral nutritional therapy.

Similac Low-Iron Liquid & Powder. (Ross) Protein 14.3 g, carbohydrates 72 g, fat 36 g, Fe 1.5 mg, with appropriate vitamins and minerals. **Liq.:** 390 mL concentrate, 240 mL and 1 qt. ready-to-use, 120 mL and 240 mL nursettes. **Pow.:** 1 lb. *OTC.*
Use: Nutritional supplement.

Similac Natural Care Human Milk Fortifier. (Ross) Liquid fortifier designed to be mixed with human milk or fed alternately with human milk to low-birth-weight infants. Supplied as 24 Cal/fl oz. Bot. 4 fl oz. *OTC.*
Use: Nutritional supplement.

Similac PM 60/40. (Ross) Milk-based formula ready-to-feed or powder with 60:40 whey to casein ratio (20 Cal/fl oz). **Bot.:** Hospital use 4 fl oz. ready-to-feed. **Pow.:** Can lb. *OTC.*
Use: Nutritional supplement.

Similac Sensitive for Fussiness & Gas. (Abbott Nutrition) Infant formula containing 2.14 g of protein (milk protein isolate), 11.1 g of carbohydrate (corn maltodextrin, sugar [sucrose], galactooligosaccharides), 5.4 g of fat (coconut oil, linoleic acid, high oleic safflower oil, soy oil), Fe 1.8 mg, Na 30 mg, K 107 mg, 100 Kcal per 148 mL, vitamins A, B_1, B_2, B_3, B_5, B_6, B_{12}, C, D, E, K, folic acid, biotin, chloride, inositol, Ca, Cu, Mg, Mn, P, Zn, I, Cl, Se. **Pow.:** 963 g *SimplePacs*, 657 g *SimplePacs*, 357 g can. **Liq.:** 946 mL (concentrated liquid), 946 mL (ready-to-feed liquid), 384 mL can (concentrated liquid), 237 mL (ready-to-feed liquid), 59 mL (ready-to-feed liquid). *OTC.*
Use: Nutritional supplement.

Similac Sensitive for Spit-Up. (Abbott Nutrition) Infant formula containing 2.14 g of protein (milk protein isolate), 10.7 g of carbohydrate (corn syrup, rice starch, sugar), 5.4 g of fat (coconut oil, high oleic safflower oil, soy oil), Fe 1.8 mg, Na 30 mg, K 107 mg, 100 Kcal per 148 mL, vitamins A, B_1, B_2, B_3, B_5, B_6, B_{12}, C, D, E, K, folic acid, biotin, inositol, Ca, Cu, Mg, Mn, P, Zn, I, Cl, Se. **Pow.:** 657 g *SimplePacs*, 349 g can. **Liq.:** 946 mL (ready-to-feed liquid). *OTC.*
Use: Nutritional supplement.

Similac Soy Isomil. (Abbott Nutrition) Infant formula containing 2.45 g of protein (soy protein isolate, L-methionine), 10.4 g of carbohydrate (corn syrup solids, sugar, fructooligosaccharides), 5.46 g of fat (coconut oil, high oleic safflower oil, soy oil), Fe 1.8 mg, Na 44 mg, K 108 mg, 100 Kcal per 148 mL, vitamins A, B_1, B_2, B_3, B_5, B_6, B_{12}, C, D, E, K, folic acid, biotin, inositol, Ca, Cu, Mg, Mn, P, Zn, I, Cl, Se. **Pow.:** 657 g *SimplePacs*, 963 g *SimplePacs*, 352 g can, 17.6 g packet. **Liq.:** 946 mL (ready-to-feed liquid), 384 mL (concentrated liquid), 237 mL (liquid), 59 mL (ready-to-feed liquid). *OTC.*
Use: Nutritional supplement.

Similac Special Care 20. (Ross) Infant formula ready-to-feed (20 Cal/fl oz). Bot. 4 fl oz. *OTC.*
Use: Nutritional supplement.

Similac Special Care 24. (Ross) Infant formula ready-to-feed (24 Cal/fl oz). Bot. 4 fl oz. *OTC.*
Use: Nutritional supplement.

Similac 13/Similac 13 with Iron. (Ross) Milk-based infant formula ready-to-feed containing 13 calories/fl oz, 1.8 mg Fe/100 calories. Bot. 4 fl. oz. *OTC.*
Use: Nutritional supplement.

Similac 24 LBW. (Ross) Low-iron infant formula, ready-to-feed, 24 calories/fl oz. Bot. 4 fl oz. *OTC.*
Use: Nutritional supplement.

Similac 24/Similac 24 with Iron. (Ross) Milk-based infant formula ready-to-feed (24 cal/fl oz), Fe 1.8 mg/100 calories. Bot. 4 fl oz. *OTC.*
Use: Nutritional supplement.

Similac 27. (Ross) Milk-based ready-to-feed infant formula (27 cal/fl oz). Bot. 4 fl oz. *OTC.*
Use: Nutritional supplement.

Similac 20/Similac with Iron 20. (Ross) Milk-based infant formula. Standard dilution (20 cal/fl oz). Similac with iron: Fe 1.8 mg/100 cal. **Pow.:** Can lb. **Concentrated Liq.:** Can 13 fl oz. **Ready-to-feed:** Can 8 fl oz, 32 fl oz. Bot. 4 fl oz, 8 fl oz. *OTC.*
Use: Nutritional supplement.

•**simotaxel.** (sim-oh-TAX-el) USAN.
Use: Antineoplastic.

Simplet. (Major) Pseudoephedrine hydrochloride 60 mg, chlorpheniramine maleate 4 mg, acetaminophen 650 mg. Tab. Bot. 100s. *OTC.*
Use: Upper respiratory combination, analgesic, antihistamine, decongestant.

Simply Cough. (McNeil) Dextromethorphan HBr 5 mg/5 mL. Corn syrup, sucralose, alcohol free, cherry berry flavor. Liq. 120 mL. *OTC.*
Use: Nonnarcotic antitussive.

Simply Saline. (Blairex) Sodium chloride. Soln. Spray bot. 44 mL. *OTC.*
Use: Nasal decongestant.

Simply Sleep. (McNeil) Diphenhydramine hydrochloride 25 mg. Tab. 24s, 48s. *OTC.*
Use: Nonprescription sleep aid.

Simply Stuffy. (McNeil) Pseudoephedrine hydrochloride 30 mg. Lactose. Tab. Pkg. 24s. *OTC.*
Use: Nasal decongestant, arylalkylamine.

Simponi. (Janssen Biotech) Golimumab 50 mg per 0.5 mL. Polysorbate 80. Preservative free. Inj., Soln. Single-dose prefilled syringe, prefilled *SmartJect* autoinjector (needle cover on the prefilled syringe and on the prefilled syringe in the autoinjector contains dry natural rubber, a derivative of latex). *Rx.*
Use: Immunologic agent, immunomodulator.

Simponi Aria. (Janssen Biotech) Golimumab 50 mg per 4 mL. Polysorbate 80. Preservative free. Inj., Soln., concentrate. Vial. *Rx.*
Use: Immunologic agent, immunomodulator.

Simron Plus. (GlaxoSmithKline) Fe 10 mg, vitamins B_{12} 3.33 mcg, C 50 mg, B_6 1 mg, folic acid 0.1 mg. Cap. Parabens. Bot. 100s. *OTC.*
Use: Mineral supplement.

•**simtrazene.** (SIM-trah-seen) USAN.
Use: Antineoplastic.

•**simtuzumab.** (sim-TOOZ-ue-mab) USAN.
Use: Fibrosis; antineoplastic.

Simulect. (Novartis) Basiliximab 200 mg, sucrose, mannitol, potassium phosphate, sodium chloride, preservative free. Pow. for Inj., lyophilized. Single-use vial. *Rx.*
Use: Immunologic, immunosuppressive.

•**simvastatin.** (SIM-vuh-STAT-in) *USP. Formerly Synvinolin.*
Use: Antihyperlipidemic, HMG-CoA reductase inhibitor.
See: Zocor.
W/Sitagliptin.
See: Juvisync.

simvastatin. (Various Mfr.) Simvastatin 5 mg (film-coated), 10 mg, 20 mg, 40 mg, 80 mg. May contain lactose. Tab. 30s, 60s (5 mg only); 90s (5 mg, 80 mg only); 500s (5 mg only); 1000s (5 mg, 80 mg only); unit-of-use 30s (80 mg only); UD 100s (except 5 mg, 80 mg). *Rx.*
Use: Antihyperlipidemic, HMG-CoA reductase inhibitor.

simvastatin/ezetimibe.
Use: Antihyperlipidemic.
See: Vytorin.

simvastatin/niacin.
Use: Antihyperlipidemic.
See: Simcor.

Sinadrin PE. (Reese) Acetaminophen 650 mg, dexbrompheniramine 2 mg, phenylephrine hydrochloride 10 mg. Dye free. Tab. 30s. *OTC.*
Use: Upper respiratory combination; decongestant, antihistamine, and analgesic combination.

•**sinapultide.** (si-na-PUL-tide) USAN.
Use: Treatment of respiratory distress syndrome (pulmonary surfactant).

Sinarest Decongestant. (Novartis) Oxymetazoline hydrochloride 0.05%. Spray. Bot. 0.5 oz. *OTC.*
Use: Decongestant.

Sinarest Extra-Strength. (Novartis) Acetaminophen 500 mg, chlorpheniramine maleate 2 mg, pseudoephedrine hydrochloride 30 mg. Tab. 24s. *OTC.*
Use: Analgesic; antihistamine; decongestant.

Sinarest No Drowsiness. (Novartis) Pseudoephedrine hydrochloride 30 mg, acetaminophen 500 mg. Tab. Pkg. 20s. *OTC.*
Use: Analgesic; decongestant.

Sinarest Sinus. (Novartis) Acetaminophen 325 mg, chlorpheniramine maleate 2 mg, pseudoephedrine hydrochloride 30 mg. Tab. Pkg. 20s, 40s, 80s. *OTC.*
Use: Analgesic; antihistamine; decongestant.

Sinarest 12 Hour. (Novartis) Oxymetazoline hydrochloride 0.05%. Nasal Spray Bot. 15 mL. *OTC.*
Use: Decongestant.

•**sincalide.** (SIN-kah-lide) USAN.
Use: Choleretic, diagnostic aid, gastrointestinal function test.
See: Kinevac.

Sine-Aid IB. (McNeil Consumer) Pseudoephedrine 30 mg, ibuprofen 200 mg. Capl. Pkg. 20s. *OTC.*
Use: Analgesic; decongestant.

Sine-Aid Sinus Headache. (McNeil Consumer) Acetaminophen 325 mg, pseudoephedrine hydrochloride 30 mg. Tab. Bot. 24s, 50s, 100s. *OTC.*
Use: Analgesic; decongestant.

Sine-Aid Sinus Headache, Extra Strength. (McNeil Consumer) Acetaminophen 500 mg, pseudoephedrine hydrochloride 30 mg. Capl. Bot. 24s, 50s. *OTC.*
Use: Analgesic; decongestant.

•**sinefungin.** (sih-neh-FUN-jin) USAN.
Use: Antifungal.

Sinemet. (Merck) Carbidopa/levodopa 10 mg/100 mg, 25 mg/100 mg, 25 mg/250 mg. Tab. 100s. *Rx.*
Use: Antiparkinson agent.

Sinemet CR. (Merck Sharp & Dohme) Carbidopa/levodopa 25 mg/100 mg, 50 mg/200 mg. ER Tab. 100s. *Rx.*
Use: Antiparkinson agent.

Sine-Off Cough/Cold. (Hogil) Phenylephrine hydrochloride 5 mg, dextromethorphan HBr 15 mg, guaifenesin 200 mg, acetaminophen 325 mg. Tab. 24s. *OTC.*
Use: Upper respiratory combination, decongestant, antihistamine, and expectorant combination.

Sine-Off Multi Symptom Relief Severe Cold. (Hogil) Acetaminophen 325 mg, guaifenesin 200 mg, phenylephrine hydrochloride 5 mg. Tab. 24s. *OTC.*
Use: Upper respiratory combination, antitussive and expectorant combination.

Sine-Off Non-Drowsy Maximum Strength. (Hogil) Phenylephrine hydrochloride 5 mg, acetaminophen 325 mg. Tab. Pkg. 12s. *OTC.*
Use: Upper respiratory combination, decongestant, analgesic.

Sine-Off Sinus/Cold. (Hogil) Phenylephrine hydrochloride 5 mg, chlorpheniramine maleate 2 mg, acetaminophen 500 mg. Tab. 24s. *OTC.*
Use: Upper respiratory combination, decongestant, antihistamine, and analgesic combination.

Singlet for Adults. (GlaxoSmithKline) Pseudoephedrine hydrochloride 60 mg, chlorpheniramine maleate 4 mg, acetaminophen 650 mg, sucrose. Tab. Bot. 100s. *OTC.*
Use: Upper respiratory combination, analgesic, antihistamine, decongestant.

Singulair. (Merck) Montelukast. **Chew. Tab.:** 4 mg (equiv. to montelukast sodium 4.2 mg), 5 mg (equiv. to montelukast sodium 5.2 mg). Aspartame, mannitol, phenylalanine 0.674 mg (4 mg only), 0.842 mg (5 mg only), cherry flavor. Unit-of-use 30s, 90s, UD 100s. **Gran.:** 4 mg/packet (equiv. to montelukast sodium 4.2 mg). Mannitol. 30 packets. **Tab.:** 10 mg (equiv. to montelukast sodium 10.4 mg). Lactose. Film-coated. Unit-of-use 30s, 90s, UD 100s, 8000s. *Rx.*
Use: Leukotriene receptor antagonist.

Sino-Eze MLT. (Global Source) Salicylamide 3.5 g, acetaminophen 100 mg, phenylephrine hydrochloride 5 mg, chlorpheniramine maleate 2 mg. Tab. Bot. 1000s. *Rx.*
Use: Upper respiratory combination, analgesic, antihistamine, decongestant.

Sinografin. (Bracco Diagnostics) Diatrizoate meglumine 527 mg, iodipamide meglumine 268 mg, iodine 380 mg/mL. EDTA. Inj. Vials. 10 mL. *Rx.*
Use: Radiopaque agent.

Sinufed Timecelle. (Roberts) Pseudoephedrine hydrochloride 60 mg, guaifenesin 300 mg. Cap. Bot. 100s. *Rx.*
Use: Upper respiratory combination, decongestant, expectorant.

Sinumist-SR. (Roberts) Guaifenesin 600 mg. Tab. Bot. 100s. *Rx.*
Use: Upper respiratory combination, expectorant.

Sinupan. (ION Laboratories, Inc.) Phenylephrine hydrochloride 40 mg, guaifenesin 200 mg. SR Cap. Bot. 100s. *Rx.*
Use: Upper respiratory combination, decongestant, expectorant.

Sinus Excedrin Extra Strength. (Bristol-Myers Squibb) Pseudoephedrine hydrochloride 30 mg, acetaminophen 500 mg. Tab or Cap. Bot. 50s. *OTC.*
Use: Upper respiratory combination, decongestant, analgesic.

Sinus Headache & Congestion. (Rugby) Pseudoephedrine hydrochloride 30 mg, chlorpheniramine maleate 2 mg, acetaminophen 500 mg. Tab. Bot. 100s, 1000s. *OTC.*
Use: Upper respiratory combination, decongestant, antihistamine, analgesic.

Sinus Pain Formula Allerest. (Medeva) Pseudoephedrine hydrochloride 30 mg, chlorpheniramine maleate 2 mg, acetaminophen 500 mg. **Cap.:** Bot. 24s, 50s. **Gelcap:** Bot. 20s, 40s. *OTC.*
Use: Upper respiratory combination, analgesic, antihistamine, decongestant.

Sinus Relief. (Major) Pseudoephedrine hydrochloride 30 mg, acetaminophen 325 mg. Tab. Bot. 24s, 100s, 1000s. *OTC.*
Use: Upper respiratory combination, decongestant, analgesic.

Sinus-Relief Maximum Strength. (Major) Pseudoephedrine hydrochloride 30 mg, acetaminophen 500 mg, dextrose. Tab. Pkg. 24s. *OTC.*
Use: Upper respiratory combination, decongestant, analgesic.

Sinus Tablets. (Walgreen) Acetaminophen 325 mg, chlorpheniramine maleate 2 mg, pseudoephedrine hydrochloride mg. Tab. Bot. 30s. *OTC.*
Use: Upper respiratory combination, analgesic, antihistamine, decongestant.

Sinustop. (Nature's Way) Pseudoephedrine hydrochloride 60 mg, echinacea purpura, ginger, goldenseal root. Cap. Pkg. 20s. *OTC.*
Use: Nasal decongestant, arylalkylamine.

Sinutab Maximum Strength Sinus Allergy. (J&J Consumer) Acetaminophen 500 mg, pseudoephedrine hydrochloride 30 mg, chlorpheniramine maleate 2 mg. Tab. or Capl. 24s. *OTC.*
Use: Upper respiratory combination, analgesic, antihistamine, decongestant.

Sinutab Sinus. (Pfizer) Phenylephrine hydrochloride 5 mg, acetaminophen 325 mg. PEG. Tab. Pkg. 24s. *OTC.*
Use: Upper respiratory combination, decongestant, analgesic.

Sinutab Sinus Maximum Strength Without Drowsiness Formula. (Pfizer) Acetaminophen 500 mg, pseudoephedrine hydrochloride 30 mg. Tab or Cap. Pack 24s. *OTC.*
Use: Upper respiratory combination, analgesic, decongestant.

Sinutab Sinus Regular Strength Without Drowsiness. (Pfizer) Pseudoephedrine hydrochloride 30 mg, acetaminophen 325 mg. Tab. Bot. 24s. *OTC.*
Use: Upper respiratory combination, analgesic, decongestant.

Sinutab Sinus Without Drowsiness Regular Strength. (Pfizer) Pseudoephedrine hydrochloride 30 mg, acetaminophen 325 mg. Tab. Pkg. 24s. *OTC.*
Use: Upper respiratory combination, decongestant, analgesic.

SINUtuss DM. (Dexo Pharma) Dextromethorphan HBr 30 mg, guaifenesin 600 mg, phenylephrine hydrochloride 15 mg. Tab. 100s. *Rx.*
Use: Upper respiratory combination, antitussive and expectorant combination.

•**siplizumab.** (sip-LIZ-oo-mab) USAN.
Use: Monoclonal antibody.
•**sipuleucel-T.** (SYE-pul-oo-sel) USAN.
Use: Investigational antineoplastic.
Siroil. (Siroil) Mercuric oleate, cresol, vegetable and mineral oil. Emulsion Bot. 8 oz. *OTC.*
Use: Antiseptic.
sir-o-lene.
Use: Emollient.
•**sirolimus.** (SER-oh-lih-muss) USAN. *Formerly Rapamycin.*
Use: Immunologic, immunosuppressive.
See: Rapamune.
sirolimus. (Various Mfr.) Sirolimus 0.5 mg, 1 mg, 2 mg. May contain lactose, PEG, sucrose. Tab. 30s (0.5 mg only), 90s (0.5 mg only), 100s, 500s (0.5 mg only), 1,000s (0.5 mg only), UD 100s (except 2 mg). *Rx.*
Use: Immunologic agent, immunosuppressive.
Sirturo. (Janssen Therapeutics) Bedaquiline 100 mg (equiv. to bedaquiline fumarate 120.89 mg). Lactose. Tab. 188s. *Rx.*
Use: Anti-infective, antituberculosis agent.
•**sirukumab.** (si-RUK-ue-mab) USAN.
Use: Antirheumatic agent.
•**sisapronil.** (sis-AP-roe-nil) USAN.
Use: Control of ectoparasites, particularly acari, on animals.
•**sisomicin.** (SIS-oh-MY-sin) USAN.
Use: Anti-infective.
•**sisomicin sulfate.** (SIS-oh-MY-sin) *USP.*
Use: Anti-infective.
Sitabs. (Canright) Lobeline sulfate 1.5 mg, benzocaine 2 mg, aluminum hydroxide-magnesium carbonate codried gel 150 mg. Loz. Bot. 100s. *OTC.*
Use: Smoking deterrent.
•**sitafloxacin.** (si-ta-FLOKS-a-sin) USAN.
Use: Antibacterial.
•**sitagliptin.** (SYE-ta-GLIP-tin) USAN.
Tall Man: sitaGLIPtin
Use: Antidiabetic.
W/Simvastatin.
See: Juvisync.
•**sitagliptin phosphate.** (SYE-ta-GLIP-tin) USAN.
Tall Man: sitaGLIPtin
Use: Antidiabetic.
See: Januvia.
W/Metformin Hydrochloride.
See: Janumet.
Janumet XR.
•**sitaxsentan sodium.** (SYE-tax-EN-tan) USAN.
Use: Congestive heart failure; ischemic deficits; hypertension; prostate cancer; investigational endothelin receptor antagonist.
•**sitogluside.** (SIGH-toe-GLUE-side) USAN.
Use: Antiprostatic hypertrophy.
Sitzmarks. (Konsyl) Radiopaque polyvinyl chloride radiopaque rings 24 (1 mm × 4.5 mm). Cap. Box. 10s. *Rx.*
Use: Radiopaque agent, miscellaneous GI contrast agent.
•**sivelestat.** (si-VEL-es-tat) USAN.
Use: Acute respiratory distress syndrome.
•**sivelestat sodium.** (si-VEL-es-tat) USAN.
Use: Acute respiratory distress syndrome.
Sixameen. (Spanner) Vitamins B_1 100 mg, B_6 100 mg/mL. Vial 10 mL. *OTC.*
Use: Vitamin supplement.
666 Cold Preparation, Maximum Strength. (Monticello) Dextromethorphan HBr 3.3 mg, pseudoephedrine hydrochloride 10 mg, acetaminophen 108.3 mg per 5 mL. Saccharin, sucrose, sodium 23.5 mg/5 mL. Liq. Bot. 118 mL, 177 mL. *OTC.*
Use: Upper respiratory combination, antitussive combination.
Skeeter Stik. (Triton) Lidocaine 4%, phenol 2%, isopropyl alcohol base. Liq. 14 mL. *OTC.*
Use: Topical local anesthetic.
Skelaxin. (King) Metaxalone 800 mg. Tab. Bot. 100s, 500s. *Rx.*
Use: Muscle relaxant.
skeletal muscle relaxants.
See: Baclofen.
Carisoprodol.
Chlorphenesin Carbamate.
Chlorzoxazone.
Cyclobenzaprine Hydrochloride.
Dantrolene Sodium.
Diazepam.
Metaxalone.
Methocarbamol.
Orphenadrine Citrate.
Tizanidine Hydrochloride.
Skelid. (Sanofi-Aventis) Tiludronate 200 mg (equiv. to tiludronate disodium 240 mg). Lactose. Tab. 56s. *Rx.*
Use: Bisphosphonates.
Skin Degreaser. (Health & Medical Techniques) Freon 100%. Bot. 2 oz, 4 oz. *OTC.*
Use: Dermatologic, degreaser.
skin protectants.
See: Zinc Oxide.
Skin Shield. (Del) Dyclonine hydrochloride 0.75%, benzethonium Cl 0.2%,

acetone, amyl acetate, castor oil, SD alcohol 40 10%. Waterproof. Liq. Bot. 13.3 mL. *OTC.*
Use: Dermatologic, protectant.

skin test antigen, multiple.
See: T.R.U.E. Test.

SK 110679. (GlaxoSmithKline)
Use: Hormone, growth. [Orphan Drug]

Skyla. (Bayer HealthCare) Levonorgestrel 13.5 mg (releases ≈ 14 mcg of levonorgestrel per day). Intrauterine device. 1 single-use T-shaped device covered by a silicone membrane w/inserter. *Rx.*
Use: Sex hormone, contraceptive hormone.

Sleep Cap. (Weeks & Leo) Diphenhydramine hydrochloride 50 mg. Cap. Bot. 25s, 50s. *OTC.*
Use: Sleep aid.

Sleep-ettes D Nighttime Sleep Aid. (Reese) Diphenhydramine 50 mg. Tab. 24s, 48s. *OTC.*
Use: Antihistamine, nonselective ethanolamine.

Sleep Tablets. (Towne) Scopolamine aminoxide HBr 0.2 mg, salicylamide 250 mg. Tab. Bot. 36s, 90s. *Rx.*
Use: Sleep aid.

Sleep II. (Walgreen) Diphenhydramine hydrochloride 25 mg. Tab. Bot. 16s, 32s, 72s. *OTC.*
Use: Sleep aid.

Slender. (Carnation) Skim milk, vegetable oils, caseinates, vitamins, minerals. **Liq.:** 220 Cal/10 oz. Can. **Pow.:** 173 or 200 Cal mixed w/6 oz skim or low fat milk. Pkg 1 oz. *OTC.*
Use: Dietary aid.

Slim-Fast. (Thompson Medical) Meal replacement powder mixed with milk to replace 1, 2 or 3 meals a day. *OTC.*
Use: Dietary aid.

Slim-Line. (Thompson Medical) Benzocaine, dextrose. Chewing gum. Box 24s. *OTC.*
Use: Dietary aid.

Slim-Tabs. (Wesley) Phendimetrazine tartrate 35 mg. Tab. Bot. 1000s. *c-III.*
Use: Anorexiant.

Slo-Niacin. (Upsher-Smith) Niacin. 250 mg, 500 mg, 750 mg. Sugar free. CR Tab. Bot. 100s. *OTC.*
Use: Water-soluble vitamin.

Slo-Salt-K. (Mission Pharmacal) KCl 150 mg, NaCl 410 mg. Tab. Bot. 1000s. Strip 100s. *OTC.*
Use: Salt substitute.

Slow Fe Slow Release Iron With Folic Acid. (Novartis) Fe 50 mg, folic acid 0.4 mg. SR Tab. Bot. 20s. *OTC.*
Use: Mineral, vitamin supplement.

Slow-Mag. (Purdue) Magnesium 143 mg, calcium 238 mg, chloride 405 mg, sodium 5 mg. Maltodextrin, mineral oil. Tab. 60s. *OTC.*
Use: Mineral.

Slow Magnesium Chloride with Calcium. (GeriCare) Calcium 106 mg, chloride 186.5 mg, magnesium 64 mg. Maltodextrin. Tab. 60s. *OTC.*
Use: Multimineral.

Slow Release Iron. (Cardinal Health) Ferrous sulfate exsiccated (dried) 160 mg (iron 50 mg). Maltodextrin, mineral oil. SR Tab. 30s. *OTC.*
Use: Mineral supplement.

SLT Tablets. (Western Research) Sodium levothyroxine 0.1 mg, 0.2 mg, 0.3 mg. Bot. 1000s.
Use: Hormone, thyroid.

Small Fry Chewable Tabs. (Health for Life Brands) Vitamins A 5000 units, D 1000 units, B_{12} 5 mcg, B_1 3 mg, B_2 2.5 mg, B_6 1 mg, C 50 mg, niacinamide 20 mg, calcium pantothenate 1 mg, E 1 unit, l-lysine 15 mg, biotin 10 mg. Chew. Tab. Bot. 100s, 250s, 365s. *OTC.*
Use: Mineral, vitamin supplement.

•**smallpox vaccine.** (SMAWL-pox-VAX-een) *USP.*
Use: Immunization.

smoking deterrents.
See: Bupropion hydrochloride.
Nicotine.
Nicotine Gum.
Nicotine Inhalation System.
Nicotine Nasal Spray.
Nicotine Polacrilex.
Nicotine Transdermal System.
Varenicline Tartrate.

snakebite antivenins.
See: Antivenin (Crotalidae) Polyvalent.
Antivenin (*Micurus fulvius*).

snake venom.
Use: Trypanosomiasis.

Snaplets-D. (Baker Norton) Pseudoephedrine hydrochloride 6.25 mg, chlorpheniramine maleate 1 mg. Pkt., taste free. Granules 30s. *OTC.*
Use: Antihistamine; decongestant.

Snaplets-FR. (Baker Norton) Acetaminophen 80 mg. Pkt. Granules. 32s packets. *OTC.*
Use: Analgesic.

Snootie by Sea & Ski. (Carter-Wallace) Padimate O. SPF 10. Lot. Bot. 30 mL. *OTC.*
Use: Sunscreen.

SN-13, 272.
See: Primaquine Phosphate.

Soakare. (Allergan) Benzalkonium Cl 0.01%, edetate disodium, NaOH to ad-

just pH, purified water. Bot. 4 fl oz. *OTC.*
Use: Contact lens care.

•**soap, green.** *USP.*
Use: Detergent.

soaps, germicidal.
See: Fostex.
pHisoHex.
Thylox.

soap substitutes.
See: Lowila Cake.
pHisoDerm.

•**sobetirome.** (SOE-be-TYE-rome) USAN.
Use: Dyslipidemia.

Sochlor. (OcuSoft) Sodium chloride, hypertonic. **Soln.:** 5%. Hydroxypropyl methylcellulose 2906, propylene glycol, methylparaben 0.023%, propylparaben 0.01%, boric acid. 15 mL. **Oint.:** 5%. Mineral oil, white petrolatum, lanolin oil. 3.5 g. *OTC.*
Use: Ophthalmic agent, ophthalmic hyperosmolar preparation.

•**soda lime.** (SOE-da-lyme) *NF.*
Use: Carbon dioxide absorbent.

Soda Mint. (Eli Lilly) Sodium bicarbonate 5 g, peppermint oil q.s. Tab. Bot. 100s. *OTC.*
Use: Antacid.

Sodasone. (Fellows) Prednisolone sodium phosphate 20 mg, niacinamide 25 mg/mL. Vial 10 mL. *Rx.*
Use: Corticosteroid.

SodiPhluor. (Kylemore) Fluoride 0.5 mg per mL (from 1.1 mg of sodium fluoride). Methylparaben, sucralose. Sugar free. Peach flavor. Drops. 50 mL. *Rx.*
Use: Trace element.

•**sodium acetate.** (SOE-dee-um ASS-eh-tate) *USP.*
Use: Pharmaceutic aid (in dialysis solutions).

sodium acetate. (Various Mfr.) Sodium acetate 2 mEq/mL, 4 mEq/mL. Preservative free. Inj., Soln., concentrate.
2 mEq/mL: 20 mL single-dose vial (contains in each mL 164 mg of sodium acetate [anhydrous], which provides 2 mEq each of sodium and acetate).
4 mEq/mL: 50 mL single-dose vial (contains 16.4 g of sodium acetate [anhydrous], which provides 200 mEq each of sodium and acetate). *Rx.*
Use: Intravenous nutritional therapy, electrolyte.

•**sodium acetate C 11 injection.** (SOE-dee-um ASS-eh-tate) *USP.*
Use: Radiopharmaceutical.

sodium acetosulfone. (SOE-dee-um ah-SEE-toe-sull-FONE)
Use: Leprostatic agent.

sodium acid phosphate.
See: Sodium Biphosphate.

sodium actinoquinol. (SOE-dee-um ack-TIH-no-kwin-OLE)
Use: Treatment of flash burns (ophthalmic).

•**sodium alginate.** (SOE-dee-um AL-jih-nate) *NF.*
Use: Pharmaceutic aid (suspending agent).

sodium aminobenzoate.
Use: Dermatomyositis and scleroderma.

sodium aminopterin. Aminopterin sodium.

sodium aminosalicylate.
See: Aminosalicylate Sodium.

sodium amobarbital. Amobarbital Sodium, USP.

•**sodium amylosulfate.** (SOE-dee-um AM-ill-oh-sull-fate) USAN.
Use: Enzyme inhibitor.

sodium anazolene. (SOE-dee-um an-AZE-oh-leen)
Use: Diagnostic aid.

sodium antimony gluconate. (Pentostam)
Use: Anti-infective.

•**sodium arsenate As 74.** (SOE-dee-um AHR-seh-nate) USAN.
Use: Radiopharmaceutical.

•**sodium ascorbate.** (SOE-dee-um ass-CORE-bate) *USP.*
Use: Water-soluble vitamin.
W/Ascorbic Acid.
See: Chewable Vitamin C.
Chew-C.
Fruit C 500.
Fruit C 100.
Fruit C 200.
Sunkist Vitamin C.
Vicks Vitamin C Drops.

sodium ascorbate. (Merit Pharmaceuticals) Sodium ascorbate 250 mg/mL. Inj.; Soln. Vial. 30 mL. *Rx.*
Use: Water-soluble vitamin.

sodium aurothiomalate.
See: Gold Sodium Thiosulfate.

•**sodium benzoate.** (SOE-dee-um BEN-zoe-ate) *NF.*
Use: Pharmaceutic aid (antifungal, preservative); antihyperammonemic.

sodium benzylpenicillin. Penicillin G Sodium, USP. Sodium Penicillin G. *Rx.*
Use: Anti-infective; penicillin.

•**sodium bicarbonate.** (SOE-dee-um by-CAR-boe-nate) *USP.*
Use: Alkalizer, systemic; antacid; electrolyte replacement.
See: Brioschi.
W/Aspirin, Citric Acid.
See: Alka-Seltzer Extra Strength with Aspirin.

Alka-Seltzer Lemon Lime.
Alka-Seltzer Original.
Zee-Seltzer.
W/Calcium Chloride, Dibasic Sodium Phosphate, Monobasic Sodium Phosphate, Silicon Dioxide, Sodium Chloride.
See: NeutraSal.
W/Citric Acid.
See: Alka-Seltzer Heartburn Relief.
W/Citric Acid, Potassium Bicarbonate.
See: Alka-Seltzer Gold.
W/Citric Acid, Simethicone.
See: E-Z Gas II.
W/Omeprazole.
See: Zegerid.
Zegerid OTC.
W/PEG 3350, Sodium Chloride, Potassium Chloride.
See: Suclear.
W/PEG 3350, Sodium Chloride, Sodium Sulfate, Potassium Chloride.
See: GaviLyte-C.
GaviLyte-G.
W/Potassium Bitartrate.
See: Ceo-Two.
W/Sodium Carboxymethylcellulose, Alginic Acid.
See: Pretts Diet Aid.

sodium bicarbonate. (American Pharmaceutical Partners) Sodium bicarbonate. **Inj.: 4.2% (0.5 mEq/mL):** 10 mL (5 mEq) *Bristoject* syringe. **7.5% (0.9 mEq/mL):** 50 mL (44.6 mEq) single-dose vials, 50 mL (44.6 mEq) *Bristoject* syringes and 200 mL (179 mEq) *MaxiVials*. **8.4% (1 mEq/mL):** 50 mL (50 mEq) vials and 10 and 50 mEq *Bristoject* syringes. **Neutralizing additive Soln.:** 4.2% (0.5 mEq/mL). 5 mL fill in 6 mL vials (2.5 mEq). *Rx.*
Use: Intravenous nutritional therapy, electrolyte.

sodium bicarbonate. (American Regent) Sodium bicarbonate 7.5% (0.9 mEq/mL), 8.4% (1 mEq/mL). Inj. 50 mL (44.6 mEq) vial (7.5%), 50 mL (50 mEq) vial (8.4%). *Rx.*
Use: Intravenous nutritional therapy, electrolyte.

sodium bicarbonate. (Baxter) Sodium bicarbonate 5% (0.6 mEq/mL). Inj. 500 mL (287.5 mEq). *Rx.*
Use: Intravenous nutritional therapy, electrolyte.

sodium bicarbonate. (Chain Drug) Sodium bicarbonate. 30 mEq (0.7 g) of sodium per ½ tsp. Pow. 113 g. *OTC.*
Use: Systemic alkalinizer.

sodium bicarbonate. (Hospira) Sodium bicarbonate. Inj. **4.2% (0.5 mEq/mL):** 10 mL (5 mEq) syringe. **5% (0.6 mEq/mL):** 500 mL (w/EDTA) (297.5 mEq). **7.5% (0.9 mEq/mL):** 50 mL (44.6 mEq) amp and 50 mL (44.6 mEq) syringe. **8.4% (1 mEq/mL):** 50 mL (50 mEq) flip-top vial and 10 mL (10 mEq) and 50 mL (50 mEq) syringe. *Rx.*
Use: Intravenous nutritional therapy, electrolyte.

sodium bicarbonate. (McGaw) Sodium bicarbonate 5% (0.6 mEq/mL). Inj. 500 mL (w/EDTA) (297.5 mEq). *Rx.*
Use: Intravenous nutritional therapy, electrolyte.

sodium bicarbonate. (Various Mfr.) Sodium bicarbonate 325 mg, 650 mg. Sodium; may contain mineral oil (650 mg only). Tab. 100s, 1,000s. *OTC.*
Use: Systemic alkalinizer.

sodium biphosphate.
Use: Cathartic.
See: Sodium Phosphate Monobasic.
W/Ammonium Biphosphate, Sodium Acid Pyrophosphate.
See: Ammonium Biphosphate, Sodium Biphosphate and Sodium Acid Pyrophosphate.
W/Hyoscyamine Sulfate, Methylene Blue, Methenamine, Phenyl Salicylate.
See: Urimax.

sodium bismuth tartrate.
See: Bismuth Sodium Tartrate.

sodium bisulfite. Sulfurous acid, monosodium salt. Monosodium sulfite.
Use: Antioxidant.

•**sodium borate.** (SO-dee-um) *NF.*
Use: Pharmaceutic aid (alkalizing agent).

sodium butabarbital.
See: Butabarbital Sodium.
Sodium Butyrate.

•**sodium butyrate.** (SO-dee-um) *USP.*

sodium calcium edetate.
See: Calcium Disodium Versenate.

•**sodium carbonate.** (SO-dee-um) *NF.*
Use: Pharmaceutic aid (alkalizing agent).

sodium carboxymethylcellulose. Carboxymethylcellulose Sodium, USP. CMC. Cellulose Gum.

sodium cellulose glycolate.
See: Carboxymethylcellulose Sodium.

sodium cephalothin. (SO-dee-um SEFF-ah-low-thin) Cephalothin Sodium, USP.
Use: Anti-infective.

•**sodium chloride.** (SO-dee-um KLOR-ide) *USP.*
Use: Pharmaceutic aid (tonicity agent); bronchodilator, diluent; nasal decongestant.
See: Afrin Moisturizing Saline Mist.
Ayr Saline.

Breathe Free.
Entsol.
HuMist.
Little Noses Sterile Saline Nasal Mist.
Mycinaire Saline Mist.
NaSal.
Nasal Moist.
Nasal Spray.
Normaline.
Ocean.
Ocean Complete.
Ocean for Kids.
Pretz Irrigation.
Pretz Moisturizing.
Rhinaris.
Simply Saline.

W/Calcium Chloride, Dibasic Sodium Phosphate, Monobasic Sodium Phosphate, Silicon Dioxide, Sodium Bicarbonate.
See: NeutraSal.

W/Dextrose.
See: Dextrose 5% with 0.45% Sodium Chloride.
Dextrose 5% with 0.9% Sodium Chloride.
Dextrose 5% with 0.3% Sodium Chloride.
Dextrose 5% with 0.33% Sodium Chloride.
Dextrose 5% with 0.2% Sodium Chloride.
Dextrose 5% and 0.225% Sodium Chloride.
Dextrose 10% with 0.45% Sodium Chloride.
Dextrose 10% and 0.9% Sodium Chloride.
Dextrose 10% with 0.2% Sodium Chloride.
Dextrose 10% with 0.225% Sodium Chloride.
Dextrose 3.3% and 0.3% Sodium Chloride.
Dextrose 2.5% with 0.45% Sodium Chloride.

W/Dextrose, Potassium Chloride.
See: Potassium Chloride in 5% Dextrose and 0.45% Sodium Chloride.
Potassium Chloride in 5% Dextrose and 0.9% Sodium Chloride.
Potassium Chloride in 5% Dextrose and 0.33% Sodium Chloride.
Potassium Chloride in 5% Dextrose and 0.2% Sodium Chloride.
Potassium Chloride in 10% Dextrose and 0.2% Sodium Chloride.
Potassium Chloride in 3.3% Dextrose and 0.3% Sodium Chloride.

W/Dibasic Sodium Phosphate, Monobasic Sodium Phosphate, Calcium Chloride.
See: Cephosol.

W/PEG 3350, Sodium Bicarbonate, Potassium Chloride.
See: Suclear.

W/PEG 3350, Sodium Bicarbonate, Sodium Sulfate, Potassium Chloride.
See: GaviLyte-C.
GaviLyte-G.

sodium chloride. (Various Mfr.) Sodium chloride 0.9%. May contain benzyl alcohol 9 mg. Inj. Vial 1 mL, 2 mL, 2.5 mL, 5 mL, 10 mL, 30 mL. *Rx.*
Use: Bronchodilator, diluent; intravenous nutritional therapy, electrolyte.

sodium chloride, calcium carbonate, and potassium chloride.
Use: Salt replacement.
See: Sustain.

sodium chloride diluents.
Use: Intravenous nutritional therapy, electrolyte.
See: Sodium Chloride 0.45%.
Sodium Chloride 0.9%.

sodium chloride, 5%. (Various Mfr.) Sodium 855 mEq/L, chloride 855 mEq/L, osmolarity 1710 mOsm/L. 500 mL. *Rx.*
Use: Intravenous nutritional therapy, electrolyte.

sodium chloride, hypertonic.
See: Sochlor.

•**sodium chloride injection.** (SOE-dee-um KLOR-ide) *USP.*
Use: Fluid and irrigation; electrolyte replacement; isotonic vehicle.

sodium chloride injection. (Abbott) Normal saline 0.9% in 150 mL, 250 mL, 500 mL, 1000 mL cont. **Partial-fill:** 50 mL in 200 mL, 50 mL in 300 mL, 100 mL in 300 mL. **Fliptop vial:** 10 mL, 20 mL, 50 mL, 100 mL. **Bacteriostatic vial:** 10 mL, 20 mL, 30 mL; 50 mEq, 20 mL in 50 mL fliptop or pintop vial; 100 mEq, 40 mL in 50 mL fliptop vial; sodium Cl 0.45%, 500 mL, 1000 mL; sodium Cl 5%, 500 mL; sodium Cl irrigating solution, 250 mL, 500 mL, 1000 mL, 3000 mL; (Pharmacia & Upjohn) sodium Cl 9 mg/mL w/benzyl alcohol 9.45 mg. Vial 20 mL (Sanofi Winthrop Pharmaceuticals). **Carpuject:** 2 mL fill cartridge, 22-gauge, 1¼-inch needle or 25-gauge, ⅝-inch needle. *Rx.*
Use: Fluid and irrigation; electrolyte replacement; isotonic vehicle.

sodium chloride injection. (Various Mfr.) Sodium chloride 14.6%, 23.4%. Inj. 20 mL (14.6% only), 30 mL (23.4% only), 40 mL (14.6% only), 100 mL (23.4% only), 200 mL. *Rx.*
Use: Intravenous nutritional therapy, electrolyte.

sodium chloride intravenous infusions for admixtures.
Use: Intravenous nutritional therapy, electrolyte.
See: Sodium Chloride, 5%.
Sodium Chloride, 3%.
Sodium Chloride, 0.45% (Half Normal Saline).
Sodium Chloride, 0.9% (Normal Saline).

•**sodium chloride Na 22.** (So-dee-um KLOR-ide) USAN.
Use: Radioactive agent.

sodium chloride substitutes.
See: Salt Substitutes.

sodium chloride tablets. (Parke-Davis) Sodium Cl 15 ½ g. Tab. Bot. 1000s. *OTC.*
Use: Normal saline.

sodium chloride, 3%. (Various Mfr.) Sodium 513 mEq/L, chloride 513 mEq/L. Osmolarity 1030 mOsm/L. 500 mL. *Rx.*
Use: Intravenous nutritional therapy, electrolyte.

sodium chloride 0.45%. (Dey) Sodium chloride 0.45%. Preservative free. Soln. Single-use vial 3 mL, 5 mL. *OTC.*
Use: Bronchodilator, diluent; intravenous nutritional therapy, electrolyte.

sodium chloride, 0.45% (half normal saline). (Various Mfr.) Sodium 77 mEq/L, chloride 77 mEq/L. Osmolarity ≈ 155 mOsm/L. 25 mL, 50 mL, 150 mL, 250 mL, 500 mL, 1000 mL. *Rx.*
Use: Intravenous nutritional therapy, electrolyte.

sodium chloride 0.9%. (Dey) Sodium chloride 0.9%. Preservative free. Soln. Vial 3 mL, 5 mL, 15 mL. *OTC.*
Use: Bronchodilator, diluent; intravenous nutritional therapy, electrolyte.

sodium chloride, 0.9% (normal saline). (Various Mfr.) Sodium 154 mEq/L, chloride 154 mEq/L. Osmolarity ≈ 310 mOsm/L. 2 mL, 3 mL, 5 mL, 10 mL, 20 mL, 25 mL, 30 mL, 50 mL, 100 mL, 150 mL, 250 mL, 500 mL, 1000 mL, 2 mL fill in 3 mL. *Rx.*
Use: Intravenous nutritional therapy, electrolyte.

sodium chlorothiazide for injection. (SOE-dee-um KLOR-oh-thigh-AZZ-ide) Chlorothiazide Sodium for Injection, USP.
Use: Diuretic.

•**sodium chromate Cr 51 injection.** (SOE-dee-um KROE-mate) *USP.*
Use: Diagnostic aid (blood volume determination); radiopharmaceutical.

•**sodium citrate.** (SOE-dee-um SIH-trate) *USP.*
Use: Alkalizer, systemic.
See: Anticoagulant Citrate Dextrose Solution.
Anticoagulant Citrate Phosphate Dextrose Solution.
W/Citric Acid.
See: Oracit.
Shohl's Modified.

sodium citrate/citric acid. (Pharmaceutical Associates) Sodium citrate dihydrate 500 mg/citric acid monohydrate 334 mg per 5 mL. PEG, propylene glycol, sodium benzoate, sorbitol. Each mL contains sodium ion 1 mEq and is equiv. to bicarbonate 1 mEq. Sugar free. Soln. 473 mL, UD 15 mL, UD 30 mL. *Rx.*
Use: Systemic alkalinizer; urinary alkalinizer.

sodium cloxacillin. (SOE-dee-um CLOX-ah-SILL-in)
See: Cloxacillin Sodium.

sodium colistimethate. Colistimethate Sodium, Sterile. Antibiotic produced by *Aerobacillus colistinus.*

sodium colistin methanesulfonate. Colistimethane Sodium, USP. The sodium methanesulfonate salt of an antibiotic substance elaborated by *Aerobacillus colistinus.*
Use: Anti-infective.

sodium copper chlorophyllin.
Use: Systemic deodorizer.
See: Ennds.

•**sodium dehydroacetate.** (SO-dee-um) *NF.*
Use: Pharmaceutic aid (antimicrobial preservative).

sodium dextrothyroxine. (SOE-dee-um DEX-troe-thigh-ROCK-seen)
Use: Anticholesteremic.

sodium diatrizoate. Diatrizoate Sodium, USP.
Use: Radiopaque medium.

sodium dichloroacetate.
Use: Treatment of lactic acidosis and familial hypercholesterolemia. [Orphan Drug]

sodium dicloxacillin. (SOE-dee-um DIE-klox-uh-SILL-in) Dicloxacillin Sodium, USP.
Use: Anti-infective.

sodium dicloxacillin monohydrate.
Use: Anti-infective.
See: Pathocil.

sodium dihydrogen phosphate.
See: Sodium Biphosphate.

sodium dimethoxyphenyl penicillin.
See: Methicillin Sodium.

sodium dioctyl sulfosuccinate.
See: Docusate Sodium.

sodium diphenylhydantoin. Phenytoin Sodium, USP. Diphenylhydantoin Sodium.
Use: Anticonvulsant.

sodium edetate. (SOE-dee-um eh-deh-TATE) Edetate Disodium, USP. Tetrasodium ethylenediaminetetraacetate.
Use: Chelating agent.
See: Vagisec Plus.

sodium ethacrynate. Ethacrynate Sodium for Injection, USP.
Use: Diuretic.

•**sodium ethasulfate.** (SOE-dee-um ETH-ah-SULL-fate) USAN.
Use: Detergent.

sodium ethyl-mercuri-thio-salicylate.
See: Merthiolate.
Thimerosal.

•**sodium ferric gluconate complex.** (FER-ik GLOO-koe-nate) USAN.
Use: Iron product.
See: Ferrlecit.
Nulecit.

sodium ferric gluconate complex. (Watson) Elemental iron 12.5 mg/mL. Benzyl alcohol 9 mg/mL, sucrose 195 mg/mL. Inj., Soln. Single-use vial. 5 mL. *Rx.*
Use: Trace element.

•**sodium fluorescein.** (SO-dee-um) *USP.* Fluorescein Sodium, USP; Resorcinolphthalein sodium.
Use: Diagnostic aid (corneal trauma indicator).

•**sodium fluoride.** (SOE-dee-um) *USP.*
Use: Dental caries agent.
See: ControlRx.
DentaGel.
EtheDent.
Fluor-A-Day.
Fluoride.
Flura-Drops.
Flura-Loz.
Karidium.
Karigel.
Listerine Tooth Defense.
Luride.
NaFeen.
OrthoWash.
PreviDent 5000 Plus.
T-Fluoride.
W/Potassium Nitrate.
See: Sensodyne Iso-Active Multi Action.
Sensodyne Iso-Active Whitening.
W/Vitamins.
See: Mulvidren-F.
W/Vitamins A, D, C.
See: Tri-Vi-Flor.

sodium fluoride. (Breckenridge) Fluoride 0.25 mg (from 0.55 mg of sodium fluoride) Sucralose, xylitol. Orange flavor. Chew. Tab. 120s. *Rx.*
Use: Trace element.

sodium fluoride. (Hi-Tech) Fluoride 0.5 mg per mL (from sodium fluoride 1.1 mg). Peach flavor. Drops. 50 mL. *Rx.*
Use: Prevention of dental caries.

•**sodium fluoride and phosphoric acid gel.** *USP.*
Use: Dental caries agent.

•**sodium fluoride F 18.** (SOE-dee-um) *USP.*
Use: Radiopharmaceutical.

sodium folate. Monosodium folate.
Use: Water-soluble, hematopoietic vitamin.

•**sodium formaldehyde sulfoxylate.** (SOE-dee-um) *NF.*
Use: Pharmaceutic aid (preservative).

•**sodium gluconate.** (SOE-dee-um) *USP.*
Use: Electrolyte, replacement.

sodium-glucose cotransporter 2 inhibitors.
Use: Antidiabetic agent.
See: Canagliflozin.
Dapagliflozin.

sodium glucosulfone injection.
Use: Leprostatic.

•**sodium glycerophosphate.** (SOE-dee-um GLIS-er-oh-FOS-fate) USAN.
Use: Intravenous nutritional therapy.

sodium glycerophosphate. Glycerol phosphate sodium salt.
Use: Pharmaceutic necessity.

sodium glycocholate.
See: Bile Salts.

•**sodium heparin.** (SO-dee-um) *USP.* Heparin Sodium.
Use: Anticoagulant.

sodium hexobarbital.
Use: Intravenous general anesthetic.

sodium hyaluronate.
Use: Ophthalmic.
See: Amvisc.
Amvisc Plus.
Euflexxa.
Healon.
Healon Endocoat.
Healon5.
Hyalgan.
HyGel.
Hylase Wound.
Hylira.
ProVisc.
Shellgel.
Supartz.
W/Chondroitin Sulfate.
See: DisCoVisc.
Viscoat.

W/Dextranomer.
See: Solesta.
•**sodium hydroxide.** (SOE-dee-um) *NF.*
Use: Pharmaceutic aid (alkalizing agent).
•**sodium hypochlorite solution.** (SOE-dee-um high-poe-KLOR-ite) *USP.*
Use: Anti-infective, local; disinfectant.
See: Antiformin.
Dakin's Solution.
Hyclorite.
HySept.
sodium hypophosphite. Sodium phosphinate.
Use: Pharmaceutic necessity.
sodium hyposulfite.
See: Sodium Thiosulfate.
•**sodium iodide.** (SOE-dee-um) *USP.*
Use: Nutritional supplement.
•**sodium iodide I 131.** (SOE-dee-um) *USP.*
Use: Antineoplastic; diagnostic aid (thyroid function determination); radiopharmaceutical; antithyroid agent.
See: Hicon.
sodium iodide I 131 therapeutic. (Mallinckrodt) **Cap.:** 0.75 to 100 mCi per capsule. **Oral Soln.:** 3.5 to 150 mCi per vial. *Rx.*
Use: Antithyroid agent.
•**sodium iodide I 125.** (SOE-dee-um) USAN.
Use: Diagnostic aid (thyroid function determination); radiopharmaceutical.
•**sodium iodide I 123.** (SOE-dee-um) *USP.*
Use: In vivo diagnostic aid, thyroid function test.
sodium iodide I-123. (Mallinckrodt Medical) Sodium iodide I^{123} 3.7 MBq, 7.4 MBq. Sucrose. Cap. Pkg. 1s, 3s, 5s. *Rx.*
Use: In vivo diagnostic aid, thyroid function test.
sodium iodipamide.
Use: Radiopaque medium.
•**sodium iodomethane sulfonate.** (SO-dee-um) *USP.* Methiodal Sodium.
•**sodium iothalamate.** (SOE-dee-um) *USP.* Iothalmate Sodium Inj.
Use: Radiopaque medium.
•**sodium ipodate.** (SOE-dee-um EYE-poe-date) *USP.* Ipodate Sodium.
Use: Radiopaque.
sodium isoamylethylbarbiturate.
See: Amytal Sodium.
•**sodium lactate injection.** (SOE-dee-um LACK-tate) *USP.*
Use: Fluid and electrolyte replacement.
sodium lactate injection. (Abbott) Sodium lactate 1/6 Molar, 250 mL, 500 mL, 1,000 mL; 50 mEq, 10 mL in 20 mL fliptop vial. *Rx.*
Use: Electrolyte replacement.
sodium lactate solution.
Use: Electrolyte replacement.
•**sodium lauryl sulfate.** (SOE-dee-um LAH-rill SULL-fate) *NF.* Sulfuric acid monododecyl ester sodium salt. Sodium monododecyl sulfate.
Use: Pharmaceutic aid (surfactant).
See: Duponol.
W/Hydrocortisone.
See: Nutracort.
sodium levothyroxine. Levothyroxine Sodium.
Use: Hormone, thyroid.
See: Synthroid.
sodium liothyronine. Liothyronine Sodium, USP.
Use: Hormone, thyroid.
sodium l-thyroxine.
See: Synthroid.
sodium lyapolate. (SOE-dee-um LIE-app-OLE-ate) Polyethylene sulfonate sodium. Peson (Hoechst Marion Roussel).
Use: Anticoagulant.
sodium malonylurea.
See: Barbital Sodium.
sodium mercaptomerin. Mercaptomerin Sodium, USP.
Use: Diuretic.
•**sodium metabisulfite.** (SOE-dee-um) *NF.*
Use: Pharmaceutic aid (antioxidant).
sodium methiodal. Methiodal Sodium, USP. Sodium monoiodomethanesulfonate. Sodium Iodomethanesulfonate, Inj.
Use: Radiopaque medium.
sodium methohexital for injection. Methohexital Sodium for Injection, USP.
Use: Anesthetic, general.
See: Brevital Sodium.
sodium methoxycellulose. Mixture of methylcellulose and sodium.
•**sodium monofluorophosphate.** (SOE-dee-um mahn-oh-flure-oh-FOSS-fate) *USP.*
Use: Dental caries agent.
See: Biotene Dry Mouth.
sodium monomercaptoundecahydro-closo-dodecaborate.
Use: Treatment of glioblastoma multiforme. [Orphan Drug]
sodium morrhuate, injection. Morrhuate Sodium Inj., USP.
Use: Sclerosing agent.
sodium nafcillin. (SOE-dee-um naff-SILL-in) Nafcillin Sodium, USP.
Use: Anti-infective.
sodium nicotinate. (Various Mfr.)
Use: IV nicotinic acid therapy.

• **sodium nitrite.** (SOE-dee-um NYE-trite) *USP.*
Use: Antidote to cyanide poisoning, antioxidant. Vasodilator and antidote-cyanide.
See: Cyanide Antidote Pkg.
sodium nitrite. (Hope) Sodium nitrite 30 mg/mL. Inj. Vials. 10 mL. *Rx.*
Use: Antidote, cyanide.
sodium nitrite/sodium thiosulfate.
Use: Detoxification agent, antidote.
See: Nithiodote.
• **sodium nitroprusside.** (SOE-dee-um NYE-troe-PRUSS-ide) *USP.*
Use: Antihypertensive.
See: Nitropress.
sodium nitroprusside. (Wyeth) Sodium nitroprusside. 50 mg. Pow. for Inj. 5 mL. *Rx.*
Use: Antihypertensive.
sodium novobiocin. Sodium salt of antibacterial substance produced by *Streptomyces niveus.* Novobiocin monosodium salt.
Use: Anti-infective.
sodium ortho-iodohippurate. Iodohippurate Sodium, I 131 Injection, USP.
See: Hipputope.
• **sodium oxybate.** (SOE-dee-um OX-ee-bate) USAN.
Use: Psychotherapeutic agent, miscellaneous.
See: Xyrem.
sodium pantothenate.
Use: Orally, dietary supplement.
sodium para-aminohippurate injection.
Use: IV, to determine kidney tubular excretion function.
sodium penicillin G. Penicillin G Sodium, Sterile, USP. Sodium benzylpenicillin.
sodium pentobarbital. Pentobarbital Sodium, USP.
Use: Hypnotic.
• **sodium perborate monohydrate.** (SOE-dee-um) USAN.
sodium peroxyborate.
See: Sodium Perborate Monohydrate.
sodium peroxyhydrate.
See: Sodium Perborate Monohydrate.
• **sodium pertechnetate Tc 99m injection.** (SOE-dee-um per-TEK-neh-tate) *USP.* Pertechnetic acid, sodium salt.
Use: Radiopharmaceutical.
See: Minitec.
sodium phenobarbital. Phenobarbital Sodium, USP.
Use: Anticonvulsant; hypnotic.
• **sodium phenylacetate.** (SOE-dee-um FEN-ill-ASS-eh-tate) USAN.
Use: Antihyperammonemic.
W/Sodium Benzoate.
See: Ammonul.
Ucephan.
sodium phenylacetate and sodium benzoate.
Use: Antihyperammonemic. [Orphan Drug]
• **sodium phenylbutyrate.** (SOE-dee-um fen-ill-BYOOT-ih-rate) USAN.
Use: Antihyperammonemic. Treatment of blood disorders. [Orphan Drug]
See: Buphenyl.
sodium phenylbutyrate. (Sigmapharm Labs) Sodium phenylbutyrate. Pow. 250 mL w/dosage spoon. *Rx.*
Use: Endocrine and metabolic agent.
sodium phenylethylbarbiturate. Phenobarbital Sodium, USP.
sodium phosphate.
Use: Buffering agent; source of phosphate; laxative.
See: OsmoPrep
W/Gentamicin Sulfate, Monosodium Phosphate, Sodium Chloride, Benzalkonium Chloride.
See: Garamycin Ophthalmic.
W/Sodium Biphosphate.
See: Fleet Enema.
Phospho-Soda.
sodium phosphate. (Abbott) Disodium hydrogen phosphate. 3 mM P and 4 mEq sodium. 15 mL in 30 mL fliptop vial. *Rx.*
Use: Intravenous nutritional therapy, mineral.
sodium phosphate. (Various Mfr.) Phosphate 3 mM, sodium 4 mEq per mL. Inj. Vials. 5 mL, 15 mL, 50 mL. *Rx.*
Use: Intravenous nutritional therapy, mineral.
• **sodium phosphate, dibasic.** (SOE-dee-um FOSS-fate) *USP.*
Use: Laxative.
See: Visicol.
W/Calcium Chloride, Monobasic Sodium Phosphate, Silicon Dioxide, Sodium Chloride, Sodium Bicarbonate.
See: NeutraSal.
W/Calcium Chloride, Monobasic Sodium Phosphate, Sodium Chloride.
See: Caphosol.
W/Monobasic Potassium Phosphate, Monobasic Sodium Phosphate Monohydrate, Phosphorus.
See: Phospha 250 Neutral.
• **sodium phosphate, dried.** (SO-dee-um) *USP.*
Use: Cathartic.
• **sodium phosphate, monobasic.** (SOE-dee-um FOSS-fate) *USP.*

Use: Cathartic.
See: Visicol.
W/Calcium Chloride, Dibasic Sodium Phosphate, Silicon Dioxide, Sodium Chloride, Sodium Bicarbonate.
See: NeutraSal.
W/Calcium Chloride, Dibasic Sodium Phosphate, Sodium Chloride.
See: Cephosol.
W/Dibasic Sodium Phosphate, Monobasic Potassium Phosphate, Phosphorus.
See: Phospha 250 Neutral.
W/Hyoscyamine Sulfate, Methenamine, Methylene Blue.
See: Uryl.
W/Hyoscyamine Sulfate, Methenamine, Methylene Blue, Phenyl Salicylate.
See: Phosphasal.
UtiCap.
Utrona-C.
W/Methenamine.
See: Uro-Phosphate.
Utac.
W/Methenamine, Phenyl Salicylate, Methylene Blue, Hyoscyamine, Alkaloid.
See: Fleet Enema.
Phospho-Soda.

•**sodium phosphate P 32 solution.** (SOE-dee-um FOSS-fate) *USP.*
Use: Antineoplastic; antipolycythemic; diagnostic aid (neoplasm); radiopharmaceutical.

•**sodium phosphates rectal solution.** (SO-dee-um) *USP.*
Use: Cathartic.

sodium phytate. (SOE-dee-um FYE-tate) Nonasodium phytate: Sodium cyclohexanehexyl (hexaphosphate).
Use: Chelating agent.
W/Citric Acid, Magnesium Oxide.
See: Prepopik.

•**sodium picosulfate.** (SOE-dee-um PI-koe-SUL-fate) USAN.
Use: Laxative.

•**sodium polyphosphate.** (SOE-dee-um pahl-ee-FOSS-fate) USAN.
Use: Pharmaceutic aid.

•**sodium polystyrene sulfonate.** (SOE-dee-um pah-lee-STYE-reen SULL-fuh-nate) *USP.*
Use: Ion exchange resin (potassium).
See: Kayexalate.
Kionex.
SPS.

sodium polystyrene sulfonate. (Crookes-Barnes) Sodium polystyrene sulfonate 5% Soln. Eye drops. *Lacrivial* 15 mL. *Rx.*
Use: Ion exchange resin (potassium).

sodium polystyrene sulfonate. (Paddock Laboratories) Sodium polystyrene sulfonate 15 g per 60 mL. Alcohol 0.2%, parabens, propylene glycol, saccharin. Sorbitol free. Raspberry flavor. Susp., oral or rectal. 480 mL, UD 60 mL. *Rx.*
Use: Potassium-removing resin.

sodium polystyrene sulfonate. (Various Mfr.) Sodium polystyrene sulfonate (finely ground) Pow. for Susp. (oral or rectal). 454 g. *Rx.*
Use: Potassium-removing resin.

•**sodium propionate.** (SOE-dee-um PRO-pee-oh-nate) *NF.*
Use: Pharmaceutic aid (preservative).

sodium psylliate.
Use: Sclerosing agent.

•**sodium pyrophosphate.** (SOE-dee-um pie-row-FOSS-fate) USAN.
Use: Pharmaceutic aid.

sodium radio chromate injection. Sodium Chromate Cr 51 Inj., USP.

sodium radio iodide solution. Sodium Iodide I-131 Solution, USP.
Use: Thyroid tumors; hyperthyroidism; cardiac dysfunction.

sodium radio-phosphate, P-32. Radio-Phosphate P 32 Solution. Sodium phosphate P 32 Solution, USP.

sodium rhodanate.
See: Sodium Thiocyanate.

sodium rhodanide.
See: Sodium Thiocyanate.

sodium saccharin. Saccharin Sodium, USP.
Use: Noncaloric sweetener.

•**sodium salicylate.** (SOE-dee-um) *USP.*
Use: Analgesic; IV, gout.
W/Combinations.
See: Apcogesic.
Bisalate.
Bufosal.
W/Phenylephrine Hydrochloride, Pheniramine Maleate, Caffeine Citrate.
See: Scot-Tussin Original Multi-Action Cold and Allergy.

sodium salicylate, natural.
Use: Analgesic.

sodium secobarbital. Secobarbital Sodium, USP.
Use: Hypnotic.

sodium secobarbital and sodium amobarbital.
Use: Sedative.
See: Tuinal.

•**sodium starch glycolate.** (SOE-dee-um) *NF.*
Use: Pharmaceutic aid (tablet excipient).

•**sodium stearate.** (SOE-dee-um) *NF.*

Use: Pharmaceutic aid (emulsifying and stiffening agent).

•**sodium stearyl fumarate.** (SO-dee-um) *NF.*
Use: Pharmaceutic aid (tablet/capsule lubricant).

sodium stibogluconate.
Use: CDC anti-infective agent.

sodium succinate.
Use: Alkalinize urine; awaken patients following barbiturate anesthesia.

sodium sulamyd.
Use: Sulfonamide, ophthalmic.
See: Sodium Sulamyd Ophthalmic.

sodium sulfabromomethazine.
Use: Anti-infective.

sodium sulfacetamide.
See: Ovace.
Seb-Prev.
Sulfacetamide Sodium.
W/Sulfur.
See: Avar-e Emollient.
Avar-e LS.
Avar-e LS cleanser.
BP Cleansing Wash.
Cerisa.
Clarifoam EF.
Claris.
Clenia.
Garimide.
Klaron.
Plexion Cleansing Cloths.
Plexion TS.
Rosaderm Kit.
SE 10-5 SS.
SSS 10-5.
SSS 10-4.
SulfaCleanse 8/4.
Sumadan.
Sumaxin.
Sumaxin CP.
Sumaxin TS.
Sumaxin Wash.
Virti-Sulf Emollient.
Zencia.

sodium sulfacetamide. (Acella Pharmaceuticals) Sodium sulfacetamide 10%. Disodium EDTA, methylparaben, PEG. Soap. 473 mL. *Rx.*
Use: Topical anti-infective, antibiotic.

sodium sulfacetamide and sulfur. (Acella Pharmaceuticals) Sodium sulfacetamide 10%, sulfur 5%. Alcohols, disodium EDTA, glyceryl, parabens, PEG, white petrolatum. Soap. 170.3 g, 340.2 g. *Rx.*
Use: Acne product combination.

sodium sulfacetamide and sulfur. (Austin Pharmaceuticals) Sodium sulfacetamide 10%, sulfur 5%. **Cream/Emollient:** Benzyl alcohol, caprylic/capric triglyceride, cetyl alcohol, disodium EDTA, glycerin, glyceryl, parabens, PEG, wax, zinc oxide. 28 g. **Susp.:** Benzyl alcohol, capric/caprylic triglyceride, cetyl alcohol, disodium EDTA, glycerin, glyceryl, parabens, PEG, zinc oxide. 30 g. *Rx.*
Use: Acne product combination.

sodium sulfacetamide and sulfur. (Biocomp) Sodium sulfacetamide 10%, sulfur 2%. Benzyl alcohol, cetyl alcohol, disodium EDTA, glycerin, glyceryl stearate, PEG, wax, zinc oxide. Cream. 57 g. *Rx.*
Use: Acne product combination.

sodium sulfacetamide and sulfur. (Rochester Pharmaceuticals) Sodium sulfacetamide 8%, sulfur 4%. Alcohols, aloe, edetate disodium, glyceryl stearate, parabens. Susp.; topical. 473 mL. *Rx.*
Use: Topical anti-infective, antibiotic agent.

sodium sulfacetamide 9%/sulfur 4.5%. (Various Mfr.) Sodium sulfacetamide 9%, sulfur 4.5%. May contain alcohols, aloe vera, disodium EDTA, glyceryl, parabens, PEG. Soap. 454 g. *Rx.*
Use: Keratolytic agent.

sodium sulfacetamide/sulfur. (Acella Pharmaceuticals) Sodium sulfacetamide/sulfur. **Cloth:** 10%/5%. Alcohols, aloe, disodium EDTA, glycerol, parabens, PEG, white petrolatum. 30s, 60s. **Soap:** 8%/4%. Alcohols, aloe, butylated hydroxytoluene, disodium EDTA, glycerol, green tea, parabens, PEG, white petrolatum. 473 mL. **Wash:** 9%/4%. Aloe, cetyl alcohol, disodium EDTA, glycerol, parabens, PEG-100, stearyl alcohol, white petrolatum. 473 mL. *Rx.*
Use: Acne product combination.

sodium sulfacetamide/sulfur. (Brookstone Pharmaceuticals) Sodium sulfacetamide 10%, sulfur 4%. Aloe, cetyl alcohol, disodium EDTA, glycerin, green tea, parabens, PEG-100, sodium metabisulfate, sodium thiosulfate, stearyl alcohol. Pad. 60s. *Rx.*
Use: Acne product combination.

sodium sulfacetamide/sulfur. (Fougera) Sodium sulfacetamide 10%/sulfur 4%. Alcohol, butylated hydroxytoluene, disodium EDTA, glyceryl, parabens, PEG. Soap. 473 mL. *Rx.*
Use: Acne product combination.

sodium sulfacetamide/sulfur. (Kylemore) Sodium sulfacetamide/sulfur. **Aer. Foam:** 10%/5%. Cetearyl alcohol, glycerin. 60 g. **Soap:** 10%/4%. Alcohols, BHT, disodium EDTA, parabens, PEG,

urea 10%. 473 mL. *Rx.*
Use: Acne product combination.
sodium sulfacetamide/sulfur. (River's Edge) Sodium sulfacetamide/sulfur 10%/5%. **Gel:** Benzyl alcohol, cetyl alcohol, dimethicone, disodium EDTA, glyceryl, methylparaben, mineral oil, PEG-100, propylene glycol, stearyl alcohol, urea 10%. 45 mL. **Wash:** Cetyl alcohol, disodium EDTA, glyceryl, parabens, PEG-100, stearyl alcohol, urea 10%. 355 mL. *Rx.*
Use: Acne product combination.
sodium sulfacetamide 10%. (A. Aarons.) Sodium sulfacetamide 10%, urea 10%. EDTA. Top. Pads. 30s. *Rx.*
Use: Keratolytic agent, acne product.
sodium sulfadiazine.
See: Sulfadiazine Sodium.
sodium sulfamerazine.
See: Sulfamerazine Sodium.
•**sodium sulfate.** (SOE-dee-um SULL-fate) *USP.*
Use: Calcium regulator.
W/Magnesium Sulfate, Potassium Sulfate.
See: Suclear.
Suprep Bowel Prep.
W/PEG 3350, Sodium Bicarbonate, Sodium Chloride, Potassium Chloride.
See: GaviLyte-C.
GaviLyte-G.
•**sodium sulfate S 35.** (SOE-dee-um SULL-fate) USAN.
Use: Radiopharmaceutical.
•**sodium sulfide.** (SO-dee-um) *USP.*
•**sodium sulfide gel.** (SO-dee-um) *USP.*
sodium sulfobromophthalein. Sulfobromophthalein Sodium, USP.
Use: Diagnostic aid (hepatic function determination).
sodium sulfocyanate.
See: Sodium Thiocyanate.
sodium sulfoxone. Sulfoxone Sodium, USP. Disodium sulfonyl-bis (p-phenyleneimino) dimethanesulfonate.
sodium suramin.
See: Suramin Hexasodium.
sodium taurocholate.
See: Bile Salts.
sodium tetradecyl sulfate.
Use: Sclerosing agent.
See: Sotradecol.
sodium tetraiodophenolphthalein.
See: Iodophthalein Sodium.
sodium thiamylal for injection. Thiamylal Sodium for Injection, USP.
Use: Anesthetic, general.
sodium thiocyanate. Sodium Sulfocyanate. Sodium Rhodanide.
sodium thiopental.
See: Thiopental Sodium.
•**sodium thiosulfate.** (SOE-dee-um thigh-oh-SULL-fate) *USP.*
Use: For argyria, cyanide, and iodine poisoning, arsphenamine reactions; prevention of spread of ringworm of feet; antidote to cyanide poisoning.
W/Salicylic Acid, Alcohol.
See: Versiclear.
W/Sodium Nitrite, Amyl Nitrite.
See: Cyanide Antidote Pkg.
sodium thiosulfate/sodium nitrite.
Use: Detoxification agent, antidote.
See: Nithiodote.
sodium tolbutamide. Tolbutamide Sodium, USP.
Use: Diagnostic aid (diabetes).
sodium triclofos. (SOE-dee-um TRY-kloe-foss) Sodium trichloroethylphosphate.
Use: Sedative; hypnotic.
•**sodium trimetaphosphate.** (SOE-dee-um try-met-AH-FOSS-fate) USAN.
Use: Pharmaceutic aid.
sodium valproate.
See: Valproate Sodium.
sodium vinbarbital injection.
Use: Sedative.
sodium warfarin. Warfarin Sodium, USP.
Use: Anticoagulant.
Sod-Late 10. (Schlicksup) Sodium salicylate 10 g. Tab. Bot. 1000s. *OTC.*
Use: Analgesic.
Sodol Compound. (Major) Carisoprodol 200 mg, aspirin 325 mg. Tab. Bot. 100s, 500s. *Rx.*
Use: Muscle relaxant.
Sofcaps. (Alton) Docusate sodium 100 mg, 250 mg. Cap. Bot. 100s, 1000s. *OTC.*
Use: Laxative.
•**sofinicline.** (soe-FIN-i-kleen) USAN.
Use: CNS agent.
•**sofinicline benzenesulfonate.** (soe-FIN-i-kleen) USAN.
Use: CNS agent.
Sof-Lax. (Fleet) Docusate sodium 100 mg. Softgel Cap. 60s. *OTC.*
Use: Laxative.
•**sofosbuvir.** (soe-FOS-bue-vir) USAN.
Use: Antiviral agent.
See: Sovaldi.
Sof/Pro-Clean. (Sherman Pharmaceuticals, Inc.) Buffered, hypertonic solution with thimerosal 0.004%, EDTA 0.1%, ethylene and propylene oxide, octylphenoxypolyethoxyethanol, lauryl sulfate salt of imidazoline. Soln. Bot. 30 mL. *OTC.*
Use: Contact lens care.

Sof/Pro Clean SA. (Sherman Pharmaceuticals, Inc.) Hypertonic solution: salt buffers, copolymers of ethylene and propylene oxide, octylphenoxypolyethoxyethanol, lauryl sulfate salt of imidazoline, sodium bisulfite 0.1%, sorbic acid 0.1%, trisodium EDTA 0.25%, thimerosal free. Bot. 30 mL. *OTC.*
Use: Contact lens care.

Soft'n Soothe. (B.F. Ascher) Benzocaine, menthol, moisturizers. Tube 50 g. *OTC.*
Use: Anesthetic, local.

Soft Sense. (Bausch & Lomb) **Hand Lot.:** Petrolatum, vitamin E, aloe, parabens. Non-greasy. Bot. 444 mL. **Body Lot.:** Petrolatum, vitamin E, parabens. Non-greasy. Bot. 444 mL. *OTC.*
Use: Emollient.

SoftWear. (Ciba Vision) Isotonic, sodium Cl, boric acid, sodium borate, sodium perborate (generating up to 0.006% hydrogen peroxide stabilized with phosphoric acid). Soln. Bot. 120 mL, 240 mL, 360 mL. *OTC.*
Use: Contact lens care.

Sojourn. (Piramal Critical Care) Sevoflurane. Liq. Inh. 250 mL. *Rx.*
Use: General anesthetic, volatile liquid.

•**solabegron hydrochloride.** (soe-la-BEG-ron) USAN.
Use: Antidiabetic.

Solaneed. (Hanlon) Vitamin A 25,000 units. Cap. Bot. 100s. *Rx.*
Use: Vitamin supplement.

•**solanezumab.** (SOE-la-NEZ-ue-mab) USAN.
Use: Alzheimer disease.

Solaquin. (Valeant) Hydroquinone 2% with sunscreens. Tube. 28.4 g. *OTC.*
Use: Dermatologic.

Solaquin Forte. (Valeant) Hydroquinone 4%, dioxybenzone, padimate O, oxybenzone, EDTA, sodium metabisulfite, cetearyl alcohol, stearyl alcohol, lactic acid. **Cream:** Vanishing cream base. Tube. 28.4 g. **Gel:** Padimate O, dioxybenzone, EDTA, alcohol, sodium metabisulfite. Tube. 28.4 g. *Rx.*
Use: Dermatologic.

Solar. (Doak Dermatologics) PABA, titanium dioxide, magnesium stearate in a flesh-colored, water-repellent base. Cream. Tube oz. *OTC.*
Use: Sunscreen.

Solaraze. (Pharmaderm) Diclofenac 3% (diclofenac sodium 30 mg/g). Benzyl alcohol. Gel. Tubes. 25 g, 50 g. *Rx.*
Use: Nonsteroidal anti-inflammatory drug, topical.

Solarcaine. (Schering-Plough) **Lot.:** Benzocaine, triclosan, mineral oil, alcohol, aloe extract, tocopheryl acetate, menthol, camphor, parabens, EDTA. 120 mL. **Aerosol:** Benzocaine 20% with triclosan 0.13%, SD alcohol 40 35%, tocopheryl acetate. 90 mL, 120 mL. *OTC.*
Use: Topical local anesthetic, ester local anesthetic.

Solarcaine Aloe Extra Burn Relief. (Schering-Plough) **Cream:** Lidocaine 0.5%. Aloe, EDTA, lanolin oil, lanolin, camphor, propylparaben, eucalyptus oil, menthol, tartrazine. 120 g. **Gel:** Lidocaine 0.5%. Aloe vera gel, glycerin, EDTA, isopropyl alcohol, menthol, diazolidinyl urea, tartrazine. 120 g, 240 g. **Spray:** Lidocaine 0.5%. Aloe vera gel, glycerin, EDTA, diazolidinyl urea, vitamin E, parabens. 135 mg. *OTC.*
Use: Topical local anesthetic, amide local anesthetic.

Solarcaine Medicated First-Aid (Schering-Plough) Benzocaine 20%. Triclosan 0.13%, alcohol. Spray. 90 mL. *OTC.*
Use: Topical local anesthetic, ester local anesthetic.

solargentum.
See: Silver Protein, Mild.

Solar Shield 15 SPF. (Akorn) Ethylhexyl p-methoxy-cinnamate 7.5%, oxybenzone in a moisturizing base 5%. PABA free. Waterproof. Lot. Bot. 120 mL. *OTC.*
Use: Sunscreen.

Solar Shield 30 SPF. (Akorn) Ethylhexyl p-methoxycinnamate 7.5%, oxybenzone 6%, 2-ethylhexyl salicylate 5%, 3-diphenylacrylate 7.5%, 2-ethylhexyl-2-cyano-3 in a moisturizing base, PABA free. Waterproof. Lot. Bot. 120 mL. *OTC.*
Use: Sunscreen.

Solbar Avo. (Person & Covey) Homosalate 8%, octinoxate 7.5%, oxybenzone 6%, avobenzone 3%, benzyl alcohol, disodium EDTA, glycerin, triethanolamine. Water resistant. Lot. 115 g. *OTC.*
Use: Sunscreen.

SolBar PF 15. (Person and Covey) Octyl methoxycinnamate 7.5%, oxybenzone 5%. SPF 15. Cream. Bot. 1 oz, 4 oz. *OTC.*
Use: Sunscreen.

SolBar PF 50. (Person and Covey) Oxybenzone, octyl methoxycinnamate, octocrylene, PABA free. Waterproof. SPF 50. Cream. Tube 120 g. *OTC.*
Use: Sunscreen.

SolBar PF Liquid. (Person and Covey) Octyl methoxycinnamate 7.5%, oxybenzone 6%, SD alcohol 40 76%, PABA

free. SPF 30. Liq. Bot. 120 mL. *OTC.*
Use: Sunscreen.

SolBar PF Paba Free 15. (Person and Covey) Oxybenzone 5%, octyl methoxycinnamate 7.5%. SPF 15. Cream. Tube 2.5 oz. *OTC.*
Use: Sunscreen.

SolBar Plus 15. (Person and Covey) Padimate 6%, oxybenzone 4%, dioxybenzone 2%. SPF 15. Cream. Tube 1 oz, 4 oz. *OTC.*
Use: Sunscreen.

Solesta. (Oceana Therapeutics) Dextranomer 50 mg per mL/sodium hyaluronate 15 mg per mL. Inj., Gel. Single-use 1 mL glass syringe (in cartons containing 4 pouches w/syringes, 5 sterile needles [*Sterican*, 21G × 4 ¾ inches, 0.8 × 120 mm], patient record labels, and package insert). *Rx.*
Use: Gastrointestinal agent.

Solfoton. (ECR) Phenobarbital 16 mg. Tab. or Cap. Bot. 100s, 500s. *c-IV.*
Use: Hypnotic; sedative.

Solfoton S/C. (ECR) Phenobarbital 16 mg. SC Tab. Bot. 100s. *c-IV.*
Use: Hypnotic; sedative.

Solia. (Prasco) Ethinyl estradiol 30 mcg, desogestrel 0.15 mg. Lactose. Tab. Blister cards. 28s with 7 inert tabs. *Rx.*
Use: Contraceptive hormone, sex hormone.

•**solifenacin succinate.** (sol-i-FEN-a-cin) USAN.
Use: Anticholinergic.
See: VESIcare.

Soliris. (Alexion) Eculizumab 10 mg/mL. Preservative free. Inj. Soln., Concentrate. Single-use vials. 30 mL. *Rx.*
Use: Monoclonal antibody.

•**solithromycin.** (soe-LITH-roe-MYE-sin) USAN.
Use: Antibiotic.

Soliwax. Docusate Sodium, USP. Docusate Sodium, Solasulfone (I.N.N.).

Solo. (Theralogix) Vitamins A 3,000 units, D 2,000 units, E 30 units, B_1 5 mg, B_2 5 mg, B_3 20 mg, B_5 10 mg, B_6 5 mg, B_{12} 30 mcg, C 100 mg, K 80 mcg, folic acid 0.4 mg, B, Ca, Cr, Cu, I, Mg, Mn, Mo, Se, V, Zn, biotin 30 mcg, choline 100 mg. Tab. 180s. *OTC.*
Use: Multivitamin with minerals (except iron).

Solodyn. (Valeant) Minocycline hydrochloride 55 mg, 65 mg, 80 mg, 90 mg, 105 mg, 115 mg. Lactose. Film coated. ER Tab. 30s. *Rx.*
Use: Anti-infective, tetracycline.

Soltamox. (Oncogenerix) Tamoxifen 10 mg per 5 mL (equiv. to tamoxifen citrate 15.2 mg per 5 mL). Ethanol, glycerol, propylene glycol, sorbitol. Sugar free. Licorice/aniseed flavor. Soln. 150 mL w/dosing cup. *Rx.*
Use: Hormone, antiestrogen.

Sōltice Quick-Rub. (Oakhurst) Menthol 5.1%, camphor 5.1%, eucalyptus oil, glycerin, methyl salicylate. Oint. 37 g, 85 g. *OTC.*
Use: Rub and liniment.

Solu-Barb 0.25. (Forest) Phenobarbital 0.25 g. Tab. Bot. 24s. *c-IV.*
Use: Hypnotic; sedative.

soluble complement receptor (recombinant human) type 1.
Use: Prevention or reduction of adult respiratory distress syndrome. [Orphan Drug]

soluble guanylate cyclase stimulators.
See: Riociguat.

Soluclenz Rx. (Obagi Medical Products) Benzoyl peroxide 5%. Benzyl benzoate. Gel. 27 mL. *Rx.*
Use: Topical anti-infective, antibiotic agent.

Solu-Cortef. (Pfizer) Hydrocortisone sodium succinate. Preservative free. Inj., Pow. for Soln. **100 mg:** Single-dose *Act-O-Vial.* 2 mL. **250 mg:** Single-dose *Act-O-Vial.* 2 mL. **500 mg:** Single-dose *Act-O-Vial.* 4 mL. **1,000 mg:** Single-dose *Act-O-Vial.* 8 mL. *Rx.*
Tall Man: Solu-CORTEF
Use: Corticosteroid.

Solu-Eze. (Forest) Hydroxyquinoline 0.12%, carbitol acetate 12.10%. Liq. Bot. 3 oz. *Rx.*
Use: Dermatologic.

Solu-Medrol. (Pfizer) **40 mg/vial:** Methylprednisolone sodium succinate. Sodium phosphate anhydrous (monobasic 1.6 mg, dibasic 17.5 mg), lactose, benzyl alcohol 9 mg. *Act-O-Vials.* 1 mL. **125 mg/vial:** Methylprednisolone sodium succinate. Sodium phosphate anhydrous (monobasic 1.6 mg, dibasic 17.4 mg), benzyl alcohol ≈ 18 mg. *Act-O-Vials.* 2 mL. **500 mg/vial:** Methylprednisolone sodium succinate. Sodium phosphate anhydrous (monobasic 6.4 mg, dibasic 69.6 mg). May contain benzyl alcohol 36 mg to 70.2 mg. Vials. 8 mL. Vials w/diluent. 8 mL. **1 g/vial:** Methylprednisolone sodium succinate. Sodium phosphate anhydrous (monobasic 12.8 mg, dibasic 139.2 mg). May contain benzyl alcohol 66.8 mg to 141 mg. Vials. 1 g. Vials with diluent. 1 g. *Act-O-Vials.* 8 mL. **2 g/vial:** Methylprednisolone sodium succinate. Vials with diluent. 2 g. Inj., Pow. for Soln. *Rx.*

Tall Man: Solu-MEDROL
Use: Adrenocortical steroid, glucocorticoid.
Solumol. (C & M Pharmacal) Petrolatum, mineral oil, cetylstearyl alcohol, sodium lauryl sulfate, glycerin, propylene glycol, sorbic acid, purified water. Jar lb. *OTC.*
Use: Pharmaceutical aid, ointment base.
Soluvite C.T. (Pharmics) Vitamins A 2500 units, D 400 units, B_1 1.05 mg, B_2 1.2 mg, B_6 1.05 mg, B_{12} 4.5 mcg, C 60 mg, $B_3$13.5 mg, E 15 units, fluoride 1 mg, folic acid 0.3 mg. Tab. Bot. 100s, 1000s. *Rx.*
Use: Mineral, vitamin supplement.
Solvisyn-A. (Towne) Water-soluble vitamin A 10,000 units, 25,000 units, 50,000 units. Cap. Bot. 100s, 1000s. *Rx-OTC.*
Use: Vitamin supplement.
•**solypertine tartrate.** (SAHL-ee-PURR-teen) USAN.
Use: Antiadrenergic.
Soma. (Wallace) Carisoprodol 350 mg. Tab. Bot. 100s, 500s, UD 500s. *c-IV.*
Use: Muscle relaxant.
Somagard. (Roberts)
See: Deslorelin.
•**somantadine hydrochloride.** (sah-MAN-tah-deen) USAN.
Use: Antiviral.
somatostatin.
Use: Digestive aid. [Orphan Drug]
somatostatin analogs.
See: Lanreotide.
Octreotide Acetate.
Pasireotide.
•**somatropin.** (SO-muh-TROE-pin) USAN. Growth hormone derived from the anterior pituitary gland.
Use: Hormone, growth.
See: Genotropin.
Genotropin MiniQuick.
Humatrope.
Norditropin.
Nutropin.
Nutropin AQ.
Omnitrope.
Saizen.
Serostim.
Tev-Tropin.
Somatuline Depot. (Ipsen Biopharmaceuticals) Lanreotide 60 mg (equiv. to lanreotide acetate 79.8 mg), 90 mg (equiv. to lanreotide acetate 116.4 mg), 120 mg (equiv. to lanreotide acetate 155.5 mg). Inj. Soln., ER. Single-use prefilled syringes. *Rx.*
Use: Somatostatin analog.
Somavert. (Pfizer) Pegvisomant 10 mg, 15 mg, 20 mg, mannitol 36 mg. Pow. for Inj., lyophilized. Vials. Single-dose. *Rx.*
Use: Acromegaly.
Sominex. (GlaxoSmithKline) Diphenhydramine hydrochloride 25 mg. Tab. 16s, 32s, 72s. *OTC.*
Use: Antihistamine, nonselective ethanolamine.
Sominex Pain Relief Formula. (GlaxoSmithKline) Diphenhydramine hydrochloride 25 mg, acetaminophen 500 mg. Tab. Blister pack 16s. Bot. 32s. *OTC.*
Use: Sleep aid; analgesic.
Somnote. (Breckenridge) Chloral hydrate 500 mg. Cap. 50s, UD 50s. *c-IV.*
Use: Sedative and hypnotic, nonbarbiturate.
Sonacide. (Wyeth) Potentiated acid glutaraldehyde. Bot. 1 gal, 5 gal. *OTC.*
Use: Disinfectant; sterilizing agent.
Sonafine. (Stratus Pharmaceuticals) Avocado oil, paraffins, parabens, propylene glycol, trolamine. Emulsion; topical. 45 g, 90 g. *Rx.*
Use: Flexible hydroactive dressing.
Sonahist DM. (Kylemore Pharmaceuticals) Chlorpheniramine maleate 1 mg, dextromethorphan hydrobromide 3 mg, phenylephrine hydrochloride 2 mg per mL. Glycerin, parabens, saccharin, sorbitol. Sweet orange vanilla flavor. Drops. 30 mL. *Rx.*
Use: Upper respiratory combination, antitussive combination.
Sonata. (King) Zaleplon 5 mg, 10 mg, lactose, tartrazine. Cap. Bot. 100s. *c-IV.*
Use: Sedative; hypnotic.
Sonekap. (Eastwood) Cap. Bot. 100s.
soneryl.
See: Butethal.
Soothaderm. (Pharmakon) Pyrilamine maleate 2.07 mg, benzocaine 2.08 mg, zinc oxide 41.35 mg/mL, camphor, menthol. Lot. Bot. 118 mL. *OTC.*
Use: Antihistamine; anesthetic, local.
Soothe. (Walgreen) Bismuth subsalicylate 100 mg. Tsp. Bot. 9 oz. *OTC.*
Use: Antidiarrheal.
Soothe & Cool. (Medline) Dimethicone 5%, zinc oxide 5%, lanolin, cetyl alcohol, vitamins A, D, and E. Cream. 118 mL. *OTC.*
Use: Diaper rash product.
Soothe & Cool Protect Moisture Barrier. (Medline) Petrolatum 98.3%, aloe extract, benzethonium chloride, corn oil, vitamins A, D, and E. Oint. 56 g. *OTC.*
Use: Skin protectant.

Soothe Hydration. (Bausch & Lomb) Povidone 1.25%, boric acid, potassium chloride, edetate disodium 0.1%, sorbic acid 0.1%, sodium chloride, sodium borate. Soln.; Ophth. 15 mL. *OTC.*
Use: Artificial tear solution.

Soothe Night Time. (Bausch & Lomb) Mineral oil 20%, white petrolatum 80%. Preservative free. Oint.; Ophth. 3.5 g. *OTC.*
Use: Ocular lubricant.

Soothe Preservative Free. (Bausch & Lomb) Glycerin 0.6%, propylene glycol 0.6%. Preservative free. Soln.; Ophth. 15 mL. *OTC.*
Use: Artificial tears.

Soothe XP. (Bausch & Lomb) Mineral oil 4.5%, light mineral oil 1%. EDTA, polysorbate 80, sodium chloride, sodium hydroxide and/or hydrochloride acid, sodium phosphate dibasic, sodium phosphate monobasic, octoxynol-40. Ophth. Soln. 15 mL. *OTC.*
Use: Artificial tears.

Soquette. (PBH Wesley Jessen) Polyvinyl alcohol w/benzalkonium Cl 0.01%, EDTA 0.2%. Bot. 4 fl oz. *OTC.*
Use: Contact lens care.

•**sorafenib.** (soe-RAF-e-nib) USAN.
Tall Man: SORAfenib
Use: Multikinase inhibitor.
See: Nexavar.

•**sorafenib tosylate.** (soe-RAF-e-nib) USAN.
Tall Man: SORAfenib
Use: Antineoplastic.

•**sorbic acid.** (SORE-bik) *NF.*
Use: Pharmaceutic aid (antimicrobial).
See: Clear Eyes Contact Lens Relief.

Sorbide T.D. (Merz) Isosorbide dinitrate 40 mg. TR Cap. Bot. 100s. *Rx.*
Use: Antianginal.

Sorbidon Hydrate. (Gordon Laboratories) Water-in-oil ointment. Jar 2 oz, 0.5 oz, 1 lb, 5 lb. *OTC.*
Use: Emollient.

sorbimacrogol oleate 300.
See: Polysorbate 80.

•**sorbinil.** (SORE-bih-nill) USAN.
Use: Enzyme inhibitor (aldose reductase).

•**sorbitan monolaurate.** (SORE-bih-tan MAHN-oh-LORE-ate) *NF.*
Use: Pharmaceutic aid (surfactant).
See: Span 20.

•**sorbitan monooleate.** (SORE-bih-tan MAHN-oh-OH-lee-ate) *NF.*
Use: Pharmaceutic aid (surfactant).
See: Span 80.

sorbitan monooleate polyoxyethylene derivatives.
See: Polysorbate 80.

•**sorbitan monopalmitate.** (SORE-bih-tan MAHN-oh-PAL-mih-tate) *NF.*
Use: Pharmaceutic aid (surfactant).
See: Span 40.

•**sorbitan monostearate.** (SORE-bih-tan MAHN-oh-STEE-ah-rate) *NF.*
Use: Pharmaceutic aid (surfactant).
See: Span 60.

sorbitans.
See: Polysorbate 80.

•**sorbitan sesquioleate.** (SORE-bih-tan SESS-kwih-OH-lee-ate) *NF.*
Use: Pharmaceutic aid (surfactant).
See: Arlacel C.

•**sorbitan trioleate.** (SORE-bih-tan TRY-OH-lee-ate) *NF.*
Use: Pharmaceutic aid, surfactant.
See: Span 85.

•**sorbitan tristearate.** (SORE-bih-tan TRY-STEE-ah-rate) USAN.
Use: Pharmaceutic aid; surfactant.
See: Span 65.

•**sorbitol.** (SOR-bi-tol) *NF.*
Use: Diuretic; dehydrating agent; humectant; pharmaceutic aid (sweetening agent, tablet excipient, flavor).
See: Numoisyn.
Sorbo.
W/Mannitol.
See: Sorbitol-Mannitol.

sorbitol. (B. Braun Medical) Sorbitol 3.3% (183 mOsm/L). Soln. 2,000 mL. *Rx.*
Use: Genitourinary irrigant, hexitol irrigant.

sorbitol. (Travenol) Sorbitol 3% (165 mOsm/L). Soln. 1,500 mL, 3,000 mL. *Rx.*
Use: Genitourinary irrigant, hexitol irrigant.

Sorbitol-Mannitol. (Hospira) Mannitol 0.54 g, sorbitol 2.7 g. Liq. Bot. 100 mL, 1500 mL, 3000 mL. *Rx.*
Use: Irrigant, genitourinary.

•**sorbitol solution.** (SOR-bi-tol) *USP.*
Use: Pharmaceutic aid (flavor, tablet excipient).

sorbitol solution. (Various Mfr.) 70% w/D-sorbitol. Soln. 454 mL. *OTC.*
Use: Laxative.

Sorbo. (AstraZeneca) Sorbitol Solution, USP.

Sorbsan. (Dow Hickam) Calcium alginate fiber 2 × 2, 3 × 3, 4 × 4, 4 × 8 inch. Box 1s. Wound packing fibers-calcium alginate fiber ¼ × 12 inch. Box 1s. *Rx.*
Use: Dermatologic, wound therapy.

Sorbutuss NR. (Teral) Dextromethorphan

hydrobromide 15 mg, guaifenesin 150 mg, potassium citrate 127.5 mg per 7.5 mL. Parabens, sorbitol, sucralose. Alcohol free, dye free, and sugar free. Grape flavor. Liq. 474 mL. *OTC.*
Use: Upper respiratory combination, antitussive with expectorant.

sorethytan (20) monooleate.
See: Polysorbate 80.

Soriatane. (GlaxoSmithKline) Acitretin 10 mg, 17.5 mg, 25 mg. Capsule shells contain gelatin, iron oxide, titanium dioxide, may also contain benzyl alcohol. Cap. 30s. *Rx.*
Use: Retinoid, second generation.

Soriatane CK. (Stiefel) **Cap.:** Acitretin 10 mg. Maltodextrin, gelatin, iron oxide, titanium dioxide. May contain benzyl alcohol. 30s. **Foam:** Cetyl alcohol, mineral oil, petrolatum. 94 g. *Rx.*
Use: Retinoid (dermatologic), second-generation retinoid.

Sorilux. (Stiefel) Calcipotriene 0.005%. Alcohol, edetate disodium, light mineral oil, propylene glycol, white petrolatum. Topical Foam. 60 g, 120 g. *Rx.*
Use: Antipsoriatic agent.

Sosegon. (Sanofi-Synthelabo) Pentazocine. Soln., Susp., Tab. *c-IV.*
Use: Analgesic.

Soss-10. (Roberts) Sodium sulfacetamide 10%. Soln. Bot. 15 mL. *Rx.*
Use: Anti-infective, ophthalmic.

•**sotagliflozin.** (SOE-ta-gli-FLOE-zin) USAN.
Use: Antidiabetic agent.

•**sotalol hydrochloride.** (SOTT-uh-lahl) *USP.*
Use: Antiadrenergic/sympatholytic, beta-adrenergic blocker.
See: Betapace.
Betapace AF.

sotalol hydrochloride. (Various Mfr.) Sotalol hydrochloride 80 mg, 120 mg, 160 mg, 240 mg, lactose. Tab. 100s, 500s, 1000s. *Rx.*
Use: Antiadrenergic/sympatholytic; beta-adrenergic blocker.

sotalol hydrochloride AF. (Apotex) Sotalol hydrochloride 80 mg, 120 mg, 160 mg. Tab. 100s. *Rx.*
Use: Beta-adrenergic blocking agent.

•**sotatercept.** (soe-TAT-er-sept) USAN.
Use: Chemotherapy-induced anemia.

•**soterenol hydrochloride.** (so-TER-en-ole) USAN.
Use: Bronchodilator.

•**sotirimod.** (soe-TIR-i-mod) USAN.
Use: Dermatologic agent.

Sotradecol. (AngioDynamics) Sodium tetradecyl sulfate 10 mg/mL, 30 mg/mL. Benzyl alcohol 0.02 mL. Inj. Vials. 2 mL. *Rx.*
Use: Sclerosing agent.

•**sotrastaurin.** (so-tra-STAW-rin) USAN.
Use: Immunomodulator.

•**sotrastaurin acetate.** (so-tra-STAW-rin) USAN.
Use: Immunomodulator.

Sotret. (Ranbaxy) Isotretinoin 10 mg, 20 mg, 30 mg, 40 mg. Parabens, EDTA. Softgel Cap. 30s, 100s. *Rx.*
Use: Retinoid, first generation.

Sovaldi. (Gilead Sciences) Sofosbuvir 400 mg. Film coated. Mannitol. Tab. 28s. *Rx.*
Use: Antiviral agent.

•**sovaprevir.** (soe-VA-pre-vir) USAN.
Use: Treatment of hepatitis C.

Soxa-Forte. (Vita Elixir) Sulfisoxazole 0.5 g, phenazopyridine 50 mg. Tab. *Rx.*
Use: Anti-infective.

Soyalac. (Mt. Vernon Foods, Inc.) Infant formula based on an extract from whole soybeans containing all-essential nutrients. **Ready to Serve Liq.:** Can 32 fl oz. **Double Strength Conc.:** Can 13 fl oz. **Pow.:** Can 14 oz. *OTC.*
Use: Nutritional supplement.

Soyalac-I. (Mt. Vernon Foods, Inc.) Soy protein isolate infant formula containing no corn derivatives and a negligible amount of soy carbohydrates. Contains all essential nutrients in various forms. **Ready to Serve Liq.:** Can 32 fl oz. **Double Strength Conc.:** Can 13 fl oz. *OTC.*
Use: Nutritional supplement.

soya lecithin. Soybean extract. 100s.
Use: Phosphorus therapy.

•**soybean oil.** (SOI-been) *USP.*
Use: Pharmaceutic aid.
See: Intralipid 30%.
Intralipid 20%.
Liposyn III.

Spabelin. (Arcum) Hyoscyamine sulfate 81 mcg, atropine sulfate 15 mcg, scopolamine HBr 5 mcg, phenobarbital 16.2 mg/5 mL. Elix. Bot. 16 oz, gal. *Rx.*
Use: Anticholinergic; antispasmodic; hypnotic; sedative.

Spabelin No. 1. (Arcum) Phenobarbital 15 mg, belladonna powdered extract ⅛ g. Tab. Bot. 100s, 1000s. *Rx.*
Use: Hypnotic; sedative.

Spabelin No. 2. (Arcum) Phenobarbital 30 mg, belladonna powdered extract ⅛ g. Tab. Bot. 100s, 1000s. *Rx.*
Use: Hypnotic; sedative.

Span C. (Freeda) Citrus bioflavonoids

300 mg, vitamin C (ascorbic acid and rose hips) 200 mg. Sugar free. Calcium carbonate, calcium stearate. Tab. Bot. 100s, 250s, 500s. *OTC.*
Use: Water-soluble vitamin.

Span 80. (AstraZeneca) Sorbitan monooleate, *NF 20.*

Span 85. (AstraZeneca) Sorbitan trioleate. Mixture of oleate esters of sorbitol and its anhydrides.
Use: Surface active agent.

Span 40. (AstraZeneca) Sorbitan Monopalmitate, *NF 20.*

Span-PD. (Lexis Laboratories) Phentermine hydrochloride 37.5 mg. Cap. Bot. 100s. *c-iv.*
Use: Anorexiant.

Span-RD. (Lexis Laboratories) d-methamphetamine hydrochloride 12 mg, dl-methamphetamine hydrochloride 6 mg, butabarbital 30 mg. Tab. Bot. 100s, 1000s. *c-iii.*
Use: Amphetamine; hypnotic; sedative.

Span 60. (AstraZeneca) Sorbitan Monostearate.

Span 65. (AstraZeneca) Sorbitan tristearate. Mixture of stearate esters of sorbitol and its anhydrides.
Use: Surface active agent.

Span 20. (AstraZeneca) Sorbitan Monolaurate.

•**sparfosate sodium.** (spar-FOSS-ate) USAN.
Use: Antineoplastic.

Sparkles Effervescent Granules. (Lafayette) Sodium bicarbonate 2000 mg, citric acid 1500 mg, simethicone. Pkt. Bot. UD 50s. *OTC.*
Use: Antacid.

Sparkles Granules. (Lafayette) Effervescent granules 4 g/Packet or 6 g/Packet. Each 6 g produces 500 mL of carbon dioxide gas. Ctn. 25 packets. Pkg. 2.
Use: Diagnostic aid.

Sparkles Tablets. (Lafayette) Effervescent tablets. Each 4.3 g of tablets produces 250 mL of carbon dioxide gas. Bot. 43 g (10 doses).
Use: Diagnostic aid.

•**sparsomycin.** (SPAR-so-MY-sin) USAN.
Use: Antineoplastic.

•**sparteine sulfate.** (SPAR-teh-een SULL-fate) USAN.
Use: Oxytocic.
W/Sodium Chloride.
See: Tocosamine.

Spasmatol. (Pharmed) Homatropine MBr 3 mg, pentobarbital 12 mg, mephobarbital 8 mg. Tab. Bot. 100s, 1000s. *Rx.*
Use: Anticholinergic; antispasmodic; hypnotic; sedative.

Spasmolin. (Various Mfr.) Phenobarbital 16.2 mg, hyoscyamine HBr sulfate 0.1037 mg, atropine sulfate 0.0194 mg, scopolamine HBr 0.0065 mg. Tab. Bot. 100s, 1000s. *Rx.*
Use: Gastrointestinal anticholinergic combination.

spasmolytic agents.
See: Antispasmodics.

Spasno-Lix. (Freeport) Phenobarbital 16.2 mg, hyoscyamine sulfate 0.1037 mg, atropine sulfate 0.0194 mg, hyoscine HBr 0.0065 mg, alcohol 21% to 23%/5 mL. Bot. 4 oz. *Rx.*
Use: Anticholinergic; antispasmodic; hypnotic; sedative.

S.P.B. (Sheryl) Therapeutic B complex formula with ascorbic acid 300 mg. Tab. Bot. 100s. *OTC.*
Use: Vitamin supplement.

SPD. (A.P.C.) Methyl salicylate, methyl nicotinate, dipropylene glycol salicylate, oleoresin capsicum, camphor, menthol. Cream. Bot. 4 oz, Tube 1.5 oz. *OTC.*
Use: Analgesic, topical.

spearmint.
Use: Flavor.

spearmint oil.
Use: Flavor.

Special Shampoo. (Del-Ray) Nonmedicated shampoo. *OTC.*
Use: Cleanser.

spectinomycin. (speck-TIN-oh-MY-sin) *Formerly Actinospectocin.* An antibiotic isolated from broth cultures of *Streptomyces spectabilis. Rx.*
Use: Anti-infective.

•**spectinomycin hydrochloride, sterile.** (speck-TIN-oh-MY-sin) *USP.*
Use: Anti-infective.

Spectracef. (Cornerstone) Cefditoren pivoxil 200 mg, 400 mg. Mannitol. Film-coated. Tab. Bot. 20s, 28s (400 mg only), 60s (200 mg only). *Rx.*
Use: Antibiotic, cephalosporin.

Spectra 360. (Parker) Salt-free electrode gel. Tube 8 oz.
Use: T.E.N.S. application, ECG pediatric, and long-term procedures.

Spectrobid. (Roerig) Bacampicill hydrochloride 400 mg (equiv. to 280 mg ampicillin), lactose. Tab. 100s. *Rx.*
Use: Anti-infective, penicillin.

Spectro-Biotic. (A.P.C.) Bacitracin 400 units, neomycin sulfate 5 mg, polymyxin B sulfate 5000 units/g Oint. Tube 0.5 oz, 1 oz. *OTC.*
Use: Anti-infective, topical.

Spectro-Jel. (Recsei) Soap free. Iodomethylcellulose, carboxypolymethylene, cetyl alcohol, sorbitan monooleate,

fumed silica, triethanolamine stearate, glycol polysiloxane, propylene glycol, glycerin, isopropyl alcohol 5%. Gel. Bot. 127.5 mL, pt, gal. *OTC.*
Use: Dermatologic, cleanser.

Spec-T Sore Throat Anesthetic. (Apothecon) Benzocaine 10 mg. Loz. Box 10s. *OTC.*
Use: Anesthetic, local.

spermaceti.
Use: Stiffening agent; pharmaceutic necessity for cold cream.

spermicides.
See: Nonoxynol-9.

spermine. Diaminopropyltetramethylene.

Sperti. (Whitehall-Robins) Live yeast cell derivative supplying 2000 units skin respiratory factor/g w/shark liver oil 3%, phenylmercuric nitrate 1:10,000. Oint. Tube oz. *OTC.*
Use: Dermatologic, wound therapy.

spider-bite antivenin.
See: Antivenin (*Latrodectus Mactans*).

Spider-Man Children's Chewable Vitamin. (NBTY) Vitamins A 2500 units, D 400 units, E 15 mg, B_1 1.05 mg, B_2 1.2 mg, B_3 13.5 mg, B_6 1.05 mg, B_{12} 4.5 mcg, C 60 mg, folic acid 0.3 mg, xylitol, sorbitol. Chew. Tab. Bot. 75s, 130s. *OTC.*
Use: Vitamin supplement.

•**spinosad.** (SPIN-oh-sad) USAN.
Use: Scabicide/Pediculicide.
See: Natroba.

spinosad. (Macoven Pharmaceuticals) Spinosad 0.9%. Alcohols, benzyl alcohol, butylated hydroxytoluene, propylene glycol. Susp. 120 mL. *Rx.*
Use: Scabicide/pediculicide.

•**spiperone.** (spih-per-OHN) USAN.
Use: Antipsychotic.

•**spiradoline mesylate.** (spy-RAH-doe-leen) USAN.
Use: Analgesic.

•**spiramycin.** (SPIH-rah-MY-sin) USAN. Antibiotic substance from cultures of *Streptomyces ambofaciens.*
Use: Anti-infective.

•**spiraprilat.** (SPY-rah-PRILL-at) USAN.
Use: ACE inhibitor.

•**spirapril hydrochloride.** (SPY-rah-prill) USAN.
Use: ACE inhibitor.
See: Renormax.

Spiriva. (Boehringer Ingelheim) Tiotropium bromide 18 mcg (equiv. to tiotropium bromide 22.5 mcg). Lactose. Pow. for Inh. UD 5s, 30s, 90s, w/*HandiHaler* device. *Rx.*
Use: Bronchodilator, anticholinergic.

•**spirogermanium hydrochloride.** (SPY-row-JER-MAY-nee-uhm) USAN.
Use: Antineoplastic.

•**spiromustine.** (SPY-row-MUSS-teen) USAN. *Formerly Spirohydantoin Mustard.*
Use: Antineoplastic.

spironazide. (Schein) Spironolactone 25 mg, hydrochlorothiazide 25 mg. Tab. 100s, 1,000s, UD 100s. *Rx.*
Use: Diuretic combination.

•**spironolactone.** (SPEER-oh-no-LAK-tone) *USP.*
Use: Diuretic, aldosterone antagonist.
See: Aldactone.
W/Hydrochlorothiazide.
See: Aldactazide.

spironolactone. (Various Mfr.) Spironolactone. Tab. **25 mg:** 60s, 100s, 500s, 1,000s. **50 mg:** 30s, 60s, 100s, 500s, 1,000s. **100 mg:** 100s, 500s. *Rx.*
Use: Diuretic.

spironolactone w/hydrochlorothiazide. (Various Mfr.) Spironolactone 25 mg, hydrochlorothiazide 25 mg. Tab. Bot. 30s, 60s, 100s, 250s, 500s, 1000s, UD 32s, 100s. *Rx.*
Use: Diuretic combination.

•**spiroplatin.** (SPY-row-PLAT-in) USAN.
Use: Antineoplastic.

spirotriazine hydrochloride.
Use: Anthelmintic.

•**spiroxasone.** (spy-ROX-ah-sone) USAN.
Use: Diuretic.

Spirozide. (Rugby) Spironolactone 25 mg, hydrochlorothiazide 25 mg. Tab. Bot. 100s, 500s, 1000s. *Rx.*
Use: Diuretic combination.

SPL-Serologic Types I and III. (Delmont) *Staphylococcus aureus* 120 to 180 million units, *Staphylococcus bacteriophage* plaque-forming 100 to 1000 million units/mL. Soln. Amp. 1 mL, Vial 10 mL. *Rx.*
Use: Anti-infective.

Sporanox. (Janssen) Itraconazole 100 mg. PEG, sucrose, sugar. Cap. 30s, UD 30s, *PulsePak* 28s. *Rx.*
Use: Antifungal, triazole.

Sporanox. (Ortho Biotech) Itraconazole 10 mg/mL. Saccharin, sorbitol. Cherry/caramel flavor. Oral Soln. Bot. 150 mL. *Rx.*
Use: Antifungal, triazole.

Sportscreme. (Thompson Medical) Triethanolamine salicylate 10% in a nongreasy base. Cream. 37.5 g, 90 g. *OTC.*
Use: Analgesic, topical.

Sports Spray Extra Strength. (Mentholatum Co.) Methyl salicylate 35%,

menthol 10%, camphor 5%, alcohol 58%, isobutane. Spray. 90 mL. *OTC.*
Use: Analgesic, topical.

Spray Skin Protectant. (Morton International) Isopropyl alcohol, polyvinylpyrrolidone, vinyl alcohol, plasticizer & propellant. Aer. Can 6 oz. *OTC.*
Use: Dermatologic, protectant.

Sprayzoin. (Geritrex) Benzoin compound, ethyl alcohol. Spray. 118 mL. *OTC.*
Use: Protectant.

spreading factor.
See: Hyaluronidase.

Sprintec. (Barr) Norgestimate 0.25 mg, ethinyl estradiol 35 mcg. Lactose. Tab. 28s with 7 inert tabs. *Rx.*
Use: Sex hormone, contraceptive hormone.

Sprix. (American Regent) Ketorolac tromethamine 15.75 mg/spray. Edetate disodium. Preservative free. Spray, Soln.; Intranasal. 1 single-day or 5 single-day 1.7 g bottles (delivers 8 sprays for a total of 126 mg of ketorolac). *Rx.*
Use: Nonsteroidal anti-inflammatory agent.

•**sprodiamide.** (sprah-DIE-ah-mide) USAN.
Use: Diagnostic aid (paramagnetic).

SPRX-105. (Reid-Provident) Phendimetrazine tartrate 105 mg. SR Cap. Bot. 28s, 500s. *c-III.*
Use: Anorexiant.

Sprycel. (Bristol-Myers Squibb) Dasatinib 20 mg, 50 mg, 70 mg, 80 mg, 100 mg, 140 mg. Film-coated. Lactose. Tab. 30s (80 mg, 100 mg, 140 mg), 60s (20 mg, 50 mg, 70 mg). *Rx.*
Use: Protein-tyrosine kinase inhibitor; treatment of leukemia.

SPS. (Carolina Medical Products) Sodium polystyrene sulfonate 15 g, sorbitol solution 21.5 mL, alcohol 0.3%/60 mL, propylene glycol, sodium saccharin, methylparaben, propylparaben. Cherry flavor. Susp. Bot. 120 mL, 473 mL, UD 60 mL. *Rx.*
Use: Potassium-removing resin.

•**squalamine lactate.** (SKWAH-la-meen) USAN.
Use: Antineoplastic.

•**squalane.** (SKWAH-lane) *NF.*
Use: Pharmaceutic aid (vehicle, oleaginous).

SRC Expectorant. (Edwards) Hydrocodone bitartrate 5 mg, pseudoephedrine hydrochloride 60 mg, guaifenesin 200 mg w/alcohol 12.5%. Bot. Pt. *c-III.*
Use: Antitussive; decongestant; expectorant.

Sronyx. (Watson Pharma) Ethinyl estradiol 20 mcg, levonorgestrel 0.1 mg. Lactose. Tab. 28s with 7 inert tablets (lactose). *Rx.*
Use: Contraceptive hormone, sex hormone.

SSD. (Dr. Reddy's Labs) Silver sulfadiazine 10 mg/g in a water-miscible base. Cetyl alcohol, white petrolatum, stearyl alcohol, methylparaben 0.3%. Cream. 25 g, 50 g, 85 g, 400 g, 1000 g. *Rx.*
Use: Topical anti-infective.

SSD AF. (Dr. Reddy's Labs) Silver sulfadiazine 10 mg/g in a water-miscible base. White petrolatum, stearyl alcohol, methylparaben 0.3%. Cream. Tube 50 g, 400 g, 1000 g. *Rx.*
Use: Topical anti-infective.

SSKI. (Upsher-Smith) Potassium iodide 1 g/mL. Soln. 30 mL, 240 mL. *Rx.*
Use: Thyroid drug.

S-Spas. (Southern States) Pentobarbital 16.2 mg, atropine sulfate 0.0194 mg, hyoscyamine sulfate 0.1037 mg, hyoscine HBr 0.0065 mg. **Liq.:** 5 mL. Bot. Pt. **Tab.:** Bot. 100s, 1000s. *Rx.*
Use: Anticholinergic; antispasmodic; hypnotic; sedative.

S.S.S. High Potency Vitamin. (S.S.S. Company) Vitamins C 300 mg, B_1 7.5 mg, B_2 7.5 mg, B_3 50 mg, Ca 100 mg, Fe 27 mg, E 50 units, B_6 2.5 mg, folic acid 200 mcg, B_{12} 12.5 mg, Mg 50 mg, Zn 12 mg, Cu 1.5 mg, biotin 22.5 mcg, pantothenic acid 10 mg. Tab. Bot. 20s, 40s, 80s. *OTC.*
Use: Vitamin, mineral supplement.

SSS 10-5. (Acella) Sodium sulfacetamide 10%, sulfur 5%. **Aer., foam:** Cetearyl alcohol, glycerin. 60 g. **Cream:** Alcohols, disodium EDTA, glyceryl monostearate, parabens, propylene glycol. 28 g. *Rx.*
Use: Topical anti-infective, antibiotic agent.

SSS 10-4. (Acella) Sodium sulfacetamide 10%, sulfur 4%. Alcohols, lactic acid, parabens, propylene glycol. Aer. Foam. 100 g. *Rx.*
Use: Topical anti-infective, antibiotic agent.

S.S.S. Vitamin and Mineral Supplement. (S.S.S. Company) Vitamins A 833 units, C 20 mg, E 10 units, B_1 1.7 mg, $B_2$0.57 mg, niacinamide 6.7 mg, B_6 0.67 mg, B_{12} 2 mcg, D_3 133 units, biotin 100 mcg, pantothenic acid 3 mg, I 50 mcg, Fe 3 mg, Zn 1 mg, Ma 0.8 mg, Cr 8 mcg, Mo 8 mcg/5 mL, alcohol 6.6%, sugar. Liq. Bot. 236 mL. *OTC.*
Use: Vitamin, mineral supplement.

Staftabs. (Modern Aids Inc.) Fine bone flour containing calcium, phosphorus, iron, iodine, vitamin D, magnesium. Tab. Bot. 85s, 160s. *OTC.*
Use: Mineral, vitamin supplement.

Stagesic. (Magna) Hydrocodone bitartrate 5 mg, acetaminophen 500 mg. Cap. Bot. 100s. *c-III.*
Use: Analgesic combination, narcotic.

Stahist. (Magna) Chlorpheniramine maleate 8 mg, hyoscyamine sulfate 0.19 mg, atropine sulfate 0.04 mg, scopolamine HBr 0.01 mg, pseudoephedrine hydrochloride 90 mg. Dye free. ER Tab. Bot. 100s. *Rx.*
Use: Upper respiratory combination, antihistamine, anticholinergic, decongestant.

Stahist AD. (Magna) Chlorcyclizine hydrochloride 25 mg, pseudoephedrine hydrochloride 60 mg. **Tab.:** 30s. **Liq.:** Parabens, potassium citrate, potassium sorbate, propylene glycol, sorbitol, sucralose. Alcohol free, gluten free, and sugar free. Grape flavor. 118 mL. *OTC.*
Use: Upper respiratory combination, decongestant and antihistamine.

stainless iodized ointment. (Day-Baldwin) Jar lb.

stainless iodized ointment with methyl salicylate 5%. (Day-Baldwin) Jar lb.

Stalevo 50. (Novartis) Carbidopa 12.5 mg, levodopa 50 mg, entacapone 200 mg, mannitol, sucrose. Tab. 100s, 250s. *Rx.*
Use: Antiparkinson agent.

Stalevo 100. (Novartis) Carbidopa 25 mg, levodopa 100 mg, entacapone 200 mg, mannitol, sucrose. Tab. 100s, 250s. *Rx.*
Use: Antiparkinson agent.

Stalevo 150. (Novartis) Carbidopa 37.5 mg, levodopa 150 mg, entacapone 200 mg, mannitol, sucrose. Tab. 100s, 250s. *Rx.*
Use: Antiparkinson agents.

Stalevo 125. (Novartis) Carbidopa 31.25 mg, entacapone 200 mg, levodopa 125 mg. Mannitol, sucrose. Film-coated. Tab. 100s. *Rx.*
Use: Antiparkinson agent.

Stalevo 75. (Novartis) Carbidopa 18.75 mg, entacapone 200 mg, levodopa 75 mg. Mannitol, sucrose. Film-coated. Tab. 100s. *Rx.*
Use: Antiparkinson agent.

Stalevo 200. (Novartis) Carbidopa 50 mg, levodopa 200 mg, entacapone 200 mg. Mannitol, sucrose. Film-coated. Tab. 100s. *Rx.*
Use: Antiparkinson agent.

•**stallimycin hydrochloride.** (stal-IH-MY-sin) USAN.
Use: Anti-infective.

•**stamulumab.** (sta-MUL-ue-mab) USAN.
Use: Muscular dystrophy.

Stamyl. (Sanofi-Synthelabo) Pancreatin. Tab.
Use: Digestive aid.

Stanback Headache. (Glaxo-SmithKline Consumer Healthcare) Aspirin 845 mg, caffeine 65 mg. Lactose, potassium 55 mg per packet. Pow. 2s, 6s, 50s. *OTC.*
Use: Nonnarcotic analgesic combination.

•**stannous chloride.** (STAN-uhs KLOR-ide) USAN.
Use: Pharmaceutic aid.

•**stannous fluoride.** (STAN-uhs FLOR-ide) *USP.*
Use: Dental caries agent.
See: Just For Kids.
PerioMed.

stannous fluoride. (Cypress) **Gel:** Stannous fluoride 0.4%, parabens, mint flavor. Tube 122 g. **Conc. Oral Rinse:** Stannous fluoride 0.63%, mint flavor. Bot. 283 g. *Rx-OTC.*
Use: Trace element.

•**stannous pyrophosphate.** (STAN-uhs PIE-row-FOSS-fate) USAN.
Use: Diagnostic aid (skeletal imaging).

•**stannous sulfur colloid.** (STAN-uhs SULL-fer KAHL-oyd) USAN.
Use: Diagnostic aid (bone, liver, and spleen imaging).

•**stanozolol.** (stan-OH-zoe-lole) *USP.*
Use: Anabolic steroid.

staphage lysate (SPL).
Use: Anti-infective.
See: SPL-Serologic Types I and III.

StaphAseptic. (Tec Labs) Benzethonium chloride 0.2%, lidocaine hydrochloride 2.5%. Disodium EDTA, glycerin, polyoxyl 35 castor oil, tea tree oil, white thyme oil. Gel. 56.7 g. *OTC.*
Use: Local anesthetic, topical; local anesthetic, topical combination.

staphylococcus bacteriophage lysate.
See: Staphage Lysate.

•**starch.** (stahrch) *NF.*
Use: Dusting powder; pharmaceutic aid.

starch glycerite.
Use: Emollient.

•**starch, pregelatinized.** (stahrch pree-jel-AT-inized) *NF.*
Use: Pharmaceutic aid (tablet excipient).

•**starch, topical.** (stahrch) *USP.*
Use: Dusting powder.

Starlix. (Novartis) Nateglinide 60 mg, 120 mg. Lactose. Tab. 100s. *Rx.*
Use: Antidiabetic, meglitinide.

Star-Otic. (Stellar) Burrows soln. nonaqueous, acetic acid, boric acid, propylene glycol. Drop Bot. 15 mL. *OTC.*
Use: Otic preparation.

•**statolon.** (STAY-toe-lone) USAN. Antiviral agent derived from *Penicillium stoloniferum.*
Use: Antiviral.

Statomin Maleate II. (Jones Pharma) Chlorpheniramine maleate 2 mg, acetaminophen 324 mg, caffeine 32 mg. Tab. Bot. 1000s. *Rx.*
Use: Antihistamine; analgesic.

•**stavudine.** (STAHV-you-deen) USAN.
Use: Antiretroviral.

stavudine. (Mylan) Stavudine 15 mg, 20 mg, 30 mg, 40 mg. Lactose. Cap. 60s, 100s, 500s. *Rx.*
Use: Antiretroviral agent, nucleoside reverse transcriptase inhibitor.

Stavzor. (Noven Therapeutics) Valproic acid 125 mg, 250 mg, 500 mg. Delayed release Cap. 100s. *Rx.*
Use: Anticonvulsant.

Sta-Wake Dextabs. (Health for Life Brands) Caffeine 1.5 g, dextrose 3 g. Tab. Bot. 36s, 1000s. *OTC.*
Use: CNS stimulant.

Staxyn. (GlaxoSmithKline) Vardenafil 10 mg (equiv. to vardenafil hydrochloride 11.85 mg). Aspartame, mannitol, phenylalanine 1.01 mg, sorbitol. Tab., orally disintegrating. UD 4s, 40s. *Rx.*
Use: Impotence agent, phosphodiesterase type 5 inhibitor.

Stay Alert. (Apothecary Prods.) Caffeine 200 mg. Tab. Bot. 24s, 48s. *OTC.*
Use: CNS stimulant

Stay Awake. (Major) Caffeine 200 mg, dextrose. Tab. Bot. 16s. *OTC.*
Use: CNS stimulant, analeptic.

Stay-Brite. (Sherman Pharmaceuticals, Inc.) EDTA 0.25%, benzalkonium Cl 0.01%. Spray. Bot. 30 mL. *OTC.*
Use: Contact lens care.

Stay Moist Lip Conditioner. Padimate O, oxybenzone, aloe vera, vitamin E, tropical fruit flavor. SPF 15. Lip Balm 48 g. *OTC.*
Use: Emollient.

Stay-Wet. (Sherman Pharmaceuticals, Inc.) Polyvinyl alcohol, hydroxyethylcellulose, povidone, sodium Cl, potassium Cl, sodium carbonate, benzalkonium Cl 0.01%, EDTA 0.025%. Soln. Bot. 30 mL. *OTC.*
Use: Contact lens care.

Stay-Wet Rewetting. (Sherman Pharmaceuticals, Inc.) Polyvinyl alcohol, hydroxyethycellulose, povidone, NaCl, KCl, sodium carbonate, benzalkonium Cl 0.01%, EDTA 0.025%. Soln. Bot. *OTC.*
Use: Lubricant-ophthalmic.

Stay-Wet 3 Wetting. (Sherman Pharmaceuticals, Inc.) Polyvinyl alcohol, hydroxyethycellulose, povidone, sodium Cl, potassium Cl, sodium carbonate, benzalkonium Cl 0.01%, EDTA 0.025%. Soln. 30 mL. *OTC.*
Use: Lubricant, ophthalmic.

Staze. (Del) Karaya gum. Tube 1.75 oz, 3.5 oz. *OTC.*
Use: Denture adhesive.

S-T Cort Cream. (Scot-Tussin) Hydrocortisone 0.5%, water-washable base, parabens. 120 g. *Rx.*
Use: Corticosteroid, topical.

S-T Cort Lotion. (Scot-Tussin) Hydrocortisone 0.5%, water-washable, lanolin alcohol, mineral oil base. 60 mL, 120 mL. *Rx.*
Use: Corticosteroid, topical.

•**stearic acid.** (STEER-ik) *NF.* Octadecanoic acid.
Use: Pharmaceutic aid (emulsion adjunct, tablet/capsule lubricant).

•**stearyl alcohol.** (STEE-rill AL-koe-hahl) *NF.*
Use: Pharmaceutic aid (emulsion adjunct).

•**steffimycin.** (steh-fih-MY-sin) USAN.
Use: Anti-infective; antiviral.

Stelara. (Janssen Biotech) Ustekinumab 90 mg per 1 mL. Sucrose 76 mg, L-histidine 1 mg, 0.04 mg of polysorbate 80. Preservative free. Inj., Soln. Single-use vial. *Rx.*
Use: Immunologic agent, immunomodulator.

stem cell mobilizers.
See: Plerixafor.

•**stenbolone acetate.** (STEEN-bow-lone) USAN.
Use: Anabolic.

Stendra. (Auxilium) Avanafil 50 mg, 100 mg, 200 mg. Mannitol. Tab. 30s, 100s. *Rx.*
Use: Impotence agent, phosphodiesterase type 5 inhibitor.

•**stenfilcon A.** (sten-FIL-kon) USAN.
Use: Contact lens polymer.

Steraject. (Merz) Prednisolone acetate 25 mg, 50 mg/mL. Inj. Vial 10 mL. *Rx.*
Use: Corticosteroid.

sterculia gum.
See: Karaya Gum.

Stericol. (Alton) Isopropyl alcohol 91%. Soln. Bot. 16 oz, 32 oz, gal. *OTC.*
Use: Anti-infective, topical.

sterile erythromycin gluceptate. Erythromycin monoglucoheptonate (salt). Erythromycin glucoheptonate (1:1) (salt).
Use: Anti-infective.

Sterile Lens Lubricant. (Blairex) Isotonic w/borate buffer system, sodium Cl, hydroxypropyl methylcellulose, glycerin, sorbic acid 0.25%, EDTA 0.1%, thimerosal free. Soln. Bot. 15 mL. *OTC.*
Use: Lubricant, ophthalmic.

Sterile Saline. (Bausch & Lomb) Sodium Cl, borate buffer, EDTA, thimerosal free. Soln. Bot. 60 mL. *OTC.*
Use: Lubricant, ophthalmic.

Sterile Talc Powder. (Bryan) Talc 5 g. Pow. Glass Bot. 100 mL. *Rx.*
Use: Antineoplastic.

sterile thiopental sodium. Thiopental sodium, USP.
See: Pentothal.

sterile water for irrigation. (Various Mfr.) Sterile water for irrigation 0.45%, 0.9%. Soln. Bot. 150 mL, 250 mL, 500 mL, 1000 mL, 1500 mL, 2000 mL, 4000 mL. *Rx.*
Use: Irrigant, genitourinary.

SteriLid. (Advanced) Allantoin, boric acid, cocamidopropyl betadine, etidronic acid, hepes acetate, linalool oil, panthenol, PEG-80, PEG-150, sodium laureth-13 carboxylate, sodium lauroampho acetate, sodium perborate monohydrate, sodium trideceth sulfate, sorbitan laurate, tea tree oil, tris-EDTA. Soap, foam; Ophth. 48 mL. *Rx.*
Use: Ophthalmic agent, ophthalmic nonsurgical adjunct.

Steri-Unna Boot. (Pedinol Pharmacal) Glycerin, gum acacia, zinc oxide, white petrolatum, amylum in an oil base. 10 yds. × 3.5 in. sterilized bandage.
Use: Treatment of leg ulcers, varicosities, sprains, strains & to reduce swelling after surgery.

steroid antibiotic combinations.
Use: Anti-inflammatory; otic preparations.
See: AntibiOtic.
Antibiotic Ear Solution.
Ciprodex.
Cipro HC Otic.
Coly-Mycin S Otic.
Cortisporin.
Cortisporin Otic.
Cortisporin-TC Otic.
Ear-Eze.
LazerSporin-C.
Maxitrol.
Octicair.
Otosporin.
Neomycin and Polymyxin B Sulfates and Dexamethasone.
Neomycin/Polymyxin B Sulfates, Hydrocortisone Otic.
Pediotic.
Poly-Pred Liquifilm.
Pred-G.
TobraDex.
Tobramycin and Dexamethasone.

steroids, intranasal.
See: Beclomethasone Dipropionate.
Budesonide.
Ciclesonide.
Flunisolide.
Fluticasone.
Mometasone Furoate Monohydrate.
Triamcinolone Acetonide.

S-T Forte 2. (Scot-Tussin) Hydrocodone bitartrate 2.5 mg, chlorpheniramine maleate 2 mg per 5 mL. Menthol, parabens. Sugar, alcohol, and dye free. Liq. Bot. 473 mL, 3.8 L. *c-III.*
Use: Upper respiratory combination, antitussive, antihistamine.

stilbamidine isethionate.
Use: Antiprotozoal.

•**stilbazium iodide.** (still-BAY-zee-uhm EYE-oh-dide) USAN.
Use: Anthelmintic.

stilbestrol.
See: Diethylstilbestrol Dipropionate.

stilbestronate.
See: Diethylstilbestrol Dipropionate.

Stilboestrol.
See: Diethylstilbestrol Dipropionate.

Stilboestrol DP.
See: Diethylstilbestrol Dipropionate.

•**stilonium iodide.** (STILL-oh-nee-uhm EYE-oh-dide) USAN.
Use: Antispasmodic.

Stilronate.
See: Diethylstilbestrol Dipropionate.

Stimate. (CSL Behring) Desmopressin acetate 1.5 mg/mL. Spray, Soln., intranasal. 2.5 mL (25 sprays of 150 mcg each). *Rx.*
Use: Hormone.

stimulant laxatives.
See: Agoral.
Aromatic Cascara Fluidextract.
Bisac-Evac.
Bisacodyl.
Bisacodyl Uniserts.
Black Draught.
Cascara Aromatic.
Cascara Sagrada.
Correctol.
Dulcolax.

ex•lax.
ex•lax Chocolated.
Feen-a-mint.
Fleet Laxative.
Fletcher's Castoria.
Maximum Relief ex•lax.
Modane.
Reliable Gentle Laxative.
Senexon.
Senna-Gen.
Sennosides.
Senokot.
SenokotXTRA.
Women's Gentle Laxative.

Sting-Eze. (Wisconsin Pharmacal Co.) Diphenhydramine hydrochloride, camphor, phenol, benzocaine, eucalyptol. Liq. Bot. 15 mL. *OTC.*
Use: Antihistamine, topical.

•**stinging nettle.** *USP.*
Use: Dietary supplement.

Sting-Kill. (Randob Labs) **Swab:** Benzocaine 20%, menthol 1%. Isopropyl alcohol 15%. 0.5 mL. **Wipes:** Benzocaine 20%, menthol 1%. Isopropyl alcohol 15%. 8s. *OTC.*
Use: Topical local anesthetic.

•**stiripentol.** (STY-rih-PEN-tole) USAN.
Use: Anticonvulsant.

Stivarga. (Bayer HealthCare Pharmaceuticals) Regorafenib 40 mg. Film coated. Tab. 28s. *Rx.*
Use: Kinase inhibitor, multikinase inhibitor.

•**St. John's wort, powdered extract.** *USP.*
Use: Dietary supplement.

St. Joseph Adult Chewable Aspirin. (Schering-Plough) Aspirin 81 mg, saccharin. Chew. Tab. Bot. 36s. *OTC.*
Use: Analgesic.

St. Joseph Aspirin for Adults. (Schering-Plough) Aspirin 5 g. Tab. Bot. 36s, 100s, 200s. *OTC.*
Use: Analgesic.

St. Joseph Aspirin-Free Elixir for Children. (Schering-Plough) Acetaminophen 160 mg/5 mL. Alcohol free. Elix. Bot. 2 oz, 4 oz. *OTC.*
Use: Analgesic.

St. Joseph Aspirin-Free for Children Chewable. (Schering-Plough) Acetaminophen 80 mg, fruit flavor. Chew. Tab. Bot. 30s. *OTC.*
Use: Analgesic.

St. Joseph Aspirin-Free Infant. (Schering-Plough) Acetaminophen 100 mg/mL. Aspirin and sugar free. Drops. Bot. w/dropper. 0.5 oz. *OTC.*
Use: Analgesic.

St. Joseph Aspirin-Free Tablets for Children. (Schering-Plough) Acetaminophen 80 mg. Tab. Bot. 30s. *OTC.*
Use: Analgesic.

St. Joseph Cough Suppressant. (Schering-Plough) Dextromethorphan HBr 7.5 mg/5 mL, alcohol free, sucrose, cherry flavor. Liq. Bot. 60 mL, 120 mL. *OTC.*
Use: Antitussive.

St. Joseph Cough Syrup for Children. (Schering-Plough) Dextromethorphan HBr 7.5 mg/5 mL. Syr. Bot. 2 oz, 4 oz. *OTC.*
Use: Antitussive.

Stomal. (Foy Laboratories) Phenobarbital 16.2 mg, hyoscyamine sulfate 0.1037 mg, atropine sulfate 0.0194 mg, scopolamine HBr 0.0065 mg. Tab. Bot. 1000s. *Rx.*
Use: Anticholinergic; antispasmodic; hypnotic; sedative.

Stool Softener. (Apothecary Prods.) Docusate calcium 240 mg. Cap. Bot. 50s. *OTC.*
Use: Laxative.

Stool Softener. (Rugby) Docusate sodium. **Cap.:** 100 mg, 250 mg lactose, tartrazine. Bot. 1000s. **Soft gel Cap.:** 250 mg, sorbitol, parabens. Bot. 100s, 1000s. *OTC.*
Use: Laxative.

Stool Softener DC. (Rugby) Docusate calcium 240 mg, sorbitol, parabens. Cap. Bot. 100s, 500s, 1000s. *OTC.*
Use: Laxative.

Stop. (Oral-B) Stannous fluoride 0.4%. Tube 2 oz. *Rx.*
Use: Dental caries agent.

Stopain Cold Pain Relieving. (Troy Healthcare) Menthol 6%. Alcohol, propylene glycol, triethanolamine. Gel. 70.8 g. *OTC.*
Use: Rub and liniment.

Stopain Cold Roll-On. (Troy Healthcare) Menthol 8%. Alcohol, eucalyptus oil, glycerin, peppermint oil, triethanolamine, *Boswellia serrata* extract. Liq., topical. 88 mL. *OTC.*
Use: Rub and liniment.

Stopain Cold Spray. (Troy Healthcare) Menthol 6%. Alcohol, eucalyptus oil, peppermint oil. Spray. 240 mL. *OTC.*
Use: Rub and liniment.

Stopayne Capsules. (Springbok) Codeine phosphate 30 mg, acetaminophen 357 mg. Cap. Bot. 100s, 500s, UD 100s. *c-III.*
Use: Analgesic; antitussive.

Stopayne Syrup. (Springbok) Acetaminophen 120 mg, codeine phosphate

12 mg/5 mL. Syr. Bot. 4 oz, 16 oz. *c-v.*
Use: Analgesic; antitussive.

Stop-Zit. (Purepac) Denatonium benzoate in a clear nail polish base. Bot. 0.75 oz. *OTC.*
Use: Nail-biting deterrent.

•**storax.** (STORE-ax) *USP.*
Use: Pharmaceutic necessity for benzoin tincture compound.

Stovarsol.
Use: Trichomonas vaginalis vaginitis; amebiasis; Vincent's angina.

Strattera. (Eli Lilly) Atomoxetine hydrochloride (as base) 10 mg, 18 mg, 25 mg, 40 mg, 60 mg, 80 mg, 100 mg. Cap. 30s. *Rx.*
Use: Psychotherapeutic agent.

Stren-Tab. (Barth's) Vitamins C 300 mg, B_1 10 mg, B_2 10 mg, niacin 33 mg, B_6 2 mg, pantothenic acid 20 mg, B_{12} 4 mcg. Tab. Bot. 100s, 300s, 500s. *OTC.*
Use: Vitamin supplement.

streptococcus immune globulin, group B.
Use: Immunization. [Orphan Drug]

Streptolysin O Test. (Laboratory Diagnostics) Reagent 6 x 10 mL, buffer 6 × 40 mL, Control Serum, 6 × 10 mL, or Kit.
Use: Diagnosis of "group A" streptococcal infections.

streptomycin calcium chloride. Streptomycin Calcium Chloride Complex.

streptomycin sulfate.
Use: Antituberculosis agent.

streptomycin sulfate. (Pfizer) Streptomycin sulfate 400 mg/mL. Inj. Amp. 2.5 mL. *Rx.*
Use: Anti-infective, parenteral aminoglycoside.

streptomycin sulfate. (Pharma-Tek) Streptomycin sulfate 200 mg/mL. Lyophilized cake/Pow. for Inj. Vial. 1 g. *Rx.*
Use: Anti-infective, parenteral aminoglycoside.

Streptonase B. (Wampole) Tube test for determination of streptococcal infection by serum DNase-B antibodies. Kit 1.
Use: Diagnostic aid.

•**streptonicozid.** (STREP-toe-nih-KOE-zid) USAN.
Use: Anti-infective.

•**streptonigrin.** (strep-toe-NYE-grin) USAN. Antibiotic isolated from both filtrates of *Streptomyces flocculus.*
Use: Antineoplastic.
See: Nigrin.

streptovaricin. An antibiotic composed of several related components derived from cultures of *Streptomyces variabilis.*

•**streptozocin.** (STREP-toe-ZOE-sin) USAN.
Use: Antineoplastic.
See: Zanosar.

Streptozyme. (Wampole) Rapid hemagglutination slide test for the qualitative detection and quantitative determination of streptococcal extracellular antigens in serum, plasma, and peripheral blood. Kit 15s, 50s, 150s.
Use: Diagnostic aid, streptococcus.

Stress B-Complex. (H.L. Moore Drug Exchange) Vitamins E 30 units, B_1 15 mg, B_2 15 mg, B_3 100 mg, B_5 20 mg, B_6 20 mg, B_{12} 12 mcg, C 500 mg, folic acid 0.4 mg, Zn 23.9 mg, Cu, biotin 45 mcg. Tab. Bot. 60s. *OTC.*
Use: Mineral, vitamin supplement.

Stress B Complex with Vitamin C. (Mission Pharmacal) Vitamins B_1 13.8 mg, B_2 10 mg, B_3 50 mg, B_6 4.1 mg, C 300 mg, Zn 15 mg. Tab. Bot. 60s. *OTC.*
Use: Mineral, vitamin supplement.

Stress-Bee. (Rugby) Vitamins B_1 10 mg, B_2 10 mg, B_3 100 mg, B_5 20 mg, B_6 2 mg, B_{12} 6 mcg, C 300 mg. Cap. Bot. 100s. *OTC.*
Use: Vitamin supplement.

Stress Formula. (Various Mfr.) Vitamins E 30 mg, B_1 15 mg, $B_2$15 mg, B_3 100 mg, B_5 20 mg, B_6 5 mg, B_{12} 12 mcg, C 600 mg, folic acid 0.4 mg, biotin 45 mcg. Cap., Tab. **Cap.:** Bot. 60s, 100s, 1000s. **Tab.:** Bot. 30s, 60s, 100s, 250s, 300s, 400s, 1000s, UD 100s. *OTC.*
Use: Vitamin supplement.

Stress Formula 600. (Vangard Labs, Inc.) Vitamins E 30 units, B_1 15 mg, B_2 10 mg, B_3 100 mg, B_5 20 mg, B_6 5 mg, B_{12} 12 mcg, C 500 mg, folic acid 0.4 mg, biotin 45 mcg. Tab. Bot. UD 100s. *OTC.*
Use: Vitamin supplement.

Stress Formula "605". (NBTY) Vitamins E 30 mg, B_1 15 mg, B_2 15 mg, B_3 100 mg, B_5 20 mg, B_6 5 mg, B_{12} 12 mcg, C 605 mg, folic acid 0.4 mg, biotin 45 mg. Tab. Bot. 60s. *OTC.*
Use: Vitamin supplement.

Stress Formula "605" with Zinc. (NBTY) Vitamins E 30 mg, B_1 20 mg, B_2 10 mg, B_3 100 mg, B_5 25 mg, B_6 5 mg, B_{12} 12 mcg, C 605 mg, folic acid 0.4 mg, Zn 23.9 mg, Cu, biotin 45 mcg. Tab. Bot. 60s. *OTC.*
Use: Mineral, vitamin supplement.

Stress Formula 600 Plus Iron. (Schein) Iron 27 mg, vitamins E 30 units, B_1 15 mg, B_2 15 mg, B_3 100 mg, B_5 20 mg, B_6 5 mg, B_{12} 12 mcg, C 600 mg, folic

acid 0.4 mg, biotin 45 mcg. Tab. Bot. 60s, 250s. *OTC.*
Use: Mineral, vitamin supplement.

Stress Formula 600 Plus Zinc. (Schein) Vitamins E 30 mg, B_1 20 mg, B_2 10 mg, B_3 100 mg, B_5 25 mg, B_6 5 mg, B_{12} 12 mcg, C 600 mg, folic acid 0.4 mg, zinc 23.9 mg, Cu, Mg, biotin 45 mcg. Tab. Bot. 60s, 250s. *OTC.*
Use: Mineral, vitamin supplement.

Stress Formula Vitamins. (Various Mfr.) Vitamins E 30 mg, B_1 10 mg, $B_2$10 mg, B_3 100 mg, B_5 20 mg, B_6 5 mg, B_{12} 12 mcg, C 500 mg, folic acid 0.4 mg, biotin 45 mcg. Cap. Bot. 100s. Tab. Bot. 60s. *OTC.*
Use: Vitamin supplement.

Stress Formula with Iron. (NBTY) Vitamins C 500 mg, B_1 10 mg, B_2 10 mg, B_3 100 mg, B_5 20 mg, B_6 5 mg, B_{12} 12 mcg, E 30 units, Fe 27 mg, folic acid 0.4 mg, biotin 45 mcg. Tab. Bot. 60s. *OTC.*
Use: Mineral, vitamin supplement.

Stress Formula with Zinc. (Towne) Vitamins E 45 units, C 600 mg, folic acid 400 mcg, B_1 20 mg, B_2 10 mg, niacinamide 100 mg, B_6 10 mg, B_{12} 25 mcg, biotin 40 mcg, pantothenic acid 25 mg, Cu 3 mg, Zn 23.9 mg. Tab. Bot. 60s. *OTC.*
Use: Mineral, vitamin supplement.

Stress Formula w/Zinc. (Various Mfr.) Vitamins E 30 units, B_1 10 mg, B_2 10 mg, B_3 100 mg, B_5 20 mg, B_6 5 mg, B_{12} 12 mcg, C 500 mg, folic acid 0.4 mg, biotin 45 mcg, Zn 23.9 mg, Cu. Tab. Bot. 60s. *OTC.*
Use: Mineral, vitamin supplement.

Stress "1000". (NBTY) Vitamins E 22 mg, B_1 15 mg, B_2 15 mg, B_3 100 mg, B_5 20 mg, B_6 5 mg, B_{12} 12 mcg, C 1000 mg. Tab. Bot. 60s. *OTC.*
Use: Vitamin supplement.

Stress 600 w/Zinc. (Nion Corp.) Vitamins E 45 units, B_1 20 mg, B_2 10 mg, B_3 100 mg, B_5 25 mg, B_6 10 mg, B_{12} 25 mcg, C 600 mg, folic acid 0.4 mg, Zn 5.5 mg, Cu, biotin 45 mcg. Tab. Bot. 60s. *OTC.*
Use: Mineral, vitamin supplement.

Stresstabs. (Wyeth) Vitamins E 30 mg, B_1 10 mg, B_2 10 mg, B_3 100 mg, B_5 20 mg, B_6 5 mg, B_{12} 12 mcg, C 500 mg, folic acid 0.4 mg, biotin 45 mcg. Tab. Bot. 60s. *OTC.*
Use: Vitamin supplement.

Stresstabs + Iron. (Wyeth) Fe 18 mg, E 30 units, B_1 10 mg, B_2 10 mg, B_3 100 mg, B_5 20 mg, B_6 5 mg, B_{12} 12 mcg, C 500 mg, folic acid 0.4 mg, biotin 45 mcg. Tab. Bot. 60s. *OTC.*
Use: Mineral, vitamin supplement.

Stresstabs + Zinc. (Wyeth) Vitamins E 30 mg, B_1 10 mg, B_2 10 mg, B_3 100 mg, B_5 20 mg, B_6 5 mg, B_{12} 12 mcg, C 500 mg, folic acid 0.4 mg, Zn 23.9 mg, Cu, biotin 45 mcg. Tab. Bot. 60s. *OTC.*
Use: Mineral, vitamin supplement.

Stresstabs 600. (Wyeth) Vitamins B_1 15 mg, B_2 10 mg, B_6 5 mg, B_{12} 12 mcg, C 600 mg, niacinamide 100 mg, vitamin E 30 units, biotin 45 mcg, folic acid 400 mcg, calcium pantothenate 20 mg. Tab. Bot. 30s, 60s, UD 10 x 10s. *OTC.*
Use: Vitamin supplement.

Stresstabs 600 with Iron. (Wyeth) Ferrous fumarate 27 mg, vitamins E 30 units, B_1 15 mg, B_2 15 mg, B_3 100 mg, B_5 20 mg, B_6 5 mg, B_{12} 12 mcg, C 600 mg, folic acid 0.4 mg, biotin 45 mcg. Tab. Bot. 30s, 60s. *OTC.*
Use: Mineral, vitamin supplement.

Stresstabs 600 with Zinc. (Wyeth) Vitamins B_1 15 mg, B_2 10 mg, B_3 100 mg, B_5 20 mg, B_6 5 mg, B_{12} 12 mcg, C 600 mg, E 30 units, folic acid 0.4 mg, biotin 45 mcg, Cu, Zn 23.9 mg. Tab. Bot. 30s, 60s. *OTC.*
Use: Mineral, vitamin supplement.

Stresstein. (Novartis) Maltodextrin, medium chain triglycerides, l-leucine, soybean oil, l-isoleucine, l-valine, l-glutamic acid, l-arginine, l-lysine acetate, l-alanine, l-threonine, l-phenylalanine, l-aspartic acid, l-histidine, l-methionine, glycine, polyglycerol esters of fatty acids, l-serine, l-proline, sodium Cl, l-tryptophan, l-cysteine, sodium citrate, vitamins and minerals. Powder 3.4 oz. packets. *OTC.*
Use: High-protein, branched chain enriched tube feeding.

Striant. (Actient Pharmaceuticals) Testosterone 30 mg. Lactose. Buccal system. Blister packs of 10 systems. *Rx.*
Use: Androgen, sex hormone.

Stribild. (Gilead Sciences) Elvitegravir 150 mg/cobicistat 150 mg/emtricitabine 200 mg/tenofovir disoproxil fumarate 300 mg (equiv. to tenofovir disoproxil 245 mg). Film coated. Lactose. Tab. 30s. *Rx.*
Use: Antiretroviral agent, miscellaneous antiretroviral combination.

Stri-dex Antibacterial Cleansing. (Bayer Consumer Care) Triclosan 1%, acetylated lanolin alcohol, EDTA. Bar. 105 g. *OTC.*
Use: Dermatologic, acne.

Stri-dex B.P. (Bayer Consumer Care)

Benzoyl peroxide 10%. in greaseless, vanishing cream base. *OTC.*
Use: Dermatologic, acne.

Stri-dex Clear. (Bayer Consumer Care) Salicylic acid 2%, SD alcohol 9.3%, EDTA. Gel. Tube. 30 g. *OTC.*
Use: Dermatologic, acne.

Stri-dex Face Wash. (Bayer Consumer Care) Triclosan 1%, glycerin, EDTA, alcohol free. Soln. Bot. 237 mL. *OTC.*
Use: Dermatologic, acne.

Stri-dex Lotion. (Bayer Consumer Care) Salicylic acid 0.5%, alcohol 28%, sulfonated alkyl benzenes, citric acid, sodium carbonate, simethicone, water. Bot. 4 oz. *OTC.*
Use: Dermatologic, acne.

Stri-dex Maximum Strength. (Bayer Consumer Care) Salicylic acid 2%, SD alcohol 44%, citric acid, menthol. Pad. Box 55s, 90s, dual-textured 32s. *OTC.*
Use: Antiacne.

Stri-dex Oil Fighting Formula. (Bayer Consumer Care) Salicylic acid 2%, citric acid, menthol, SD alcohol 54%. Super Scrub Pads. Box 55s. *OTC.*
Use: Dermatologic, acne.

Stri-dex Regular Strength. (Bayer Consumer Care) Salicylic acid 0.5%, SD alcohol 28%, citric acid, menthol. Pad. Box 55s. *OTC.*
Use: Dermatologic, acne.

Stri-dex Sensitive Skin. (Bayer Consumer Care) Salicylic acid 0.5%, citric acid, aloe vera gel, menthol, SD alcohol 28%. Pad. Box 50s, 90s. *OTC.*
Use: Dermatologic, acne.

Stromectol. (Merck & Co.) Ivermectin 3 mg. Tab. UD 20s. *Rx.*
Use: Anthelmintic.

strong iodine solution (Lugol's Solution). (Various Mfr.) Iodine 5% (50 mg/mL)/potassium iodide 10% (100 mg/mL). Soln. 120 mL, 437 mL, gal. *Rx.*
Use: Thyroid drug.

strong iodine tincture. (Various Mfr.) Iodine 7%, potassium iodide 5%, alcohol 83%. Soln. Bot. 500 mL, 4000 mL. *OTC.*
Use: Antimicrobial; antiseptic.

StrongStart. (Savage) Ca 200 mg, Fe 29 mg, vitamin A 1000 units, D 400 units, E 30 units, B_1 3 mg, B_2 3 mg, B_3 15 mg, B_5 7 mg, B_6 20 mg, B_{12} 12 mcg, C 100 mg, folic acid 1 mg, Zn 20 mg; docusate sodium 25 mg (Tab only). Tab., Chew. Tab. Bot. 30s, 100s. *Rx.*
Use: Vitamin, mineral supplement

strontium bromide. (Various Mfr.) Strontium bromide Cryst. or Granule, Bot. 0.25 lb, 1 lb. Amp. 1 g/10 mL. *Rx.*
Use: Antiepileptic; sedative.

•**strontium chloride Sr 85.** (STRAHN-shee-uhm) USAN.
Use: Radiopharmaceutical.

•**strontium chloride Sr 89 injection.** (STRAHN-shee-uhm) *USP.*
Use: Antineoplastic; radiopharmaceutical.
See: Metastron.

•**strontium nitrate Sr 85.** (STRAHN-shee-uhm) USAN.
Use: Radiopharmaceutical.

strontium Sr 85 injection.
Use: Diagnostic aid (bone scanning).

Strovite. (Everett) Vitamins B_1 15 mg, B_2 15 mg, B_3 100 mg, B_5 18 mg, B_6 4 mg, B_{12} 5 mcg, C 500 mg, folic acid 0.5 mg. Tab. Bot. 100s. *OTC.*
Use: Mineral, vitamin supplement.

Strovite Advance. (Everett) Vitamin D_3 400 units, E 100 units, B_1 20 mg, B_2 5 mg, B_3 25 mg, B_5 15 mg, B_6 25 mg, B_{12} 50 mcg, C 300 mg, folic acid 1 mg, Zn 25 mg, carotenoids 3000 units, biotin 100 mcg, alpha lipoic acid 15 mg, lutein 5 mg, Cr, Cu, Mg, Mn, Se, mineral oil. Tab. Bot. 100s. *Rx.*
Use: Vitamin, mineral supplement.

Strovite Forte. (Everett) Fe 10 mg, vitamins A 3000 units (acetate), A 1000 units (beta-carotene), E 60 units, D_3 400 units, folic acid 1 mg, C 500 mg, B_1 20 mg, B_2 20 mg, B_6 25 mg, B_{12} 50 mcg, B_3 100 mg, biotin 0.15 mg, B_5 25 mg, Se 50 mcg, Mg 50 mg, Zn 15 mg, Mo 20 mcg, Cu 3 mg, Cr 0.05 mg. Tab. Bot. 100s. *Rx.*
Use: Vitamin, mineral supplement.

Strovite One. (Everett) Vitamin A (as carotenoids) 3,000 units, E 100 units, D_3 1,000 units, C 300 mg, B_1 20 mg, B_2 5 mg, B_3 25 mg, B_6 25 mg, B_{12} 50 mcg, biotin 100 mcg, folic acid 1 mcg, alpha-lipoic acid 15 mg, lutein 5 mg, pantothenic acid 15 mg, Cr, Cu, Mg, Mn, Se, Zn. Maltodextrin, soybean oil, sucrose. Tab. 90s. *Rx.*
Use: Multivitamin with minerals.

Strovite Plus. (Everett) Vitamins A 5000 units, E 30 mg, B_1 20 mg, B_2 20 mg, B_3 100 mg, B_5 25 mg, B_6 25 mg, B_{12} 50 mcg, C 500 mg, Fe 9 mg, folic acid 0.8 mg, Zn 22.5 mg, biotin 150 mcg, Cr, Cu, Mg, Mn. Bot. 100s. *OTC.*
Use: Mineral, vitamin supplement.

S.T. 37. (Numark Labs) Hexylresorcinol 0.1% in glycerin aqueous soln. Bot. 5.5 oz, 12 oz. *OTC.*
Use: Antiseptic, topical.

Stuart Formula. (J & J Merck Consumer Pharm.) Vitamins A 5000 units, B_1 1.5 mg, B_2 1.7 mg, B_3 20 mg, B_6 1 mg, B_{12} 3 mcg, C 50 mg, D 400 units, E 10 units, Fe 5 mg, Cu, folic acid 0.4 mg, Ca, I, P. Tab. Bot. 100s. *OTC.*
Use: Mineral, vitamin supplement.

StuartNatal Plus 3. (Integrity) Ca 200 mg, Fe (as ferrous fumarate) 28 mg, vitamin A 3000 units, D 400 units, E (as dl-alpha tocopheryl acetate) 22 mg, B_1 1.8 mg, B_2 4 mg, B_3 20 mg, B_6 25 mg, B_{12} 12 mcg, C 120 mg, folic acid 1 mg, Cu, Mg, Zn 25 mg. Tab. Bot. 100s. *Rx.*
Use: Vitamin, mineral supplement.

Stuart One. (Everett) Folic acid 0.8 mg, iron 27 mg, vitamins A 1,100 units, D 1,000 units, E 10 units, B_1 1.6 mg, B_2 1.8 mg, B_3 10 mg, B_6 2.5 mg, B_{12} 12 mcg, C 6 mg, Cu, I, Zn, DHA 200 mg. Glycerin, sorbitol, soy lecithin, soybean oil, sunflower oil. Cap., softgel. 30s. *OTC.*
Use: Prenatal vitamin with minerals.

Stuart Prenatal. (Integrity) Vitamins A (100% as beta carotene) 4000 units, B_1 1.8 mg, B_2 1.7 mg, B_3 20 mg, B_6 2.6 mg, B_{12} 8 mcg, C 120 mg, D 400 units, E (dl-alpha tocopheryl acetate) 30 units, Fe (as ferrous fumarate) 28 mg, Ca 200 mg, Zn 25 mg, folic acid 800 mcg. Tab. Bot. 100s. *OTC.*
Use: Mineral, vitamin supplement.

Stuart Prenatal + DHA. (Xanodyne) Folic acid 0.8 mg, Ca 200 mg, Fe 28 mg, vitamins A 4,000 units, D 400 units, E 30 units, B_1 1.8 mg, B_2 1.7 mg, B_3 20 mg, B_6 2.6 mg, B_{12} 8 mcg, C 120 mg, Zn. **Tab.:** PEG, glucose, sucrose, sodium benzoate, polysorbate 80, wax. 60s. **Gelcaps:** Vitamin E 3 units, fish oil 656 mg (EPA 98 mg, DHA 262 mg, other omega-3 14 mg). Enteric coated. Coconut oil, glycerin, oleic acid. 60s. *OTC.*
Use: Prenatal vitamin with minerals.

Stulex. (Jones Pharma) Docusate sodium 250 mg. Tab. Bot. 100s, 1000s. *OTC.*
Use: Fecal softener.

S2. (Nephron) Racepinephrine hydrochloride 2.25% (epinephrine base 1.125%). Edetate disodium. Soln. for Inh. Single-use vial. 0.5 mL. *OTC.*
Use: Bronchodilator, sympathomimetic; vasopressor.

Stye. (Del) White petrolatum 57.7%, mineral oil 31.9%. Wheat germ oil. Ophth. Oint. Bot. 3.5 g. *OTC.*
Use: Lubricant, ophthalmic.

Stypt-Aid. (Pharmakon) Benzocaine 28.71 mg, methylbenzethonium hydrochloride 9.95 mg, aluminum Cl hexahydrate 55.43 mg, ethyl alcohol 70.97%/mL in a glycerin, menthol base. Spray. 60 mL. *OTC.*
Use: Anesthetic, local.

styptirenal.
See: Epinephrine.

Stypto-Caine. (Pedinol Pharmacal) Hydroxyquinoline sulfate, tetracaine hydrochloride, aluminum Cl, aqueous glycol base. Soln. Bot. 2 oz. *Rx.*
Use: Hemostatic solution.

styrene polymer, sulfonated, sodium salt. Sodium Polystyrene Sulfonate, USP.

styronate resins. Ammonium and potassium salts of sulfonated styrene polymers.
Use: Conditions requiring sodium restriction.

Sublimaze. (Akorn) Fentanyl 50 mcg/mL. Preservative free. Inj., Soln. Amp. 2 mL, 5 mL, 10 mL, 20 mL. *c-II.*
Use: Opioid analgesic.

Sublingual B Total. (Pharmaceutical Labs) Vitamins B_2 1.7 mg, B_3 20 mg, B_5 30 mg, B_6 2 mg, B_{12} 1000 mcg, C 60 mg. Liq. Bot. 30 mL. *OTC.*
Use: Vitamin supplement.

Suboxone. (Reckitt Benckiser) Buprenorphine hydrochloride/naloxone hydrochloride 2 mg/0.5 mg, 8 mg/2 mg. Acesulfame K, maltitol, lime flavoring. Film; sublingual. 30s. *c-III.*
Use: Analgesic.

substituted ureas.
Use: Antisickling agent.
See: Hydrea.
Hydroxyurea.

Subsys. (Insys Therapeutics) Fentanyl 100 mcg, 200 mcg, 400 mcg, 600 mcg, 800 mcg. Alcohol 63.6%, propylene glycol, xylitol. Spray; sublingual. Single-spray units in blister packages. UD 6s, UD 14s, UD 28s. *c-II.*
Use: Opioid analgesic.

•**succimer.** (SUX-ih-mer) USAN.
Use: Diagnostic aid; cystine kidney stones, mercury and lead poisoning. [Orphan Drug]
See: Chemet.

succinimides.
Use: Anticonvulsant
See: Methsuximide.

•**succinobucol.** (sux-in-oh-BUE-kol) USAN.
Use: Cardiovascular agent.

•**succinylcholine chloride.** (suck-sin-ill-KOE-leen KLOR-ide) *USP.*

Use: Neuromuscular blocker.
See: Anectine.
Quelicin.
Sucostrin.

succinylsulfathiazole.
Use: Anti-infective, intestinal.

Suclear. (Braintree Labs) **Soln.:** Sodium sulfate 17.5 g, potassium sulfate 3.13 g, magnesium sulfate 1.6 g. Sodium benzoate, sucralose. 180 mL w/mixing container. **Pow. for Soln.:** PEG 3350 210 g, sodium chloride 5.6 g, sodium bicarbonate 2.86 g, potassium chloride 0.74 g. Cherry, lemon-lime, orange, and pineapple flavors. 2 L bottle. *Rx.*
Use: Laxative, bowel evacuant.

Sucostrin. (Apothecon) Succinylcholine Cl 20 mg/mL Inj. Vial 10 mL. *Rx.*
Use: Neuromuscular blocker.

Sucostrin Chloride. (Marsam) Succinylcholine Cl 20 mg/mL w/methylparaben 0.1%, propylparaben 0.01%. Vial 10 mL; High potency 100 mg/mL. Vial 10 mL. *Rx.*
Use: Muscle relaxant.

Sucraid. (Orphan Medical) Sacrosidase 8500 units/mL. Soln. Bot. 118 mL. *Rx.*
Use: Nutritional therapy.

•**sucralfate.** (sue-KRAL-fate) *USP.*
Use: Antiulcerative; oral complications of chemotherapy. [Orphan Drug]
See: Carafate.
Orafate.
ProThelial.

sucralfate. (Precision Dose) Sucralfate 1 g/10 mL. Methylparaben, sorbitol. Susp. Unit dose cups. 10 mL. *Rx.*
Use: Antiulcerative.

sucralfate. (Various Mfr.) Sucralfate 1 g. Tab. Bot. 100s, 500s. *Rx.*
Use: Antiulcerative.

Sucrets Children's Formula. (Insight) Dyclonine hydrochloride 1.2 mg. Corn syrup, sucrose, cherry flavor. Loz. Tin 24s. *OTC.*
Use: Sore throat treatment for children 3 years and older.

Sucrets Complete. (Insight) Dyclonine hydrochloride 3 mg, menthol 6 mg. Acesulfame K, corn syrup, sucrose. Cherry and cool citrus flavors. Loz. 18s. *OTC.*
Use: Mouth and throat product.

Sucrets DM Cough Formula. (Insight) Dextromethorphan HBr 10 mg. Corn syrup, hydrogenated palm oil, sugar (honey lemon flavor only); menthol, sucrose (cherry flavor only). Honey lemon and cherry flavors. Loz. 18s. *OTC.*
Use: Nonnarcotic antitussive.

Sucrets DM Cough Suppressant. (Insight) Dextromethorphan HBr 10 mg. Corn syrup, menthol, sucrose. Cherry flavor. Loz. 6s. *OTC.*
Use: Nonnarcotic antitussive.

Sucrets Maximum Strength Sore Throat. (Insight) Dyclonine hydrochloride 3 mg. Loz. Corn syrup, menthol, sucrose. Loz. Tin 24s, 48s, 55s. *OTC.*
Use: Mouth and throat preparation.

Sucrets Original Formula Sore Throat. (Insight) Hexylresorcinol 2.4 mg. Corn syrup, menthol, sucrose. Mint flavor. Loz. 18s. *OTC.*
Use: Mouth and throat preparation.

Sucrets Original Formula Sore Throat Wild Cherry. (Insight) Dyclonine hydrochloride 2 mg. Corn syrup, menthol, sucrose. Cherry flavor. Loz. 24s. *OTC.*
Use: Mouth and throat product.

Sucrets Throat Spray. (Insight) Dyclonine hydrochloride 0.1%, alcohol 10%, sorbitol. Spray. Bot. 90 mL, 120 mL. *OTC.*
Use: Mouth and throat preparation.

•**sucroferric oxyhydroxide.** (soo-kroe-FER-ik OX-ee-hye-DROX-ide)
Use: Trace element.

•**sucrose.** (SUE-krose) *NF.*
Use: IV; diuretic & dehydrating agent; pharmaceutic aid (flavor, tablet excipient).

•**sucrose octaacetate.** (SUE-krose) *NF.*
Use: Pharmaceutic aid (alcohol denaturant).

•**sucrosofate potassium.** (sue-KROE-so-FATE) USAN.
Use: Antiulcerative.

Sudafed. (McNeil) Pseudoephedrine hydrochloride. 30 mg, 60 mg. **30 mg:** Box 24s, 48s. Bot. 100s, 1000s. **60 mg:** Bot. 100s, 1000s. *OTC.*
Use: Decongestant.

Sudafed Children's Non-Drowsy. (McNeil) Pseudoephedrine hydrochloride 15 mg/5 mL, EDTA, saccharin, sorbitol, grape flavor, alcohol free. Liq. 118 mL. *OTC.*
Use: Nasal decongestant, arylalkylamine.

Sudafed Cold & Sinus Non-Drowsy. (McNeil) Pseudoephedrine hydrochloride 30 mg, acetaminophen 325 mg, sorbitol. Liqui-Caps. Pkg. 10s, 20s. *OTC.*
Use: Upper respiratory combination, decongestant, analgesic.

Sudafed Maximum Strength Non-Drowsy Non-Drying Sinus. (McNeil) Pseudoephedrine hydrochloride 30 mg,

guaifenesin 200 mg. Glycerin, PEG, sorbitol. Cap. 24s. *OTC.*
Use: Upper respiratory combination, decongestant and expectorant combination.

Sudafed Multi-Symptom Cold & Cough. (McNeil) Dextromethorphan HBr 10 mg, guaifenesin 100 mg, pseudoephedrine hydrochloride 30 mg, acetaminophen 250 mg, sorbitol. Liquicaps. Pkg. 20s. *OTC.*
Use: Upper respiratory combination, antitussive, expectorant, decongestant, analgesic.

Sudafed Non-Drowsy Maximum Strength. (McNeil) Pseudoephedrine hydrochloride 30 mg, lactose, sucrose. Tab. Bot. 24s, 96s. *OTC.*
Use: Nasal decongestant, arylalkylamine.

Sudafed Non-Drowsy 12 Hour Long-Acting. (McNeil) Pseudoephedrine hydrochloride 120 mg. ER Tab. Pkg. 10s. *OTC.*
Use: Nasal decongestant, arylalkylamine.

Sudafed Non-Drowsy 24 Hour Long-Acting. (McNeil) Pseudoephedrine hydrochloride 240 mg (immediate-release 60 mg, controlled-release 180 mg). CR Tab. Pkg. 10s. *OTC.*
Use: Nasal decongestant, arylalkylamine.

Sudafed PE. (McNeil) Phenylephrine hydrochloride 10 mg. Acesulfame K. Tab. 18s. *OTC.*
Use: Nasal decongestant.

Sudafed PE Day & Night. (McNeil) Tab. **Day:** Phenylephrine hydrochloride 10 mg. PEG. 18s. **Night:** Diphenhydramine hydrochloride 25 mg, phenylephrine hydrochloride 10 mg. PEG. 12s. *OTC.*
Use: Upper respiratory combination, decongestant and antihistamine.

Sudafed PE Maximum Strength Nasal Decongestant. (McNeil) Phenylephrine hydrochloride 10 mg. Acesulfame K, PEG. Tab. 18s, 36s, 72s. *OTC.*
Use: Nasal decongestant.

Sudafed PE Multi-Symptom Cold and Cough. (McNeil) Dextromethorphan HBr 10 mg, guaifenesin 100 mg, phenylephrine hydrochloride 5 mg, acetaminophen 325 mg. PEG. Tab. 20s. *OTC.*
Use: Antitussive and expectorant combination, upper respiratory combination.

Sudafed PE Multi-Symptom Severe Cold. (McNeil) Phenylephrine hydrochloride 5 mg, diphenhydramine hydrochloride 12.5 mg, acetaminophen 325 mg. PEG. Tab. 12s, 24s. *OTC.*
Use: Decongestant, antihistamine, and analgesic, upper respiratory combination.

Sudafed PE Nighttime Cold Maximum Strength. (McNeil) Phenylephrine hydrochloride 5 mg, diphenhydramine hydrochloride 25 mg, acetaminophen 325 mg. Tab. 20s. *OTC.*
Use: Decongestant, antihistamine, and analgesic combination, upper respiratory combination.

Sudafed PE Non-Drying Sinus. (McNeil) Phenylephrine hydrochloride 5 mg, guaifenesin 200 mg. PEG. Caps. Pkg. 24s. *OTC.*
Use: Upper respiratory combination, decongestant, expectorant.

Sudafed PE Sinus Headache Maximum Strength. (McNeil) Phenylephrine hydrochloride 5 mg, acetaminophen 325 mg. PEG. Tab. 24s, 48s, 72s. *OTC.*
Use: Decongestant and analgesic combination.

Sudafed Sinus & Allergy. (McNeil) Pseudoephedrine hydrochloride 60 mg, chlorpheniramine maleate 4 mg. Lactose. Tab. Pkg. 24s. *OTC.*
Use: Upper respiratory combination, decongestant, antihistamine.

Sudafed 12 Hour. (McNeil) Pseudoephedrine hydrochloride 120 mg. SA Cap. Box 10s, 20s, 40s. *OTC.*
Use: Decongestant.

SudaHist. (Larken Laboratories) Chlorpheniramine maleate 12 mg, pseudoephedrine hydrochloride 120 mg. Lactose. ER Tab. 100s. *Rx.*
Use: Upper respiratory combination, decongestant and antihistamine.

Sudal-DM. (Atley) Dextromethorphan HBr 30 mg, guaifenesin 500 mg, dye free. SR Tab. Bot. 100s. *Rx.*
Use: Upper respiratory combination, antitussive, expectorant.

Sudal 120/600. (Atley) Pseudoephedrine hydrochloride 120 mg, guaifenesin 600 mg. SR Tab. Bot. 100s. *Rx.*
Use: Upper respiratory combination, decongestant, expectorant.

Sudal-12 Tannate. (Atley) Pseudoephedrine polistirex (equiv. to pseudoephedrine hydrochloride 30 mg), chlorpheniramine polistirex (equiv. to chlorpheniramine maleate 6 mg) per 5 mL. Corn syrup, parabens. Strawberry flavor. ER Susp. 473 mL. *Rx.*
Use: Decongestant and antihistamine.

Sudanyl. (Dover Pharmaceuticals) Pseudoephedrine hydrochloride. Tab.

Sugar, lactose, and salt free. UD Box 500s.
Use: Decongestant.

SudaTrate. (Larken) Methscopolamine nitrate 2.5 mg, pseudoephedrine hydrochloride 120 mg. ER Tab. 100s. *Rx.*
Use: Upper respiratory combination; decongestant, antihistamine, and anticholinergic combination.

Sudatuss-2 DF. (PGD) Codeine phosphate 10 mg, guaifenesin 100 mg, pseudoephedrine hydrochloride 30 mg per 5 mL. Alcohol free. Parabens, aspartame, phenylalanine. Cherry flavor. Liq. 473 mL. *c-v.*
Use: Antitussive and expectorant.

Sudden Tan Lotion. (Schering-Plough) Padimate O, dihydroxyacetone, Bot. 4 oz. *OTC.*
Use: Artificial tanning; moisturizer; sunscreen.

SudoGest Non-Drowsy. (Major) Pseudoephedrine hydrochloride 30 mg. PEG, sugar. Tab. 100s. *Rx.*
Use: Nasal decongestant, arylalkylamine.

SudoGest Sinus & Allergy Maximum Strength. (Major) Chlorpheniramine maleate 4 mg, pseudoephedrine hydrochloride 60 mg. Lactose. Tab. 48s. *OTC.*
Use: Upper respiratory combination, decongestant and antihistamine.

SudoGest Sinus Maximum Strength. (Major) Pseudoephedrine hydrochloride 30 mg, acetaminophen 500 mg, dextrose. Tab. Pkg. 24s. *OTC.*
Use: Upper respiratory combination, decongestant, analgesic.

•**sudoxicam.** (sue-DOX-ih-kam) USAN.
Use: Anti-inflammatory.

Sudrin. (Jones Pharma) Pseudoephedrine hydrochloride 30 mg. Tab. Bot. 100s, 1000s. *OTC.*
Use: Decongestant.

Sufenta. (Akorn) Sufentanil citrate (as base) 50 mcg/mL. Preservative free. Inj. Amp. 1 mL, 2 mL, 5 mL. *c-II.*
Use: Opioid analgesic.

•**sufentanil.** (sue-FEN-tuh-nill) USAN.
Tall Man: SUFentanil
Use: Analgesic.

•**sufentanil citrate.** (sue-FEN-tuh-nill SIH-trate) *USP.*
Tall Man: SUFentanil
Use: Opioid analgesic.
See: Sufenta.

•**sufentanil citrate injection.** (sue-FEN-tuh-nill SIH-trate) *USP.*
Tall Man: SUFentanil
Use: Analgesic; narcotic.

•**sufotidine.** (sue-FOE-tih-DEEN) USAN.
Use: Antiulcerative.

Sufrex. (Janssen) Ketanserin tartrate. *Rx.*
Use: Serotonin antagonist.

•**sugammadex sodium.** (soo-GAM-ma-dex) USAN.
Use: CNS agent.

•**sugar, compressible.** (SHUG-er) *NF.*
Use: Pharmaceutic aid (flavor; tablet excipient).

•**sugar, confectioner's.** (SHUG-er) *NF.*
Use: Pharmaceutic aid (flavor; tablet excipient).

•**sugar, invert, injection.** (SHUG-er) *USP.*
Use: Replenisher (fluid and nutrient).

•**sugar spheres.** (SHUG-er) *NF.*
Use: Pharmaceutic aid (vehicle, solid carrier).

•**sulamserod hydrochloride.** (sul-AM-se-rod) USAN.
Use: Urge incontinence; atrial fibrillations.

Sular. (Sciele Pharma) Nisoldipine 8.5 mg, 17 mg, 34 mg. Tartrazine (17 mg only), lactose, polyethylene glycol. Film coated. ER Tab. 100s. *Rx.*
Use: Calcium channel blocker.

•**sulazepam.** (sull-AZE-eh-pam) USAN.
Use: Anxiolytic.

Sulazo. (Freeport) Sulfisoxazole 500 mg, phenylazodiaminopyridine hydrochloride 50 mg. Tab. Bot. 1000s. *Rx.*
Use: Analgesic; anti-infective.

•**sulbactam benzathine.** (sull-BACK-tam BENZ-ah-theen) USAN.
Use: Synergistic (penicillin/cephalosporin); inhibitor (β-lactamase).

•**sulbactam pivoxil.** (sull-BACK-tam pihv-OX-ill) USAN.
Use: Inhibitor (β-lactamase); synergist (penicillin/cephalosporin).

sulbactam sodium/ampicillin sodium.
Use: Anti-infective; penicillin.
See: Unasyn.

•**sulbactam sodium sterile.** (sull-BACK-tam) *USP.*
Use: Inhibitor (β-lactamase); synergist (penicillin/cephalosporin).

•**sulconazole nitrate.** (SULL-CONE-ah-zole) *USP.*
Use: Antifungal.
See: Exelderm.

•**sulesomab.** (sue-LEH-so-mab) USAN.
Use: Monoclonal antibody (diagnostic aid for detection of infectious lesions).

•**sulfabenz.** (SULL-fah-benz) USAN.
Use: Anti-infective.

•**sulfabenzamide.** (SULL-fah-BENZ-ah-mid) *USP.*
Use: Anti-infective.

sulfabromethazine sodium.
Use: Anti-infective.
Sulfacet. (Dermik)
See: Sulfacetamide.
•**sulfacetamide.** (sull-fah-SEE-tah-mide) *USP.*
Use: Anti-infective.
W/Combinations.
See: Acet-Dia-Mer Sulfonamides.
Chero-Trisulfa-V.
Sulfa-10 Ophthalmic.
•**sulfacetamide sodium.** (sull-fah-SEE-tah-mide) *USP.*
Use: Anti-infective.
See: AK-Sulf.
Bleph 10.
Klaron.
Klaron 10%.
Ovace.
Ovace Plus.
Seb-Prev.
Seb-Prev Wash.
Sulster.
W/Prednisolone Acetate.
See: Blephamide.
Blephamide S.O.P.
Metimyd.
Predsulfair.
Vasocidin.
W/Sulfur.
See: Novacet.
Plexion.
Plexion SCT.
Rosanil.
Sulfacet-R.
Vanocin.
Zetacet.
sulfacetamide sodium. (Fera Pharmaceuticals) Sulfacetamide sodium 10%. White petrolatum, mineral oil. Oint.; Ophth. 3.5 g. *Rx.*
Use: Ophthalmic antibiotic.
sulfacetamide sodium. (Various Mfr.) Sulfacetamide sodium. **Lot.:** 10%. May contain disodium EDTA, PEG 400, methylparaben, urea. 89 g, 118 mL. **Soln.:** 10%. 15 mL. **Oint.:** 10%. Tube 3.5 g.
Use: Anti-infective.
sulfacetamide sodium and prednisolone sodium phosphate. (Schein) Sulfacetamide sodium 10%, prednisolone sodium phosphate 0.25%. Thimerosal 0.01%, EDTA, boric acid. Soln. 5 mL, 10 mL. *Rx.*
Use: Anti-infective, ophthalmic.
sulfacetamide sodium 10%. (Fougera) Sulfacetamide sodium 100 mg per mL. Methylparaben, EDTA. Top. Susp. 118 mL. *Rx.*
Use: Acne product.
sulfacetamide sodium 10% and sulfur 5%. (Glades) Sulfur 5%, sodium sulfacetamide 10%, cetyl alcohol, benzyl alcohol, EDTA. Bot. 25 mL. Tube 30 mL. *Rx.*
Use: Dermatologic, acne.
sulfacetamide, sulfadiazine, and sulfamerazine.
See: Acet-Dia-Mer-Sulfonamide.
Sulfacet-R. (Dermik) Sulfur 5%, sulfacetamide sodium 10%, parabens. Lot. Bot. 25 mL. *Rx.*
Use: Dermatologic, acne.
sulfacitine. *See:* Sulfacytine.
SulfaCleanse 8/4. (PruGen) Sodium sulfacetamide 8%, sulfur 4%. Alcohols, aloe, butylated hydroxytoluene, edetate disodium, glyceryl, green tea, parabens, PEG. Soap. 473 mL. *Rx.*
Use: Acne product combination.
•**sulfacytine.** (SULL-fah-SIGH-teen) USAN.
Use: Anti-infective.
sulfadiasulfone sodium. Acetosulfone sodium.
•**sulfadiazine.** (SULL-fah-DIE-ah-zeen) *USP.*
Tall Man: sulfADIAZINE
Use: Anti-infective. [Orphan Drug]
W/Combinations.
See: Acet-Dia-Mer-Sulfonamide.
Chemozine.
Chero-Trisulfa-V.
Meth-Dia-Mer Sulfonamides.
Silvadene.
Triple Sulfa.
sulfadiazine. (Sandoz) Sulfadiazine 500 mg. Tab. 100s, 1000s. *Rx.*
Use: Anti-infective.
sulfadiazine and sulfamerazine. Citrasulfas.
•**sulfadiazine, silver.** (sull-fah-DIE-ah-zeen) *USP.*
Tall Man: sulfADIAZINE
Use: Anti-infective, topical.
•**sulfadiazine sodium.** (SULL-fah-DIE-ah-zeen) *USP.*
Tall Man: sulfADIAZINE
Use: Anti-infective.
•**sulfadiazine sodium injection.** (SULL-fah-DIE-ah-zeen) *USP.*
Use: Anti-infective.
sulfadiazine, sulfamerazine, and sulfacetamide.
See: Acet-Dia-Mer-Sulfonamide.
•**sulfadimethoxine.** (SUL-fa-DYE-meth-OX-een) *USP.*
Use: Antibiotic (veterinary).
•**sulfadimethoxine sodium.** (SUL-fa-DYE-meth-OX-een) *USP.*
Use: Antibiotic (veterinary).

sulfadimidine.
See: Sulfamethazine.
sulfadine.
See: Sulfadimidine.
Sulfamethazine.
Sulfapyridine.
•**sulfadoxine.** (SULL-fah-DOX-een) *USP.*
Use: Anti-infective.
sulfaguanidine.
Use: GI tract infections.
Sulfair 15. (Bausch & Lomb) Sodium sulfacetamide 15%. Soln. Bot. 15 mL. *Rx.*
Use: Anti-infective, ophthalmic.
•**sulfalene.** (SULL-fah-leen) USAN.
Use: Anti-infective.
•**sulfamerazine.** (sull-fah-MER-ah-zeen)
Use: Anti-infective.
W/Combinations
See: Chemozine.
Chero-Trisulfa-V.
sulfamerazine sodium.
Use: Anti-infective.
sulfamerazine, sulfadiazine, and sulfamethazine.
Use: Anti-infective.
See: Meth-Dia-Mer Sulfonamides.
sulfamerazine, sulfadiazine, and sulfathiazole.
Use: Anti-infective.
•**sulfameter.** (SULL-fam-EE-ter) USAN.
Use: Anti-infective.
•**sulfamethazine.** (sull fa-METH-ah-zeen) *USP.*
Use: Anti-infective.
W/Sulfadiazine, Sulfamerazine.
See: Triple Sulfa.
•**sulfamethizole.** (sul-fa-METH-i-zole) USAN.
Use: Anti-infective.
sulfamethoprim. (Par Pharmaceuticals) Sulfamethoxazole 400 mg, trimethoprim 80 mg. Tab. 100s, 500s. *Rx.*
Use: Anti-infective.
•**sulfamethoxazole.** (sull-fah-meth-OX-ah-zole) *USP.*
Use: Anti-infective.
W/Trimethoprim.
See: Bactrim.
sulfamethoxazole and phenazopyridine hydrochloride.
Use: Anti-infective, urinary.
•**sulfamethoxazole and trimethoprim injection.** (SULL-fah-meth-OX-ah-zole and try-METH-oh-prim) *USP.*
Use: Anti-infective, urinary.
sulfamethoxazole and trimethoprim oral suspension. (Various Mfr.) Trimethoprim 40 mg, sulfamethoxazole 200 mg/5 mL. Bot. 150 mL, 200 mL, 480 mL. *Rx.*
Use: Anti-infective, urinary.
sulfamethoxazole and trimethoprim tablets. (Various Mfr.) Trimethoprim 80 mg, sulfamethoxazole 400 mg. Tab. Bot. 100s, 500s. *Rx.*
Use: Anti-infective, urinary.
sulfamethoxazole/trimethoprim DS. (Various Mfr.) Trimethoprim 160 mg, sulfamethoxazole 800 mg. Tab, double-strength. Bot. 100s, 500s. *Rx.*
Use: Anti-infective.
sulfamethoxydiazine. Sulfameter.
Use: Anti-infective.
sulfamethoxypyridazine acetyl.
Use: Anti-infective.
sulfamethylthiadiazole.
Use: Anti-infective.
sulfametin. *Formerly Sulfamethoxydiazine.*
Use: Anti-infective.
sulfamezanthene.
Use: Anti-infective.
See: Sulfamethazine.
Sulfamide. (Rugby) Prednisolone acetate 0.5%, sodium sulfacetamide, hydroxypropyl methylcellulose, polysorbate 80, sodium thiosulfate, benzalkonium Cl 0.01%. Susp. Bot. 5 and 15 mL. *Rx.*
Use: Anti-infective, ophthalmic.
•**sulfamonomethoxine.** (SULL-fah-mahn-oh-meh-THOCK-seen) USAN.
Use: Anti-infective.
•**sulfamoxole.** (sull-fah-MOX-ole) USAN.
Use: Anti-infective.
p-sulfamoylbenzylamine hydrochloride. Sulfbenzamide.
Sulfamylon. (UDL) **Cream:** Mafenide 85 mg/g (as acetate). EDTA, cetyl alcohol, stearyl alcohol, parabens, sodium metabisulfite. 56.7 g, 113.4 g, 453.6 g. **Top. Soln.:** Mafenide acetate 5%. Packets. 50 g for reconstitution. *Rx.*
Use: Topical anti-infective.
2-sulfanilamidopyridine. Sulfadiazine, USP.
Use: Anti-infective.
•**sulfanilate zinc.** (sull-FAN-ih-late) USAN.
Use: Anti-infective.
n-sulfanilylacetamide.
Use: Anti-infective.
See: Sulfacetamide.
sulfanilylbenzamide.
Use: Anti-infective.
See: Sulfabenzamide.
•**sulfanitran.** (SULL-fah-NYE-tran) USAN.
Use: Anti-infective.
•**sulfapyridine.** (sull-fah-PEER-ih-deen) *USP.*
Use: Dermatitic herpetiformis suppressant. [Orphan Drug]

•**sulfasalazine.** (SULL-fuh-SAL-uh-zeen) *USP. Formerly Salicylazosulfapyridine.*
Tall Man: sulfaSALAzine
Use: Anti-infective; antirheumatic.
See: Azulfidine.
Azulfidine EN-tabs.
Sulfazine.
Sulfazine EC.

sulfasalazine. (Greenstone) Sulfasalazine 500 mg. Enteric coated. DR Tab. 100s, 300s. *Rx.*
Use: Anti-infective; antirheumatic.

sulfasalazine. (Various Mfr.) Sulfasalazine 500 mg. Tab. 100s, 300s, 500s, 1000s. *Rx.*
Use: Anti-infective; antirheumatic.

•**sulfasomizole.** (SULL-fah-SAHM-ih-zole) USAN.
Use: Antibacterial; anti-infective; sulfonamide.

sulfasymasine.
Use: Anti-infective sulfonamide.

Sulfa-10 Ophthalmic. (Maurry) Sodium sulfacetamide 10%, hydroxyethylcellulose, sodium borate, boric acid, disodium edetate, sodium metabisulfite, sodium thiosulfate 0.2%, chlorobutanol 0.2%, methylparaben 0.015%. Bot. 15 mL. *Rx.*
Use: Anti-infective, ophthalmic.

Sulfa-Ter-Tablets. (A.P.C.) Trisulfapyrimidines. Tab. Bot. 1000s.

•**sulfathiazole.** (sull-fah-THIGH-ah-zole) *USP.*
Use: Anti-infective.

Sulfatrim. (Activis MidAtlantic) Trimethoprim 40 mg, sulfamethoxazole 200 mg/5 mL. Alcohol < 0.5%, parabens, saccharin, sucrose. Fruit licorice and cherry flavors. Susp. 473 mL. *Rx.*
Use: Anti-infective.

Sulfatrim DS. (Ivax) Trimethoprim 800 mg, sulfamethoxazole 160 mg. Tab. Bot. 100s, 500s. *Rx.*
Use: Anti-infective.

Sulfatrim SS. (Ivax) Trimethoprim 400 mg, sulfamethoxazole 80 mg. Tab. Bot. 100s. *Rx.*
Use: Anti-infective.

Sulfa-Trip. (Major) Sulfathiazole 3.42%, sulfacetamide 2.86%, sulfabenzamide 3.7%, urea 0.64%. Cream. Tube 82.5 g. *Rx.*
Use: Anti-infective, vaginal.

Sulfa Triple No. 2. (Global Source) Sulfadiazine 162 mg, sulfamerazine 162 mg, sulfamethazine 162 mg. Tab. Bot. 1000s. *Rx.*
Use: Anti-infective.

•**sulfazamet.** (sull-FAZE-ah-MET) USAN.
Use: Anti-infective.

Sulfazine. (Qualitest) Sulfasalazine 500 mg. Tab. 100s, 180s, 500s, 1,000s. *Rx.*
Use: Gastrointestinal agent.

Sulfazine EC. (Qualitest) Sulfasalazine 500 mg. Tab., delayed release. 100s, 300s. *Rx.*
Use: Gastrointestinal agent.

•**sulfinalol hydrochloride.** (SULL-FIN-ah-lahl) USAN.
Use: Antihypertensive.

•**sulfinpyrazone.** (sull-fin-PEER-uh-zone) *USP.*
Use: Uricosuric.

•**sulfisoxazole.** (sull-fih-SOX-uh-zole) *USP.*
Tall Man: sulfiSOXAZOLE
Use: Anti-infective.
See: Gantrisin Pediatric.
Soxa.
Sulfisoxazole.

•**sulfisoxazole, acetyl.** (sull-fih-SOX-uh-zole, ASS-eh-till) *USP.*
Tall Man: sulfiSOXAZOLE
Use: Anti-infective.

sulfisoxazole diethanolamine. Sulfisoxazole Diolamine.

•**sulfisoxazole diolamine.** (sull-fih-SOX-uh-zole die-OLE-ah-meen) *USP.*
Tall Man: sulfiSOXAZOLE
Use: Anti-infective.

Sulfoam. (Doak) Sulfur 2%, parabens. Shampoo. Bot. 237 mL. *OTC.*
Use: Control dandruff.

sulfobromophthalein sodium. *USP.*
Use: Liver function test.

sulfocarbolates. Salts of Phenolsulfonic Acid, Usually Ca, Na, K, Cu, Zn.

•**sulfocon B.** (sul-FOE-kon) USAN.
Use: Hydrophobic.

sulfocyanate.
See: Potassium Thiocyanate.

Sulfo-Ganic. (Marcen) Thioglycerol 20 mg, sodium citrate 5 mg, phenol 0.5%, benzyl alcohol 0.5%/mL. Inj. Vial 10 mL, 30 mL.
Use: Antiarthritic.

Sulfolax. (Major) Docusate calcium 240 mg. Parabens, sorbitol. Soft Gel Cap. Bot. 100s. *OTC.*
Use: Laxative.

Sulfo-Lo. (Whorton Pharmaceuticals, Inc.) Sublimed sulfur, freshly precipitated polysulfides of zinc, potassium, sulfate, and calamine in aqueous-alcoholic suspension. **Lotion:** Bot. 4 oz, 8 oz. **Soap:** 3 oz. *OTC.*
Use: Dermatologic, acne.

•**sulfomyxin.** (SULL-foe-MIX-in) USAN.
Use: Anti-infective.

sulfonamides.
Use: Anticonvulsants.
See: Sulfacetamide Sodium.
Sulfadiazine.
Sulfamethoxazole.
Sulfisoxazole.
Sulfisoxazole Diolamine.
Zonisamide.

sulfonamides, triple.
See: Acet-Dia-Mer Sulfonamide.
Meth-Dia-Mer Sulfonamides.

sulfones.
See: Dapsone.
Glucosulfone Sodium.

•**sulfonterol hydrochloride.** (sull-FAHN-teer-ole) USAN.
Use: Bronchodilator.

sulfonylureas.
See: Chlorpropamide.
Glimepiride.
Glipizide.
Glyburide.
Tolazamide.
Tolbutamide.

Sulforcin. (Galderma) Sulfur 5%, resorcinol 2%, SD alcohol 40 11.65%, methylparaben. Lot. Bot. 120 mL. *OTC.*
Use: Dermatologic.

sulformethoxine. *Name used for Sulfadoxine.*

sulforthomidine. *Name used for Sulfadoxine.*

sulfosalicylate with methenamine.
See: Hexalen.

sulfosalicylic acid. Salicylsulphonic acid.

sulfur.
Use: Antiseborrheic.
See: Sulfoam.
W/Benzocaine.
See: Chigg Away.
W/Benzoyl Peroxide.
See: NuOx.
W/Salicylic Acid.
See: Exoderm.
W/Sodium Sulfacetamide.
See: Avar-e Emollient.
Avar-e LS.
Avar LS Cleanser.
BP Cleansing Wash.
Cerisa.
Clarifoam EF.
Claris.
Garimide.
Rosaderm Kit.
SE 10-5 SS.
SSS 10-5.
SSS 10-4.
SulfoCleanse 8/4.
Sumadan.
Sumaxin.
Sumaxin CP.
Sumaxin TS.
Sumaxin Wash.
Virti-Sulf Emollient.
Zencia.

sulfurated lime topical solution.
Vleminckx Lotion.
Use: Scabicide; parasiticide.

sulfur combinations.
See: Aveenobar Medicated.
Acnomel.
Acnotex.
Adult Acnomel.
Akne.
Avar.
Avar-e Emollient.
Avar-e Green.
Clearasil Adult Care.
Clenia.
Liquimat.
Pernox.
Plexion.
Plexion Cleansing Cloths.
Plexion SCT.
Plexion TS.
Rezamid.
SAStid Soap.
Sebulex with Conditioners.
Sulfacet-R.
Sulfo-lo.
Sulforcin.
Sulfur-8.
Sulpho-Lac.
Vanocin.

•**sulfur dioxide.** (SULL-fer die-OX-ide) *NF.*
Use: Pharmaceutic aid (antioxidant).

Sulfur-8 Hair & Scalp Conditioner. (Schering-Plough) Sulfur 2%, menthol 1%, triclosan 0.1%. Cream. Jar 2 oz, 4 oz, 8 oz. *OTC.*
Use: Antiseborrheic.

Sulfur-8 Light Formula Hair & Scalp Conditioner. (Schering-Plough) Sulfur, triclosan, menthol. Cream. Jar 2 oz, 4 oz. *OTC.*
Use: Antiseborrheic.

Sulfur-8 Shampoo. (Schering-Plough) Triclosan 0.2%. Bot. 6.85 oz, 10.85 oz. *OTC.*
Use: Antiseborrheic.

•**sulfur hexafluoride.** (SUL-fur) USAN.
Use: Diagnostic aid (ultrasound).

•**sulfuric acid.** (sul-FURE-ik) *NF.*
Use: Pharmaceutic aid (acidifying agent).

sulfuric acid/sulfonated phenolics.
Use: Mouth and throat product.
See: Debacterol.

sulfur ointment.
Use: Scabicide; parasiticide.

•**sulfur, precipitated.** (SUL-fur pree-SIP-a-TAY-ted) *USP.*
Use: Scabicide; parasiticide.
See: SAStid Soap.
Sulfur Soap.

sulfur, salicyl diasporal. (Doak Dermatologics)
See: Diasporal.

sulfur soap. (GlaxoSmithKline) Precipitated sulfur 10%, EDTA. Cake 116 g. *OTC.*
Use: Dermatologic, acne.

•**sulfur, sublimed.** (SUL-fur) *USP.* Flowers of Sulfur.
Use: Parasiticide; scabicide.

sulfur, topical.
See: Thylox.

•**sulindac.** (sull-IN-dak) *USP.*
Use: Nonsteroidal anti-inflammatory agent.
See: Clinoril.

sulindac. (Various Mfr.) Sulindac 150 mg, 200 mg. Tab. Bot. 100s, 500s, 1000s, UD 100s. *Rx.*
Use: Anti-inflammatory; NSAID.

•**sulisobenzone.** (sul-EYE-so-BEN-zone) USAN.
Use: Ultraviolet screen.
See: Uvinul MS-40.

•**sulmarin.** (SULL-mah-rin) USAN.
Use: Hemostatic.

Sulmasque. (C & M Pharmacal) Sulfur 6.4%, isopropyl alcohol 15%, methylparaben. Mask 150 g. *OTC.*
Use: Dermatologic, acne.

Sulnac. (Alra) Sulfathiazole 3.42%, sulfacetamide 2.86%, sulfabenzamide 3.7%, urea 0.64% in cream base. Tube 2.75 oz. *Rx.*
Use: Anti-infective.

•**sulnidazole.** (sull-NIH-dah-zole) USAN.
Use: Antiprotozoal (trichomonas).

•**suloctidil.** (sull-OCK-tih-dill) USAN.
Use: Vasodilator (peripheral).

•**sulofenur.** (SUE-low-FEN-ehr) USAN.
Use: Antineoplastic.

•**sulopenem.** (soo-loe-PEN-em) USAN.
Use: Anti-infective.

•**sulopenem etzadroxil.** (soo-loe-PEN-em et-za-DROX-il) USAN.
Use: Antibiotic.

•**sulotroban.** (suh-LOW-troe-ban) USAN.
Use: Treatment of glomerulonephritis.

•**suloxifen oxalate.** (sull-OX-ih-fen OX-ah-late) USAN.
Use: Bronchodilator.

sulphabenzide.
See: Sulfabenzamide.

Sulpho-Lac Acne Medication. (Doak Dermatologics) Sulfur 5%, zinc sulfate 27%, Vleminckx's Soln. 53%. Cream. Tube 28.35 g, 50 g. *OTC.*
Use: Dermatologic, acne.

Sulpho-Lac Soap. (Doak Dermatologics) Sulfur 5%, a coconut and tallow oil soap base. Bar 85 g. *OTC.*
Use: Dermatologic, acne.

•**sulpiride.** (SULL-pih-ride) USAN.
Use: Antidepressant.

•**sulprostone.** (sull-PRAHST-ohn) USAN.
Use: Prostaglandin.

Sul-Ray Acne. (Last) Sulfur 2% in cream base. Cream. Jar 1.75 oz, 6.75 oz, 20 oz. *OTC.*
Use: Dermatologic, acne.

Sul-Ray Aloe Vera Analgesic Rub. (Last) Camphor 3.1%, menthol 1.25%. Bot. 4 oz, 8 oz. *OTC.*
Use: Analgesic, topical.

Sul-Ray Aloe Vera Skin Protectant. (Last) Zinc oxide 1%, allantoin 0.5%. Cream. Jar 1 oz. *OTC.*
Use: Dermatologic, protectant.

Sul-Ray Shampoo. (Last) Sulfur shampoo 2%. Bot. 8 oz. *OTC.*
Use: Antidandruff.

Sul-Ray Soap. (Last) Sulfur soap. Bar 3 oz. *OTC.*
Use: Dermatologic, acne.

Sulster. (Akorn) Sulfacetamide sodium 1%. Soln. 5 mL, 10 mL. *Rx.*
Use: Ophthalmic antibiotic.

•**sultamicillin.** (SULL-TAM-ih-sill-in) USAN.
Use: Anti-infective.

•**sulthiame.** (sull-THIGH-aim) USAN.
Use: Anticonvulsant.

•**sulukast.** (suh-LOO-kast) USAN.
Use: Antiasthmatic (leukotriene antagonist).

Sumacal. (Biosearch Medical Products) CHO 95 g, 380 Cal., Na 100 mg, chloride 210 mg, K < 39 mg, Ca 20 mg/100 g. Pow. Bot. 400 g. *OTC.*
Use: Glucose polymer.

Sumadan. (Medimetriks) Sodium sulfacetamide 9%, sulfur 4.5%. Alcohols, aloe, edetate disodium, glyceryl, green tea, parabens, PEG. Soap. 473 mL. *Rx.*
Use: Anti-infective, antibiotic combination.

Sumadan XLT Wash. (Medimetriks) Sodium sulfacetamide 9%, sulfur 4.5%. Alcohols, edetate disodium, glyceryl, lemon oil, PEG, propylene glycol. Soap. 473 mL w/*Niseko* sunscreen SPF 25. Avobenzone 3%, octinoxate 7.5%, octisalate 5%. Alcohols, edetate disodium, glycerin, glyceryl, isoparaffin, methylparaben. 90 mL. *Rx.*

Use: Topical anti-infective, antibiotic agent.

•**sumarotene.** (sue-MAHR-oh-teen) USAN.
Use: Keratolytic.

•**sumatriptan.** (SUE-muh-TRIP-tan) *USP.*
Tall Man: SUMAtriptan
Use: Agent for migraine, serotonin 5-HT_1 receptor agonist.
See: Imitrex.

sumatriptan. (Sandoz) Sumatriptan 5 mg, 20 mg. Soln., intranasal. 100 mcL unit-dose spray device. 6s. *Rx.*
Use: Agent for migraine, serotonin 5-HT_1 receptor agonist.

sumatriptan. (Various Mfr.) Sumatriptan succinate 25 mg, 50 mg, 100 mg. May contain lactose, PEG. Tab. 9s, 100s, UD 9s. *Rx.*
Use: Agent for migraine, serotonin 5-HT_1 receptor agonist.

•**sumatriptan succinate.** (SUE-muh-TRIP-tan SOOS-in-ate) USAN.
Tall Man: SUMAtriptan
Use: Antimigraine agent, serotonin 5-HT_1 receptor agonist.
See: Alsuma.
Imitrex.
Sumavel.
Zecuity.

sumatriptan succinate. (Sandoz) Sumatriptan. Inj., Soln. **6 mg per 0.5 mL:** Sodium chloride 3.5 mg. Single-dose prefilled syringe cartridge. 6 mg. **4 mg per 0.5 mL:** Sodium chloride 3.8 mg. Single-dose vial. 4 mg. *Rx.*
Use: Agent for migraine, serotonin 5-HT_1 receptor agonist.

Sumavel. (Zogenix) Sumatriptan succinate 6 mg per 0.5 mL. Sodium chloride 3.5 mg. Inj., Soln. Single-dose, prefilled, needle-free *DosePro* system. *Rx.*
Use: Agent for migraine, serotonin 5-HT_1 receptor agonist.

Sumaxin. (Medimetriks) Sodium sulfacetamide 10%, sulfur 4%. Aloe, cetyl alcohol, edetate disodium, glycerin, glyceryl stearate, green tea, parabens, PEG-100, stearyl alcohol. Pad. 60s. *Rx.*
Use: Acne product combination.

Sumaxin CP. (Medimetriks) Sodium sulfacetamide 10%, sulfur 4%. Alcohols, aloe, BHT, edetate disodium, glycerin, glyceryl, green tea, parabens, PEG. Pads. Kit w/60 pads and 473 mL of *Rehyla Wash. Rx.*
Use: Acne product combination.

Sumaxin TS. (Medimetriks) Sodium sulfacetamide 8%, sulfur 4%. Aloe, cetyl alcohol, edetate disodium, glyceryl, green tea, parabens, PEG-100, stearyl alcohol. Susp., topical. 473 mL. *Rx.*
Use: Acne product combination.

Sumaxin Wash. (Medimetriks) Sodium sulfacetamide 9%, sulfur 4%. Aloe, cetyl alcohol, edetate disodium, glyceryl, green tea, parabens, PEG-100, stearyl alcohol. Liq. 473 mL. *Rx.*
Use: Acne product combination.

Summer's Eve Disposable Douche. (C.B. Fleet) **Soln.:** Vinegar. 135 mL (1s, 2s). **Soln. Reg.:** Citric acid, sodium benzoate. **Soln. Scented:** Citric acid, sodium benzoate, octoxynol-9, EDTA. 135 mL (1s, 2s, 4s). *OTC.*
Use: Douche.

Summer's Eve Disposable Douche Extra Cleansing. (C.B. Fleet) Vinegar, sodium Cl, benzoic acid. Soln. 135 mL (1s, 2s, 4s). *OTC.*
Use: Douche.

Summer's Eve Feminine Bath. (C.B. Fleet) Ammonium laureth sulfate, EDTA. Liq. Bot. 45 mL, 345 mL. *OTC.*
Use: Vaginal preparation.

Summer's Eve Feminine Powder. (C.B. Fleet) Cornstarch, octoxynol-9, benzethonium chloride. Pow. Bot. 30 g, 210 g. *OTC.*
Use: Vaginal preparation.

Summer's Eve Feminine Wash. (C.B. Fleet) **Wipes:** Octoxynol-9, EDTA. Box 16s. **Liq.:** Ammonium laureth sulfate, PEG-75, lanolin, EDTA. Bot. 60 mL, 240 mL, 450 mL. *Rx.*
Use: Vaginal preparation.

Summer's Eve Medicated Disposable Douche. (C.B. Fleet) Contains povidone-iodide 0.3%. Single or twin 135 mL disposable units. *OTC.*
Use: Temporary relief of minor vaginal irritation and itching.

Summer's Eve Post Menstrual Disposable Douche. (C.B. Fleet) Sodium lauryl sulfate, parabens, monosodium and disodium phosphates, EDTA. Soln. 135 mL (2s). *OTC.*
Use: Douche.

Summit Extra Strength. (Pfeiffer) Acetaminophen 250 mg, aspirin 250 mg, caffeine 65 mg. Capl. Bot. 50s. *OTC.*
Use: Analgesic combination.

•**suncillin sodium.** (SUN-SILL-in SOE-dee-um) USAN.
Use: Anti-infective.

Sundown. (Johnson & Johnson) A series of products marketed under the Sundown name including: **Moderate:** (SPF 4) Padimate O, oxybenzone. **Extra:** (SPF 6) Oxybenzone, padimate O. **Maximal:** (SPF 8) Oxybenzone,

padimate O. **Ultra:** (SPF 15, 30) oxybenzone, padimate O, octyl methoxycinnamate. *OTC.*
Use: Sunscreen.

Sundown Sport Sunblock. (Johnson & Johnson) Titanium dioxide, zinc oxide. PABA free. Waterproof. SPF 15. Lot. 90 mL. *OTC.*
Use: Sunscreen.

Sundown Sunblock Cream Ultra SPF 24. (Johnson & Johnson) Padimate O, oxybenzone. *OTC.*
Use: Sunscreen.

Sundown Sunblock Stick SPF 15. (Johnson & Johnson) Octyl dimethyl PABA, oxybenzone. Stick 0.35 oz. *OTC.*
Use: Sunscreen.

Sundown Sunblock Stick SPF 20. (Johnson & Johnson) Octyl dimethyl PABA, octyl methoxycinnamate, oxybenzone, titanium dioxide. *OTC.*
Use: Sunscreen.

Sundown Sunblock Ultra Lotion 30 SPF. (Johnson & Johnson) Octyl methoxycinnamate, octyl salicylate, oxybenzone, titanium dioxide, cetyl alcohol, PABA free. Waterproof. Lot. Bot. 120 mL. *OTC.*
Use: Sunscreen.

Sundown Sunblock Ultra SPF 20. (Johnson & Johnson) Octyl dimethyl PABA, octyl methoxycinnamate, oxybenzone, titanium dioxide. *OTC.*
Use: Sunscreen.

Sundown Sunscreen Stick SPF 8. (Johnson & Johnson) Octyl dimethyl PABA, oxybenzone. Stick 0.35 oz. *OTC.*
Use: Sunscreen.

Sundown Sunscreen Ultra. (Johnson & Johnson) Octyl methoxycinnamate, octyl salicylate, oxybenzone, titanium dioxide, stearyl alcohol, cetyl alcohol, PABA free. Waterproof. SPF 15. Cream. Tube 60 g. *OTC.*
Use: Sunscreen.

•**sunepitron hydrochloride.** (soo-NE-pi-tron) USAN.
Use: Anxiolytic; antidepressant.

Sunice. (Citroleum) Allantoin 0.25%, menthol 0.25%, methyl salicylate 10%. Cream. Jar 3 oz. *OTC.*
Use: Burn therapy.

•**sunitinib malate.** (sue-NIH-tih-nib) USAN.
Tall Man: SUNItinib
Use: Protein-tyrosine kinase inhibitor.
See: Sutent.

Sunkist Multivitamins Complete, Children's. (Novartis) Fe 18 mg, vitamin A 5000 units, D_3 400 units, E 30 units, B_1 1.5 mg, B_2 1.7 mg, B_3 20 mg, B_5 10 mg, B_6 2 mg, B_{12} 6 mcg, C 60 mg, folic acid 400 mcg, Ca 100 mg, Cu, I, K, Mg, Mn, P, Zn 10 mg, biotin 40 mcg, K_1 10 mcg. Sorbitol, aspartame, phenylalanine, tartrazine. Chew. Tab. Bot. 60s. *OTC.*
Use: Mineral, vitamin supplement.

Sunkist Multivitamins + Extra C, Children's. (Novartis) Vitamin A 2500 units, E 15 units, D_3 400 units, B_1 1.05 mg, B_2 1.2 mg, B_3 13.5 mg, B_6 1.05 mg, B_{12} 4.5 mcg, C 250 mg, folic acid 0.3 mg, vitamin K 5 mcg, sorbitol, aspartame, phenylalanine. Chew. Tab. Bot. 60s. *OTC.*
Use: Vitamin supplement.

Sunkist Vitamin C. (Novartis) Vitamin C (as ascorbic acid and sodium ascorbate) 60 mg, 250 mg, 500 mg. Fructose (except 60 mg), sorbitol, sucrose, lactose, orange flavor. Chew. Tab. Bot. 11s (60 mg only), 60s (250 mg only), 75s (500 mg only). *OTC.*
Use: Water-soluble vitamin.

SUNPRuF 15. (C & M Pharmacal) Octyl methoxycinnamate 7.5%, benzopherone-3 5%. PABA free. Waterproof. SPF 15. Lot. Bot. 240 mL. *OTC.*
Use: Sunscreen.

SUNPRuF 17. (C & M Pharmacal) Octyl methoxycinnamate 7.8%, octyl salicylate 5.2%, oil-free, water-resistant. SPF 17. Lot. Bot. 120 g. *OTC.*
Use: Sunscreen.

Sunshine Chewable Tablets. (Fibertone) Fe 5 mg, vitamins A 5000 units, D 400 units, E 67 mg, B_1 15 mg, B_2 15 mg, B_3 25 mg, B_5 20 mg, B_6 15 mg, B_{12} 15 mcg, C 150 mg, folic acid 0.1 mg, Ca, Cu, Mn, Zn, K, iodide, biotin, betaine, PABA, choline bitartrate, inositol, lecithin, hesperidin, rutin, bioflavonoids. Sorbitol, aspartame. Citrus flavor. Bot. 60s. *OTC.*
Use: Mineral, vitamin supplement.

Sunstick. (Rydelle) Lip and face protectant containing digalloyl trioleate 2.5% in emollient base. Stick Plas. swivel container 0.14 oz. *OTC.*
Use: Lip protectant.

SU-101.
Use: Malignant glioma. [Orphan Drug]

Supartz. (Bioventus) Sodium hyaluronate 10 mg/mL. Inj. Prefilled syringes. 2.5 mL. *Rx.*
Use: Physical adjunct.

Super Aytinal. (Walgreen) Vitamins A 7000 units, B_1 5 mg, B_2 5 mg, B_5 10 mg, B_6 3 mg, B_{12} 9 mcg, C 90 mg, pantothenic acid 10 mg, D 400 units, E 30 units, niacin 30 mg, biotin 55 mcg, folic acid 0.4 mg, Fe 30 mg, Ca 162 mg,

P 125 mg, I 150 mcg, Cu 3 mg, Mn 7.5 mg, Mg 100 mg, K 7.7 mg, Zn 24 mg, Cl 7 mg, Cr 15 mcg, Se 15 mcg, choline bitartrate 1000 mcg, inositol 1000 mcg, PABA 1000 mcg, rutin 1000 mcg, yeast 12 mg. Bot. 50s, 100s, 365s. *OTC.*
Use: Mineral, vitamin supplement.

Super-B. (Towne) Vitamins B_1 50 mg, B_2 20 mg, B_6 5 mg, B_{12} 15 mcg, C 300 mg, liver desiccated 100 mg, dried yeast 100 mg, niacinamide 25 mg, Ca pantothenate 5 mg, Fe 10 mg. Captab. Bot. 50s, 100s, 150s, 250s. *OTC.*
Use: Mineral, vitamin supplement.

Super Calcium 600 + D_3 400. (Mason) Vitamin D_3 400 units, calcium carbonate 600 mg. Maltodextrin, mineral oil, soy. Preservative free. Tab. 400s. *OTC.*
Use: Nutritional supplement.

Super Calcium 1200. (Schiff Products/ Weider Nutrition Intl.) Calcium carbonate 1512 mg (600 mg calcium). Cap. Bot. 60s, 120s. *OTC.*
Use: Mineral supplement.

Super Calicaps M-Z. (Nion Corp.) Ca 1200 mg, Mg 400 mg, Zn 15 mg, vitamins A 5000 units, D 400 units, Se 15 mcg. 3 Tabs. Bot. 90s. *OTC.*
Use: Mineral, vitamin supplement.

Super D Perles. (Pharmacia) Vitamins A 10,000 units, D 400 units. Cap. Bot. 100s. *OTC.*
Use: Vitamin supplement.

SuperEPA. (Advanced Nutritional Technology) Omega-3 polyunsaturated fatty acids 1200 mg. Cap. containing EPA 360 mg, DHA 240 mg. Bot. 60s, 90s. *OTC.*
Use: Nutritional supplement.

SuperEPA 2000. (Advanced Nutritional Technology) EPA 563 mg, DHA 312 mg, vitamin E 20 units. Cap. Bot. 30s, 60s, 90s. *OTC.*
Use: Nutritional supplement.

Supere-Pect. (Barth's) Alpha tocopherol 400 units, apple pectin 100 mg. Cap. Bot. 50s, 100s, 250s. *OTC.*
Use: Nutritional supplement.

Super Hi Potency. (Nion Corp.) Vitamins A 10,000 units, D 400 units, E 150 units, B_1 75 mg, B_2 75 mg, B_3 75 mg, B_5 75 mg, B_6 75 mg, B_{12} 75 mcg, C 250 mg, folic acid 0.4 mg, Zn 15 mg, betaine, biotin 75 mcg, Ca, Fe, hesperidin, I, K, Mg, Mn, Se. Tab. Bot. 100s. *OTC.*
Use: Mineral, vitamin supplement.

Super Hydramin Protein Powder. (Nion Corp.) Protein 41%, carbohydrate 21.8%, fat 1% in powder form. Can 1 lb. *OTC.*
Use: Nutritional supplement.

superinone. Tyloxapol.

Super Nutri-Vites. (Faraday) Vitamins A 36,000 units, D 400 units, B_1 25 mg, B_2 25 mg, B_6 50 mg, B_{12} 50 mcg, niacinamide 50 mg, Ca pantothenate 12.5 mg, choline bitartrate 150 mg, inositol 150 mg, betaine hydrochloride 25 mg, PABA 15 mg, glutamic acid 25 mg, desiccated liver 50 mg, C 150 mg, E 12.5 units, Mn gluconate 6.15 mg, bone meal 162 mg, Fe gluconate 50 mg, Cu gluconate 0.25 mg, Zn gluconate 2.2 mg, K iodide 0.1 mg, Ca 53.3 mg, P 24.3 mg, Mg gluconate 7.2 mg. Protein-coated Tab. Bot. 60s, 100s. *OTC.*
Use: Mineral, vitamin supplement.

superoxide dismutase (recombinant human).
Use: Protection of donor organ tissue. [Orphan Drug]

Super Plenamins Multiple Vitamins and Minerals. (Rexall Group) Vitamins A 8000 units, D_2 400 units, vitamins B_1 2.5 mg, B_2 2.5 mg, C 75 mg, niacinamide 20 mg, B_6 1 mg, B_{12} 3 mcg, biotin 20 mcg, E 10 units, pantothenic acid 3 mg, liver conc. 100 mg, Fe 30 mg, Ca 75 mg, P 58 mg, I 0.15 mg, Cu 0.75 mg, Mn 1.25 mg, Mg 10 mg, Zn 1 mg. Tab. Bot. 36s, 72s, 144s, 288s, 365s. *OTC.*
Use: Mineral, vitamin supplement.

Superplex T. (Major) Vitamins B_1 15 mg, B_2 10 mg, B_3 100 mg, B_5 20 mg, B_6 5 mg, B_{12} 10 mcg, C 500 mg. Tab. Bot. 100s. *OTC.*
Use: Vitamin supplement.

Super Poli-Grip/Wernet's Cream. (Block Drug) Carboxymethylcellulose gum, ethylene oxide polymer, petrolatum-mineral oil base. Tube 0.7 oz, 1.4 oz, 2.4 oz. *OTC.*
Use: Denture adhesive.

Super Quints-50. (Freeda) Vitamins B_1 50 mg, B_2 50 mg, B_3 50 mg, B_5 50 mg, B_6 50 mg, B_{12} 50 mcg, folic acid 0.4 mg, PABA 30 mg, d-biotin 50 mcg, inositol 50 mg. Tab. Bot. 100s, 250s, 500s. *OTC.*
Use: Vitamin supplement.

Super Shade SPF-25. (Schering-Plough) Ethylhexyl p-methoxycinnamate, padimate O oxybenzone. SPF 25. Lot. Bot. 4 fl. oz. *OTC.*
Use: Sunscreen.

Super Shade Sunblock Stick SPF-25. (Schering-Plough) Ethylhexyl p-methoxycinnamate, oxybenzone, padimate O in stick. SPF 25. Tube 0.43 oz.

OTC.
Use: Sunscreen.
Super Strength D-2000 IU. (Nature's Bounty) Vitamin D_3 (cholecalciferol) 2,000 units. Calcium 142 mg. Gluten free, preservative free, and sugar free. Tab. 100s. *OTC.*
Use: Fat-soluble vitamin.
Super Stress. (Towne) Vitamins C 600 mg, E 30 units B_1 15 mg, B_2 15 mg, niacin 100 mg, B_6 5 mg, B_{12} 12 mcg, pantothenic acid 20 mg. Tab. Bot. 60s. *OTC.*
Use: Vitamin supplement.
Super Troche. (Weeks & Leo) Benzocaine 5 mg, cetalkonium Cl 1 mg. Loz. Bot. 15s, 30s. *OTC.*
Use: Mouth and throat preparation.
Super Troche Plus. (Weeks & Leo) Benzocaine 10 mg, cetalkonium Cl 2 mg. Loz. Bot. 12s. *OTC.*
Use: Mouth and throat preparation.
Super-T with Zinc. (Towne) Vitamins A 10,000 units, D 400 units, E 15 units, C 200 mg, B_1 10 mg, B_2 10 mg, B_6 5 mg, B_{12} 6 mcg, niacinamide 50 mg, Fe 18 mg, I 0.1 mg, Cu 2 mg, Mn 1 mg, Zn 15 mg. Cap. Bot. 130s. *OTC.*
Use: Mineral, vitamin supplement.
Supervim. (US Ethicals) Vitamins and minerals. Tab. Bot. 100s.
Use: Mineral, vitamin supplement.
Super Wernet's Powder. (Block Drug) Carboxymethylcellulose gum, ethylene oxide polymer. Bot. 0.63 oz, 1.75 oz, 3.55 oz. *OTC.*
Use: Denture adhesive.
Suplena. (Abbot Nutrition) Protein (L-carnitine, milk protein, taurine) 45 g, carbohydrates (corn maltodextrin, maltitol syrup, sucrose) 205 g, fat (fructooligosaccharides, high oleic safflower oil, canola oil, soy lecithin) 96/L. Sodium 785 mg/L, potassium 1120 mg/L, 600 mOsm/kg H_2O, 1.8 cal/mL. Vitamins A, B_1, B_2, B_3, B_5, B_6, B_7, B_{12}, C, D, E, K, Ca, choline, Cl^-, Cr, Cu, Fe, folic acid, I, Mg, Mn, Mo, P, Se, Zn. Gluten and lactose free. Vanilla flavor. Liq. 240 mL. *OTC.*
Use: Enteral nutritional therapy, defined formula diets.
Suplical. (Parke-Davis) Calcium 600 mg/Square. Bot. 30s, 60s. *OTC.*
Use: Mineral supplement.
Supprelin LA. (Indevus) Histrelin acetate 50 mg. Implant, Subcutaneous. In carton with implantation kit. *Rx.*
Use: Hormone, gonadotropin-releasing hormone analog.
Suppress. (Ferndale) Dextromethorphan HBr 7.5 mg. Loz. 1000s. *OTC.*
Use: Antitussive.
Supra Min. (Towne) Vitamins A 10,000 units, D 400 units, E 30 units, C 250 mg, folic acid 0.4 mg, B_1 10 mg, B_2 10 mg, niacin 100 mg, B_6 5 mg, B_{12} 6 mcg, pantothenic acid 20 mg, I 150 mcg, Fe 100 mg, Mg 2 mg, Cu 20 mg, Mn 1.25 mg. Tab. Bot. 130s. *OTC.*
Use: Mineral, vitamin supplement.
Suprane. (Baxter) Desflurane. 240 mL. Volatile Liq. Bot. *Rx.*
Use: Anesthetic, general.
Suprarenal. Dried, partially defatted and powdered adrenal gland of cattle, sheep, or swine.
Suprax. (Lupin Pharma) Cefixime. **Tab.:** 400 mg. Film coated. Lactose, PEG. 10s, 50s, 100s. **Chew. Tab.:** 100 mg, 150 mg, 200 mg. Aspartame; mannitol; phenylalanine 3.3 mg (100 mg), 5 mg (150 mg), 6.7 mg (200 mg); tutti frutti flavoring. 10s. 50s, UD 60s. **Cap.:** 400 mg. Mannitol. 50s. **Pow. for Oral Susp.:** 100 mg/5 mL, 200 mg/5 mL, 500 mg/5 mL. Sodium benzoate, sucralose (500 mg/5 mL only), sucrose. Strawberry flavored. 10 mL, 20 mL (500 mg/5 mL); 25 mL, 37.5 mL, 50 mL, 75 mL, 100 mL (200 mg/5 mL); 50 mL (100 mg/5 mL). *Rx.*
Use: Anti-infective, cephalosporin.
Suprazine. (Major) Trifluoperazine 1 mg, 2 mg, 5 mg, 10 mg. Tab. Bot. 100s, 250s, 1000s, UD 100s (2 mg only). *Rx.*
Use: Anxiolytic.
Suprenza. (Akrimax) Phentermine hydrochloride 15 mg (equiv. to 12 mg phentermine base), 30 mg (equiv. to 24 mg phentermine base), 37.5 mg (equiv. to 30 mg phentermine base). Mannitol, sucralose. Peppermint flavor. Tab., disintegrating. 30s. *c-iv.*
Use: CNS stimulant, sympathomimetic anorexiant.
Suprep Bowel Prep. (Braintree Labs) Sodium sulfate 17.5 g, potassium sulfate 3.13 g, magnesium sulfate 1.6 g per 180 mL. Sodium benzoate, sucralose. Soln. Kit w/2s and mixing container. *Rx.*
Use: Laxative, miscellaneous bowel evacuant.
Suprins. (Towne) Vitamins A palmitate 10,000 units, D 400 units, B_1 10 mg, B_2 10 mg, B_6 5 mg, B_{12} 6 mcg, C 250 mg, calcium pantothenate 20 mg, niacinamide 100 mg, biotin 25 mcg, E 15 units, Ca 103 mg, P 80 mg, Fe 10 mg, I 0.1 mg, Cu 1.0 mg, Zn 20 mg, Mn 1.25 mg. Captab. Bot. 100s. *OTC.*
Use: Mineral, vitamin supplement.

•**suproclone.** (SUH-pro-klone) USAN.
Use: Sedative; hypnotic.
•**suprofen.** (sue-PRO-fen) *USP.*
Use: Anti-inflammatory.
•**suramin hexasodium.** (SOOR-ah-min hex-ah-SOE-dee-um) USAN.
Use: Antineoplastic.
Surbex Filmtab. (Abbott) Vitamins B_1 6 mg, B_2 6 mg, B_3 30 mg, B_6 2.5 mg, B_5 10 mg, B_{12} 5 mcg. Filmtab. Bot. 100s. *OTC.*
Use: Mineral, vitamin supplement.
Surbex 750 with Iron. (Abbott) Vitamins B_1 15 mg, B_2 15 mg, B_6 25 mg, B_{12} 12 mcg, C 750 mg, B_5 20 mg, E 30 units, B_3 100 mg, Fe 27 mg, folic acid 0.4 mg. Tab. Bot. 50s. *OTC.*
Use: Mineral, vitamin supplement.
Surbex 750 with Zinc. (Abbott) B_1 15 mg, B_2 15 mg, B_6 20 mg, B_{12} 12 mcg, C 750 mg, E 30 units, B_5 20 mg, niacin 100 mg, folic acid 0.4 mg, Zn 22.5 mg. Tab. Bot. 50s. *OTC.*
Use: Mineral, vitamin supplement.
Surbex-T Filmtab. (Abbott) Vitamins B_1 15 mg, B_2 10 mg, B_3 100 mg, B_6 5 mg, B_{12} 10 mcg, B_5 20 mg, C 500 mg. Filmtab. Bot. 100s. *OTC.*
Use: Mineral, vitamin supplement.
Surbex with C Filmtabs. (Abbott) Vitamins B_1 6 mg, B_2 6 mg, B_3 30 mg, B_5 10 mg, B_6 2.5 mg, B_{12} 5 mg, C 500 mg. Film-coated. Tab. Bot. 100s. *OTC.*
Use: Vitamin supplement.
Surbu-Gen-T. (Ivax) Vitamins B_1 15 mg, B_2 10 mg, B_3 100 mg, B_5 20 mg, B_6 5 mg, B_{12} 10 mcg, C 500 mg. Tab. Bot. 100s. *OTC.*
Use: Vitamin supplement.
SureCell HCG-Urine Test. (Kodak Dental) Polyclonal/monoclonal antibody sandwich-based ELISA to detect human chorionic gonadotropin in urine. Kit 10s, 25s, 100s.
Use: Diagnostic aid.
SureCell Herpes (HSV) Test. (Kodak Dental) Monoclonal antibody-based ELISA to detect HSV 1 & 2 antigens from lesions. Kit 10s, 25s.
Use: Diagnostic aid.
SureCell Strep A Test. (Kodak Dental) ELISA to detect group A streptococci. Kit 10s, 25s, 100s.
Use: Diagnostic aid.
SureLac. (Caraco) 3000 FCC lactase units, sorbitol, mannitol. Chew. Tab. Bot. 60s. *OTC.*
Use: Nutritional supplement.
surface active extract of saline lavage of bovine lungs.
Use: Respiratory failure in preterm infants. [Orphan Drug]
surfactant, natural lung.
Use: Surfactant replacement therapy in neonatal respiratory distress syndrome.
See: Survanta.
surfactant, synthetic lung.
Use: Surfactant replacement therapy in neonatal respiratory distress syndrome.
Surfak Stool Softener. (Chattem) Docusate calcium 240 mg. Corn oil, glycerin, propylene glycol, sorbitol. Cap., soft gel. 10s. *OTC.*
Use: Laxative, fecal softener/surfactant.
Surfaxin. (Discovery Laboratories) Lucinactant 30 mg phospholipids per mL. Dipalmitoylphosphatidylcholine 22.5 mg, palmitoyloleoylphosphatidylglycerol, sodium salt 7.5 mg, palmitic acid 4.05 mg, sinapultide 0.862 mg. Preservative free. Susp., intratracheal. Single-use vial. 8.5 mL. *Rx.*
Use: Lung surfactant.
•**surfilcon A.** (SER-FILL-kahn A) USAN.
Use: Hydrophilic contact lens material.
Surfol Post-Immersion Bath Oil. (Stiefel) Mineral oil, isopropyl myristate, isostearic acid, PEG-40, sorbitan peroleate. Bot. 8 oz. *OTC.*
Use: Dermatologic.
•**surfomer.** (SER-foe-mer) USAN.
Use: Hypolipidemic.
Surgasoap. (Wade) Castile vegetable oils. Bot. Qt., gal. *OTC.*
Use: Dermatologic, cleanser.
Surgel. (Ulmer Pharmacal) Propylene glycol, glycerin. Gel. Bot. 120 mL, 240 mL, gal. *OTC.*
Use: Lubricant.
Surgel Liquid. (Ulmer Pharmacal) Patient lubricant fluid. Bot. 4 oz, 8 oz, gal.
Use: Lubricant.
•**surgibone.** (SER-jih-bone) USAN. Bone and cartilage obtained from bovine embryos and young calves.
Use: Prosthetic aid (internal bone splint).
Surgical Simplex P. (Howmedica) Methyl methacrylate 20 mL poly 6.7 g, methyl methacrylate-styrene copolymer 33.3 g. **Pow.:** 40 g. **Liq.:** 20 mL. Bot.
Use: Bone cement.
Surgical Simplex P Radiopaque. (Howmedica) Methyl methacrylate 20 mL, poly 6 g, methyl methacrylate-styrene copolymer 30 g. **Pow.:** 40 g. **Liq.:** 20 mL. Bot.
Use: Bone cement.
Surgicel. (Johnson & Johnson) Sterile absorbable knitted fabric prepared by

controlled oxidation of regenerated cellulose. Sterile strips 2 × 14, 4 × 8, 2 × 3, 0.5 × 2 inches. Surgical Nu-knit: 1 × 1, 3 × 4, 6 × 9 inches. Box 1s. *Rx.*
Use: Hemostatic.

Surgidine. (Continental Consumer Products) Iodine 0.8% in iodine complex. Germicide. Bot. 8 oz, gal. Foot operated dispenser 8 oz, gal. *OTC.*
Use: Antiseptic.

Surgi-Kleen. (Sween) Bot. 2 oz, 8 oz, 16 oz, 21 oz, gal, 5 gal, 30 gal, 55 gal.
Use: Dermatologic, cleanser.

Surgilube. (E. Fougera) Sterile surgical lubricant. Foilpac 3 g, 5 g. Tube 5 g, 2 oz, 4.25 oz.
Use: Lubricant.

Surgilube. (Savage) Chlorhexidine gluconate. Jelly; vaginal. 5 g, 120.49 g. *OTC.*
Use: Miscellaneous vaginal preparation.

•**suricainide maleate.** (ser-ih-CANE-ide) USAN.
Use: Cardiovascular agent (antiarrhythmic).

•**suritozole.** (suh-RIH-tah-ZOLE) USAN.
Use: Antidepressant.

Surmontil. (Barr/Duramed) Trimipramine maleate 25 mg, 50 mg, 100 mg. Lactose. Cap. Bot. 100s, UD 100s (50 mg only). *Rx.*
Use: Antidepressant.

surofene. Hexachlorophene.

•**suronacrine maleate.** (SUE-row-NAH-kreen) USAN.
Use: Cholinergic; cholinesterase inhibitor.

•**surotomycin.** (sur-OH-toe-MYE-sin) USAN.
Use: Antibacterial.

Surpass. (Wrigley) Calcium carbonate 300 mg (elemental calcium 120 mg). Aspartame, sorbitol, phenylalanine 3.9 mg. Wintergreen flavor. Gum. Box. 10s. *OTC.*
Use: Mineral supplement; antacid.

Surpass Extra Strength. (Wrigley) Calcium carbonate 450 mg (elemental calcium 180 mg). Aspartame, sorbitol, phenylalanine 3.9 mg. Fruit flavor. Gum. Box. 10s. *OTC.*
Use: Mineral supplement; antacid.

Survanta. (Ross Labs) Beractant 25 mg/mL, sodium chloride solution 0.9%, triglycerides 0.5 to 1.75 mg, free fatty acids 1.4 to 3.5 mg, protein < 1 mg/mL. Susp. Single-use vial containing 8 mL suspension. *Rx.*
Use: Lung surfactant.

Suspen. (Circle) Penicillin V potassium 250 mg/5 mL. Bot. 100 mL. *Rx.*
Use: Anti-infective, penicillin.

•**suspension structured vehicle.** *NF.*
Use: Pharmaceutical vehicle.

Sustacal Basic. (Bristol-Myers Squibb) A vanilla, strawberry, or chocolate flavored liquid containing 36.6 g protein, 34.6 g fat, 145.8 g carbohydrate, 833 mg Na, 1583 mg K/L. 1.04 Cal/mL, with appropriate vitamin and mineral levels to meet 100% of the US RDAs. Liq. Can 240 mL. *OTC.*
Use: Nutritional supplement.

Sustacal HC. (Bristol-Myers Squibb) High calorie nutritionally complete food. Protein 16%, fat 34%, carbohydrate 50%. Can 8 oz. Vanilla, chocolate, or eggnog. *OTC.*
Use: Nutritional supplement.

Sustacal Plus. (Bristol-Myers Squibb) A vanilla, eggnog, or chocolate flavored liquid containing 61 g protein, 58 g fat, 190 g carbohydrate, 15.2 mg Fe, 850 mg Na, 1480 mg K, 1520 cal/L, with appropriate vitamin and mineral levels to meet 100% of the US RDAs. Liq. Bot. 237 mL, 960 mL. *OTC.*
Use: Nutritional supplement.

Sustacal Powder. (Bristol-Myers Squibb) Caloric distribution and nutritional value when added to milk are similar to that of Sustacal liquid except lactose. Contains vanilla: Pow. 1.9 oz. packets 4s, 1 lb. can; Chocolate 1.9 oz. packets 4s. *OTC.*
Use: Nutritional supplement.

Sustacal Pudding. (Bristol-Myers Squibb) Ready-to-eat fortified pudding containing at least 15% of the US RDAs for protein, vitamins and minerals, in a 240 calorie serving. As a % of the calories, protein 11%, fat 36%, carbohydrate 53%. Flavors: Chocolate, vanilla, and butterscotch. Tins, 5 oz, 110 oz. *OTC.*
Use: Nutritional supplement.

Sustagen. (Bristol-Myers Squibb) High-calorie, high-protein supplement containing as a % of the calories, 24% protein, 8% fat, 68% carbohydrate. Contains all known essential vitamins and minerals. Prepared from nonfat milk, corn syrup solids, powdered whole milk, calcium caseinate, and dextrose. Vanilla: Can 1 lb, 5 lb. Chocolate: Can 1 lb. *OTC.*
Use: Nutritional supplement.

Sustain. (Zee Medical) Sodium chloride 220 mg, calcium carbonate 18 mg, potassium chloride 15 mg. Tab. 24s. *Rx.*
Use: Salt replacement.

Sustenex. (Ganeden) *B. coagulans* 2 billion viable cells. Lactose free. Cap. 30s. *OTC.*
Use: Probiotic.

Sustiva. (Bristol-Myers Squibb) Efavirenz. **Cap:** 50 mg, 200 mg. Lactose. Bot. 30s (50 mg), 90s (200 mg). **Tab:** 600 mg. Lactose. Bot. 30s. *Rx.*
Use: Antiretroviral, non-nucleoside reverse transcriptase inhibitor.

Sutent. (Pfizer) Sunitinib malate (as base) 12.5 mg, 25 mg, 50 mg. Cap. 28s. *Rx.*
Use: Protein-tyrosine kinase inhibitor.

•**sutezolid.** (soo-TEZ-oh-lid) USAN.
Use: Antituberculosis agent.

•**suture, absorbable surgical.** (SOO-chur) *USP.*
Use: Surgical aid.

•**suture, nonabsorbable surgical.** (SOO-chur) *USP.*
Use: Surgical aid.

Suvaplex. (Tennessee Pharmaceutic) Vitamins A 5000 units, D 500 units, B_1 2.5 mg, B_2 2.5 mg, B_6 0.5 mg, B_{12} 1 mcg, C 37.5 mg, Ca pantothenate 5 mg, niacinamide 20 mg, folic acid 0.1 mg. Tab. Bot. 100s. *OTC.*
Use: Mineral, vitamin supplement.

•**suvorexant.** (SOO-voe-REX-ant) USAN.
Use: CNS agent.

•**suxemerid sulfate.** (sux-EM-er-rid) USAN.
Use: Antitussive.

swamp root. Compound of various organic roots in an alcohol base.
Use: Diuretic to the kidney.

Sween-A-Peel. (Sween) Wafer 4 × 4. Box 5s, 20s; Sheets 1212. Box 2s, 12s. *OTC.*
Use: Dermatologic, protectant.

Sween Cream. (Coloplast) Beeswax, cetyl alcohol, cod liver oil (vitamins A and D), lanolin oil, stearyl alcohol. Cream. 340 g. *OTC.*
Use: Emollient.

Sween Kind Lotion. (Sween) Bot. 21 oz, gal. *OTC.*
Use: Dermatologic, cleanser.

Sween Prep. (Sween) Box wipes 54s. Dab-o-matic 2 oz. Spray Top 4 oz. *OTC.*
Use: Dermatologic, protectant, medicated.

Sween Soft Touch. (Sween) Bot. 2 oz, 16 oz, 21 oz, 32 oz, 1 gal., 5 gal. *OTC.*
Use: Dermatologic, protectant, medicated.

Sweeta. (Bristol-Myers Squibb) Saccharin sodium, sorbitol. Bot. 24 mL, 2 oz, 4 oz. *OTC.*
Use: Sweetening agent.

Sweetaste. (Purepac) Saccharin 0.25 g, 0.5 g, 1 g. Tab. w/Sodium bicarbonate. Bot. 1000s. *OTC.*
Use: Sugar substitute.

sweetening agents.
See: Saccharin.
Sweetaste.

Swiss Kriss. (Modern Aids Inc.) Senna leaves, herbs. Coarse cut mixture. Can 1.5 oz, 3.25 oz, Tab. 24s, 120s, 250s. *OTC.*
Use: Laxative.

Syeda. (Sandoz) Drospirenone 3 mg, ethinyl estradiol 30 mcg. Film coated. Lactose, PEG. Tab. Blister card 28s (w/7 inert tablets). *Rx.*
Use: Oral contraceptive.

Sylatron. (Schering) Peginterferon alfa-2b 40 mcg per 0.1 mL, 60 mcg per 0.1 mL, 120 mcg per 0.1 mL (when reconstituted). Inj., lyophilized Pow. for Soln. Single-use vial (contains dibasic sodium phosphate anhydrous 1.11 mg, monobasic sodium phosphate dihydrate 1.11 mg, 0.074 mg of polysorbate 80, sucrose 59.2 mg) w/1.25 mL diluent vial, BD *Safety Lok* syringe, and alcohol swabs. *Rx.*
Use: Immunomodulator.

Syllact. (Wallace) Psyllium seed husks 3.3 g, 14 cal/rounded tsp, dextrose, parabens, fruit flavor, saccharin. Pow. Bot. 284 g. *OTC.*
Use: Laxative.

Sylvant. (Janssen Biotech) Siltuximab 100 mg, 400 mg. L-histidine 3.7 mg (100 mg), 14.9 mg (400 mg), polysorbate 80, sucrose. Preservative free. Inj., lyophilized Pow. for Soln. Single-use vial. *Rx.*
Use: Monoclonal antibody.

Symax Duotab. (Capellon) Hyoscyamine sulfate 0.375 mg (0.125 mg immediate release, 0.25 mg extended release). ER Tab. 90s. *Rx.*
Use: Gastrointestinal anticholinergic/antispasmodic.

Symax FasTab. (Capellon) Hyoscyamine sulfate 0.125 mg. Lactose, mannitol. Peppermint flavor. Chew. Tab., dispersible. 100s. *Rx.*
Use: Gastrointestinal anticholinergic/antispasmodic.

Symax-SL. (Capellon) Hyoscyamine sulfate 0.125 mg. Lactose, mannitol. Peppermint flavor. Sublingual Tab. 100s. *Rx.*
Use: Anticholinergic, antispasmodic, belladonna alkaloid.

Symax-SR. (Capellon) Hyoscyamine sulfate 0.375 mg. SR Tab. 100s. *Rx.*

Use: Anticholinergic, antispasmodic, belladonna alkaloid.

Symbicort. (AstraZeneca) Budesonide/formoterol 80 mcg/4.5 mcg, 160 mcg/4.5 mcg per actuation. Formoterol 3.7 mcg as the free base, equiv. to formoterol fumarate dihydrate 4.5 mcg. Inh. Aerosol. Canisters 6 g (60 actuations) (160 mcg/4.5 mcg) 6.9 g (60 actuations) (80 mcg/4.5 mcg), 10.2 g (120 a ctuations) with actuator. *Rx.*
Use: Respiratory agent.

Symbyax. (Eli Lilly) Olanzapine/fluoxetine hydrochloride 3 mg/25 mg, 6 mg/25 mg, 6 mg/50 mg, 12 mg/25 mg, 12 mg/50 mg. Cap. 30s; 100s, 1000s, blister UD 100s (except 3 mg/25 mg). *Rx.*
Use: Psychotherapeutic agent.

•**symclosene.** (SIM-kloe-seen) USAN.
Use: Anti-infective, topical.

•**symetine hydrochloride.** (SIM-eh-teen) USAN.
Use: Antiamebic.

Symlin. (Amylin Pharmaceuticals, Inc.) Pramlintide acetate 0.6 mg/mL, 1 mg/mL. Soln. for Inj. Vials. 5 mL (0.6 mg/mL only). Multidose pen injectors (1 mg/mL only). 1.5 mL, 2.7 mL. *Rx.*
Use: Antidiabetic agent, amylin analog.

Symmetrel. (Endo) Amantadine hydrochloride. **Tab:** 100 mg. 100s, 500s. **Syrup:** 50 mg/5 mL. Sorbitol, parabens. 480 mL. *Rx.*
Use: Antiviral; antiparkinsonian; treatment of drug-induced extrapyramidal symptoms.

SymPak PDX. (Dexo) Tab. **Day (Ah-Chew Ultra):** Chlorpheniramine maleate 2 mg (as chlorpheniramine tannate), methscopolamine nitrate 1.5 mg, phenylephrine hydrochloride 10 mg (as phenylephrine tannate). Saccharin, sugar. Blister card for 14-day dosing regimen. 2s. **Night (Dexodryl):** Chlorpheniramine maleate 2 mg (as chlorpheniramine tannate), methscopolamine nitrate 1.5 mg. Saccharin, sugar. Blister card for 14-day dosing regimen. 2s. *Rx.*
Use: Upper respiratory combination; decongestant, antihistamine, and anticholinergic combination.

SymPak II. (Dexo) Tab. **Day (Sinuhist):** Brompheniramine maleate 6 mg, pseudoephedrine hydrochloride 45 mg. Blister card for 14-day dosing regimen. 2s. **Night (Omnihist II LA):** Chlorpheniramine maleate 8 mg, methscopolamine nitrate 2.5 mg, phenylephrine hydrochloride 25 mg. Blister card for 14-day dosing regimen. 2s. *Rx.*
Use: Upper respiratory combination; decongestant, antihistamine, and anticholinergic combination.

sympatholytic agents.
See: Antiadrenergics/sympatholytics.

sympathomimetic agents.
See: Albuterol.
Arfomoterol Tartrate.
Bitolterol Mesylate.
Ephedrine Sulfate.
Epinephrine.
Formoterol Fumarate.
Indacaterol.
Isoetharine Hydrochloride.
Isoproterenol Hydrochloride.
Levalbuterol Hydrochloride.
Metaproterenol Sulfate.
Pirbuterol Acetate.
Salmeterol Xinafoate.
Terbutaline Sulfate.

Syna-Clear. (Pruvo) Decongestant plus Vitamin C. 25 mg. Tab. Bot. 12s, 30s.
Use: Decongestant.

Synacort. (Roche) Hydrocortisone cream. **1%:** Tube 15 g, 30 g, 60 g. **2.5%:** Tube 30 g. *Rx.*
Use: Corticosteroid, topical.

Synagis. (MedImmune) Palivizumab 100 mg/mL. Preservative free. Inj., Soln. Single-dose vial. 0.5 mL (w/histidine 1.9 mg, glycine 0.06 mg/mL), 1 mL (histidine 3.9 mg, glycine 0.1mg/mL). *Rx.*
Use: Monoclonal antibody.

Synalar. (Medimetriks Pharmaceuticals) Fluocinolone acetonide. **Oint.:** 0.025%. 60 g and 120 g and kits w/*Keraden cream* (white petrolatum), 255 g (alcohols, beeswax, caprylic/capric triglyceride, cholesterol, edetate disodium, glycerin, linoleic acid, linolenic acid, methylparaben, olive fruit oil, olive oil, paraffin, petrolatum, sodium hyaluronate, triethanolamine, wax, white petrolatum). **Cream:** 0.025%. 60 g and 120 g and kits w/*Keraden cream* (alcohols, beeswax, edetate disodium, mineral oil, parabens, propylene glycol), 255 g (alcohols, beeswax, caprylic/capric triglyceride, cholesterol, edetate disodium, glycerin, linoleic acid, linolenic acid, methylparaben, olive fruit oil, olive oil, paraffin, petrolatum, sodium hyaluronate, triethanolamine, wax). **Soln.; topical:** Propylene glycol. 60 mL and 90 mL w/applicator. *Rx.*
Use: Anti-inflammatory agent, topical corticosteroid.

Synalar TS Kit. (Medimetriks Pharmaceuticals) Fluocinolone acetonide 0.01%. Propylene glycol. 90 mL.

W/*Rehyla Hair and Body Cleanser.* Cetyl alcohol, cholesterol, edetate disodium, glycerin, glyceryl, PEG, propylene glycol, salicylic acid, sodium hyaluronate, titanium dioxide. Soln.; topical. 454 g. *Rx.*
Use: Anti-inflammatory agent, topical corticosteroid.

Synalgos-DC. (Caraco Pharma) Dihydrocodeine bitartrate 16 mg, aspirin 356.4 mg, caffeine 30 mg. Cap. Bot. 100s, 500s. *c-III.*
Use: Analgesic combination; narcotic.

Synarel. (Pfizer) Nafarelin acetate 2 mg/mL (as nafarelin base). Nasal solution. Bot. 10 mL with metered pump spray. *Rx.*
Use: Endometriosis.

Syncaine.
See: Procaine Hydrochloride.

Syncort.
See: Desoxycorticosterone Acetate.

Syncortyl.
See: Desoxycorticosterone Acetate.

Synemol. (Roche) Fluocinolone acetonide 0.025% in water-washable aqueous emollient base. Tube 15 g, 30 g, 60 g, 120 g. *Rx.*
Use: Corticosteroid, topical.

Synera. (Galen US) Lidocaine 70 mg, tetracaine 70 mg. Polyvinyl alcohol, parabens, sorbitan monopalmitate. Patch. 2s, 10s. *Rx.*
Use: Topical local anesthetic.

Synercid. (Monarch) Quinupristin 150 mg, dalfopristin 350 mg/10 mL. Inj. lyophilized. Vial 10 mL. *Rx.*
Use: Streptogramin

Synophylate. (Schwarz Pharma) Theophylline sodium glycinate. **Elix.:** Theophylline 165 mg/15 mL w/alcohol 20%. Bot. Pt, gal. **Tab.:** Theophylline 165 mg. Tab. Bot. 100s, 1000s. *Rx.*
Use: Bronchodilator.

Synribo. (Teva) Omacetaxine mepesuccinate 3.5 mg. Mannitol. Preservative free. Inj., lyophilized Pow. for Soln. Single-use vial. *Rx.*
Use: Antineoplastic, protein synthesis inhibitor.

Syn-Rx. (Medeva) **AM:** Pseudoephedrine hydrochloride 60 mg, guaifenesin 600 mg. CR Tab. Bot. 28s. **PM:** Guaifenesin 600 mg. CR Tab. Bot. 28s. In 14-day treatment regimen of 56 tablets. *Rx.*
Use: Upper respiratory combination, decongestant, expectorant.

Synsorb Pk.
Use: Verocytotoxogenic *E. coli* infections. [Orphan Drug]

Synthaloids. (Buffington) Benzocaine, calcium-iodine complex. Loz. Salt free. Bot. 100s, 1000s. Unit boxes 8s, 16s. Box 24s. *Dispens-a-Kit* 500s. *Aidpaks* 100s. *Medipaks* 200s. *OTC.*
Use: Sore throat relief.

synthetic conjugated estrogens, A.
Use: Estrogen.
See: Cenestin.

•**synthetic conjugated estrogens, B.** (ES-troe-jens) USAN.
Use: Hormone replacement therapy, estrogen therapy.

synthetic lung surfactant.
See: Exosurf Neonatal.

synthoestrin.
See: Diethylstilbestrol Dipropionate.

Synthroid. (Abbott) Sodium levothyroxine 0.025 mg, 0.05 mg, 0.075 mg, 0.088 mg, 0.1 mg, 0.112 mg, 0.125 mg, 0.137 mg, 0.15 mg, 0.175 mg, 0.2 mg, 0.3 mg. Lactose, sugar. Tab. Bot. 100s, 1000s, UD 100s (0.05 mg, 0.075 mg, 0.1 mg, 0.125 mg, 0.15 mg, 0.2 mg). *Rx.*
Use: Hormone, thyroid.

Synthroid Injection. (Abbott) Lyophilized sodium levothyroxine 200 mcg, 500 mcg. Vial. 10 mL (100 mcg/mL when reconstituted.) *Rx.*
Use: Hormone, thyroid.

Synvisc. (Genzyme) Hylan polymers 8 mg/mL. Inj. Prefilled syringe. 2 mL. *Rx.*
Use: Physical adjunct.

Synvisc-One. (Genzyme) Hylan polymers 8 mg/mL. Sodium chloride 8.5 mg/mL. Inj. Prefilled syringe. 6 mL. *Rx.*
Use: Physical adjunct.

Syphilis (FTA-ABS) Fluoro Kit. (Clinical Sciences)
Use: Test for syphilis.

Syprine. (Aton Pharma) Trientine hydrochloride 250 mg. Cap. Bot. 100s. *Rx.*
Use: Chelating agent.

Syracol CF. (Roberts) Dextromethorphan HBr 15 mg, guaifenesin 200 mg. Tab. Bot. 500s. *OTC.*
Use: Antitussive; expectorant.

Syroxine. (Major) Sodium levothyroxine 0.1 mg, 0.2 mg, 0.3 mg. Tab. Bot. 100s, 250s, 1000s, UD 100s. (3 mg 1000s). *Rx.*
Use: Hormone, thyroid.

Syrpalta. (Emerson) Syr. containing comb. of fruit flavors. Bot. Pt, gal. *OTC.*
Use: Pharmaceutical aid.

•**syrup.** (SIR-up) *NF.*
Use: Pharmaceutic aid (flavor).

Syrvite. (Various Mfr.) Vitamins A 2500 units, D 400 units, E 15 mg, B_1 1.05 mg, B_2 1.2 mg, B_3 13.5 mg, B_6 1.05 mg, B_{12} 4.5 mcg, C 60 mg/5 mL

Liq. Bot. 480 mL. *OTC.*
Use: Vitamin supplement.

Systane. (Alcon) PEG-400 0.4%, propylene glycol 0.3%. Soln., Ophth. 20 mL. *OTC.*
Use: Artificial tear solution.

Systane Balance. (Alcon) Propylene glycol 0.6%, boric acid, edetate disodium, mineral oil, polyquaternium-1 0.001%. Soln., Ophth. 10 mL. *OTC.*
Use: Artificial tears.

Systane Nighttime. (Alcon) Mineral oil 3%, white petrolatum 94%. Lanolin. Preservative free. Oint., Ophth. 3.5 g. *OTC.*
Use: Ocular lubricant.

Systane Ultra. (Alcon) Propylene glycol 0.3%, PEG 400 0.4%. Soln.; Ophth. 10 mL. *OTC.*
Use: Artificial tears.

systemic deodorizers.
See: Chlorophyllin Copper Complex.
Sodium Copper Chlorophyllin.

T

TA. (C & M Pharmacal) Triamcinolone acetonide 0.025%, 0.05%. Cream. Jar 2 oz, 8 oz, 1 lb. *Rx.*
Use: Corticosteroid, topical.

TA. (Wampole) Antithyroid antibodies by IFA. Test 48s.
Use: Diagnostic aid, thyroid.

•**tabalumab.** (ta-BAL-ue-mab) USAN.
Use: Autoimmune diseases and B cell malignancies.

Tabasyn. (Freeport) Chlorpheniramine maleate 2 mg, phenylephrine hydrochloride 10 mg, acetaminophen 5 g, salicylamide 5 g. Tab. Bot. 1000s. *Rx.*
Use: Analgesic, antihistamine, decongestant.

Tab-A-Vite. (Major) Vitamins A 3,000 units, D 400 units, E 30 units, B_1 1.5 mg, B_2 1.7 mg, B_3 20 mg, B_5 10 mg, B_6 2 mg, B_{12} 6 mcg, C 60 mg, folate 0.4 mg, Ca 45 mg. Gluten free, lactose free, and preservative free. Tab. UD 100s. *OTC.*
Use: Multivitamin.

Tab-A-Vite Maximum. (Major) Vitamins A 2,500 units, D 400 units, E 30 units, B_1 1.5 mg, B_2 1.7 mg, B_3 20 mg, B_5 10 mg, B_6 2 mg, B_{12} 6 mcg, C 60 mg, K, Fe 18 mg, Ca 162 mg, folate 0.4 mg, B, Cl, Cr, Cu, I, K, Mg, Mn, Mo, Ni, P, Se, Si, Sn, V, Zn, biotin. Lactose free and sugar free. Tab. 60s. *OTC.*
Use: Multivitamin.

Tab-A-Vite + Iron. (Major) Fe 18 mg, vitamins A 5000 units, D 400 units, E 30 units, B_1 1.5 mg, B_2 1.7 mg, B_3 20 mg, B_5 10 mg, B_6 2 mg, B_{12} 6 mcg, C 60 mg, FA 0.4 mg, tartrazine. Tab. Bot. 100s. *OTC.*
Use: Mineral, vitamin supplement.

Tab-A-Vite with Beta-Carotene. (Major) Vitamins A 5000 units, D 400 units, E 30 units, B_1 1.5 mg, B_2 1.7 mg, B_3 20 mg, B_5 10 mg, B_6 2 mg, B_{12} 6 mcg, C 60 mg, FA 0.4 mg. Tab. 100s. *OTC.*
Use: Mineral, vitamin supplement.

Tab-A-Vite Women's. (Major) Vitamins A 2,500 units, D 400 units, E 30 units, B_1 15 mg, B_2 1.7 mg, B_3 10 mg, B_5 5 mg, B_6 2 mg, B_{12} 6 mcg, C 60 mg, Fe 18 mg, Ca 450 mg, folate 0.4 mg, Mg, Zn. Mannitol. Lactose free, preservative free, and sugar free. Tab. 60s. *OTC.*
Use: Multivitamin.

Tabloid. (Prasco) Thioguanine 40 mg. Lactose. Tab. 25s. *Rx.*
Use: Antineoplastic.

Tacaryl. (Bristol-Myers Squibb) Methdilazine 3.6 mg. Chew. Tab. Bot. 100s. *Rx.*
Use: Antipruritic.

•**tacedinaline.** (ta-see-DYE-na-leen) USAN.
Use: Cancer agent.

TachoSil. (Baxter) Human fibrinogen 3.6 to 7.4 mg (5.5 mg), human thrombin 1.3 to 2.7 units (2 units) per cm^2. Albumin (human), equine collagen. Patch; Top. 1s and 2s (packages of 1s in 9.5 cm × 4.8 cm, package of 2s in 4.8 cm × 4.8 cm). *Rx.*
Use: Fibrin sealant (human).

tachysterol.
See: Dihydrotachysterol.

Tacitin. (Novartis) Under study. Benzoctamine, B.A.N.

•**taclamine hydrochloride.** (TACK-lah-meen) USAN.
Use: Anxiolytic.

Taclonex. (Leo Pharma) Calcipotriene 0.005%, betamethasone dipropionate 0.064%. Mineral oil, white petrolatum. Oint. 60 g, 100 g. *Rx.*
Use: Antipsoriatic agent.

Taclonex Scalp. (Leo Pharma) Calcipotriene hydrate 0.005%, betamethasone dipropionate 0.064%. Castor oil, mineral oil. Susp. 15 g, 30 g, 60 g. *Rx.*
Use: Antipsoriatic agent.

•**tacrine hydrochloride.** (TACK-reen) USAN.
Use: Cognition adjuvant.

•**tacrolimus.** (tak-ROE-li-mus) USAN.
Use: Immunomodulator, topical; immunologic agent; immunosuppressive.
See: Astagraf XL.
Prograf.
Protopic.

tacrolimus. (Sandoz) Tacrolimus 0.5 mg, 1 mg, 5 mg. Lactose. Cap. 100s. *Rx.*
Use: Immunologic agent, immunosuppressive.

Tac-3. (Allergan) Triamcinolone acetonide 3 mg/mL. Susp. Vial 5 mL. *Rx.*
Use: Corticosteroid.

•**tadalafil.** (tah-DA-la-fil) USAN.
Use: Erectile dysfunction.
See: AdCirca.
Cialis.

•**tafamidis.** (TA-fam-id-is) USAN.
Use: Transthyretin-associated amyloidosis.

•**tafamidis meglumine.** (TA-fam-id-is) USAN.
Use: Transthyretin-associated amyloidosis.

•**tafenoquine.** (ta-FEN-oh-kwin) USAN.
Use: Antimalarial.

•**tafenoquine succinate.** (ta-FEN-oh-kwin) USAN.
Use: Antimalarial.

Tafinlar. (GlaxoSmithKline) Dabrafenib 50 mg (equiv. to dabrafenib mesylate 59.25 mg), 75 mg (equiv. to dabrafenib mesylate 88.88 mg). Cap. 120s. *Rx.*
Use: Kinase inhibitor, BRAF inhibitor.

•**tafluprost.** (TA-floo-prost) USAN.
Use: Ophthalmic agent.
See: Zioptan.

Tagamet. (GlaxoSmithKline) Cimetidine. Tab. **400 mg:** Bot. 60s. **800 mg:** Bot. 30s. *Rx.*
Use: Histamine H_2 antagonist.

Tagamet HB 200. (GlaxoSmithKline Consumer) Cimetidine 200 mg. Tab. Bot. 6s, 30s, 50s. *OTC.*
Use: Histamine H_2 antagonist.

•**talabostat.** (tal-AB-oh-stat) USAN.
Use: Antineoplastic.

•**talabostat mesylate.** (tal-AB-oh-stat) USAN.
Use: Antineoplastic.

•**talactoferrin alfa.** (ta-LAK-toe-FER-in) USAN.
Use: Anti-infective.

•**taladegib.** (TAL-a-DEG-ib) USAN.
Use: Antineoplastic.

•**talampicillin hydrochloride.** (TAL-AM-pih-sill-in) USAN.
Use: Anti-infective.

•**talaporfin sodium.** (tal-a-PORE-fin) USAN.
Use: Photosensitizer.

•**talc.** (talk) *USP.* A native hydrous magnesium silicate.
Use: Dusting powder, pharmaceutic aid (tablet/capsule lubricant).
W/Zinc Oxide.
See: Caldesene.

talc powder, sterile.
Use: Antineoplastic.
See: Sclerosol.

•**taleranol.** (TAL-ehr-ah-nole) USAN.
Use: Enzyme inhibitor (gonadotropin).

•**taliglucerase alfa.** (TAL-i-GLOO-ser-ase AL-fa) USAN.
Use: Gaucher disease.
See: Elelyso.

•**talimogene laherparepvec.** (tal-IM-oh-jeen la-HER-pa-REP-vek) USAN.
Use: Antineoplastic.

•**talisomycin.** (TAL-i-soe-MYE-sin) USAN.
Formerly Tallysomycin A.
Use: Antineoplastic.

•**talizumab.** (tal-IZ-ue-mab) USAN.
Use: Anaphylaxis.

•**talmetacin.** (TAL-MET-ah-sin) USAN.
Use: Analgesic, antipyretic, anti-inflammatory.

•**talniflumate.** (tal-NYE-FLEW-mate) USAN.
Use: Anti-inflammatory, analgesic.

•**talopram hydrochloride.** (TAY-low-pram) USAN.
Use: Potentiator (catecholamine).

•**talosalate.** (TAL-oh-SAL-ate) USAN.
Use: Analgesic, anti-inflammatory.

•**talotrexin ammonium.** (tal-oh-TREX-in) USAN.
Use: Antineoplastic.

•**talsaclidine fumarate.** (tale-SACK-lih-deen) USAN.
Use: Alzheimer disease treatment (muscarinic M_1-agonist).

•**taltobulin.** (tal-toe-BUE-lin) USAN.
Use: Antineoplastic.

Talwin. (Abbott Hospital Products) Pentazocine lactate 30 mg/mL. Inj. **Vials:** With acetone sodium bisulfite 2 mg and methylparaben 1 mg/mL. 10 mL. **Uni-Amps:** 1 mL. **Uni-Nest amps:** 1 mL. **Carpujects:** With acetone sodium bisulfite 1 mg. 1 mL, 2 mL. *c-iv.*
Use: Narcotic agonist-antagonist analgesic.

Tambocor. (Medicis) Flecainide acetate 50 mg, 100 mg, 150 mg. Tab. 100s, UD 100s (except 150 mg). *Rx.*
Use: Antiarrhythmic agent.

•**tametraline hydrochloride.** (tah-MET-rah-leen) USAN.
Use: Antidepressant.

Tamiflu. (Genentech) Oseltamivir phosphate. **Cap.:** 30 mg, 45 mg, 75 mg. UD 10s. **Pow. for Oral Susp.:** 6 mg/mL after reconstitution. Sorbitol, saccharin, sodium benzoate, tutti-frutti flavor. 60 mL w/bottle adapter and oral dispenser. *Rx.*
Use: Antiviral.

•**tamoxifen citrate.** (ta-MOX-ih-fen) *USP.*
Use: Treatment of mammary carcinoma, antiestrogen.
See: Soltamox.

tamoxifen citrate. (Various Mfr.) Tamoxifen citrate (as base) 10 mg, 20 mg. Tab. Bot. 60s, 180s, 500s, 1000s, UD 100s (10 mg only); 30s, 90s, 100s, 500s, 1000s, UD 100s (20 mg only). *Rx.*
Use: Antineoplastic, antiestrogen.

•**tampramine fumarate.** (TAM-prah-MEEN) USAN.
Use: Antidepressant.

Tamp-R-Tel. (Wyeth) A tamper-resistant package for narcotic drugs which includes the following: **Codeine phosphate:** 30 mg, 60 mg/mL. **Hydromorphone hydrochloride:** 1 mg, 2 mg, 3 mg, 4 mg/*Tubex.* **Meperidine hydrochloride:** 25 mg/mL. **Promethazine**

hydrochloride: 25 mg/mL, 2 mL. **Meperidine hydrochloride:** 25 mg/mL, 50 mg/mL, 75 mg/mL, 100 mg/mL. **Morphine Sulfate:** 2 mg, 4 mg, 8 mg, 10 mg, 15 mg/mL. **Pentobarbital, Sodium:** 100 mg/2 mL. **Phenobarbital, Sodium:** 30 mg, 60 mg, 130 mg/mL. **Secobarbital, Sodium:** 100 mg/2 mL.

•**tamsulosin hydrochloride.** (tam-SOO-loe-sin) USAN.
Use: Benign prostatic hyperplasia therapy; antiadrenergic.
See: Flomax.
W/Dutasteride.
See: Jalyn.

tamsulosin hydrochloride. (Various Mfr.) Tamsulosin hydrochloride 0.4 mg. May contain sugar spheres. Cap. 30s, 100s, 500s, 1,000s, UD 16s, UD 30s. *Rx.*
Use: Antiadrenergic agent, peripherally acting; alpha-1 adrenergic blocker.

Tanac Gel. (Del) Dyclonine hydrochloride 1%, allantoin 0.5%, petrolatum, lanolin. Tube 9.45 mL. *OTC.*
Use: Cold sores, fever blisters, moisturizer.

Tanac Liquid. (Del) Benzocaine 10%. Benzalkonium chloride 0.12%, saccharin. 13 mL. *OTC.*
Use: Mouth and throat preparation.

TanaCof-DM. (Larken) Dextromethorphan tannate 25 mg, dexchlorpheniramine tannate 2.5 mg, pseudoephedrine tannate 75 mg per 5 mL. Parabens, aspartame, phenylalanine. Cotton candy flavor. Susp. 118 mL, 473 mL. *Rx.*
Use: Antitussive combination.

Tanac Roll-On. (Del) Benzocaine 5%. Benzalkonium chloride 0.12%, saccharin. Liq.; dental. 8.8 mL. *OTC.*
Use: Topical local anesthetic, ester local anesthetic.

Tanac Stick. (Del) Benzocaine 7.5%, tannic acid 6%, octyl dimethyl PABA 0.75%, allantoin 0.2%, benzalkonium chloride. 7.5%. Saccharin. Stick 0.1 oz. *OTC.*
Use: Cold sores, fever blisters, moisturizer.

Tanadex. (Del) Tannic acid 2.86%, phenol 1.05%, benzocaine 0.47%. Liq. Bot. 3 oz. *OTC.*
Use: Throat preparation.

Tan-a-Dyne. (Archer-Taylor) Tannic acid compound w/iodine. Liq. Bot. 4 oz., pt., gal. *OTC.*
Use: Gargle.

Tanafed DMX. (First Horizon) Dextromethorphan tannate 25 mg, dexchlorpheniramine tannate 2.5 mg, pseudoephedrine tannate 75 mg per 5 mL. Methylparaben, saccharin, sucrose, cotton candy flavor. Susp. 20 mL, 118 mL, 473 mL. *Rx.*
Use: Antitussive combination.

Tanafed DP. (First Horizon) Pseudoephedrine tannate 75 mg, dexchlorpheniramine tannate 2.5 mg/5 mL, methylparaben, saccharin, sucrose, strawberry-banana flavor. Susp. 20 mL, 118 mL, 473 mL. *Rx.*
Use: Decongestant and antihistamine.

TanaHist-D Pediatric. (Larken Laboratories) Chlorpheniramine tannate 2 mg, phenylephrine tannate 6 mg per mL. Methylparaben, saccharin, sorbitol. Cotton candy flavor. Soln., Conc. 60 mL w/dropper. *Rx.*
Use: Upper respiratory combination, decongestant and antihistamine.

TanaHist PD. (Larken Laboratories) Chlorpheniramine tannate 2 mg/mL. **Susp.:** Methylparaben, saccharin, sorbitol. Cotton candy flavor. 60 mL. **Drops:** Glycerin, methylparaben, saccharin, sodium benzoate, sorbitol. Cotton Candy flavor. 59 mL w/dropper. *Rx.*
Use: Antihistamine, nonselective alkylamine.

•**tanaproget.** (tan-a-PRO-jet) USAN.
Use: Contraceptive.

Tanavan. (Scientific Laboratories) Phenylephrine tannate 12.5 mg, pyrilamine tannate 30 mg per 5 mL. Grape flavor. Susp. 118 mL, 473 mL. *Rx.*
Use: Decongestant and antihistamine.

tanbismuth.
See: Bismuth Tannate.

•**tandamine hydrochloride.** (TAN-dah-meen) USAN.
Use: Antidepressant.

Tandem. (US Pharmaceutical) Elemental Fe 106 mg (ferrous fumarate 162 mg, polysaccharide iron complex 115.2 mg). Cap. Blister pack 90s. *Rx.*
Use: Dietary supplement.

Tandem DHA. (US Pharmaceutical) Vitamin B_6 25 mg, C 20 mg, folic acid 1 mg, Fe 30 mg, DHA 215.2 mg, EPA 53.46 mg. Cap. 90s. *Rx.*
Use: Multivitamin with iron.

Tandem F. (US Pharmaceutical) Fe 106 mg, folic acid 1 mg. Cap. 90s. *Rx.*
Use: Iron with vitamins.

Tandem OB. (US Pharmaceutical) Vitamin B_1 10 mg, B_2 6 mg, B_3 30 mg, B_5 10 mg, B_6 5 mg, B_{12} 15 mcg, C 200 mg, folic acid 1 mg, Cu 0.8 mg, Fe 106 mg, Mg 6.9 mg, Mn 1.3 mg, Zn 18.2 mg. Cap. 90s. *Rx.*
Use: Multivitamin with iron and other mineral.

Tandem Plus. (US Pharmaceutical) Vitamin B_1 10 mg, B_2 6 mg, B_3 30 mg, B_5 10 mg, B_6 5 mg, B_{12} 15 mcg, C 200 mg, folic acid 1 mg, Cu 0.8 mg, Fe 106 mg, Mn 1.3 mg, Zn 18.2 mg. Cap. 90s. *Rx.*
Use: Multivitamin with iron and other minerals.

•**tandospirone citrate.** (TAN-doe-SPYE-rone) USAN.
Use: Anxiolytic.

•**tandutinib.** (tan-DOO-ti-nib) USAN.
Use: Cardiovascular agent.

Tannate Pediatric. (Amneal Pharmaceuticals) Chlorpheniramine tannate 4.5 mg, phenylephrine tannate 5 mg per 5 mL. Methylparaben, saccharin, sucrose. Susp. 118 mL, 473 mL. *Rx.*
Use: Upper respiratory combination, antihistamine and decongestant.

•**tannic acid.** (TAN-ik) *USP.* Gallotannic acid. Glycerite. Tannin.
Use: Astringent.
See: Zilactin Medicated.

Tannic Spray. (Gebauer) Tannic acid 4.5%, chlorobutanol 1.3%, menthol < 1%, benzocaine < 1%, propylene glycol 33%, ethanol 60%. Liq. Bot. 2 oz. 4 oz. *OTC.*
Use: Relief of sunburn and other minor burns.

Tannic-12 S. (Cypress) Carbetapentane tannate 30 mg, chlorpheniramine tannate 4 mg per 5 mL. Methylparaben, saccharin, sucrose. Strawberry flavor. Susp. 118 mL. *Rx.*
Use: Upper respiratory combination, antitussive combination.

•**tanomastat.** (ta-NOE-ma-stat) USAN.
Use: Osteoarthritis; oncology.

Tanoral. (Pharmed) Phenylephrine tannate 25 mg, chlorpheniramine tannate 8 mg, pyrilamine tannate 25 mg. Tab. Bot. 100s. *Rx.*
Use: Antihistamine, decongestant.

Tanzeum. (GlaxoSmithKline) Albiglutide 30 mg, 50 mg. Mannitol, polysorbate 80. Preservative free. Inj., lyophilized Pow. for Soln. Single-dose pen. *Rx.*
Use: Antidiabetic agent, glucagonlike peptide 1 receptor agonist.

•**tanzisertib.** (TAN-zi-SER-tib) USAN.
Use: Treatment of idiopathic pulmonary fibrosis.

Tapar. (Warner Chilcott) Acetaminophen 325 mg. Tab. Bot. 100s. *OTC.*
Use: Analgesic.

Tapazole. (Monarch) Methimazole 5 mg, 10 mg. Tab. Bot. 100s. *Rx.*
Use: Hyperthyroidism.

•**tape, adhesive.** (tape) *USP.*
Use: Surgical aid.

•**tapentadol.** (ta-PEN-ta-dol) USAN.
Use: Analgesic.
See: Nucynta.
Nucynta ER.

Ta-Poff. (Ulmer Pharmacal) Adhesive tape remover. Liq. Bot. 1 pt. Aerosol. Can 6 oz. *OTC.*

•**taprenepag.** (ta-PREN-e-pag) USAN.
Use: Ophthalmic agent.

•**taprenepag isopropyl.** (ta-PREN-e-pag) USAN.
Use: Ophthalmic agent.

Tapuline. (Wesley) Activated attapulgite 600 mg, pectin 60 mg, homatropine methylbromide 0.5 mg. Chew. Tab. Bot. 100s, 1000s. *OTC.*
Use: Antidiarrheal.

tar.
See: Coal Tar.

Tarabine PFS. (Adria) Cytarabine 20 mg/mL, preservative free. Inj. Single vial 5 mL, bulk package vial 50 mL. *Rx.*
Use: Antimetabolite.

Taraphilic. (Medco) Coal tar distillate 1%, stearyl alcohol, petrolatum, parabens. Oint. 454 g. *OTC.*
Use: Dermatologic.

Tarceva. (Genentech Inc.) Erlotinib 25 mg, 100 mg, 150 mg. Lactose. Film-coated. Tab. 30s. *Rx.*
Use: Epidermal growth factor receptor inhibitor.

tar-containing products.
Use: Dermatologic.
See: Balnetar.
Coal Tar.
Cutar Emulsion.
Doak Tar.
Fototar.
Medotar.
MG 217 Medicated Tar.
Oxipor VHC.
Packer's Pine Tar.
Pine Tar Oils.
Polytar.
PsoriGel.
Taraphilic.

tar derivatives, shampoo.
Use: Dermatologic.
See: Creamy Tar.
DHS Tar.
Doak Tar.
Ionil T Plus.
MG 217 Medicated Tar.
Neutrogena T/Gel Original.
Polytar.
Zetar.

Targretin. (Valeant) Bexarotene. **Soft Gelatin Cap.:** 75 mg. Bot. 100s.

Gel: 1%, dehydrated alcohol. Tube 60 g. *Rx.*
Use: Rexinoid.

•**tariquidar.** (tar-I-kwi-dar) USAN.
Use: Chemotherapeutic aid.

Tarka. (Abbott) Trandolapril maleate/verapamil hydrochloride 1 mg/240 mg, 2 mg/180 mg, 2 mg/240 mg, 4 mg/240 mg. Lactose. Film-coated. Tab. Bot. 100s. *Rx.*
Use: Antihypertensive.

Tarnphilic. (Medco Lab) Coal tar 1%, polysorbate 0.5% in aquaphilic base. Jar 16 oz. *OTC.*
Use: Dermatologic.

Taron-Crystals. (Trigen) Potassium citrate monohydrate 3,300 mg, citric acid monohydrate 1,002 mg per packet. Each packet contains potassium ion 30 mEq and is equiv. to bicarbonate 30 mEq. Sucralose. Blueberry flavor. Pow. for Soln., oral. UD packet. *Rx.*
Use: Systemic alkalinizer.

Tarpaste. (Doak Dermatologics) Coal tar distilled 5% in zinc paste. Tube 1 oz, Jar 4 oz, w/Hydrocortisone 0.5%. Tube 1 oz. *OTC.*
Use: Dermatitis.

Tarsum Shampoo/Gel. (Summers) Coal tar 10%, salicylic acid 5% in shampoo base. Bot. 4 oz. *OTC.*
Use: Antiseborrheic, dermatologic, hair, and scalp.

tartar emetic.
See: Antimony Potassium Tartrate.

•**tartaric acid.** (tar-TAR-ik-AS-id) *NF.*
Use: Pharmaceutic aid (buffering agent).

Tashan. (Block Drug) Skin Cream. Vitamins A palmitate, D_2, D-panthenol, E. Tube 1 oz. *OTC.*
Use: Emollient.

•**tasidotin hydrochloride.** (TA-si-DOE-tin) USAN.
Use: Antineoplastic.

Tasigna. (Novartis) Nilotinib 150 mg, 200 mg (as nilotinib hydrochloride). Lactose. Cap. UD 28s. *Rx.*
Use: Protein-tyrosine kinase inhibitor.

•**tasimelteon.** (TAS-i-MEL-tee-on) USAN.
Use: Sedative and hypnotic, nonbarbiturate; melatonin receptor agonist.

Tasmar. (Valeant) Tolcapone 100 mg, 200 mg, lactose. Tab. Bot. 90s. *Rx.*
Use: Antiparkinson agent.

•**tasosartan.** (tass-OH-sahr-tan) USAN.
Use: Antihypertensive.

•**taspoglutide.** (tas-poe-GLUE-tide) USAN.
Use: Antidiabetic.

Taste Function Test, Accusens T. (Westport Pharmaceuticals, Inc.) Tastant 60 mL. Kit. 15 Bot.
Use: Diagnostic aid.

•**tavaborole.** (TA-va-BOR-ole) USAN.
Use: Antifungal agent.

Ta-Verm. (Table Rock) Piperazine citrate 100 mg/mL Syr. Bot. 1 pt, 1 gal. 500 mg Tab. Bot. 100s, 500s. *Rx.*
Use: Anthelmintic.

Tavilen Plus. (Table Rock) Liver solution 1 g, ferric pyrophosphate soluble 500 mg, vitamins B_1 6 mg, B_2 7.2 mg, B_6 3 mg, B_{12} 24 mcg, panthenol 3 mg, niacinamide 60 mg, l-lysine hydrochloride 300 mg, 5% alcohol/mL. Bot. 16 oz., 1 gal. *OTC.*
Use: Hematinic.

Tavist. (Novartis) Clemastine fumarate.
Tab.: 2.68 mg. Bot. 100s. **Syrup:** 0.67 mg/5 mL. Bot. 118 mL. *Rx.*
Use: Antihistamine.

Tavist Allergy. (Novartis Consumer Health) Clemastine fumarate 1.34 mg, lactose.Tab. Pkg. 8s. *OTC.*
Use: Antihistamine, nonselective ethanolamine.

Tavist Allergy/Sinus/Headache. (Novartis) Pseudoephedrine hydrochloride 30 mg, clemastine fumarate 0.335 mg, acetaminophen 500 mg, methylparaben. Tab. Bot. 24s, 48s. *OTC.*
Use: Upper respiratory combination, decongestant, antihistamine, analgesic.

Tavist Sinus Maximum Strength. (Novartis) Pseudoephedrine hydrochloride 30 mg, acetaminophen 500 mg, lactose, dextrose, methylparaben. Tab. Pkg. 24s. *OTC.*
Use: Upper respiratory combination, decongestant, analgesic.

taxoids.
Use: Antimitotic.
See: Cabazitaxel.
Docetaxel.
Paclitaxel.

Taxotere. (Aventis) Docetaxel 20 mg/mL. Alcohol, polysorbate 80. Inj., Soln., concentrate. Single-use vial. 1 mL, 4 mL. *Rx.*
Use: Antimitotic, taxoid.

•**tazadolene succinate.** (TAZZ-ah-DOE-leen) USAN.
Use: Analgesic.

•**tazarotene.** (tazz-AHR-oh-teen) USAN.
Use: Antiacne, antipsoriatic, retinoid.
See: Fabior.
Tazorac.

Tazicef. (Hospira) Ceftazidime.
Inj.: 1 g, 2 g. *Galaxy* containers.

Pow. for Inj.: 1 g, 2 g, 6 g. Sodium 2.3 mEq/g. Vials. *ADD-Vantage* vials. Piggyback vials (1 g, 2 g only). Bulk package (6 g only). *Rx.*
Use: Anti-infective, cephalosporin.

•**tazifylline hydrochloride.** (TAY-zih-FIH-lin) USAN.
Use: Antihistamine.

•**tazobactam.** (TAZZ-oh-BACK-tam) USAN.
Use: Inhibitor (beta-lactamase).

•**tazobactam sodium.** (TAZZ-oh-BACK-tam) USAN.
Use: Inhibitor (beta-lactamase).

tazobactam sodium/piperacillin.
Use: Extended-spectrum penicillin.
See: Zosyn.

•**tazofelone.** (TAY-zah-feh-lone) USAN.
Use: Suppressant (inflammatory bowel disease).

•**tazolol hydrochloride.** (TAY-zoe-lole) USAN.
Use: Cardiotonic.

•**tazomeline citrate.** (tazz-OH-meh-leen) USAN.
Use: Alzheimer disease treatment (cholinergic agonist).

Tazorac. (Allergan) Tazarotene. **Cream:** 0.05%, 0.1%, benzyl alcohol 1%, EDTA, medium chain triglycerides, mineral oil. Cream. Tube 15 g, 30 g, 60 g. **Gel:** 0.05%, 0.1%, benzyl alcohol 1%, EDTA. Tube. 30 g, 100 g. *Rx.*
Use: Antiacne, antipsoriatic, retinoid.

Taztia XT. (Andrx Pharmaceuticals) Diltiazem hydrochloride 120 mg, 180 mg, 240 mg, 300 mg, 360 mg. ER Cap. 30s, 90s. *Rx.*
Use: Calcium channel blocker.

TBA-Pred. (Keene Pharmaceuticals) Prednisolone tebutate 10 mg/mL Susp. Vial 10 mL. *Rx.*
Use: Corticosteroid.

tbo-filgrastim.
Use: Granulocyte colony-stimulating factor.
See: Granix.

TC Suspension. (Aventis) Aluminum hydroxide 600 mg, magnesium hydroxide 300 mg/5 mL, sorbitol, sodium 0.8 mg/5 mL. Liq. In UD 15 mL, 30 mL (100s). *OTC.*
Use: Antacid.

T/Derm Tar Emollient. (Neutrogena) Neutar solubilized coal tar extract 5% in oil base. Bot. 4 oz. *OTC.*
Use: Antipsoriatic, antipruritic.

T-Dry. (Jones Pharma) Pseudoephedrine hydrochloride 120 mg, chlorpheniramine maleate 12 mg. SR Cap. Bot. 100s. *Rx.*
Use: Antihistamine, decongestant.

T-Dry Jr. (Jones Pharma) Pseudoephedrine hydrochloride 60 mg, chlorpheniramine maleate 4 mg. SR Cap. Bot. 100s. *OTC.*
Use: Antihistamine, decongestant.

TDX Cortisol. (Abbott Diagnostics) Fluorescence polarization immunoassay for the quantitative determination of cortisol in serum, plasma, or urine.
Use: Diagnostic aid.

TDX Thyroxine. (Abbott Diagnostics) Automated assay for quantitation of unsaturated thyroxine-binding sites in serum or plasma.
Use: Diagnostic aid.

TDX Total Estriol. (Abbott Diagnostics) Fluorescence polarization immunoassay for the quantitative determination of total estriol in serum, plasma, or urine.
Use: Diagnostic aid.

TDX Total T3. (Abbott Diagnostics) Automated assay for quantitation of total circulating triiodothyronine (T3) in serum or plasma.
Use: Diagnostic aid.

TDX T-Uptake. (Abbott Diagnostics) Automated assay for the determination of thyroxine-binding capacity in serum or plasma.
Use: Diagnostic aid.

Te Anatoxal Berna. (Berna) Tetanus toxoid adsorbed, 10 Lf units/0.5 mL. Vial 5 mL, Syringe. 0.5 mL. *Rx.*
Use: Immunization.

Tear Drop. (Parmed Pharmaceuticals, Inc.) Benzalkonium chloride 0.01%, polyvinyl alcohol, NaCl, EDTA. Soln. Drops. Bot. 15 mL. *OTC.*
Use: Artificial tears.

Tearisol. (Novartis Ophthalmic) Hydroxypropyl methylcellulose 0.5%, edetate disodium, benzalkonium chloride 0.01%, boric acid, potassium chloride. Bot. 15 mL. *OTC.*
Use: Artificial tears.

Tears Again. (Altaire) White petrolatum, mineral oil. Oint.; Ophth. 3.5 g. *OTC.*
Use: Ocular lubricant.

Tears Again. (OcuSOFT) **Soln.; Ophth.:** Hydroxypropyl methylcellulose 0.3%, boric acid, phosphoric acid, potassium chloride, sodium chloride *Dissipate* as a preservative. 15 mL. **Soln., gel forming:** Carboxymethylcellulose sodium 0.7%, boric acid, phosphoric acid, potassium chloride, sodium chloride. 15 mL. *OTC.*
Use: Artificial tears.

Tears Again Advanced. (OcuSOFT) Retinyl palmitate, tocopheryl acetate, magnesium ascorbyl phosphate, polysorbate 80, sodium chloride, sodium hydroxide, phenoxyethanol, alcohol, disodium EDTA, PEG-12, glyceryl. Spray, Soln.; Ophth. 15 mL. *OTC.*
Use: Ocular lubricant.

Tears Again MC. (OcuSOFT) Hydroxypropyl methylcellulose 0.3%, boric acid, phosphoric acid, potassium chloride, sodium chloride *Dissipate* as a preservative. Drops. 15 mL. *OTC.*
Use: Artificial tears.

Tears Again Night & Day. (OcuSOFT) Carboxymethylcellulose 1.5%, polyvinylpyrrolidone 0.1%. Gel; Ophth. 3.5 g. *OTC.*
Use: Ocular lubricant.

TearSaver. (FCI) Collagen implant. Implant. 0.2 mm, 0.3 mm, 0.4 mm. *Rx.*
Use: Ophthalmic collagen implant.

Tears Naturale. (Alcon) Dextran 70 0.1%, benzalkonium chloride 0.01%, hydroxypropyl methylcellulose 0.3%, sodium chloride, EDTA, hydrochloric acid, sodium hydrochloride, potassium chloride. Soln. Bot. 15 mL, 30 mL. *OTC.*
Use: Artificial tears.

Tears Naturale Forte. (Alcon) Dextran 70 0.1%, hydroxypropyl methylcellulose 0.3%, glycerin 0.2%, polyquaternium-1 0.001%, NaCl, KCl, sodium borate. Soln. 15 mL, 30 mL. *OTC.*
Use: Artificial tears.

Tears Naturale Free. (Alcon) Hydroxypropyl methylcellulose 2910 0.3%, dextran 70 0.1%, NaCl, KCl, sodium borate. Soln. Single-use containers 0.6 mL. *OTC.*
Use: Artificial tears.

Tears Naturale P.M. (Alcon) White petrolatum 94%, mineral oil 3%, lanolin. Preservative free. Oint.; Ophth. 3.5 g. *OTC.*
Use: Ocular lubricant.

Tears Naturale II. (Alcon) Dextran 70 0.1%, hydroxypropyl methylcellulose 2910 0.3%, polyquaternium-1 0.001%, sodium chloride, potassium chloride, sodium borate. Soln. *Drop-tainer* 15 mL, 30 mL. *OTC.*
Use: Artificial tears.

Tears Plus. (Allergan) Polyvinyl alcohol 1.4%, NaCl, povidone 0.6%, chlorobutanol 0.5%. *OTC.*
Use: Artificial tears.

tear test strips.
Use: Ophthalmic diagnostic product.
See: Schirmer Tear Test.

tea tree oil. (Metabolic Prod.) Australian oil of *Melaleuca alternifolia* 100% pure. Bot. 1 oz, 4 oz, 8 oz, 16 oz. **Cream:** Bot. 8 oz. **Oint.:** Tube 1 oz, 3 oz. *OTC.*
Use: Antiseptic, antifungal, topical.

•**tebanicline tosylate.** (te-BAN-i-kleen) USAN.
Use: Analgesic.

•**tebufelone.** (teh-BYOO-feh-LONE) USAN.
Use: Analgesic, anti-inflammatory.

•**tebuquine.** (TEH-buh-KWIN) USAN.
Use: Antimalarial.

T.E.C. (Invenex) Zn 1 mg, Cu 0.4 mg, Cr 4 mcg, Mn 0.1 mg. Vial 10 mL. *Rx.*
Use: Trace element supplement.

•**tecadenoson.** (tek-a-DEN-o-son) USAN.
Use: Cardiovascular agent.

•**tecalcet hydrochloride.** (TE-kal-set) USAN.
Use: Hyperparathyroidism.

•**tecarfarin.** (TEK-ar far-in) USAN.
Use: Anticoagulant.

•**tecarfarin sodium.** (TEK-ar far-in) USAN.
Use: Anticoagulant.

•**tecastemizole.** (tek-a-STEM-mi-zole) USAN.
Use: Antihistamine.

•**teceleukin.** (teh-see-LOO-kin) USAN.
Use: Immunostimulant.

•**tecemotide.** (TEK-e-MOE-tide) USAN.
Use: Antineoplastic.

Tecfidera. (Biogen Idec) Dimethyl fumarate 120 mg, 240 mg. Cap., delayed release. Starter pack (30-day starter pack contains 14 of the 120 mg capsules and 46 of the 240 mg capsules), 14s (120 mg only), 60s (240 mg only). *Rx.*
Use: Immunomodulator.

Techneplex. (Bristol-Myers Squibb) Technetium Tc 99m pentetate kit. 10 vials/kit.
Use: Radiopaque agent.

TechneScan MAA. (Mallinckrodt) Aggregated albumin (human).
Use: Preparation of Tc 99m Aggregated Albumin (Human).

•**technetium Tc 99m albumin aggregated injection.** (tek-NEE-shee-uhm Tc 99m al-BYOO-min AGG-reh-GAY-tuhd) *USP.*
Use: Diagnostic aid (lung imaging), radioactive agent.

•**technetium Tc 99m albumin colloid injection.** (tek-NEE-shee-uhm Tc 99m al-BYOO-min) *USP.*
Use: Radiopharmaceutical.

•**technetium Tc 99m albumin injection.** (tek-NEE-shee-uhm Tc 99m al-BYOO-min) *USP.*
Use: Radiopharmaceutical.

•**technetium Tc 99m albumin microaggregated.** (tek-NEE-shee-uhm Tc 99m al-BYOO-min) USAN.
Use: Radiopharmaceutical.

technetium Tc 99m antimelanoma murine monoclonal antibody.
Use: Diagnostic aid. [Orphan Drug]

•**technetium Tc 99m antimony trisulfide colloid.** (tek-NEE-shee-uhm) USAN.
Use: Radiopharmaceutical.

•**technetium Tc 99m apcitide.** (tek-NEE-shee-uhm APP-sih-tide) *USP.*
Use: Radiopharmaceutical.

•**technetium Tc 99m arcitumomab injection.** (tek-NEE-shee-uhm AR-si-TOOM-oh-mab) USAN.
Use: Radiopharmaceutical.

•**technetium Tc 99m bicisate.** (tek-NEE-shee-uhm Tc 99m bye-SIS-ate) USAN.
Use: Diagnostic aid (brain imaging), radiopharmaceutical.

•**technetium Tc 99m depreotide injection.** (tek-NEE-shee-uhm) *USP.*
Use: Radiopharmaceutical.

•**technetium Tc 99m disofenin injection.** (tek-NEE-shee-uhm) *USP.*
Use: Radiopharmaceutical; diagnostic aid (hepatobiliary function determination).

•**technetium Tc 99m etarfolatide.** (tek-NEE-shee-uhm) USAN.
Use: Diagnostic aid.

•**technetium Tc 99m etidronate injection.** (tek-NEE-shee-uhm) *USP.*
Use: Radiopharmaceutical.

•**technetium Tc 99m exametazime injection.** (tek-NEE-shee-uhm Tc 99m ex-ah-MET-ah-zeem) *USP.*
Use: Radiopharmaceutical.

•**technetium Tc 99m fanolesomab.** (tek-NEE-shee-uhm fa-noe-LES-oh-mab) USAN.
Use: Diagnostic aid (polymorphonuclear neutrophil accumulation); radiopharmaceutical.

technetium Tc 99m ferpentetate injection.
Use: Radiopharmaceutical.

•**technetium Tc 99m furifosmin.** (tek-NEE-shee-uhm Tc 99m fyoor-ih-FOSS-min) USAN.
Use: Diagnostic aid (radioactive, cardiac disease), radiopharmaceutical.

technetium Tc 99m generator solution. (New England Nuclear) Pertechnetate sodium Tc 99m.
Use: Radiopharmaceutical, radiopaque agent.

•**technetium Tc 99m glucepate injection.** (tek-NEE-shee-uhm) *USP. Formerly Technetium Tc 99m Sodium Gluceptate.*
Use: Radiopharmaceutical.

•**technetium Tc 99m lidofenin injection.** (tek-NEE-shee-uhm) *USP.*
Use: Radiopharmaceutical.

technetium Tc-99m mebrofenin. (CIS-US) Mebrofenin 45 mg. When sodium pertechnetate Tc-99m injection is added to the vial, the diagnostic agent technetium Tc-99m mebrofenin is formed containing up to 3,700 MBq (100 millicuries) of Tc-99m. Also contains stannous fluoride dihydrate (minimum) and total tin 1.03 mg maximum (as stannous fluoride dihydrate). May contain parabens. Inj., Lyophilized Pow. for Soln. Kits of 5 and 30 multidose vials. *Rx.*
Use: Radiopaque agent.

•**technetium Tc 99m mebrofenin injection.** (tek-NEE-shee-uhm) *USP.*
Use: Radiopharmaceutical.
See: Choletec.

•**technetium Tc 99m medronate disodium.** (tek-NEE-shee-uhm) USAN.
Use: Radiopharmaceutical.

•**technetium Tc 99m medronate injection.** (tek-NEE-shee-uhm) *USP.*
Use: Diagnostic aid (skeletal imaging), radiopharmaceutical.
See: Macrotec.

•**technetium Tc 99m mertiatide injection.** (tek-NEE-shee-uhm Tc 99m MEER-TIE-ah-tide) *USP.*
Use: Diagnostic aid (renal function); radiopharmaceutical.

technetium Tc 99m murine monoclonal antibody (IgG2a) to B cell.
Use: Diagnostic aid. [Orphan Drug]

technetium Tc 99m murine monoclonal antibody to hCG.
Use: Diagnostic aid. [Orphan Drug]

technetium Tc 99m murine monoclonal antibody to human alpha-fetoprotein.
Use: Diagnostic aid. [Orphan Drug]

•**technetium Tc 99m nitridocade.** (tek-NEE-shee-uhm Tc 99m nye-TRID-oh-kade) USAN.
Use: Diagnostic aid (coronary artery disease); radiopharmaceutical.

•**technetium Tc 99m nofetumomab merpentan injection.** (tek-NEE-shee-uhm Tc 99m no-fe-TUE-mo-mab) *USP.*
Use: Radiopharmaceutical.

•**technetium Tc 99m oxidronate injection.** (tek-NEE-shee-uhm) *USP.*
Use: Diagnostic aid (skeletal imaging), radiopharmaceutical.

•**technetium Tc 99m pentetate calcium trisodium.** (tek-NEE-shee-uhm KAL-see-uhm try-so-dee-uhm) USAN.
Use: Radiopharmaceutical.

•**technetium Tc 99m pentetate injection.** (tek-NEE-shee-uhm) *USP. Formerly Technetium Tc 99m Pentetate Sodium.*
Use: Radiopharmaceutical.

•**technetium Tc 99m (pyro- and trimeta-) phosphates injection.** (tek-NEE-shee-uhm) *USP.*
Use: Radiopharmaceutical.

•**technetium Tc 99m pyrophosphate injection.** (tek-NEE-shee-uhm) *USP.*
Use: Radiopharmaceutical.

•**technetium Tc 99m red blood cells injection.** (tek-NEE-shee-uhm) *USP.*
Use: Radiopharmaceutical.

•**technetium Tc 99m sestamibi.** (tek-NEE-shee-uhm SES-ta-MIB-ee) *USP.*
Use: Diagnostic aid (radiopaque medium, cardiac perfusion); radiopharmaceutical.

•**technetium Tc 99m siboroxime.** (tek-NEE-shee-uhm Tc 99m sih-boe-ROX-eem) USAN.
Use: Diagnostic aid (brain imaging), radiopharmaceutical.

•**technetium Tc 99m succimer injection.** (tek-NEE-shee-uhm) *USP.*
Use: Radiopharmaceutical, diagnostic aid (renal function determination).

•**technetium Tc 99m sulfur colloid injection.** (tek-NEE-shee-uhm) *USP.*
Use: Radiopharmaceutical.

technetium Tc 99m sulfur colloid kit.
Use: Radiopharmaceutical.
See: Tesuloid.

•**technetium Tc 99m teboroxime.** (tek-NEE-shee-uhm Tc 99m teh-boe-ROX-eem) USAN.
Use: Diagnostic aid (radiopaque medium, cardiac perfusion), radiopharmaceutical.

•**technetium Tc 99m tilmanocept.** (tek-NEE-shee-um til-MAN-oh-sept) USAN.
Use: Radiopharmaceutical.
See: Lymphoseek.

teclosine. Under study.
Use: Amebicide.

•**teclozan.** (TEH-kloe-zan) USAN.
Use: Antiamebic.
See: Falmonox.

Tecnu First Aid. (Tec Labs) Lidocaine hydrochloride 2.5%, benzethonium chloride 0.2%, disodium EDTA, glycerin, castor oil, tea tree oil, white thyme oil. Gel. 56.7 g. *OTC.*
Use: Topical local anesthetic.

Tecnu Outdoor Skin Cleanser. (Tec Labs) Deodorized mineral spirits, propylene glycol, octylphenoxypolyethoxyethanol, mixed fatty acid soap. Lot. 118 mL, 355 mL. *OTC.*
Use: Poison ivy prevention.

•**tecogalan sodium.** (TEE-koe-gay-lan) USAN.
Use: Antineoplastic adjunct.

•**tecovirimat.** (tek-oh-VIR-i-mat) USAN.
Use: Treatment of smallpox.

•**tedatioxetine.** (TE-da-tye-OX-e-teen) USAN.
Use: Antidepressant.

•**tedatioxetine hydrobromide.** (TE-da-tye-OX-e-teen) USAN.
Use: Antidepressant.

•**tedisamil.** (te-DIS-a-mil) USAN.
Use: Investigational antiarrhythmic agent.

•**tedisamil sesquifumarate.** (te-DIS-a-mil SES-kwi-FUE-ma-rate) USAN.
Use: Antiarrhythmic agent.

•**tedizolid.** (TED-eye-ZOE-lid) USAN.
Use: Antibiotic.

•**tedizolid phosphate.** (TED-eye-ZOE-lid) USAN.
Use: Treatment of complicated skin and skin structure infections.

Tedral. (Parke-Davis) **Elix.:** Theophylline 32.5 mg, ephedrine hydrochloride 6 mg, phenobarbital 2 mg/5 mL. Alcohol 15%. Pediatric. Bot. Pt. **Tab.:** Theophylline 118 mg, ephedrine hydrochloride 24 mg, phenobarbital 8 mg. Tab. Bot. 24s, 100s, 1000s. UD 100s. **Susp. (Pediatric Pharmaceuticals):** Theophylline 65 mg, ephedrine hydrochloride 12 mg, phenobarbital 4 mg/5 mL. Bot. 8 oz. *Rx.*
Use: Antiasthmatic.

Tedral-SA. (Parke-Davis) Theophylline 180 mg, ephedrine hydrochloride 48 mg, phenobarbital 25 mg. SA Tab. Bot. 100s, 1000s. *Rx.*
Use: Antiasthmatic.

•**teduglutide.** (te-DUE-gloo-tide) USAN.
Use: Gastrointestinal disease.
See: Gattex.

Teebacin. (CMC) Sod. p-aminosalicylate. **Tab.:** 0.5 g Bot. 1000s. **Pow.:** Bot. lb. *Rx.*
Use: Antituberculosal.

Teebaconin. (CMC) Isoniazid 50 mg, 100 mg, 300 mg. Tab. Bot. 100s, 1000s. *Rx.*
Use: Antituberculosal.

Teebaconin w/Vitamin B_6. (CMC) Isoniazid 100 mg, 10 mg pyridoxine hydrochloride. Tab. Bot. 100s, 500s, 1000s. Isoniazid 300 mg, 30 mg pyridoxine

hydrochloride. Tab. Bot. 100s, 1000s. *Rx.*
Use: Antituberculosal.

Teev. (Keene Pharmaceuticals) Estradiol valerate 4 mg, testosterone enanthate 90 mg/mL. Inj. Vial 10 mL. *Rx.*
Use: Androgen, estrogen combination.

•**tefibazumab.** (tef-ee-BA-zoo-mab) USAN.
Use: Anti-infective.

Teflaro. (Forest Pharmaceuticals) Ceftaroline fosamil (as ceftaroline fosamil monoacetate) 400 mg, 600 mg. Inj., Pow. for Soln. Single-use vial. *Rx.*
Use: Anti-infective, cephalosporin and related antibiotic.

•**teflurane.** (TEH-flew-rane) USAN.
Use: Anesthetic, general.

tegacid.
See: Glyceryl Monostearate.

•**tegafur.** (TEH-gah-fer) USAN.
Use: Antineoplastic.

Tegamide. (G & W) Trimethobenzamide hydrochloride 100 mg, 200 mg. Supp. Box. 10s, 50s. *Rx.*
Use: Antiemetic.

•**tegaserod maleate.** (teg-a-SER-od) USAN.
Note: Available through investigational limited access program.
Use: Gastrointestinal motility disorders.

•**teglarinad chloride.** (teg-LAR-i-nad klor-ide) USAN.
Use: Antineoplastic.

•**tegobuvir.** (TEG-oh-BUE-vir) USAN.
Use: Hepatitis C.

Tegretol. (Novartis) Carbamazepine. **Tab.:** 200 mg. 100s. **Susp.:** 100 mg/5 mL. Sorbitol, sucrose. Citrus/vanilla flavor. 450 mL. *Rx.*
Tall Man: TEGretol
Use: Anticonvulsant.

Tegretol-XR. (Novartis) Carbamazepine 100 mg, 200 mg, 400 mg. Mannitol, PEG. Film coated. ER Tab. 100s. *Rx.*
Tall Man: TEGretol
Use: Anticonvulsant.

Tegrin. (Block Drug) Allantoin 2%, coal tar extract 5% in cream base. Cream. Tube 2 oz, 4.4 oz. *OTC.*
Use: Antipsoriatic.

T.E.H. Compound. (Various Mfr.) Theophylline 130 mg, ephedrine sulfate 25 mg, hydroxyzine hydrochloride 10 mg. Tab. Bot. 100s, 500s. *Rx.*
Use: Antiasthmatic.

•**teicoplanin.** (teh-kah-PLAN-in) USAN.
Use: Anti-infective.

Tekamlo. (Novartis) Amlodipine besylate/aliskiren (as aliskiren hemifumarate) 5 mg/150 mg, 10 mg/150 mg, 5 mg/300 mg, 10 mg/300 mg. Film coated. PEG. Tab. 30s, 90s, UD 100s. *Rx.*
Use: Antihypertensive combination.

Tekral. (Capellon Pharmaceutical) Diphenhydramine hydrochloride 100 mg, pseudoephedrine hydrochloride 120 mg. Lactose. Tab. 90s. *Rx.*
Use: Upper respiratory combination, decongestant, antihistamine.

Tekturna. (Novartis) Aliskiren 150 mg, 300 mg. Film-coated. Tab. 30s, 90s, UD 100s. *Rx.*
Use: Renin angiotensin system antagonist, direct renin inhibitor.

Tekturna HCT. (Novartis) Aliskiren/hydrochlorothiazide 150 mg/12.5 mg, 150 mg/25 mg, 300 mg/12.5 mg, 300 mg/25 mg. Lactose. Film-coated. Tab. 30s, 90s, blister pack 100s. *Rx.*
Use: Antihypertensive combination.

Telachlor TD Caps. (Major) Chlorpheniramine maleate 8 mg, 12 mg. TD Tab. Bot. 1000s. *Rx.*
Use: Antihistamine.

•**telaprevir.** (tel-A-pre-vir) USAN.
Use: Antiviral.
See: Incivek.

•**telapristone acetate.** (TEL-a-PRIS-tone) USAN.
Use: Female reproductive disorders.

•**telavancin hydrochloride.** (tel-a-VAN-sin) USAN.
Use: Antibacterial agent.
See: Vibativ.

•**telbivudine.** (tel-BI-vyoo-deen) USAN.
Use: Antiretroviral, nucleoside reverse transcriptase inhibitor.
See: Tyzeka.

•**telcagepant.** (tel-KA-je-pant) USAN.
Use: Treatment of migraine.

•**telcagepant potassium.** (tel-KA-je-pant) USAN.
Use: Treatment of migraine.

•**telinavir.** (teh-LIN-ah-veer) USAN.
Use: Antiviral.

•**telithromycin.** (tel-ITH-roe-MYE-sin) USAN.
Use: Anti-infective.
See: Ketek.

•**telmapitant.** (tel-MA-pi-tant) USAN.
Use: Antiemetic.

•**telmisartan.** (tell-mih-SAHR-tan) USAN.
Use: Angiotensin II receptor antagonist; antihypertensive.
See: Micardis.
W/Hydrochlorothiazide.
See: Micardis HCT.

telmisartan. (Various Mfr.) Telmisartan 20 mg, 40 mg, 80 mg. May contain

sorbitol. Tab. UD 30s. *Rx.*
Use: Renin angiotensin system antagonist, angiotensin II receptor antagonist.

telmisartan/amlodipine. (Various Mfr.) Telmisartan/amlodipine besylate 40 mg/5 mg, 40 mg/10 mg, 80 mg/5 mg, 80 mg/10 mg. May contain mannitol. Tab. 30s, 90s, 100s, UD 100s. *Rx.*
Use: Antihypertensive combination.

telmisartan/hydrochlorothiazide. (Various Mfr.) Telmisartan/hydrochlorothiazide 40 mg/12.5 mg, 80 mg/12.5 mg, 80 mg/25 mg. May contain lactose, mannitol. Tab. 30s, 90s, 100s, 500s, UD 100s. *Rx.*
Use: Antihypertensive combination.

•**telotristat.** (tel-OH-tri-stat) USAN.
Use: Carcinoid syndrome.

•**telotristat ethyl.** (tel-OH-tri-stat) USAN.
Use: Carcinoid syndrome.

•**telotristat etiprate.** (tel-OH-tri-stat) USAN.
Use: Carcinoid syndrome.

•**teloxantrone hydrochloride.** (teh-LOX-an-trone) USAN.
Use: Antineoplastic.

•**teludipine hydrochloride.** (teh-LOO-dih-peen) USAN.
Use: Antihypertensive, calcium channel antagonist.

•**temafloxacin hydrochloride.** (teh-mah-FLOX-ah-SIN) USAN.
Use: Anti-infective (microbial DNA topoisomerase inhibitor).

•**temanogrel.** (tem-AN-oh-grel) USAN.
Use: Anti-platelet agent.

•**temanogrel hydrochloride.** (tem-AN-oh-grel) USAN.
Use: Anti-platelet agent.

•**tematropium methylsulfate.** (teh-mah-TROE-pee-UHM METH-ill-SULL-fate) USAN.
Use: Anticholinergic.

•**temazepam.** (tem-AZE-uh-pam) *USP.*
Use: Sedative/hypnotic, nonbarbiturate.
See: Restoril.

temazepam. (Various Mfr.) Temazepam 7.5 mg, 15 mg, 22.5 mg, 30 mg. Lactose. Cap. 30s (22.5 mg only); 100s (except 22.5 mg); 500s (15 mg and 30 mg only). *c-IV.*
Use: Sedative/hypnotic, nonbarbiturate.

•**temelastine.** (teh-mell-ASS-teen) USAN.
Use: Antihistamine.

•**temocapril hydrochloride.** (teh-MOE-cap-RILL) USAN.
Use: Antihypertensive.

•**temocillin.** (TEE-moe-SIH-lin) USAN.
Use: Anti-infective.

Temodar. (Schering) Temozolomide. **Cap.:** 5 mg, 20 mg, 100 mg, 140 mg, 180 mg, 250 mg. Lactose. 5s, 14s (except 250 mg). **Inj., lyophilized Pow. for Soln.:** 100 mg. Single-use vial. *Rx.*
Use: Antineoplastic.

•**temoporfin.** (teh-moe-PORE-fin) USAN.
Use: Antineoplastic.

Temovate. (Pharmaderm) **Cream:** Clobetasol propionate 0.05%. Tube 15 g, 30 g, 45 g. **Emollient:** Clobetasol propionate 0.05%. Tube 15 g, 30 g, 60 g. **Gel:** Clobetasol propionate 0.05%. Tube 15 g, 30 g, 60 g. **Oint.:** Clobetasol propionate 0.05%. Tube 15 g, 30 g, 45 g. *Rx.*
Use: Corticosteroid, topical.

•**temozolomide.** (TEM-oh-ZOE-loe-mide) USAN.
Use: Antineoplastic.
See: Temodar.

temozolomide. (Various Mfr.) Temozolomide 5 mg, 20 mg, 100 mg, 140 mg, 180 mg, 250 mg. May contain lactose. Cap. 5s, 14s (except 250 mg). *Rx.*
Use: Antineoplastic, imidazotetrazine derivative.

Tempo. (Thompson Medical) Calcium carbonate 414 mg, aluminum hydroxide 133 mg, magnesium hydroxide 81 mg, simethicone 20 mg. Chew. Tab. Bot. 10s, 30s, 60s. *OTC.*
Use: Antacid, antiflatulent.

Temporary Punctal/Canalicular Collagen Implant. (Eagle Vision) 0.2 mm, 0.3 mm, 0.4 mm, 0.5 mm, 0.6 mm. Box 72s. *Rx.*
Use: Collagen implant, ophthalmic.

Temp Tab. (National Vitamin) Chloride (as sodium and potassium chloride) 287 mg, sodium (as chloride) 180 mg, potassium (as chloride) 15 mg. Tab. Preservative-free. 100s. *OTC.*
Use: Electrolyte.

•**temsirolimus.** (TEM-sir-OH-li-mus) USAN.
Use: Antineoplastic, protein-tyrosine kinase inhibitor, mTor inhibitor.
See: Torisel.

•**temurtide.** (teh-MER-TIDE) USAN.
Use: Vaccine adjuvant.

Tenar PSE. (Centrix) Guaifenesin 200 mg, pseudoephedrine hydrochloride 40 mg. Sorbitol, sucralose. Grape flavor. Liq. 473 mL. *Rx.*
Use: Upper respiratory combination, decongestant and expectorant combination.

Tencet. (Roberts) Acetaminophen

500 mg, butalbital 50 mg, caffeine 40 mg. Cap. Bot. 100s, UD 1000s. *Rx.*
Use: Analgesic, hypnotic, sedative.

Tencon. (International Ethical Labs) Acetaminophen 650 mg, butalbital 50 mg. Tab. Bot. 100s. *Rx.*
Use: Analgesic, hypnotic, sedative.

•**tenecteplase.** (teh-NECK-teh-place) USAN.
Use: Thrombolytic agent, tissue plasminogen activator.
See: TNKase.

•**teneliximab.** (ten-el-IKS-i-mab) USAN.
Use: Monoclonal antibody.

Tenex. (Promius Pharma) Guanfacine hydrochloride 1 mg, 2 mg. Lactose. Tab. 100s, 500s (1 mg only). *Rx.*
Use: Antihypertensive.

•**tenifatecan.** (TEN-i-fa-TEK-an) USAN.
Use: Antineoplastic.

•**teniposide.** (TEN-ih-POE-side) USAN.
Use: Antineoplastic. [Orphan Drug]
See: Vumon.

teniposide. (Various Mfr.) Teniposide 10 mg/mL (50 mg per 5 mL). May contain alcohol, benzyl alcohol, castor oil. Inj., Soln., concentrate. 5 mL amp. *Rx.*
Use: Antineoplastic, epipodophyllotoxin, podophyllotoxin derivative.

Tenivac. (Sanofi Pasteur) Diphtheria 2 Lf units, tetanus 5 Lf units per 0.5 mL dose. Aluminum phosphate 1.5 mg (aluminum 0.33 mg), formaldehyde ≤ 5 mcg. Single-dose vial or syringe. 0.5 mL. *Rx.*
Use: Agent for active immunization.

•**tenivastatin calcium.** (te-NI-va-sta-tin) USAN.
Use: Antihyperlipidemic; HMG-CoA reductase inhibitor.

Ten-K. (Novartis) Potassium chloride 750 mg (10 mEq). CR Cap. Bot. 100s, 500s. UD, blister pak 100s. *Rx.*
Use: Electrolyte supplement.

•**tenofovir.** (te-NOE-fo-veer) USAN.
Use: Antiviral.

•**tenofovir alafenamide.** (ten-OF-oh-vir AL-a-FEN-a-mide) USAN.
Use: Antiretroviral agent.

•**tenofovir alafenamide fumarate.** (ten-OF-oh-vir AL-a-FEN-a-mide) USAN.
Use: Antiretroviral agent.

•**tenofovir disoproxil fumarate.** (te-NOE-fo-veer dye-soe-PROX-il) USAN.
Use: Antiretroviral, nucleotide analog reverse transcriptase inhibitor.
See: Viread.
W/Cobicistat, Elvitegravir, Emtricitabine.
See: Stribild.
W/Efavirenz, Emtricitabine.
See: Atripla.
W/Emtricitabine.
See: Truvada.
W/Emtricitabine, Rilpivirine.
See: Complera.

Tenol. (Vortech Pharmaceuticals) **Liq.:** Acetaminophen 120 mg, NAPA alcohol 7%/5 mL. Bot. 3 oz, 4 oz, gal. **Tab.:** Acetaminophen 325 mg. Bot. 1000s. *OTC.*
Use: Analgesic.

Tenol-Plus. (Vortech Pharmaceuticals) Acetaminophen 250 mg, aspirin 250 mg, caffeine 65 mg. Tab. Bot. 1000s. *OTC.*
Use: Analgesic.

Tenoretic. (AstraZeneca) Atenolol/chlorthalidone 50 mg/25 mg, 100 mg/25 mg. Tab. Bot. 100s. *Rx.*
Use: Antihypertensive, diuretic.

Tenormin. (AstraZeneca) Atenolol 25 mg, 50 mg, 100 mg. Tab. 100s. *Rx.*
Use: Antiadrenergic/sympatholytic, beta-adrenergic blocker.

•**tenoxicam.** (ten-OX-ih-kam) USAN.
Use: Anti-inflammatory.

Tensive Conductive Adhesive Gel. (Parker) Nonflammable conductive adhesive electrode gel, eliminates tape and tape irritation. Tube 60 g.
Use: Therapeutic aid.

Tensocaine. (Sanofi-Synthelabo) Acetaminophen. Tab. *OTC.*
Use: Analgesic.

Tensolate. (Apco) Phenobarbital 0.25 g, hyoscyamine sulfate 0.1037 mg, atropine sulfate 0.0194 mg, hyoscine HBr 0.0065 mg. Tab. Bot. 100s. *Rx.*
Use: Antispasmodic.

Tensolax. (Sanofi-Synthelabo) Chlormezanone. Tab. *Rx.*
Use: Muscle relaxant.

Tensopin. (Apco) Phenobarbital 0.25 g, homatropine methylbromide 2.5 mg. Tab. Bot. 100s. *Rx.*
Use: Antispasmodic.

T.E.P. (Geneva) Phenobarbital 8 mg, theophylline 130 mg, ephedrine hydrochloride 24 mg. Tab. Bot. 100s. *Rx.*
Use: Antiasthmatic combination.

Tepanil. (3M) Diethylpropion hydrochloride 25 mg. Tab. Bot. 100s. *c-IV.*
Use: Anorexiant.

Tepanil Ten-Tab. (3M) Diethylpropion 75 mg. Tab. Bot. 30s, 100s, 250s. *c-IV.*
Use: Anorexiant.

•**tepoxalin.** (teh-POX-ah-lin) USAN.
Use: Antipsoriatic.

•**teprotide.** (TEH-pro-tide) USAN.

Use: Angiotensin-converting enzyme inhibitor.

•**teprotumumab.** (TEP-roe-TOOM-oo-mab) USAN.
Use: Antineoplastic.

tequinol sodium. *Name used for Actinoquinol Sodium.*

Tera-Gel. (Geritrex) Coal tar 0.5%. EDTA, parabens. Shampoo. 114 mL. *OTC.*
Use: Photochemotherapy.

Terazol 7. (Janssen Pharmaceuticals) Terconazole 0.4%, cetyl alcohol, stearyl alcohol. Vag. Cream. Tube 45 g w/1 measured-dose applicator. *Rx.*
Use: Antifungal, vaginal.

Terazol 3. (Janssen Pharmaceuticals) **Cream, vaginal:** Terconazole 0.8%. Tube 20 g with 1 measured-dose applicator. **Supp., vaginal:** Terconazole 80 mg, coconut oil/palm kernel oil. 2.5 g. 3s. *Rx.*
Use: Antifungal, vaginal.

•**terazosin hydrochloride.** (ter-AZ-oh-sin) *USP.*
Use: Antihypertensive, antiadrenergic.
See: Hytrin.

terazosin hydrochloride. (Geneva) Terazosin 1 mg, 2 mg, 5 mg, 10 mg (as base). Tab. Bot. 100s, 1000s. *Rx.*
Use: Antiadrenergic.

terazosin hydrochloride. (Various Mfr.) Terazosin hydrochloride 1 mg, 2 mg, 5 mg, 10 mg (as base), may contain lactose. Cap. Bot. 100s, 500s. *Rx.*
Use: Antiadrenergic.

•**terbinafine.** (TER-bin-ah-feen) USAN.
Use: Antifungal.
See: Terbinex.

terbinafine hydrochloride.
Use: Antifungal, allylamine.
See: Lamisil.
Lamisil AT.
Lamisil AT Jock Itch.

terbinafine hydrochloride. (Taro) Terbinafine hydrochloride 1%. Benzyl alcohol, cetyl alcohol, stearyl alcohol. Cream. 24 g. *OTC.*
Use: Topical anti-infective, antifungal agent.

terbinafine hydrochloride. (Various Mfr.) Terbinafine hydrochloride 250 mg. May contain lactose. Tab. 30s, 90s, 100s, 500s. *Rx.*
Use: Antifungal agent, allylamine antifungal.

Terbinex. (JSJ Pharmaceuticals) Terbinafine 250 mg. Tab. Kit w/ 42 tablets and 12 mL topical Eco Formula.
Use: Antifungal agent, allylamine antifungal.

•**terbutaline sulfate.** (ter-BYOO-tuh-leen) *USP.*
Use: Bronchodilator, sympathomimetic.

terbutaline sulfate. (Global) Terbutaline sulfate 2.5 mg, 5 mg. Tab. Bot. 100s. *Rx.*
Use: Bronchodilator, sympathomimetic.

terbutaline sulfate. (Various Mfr.) Terbutaline sulfate 1 mg/mL. Inj. Vials. 1 mL single-use. *Rx.*
Use: Bronchodilator, sympathomimetic.

Tercodryl. (Health for Life Brands) Codeine phos. 0.75 g, pyrilamine maleate 25 mg/fl. oz. Bot. 4 oz. *c-v.*
Use: Antihistamine, antitussive.

•**terconazole.** (ter-CONE-uh-zole) USAN. *Formerly triaconazole.*
Use: Antifungal.
See: Terazol 7.
Terazol 3.

terconazole. (Perrigo) Terconazole 80 mg. Vag. Supp. 3s with applicator. *Rx.*
Use: Vaginal antifungal agent.

terconazole. (Various Mfr.) Terconazole 0.4%, 0.8%. Alcohols. Vaginal cream. Tube. 20 g (0.8 % only), 45 g (0.4% only). *Rx.*
Use: Vaginal antifungal agent.

Terg-A-Zyme. (Alconox) Detergent with enzyme action. Box 4 lb Ctn. 9 × 4 lb, 25 lb, 50 lb, 100 lb, 300 lb. *OTC.*
Use: Biodegradable detergent and wetting agent.

•**tergenpumatucel-L.** (TER-jen-pum-a-too-sel-el) USAN.
Use: Antineoplastic.

Teridol Jr. (Health for Life Brands) Terpin hydrate, cocillana, potassium guaiacol sulfonate, ammonium chloride. Bot. 3 oz. *OTC.*
Use: Expectorant.

•**teriflunomide.** (TER-i-FLOO-noe-mide) USAN.
Use: Treatment of multiple sclerosis.
See: Aubagio.

•**teriparatide.** (ter-i-PAR-a-tide) USAN.
Use: Parathyroid hormone.
See: Forteo.

•**terlakiren.** (ter-lah-KIE-ren) USAN.
Use: Antihypertensive.

•**terlipressin.** (TER-li-PRES-in) USAN.
Use: Investigational posterior pituitary hormone; treatment of bleeding esophageal varices; vasoconstrictor. [Orphan Drug]
See: Glypressin.

Terocin. (Alexso) **Lot.:** Capsaicin 0.025%, lidocaine 2.5%, menthol 10%, methyl salicylate 25%. Aloe, borago

seed oil, cetyl alcohol, parabens, PEG, propylene glycol, triethanolamine. 120 mL. **Patch; topical:** Lidocaine 4%, menthol 4%. Aloe, EDTA disodium, glycerin, lemon peel oil, parabens, polysorbate 80, urea. 10s. *OTC.*
Use: Topical local anesthetic combination.

•**terodiline hydrochloride.** (TEH-row-DIE-leen) USAN.
Use: Vasodilator, coronary.

•**teroxalene hydrochloride.** (ter-OX-ah-leen) USAN.
Use: Antischistosomal.

•**teroxirone.** (TER-OX-ih-rone) USAN.
Use: Antineoplastic.

Terpex Jr. (Health for Life Brands) d-Methorphan 25 mg, terpin hydrate, potassium guaiacol sulfonate, cocillana, ammonium chloride. Bot. 4 oz. *OTC.*
Use: Expectorant.

Terphan. (Pal-Pak, Inc.) Terpin hydrate 85 mg, dextromethorphan hydrobromide 10 mg/5 mL w/alcohol 40% Elix. Bot. Gal. *OTC.*
Use: Antitussive, expectorant.

•**terpin hydrate and codeine oral solution.** (TER-pin) *USP.*
Use: Expectorant, antitussive.

•**terpin hydrate oral solution.** (TER-pin) *USP.*
Use: Expectorant.

Terra-Cortril. (Pfizer) Hydrocortisone 1.5%, oxytetracycline hydrochloride 0.5%. Ophth. Susp. Bot. 5 mL. *Rx.*
Use: Anti-infective, corticosteroid, ophthalmic.

Terrell. (Piramal Critical Care) Isoflurane. Liq. for Inh. 100 mL, 250 mL. *Rx.*
Use: General anesthetic.

Tersaseptic. (Doak Dermatologics) DEA-lauryl sulfate, lauramide DEA, propylene glycol, ethoxydiglycol, PEG-12 distearate, EDTA, triclosan, citric acid/ Shampoo/cleanser. Soapless. 473 mL. *OTC.*
Use: Dermatologic, acne.

tersavid.
Use: Monoamine oxidase inhibitor.

tertiary amyl alcohol.
See: Amylene Hydrate.

•**tesamorelin.** (TES-ah-moe-REL-in) USAN.
Use: Growth hormone–releasing factor.
See: Egrifta.

•**tesicam.** (TESS-ih-kam) USAN.
Use: Anti-inflammatory.

•**tesimide.** (TESS-ih-mide) USAN.
Use: Anti-inflammatory.

Tesogen. (Sigma-Tau) Testosterone 25 mg, estrone 2 mg/mL. Vial 10 mL. *c-III.*
Use: Androgen.

Tesogen L.A. (Sigma-Tau) Testosterone enanthate 180 mg, 90 mg, 50 mg, estradiol valerate 8 mg, 4 mg, 2 mg, respectively/mL. Vial 10 mL. *Rx.*
Use: Androgen, estrogen combination.

tespa.
Use: Antineoplastic.
See: Thiotepa.

Tessalon. (Pfizer) Benzonatate 200 mg. Parabens. Cap. Bot. 100s, 500s. *Rx.*
Use: Nonnarcotic antitussive.

Tessalon Perles. (Pfizer) Benzonatate 100 mg. Parabens. Cap. Bot. 100s, 500s. *Rx.*
Use: Nonnarcotic antitussive.

Testamone. (Oxypure) Testosterone 100 mg/mL. Inj. Vial 10 mL. *c-III.*
Use: Androgen.

Testex. (Taylor Pharmaceuticals) Testosterone propionate 50 mg, 100 mg/mL in sesame oil. Vial 10 mL. *c-III.*
Use: Androgen.

Testim. (Auxilium Pharm) Testosterone 1%. Ethanol 74%, glycerin. Gel. 5 g. *c-III.*
Use: Sex hormone, androgen.

Testoject-50. (Merz) Testosterone 50 mg/mL. Vial 10 mL. *c-III.*
Use: Androgen.

Testoject-LA. (Merz) Testosterone cypionate 200 mg/mL in oil. Vial 10 mL. *c-III.*
Use: Androgen.

•**testolactone.** (TESS-toe-LAK-tone) *USP.*
Use: Antineoplastic; sex hormone, androgen.

Testolin. (Taylor Pharmaceuticals) Testosterone suspension 25 mg, 50 mg, 100 mg/mL. Vial 10 mL 25 mg/mL. Vial 30 mL. *c-III.*
Use: Androgen.

Testopel. (Slate Pharmaceuticals) Testosterone 75 mg for subcutaneous administration. Pellets. 1 Pellet/Vial. Box 3s, 10s, 100s. *c-III.*
Use: Sex hormone, androgen.

•**testosterone.** (tess-TAHS-ter-ohn) *USP.*
Use: Androgen, sex hormone.
See: Androderm.
AndroGel 1%.
Andronaq-50.
Fortesta.
Homogene-S.
Malotrone.
Striant.
Testim.
Testolin.
Testopel.

W/Combinations.
See: Andesterone.
Angen.
Tesogen.

testosterone. 2%. Oint.
Use: Vulvar dystrophies. [Orphan Drug]

testosterone, buccal.
Use: Androgen, sex hormone.
See: Striant.

testosterone cyclopentane propionate. Testosterone Cypionate.

•**testosterone cypionate.** (tess-TAHS-ter-ohn) *USP.*
Use: Androgen, sex hormone.
See: Depo-Testosterone.
W/Combinations.
See: Depo-Testadiol.
Menoject L.A.

testosterone cypionate. (Sandoz) Testosterone cypionate 100 mg/mL. Benzyl alcohol 9.45 mg, benzyl benzoate 0.1 mL, cottonseed oil 736 mg. Inj. Vials. 10 mL. *c-III.*
Use: Sex hormone, androgen.

testosterone cypionate. (Various Mfr.) Testosterone cypionate 200 mg/mL. Benzyl alcohol, cottonseed oil. Inj. Vials. 1 mL, 10 mL. *c-III.*
Use: Sex hormone, androgen.

•**testosterone enanthate.** (tess-TAHS-ter-ohn) *USP.*
Use: Sex hormone, androgen.
W/Estradiol Valerate.
See: Valertest.

testosterone enanthate. (Paddock) Testosterone enanthate 200 mg/mL. Sesame oil. Inj. Multiple-dose vials. 5 mL. *c-III.*
Use: Androgen, sex hormone.

testosterone heptanoate.
Use: Androgen.
See: Testosterone Enanthate.

•**testosterone ketolaurate.** (tess-TAHS-ter-ohn KEY-toe-LORE-ate) USAN.
Use: Androgen.

•**testosterone phenylacetate.** (tess-TAHS-ter-ohn fen-ill-ASS-ah-tate) USAN. Perandren phenylacetate.
Use: Androgen.

•**testosterone propionate.** (tess-TAHS-ter-ohn) *USP.*
Use: Androgen.

testosterone, transdermal.
Use: Sex hormone, androgen.
See: Androderm.

•**testosterone undecanoate.** (tess-TAHS-ter-ohn un-DEK-a-NOE-ate) USAN.
Use: Androgen.
See: Aveed.

Testred. (Valeant) Methyltestosterone 10 mg. Cap. Bot. 100s. *c-III.*
Use: Sex hormone, androgen.

Testuria. (Wyeth) Combination kit containing 5 × 20 sterile dip strips and 5 × 20 culture trays of trypticase soy agar.
Use: Diagnostic aid.

Tesuloid. (Bristol-Myers Squibb) Technetium Tc 99m sulfur colloid. 5 Vials. Kit.
Use: Radiopaque agent.

•**tetanus and diphtheria toxoids adsorbed for adult use.** (TET-ah-nus and diff-THEER-ee-uh TOX-oyds) *USP.*
Use: Immunization.
See: Decavac.

tetanus and diphtheria toxoids adsorbed purogenated. (Wyeth) Tetanus and diphtheria toxoids adsorbed purogenated. Adult *Lederject* disposable syringe 10 × 0.5 mL. Vial 5 mL, new package. *Rx.*
Use: Immunization.

tetanus and diphtheria toxoids and acellular pertussis vaccine, adsorbed.
Use: Immunization.
See: Adacel.
Boostrix.
Daptacel.
Infanrix.
TriHIBit.

tetanus, diphtheria, acellular pertussis, Haemophilus influenzae type B conjugate vaccine.
Use: Immunization.
See: TriHIBit.

tetanus, diphtheria toxoids, and aluminum phosphate adsorbed. (Wyeth) Tetanus, diphtheria toxoids, and aluminum phosphate adsorbed. Inj. Vial 5 mL, *Tubex* 0.5 mL. *Rx.*
Use: Immunization.

•**tetanus immune globulin.** (TET-ah-nus ih-MYOON GLAH-byoo-lin) *USP. Formerly Tetanus Immune Human Globulin.* Gamma globulin fraction of the plasma of persons who have been hyperimmunized with tetanus toxoid, 16.5%. Vial 250 units.
Use: Prophylaxis of injured, against tetanus (passive immunizing agent).
See: HyperTET S/D.

•**tetanus toxoid.** (TET-n-us TOX-oyd) *USP.*
Use: Immunization.

•**tetanus toxoid, adsorbed.** (TET-n-us TOX-oyd) *USP.*
Use: Immunization.

tetanus toxoid, aluminum phosphate adsorbed. *Rx.*
Use: Immunization.
Tetcaine. (Ocusoft) Tetracaine hydrochloride 0.5%. Chlorobutanol 0.4%, sodium chloride 0.75%. Soln. 15 mL. *Rx.*
Use: Ophthalmic local anesthetic.
tetiothalein sodium.
See: Iodophthalein Sodium.
Tetrabead. (Abbott Diagnostics) Solid phase radioimmunoassay for the quantitative measurement of total circulating serum thyroxine.
Use: Diagnostic aid.
Tetrabead-125. (Abbott Diagnostics) T-3 uptake radioassay for the measurement of thyroid function by indirectly determining the degree of saturation of serum thyroxine binding globulin (TBG).
Use: Diagnostic aid.
tetrabenazine.
See: Xenazine.
•**tetracaine.** (TEH-trah-cane) *USP.*
Use: Anesthetic (topical).
W/Lidocaine.
See: Pliaglis.
Synera.
tetracaine. (Akorn) Tetracaine hydrochloride 1%. Sodium chloride 7.5 mg. Preservative free. Inj., Soln. Amp. 2 mL. *Rx.*
Use: Injectable local anesthetic, ester local anesthetic.
tetracaine and menthol ointment.
Use: Anesthetic, local.
•**tetracaine hydrochloride.** (TEH-trah-cane) *USP.*
Use: Anesthetic, injectable local ester; ophthalmic local anesthetic.
See: Altacaine.
Pontocaine.
Pontocaine Hydrochloride.
W/Benzocaine, Butamben, Benzalkonium Chloride.
See: Cetacaine.
tetracaine hydrochloride. (Various Mfr.) Tetracaine hydrochloride 0.5%. Soln. 1 mL, 2 mL, 15 mL. *Rx.*
Use: Anesthetic; ophthalmic.
Tetracap. (Circle) Tetracycline hydrochloride 250 mg. Cap. Bot. 100s. *Rx.*
Use: Anti-infective, tetracycline.
tetrachlorethylene. Perchloroethylene, tetrachlorethylene.
Use: Anthelmintic (hookworms and some trematodes).
Tetracon. (Professional Pharmacal) Tetrahydrozoline hydrochloride 0.5 mg, disodium edetate 1 mg, boric acid 12 mg, benzalkonium chloride 0.1 mg, sodium chloride 2.2 mg, sodium borate 0.5 mg/mL w/water. Liq. Bot. 15 mL. *OTC.*
Use: Anti-irritant; ophthalmic.
tetracyclic compounds.
Use: Antidepressant.
See: Maprotiline Hydrochloride.
Mirtazapine.
•**tetracycline and amphotericin B.** (teh-trah-SIGH-kleen) *USP.*
•**tetracycline hydrochloride.** (teh-trah-SIGH-kleen) *USP.*
Use: Anti-infective; antiamebic; antirickettsial.
See: Bicycline.
Cyclopar.
Panmycin.
Tetracap.
Tetracyn.
W/Bismuth Subcitrate Potassium, Metronidazole.
See: Pylera.
W/Diphenhydramine Hydrochloride, Hydrocortisone, Nystatin.
See: First Mary's Mouthwash.
tetracycline hydrochloride. (Various Mfr.) Tetracycline hydrochloride 250 mg. 500 mg. Cap. Bot. 100s, 1000s, UD 100s. *Rx.*
Use: Anti-infective, antiamebic, antirickettsial.
•**tetracycline oral suspension.** (teh-trah-SIGH-kleen) *USP.*
Use: Anti-infective, tetracycline.
•**tetracycline phosphate complex.** (teh-trah-SIGH-kleen) *USP.*
Use: Anti-infective.
tetracyclines.
See: Demeclocycline Hydrochloride.
Doxycycline.
Doxycycline Hyclate.
Minocycline Hydrochloride.
Oxytetracycline.
Tetracycline Hydrochloride.
tetracycline with n-acetyl-para-aminophenol, phenyltoloxamine citrate. (Roberts) Paltet, Cap.
Use: Anti-infective, tetracycline.
Tetracyn. (Pfizer) Tetracycline hydrochloride. Cap. **250 mg:** Bot. 1000s. **500 mg:** Bot. 100s. *Rx.*
Use: Anti-infective, tetracycline.
tetradecyl sulfate, sodium.
Use: Sclerosing agent.
See: Sotradecol.
tetraethyl ammonium bromide (TEAB).
Use: Diagnostic & therapeutic agent in peripheral vascular disorders. Diagnostic in hypertension.
tetraethylammonium chloride.
Use: Ganglionic blocking.
tetraethylthiuram disulfide.
See: Disulfiram.

•**tetrafilcon A.** (teh-trah-FILL-kahn) USAN.
Use: Contact lens material (hydrophilic).

tetrafluoroethane.
W/Pentafluoropropane.
See: Gebauer's Spray and Stretch.

Tetra-Formula. (Reese Pharm) Dextromethorphan HBr 10 mg, benzocaine 15 mg. Sucrose, glucose, dextrose. Loz. Pkg. 10s. *OTC.*
Use: Nonnarcotic antitussive.

tetrahydroaminoacridine.
Use: Cholinergic agent for Alzheimer disease.
See: Cognex.

tetrahydrophenobarbital calcium.
See: Cyclobarbital Calcium.

tetrahydroxyquinone. *Name used for tetroquinone.*

•**tetrahydrozoline hydrochloride.** (teh-trah-high-DRAHZ-ah-leen) *USP.*
Use: Adrenergic (vasoconstrictor); nasal decongestant, imidazoline; ophthalmic decongestant.
See: Altazine.
Murine Plus.
Opti-Clear.
Optigene 3.
Tyzine.
Tyzine Pediatric.
Visine.
Visine Advanced Relief.
Visine Maximum Redness Relief.

tetrahydrozoline hydrochloride. (Various Mfr.) Tetrahydrozoline hydrochloride 0.05%. Ophth. Soln. 15 mL. *OTC.*
Use: Ophthalmic decongestant.

tetraiodophenolphthalein sodium.
See: Iodophthalein Sodium.

tetraiodophthalein sodium.
See: Iodophthalein Sodium.

tetramethylene dimethanesulfonate. Busulfan.

tetramethylthiuram disulfide. Thiram.
Use: Anti-infective; antifungal.

•**tetramisole hydrochloride.** (teh-TRAM-ih-sole) USAN.
Use: Anthelmintic.

Tetraneed. (Hanlon) Pentaerythritol tetranitrate 80 mg. Time Cap. Bot. 100s. *Rx.*
Use: Antianginal.

tetrantoin.
Use: Anticonvulsant.

tetrastarch.
Use: Plasma expander.
See: Voluven.

Tetratab. (Freeport) Pentaerythritol tetranitrate 10 mg. Tab. Bot. 1000s. *Rx.*
Use: Antianginal.

Tetratab No. 1. (Freeport) Pentaerythritol tetranitrate 20 mg. Tab. Bot. 1000s. *Rx.*
Use: Antianginal.

•**tetraxetan.** (te-TRAX-e-tan) USAN.
Use: Chelating agent.

•**tetrazolast meglumine.** (teh-TRAZZ-oh-last meh-GLUE-meen) USAN.
Use: Antiallergic; antiasthmatic.

Tetrazyme. (Abbott Diagnostics) Test kit 100s, 500s.
Use: Enzyme immunoassay for quantitative measurement of total circulating serum thyroxine (free and protein bound).

Tetrix. (Coria) Aluminum magnesium hydroxide stearate, cetyl dimethicone copolyol, cyclomethicone, dimethicone, hexyl laurate, polyglyceryl-4 isostearate, sodium chloride. Propylparabens. Cream. Kit w/two 56.7 g tubes and two 56.7 g tubes of *CaraVe* moisturizing cream. *Rx.*
Use: Miscellaneous topical combination.

•**tetrofosmin.** (teh-troe-FOSS-min) USAN.
Use: Diagnostic aid.

•**tetroquinone.** (TEH-troe-kwih-NOHN) USAN.
Use: Treat keloids, keratolytic (systemic).

•**tetroxoprim.** (tet-ROX-oh-prim) USAN.
Use: Anti-infective.

•**tetrydamine.** (teh-TRID-ah-meen) USAN.
Use: Analgesic; anti-inflammatory.

Tetterine. (S.S.S. Company) Miconazole nitrate 2%. Petrolatum. Oint. 28.4 g. *OTC.*
Use: Topical anti-infective, antifungal agent.

Teveten. (Abbott) Eprosartan mesylate 400 mg, 600 mg. Lactose, PEG. Film-coated. Tab. 100s. *Rx.*
Use: Antihypertensive.

Teveten HCT. (Abbott) Eprosartan/hydrochlorothiazide 600 mg/12.5 mg, 600 mg/25 mg. Lactose. Film coated. Tab. 100s. *Rx.*
Use: Antihypertensive combination.

Tev-Tropin. (Gate) Somatropin 5 mg (≈ 15 units)/vial. Mannitol 30 mg. Pow. for Inj., lyophilized. Vials w/5 mL diluent (bacteriostatic sodium chloride 0.9% for injection w/benzyl alcohol 0.9%). *Rx.*
Use: Growth hormone.

Texacort. (Mission) Hydrocortisone 2.5%. Alcohol. Lipid free. Soln. 30 mL. *Rx.*
Use: Corticosteroid.

tezacitabine.
Use: Antineoplastic.

•**tezampanel.** (tez-AM-pan-el) USAN.
Use: Treatment of migraines.

tezosentan.
Use: Dual endothelin receptor antagonist.

T-Fluoride. (Tennessee Pharmaceutic) Sodium fluoride 2.21 mg. Tab. Bot. 100s, 1000s. *Rx.*
Use: Dental caries preventative.

T4. Levothyroxine Sodium.

T4 endonuclease V, liposome encapsulated.
Use: Xeroderma pigmentosum. [Orphan Drug]

T-4 RIA (PEG). (Abbott Diagnostics) Diagnostic kit 50s, 100s, 500s. *Rx.*
Use: For quantitative measurement of total circulating serum thyroxine.

T4, soluble, human recombinant. (Biogen) Phase I/II HIV.
Use: Antiviral.

TG.
Use: Antineoplastic.
See: Thioguanine.

T/Gel Scalp. (Neutrogena) Neutar coal tar extract 2%, salicylic acid 2%. Soln. Bot. 2 oz. *OTC.*
Use: Antipsoriatic; antiseborrheic.

T/Gel Therapeutic Conditioner. (Neutrogena) Neutar coal tar extract 1.5% in oil free conditioner base. Liq. Bot. 1.4 oz. *OTC.*
Use: Antipsoriatic; antiseborrheic.

T/Gel Therapeutic Shampoo. (Neutrogena) Neutar coal tar extract 2% in mild shampoo base. Bot. 4.4 oz., 8.5 oz. *OTC.*
Use: Antipsoriatic; antiseborrheic.

T-Gesic. (T.E. Williams Pharmaceuticals) Hydrocodone bitartrate 5 mg, acetaminophen 500 mg. Cap. Bot. 100s. *c-III.*
Use: Analgesic combination; narcotic; hypnotic; sedative.

TG45PSE/400GFN. (TG United Pharmaceuticals) Guaifenesin 400 mg, pseudoephedrine hydrochloride 45 mg. Tab. 60s. *OTC.*
Use: Upper respiratory combination, decongestant and expectorant combination.

TGQ 15DM/5PEH/2CPM. (TG United Pharmaceuticals) Chlorpheniramine maleate 2 mg, dextromethorphan hydrobromide 15 mg, phenylephrine hydrochloride 5 mg. Parabens, potassium citrate, potassium sorbate, propylene glycol, sorbitol, sucralose. Strawberry flavor. Liq. 473 mL. *Rx.*
Use: Upper respiratory combination, antitussive combination.

TGQ 50PSE/3BRM/30DM. (TG United Pharmaceuticals) Brompheniramine maleate 3 mg, dextromethorphan hydrobromide 30 mg, pseudoephedrine hydrochloride 50 mg per 5 mL. Parabens, potassium sorbate, propylene glycol, sorbitol, sucralose. Berry-vanilla flavor. Syrup. 473 mL. *Rx.*
Use: Upper respiratory combination, antitussive combination.

TGQ 40PSE/4BRM/20DM. (TG United Pharmaceuticals) Brompheniramine maleate 4 mg, dextromethorphan hydrobromide 20 mg, pseudoephedrine hydrochloride 40 mg. Tab. 100s. *Rx.*
Use: Upper respiratory combination, antitussive combination.

TGQ 7.5PEH/4BRM/15DM. (TG United Pharmaceuticals) Brompheniramine maleate 4 mg, dextromethorphan hydrobromide 15 mg, phenylephrine hydrochloride 7.5 mg per 5 mL. Parabens, potassium sorbate, propylene glycol, sorbitol, sucralose. Strawberry flavor. Liq. 473 mL. *Rx.*
Use: Upper respiratory combination, antitussive combination.

TGQ 30PSE/150GFN/15DM. (TG United Pharmaceuticals) Dextromethorphan hydrobromide 15 mg, guaifenesin 150 mg, pseudoephedrine hydrochloride 30 mg. Saccharin, sorbitol. Alcohol free. Mint flavor. Liq. 30 mL, 473 mL. *Rx.*
Use: Upper respiratory combination, antitussive and expectorant combination.

TGQ 30PSE/3BRM/15DM. (TG United Pharmaceuticals) Brompheniramine maleate 3 mg, dextromethorphan hydrobromide 15 mg, pseudoephedrine hydrochloride 30 mg per 5 mL. Parabens, potassium sorbate, propylene glycol, sorbitol, sucralose. Berry-vanilla flavor. Liq. 473 mL. *Rx.*
Use: Upper respiratory combination, antitussive combination.

TG10PEH/380GFN. (TG United Pharmaceuticals) Guaifenesin 380 mg, phenylephrine hydrochloride 10 mg. Tab. 60s. *OTC.*
Use: Upper respiratory combination, decongestant and expectorant combination.

•**thalidomide.** (the-LID-oh-mide) USAN.
Use: Anti-infective; hypnotic; sedative; immunomodulator.
See: Thalomid.

Thalitone. (Monarch) Chlorthalidone 15 mg. Lactose. Tab. Bot. 100s. *Rx.*
Use: Diuretic.

•**thallous chloride Tl 201 injection.** (THAL-uhs) *USP.*
Use: Diagnostic aid (radiopaque medium); radioactive agent.

Thalomid. (Celgene) Thalidomide 50 mg, 100 mg, 150 mg, 200 mg. Cap. UD 28s, UD 84s (200 mg only), UD 112s (150 mg only), UD 140s (100 mg only), UD 280s (50 mg only). *Rx.*
Note: Available only to be prescribed and dispensed under the terms of the System for Thalidomide Education and Prescribing Safety (S.T.E.P.S.) restricted distribution program.
Use: Immunomodulator.

Tham. (Abbott) Tromethamine 18 g, acetic acid 2.5 g single-dose container. Soln. *Rx.*
Use: Nutritional supplement.

Tham-E. (Abbott) Tromethamine 36 g, NaCl 30 mEq/L, KCl 5 mEq/L, Cl 35 mEq/L. Total osmolarity 367 mOsm/L. Single-dose container 150 mL. *Rx.*
Use: Nutritional supplement.

theamin. Monoethanolamine salt of theophylline.

thenalidine tartrate.
Use: Antihistamine; antipruritic.

thenyldiamine hydrochloride.
Use: Antihistamine.

theobroma oil. Cocoa Butter.
Use: Pharmaceutical aid; suppository base.

theobromine sodium acetate. Theobromine calcium salt mixture with calcium salicylate.
Use: Diuretic; muscle relaxant.

Theochron. (Forest) Theophylline 100 mg, 200 mg, 300 mg, 450 mg. ER Tab. 100s, 500s (200 mg, 300 mg, 450 mg), 1,000s. *Rx.*
Use: Bronchodilator.

•**theofibrate.** (thee-oh-FYE-brate) USAN.
Use: Antihyperlipoproteinemic.

Theogen. (Sigma-Tau) Conjugated estrogens 2 mg/mL. Vial 10 mL, 30 mL. *Rx.*
Use: Estrogen.

Theogen I.P. (Sigma-Tau) Estrone 2 mg, potassium estrone sulfate 1 mg/mL. Inj. Vial 10 mL. *Rx.*
Use: Estrogen.

Theophenyllin. (H.L. Moore Drug Exchange) Theophylline 130 mg, ephedrine hydrochloride 24 mg, phenobarbital 8 mg. Tab. Bot. 1000s. *Rx.*
Use: Antiasthmatic.

•**theophylline.** (thee-AHF-ih-lin) *USP.*
Use: Bronchodilator; coronary vasodilator, diuretic; pharmaceutic necessity for Aminophylline Injection.
See: Elixophyllin.
Theo-24.
Theochron.
Uniphyl.
W/Guaifenesin.
See: Ed-Bron G.
W/Guaifenesin, Pseudoephedrine Hydrochloride.
See: Broncomar.
W/Combinations.
See: Ceepa.
Co-Xan.
Neoasma.
Quibron Plus.
Tedral SA.

theophylline. (Inwood) Theophylline 125 mg, 200 mg. ER Cap. 100s. *Rx.*
Use: Bronchodilator.

theophylline. (Various Mfr.) Theophylline 100 mg, 200 mg, 300 mg, 450 mg. ER Tab. 100s, 500s (200 mg, 300 mg), 1,000s (200 mg, 450 mg). *Rx.*
Use: Bronchodilator.

theophylline aminoisobutanol. Theophylline w/2-amino-2-methyl-1-propanol.
See: Butaphyllamine.

theophylline, 8-chloro, diphenhydramine. Dimenhydrinate.
See: Dramamine.

theophylline ethylenediamine.
See: Aminophylline.

theophylline in dextrose 5%. (Various Mfr.) Theophylline 0.8 mg/mL, 1.6 mg/mL, 2 mg/mL, 3.2 mg/mL, 4 mg/mL. Inj., Soln. 50 mL (4 mg/mL), 100 mL (2 mg/mL, 4 mg/mL), 250 mL (1.6 mg/mL, 3.2 mg/mL), 500 mL (0.8 mg/mL, 1.6 mg/mL), 1,000 mL (0.8 mg/mL). *Rx.*
Use: Bronchodilator.

theophylline olamine. Theophylline compound with 2-amino-ethanol (1:1).
Use: Bronchodilator.

theophylline reagent strips. (Bayer Consumer Care) Seralyzer reagent strip. Bot. 25s.
Use: Diagnostic aid; theophylline.

•**theophylline sodium glycinate.** (thee-AHF-ih-lin) *USP.*
Use: Bronchodilator.
See: Synophylate.

Theo-24. (UCB Pharma) Theophylline 100 mg, 200 mg, 300 mg, 400 mg. Sucrose. ER Cap. Bot. 100s, 500s (200 mg and 300 mg only). *Rx.*
Use: Antiasthmatic; bronchodilator.

Thera Bath. (Walgreen) Mineral oil 90%. Bot. 16 oz. *OTC.*
Use: Emollient.

Thera Bath with Vitamin E. (Walgreen) Mineral oil 91%, Vit. E 2000 units/16 oz. *OTC.*
Use: Emollient.

Therabid. (Mission Pharmacal) Vitamins C 500 mg, B_1 15 mg, B_2 10 mg, B_3

100 mg, B_5 20 mg, B_6 10 mg, B_{12} 5 mcg, A 5000 units, D 200 units, E 30 mg. Tab. Bot. 60s. *OTC.*
Use: Mineral, vitamin supplement.

Therabrand. (Health for Life Brands) Vitamins A 25,000 units, D 1000 units, B_1 10 mg, B_2 10 mg, niacinamide 100 mg, C 200 mg, B_6 5 mg, calcium pantothenate 20 mg, B_{12} 5 mcg. Cap. Bot. 100s, 1000s. *OTC.*
Use: Mineral, vitamin supplement.

Therabrand-M. (Health for Life Brands) Vitamins A 25,000 units, D 1000 units, C 200 mg, B_1 10 mg, B_2 10 mg, B_6 5 mg, niacinamide 100 mg, calcium pantothenate 20 mg, E 5 units, B_{12} 5 mcg, I 0.15 mg, Fe 15 mg, Cu 1 mg, Ca 125 mg, Mn 1 mg, Mg 6 mg, Zn 1.5 mg. Cap. Bot. 100s, 1000s. *OTC.*
Use: Mineral, vitamin supplement.

TheraCal D4000. (Theralogix) Vitamins D 1,000 units, K 25 mcg, Ca, Mg, Sr, B. Tab. 360s. *OTC.*
Use: Multivitamin with minerals.

TheraCal D2000. (Theralogix) Vitamins D 500 units, K 25 mcg, Ca, Mg, Sr, B. Tab. 360s. *OTC.*
Use: Multivitamin with minerals.

Theracap. (Arcum) Vitamins A 10,000 units, D 400 units, B_1 10 mg, B_2 5 mg, niacinamide 150 mg, C 150 mg. Cap. Bot. 100s, 1000s. *OTC.*
Use: Vitamin supplement.

Thera-Combex H-P. (Parke-Davis) Vitamins C 500 mg, B_1 25 mg, B_2 15 mg, B_{12} 5 mcg, niacinamide 100 mg, panthenol 20 mg. Cap. Bot. 100s. *OTC.*
Use: Vitamin supplement.

TheraCys. (Sanofi Pasteur) BCG live (for intravesical administration) 10.5 $\pm$ 8.7 $\times 10^8$ CFU (equivalent to $\approx$ 81 mg dry weight). Monosodium glutamate. Preservative free. Inj., Lyophilized, Pow. for Susp. Vials. 81 mg w/3 mL diluent vial. *Rx.*
Use: Biological response modifier.

TheraDerm. (Major) Castor oil, cetyl alcohol, disodium EDTA, lanolin, mineral oil, parabens, PEG, petrolatum, triethanolamine. Lot. 236 mL. *OTC.*
Use: Emollient.

Thera-D 4000. (Theralogix) Vitamin D_3 4,000 units. Tab. 90s. *OTC.*
Use: Fat-soluble vitamin.

Thera-D 2000. (Theralogix) Vitamin D_3 2,000 units. Tab. 180s. *OTC.*
Use: Fat-soluble vitamin.

Theraflu Cold & Cough. (Novartis) Dextromethorphan HBr 20 mg, pheniramine maleate 20 mg, phenylephrine hydrochloride 10 mg. Acesulfame K, maltodextrin, sodium 43 mg. Pow. Pkt. 6s. *Rx.*
Use: Upper respiratory combination, antitussive combination.

Theraflu Cold & Sore Throat. (Novartis) Phenylephrine hydrochloride 10 mg, pheniramine maleate 20 mg, acetaminophen 325 mg. Acesulfame K, sucrose, sodium 44 mg. Lemon flavor. Pow. 6s. *OTC.*
Use: Upper respiratory combination, decongestant, antihistamine, and analgesic.

Theraflu Daytime Severe Cold & Cough. (Novartis) **Cap.:** Acetaminophen 325 mg, dextromethorphan HBr 10 mg, phenylephrine hydrochloride 5 mg. PEG. 24s. **Pow.:** Acetaminophen 650 mg, dextromethorphan hydrobromide 20 mg, phenylephrine hydrochloride 10 mg. Acesulfame K, aspartame, maltodextrin, phenylalanine 14 mg, sucrose. Berry infused with menthol and green tea flavor. 6s. *OTC.*
Use: Upper respiratory combination, analgesic, antitussive, decongestant combination.

Theraflu Flu & Chest Congestion. (Novartis) Guaifenesin 400 mg, acetaminophen 1,000 mg. Acesulfame K, aspartame, maltodextrin, phenylalanine 24 mg/packet, sodium 15 mg/packet, sucrose. Citrus flavor. Pow. 6s. *OTC.*
Use: Upper respiratory combination, expectorant with analgesic combination.

Theraflu Flu & Sore Throat. (Novartis) Phenylephrine hydrochloride 10 mg, pheniramine maleate 20 mg, acetaminophen 650 mg. Acesulfame K, sucrose, sodium 51 mg. Apple cinnamon flavor. Pow. 6s. *OTC.*
Use: Upper respiratory combination, decongestant, antihistamine, and analgesic.

Theraflu Nighttime Severe Cold. (Novartis) Acetaminophen 325 mg, chlorpheniramine maleate 2 mg, dextromethorphan HBr 10 mg, phenylephrine hydrochloride 5 mg. Acesulfame potassium, PEG. Tab. 24s. *OTC.*
Use: Upper respiratory combination, decongestant, analgesic, antihistamine, antitussive combination.

Theraflu Nighttime Severe Cough & Cold. (Novartis) Acetaminophen 650 mg, diphenhydramine hydrochloride 25 mg, phenylephrine hydrochloride 10 mg. Acesulfame K, aspartame, maltodextrin, phenylalanine 13 mg, sucrose. Honey lemon flavor infused with chamomile and white tea. Pow. 6s. *OTC.*

Use: Upper respiratory combination; decongestant, antihistamine, and analgesic combination.

Thera-Flur. (Colgate Oral Pharmaceuticals) Fluoride 0.5% (from sod. fluoride 1.1%). pH 4.5. Gel-Drops. Bot. 24 mL, 60 mL. *Rx.*

Use: Dental caries agent.

Thera-Flur-N. (Colgate Oral Pharmaceuticals) Neutral sodium fluoride 1.1%. Liq. Bot. 24 mL, 60 mL. *Rx.*

Use: Dental caries agent.

Theraflu Severe Cold & Cough Daytime/Nighttime. (Novartis) Pow. for Soln. **Daytime:** Acetaminophen 650 mg, dextromethorphan hydrobromide 20 mg, phenylephrine hydrochloride 10 mg per packet. Acesulfame K, aspartame, maltodextrin, sucrose, phenylalanine 14 mg, potassium 10 mg, sodium 20 mg. Berry infused with menthol and green tea flavor. 6s. **Nighttime:** Acetaminophen 650 mg, diphenhydramine hydrochloride 25 mg, phenylephrine hydrochloride 10 mg per packet. Acesulfame K, aspartame, maltodextrin, sucrose, phenylalanine 13 mg, potassium 10 mg, sodium 23 mg. Honey-lemon infused with chamomile and white tea flavor. 18s. *OTC.*

Use: Upper respiratory combination; decongestant, antihistamine, and analgesic combination.

Theraflu Sugar-Free Nighttime Severe Cough & Cold. (Novartis) Acetaminophen 650 mg, diphenhydramine hydrochloride 25 mg, phenylephrine hydrochloride 10 mg. Acesulfame K, aspartame, maltodextrin, phenylalanine 13 mg. Sugar free. Honey lemon flavor. Pow. 6s. *OTC.*

Use: Upper respiratory combination; decongestant, antihistamine, and analgesic combination.

Theraflu Thin Strips Daytime Cough & Cold. (Novartis) Dextromethorphan HBr 20 mg, phenylephrine hydrochloride 10 mg. Alcohol < 5%, mannitol, sucralose. Cherry menthol flavor. Oral Strips. 12s. *OTC.*

Use: Upper respiratory combination, antitussive combination.

Theraflu Thin Strips Multi Symptom. (Novartis) Diphenhydramine hydrochloride 25 mg. Alcohol (less than 5%), sorbitol, sucralose. Cherry flavor. Orally Disintegrating Strips. 12s. *OTC.*

Use: Nonnarcotic antitussive.

Theraflu Thin Strips Nighttime Cold & Cough. (Novartis) Diphenhydramine hydrochloride 25 mg, phenylephrine hydrochloride 10 mg. Alcohol (less than 5%), mannitol, PEG, sucralose. Peppermint flavor. Orally Disintegrating Strips. 12s. *OTC.*

Use: Upper respiratory combination, decongestant and antihistamine.

Theraflu Warming Relief Daytime Multi-Symptom Cold. (Novartis) Acetaminophen 325 mg, dextromethorphan hydrobromide 10 mg, phenylephrine hydrochloride 5 mg. Benzoic acid, menthol, PEG, sucralose. Tab. 24s. *OTC.*

Use: Upper respiratory combination, antitussive combination.

Theraflu Warming Relief Flu & Sore Throat. (Novartis) Acetaminophen 108.3 mg, diphenhydramine hydrochloride 4.16 mg, phenylephrine hydrochloride 1.67 mg. Acesulfame K, alcohol 10%, edetate disodium, glycerin, maltitol, propylene glycol, sodium 2.3 mg, sodium benzoate. Cherry flavor. Liq. 245.5 mL. *OTC.*

Use: Upper respiratory combination; decongestant, antihistamine, and analgesic combination.

Therafortis. (General Vitamin) Vitamins A 12,500 units, D 1000 units, B_1 5 mg, B_2 5 mg, B_6 1 mg, B_{12} 3 mcg, niacinamide 50 mg, pantothenic acid salt 10 mg, C 150 mg, folic acid 0.5 mg. Cap. Bot. 100s, 1000s. *OTC.*

Use: Vitamin supplement.

Theragenerix. (Ivax) Vitamins A 5500 units, D 400 units, E 30 mg, B_1 3 mg, B_2 3.4 mg, B_3 30 mg, B_5 10 mg, B_6 3 mg, B_{12} 9 mcg, C 120 mg, folic acid 0.4 mg, biotin 15 mcg, beta-carotene 2500 units. Tab. Bot. 130s, 1000s. *OTC.*

Use: Vitamin supplement.

Theragenerix-H. (Ivax) Fe 66.7 mg, vitamins A 8333 units, D 133 units, E 5 units, B_1 3.3 mg, B_2 3.3 mg, B_3 33.3 mg, B_5 11.7 mg, B_6 3.3 mg, B_{12} 50 mcg, C 100 mg, folic acid 0.33 mg, Cu, Mg. Tab. Bot. 100s, 1000s. *OTC.*

Use: Mineral, vitamin supplement.

Theragenerix-M. (Ivax) Fe 27 mg, vitamins A 5000 units, D 400 units, E 30 mg, B_1 3 mg, B_2 3.4 mg, B_3 30 mg, B_5 10 mg, B_6 3 mg, B_{12} 9 mcg, C 120 mg, folic acid 0.4 mg, Ca, Cl, Cr, Cu, I, K, biotin 15 mcg, Mg, Mn, Mo, P, Se, Zn 15 mg, beta-carotene 2500 units. Tab. Bot. 130s, 1000s. *OTC.*

Use: Mineral, vitamin supplement.

Thera-Gesic. (Mission Pharmacal) Methyl salicylate, menthol. Balm. Tube 90 g, 150 g. *OTC.*

Use: Analgesic, topical.

Theragran. (Bristol-Myers Squibb) **Capl.:** Vitamins A 5000 units, D 400 units, E 30 units, B_1 3 mg, $B_2$3.4 mg, B_3 20 mg, B_5 10 mg, B_6 3 mg, B_{12} 9 mcg, C 90 mg, folic acid 0.4 mg, biotin 30 mcg. Bot. 100s. **Liq.:** Vitamins A 5000 units, D 400 units, B_1 10 mg, B_2 10 mg, B_3 100 mg, B_5 21.4 mg, B_6 4.1 mg, B_{12} 5 mcg, C 200 mg/5 mL. Liq. Bot. 120 mL. *OTC.*
Use: Vitamin supplement.

Theragran AntiOxidant. (Bristol-Myers Squibb) Vitamins A 5000 units, C 250 mg, E 200 units, Mn, Cu, Zn, Se. Softgel Cap. Bot. 50s. *OTC.*
Use: Mineral, vitamin supplement.

Theragran Jr. with Iron. (Bristol-Myers Squibb) Fe 18 mg, vitamins A 5000 units, D 400 units, E 30 mg, B_1 1.5 mg, B_2 1.7 mg, B_3 20 mg, B_6 2 mg, B_{12} 6 mcg, C 60 mg, folic acid 0.4 mg w/tartrazine. Tab. Bot. 75s. *OTC.*
Use: Mineral, vitamin supplement.

Theragran Stress Formula. (Bristol-Myers Squibb) Fe 27 mg, vitamins E 30 units, B_1 15 mg, B_2 15 mg, B_3 100 mg, B_5 20 mg, B_6 25 mg, B_{12}12 mcg, C 600 mg, folic acid 0.4 mg, biotin 45 mcg. Tab. Bot. 75s. *OTC.*
Use: Mineral, vitamin supplement.

Thera Hematinic. (Major) Fe 66.7 mg, A 8333 units, D 133 units, E 5 units, B_1 3.3 mg, B_2 3.3 mg, B_3 33.3 mg, B_5 11.7 mg, B_6 3.3 mg, B_{12} 50 mcg, C 100 mg, folic acid 0.33 mg, Cu, Mg. Tab. Bot. 250s, 1000s. *OTC.*
Use: Mineral, vitamin supplements.

Thera-Hist Cold & Allergy. (Major) Pseudoephedrine hydrochloride 15 mg, chlorpheniramine maleate 1 mg/5 mL, sorbitol, sucrose. Syr. Bot. 118 mL. *OTC.*
Use: Upper respiratory combination, decongestant, antihistamine.

Thera-Hist Cold & Cough. (Major) Pseudoephedrine hydrochloride 15 mg, chlorpheniramine maleate 1 mg, dextromethorphan HBr 5 mg per 5 mL. Sorbitol, sucrose, cherry flavor. Syr. Bot. 118 mL. *OTC.*
Use: Upper respiratory combination, decongestant, antihistamine, antitussive.

Thera-M. (Various Mfr.) Vitamins A 5000 units, B_1 3 mg, B_2 3.4 mg, B_3 20 mg, B_5 10 mg, B_6 3 mg, B_{12} 9 mcg, C 90 mg, D 400 units, E 30 units, Fe 27 mg, folic acid 0.4 mg, biotin 30 mcg, P, Ca, Cu, Cr, Se, Mo, K, Cl, I, Mg, Mn, Zn 15 mg. Tab. Bot. 130s, 1000s. *OTC.*
Use: Mineral, vitamin supplement.

Thera M Plus. (Major) Iron 9 mg, calcium 30 mg, vitamins A 5,000 units, D 400 units, E 60 units, B_1 3 mg, B_2 3.4 mg, B_3 20 mg, B_5 10 mg, B_6 6 mg, B_{12} 12 mcg, C 90 mg, K 28 mcg, folic acid 0.4 mg, B, Cl, Cr, Cu, I, K, Mg, Mn, Mo, Ni, P, Se, Si, Sn, V, Zn, biotin. Maltodextrin, mannitol. Lactose free, preservative free, sugar free. Tab. UD 100s. *OTC.*
Use: Multivitamin with minerals (including iron).

Thera Multi-Vitamin. (Major) Vitamins A 10,000 units, D 400 units, B_1 10 mg, B_2 10 mg, B_3 100 mg, B_5 21.4 mg, B_6 4.1 mg, B_{12} 5 mcg, C 200 mg/5 mL. Liq. Bot. 118 mL. *OTC.*
Use: Vitamin supplement.

Thera Natal Complete. (Theralogix) Vitamins A 3,000 units, C 100 mg, D_3 2,000 units, E 30 mg, B_1 1.5 mg, B_2 1.7 mg, B_3 20 mg, B_5 6 mg, B_6 12 mg, B_{12} 12 mcg, folate 1 mg, Ca 140 mg, Fe 27 mg, I, Mg, Zn, Cu, Se, Cr, Mo. **Tab.:** Biotin 30 mcg, choline 50 mg. 91s. **Softgels:** Vitamins D_3 500 units, B_6 9 mg, DHA 150 mg, choline 75 mg. 182s. *Rx.*
Use: Prenatal vitamin with minerals.

Thera Natal Core Nutrition. (Theralogix) Vitamins A 3,000 units, C 100 mg, D_3 2,000 units, E 30 units, B_1 1.5 mg, B_2 1.7 mg, B_3 20 mg, B_5 6 mg, B_6 12 mg, B_{12} 12 mcg, folic acid 1 mg, biotin 30 mcg, choline 50 mg, Fe 27 mg, Ca 140 mg, Zn, Cu, I, Mg, Cr, Mo, Se. Tab. 90s. *Rx.*
Use: Prenatal vitamin with minerals.

Theraneed. (Hanlon) Vitamins A 16,000 units, B_1 10 mg, B_2 10 mg, B_6 2 mg, C 300 mg, calcium pantothenate 10 mg, niacinamide 10 mg, B_{12} 10 mcg. Cap. Bot. 100s. *OTC.*
Use: Mineral, vitamin supplement.

Therapals. (Faraday) Vitamins A 25,000 units, D 400 units, B_1 10 mg, B_2 5 mg, niacinamide 150 mg, B_6 0.5 mg, E 5 units, C 150 mg, B_{12}10 mcg, Ca 103 mg, cobalt 0.1 mg, Cu 1 mg, K 0.15 mg, Mg 6 mg, Mn 1 mg, Mo 0.2 mg, P 80 mg, K 5 mg, Zn 1.2 mg. Tab. Bot. 100s, 250s, 1000s. *OTC.*
Use: Mineral, vitamin supplement.

TheraPatch Cold Sore. (LecTec) Lidocaine hydrochloride 4%, camphor 0.5%, aloe vera, eucalyptus oil, glycerin. Patch. Box 21s. *OTC.*
Use: Anesthetic, local.

TheraPatch Vapor Patch for Kids Cough Suppressant. (LecTec Corp.) Camphor 4.7%, menthol 2.6%. Glycerin, cherry scent. Patch. Box. 7s. *OTC.*

Use: Upper respiratory combination, topical.

Therapeutic. (Ivax) Vitamins A 5000 units, D 400 units, E 30 units, B_1 3 mg, B_2 3.4 mg, B_3 20 mg, B_5 10 mg, B_6 3 mg, B_{12} 9 mcg, C 90 mg, folic acid 0.4 mg, d-biotin 30 mcg. Tab. Bot. 100s, 130s. *OTC.*
Use: Vitamin supplement.

Therapeutic-H. (Ivax) Fe 66.7 mg, A 8333 units, D 133 units, E 5 units, B_1 3.3 mg, B_2 3.3 mg, B_3 33.3 mg, B_5 11.7 mg, B_6 3.3 mg, B_{12} 50 mcg, C 100 mg, folic acid 0.33 mg, Cu, Mg. Tab. Bot. 100s. *OTC.*
Use: Mineral, vitamin supplement.

Therapeutic-M. (Ivax) Fe 27 mg, vitamins A 5000 units, D 400 units, E 30 units, B_1 3 mg, B_2 3.4 mg, B_3 20 mg, B_5 10 mg, B_6 3 mg, B_{12} 9 mcg, C 90 mg, folic acid 0.4 mg, Ca, Cl, Cr, Cu, I, K, Mg, Mn, Mo, P, Se, Zn 15 mg, biotin 30 mcg. Tab. Bot. 1000s. *OTC.*
Use: Mineral, vitamin supplement.

Therapeutic Mineral Ice. (Novartis Consumer Health) Menthol 2%, ammonium hydroxide, carbomer 934, cupric sulfate, isopropyl alcohol, magnesium sulfate, thymol. Gel. Tube 105 mL, 240 mL, 480 mL. *OTC.*
Use: Liniment.

Therapeutic V & M. (Whiteworth Towne) Vitamins A 10,000 units, D 400 units, B_1 10 mg, B_2 10 mg, B_6 5 mg, B_{12} 5 mcg, niacinamide 100 mg, calcium pantothenate 20 mg, C 200 mg, E 15 units, I 0.15 mg, Fe 12 mg, Cu 2 mg, Mn 1 mg, Mg 60 mg, Zn 1.5 mg. Tab. *OTC.*
Use: Mineral, vitamin supplement.

Theraphon. (Health for Life Brands) Vitamins A 25,000 units, D 1000 units, B_1 10 mg, B_2 5 mg, C 150 mg, niacinamide 150 mg. Cap. Bot. 100s, 1000s. *OTC.*
Use: Vitamin supplement.

Thera-Plus. (Hi-Tech) Vitamins A 5,000 mg, D 400 mg, B_1 10 mg, B_2 10 mg, B_3 100 mg, B_5 21.4 mg, B_{12} 5 mcg, C 200 mg per 5 mL. Cherry flavoring, glycerin, methylparaben, sodium benzoate, sugar. Liq. 118 mL. *OTC.*
Use: Nutritional supplement, vitamin.

Therapy Ice. (Major) Menthol 2%. Isopropyl alcohol. Gel. 226.8 g. *OTC.*
Use: Emollient.

TheraSeal Hand Protection. (Coria Labs) Dimethicone 1%. Cyclomethicone, cyclomethicone aluminum magnesium hydroxide stearate, cetyl dimethicone copolyol and polyglyceryl-4-isostearate and hexyl laurate, sodium chloride, imidurea. Cream. 180 g. *OTC.*
Use: Skin protectant.

Thera-Tabs M. (Geri-Care Pharmaceuticals) Iron 27 mg, calcium 40 mg, vitamins A 5,000 units, D 400 units, E 30 units, B_1 3 mg, B_2 3.4 mg, B_3 20 mg, B_5 10 mg, B_6 3 mg, B_{12} 9 mcg, C 90 mg, folate 0.4 mg, chloride, Cr, Cu, I, K, Mg, Mn, Mo, P, Se, Zn, biotin. Mineral oil, PEG, sucrose. Caplet. 1,000s. *OTC.*
Use: Multivitamin w/minerals.

TheraTears. (Advanced Vision Research) **Gel.:** Carboxymethylcellulose sodium 1%, KCl, sodium bicarbonate, NaCl, sodium phosphate. UD 28s. **Soln.:** Carboxymethylcellulose sodium 0.25%, borate buffers, calcium chloride, KCl, magnesium chloride, NaCl, sodium bicarbonate, sodium phosphate. Preservative free. 15 mL, 30 mL. *OTC.*
Use: Artificial tears.

Theravee Hematinic Vitamin. (Vangard Labs, Inc.) Fe 66.7 mg, A 8333 units, D 133 units, E 5 units, B_1 3.3 mg, B_2 3.3 mg, B_3 33.3 mg, B_5 11.7 mg, B_6 3.3 mg, B_{12} 50 mcg, C 100 mg, folic acid 0.33 mg, Cu, Mg. Tab. Bot. UD 100s. *OTC.*
Use: Mineral, vitamin supplement.

Theravee-M. (Vangard Labs, Inc.) Fe 27 mg, vitamins A 5000 units, D 400 units, E 30 units, B_1 3 mg, B_2 3.4 mg, B_3 30 mg, B_5 10 mg, B_6 3 mg, B_{12} 9 mcg, C 120 mg, folic acid 0.4 mg, Ca, Cl, Cr, Cu, K, I, Mg, Mn, Mo, Se, Zn 15 mcg, biotin 15 mcg, beta-carotene 2500 units. Tab. Bot. 100s, 1000s, UD 100s. *OTC.*
Use: Mineral, vitamin supplement.

Theravee Vitamin. (Vangard Labs, Inc.) Vitamins A 5500 units, D 400 units, E 30 units, B_1 3 mg, B_2 3.4 mg, B_3 30 mg, B_5 10 mg, B_6 3 mg, B_{12} 9 mcg, C 120 mg, folic acid 0.4 mg, biotin 15 mcg. Tab. Bot. 100s. UD 100s. *OTC.*
Use: Vitamin supplement.

Theravim. (NBTY) Vitamins A 5000 units, D 400 units, E 30 units, B_1 3 mg, B_2 3.4 mg, B_3 30 mg, B_5 10 mg, B_6 3 mg, B_{12} 9 mcg, C 90 mg, folic acid 0.4 mg, beta-carotene 1250 units, biotin 35 mcg. Tab. Bot. 130s. *OTC.*
Use: Vitamin supplement.

Theravim-M. (NBTY) Fe 27 mg, vitamins A 5000 units, D 400 units, E 30 mg, B_1 3 mg, B_2 3.4 mg, B_3 20 mg, B_5 10 mg, B_6 3 mg, B_{12} 9 mcg, C 90 mg, folic acid 0.4 mg, Ca, Cl, Cr, Cu, I, K, Mg, Mn, Mo, P, Se, Zn 15 mg, biotin 30 mcg. Tab. Bot. 130s. *OTC.*
Use: Mineral, vitamin supplement.

Theravite. (Alra) Vitamins A 10,000 units, D 400 units, B_1 10 mg, B_2 10 mg, B_3 100 mg, B_5 21.4 mg, B_6 4.1 mg, B_{12} 5 mcg, C 200 mg/5 mL. Liq. Bot. 118 mL. *OTC.*
Use: Vitamin supplement.

Therems. (Rugby) Vitamins A 5000 units, D 400 units, E 30 mg, B_1 3 mg, B_2 3.4 mg, B_3 30 mg, B_5 10 mg, B_6 3 mg, B_{12} 9 mcg, C 120 mg, folic acid 0.4 mg, beta-carotene 1250 units, biotin 15 mcg. Tab. Bot. 130s, 1000s. *OTC.*
Use: Vitamin supplement.

Therems-H. (Rugby) Vitamins A 1,400 units, C 100 mg, D 140 units, E 5 units, B_1 3.3 mg, B_2 3.3 mg, B_3 33.3 mg, B_5 11.7 mg, B_6 3.3 mg, B_{12} 50 mcg, folic acid 330 mcg, sodium 12 mg, Ca 130 mg, Fe, Mg, Cu. Film coated. PEG, mineral oil. Tab. 90s. *OTC.*
Use: Multivitamin.

Therems-M. (Rugby) Vitamins A 5,000 units, C 90 mg, D 400 units, E 60 units, K 28 mcg, B_1 3 mg, B_2 3.4 mg, B_3 20 mg, B_5 10 mg, B_6 6 mg, B_{12} 12 mcg, biotin 30 mcg, folic acid 400 mcg, Ca 40 mg, Fe, P, I, Mg, Zn, Se, Cu, Mn, Cr, Mo, Cl, K, B, Ni, Sn, V, Tn. Mannitol, sucrose, soy. Tab. 130s, 1,000s. *OTC.*
Use: Multivitamin.

Therevac. (Jones Pharma) Docusate potassium 283 mg, benzocaine 20 mg w/soft soap in PEG 400 and glycerin base. Unit 4 mL, Cap. Pkgs. 4s, 12s, 50s. *OTC.*
Use: Bowel evacuant.

Therevac Plus. (Jones Pharma) Docusate sodium 283 mg, benzocaine 20 mg, glycerin 275 mg in a base of soft soap, polyethylene glycol, per 4 mL ampule. Disposable enema. Box 50s, UD 30s. *OTC.*
Use: Laxative.

Therevac-SB. (Jones Pharma) Docusate sodium 283 mg in a base of soft soap, polyethylene glycol, glycerin 275 mg per 4 mL ampule. Disposable enema. UD 30s. *OTC.*
Use: Laxative.

Therex-M. (Halsey Drug) Vitamins A 10,000 units, D 400 units, E 15 units, C 200 mg, B_1 10 mg, B_2 10 mg, niacinamide 100 mg, B_6 5 mg, B_{12} 5 mcg, calcium pantothenate 20 mg, I 150 mcg, Fe 12 mg, Mg 65 mg, Cu 2 mg, Zn 1.5 mg, Mn 1 mg. Tab. Bot. 100s. *OTC.*
Use: Mineral, vitamin supplement.

Therex No. 1. (Halsey Drug) Vitamins A 10,000 units, D 400 units, E 15 units, C 200 mg, B_1 10 mg, B_2 10 mg, niacinamide 100 mg, B_6 5 mg, B_{12} 5 mcg, calcium pantothenate 20 mg. Tab. Bot. 100s. *OTC.*
Use: Vitamin, mineral supplement.

Therex-Z. (Halsey Drug) Vitamins A 10,000 units, D 400 units, E 15 units, C 200 mg, B_1 10 mg, B_2 10 mg, niacinamide 100 mg, B_{12} 5 mcg, B_6 5 mg, Ca pantothenate 20 mg, I 150 mcg, Cu 2 mg, Fe 12 mg, Zn 22.5 mg. Tab. Bot. 100s. *OTC.*
Use: Mineral, vitamin supplement.

Therma-Kool. (Nortech Laboratories) Compresses in following sizes: 3" × 5", 4" × 9", 8.5" × 10.5".
Use: Cold, hot compress.

Thermazene. (Ascend Labs) Silver sulfadiazine 10 mg/g in a water-miscible base. White petrolatum, stearyl alcohol, methylparaben 0.3%. Cream. Tube 50 g, 400 g, 1000 g. *Rx.*
Use: Topical anti-infective.

Thermodent. (Mentholatum Co.) Strontium chloride 10%. Tube. *OTC.*
Use: Dentrifice.

Theroal. (Vangard Labs, Inc.) Theophylline 24 mg, ephedrine hydrochloride 24 mg, phenobarbital 8 mg. Tab. Bot. 100s, 1000s. *Rx.*
Use: Antiasthmatic combination.

Theroxide Wash. (Medicis) Benzoyl peroxide 10%. Liq. Bot. 120 mL. *Rx.*
Use: Dermatologic, acid.

ThexForte. (KM Lee) Vitamins B_1 25 mg, B_2 15 mg, B_3 100 mg, B_5 10 mg, B_6 5 mg, C 500 mg. Cap. Bot. 75s. *OTC.*
Use: Vitamin supplement.

Thia. (Sigma-Tau) Thiamine hydrochloride 100 mg/mL. Inj. Vial 30 mL. *Rx.*
Use: Vitamin supplement.

•**thiabendazole.** (THIGH-uh-BEND-uh-zole) *USP.*
Use: Anthelmintic.

thiacetarsamide sodium. Sodium mercaptoacetate S, S-diester with p-carbamoyl dithiobenzene arsonous acid.
Use: Antitrichomonal.

Thia-Dia-Mer-Sulfonamides. Sulfadiazine w/sulfamerazine & sulfathiazole.

Thiamilate. (Tyson) Thiamin (B_1) 20 mg. Enteric-coated Tab. Bot. 100s. *OTC.*
Use: Water-soluble vitamin.

thiamin (B_1).
Use: Water-soluble vitamin.
See: Thiamilate.
Thiamine Hydrochloride.

•**thiamine hydrochloride.** (THIGH-uh-min) *USP.*
Use: Enzyme co-factor vitamin.
See: Betalin S.
Thia.

thiamine hydrochloride. (Various Mfr.) Thiamin (B_1). **Tab.:** 50 mg, 100 mg, 250 mg. Bot. 100s, 250s; 1000s, UD 100s (100 mg only). **Inj.:** 100 mg/mL. Benzyl alcohol ≤ 9 mg. *Tubex* 1 mL in 2 mL. Multiple-dose vials. 2 mL. *Rx-OTC.*
Use: Water-soluble vitamin.

•**thiamine mononitrate.** (THIGH-uh-min) *USP.*
Use: Enzyme cofactor vitamin.

•**thiamiprine.** (thigh-AM-ih-preen) USAN.
Use: Antineoplastic.

•**thiamphenicol.** (THIGH-am-FEN-ih-kahl) USAN.
Use: Anti-infective.

•**thiamylal.** (thigh-AM-ih-lahl) *USP.*
Use: Anesthetic (intravenous).

•**thiamylal sodium for injection.** (thigh-AM-ih-lahl) *USP.*
Use: Anesthetic (intravenous).

thiazesim.
Use: Antidepressant.

•**thiazesim hydrochloride.** (thye-AZ-e-sim) USAN.
Use: Antidepressant.

•**thiazinamium chloride.** (THIGH-ah-ZIN-am-ee-uhm) USAN.
Use: Antiallergic.

thiazolidinediones.
Use: Antidiabetic.
See: Pioglitazone Hydrochloride. Rosiglitazone Maleate.

thiethylene thiophosphoramide.
See: Thiotepa.

•**thiethylperazine.** (THIGH-eth-ill-PURR-ah-zeem) USAN.
Use: CNS depressant; antiemetic.

•**thiethylperazine maleate.** (THIGH-eth-ill-PURR-ah-zeen) *USP.*
Use: Antiemetic.

thihexinol methylbromide.
Use: Anticholinergic.

•**thimerfonate sodium.** (thigh-MER-foe-nate) USAN.
Use: Anti-infective, topical.

•**thimerosal.** (thigh-MER-oh-sal) *USP.*
Use: Anti-infective, topical; pharmaceutic aid (preservative).
W/Trifluridine.
See: Viroptic.

thiocarbanidin. Under study.
Use: Tuberculosis.

thiocyanate sodium. Sodium thiocyanate.
Use: Antihypertensive.

thiodinone. Name used for Nifuratel.

thiodiphenylamine.
See: Phenothiazine.

thioglycerol.
W/Sodium Citrate, Phenol, Benzyl Alcohol.
See: Sulfo-ganic.

•**thioguanine.** (THIGH-oh-GWAHN-een) *USP.*
Use: Antineoplastic.
See: Tabloid.

thiohexamide.
Use: Blood sugar-lowering compound.

thioisonicotinamide. Under study.
Use: Antituberculosal.

Thiola. (Mission Pharmacal) Tiopronin 100 mg. Tab. Bot. 100s. *Rx.*
Use: Anticholelithiasis.

•**thiopental sodium.** (thigh-oh-PEN-tahl) *USP.*
Use: Anesthetic (intravenous); anticonvulsant.

thiophosphoramide.
See: Thiotepa.

Thioplex. (Amgen) Thiotepa 15 mg. Powd. for Inj. Vials. *Rx.*
Use: Antineoplastic.

thiopropazate hydrochloride.
Use: Anxiolytic.

thioproperazine mesylate.
Use: CNS depressant; antiemetic.

•**thioridazine.** (THIGH-oh-RID-uh-zeen) *USP.*
Use: Antipsychotic; hypnotic; sedative.

•**thioridazine hydrochloride.** (THIGH-oh-RID-ah-zeen) *USP.*
Use: Antipsychotic; hypnotic; sedative.

thioridazine hydrochloride. (Various Mfr.) Thioridazine hydrochloride 10 mg, 25 mg, 50 mg, 100 mg. Tab. 60s, 100s, 1,000s, UD 100s. *Rx.*
Use: Antipsychotic.

thioridazine hydrochloride concentrate. (Various Mfr.) Thioridazine hydrochloride. **30 mg/mL:** Bot. 120 mL. **100 mg/mL:** Bot. 120 mL, 3.4 mL (UD 100s). *Rx.*
Use: Antipsychotic.

•**thiosalan.** (THIGH-oh-sal-AN) USAN.
Use: Disinfectant.

•**thiotepa.** (thigh-oh-TEP-uh) *USP.*
Use: Antineoplastic.
See: Thioplex.

thiotepa. (Bedford) Thiotepa 15 mg. Pow. for Inj, lyophilized. Single-dose vial. *Rx.*
Use: Antineoplastic.

thiotepa. (Sicor) Thiotepa 30 mg. Pow. for Inj., lyophilized. Single-dose vials. *Rx.*
Use: Antineoplastic.

thiotepa. (Wyeth) Thiotepa powder 15 mg, sodium chloride 80 mg, sodium bicarbonate 50 mg. Vial. Pow. for

Recon. Vial 15 mg. *Rx.*
Use: Antineoplastic.

•**thiothixene.** (THIGH-oh-THIX-een) *USP.*
Use: Antipsychotic.
See: Navane.

thiothixene. (Various Mfr.) Thiothixene 1 mg, 2 mg, 5 mg, 10 mg. May contain lactose. Cap. 100s, 1000s, UD 100s (2 mg, 5 mg only). *Rx.*
Use: Antipsychotic.

•**thiothixene hydrochloride.** (THIGH-oh-THIX-een) *USP.*
Use: Antipsychotic.

thiouracil. 2-Thiouracil.
Use: Treatment of hyperthyroidism, antianginal, congestive heart failure.

thioxanthene derivatives.
See: Thiothixene.

•**thiphenamil hydrochloride.** (thigh-FEN-ah-mill) USAN.
Use: Muscle relaxant.

•**thiphencillin potassium.** (thigh-fen-SILL-in) USAN.
Use: Anti-infective.

•**thiram.** (THIGH-ram) USAN.
Use: Antifungal.

Thixo-Flur. (Colgate Oral) Acidulated phosphate sodium fluoride in gel base 1.2%. Gel. Bot. 4 oz, 8 oz., 32 oz.
Use: Dental caries agent.

•**thonzonium bromide.** (thahn-ZOE-nee-uhm) *USP.*
Use: Detergent.
W/Colistin Sulfate, Neomycin Sulfate, Hydrocortisone Acetate.
See: Coly-Mycin-S Otic.
Cortisporin-TC.

•**thonzylamine hydrochloride.** (thon-ZIL-a-meen) USAN.
Use: Antihistamine.
W/Chlophedianol Hydrochloride, Phenylephrine Hydrochloride.
See: Vanacof APE.
W/Phenylephrine Hydrochloride.
See: NasOpen PE.

Thorets. (Buffington) Benzocaine lozenge. *Dispens-A-Kits* 500s. Sugar, lactose, and salt free. *OTC.*
Use: Sore throat relief.

Thor-Prom. (Major) Chlorpromazine 10 mg, 25 mg, 50 mg, 100 mg, 200 mg. Tab. Bot. 100s, 1000s (except 200 mg). Tab. Bot. 250s, 1000s (200 mg only). *Rx.*
Use: Antiemetic; antipsychotic.

•**thozalinone.** (thoe-ZAL-ah-nohn) USAN.
Use: Antidepressant.

3 Day Vaginal. (Taro) Clotrimazole 2%. Benzyl alcohol. Cream; vaginal. 21 g tube w/3 disposable applicators. *OTC.*
Use: Vaginal antifungal agent.

357 HR Magnum. (BDI) Caffeine 200 mg. Tab. Bot. 36s, 100s, 500s. *OTC.*
Use: CNS stimulant, analeptic.

•**threonine.** (THREE-oh-neen) *USP.*
Use: Amino acid.
See: Threostat.

l-threonine.
Use: Antispasmodic. [Orphan Drug]

threonine. (Freeda) Threonine 500 mg. Tab. 100s, 250s. *OTC.*
Use: Nutritional supplement.

Threostat. (Tyson) *Rx.*
Use: Antispasmodic.
See: Threonine.

Thrive. (Novartis) Nicotine polacrilex 2 mg, 4 mg. Acesulfame K, glycerin, maltitol, saccharin, sodium 11 mg, sorbitol. Mint flavor. Gum. 110s. *OTC.*
Use: Smoking deterrent, nicotine.

Throat Discs. (GlaxoSmithKline) Capsicum, peppermint, mineral oil, sucrose. Box 60s. *OTC.*
Use: Throat preparation.

Throat-Eze. (Faraday) Cetylpyridinium chloride 1:3000, cetyl dimethylbenzyl ammonium chloride 1:3000, benzocaine 10 mg. Wafer. Loz., foil wrapped. Vial 15. *OTC.*
Use: Anesthetic, local.

Thrombate III. (Talecris) Antithrombin III (human) 500 units, 1000 units. Pow. for Inj., lyophilized. Single-use vial w/10 mL (500 mL units only), 20 mL (1000 units only). Sterile water for injection. *Rx.*
Use: Antithrombin.

Thrombi-Gel 40. (King Pharmaceuticals) Thrombin (bovine origin) 1,000 units. Residual formaldehyde ≤ 0.2 mg. Preservative free. Pad, lyophilized; top. Single-use 5s. *Rx.*
Use: Topical hemostatic.

Thrombi-Gel 100. (King Pharmaceuticals) Thrombin (bovine origin) 20,000 units. Residual formaldehyde ≤ 0.2 mg. Preservative free. Pad, lyophilized; top. Single-use 5s. *Rx.*
Use: Topical hemostatic.

Thrombi-Gel 10. (King Pharmaceuticals) Thrombin (bovine origin) 1,000 units. Residual formaldehyde ≤ 0.2 mg. Preservative free. Pad, lyophilized; top. Single-use 10s. *Rx.*
Use: Topical hemostatic.

•**thrombin.** (THROM-bin) *USP.* Thrombin, topical, mammalian origin.
Use: Hemostatic.
See: Evithrom.
Recothrom.
Thrombi-Gel 40.

Thrombi-Gel 100.
Thrombi-Gel 10.
Thrombin-JMI.
Thrombi-Pad 3 × 3.
W/Calcium Chloride, Fibrinogen, Fibrinolysis Inhibitor, Protein.
See: Tisseel.
W/Fibrinogen.
See: Evarrest.

•**thrombin alfa.** (THROM-bin AL-fa) USAN.
Use: Hemostatic.

thrombin inhibitors.
Use: Anticoagulant.
See: Argatroban.
Bivalirudin.
Dabigatrin Etexilate.
Desirudin.
Lepirudin.

Thrombin-JMI. (King Pharmaceuticals) Thrombin 1,000 units/mL. Preservative free. Pow. for Soln., lyophilized; top. 5,000 unit vials and Epistaxis Kit w/diluent; 20,000 unit vials, Pump Spray Kit, and Syringe Spray Kit w/diluent. *Rx.*
Use: Topical hemostatic.

Thrombi-Pad 3 x 3. (King Pharmaceuticals) Thrombin (bovine origin) 200 units. Preservative free. Pad, lyophilized; top. Single-use 1s. *Rx.*
Use: Topical hemostatic.

thrombolytic agents.
See: Human Protein C.
Tissue Plasminogen Activators.
Thrombolytic Enzymes.

thrombolytic enzymes.
See: Streptokinase.
Urokinase.

thromboplastin.
Use: Diagnostic aid (prothrombin estimation).

thrombopoietin receptor agonists.
See: Eltrombopag.

Thylox. (C.S. Dent & Co.) Medicated bar soap w/absorbable sulfur. Bar 3.4 oz. *OTC.*
Use: Cleanser.

•**thymalfasin.** (thigh-MAL-fah-sin) USAN. *Formerly Thymosin.*
Use: Antineoplastic; vaccine enhancement; hepatitis, infectious disease treatment.

Thymoglobulin. (SangStat) Antithymocyte globulin (rabbit) 25 mg. Glycine 50 mg, mannitol 50 mg, sodium chloride 10 mg. Pow. for Inj., lyophilized. Vial 7 mL w/diluent vial 5 mL. *Rx.*
Use: Immune globulin.

•**thymol.** (THIGH-mole) *NF.*
Use: Antifungal; anti-infective; anesthetic, local; antitussive; decongestant; pharmaceutic aid (stabilizer).
W/Combinations.
See: Listerine, Natural Citrus.
Listerine, Tartar Control.

thymol. (Various Mfr.) Thymol 0.25 lb, 1 lb.
Use: Antifungal; anti-infective; anesthetic, local; antitussive; decongestant; pharmaceutic aid (stabilizer).

thymol iodide.
Use: Antifungal; anti-infective.

•**thymopentin.** (THIGH-moe-PEN-tin) USAN. *Formerly Thymopoietin 32-36.*
Use: Immunoregulator.

thyodatil. *Name used for nifuratel.*

Thyrogen. (Genzyme) Thyrotropin alfa 1.1 mg (4 to 12 units/mg). Mannitol, sodium chloride. Inj., Lyophilized, Pow. for Soln. Kits w/diluent. *Rx.*
Use: In vivo diagnostic aid, thyroid function test.

•**thyroid.** (THIGH-royd) *USP.*
Use: Hormone, thyroid.
See: Arco Thyroid.

thyroid combinations.
See: Henydin.

thyroid desiccated.
Use: Hormone, thyroid.
See: Armour Thyroid.
Bio-Throid.
Nature Throid.
Thyroid USP.
Westhroid.
Westhroid-P.

thyroid drugs.
See: Antithyroid agents.
Methimazole.
Potassium Iodide.
Propylthiouracil.
Sodium Iodide I 131.

thyroid function tests.
Use: In vivo diagnostic aid.
See: Sodium Iodide I 123.
Sodium Iodide I 125.
Sodium Iodide I 131.
Thyrogen.
Thyrotropin Alfa.
Thytropar.

thyroid hormones.
See: Levothyroxine Sodium.
Liothyronine Sodium.
Liotrix.
Thyroid Desiccated.

Thyroid USP. (Various Mfr.) Thyroid desiccated 32.5 mg (½ gr), 65 mg (1 gr), 130 mg (2 gr), 195 mg (3 gr). Tab. Bot. 100s, 1000s. *Rx.*
Use: Hormone, thyroid.

Thyrolar. (Forest) Liotrix 0.25 gr, 0.5 gr, 1 gr, 2 gr, 3 gr, lactose. Tab. Bot. 100s.

Rx.
Use: Hormone, thyroid.

•**thyromedan hydrochloride.** (thigh-ROW-meh-dan) USAN.
Use: Thyromimetic.

thyropropic acid. (Warner Chilcott) Triopron.
Use: Anticholesteremic.

ThyroSafe. (Recip) Potassium iodide 65 mg. Lactose. Tab. 10s, 20s. *OTC.*
Use: Thyroid drug.

ThyroShield. (Fleming) Potassium iodide 65 mg/mL. Parabens, saccharin, sucrose. Black-raspberry flavor. Soln. 30 mL. *OTC.*
Use: Thyroid drug.

Thyro-Tabs. (Lloyd) Levothyroxine sodium 0.025 mg, 0.05 mg, 0.075 mg, 0.088 mg, 0.1 mg, 0.112 mg, 0.125 mg, 0.15 mg, 0.175 mg, 0.2 mg, 0.3 mg. Tab. Bot. 100s, 1000s. *Rx.*
Use: Hormone, thyroid.

thyrotropic hormone.
Use: In vivo diagnostic aid.
See: Thytropar.

thyrotropic principle of bovine anterior pituitary glands.
See: Thytropar.

thyrotropin.
Use: Diagnostic aid.
See: Thytropar.

•**thyrotropin alfa.** (thye-roh-TROH-pin) USAN.
Use: In vivo diagnostic aid, thyroid function test.
See: Thyrogen.

thyrotropin-releasing hormone.
Use: Diagnostic aid.

•**thyroxine I 131.** (thigh-ROX-een) USAN.
Use: Radiopharmaceutical.

•**thyroxine I 125.** (thigh-ROX-een) USAN.
Use: Radiopharmaceutical.

thyrozyme-II A. (Abbott Diagnostics) T-4 diagnostic kit. 100, 500 test units.
Use: Diagnostic aid, thyroid.

Thytropar. (Centeon) Thyrotropin from bovine anterior pituitary glands. Thyrotropin. Vial 10 units.
Use: Thyroid agent.

•**tiacrilast.** (TIE-ah-KRILL-ast) USAN.
Use: Antiallergic.

•**tiacrilast sodium.** (TIE-ah-KRILL-ast) USAN.
Use: Antiallergic.

•**tiagabine hydrochloride.** (tye-AG-a-been) USAN.
Tall Man: tiaGABine
Use: Anticonvulsant.
See: Gabitril.

tiagabine hydrochloride. (Sun Pharmaceuticals) Tiagabine hydrochloride 2 mg, 4 mg. Film coated. Lactose, PEG, vegetable oil. Tab. 30s, 100s (4 mg only), 1,000s. *Rx.*
Use: Anticonvulsant.

•**tiamenidine.** (TIE-ah-MEN-ih-DEEN) USAN.
Use: Antihypertensive.

•**tiamenidine hydrochloride.** (TIE-ah-MEN-ih-DEEN) USAN.
Use: Antihypertensive.

•**tiapamil hydrochloride.** (tie-APP-ah-mill) USAN.
Use: Calcium antagonist.

•**tiaramide hydrochloride.** (TIE-ar-ah-MIDE) USAN.
Use: Antiasthmatic.

Tiazac. (Forest) Diltiazem hydrochloride 120 mg, 180 mg, 240 mg, 300 mg, 360 mg, 420 mg. Sucrose. ER Cap. Bot. 7s, 30s, 90s, 1000s. *Rx.*
Use: Calcium channel blocker.

•**tiazofurin.** (tye-AZ-oh-FURE-in) USAN.
Use: Antineoplastic.

TI-Baby Natural. (Fischer) Titanium dioxide 5%. SPF 16. Lot. Bot. 120 mL. *OTC.*
Use: Sunscreen.

•**tibenelast sodium.** (TIE-ben-ell-ast) USAN.
Use: Antiasthmatic; bronchodilator.

•**tibolone.** (TIH-bole-ohn) USAN.
Use: Menopausal symptoms suppressant.

•**tibric acid.** (TIE-brick) USAN.
Use: Antihyperlipoproteinemic.

•**tibrofan.** (TIE-broe-fan) USAN.
Use: Disinfectant.

•**ticabesone propionate.** (tie-CAB-eh-sone) USAN.
Use: Corticosteroid, topical.

•**ticagrelor.** (tye-KA-grel-or) USAN.
Use: Aggregation inhibitor.
See: Brilinta.

•**ticarbodine.** (tie-CAR-boe-deen) USAN.
Use: Anthelmintic.

ticarcillin/clavulanate.
Use: Extended-spectrum penicillin.
See: Timentin.

•**ticarcillin cresyl sodium.** (tie-CAR-SIH-lin KREH-sill) USAN.
Use: Anti-infective.

•**ticarcillin disodium.** (tie-CAR-SIH-lin) *USP.*
Use: Extended-spectrum penicillin.

ticarcillin disodium and clavulanate potassium, sterile.
Use: Anti-infective; inhibitor (β-lactamase).
See: Timentin.

•**ticarcillin monosodium.** (tie-CAR-SIH-lin) *USP.*
Use: Anti-infective.

Tice BCG. (Organon) BCG live for intravesical administration. 1 to 8 × 10^8 CFU (equivalent to ≈ 50 mg wet weight). Preservative free. Inj. Lyophilized. Pow. for Susp. Vials. ≈ 50 mg. *Rx.*
Use: Biological response modifier.

•**ticilimumab.** (tis-i-LIM-ue-mab) USAN.
Use: Antineoplastic.

•**ticlatone.** (TIE-klah-tone) USAN.
Use: Anti-infective; antifungal.

Ticlid. (Roche) Ticlopidine hydrochloride 250 mg. Tab. Bot. 30s, 60s, 500s. *Rx.*
Use: Antiplatelet.

•**ticlopidine hydrochloride.** (tie-KLOE-pih-DEEN) USAN.
Use: Platelet inhibitor.
See: Ticlid.

ticlopidine hydrochloride. (Various Mfr.) Ticlopidine hydrochloride 250 mg. Tab. Bot. 30s, 60s, 100s, 500s, 1000s. *Rx.*
Use: Platelet inhibitor.

•**ticolubant.** (tih-kahl-YOU-bant) USAN.
Use: Antipsoriatic.

Ticon. (Hauck) Trimethobenzamide hydrochloride 100 mg/mL, phenol. Inj. Vial 20 mL. *Rx.*
Use: Antiemetic; antivertigo.

•**ticrynafen.** (TIE-krin-ah-fen) USAN.
Use: Diuretic; uricosuric; antihypertensive.

Tidafen DM. (Tiber) Dextromethorphan HBr 60 mg, guaifenesin 800 mg, pseudoephedrine hydrochloride 90 mg. ER Tab. 100s. *Rx.*
Use: Upper respiratory combination, antitussive and expectorant combination.

tidembersat.
Use: Antimigraine.

Tidex. (Allison) Dextroamphetamine sulfate 5 mg. Tab. Bot. 100s, 1000s. *c-II.*
Use: Antiobesity agent.

Tidexsol. (Sanofi-Synthelabo) Acetaminophen. Tab. *OTC.*
Use: Analgesic.

•**tifurac sodium.** (TIE-fyoor-ak) USAN.
Use: Analgesic.

Tigan. (Monarch) Trimethobenzamide hydrochloride 300 mg. Cap. 100s. *Rx.*
Use: Antiemetic.

Tigan. (JHP Pharm) Trimethobenzamide hydrochloride 100 mg/mL. Amps (with methyl- and propylparabens). Inj. 2 mL. Vials (with phenol). 20 mL. Syringe (with phenol and EDTA). 2 mL. *Rx.*
Use: Antiemetic.

•**tigapotide triflutate.** (TYE-gah-POE-tide) USAN.
Use: Antineoplastic.

•**tigecycline.** (tye-ge-SYE-kleen) USAN.
Use: Anti-infective, glycylcycline.
See: Tygacil.

•**tigemonam dicholine.** (TIE-jem-OH-nam die-KOE-leen) USAN.
Use: Antimicrobial.

Tiger Balm. (Prince of Peace) Menthol 8%, camphor 11%. Cajuput oil, clove oil, mint oil, petrolatum. Oint. 18 g. *OTC.*
Use: Rub and liniment.

•**tigestol.** (tie-JESS-tole) USAN.
Use: Hormone, progestin.

Tigo. (Burlington) Polymyxin B sulfate 5000 units, zinc bacitracin 400 units, neomycin sulfate 5 mg/g Oint. Tube 0.5 oz. *OTC.*
Use: Anti-infective, topical.

Tihist-DP. (Vita Elixir) Dextromethorphan HBr 10 mg, pyrilamine maleate 16 mg, sodium citrate 3.3 g/5 mL. *OTC.*
Use: Antitussive; antihistamine.

Tihist Nasal Drops. (Vita Elixir) Pyrilamine maleate 0.1%, phenylephrine hydrochloride 0.25%, sodium bisulfite 0.2%, methylparaben 0.02%, propylparaben 0.01%/30 mL. Bot. *OTC.*
Use: Antihistamine; decongestant.

Tija. (Vita Elixir) Oxytetracycline hydrochloride. **Syrup:** 125 mg/5 mL. **Tab.:** 250 mg. *Rx.*
Use: Anti-infective, tetracycline.

Tikosyn. (Pfizer) Dofetilide 125 mcg, 250 mcg, 500 mcg. Cap. Bot. 14s, 60s, UD 40s. *Rx.*
Use: Antiarrhythmic.

•**tildipirosin.** (TIL-di-PIR-oh-sin) USAN.
Use: Respiratory agent.

•**tildrakizumab.** (TIL-dra-KIZ-ue-mab) USAN.
Use: Monoclonal antibody.

•**tiletamine hydrochloride.** (tie-LET-ah-meen) *USP.*
Use: Anesthetic; anticonvulsant.

Tilia Fe. (Watson) **Phase 1:** Norethindrone acetate 1 mg, ethinyl estradiol 20 mcg (5 tabs.). **Phase 2:** Norethindrone acetate 1 mg, ethinyl estradiol 30 mcg (7 tabs.). **Phase 3:** Norethindrone acetate 1 mg, ethinyl estradiol 35 mcg (9 tabs.). Ferrous fumarate 75 mg (7 tabs.). Lactose. Tab. 28s. *Rx.*
Use: Sex hormone, contraceptive hormone.

•**tilidine hydrochloride.** (TIH-lih-DEEN) USAN.
Use: Analgesic.

Tl-lite. (Fischer) Ethylhexyl p-methoxycinnamate 7.5%, titanium dioxide 2%,

cetyl alcohol, phenethyl alcohol, parabens, EDTA. Cream 60 g. *OTC.*
Use: Sunscreen.

•**tilmacoxib.** (til-ma-KOX-ib) USAN.
Use: Cox-2 inhibitor.

•**tilomisole.** (TILL-oh-mih-sahl) USAN.
Use: Immunoregulator.

•**tilorone hydrochloride.** (TIE-lore-ohn) USAN.
Use: Antiviral.

•**tiludronate disodium.** (tie-LOO-droe-nate) USAN.
Use: Bisphosphonate.
See: Skelid.

•**timefurone.** (tie-MEH-fyoor-OHN) USAN.
Use: Antiatherosclerotic.

Time-Hist QD. (AMBI) Pseudoephedrine hydrochloride 120 mg, chlorpheniramine maleate 6 mg. PEG. ER Tab. Bot. 100s. *Rx.*
Use: Upper respiratory combination, decongestant, antihistamine, anticholinergic.

Timentin. (GlaxoSmithKline) **Inj., Pow. for Reconstitution:** Ticarcillin 3 g, clavulanic acid 0.1 g. Sodium 4.51 mEq, potassium 0.15 mEq/g. Vials. 3.1 g. *ADD-Vantage* vials. Pharmacy bulk pkg. (ticarcillin disodium 30 g, clavulanic acid 1 g). **Inj. Soln.:** Ticarcillin 3 g, clavulanic acid 0.1 g per 100 mL. Sodium 18.7 mEq, potassium 0.5 mEq/100 mL. Premixed, frozen *Galaxy* plastic cont. 100 mL. *Rx.*
Use: Extended-spectrum penicillin.

•**timobesone acetate.** (tie-MOE-beh-sone) USAN.
Use: Adrenocortical steroid, topical.

•**timolol.** (TI-moe-lahl) USAN.
Use: Antiadrenergic (β-receptor).

timolol/brimonidine tartrate.
Use: Agent for glaucoma.
See: Combigen.

•**timolol maleate.** (TI-moe-lahl) *USP.*
Use: Agent for glaucoma; antiadrenergic/sympatholytic, beta-adrenergic blocker.
See: Blocadren.
Betimol.
Istalol.
Timoptic.
Timoptic-XE.

timolol maleate. (Falcon Ophthalmics) Timolol maleate 0.25%, 0.5%. Gel-forming Soln. Bot. 2.5 mL, 5 mL. *Rx.*
Use: Agent for glaucoma; beta-adrenergic blocker.

timolol maleate. (Various Mfr.) Timolol maleate **Ophth. Soln.:** 0.25%, 0.5%. Bot. 2.5 mL, 5 mL, 10 mL, 15 mL. **Tab.:** 5 mg, 10 mg, 20 mg. Bot. 100s. *Rx.*
Use: Agent for glaucoma; antiadrenergic/sympatholytic; beta-adrenergic blocker.

timolol maleate/dorzolamide hydrochloride.
Use: Agent for glaucoma.
See: Cosopt.

timolol maleate ophthalmic. (Various Mfr.) Timolol maleate 3.4 mg/0.25 mL and 6.8 mg/0.5 mL. Soln. Bot. 2.5 mL, 5 mL, 10 mL, 15 mL. *Rx.*
Use: Antiglaucoma agent.

Timoptic. (Valeant) Timolol maleate 0.25%, 0.5%. Ophth. Soln. *Ocumeter* 2.5 mL, 5 mL, 10 mL, 15 mL; *Ocudose* UD 60s. *Rx.*
Use: Antiglaucoma agent; beta-adrenergic blocker.

Timoptic-XE. (Valeant) Timolol maleate 0.25%, 0.5%. Gel-forming Soln. *Ocumeter* 2.5 mL, 5 mL. *Rx.*
Use: Antiglaucoma agent; beta-adrenergic blocker.

•**tinabinol.** (tie-NAB-ih-NOLE) USAN.
Use: Antihypertensive.

Tinactin. (Schering-Plough) **Cream 1%:** Tolnaftate (10 mg/g) in homogeneous, nonaqueous vehicle of PEG-400, propylene glycol, carboxypolymethylene, monoamylamine, titanium dioxide, butylated hydroxytoluene. Tube 15 g, 30 g, UD 0.7 g. **Pow. 1%:** Tolnaftate w/corn starch, talc. Plastic container 45 g, 90 g. **Aerosol Pow. 1%:** Tolnaftate w/butylated hydroxytoluene, talc, polyethylene-polypropylene glycol monobutyl ether, denatured alcohol and inert propellant of isobutane. Spray Can 100 g. **Aerosol Liq. 1%:** Tolnaftate w/butylated hydroxytoluene, polyethylene-polyproplyene glycol monobutyl ether, 36% alcohol, and inert propellant of isobutane. Spray Can 120 mL. *OTC.*
Use: Antifungal.

Tinastat. (Vita Elixir) Sodium hyposulfite, benzethonium chloride/2 oz. *OTC.*
Use: Keratolytic.

Tinaval. (Pal-Pak, Inc.) Tolnaftate 1%. Pow. Bot. 45 g. *OTC.*
Use: Antifungal for jock itch, athlete's foot.

Tindamax. (Mission Pharmacal) Tinidazole 250 mg, 500 mg. Tab. 20s (500 mg only), 40s (250 mg only), 60s (500 mg only). *Rx.*
Use: Antiprotozoal.

tine test, old tuberculin. (Wyeth) Box of 25, 100, 250 test applicators.
See: Tuberculin Tine Test.

tine test, purified protein derivative. (Wyeth) Box of 25 or 100 test applicators.
See: Tuberculin Tine Test.

•**tin fluoride.** *USP.* Stannous Fluoride.

•**tinidazole.** (tie-NIH-dah-zole) USAN.
Use: Antiprotozoal.
See: Tindamax.

tinidazole. (BioComp Pharma) Tinidazole 250 mg, 500 mg. PEG, polydextrose. Tab. 20s (500 mg), 40s (250 mg), 60s (500 mg). *Rx.*
Use: Anti-infective agent, antiprotozoal.

Tinset. (Janssen) Oxatomide.
Use: Antiallergic; antiasthmatic.

•**tinzaparin sodium.** (tin-ZAP-ah-rin) USAN.
Use: Anticoagulant; low molecular weight heparin.

•**tioconazole.** (TIE-oh-KOE-nah-zole) *USP.*
Use: Antifungal.
See: Monistat 1.
Vagistat-1.

•**tiodazosin.** (TIE-oh-DAY-zoe-sin) USAN.
Use: Antihypertensive.

•**tiodonium chloride.** (TIE-oh-doe-nee-uhm) USAN.
Use: Anti-infective.

•**tiomolibdate diammonium.** (TYE-oh-moe-LIB-date) USAN.
Use: Alzheimer disease.

•**tioperidone hydrochloride.** (tie-oh-PURR-ih-dohn) USAN.
Use: Antipsychotic.

•**tiopinac.** (tie-OH-pin-ACK) USAN.
Use: Anti-inflammatory; analgesic, antipyretic.

tiopronin.
Use: Homozygous cystinuria. [Orphan Drug]
See: Thiola.

•**tiospirone hydrochloride.** (tie-OH-spih-rone) USAN.
Use: Antipsychotic.

•**tiotidine.** (TIE-OH-tih-deen) USAN.
Use: Antiulcerative.

tiotropium bromide.
Use: Bronchodilator, anticholinergic.
See: Spiriva.

•**tioxidazole.** (tie-OX-ih-DAH-zole) USAN.
Use: Anthelmintic.

•**tipapkinogene sovacivec.** (TIP-a-KIN-oh-jeen soe-VAS-i-vek) USAN.
Use: Antineoplastic.

•**tipelukast.** (TYE-pe-LOO-kast) USAN.
Use: Respiratory agent.

•**tipentosin hydrochloride.** (TIE-pin-toe-SIN) USAN.
Use: Antihypertensive.

•**tipifarnib.** (tip-ee-FAR-nib) USAN.
Use: Cancer.

•**tiplasinin.** (ti-PLAS-in-in) USAN.
Use: Hematologic.

Tipramine Tabs. (Major) Imipramine. Tab. **10 mg:** Bot. 250s. **25 mg, 50 mg:** Bot. 250s, 1000s. *Rx.*
Use: Antidepressant.

•**tipranavir.** (tip-RA-na-veer) USAN.
Use: Antiretroviral, protease inhibitor.
See: Aptivus.

•**tipredane.** (tie-PRED-ANE) USAN.
Use: Adrenocortical steroid, topical.

•**tiprenolol hydrochloride.** (tie-PREH-no-lole) USAN.
Use: Antiadrenergic (β-receptor).

•**tiprinast meglumine.** (TIE-prih-nast meh-GLUE-meen) USAN. Under study.
Use: Antiallergic.

•**tipropidil hydrochloride.** (TIE-PRO-pih-dill) USAN.
Use: Vasodilator.

•**tiqueside.** (TIE-kweh-side) USAN.
Use: Antihyperlipidemic.

•**tiquinamide hydrochloride.** (tie-KWIN-ah-mide) USAN.
Use: Anticholinergic (gastric).

•**tirapazamine.** (tie-rah-PAZZ-ah-meen) USAN.
Use: Antineoplastic.

•**tirasemtiv.** (TYE-ra-SEM-tiv) USAN.
Use: Musculoskeletal agent.

tiratricol.
Use: Antineoplastic. [Orphan Drug]

•**tirilazad mesylate.** (tie-RIH-lah-zad) USAN.
Use: Antioxidant.
See: Freedox.

•**tirofiban hydrochloride.** (tie-rah-FIE-ban) USAN.
Use: Antiplatelet, glycoprotein IIb/IIIa inhibitor.
See: Aggrastat.

TI-Screen. (Pedinol Pharmacal) **Gel:** SPF 20+, ethylhexyl p-methoxycinnamate 7.5%, oxybenzone 5%, 2-ethylhexyl salicylate 5%, SD alcohol 40 71%. 120 g. **Lip Balm:** SPF 8+, ethylhexyl p-methoxycinnamate 7.5%, oxybenzone 5%, petrolatum. 4.5 g. **Lot.:** SPF 8, ethylhexyl p-methoxycinnamate 6%, oxybenzone 2%. Bot. 120 mL. *OTC.*
Use: Sunscreen.

TI-Screen Natural. (Pedinol Pharmacal) Titanium dioxide 5%. Lot. Bot. 120 mL. *OTC.*
Use: Sunscreen.

TI-Screen Sports. (Pedinol Pharmacal)

Octinoxate 7.5%, oxybenzone 6%, octisalate 5%, avobenzone 2%. Alcohol 70%. Gel. 120 mL. *OTC.*
Use: Sunscreen.

TI-Screen Sunless. (Pedinol Pharmacal) Octyl methoxycinnamate 7.5%, benzophene-3 3%, mineral oil, alcohols, PEG-100, parabens. SPF 17 or 23. Cream. Tube 118 mL. *OTC.*
Use: Sunscreen.

•**tisilfocon A.** (tih-sill-FOE-kahn) USAN.
Use: Contact lens material (hydrophobic).

Tisit. (Pfeiffer) **Gel:** Pyrethrins 0.3%, piperonyl butoxide 3%. 30 mL. **Lot.:** Pyrethrins 0.3%, piperonyl butoxide 2% (petroleum distillate and piperonyl butoxide equiv. to 1.6% ether). 59 mL, 118 mL. **Shampoo:** Pyrethrins 0.33%, piperonyl butoxide 4%. Bot. 59 mL, 118 mL. With comb. *OTC.*
Use: Pediculicide.

•**tisocalcitate.** (ti-soe-KAL-si-tate) USAN.
Use: Psoriasis.

TiSol. (Parnell) Benzyl alcohol 1%, menthol 0.04%, isotonic sodium chloride 0.9%, sorbitol, EDTA. Soln. Bot. 237 mL. *OTC.*
Use: Throat preparation.

Tisseel. (Baxter) **Pow. for Soln., lyophilized; Top.:** Total protein 96 to 125 mg/mL, fibrinogen 67 to 106 mg/mL, fibrinolysis inhibitor (synthetic) 2,250 to 3,750 kallikrein-inhibiting units/mL, thrombin (human) 400 to 625 units/mL, calcium chloride 36 to 44 mcmol/mL (when reconstituted). Polysorbate 80, albumin (human). In 2, 4, 10 mL kits (single-use vials with or without *Duploject* system). **Soln.; Top.:** Total protein 96 to 125 mg/mL, fibrinogen 67 to 106 mg/mL, fibrinolysis inhibitor (synthetic) 2,250 to 3,750 kallikrein-inhibiting units/mL, thrombin (human) 400 to 625 units/mL, calcium chloride 36 to 44 mcmol/mL. Polysorbate 80, albumin (human). In 2, 4, and 10 mL single-use prefilled (frozen) syringe with *DUO Set. Rx.*
Use: Fibrin sealant (human).

tissue fixative and wash solution. (Wampole) A modified Michel's tissue fixative and buffered wash solution.
Use: Tissue specimen fixative.

tissue plasminogen activators.
See: Alteplase, Recombinant.
Reteplase, Recombinant.
Tenecteplase.

tissue respiratory factor (TRF). (International Hormone) RSF, SRF, LYCD, PCO, Procytoxid marketed as 2000 units. Supplied as bulk liquid concentrate. *Rx.*
Use: Promotion of cellular oxidation.

Tis-U-Sol. (Baxter PPI) Pentalyte irrigation containing NaCl 800 mg, KCl 40 mg, magnesium sulfate 20 mg, sodium phosphate 8.75 mg, 6.25 mg monobasic potassium phosphate/100 mL. Bot. 250 mL, 1000 mL. *Rx.*
Use: Irrigant.

•**titanium dioxide.** (tie-TANE-ee-uhm die-OX-ide) *USP.*
Use: Solar ray protectant, topical.
W/Avobenzone, Ecamsule, Octocrylene.
See: Capital Soleil 20.

Titralac. (3M) Calcium carbonate 420 mg, saccharin, Na 0.3 mg. Chew. Tab. Bot. 40s, 100s, 1000s. *OTC.*
Use: Antacid.

Titralac Plus. (3M) **Chew. Tab.:** Calcium carbonate 420 mg, simethicone 21 mg, saccharin, sodium 1.1 mg. Bot. 100s. **Liq.:** Calcium carbonate 500 mg, simethicone 20 mg, saccharin, sorbitol, sodium 0.15 mg. Bot. 360 mL. *OTC.*
Use: Antacid.

•**tivantinib.** (tye-VAN-ti-nib) USAN.
Use: Antineoplastic.

Tivicay. (GlaxoSmithKline) Dolutegravir 50 mg. Film coated. Mannitol. Tab. 30s. *Rx.*
Use: Antiretroviral agent, integrase inhibitor.

Tivorbex. (Iroko Pharmaceuticals) Indomethacin 20 mg, 40 mg. Lactose. Cap. 30s, 90s. *Rx.*
Use: Nonsteroidal anti-inflammatory agent.

•**tivozanib.** (ti-VOE-za-nib) USAN.
Use: Antineoplastic.

•**tivozanib hydrochloride.** (ti-VOE-za-nib) USAN.
Use: Antineoplastic.

•**tixanox.** (TIX-ah-nox) USAN.
Use: Antiallergic.

•**tixocortol pivalate.** (tix-OH-kahr-tole PIH-vah-late) USAN.
Use: Anti-inflammatory, topical.

•**tizanidine hydrochloride.** (tie-ZAN-ih-deen) USAN.
Tall Man: tiZANidine
Use: Antispasmodic.
See: Zanaflex.

tizanidine hydrochloride. (Various Mfr.) Tizanidine. **Tab.:** 2 mg, 4 mg (may contain lactose). 30s (4 mg only), 150s, 300s (4 mg only), 500s, 1,000s, UD 100s (4 mg only). **Cap.:** 2 mg, 4 mg, 6 mg. May contain sugar. 150s. *Rx.*
Use: Antispasmodic.

TL-DEX DM. (Trigen Labs) Dextromethorphan hydrobromide 15 mg, guaifenesin

200 mg, pseudoephedrine hydrochloride 32 mg per 5 mL. Potassium sorbate, parabens, propylene glycol, sorbitol, sucralose. Grape flavor. Liq. 473 mL. *Rx.*
Use: Upper respiratory combination, antitussive and expectorant combination.

TL-Hist CM. (Trigen Labs) Chlorpheniramine maleate 2 mg, codeine phosphate 10 mg per 5 mL. Sorbitol, sucralose, parabens, potassium citrate, potassium sorbate. Cotton candy flavor. Liq. 473 mL. *c-v.*
Use: Upper respiratory combination, antitussive combination.

TL-Hist DM. (Trigen Labs) Brompheniramine maleate 4 mg, dextromethorphan hydrobromide 15 mg, phenylephrine hydrochloride 7.5 mg per 5 mL. Parabens, potassium sorbate, propylene glycol, sorbitol, sucralose. Strawberry flavor. Liq. 473 mL. *Rx.*
Use: Upper respiratory combination, antitussive combination.

TL Icon. (Trigen Laboratories) Fe 110 mg, folic acid 0.5 mg, intrinsic factor 240 mg, vitamin B_{12} 15 mcg, vitamin C 75 mg. Cap. 60s. *Rx.*
Use: Trace element.

TMP-SMZ. Trimethoprim-Sulfamethoxazole. *Rx.*
Use: Anti-infective.
See: Bactrim.
Bethaprim.
Cotrim.
Septra.
Sulfatrim.

TNKase. (Genentech) Tenecteplase 50 mg. L-arginine 0.55 g, phosphoric acid 0.17 g, polysorbate 20 4.3 mg. Inj., Lyophilized, Pow. for Soln. Vial w/one 10-mL vial of Sterile Water for Injection and syringe. *Rx.*
Use: Thrombolytic agent; tissue plasminogen activator.

TOBI. (Novartis) Tobramycin 300 mg per 5 mL. Preservative free. Soln. for Inhal. Amp. 5 mL (w/sodium chloride, sulfuric acid, sodium hydroxide). *Rx.*
Use: Cystic fibrosis.

TOBI Podhaler. (Novartis) Tobramycin 28 mg. Cap.; oral inhal. UD 224s w/*Podhaler* device. *Rx.*
Use: Anti-infective, parenteral aminoglycoside.

•**toborinone.** (toe-BORE-ih-nohn) USAN.
Use: Cardiotonic.

Tobrades. (Alcon) Dexamethasone 0.1%, tobramycin 0.3%, thimerosal 0.001%, alcohol 0.5%, propylene glycol, polyoxyethylene, polyoxypropylene. Susp. 2.5 mL, 5 mL. *Rx.*
Use: Anti-infective; corticosteroid.

TobraDex. (Alcon) **Ophth. Oint.:** Dexamethasone 0.1%, tobramycin 0.3%, chlorobutanol 0.5%, mineral oil, white petrolatum. 3.5 g. **Ophth. Susp.:** Tobramycin 0.3%, dexamethasone 0.1%, benzalkonium chloride 0.01%, EDTA, sodium chloride, tyloxapol. *Drop-Tainers.* 3.5 mL. *Rx.*
Use: Anti-infective; corticosteroid; ophthalmic.

TobraDex ST. (Alcon) Dexamethasone 0.05%, tobramycin 0.3%. Benzalkonium chloride 0.1 mg, edetate disodium, xanthan gum, sodium chloride, tyloxapol, propylene glycol. Ophth. Susp. *Drop-Tainer.* 2.5 mL, 5 mL, 10 mL. *Rx.*
Use: Ophthalmic steroid antibiotic combination.

•**tobramycin.** (TOE-bruh-MY-sin) *USP.* An antibiotic obtained from cultures of *Streptomyces tenebrarius.*
Use: Anti-infective, ophthalmic.
See: AkTob.
Bethkis.
TOBI.
TOBI Podhaler.
Tobrex.
W/Dexamethasone.
See: TobraDex.
TobraDex ST.
W/Loteprednol.
See: Zylet.

tobramycin. (Akorn) Tobramycin 0.3%. Benzalkonium chloride 0.01%, boric acid, sodium sulfate. Soln. 5 mL. *Formerly AKTob. Rx.*
Use: Anti-infective, ophthalmic.

tobramycin. (Various Mfr.) Tobramycin. **Soln.:** 0.3%. Benzalkonium chloride 0.01%, boric acid. 5 mL. **Soln.; Inhal.:** 300 mg per 5 mL. Sodium chloride, sodium hydroxide, sulfuric acid. Preservative free. Single-use ampule. 5 mL. *Rx.*
Use: Anti-infective, ophthalmic.

tobramycin and dexamethasone. (Various Mfr.) Dexamethasone 0.1%, tobramycin 0.3%. Benzalkonium chloride 0.01%, edetate disodium. Susp., Ophth. *Drop-tainers.* 2.5 mL, 5 mL, 10 mL. *Rx.*
Use: Ophthalmic steroid antibiotic combination.

•**tobramycin and dexamethasone ophthalmic ointment.** (TOE-bruh-MY-sin) *USP.*
Use: Anti-infective, ophthalmic.

tobramycin in 0.9% sodium chloride. (Hospira) Tobramycin (as sulfate) 0.8 mg/mL, 1.2 mg/mL. Inj. Single-dose flexible containers. 50 mL (1.2 mg/mL only), 100 mL (0.8 mg/mL only). *Rx.*
Use: Aminoglycoside.

•**tobramycin sulfate.** (TOE-bruh-MY-sin) *USP.*
Use: Anti-infective; aminoglycoside.

tobramycin sulfate. (Various Mfr.) Tobramycin sulfate. **Inj., Pow for Soln.:** 1.2 g (40 mg/mL after reconstitution). Preservative free. Pharmacy bulk package vial. 50 mL. **Inj., Soln.:** 10 mg/mL, 40 mg/mL, 1.2 g per 30 mL. May contain edetate disodium, sodium bisulfate, sodium metabisulfate. Vial. 2 mL (except 1.2 g per 30 mL), 30 mL (except 10 mg/mL), 50 mL (40 mg/mL only). **Soln., Inhal.:** 300 mg per 5 mL. Sodium chloride. Preservative free. Ampule. 5 mL. *Rx.*
Use: Parenteral aminoglycoside.

Tobrex. (Alcon) Tobramycin. **Oint.:** 3 mg/g. White petrolatum, mineral oil, chlorobutanol 0.05%. 3.5 g. **Soln.:** 0.3%. Benzalkonium chloride 0.01%, tyloxapol, boric acid. Bot. 5 mL *Drop-Tainer. Rx.*
Use: Anti-infective, ophthalmic.

•**tocamphyl.** (toe-KAM-fill) USAN.
Use: Choleretic.

•**tocilizumab.** (toe-si-LIZ-oo-mab) USAN.
Use: Immune globulin.
See: Actemra.

•**tocladesine.** (toe-CLA-de-seen) USAN.
Use: Antineoplastic; immunomodulator.

•**tocopherols excipient.** (toe-KAHF-ehr-ols) *NF.*
Use: Pharmaceutic aid (antioxidant).

•**tocophersolan.** (toe-KAHF-ehr-SO-lan) USAN.
Use: Vitamin supplement.

dl-alpha tocopheryl. Vitamin E.

dl-alpha tocopheryl acetate. Vitamin E.
See: GRX Vitamin E.

Tocosamine. (Trent) Sparteine sulfate 150 mg, sodium chloride 4.5 mg/mL. Amps. 1 mL. Box 12s, 100s. *Rx.*
Use: Oxytocic.

Today Sponge. (Mayer Laboratories) 1,000 mg of nonoxynol 9. Benzoic acid, sodium metabisulfite. Sponge; vaginal. 3s. *OTC.*
Use: Spermicide.

Toetal Fresh. (Medimetriks) Camphor, edetate disodium, eucalyptol, menthol, propylene glycol, urea. Soln.; Top. 28 mL w/applicator brush. *OTC.*
Use: Miscellaneous topical combination.

•**tofacitinib.** (TOE-fa-SYE-ti-nib) USAN.
Use: Immunological disorders.
See: Xeljanz.

•**tofacitinib citrate.** (TOE-fa-SYE-ti-nib) USAN.
Use: Immunological disorders.

•**tofenacin hydrochloride.** (tah-FEN-ah-sin) USAN.
Use: Anticholinergic.

•**tofimilast.** (toe-FIM-i-last) USAN.
Use: Chronic obstructive disease; asthma.

•**tofogliflozin.** (TOE-foe-gli-FLOE-zin) USAN.
Use: Treatment of diabetes mellitus.

Tofranazine. (Novartis) Combination of imipramine and promazine. Pending release.

Tofranil. (Mallinckrodt) Imipramine hydrochloride 10 mg, 25 mg, 50 mg. Tab. Bot. 100s. *Rx.*
Use: Antidepressant; antineuritic.

Tofranil-PM. (Mallinckrodt) Imipramine pamoate 75 mg, 100 mg, 125 mg, 150 mg, parabens. Cap. Bot. 30s, 100s. *Rx.*
Use: Antidepressant.

•**tolamolol.** (tahl-AIM-oh-lahl) USAN.
Use: Beta-adrenergic receptor blocker; coronary vasodilator; cardiovascular agent (antiarrhythmic).

•**tolazamide.** (tole-AZE-uh-mid) *USP.*
Tall Man: TOLAZamide
Use: Hypoglycemic; antidiabetic.

tolazamide. (Various Mfr.) Tolazamide 100 mg, 250 mg, 500 mg. Tab. 100s, 200s (250 mg only), 250s (except 250 mg), 500s (except 100 mg), 1000s (250 mg only). *Rx.*
Use: Antidiabetic.

•**tolbutamide.** (tole-BYOO-tuh-mide) *USP.*
Tall Man: TOLBUTamide
Use: Hypoglycemic; antidiabetic.

tolbutamide. (Various Mfr.) Tolbutamide 500 mg. Tab. 100s, 500s. *Rx.*
Use: Antidiabetic.

•**tolbutamide sodium.** (tole-BYOO-tuh-mide) *USP.*
Tall Man: TOLBUTamide
Use: In vivo diagnostic aid.

•**tolcapone.** (TOLE-kah-pone) USAN.
Use: Antiparkinsonian.
See: Tasmar.

•**tolciclate.** (tole-SIGH-klate) USAN.
Use: Antifungal.

Tolerex. (Procter & Gamble) Protein 20.6 g, carbohydrate 226.3 g, fat 1.45 g, Na 468 mg, K 1172 mg, mOsm/Kg H_2O 550, cal/mL 1, vitamins A, B_1, B_2, B_3, B_5, B_6, B_{12}, C, D, E, K, folic acid, bio-

tin, choline, Ca, P, I, Fe, Mg, Cu, Zn, Mn, Se, Mo, Cr. Assorted flavors Pow. Pkts. 80 g. *OTC.*
Use: Mineral, vitamin supplement.

•**tolevamer potassium sodium.** (toe-LEV-a-mer) USAN.
Use: Antidiarrheal.

•**tolevamer sodium.** (toe-LEV-a-mer) USAN.
Use: Antidiarrheal.

•**tolfamide.** (TAHL-fah-MIDE) USAN.
Use: Enzyme inhibitor (urease).

Tolfrinic. (B.F. Ascher) Ferrous fumarate 200 mg, vitamins B_{12} 25 mcg, C 100 mg. Tab. Bot. 100s. *OTC.*
Use: Mineral, vitamin supplement.

•**tolgabide.** (TOLE-gah-bide) USAN.
Use: Antiepileptic (control of abnormal movements).

•**tolimidone.** (TAHL-IH-mih-dohn) USAN.
Use: Antiulcerative.

•**tolindate.** (TOLE-in-DATE) USAN.
Use: Antifungal.

•**tolmetin.** (TOLE-meh-tin) USAN.
Use: Anti-inflammatory.

•**tolmetin sodium.** (TOLE-meh-tin) *USP.*
Use: Anti-inflammatory.

tolmetin sodium. (Various Mfr.) Tolmetin sodium. **Tab.:** 200 mg, 600 mg. Bot. 100s, 500s (600 mg only), UD 100s (600 mg only). **Cap.:** 400 mg. Bot. 100s, 500s, 1000s, UD 100s. *Rx.*
Use: Anti-inflammatory.

•**tolnaftate.** (tahl-NAFF-tate) *USP.*
Use: Antifungal.
See: Blis-To-Sol.
Breezee Mist Antifungal.
Dr. Scholl's.
Lamisil AF Defense.
Micocide NS.
Tinactin.

•**tolofocon A.** (TOE-low-FOE-kahn A) USAN.
Use: Contact lens material (hydrophobic).

toloxychlorinal.
Use: Sedative.

•**tolpovidone I 131.** (tahl-POE-vih-dohnl 131) USAN.
Use: Diagnostic aid (hypoalbuminemia); radiopharmaceutical.

•**tolpyrramide.** (tole-PIR-a-mide) USAN.
Use: Oral hypoglycemic; antidiabetic.

•**tolterodine.** (tole-TEH-roe-deen) USAN.
Use: Treatment of urinary incontinence.

tolterodine tartrate.
Use: Anticholinergic.
See: Detrol.
Detrol LA.

tolterodine tartrate. (Various Mfr.) Tolterodine tartrate. **ER Cap.:** 2 mg, 4 mg. May contain sucrose. 30s, 90s, 500s. **Tab.:** 1 mg, 2 mg. Film coated. 60s, 500s, UD 140s. *Rx.*
Use: Urinary anticholinergic.

•**tolu balsam.** (toe-LOO BALL-sam) *USP.*
Use: Pharmaceutic necessity for Compound Benzoin Tincture; expectorant.

tolu balsam. (Eli Lilly) Syr. Bot. 16 fl. oz.
Use: Vehicle.

•**tolu balsam tincture.** (toe-LOO BALL-sam) *NF.*
Use: Flavor.

toluidine blue o. Tolonium chloride.

Tolu-Sed. (Scherer) Codeine phosphate 10 mg, guaifenesin 100 mg/5 mL w/alcohol 10%. Sugar free. Bot. 4 oz., pt. *c-v.*
Use: Antitussive; expectorant.

Tolu-Sed DM. (Scherer) Dextromethorphan HBr 10 mg, guaifenesin 100 mg per 5 mL. Alcohol 10%. Sugar free. Liq. Bot. 118 mL *OTC.*
Use: Upper respiratory combination, antitussive, expectorant.

•**tolvaptan.** (TOLE-vap-tan) USAN.
Use: Congestive heart failure; hyponatremia.
See: Samsca.

•**tomelukast.** (tah-MELL-you-KAST) USAN.
Use: Antiasthmatic (leukotriene antagonist).

Tomocat. (Mallinckrodt) Barium sulfate 5%. Simethicone, sorbitol, strawberry flavor. Conc. Susp. Bot. 145 mL (480 mL for dilution), 225 mL (1000 mL for dilution); enema kit in 110 mL with 480 mL bot. for dilution with flexible tubing, clamp, and enema tip. *Rx.*
Use: Radiopaque agent, miscellaneous gastrointestinal contrast agent.

Tomocat 1000. (Lafayette) Barium sulfate suspension concentrate 5% w/v. Bot. for dilution to 1.5% w/v at time of use. Bot. 225 mL w/1000 mL dilution Bot. Case 24 Bot. and 2 Dilution Bot.
Use: Radiopaque medium used to mark the GI tract during CT scans.

•**tomopenem.** (TOE-moe-PEN-em) USAN.
Use: Antibiotic.

tomoxetine hydrochloride. (TOE-MOX-eh-teen)
See: Atomoxetine Hydrochloride.

Tom's of Maine Natural Cough & Cold Rub Cough Suppressant. (Tom's of Maine) Camphor 4.8%, menthol 2.6%. Rub. Tube 92.4 g. *OTC.*
Use: Upper respiratory combination, topical.

•**tonapofylline.** (TOE-na-POF-i-lin) USAN.
Use: Heart failure.

Tonavite-M. (Ivax) Elix. Bot. 12 oz, pt., gal.
Use: Dietary supplement.

•**tonazocine mesylate.** (toe-NAZ-oh-seen) USAN.
Use: Analgesic.

Tono-B Pediatric. (Pal-Pak, Inc.) Fe 5 mg, thiamine hydrochloride 0.167 mg, riboflavin 0.133 mg. Tab. Bot. 1000s. *OTC.*
Use: Mineral, vitamin supplement.

Tonopaque. (Mallinckrodt) Barium sulfate 95%. Simethicone. Pow. for Susp. Kits. 340 g, 454 g. *Rx.*
Use: Radiopaque agent, GI contrast agent.

Tonsiline. (Oakhurst) Alcohol 4%, glycerin, sucrose, iron chloride, magnesium carbonate, tolu balsam, sodium saccharin. Mouthwash. 118 mL. *OTC.*
Use: Mouth and throat product.

Toothache Gel. (Roberts Med) Benzocaine. Benzyl alcohol, oil of cloves, propylene glycol. Gel; dental. 15 g. *OTC.*
Use: Topical local anesthetic, ester local anesthetic.

Toothache Relief-3 in 1. (C.S. Dent & Co.) Benzocaine. Gum, Liq., Lot./Gel; dental. *OTC.*
Use: Analgesic, topical.

Topamax. (Janssen) Topiramate **Tab.:** 25 mg, 50 mg, 100 mg. Lactose. 60s. **Sprinkle Cap.:** 15 mg, 25 mg. Sucrose. 60s. *Rx.*
Use: Anticonvulsant.

Top Brass ZP-11. (Revlon) Zinc pyrithione 0.5% in cream base. *OTC.*
Use: Antidandruff.

Top-Form. (Colgate Oral) Topical form-fitting gel applicators. Disposable trays for topical fluoride office treatments, plus permanent trays for topical fluoride home self-treatments. Box 100s. *Rx.*
Use: Topical fluoride applications in home or office.

Topic. (Roche) 5% benzyl alcohol in greaseless gel base containing camphor, menthol, w/30% isopropyl alcohol. Tube 2 oz. *OTC.*
Use: Antipruritic.

Topicaine. (ESBA Labs) Lidocaine hydrochloride 4%. Alcohol, aloe, benzyl alcohol, disodium EDTA, glycerin, glyceryl, jojoba oil. Gel. 10 g, 30 g, 113 g. *OTC.*
Use: Topical local anesthetic, amide local anesthetic.

Topicaine 5. (ESBA Labs) Lidocaine hydrochloride 5%. Aloe vera oil, benzyl alcohol, EDTA, ethanol, glycerin, glyceryl, jojoba oil, shea butter. Gel. 10 g, 30 g, 113 g. *OTC.*
Use: Topical local anesthetic, amide local anesthetic.

topical anesthetics, miscellaneous.
See: Ethyl Chloride.
Fluro-Ethyl.

Topical Fluoride. (Pacemaker) Acidulated phosphate fluoride. Flavors: Orange, bubble gum, lime, raspberry, grape, cinnamon. Liq. Bot. 4 oz, pt. *Rx.*
Use: Corticosteroid, topical.

Topicort. (Taro) Desoximetasone. **Cream:** 0.25% emollient cream consisting of isopropyl myristate, cetyl stearyl alcohol, white petrolatum, mineral oil, lanolin alcohol, purified water. Tube 15 g, 60 g, 120 g. **Gel:** 0.05% in gel base. 20% alcohol. Tube 15 g, 60 g. **Oint.:** 0.05%, 0.25%. Tube 15 g, 60 g. **Spray; topical:** 0.25%. Glyceryl oleate, isopropyl alcohol 23.4%, menthol, mineral oil. 100 mL. *Rx.*
Use: Corticosteroid, topical.

Topicort LP. (Taro) Desoximetasone 0.05%. Cream. Tube 15 g, 60 g. *Rx.*
Use: Corticosteroid, topical.

Topiragen. (Upsher-Smith) Topiramate 25 mg, 50 mg, 100 mg, 200 mg. Lactose, PEG. Tab. 60s. *Rx.*
Use: Anticonvulsant.

•**topiramate.** (toe-PIRE-ah-MATE) USAN.
Use: Anticonvulsant.
See: Qudexy XR.
Topamax.
Topiragen.
Trokendi XR.
W/Phentermine Hydrochloride.
See: Qsymia.

topiramate. (Various Mfr.) Topiramate. **Cap., sprinkle:** 15 mg, 25 mg. PEG, sugar. 60s, 500s. **Tab.:** 25 mg, 50 mg, 100 mg, 200 mg. May contain lactose and PEG. 30s (25 mg and 50 mg only), 60s, 90s (100 mg only), 100s, 500s, 1,000s, UD 30s (200 mg only), UD 80s (200 mg only), UD 100s. *Rx.*
Use: Anticonvulsant.

•**topixantrone.** (toe-PIX-an-trone) USAN.
Use: Antineoplastic.

Toposar. (Novaplus/Sicor) Etoposide 20 mg, benzyl alcohol 30 mg, alcohol 30.5%/mL. Inj. Multiple-dose vial. 5 mL, 25 mL, 50 mL. *Rx.*
Use: Antineoplastic.

•**topotecan hydrochloride.** (toe-poe-TEE-kan) USAN.
Use: DNA topoisomerase inhibitor.
See: Hycamtin.

topotecan hydrochloride. (Various Mfr.) Topotecan hydrochloride 4 mg. May

contain mannitol. Preservative free. Inj., lyophilized Pow. for Soln. Single-dose vial. *Rx.*
Use: Antineoplastic, DNA topoisomerase inhibitor.

Toprol XL. (AstraZeneca) Metoprolol succinate 23.75 mg (equivalent to metoprolol tartrate 25 mg), 47.5 mg (equivalent to metoprolol tartrate 50 mg), 95 mg (equivalent to metoprolol tartrate 100 mg), 190 mg (equivalent to metoprolol tartrate 200 mg). ER Tab. Bot. 100s. *Rx.*
Use: Antihypertensive; antiadrenergic/sympatholytic, beta-adrenergic blocker.

•**topsalysin.** (TOP-sa-LYE-sin) USAN.
Use: Antineoplastic.

•**topterone.** (TOP-ter-ohn) USAN.
Use: Antiandrogen.

•**toquizine.** (TOE-kwih-zeen) USAN.
Use: Anticholinergic.

•**toralizumab.** (toe-ra-LYE-zyoo-mab) USAN.
Use: Monoclonal antibody.

•**torapsel.** (tore-AP-sel) USAN.
Use: Hematologic agent.

•**torcetrapib.** (tore-SET-ra-pib) USAN.
Use: Cardiovascular agent.

•**torcitabine.** (tore-SITE-a-been) USAN.
Use: Polymerase inhibitor (hepatitis B).

•**toremifene citrate.** (TORE-EM-ih-feen) USAN.
Use: Antiestrogen; antineoplastic.
See: Fareston.

•**torezolid.** (toe-REZ-oh-lid) USAN.
Use: Antibiotic.

•**torezolid phosphate.** (tore-EZ-oh-lid) USAN.
Use: Antibiotic.

Torisel. (Wyeth) Temsirolimus 25 mg/mL. Alcohol, polysorbate 80. Concentrated Soln. for Inj. 2-vial kits. *Rx.*
Use: Antineoplastic, protein-tyrosine kinase inhibitor, mTOR inhibitor.

•**torsemide.** (TORE-suh-MIDE) *USP.*
Use: Diuretic.
See: Demadex.

torsemide. (Teva) Torsemide 5 mg, 10 mg, 20 mg, 100 mg. Lactose. Tab. 100s. *Rx.*
Use: Diuretic.

torula yeast, dried. Obtained by growing *Candida (torulopsis) utilis* yeast on wood pulp wastes.
Use: Natural source of protein and Vitamin B-complex vitamins.

•**tosagestin.** (TOE-sa-jes-tin) USAN.
Use: Hormone replacement therapy.

•**tosedostat.** (toe-SED-oh-stat) USAN.
Use: Antineoplastic.

•**tosifen.** (TOE-sih-fen) USAN.
Use: Antianginal.

•**tosufloxacin.** (toe-SUE-FLOX-ah-sin) USAN.
Use: Anti-infective.

Totacillin. (GlaxoSmithKline) Ampicillin trihydrate equivalent to: **Cap.:** 250 mg, 500 mg. Bot. 500s. **Pow. for Oral Susp.:** 125 mg/5 mL, 250 mg/5 mL. Bot. 100 mL, 200 mL. *Rx.*
Use: Anti-infective, penicillin.

Total. (Allergan) Polyvinyl alcohol, edetate disodium, benzalkonium chloride in a sterile, buffered, isotonic solution. Soln. Bot. 60 mL, 120 mL. *OTC.*
Use: Contact lens care.

TotalDay. (Nature's Blend) Vitamins A 25,000 units, D 1,000 units, E 100 units, B_1 100 mg, B_2 100 mg, B_3 100 mg, B_5 100 mg, B_6 100 mg, B_{12} 100 mcg, C 500 mg, folate 1 mg, Fe 18 mg, Ca 250 mg, Cl, Cr, Cu, I, K, Mg, Mn, Mo, P, Se, Zn, biotin, choline, citrus bioflavonoids complex, inositol, PABA, rutin. Maltodextrin, polydextrose. Tab., timed release. 120s. *OTC.*
Use: Multivitamin with minerals.

Total Eclipse Cooling Alcohol. (Novartis) Padimate O, oxybenzone, glyceryl PABA, alcohol 77%. SPF 15. Lot. Bot. 120 mL. *OTC.*
Use: Sunscreen.

Total Eclipse Moisturizing. (Novartis) Padimate O, oxybenzone, octyl salicylate. Moisturizing base. SPF 15. Lot. Bot. 120 mL. *OTC.*
Use: Sunscreen.

Total Eclipse Oil & Acne Prone Skin Sunscreen. (Novartis) Padimate O, oxybenzone, glyceryl PABA, alcohol 77%. SPF 15. Lot. Bot. 120 mL. *OTC.*
Use: Sunscreen.

Total Formula. (Vitaline) Fe 20 mg, vitamins A 10,000 units, D 400 units, E 30 units, B_1 15 mg, B_2 15 mg, B_3 25 mg, B_5 25 mg, B_6 25 mg, B_{12} 25 mcg, C 100 mg, folic acid 0.4 mg, Ca, Cr, Cu, I, K, Mg, Mn, Mo, P, Se, Si, V, vitamin K, biotin 300 mcg, Zn 30 mg, choline, bioflavonoids, hesperidin, inositol, PABA, rutin. Tab. Bot. 90s, 100s. *OTC.*
Use: Mineral, vitamin supplement.

Total Formula-2. (Vitaline) Fe 20 mg, vitamins A 10,000 units, D 400 units, E 30 units, B_1 15 mg, B_2 15 mg, B_3 25 mg, B_5 25 mg, B_6 25 mg, B_{12} 25 mcg, C 100 mg, folic acid 0.4 mg, Ca, Cr, Cu, I, K, Mg, Mn, Mo, P, Se, Si, V, vitamin K, biotin 300 mcg, Zn 30 mg, choline, bio-

flavonoids, hesperidin, inositol, PABA, rutin. Tab. with boron. Bot. 60s. *OTC.*
Use: Mineral, vitamin supplement.

totaquine. Alkaloids from *Cinchona* bark, 7% to 12% quinine anhydrous, 70% to 80% total alkaloids (cinchonidine, cinchonine, quinidine & quinine).

Totect. (TopoTarget) Dexrazoxane 500 mg (equiv. to dexrazoxane hydrochloride 589 mg). Preservative free. Inj. Lyophilized Pow. for Soln. Single-use vials with 50 mL sodium lactate injection. *Rx.*
Use: Cytoprotective agent.

totomycin hydrochloride. Tetracycline.

Touro A & D. (Dartmouth) Chlorpheniramine maleate 4 mg, phenyltoloxamine citrate 50 mg, phenylephrine hydrochloride 20 mg. SR Cap. Bot. 100s. *Rx.*
Use: Antihistamine; decongestant.

Touro CC. (Dartmouth) Guaifenesin 575 mg, pseudoephedrine hydrochloride 60 mg, dextromethorphan HBr 30 mg. Dye free. ER Tab. Bot. 100s. *Rx.*
Use: Upper respiratory combination, antitussive and expectorant combination.

Touro CC-LD. (Dartmouth) Dextromethorphan HBr 30 mg, guaifenesin 575 mg, pseudoephedrine 25 mg. Dye free. SR Tab. 100s. *Rx.*
Use: Antitussive and expectorant.

Touro HC. (Dartmouth) Hydrocodone bitartrate 5 mg, guaifenesin 575 mg. Dye free. ER Tab. 100s. *c-III.*
Use: Antitussive with expectorant.

•**tovetumab.** (toe-VET-ue-mab) USAN.
Use: Antineoplastic.

Toviaz. (Pfizer) Fesoterodine fumarate 4 mg, 8 mg. Lactose, PEG, polyvinyl alcohol. Film-coated. ER Tab. 30s, 90s, UD 100s. *Rx.*
Use: Renal and genitourinary agent, anticholinergic.

Toxo. (Wampole) *Toxoplasma* antibody test system. Tests 120s.
Use: An IFA test system for the detection of antibodies to *Toxoplasma gondii.*

toxoid, diphtheria.
Use: Immunization.
See: Diphtheria and Tetanus Toxoids, Acellular Pertussis and Haemophilus Influenzae Type B Conjugate Vaccine.
Diphtheria and Tetanus Toxoids, Adult.
Diphtheria and Tetanus Toxoids, and Acellular Pertussis Adsorbed, Hepatitis B (Recombinant) and Inactivated Poliovirus Vaccine Combined.
Diphtheria and Tetanus Toxoids and Acellular Pertussis Vaccine, Adsorbed.
Diphtheria and Tetanus Toxoids, Pediatric.
Tetanus and Diphtheria Toxoids Adsorbed for Adult Use.

toxoid, tetanus. *Rx.*
Use: Immunization.
See: Diphtheria and Tetanus Toxoids, Acellular Pertussis and Haemophilus Influenzae Type B Conjugate Vaccine.
Diphtheria and Tetanus Toxoids, Adult.
Diphtheria and Tetanus Toxoids and Acellular Pertussis Adsorbed, Hepatitis B (Recombinant) and Inactivated Poliovirus Vaccine Combined.
Diphtheria and Tetanus Toxoids and Acellular Pertussis Vaccine, Adsorbed.
Diphtheria and Tetanus Toxoids, Pediatric.
Tetanus and Diphtheria Toxoids Adsorbed for Adult Use.
Tetanus Toxoid.
Tetanus Toxoid, Adsorbed.
Tetanus Toxoid, Adsorbed, Purogenated.

toxoplasmosis test.
Use: Diagnostic aid.
See: TPM Test.

•**tozadenant.** (toe-ZA-de-nant) USAN.
Use: Antiparkinson agent.

•**tozasertib.** (TOE-za-SER-tib) USAN.
Use: Antineoplastic agent.

•**tozasertib lactate.** (TOE-za-SER-tib) USAN.
Use: Antineoplastic agent.

t-PA.
Use: Tissue plasminogen activator.
See: Activase.

TPM-Test. (Wampole) Indirect hemagglutination test for the qualitative and quantitative determination of antibodies to *Toxoplasma gondii* in serum. Kit 120s.
Use: Diagnostic aid, toxoplasmosis.

TPN Electrolytes. (Hospira) Na^+ 35 mEq, K^+ 20 mEq, Ca^{++} 4.5 mEq, Mg^{++} 5 mEq, Cl^- 35 mEq, acetate 29.5 mEq/20 mL, osmolarity 6220 mOsm/L. Soln. Pharmacy bulk packaging vial 100 mL. *Rx.*
Use: Intravenous nutritional therapy, intravenous replenishment solution.

TPN Electrolytes III. (Hospira) Na 25 Eq, K 40.6 mEq, Ca 5 mEq, Mg 8 mEq, Cl 33.5 mEq, acetate 40.6 mEq, gluconate 5 mEq/20 mL, osmolarity 7520 mOsm/L. Soln. Pharmacy bulk pkg. Vial 100 mL. *Rx.*
Use: Intravenous nutritional therapy, intravenous replenishment solution.

TPN Electrolytes II. (Hospira) Na 18 mEq, K 18 mEq, Ca 4.5 mEq, Mg 5 mEq, Cl 35 mEq, acetate 10.5 mEq/20 mL, osmolarity 4320 mOsm/L. Soln. Single-dose and additive syr. 20 mL *Rx.*
Use: Intravenous nutritional therapy, intravenous replenishment solution.

•**trabectedin.** (tra-BEK-te-din) USAN.
Use: Antineoplastic.

•**tracazolate.** (trak-AZ-oh-late) USAN.
Use: Sedative; hypnotic.

Trace. (Young Dental) Erythrosine conc. soln. Squeeze Bot. 30 mL, 60 mL. Dispenser Packets 200s. *OTC.*
Use: Diagnostic aid, disclose dental plaque.

trace elements.
Use: Mineral supplement.
See: Carbonyl Iron.
Complex Zinc Carbonates.
Copper Gluconate.
Ferric Carboxymaltose.
Ferrous Fumarate.
Ferrous Gluconate.
Ferrous Sulfate.
Ferrous Sulfate Exsiccated (Dried).
Fluoride.
Iron.
Iron Dextran.
Iron/Liver Combination.
Iron Sucrose.
Iron with Vitamin B_{12} and IFC.
Iron with Vitamin C.
Iron with Vitamins.
Manganese.
Polysaccharide-Iron Complex.
Sodium Ferric Gluconate Complex.
Sucroferric Oxyhydroxide.
Zinc Acetate.
Zinc Gluconate.
Zinc Sulfate.

Trace Elements 4 Pediatric. (American Regent) Chromium (as chloride) 1 mcg, copper (as sulfate) 0.1 mg, manganese (as sulfate) 0.03 mg, zinc (as sulfate) 0.5 mg. Benzyl alcohol 0.9%. Inj. Multidose vial. 10 mL. *Rx.*
Use: Trace metal combination.

trace metals.
See: Chromic Chloride.
Zinc Sulfate.

Traceplex. (Enzyme Process) Fe 30 mg, I 0.1 mg, Cu 0.5 mg, Mg 40 mg, Zn 10 mg, B_{12} 5 mcg/4 Tabs. Bot. 100s, 250s. *OTC.*
Use: Mineral supplement.

Tracer bG. (Boehringer Mannheim) Reagent strips. Kit. 25s, 50s.
Use: Diagnostic aid.

Trace 28. (Young Dental) **Liq.:** FD&C Red No. 28 in aqueous soln. Bot. 30 mL, 60 mL. **Tab.:** FD&C Red No. 28. Box 30s, 180s, 700s. *OTC.*
Use: Diagnostic aid, disclose dental plaque.

Tracleer. (Actelion Pharm) Bosentan 62.5 mg, 125 mg. Tab. Bot. 60s. *Rx.*
Use: Vasodilator, endothelin receptor antagonist.

Tracrium Injection. (GlaxoSmithKline) Atracurium besylate 10 mg/mL Amp. 5 mL. Box 10s; 10 mL MDV. Box 10s. *Rx.*
Use: Muscle relaxant.

Tradjenta. (Boehringer Ingelheim) Linagliptin 5 mg. Film coated. Mannitol. Tab. 30s, 90s, 1,000s, UD 100s. *Rx.*
Use: Antidiabetic agent, dipeptidyl peptidase-4 inhibitor.

•**trafermin.** (trah-FUR-min) USAN.
Use: Treatment of stroke and coronary artery disease.

•**tragacanth.** (TRAG-ah-kanth) *NF.*
Use: Pharmaceutic aid (suspending agent).

•**tralokinumab.** (TRAL-oh-KIN-ue-mab) USAN.
Use: Respiratory agent.

•**tralonide.** (TRAL-oh-nide) USAN.
Use: Corticosteroid, topical.

tramadol. (Various Mfr.) Tramadol hydrochloride 50 mg. Tab. 100s, 500s, 1,000s. *Rx.*
Use: Opioid analgesic.

tramadol and acetaminophen. (Par) Tramadol hydrochloride 37.5 mg, acetaminophen 325 mg. Tab. 20s, 100s, 500s. *Rx.*
Use: Narcotic analgesic combination.

•**tramadol hydrochloride.** (TRAM-uh-dole) USAN.
Tall Man: traMADol
Use: Opioid analgesic.
See: ConZip.
Rybix ODT.
Ultram.
Ultram ER.
W/Acetaminophen.
See: Ultracet.

tramadol hydrochloride. (KLE 2) Tramadol hydrochloride 150 mg (total dose of 150 mg in a combination of 37.5 mg immediate-release and 112.5 mg extended-release tramadol). May contain lactose, sucrose. ER Cap. 500s, 1,000s. *Rx.*
Use: Opioid analgesic.

tramadol hydrochloride. (Various Mfr.) Tramadol hydrochloride. **Tab.:** 50 mg. May contain lactose, PEG. 100s, 500s,

1,000s, UD 30s, UD 100s, UD 300s. **ER Tab.:** 100 mg, 200 mg, 300 mg. 30s, 90s, 500s. *Rx.*
Use: Opioid analgesic.

•**tramazoline hydrochloride.** (tram-AZ-oh-leen) USAN.
Use: Adrenergic.

•**trametinib.** (tra-ME-ti-nib) USAN.
Use: Antineoplastic.
See: Mekinist.

•**trametinib dimethyl sulfoxide.** (tra-ME-ti-nib) USAN.
Use: Antineoplastic.

•**tramiprosate.** (tram-IP-roe-sate) USAN.
Use: Alzheimer disease.

Trandate. (Faro Pharmaceuticals) Labetalol hydrochloride 100 mg, 200 mg, 300 mg. Tab. 100s, 500s, UD 100s. *Rx.*
Use: Antiadrenergic/sympatholytic, alpha/beta-adrenergic blocker.

•**trandolapril.** (tran-DOL-a-pril) *USP.*
Use: Antihypertensive.
See: Mavik.
W/Verapamil Hydrochloride.
See: Tarka.

trandolapril. (Teva) Trandolapril 1 mg, 2 mg, 4 mg. May contain lactose. Tab. 30s (1 mg only), 90s (except 1 mg), 100s. *Rx.*
Use: Antihypertensive.

trandolapril/verapamil hydrochloride. (Glenmark Pharmaceuticals) Trandolapril/verapamil hydrochloride 1 mg/240 mg, 2 mg/180 mg, 2 mg/240 mg, 4 mg/240 mg. Film coated. Lactose. ER Tab. 100s. *Rx.*
Use: Antihypertensive combination.

•**tranexamic acid.** (tran-ex-AM-ik) USAN.
Use: Hemostatic. [Orphan Drug]
See: Cyklokapron.
Lysteda.

tranexamic acid. (American Regent) Tranexamic acid 100 mg/mL. Inj., Soln. Single-dose vial. 10 mL. *Rx.*
Use: Systemic hemostatic.

tranexamic acid. (Watson Pharma) Tranexamic acid 650 mg. May contain glyceryl, lactose, PEG. Tab. 30s, 1,000s. *Rx.*
Use: Systemic hemostatic.

•**tranilast.** (TRAN-ill-ast) USAN.
Use: Antiasthmatic.

tranquilizers.
See: Compazine.
Fenarol.
Librium.
Loxitane.
Meprobamate.
Miltown.
Permitil.
Prolixin.
Tranxene.
Trilafon.
Valium.
Vistaril.

Tranquils. (Halsey Drug) **Cap.:** Pyrilamine maleate 25 mg. Bot. 30s. **Tab.:** Acetaminophen 300 mg, pyrilamine maleate 25 mg. Bot. 30s. *OTC.*
Use: Sleep aid.

•**transcainide.** (trans-CANE-ide) USAN.
Use: Antiarrhythmic, cardiovascular agent.

Transderm-Nitro. (Summit) Nitroglycerin 12.5 mg, 25 mg, 50 mg, 75 mg, 100 mg. Patch. Box 30s, UD 30s (except 75 mg), 100s (except 75 mg, 100 mg). *Rx.*
Use: Antianginal.

Transderm-Scōp. (Baxter) Scopolamine 1.5 mg (delivers scopolamine ≈ 1 mg over 3 days). Transdermal Patch. 10s, 24s. *Rx.*
Use: Antiemetic/antivertigo agent.

transforming growth factor-beta 2. (Celtrix)
Use: Immunomodulator. [Orphan Drug]

Transthyretin EIA. (Abbott Diagnostics) Test kits 100s.
Use: Diagnostic aid.

Trans-Ver-Sal AdultPatch. (Doak Dermatologics) Salicylic acid 15%. Transdermal patch. 6 mm, 12 mm. 40s. Securing tape and cleaning file. *OTC.*
Use: Keratolytic.

Trans-Ver-Sal PediaPatch. (Doak Dermatologics) Salicylic acid 15%. Transdermal patch. 6 mm. 20s. Securing tape and cleaning file. *OTC.*
Use: Keratolytic.

Trans-Ver-Sal PlantarPatch. (Doak Dermatologics) Salicylic acid 15%. Transdermal patch. 20 mm patches, 25s. Securing tapes, cleaning file. *OTC.*
Use: Dermatologic, wart therapy.

Tranxene T-tab. (Recordati Rare Diseases) Clorazepate dipotassium 3.75 mg, 7.5 mg, 15 mg. Tab. 100s, 500s, UD 100s. *c-iv.*
Use: Anxiolytic.

tranylcypromine. (Par) Tranylcypromine sulfate 10 mg. Film-coated. Tab. 100s. *Rx.*
Use: Antidepressant, monoamine oxidase inhibitor.

•**tranylcypromine sulfate.** (tran-ill-SIP-row-meen) *USP.*
Use: Antidepressant, monoamine oxidase inhibitor.
See: Parnate.

•**trastuzumab.** (tras-TOOZ-oo-mab) USAN.
Use: Monoclonal antibody.
See: Herceptin.

•**trastuzumab emtansine.** (tras-TOOZ-oo-mab em-TAN-seen) USAN.
Use: Antineoplastic.
See: Kadcyla.

Trasylol. (Bayer Consumer Care) Aprotinin 1.4 mg/mL. Inj. Vial 100 mL, 200 mL. *Rx.*
Use: Antihemophilic.

T-Rau. (Tennessee Pharmaceutic) Rauwolfia serpentina 50 mg or 100 mg. Tab. Bot. 100s, 1000s. *Rx.*
Use: Hypotensive.

Travamulsion 10% Intravenous Fat Emulsion. (Baxter PPI) 1.1 kcal/mL 270 mOsm/L. Bot. 500 mL. *Rx.*
Use: Nutritional supplement, parenteral.

Travamulsion 20% Intravenous Fat Emulsion. (Baxter PPI) 2 kcal/mL 300 mOsm/L. Bot. 500 mL. *Rx.*
Use: Nutritional supplement, parenteral.

Travasol. (Baxter Medication Delivery) Crystalline L-amino acids 8.5%. Inj. 500 mL, 1,000 mL, 2,000 mL. *Rx.*
Use: Nutritional supplement, parenteral.

Travasol 10%. (Baxter Medication Delivery) Crystalline L-amino acids 10%. Inj. Bot. 200 mL, 500 mL, 1000 mL, 2000 mL. *Rx.*
Use: Nutritional supplement, parenteral.

Travasol 3.5% M Injection with Electrolyte #45. (Baxter Medication Delivery) Crystalline L-amino acids 3.5%. Soln. Bot. IV 500 mL, 1000 mL. *Rx.*
Use: Nutritional supplement, parenteral.

Travasorb HN Peptide Diet. (Baxter PPI) High-nitrogen defined peptide 333 kcal. Pkt. 6 pkt. Carton. *OTC.*
Use: Nutritional supplement.

Travasorb MCT Liquid Diet. (Baxter PPI) Digestible protein medium-chain triglyceride diet. 89 g packets. *OTC.*
Use: Nutritional supplement.

Travasorb MCT Powder Diet. (Baxter PPI) Digestible protein medium-chain triglyceride diet 400 kcal. Pkt. 6 pkt. Carton. *OTC.*
Use: Nutritional supplement.

Travasorb Renal Diet. (Baxter PPI) 467 kcal. Pkt. 6 pkt. Carton. 112 g packets. *OTC.*
Use: Nutritional supplement.

Travasorb Standard Diet. (Baxter PPI) Defined peptide diet, 333 kcal. pkt. 6 packets. Ctn. *OTC.*
Use: Nutritional supplement.

Travasorb Whole Protein Liquid Diet. (Baxter PPI) Lactose free complete nutrition 250 kcal. Can. 8 oz. *OTC.*
Use: Nutritional supplement.

Travatan Z. (Alcon) Travoprost 0.004%. Polyoxyl 40 hydrogenated castor oil, *sofZia* as a preservative. Ophth. Soln. *Drop-Tainers.* 2.5 mL, 5 mL. *Rx.*
Use: Agent for glaucoma; prostaglandin agonist.

Travel Aids. (Faraday) Dimenhydrinate 50 mg. Tab. Bot. 30s. *OTC.*
Use: Antiemetic; antivertigo.

Travel-Eze. (Health for Life Brands) Pyrilamine maleate 25 mg, hyoscine hydrobromide 0.325 mg. Tab. Pkg. 20s. *OTC.*
Use: Antiemetic; antivertigo.

Travel Sickness. (Various Mfr.) Meclizine 25 mg. May contain aspartame, dextrose, phenylalanine, sugar. Chew. Tab. 100s. *OTC.*
Use: Antiemetic/antivertigo agent, anticholinergic.

Traveltabs. (Armenpharm Ltd.) Dimenhydrinate 50 mg. Tab. Bot. 100s. *OTC.*
Use: Antiemetic; antivertigo.

Travert. (Baxter PPI) Invert sugar injection 10% in water or saline. Plastic Bot. 500 mL, 1000 mL, electrolyte No. 2 Bot. 500 mL, 1000 mL, electrolyte No. 4 Bot. 250 mL, 500 mL Soln. (10%). *Rx.*
Use: Fluid, electrolyte replacement.

5% Travert and Electrolyte No. 2. (Baxter PPI) Invert sugar 50 g/L, calories 196 Cal/L, Na 56 mEq/L, K 25 mEq/L, Mg 6 mEq/L, Cl 56 mEq/L, phosphate 12.5 mEq/L, lactate 25 mEq/L, osmolarity 449 mOsm/L. 1000 mL. *Rx.*
Use: Nutritional supplement, parenteral.

10% Travert and Electrolyte No. 2. (Baxter PPI) Invert sugar 100 g/L, calories 384 Cal/L, Na 56 mEq/L, K 25 mEq/L, Mg 6 mEq/L, Cl 56 mEq/L, phosphate 12.5 mEq/L, lactate 25 mEq/L, osmolarity 726 mOsm/L. 1000 mL. *Rx.*
Use: Nutritional supplement, parenteral.

•**travoprost.** (TRA-voe-prost) USAN.
Use: Antiglaucoma; prostaglandin agonist.
See: Travatan Z.

travoprost. (Various Mfr.) Travoprost 0.004%. Benzalkonium chloride 0.15 mg/mL, boric acid, edetate disodium. Soln.; Ophth. Dropper bottles. 2.5 mL, 5 mL. *Rx.*
Use: Agent for glaucoma, prostaglandin agonist.

•**trazodone hydrochloride.** (TRAY-zoe-dohn) *USP.*
Tall Man: traZODone
Use: Antidepressant.
See: Oleptro.

trazodone hydrochloride. (Barr) Trazodone hydrochloride 300 mg. Tab. Bot. 100s, 500s. *Rx.*
Use: Antidepressant.

trazodone hydrochloride. (Various Mfr.). Trazodone hydrochloride 50 mg, 100 mg, 150 mg. Tab. 100s, 500s, 1000s. UD 100s (except 150 mg). *Rx.*
Use: Antidepressant.

Treagan. (Trigen Labs) Antipyrine 5.4%, benzocaine 1.4%, u-polycosanol 410 0.0097%, acetic acid, glycerin. Soln., otic. 15 mL w/dropper. *Rx.*
Use: Miscellaneous otic preparation.

Treanda. (Cephalon) Bendamustine hydrochloride 25 mg, 100 mg. Preservative free. Mannitol 170 mg (100 mg), 42.5 mg (25 mg). Inj., Lyophilized, Pow. for Soln. Single-use vials. 20 mL (100 mg), 8mL (25 mg). *Rx.*
Use: Antineoplastic.

Treanda. (Teva) Bendamustine hydrochloride 90 mg/mL. Inj., Soln., concentrate. Single-use vial. 0.5 mL, 2 mL. *Rx.*
Use: Antineoplastic.

•**trebananib.** (tre-BAN-a-nib) USAN.
Use: Antineoplastic.

•**trebenzomine hydrochloride.** (TRAY-BEN-zoe-meen) USAN.
Use: Antidepressant.

Trecator. (Wyeth) Ethionamide 250 mg. Film-coated. Tab. Bot. 100s. *Rx.*
Use: Antituberculosis agent.

•**trecovirsen sodium.** (treh-koe-VEER-sin) USAN.
Use: Antiviral.

•**trefentanil hydrochloride.** (treh-FEN-tah-nill) USAN.
Use: Analgesic.

•**trelagliptin.** (TREL-a-GLIP-tin) USAN.
Use: Antidiabetic agent.

•**trelagliptin succinate.** (TREL-a-GLIP-tin) USAN.
Use: Antidiabetic agent.

•**treloxinate.** (trell-OX-ih-nate) USAN.
Use: Antihyperlipoproteinemic.

Trelstar. (Watson) Triptorelin pamoate 3.75 mg, 11.25 mg, 22.5 mg. Mannitol, polysorbate 80. Inj., lyophilized microgranules for Susp. Single-dose vial and in *Mixject* delivery system w/2 mL of diluent.

Trelstar Depot. (Watson) Triptorelin pamoate equivalent to 3.75 mg triptorelin peptide base, mannitol. Microgranules for Inj., lyophilized. Single-dose vial. *Rx.*
Use: Hormone; gonadotropin-releasing hormone analog.

Trelstar LA. (Watson) Triptorelin pamoate equivalent to 11.25 mg triptorelin peptide base, mannitol. Microgranules for Inj., lyophilized. Single-dose vial. *Rx.*
Use: Hormone; gonadotropin-releasing hormone analog.

•**trenonacog alfa.** (tre-NOE-na-kog) USAN.
Use: Treatment of hemophilia B.

Trental. (Hoechst Marion Roussel) Pentoxifylline 400 mg. Film-coated. CR Tab. Bot. 100s. Bulk pack. 5000s. *Rx.*
Tall Man: TRENtal
Use: Hemorrheologic agent.

Treo. (Biopharmaceutics) **SPF 8:** Octocrylene, octyl methoxycinnamate, benzophenone-3, octyl salicylate, isostearyl alcohol, diazolidinyl urea, propylparabens, citronella oil 0.05% (as insect repellant). Lot. Bot. 118 mL. **SPF 15:** Octocrylene, octyl methoxycinnamate, benzophenone-3, octyl salicylate, isostearyl alcohol, diazolidinyl urea, propylparaben, citronella oil 0.05% (as insect repellant). Lot. Bot. 118 mL. **SPF 30:** Octocrylene, octyl methoxycinnamate, benzophenone-3, octyl salicylate, isostearyl alcohol, diazolidinyl urea, propylparaben, citronella oil 0.05% (as insect repellant). Lot. Bot. 118 mL. *OTC.*
Use: Sunscreen.

treosulfan.
Use: Antineoplastic. [Orphan Drug]
See: Ovastat.

•**trepipam maleate.** (TREH-pih-pam MAL-ee-ate) USAN. *Formerly Trimopam Maleate.*
Use: Sedative; hypnotic.

•**treprostinil diolamine.** (tre-PROST-i-nil) USAN.
Use: Antihypertensive agent.

•**treprostinil sodium.** (treh-PRAHST-in-ill SO-dee-uhm) USAN.
Use: Vasodilator.
See: Orenitram.
Remodulin.
Tyvaso.

•**trestolone acetate.** (TRESS-toe-lone) USAN.
Use: Antineoplastic; androgen.

trethocanoic acid.
Use: Anticholesteremic.

•**tretinoin.** (TREH-tih-NO-in) *USP.*
Use: Retinoid.
See: Atradin.
Avita.
Refissa.
Renova.
Retin-A.
Tretinoin Microsphere.
Tretin-X.

W/Clindamycin Phosphate.
See: Ziana.
W/Fluocinolone Acetonide, Hydroquinone.
See: Tri-Luma.

tretinoin. (Alpharma, Spear Dermatology) Tretinoin 0.025%, may contain stearyl alcohol. Cream. Tube. 20 g, 45 g. *Rx.*
Use: Retinoid.

tretinoin. (Barr) Tretinoin 10 mg. Cap. 100s. *Rx.*
Use: Retinoid.

tretinoin. (Spear Dermatology.) Tretinoin. **Cream:** 0.05%, 0.1%, stearyl alcohol. Tube. 20 g, 45 g. **Gel:** 0.01%, 0.025%, alcohol. Tube. 15 g, 45 g. *Rx.*
Use: Retinoid.

tretinoin microsphere. (Oceanside Pharmaceuticals) Tretinoin 0.04%, 0.1%. May contain benzyl alcohol, disodium EDTA, glycerin, propylene glycol, trolamine. Gel. 20 g and 45 g tubes, 50 g pump. *Rx.*
Use: First-generation retinoid.

Tretin-X. (Onset Dermatologics) Tretinoin. **Cream:** 0.025%, 0.05%, 0.0375%, 0.075%, 0.1%. Stearyl alcohol. Hydrophilic vehicle. 35 g. **Gel:** 0.01%, 0.025%. Alcohol 90%. 35 g. *Rx.*
Use: Retinoid.

Tretten. (Novo Nordisk) Coagulation factor XIII A-subunit (recombinant) 2,000 to 3,125 units (actual amount in units stated on each vial). Sodium chloride, sucrose. Preservative free. Inj., lyophilized Pow. for Soln. Single-use vial w/diluent (after reconstitution with provided diluent, each vial contains recombinant coagulation factor XIII A-subunit 667 to 1,042 units/mL). *Rx.*
Use: Antihemophilic agent.

Trexall. (Barr) Methotrexate 5 mg, 7.5 mg, 10 mg, 15 mg. Film-coated. Lactose. Tab. 30s, 60s, 100s. *Rx.*
Use: Antimetabolite, folic acid antagonist.

Trexan. (DuPont) Naltrexone hydrochloride 50 mg. Tab. Bot. 50s. *Rx.*
Use: Opioid antagonist.

Treximet. (GlaxoSmithKline) Naproxen sodium 500 mg, sumatriptan 85 mg. Dextrose, sodium 61.2 mg. Film-coated. Tab. 9s. *Rx.*
Use: Agent for migraine, migraine combination.

Trezix. (Wraser Pharmaceuticals) Acetaminophen 356.4 mg, caffeine 30 mg, dihydrocodeine bitartrate 16 mg. Cap. 100s. *c-III.*
Use: Opioid analgesic combination.

Triac. (Eon Labs) Triprolidine hydrochloride 2.5 mg, pseudoephedrine hydrochloride 60 mg. Tab. Bot. 100s, 1000s. *Rx.*
Use: Antihistamine; decongestant.

Triacet. (Teva) Triamcinolone acetonide 0.1%. Cream. Tube 15 g, 80 g. *Rx.*
Use: Corticosteroid, topical.

•**triacetin.** (try-ah-SEE-tin) *USP. Formerly glyceryl triacetate.*
Use: Antifungal, topical.

Triacin-C Cough. (Alpharma) Pseudoephedrine hydrochloride 30 mg, triprolidine hydrochloride 1.25 mg, codeine phosphate 10 mg per 5 mL. Alcohol 4.3%, methylparaben, caramel flavor. Syrup. Bot. 118 mL, 473 mL, 3.8 L. *c-v.*
Use: Upper respiratory combination, antihistamine, antitussive, decongestant.

Triact. (Sanofi-Synthelabo) Aluminum, magnesium hydroxide, simethicone. Liq., Tab. *OTC.*
Use: Antacid; antiflatulent.

Triacting Cold & Allergy. (AmerisourceBergen) Pseudoephedrine hydrochloride 15 mg, chlorpheniramine maleate 1 mg/5 mL, sorbitol, sucrose, orange flavor, alcohol free. Liq. Bot. 118 mL. *OTC.*
Use: Upper respiratory combination, decongestant, antihistamine.

Tri-Acting Cold & Allergy. (Topco) Pseudoephedrine hydrochloride 15 mg, chlorpheniramine maleate 1 mg/5 mL, sorbitol, sucrose, orange flavor, alcohol free. Syr. Bot. 118 mL. *OTC.*
Use: Upper respiratory combination, decongestant, antihistamine.

Tri-Acting Cold & Cough. (Topco) Pseudoephedrine hydrochloride 15 mg, chlorpheniramine maleate 1 mg, dextromethorphan HBr 5 mg per 5 mL. Sorbitol, sucrose, cherry flavor, alcohol free. Syr. Bot. 118 mL. *OTC.*
Use: Upper respiratory combination, decongestant, antihistamine, antitussive.

Triad. (Forest) Butalbital 50 mg, acetaminophen 325 mg, caffeine 40 mg. Cap. Bot. 100s. *Rx.*
Use: Analgesic; hypnotic; sedative.

•**triafungin.** (TRY-ah-FUN-jin) USAN.
Use: Antifungal.

Trial AG. (Zee Medical) Aluminum hydroxide 200 mg, magnesium hydroxide 200 mg, simethicone 25 mg. Sucrose, mannitol. Lemon flavor. Tab. 20s. *OTC.*
Use: Antacid.

Trial Antacid. (Zee Medical) Calcium carbonate 420 mg (elemental calcium 168 mg). Sorbitol. Spearmint flavor. Chew. Tab. 24s. *OTC.*
Use: Mineral supplement; antacid.

Triall. (Breckenridge) Chlorpheniramine maleate 2 mg, methscopolamine nitrate 0.75 mg, phenylephrine hydrochloride 8 mg. Sorbitol. Alcohol free. Grape flavor. Syrup. 473 mL. *Rx.*
Use: Upper respiratory combination; decongestant, antihistamine, and anticholinergic combination.

•**triamcinolone.** (TRY-am-SIN-oh-lone) *USP.*
Use: Corticosteroid, topical.

•**triamcinolone acetonide.** (TRY-am-SIN-oh-lone ah-SEE-toe-nide) *USP.*
Use: Corticosteroid, topical; anti-inflammatory, topical; respiratory inhalant, corticosteroid; adrenocortical steroid, glucocorticoid; ophthalmic corticosteroid.
See: Dermasorb TA.
Kenalog.
Nasacort Allergy 24 HR.
Triacet.
Trianex.
Triderm.
Triesence.
Tri-Nasal.
Trivaris.
W/Nystatin.
See: Mycolog-II.

triamcinolone acetonide. (Barr Labs) Triamcinolone acetonide 55 mcg/actuation. Benzalkonium chloride, dextrose, edentate disodium. Spray; Susp.; intranasal. Bot. w/ metered-dose pump unit and nasal adapter. 16.5 g (providing 120 actuations). *Rx.*
Use: Respiratory inhalant product, intranasal steroid.

triamcinolone acetonide. (Various Mfr.) Triamcinolone acetonide. **Cream: 0.025%, 0.1%:** Tube 15 g, 80 g, 454 g. **0.5%:** 15 g. **Lot.:** 0.025%, 0.1%. Bot. 60 mL. **Oint.: 0.025%, 0.1%:** Tube 15 g, 80 g, 454 g. **0.5%:** Tube 15 g. **Paste:** 0.1%.
Use: Corticosteroid, topical; anti-inflammatory, topical.

•**triamcinolone acetonide sodium phosphate.** (TRY-am-SIN-oh-lone ah-SEE-toe-nide) USAN.
Use: Corticosteroid, topical.

•**triamcinolone hexacetonide.** (TRY-am-SIN-ole-ohn HEX-ah-SEE-tone-ide) *USP.*
Use: Adrenocortical steroid, glucocorticoid.
See: Aristospan.

triamcinolone-16,17-acetonide.
See: Triamcinolone acetonide.

Triaminic AllerChews. (Novartis) Loratadine 10 mg. Mannitol. Orally Disintegrating Tab. 8s. *OTC.*
Use: Antihistamine, peripherally selective piperidine.

Triaminic AM Cough and Decongestant Formula. (Novartis) Pseudoephedrine hydrochloride 15 mg, dextromethorphan HBr 7.5 mg/5 mL, sorbitol, sucrose, orange flavor. Alcohol and dye free. Liq. Bot. 118 mL, 237 mL. *OTC.*
Use: Antitussive; decongestant.

Triaminic AM Decongestant Formula. (Novartis) Pseudoephedrine hydrochloride 15 mg/5 mL, sorbitol, sucrose, orange flavor, alcohol and dye free. Syr. Bot. 118 mL, 237 mL. *OTC.*
Use: Decongestant.

Triaminic AM Non-Drowsy Cough & Decongestant. (Novartis) Pseudoephedrine hydrochloride 15 mg, dextromethorphan HBr 7.5 mg per 5 mL. EDTA, sorbitol, sucrose, orange/strawberry flavor. Liq. Bot. 118 mL. *OTC.*
Use: Upper respiratory combination, decongestant, antitussive.

Triaminic Chest & Nasal Congestion. (Novartis Consumer Health) Phenylephrine hydrochloride 2.5 mg, guaifenesin 50 mg per 5 mL. Acesulfame K, sodium 3 mg. Tropical flavor. Liq. Bot. 118 mL. *OTC.*
Use: Upper respiratory combination, decongestant, expectorant.

Triaminic Children's Thin Strips Day Time Cold & Cough. (Novartis Consumer Health) Dextromethorphan HBr 5 mg, phenylephrine hydrochloride 2.5 mg. Alcohol < 0.5%. PEG, sucralose. Wild berry flavor. Oral Strips. 14s. *OTC.*
Use: Upper respiratory combination, antitussive combination.

Triaminic Children's Thin Strips Night Time Cold & Cough. (Novartis Consumer Health) Diphenhydramine hydrochloride 12.5 mg, phenylephrine hydrochloride 5 mg. Maltodextrin, mannitol, PEG, sucralose. Grape flavor. Oral Strips. 14s. *OTC.*
Use: Upper respiratory combination, decongestant and antihistamine.

Triaminic Cough & Runny Nose. (Novartis Consumer Health) **Orally Disintegrating Strips:** Diphenhydramine hydrochloride 12.5 mg. Alcohol less than 5%, sorbitol, sucralose. Grape flavor. 6s. **Soft-chews:** Chlorpheniramine maleate 1 mg, dextromethorphan hydrobromide 5 mg. Aspartame, maltodextrin, mannitol, phenylalanine 17.6 mg, sodium 5 mg, sorbitol, sucrose. Cherry

flavor Tab., soft chews. 18s. *OTC.*
Use: Antihistamine, upper respiratory combination, antitussive combination.
Triaminic Cough & Sore Throat. (Novartis Consumer Health) Dextromethorphan hydrobromide 5 mg, acetaminophen 160 mg per 5 mL. EDTA, sucrose, sorbitol, sodium 5 mg/5 mL, grape flavor, alcohol free. Liq. 118 mL. *OTC.*
Use: Upper respiratory combination, antitussive combination.
Triaminic Daytime Cold & Cough. (Novartis Consumer Health) Phenylephrine hydrochloride 2.5 mg, dextromethorphan HBr 5 mg per 5 mL. Sorbitol, sucrose, cherry flavor, alcohol free. Liq. Bot. 118 mL. *OTC.*
Use: Upper respiratory combination, antitussive combination.
Triaminic-D Children's. (Novartis Consumer Health) Chlorpheniramine maleate 1 mg, dextromethorphan hydrobromide 7.5 mg, pseudoephedrine hydrochloride 15 mg per 5 mL. Disodium edetate, propylene glycol, sodium 6 mg, sorbitol, sucrose. Alcohol free. Grape flavor. Syrup. 118 mL. *OTC.*
Use: Upper respiratory combination, antitussive combination.
Triaminic Flu, Cough & Fever. (Novartis Consumer Health) Chlorpheniramine maleate 1 mg, dextromethorphan HBr 7.5 mg, acetaminophen 160 mg per 5 mL. EDTA, sorbitol, sucrose, sodium 6 mg/5 mL. Bubble gum flavor. Liq. Bot. 118 mL. *OTC.*
Use: Upper respiratory combination, antitussive combination.
Triaminic Infants' Fever Reducer/Pain Reliever. (Novartis Consumer Health) Acetaminophen 100 mg/mL. Butylparaben, corn syrup, glycerin, propylene glycol, sodium benzoate, sorbitol. Alcohol free. Cherry and grape flavor. Soln., concentrate. 15 mL w/dropper. *OTC.*
Use: CNS agent.
Triaminic Long Acting Cough. (Novartis Consumer Health) Dextromethorphan HBr 7.5 mg per 5 mL. Dye free. EDTA, sorbitol, sucrose. Berry punch flavor. Liq. 118 mL. *OTC.*
Use: Nonnarcotic antitussive.
Triaminic Night Time Cold & Cough. (Novartis Consumer Health) Diphenhydramine hydrochloride 6.25 mg, phenylephrine hydrochloride 2.5 mg per 5 mL. Alcohol free. Acesulfame K, EDTA, mannitol. Grape flavor. Liq. 118 mL with dosage cup. *OTC.*
Use: Upper respiratory combination, decongestant and antihistamine combination.
Triaminic Thin Strips Cold with Stuffy Nose. (Novartis Consumer Health) Phenylephrine hydrochloride 2.5 mg. Maltodextrin, sucralose. Raspberry flavor. Orally Disintegrating Strips. 16s. *OTC.*
Use: Nasal decongestant, arylalkylamine.
Triaminic Thin Strips Cough & Runny Nose. (Novartis Consumer Health) Diphenhydramine hydrochloride 12.5 mg. Alcohol (less than 5%), sorbitol, sucralose. Grape flavor. Orally Disintegrating Strips. 16s. *OTC.*
Use: Nonnarcotic antitussive.
Triaminic Thin Strips Long Acting Cough. (Novartis Consumer Health) Dextromethorphan hydrobromide 7.5 mg. Alcohol (less than 5%), sorbitol, sucralose. Cherry flavor. Orally Disintegrating Strips. 16s. *OTC.*
Use: Nonnarcotic antitussive.
Triamolone 40. (Forest) Triamcinolone diacetate 40 mg/mL. Vial 5 mL. *Rx.*
Use: Corticosteroid.
•**triampyzine sulfate.** (TRY-AM-pih-zeen) USAN.
Use: Anticholinergic.
•**triamterene.** (try-AM-tur-een) *USP.*
Use: Diuretic.
See: Dyrenium.
W/Hydrochlorothiazide
See: Dyazide.
triamterene/hydrochlorothiazide. (Various Mfr.) **Cap.:** Triamterene 37.5 mg, 50 mg, hydrochlorothiazide 25 mg, may contain lactose. Bot. 100s, 1000s. **Tab.:** Triamterene 37.5 mg, hydrochlorothiazide 25 mg. Bot. 100s, 500s, 1000s; triamterene 75 mg, hydrochlorothiazide 50 mg. Bot. 100s, 250s, 500s, 1000s. *Rx.*
Use: Diuretic combination.
Trianex. (Upsher-Smith) Triamcinolone acetonide 0.05%. Lanolin alcohol, mineral oil, wax, white petrolatum. Oint. 17 g, 85 g. *Rx.*
Use: Anti-inflammatory agent, topical corticosteroid.
Trianide. (Seatrace) Triamcinolone acetonide 40 mg/mL. Vial 5 mL. *Rx.*
Use: Corticosteroid.
Tri-A-Vite F. (Major) F_1 0.5 mg, vitamins A 1500 units, D 400 units, C 35 mg/mL Drops. Bot. 50 mL. *Rx.*
Use: Vitamin supplement.
Triaz. (Medicis) Benzoyl peroxide. **Cloths:** 3%, 6%, 9%. Cetyl alcohol, glycerine, glycolic acid, zinc. 60s. **Gel:** 3%, 6%, 9%. Glycerin (except 9%), zinc lactase, EDTA, cetyl stearyl alcohol (ex-

cept 3%), glycolic acid (9% only). Tube 42.5 g. **Lot.:** 3%, 6%, 10%. Glycerin, glycolic acid, petrolatum, menthol, zinc lactate. 85.1 g (10% only), 170.3 g, 340.2 g (except 10%). *Rx.*
Use: Antiacne.

triazenes.
Use: Alkylating agents.
See: Dacarbazine.

•**triazolam.** (trye-AZ-oh-lam) *USP.*
Use: Sedative/hypnotic, nonbarbiturate.
See: Halcion.

triazolam. (Various Mfr.) Triazolam 0.125 mg, 0.25 mg. Tab. Bot. 10s, 100s, 500s, UD 100s. *c-IV.*
Use: Sedative/hypnotic, nonbarbiturate.

triazole antifungals.
Use: Antifungal agents.
See: Fluconazole.
Itraconazole.
Posaconazole.
Voriconazole.

•**tribenoside.** (try-BEN-oh-SIDE) USAN. Not available in US.
Use: Sclerosing agent.

Tri-Biozene. (Reese) Polymyxin B sulfate 10,000 units, neomycin 3.5 mg, bacitracin zinc 500 units, pramoxine hydrochloride 10 mg per g. White petrolatum. Oint. Tubes. 15 g. *OTC.*
Use: Anti-infective, antibiotic, topical.

tribromoethanol.
Use: Anesthetic (inhalation).

tribromomethane. Bromoform.

•**tribromsalan.** (trye-BROM-sa-lan) USAN.
Use: Disinfectant.

tricalcium phosphate.
Use: Mineral supplement.
See: Calcium Phosphate, Tribasic.

TriCare Prenatal Compleat. (Medecor Pharma) Folic acid 1 mg, calcium 200 mg, iron 27 mg, vitamins D 400 units, E 30 units, B_1 1.6 mg, B_2 1.6 mg, B_3 20 mg, B_6 3.1 mg, B_{12} 12 mcg, C 100 mg, Cu, Zn. **Tab.:** Film coated. 30s. **Cap., softgel:** DHA 135 mg, EPA 33.8 mg, other omega-3s 71.2 mg. Coconut oil, orange oil, sucralose, xylitol. Fruit flavor. 30s. *Rx.*
Use: Prenatal vitamin with minerals.

•**tricetamide.** (trye-SET-a-mide) USAN.
Use: Hypnotic; sedative.

Tri-Chlor. (Gordon Laboratories) Trichloroacetic acid 80%. Bot. 15 mL. *Rx.*
Use: Cauterizing agent.

trichlorfon.
See: Metrifonate.

trichloroacetic acid. Acetic acid, trichloro.
Use: Topical, as a caustic.

trichlorobutyl alcohol.
See: Chlorobutanol.

•**trichloromonofluoromethane.** (try-klor-oh-mahn-oh-flure-oh-METH-ane) *NF.*
Use: Pharmaceutic aid (aerosol propellant).
W/Dichlorodifluoromethane.
See: Aerofreeze.

Trichotine. (Schwarz Pharma) **Pow.:** Sodium lauryl sulf., sod. perborate, monohydrate silica. Pkg. 150 g, 360 g. **Liq.:** Sodium lauryl sulfate, sodium borate, SD alcohol 40 8%, SD alcohol 23-A, EDTA. Bot. 120 mL, 240 mL. *OTC.*
Use: Feminine hygiene.

•**triciribine phosphate.** (TRY-SIH-bean) USAN. *Formerly Phosphate Salt of Tricyclic Nucleoside.*
Use: Antineoplastic.

•**tricitrates oral solution.** (TRY-SIH-trates) *USP.*
Use: Alkalizer (systemic, urinary); antiurolithic (cystine calculi, uric acid calculi); buffer (neutralizing).

triclobisonium. (Roche) Triburon, Oint.

triclobisonium chloride.
Use: Anti-infective, topical.

•**triclocarban.** (TRY-kloe-CAR-ban) USAN.
Use: Disinfectant.
See: Artra Beauty Bar.

•**triclofenol piperazine.** (TRY-kloe-FEE-nole pih-PURR-ah-zeen) USAN.
Use: Anthelmintic.

•**triclofos sodium.** (TRY-kloe-foss) USAN.
Use: Hypnotic; sedative.

•**triclonide.** (TRY-kloe-nide) USAN.
Use: Anti-inflammatory.

•**triclosan.** (TRY-kloe-san) *USP.*
Use: Anti-infective; disinfectant.
See: AmeriWash.
ASC Lotionized.
Ca-Rezz.
Clean and Clear Foaming Facial Cleanser.
Clearasil Daily Face Wash.
Sarna.
Stridex Face Wash.

Tricodene Sugar Free. (Pfeiffer) Chlorpheniramine maleate 2 mg, dextromethorphan HBr 10 mg per 5 mL. Menthol, saccharin, sorbitol, mannitol, alcohol free, sugar free. Liq. Bot. 120 mL. *OTC.*
Use: Upper respiratory combination, antihistamine, antitussive.

Tricodene Syrup. (Pfeiffer) Pyrilamine maleate 4.17 mg, codeine phosphate 8.1 mg, terpin hydrate, menthol/5 mL.

Syr. Bot. 120 mL. *c-v.*
Use: Antihistamine; antitussive.

Tricof. (Scientific Laboratories) Dihydrocodeine bitartrate 7.5 mg, chlorpheniramine maleate 2 mg, pseudoephedrine hydrochloride 15 mg per 5 mL. Sugar, alcohol, and dye free. Grape flavor. Syrup. 473 mL. *c-III.*
Use: Antitussive combination.

Tricof EXP. (Scientific Laboratories) Dihydrocodeine bitartrate 7.5 mg, guaifenesin 100 mg, pseudoephedrine hydrochloride 15 mg per 5 mL. Sugar and alcohol free. Vanilla-fruit flavor. Syrup. 473 mL. *c-III.*
Use: Antitussive and expectorant combination.

Tricof PD. (Scientific Laboratories) Dihydrocodeine bitartrate 3 mg, chlorpheniramine maleate 2 mg, phenylephrine hydrochloride 7.5 mg per 5 mL. Grape flavor. Syrup. 473 mL. *c-v.*
Use: Antitussive combination.

TriCor. (AbbVie) Fenofibrate 48 mg, 145 mg. Lactose, sucrose. Tab. Bot. 90s. *Rx.*
Use: Antihyperlipidemic; fibric acid derivatives.

Tricosal. (Invamed) Choline magnesium trisalicylate 500 mg, 750 mg, 1000 mg. Tab. Bot. 100s, 500s. *Rx.*
Use: Salicylate.

tricyclic antidepressants.
Use: Antidepressant.
See: Amitriptyline Hydrochloride.
Amoxapine.
Clomipramine Hydrochloride.
Desipramine Hydrochloride.
Doxepin Hydrochloride.
Imipramine Hydrochloride.
Imipramine Pamoate.
Nortriptyline Hydrochloride.
Protriptyline Hydrochloride.
Trimipramine Maleate.

Tridal. (Scientific Laboratories) Codeine phosphate 12.5 mg, guaifenesin 125 mg, phenylephrine hydrochloride 4 mg per 5 mL. Sugar, alcohol, and dye free. Syrup. 473 mL. *c-v.*
Use: Antitussive and expectorant combination.

Tridal HD. (Scientific Laboratories) Hydrocodone bitartrate 2 mg, chlorpheniramine maleate 2 mg, phenylephrine hydrochloride 5 mg per 5 mL. Sugar and alcohol free. Cherry flavor. Susp. 473 mL. *c-III.*
Use: Antitussive combination.

Tridal HD Plus. (Scientific Laboratories) Hydrocodone bitartrate 3.5 mg, chlorpheniramine maleate 2 mg, phenylephrine hydrochloride 7.5 mg per 5 mL. Sugar free. Black raspberry flavor. Syrup. 473 mL. *c-III.*
Use: Antitussive combination.

Triderm. (Del-Ray) Triamcinolone acetonide 0.1%. Cream. Tube 30 g, 90 g. *Rx.*
Use: Corticosteroid.

Tridesilon Otic. (Bayer Consumer Care) Desonide 0.05%, acetic acid 2% in vehicle. Bot. 10 mL. *Rx.*
Use: Otic.

Tridrate Bowel Cleansing System. (Lafayette) Magnesium citrate 19 g. Bisacodyl tablets 5 mg each (3s). Bisacodyl suppository 10 mg (1s). Kit. *OTC.*
Use: Laxative.

•**trientine hydrochloride.** (TRY-en-TEEN) *USP.*
Use: Chelating agent; Wilson disease therapy adjunct.
See: Cuprid.
Syprine.

Triesence. (Alcon Laboratories) Triamcinolone acetonide 40 mg/mL. Sodium chloride, carboxymethylcellulose sodium 0.5%, polysorbate 80 0.015%, potassium chloride, sodium acetate, sodium citrate. Inj., Susp., Intravitreal. Single-use vials. 1 mL. *Rx.*
Use: Corticosteroid.

Tri-Estarylla. (Sandoz) Ethinyl estradiol/norgestimate. Tab. **Phase 1:** 35 mcg/0.18 mg (7 tablets). **Phase 2:** 35 mcg/0.215 mg (7 tablets). **Phase 3:** 35 mcg/0.25 mg (7 tablets).Lactose. Tab. 28s w/7 inert tablets. *Rx.*
Use: Triphasic oral contraceptive.

triethanolamine.
See: Trolamine.

triethanolamine salicylate.
See: Aspercreme.
Myoflex.

triethanolamine trinitrate biphosphate.
Trolnitrate Phosphate.

•**triethyl citrate.** (trye-ETH-il) *NF.*
Use: Pharmaceutic aid (plasticizer).

triethylenemelamine. Tretamine TEM.
Use: Antineoplastic.

triethylenethiophosphoramide.
See: Thiotepa.

Trifed-C. (Geneva) Pseudoephedrine hydrochloride 30 mg, triprolidine hydrochloride 1.25 mg, codeine phosphate 10 mg/5 mL, alcohol 4.3%. Syrup. Bot. Pt., gal. *c-v.*
Use: Antihistamine; antitussive; decongestant.

•**trifenagrel.** (try-FEN-ah-GRELL) USAN.
Use: Antithrombotic.

•**triflocin.** (try-FLOW-sin) USAN.
Use: Diuretic.
Tri-Flor-Vite with Fluoride. (Everett) Fluoride 0.25 mg, vitamins A 1500 units, D 400 units, C 35 mg/mL. Drops. 50 mL. *Rx.*
Use: Fluoride, vitamin supplement.
•**triflubazam.** (try-FLEW-bah-zam) USAN.
Use: Anxiolytic.
•**triflumidate.** (try-FLEW-mih-DATE) USAN.
Use: Anti-inflammatory.
•**trifluoperazine hydrochloride.** (try-flew-oh-PURR-uh-zeen) *USP.*
Use: Antipsychotic; anxiolytic; hypnotic; sedative.
trifluoperazine hydrochloride. (Various Mfr.) Trifluoperazine hydrochloride 1 mg, 2 mg, 5 mg, 10 mg. Tab. Bot. 100s, 500s, 1000s, UD 100s. *Rx.*
Use: Antipsychotic.
trifluorothymidine. *Rx.*
Use: Ophthalmic.
See: Viroptic.
•**trifluperidol.** (TRY-flew-PURR-ih-dahl) USAN.
Use: Antipsychotic.
•**trifluridine.** (try-FLEW-RIH-deen) *USP.*
Use: Antiviral used to treat herpes simplex eye infections.
See: Viroptic.
trifluridine. (Falcon Ophthalmics) Trifluridine 1%, in aqueous solution with NaCl, thimerosal 0.001%. Ophth. Soln. Bot. 7.5 mL. *Rx.*
Use: Antiviral.
Triglide. (Shionogi Pharma) Fenofibrate 50 mg, 160 mg. Lactose. Tab. 30s. *Rx.*
Use: Antihyperlipidemic agent, fibric acid derivative.
triglyceride reagent strip. (Bayer Consumer Care) *Seralyzer* reagent strip. Bot. 25s.
Use: Diagnostic aid, triglycerides.
triglycerides, medium chain.
Use: Nutritional supplement.
See: MCT Oil.
Trigofen DM. (Trigen Laboratories) Chlorpheniramine maleate 1 mg, dextromethorphan hydrobromide 3 mg, phenylephrine hydrochloride 2 mg. Parabens, potassium citrate, potassium sorbate, propylene glycol, sorbitol, sucralose. Alcohol free, dye free, and sugar free. Orange-vanilla flavor. Liq. 30 mL w/dropper. *Rx.*
Use: Upper respiratory combination, antitussive combination.
Trihexane. (Rugby) Trihexyphenidyl 2 mg. Tab. Bot. 100s, 1000s. *Rx.*
Use: Anticholinergic; antiparkinsonian.
Trihexidyl. (Schein) Trihexyphenidyl 2 mg. Tab. Bot. 100s, 1000s. *Rx.*
Use: Anticholinergic; antiparkinsonian.
Trihexy-5. (Geneva) Trihexyphenidyl 5 mg. Tab. Bot. 100s, 1000s. *Rx.*
Use: Anticholinergic; antiparkinsonian.
•**trihexyphenidyl hydrochloride.** (try-hex-ee-FEN-in-dill) *USP.*
Use: Anticholinergic; antiparkinsonian.
trihexyphenidyl hydrochloride. (VersaPharm) Trihexyphenidyl hydrochloride 2 mg per 5 mL. Alcohol 5%, parabens, sorbitol. Lime-peppermint flavor. Elix. 473 mL. *Rx.*
Use: Antiparkinson agent.
Trihexy-2. (Geneva) Trihexyphenidyl 2 mg. Tab. Bot. 100s, 1000s. *Rx.*
Use: Anticholinergic; antiparkinsonian.
Tri-Histin. (Recsei) **Cap.:** Bot. 100s, 500s, 1000s. **Liq.:** Pyrilamine maleate 5 mg, chlorpheniramine maleate 0.5 mg/5 mL. Bot. Pt., gal. **SA Cap.: 100 mg:** Pyrilamine maleate 40 mg, pheniramine maleate 25 mg. **Tab.: 25 mg:** Pyrilamine maleate 10 mg, chlorpheniramine maleate 1 mg. Bot. 100s, 500s, 1000s. **50 mg:** Pyrilamine maleate 20 mg, methapyrilene hydrochloride 15 mg, chlorpheniramine maleate 2 mg. Bot. 1000s. *Rx-OTC.*
Use: Antihistamine combination.
Trihydroxyethylamine. Triethanolamine.
l-triiodothyronine sodium.
Use: Hormone, thyroid.
See: Cytomel.
Liothyronine sodium.
Tri-K. (Century) Potassium acetate 0.5 g, potassium bicarbonate 0.5 g, potassium citrate 0.5 g/fl. oz. Saccharin. Bot. Pt., gal. *Rx.*
Use: Electrolyte supplement.
•**trikates oral solution.** (TRY-kates) *USP.*
Use: Replenisher (electrolyte).
Tri-Legest Fe. (Barr Labs) **Phase 1:** Ethinyl estradiol 20 mcg, norethindrone acetate 1 mg. **Phase 2:** Ethinyl estradiol 30 mcg, norethindrone acetate 1 mg. **Phase 3:** Ethinyl estradiol 35 mcg, norethindrone acetate 1 mg.Lactose. Tab. 28s w/7 inert tablets (ferrous fumarate 75 mg per tablet). *Rx.*
Use: Triphasic oral contraceptive.
Trileptal. (Novartis) Oxcarbazepine. **Tab.:** 150 mg, 300 mg, 600 mg. Bot. 100s, UD 100s. **Susp.:** 60 mg/mL. Saccharin, sorbitol, ethanol. Bot. 250 mL with dosing syr. and adapter. *Rx.*
Use: Anticonvulsant.
Tri-Linyah. (Northstar) **Phase 1:** Ethinyl estradiol 35 mcg, norgestimate

0.18 mg. 7s. **Phase 2:** Ethinyl estradiol 35 mcg, norgestimate 0.215 mg. 7s. **Phase 3:** Ethinyl estradiol 35 mcg, norgestimate 0.25 mg. 7s. PEG, lactose. Tab. 28s (w/7 inert tablets). *Rx.*
Use: Triphasic oral contraceptive.

Trilipix. (Abbott Laboratories) Fenofibrate 45 mg, 135 mg (as fenofibric acid). Cap., delayed release. 30s, 90s. *Rx.*
Use: Antihyperlipidemic agent, fibric acid derivative.

•**trilostane.** (TRY-low-stane) USAN.
Use: Adrenocortical suppressant.

Tri-Luma. (Galderma) Fluocinolone acetonide 0.01%, hydroquinone 4%, tretinoin 0.05%, cetyl alcohol, glycerin, parabens, sodium metabisulfite, stearyl alcohol. Cream. Tube 30 g. *Rx.*
Use: Treatment of melasma.

Trimahist. (Tennessee Pharmaceutic) Phenylephrine hydrochloride 5 mg, prophenpyridamine maleate 12.5 mg, l-menthol 1 mg, alcohol 5%/5 mL. Elix. Bot. Pt., gal. *Rx.*
Use: Antihistamine; decongestant.

Trimax. (Sanofi-Synthelabo) Aluminum, magnesium hydroxide, simethicone. Gel. Tab. *OTC.*
Use: Antacid; antiflatulent.

trimazinol.
Use: Anti-inflammatory.

•**trimazosin hydrochloride.** (try-MAY-zoe-sin) USAN.
Use: Antihypertensive.

•**trimegestone.** (try-meh-JESS-tone) USAN.
Use: Hormone, progestin.

•**trimeprazine tartrate.** (trye-MEP-ra-zeen) USAN.
Use: Antipruritic.

trimetamide. Trimethamide.

trimethamide.
Use: Antihypertensive.

trimethobenzamide. (Various Mfr.) Trimethobenzamide hydrochloride 300 mg. Cap. Bot. 100s, 250s, 500s, 1,000s, UD 30s, UD 60s. *Rx.*
Use: Antiemetic/antivertigo agent.

•**trimethobenzamide hydrochloride.** (try-meth-oh-BEN-zuh-mide) *USP.*
Use: Antiemetic.
See: Tigan.

trimethobenzamide hydrochloride. (Various Mfr.) Trimethobenzamide hydrochloride 100 mg/mL. Amp. 2 mL. Vials. 20 mL. *Rx.*
Use: Antiemetic/antivertigo agent.

•**trimethoprim.** (try-METH-oh-prim) *USP.*
Use: Anti-infective.
See: Proloprim.
Trimpex.
W/Polymyxin B Sulfate.
See: Polytrim.
W/Sulfamethoxazole.
See: Bactrim.

trimethoprim and sulfamethoxazole. (Various Mfr.) **Tab.:** Trimethoprim 80 mg, sulfamethoxazole 400 mg. Bot. 100s, 500s. **Susp.:** Trimethoprim 40 mg, sulfamethoxazole 200 mg/5 mL. Alcohol 0.26%, methylparaben, saccharin, sorbitol. Grape and cherry flavors. 473 mL. **Inj.:** Sulfamethoxazole 80 mg/mL, trimethoprim 16 mg/mL. May contain alcohol, benzyl alcohol, metabisulfite. Single-use vial. 5 mL. Multiple-use vial. 10 mL, 30 mL. *Rx.*
Use: Anti-infective combination.

trimethoprim and sulfamethoxazole DS. (Various Mfr.) Trimethoprim 160 mg, sulfamethoxazole 800 mg. Tab. Bot. 100s, 500s. *Rx.*
Use: Anti-infective combination.

trimethoprim hydrochloride.
Use: Anti-infective.
See: Primsol.

•**trimethoprim sulfate.** (try-METH-oh-prim) USAN.
Use: Anti-infective.

trimethoprim sulfate and polymyxin B sulfate ophthalmic. (Various Mfr.) Trimethoprim 1 mg, polymyxin B sulfate 10,000 units/mL. Soln. Bot. 10 mL. *Rx.*
Use: Anti-infective, ophthalmic.

trimethylene. Cyclopropane.

•**trimetozine.** (try-MET-oh-zeen) USAN.
Use: Hypnotic; sedative.

•**trimetrexate.** (TRY-meh-TREK-sate) USAN.
Use: Antineoplastic.

•**trimetrexate glucuronate.** (TRY-meh-TREK-sate glue-CURE-uh-nate) USAN.
Use: Antineoplastic.

•**trimipramine.** (TRY-MIH-prah-meen) USAN.
Use: Antidepressant.

•**trimipramine maleate.** (TRY-MIH-prah-meen) USAN.
Use: Antidepressant.
See: Surmontil.

trimipramine maleate. (Actavis) Trimipramine maleate 25 mg, 50 mg, 100 mg. Lactose. Cap. 30s; 90s, 270s (except 100 mg). *Rx.*
Use: Antidepressant, tricyclic antidepressant.

Trimixin. (Hance) Bacitracin 200 units, polymyxin B sulfate 4000 units, neomycin sulfate 3 mg/g Oint. Tube 0.5 oz. *OTC.*
Use: Anti-infective, topical.

•**trimoprostil.** (TRY-moe-PRAHS-till) USAN.
Use: Gastric antisecretory.

Trimo-San. (Cooper Surgical) Oxyquinoline sulfate 0.025%, boric acid 1%, sodium borate 0.7%, sodium lauryl sulfate 0.1%, glycerin, methylparaben. Jelly. 120 g w/applicator, 120 g refill. *OTC.*
Use: Vaginal agent.

Trimox. (Sandoz) Amoxicillin 125 mg/5 mL when reconstituted. Sucrose. Raspberry-strawberry flavor. Pow. for Oral Susp. Bot. 80 mL, 100 mL, 150 mL. *Rx.*
Use: Penicillin, aminopenicillin.

•**trimoxamine hydrochloride.** (TRY-MOX-am-een) USAN.
Use: Antihypertensive.

Trimox Pediatric Drops. (Apothecon) Amoxicillin trihydrate 50 mg/mL when reconstituted, sucrose. Pow. for Oral Susp. Bot. 15 mL. *Rx.*
Use: Anti-infective, penicillin.

Trimpex. (Roche) *Tel-E-Dose* 100s. *Rx.*
Use: Anti-infective, urinary.

Trim-Qwik. (Columbia) Powder-based meal food supplement. Can 10 oz. *OTC.*
Use: Nutritional supplement.

Trimstat. (Laser) Phendimetrazine tartrate 35 mg. Tab. Bot. 100s, 1000s. *c-III.*
Use: Anorexiant.

Trim-Sulfa. *Rx.*
Use: Anti-infective.
See: Proloprim.
Trimethoprim.
Trimpex.

Trim Sulf D/S. (Lexis Laboratories) Sulfamethoxazole 800 mg, trimethoprim 160 mg. Tab. Bot. 100s, 500s. *Rx.*
Use: Anti-infective.

Trim Sulf S/S. (Lexis Laboratories) Sulfamethoxazole 400 mg, trimethoprim 80 mg. Tab. Bot. 100s, 500s. *Rx.*
Use: Anti-infective.

Tri-Nasal. (Muro) Triamcinolone acetonide 50 mcg/spray, EDTA, benzalkonium chloride 0.01%. Spray. Bot. 15 mL with triamcinolone acetonide 7.5 mg/bot. (120 metered sprays) with nasal applicator. *Rx.*
Use: Respiratory inhalant, intranasal steroid.

Trinate. (Cypress) Ca 200 mg, Fe 28 mg, vitamin A 3000 units, D 400 units, E (dl-alpha tocopheryl acetate) 22 mg, B_1 1.8 mg, B_2 4 mg, B_3 20 mg, B_6 25 mg, B_{12} 12 mcg, C 120 mg, folic acid 1 mg, Zn 25 mg, Cu, Mg. Tab. Bot. 100s. *Rx.*
Use: Mineral, vitamin, supplement.

•**trinecol.** (TRI-ne-kol) USAN. (Pullus)
Use: Oral tolerance therapy.

TriNessa. (Watson) **Phase 1:** Norgestimate 0.18 mg, ethinyl estradiol 35 mcg. 7 tabs. **Phase 2:** Norgestimate 0.215 mg, ethinyl estradiol 35 mcg. 7 tabs. **Phase 3:** Norgestimate 0.25 mg, ethinyl estradiol 35 mcg. 7 tabs. Tab. 28s with 7 inert tabs. *Rx.*
Use: Contraceptive hormone, sex hormone.

trinitrin tablets.
See: Nitroglycerin.

Tri-Norinyl. (Watson) **Phase 1:** Norethindrone 0.5 mg, ethinyl estradiol 35 mcg (7 tabs.). **Phase 2:** Norethindrone 1 mg, ethinyl estradiol 35 mcg (9 tabs.). **Phase 3:** Norethindrone 0.5 mg, ethinyl estradiol 35 mcg (5 tabs.). Lactose. *Wallette* 28s with 7 inert tabs. *Rx.*
Use: Sex hormone, contraceptive hormone.

Trinotic. (Forest) Secobarbital 65 mg, amobarbital 40 mg, phenobarbital 25 mg. Tab. Bot. 1000s. *c-II.*
Use: Hypnotic.

Triofed. (Alra) Pseudoephedrine hydrochloride 30 mg, triprolidine hydrochloride 1.25 mg/5 mL. Syr. Bot. 118 mL, 473 mL. *OTC.*
Use: Antihistamine, decongestant.

•**triolein I 131.** (TRY-oh-leen) USAN.
Use: Radiopharmaceutical.

•**triolein I 125.** (TRY-oh-leen) USAN.
Use: Radiopharmaceutical.

Triostat. (JHP Pharmaceuticals) Liothyronine sodium 10 mcg/mL, w/ammonia 2.19 mg/mL, alcohol 6.8%. Inj. Vial 1 mL. *Rx.*
Use: Hormone, thyroid.

trioxane.
See: Trioxymethylene.

•**trioxifene mesylate.** (TRY-OX-ih-feen) USAN.
Use: Antiestrogen.

TriOxin. (Vertical Pharmaceuticals) Benzocaine 15 mg, chloroxylenol 1 mg, hydrocortisone acetate 10 mg per mL. Isopropyl alcohol, PEG-12, PEG-40. Susp., Otic. 15 mL. *Rx.*
Use: Ophthalmic and otic agent, miscellaneous otic preparation.

trioxymethylene. Name is incorrectly used to denote paraformaldehyde in some pharmaceuticals.
See: Paraformaldehyde.

Tri-Pain. (Ferndale) Acetaminophen 162 mg, aspirin 162 mg, salicylamide 162 mg, caffeine 16.2 mg. Tab. Bot. 100s. *OTC.*
Use: Analgesic combination.

•**tripamide.** (TRIP-ah-mide) USAN.
Use: Antihypertensive; diuretic.

Tri-Pase 8. (Acella) Lipase 8,000 units, protease 30,000 units, amylase 30,000 units. Lactose. Tab. 100s. *Rx.*
Use: Digestive enzyme.

Tri-Pase 16. (Acella) Lipase 16,000 units, protease 60,000 units, amylase 60,000 units. Lactose. Tab. 100s. *Rx.*
Use: Digestive enzyme.

•**tripelennamine citrate.** (trih-pell-EN-au-meen SIH-trate) *USP.*
Use: Antihistamine.

•**tripelennamine hydrochloride.** (trih-pell-EN-au-meen) *USP.*
Use: Antihistamine.
See: PBZ.
Pyribenzamine.

triphenylmethane dyes.
See: Fuchsin, Basic.
Methylrosaniline Chloride.

triphenyltetrazolium chloride. TTC.

tripiperazine dicitrate, hydrous.
See: Piperazine Citrate.

triple antibiotic. (Various Mfr.) Polymyxin B sulfate 5,000 units, neomycin 3.5 mg, bacitracin zinc 400 units per g. Oint. Tubes. 15 g, 30 g, 454 g. *OTC.*
Use: Anti-infective, antibiotic, topical.

triple antibiotic ophthalmics. (Various Mfr.) Polymyxin B sulfate 10,000 units/g, neomycin sulfate 3.5 mg/g, bacitracin 400 units. Oint. 3.5 g. *Rx.*
Use: Anti-infective; ophthalmic.

triple barbiturate elixir. (CMC) Phenobarbital 0.25 g, butabarbital 0.125 g, pentobarbital g/5 mL. Bot. Pt., gal. *c-II.*
Use: Sedative.

Triple Cream. (Summers Labs) Avena sativa, beeswax, benzyl alcohol, white petrolatum. Cream. 114 g. OTC. Miscellaneous emollient.

Triple Dye. (Kerr Drug) Gentian violet, proflavine, hemisulfate, brilliant green in water. Dispensing Bot. 15 mL. Single-Use *Dispos-A-Swab* 0.65 mL. Box 10s. Case 10 × 50 Box.
Use: Antiseptic.

Triple Dye. (Xttrium) Brilliant green 2.29 mg, proflavine hemisulfate 1.14 mg, gentian violet 2.29 mg/mL. Bot. 30 mL.
Use: Disinfectant.

Triple-Gen. (Ivax) Hydrocortisone 1%, neomycin sulfate 0.35%, polymyxin B sulfate 10,000 units/mL, benzalkonium chloride, cetyl alcohol, glyceryl monostearate, polyoxyl 40 stearate, propylene glycol, mineral oil. Susp. Bot. 7.5 mL. *Rx.*
Use: Anti-infective; corticosteroid; ophthalmic.

Triplen. (Henry Schein) Tripelennamine hydrochloride 50 mg. Tab. Bot. 100s, 1000s. *Rx.*
Use: Antihistamine.

Triple Paste AF. (Summers) Miconazole nitrate 2%. Beeswax, lanolin, stearyl alcohol, white petrolatum, zinc oxide. Oint. 56.7 g. *OTC.*
Use: Topical antifungal agent.

•**triple sulfa.** (TRIP-el-SUL-fa) *USP.* Sulfathiazole, sulfacetamide, and sulfabenzamide.
Use: Anti-infective.

Triple Sulfoid. (Pal-Pak, Inc.) Sulfadiazine 167 mg, sulfamerazine 167 mg, sulfamethazine 167 mg/5 mL. **Liq.:** Bot. Pt., 2 oz. 12s. **Tab.:** Bot. 100s, 1000s. *Rx.*
Use: Anti-infective, sulfonamide.

triple sulfonamide. Dia-Mer-Thia Sulfonamides. Meth-Dia-Mer Sulfonamides.
Use: Anti-infective, sulfonamide.

Triple Vita. (Rosemont) Vitamins A 1500 units, D 400 units, C 35 mg/mL, alcohol free. Drops. Bot. 50 mL. *OTC.*
Use: Vitamin supplement.

Triple Vita-Flor. (Rosemont) Fluoride 0.5 mg, vitamins A 1500 units, D 400 units, C 35 mg/mL, alcohol free. Drops. Bot. 50 mL. *Rx.*
Use: Dental caries agent; vitamin supplement.

Triple Vitamin ADC w/Fluoride. (Nilor Pharm) Fluoride 0.5 mg, vitamins A 1500 units, D 400 units, C 35 mg/mL. Drops. Bot. 50 mL. *Rx.*
Use: Mineral, vitamin supplement; dental caries agent.

Triple Vitamins w/Fluoride. (Major) Vitamin A 2500 units, D 400 units, C 60 mg, fluoride 1 mg, dextrose, sucrose. Chew. Tab. Bot. 100s. *Rx.*
Use: Vitamin supplement; dental caries agent.

Triplevite w/Fluoride. (Geneva) Fluoride. **0.25 mg/mL:** Vitamins A 1500 units, D 400 units, C 35 mg, alcohol free. Drops. Bot. 50 mL. **0.5 mg/mL:** Vitamins A 1500 units, D 400 units, C 35 mg/mL, alcohol free, cherry flavor. Drops. Bot. 50 mL. *Rx.*
Use: Dental caries agent; vitamin supplement.

Tripodrine. (Schein) Pseudoephedrine hydrochloride 60 mg, triprolidine hydrochloride 2.5 mg. Tab. Bot. 100s, UD 100s. *Rx.*
Use: Antihistamine; decongestant.

Triposed Syrup. (Halsey Drug) **Syr.:** Triprolidine hydrochloride 1.25 mg, pseudoephedrine hydrochloride 30 mg/5 mL. Bot. 120 mL, 240 mL, 473 mL,

gal. **Tab.:** Triprolidine hydrochloride 2.5 mg, pseudoephedrine hydrochloride 60 mg. Bot. 100s, 1000s. *OTC.*
Use: Antihistamine; decongestant.

tripotassium citrate.
See: Potassium Citrate.

Tri-Previfem. (Qualitest) **Phase 1:** Norgestimate 0.18 mg, ethinyl estradiol 35 mcg. 7 tabs. **Phase 2:** Norgestimate 0.215 mg, ethinyl estradiol 35 mcg. 7 tabs. **Phase 3:** Norgestimate 0.25 mg, ethinyl estradiol 35 mcg. 7 tabs. Lactose. Tab. 28s with 7 inert tabs. *Rx.*
Use: Sex hormone, contraceptive hormone.

•**triprolidine hydrochloride.** (try-PRO-lih-deen) *USP.*
Use: Antihistamine, nonselective alkylamine.
See: VanaHist PD.
W/Chlophedianol Hydrochloride.
See: ProHist CF.
W/Codeine Phosphate, Pseudoephedrine Hydrochloride.
See: Poly Hist NC.
W/Pseudoephedrine Hydrochloride.
See: Altafed.
Aprodine.
Ed A-Hist PSE.
Entre-Hist PSE.
Genac.
Hist PSE.
Silafed.

triprolidine hydrochloride and pseudoephedrine hydrochloride. (Various Mfr.) Triprolidine hydrochloride 1.25 mg, pseudoephedrine hydrochloride 30 mg/5 mL. Syr. Bot. 118 mL. *OTC.*
Use: Upper respiratory combination, antihistamine, decongestant.

Triptifed. (Weeks & Leo) Triprolidine hydrochloride 2.5 mg, pseudoephedrine hydrochloride 60 mg. Tab. Bot. 36s, 100s. *Rx.*
Use: Antihistamine; decongestant.

Triptone. (Del Pharmaceuticals) Dimenhydrinate 50 mg. Tab. Bot. 12s. *OTC.*
Use: Antiemetic; antivertigo.

•**triptorelin.** (TRIP-toe-RELL-in) USAN.
Use: Antineoplastic.

•**triptorelin pamoate.** (TRIP-toe-RELL-in) USAN.
Use: Antineoplastic; hormone, gonadotropin-releasing hormone analog.
See: Trelstar.
Trelstar Depot.
Trelstar LA.

trisaccharides A and B.
Use: Hemolytic disease of the newborn. [Orphan Drug]

Trisenox. (Cephalon) Arsenic trioxide 1 mg/mL, preservative free. Inj. Box 10s. *Rx.*
Use: Antineoplastic.

trisodium citrate concentration.
Use: Leukapheresis procedures. [Orphan Drug]

Trisol. (Buffington) Borax, sodium chloride, boric acid. Irrig. Bot. oz, 4 oz. *OTC.*
Use: Artificial tears.

Trispec PSE. (Deliz) Dextromethorphan hydrobromide 15 mg, guaifenesin 125 mg, pseudoephedrine hydrochloride 30 mg. Glycerin, saccharin, sodium 17 mg per 5 mL, sodium benzoate, sorbitol. Alcohol free, dye free, and sugar free. Grape flavor. Liq. 118 mL. *OTC.*
Use: Upper respiratory combination, antitussive and expectorant combination.

Trispec PSE Pediatric. (Deliz) Dextromethorphan HBr 15 mg, guaifenesin 25 mg, pseudoephedrine hydrochloride 30 mg per 5 mL. Sugar, alcohol, and dye free. Saccharin, sorbitol. Grape flavor. Liq. Drops. 30 mL. *Rx.*
Use: Antitussive and expectorant combination.

Tri-Sprintec. (Barr) **Phase 1:** Norgestimate 0.18 mg, ethinyl estradiol 35 mcg. 7 tabs. **Phase 2:** Norgestimate 0.215 mg, ethinyl estradiol 35 mcg. 7 tabs. **Phase 3:** Norgestimate 0.25 mg, ethinyl estradiol 35 mcg. 7 tabs. Lactose. Tab. 28s. 7 inert tablets. *Rx.*
Use: Contraceptive hormone, sex hormone.

Tri-Statin. (Rugby) Triamcinolone acetonide 0.1%, neomycin sulfate 0.25%, gramicidin 0.25 mg, nystatin 100,000 units/g Cream. Tube 15 g, 30 g, 60 g, 120 g, 480 g. *Rx.*
Use: Anti-infective; corticosteroid, topical.

Tri-Statin II. (Rugby) Triamcinolone acetonide 0.1%, 100,000 units nystatin per g, white petrolatum, parabens. Cream. Tube 15 g, 30 g, 60 g, 120 g, 480 g. *Rx.*
Use: Antifungal; corticosteroid, topical.

trisulfapyridmines.
Use: Anti-infective, sulfonamide.
See: Triple Sulfa.

•**trisulfapyrimidines oral suspension.** (try-SOLL-fah-peer-IH-mih-deenz) *USP.*
Use: Anti-infective.
See: Meth-Dia-Mer Sulfonamides.

Tri-Super Flavons 1000. (Freeda) Bioflavonoids 1000 mg. Tab. Bot. 100s, 250s, 500s. *OTC.*
Use: Water-soluble vitamin.

Trital SR. (Breckenridge) Acetaminophen 325 mg, chlorpheniramine maleate 8 mg, phenylephrine hydrochloride 40 mg, phenyltoloxamine citrate 50 mg. Tartrazine. Tab. 100s. *Rx.*
Use: Upper respiratory combination; decongestant, antihistamine, and analgesic combination.

Tritan. (Eon Labs) Phenylephrine tannate 25 mg, chlorpheniramine tannate 8 mg, pyrilamine tannate 25 mg. Tab. Bot. 100s, 250s, 1000s. *Rx.*
Use: Antihistamine; decongestant.

Tri-Tannate. (Rugby) Phenylephrine tannate 25 mg, chlorpheniramine tannate 8 mg, pyrilamine tannate 25 mg. Tab. Bot. 100s, 250s. *Rx.*
Use: Antihistamine; decongestant.

Tri-Tannate Pediatric. (Rugby) Phenylephrine tannate 5 mg, chlorpheniramine tannate 2 mg, pyrilamine tannate 12.5 mg. Susp. Bot. 473 mL. *Rx.*
Use: Antihistamine; decongestant.

Tri-Tannate Plus Pediatric Suspension. (Rugby) Phenylephrine tannate 5 mg, ephedrine tannate 5 mg, chlorpheniramine tannate 4 mg, carbetapentane tannate 30 mg/5 mL. Bot. 480 mL. *Rx.*
Use: Antihistamine; antitussive; decongestant.

•**tritiated water.** (TRIT-ee-ay-ted WA-ter) USAN.
Use: Radiopharmaceutical.

Tri-Tinic. (Vortech Pharmaceuticals) Liver desiccated 75 mg, stomach 75 mg, Vitamins B_{12} 15 mcg, Fe 110 mg, folic acid 1 mg, ascorbic acid 75 mg. Cap. Bot. 100s. *Rx.*
Use: Mineral, vitamin supplement.

TriTuss. (Everett) Dextromethorphan HBr 25 mg, guaifenesin 175 mg, phenylephrine hydrochloride 12.5 mg per 5 mL. Sugar and alcohol free. Saccharin, sorbitol. Strawberry flavor. Syrup. 473 mL. *Rx.*
Use: Upper respiratory combination, antitussive and expectorant combination.

TriTuss-A. (Everett) Phenylephrine hydrochloride 2 mg, carbinoxamine maleate 1 mg, dextromethorphan HBr 2 mg per 1 mL. Sugar free. Parabens, saccharin, sorbitol. Cherry flavor. Oral Drops. Bot. 30 mL with calibrated dropper. *Rx.*
Use: Pediatric antitussive combination.

TriTuss-ER. (Everett) Dextromethorphan HBr 30 mg, guaifenesin 600 mg, phenylephrine hydrochloride 10 mg. ER Tab. 100s. *Rx.*
Use: Upper respiratory combination, antitussive and expectorant combination.

Tritussin. (Scientific Laboratories) Hydrocodone bitartrate 5 mg, chlorpheniramine maleate 2 mg, phenylephrine hydrochloride 5 mg per 5 mL. Sugar and alcohol free. Candy apple flavor. Syrup. 473 mL. *c-III.*
Use: Antitussive combination.

Tritussin Cough. (Towne) Pyrilamine maleate 40 mg, pheniramine maleate 20 mg, citric acid 100 mg, codeine phosphate 58 mg/fl. oz. w/menthol and glycerin in flavored base. Syr. Bot. 4 oz. *c-V.*
Use: Antihistamine; antitussive; expectorant.

Trivaris. (Allergan) Triamcinolone acetonide 80 mg/mL. Sodium hyaluronate 2.3%. Preservative free. Inj., Gel Susp. Single-use glass syringe. *Rx.*
Use: Adrenocortical steroid, glucocorticoid.

Triveen-PRx RNF. (Trigen Labs) Folic acid 1.2 mg, Ca 160 mg, Fe 26 mg, vitamins D 400 units, E 30 units, B_6 25 mg, C 28 mg, DHA 300 mg, docusate sodium 55 mg. Beeswax, glycerin, soybean oil. Softgels. 30s, 60s. *Rx.*
Use: Prenatal vitamin with minerals.

Triveen-Ten. (Trigen Labs) Folic acid 0.5 mg, Fe 15 mg, vitamins A 1,250 units, D 120 units, E 15 units, B_1 1 mg, B_2 1.7 mg, B_{12} 1 mcg, C 30 mg, Cu, Se, Mg, Zn, CoQ10 50 mg, DHA 50 mg, lycopene 5 mg. Glycerin, lemon oil, polysorbate 80. Tab. 60s. *Rx.*
Use: Prenatal vitamin with minerals.

Tri-Vert. (T.E. Williams Pharmaceuticals) Dimenhydrinate 25 mg, niacin 50 mg, pentylenetetrazol 25 mg. Cap. Bot. 100s. *OTC.*
Use: Motion sickness.

Tri-Vi-Flor. (Zylera) Fluoride 0.25 mg, 0.5 mg. L-methylfolate calcium 0.2 mg, vitamins A 1,125 units, D 300 units, C 25 mg. Biphasic enteric-coated microbead suspension. Potassium sorbate, sodium benzoate, sucrose. Fruit flavor. Susp., concentrate. 50 mL w/dropper. *Rx.*
Use: Multivitamin with fluoride.

Tri-Vi-Floro. (Deston Therapeutics) Fluoride 0.25 mg, vitamins A 1,125 units, C 25 mg, D 300 units, L-methylfolate calcium 200 mcg per 1 mL. Biphasic microbead suspension. Potassium sorbate, sodium benzoate, sucrose. Susp., concentrate. 50 mL w/dropper. *OTC.*
Use: Multivitamin w/fluoride.

Tri-Vi-Flor 1.0 mg. (Bristol-Myers Squibb) Fluoride 1 mg, vitamins A 2500 units, D 400 units, C 60 mg, sucrose. Tab. Bot.

100s, 1000s. *Rx.*
Use: Dental caries agent; nutritional supplement.

Tri-Vi-Flor 0.5 mg. (Bristol-Myers Squibb) Fluoride 0.5 mg, vitamins A 1500 units, D 400 units, C 35 mg/mL. Drops. Bot. 50 mL. *Rx.*
Use: Dental caries agent; nutritional supplement.

Tri-Vi-Flor 0.25 mg. (Bristol-Myers Squibb) Fluoride 0.25 mg, vitamins A 1500 units, D 400 units, C 35 mg/1 mL. Drops. Bot. 50 mL. *Rx.*
Use: Dental caries agent; nutritional supplement.

Tri-Vi-Flor 0.25 mg with Iron. (Bristol-Myers Squibb) Fluoride 0.25 mg, vitamins A 1500 units, D 400 units, C 35 mg, Fe 10 mg/1 mL. Drops. Bot. 50 mL. *Rx.*
Use: Dental caries agent; nutritional supplement.

Tri-Vi-Sol. (Bristol-Myers Squibb) Vitamin A 1500 units, D 400 units, C 35 mg/1 mL. Drops. Bot. 50 mL with calibrated safety-dropper. *OTC.*
Use: Vitamin supplement.

Tri-Vita. (Major) Vitamins A 1,500 units, D 400 units, C 35 mg per mL. Glycerin, polysorbate 80, potassium sorbate, propylene glycol, sodium benzoate. Alcohol free, sugar free. Fruit flavor. Drops. 50 mL w/dropper. *OTC.*
Use: Multivitamin.

Trivitamin Fluoride. (Schein) **Drops:** Fluoride 0.25 mg or 0.5 mg, vitamins A 1500 units, D 400 units, C 35 mg/mL. Bot. 50 mL. **Chew. Tab.:** Fluoride 0.5 mg, vitamins A 2500 units, D 400 units, C 60 mg, sucrose. Bot. 100s. *Rx.*
Use: Fluoride, vitamin supplement; dental caries agent.

Tri-Vitamin With Fluoride. (Rugby) Fluoride 0.5 mg, Vitamins A 1500 units, D 400 units, C 35 mg/mL Drops. Bot. 50 mL. *Rx.*
Use: Mineral, vitamin supplement.

Tri-Vitamin With Fluoride 0.5 mg. (Sancilio) Fluoride 0.5 mg, vitamins A 1,500 units, D 400 units, C 35 mg. Fruit flavoring, glycerin, parabens, polysorbate 80, propylene glycol, sucralose. Dye free, gluten free, and sugar free. Drops. 50 mL w/dropper. *Rx.*
Use: Multivitamin with fluoride.

Tri-Vitamin With Fluoride 0.25 mg. (Sancilio) Fluoride 0.25 mg, vitamins A 1,500 units, D 400 units, C 35 mg. Fruit flavoring, glycerin, parabens, polysorbate 80, propylene glycol, sucralose. Dye free, gluten free, and sugar free. Drops. 50 mL w/dropper. *Rx.*
Use: Multivitamin with fluoride.

Tri-Vite. (Foy Laboratories) Thiamine hydrochloride 100 mg, pyridoxine hydrochloride 100 mg, cyanocobalamin 1000 mcg/mL. Vial 10 mL. *Rx.*
Use: Vitamin supplement.

Trivora. (Watson) **Phase 1:** Levonorgestrel 0.05 mg, ethinyl estradiol 30 mcg (6 tablets). **Phase 2:** Levonorgestrel 0.075 mg, ethinyl estradiol 40 mcg (5 tablets). **Phase 3:** Levonorgestrel 0.125 mg, ethinyl estradiol 30 mcg (10 tablets). Lactose. Pack. 28s with 7 inert tablets. *Rx.*
Use: Sex hormone, contraceptive hormone.

Tri-zel. (Rochester Pharmaceuticals) Vitamins B_3 600 mg, B_6 5 mg, folic acid 0.5 mg, Cu, Zn, azelaic acid 5 mg. Tab. 60s. *Rx.*
Use: Multivitamin with minerals (except iron).

Trizivir. (ViiV Healthcare) Abacavir sulfate 300 mg, lamivudine 150 mg, zidovudine 300 mg. Film-coated. Tab. Bot. 60s. *Rx.*
Use: Antiretroviral, nucleoside analog reverse transcriptase inhibitor combination.

Trocaine. (Roberts) Benzocaine 10 mg. Loz. UD 4s, 500s. *OTC.*
Use: Dietary aid.

•**troclosene potassium.** (TROE-kloe-seen) USAN.
Use: Anti-infective, topical.

•**trodusquemine.** (troe-DOO-skwe-meen) USAN.
Use: Obesity.

•**troglitazone.** (TROE-glih-tazz-ohn) USAN.
Use: Antidiabetic.

Trokendi XR. (Supernus Pharmaceuticals) Topiramate 25 mg, 50 mg, 100 mg, 200 mg. Mannitol, PEG, sodium benzoate, sugar. ER Cap. 100s, UD 30s. *Rx.*
Use: Anticonvulsant.

•**trolamine.** (TROLE-ah-meen) *NF. Formerly Triethanolamine.*
Use: Pharmaceutic aid (alkalizing agent), analgesic.

trolamine salicylate.
Use: Rub and liniment.
See: Analgesic Creme Rub.
Aspercreme with Aloe.
Flex-Power Performance Sports.

tromal.
Use: Analgesic; antidepressant agent.

•**tromethamine.** (TROE-meth-ah-meen) *USP.*
Use: Alkalizer.

Tronolane. (Monticello) **Cream:** Pramoxine hydrochloride 1%, zinc oxide 5%, cetyl alcohol, parabens. Tube 30 g, 60 g. **Supp.:** Hard fat 88.7%, phenylephrine hydrochloride 0.25%. Parabens. 12s. *OTC.*
Use: Anorectal preparation.

Tropamine+. (NeuroGenesis/Matrix Tech.) Vitamins D 250 mg, l-phenylalanine, l-tyrosine 150 mg, l-glutamine 50 mg, B_1 1.67 mg, B_2 2.5 mg, B_3 16.7 mg, B_5 15 mg, B_6 3.3 mg, B_{12} 5 mcg, folic acid 0.067 mg, C 100 mg, Ca 25 mg, Cr 0.01 mg, Fe 1.5 mg, Mg 25 mg, Zn 5 mg, yeast and preservative free. Cap. Bot. 42s, 180s. *OTC.*
Use: Nutritional supplement.

•**tropanserin hydrochloride.** (troe-PAN-ser-in) USAN.
Use: Serotonin receptor antagonist (specific in migraine).

TrophAmine Injection. (McGaw) Nitrogen 4.65 g, amino acids 30 g, protein 29 g/500 mL. Bot. 500 mL IV infusion. *OTC.*
Use: Nutritional supplement.

Troph-Iron. (GlaxoSmithKline Consumer) Vitamins B_{12} 25 mcg, B_1 10 mg, Fe 20 mg/5 mL. Saccharin. Bot. 4 fl. oz. *OTC.*
Use: Mineral, vitamin supplement.

Trophite (Iron). (Menley & James Labs, Inc.) Fe 60 mg, B_1 30 mg, B_{12} 75 mcg. Liq. Bot. 120 mL. *OTC.*
Use: Mineral, vitamin supplement.

Tropicacyl. (Akorn) Tropicamide 0.5%. Benzalkonium chloride 0.1%, EDTA. Soln.; Ophth. 15 mL. *Rx.*
Use: Cycloplegic; mydriatic.

Tropical Blend. (Schering-Plough) A series of products is marketed under the *Tropical Blend* name including: *Hawaii Blend Oil* SPF 2 (Bot. 8 oz.); *Hawaii Blend Lotion* SPF 2 (Bot. 8 oz.); *Rio Blend Oil* SPF 2 (Bot. 8 oz.); *Rio Blend Lotion* SPF 2 (Bot. 8 oz.); *Jamaica Blend Oil* SPF 2 (Bot. 8 oz.); *Jamaica Blend Lotion* SPF 2 (Bot. 8 oz.). All contain homosalate in various oil and lotion bases. *OTC.*
Use: Sunscreen.

Tropical Blend Dark Tanning. (Schering-Plough) **SPF 2:** Homosalate. **Oil:** Padimate O, oxybenzone. Bot. 180 mL, 240 mL. **Lot.:** Bot. 240 mL. **SPF 4:** Ethylhexyl p-methoxycinnamate, oxybenzone. Bot. 240 mL. *OTC.*
Use: Sunscreen.

Tropical Blend Dry Oil. (Schering-Plough) Homosalate, oxybenzone. Oil. Bot. 180 mL. *OTC.*
Use: Sunscreen.

Tropical Blend Tan Magnifier. (Schering-Plough) Triethanolamine salicylate. Oil. Bot. 240 mL. *OTC.*
Use: Sunscreen.

Tropical Gold Dark Tanning Lotion. (Ivax) SPF 4. Ethylhexyl p-methoxycinnamate, oxybenzone, benzyl alcohol, parabens, aloe extract, jojoba oil, vitamin E, EDTA. PABA free. Waterproof. Lot. Bot. 240 mL. *OTC.*
Use: Sunscreen.

Tropical Gold Dark Tanning Oil. (Ivax) SPF 2. Ethylhexyl p-methoxycinnamate, octyldimethyl PABA, mineral oil, coconut oil, cocoa butter, aloe, lanolin, eucalyptus oil, oils of plumeria, manako (mango), kuawa (guava), mikara (papaya), liliko (passion fruit), taro, kukui. Oil. Bot. 240 mL. *OTC.*
Use: Sunscreen.

Tropical Gold Sport Sunblock. (Ivax) SPF 15. Ethylhexyl p-methoxycinnamate, oxybenzone, diazolidinyl urea, parabens, aloe extract, jojoba oil, vitamin E, EDTA. PABA free. Perspiration-proof. Lot. Bot. 180 mL. *OTC.*
Use: Sunblock.

Tropical Gold Sunblock. (Ivax)
Lot: SPF 15: Ethylhexyl p-methoxycinnamate, oxybenzone, vegetable oil, benzyl alcohol, parabens, imidazolidinyl urea, vitamin E, aloe extract, jojoba oil, EDTA. PABA free. Waterproof. Bot. 118 mL.
SPF 17: Ethylhexyl p-methoxycinnamate, 2-ethylhexyl salicylate, homosalate, oxybenzone, aloe extract, vitamin E, vegetable and jojoba oils, benzyl alcohol, imidazolidinyl urea, parabens, EDTA. PAPA free. Waterproof. Bot. 118 mL. **SPF 30:** Ethylhexyl p-methoxycinnamate, 2-ethylhexyl salicylate, homosalate, oxybenzone, aloe extract, vitamin E, vegetable and jojoba oils, benzyl alcohol, imidizolidinyl urea, parabens, EDTA. PABA free. Waterproof. 118 mL. *OTC.*
Use: Sunblock.

Tropical Gold Sunscreen. (Ivax) SPF 8. Ethylhexyl p-methoxycinnamate, oxybenzone, benzyl alcohol, parabens, aloe extract, jojoba oil, vitamin E, EDTA. PABA free. Waterproof. Lot. Bot. 118 mL. *OTC.*
Use: Sunscreen.

•**tropicamide.** (troe-PIK-a-mide) *USP.*
Use: Anticholinergic (ophthalmic).
See: Mydral.

Mydriacyl.
Tropicacyl.

tropicamide. (Various Mfr.) Tropicamide 0.5%, 1%. Benzalkonium chloride, EDTA. Soln.; Ophth. 2 mL (0.5%), 15 mL.
Use: Anticholinergic (ophthalmic).

tropine benzhydryl ester methanesulfonate. Also named benztropine methane-sulfonate.

•**trospectomycin.** (TROE-speck-toe-MY-sin) USAN.
Use: Anti-infective.

•**trospium chloride.** (TROSE-pee-um) USAN.
Use: Anticholinergic.
See: Sanctura.

trospium chloride. (Watson) Trospium chloride 60 mg. PEG, polyvinyl alcohol, sucrose. ER Cap. 30s, 60s, 500s. *Rx.*
Use: Urinary anticholinergic.

trospium chloride. (Various Mfr.) Trospium chloride 20 mg. Film coated. Lactose. Tab. 60s. *Rx.*
Use: Anticholinergic.

Trovit. (Sigma-Tau) Vitamins B_2 0.3 mg, B_6 1 mg, choline chloride 25 mg, panthenol 2 mg, dl-methionine 10 mg, inositol 20 mg, niacinamide 50 mg, vitamins B_{12} 10 mcg/mL. Vial 30 mL. *Rx.*
Use: Vitamin B supplement.

T.R.U.E. Test. (GlaxoSmithKline) Allergen-containing patches. Test in multipak cartons (5s). *Rx.*
Use: Diagnostic aid, allergic.

TruNature Chewable Probiotic. (TruNature) 1.5 billion CFU blend of *L. acidophilus* and *B. lactis*. Dextrose, mannitol, sucralose, xylitol. Grape or vanilla flavor. Chew. Tab. 60s. *OTC.*
Use: Probiotic.

TruNature Digestive Probiotic. (TruNature) 10 billion CFU blend of *L. acidophilus* and *B. lactis*. Gluten free. Cap. 100s. *OTC.*
Use: Probiotic.

Trusopt. (Merck) Dorzolamide (as base) 2%. Benzalkonium chloride 0.0075%, hydroxyethylcellulose, sodium hydroxide, mannitol. Soln. *Ocumeters.* 5 mL, 10 mL. *Rx.*
Use: Antiglaucoma.

Truvada. (Gilead) Emtricitabine 200 mg/tenofovir disoproxil fumarate 300 mg (equiv. to tenofovir disoproxil 245 mg). Lactose. Film-coated. Tab. 30s. *Rx.*
Use: Antiretroviral.

trypan blue.
Use: Ophthalmic surgery aid.
See: MembraneBlue.
VisionBlue.

•**trypsin, crystallized.** (TRIP-sin) *USP.*
Use: Proteolytic enzyme.
W/Castor Oil.
See: Granulex.
W/Combinations.
See: Xenaderm.

tryptizol hydrochloride. Amitriptyline hydrochloride.

•**tryptophan.** (TRIP-toe-FAN) *USP.*
Use: Amino acid.

T/Scalp. (Neutrogena) Hydrocortisone 1%. Liq. Greaseless. Bot. 60 mL, 105 mL. *OTC.*
Use: Antipruritic; corticosteroid, topical.

TSPA.
Use: Antineoplastic.
See: Thiotepa.

TTC. Triphenyltetrazolium Chloride.

T-3 RIAbead. (Abbott Diagnostics) Test kit 50s, 100s.
Use: Diagnostic aid, thyroid.

tuaminoheptane sulfate.
Use: Adrenergic.

•**tuberculin.** (too-BURR-kyoo-lin) *USP.*
Use: Diagnostic aid (dermal reactivity indicator).
See: Aplisol.
Aplitest.
Tubersol.

Tuberculin, Mono-Vacc Test. (Lincoln Diagnostics) Mono-Vacc test is a sterile, disposable multiple puncture scarifier with liquid Old Tuberculin on the points. Box 25 tests. *Rx.*
Use: Diagnostic aid.

Tuberculin, Old Monovacc Test. (Wyeth) 5 TU activity test. Soln. of Old Tuberculin containing acacia 7%, lactose 8.5%. Test. Kits 25s, 100s, 250s. *Rx.*
Use: Diagnostic aid.

Tuberculin, Old, Tine Test. (Wyeth) 5 TY activity per test. Soln. of Old Tuberculin, containing acacia 7%, lactose 8.5%. Test. Kits 25s, 100s, 250s.
Use: Diagnostic aid.

tuberculin purified protein derivative.
Use: Diagnostic aid.
See: Aplisol.
Tubersol.

tuberculin tests.
Use: Diagnostic aid.
See: Aplisol.
Aplitest.
Tine Test PPD.
Tuberculin, Old MonoVacc Test.
Tuberculin, Old, Tine Test.
Tubersol.

tuberculin tine test. (Wyeth) **Old Tuberculin (OT):** Each disposable test unit consists of a stainless steel disc, with 4 tines (or prongs) 2 mm long, attached to a plastic handle. The tines have been dip-dried with antigenic material. The entire unit is sterilized by ethylene oxide gas. The test has been standardized by comparative studies, utilizing 0.05 mg US Standard Old Tuberculin 5 units or 0.0001 mg US Standard 5 units by the Mantoux technique. Reliability appears to be comparable to the standard Mantoux. Tests in a jar 25s. Package 100s. Bin Package 250s. **Purified Protein Derivative (PPD):** Equivalent to or more potent than 5 TU PPD Mantoux test. Tests in a jar 25s. Package 100s.
Use: Diagnostic aid.

tuberculosis vaccine.
Use: Immunization.
See: Tice BCG.

Tubersol. (Aventis Pasteur) Tuberculin purified protein derivative (Mantoux) 5 TU/0.1 mL, potassium and sodium phosphates, phenol 0.35%, polysorbate 80. Vial 1 mL (10 tests), 5 mL (50 tests). *Rx.*
Use: Diagnostic aid, tuberculosis.

•**tubocurarine chloride.** (too-boe-cure-AHR-een) *USP.*
Use: Neuromuscular blocker.

tubocurarine chloride, dimethyl. Dimethylether of d-tubocurarine chloride.

tubocurarine chloride hydrochloride pentahydrate. Tubocurarine Chloride.

tubocurarine iodide, dimethyl. Dimethyl ether of d-tubocurarine iodide.
Use: Muscle relaxant.

•**tubulozole hydrochloride.** (too-BYOO-lah-ZAHL) USAN.
Use: Antineoplastic (microtubule inhibitor).

Tucks. (Pfizer Consumer Health) Pramoxine hydrochloride 1%. Zinc oxide 12.5%, mineral oil 46.6%, cocoa butter. Oint. 30 g with applicator. *OTC.*
Use: Anorectal preparation.

Tucks Ointment. (Pfizer Consumer Health) Hydrocortisone 1%, diazolidinyl urea, parabens, mineral oil, sorbitan sesquioleate, white petrolatum. Oint. Tube 21 g. *OTC.*
Use: Corticosteroid, topical.

Tucks Suppositories. (Pfizer Consumer Health) Topical starch 51%, benzyl alcohol, soybean oil, tocopheryl acetate. Supp. Pkg. 12s. *OTC.*
Use: Anorectal preparation.

Tucks Take-Alongs. (Parke-Davis) Non-woven wipes saturated with solution of witch hazel 50%, glycerine 10%, benzalkonium chloride 0.003%. Box 12s. *OTC.*
Use: Anorectal preparation.

•**tucotuzumab celmoleukin.** (TOO-koe-TOOZ-oo-mab SEL-moe-LOO-kin) USAN.
Use: Immune globulin.

Tudorza Pressair. (Forest Pharmaceuticals) Aclidinium bromide 400 mcg/actuation. Lactose. Pow.; Inhal. Inhalation device w/60 metered doses. *Rx.*
Use: Bronchodilator, anticholinergic.

tumor necrosis factor-binding protein I. Serono *Rx.*
Use: Treatment of AIDS. [Orphan Drug]

tumor necrosis factor-binding protein II. Serono *Rx.*
Use: Treatment of AIDS. [Orphan Drug]

Tums Calcium for Life Bone Health. (GlaxoSmithKline Consumer) Calcium carbonate 1250 mg (elemental calcium 500 mg). Chew. Tab. Bot. 90s. *OTC.*
Use: Mineral supplement; antacid.

Tums Calcium for Life PMS. (GlaxoSmithKline Consumer) Calcium carbonate 750 mg (elemental calcium 300 mg). Sucrose. Strawberry flavor. Chew. Tab. Bot. 120s. *OTC.*
Use: Mineral supplement; antacid.

Tums Dual Action. (GlaxoSmithKline Consumer) Famotidine 10 mg, calcium carbonate 800 mg, magnesium hydroxide 165 mg. Aspartame, glyceryl, lactose, phenylalanine 2.2 mg, polysorbate 80. Berry flavor. Chew. Tab. 25s. *OTC.*
Use: Histamine H_2 antagonist combination.

Tums E-X. (GlaxoSmithKline Consumer) Calcium carbonate 750 mg (elemental calcium 300 mg). Sucrose, talc. Mixed berry, assorted fruit and sugar free orange (aspartame, phenylalanine < 1 mg, sorbitol) flavors. Chew. Tab. Bot. 96s. *OTC.*
Use: Mineral supplement; antacid.

Tums Freshers. (GlaxoSmithKline Consumer) Calcium carbonate 500 mg (200 mg of elemental calcium). Maltodextrin, mint flavoring, sorbitol, sucralose, sucrose. Chew. Tab. 50s. *OTC.*
Use: Mineral.

Tums Kids. (GlaxoSmithKline Consumer) Calcium carbonate 750 mg (elemental calcium 300 mg). Dextrose, gluten, maltodextrin, sorbitol, sucrose. Cherry flavor. Chew. Tab. 36s. *OTC.*
Use: Mineral supplement; antacid.

Tums Plus. (GlaxoSmithKline Consumer) Calcium carbonate 500 mg, (elemental

calcium 200 mg), simethicone 20 mg. Sucrose, sodium. Assorted fruit and mint flavors. Chew. Tab. Bot. 48s. *OTC.*
Use: Mineral supplement; antacid.

Tums Quik Pak. (GlaxoSmithKline Consumer) Calcium carbonate 1,000 mg. Dextrose, maltodextrin, sorbitol, sucrose. Berry flavor. Pow. 24s. *OTC.*
Use: Mineral supplement; antacid.

Tums Smooth Dissolve. (GlaxoSmithKline Consumer) Calcium carbonate 750 mg (elemental calcium 300 mg). Sorbitol, dextrose, sucrose (2 g sugar). Peppermint and assorted fruit flavors. Chew. Tab. 45s. *OTC.*
Use: Mineral supplement; antacid.

Tums Smoothies. (GlaxoSmithKline Consumer) Calcium carbonate 750 mg (elemental calcium 300 mg). Dextrose, maltodextrin, sorbitol, sucrose. Peppermint flavor. Chew. Tab. 60s. *OTC.*
Use: Mineral.

Tums Ultra. (GlaxoSmithKline Consumer) Calcium carbonate 1000 mg (elemental calcium 400 mg). Sucrose, talc. Mint flavor. Chew. Tab. Bot. 86s. *OTC.*
Use: Mineral supplement; antacid.

Tur-Bi-Kal Nasal Drops. (Emerson) Phenylephrine hydrochloride in a saline solution. Drops. Bot. oz., 12s. *OTC.*
Use: Decongestant.

Turbinaire.
See: Decadron Phosphate.

Turbinaire Decadron Phosphate. (Merck & Co.) Each metered spray delivers dexamethasone sodium phosphate equivalent to dexamethasone ≈ 84 mcg (170 sprays per cartridge), alcohol 2%. Aerosol. 12.6 g w/adapter or 12.6 g refill. *Rx.*
Use: Corticosteroid, topical.

•**turofexorate isopropyl.** (TUR-oh-FEX-or-ate) USAN.
Use: Treatment of lipid disorders.

Tusibron. (Kenwood) Guaifenesin 100 mg/5 mL, alcohol 3.5%. Liq. Bot. 118 mL. *OTC.*
Use: Expectorant.

Tusnel. (Llorens) Dextromethorphan HBr 15 mg, guaifenesin 200 mg, pseudoephedrine hydrochloride 30 mg per 5 mL. Alcohol, sugar, and dye free. Aspartame, parabens, phenylalanine 16.9 mg/5 mL. Liq. 178 mL. *OTC.*
Use: Upper respiratory combination, antitussive and expectorant combination.

Tusnel C. (Llorens) Codeine phosphate 10 mg, guaifenesin 100 mg, pseudoephedrine hydrochloride 30 mg per 5 mL. Propylene glycol, saccharin, sodium 2 mg per 5 mL, sodium benzoate, sorbitol. Alcohol free and sugar free. Syrup. 473 mL. *c-v.*
Use: Upper respiratory combination, antitussive and expectorant combination.

Tusnel-DM Pediatric. (Llorens) Dextromethorphan hydrobromide 2.5 mg, guaifenesin 25 mg, pseudoephedrine hydrochloride 7.5 mg. Glycerin, propylene glycol, saccharin, sodium benzoate. Drops. 60 mL. *OTC.*
Use: Upper respiratory combination, antitussive and expectorant combination.

Tusnel Pediatric. (Llorens) Dextromethorphan HBr 5 mg, guaifenesin 50 mg, pseudoephedrine hydrochloride 15 mg per 5 mL. Alcohol free. Aspartame, corn syrup, parabens, phenylalanine. Liq. 118 mL, 3,780 mL. *OTC.*
Use: Upper respiratory combination, antitussive and expectorant combination.

Tussabar. (Tennessee Pharmaceutic) Acetaminophen 400 mg, salicylamide 500 mg, potassium guaiacolsulfonate 120 mg, pyrilamine maleate 30 mg, ammonium chloride 500 mg, sodium citrate 500 mg, phenylephrine hydrochloride 30 mg/oz. Bot. Pt., gal. *Rx.*
Use: Analgesic; antihistamine; decongestant; expectorant.

Tussabid. (ION Laboratories, Inc.) Guaifenesin 200 mg, dextromethorphan HBr 30 mg. Cap. Bot. 24s, 100s. *OTC.*
Use: Antihistamine; expectorant.

Tussafed. (Everett) **Drops:** Carbinoxamine maleate 2 mg, pseudoephedrine hydrochloride 25 mg, dextromethorphan HBr 4 mg/mL. Bot. 30 mL with calibrated dropper. **Syrup:** Dextromethorphan HBr 15 mg, pseudoephedrine hydrochloride 60 mg, carbinoxamine maleate 4 mg per 5 mL. Menthol, grape flavor, alcohol free, sugar free. Bot. 120 mL, 480 mL. *Rx.*
Use: Upper respiratory combination, antihistamine, antitussive, decongestant.

Tussafed EX. (Everett Laboratories) Dextromethorphan HBr 30 mg, guaifenesin 200 mg, phenylephrine hydrochloride 10 mg per 5 mL. EDTA, saccharin, sorbitol, cherry-vanilla flavor, alcohol free. Syr. Bot. 473 mL. *Rx.*
Use: Upper respiratory combination, antitussive, expectorant, decongestant.

Tussafin Expectorant. (Rugby) Pseudoephedrine hydrochloride 60 mg, hydrocodone bitartrate 5 mg, guaifenesin 200 mg/5 mL, alcohol 2.5%. Liq. Bot.

480 mL. *c-III.*
Use: Antitussive; decongestant; expectorant.

Tussanil DH. (Edwards) Phenylephrine hydrochloride 10 mg, chlorpheniramine maleate 4 mg, hydrocodone bitartrate 2.5 mg/5 mL w/alcohol 5%. Syrup. Bot. Pt. *c-III.*
Use: Antihistamine; antitussive; decongestant.

Tussanil Expectorant. (Edwards) Hydrocodone bitartrate 2.5 mg, phenylephrine hydrochloride 10 mg, guaifenesin 100 mg/5 mL w/alcohol 5%. Syrup. Bot. Pt. *c-III.*
Use: Antitussive; decongestant; expectorant.

Tussanol. (Tyler) Pyrilamine maleate ¾ g, codeine phosphate 1 g, ammonium chloride 7.5 g, sodium citrate 5 g, menthol g/fl. oz. Bot. 4 fl. oz, pt, gal. *c-v.*
Use: Antihistamine; antitussive; expectorant.

Tussanol with Ephedrine. (Tyler) Ephedrine sulfate 2 g, pyrilamine maleate 0.75 g, codeine phosphate 1 g, ammonium chloride 7.5 g, sodium citrate 5 g, menthol g/30 mL. Bot. 16 fl. oz. *c-v.*
Use: Bronchodilator; antihistamine; antitussive; expectorant.

Tussar DM. (Aventis) Dextromethorphan HBr 15 mg, chlorpheniramine maleate 2 mg, phenylephrine hydrochloride 5 mg/5 mL w/methylparaben 0.1% Bot. 4 oz., pt. *Rx.*
Use: Antihistamine; antitussive; expectorant.

Tussar SF. (Aventis) Codeine phosphate 10 mg, guaifenesin 100 mg, pseudoephedrine hydrochloride 30 mg/5 mL, alcohol 2.5%. Bot. 120 mL, 473 mL. *c-v.*
Use: Antitussive; decongestant; expectorant.

Tussar-2. (Aventis) Codeine phosphate 10 mg, guaifenesin 100 mg, pseudoephedrine hydrochloride 30 mg/5 mL, alcohol 2.5%. Syrup. Bot. 473 mL. *c-v.*
Use: Antitussive; expectorant; decongestant.

Tussend. (Monarch) **Syr.:** Hydrocodone bitartrate 2.5 mg, pseudoephedrine hydrochloride 30 mg, chlorpheniramine maleate 2 mg per 5 mL. Alcohol 5%, corn syrup, parabens, saccharin, sucrose, banana flavor. Bot. 473 mL. **Tab.:** Hydrocodone bitartrate 5 mg, chlorpheniramine maleate 4 mg, pseudoephedrine hydrochloride 60 mg. Lactose. Bot. 100s. *c-III.*
Use: Upper respiratory combination, antitussive, antihistamine, decongestant.

Tussgen. (Ivax) Pseudoephedrine hydrochloride 60 mg, hydrocodone bitartrate 5 mg/5 mL. Liq. Bot. 100s, 1000s. *c-III.*
Use: Antitussive; decongestant.

TussiCaps Full Strength. (ECR Pharmaceuticals) Chlorpheniramine maleate 8 mg (as chlorpheniramine polistirex), hydrocodone bitartrate 10 mg (as hydrocodone polistirex). Butyl alcohol, dehydrated alcohol, isopropyl alcohol, SDA3A alcohol, SD-45 alcohol. ER Cap. 20s, 100s. *c-III.*
Use: Upper respiratory combination, antitussive combination.

TussiCaps Half Strength. (ECR Pharmaceuticals) Chlorpheniramine maleate 4 mg (as chlorpheniramine polistirex), hydrocodone bitartrate 5 mg (as hydrocodone polistirex). Butyl alcohol, dehydrated alcohol, isopropyl alcohol, SDA3A alcohol, SD-45 alcohol. ER Cap. 20s, 100s. *c-III.*
Use: Upper respiratory combination, antitussive combination.

Tussigon. (Monarch) Hydrocodone bitartrate 5 mg, homatropine methylbromide 1.5 mg. Tab. Bot. 100s, 500s. *c-III.*
Use: Upper respiratory combination, antitussive combination.

TussiNATE. (Pediamed) Hydrocodone bitartrate 3.5 mg, diphenhydramine hydrochloride 12.5 mg, phenylephrine hydrochloride 5 mg per 5 mL. Alcohol free. Saccharin, sucrose. Black raspberry flavor. Syrup. 473 mL. *c-III.*
Use: Antitussive combination.

Tussionex Pennkinetic. (CellTech) Hydrocodone polistirex 10 mg, chlorpheniramine polistirex 8 mg per 5 mL. Parabens, sucrose, corn syrup, PEG. ER Susp. Bot. 473 mL. *c-III.*
Use: Upper respiratory combination, antitussive combination.

Tussi-Organidin-S NR. (Victory Pharma) Codeine phosphate 10 mg, guaifenesin 300 mg per 5 mL. Alcohol and sugar free. PEG, saccharin, sorbitol. Liq. 118 mL with dosing syringe. *c-v.*
Use: Upper respiratory combination, antitussive with expectorant.

Tussi-Pres. (Kramer-Novis) Dextromethorphan hydrobromide 15 mg, guaifenesin 200 mg, phenylephrine hydrochloride 5 mg per 5 mL. Alcohol and sugar free. Phenylalanine 15 mg/5 mL, aspartame, parabens. Cherry flavor. Liq. 474 mL. *Rx.*
Use: Upper respiratory combination, antitussive and expectorant combination.

Tussi-Pres Pediatric. (Kramer-Novis) Phenylephrine hydrochloride 2.5 mg, dextromethorphan HBr 5 mg, guaifenesin 75 mg per 5 mL. Sugar, alcohol, and dye free. Parabens, aspartame, phenylalanine 14 mg per 5 mL. Orange flavor. Liq. 473 mL. *Rx.*
Use: Upper respiratory combination, antitussive and expectorant combination.

Tussi-12. (Meda Pharmaceuticals) Carbetapentane tannate 30 mg, chlorpheniramine tannate 4 mg, phenylephrine tannate 5 mg/mL, glycerin, methylparaben, saccharin, sucrose. Susp. Pt. *Rx.*
Use: Upper respiratory combination, antihistamine, antitussive, decongestant.

Tussi-12 DS. (Meda Pharmaceuticals) Carbetapentane tannate 60 mg, pyrilamine tannate 40 mg, phenylephrine tannate 10 mg. Tab. 100s. *Rx.*
Use: Upper respiratory combination, antitussive combination.

Tuss-LA. (Hyrex) Pseudoephedrine hydrochloride 120 mg, guaifenesin 500 mg. LA Tab. Bot. 100s. *Rx.*
Use: Decongestant; expectorant.

Tusso DM. (Everett) Dextromethorphan HBr 23 mg (8 mg immediate release/ 15 mg extended release), guaifenesin 600 mg (200 mg immediate release/ 400 mg extended release), phenylephrine hydrochloride 9 mg (extended release). Lactose. ER Tab. 100s. *Rx.*
Use: Upper respiratory combination, antitussive with expectorant.

Tusso DMR. (Everett Labs) Dextromethorphan hydrobromide 14 mg, guaifenesin 288 mg, phenylephrine hydrochloride 7 mg. Maltodextrin. Cap. 100s. *Rx.*
Use: Upper respiratory combination, antitussive and expectorant combination.

Tusso XR. (Everett) Dextromethorphan HBr 20 mg, guaifenesin 100 mg, phenylephrine hydrochloride 10 mg per 5 mL. Acesulfame K, aspartame, methylparaben, phenylalanine 25.26 mg/ 5 mL. Grape flavor. Susp. 473 mL. *Rx.*
Use: Upper respiratory combination, antitussive and expectorant combination.

Tussplex. (Breckenridge) Hydrocodone bitartrate 6 mg, pyrilamine maleate 12 mg, phenylephrine hydrochloride 5 mg per 5 mL. Alcohol and sugar free. Saccharin, sorbitol. Black cherry flavor. Syrup. 473 mL. *c-III.*
Use: Upper respiratory combination, antitussive combination.

Tusstat. (Century) Diphenhydramine hydrochloride 12.5 mg/5 mL, alcohol 5%. Syrup. Bot. 30 mL, 118 mL, 473 mL, 3.8 L. *Rx.*
Use: Antihistamine, nonselective ethanolamine; antitussive.

Tusstat Expectorant. (Century) Diphenhydramine hydrochloride 80 mg, ammonium chloride 12 g, sodium citrate 5 g, menthol 0.13 g, alcohol 5%/oz. Bot. 4 fl. oz, pt, gal. *Rx.*
Use: Antihistamine; expectorant.

•**tuvirumab.** (tuh-VIE-roo-mab) USAN.
Use: Monoclonal antibody (antiviral).

T-Vites. (Freeda) Vitamins B_1 25 mg, B_2 25 mg, B_3 150 mg, B_5 25 mg, B_6 25 mg, C 100 mg, biotin 30 mcg, PABA, K, Mg, Mn carbonate 2 mg, Zn gluconate 20 mg. Tab. Bot. 100s. *OTC.*
Use: Mineral, vitamin supplement.

Tween 20, 40, 60, 80. *NF.* (AstraZeneca) Polysorbates.
Use: Surface active agents.

12-Hour Antihistamine Nasal Decongestant. (United Research Laboratories) Pseudoephedrine sulfate 120 mg, dexbrompheniramine maleate 6 mg, sugar, sucrose. SR Tab. Bot. 10s. *OTC.*
Use: Decongestant.

12-Hour Cold. (Ivax) Dexbrompheniramine maleate 6 mg, pseudoephedrine sulfate 120 mg. SR Tab. Pkg. 10s, 20s. *OTC.*
Use: Antihistamine; decongestant.

12-Hour Nasal. (Various Mfr.) Oxymetazoline hydrochloride 0.05%. Soln. Spray Bot. 15 mL. *OTC.*
Use: Nasal decongestant, imidazoline.

Twelve Resin-K. (Key Company) Vitamin B_{12} 1,000 mcg on resin. Tab. 60s, 250s, 1000s. *OTC.*
Use: Water-soluble vitamin.

20% ProSol. (Baxter Healthcare) Amino acids 20 g, total nitrogen 3.21 g/ 100 mL, lysine acetate, glacial acetic acid. Sulfite free. Inj. *Vialflex* Cont. 500 mL, 1000 mL, 2000 mL. *Rx.*
Use: Nutritional therapy, intravenous.

20-20. (BDI) Caffeine 200 mg. Tab. Bot. 100s, 500s. *OTC.*
Use: CNS stimulant, analeptic.

20/20 Eye Drops. (S.S.S. Company) Naphazoline hydrochloride 0.012%. Benzalkonium chloride, EDTA, glycerin 0.2%. Ophth. Drops. 15 mL. *OTC.*
Use: Ophthalmic decongestant.

Twice-a-Day 12-Hour Nasal. (Major) Oxymetazoline 0.05%, EDTA, benzalkonium chloride, benzyl alcohol. Soln. Spray bot. 15 mL, 30 mL. *OTC.*
Use: Nasal decongestant, imidazoline.

Twinject. (Sciele) Epinephrine 1:1,000 (0.15 mg per 0.15 mL), 1:1,000 (0.3 mg per 0.3 mL). Chlorobutanol, sodium bisulfite. Latex free. Dual-dose autoinjector (contains a total of epinephrine 2 mL). *Rx.*
Use: Vasopressor used in shock.

Twinrix. (GlaxoSmithKline) Inactivated hepatitis A 720 ELU (ELISA [enzyme-linked immunosorbent assay] units), recombinant HBsAg (hepatitis B surface antigen) protein 20 mcg/mL. Preservative free. Inj. Single-dose vials. Single-dose prefilled, disposable *TIP-LOK* syringes. *Rx.*
Use: Active immunization, viral vaccine.

TwoCal HN High Nitrogen Liquid Nutrition. (Ross) High-nitrogen liquid nutrition (2 calories/mL). 1900 calories (1 quart), provides 100% US RDA for vitamins and minerals for adults and children over 4 yrs. Can 8 fl. oz. *OTC.*
Use: Nutritional supplement.

2-Tone Disclosing Solution. (Young Dental) Dropper Bot. 2 oz.
Use: Disclosing solution.

Twynsta. (Boehringer Ingelheim) Amlodipine besylate/telmisartan. 5 mg/40 mg, 10 mg/40 mg, 5 mg/80 mg, 10 mg/80 mg. Sorbitol. Tab. Blisters. 30s, 90s. *Rx.*
Use: Antihypertensive.

•**tybamate.** (TIE-bam-ate) USAN.
Use: Anxiolytic.

Ty-Cold. (Major) 30 mg pseudoephedrine, 2 mg chlorpheniramine maleate, 15 mg dextromethorphan HBr, 325 mg acetaminophen. Tab. Pkg. 24s. *OTC.*
Use: Analgesic; antihistamine; antitussive; decongestant.

Tygacil. (Wyeth) Tigecycline 50 mg. Lactose. Preservative free. Pow. for Inj., lyophilized. Single-dose vial. 10 mL. *Rx.*
Use: Anti-infective, glycylcycline.

Tykerb. (GlaxoSmithKline) Lapatinib 250 mg (equiv. to lapatinib ditosylate 398 mg). Film coated. Tab. 150s. *Rx.*
Use: Tyrosine kinase inhibitor, antineoplastic.

Tylenol Allergy Multi-Symptom. (McNeil Consumer) Phenylephrine hydrochloride 5 mg, chlorpheniramine maleate 2 mg, acetaminophen 325 mg. 24s. **Capl.:** PEG, sucralose. **Gelcaps:** Benzyl alcohol, parabens. *OTC.*
Use: Upper respiratory combination, decongestant, antihistamine, analgesic.

Tylenol Allergy Multi-Symptom Convenience Pack. (McNeil Consumer) **Day:** Phenylephrine hydrochloride 5 mg, chlorpheniramine maleate 2 mg, acetaminophen 325 mg. Sucralose. Capl. 24s. **Night:** Phenylephrine hydrochloride 5 mg, diphenhydramine hydrochloride 25 mg, acetaminophen 325 mg. Sucralose. Capl. 24s. *OTC.*
Use: Upper respiratory combination, decongestant, antihistamine, analgesic.

Tylenol Allergy Multi-Symptom Nighttime. (McNeil Consumer) Phenylephrine hydrochloride 5 mg, diphenhydramine hydrochloride 25 mg, acetaminophen 325 mg. Sucralose. Capl. 24s. *OTC.*
Use: Upper respiratory combination, decongestant, antihistamine, analgesic.

Tylenol Arthritis Pain. (McNeil Consumer) Acetaminophen 650 mg. **ER Capl.:** 24s, 50s, 100s, 150s, 225s. **ER Gelltabs:** Parabens. 20s, 40s, 80s. *OTC.*
Use: Analgesic.

Tylenol Chest Congestion. (McNeil Consumer) **Capl.:** Acetaminophen 325 mg, guaifenesin 200 mg. Mannitol, PEG, polyvinyl alcohol, sucralose. Cool burst flavor. 24s. **Liq.:** Acetaminophen 166.67 mg, guaifenesin 66.67 mg per 5 mL. PEG, sorbitol, sucralose, sucrose. Cool burst flavor. Bot. 240 mL. *OTC.*
Use: Upper respiratory combination, analgesic, expectorant.

Tylenol Children's. (McNeil Consumer) Acetaminophen. **Meltaways (Chew. Tab./Dispersible):** 80 mg. Dextrose, sucralose. Bubble gum, grape, and watermelon flavors. 30s. **Susp.:** 160 mg/5 mL. Sodium 2 mg/5 mL. Cherry, grape, bubblegum flavors (alcohol free, dye free, butylparaben, corn syrup, sorbitol); strawberry flavor (butylparaben, corn syrup, sorbitol, sucralose); cherry flavor (dye free, parabens, sorbitol, sucralose, sucrose). Bot. 60 mL, 120 mL. *OTC.*
Use: Analgesic.

Tylenol Cold Head Congestion Daytime. (McNeil Consumer) Dextromethorphan 10 mg, phenylephrine hydrochloride 5 mg, acetaminophen 325 mg. Sucralose. Cool burst flavor. Capl. 24s. *OTC.*
Use: Upper respiratory combination, antitussive combination.

Tylenol Cold Head Congestion Nighttime. (McNeil Consumer) Dextromethorphan 10 mg, chlorpheniramine 2 mg, phenylephrine hydrochloride 5 mg, acetaminophen 325 mg. Sucralose. Cool burst flavor. Capl. 24s. *OTC.*
Use: Upper respiratory combination, antitussive combination.

Tylenol Cold Multi-Symptom Daytime. (McNeil Consumer) **Capl.:** Dextromethorphan 10 mg, phenylephrine hydrochloride 5 mg, acetaminophen 325 mg. Sucralose. Cool burst flavor. 24s. **Gel cap:** Dextromethorphan 10 mg, phenylephrine hydrochloride 5 mg, acetaminophen 325 mg. Benzyl alcohol, EDTA, parabens. 24s. **Liq.:** Dextromethorphan 3.33 mg, phenylephrine hydrochloride 1.67 mg, acetaminophen 108.33 mg per 5 mL. Ethanol, sodium 1.67 mg per 5 mL, sorbitol, sucralose. Citrus burst flavor. Bot. 240 mL. *OTC.*
Use: Upper respiratory combination, antitussive combination.

Tylenol Cold Multi-Symptom Nighttime. (McNeil Consumer) **Capl.:** Dextromethorphan 10 mg, chlorpheniramine maleate 2 mg, phenylephrine hydrochloride 5 mg, acetaminophen 325 mg. Sucralose. Cool burst flavor. 24s. **Liq.:** Dextromethorphan 3.33 mg, doxylamine succinate 2.08 mg, phenylephrine hydrochloride 1.67 mg, acetaminophen 108.33 mg per 5 mL. Sodium, sorbitol, sucralose. Cool burst flavor. Bot. 240 mL. *OTC.*
Use: Upper respiratory combination, antitussive combination.

Tylenol Cold Severe Congestion Daytime. (McNeil Consumer) Dextromethorphan HBr 15 mg, guaifenesin 200 mg, pseudoephedrine hydrochloride 30 mg, acetaminophen 325 mg. Mannitol, sodium 3 mg, sucralose. Cool burst flavor. Capl. 100s. *OTC.*
Use: Upper respiratory combination, antitussive and expectorant combination.

Tylenol Cough & Sore Throat Nighttime. (McNeil Consumer) Dextromethorphan HBr 5 mg, doxylamine succinate 2.08 mg, acetaminophen 166.7 mg per 5 mL. Sodium 3.67 mg per 5 mL, sorbitol, sucralose. Cool burst flavor. Liq. Bot. 240 mL. *OTC.*
Use: Upper respiratory combination, antitussive combination.

Tylenol 8 Hour. (McNeil Consumer) Acetaminophen 650 mg. Polyvinyl alcohol, sucralose. ER Capl. 24s, 50s, 100s, 150s. *OTC.*
Use: Analgesic.

Tylenol Extra Strength. (McNeil Consumer) Acetaminophen. **Capl.:** 500 mg. Castor oil, sucralose. Regular and cool flavors. Bot. 50s, 100s. **Chew Tab. (GoTabs):** 500 mg. Acesulfame K, dextrose, sucralose. Spearmint ice flavors. 6s. **Liq.:** 166.6 mg/5 mL. Corn syrup, saccharin, sorbitol. 240 mL with dosage cup. **Rapid Release Tab.:** 500 mg. Benzyl alcohol, parabens. 24s, 50s, 100s, 225s. **Tab. (EZ Tab):** 500 mg. Sucralose. 50s, 100s, 225. *OTC.*
Use: Analgesic.

Tylenol Extra Strength GoTabs. (McNeil Consumer) Acetaminophen 500 mg. Acesulfame, potassium, sucralose. Spearmint ice flavor. Chew. Tab. 6s. *OTC.*
Use: Analgesic.

Tylenol, Infants'. (McNeil Consumer) Acetaminophen 100 mg/mL. Cherry and grape flavors (corn syrup, sorbitol), cherry flavor (dye free, parabens, sorbitol, sucralose). Soln. Conc. Oral. 15 mL, 30 mL with 0.8 mL dropper. *OTC.*
Use: Analgesic.

Tylenol Meltaways, Jr. (McNeil Consumer) Acetaminophen 160 mg. Dextrose, sucralose. Bubble gum and grape punch flavors. Chew. Tab./Dispersible. 24s. *OTC.*
Use: Analgesic.

Tylenol Plus Children's Cold & Allergy. (McNeil Consumer) Acetaminophen 160 mg, diphenhydramine hydrochloride 12.5 mg, phenylephrine hydrochloride 2.5 mg. Sorbitol, sucralose, sucrose. Bubble gum flavor. Susp. 118.3 mL. *OTC.*
Use: Upper respiratory combination; decongestant, antihistamine, and analgesic combination.

Tylenol Plus Cold, Children's. (McNeil Consumer) Phenylephrine hydrochloride 2.5 mg, chlorpheniramine maleate 1 mg, acetaminophen 160 mg per 5 mL. Sorbitol, sucrose. Grape flavor. Susp. Bot. 118 mL. *OTC.*
Use: Upper respiratory combination, decongestant, antihistamine, analgesic.

Tylenol Plus Cough & Runny Nose, Children's. (McNeil Consumer) Dextromethorphan HBr 5 mg, chlorpheniramine maleate 1 mg, acetaminophen 160 mg per 5 mL. Acesulfame K, corn syrup, sorbitol. Cherry flavor. Susp. Bot. 120 mL. *OTC.*
Use: Upper respiratory combination, antitussive combination.

Tylenol Plus Cough & Sore Throat, Children's. (McNeil Consumer) Dextromethorphan HBr 5 mg, acetaminophen 160 mg per 5 mL. Acesulfame K, corn syrup, sorbitol. Cherry flavor. Susp. Bot. 120 mL. *OTC.*
Use: Upper respiratory combination, antitussive combination.

Tylenol Plus Flu, Children's. (McNeil Consumer) Dextromethorphan HBr 5 mg, chlorpheniramine maleate 1 mg, phenylephrine hydrochloride 2.5 mg, acetaminophen 160 mg per 5 mL. Sorbitol, sucrose. Bubble gum flavor. Susp. Bot. 120 mL. *OTC.*
Use: Upper respiratory combination, antitussive combination.

Tylenol Plus Multi-Symptom Cold, Children's. (McNeil Consumer) Dextromethorphan HBr 5 mg, chlorpheniramine maleate 1 mg, phenylephrine hydrochloride 2.5 mg, acetaminophen 160 mg per 5 mL. Sorbitol, sucrose. Grape flavor. Susp. Bot. 120 mL. *OTC.*
Use: Upper respiratory combination, antitussive combination.

Tylenol PM. (McNeil Consumer) Acetaminophen 500 mg, diphenhydramine 25 mg. Tab. Bot. 24s, 50s, 100s, 150s. Gelcap. Parabens. Bot. 50s. Geltab. Parabens. Bot. 50s, 100s. *OTC.*
Use: Upper respiratory combination, analgesic, antihistamine.

Tylenol PM Extra Strength. (McNeil Consumer) Acetaminophen 500 mg, diphenhydramine hydrochloride 25 mg. Tab. 24s, 50s. *OTC.*
Use: Nonprescription sleep aid.

Tylenol Regular Strength. (McNeil Consumer) Acetaminophen 325 mg. Tab. 100s. *OTC.*
Use: Analgesic.

Tylenol Severe Allergy. (McNeil Consumer) Diphenhydramine hydrochloride 12.5 mg, acetaminophen 500 mg. Tab. 24s. *OTC.*
Use: Upper respiratory combination, analgesic, antihistamine.

Tylenol Sinus Congestion & Pain Daytime. (McNeil Consumer) Acetaminophen 325 mg, phenylephrine hydrochloride 5 mg. **Caplets:** PEG, sucralose. Cool burst flavor. 24s, 48s. **Gelcaps:** EDTA, parabens. 24s, 48s. *OTC.*
Use: Upper respiratory combination, decongestant and analgesic combination.

Tylenol Sinus Congestion & Pain Nighttime. (McNeil Consumer) Phenylephrine 5 mg, chlorpheniramine maleate 2 mg, acetaminophen 325 mg. Sucralose. Cool burst flavor. Tab. 24s. *OTC.*
Use: Upper respiratory combination, decongestant, antihistamine, and analgesic combination.

Tylenol Sinus Congestion & Pain Severe Daytime. (McNeil Consumer) Phenylephrine hydrochloride 5 mg, guaifenesin 200 mg, acetaminophen 325 mg. Sucralose. Cool burst flavor. Tab. 24s. *OTC.*
Use: Upper respiratory combination, decongestant and expectorant combination.

Tylenol Sinus Severe Congestion. (McNeil Consumer) Pseudoephedrine hydrochloride 30 mg, guaifenesin 200 mg, acetaminophen 325 mg. Mannitol, sucralose. Cool burst flavor. Tab. 24s. *OTC.*
Use: Upper respiratory combination, decongestant, expectorant, analgesic.

Tylenol Sore Throat Daytime. (McNeil Consumer) Acetaminophen 166.6 mg/5 mL. Sucralose, sucrose, sorbitol. Cool burst flavor. Liq. Bot. 240 mL. *OTC.*
Use: Analgesic.

Tylenol Sore Throat Nighttime. (McNeil Consumer) Diphenhydramine hydrochloride 8.3 mg, acetaminophen 166.6 mg per 5 mL. Sodium 3.6 mg per 5 mL, sorbitol, sucralose, sucrose. Cool burst flavor. Liq. 240 mL. *OTC.*
Use: Upper respiratory combination, antihistamine, analgesic.

Tylenol with Codeine. (Janssen) **Tab.:** Acetaminophen 300 mg with codeine phosphate. Tab. **No. 3:** Codeine phosphate 30 mg. 100s, 500s, 1000s, UD 100s. **No. 4:** Codeine phosphate 60 mg. 100s, 500s, UD 500s. *c-III.*
Use: Analgesic combination; narcotic.

Tylenol with Flavor Creator Children's. (McNeil Consumer Health) Acetaminophen 160 mg/5 mL. Sugar free. Butylparaben, corn syrup, sorbitol, sucralose. Apple, bubble gum, chocolate, and strawberry flavors. Oral Susp. 120 mL. *OTC.*
Use: Analgesic.

Tyler Panplex 2-Phase. (Integrative Therapeutics) Amylase 12,600 units, lipase 1,008 units, protease 12,600 units. Cottonseed oil. Gluten free and preservative free. Tab. 60s, 180s. *OTC.*
Use: Digestive enzyme.

Tyler Prenatal. (Integrative Therapeutics) Folic acid 0.1 mg, Ca 125 mg, Fe 5 mg, vitamins A 1,250 units, D 25 units, E 25 units, B_1 6.25 mg, B_2 6.25 mg, B_3 7.5 mg, B_5 6.25 mg, B_6 10.5 mg, B_{12} 25 mcg, C 62.5 mg, potassium 12.5 mg, Mg, Zn, Se, Cu, Mn, Cr, Mo, K, V, biotin 37.5 mg, citrus bioflavonoids complex 9.25 mg, choline 6.25 mg, betaine hydrochloride 6.25 mg, inositol 6.25 mg, L-glutamic acid hydrochloride 6.25 mg, PABA 3 mg, hesperidin complex 2.5 mg, rutin 2.5 mg. Gluten free, preservative

free. Soybean oil. Cap. 240s. *OTC.*
Use: Prenatal vitamin with minerals.

Tyler Similase Jr. (Integrative Therapeutics) Amylase 3,350 units, lipase 465 units, protease 7,250 units. Preservative free. Cap. 90s. *OTC.*
Use: Digestive enzyme.

Tylosterone. (Eli Lilly) Diethylstilbestrol 0.25 mg, methyltestosterone 5 mg. Tab. Bot. 100s. *Rx.*
Use: Androgen, estrogen combination.

•**tyloxapol.** (till-OX-ah-pahl) *USP.*
Use: Detergent, ophthalmic; cystic fibrosis. [Orphan Drug]
See: Enuclene.

Typhim Vi. (Aventis Pasteur) Typhoid purified Vi polysaccharide vaccine 25 mcg/0.5 mL, sodium chloride 4.15 mg, disodium phosphate 0.065 mg, monosodium phosphate 0.023 mg, Sterile Water for Injection 0.5 mL. Inj. Syringes 0.5 mL, vial 20 dose, 50 dose. *Rx.*
Use: Immunization, typhoid.

typhoid vaccine.
Use: Immunization.
See: Vivotif Berna.

typhoid Vi polysaccharide vaccine.
Use: Immunization.
See: Typhim Vi.

Tyrex-2. (Ross) Protein 30 g, fat 15.5 g, carbohydrates 30 g, Na 880 mg, K 1370 mg, Cal 410/100 g. With appropriate vitamins and minerals. Phenylalanine and tyrosine free. Pow. Can 325 g. *OTC.*
Use: Nutritional supplement.

Tyrodone. (Major) Hydrocodone bitartrate 5 mg, pseudoephedrine hydrochloride 60 mg/5 mL, alcohol 5%. Liq. Bot. 473 mL. *c-III.*
Use: Antitussive; decongestant.

Tyromex-1. (Ross) Protein 15 g, fat 23.9 g, carbohydrates 46.3 g, linoleic acid 1800 mg, Fe 9 mg, Na 190 mg, K 675 mg, Cal 480/100 g. With appropriate vitamins and minerals. Phenylalanine, tyrosine, and methionine free. Pow. Can 350 g. *OTC.*
Use: Nutritional supplement.

•**tyropanoate sodium.** (TIE-row-PAN-oh-ate) *USP.*
Use: Diagnostic aid (radiopaque medium, cholecystographic).

tyropaque caps. (Sanofi-Synthelabo) Tyropanoate sodium. *Rx.*
Use: Oral cholecystographic medium.

•**tyrosine.** (TIE-row-SEEN) *USP.* L-Tyrosine.
Use: Amino acid.

tyrosine hydroxylase inhibitor.
Use: Antihypertensive.
See: Demser.

tyrosine kinase inhibitors.
Use: Antineoplastic.
See: Axitinib.
Bosutinib.
Cabozantinib.
Ceritinib.
Crizotinib.
Ibrutinib.
Lapatinib.
Pazopanib.
Ponatinib.
Vandetanib.
Ziv-Aflibercept.

Tyrosum Skin Cleanser. (Summers) Isopropanol 50%, polysorbate 80 2%, and acetone 10%. Bot. 120 mL, pt. Towelettes 24s, 50s. *OTC.*
Use: Dermatologic, cleanser.

Tysabri. (Biogen Idec) Natalizumab 300 mg per 15 mL. Polysorbate 80. Preservative free. Inj., Soln., Conc. Single-use vial. 15 mL. *Rx.*
Note: Only available through a special restricted distribution program (the TOUCH prescribing program).
Use: Immunologic agent, immunomodulator.

Tyvaso. (United Therapeutics) Treprostinil 0.6 mg/mL. Soln.; Inhal. Ampule. 2.9 mL. *Rx.*
Use: Vasodilator, peripheral vasodilator.

Tyzeka. (Novartis) Telbivudine. **Tab.:** 600 mg. Film-coated. 30s. **Soln.:** 100 mg per 5 mL. Saccharin, sodium 47 mg per 30 mL. Passion fruit flavor. Bot. 300 mL. *Rx.*
Use: Antiretroviral, nucleoside reverse transcriptase inhibitor.

Tyzine. (Kenwood) Tetrahydrozoline hydrochloride 0.1%, benzalkonium chloride, EDTA. Soln. Bot. 30 mL with dropper. Spray bot. 15 mL. *Rx.*
Use: Nasal decongestant, imidazoline.

Tyzine Pediatric. (Kenwood) Tetrahydrozoline hydrochloride 0.05%, benzalkonium chloride, EDTA. Soln. Dropper bot. 15 mL. *Rx.*
Use: Nasal decongestant, imidazoline.

U

UAA. (Econo Med Pharmaceuticals) Methenamine 40.8 mg, phenyl salicylate 18.1 mg, methylene blue 5.4 mg, benzoic acid 4.5 mg, atropine sulfate 0.03 mg, hyoscyamine 0.03 mg. Tab. Bot. 100s, 1000s. *Rx.*
Use: Anti-infective, urinary.

UAD Cream. (Forest) Clioquinol 3%, hydrocortisone 1%, ceresin, glyceryl oleate, propylene glycol, parabens, mineral oil, pramoxine hydrochloride. Cream. Tube. 15 g. *Rx.*
Use: Corticosteroid; anesthetic, local.

UAD Lotion. (Forest) Clioquinol 0.75%, hydrocortisone 0.25%, cetyl alcohol, glyceryl stearate, lanolin, parabens, mineral oil, pramoxine hydrochloride, propylene glycol. Lot. Bot. 20 mL. *Rx.*
Use: Corticosteroid; anesthetic, local.

•**ubidecarenone.** *NF.*
Use: Dietary supplement.

•**ubrogepant.** (ue-BROE-je-pant) USAN.
Use: Agent for migraine.

UBT. (Biomerica) For detection of blood in the urine.
Use: Diagnostic aid.

Uceris. (Santarus) Budesonide 9 mg. Lactose. ER Tab. 30s. *Rx.*
Use: Adrenocortical steroid, glucocorticoid.

UCG-Beta Slide Monoclonal II. (Wampole) Two-minute latex agglutination inhibition slide test for the qualitative detection of B-hCG/hCG (sensitivity 0.5 units hCG/mL) in urine. Kit 50s, 100s, 300s.
Use: Diagnostic aid.

UCG-Beta Stat. (Wampole) One-hour passive hemagglutination inhibition tube test for the qualitative detection and quantitative determination of B-hCG/hCG (sensitivity 0.2 units hCG/mL) in urine. Kit 50s, 300s.
Use: Diagnostic aid.

UCG-Lyphotest. (Wampole) One-hour passive hemagglutination inhibition tube test for the qualitative or quantitative determination of human chorionic gonadotropin (sensitivity 0.5-1 units hCG/mL) in urine. Kit 10s, 50s, 300s.
Use: Diagnostic aid.

UCG-Slide Test. (Wampole) Rapid latex agglutination inhibition slide test for the qualitative detection of human chorionic gonadotropin (Sensitivity: 2 units hCG/mL) in urine. Kit 30s, 100s, 300s, 1000s.
Use: Diagnostic aid.

UCG-Test. (Wampole) Two-hour hemagglutination inhibition tube test for the determination of human chorionic gonadotropin (sensitivity 0.5 units hCG/mL undiluted specimen; 1.5 units hCG/mL 1:3 diluted specimen) in urine and serum. Kit 10s, 25s, 100s, 300s.
Use: Diagnostic aid.

UCG-Titration Set. (Wampole) Two-hour hemagglutination inhibition tube test for the determination of human chorionic gonadotropin (sensitivity 1 units hCG/mL) in urine or serum. Kit 45s.
Use: Diagnostic aid.

U-cort. (Taro) Hydrocortisone acetate 1%. Urea 10%, alcohol, EDTA. Cream. 28.35 g, 7 g. *Rx.*
Use: Anti-inflammatory.

Udamin. (Poly Pharmaceuticals) Vitamins B_{12} 500 mcg, B_6 25 mg, E 150 units (as d-alpha tocopheryl acid succinate) and 34 mg (as d-gamma, d-delta, d-beta tocopheryls), Se, Zn, folic acid 2,000 mcg. Lycopene complex 5 mg. Coconut oil, maltodextrin, polydextrose, PEG, soy protein. Film coated. Tab. 100s. *Rx.*
Use: Multivitamin with minerals (except iron).

Udamin SP. (Poly Pharmaceuticals) Vitamins B_{12} 250 mcg, B_6 12.5 mg, E 75 units (as d-alpha tocopheryl acid succinate) and 17 mg (as d-gamma, d-delta, d-beta tocopheryls), Se, Zn, folic acid 1,000 mcg. Lycopene complex 2.5 mcg, saw palmetto extract 320 mg. Maltodextrin, polydextrose, PEG, soy protein. Film coated. Tab. 100s. *Rx.*
Use: Multivitamin with minerals (except iron).

Udderly Smooth. (Redex) Dimethicone, isopropyl myristate, lanolin oil, mineral oil, parabens, PEG-2, urea. Cream 227 g. *OTC.*
Use: Emollient.

•**udenafil.** (ue-DEN-a-fil) USAN.
Use: Erectile dysfunction.

Uendex. Dextran sulfate, inhaled, aerosolized.
Use: Cystic fibrosis treatment. [Orphan Drug]

Ulcerease. (Med-Derm) Liquified phenol 0.6%, glycerin, sugar free. Liq. Bot. 180 mL. *OTC.*
Use: Anesthetic, local.

Ulcerin. (Sanofi-Synthelabo) Aluminum hydroxide. Tab. *OTC.*
Use: Antacid.

Ulcerin P. (Sanofi-Synthelabo) Aluminum hydroxide. Tab. *OTC.*
Use: Antacid.

•**uldazepam.** (ul-DAZ-e-pam) USAN.
Use: Hypnotic; sedative.

Ulesfia. (Shionogi Inc) Benzyl alcohol 5%. Mineral oil, polysorbate 80, trolamine. Lot. 240 mL and in kits (two 240 mL bottles w/nit comb). *Rx.*
Use: Scabicide/pediculicide.

•**ulimorelin.** (UE-li-moe-REL-in) USAN.
Use: Gastrointestinal agent.

•**ulimorelin hydrochloride.** (UE-li-moe-REL-in) USAN.
Use: Gastrointestinal agent.

•**ulipristal.** (UE-li-PRIS-tal) USAN.
Use: Contraceptive agent.

•**ulipristal acetate.** (UE-li-PRIS-tal) USAN.
Use: Contraceptive agent.

•**ulocuplumab.** (UE-loe-KUP-lue-mab) USAN.
Use: Antineoplastic.

•**ulodesine.** (ue-LOE-de-seen) USAN.
Use: Agent for gout.

•**ulodesine succinate.** (ue-LOE-de-seen) USAN.
Use: Agent for gout.

Uloric. (Takeda Pharmaceuticals America) Febuxostat 40 mg, 80 mg. Lactose. Tab. 30s, 90s (40 mg), 100s (80 mg), 500s (40 mg), 1000s (80 mg), UD 100s. *Rx.*
Use: Agent for gout, xanthine oxidase inhibitor.

Ulpax. (Roche) Ablukast sodium.
Use: Antiasthmatic (leukotriene antagonist).

Ultane. (Abbott) Sevoflurane. Bot. 250 mL. *Rx.*
Use: Anesthetic, general, volatile liquid.

Ultimate OB DHA. (Trigen Labs) Vitamin D_3 400 units, E 10 mg, B_1 1.5 mg, B_2 1.6 mg, B_3 17 mg, B_5 10 mg, B_6 50 mg, B_{12} 12 mcg, folic acid 1 mg, Fe 28 mg, I, Zn, Se, Cu. **Tab.:** Biotin 30 mcg. PEG. UD 30s. **Softgel Cap.:** DHA 200 mg. Glycerin, vitamin E oil. UD 30s. *Rx.*
Use: Prenatal vitamin with minerals.

Ultimate Probiotic Formula Acidophilus. (Rexall Sundown) *L. acidophilus* 2 billion CFU. Gluten free, lactose free, preservative free, and sugar free. Tab. 60. *OTC.*
Use: Probiotic.

Ultiva. (Bionich Pharma Group) Remifentanil hydrochloride (as base) 1 mg (3 mL vials), 2 mg (5 mL vials), 5 mg (10 mL vials), preservative free. Glycine 15 mg. Pow. for Inj. *c-II.*
Use: Opioid analgesic.

UltraBag Dianeal PD-2 w/4.25% Dextrose. (Baxter) Dextrose 4.25 g/L, Na^+ 132 mEq/L, Ca^{++} 3.5 mEq/L, Mg^{++} 0.5 mEq/L, Cl^- 96 mEq/L, lactate 40 mEq/L, osmolarity 485 mOsm/L. Preservative free. Inj., Soln. *UltraBag* container. 1,500 mL, 2,000 mL, 2,500 mL, 3,000 mL. *Rx.*
Use: Electrolyte, peritoneal dialysis solution.

UltraBag Dianeal PD-2 w/1.5% Dextrose. (Baxter) Dextrose 1.5 g/L, Na^+ 132 mEq/L, Ca^{++} 3.5 mEq/L, Mg^{++} 0.5 mEq/L, Cl^- 96 mEq/L, lactate 40 mEq/L, osmolarity 346 mOsm/L. Preservative free. Inj., Soln. *UltraBag* container. 1,500 mL, 2,000 mL, 2,500 mL, 3,000 mL. *Rx.*
Use: Electrolyte, peritoneal dialysis solution.

UltraBag Dianeal PD-2 w/2.5% Dextrose. (Baxter) Dextrose 2.5 g/L, Na^+ 132 mEq/L, Ca^{++} 3.5 mEq/L, Mg^{++} 0.5 mEq/L, Cl^- 96 mEq/L, lactate 40 mEq/L, osmolarity 396 mOsm/L. Preservative free. Inj., Soln. *UltraBag* container. 1,500 mL, 2,000 mL, 2,500 mL, 3,000 mL. *Rx.*
Use: Electrolyte, peritoneal dialysis solution.

Ultrabex. (Health for Life Brands) Vitamins B_1 20 mg, C 50 mg, B_2 2 mg, B_6 0.5 mg, niacinamide 35 mg, calcium pantothenate 0.5 mg, wheat germ oil 30 mg, B_{12} 20 mcg, liver desiccated 150 mg, iron 11.58 mg, calcium 29 mg, phosphorus 23 mg, dicalcium phosphate 100 mg, magnesium 1.11 mg, manganese 1.3 mg, potassium 2.24 mg, zinc 0.68 mg, choline 25 mg, inositol 25 mg, pepsin 32.5 mg, diastase 32.5 mg, hesperidin 25 mg, biotin 20 mcg, hydrolyzed yeast 81.25 mg, protein digest 47.04 mg, amino acids 34.21 mg. Cap. Bot. 50s, 100s, 1000s. *OTC.*
Use: Mineral, vitamin supplement.

Ultra B-50. (NBTY) Vitamins B_1 50 mg, B_2 50 mg, B_3 50 mg, B_5 50 mg, B_6 50 mg, B_{12} 50 mcg, folic acid 0.1 mg, PABA 50 mg, inositol 50 mg, biotin 50 mcg, choline 50 mg, lecithin 50 mg. Tab. Bot. 60s, 180s. *OTC.*
Use: Vitamin supplement.

Ultra B-100. (NBTY) Vitamins B_1 100 mg, B_2 100 mg, B_3 100 mg, B_5 100 mg, B_6 100 mg, B_{12} 100 mcg, folic acid 0.1 mg, PABA 100 mg, inositol 100 mg, biotin 100 mcg, choline bitartrate 100 mg. TR Tab. Bot. 50s. *OTC.*
Use: Vitamin supplement.

ULTRAbrom PD. (WE Pharmaceuticals) Brompheniramine maleate 6 mg, pseudoephedrine 60 mg. ER Cap. Bot.

100s. *Rx.*
Use: Upper respiratory combination, antihistamine, decongestant.

Ultracal. (Bristol-Myers Squibb) Protein 44 g, carbohydrate 123 g, fat 45 g, Na 930 mg, K 1610 mg, mOsm 310 kg H_2O, 1.06 cal/mL, vitamins A, B_1, B_2, B_3, B_5, B_6, B_{12}, C, D, E, K, folic acid, choline, biotin, Ca, P, I, Fe, Mg, Cu, Zn, Mn, Cl, Se, Cr, Mo. Liq. Can. 8 oz. *OTC.*
Use: Nutritional supplement.

Ultra Cap. (Weeks & Leo) Acetaminophen 300 mg, guaifenesin 100 mg, chlorpheniramine maleate 4 mg, phenylephrine hydrochloride 10 mg, dextromethorphan HBr 6 mg. Cap. Vial 18s. *Rx.*
Use: Analgesic; antihistamine; antitussive; decongestant; expectorant.

Ultra-Care. (Allergan) **Disinfecting Soln.:** Hydrogen peroxide 3%, sodium stannate, sodium nitrate, phosphate buffer. Bot. 120 mL, 360 mL. **Neutralizer Tab.:** Catalase, hydroxypropyl methylcellulose, buffering agents. Pkg. 12s, 36s w/cup. *OTC.*
Use: Contact lens disinfection system.

Ultracet. (Ortho-McNeil) Tramadol hydrochloride 37.5 mg, acetaminophen 325 mg. Film-coated. Tab. Bot. 20s, 100s, 500s, UD 100s. *Rx.*
Use: Nonnarcotic analgesic combination.

Ultracin. (Cal Pharma) Capsaicin 0.025%, menthol 10%, methyl salicylate 28%. Alcohols, aloe, glyceryl, methylisothiazolinone, PEG, propylene glycol, soya lecithin. Lot. 120 mL. *OTC.*
Use: Rub and liniment.

Ultracortinol. (Novartis) Agent to suppress overactive adrenal glands. Pending release.

Ultra Freeda. (Freeda) Vitamins A 4166 units, D 133 units, E 66.7 mg, B_1 16.7 mg, B_2 16.7 mg, B_3 33 mg, B_5 33 mg, B_6 16.7 mg, B_{12} 33 mcg, C 333 mg, folic acid 0.27 mg, iron 2 mg, calcium 27 mg, zinc 1.1 mg, choline, inositol, bioflavonoids, PABA, biotin 100 mcg, Cr, I, K, Mg, Mn, Mo, Se. Tab. Bot. 90s, 180s, 270s. *OTC.*
Use: Mineral, vitamin supplement.

Ultra Freeda Iron Free. (Freeda) Vitamins A 4166 units, D 133 units, E_2 66.7 mg, B_1 16.7 mg, B_2 16.7 mg, B_3 33 mg, B_5 33 mg, B_6 16.7 mg, B_{12} 33 mcg, C 333 mg, FA 0.27 mg, Ca 27 mg, Zn 1.1 mg, choline, inositol, bioflavonoids, PABA, biotin 100 mcg, Cr, I, K, Mg, Mn, Mo, Se. Tab. Bot. 90s, 180s, 270s. *OTC.*
Use: Mineral, vitamin supplement.

Ultragesic. (Stewart-Jackson Pharmacal) Acetaminophen 500 mg, hydrocodone bitartrate 5 mg. Cap. Bot. 100s. *c-III.*
Use: Analgesic combination; narcotic.

Ultralan. (Elan) Protein 60 g, fat 50 g, carbohydrates 202 g, Na 1.035 g, K 1.755 g/L. Lactose free. With appropriate vitamins and minerals. Liq. In 1000 mL *New Pak* systems w/ and w/o *ColorCheck. OTC.*
Use: Nutritional supplement.

ultralente insulin.
See: Iletin.

Ultram. (Janssen) Tramadol hydrochloride 50 mg. Lactose, PEG. Film-coated. Tab. Bot. 100s. *Rx.*
Use: Opioid analgesic.

Ultram ER. (Janssen) Tramadol hydrochloride 100 mg, 200 mg, 300 mg. Polyvinyl alcohol. ER Tab. 30s. *Rx.*
Use: Opioid analgesic.

Ultra Mide 25. (Ivax) Bot. 8 oz. *OTC.*
Use: Emollient.

Ultra-Natal. (Ethex) Iron (carbonyl iron) 90 mg, iodine (potassium iodide) 150 mcg, calcium citrate 200 mg, cupric oxide 2 mg, zinc oxide 25 mg, folic acid 1 mg, vitamins A 2700 units, D_3 400 units, E 30 units, C 120 mg, B_1 3 mg, B_2 3.4 mg, B_6 20 mg, B_{12} 12 mcg, niacinamide 20 mg, docusate sodium. Dye free. Tab. UD 100s. *Rx.*
Use: Vitamin, mineral supplement.

Ultra-NatalCare. (Ethex) Ca 200 mg, Fe (as carbonyl iron) 90 mg, vitamin A 2700 units, D_3 400 units, E (dl-alpha-tocopheryl acetate) 30 units, B_1 3 mg, B_2 3.4 mg, B_3 20 mg, B_6 20 mg, B_{12} 12 mcg, C 120 mg, folic acid 1 mg, Zn 25 mg, Cu, I, docusate sodium 50 mg. Tab. UD 100s. *Rx.*
Use: Vitamin, mineral supplement.

Ultrapred. (Horizon) Prednisolone acetate 1%. Susp. Bot. 5 mL. *Rx.*
Use: Corticosteroid, ophthalmic.

UltraSal-ER. (Elorac) Salicylic acid 28.5% Film forming. Carthamus tinctorius seed oil, isopropyl alcohol, olea europaea fruit oil, polysorbate 80. ER Soln.; topical. 10 mL w/brush applicator. *Rx.*
Use: Keratolytic agent.

Ultrasone. (Gordon Laboratories) Ultrasound aid. Bot. Qt, gal. Plastic Bot. 8 oz.
Use: Ultrasound contact cream.

Ultra Strength D2000. (Mason Natural) Vitamin D_3 (cholecalciferol) 2000 units. Cap. 60s. *OTC.*
Use: Vitamin, fat-soluble vitamin.

Ultra Strength Vitamin D3. (Nature's Blend) Cholecalciferol 5,000 units per

mL. Soybean oil, vitamin E. Gluten free. Drops. 52.5 mL. *OTC.*
Use: Fat-soluble vitamin.

Ultravate. (Ranbaxy) Halobetasol propionate. *Rx.*
Use: Corticosteroid, topical.

Ultravate X. (Ranbaxy) Halobetasol propionate 0.05%. **Cream:** Cetyl alcohol, glycerin, urea. 50 g w/225 g of *Lac-Hydrin Ten Plus* moisturizing cream. **Oint.:** Beeswax, petrolatum, propylene glycol. 50 g w/225 g of *Lac-Hydrin Ten Plus* moisturizing cream. *Rx.*
Use: Anti-inflammatory agent, topical corticosteroid.

Ultravist 150. (Baxter) Iopromide 311.7 mg, iodine 150 mg/mL. EDTA. Inj. Vials. 50 mL. *Rx.*
Use: Radiopaque, parenteral.

Ultravist 300. (Baxter) Iopromide 623.4 mg, iodine 300 mg/mL. EDTA. Inj. Vials. 50 mL, 100 mL, 150 mL. *Rx.*
Use: Radiopaque, parenteral.

Ultravist 370. (Baxter) Iopromide 768.86 mg, iodine 370 mg/mL. EDTA. Inj. Vials. 50 mL, 100 mL, 150 mL. 200 mL fill in 250 mL vial. *Rx.*
Use: Radiopaque, parenteral.

Ultravist 240. (Baxter) Iopromide 498.72 mg, iodine 240 mg/mL. EDTA. Inj. Vials. 50 mL, 100 mL fill in 250 mL vial. *Rx.*
Use: Radiopaque, parenteral.

Ultra Vitamin A & D. (NBTY) Vitamins A 25,000 units, D 1000 units. Tab. Bot. 100s. *OTC.*
Use: Vitamin supplement.

Ultra Vita Time. (NBTY) Iron 6 mg, vitamins A 10,000 units, D 400 units, E 13 units, B_1 25 mg, B_2 25 mg, B_3 50 mg, B_5 12.5 mg, B_6 15 mg, B_{12} 50 mcg, C 150 mg, folic acid 0.4 mg, B, Ca, Cr, Cu, I, K, Mg, Mn, Mo, P, Se, Zn 5 mg, biotin 1 mg, bioflavonoids, bone meal, PABA, choline bitartrate, betaine, inositol, lecithin, desiccated liver, rutin. Tab. Bot. 100s. *OTC.*
Use: Mineral, vitamin supplement.

Ultrazyme Enzymatic Cleaner. (Allergan) Subtilisin A, effervescing, buffering, and tableting agents for dilution in hydrogen peroxide 3%. Tab. Pkg. 5s, 10s, 15s, 20s. *OTC.*
Use: Contact lens care.

Ultresa. (Aptalis Pharma US) Lipase/protease/amylase 13,800 units/27,600 units/27,600 units, 20,700 units/41,400 units/41,400 units, 23,000 units/46,000 units/46,000 units. Castor oil. Cap., delayed release. 100s, 500s (23,000 units/46,000 units/46,000 units only). *Rx.*
Use: Digestive enzyme.

Ultrum. (Towne) Vitamins A 5000 units, E 30 units, C 90 mg, folic acid 400 mcg, B_1 2.25 mg, B_2 2.6 mg, niacinamide 20 mg, B_6 3 mg, B_{12} 9 mcg, biotin 45 mcg, D 400 units, pantothenic acid 10 mg, calcium 162 mg, phosphorus 125 mg, iodine 150 mcg, iron 27 mg, magnesium 100 mg, copper 3 mg, manganese 7.5 mg, potassium 7.5 mg, zinc 22.5 mg. Tab. Bot. 100s. *OTC.*
Use: Mineral, vitamin supplement.

Ultrum with Selenium. (Towne) Vitamins A 5000 units, E 30 units, C 90 mg, folic acid 2.25 mg, B_1 2.25 mg, B_2 2.6 mg, niacinamide 20 mg, B_6 3 mg, B_{12} 9 mcg, D 400 units, biotin 45 mcg, pantothenic acid 10 mg, calcium 162 mg, phosphorus 125 mg, iodine 150 mcg, iron 27 mg, magnesium 100 mg, copper 3 mg, manganese 7.5 mg, potassium 7.7 mg, chloride 7 mg, molybdenum 15 mcg, selenium 15 mcg, zinc 22.5 mg. Tab. Bot. 130s. *Rx.*
Use: Mineral, vitamin supplement.

•**umeclidinium.** (ue-MEK-li-DIN-ee-um) USAN.
Use: Treatment of chronic obstructive pulmonary disorder.
W/Vilanterol.
See: Anoro Ellipta.

•**umeclidinium bromide.** (ue-MEK-li-DIN-ee-um) USAN.
Use: Treatment of chronic obstructive pulmonary disorder.

Umecta. (Innocutis) Urea. **Emulsion:** 40%. Helianthus annuus oil, EDTA. 113.5 g. **Nail Film:** 40%. EDTA, PEG-6 caprylic/capric glycerides. 18 mL with applicator. **Top. Aerosol:** 40%. Glycine, shea butter oil, sunflower oil. 114 g. **Top. Susp.:** 40%. Helianthus annuus oil, EDTA. 283.4 g. *Rx.*
Use: Emollient.

Umecta 40%. (Innocutis) Urea 40%. EDTA, glycerin, PEG-6. Susp. 18 mL with applicator. *Rx.*
Use: Emollient.

Umecta PD. (Innocutis) **Emulsion:** Urea 40%. EDTA, shea butter oil, sunflower oil. 142 g, 200 g. **Susp.:** Urea 40%. EDTA, shea butter oil, sunflower oil. 257 g. *Rx.*
Use: Emollient.

•**umirolimus.** (UE-mir-OH-li-mus) USAN.
Use: Prevention of restenosis.

UN-Aspirin, Extra Strength. (Zee Medical) Acetaminophen 500 mg. Castor oil. Tab. 250s. *OTC.*
Use: Analgesic.

Unasyn. (Roerig) Ampicillin sodium/sulbactam sodium 1 g/0.5 g, 10 g/5 g. Inj., Pow. for Soln. Vial (1 g/0.5 g), bulk pkg (10 g/5 g). *Rx.*
Use: Penicillin, aminopenicillin.

•**undecanoate.** (un-DEK-a-NOE-ate) USAN.
Use: Antifungal.

10-undecenoic acid. Undecylenic acid.
Use: Antifungal, topical.

10-undecenoic acid, zinc (2+) salt. Zinc undecylenate.
Use: Antifungal, topical.

undecoylium chloride-iodine. (Ruson) Virac, preps.
Use: Anti-infective, topical.

•**undecylenic acid.** (un-deh-sill-EN-ik) *USP.*
Use: Antifungal, topical.
See: DiabetiDerm.
Elon Dual Defense Antifungal Formula.
Fungi Cure Maximum Strength.
Gordochom.

undecylenic acid salts. Calcium, copper, zinc.

Undelenic Ointment. (Gordon Laboratories) Undecylenic acid 5%, zinc undecylenate 20%. Jar oz, lb. *OTC.*
Use: Antifungal, topical.

Undelenic Tincture. (Gordon Laboratories) Undecylenic acid 10%, chloroxylenol 0.5%. Brush Bot. oz. Bot. pt. *OTC.*
Use: Antifungal, topical.

Unguentine. (Lee) Phenol 1% in ointment base. Tube oz. *OTC.*
Use: Dermatologic; counterirritant.

Unguentine Maximum Strength. (Lee) Benzocaine 5%, resorcinol 2%. Alcohols, methylparaben, mineral oil. Cream. 28.3 g. *OTC.*
Use: Local anesthetic, topical.

Unibase. (Gallipot) Proprietary blend of emulsifiers and preservative cream; conc. 500g. *Rx.*
Use: Ointment and Lotion base.

Unicap. (Pfizer) **Cap.:** Vitamins A 5000 units, D 400 units, E 30 units, B_1 1.5 mg, B_2 1.7 mg, B_3 20 mg, B_6 2 mg, B_{12} 6 mcg, C 60 mg, FA 0.4 mg. Bot. 120s. **Tab.:** Vitamins A 5000 units, D 400 units, E 15 units, B_1 1.5 mg, B_2 1.7 mg, B_3 20 mg, B_6 2 mg, B_{12} 6 mcg, C 60 mg, FA 0.4 mg. Tab. Bot. 120s. *OTC.*
Use: Vitamin supplement.

Unicap Jr. Chewable. (Pfizer) Vitamins A 5000 units, D 400 units, E 15 units, C 60 mg, folic acid 400 mcg, B_1 1.5 mg, B_2 1.7 mg, B_3 20 mg, B_6 2 mg, B_{12} 6 mcg. Tab. Bot. 120s. *OTC.*
Use: Vitamin supplement.

Unicap M. (Pfizer) Iron 18 mg, vitamins A 5000 units, D 400 units, E 30 units, B_1 1.5 mg, B_2 1.7 mg, B_3 20 mg, B_5 10 mg, B_6 2 mg, B_{12} 6 mcg, C 60 mg, folic acid 0.4 mg, Ca, Cu, I, K, Mn, P, Zn 15 mg, tartrazine. Tab. Bot. 120s. *OTC.*
Use: Mineral, vitamin supplement.

Unicap Plus Iron. (Pfizer) Vitamins A 5000 units, D 400 units, E 30 units, C 60 mg, folic acid 0.4 mg, B_1 1.5 mg, B_2 1.7 mg, B_3 20 mg, B_5 10 mg, B_6 2 mg, B_{12} 6 mcg, iron 22.5 mg, Ca. Tab. Bot. 120s. *OTC.*
Use: Mineral, vitamin supplement.

Unicap Sr. (Pfizer) Iron 10 mg, vitamins A 5000 units, D 200 units, E 15 units, B_1 1.2 mg, B_2 1.4 mg, $B_3$16 mg, B_5 10 mg, B_6 2.2 mg, B_{12} 3 mcg, C 60 mg, folic acid 0.4 mg, Ca, Cu, I, K, Mg, Mn, P, Zn 15 mg. Tab. Bot. 120s. *OTC.*
Use: Mineral, vitamin supplement.

Unicap T. (Pfizer) Iron 18 mg, vitamins A 5000 units, D 400 units, E 30 units, B_1 10 mg, B_2 20 mg, B_3 100 mg, B_5 25 mg, B_6 6 mg, B_{12} 18 mcg, C 500 mg, folic acid 0.4 mg, Cu, I, K, Mn, Se, Zn 15 mg, tartrazine. Tab. Bot. 60s. *OTC.*
Use: Mineral, vitamin supplement.

Unicomplex-M. (Rugby) Vitamins A 5,000 units, D 400 units, E 30 units, B_1 1.5 mg, B_2 1.7 mg, B_3 20 mg, B_5 10 mg, B_6 2 mg, B_{12} 6 mcg, C 60 mg, folic acid 0.4 mg, Ca 60 mg, Cu, Fe, I, K, Mn, P, Zn. Maltodextrin, tartrazine. Tab. 90s. *OTC.*
Use: Mineral, vitamin supplement.

Unicomplex-T & M. (Rugby) Iron 18 mg, vitamins A 5000 units, D 400 units, E 30 mg, B_1 10 mg, B_2 10 mg, B_3 100 mg, B_5 25 mg, B_6 6 mg, B_{12} 18 mcg, C 500 mg, FA 0.4 mg, Ca, Cu, I, K, Mn, Zn 15 mg. Tab. Bot. 60s. *OTC.*
Use: Mineral, vitamin supplement.

Unicomplex-T with Minerals. (Rugby) Iron 10 mg, vitamins A 5000 units, D 400 units, E 15 mg, B_1 10 mg, B_2 10 mg, B_3 100 mg, B_5 20 mg, B_6 2 mg, B_{12} 4 mcg, C 300 mg, folic acid 0.4 mg, Ca, Cu, I, K, Mg, Mn. Tab. Bot. 60s. *OTC.*
Use: Mineral, vitamin supplement.

Unifed. (Altaire) Pseudoephedrine hydrochloride 30 mg per 5 mL. Methylparaben, glycerin, sorbitol, sucrose. Liq. 118 mL. *OTC.*
Use: Nasal decongestant.

Unifiber. (Niche) Powdered cellulose. Pow. Bot. 150 g, 270 g, 480 g. *OTC.*
Use: Laxative.

•**unifocon A.** (you-nih-FOE-kahn A) USAN.
Use: Contact lens material (hydrophic).

Uniphyl. (Purdue) Theophylline. CR Tab. **400 mg:** 100s, 500s. **600 mg:** 100s. *Rx.*
Use: Bronchodilator.

Uniretic. (Schwarz Pharma) Moexipril hydrochloride/hydrochlorothiazide 7.5 mg/12.5 mg, 15 mg/12.5 mg. Film coated. Lactose. Tab. 100s. *Rx.*
Use: Antihypertensive.

Unisol. (Alcon) Buffered isotonic solution with sodium Cl, boric acid, sodium borate. Bot. 15 mL (25s), 120 mL (2s, 3s). *OTC.*
Use: Contact lens care.

Unisol 4 Sterile Saline. (Alcon) Buffered isotonic solution with sodium Cl, boric acid, sodium borate. Bot. 120 mL. *OTC.*
Use: Contact lens care.

Unisol Plus. (Alcon) Buffered isotonic solution w/NaCl, boric acid, sodium borate. Aerosol Bot. 240 mL, 360 mL. *OTC.*
Use: Contact lens care.

Unisom PM Pain. (Chattem) Acetaminophen 325 mg, diphenhydramine hydrochloride 50 mg. Mineral oil. Tab. 30s. *OTC.*
Use: Nonprescription sleep aid combination.

Unisom SleepGels. (Chattem) Diphenhydramine hydrochloride 50 mg. Glycerin, PEG, propylene glycol, sorbitol. Cap., softgels. 8s, 16s, 32s. *OTC.*
Use: Antihistamine, nonselective ethanolamine.

Unisom SleepMelts. (Chattem) Diphenhydramine hydrochloride 25 mg. Mannitol, sucralose, sucrose. Cherry flavor. Tab., Orally disintegrating. 24s. *OTC.*
Use: Nonprescription sleep aid.

Unisom SleepTabs. (Chattem) Doxylamine succinate 25 mg. Tab. 8s, 16s, 32s, 48s. *OTC.*
Use: Antihistamine, nonselective ethanolamine.

Unithroid Direct. (Lannett) Levothyroxine sodium 0.025 mg, 0.05 mg, 0.075 mg, 0.088 mg, 0.1 mg, 0.112 mg, 0.125 mg, 0.15 mg, 0.175 mg, 0.2 mg, 0.3 mg, lactose. Tab. Bot. 100s, 1000s. *Rx.*
Use: Hormone, thyroid.

Uni-Tussin DM. (United Research Laboratories) Dextromethorphan HBr 10 mg, guaifenesin 100 mg/5 mL. Syr. Bot. 118 mL. *OTC.*
Use: Antitussive; expectorant.

Univasc. (Schwarz Pharma) Moexipril hydrochloride 7.5 mg, 15 mg. Film coated. Lactose. Tab. 100s. *Rx.*
Use: Antihypertensive; renin angiotensin system antagonist; angiotensin-converting enzyme inhibitor.

Unna's boot.
See: Zinc Gelatin.

unoprostone isopropyl. (ue-noe-PROST-one)
Use: Agent for glaucoma.
See: Rescula.

Unproco Capsules. (Solvay) Dextromethorphan HBr 30 mg, guaifenesin 200 mg. Cap. Bot. 100s. *OTC.*
Use: Antitussive; expectorant.

UpCal D. (Global Health) **Chew. Tab.:** Vitamin D_3 125 units, Ca, Mg. Sucralose. Fruit punch and cinnamon flavors. 120s. **Pow.:** Vitamin D_3 250 units per packet/scoop, Ca. Dextrose. Single-use packet. 454 g, 2.5 g. *OTC.*
Use: Multivitamin with minerals.

Uplex. (Arcum) Vitamins A 5000 units, D 400 units, B_1 3 mg, B_2 3 mg, B_6 1 mg, B_{12} 2.5 mcg, nicotinamide 20 mg, calcium pantothenate 5 mg, C 50 mg. Cap. Bot. 100s, 1000s. *OTC.*
Use: Mineral, vitamin supplement.

Uplex No. 2. (Arcum) Vitamins A palmitate 10,000 units, D 400 units, B_1 5 mg, B_2 5 mg, C 100 mg, B_6 2 mg, B_{12} 3 mcg, E 2.5 units, niacinamide 25 mg, calcium pantothenate 5 mg. Cap. Bot. 100s, 1000s. *OTC.*
Use: Mineral, vitamin supplement.

u-polycosanol 410.
W/Antipyrine, Benzocaine.
See: Treagan.

upper respiratory combinations.
See: Antihistamine and Analgesic Combinations.
Antitussive and Expectorant Combinations.
Antitussive Combinations.
Antitussives with Expectorants.
Decongestant and Analgesic Combinations.
Decongestant and Antihistamine Combinations.
Decongestant, Antihistamine, and Analgesic Combinations.
Decongestant, Antihistamine, and Anticholinergic Combinations.
Decongestant, Antihistamine, and Expectorant Combinations.
Decongestant and Expectorant Combinations.
Expectorants with Analgesics.
Topical Combinations.

Urabeth Tabs. (Major) Bethanechol 5 mg, 10 mg, 25 mg, 50 mg. Tab. **5 mg:** Bot. 100s. **10 mg:** Bot. 250s. **25 mg:** Bot. 250s, 1000s. **50 mg:** Bot. 100s, UD 100s. *Rx.*
Use: Genitourinary.

Uracid. (Wesley) dl-Methionine 0.2 g.

Cap. Bot. 100s, 1000s. *Rx.*
Use: Diaper rash preparation.
•**uracil.** (YOUR-ah-sil) USAN.
Use: Potentiator in tegafur therapy.
uradal.
See: Carbromal.
Uramaxin. (Medimetriks Pharmaceuticals) Urea. **Cream:** 45%. Camphor, edetate disodium, eucalyptus oil, menthol. 255 g. **Lot.:** 45%. Camphor, edetate disodium, ethyl alcohol, eucalyptus oil, menthol, titanium dioxide. 473 mL. *Rx.*
Use: Emollient.
Uramaxin GT. (Medimetriks) Urea 45%. Camphor, edetate disodium, eucalyptus oil, menthol, propylene glycol. Soln. 20 mL prefilled applicator. *Rx.*
Use: Emollient.
•**urea.** (your-EE-a) *USP.*
Use: Topically for dry skin; diuretic.
See: Aluvea.
Aquacare.
Aquacare-HP.
Atrac-Tain.
BP-50.
Dermal Therapy Finger Care.
Dermasorb XM.
Flexitol Heel Balm.
Gordon's Urea.
Gormel.
Hydro 40.
Hydro 35.
Kerafoam.
Kerafoam 42.
Keralac.
Latrix XM.
Nutraplus.
Rea-lo.
RE Urea 50.
Umecta.
Umecta PD.
Uramaxin.
Uramaxin GT.
Urea 50%.
Urea 40.
Urea 45%.
Urea 42%.
Utopic.
W/Combinations.
See: Amino-Cerv.
Akne Drying Lotion.
W/Hydrocortisone Acetate.
See: Carmol HC.
W/Micronized Hydrocortisone Acetate.
See: Carmol-HC.
W/Papain.
See: Pap-Urea.
urea. (Austin Pharmaceuticals) Urea 39%. Cetyl alcohol, glyceryl, mineral oil, petrolatum, propylene glycol. Cream. 227 g. *Rx.*
Use: Emollient.
urea. (Clay Park) Urea 40%. Glycerin, EDTA. Gel. 15 mL. *Rx.*
Use: Emollient.
urea. (Exact-Rx) Urea. **Cream: 45%:** Alcohol, camphor, edetate disodium, eucalyptus oil, menthol, titanium dioxide. 255 g. **50%:** Disodium EDTA, glycerin, lactic acid, mineral oil, zinc. 142 g, 255 g. **Emulsion:** 50%. Cetyl alcohol, disodium EDTA, glycerin, lactic acid, linoleic acid, mineral oil, PEG, titanium dioxide, zinc. 283.5 g. **Lot.:** 45%. Alcohol, camphor, disodium EDTA, eucalyptus oil, menthol. 453.5 g. **Susp., Top.:** 50%. Caprylic/capric triglyceride, cetyl alcohol, edetate disodium, glycerin, lactic acid, linoleic acid, PEG, propylene glycol, salicylic acid, titanium dioxide, vitamin E. 283.5 g. *Rx.*
Use: Emollient.
urea. (Hi-Tech) Urea. **Cream:** 40%. Mineral oil, petrolatum, cetyl alcohol. 28.35 g, 198.6 g. **Lot.:** 40%. Mineral oil, petrolatum, cetyl alcohol. 236.6 mL. *Rx.*
Use: Emollient.
urea. (Prasco) Urea. **Emulsion:** 40%. EDTA, glycerin, sunflower oil. 114 g, 228 g. **Susp.:** 40%. EDTA, glycerin, sunflower oil. 285 g. *Rx.*
Use: Emollient.
urea. (River's Edge) Urea 35%. Cetyl alcohol, EDTA, lactic acid. Lot. 207 mL, 325 mL. *Rx.*
Use: Emollient.
urea. (Various Mfr.) Urea 50%. May contain caprylic/capric triglyceride, cetyl alcohol, edetate disodium, glycerin, lactic acid, linoleic acid, PEG-6, propylene glycol, salicylic acid, titanium dioxide, triethanolamine, vitamin E. Susp., Top. Tube. 284 g. *Rx.*
Use: Emollient.
•**urea C 14.** (yoor-EE-a) *USP.*
Ureacin-10. (Pedinol Pharmacal) Urea 10%. Lot. Bot. 8 oz. *OTC.*
Use: Emollient.
Ureacin-20 Creme. (Pedinol Pharmacal) Urea 20%. Cream. Jar 2.5 oz. *OTC.*
Use: Emollient.
•**urea C 13.** (yoor-EE-a) *USP.*
Urea 50%. (Acella Pharmaceuticals) Urea 50%. Caprylic/capril triglycerides, cetyl alcohol, disodium EDTA, glycerin, lactic acid, linoleic acid, PEG-6, polysorbate 60, propylene glycol, titanium dioxide, triethanolamine, vitamin E, zinc. Emuls. 295 mL. *Rx.*
Use: Emollient.
Urea 50%. (E. Fougera) Urea 50%. Cetyl alcohol, disodium EDTA, glycerin, lactic

acid, PEG 6, vitamin E, zinc pyrithione. Oint. 45 g. *Rx.*
Use: Emollient.

Urea 40. (Kylemore) Urea 40%. Disodium EDTA, glycerin, PEG. Gel. 15 mL w/applicator brush. *Rx.*
Use: Emollient.

Urea 45%. (River's Edge) Urea 45%. Camphor, edentate disodium, ethyl alcohol, eucalyptus oil, menthol, titanium dioxide. Cream. 255 g. *Rx.*
Use: Emollient.

Urea 42%. (River's Edge) Urea (carbamide) 42%. Disodium EDTA, glycerine, lactic acid. Cloth, Top. 30s. *Rx.*
Use: Emollient.

urea peroxide.
See: Gly-Oxide.
Proxigel.

urea topical suspension 50%. (A. Aarons) Urea 50%. Cetyl alcohol, EDTA, glycerin, lactic acid, PEG, titanium dioxide. Top. Susp. 284 g. *Rx.*
Use: Emollient.

Urecholine. (Barr/Duramed) Bethanechol chloride 5 mg, 10 mg, 25 mg, 50 mg. Lactose. Tab. 100s. *Rx.*
Use: Urinary cholinergic.

•**uredepa.** (YOU-ree-DEH-pah) USAN.
Use: Antineoplastic.
See: Avinar.

p-ureidobenzenearsonic acid.
See: Carbarsone.

Urelief. (Rocky Mtn.) Methenamine 2 g, salol 0.5 g, methylene blue 1/10 g, benzoic acid g, hyoscyamine sulfate g, atropine sulfate g. Tab. Bot. 100s. *Rx.*
Use: Anti-infective, urinary.

Urelle. (Pharmelle) Methenamine 81 mg, sodium phosphate monobasic 40.8 mg, phenyl salicylate 32.4 mg, methylene blue 10.8 mg, hyoscyamine sulfate 0.12 mg, sugar, mineral oil. Tab. 90s. *Rx.*
Use: Anti-infective, urinary.

•**urelumab.** (ue-REL-ue-mab) USAN.
Use: Antineoplastic.

Urese.
See: Benzthiazide.

urethan. Ethyl Carbamate, Ethyl Urethan, Urethane.
Use: Antineoplastic.

Uretron D/S. (Marin) Methenamine 120 mg, sodium biphosphonate 40.8 mg, phenyl salicylate 36.2 mg, methylene blue 10.8 mg, hyoscyamine sulfate 0.12 mg, parabens, sucrose. Tab. 100s. *Rx.*
Use: Anti-infective, urinary.

Urex. (3M) Methenamine hippurate 1 g. Tab. Bot. 100s. *Rx.*
Use: Anti-infective, urinary.

Uric Acid Reagent Strips. (Bayer Consumer Care) *Seralyzer* reagent strip. For uric acid in serum or plasma. Bot. 25s.
Use: Diagnostic aid.

uricosuric agents.
See: Anturane.
Benemid.

Uricult. (Orion) Urine culture test to detect bacteria and identify uropathogens. Bot. 10s.
Use: Diagnostic aid.

uridine. Idoxuridine.
Use: Reagent.

•**uridine triacetate.** (URE-i-deen trye-AS-e-tate) USAN.
Use: Antidote for 5-fluorouracil toxicity.

Urifon-Forte. (T.E. Williams Pharmaceuticals) Sulfamethizole 450 mg, phenazopyridine hydrochloride 50 mg. Cap. Bot. 100s, 1000s. *Rx.*
Use: Anti-infective, urinary.

Urigen. (Fellows) Calcium mandelate 0.2 g, methenamine 0.2 g, phenazopyridine hydrochloride 50 mg, sodium phosphate 80 mg. Cap. Bot. 100s, 1000s. *Rx.*
Use: Anti-infective, urinary.

Urimar-T. (Marnel) Methenamine 120 mg, sodium phosphate monobasic 40.8 mg, phenyl salicylate 36.2 mg, methylene blue 10.8 mg, hyoscyamine sulfate 0.12 mg. Sugar-coated. Tab. Bot. 4s, 100s. *Rx.*
Use: Anti-infective, urinary.

Urimax. (Xanodyne) Methenamine 81.6 mg, sodium biphosphate 40.8 mg, phenyl salicylate 36.2 mg, methylene blue 10.8 mg, hyoscyamine sulfate 0.12 mg. Magenta. Film-coated. DR Tab. 100s. *Rx.*
Use: Treatment of urinary tract infections.

Urinary Antiseptic #3 S.C.T. (Teva) Atropine sulfate 0.06 mg, hyoscyamine sulfate 0.03 mg, methenamine 120 mg, methylene blue 6 mg, phenyl salicylate 30 mg, benzoic acid 7.5 mg. Tab. Bot. 100s, 1000s. *Rx.*
Use: Anti-infective, urinary.

Urinary Antiseptic #2. (Various Mfr.) Atropine sulfate 0.03 mg, hyoscyamine 0.03 mg, methenamine 40.8 mg, methylene blue 5.4 mg, phenyl salicylate 18.1 mg, benzoic acid 4.5 mg. Tab. Bot. 100s, 1000s. *Rx.*
Use: Anti-infective, urinary.

Urinary Antiseptic #2 S.C.T. (Teva) Atropine sulfate 0.03 mg, hyoscyamine sulfate 0.03 mg, methenamine 40.8 mg,

methylene blue 5.4 mg, phenyl salicylate 18.1 mg, benzoic acid 4.5 mg. Tab. Bot. 100s, 1000s. *Rx.*
Use: Anti-infective, urinary.

urinary cholinergics.
See: Bethanechol Chloride.
Neostigmine Methylsulfate.

urine sugar test.
See: Clinistix.

urine tests.
See: Diagnostic Agents.

Urin-Tek. (Bayer Consumer Care) Tubes, plastic caps, adhesive labels, collection cups, and disposable tube holder. Package 100 × 5.

Urisan-P. (Sandia) Atropine sulfate 0.03 mg, hyoscyamine 0.03 mg, gelsemium 6.1 mg, methenamine 40.8 mg, salol 18.1 mg, benzoic acid 4.5 mg, methylene blue 5.4 mg, phenylazo diamino pyridine hydrochloride 100 mg. Tab. Bot. 100s, 1000s. *Rx.*
Use: Anti-infective, urinary.

Urisedamine. (PolyMedica) Methenamine mandelate 500 mg, l-hyoscyamine 0.15 mg. Tab. Bot. 100s. *Rx.*
Use: Anti-infective, urinary.

Uriseptic. (SDA Labs) Methenamine 40.8 mg, phenyl salicylate 18.1 mg, methylene blue 5.4 mg, benzoic acid 4.5 mg, atropine sulfate 0.03 mg, hyoscyamine sulfate 0.03 mg. Tab. 100s. *Rx.*
Use: Anti-infective, urinary.

Urispas. (Ortho-McNeil) Flavoxate hydrochloride 100 mg, castor oil. Tab. Bot. 100s, UD 100s. *Rx.*
Use: Anticholinergic.

Uristix. (Siemens Medical) Urine test for glucose and protein. Reagent strips. 100s.
Use: Diagnostic aid.

Uristix 4 Reagent Strips. (Bayer Consumer Care) Urinalysis reagent strip test for glucose, protein, nitrite, leukocytes. Bot. 100s.
Use: Diagnostic aid.

Uristix Reagent Strips. (Bayer Consumer Care) Urinalysis reagent strip test for protein and glucose. Bot. 100s.
Use: Diagnostic aid.

Uritact DS. (Cypress) Hyoscyamine sulfate 0.06 mg, methenamine 81.6 mg, phenyl salicylate 36.2 mg, atropine sulfate 0.06 mg, methylene blue 10.8 mg, benzoic acid 9 mg. Alcohol free and sugar free. Tab. 100s. *Rx.*
Use: Anti-infective, urinary.

Uritin. (Global Source) Methenamine 40.8 mg, atropine sulfate 0.03 mg, hyoscyamine sulfate 0.03 mg, salol 18.1 mg, benzoic acid 4.5 mg, methylene blue 5.4 mg, gelsemium 6.1 mg. Tab. Bot. 1000s. *Rx.*
Use: Anti-infective, urinary.

Uritin Formula. (Various Mfr.) Atropine sulfate 0.03 mg, hyoscyamine 0.03 mg, methenamine 40.8 mg, methylene blue 5.4 mg, phenyl salicylate 18.1 mg, benzoic acid 4.5 mg. Tab. Bot. 1000s. *Rx.*
Use: Anti-infective, urinary.

Urobak. (Shire US) Sulfamethoxazole 500 mg. Tab. Bot. 100s, 1000s. *Rx.*
Use: Anti-infective, sulfonamide.

Uro Blue. (R.A. McNeil) Methenamine 120 mg, sodium phosphate monobasic 40.8 mg, phenyl salicylate 36.2 mg, methylene blue 10.8 mg, hyoscyamine sulfate 0.12 mg, sugar. Tab. 100s. *Rx.*
Use: Anti-infective, urinary.

Urocit-K. (Mission Pharmacal) Potassium citrate 5 mEq, 10 mEq, 15 mEq. Wax matrix. ER Tab. 100s. *Rx.*
Use: Genitourinary.

•**urofollitropin.** (YOUR-oh-fahl-ih-TROE-pin) USAN.
Use: Sex hormone, ovulation stimulant.
See: Bravelle.

urogastrone. (Chiron Vision)
Use: Corneal transplant surgery. [Orphan Drug]

Urogesic. (Edwards) Phenazopyridine hydrochloride 100 mg. Tab. Bot. 100s. *Rx.*
Use: Interstitial cystitis agent.

Urogesic Blue. (Edwards) Methenamine 81.6 mg, monobasic sodium phosphate 40.8 mg, methylene blue 10.8 mg, hyoscyamine (as sulfate) 0.12 mg. Mannitol. Tab. 100s. *Rx.*
Use: Anti-infective, urinary.

urography agents.
See: Iodohippurate Sodium.
Iodopyracet.
Iodopyracet Compound.
Renografin.
Renovist.
Renovue.

•**urokinase.** (YOUR-oh-KIN-ace) USAN.
Use: Plasminogen activator; thrombolytic agent; thrombolytic enzyme.

•**urokinase alfa.** (YOUR-oh-KIN-ace) USAN.
Use: Thrombolytic (plasminogen activator).

Uro-KP-Neutral. (Star) Phosphorus 250 mg, potassium 49.4 mg, sodium 250.5 mg. Film-coated. Tab. Bot. 100s. *Rx.*
Use: Mineral supplement.

Urologic Sol G. (Abbott Hospital

Products) Bot. 1000 mL.
Use: Irrigant, ophthalmic.

Uro-Mag. (Blaine) Magnesium oxide 140 mg (elemental Mg 84.5 mg). Cap. Bot. 100s, 1000s, UD 100s. *OTC.*
Use: Mineral.

uronal.
See: Barbital.

Uro-Phosphate. (ECR) Sodium biphosphate 434.78 mg, methenamine 300 mg. Film-coated Tab. Bot. 100s. *Rx.*
Use: Anti-infective, urinary.

Uroplus DS. (Shire US) Trimethoprim 160 mg, sulfamethoxazole 800 mg. Tab. Bot. 100s, 500s. *Rx.*
Use: Anti-infective.

Uroplus SS. (Shire US) Trimethoprim 80 mg, sulfamethoxazole 800 mg. Tab. Bot. 100s, 500s. *Rx.*
Use: Anti-infective.

Uroquid-Acid No. 2. (Beach) Methenamine mandelate 500 mg, sodium acid phosphate monohydrate 500 mg. Tab. Bot. 100s. *Rx.*
Use: Anti-infective, urinary.

urotropin new. (Various Mfr.) Methenamine anhydromethylene citrate.

Urovist Cysto. (Berlex) Diatrizoate meglumine 300 mg, edetate calcium disodium 0.05 mg/mL. Dilution Bot. 500 mL w/300 mL. *Rx.*
Use: Radiopaque agent.

Urovist Cysto Pediatric. (Berlex) Diatrizoate meglumine 300 mg, edetate calcium disodium 0.1 mg/mL. Dilution bot. 300 mL w/100 mL soln. *Rx.*
Use: Radiopaque agent.

Urovist Meglumine DIU/CT. (Berlex) Diatrizoate meglumine 300 mg, edetate calcium disodium 0.05 mg/mL. Soln. Bot. 300 mL. Ctn. 10s. *Rx.*
Use: Radiopaque agent.

Urovist Sodium 300. (Berlex) Diatrizoate sodium 500 mg, edetate calcium disodium 0.1 mg/mL. Soln. Vial 50 mL, Box 10s. *Rx.*
Use: Radiopaque agent.

Uroxatral. (Covis) Alfuzosin hydrochloride 10 mg. Mannitol. ER Tab. 30s, 100s, UD 100s. *Rx.*
Use: Antihypertensive, antiadrenergic.

Ursinus Inlay-Tabs. (Novartis) Pseudoephedrine hydrochloride 30 mg, aspirin 325 mg. Tab. Bot. 24s. *OTC.*
Use: Decongestant; analgesic.

URSO. (Novartis) Ursodiol.
Use: Management and treatment of primary biliary cirrhosis. [Orphan Drug]

ursodeoxycholic acid, buffered.
Use: Primary biliary cirrhosis. [Orphan Drug]

•**ursodiol.** (UR-so-DIE-ol) *USP.* Ursodeoxycholic acid.
Use: Anticholelithogenic; urolithic. Management and treatment of primary biliary cirrhosis, gallstone solubilizing agent.
See: Actigall.
URSO.

ursodiol. (Teva) Ursodiol 250 mg, 500 mg. Film-coated. Tab. 100s. *Rx.*
Use: GI agent, gallstone solubilizing agent.

ursodiol. (Watson) Ursodiol 300 mg. Cap. 100s. *Rx.*
Use: Anticholelithogenic; urolithic; gallstone solubilizing agent.

Urso Forte. (Aptalis Pharma US) Ursodiol 500 mg. Film-coated. Tab. 100s, 500s. *Rx.*
Use: Gallstone solubilizing agent.

Urso 250. (Aptalis Pharma US) Ursodiol 250 mg. Film-coated. Tab. 100s, 500s. *Rx.*
Use: Gallstone solubilizing agent.

Uryl. (Portal Pharmaceutical) Hyoscyamine sulfate 0.12 mg, methenamine 81.6 mg, methylene blue 10.8 mg, monobasic sodium phosphate 40.8 mg. Mannitol. Tab. 100s. *Rx.*
Use: Anti-infective, methenamine combination.

•**usistapide.** (ue-SIS-ta-pide) USAN.
Use: Treatment of obesity and type 2 diabetes.

•**ustekinumab.** (US-te-KIN-ue-mab) USAN.
Use: Immunomodulator.
See: Stelara.

Ustell. (Biocomp Pharma) Methenamine 120 mg, methylene blue 10 mg, phenyl salicylate 36 mg, sodium phosphate monobasic 40.8 mg, hyoscyamine sulfate 0.12 mg. Ammonium hydroxide, propylene glycol. Cap. 100s. *Rx.*
Use: Anti-infective agent, methenamine combination.

Utac. (Breckenridge) Methenamine mandelate 500 mg, sodium acid phosphate monobasic monohydrate 500 mg. Film-coated. Tab. 100s. *Rx.*
Use: Anti-infective, methenamine.

uterine-active agents.
See: Abortifacients.
Cervical Ripening Agents.
Methylergonovine Maleate.
Oxytocics.
Uterine Relaxant.

uterine relaxant.
See: Ritodrine.

uterine stimulants.
See: Ergonovine Maleate.
Methylergonovine Maleate.

Uticap. (Cypress) Methenamine 120 mg, methylene blue 10 mg, phenyl salicylate 36 mg, sodium phosphate monobasic 40.8 mg, hyoscyamine sulfate 0.12 mg. Cap. 100s. *Rx.*
Use: Anti-infective agent, methenamine.

Utimox. (Parke-Davis) Amoxicillin trihydrate. **Cap.:** 250 mg Bot. 100s, 500s, UD 100s; 500 mg Bot. 100s, UD 100s. **Oral Susp.:** 125 mg or 250 mg/5 mL Bot. 80 mL, 100 mL, 150 mL, 200 mL. *Rx.*
Use: Anti-infective, penicillin.

UTI Relief. (Consumers Choice Systems) Phenazopyridine hydrochloride 97.2 mg. Tab. 12s. *Rx.*
Use: Interstitial cystitis agent.

Utopic. (Artesa Labs) Urea 41%. Cetyl alcohol, glyceryl stearate, mineral oil, petrolatum, propylene glycol. Cream. 227 g. *Rx.*
Use: Emollient.

Utrona-C. (Cypress Pharmaceutical) Hyoscyamine sulfate 0.12 mg, methenamine 81.6 mg, methylene blue 10.8 mg, phenyl salicylate 36.2 mg, sodium phosphate monobasic 40.8 mg. Mineral oil, PEG, sugar. Tab. 100s. *Rx.*
Use: Anti-infective, methenamine combination.

Uvadex. (Therakos) Methoxsalen 20 mcg/mL, alcohol 0.05 mL. Soln. Vial 10 mL. *Rx.*
Use: Cutaneous T-cell lymphoma; sclerosis treatment; cardiac allograft rejection prevention; psoralens.

Uvasal. (Sanofi-Synthelabo) Sodium bicarbonate, tartaric acid. Pow. Bot. *OTC.*
Use: Antacid.

uva ursi. (Sherwood Davis & Geck) Leaves. Fluid extract. Bot. pt, gal.

Uvinul MS-40. (General Aniline & Film) *See:* Sulisobenzone.

UV Protective. (Kiehl's) Avobenzone 2%, ecamsule 2%, octocrylene 10%. EDTA, glycerin, parabens, stearyl alcohol. Fragrance free. SPF 15. Cream. 100 g. *OTC.*
Use: Sunscreen.

V

•**vabicaserin hydrochloride.** (va-BIK-a-SER-in) USAN.
Use: Antipsychotic.
vaccine, adenovirus. *Rx.*
Use: Immunization.
See: Adenovirus Vaccine.
vaccine, anthrax. *Rx.*
Use: Immunization.
See: Anthrax Vaccine.
vaccine, BCG. *Rx.*
Use: Immunization.
See: BCG Vaccine.
TheraCys.
Tice BCG.
vaccine, Haemophilus b conjugate. *Rx.*
Use: Immunization.
See: ActHIB.
HibTITER.
Liquid PedvaxHIB.
W/Hepatitis B.
See: Comvax.
vaccine, hepatitis A. *Rx.*
Use: Immunization.
See: Havrix.
Vaqta.
vaccine, hepatitis B, recombinant. *Rx.*
Use: Immunization.
See: Engerix-B.
Recombivax HB.
vaccine, influenza A & B. *Rx.*
Use: Immunization.
See: Fluarix.
FluMist.
Fluvirin.
Fluzone.
vaccine, Japanese encephalitis. *Rx.*
Use: Immunization.
See: JE-Vax.
vaccine, measles. *Rx.*
Use: Immunization.
See: Attenuvax.
W/Mumps and Rubella Vaccines.
See: M-M-R II.
vaccine, meningococcal polysaccharide. *Rx.*
Use: Immunization.
See: Menomune A/C/Y/W-135.
vaccine, mumps. Mumps Virus Vaccine Live.
Use: Immunization.
See: Mumpsvax.
vaccine, papillomavirus. *Rx.*
Use: Immunization.
See: Gardasil.
vaccine, pertussis. Pertussis Vaccine. *Rx.*
Use: Immunization.
See: ActHIB/DTP.
Diphtheria and Tetanus Toxoids, Acellular Pertussis and Haemophilus Influenzae Type B Conjugate Vaccine.
Diphtheria and Tetanus Toxoids and Acellular Pertussis Vaccine, Adsorbed.
Tripedia.
vaccine, pneumococcal polyvalent. *Rx.*
Use: Immunization.
See: Pneumovax 23.
vaccine, pneumococcal 7-valent conjugate. *Rx.*
Use: Immunization.
See: Prevnar.
vaccine, poliovirus. *Rx.*
Use: Immunization.
See: IPOL.
Poliovirus Vaccine, Inactivated.
vaccine, rabies. Rabies Vaccine. *Rx.*
Use: Immunization.
See: Imovax Rabies.
RabAvert.
Rabies Vaccine Adsorbed.
vaccines, bacterial.
Use: Immunization.
See: Anthrax Vaccine.
BCG Vaccine.
Haemophilus b Conjugate Vaccine.
Haemophilus b Conjugate Vaccine with Hepatitis B Vaccine.
Meningococcal Vaccine.
Pneumococcal Conjugate Vaccine.
Pneumococcal 7-Valent Conjugate Vaccine.
Pneumococcal Vaccine, Polyvalent.
Typhoid Vaccine.
vaccine, smallpox. *Rx.*
Use: Immunization.
See: Dryvax
vaccine, typhoid. *Rx.*
Use: Immunization.
See: Typhim Vi.
Vivotif Berna.
vaccine, varicella. *Rx.*
Use: Immunization.
See: Varivax.
vaccines, viral. *Rx.*
Use: Immunization.
See: Hepatitis A, Inactivated and Hepatitis B, Recombinant Vaccine.
Hepatitis A Vaccine, Inactivated.
Hepatitis B Vaccine, Recombinant.
Human Papillomavirus Recombinant Vaccine, Bivalent.
Human Papillomavirus Recombinant Vaccine, Quadrivalent.
Influenza A and B Vaccine.
Influenza A (H5N1) Virus Vaccine, Adjuvanted.
Influenza A Virus Vaccine, H5N1.
Influenza Virus Vaccine.

Japanese Encephalitis Virus Vaccine.
Measles, Mumps, and Rubella Virus Vaccine, Live.
Measles, Mumps, Rubella, and Varicella Virus Vaccine, Live, Attenuated.
Poliovirus Vaccine, Inactivated.
Rotavirus Vaccine Live.
Rubella and Mumps Virus Vaccine, Live.
Smallpox Vaccine.
Varicella Virus Vaccine.
Yellow Fever Vaccine.
Zoster Vaccine Live.

vaccine, whooping cough. Pertussis Vaccine. *Rx.*
Use: Immunization.
See: Acel-Imune.
ActHIB/DTP.
Diphtheria and Tetanus Toxoids, Acellular Pertussis and Haemophilus Influenzae Type B Conjugate Vaccine.
Diphtheria and Tetanus Toxoids and Acellular Pertussis Vaccine, Adsorbed.
Tripedia.

vaccine, yellow fever. *Rx.*
Use: Immunization.
See: YF-Vax.

vaccine, zoster. *Rx.*
Use: Immunization.
See: Zostavax.

•**vaccinia immune globulin intravenous.** (vax-IN-ee-ah) *USP. Formerly Vaccinia Immune Human Globulin.*
Use: Immunization.

vaccinia immune globulin intravenous (human). (Dynport Vaccine Company LLC) Vaccinia immune globulin 50 mcg/mL (immunoglobulin 2,500 mg/vial). Sucrose 5%, albumin (human) 1%. Soln. for Inj. Vials. *Rx.*
Use: Immunization.

vacocin. Under study.
Use: Anti-infective.

Vademin-Z. (Roberts) Vitamin A 12,500 units, D 50 units, E 50 mg, B_1 10 mg, B_2 5 mg, B_3 25 mg, B_5 10 mg, B_6 2 mg, C 150 mg, Zn 2.6 mg, Mg, Mn. Cap. Bot. 60s. *OTC.*
Use: Mineral, vitamin supplement.

Vagifem. (Novo Nordisk) Estradiol 10 mcg (equiv. to hemihydrate 10.3 mcg), 25 mcg (equiv. to hemihydrate 25.8 mcg). Lactose. Film-coated. Vaginal Tab. Single-use applicator. 8s, 18s. *Rx.*
Use: Estrogen, sex hormone.

Vagi-Gard Advanced Sensitive Formula. (Lake Consumer) Benzocaine 5%, resorcinol, methylparaben, sodium sulfite, EDTA, mineral oil. Cream. Tube 45 g. *OTC.*
Use: Vaginal agent.

Vagi-Gard Maximum Strength. (Lake Consumer) Benzocaine 20%, resorcinol 3%, methylparaben, sodium sulfite, EDTA, mineral oil. Cream. Tube 45 g. *OTC.*
Use: Vaginal agent.

vaginal antifungal agents.
See: Butoconazole Nitrate.
Clotrimazole.
Miconazole Nitrate.
Nystatin.
Terconazole.
Tioconazole.

vaginal preparations.
See: Butoconazole Nitrate.
Chlorhexidine Gluconate
Clindamycin Phosphate.
Clotrimazole.
Metronidazole.
Miconazole Nitrate.
Nystatin.
Sulfonamides.
Terconazole.
Tioconazole.
Vaginal Antifungal Agents.

Vagisec Plus. (Durex) Polyoxyethylene nonylphenol 5.25 mg, sodium edetate 0.66 mg, docusate sodium 0.07 mg, aminoacridine hydrochloride 6 mg. Supp. Box 28s. *Rx.*
Use: Vaginal agent.

Vagisil. (Combe) Benzocaine 5%, resorcinol 2%. Aloe, cetearyl alcohol, corn oil, lanolin alcohol, methylparaben, mineral oil, PEG-100, triethanolamine, trisodium EDTA, vitamins A, D_3, E. Cream. 28 g. *OTC.*
Use: Vaginal agent.

Vagisil Maximum Strength. (Combe) Pramoxine hydrochloride 1%. Aloe, disodium edetate, glycerin, parabens, PEG-7. Wipes. 12s. *OTC.*
Use: Topical local anesthetic.

Vagisil Powder. (Combe) Cornstarch, aloe, mineral oil, benzethonium chloride, magnesium stearate, silica, fragrance. Pow. 198 g, 312 g. *OTC.*
Use: Vaginal agent.

Vagistat-1. (Novartis Consumer Health) Tioconazole 6.5%, white petrolatum. Vaginal Oint. Prefilled single-dose applicator 300 mg. *OTC.*
Use: Antifungal; vaginal.

Vagistat-3 Combination Pack. (Novartis Consumer Health) Miconazole nitrate.
Top. Cream: 2%. Mineral oil. 9 g.
Vag. Supp.: 200 mg. Hydrogenated

vegetable oil. 3s with 3 disposable applicators. *OTC.*
Use: Vaginal preparation.

Valacet. (Pal-Pak, Inc.) Hyoscyamus 10.8 mg, aspirin 259.2 mg, caffeine anhydrous 16.2 mg, gelsemium extract 0.6 mg. Tab. Cap. Bot. 100s, 1000s, 5000s. *Rx.*
Use: Analgesic; anticholinergic; antispasmodic.

•**valacyclovir hydrochloride.** (val-lay-SIGH-kloe-vihr) USAN.
Tall Man: valACYclovir
Use: Antiviral, antiherpes virus agent.
See: Valtrex.

valacyclovir hydrochloride. (Ranbaxy) Valacyclovir hydrochloride 500 mg, 1 g. Film-coated. PEG 400, PEG 6,000. Tab. 10s, 30s, 500s. *Rx.*
Use: Antiviral, antiherpes virus agent.

•**valategrast hydrochloride.** (val-A-te-grast) USAN.
Use: Asthma.

•**valbenazine.** (val-BEN-a-zeen) USAN.
Use: Treatment of hyperkinetic movement disorders.

Valchlor. (Ceptaris) Mechlorethamine 0.016% (equiv. to mechlorethamine hydrochloride 0.02%). Edetate disodium, glycerin, isopropyl alcohol, lactic acid, menthol, propylene glycol. Gel. 60 g. *Rx.*
Use: Alkylating agent, nitrogen mustard.

Valcyte. (Roche) Valganciclovir. **Tab.:** 450 mg (equiv. to valganciclovir hydrochloride). Film-coated. 60s. **Pow. for Soln.:** 50 mg/mL. Mannitol, Saccharin. Tutti-frutti flavor. Glass bot. w/bot. adapter and 2 oral dispensers. 100 mL. *Rx.*
Use: Antiviral.

Valentine. (BDI) Caffeine 200 mg. Tab. Bot. 100s, 500s. *OTC.*
Use: CNS stimulant, analeptic.

Valergen 20. (Hyrex) Estradiol Valerate in oil 20 mg/mL, castor oil, benzyl benzoate, benzyl alcohol. Inj. Multi-dose vial 10 mL. *Rx.*
Use: Estrogen.

•**valerian.** (va-LAR-ee-an) *NF.*
Use: Dietary supplement.

valerian. (Eli Lilly) Tincture, alcohol 68%. Bot. 4 fl oz, 16 fl oz. *Rx.*

•**valerian extract, powdered.** (va-LAR-ee-an) *NF.*
Use: Pharmaceutical vehicle.

Valertest. (Hyrex) **No. 1:** Estradiol valerate 4 mg, testosterone enanthate 90 mg/mL. Vial 10 mL. **No. 2:** Double strength. Vial 10 mL. Amp. 2 mL, 10s. *Rx.*
Use: Androgen, estrogen combination.

valethamate bromide.
Use: Anticholinergic.

•**valganciclovir hydrochloride.** (val-gan-SIGH-kloe-veer) USAN.
Tall Man: valGANciclovir
Use: Antiviral.
See: Valcyte.

•**valine.** (VAY-leen) *USP.*
Use: Amino acid.

valine, isoleucine, and leucine.
Use: Hyperphenylalaninemia. [Orphan Drug]
See: VIL.

Valisone. (Schering-Plough) Betamethasone valerate. **Cream:** 1 mg hydrophilic cream of water, mineral oil, petrolatum, polyethylene glycol 1000 monocetyl ether, cetostearyl alcohol, monobasic sodium phosphate, phosphoric acid, 4-chloro-m-cresol as preservative. Tube 15 g, 45 g, 110 g. Jar 430 g. **Oint.:** 1 mg/g base of liquid and white petrolatum and hydrogenated lanolin. Tube 15 g, 45 g. **Lot.:** 1 mg/g w/isopropyl alcohol 47.5%, water slightly thickened w/carboxyvinyl polymer, pH adjusted w/sodium hydroxide. Bot. 20 mL, 60 mL. **Reduced Strength Cream 0.01%:** Hydrophilic cream of water, mineral oil, petrolatum, polyethylene glycol 1000 monocetyl ether, cetostearyl alcohol, monobasic sodium phosphate, phosphoric acid, 4-chloro-m-cresol as preservative. Tube 15 g, 60 g. *Rx.*
Use: Corticosteroid, topical.

Valium. (Genentech) Diazepam 2 mg, 5 mg, 10 mg. Lactose. Tab. Bot. 100s, 500s. *c-IV.*
Use: Anxiolytic; anticonvulsant.

Valium Injection. (Genentech) Diazepam 5 mg/mL, propylene glycol 40%, ethyl alcohol 10%, sodium benzoate 5%, benzoic acid, benzyl alcohol 1.5%. Amp. 2 mL. Vial 10 mL. *Tel-E-Ject.* (Disposable syringe) 2 mL. *c-IV.*
Use: Anxiolytic; anticonvulsant.

vallergine.
See: Promethazine Hydrochloride.

Valnac Cream. (Alra) Betamethasone valerate 0.1%. Cream. Oint. Tube 15 g, 45 g. *Rx.*
Use: Corticosteroid, topical.

•**valnoctamide.** (val-NOCK-tah-mid) USAN.
Use: Anxiolytic.

•**valomaciclovir stearate.** (val-oh-ma-SYE-kloe-veer) USAN.

Use: Herpes zoster (inhibitor of DNA polymerase).

•**valopicitabine dihydrochloride.** (val-OH-pi-SYE-ta-been) USAN.
Use: Hepatitis.

Valorin. (Otis Clapp) Acetaminophen 325 mg, 500 mg. Sugar free. Tab. 300s (325 mg only), UD 300s (500 mg only). *OTC.*
Use: Analgesic.

valproate.
Use: Anticonvulsant.
See: Depacon.

valproate. (Various Mfr.) Valproate sodium 100 mg/mL. May contain EDTA. May be preservative free. Inj., Conc. Single-dose vials. 5 mL. *Rx.*
Use: Anticonvulsant.

•**valproate sodium.** (VAL-pro-ate) USAN.
Use: Anticonvulsant.
See: Depacon.

•**valproic acid.** (VAL-pro-ik) *USP.*
Use: Anticonvulsant; antimigraine.
See: Depakene.
Stavzor.

valproic acid. (Various Mfr.) Valproic acid. **Cap.:** 250 mg. May contain corn oil, parabens, peanut oil. 100s, UD 80s, UD 100s, UD 300s, UD 750s. **Soln.:** 250 mg/5 mL. May contain alcohol, glycerin, parabens, sorbitol, sucrose. 473 mL, UD 5 mL. *Rx.*
Use: Anticonvulsant.

•**valrocemide.** (val-ROE-se-mide) USAN.
Use: Antiepileptic, anticonvulsant.

•**valsartan.** (VAL-sahr-tan) USAN.
Use: Renin angiotensin system antagonist, angiotensin II receptor antagonist.
See: Diovan.
W/Amlodipine Besylate.
See: Exforge.
W/Amlodipine/Hydrochlorothiazide.
See: Exforge HCT.
W/Hydrochlorothiazide.
See: Diovan HCT.

valsartan and hydrochlorothiazide. (Various Mfr.) Valsartan/hydrochlorothiazide 80 mg/12.5 mg, 160 mg/12.5 mg, 160 mg/25 mg, 320 mg/12.5 mg, 320 mg/25 mg. May contain lactose, PEG, polydextrose. Tab. 90s, 500s, 1,000s, 3,500s (320 mg/12.5 mg and 320 mg/25 mg only), 7,000s (160 mg/12.5 mg and 160 mg/25 mg only), 14,000s (80 mg/12.5 mg only), UD 30s (except 80 mg/12.5 mg). *Rx.*
Use: Antihypertensive combination.

•**valspodar.** (VAL-spoh-dar) USAN.
Use: Antineoplastic; multidrug resistance inhibitor.

•**valtorcitabine dihydrochloride.** (val-tore-SITE-ah-been) USAN.
Use: Antifungal.

Valtrex. (GlaxoSmithKline) Valacyclovir hydrochloride (as base) 500 mg, 1 g. Film-coated. Tab. Bot. 21s (1 g only); 30s, UD 100s (500 mg only). *Rx.*
Use: Antiviral, antiherpes virus agent.

Valturna. (Novartis) Aliskiren/valsartan 150 mg/160 mg, 300 mg/320 mg. Film-coated. Tab. 30s, 90s, UD 100s. *Rx.*
Use: Antihypertensive combination.

Valuphed. (H.L. Moore Drug Exchange) Pseudoephedrine hydrochloride 60 mg, triprolidine hydrochloride 2.5 mg. Tab. Pkg. 24s. *OTC.*
Use: Antihistamine, decongestant.

Vamate. (Major) Hydroxyzine pamoate 50 mg. Cap. Bot. 100s, 250s, 500s, UD 100s. *Rx.*
Use: Anxiolytic.

Vanacof APE. (GM Pharmaceuticals) Chlophedianol hydrochloride 8.3 mg, phenylephrine hydrochloride 3.3 mg, thonzylamine hydrochloride 16.7 mg. Glycerin, maltitol, propylene glycol, saccharin, sodium 2.3 mg per 5 mL, sorbitol. Alcohol free, gluten free, and sugar free. Tutti-frutti flavor. Liq. 118 mL. *OTC.*
Use: Upper respiratory combination, antitussive combination.

Vanacof DM. (GM Pharmaceuticals) Dextromethorphan hydrobromide 6 mg, guaifenesin 66.7 mg, phenylephrine hydrochloride 3.3 mg. Glycerin, methylparaben, sucralose, xylitol. Alcohol free, dye free, gluten free, sugar free. Raspberry flavor. Liq. 240 mL. *OTC.*
Use: Upper respiratory combination, antitussive and expectorant combination.

Vanacof Dx. (GM Pharmaceuticals) Chlophedianol hydrochloride 12.5 mg, guaifenesin 100 mg, pseudoephedrine hydrochloride 30 mg per 5 mL. Glycerin, propylene glycol, saccharin, sorbitol. Alcohol free, dye free, and sugar free. Raspberry flavor. Liq. 473 mL. *OTC.*
Use: Upper respiratory combination, antitussive and expectorant combination.

Vanacof-8. (GM Pharmaceuticals) Chlophedianol hydrochloride 8.3 mg, pyrilamine maleate 16.7 mg. Glycerin, maltitol, propylene glycol, saccharin, sodium 2.3 mg per 5 mL, sorbitol, sucralose. Alcohol free, gluten free, sugar free. Green apple flavor. Liq. 118 mL. *OTC.*
Use: Upper respiratory combination, antitussive combination.

Vanacof GPE. (GM Pharmaceuticals) Chlophedianol hydrochloride 8.3 mg,

guaifenesin 66.7 mg, phenylephrine hydrochloride 3.3 mg. Glycerin, maltitol, propylene glycol, saccharin, sorbitol, sucralose. Alcohol free, gluten free, and sugar free. Raspberry flavor. Liq. 118 mL. *OTC.*
Use: Upper respiratory combination, antitussive and expectorant combination.

Vanadryx TR. (Vangard Labs, Inc.) Dexbrompheniramine maleate 6 mg, pseudoephedrine sulfate 120 mg. Tab. Bot. 100s, 500s. *Rx.*
Use: Antihistamine, decongestant.

VanaHist PD. (GM Pharmaceuticals) Triprolidine hydrochloride 0.625 mg/mL. Glycerin, sucralose, xylitol. Strawberry-banana flavor. Liq. 30 mL. *OTC.*
Use: Antihistamine, nonselective alkylamine.

Vancocin. (ViroPharma) Vancomycin 125 mg, 250 mg. PEG. Cap. *Identi-Dose.* 20s. *Rx.*
Use: Anti-infective agent.

•**vancomycin.** (van-koe-MY-sin) *USP.*
Use: Anti-infective.

•**vancomycin hydrochloride.** (van-koe-MY-sin) *USP.* An antibiotic from *Streptomyces orientalis.*
Use: (IV) Gram-positive (staph.) infection; anti-infective.
See: Vancocin.
Vancoled.

vancomycin hydrochloride. (American Pharmaceutical Partners) Vancomycin 5 g, 10 g. Inj., Pow. for Soln. Pharmacy bulk package. 100 mL. *Rx.*
Use: Anti-infective.

vancomycin hydrochloride. (Baxter) Vancomycin 500 mg, 1 g. Inj., Soln. *Galaxy* container. 100 mL (500 mg only), 200 mL (1 g only). *Rx.*
Use: Anti-infective.

vancomycin hydrochloride. (Various Mfr.) Vancomycin 125 mg, 250 mg. PEG. Cap. Identi-Dose. 20s. *Rx.*
Use: Anti-infective

Vancor Intravenous. (Pharmacia) Vancomycin hydrochloride 500 mg, 1 g. Pow. for Inj. Vials.
Use: Anti-infective.

Vandazole. (Upsher-Smith Laboratories, Inc.) Metronidazole 0.75%. EDTA, parabens. Vaginal Gel. Tube. 70 g with 5 applicators. *Rx.*
Use: Vaginal preparation, anti-infective.

•**vandetanib.** (van-DET-a-nib) USAN.
Use: Antineoplastic.
See: Caprelsa.

Vanex Expectorant. (Jones Pharma) Pseudoephedrine hydrochloride 30 mg, hydrocodone bitartrate 2.5 mg, guaifenesin 100 mg/5 mL. Alcohol 5%, glucose, saccharin, sorbitol, sucrose, tartrazine. Tropical fruit punch flavor. Liq. Bot. 473 mL. *c-III.*
Use: Antitussive, decongestant, expectorant.

Vanicream. (Pharmaceutical Specialties) BHT, ceteareth-20, cetearyl alcohol, glyceryl, PEG, propylene glycol, simethicone, sorbitol, white petrolatum. Dye free and fragrance free. Cream. 453 g. *OTC.*
Use: Pharmaceutical aid; ointment and lotion base.

Vanicream Sunscreen SPF 30. (Pharmaceutical Specialties) Titanium dioxide 5%, zinc oxide 5%, caprylic/capric triglyceride, cetyl alcohol, PEG-12, PEG-30, etrasodium EDTA, vitamin E. PABA free. Cream. 113 g. *OTC.*
Use: Sunscreen.

Vanicream Sunscreen SPF 35. (Pharmaceutical Specialties) Octinoxate 7.5%, zinc oxide 8%, glycerin, PEG-30, castor oil, vitamin E. PABA free. Cream. 113 g. *OTC.*
Use: Sunscreen.

•**vanilla.** (va-NIL-a) *NF.*
Use: Pharmaceutic aid (flavor).

vanillal.
See: Ethyl Vanillin.

•**vanilla tincture.** (va-NIL-a) *NF.*
Use: Pharmaceutic aid (flavor).

•**vanillin.** (vah-NILL-in) *NF.*
Use: Pharmaceutical aid (flavor).

•**vaniprevir.** (van-I-pre-vir) USAN.
Use: Hepatitis C.

Vaniqa. (SkinMedica) Eflornithine hydrochloride 13.9%. Parabens, mineral oil, alcohols. Cream. 30 g. *Rx.*
Use: Dermatological agent.

vanirome.
See: Ethyl Vanillin.

Vanocin. (ViroPharma) Sodium sulfacetamide 10%, sulfur 5%, benzyl alcohol, cetyl alcohol, EDTA, parabens, stearyl alcohol. Lot. Bot. 30 g, 60 g. *Rx.*
Use: Anti-infective.

Vanos. (Medicis) Fluocinonide 0.1%. Cream. 30 g, 60 g. *Rx.*
Use: Anti-inflammatory agent, topical corticosteroid.

Vanoxide HC. (Summers Laboratories) Benzoyl peroxide 5%, hydrocortisone 0.5%. Cetyl alcohol, lanolin oil, mineral oil, parabens, tetrasodium EDTA. Lot. 25 g and kits with *Benzoyl-Pak* and *ABC Lotion. Rx.*
Use: Dermatologic, acne.

Vanquish. (Bayer Consumer Care) Aspirin 227 mg, acetaminophen 194 mg, caffeine 33 mg, aluminum hydroxide 25 mg, magnesium hydroxide 50 mg. Capl. Bot. 60s, 100s. *OTC.*
Use: Analgesic combination; antacid.

Vantas. (Endo Pharmaceuticals) Histrelin acetate 50 mg. Implant, Subcutaneous. In carton with implantation kit. *Rx.*
Use: Hormone, gonadotropin-releasing hormone analog.

•**vantictumab.** (van-TIK-tue-mab) USAN.
Use: Antineoplastic.

Vantin. (Pharmacia & Upjohn) Cefpodoxime proxetil 100 mg, 200 mg. Lactose. Film-coated. Tab. Bot. 20s, 100s, UD 100s. *Rx.*
Use: Anti-infective.

•**vapiprost hydrochloride.** (VAP-ih-prahst) USAN.
Use: Antagonist (thromboxane A_2).

•**vapitadine dihydrochloride.** (va-PI-ta-deen) USAN.
Use: Atopic dermatitis.

Vapocet. (Major) Hydrocodone 5 mg, acetaminophen 500 mg. Tab. Bot. 100s. *c-III.*
Use: Analgesic combination; narcotic.

Vaponefrin. (Medeva) A 2.25% solution of bioassayed racemic epinephrine as hydrochloride, chlorobutanol 0.5%. Soln. Vial 7.5 mL, 15 mL, 30 mL. *OTC.*
Use: Bronchodilator.

Vaporizer in a Bottle. (Columbia) Wick-dispensed medicated vapors.
Use: Cough, cold, sinus, hay fever preparation.

•**vapreotide.** (vap-REE-oh-tide) USAN.
Use: Antineoplastic.

•**vapreotide acetate.** (vap-REE-oh-tide) USAN.
Use: Esophageal bleeding.

Vaprino A-D. (Boehringer Ingelheim) Loperamide hydrochloride 2 mg. Tab. 12s, 48s. *OTC.*
Use: Antidiarrheal.

Vaprisol Premixed in Dextrose 5%. (Cumberland) Conivaptan hydrochloride 0.2 mg/mL. Dextrose 5 g. Inj., Soln. *Intravia* plastic container. 100 mL. *Rx.*
Use: Vasopressin receptor antagonist.

Vaqta. (Merck) **Adult:** Hepatitis A virus antigen 50 U/mL. **Pediatric/Adolescent:** Hepatitis A virus antigen 25 U/0.5 mL, Inj. Single-dose vial, prefilled syringe. *Rx.*
Use: Active immunization agent, viral vaccine.

•**vardenafil dihydrochloride.** (var-DEN-a-fil) USAN.
Use: Erectile dysfunction.

vardenafil hydrochloride.
Use: Impotence agent.
See: Levitra.
Staxyn.

•**varenicline tartrate.** (var-e-NI-kleen) USAN.
Use: Smoking cessation.
See: Chantix.

•**varespladib.** (va-res-PLA-dib) USAN.
Use: Treatment of dyslipidemia.

•**varespladib methyl.** (va-res-PLA-dib) USAN.
Use: Treatment of dyslipidemia.

Varibar Honey. (Bracco Diagnostics) Barium sulfate 40%. Apple flavoring, glycerin, polysorbate 80, potassium sorbate, saccharin, simethicone, sodium benzoate, xylitol. Susp. 250 mL. *Rx.*
Use: Radiopaque agent, miscellaneous GI contrast agent.

Varibar Nectar. (Bracco Diagnostics) Barium sulfate 40%. Apple flavoring, glycerin, maltodextrin, polysorbate 80, potassium sorbate, saccharin, simethicone, sodium benzoate, xylitol. Susp. 240 mL. *Rx.*
Use: Radiopaque agent, miscellaneous GI contrast agent.

Varibar Pudding. (Bracco Diagnostics) Barium sulfate 40%. Glycerin, maltodextrin, polysorbate 80, potassium sorbate, saccharin, simethicone, sodium benzoate, vanilla flavoring, xylitol. Paste. 230 mL. *Rx.*
Use: Radiopaque agent, miscellaneous GI contrast agent.

Varibar Thin Honey. (Bracco Diagnostics) Barium sulfate 40%. Apple flavoring, glycerin, polysorbate 80, potassium sorbate, saccharin, simethicone, sodium benzoate, xylitol. Susp. 250 mL. *Rx.*
Use: Radiopaque agent, miscellaneous GI contrast agent.

Varibar Thin Liquid. (Bracco Diagnostics) Barium sulfate 40%. Apple flavoring, maltodextrin, polysorbate 80, saccharin, simethicone, xylitol. Pow. for Susp. 148 g. *Rx.*
Use: Radiopaque agent, miscellaneous GI contrast agent.

varicella virus vaccine.
Use: Immunization, viral vaccine.
See: Varivax.
Zostavax.

varicella-zoster IgG IFA test system. (Wampole) Test for the qualitative or semi-qualitative detection of VZ IgG antibody in human serum. Test kit 100s.
Use: Diagnostic aid.

•**varicella-zoster immune globulin.** (var-i-SEL-a ZOS-ter) *USP.*
Use: Immunization.

Vari-Flavors. (Ross) Flavor packets to provide flavor variety for patients on liquid diets. Dextrose, artificial flavor, artificial color. Packet 1 g, Ctn. 24s. *Rx.*
Use: Flavoring.

Variplex-C. (NBTY) Vitamins B_1 15 mg, B_2 10 mg, B_3 100 mg, B_5 20 mg, B_6 5 mg, B_{12} 10 mcg, C 500 mg. Tab. Bot. 100s. *OTC.*
Use: Vitamin supplement.

Varithena. (Biocompatibles) Polidocanol 10 mg/mL. Ethanol 4.2%. Inj., foam. 303 mL w/pressurized oxygen canister and administration kit. *Rx.*
Use: Sclerosing agent.

Varivax. (Merck & Co.) Varicella virus vaccine. 1350 PFU of Oka/Merck varicella virus (live), sucrose. Pow. for Inj. Single-dose vials 1s, 10s. *Rx.*
Use: Immunization, viral vaccine.

Varizig. (Cangene Corporation) Varicella-zoster immune globulin (human) 125 units. Polysorbate 80. Preservative free. Inj., lyophilized Pow. for Soln. Single-use vial w/diluent. *Rx.*
Use: Immune globulin.

•**varlitinib.** (var-li-TIN-ib) USAN.
Use: Antineoplastic.

•**varlitinib tosylate.** (var-LI-ti-nib) USAN.
Use: Antineoplastic.

Vascepa. (Amarin Pharma) Icosapent ethyl 1 g. Glycerin, maltitol, sorbitol. Cap., softgel. 120s. *Rx.*
Use: Antihyperlipidemic agent.

Vascunitol. (Apco) Mannitol hexanitrate 0.5 g. Tab. Bot. 100s. *Rx.*
Use: Vasodilator.

Vascused. (Apco) Mannitol hexanitrate 0.5 g, phenobarbital 0.25 g. Tab. Bot. 100s. *Rx.*
Use: Vasodilator.

Vaseline Dermatology Formula Cream. (Chesebrough-Ponds USA) Petrolatum, mineral oil, dimethicone. Jar 3 oz, 5.25 oz. *OTC.*
Use: Emollient.

Vaseline Dermatology Formula Lotion. (Chesebrough-Ponds USA) Petrolatum, mineral oil, dimethicone. Bot. 5.5 oz, 11 oz, 16 oz. *OTC.*
Use: Emollient.

Vaseline First Aid Carboxylated Petroleum Jelly. (Chesebrough-Ponds USA) Petrolatum, chloroxylenol. Plastic Jar 1.75 oz, 3.75 oz. Plastic Tube 1 oz, 2.5 oz. *OTC.*
Use: Medicated anti-infective.

Vaseline Intensive Care Active Sport. (Chesebrough-Ponds USA) Ethylhexyl p-methoxycinnamate, oxybenzone. PABA free. **SPF 8:** Lot. Bot. 120 mL. **SPF 15:** Lot. Bot. 120 mL. *OTC.*
Use: Sunscreen.

Vaseline Intensive Care Baby SPF 15. (Chesebrough-Ponds USA) Titanium dioxide. PABA free. Waterproof. Lot. Bot. 120 mL. *OTC.*
Use: Sunscreen.

Vaseline Intensive Care Baby SPF 30. (Chesebrough-Ponds USA) Ethylhexyl p-methoxycinnamate, oxybenzone, 2-ethylhexyl salicylate, titanium dioxide, C12-15 alkyl benzoate, glycerin, aloe vera gel, vitamin E, cetyl alcohol, parabens, EDTA. Lot. Bot. 118 mL. *OTC.*
Use: Sunscreen.

Vaseline Intensive Care Blockout SPF 40+. (Chesebrough-Ponds USA) Padimate O, ethylhexyl p-methoxycinnamate, oxybenzone, 2-ethylhexyl salicylate, titanium dioxide. Waterproof. Lot. Bot. 120 mL. *OTC.*
Use: Sunscreen.

Vaseline Intensive Care Blockout SPF 30. (Chesebrough-Ponds USA) Ethylhexyl p-methoxycinnamate, oxybenzone, 2-ethylhexyl salicylate, titanium dioxide. Waterproof. Lot. Bot. 120 mL. *OTC.*
Use: Sunscreen.

Vaseline Intensive Care Moisturizing Sunscreen. (Chesebrough-Ponds USA) Ethylhexyl p-methoxycinnamate, oxybenzone, C12-15 alkyl octanoate, glycerin, aloe vera gel, cetyl alcohol, petrolatum, vitamin E, parabens, EDTA. SPF 4, SPF 8: Lot. Bot. 117 mL. *OTC.*
Use: Sunscreen.

Vaseline Intensive Care No Burn No Bite SPF 8. (Chesebrough-Ponds USA) Ethylhexyl p-methoxycinnamate, oxybenzone. PABA free. Waterproof. Lot. Bot. 180 mL. *OTC.*
Use: Sunscreen.

Vaseline Intensive Care Sport Sunblock. (Chesebrough-Ponds USA) Ethylhexyl p-methoxycinnamate, oxybenzone, C12-15 alkyl benzoate, aloe vera gel, vitamin E, EDTA. Lot. Bot. 118 mL. *OTC.*
Use: Sunscreen.

Vaseline Intensive Care Sunblock. (Chesebrough-Ponds USA) Ethylhexyl p-methoxycinnamate, oxybenzone, 2-ethylhexyl salicylate. PABA free. Waterproof. **SPF 4:** Lot. Bot. 180 mL; **SPF 8:** Lot. Bot. 120 mL, 180 mL; **SPF 15:** Lot. Bot. 120 mL, 180 mL; **SPF 25:** Lot.

Bot. 120 mL, 180 mL. *OTC.*
Use: Sunscreen.

Vaseline Intensive Care Ultra Violet Daily Defense. (Chesebrough-Ponds USA) Ethylhexyl p-methoxycinnamate, oxybenzone, vitamin E, cetyl alcohol, acetylated lanolin, alcohol, parabens, EDTA. SPF 15. Lot. Bot. 118 mL. *OTC.*
Use: Sunscreen.

Vaseline Pure Petroleum Jelly Skin Protectant. (Chesebrough-Ponds USA) White petrolatum. Tube 1 oz, 2.5 oz. Jar 1.75 oz, 3.75 oz, 7.75 oz, 13 oz. *OTC.*
Use: Dermatologic; counterirritant.

Vaseretic. (Valeant) Enalapril maleate/hydrochlorothiazide 10 mg/25 mg. Lactose. Tab. 100s. *Rx.*
Use: Antihypertensive.

Vasimid.
See: Tolazoline Hydrochloride.

vasoactive intestinal polypeptide. (Research Triangle Pharmaceuticals)
Use: Treatment of acute esophageal food impaction. [Orphan Drug]

Vasoderm. (Taro) Fluocinonide 0.05%, anhydrous glycerin base. Cream. Tube 15 g, 30 g, 60 g. *Rx.*
Use: Corticosteroid, topical.

Vasoderm-E. (Taro) Fluocinonide 0.05%, emollient mineral oil and white petrolatum base. Cream. Tube 15 g, 30 g, 60 g, 120 g. *Rx.*
Use: Corticosteroid, topical.

Vasodilan. (Mead Johnson) Isoxsuprine hydrochloride 10 mg, 20 mg. Tab. 100s, 1000s, UD 100s (10 mg only). *Rx.*
Use: Vasodilator.

vasodilator combinations.
See: Isosorbide Dinitrate/Hydralazine Hydrochloride.

vasodilator combinations, peripheral.
See: Lipo-Nicin.

vasodilators.
See: Amyl Nitrite.
Endothelin Receptor Antagonists.
Human B-Type Natriuretic Peptides.
Nitrates.
Prostacyclin Analog.
Soluble Guanylate Cyclase Stimulators.
Vasodilator Combinations.
Vasodilator Combinations, Peripheral.
Vasodilators, Peripheral.

vasodilators, coronary.
See: Glyceryl Trinitrate.
Isordil.
Khellin.
Papaverine Hydrochloride.
Pentaerythritol Tetranitrate.
Peritrate.

vasodilators, peripheral.
See: Epoprostenol Sodium.
Ethaverine Hydrochloride.
Hydralazine Hydrochloride.
Isoxsuprine Hydrochloride.
Minoxidil.
Papaverine Hydrochloride.
Treprostinil Sodium.
Vasodilator Combinations, Peripheral.

Vasoflo. (Roberts) Papaverine hydrochloride 150 mg. Cap. Bot. 100s. *Rx.*
Use: Vasodilator.

Vasolate. (Parmed Pharmaceuticals, Inc.) Pentaerythritol tetranitrate 30 mg. Cap. Bot. 100s, 1000s. *Rx.*
Use: Antianginal.

Vasolate-80. (Parmed Pharmaceuticals, Inc.) Pentaerythritol tetranitrate 80 mg. Cap. Bot. 100s, 1000s. *Rx.*
Use: Antianginal.

Vasolex. (Stratus) Balsam peru 87 mg, castor oil 788 mg, trypsin 90 units. White petrolatum. Oint. 5 g, 30 g, 60 g. *Rx.*
Use: Dermatologic, enzyme preparation.

•**vasopressin.** (VAY-so-PRESS-in) *USP.*
Use: Posterior pituitary hormone.
See: Pitressin Synthetic.

vasopressin. (Various Mfr.) Vasopressin 20 pressor units/mL. Chlorobutanol 0.5%. Inj. Vial. 0.5 mL, 1 mL, 10 mL. *Rx.*
Use: Posterior pituitary hormone.

vasopressin receptor antagonist.
See: Conivaptan Hydrochloride.
Tolvaptan.

vasopressors.
See: Dobutamine.
Dobutamine Hydrochloride in 5% Dextrose Injection.
Dopamine Hydrochloride.
Droxidopa.
Ephedrine.
Epinephrine.
Isoproterenol Hydrochloride.
Metaraminol.
Midodrine Hydrochloride.
Norepinephrine Bitartrate.
Phenylephrine Hydrochloride.

Vasotec. (Biovail) Enalapril maleate 2.5 mg, 5 mg, 10 mg, 20 mg. Lactose. Tab. 30s, 90s, 1,000s (except 2.5 mg). *Rx.*
Use: Renin angiotensin system antagonist, angiotensin-converting enzyme inhibitor.

Vasotus. (Sheryl) Codeine phosphate 1/6 g, phenylephrine hydrochloride, prophenpyridamine maleate. Liq. Bot. 473 mL. *c-v.*
Use: Antihistamine, antitussive, decongestant.

•**vatiquinone.** (va-TI-kwi-NONE) USAN.
Use: Treatment of inherited mitochondrial respiratory chain diseases.

Vaxsyn HIV-1. (MicroGeneSys) T-Lymphotropic Virus Type III GP 160 Antigen.
Use: AIDS. [Orphan Drug]

Vazobid-PD. (Wraser) Brompheniramine maleate 1.2 mg, phenylephrine hydrochloride 2 mg. Acesulfame, aspartame, glycerin, methylparaben, sodium benzoate. Bubble gum flavor. Susp. 118 mL. *OTC.*
Use: Upper respiratory combination, decongestant and antihistamine.

Vazosan. (Sandia) Papaverine hydrochloride 150 mg. Tab. Bot. 100s, 1000s. *Rx.*
Use: Vasodilator.

Vazotab. (Gentex Pharma) Phenylephrine hydrochloride 10 mg, pyrilamine maleate 25 mg. Tab. 100s. *OTC.*
Use: Upper respiratory combination, decongestant and antihistamine.

Vazotan. (Gentex Pharma) Phenylephrine hydrochloride 10 mg, brompheniramine maleate 6 mg, carbetapentane citrate 25 mg per 5 mL. Methylparaben, phenylalanine 8.419 mg/5 mL. Bubble gum flavor. Oral Susp. 120 mL. *Rx.*
Use: Antitussive combination.

V-Cillin K. (Eli Lilly) Penicillin V potassium 125 mg, 250 mg, 500 mg. Tab. **125 mg:** Bot. 100s. **250 mg:** Bot. 100s, 500s. **500 mg:** Bot. 24s, 100s, 500s. *Rx.*
Use: Anti-infective; penicillin.

V-Cillin K for Oral Solution. (Eli Lilly) Penicillin V potassium 125 mg, 250 mg/ 5 mL. **125 mg:** Bot. 100 mL, 150 mL, 200 mL, UD 5 mL. **250 mg:** Bot. 100 mL, 150 mL, 200 mL. *Rx.*
Use: Anti-infective; penicillin.

V-Cof. (Macoven Pharmaceuticals) Brompheniramine maleate 6 mg, carbetapentane citrate 25 mg, phenylephrine hydrochloride 10 mg per 5 mL. Acesulfame, aspartame, glycerin, methylparaben, sodium benzoate. Bubble gum flavor. Susp. 118 mL. *Rx.*
Use: Upper respiratory combination, antitussive combination.

V-Dec-M. (Seatrace) Pseudoephedrine hydrochloride 120 mg, guaifenesin 500 mg. SR Tab. Bot. 12s, 100s. *Rx.*
Use: Upper respiratory combination; decongestant, expectorant.

VDRL Antigen. (Laboratory Diagnostics) VDRL antigen with buffered saline. Blood test in diagnosis of syphilis. **Vial:** Sufficient for 500 tests. **Amp.:** 10 × 0.5 mL sufficient for 500 tests.
Use: Diagnostic aid.

VDRL Slide Test. (Laboratory Diagnostics) VDRL antigen. Slide flocculation and spinal fluid test for syphilis. Vial 5 mL Complete kit, reactive control, nonreactive control, 5 mL.
Use: Diagnostic aid.

Vectibix. (Amgen) Panitumumab 20 mg/ mL. Preservative free. Sodium acetate, sodium chloride. Soln. for Inj. Single-use vials. 5 mL, 10 mL, 20 mL. *Rx.*
Use: Monoclonal antibody.

Vectical. (Galderma) Calcitriol 0.0003%. Mineral oil, white petrolatum. Oint. Tube. 5 g, 100 g. *Rx.*
Use: Antipsoriatic agent.

Vectrin. (Warner Chilcott) Minocycline 50 mg, 100 mg. Cap. Bot. 50s (100 mg only), 100s (50 mg only), 1000s. *Rx.*
Use: Anti-infective.

•**vecuronium bromide.** (veh-CUE-row-nee-uhm) *USP.*
Use: Neuromuscular blocker.

vecuronium bromide. (Marsam) Vecuronium bromide 10 mg, 20 mg. Inj. Vial 10 mL (with and without diluent), 20 mL (without diluent). *Rx.*
Use: Neuromuscular blocker.

vecuronium bromide. (Various Mfr.) Vecuronium bromide 10 mg, 20 mg. May contain mannitol. Pow. for Inj. Vials. 10 mL (10 mg only), 20 mL (20 mg only). *Rx.*
Use: Neuromuscular blocker.

•**vedolizumab.** (VE-doe-LIZ-ue-mab) USAN.
Use: Immunomodulator.

•**vedotin.** (ve-DOE-tin) USAN.
Use: Antineoplastic.

•**vedroprevir.** (ved-ROE-pre-vir) USAN.
Use: Treatment of hepatitis C.

VE-400. (Western Research) Vitamin E 400 units. Cap. Bot. 1008s. *OTC.*
Use: Vitamin supplement.

•**vegetable oil, hydrogenated.** *NF.*
Use: Pharmaceutical aid (tablet/capsule lubricant).

vehicle/n and vehicle/n mild. (Neutrogena) Topical vehicle system for compounding. *Appliderm* Applicator Bot. oz. *OTC.*
Use: Pharmaceutical aid.

velacycline.
Use: Anti-infective; tetracycline.

•**velafermin.** (VEL-a-FER-min) USAN.
Use: Mucositis.

•**velaglucerase alfa.** (VEL-a-GLOO-ser-ase) USAN.
Use: Endocrine and metabolic agent.
See: VPRIV.

Velban. (Lilly) Vinblastine sulfate 10 mg. Pow. for Inj. Vial. *Rx.*
Use: Antineoplastic.

Velcade. (Millenium) Bortezomib 3.5 mg. Mannitol 35 mg. Preservative free. Pow. for Inj., lyophilized. Single-dose vials. *Rx.*
Use: Proteasome inhibitor.

•**velcalcetide.** (vel-KAL-se-tide) USAN.
Use: Treatment of secondary hyperparathyroidism associated with chronic kidney disease.

•**velcalcetide hydrochloride.** (vel-KAL-se-tide) USAN.
Use: Treatment of secondary hyperparathyroidism associated with chronic kidney disease.

•**veledimex.** (vel-ED-i-mex) USAN.
Use: Immunostimulant; antineoplastic.

Veletri. (Actelion) Epoprostenol 0.5 mg, 1.5 mg (as epoprostenol sodium). Sucrose. Inj., lyophilized Pow. for Soln. Single-use vial. *Rx.*
Use: Peripheral vasodilator.

•**veliflapon.** (VEL-i-FLAP-on) USAN.
Use: Cardiovascular agent.

•**veliparib.** (veli-PAR-ib) USAN.
Use: Antineoplastic.

Velivet. (Barr) **Phase 1:** Desogestrel 0.1 mg, ethinyl estradiol 25 mcg. 7 tabs. **Phase 2:** Desogestrel 0.125 mg, ethinyl estradiol 25 mcg. 7 tabs. **Phase 3:** Desogestrel 0.15 mg, ethinyl estradiol 25 mcg. 7 tabs. Tab. 28s with 7 inert tabs. *Rx.*
Use: Sex hormone, contraceptive hormone.

•**velnacrine maleate.** (VELL-NAH-kreen) USAN.
Use: Inhibitor (cholinesterase).

•**velneperit.** (vel-NEP-er-it) USAN.
Use: Treatment of clinical obesity.

Velphoro. (Fresenius) Sucroferric oxyhydroxide 500 mg (equiv. to sucroferric oxyhydroxide 2,500 mg). Sucrose, woodberry flavoring. Chew. Tab. 90s. *Rx.*
Use: Trace element, iron-containing product.

•**velusetrag.** (vel-u-SET-rag) USAN.
Use: Treatment of constipation.

•**velusetrag hydrochloride.** (vel-u-SET-rag) USAN.
Use: Treatment of constipation.

Velvachol. (Valeant) Hydrophilic ointment base petrolatum, mineral oil, cetyl alcohol, cholesterol, parabens, stearyl alcohol, purified water, sodium lauryl sulfate. Jar lb. *OTC.*
Use: Pharmaceutical aid; ointment base.

•**vemurafenib.** (VEM-ue-RAF-e-nib) USAN.
Use: Antineoplastic.
See: Zelboraf.

Venelex. (Stratus) Balsam peru 87 mg, castor oil 788 mg, white petrolatum. Oint. 60 g. *Rx.*
Use: Emollient.

venesetic.
See: Amobarbital Sodium.

venlafaxine. (Upstate Pharma) Venlafaxine 37.5 mg, 75 mg, 150 mg, 225 mg. May contain lactose and mannitol. ER Tab. 30s, 90s. *Rx.*
Use: Antidepressant, serotonin and norepinephrine reuptake inhibitor.

•**venlafaxine hydrochloride.** (VEN-lah-fax-EEN) USAN.
Use: Antidepressant.
See: Effexor XR.

venlafaxine hydrochloride. (Various Mfr.) Venlafaxine. **Tab.:** 25 mg, 37.5 mg, 50 mg, 75 mg, 100 mg. May contain lactose, mannitol, PEG. 30s, 60s, 90s, 100s, 500s, 1,000s, UD 100s **ER Cap.:** 37.5 mg, 75 mg, 150 mg. May contain sugar spheres. 30s, 90s. *Rx.*
Use: Antidepressant.

Venofer. (Fresenius) Elemental iron 20 mg/mL, preservative free, sucrose 300 mg/mL. Inj. Single-dose vial. 2.5 mL, 5 mL, 10 mL. *Rx.*
Use: Trace element.

Venomil. (Bayer Consumer Care) Freeze-dried venom or venom protein. Vials of 12 mcg or 120 mcg for honey bee, white-faced hornet, yellow hornet, yellow jacket, or wasp. Vials of 36 mcg or 360 mcg for mixed vespids (white-faced hornet, yellow hornet, yellow jacket). Diagnostic 1 mcg/mL. Maintenance 100 mcg/mL. Individual patient kit. *Rx.*
Use: Antivenin.

Venstat. (Seatrace) Brompheniramine maleate 10 mg/mL. Vial 10 mL. *Rx.*
Use: Antihistamine.

Ventavis. (CoTherix) Iloprost 10 mcg/mL, 20 mcg/mL. Ethanol 0.81 mg (10 mcg/mL), 1.62 mg (20 mcg/mL). Preservative free. Soln. for Inh. Single-dose ampules. 1 mL. *Rx.*
Use: Treatment of pulmonary hypertension.

Ventolin. (GlaxoSmithKline) Albuterol. **Syr.:** Albuterol sulfate 2 mg/5 mL, saccharin, strawberry flavor. Bot. 480 mL. **Tab.:** Albuterol sulfate 2 mg, 4 mg. Bot. 100s, 500s. *Rx.*
Use: Bronchodilator, sympathomimetic.

Ventolin HFA. (GlaxoSmithKline) Albuterol sulfate 90 mcg/actuation. Aerosol.

Can. 18 g (200 inhalations). Contains no chlorofluorocarbons. *Rx.*
Use: Bronchodilator, sympathomimetic.

Ventolin Inhalation Solution. (GlaxoSmithKline) Albuterol sulfate 0.5%. Bot. 20 mL w/calibrated dropper. *Rx.*
Use: Bronchodilator.

Ventolin Nebules. (GlaxoSmithKline) Albuterol sulfate 0.083%, sulfuric acid. Soln. for Inh. In 3 mL unit-dose nebules. *Rx.*
Use: Bronchodilator.

Ventolin Rotacaps. (GlaxoSmithKline) Microfine albuterol sulfate 200 mg, lactose. Cap. for Inh. Bot. 100s, UD 24s. For use with the *Rotahaler* inhalation device. *Rx.*
Use: Bronchodilator.

•**veradoline hydrochloride.** (VEER-aid-OLE-een) USAN.
Use: Analgesic.

Veramyst. (GlaxoSmithKline) Fluticasone furoate 27.5 mcg/actuation. Dextrose 0.015% w/w benzalkonium chloride, polysorbate 80, EDTA. Spray, Susp. Intranasal. 10 g (120 actuations) brown glass bottles with metering atomizing pump and nasal adaptor. *Rx.*
Use: Intranasal steroid, respiratory inhalant.

•**verapamil.** (veh-RAP-ah-mill) USAN.
Use: Vasodilator (coronary).

•**verapamil hydrochloride.** (veh-RAP-ah-mill) *USP.*
Use: Antianginal, antiarrhythmic, antihypertensive, calcium channel blocker.
See: Calan.
Calan SR.
Covera-HS.
Isoptin SR.
Verelan.
Verelan PM.
W/Trandolapril.
See: Tarka.

verapamil hydrochloride. (Various Mfr.) Verapamil hydrochloride. **40 mg. Tab.:** May contain lactose. Bot. 30s, 100s, 500s, 1000s. **80 mg, 120 mg. Tab.:** May contain lactose. 100s, 250s, 500s, 1000s, 4000s (120 mg only), 7000s (80 mg only), UD 100s. **2.5 mg/mL. Inj.:** May contain sodium chloride. 2 mL, 4 mL vials, amps, and syringes; single-use 2 mL fills; *Carpuject* syringe 2 mL; 2 mL fill in single-use 2 mL *Carpuject Interlink* syringe. **ER Cap.:** 100 mg, 200 mg, 300 mg. May contain maltodextrin, sugar spheres. 30s, 100s, 500s. *Rx.*
Use: Antianginal; antiarrhythmic; antihypertensive; calcium channel blocker.

verapamil hydrochloride extended release. (Various Mfr.) Verapamil hydrochloride. **ER Cap.:** 120 mg, 180 mg, 240 mg. May be pellet-filled. May contain sugar. Bot. 100s, 500s, UD 100s. **ER Tab.:** 120 mg, 180 mg, 240 mg. 100s, 500s. *Rx.*
Use: Antianginal; antiarrhythmic; antihypertensive; calcium channel blocker.

verapamil hydrochloride extended release. (Watson) Verapamil hydrochloride 360 mg. Pellet-filled. ER Cap. 100s. *Rx.*
Use: Calcium channel blocker.

verapamil hydrochloride SR. (Schein) Verapamil hydrochloride 120 mg, 180 mg, 240 mg, 360 mg, parabens. SR Cap. Bot. 100s. *Rx.*
Use: Antianginal; antiarrythmic; antihypertensive.

Verazeptol. (Femco) Chlorothymol, eucalyptol, menthol, phenol, boric acid, zinc sulfate. Pow. Bot. 3 oz, 6 oz, 10 oz. *OTC.*
Use: Vaginal agent.

Verazinc. (Forest) Zinc sulfate 220 mg. Cap. Bot. 100s, 1000s. *OTC.*
Use: Mineral supplement.

•**vercirnon.** (ver-SIR-non) USAN.
Use: Immunomodulator.

•**vercirnon sodium.** (ver-SIR-non) USAN.
Use: Immunomodulator.

Verdeso. (Aqua Pharmaceuticals) Desonide 0.05%. Cetyl alcohol, light mineral oil, propylene glycol, white petrolatum. Aer., foam. 100 g. *Rx.*
Use: Anti-inflammatory agent, topical corticosteroid.

Veregen. (Doak Dermatologics) Kunecatechins 15%. Gallic acid, caffeine, and theobromine constitute ≈ 2.5% of the product. Isopropyl myristate, oleyl alcohol. Oint. Tube. 15 g. *Rx.*
Use: Catechin, treatment of external genital and perianal warts.

Verelan. (Kremers Urban) Verapamil hydrochloride 120 mg, 180 mg, 240 mg, 360 mg. Sugar, parabens. Pellet-filled. ER Cap. Bot. 100s. *Rx.*
Use: Calcium channel blocker.

Verelan PM. (Kremers Urban) Verapamil hydrochloride 100 mg, 200 mg, 300 mg. Sugar. Pellet-filled. ER Cap. Bot. 100s. *Rx.*
Use: Calcium channel blocker.

Vergo. (Daywell Laboratories, Inc.) Calcium pantothenate 8%, ascorbic acid 2%, starch. Oint. Tube 0.5 oz. *Rx.*
Use: Keratolytic.

•**verilopam hydrochloride.** (veh-RILL-OH-pam) USAN.
Use: Analgesic.

Veripred 20. (Hawthorn Pharmaceuticals) Prednisolone 20 mg per 5 mL. Equiv. to prednisolone sodium phosphate 26.9 mg. Corn syrup, edetate disodium, methylparaben, saccharin. Grape flavor. Soln., Oral. 237 mL. *Rx.*
Use: Adrenocortical steroid, glucocorticoid.

•**verlukast.** (ver-LOO-kast) USAN.
Use: Antiasthmatic (leukotriene antagonist).

Verluma. (NeoRx; DuPont) Nofetumomab merpentan 10 mg for conjugation w/technetium 99m. Kit. *Rx.*
Use: Radioimmunoscintigraphy agent.

Vermox. (Janssen) Mebendazole 100 mg. Tab. Box 12s. *Rx.*
Use: Anthelmintic.

vernamycins. Under study.
Use: Anti-infective.

vernolepin. A sesquiterpene dilactone. Under study.
Use: Antineoplastic.

•**verofylline.** (VER-OH-fill-in) USAN.
Use: Antiasthmatic; bronchodilator.

veronal sodium.
See: Barbital Sodium.

•**verpasep caltespen.** (VER-pa-sep kal-TES-pen) USAN.
Use: Human papillomavirus.

Versa Alcohol Base. (Humco) Aloe, ethylhexylglycerin, SD alcohol 40, polyacrylamide, laureth-7, phenoxyethanol. Fragrance, oil, and dye free. Gel. 1 lb, 10 lb, 20 lb, 40 lb. *OTC.*
Use: Ointment and lotion base.

Versa Aqua Base. (Humco) DMDM hydantoin, iodoproyl butylcarbamate, PEG-18 palmitate, PPG-18 butyl ether, propylene glycol, SD alcohol 40, triethanolamine. Fragrance and dye free. Gel. 1 lb, 10 lb, 20 lb, 40 lb. *OTC.*
Use: Ointment and lotion base.

Versacaps. (Seatrace) Pseudoephedrine hydrochloride 60 mg, guaifenesin 300 mg, benzyl alcohol, EDTA, parabens, sucrose. SR. Cap. Bot. 100s. *Rx.*
Use: Upper respiratory combination; decongestant, expectorant.

Versacloz. (Jazz Pharmaceuticals) Clozapine 50 mg/mL. Glycerin, parabens, sorbitol. Susp. 100 mL. *Rx.*
Use: Antipsychotic agent, dibenzapine derivative.

Versa HRT Base Botanical. (Humco) Almond, aloe, carbomer, cetyl alcohol, folic acid, glycerin, glyceryl stearate, grape, MSM, PEG-100 stearate, phenoxyethanol, primrose, red clover, salicylic acid, selenium, stearic acid, triethanolamine, wheat, and vitamins A,C,D, and E. Cream. 1 lb, 10 lb, 20 lb, 40 lb. *OTC.*
Use: Ointment and lotion base.

Versa HRT Base Heavy. (Humco) Almond, C12–15 alkyl benzoate, caprylic/capric triglyceride, carbomer, cetyl alcohol, dimethicone, glyceryl stearate, olive, PEG-100 stearate, propylene glycol, stearic acid, triethanolamine, wheat, and vitamins A and E. Cream. 1 lb, 10 lb, 20 lb, 40 lb. *OTC.*
Use: Ointment and lotion base.

Versa HRT Base Natural. (Humco) Almond, carbomer, cetyl alcohol, glycerin, glyceryl stearate, PEG-100 stearate, phenoxyethanol, salicylic acid, stearic acid, triethanolamine, wheat, and vitamins A, C, and E. Cream. 1 lb, 10 lb, 20 lb, 40 lb. *OTC.*
Use: Ointment and lotion base.

Versal. (Suppositoria Laboratories, Inc.) Bismuth subgallate, balsam peru, zinc oxide, benzyl benzoate. Supp. Box 12s, 100s, 1000s. *OTC.*
Use: Anorectal preparation.

Versa LipoBase Heavy. (Humco) Ceteareth-12, ceteareth-20, cetearyl alcohol, cetearyl isononanoate, cetyl palmitate, glycerin, glyceryl stearate, lecithin, honeysuckle, perilla, polyquaternium-37, PPG-1, trideceth-7, propylene glycol dicaprylate/dicaprate, tea tree, vitamin E. Water and oil soluble. Cream. 1 lb, 10 lb, 20 lb, 40 lb. *OTC.*
Use: Ointment and lotion base.

Versa LipoBase Regular. (Humco) Almond, aloe, C12-15 alkyl benzoate, cetearyl alcohol, cetearyl glucoside, cetyl alcohol, dimethicone, glycerin, glyceryl stearate, grape, hydroxymethylglycinate, lecithin, perilla, phenoxyethanol, polyacrylamide, silicate, wheat, xanthan, and vitamins A, C, and E. Water and oil soluble. Cream. 1 lb, 10 lb, 20 lb, 40 lb. *OTC.*
Use: Ointment and lotion base.

Versa PLO20. (Humco) Isopropyl palmitate, pluronic lecithin 20%, poloxamer 407. Gel. In flowable (with SD alcohol 40) and regular. 1 lb. *OTC.*
Use: Ointment and lotion base.

Versa VaniBase. (Humco) Caprylic/capric triglyceride, ceteareth-20, cetearyl alcohol, dimethicone, ethylhexylglycerin, glyceryl stearate, isopropyl palmitate, octydodecanol, PEG-100 stearate, phenoxyethanol, propylene glycol, triethanolamine. Fragrance and dye free. Cream. 1 lb. *OTC.*
Use: Ointment and lotion base.

versenate, calcium disodium.
See: Calcium Disodium Versenate.

versenate disodium.
See: Disodium Versenate.

•**versetamide.** (ver-SET-ah-mide) USAN.
Use: Pharmaceutical aid.

Versiclear. (Hope) Sodium thiosulfate 25%, salicylic acid 1%, isopropyl alcohol 10%, propylene glycol, menthol, EDTA. Lot. 120 mL. *Rx.*
Use: Anti-infective, topical.

versidyne.
Use: Analgesic.

Verstran. (Parke-Davis) Prazepam.
Use: Anxiolytic.

•**verteporfin.** (ver-teh-PORE-fin) USAN.
Use: Antineoplastic; ophthalmic phototherapy.
See: Visudyne.

•**verubulin.** (VER-ue-BUE-lin) USAN.
Use: Antineoplastic.

•**verubulin hydrochloride.** (VER-ue-BUE-lin) USAN.
Use: Antineoplastic.

•**verucerfont.** (VER-ue-SER-font) USAN.
Use: CNS agent.

Verukan-20. (Syosset Laboratories Co., Inc.) Salicylic acid 16.7%, lactic acid in flexible collodion 16.7%. Bot. 15 mL. *OTC.*
Use: Keratolytic.

Verv Alertness. (A.P.C.) Caffeine 200 mg. Cap. Vial 15s. *OTC.*
Use: CNS stimulant.

•**vesencumab.** (ve-SENK-ue-mab) USAN.
Use: Antineoplastic.

VESIcare. (Astellas) Solifenacin succinate 5 mg, 10 mg. Film-coated. Tab. 30s, 90s, UD 100s. *Rx.*
Use: Anticholinergic.

•**vesnarinone.** (VESS-nah-rih-NOHN) USAN.
Use: Cardiovascular agent.

•**vestipitant mesylate.** (ves-tee-PIT-ant) USAN.
Use: CNS agent.

Vestura. (Watson) Ethinyl estradiol 20 mcg, drospirenone 3 mg. Lactose. Tab. Blister pack 28s w/4 inert tablets. *Rx.*
Use: Oral monophasic contraceptive.

Vexol. (Alcon) Rimexolone 1%. Benzalkonium chloride 0.01%, polysorbate 80, EDTA, sodium chloride. Ophth. Susp. *Drop-Tainers.* 5 mL, 10 mL. *Rx.*
Use: Corticosteroid, ophthalmic.

Vfend. (Roerig) Voriconazole. **Tab.:** 50 mg, 200 mg. Lactose. Film-coated. Bot. 30s. **Pow. for Inj., lyophilized:** 200 mg, sulfobutyl ether beta-cyclodextrin sodium 3200 mg. Preservative free. Single-use vials. **Pow. for Oral Susp.:** 45 g (40 mg/mL after reconstitution). Sodium benzoate, sucrose. Orange flavor. 100 mL w/5 mL oral dispenser. *Rx.*
Use: Antifungal.

Viacaps. (Manne) Vitamins A (soluble) 45,000 units, C 500 mg. Cap. Bot. 60s, 120s, 1000s. *OTC.*
Use: Vitamin supplement.

Viactiv Multi-Vitamin Flavor Glides. (McNeil Nutritionals) Biotin 30 mcg, calcium 200 mg, chromium 12 mcg, copper 2 mg, iodine 38 mcg, iron 18 mg, lutein 250 mg, magnesium 40 mg, manganese 2 mg, molybdenum 75 mcg, pantothenic acid 10 mg, potassium 40 mg, selenium 55 mcg, vitamin A 2,500 units, vitamin B_1 1.5 mg, vitamin B_2 1.7 mg, vitamin B_3 15 mg, vitamin B_6 2 mg, folic acid 400 mcg, vitamin B_{12} 6 mcg, vitamin C 60 mg, vitamin D 400 units, vitamin E 33 units, vitamin K 20 mcg, zinc 15 mg. Glucose, maltodextrin, polydextrose, sucralose. Berry flavor. Tab. 50s. *OTC.*
Use: Nutritional supplement.

Viagra. (Pfizer) Sildenafil citrate 25 mg, 50 mg, 100 mg (except 25 mg), lactose. Film-coated. Tab. Bot. 30s, 100s. *Rx.*
Use: Anti-impotence.

Vianain. (Genzyme) Ananain, comosain.
Use: Burn treatment. [Orphan Drug]

Vi antigen.
Use: Immunization.
See: Typhim Vi.

Vibativ. (Theravance) Telavancin 250 mg, 750 mg. Hydroxypropyl-beta-cyclodextrin 2,500 mg (250 mg), 7,500 mg (750 mg), mannitol 312.5 (250 mg), 937.5 mg (750 mg). Preservative free. Inj., lyophilized Pow. for Soln. Single-dose vial. *Rx.*
Use: Anti-infective agent, lipoglycopeptide.

•**vibegron.** (vye-BEG-ron) USAN.
Use: Genitourinary agent.

vibesate. Polvinate 9.3%, molrosinol 3.1% with propellant.

Vibramycin. (Pfizer) **Cap.:** Doxycycline hyclate 100 mg. 50s. **Pow. for Oral Susp.:** Doxycycline monohydrate 25 mg/5 mL. Parabens, sucrose. Raspberry flavor. 60 mL. **Syrup:** Doxycycline calcium 50 mg/5 mL. Glycerin, parabens, sodium metabisulfite, sorbitol. Apple-raspberry flavor. 473 mL. *Rx.*
Use: Anti-infective; tetracycline.

Vibramycin IV. (Pfizer) Doxycycline (as hyclate) 200 mg. Powder for Inj. Vial. *Rx.*
Use: Anti-infective; tetracycline.

Vicam IV. (Keene Pharmaceuticals) Vitamins B_1 50 mg, B_2 5 mg, B_{12} 1000 mcg, B_6 5 mg, dexpanthenol 6 mg, niacinamide 125 mg, C 50 mg/mL, benzyl alcohol 1% as preservative in water for injection. Vial, multiple-dose. *Rx.*
Use: Nutritional supplement; parenteral.

Vicks Children's NyQuil Cold & Cough. (Procter & Gamble) Dextromethorphan HBr 5 mg, chlorpheniramine maleate 0.67 mg per 5 mL. Alcohol free. Sucrose, sodium 23.7 mg/5 mL. Liq. 118 mL. *OTC.*
Use: Upper respiratory combination; antitussive combination.

Vicks DayQuil Cold & Flu Relief. (Procter & Gamble) **Liq.:** Dextromethorphan HBr 3.33 mg, phenylephrine hydrochloride 1.67 mg, acetaminophen 108.33 mg per 5 mL. Alcohol free. Disodium EDTA, glycerin, propylene glycol, saccharin, sodium 50 mg, sorbitol, sucralose. Original and cherry flavors. Liq. 177 mL, 295 mL. **Liquid-filled Cap.:** Dextromethorphan HBr 10 mg, phenylephrine hydrochloride 5 mg, acetaminophen 325 mg. Sorbitol. 12s, 20s. *OTC.*
Use: Upper respiratory combination, antitussive combination.

Vicks DayQuil Sinex. (Proctor & Gamble) Acetaminophen 325 mg, phenylephrine hydrochloride 5 mg. Glycerin, PEG, sorbitol. Cap., liquid filled. 20s. *OTC.*
Use: Upper respiratory combination, decongestant and analgesic combination.

Vicks Nature Fusion Cough. (Procter & Gamble) Dextromethorphan 5 mg per 5 mL. Corn syrup, glycerin, honey, PEG, propylene glycol, sodium 6 mg. Alcohol free, dye free, and gluten free. Liq. 236 mL. *OTC.*
Use: Nonnarcotic antitussive.

Vicks NyQuil Cold/Flu Relief. (Procter & Gamble) **Liq.:** Dextromethorphan HBr 5 mg, doxylamine succinate 2.08 mg, acetaminophen 108.33 mg per 5 mL. Acesulfame, alcohol, corn syrup, propylene glycol, saccharin, sodium. Original, cherry, or vanilla-cherry flavors. 240 mL, 260 mL. **Liquid-filled Cap.:** Dextromethorphan HBr 15 mg, doxylamine succinate 6.25 mg, acetaminophen 325 mg. Glycerin, propylene glycol, sorbitol. 16s, 24s, 48s, 72s. *OTC.*
Use: Upper respiratory combination; antitussive combination.

Vicks NyQuil Cough. (Procter & Gamble) Dextromethorphan HBr 5 mg, doxylamine succinate 2.08 mg per 5 mL. Alcohol, corn syrup, saccharin, sodium 6 mg/5 mL. Liq. 240 mL, 360 mL. *OTC.*
Use: Upper respiratory combination; antitussive combination.

Vicks NyQuil Sinex Nighttime Sinus Relief. (Proctor & Gamble) Acetaminophen 325 mg, doxylamine succinate 6.25 mg, phenylephrine hydrochloride 5 mg. Glycerin, PEG, sorbitol. Cap., liquid filled. 20s. *OTC.*
Use: Upper respiratory combination; decongestant, antihistamine, and analgesic combination.

Vicks Sinex 12 Hour. (Procter & Gamble) Oxymetazoline hydrochloride 0.05%, camphor, menthol, eucalyptol, EDTA, benzalkonium chloride, chlorhexidine, gluconate, sodium chloride, tyloxapol. Soln. Spray Bot. 15 mL. *OTC.*
Use: Nasal decongestant, imidazoline.

Vicks Sinex 12 Hour UltraFine Mist. (Procter & Gamble) Oxymetazoline hydrochloride 0.05%, aromatic vapors (camphor, eucalyptus, menthol), tyloxapol, disodium EDTA, benzalkonium chloride, sodium chloride. Soln. Spray Bot. 15 mL. *OTC.*
Use: Nasal decongestant, imidazoline.

Vicks VapoDrops Cough Relief. (Procter & Gamble) **Menthol flavor:** Menthol 3.3 mg. Eucalyptus oil, corn syrup, sucrose. **Cherry flavor:** Menthol 1.7 mg. Eucalyptus oil, corn syrup, sucrose, citric acid. Loz. Pkg. 20s. *OTC.*
Use: Mouth and throat preparation.

Vicks Vapor Inhaler. (Procter & Gamble) Levmetamfetamine 50 mg. Menthol, camphor, lavender oil. Inhaler. Single plastic inhaler. *OTC.*
Use: Nasal decongestant, imidazoline.

Vicks VapoRub. (Procter & Gamble) **Oint.:** Camphor 4.8%, menthol 2.6%, eucalyptus oil 1.2%. Cedarleaf oil, nutmeg oil, petrolatum, turpentine oil. 50 g, 100 g, 170 g. **Cream:** Camphor 5.2%, menthol 2.8%, eucalyptus oil 1.2%. EDTA, glycerin, cetyl alcohol, parabens, stearyl alcohol, cedarleaf oil, nutmeg oil, turpentine oil. 88 mL. *OTC.*
Use: Upper respiratory topical combination.

Vicks VapoSteam. (Procter & Gamble) Camphor 6.2%. Alcohol 78%, eucalyptus oil, menthol, cedar leaf oil, nutmeg oil. 8 oz. *OTC.*
Use: Antitussive, decongestant.

Vicodin. (AbbVie) Hydrocodone bitartrate 5 mg, acetaminophen 300 mg. Tab. 100s, 500s. *c-III.*
Use: Analgesic combination; narcotic.

Vicodin ES. (AbbVie) Hydrocodone bitartrate 7.5 mg, acetaminophen 300 mg.

Tab. 100s, 500s. *c-III.*
Use: Analgesic combination; narcotic.

Vicodin HP. (AbbVie) Hydrocodone bitartrate 10 mg, acetaminophen 300 mg. Tab. 100s, 500s. *c-III.*
Use: Analgesic combination; narcotic.

Vicon Forte. (UCB) Vitamins A 8000 units, E 50 units, C 150 mg, B_3 25 mg, B_1 10 mg, B_5 10 mg, B_2 5 mg, B_6 2 mg, B_{12} 10 mcg, folic acid 1 mg, zinc sulfate 18 mg, Mg, Mn. Lactose. Cap. Bot. 60s, 500s, UD 100s. *Rx.*
Use: Mineral, vitamin supplement.

Vicon Plus. (UCB) Vitamins A 4000 units, E 50 units, C 150 mg, B_3 25 mg, B_1 10 mg, B_5 10 mg, B_2 5 mg, zinc sulfate 18 mg, Mg, Mn, B_6 2 mg. Lactose. Cap. Bot. 60s. *OTC.*
Use: Mineral, vitamin supplement.

Vicoprofen. (Abbott) Hydrocodone bitartrate 7.5 mg, ibuprofen 200 mg. Tab. Bot. 100s, 500s, UD 100s. *c-III.*
Use: Analgesic; narcotic.

•**vicriviroc maleate.** (VI-kri-VIR-ok) USAN.
Use: Antiviral.

Victors. (Procter & Gamble) Special Vicks Medication (menthol, eucalyptus oil) in a soothing Vicks sugar base. Regular or cherry flavor drops. Stick-Pack 10s, Bag 40s. *OTC.*
Use: Anesthetic, local.

Victoza. (Novo Nordisk) Liraglutide 6 mg/mL. Propylene glycol. Inj., Soln. Prefilled, multidose pen. 3 mL. *Rx.*
Use: Antidiabetic agent, glucagon-like peptide 1 receptor agonist.

Victrelis. (Schering) Boceprevir 200 mg. Cap. 12s. *Rx.*
Use: Anti-infective agent, antiviral agent.

•**vidarabine.** (vih-DAR-ah-BEAN) *USP.*
Use: Antiviral.

•**vidarabine sodium phosphate.** (vih-DAR-ah-BEAN) USAN.
Use: Antiviral.

Vi-Daylin ADC Drops. (Ross) Vitamins A 1500 units, C 35 mg, D 400 units/mL. Bot. 30 mL, 50 mL w/dropper. *OTC.*
Use: Vitamin supplement.

Vi-Daylin ADC Vitamin + Iron Drops. (Ross) Vitamins A 1500 units, C 35 mg, D 400 units, Fe 10 mg/mL. Methylparaben. Bot. 50 mL. *OTC.*
Use: Mineral, vitamin supplement.

Vi-Daylin Chewable. (Ross) Vitamins A 2500 units, D 400 units, E 15 units, C 60 mg, folic acid 0.3 mg, B_1 1.05 mg, B_2 1.2 mg, niacin 13.5 mg, B_6 1.05 mg, B_{12} 4.5 mcg. Tab. Bot. 100s. *OTC.*
Use: Vitamin supplement.

Vi-Daylin Drops. (Ross) Vitamins A 1500 units, D 400 units, E 5 units, C 35 mg, B_1 0.5 mg, B_2 0.6 mg, niacin 8 mg, B_6 0.4 mg, B_{12} 1.5 mcg/mL. Bot. 50 mL. *OTC.*
Use: Vitamin supplement.

Vi-Daylin/F ADC + Iron Drops. (Ross) Vitamins A 1500 units, C 35 mg, D 400 units, Fe 10 mg, fluoride 0.25 mg/mL. Methylparaben. Bot. 50 mL. *Rx.*
Use: Dental caries agent; mineral, vitamin supplement.

Vi-Daylin/F ADC Vitamins Drops. (Ross) Vitamins A 1500 units, D 400 units, C 35 mg, fluoride 0.25 mg/mL. Alcohol ≈ 0.3%, parabens. Bot. 50 mL. *Rx.*
Use: Dental caries agent; vitamin supplement.

Vi-Daylin/F Drops. (Ross) Vitamins A 1500 units, D 400 units, E 5 units, C 35 mg, B_1 0.5 mg, B_2 0.6 mg, B_3 8 mg, B_6 0.4 mg, fluoride 0.25 mg/mL. Methylparaben. Bot. 50 mL. *Rx.*
Use: Dental caries agent; vitamin supplement.

Vi-Daylin/F Multivitamin + Iron. (Ross) Fluoride 0.25 mg, vitamins A 1500 units, D 400 units, E 4.1 mg, B_1 0.5 mg, B_2 0.6 mg, B_3 8 mg, B_6 0.4 mg, C 35 mg, Fe 10 mg/mL. Alcohol < 0.1%, methylparaben. Drops. Bot. 50 mL. *Rx.*
Use: Dental caries agent; mineral, vitamin supplement.

Vi-Daylin Liquid. (Ross) Vitamins A 2500 units, B_1 1.05 mg, B_2 1.2 mg, B_6 1.05 mg, B_{12} 4.5 mcg, C 60 mg, D 400 units, E 20.4 mg (as d-alpha tocopheryl acetate), niacin 13.5 mg/5 mL. Bot. 8 oz, 473 mL. *OTC.*
Use: Vitamin supplement.

Vi-Daylin Multivitamin Drops. (Ross) Vitamins A 1500 units, D 400 units, E 5 mg, B_1 0.5 mg, B_2 0.6 mg, B_3 8 mg, B_6 0.4 mg, B_{12} 1.5 mcg, C 35 mg/mL. Alcohol < 0.5%. Bot. 50 mL. *OTC.*
Use: Vitamin supplement.

Vi-Daylin Multivitamin Liquid. (Ross) Vitamins A 2500 units, D 400 units, E 15 mg, B_1 1.05 mg, B_2 1.2 mg, B_3 13.5 mg, B_6 1.05 mg, B_{12} 4.5 mcg, C 60 mg/5 mL. Alcohol < 0.5%. Bot. 240 mL, 480 mL. *OTC.*
Use: Vitamin supplement.

Vi-Daylin Multivitamin Plus Iron Chewable. (Ross) Vitamins A 2500 units, D 400 units, E 15 units, C 60 mg, folic acid 0.3 mg, B_1 1.05 mg, B_2 1.2 mg, B_3 13.5 mg, B_6 1.05 mg, B_{12} 4.5 mcg, iron 12 mg. Tab. Bot. 100s. *OTC.*
Use: Mineral, vitamin supplement.

Vi-Daylin Multivitamin + Iron Drops. (Ross) Fe 10 mg, vitamins A 1500 units,

D 400 units, E 5 mg, B_1 0.5 mg, B_2 0.6 mg, B_3 8 mg, B_6 0.4 mg, C 35 mg. Alcohol < 0.5%, methylparaben. Bot. 50 mL. *OTC.*
Use: Mineral, vitamin supplement.

Vi-Daylin Multivitamin Plus Iron Liquid. (Ross) Vitamins A 2500 units, D 400 units, C 60 mg, E 15 units, B_1 1.05 mg, B_2 1.2 mg, B_3 13.5 mg, B_6 1.05 mg, B_{12} 4.5 mcg, Fe 10 mg/tsp. ≤ 0.5% alcohol, glucose, sucrose, parabens. 237 mL, 473 mL. *OTC.*
Use: Mineral, vitamin supplement.

Vidaza. (Celgene) Azacitidine 100 mg. Mannitol 100 mg. Preservative free. Pow. for Inj., lyophilized. Single-use vials. *Rx.*
Use: DNA demethylation agent.

Videcon. (Vita Elixir) Vitamin D 50,000 units. Cap. *Rx.*
Use: Vitamin supplement.

Vi-Derm Soap. (Arthrins) Extract of Amaryllis 10%. Cake. Pkg. 1s. Bar 3.5 oz. *OTC.*
Use: Dermatologic; cleanser.

Videx. (Bristol-Myers Squibb) Didanosine 2 g, 4 g. Pow. for Oral Soln. 100 mL (after reconstitution), 200 mL (after reconstitution). *Rx.*
Use: Antiretroviral, nucleoside reverse transcriptase inhibitor.

Videx EC. (Bristol-Myers Squibb) Didanosine 125 mg, 200 mg, 250 mg, 400 mg. DR Cap. (with enteric-coated beadlets) 30s. *Rx.*
Use: Antiretroviral, nucleoside reverse transcriptase inhibitor.

•**vidupiprant.** (vye-DUE-pi-prant) USAN.
Use: Treatment of asthma.

•**vifilcon A.** (vie-FILL-kahn A) USAN.
Use: Contact lens material (hydrophilic).

•**vifilcon B.** (vie-FILL-kahn B) USAN.
Use: Contact lens material (hydrophilic).

Vifluorineed. (Hanlon) Vitamins A 5000 units, D 400 units, C 75 mg, B_1 2 mg, B_2 3 mg, niacinamide 20 mg, fluoride 1 mg. Chew. Tab. Bot. 100s. *Rx.*
Use: Mineral, vitamin supplement.

•**vigabatrin.** (vie-GAB-at RIN) USAN.
Use: Anticonvulsant (tardive dyskinesia).
See: Sabril.

Vigamox. (Alcon) Moxifloxacin hydrochloride 0.5% (5 mg/mL). Boric acid, sodium chloride, purified water. Soln. *Drop-Tainer* 3 mL. *Rx.*
Use: Antibiotic, ophthalmic.

Vigomar Forte. (Marlop) Fe 12 mg, vitamins A 10,000 units, D 400 units, E 15 units, B_1 10 mg, B_2 10 mg, B_3 100 mg, B_5 20 mg, B_6 5 mg, B_{12} 5 mcg, C 200 mg, I, Mg, Mn, Cu, Zn 1.5 mg. Tab. Bot. 100s. *OTC.*
Use: Mineral, vitamin supplement.

Viibryd. (Forest Pharmaceuticals) Vilazodone hydrochloride 10 mg, 20 mg, 40 mg. Lactose, PEG. Tab. 30s, 90s, 500s, UD 100s. *Rx.*
Use: Selective serotonin reuptake inhibitor, 5-HT_{1A} receptor agonist.

Viibryd Patient Starter Kit. (Forest Pharmaceuticals) Vilazodone hydrochloride 10 mg, 20 mg, 40 mg. Lactose, PEG. Tab. UD 30s (30-tablet blister card containing seven 10 mg tablets, seven 20 mg tablets, and sixteen 40 mg tablets). *Rx.*
Use: Selective serotonin reuptake inhibitor, 5-HT_{1A} receptor agonist.

VIL. (Leas Research)
Use: Hyperphenylalaninemia. [Orphan Drug]

•**vilanterol.** (vye-LAN-ter-ol) USAN.
Use: Respiratory agent.
W/Fluticasone Furoate.
See: BreoEllipta.
W/Umeclidinium.
See: Anoro Ellipta.

•**vilanterol trifenatate.** (vye-LAN-ter-ol trye-FEN-a-tate) USAN.
Use: Respiratory agent.

•**vilazodone.** (vil-AZ-oh-done) USAN.
Use: Antidepressant.

•**vilazodone hydrochloride.** (vil-AZ-oh-done) USAN.
Use: Antidepressant.
See: Viibryd.
Viibryd Patient Starter Kit.

•**vildagliptin.** (VIL-da-GLIP-tin) USAN.
Use: Antidiabetic.

Vilex. (Oxypure) Vitamin B_1 100 mg, riboflavin phosphate sodium 1 mg, B_6 10 mg, panthenol 5 mg, niacinamide 100 mg/mL. Amp. 30 mL. *Rx.*
Use: Vitamin supplement.

Viliva. (Vita Elixir) Ferrous fumarate 3 g. *OTC.*
Use: Mineral supplement.

ViloFane-Dp. (Seton Pharmaceuticals) L-methylfolate 7.5 mg. Tab. 30s, 90s. *Rx.*
Use: Water-soluble vitamin.

•**viloxazine.** (vih-LOX-ah-zeen) USAN.
Use: Antidepressant.
See: Catatrol.

Viminate. (Various Mfr.) Vitamins B_1 2.5 mg, B_2 1.25 mg, B_3 25 mg, B_5 5 mg, B_6 0.5 mg, B_{12} 0.5 mcg, Fe 7.5 mg, Zn 1 mg, choline, I, Mg, Mn 5 mL. Alcohol 18%. Liq. Bot. 480. *OTC.*
Use: Mineral, vitamin supplement.

Vi-Min-for-All. (Barth's) Vitamins A 3 mg,

D 10 mcg, C 120 mg, B_1 35 mg, B_{12} 15 mcg, biotin, niacin 2.33 mg, E 30 units, B_6, pantothenic acid, Ca 375 mg, P 180 mg, Fe 20 mg, I 0.1 mg, rutin 10 mg, hesperidin-lemon bioflavonoid complex 10 mg, choline, inositol 2.4 mg, Cu 10 mcg, Mn 2 mg, Zn 110 mcg, silicone 210 mcg. Tab. Bot. 100s, 500s. *OTC.*
Use: Mineral, vitamin supplement.

Vimizim. (BioMarin Pharmaceutical Inc) Elosulfase alfa 1 mg/mL. Preservative free. Soln., concentrate; Inj. Vial. 5 mL. *Rx.*
Use: Endocrine and metabolic agent.

Vimovo. (Horizon Pharma) Naproxen/esomeprazole 375 mg/20 mg (as esomeprazole magnesium trihydrate 22.3 mg), 500 mg/20 mg (as esomeprazole magnesium trihydrate 22.3 mg). Enteric-coated. Glyceryl monostearate, polydextrose, polyethylene glycol, polysorbate 80, propylparaben. Tab., delayed release. 60s, 500s, UD 100s (500 mg/20 mg only). *Rx.*
Use: Nonnarcotic analgesic combination.

Vimpat. (Schwarz Pharma) Lacosamide. **Soln., oral:** 10 mg/mL. Acesulfame K, aspartame, glycerin, parabens, PEG, phenylalanine 0.016 mg/mL, propylene glycol, sorbitol. Strawberry flavor. 465 mL. **Tab.:** 50 mg, 100 mg, 150 mg, 200 mg. PEG. Film-coated. 60s, 180s. **Inj., Soln.:** 10 mg/mL. Single-use glass vial. 20 mL. *c-v.*
Use: Anticonvulsant.

Vinactane Sulfate. (Novartis) Viomycin Sulfate.

•**vinafocon A.** (VIE-nah-FOE-kahn A) USAN.
Use: Contact lens material (hydrophobic).

Vinate DHA. (Breckenridge) Folate 1.53 mg, calcium 75 mg, iron 27 mg, vitamins E 30 units, B_6 25 mg, B_{12} 1,000 mcg, C 40 mg, algal oil and soy lecithin blend 687 mg. Glycerin, soy. Cap. 30s. *Rx.*
Use: Prenatal vitamin with minerals.

Vinate DHA RF. (Breckenridge) Folate 1.13 mg, calcium 110 mg, iron 27 mg, vitamins D 200 units, E 21 units, B_1 1.4 mg, B_2 1.4 mg, B_3 18 mg, B_6 25 mg, B_{12} 1,000 mcg, C 85 mg, I, Mg, Se. Algal oil blend (omega 3, 6, and 9) 581.28 mg. Glycerin, sorbitol, soy lecithin. Cap. 90s. *Rx.*
Use: Prenatal vitamin with minerals.

Vinate Good Start Chewable Prenatal Formula. (Breckenridge) Ca 200 mg, Fe 29 mg, vitamin A 1000 units, D 400 units, E 30 units, B_1 3 mg, B_2 3 mg, B_3 15 mg, B_5 7 mg, B_6 20 mg, B_{12} 12 mcg, C 100 mg, folic acid 1 mg, Zn 20 mg. Chew. Tab. 100s. *Rx.*
Use: Prenatal vitamin.

Vinate GT. (Breckenridge) Ca 200 mg, Fe 90 mg, vitamin A 2700 units, D_3 400 units, E 10 units, B_1 3 mg, B_2 3.4 mg, B_3 20 mg, B_5 6 mg, B_6 20 mg, B_{12} 12 mcg, C 120 mg, folic acid 1 mg, biotin 30 mcg, docusate sodium 50 mg, Zn 15 mg, Cu, Mg. Tab. UD 90s. *Rx.*
Use: Vitamin supplement.

vinbarbital.
Use: Hypnotic, sedative.

vinbarbital sodium.
Use: Hypnotic, sedative.

•**vinblastine sulfate.** (vin-BLAST-een) *USP.* Vincaleukoblastine. Alkaloid extracted from *Vinca rosea* Linn.
Tall Man: vinBLAStine
Use: Antineoplastic.
See: Velban.

vinblastine sulfate. (Various Mfr.) Vinblastine sulfate. **Pow. for Inj.:** 10 mg. Vial. **Inj.:** 1 mg/mL, benzyl alcohol 0.9%. Vial 10 mL, 25 mL. *Rx.*
Use: Antineoplastic.

vinca alkaloids.
Use: Antimitotic agent.
See: Vinblastine Sulfate.
Vincristine Sulfate.
Vincristine Sulfate Liposome.
Vinorelbine Tartrate.

vincaleukoblastine, 22-oxo-sulfate (1:1) (salt). Vincristine Sulfate.

Vincasar PFS. (Gensia Sicor) Vincristine sulfate 1 mg/mL. Vial 1 mL. *Rx.*
Use: Antineoplastic.

•**vincofos.** (VIN-koe-foss) USAN.
Use: Anthelmintic.

•**vincristine sulfate.** (vin-KRISS-teen) *USP.*
Tall Man: vinCRIStine
Use: Antineoplastic.
See: Vincasar PFS.

vincristine sulfate liposome.
Use: Vinca alkaloid.
See: Marqibo.

•**vindesine.** (VIN-deh-seen) USAN.
Use: Antineoplastic.

•**vindesine sulfate.** (VIN-deh-seen) USAN.
Use: Antineoplastic.

•**vinepidine sulfate.** (VIN-eh-pih-DEEN) USAN.
Use: Antineoplastic.

•**vinflunine ditartrate.** (vin-FLOO-neen) USAN.
Use: Treatment of cancer.

•**vinglycinate sulfate.** (vin-GLIE-sin-ate) USAN.
Use: Antineoplastic.

•**vinleurosine sulfate.** (vin-LOO-row-seen) USAN. Sulfate salt of an alkaloid extracted from *Vinca rosea* Linn. Also see Vinblastine.
Use: Antineoplastic.

•**vinorelbine tartrate.** (vih-NORE-ell-bean) USAN. Sulfate salt of an alkaloid extracted from *Vinca rosea* Linn.
Use: Antineoplastic.
See: Navelbine.

vinorelbine tartrate. (Gensia Sicor) Vinorelbine tartrate 10 mg/mL. Inj. Vials. 1 mL, 5 mL. *Rx.*
Use: Antineoplastic.

•**vinpocetine.** (VIN-poe-SEH-teen) USAN.
Use: Antineoplastic.

•**vinrosidine sulfate.** (vin-ROW-sih-deen) USAN. Sulfate salt of an alkaloid extracted from *Vinca rosea* Linn.
Use: Antineoplastic.
See: Vinblastine.

•**vintafolide.** (vin-TAF-oh-lide) USAN.
Use: Antineoplastic.

vinyl ether. (VYE-nil)
Use: Anesthetic, general.

vinyzene. Bromchlorenone.
Use: Fungicide.

•**vinzolidine sulfate.** (VIN-ZOLE-ih-deen) USAN.
Use: Antineoplastic.

Vio-Bec. (Solvay) Vitamins B_1 25 mg, B_2 25 mg, niacinamide 100 mg, calcium pantothenate 40 mg, B_6 25 mg, C 500 mg. Cap. Bot. 100s. *OTC.*
Use: Mineral, vitamin supplement.

Viodo HC. (Alra) Iodochlorhydroxyquin 3%, hydrocortisone 1% in cream base. Tube 20 g. *OTC.*
Use: Antifungal; corticosteroid, topical.

Viogen-C. (Ivax) Vitamins B_1 20 mg, B_2 10 mg, B_3 100 mg, B_5 20 mg, B_6 5 mg, C 300 mg, Mg, zinc sulfate 50 mg. Tartrazine. Cap. Bot. 100s. *OTC.*
Use: Mineral, vitamin supplement.

Viokace. (Aptalis Pharma US) Lipase/protease/amylase 10,440 units/39,150 units/39,150 units, 20,880 units/78,300 units/78,300 units. Lactose. Tab. 100s. *Rx.*
Use: Digestive enzyme.

Viorele. (Glenmark Pharmaceuticals) **Phase 1:** Desogestrel 0.15 mg, ethinyl estradiol 20 mcg. Film coated. Lactose. Tab. 21s. **Phase 2:** Ethinyl estradiol 10 mcg. Film coated. Tab. 5s w/2 green inert tab. *Rx.*
Use: Oral contraceptive hormone, biphasic contraceptive.

•**vipadenant.** (vye-PA-de-nant) USAN.
Use: Parkinson disease.

•**viprostol.** (vie-PRAHST-ole) USAN.
Use: Hypotensive; vasodilator.

Vi-Q-Tuss. (Vintage) Hydrocodone bitartrate 5 mg, guaifenesin 100 mg per 5 mL. Sugar, alcohol, and dye free. Menthol, parabens, saccharin, sorbitol. Cherry flavor. Syrup. 30 mL, 120 mL, 473 mL, 3785 mL. *c-III.*
Use: Antitussive with expectorant.

Virac. (Ruson) Undecoylium Cl-iodine. Iodine complexed with a cationic detergent. Surgical Soln. Bot. 2 oz, 8 oz, 1 gal. *OTC.*
Use: Antiseptic.

Viracept. (Pfizer) Nelfinavir mesylate 250 mg. Tab. 270s, 300s. *Rx.*
Use: Antiviral.

Viracil. (Health for Life Brands) Phenylephrine hydrochloride 5 mg, hesperidin 50 mg, thenylene hydrochloride 12.5 mg, pyrilamine maleate 12.5 mg, vitamin C 50 mg, salicylamide 2.5 g, caffeine 0.5 g, sodium salicylate 1.25 g. Cap. Bot. 16s, 36s. *OTC.*
Use: Analgesic, antihistamine, decongestant, vitamin supplement.

Viramisol. (Seatrace) Adenosine phosphate 25 mg/mL. Vial 10 mL. *OTC.*
Use: Relief of varicose vein complications.

Viramune. (Boehringer Ingelheim) Nevirapine. **Tab.:** 200 mg. Lactose. 60s. **Oral Susp.:** 50 mg/5 mL (as nevirapine hemihydrate), parabens, sorbitol, sucrose. 240 mL. *Rx.*
Use: Antiviral.

Viramune XR. (Boehringer Ingelheim) Nevirapine 100 mg, 400 mg. Lactose. ER Tab. 30s (400 mg), 90s (100 mg). *Rx.*
Use: Antiviral.

Viranol. (Aventis) Salicylic acid in collodion gel w/lactic acid, camphor, pyroxylin, ethyl alcohol, ethyl acetate. Gel. Tube 8 g. *OTC.*
Use: Dermatologic; wart therapy.

Virasal. (Elorac) Salicylic acid 27.5%. Isopropyl alcohol. Liq. 10 mL w/brush applicator. *Rx.*
Use: Keratolytic agent.

Viravan-DM. (PediaMed) **Chew. Tab.:** Dextromethorphan tannate 25 mg, pyrilamine tannate 30 mg, phenylephrine tannate 25 mg. Sugar, sucralose. Dye free. Grape flavor. 100s. **Susp.:** Dextromethorphan tannate 25 mg, pyrilamine tannate 30 mg, phenylephrine tannate

12.5 mg per 5 mL. Methylparaben, sucralose, sucrose. Grape flavor. 473 mL. *Rx.*
Use: Pediatric antitussive.

Viravan-T. (PediaMed) Phenylephrine tannate 25 mg, pyrilamine tannate 30 mg. Sugar, saccharin. Dye free. Grape flavor. Chew. Tab. 100s. *Rx.*
Use: Decongestant and antihistamine.

Virazole. (ICN) Ribavirin 6 g per vial. Contains 20 mg/mL when reconstituted w/300 mL sterile water. Pow. for Soln., Lyophilized, Inh. Vials. *Rx.*
Use: Antiviral.

Virdec. (Virtus) Chlorpheniramine maleate 1 mg, phenylephrine hydrochloride 3.5 mg. Glycerin, parabens, potassium citrate, potassium sorbate, propylene glycol, sucralose. Alcohol free, gluten free, and sugar free. Raspberry flavor. Drops. 30 mL w/dropper. *OTC.*
Use: Upper respiratory combination, decongestant and antihistamine.

Virdec DM. (Virtus) Chlorpheniramine maleate 1 mg, dextromethorphan hydrobromide 3 mg, phenylephrine hydrochloride 3.5 mg per mL. Glycerin, parabens, potassium citrate, potassium sorbate, propylene glycol, sucralose. Alcohol free, gluten free, and sugar free. Grape flavor. Syrup. 30 mL w/dropper. *OTC.*
Use: Upper respiratory combination, antitussive combination.

Viread. (Gilead Sciences) Tenofovir disoproxil fumarate. **Tab.:** 150 mg (equiv. to tenofovir disoproxil 123 mg), 200 mg (equiv. to tenofovir disoproxil 163 mg), 250 mg (equiv. to tenofovir disoproxil 204 mg), 300 mg (equiv. to tenofovir disoproxil 245 mg). Lactose. Film coated. 30s. **Pow.:** 40 mg/g (equiv. to tenofovir disoproxil 33 mg). Mannitol. Multiuse bot. 60 g w/dosing scoop. *Rx.*
Use: Antiretroviral agent, nucleotide analog reverse transcriptase inhibitor.

•**virginiamycin.** (vihr-JIH-nee-ah-MY-sin) USAN. An antibiotic produced by *Streptomyces virgina.*
Use: Anti-infective.

•**viridofulvin.** (vih-RID-oh-FULL-vin) USAN.
Use: Antifungal.

Virilon. (Star) Methyltestosterone 10 mg. Cap. Bot. 100s, 1000s. *c-III.*
Use: Sex hormone, androgen.

Virogen Herpes Slide Test. (Wampole) Latex agglutination slide test for the detection of herpes simplex virus antigens directly from lesions or cell culture. Test kit 100s.
Use: Diagnostic aid.

Virogen Rotatest. (Wampole) Latex agglutination slide test for the qualitative detection of rotavirus in fecal specimens. Test kit 50s.
Use: Diagnostic aid.

Virogen Rubella Microlatex Test. (Wampole) Latex agglutination microlatex test for the detection of rubella virus antibody in serum. Test kit 500s, 5000s.
Use: Diagnostic aid.

Virogen Rubella Slide Test. (Wampole) Latex agglutination slide test for the detection of rubella virus antibody in serum. Test kit 100s, 500s, 5000s.
Use: Diagnostic aid.

Virogen Rubella Slide Test with Fast Trak Slides. (Wampole) Latex agglutination slide test for the detection of rubella virus antibody in serum.
Use: Diagnostic aid.

Viroptic. (Monarch) Trifluridine 1%, thimerosal 0.001%. Soln. Drop-Dose 7.5 mL. *Rx.*
Use: Antiviral; ophthalmic.

•**viroxime.** (vie-ROX-eem) USAN.
Use: Antiviral.

Virozyme Injection. (Marcen) Sodium nucleate 2.5%, phenol 0.5%, protein hydrolysate 2.5%, benzyl alcohol 0.2%. Vial 5 mL, 10 mL. *Rx.*
Use: Immunomodulator.

Virt-Bal DHA. (Virtus Pharmaceuticals) Folic acid 1 mg, Ca 219 mg, Fe 26 mg, vitamins A 2,850 mg, D 840 units, E 3 units, B_1 1.8 mg, B_2 4 mg, B_3 20 mg, B_6 50 mg, B_{12} 12 mcg, C 120 mg. Cu, I, Mg, Zn. Gluten free. **Cap., softgel:** Omega-3 fatty acids ≥ 374 mg (as DHA ≥ 262 mg, other omega-3 fatty acids ≥ 112 mg), glycerin, vitamin E oil. UD 5s. **Tab.:** UD 5s. *Rx.*
Use: Prenatal vitamin with minerals.

Virt-Bal DHA Plus. (Virtus Pharmaceuticals) Folic acid 1 mg, Ca 219 mg, Fe 27 mg, vitamins A 2,850 mg, D 840 units, E 3 units, B_1 1.8 mg, B_2 4 mg, B_3 20 mg, B_6 50 mg, B_{12} 12 mcg, C 120 mg. Cu, I, Mg, Zn. Gluten free. **Cap., softgel:** Enteric coated. Omega-3 fatty acids ≥ 380 mg (as DHA ≥ 262 mg, other omega-3 fatty acids ≥ 112 mg), glycerin, vitamin E oil. UD 30s. **Tab.:** UD 30s. *Rx.*
Use: Prenatal vitamin with minerals.

Virti-Sulf Emollient. (Virtus Pharmaceuticals) Sodium sulfacetamide 10%, sulfur 5%. Cetyl alcohol, disodium EDTA, glycerin, glyceryl, parabens, PEG, propylene glycol. Cream. 28 g. *Rx.*
Use: Acne product combination.

Virt-PN DHA. (Virtus Pharmaceuticals) Folic acid 1 mg, Ca 140 mg, Fe 27 mg, vitamins D 200 units, E 10 units, B_6 25 mg, B_{12} 12 mcg, C 85 mg, DHA 300 mg. Mg. Beeswax, glycerin, soybean oil. Cap., softgel. 30s. *Rx.*
Use: Prenatal vitamin with minerals.

Virt-Select. (Virtus Pharmaceuticals) Folic acid 1.25 mg, calcium 160 mg, iron 29 mg, vitamins D 800 units, E 30 units, B_6 25 mg, C 28 mg, DHA 325 mg, docusate sodium 55 mg. Beeswax, glycerin, soy lecithin, soybean oil. Cap., softgel. 30s. *Rx.*
Use: Prenatal vitamin with minerals.

Virtussin A/C. (Virtus Pharmaceuticals) Codeine phosphate 10 mg, guaifenesin 100 mg. Cherry flavoring, parabens, potassium citrate, potassium sorbate, propylene glycol, sorbitol, sucralose. Liq. 473 mL. *c-v.*
Use: Upper respiratory combination, antitussive with expectorant.

Virt-Vite. (Virtus Pharmaceuticals) Vitamins B_6 25 mg, B_{12} 1,000 mcg, folate 2.5 mg. Tab. 90s. *Rx.*
Use: Multivitamin.

Virt-Vite Forte. (Virtus Pharmaceuticals) Vitamin B_6 25 mg, B_{12} 2,000 mcg, folate 2.5 mg. Tab. 90s. *Rx.*
Use: Multivitamin.

Virt-Vite Plus. (Virtus Pharmaceuticals) Vitamins B_1 1.5 mg, B_2 1.5 mg, B_3 20 mg, B_5 10 mg, B_6 50 mg, B_{12} 1,000 mcg, C 60 mg, folate 5 mg, biotin 300 mcg. Tab. 90s. *Rx.*
Use: Multivitamin.

Virugon. Under study. Anhydro bis-(beta-hydroxyethyl) biguanide derivative.
Use: Treatment of influenza, mumps, measles, chickenpox, and shingles.

Viscoat. (Alcon) Sodium chondroitin sulfate 40 mg, sodium hyaluronate 30 mg, sodium dihydrogen phosphate hydrate 0.45 mg, disodium hydrogen phosphate 2 mg, sodium chloride 4.3 mg/mL. Soln. Disposable Syr. 0.5 mL. *Rx.*
Use: Viscoelastic.

viscum album, extract. Visnico.
Use: Vasodilator.

Visicol. (Salix) Sodium phosphate monobasic monohydrate 1.102 g, sodium phosphate dibasic anhydrous 0.398 g. Gluten free. Tab. 40s, 100s. *Rx.*
Use: Bowel cleansing agent.

•**visilizumab.** (vye-si-loo-zoo-mab) USAN.
Use: Treatment of organ transplantation rejection and other T lymphocyte-mediated diseases and disorders.

Visine. (J & J Healthcare) Tetrahydrozoline hydrochloride 0.05%. Benzalkonium chloride, boric acid, EDTA, sodium borate. Ophth. Soln. 15 mL, 30 mL. *OTC.*
Use: Ophthalmic decongestant.

Visine-A. (J & J Healthcare) Naphazoline hydrochloride 0.025%, pheniramine maleate 0.3%. EDTA. Soln., Ophth. 15 mL. *OTC.*
Use: Ophthalmic decongestant/antihistamine combination.

Visine A.C. (J & J Healthcare) Tetrahydrozoline hydrochloride 0.05%. Benzalkonium chloride, boric acid, edetate disodium, sodium chloride, sodium citrate, zinc 0.25%. Soln., Ophth. 15 mL, 30 mL. *OTC.*
Use: Ophthalmic and otic agent, ophthalmic antihistamine.

Visine Advanced Relief. (J & J Healthcare) Tetrahydrozoline hydrochloride 0.05%. Dextran 70 0.1%, 1% of polyethylene glycol 400, povidone 1%, benzalkonium chloride, boric acid, EDTA, sodium borate. Ophth. Soln. 30 mL. *OTC.*
Use: Ophthalmic decongestant.

Visine All Day Eye Itch Relief. (J & J Healthcare) Ketotifen 0.025% (as ketotifen fumarate). May contain glycerol, sodium hydroxide and/or hydrochloric acid, benzalkonium chloride 0.01%. Soln., Ophth. 5 mL. *OTC.*
Use: Ophthalmic and otic agent, ophthalmic antihistamine.

Visine for Contacts. (J & J Healthcare) Sterile isotonic solution with borate buffer system, hypromellose, glycerin. EDTA. Soln.; Ophth. 15 mL, 30 mL. *OTC.*
Use: Artificial tears.

Visine LR. (J & J Healthcare) Oxymetazoline hydrochloride 0.025%. Benzalkonium chloride, boric acid, sodium borate, sodium chloride, EDTA. Ophth. Soln. 15 mL. *OTC.*
Use: Mydriatic; vasoconstrictor; ophthalmic decongestant.

Visine Maximum Redness Relief. (J & J Healthcare) Tetrahydrozoline hydrochloride 0.05%. Benzalkonium chloride, boric acid, edetate disodium, glycerin, hypromellose 0.36%, PEG, sodium chloride, sodium citrate. Soln., Ophth. 15 mL. *OTC.*
Use: Ophthalmic and otic agent, ophthalmic decongestant.

Visine Pure Tears. (J & J Healthcare) Glycerin 0.2%, hypromellose 0.2%, polyethylene glycol 400 1%. Soln.; Ophth. Single-drop dispenser. 9.5 mL. *OTC.*
Use: Artificial tears.

Visine Tears. (J & J Healthcare) Glycerin 0.2%, hypromellose 0.2%, 1% of polyethylene glycol 400. Soln., Ophth. 15 mL, 30 mL. *OTC.*
Use: Artificial tears.

Visine Tears Dry Eye Relief. (J & J Healthcare) Glycerin 0.2%, hypromellose 0.2%, 1% of polyethylene glycol 400. Drops. Single-drop dispenser. 15 mL, 30 mL. *OTC.*
Use: Artificial tears.

Visine Tears Preservative free. (J & J Healthcare) Glycerin 0.2%, hypromellose 0.2%, polyethylene glycol 400 1%. Soln.; Ophth. Preservative free. Single-use container. 0.4 mL. *OTC.*
Use: Artificial tears.

Visine Tired Eye Relief. (J & J Healthcare) Glycerin 0.2%, hypromellose 0.36%, 1% of polyethylene glycol 400. PEG, benzalkonium chloride, boric acid, glycine, magnesium chloride, potassium chloride, sodium borate, sodium chloride, sodium citrate, sodium lactate, sodium phosphate dibasic. Soln., Ophth. 15 mL. *OTC.*
Use: Artificial tears.

Visine Totality Multi-Symptom Relief. (J & J Healthcare) Tetrahydrozoline hydrochloride 0.05%. Benzalkonium chloride, boric acid, edetate disodium, glycerin, hypromellose 0.36%, PEG, sodium chloride, sodium citrate, zinc sulfate 0.25%. Soln., Ophth. 15 mL. *OTC.*
Use: Ophthalmic and otic agent, ophthalmic decongestant.

VisionBlue. (Dutch Ophthalmic) Trypan blue 0.06%. Ophthalmic Soln. 0.5 mL in 2.25 mL single-use *Luer Lok* syringe. *Rx.*
Use: Ophthalmic surgery aid.

Visipaque 320. (Nycomed Amersham) Iodixanol 652 mg, iodine 320 mg/mL, EDTA. Inj. Vial 50 mL. Bot. 50 mL, 100 mL, 200 mL, 150 mL fill in 200 mL bot. Flexible containers 100 mL, 150 mL, 200 mL. *Rx.*
Use: Radiopaque agent, parenteral.

Visipaque 270. (Nycomed Amersham) Iodixanol 550 mg, iodine 270 mg/mL, EDTA. Inj. Vial 50 mL. Bot. 50 mL, 100 mL, 200 mL, 150 mL fill in 200 mL bot. Flexible containers 100 mL, 150 mL, 200 mL. *Rx.*
Use: Radiopaque agent, parenteral.

Visken. (Novartis) Pindolol 5 mg, 10 mg. Tab. Bot. 100s. *Rx.*
Use: Antiadrenergic/sympatholytic, beta-adrenergic blocker.

•**vismodegib.** (VIS-moe-DEG-ib) USAN.
Use: Antineoplastic.
See: Erivedge.

VisRx Dose Pack. (Vision Pharma) **Day:** Methscopolamine nitrate 2.5 mg, pseudoephedrine hydrochloride 120 mg. **Night:** Chlorpheniramine maleate 8 mg, methscopolamine nitrate 2.5 mg.Tab., controlled release. 20s (10 day, 10 night), 60s (30 day, 30 night). *Rx.*
Use: Upper respiratory combination; decongestant, antihistamine, and anticholinergic combination.

Vistacon. (Roberts) Hydroxyzine hydrochloride 50 mg/mL. Inj. 25 mg/mL, 50 mg/mL, benzyl alcohol. Vial 10 mL; UD Vial 1 mL, 2 mL (50 mg/mL only). *Rx.*
Use: Antihistamine; anxiolytic.

Vistaril. (Pfizer) Hydroxyzine pamoate equivalent to hydroxyzine hydrochloride 25 mg, 50 mg, 100 mg. Sucrose. Cap. Bot. 100s. *Rx.*
Use: Anxiolytic; antihistamine, nonselective piperazine.

Vistide. (Gilead Sciences) Cidofovir 75 mg/mL. Preservative free. Inj. Single-use vial 5 mL. *Rx.*
Use: Antiviral.

Visudyne. (QLT Phototherapeutics/Novartis Ophthalmics) Verteporfin 15 mg (reconstituted to 2 mg/mL), egg phosphatidylglycerol. Lyophilized Cake for Inj. Single-use Vial. *Rx.*
Use: Ophthalmic phototherapy.

Vita-Bee with C Caplets. (Rugby) Vitamins B_1 15 mg, B_2 10.2 mg, B_3 50 mg, B_5 10 mg, B_6 5 mg, C 300 mg. TR Cap. Bot. 100s, 1000s. *OTC.*
Use: Vitamin supplement.

Vitabix. (Spanner) Vitamins B_1 100 mg, B_2 2 mg, B_6 5 mg, B_{12} 30 mcg, niacinamide 100 mg, panthenol 10 mg/mL. Vial 10 mL. Multiple-dose vial 30 mL. *Rx.*
Use: Vitamin supplement.

Vita-Bob Softgel Capsules. (Scot-Tussin) Vitamins A 5000 units, D 400 units, E 30 mg, B_1 1.5 mg, B_2 1.7 mg, B_3 20 mg, B_6 2 mg, B_{12} 6 mcg, C 60 mg, folic acid 0.4 mg. Cap. Bot. 100s. *OTC.*
Use: Vitamin supplement.

Vita-C. (Freeda) Ascorbic acid 1,000 mg per ¼ tsp. Gluten free, lactose free, and sugar free. Pow. 120 g, 1 lb. *OTC.*
Use: Water-soluble vitamin.

Vitacarn. (McGaw) L-carnitine 1 g/10 mL. UD Box 50s, 100s. *Rx.*
Use: L-carnitine supplement.

VitaCirc-B. (Macoven) Vitamin B_{12} 2,000 mcg (as methylcobalamin), L-methylfolate calcium 3 mg, B_6 35 mg (as

pyridoxal-5' phosphate). PEG. Tab. 90s. *Rx.*
Use: Multivitamin.

Vit-A-Drops. (Vision Pharmaceuticals) Vitamin A 5000 units, polysorbate 80. Bot. 10 mL, 15 mL. *OTC.*
Use: Lubricant; ophthalmic.

Vitadye. (AstraZeneca) FD&C yellow No. 5, FD&C red No. 40, FD&C blue No. 1 dyes and dihydroxyacetone 5%. Bot. 0.5 oz, 2 oz. *OTC.*
Use: Cosmetic for hyperpigmentation.

Vitafol Caplets. (Everett) Fe 65 mg, vitamins A 6000 units, D 400 units, E 30 mg, B_1 1.1 mg, B_2 1.8 mg, B_3 15 mg, B_6 2.5 mg, B_{12} 5 mcg, C 60 mg, folic acid 1 mg, calcium. Tab. Bot. 100s, 1000s. *Rx.*
Use: Mineral, vitamin supplement.

Vitafol-Nano. (Everett) Folate 1 mg, iron 18 mg, vitamins D 1,000 units, B_6 2.5 mg, B_{12} 12 mcg, I. Soy, sucrose. Coated. Tab. UD 30s. *Rx.*
Use: Prenatal vitamin with minerals.

Vitafol-One. (Everett) Vitamins A 1,100 units, B_1 1.6 mg, B_2 1.8 mg, B_3 15 mg, B_6 2.5 mg, B_{12} 12 mcg, C 30 mg, D_3 1,000 units, E 20 units, folic acid 1 mg, DHA 200 mg, I, Mg, Zn, Cu, Fe 29 mg. Glycerin, sorbitol, soybean oil, vegetable oil, sunflower oil. Cap., softgel. UD 30s. *Rx.*
Use: Prenatal vitamin with minerals.

Vitafol-Plus. (Everett) Folic acid 1 mg, Fe 27 mg, vitamins A 1,100 units, D_3 1,000 units, E 10 units, B_1 1.6 mg, B_2 1.8 mg, B_3 15 mg, B_6 2.5 mg, B_{12} 12 mcg, C 12 mg, DHA 200 mg, lauric acid 60 mg. Cu, I, Mg, Zn. Beeswax, glycerin, sorbitol, soy, soybean oil, sunflower oil. Cap., softgel. UD 30s. *Rx.*
Use: Prenatal vitamin with minerals.

Vitafol-PN. (Everett) Ca 125 mg, Fe 65 mg, vitamins A 1700 units, D 400 units, C 60 mg, E 30 units, folic acid 1 mg, B_1 1.6 mg, B_2 1.8 mg, B_6 2.5 mg, B_{12} 5 mcg, B_3 15 mg, Mg 25 mg, Zn 15 mg. Tab. UD 100s. *Rx.*
Use: Mineral, vitamin supplement.

Vitafol Syrup. (Everett) Fe 90 mg, B_3 39.9 mg, B_6 6 mg, B_{12} 25.02 mcg, folic acid 0.75 mg. Bot. 473 mL. *Rx.*
Use: Mineral, vitamin supplement.

Vitafol-Ultra. (Everett) Folic acid 1 mg, iron 29 mg, vitamins A 1,100 units, D 1,000 units, E 20 units, B_1 1.6 mg, B_2 1.8 mg, B_3 15 mg, B_6 2.5 mg, B_{12} 12 mcg, C 30 mg, Cu, I, Mg, Zn, algal oil blend providing DHA 200 mg. Beeswax, corn oil, glycerin, lactose, sorbitol, soybean oil, sunflower oil. Cap., softgel. UD 30s. *Rx.*
Use: Prenatal vitamin with minerals.

Vitagen Advance. (Midlothian) Vitamin B_{12} 10 mcg, desiccated stomach substance 50 mg, Fe 70 mg (from ferrous asparto glycinate), medium chain triglycerides, succinic acid 75 mg, vitamin C 152 mg (as calcium ascorbate and calcium threonate). Lactose, maltodextrin, polydextrose. Film-coated. Tab. 90s. *Rx.*
Use: Trace element, iron.

Vita-Iron Formula. (Barth's) Fe 120 mg, vitamins B_1 5 mg, B_2 10 mg, C 20 mg, niacin 2 mg, B_{12} 25 mcg, lysine, desiccated liver 200 mg, bromelains. Tab. Bot. 100s, 500s. *OTC.*
Use: Mineral, vitamin supplement.

Vita-Kaps Filmtabs. (Abbott) Vitamins A 5000 units, D 400 units, B_1 3 mg, B_2 2.5 mg, nicotinamide 20 mg, B_6 1 mg, C 50 mg, B_{12} 3 mcg. Bot. 100s, 1000s. *OTC.*
Use: Vitamin supplement.

Vitakaps-M. (Abbott) Vitamins A 5000 units, D 400 units, B_1 3 mg, B_2 2.5 mg, nicotinamide 20 mg, B_6 1 mg, B_{12} 3 mcg, C 50 mg, Fe 10 mg, Cu 1 mg, I 0.15 mg, Mn 1 mg, Zn 7.5 mg. Filmtab. Bot. 100s. *OTC.*
Use: Mineral, vitamin supplement.

Vita-Kid Chewable Wafers. (Solgar) Vitamins A 10,000 units, D 400 units, E 10 mg, B_1 2 mg, B_2 2 mg, B_3 10 mg, B_6 2 mg, B_{12} 5 mcg, C 100 mg, FA 0.3 mg, orange flavor. Bot. 50s, 100s. *OTC.*
Use: Vitamin supplement.

Vitalax. (Vitalax) Candy base, gumdrop flavor. Pkg. 20s. *OTC.*
Use: Laxative.

Vital B-50. (Ivax) Vitamins B_1 50 mg, B_2 50 mg, B_3 50 mg, B_5 50 mg, B_6 50 mg, B_{12} 50 mcg, folic acid 0.1 mg, biotin 50 mcg, PABA, choline bitartrate, inositol. TR Tab. Bot 60s. *OTC.*
Use: Vitamin supplement.

Vitalee. (MedChem) Vitamins A 3,000 units, D 400 units, E 30 units, B_1 1.5 mg, B_2 1.7 mg, B_3 20 mg, B_5 10 mg, B_6 2 mg, B_{12} 6 mcg, C 60 mg, folate 0.4 mg. PEG, sucrose. Tab. 30s. *OTC.*
Use: Multivitamin.

Vitalets. (Freeda) Fe 10 mg, vitamins A 5000 units, D 400 units, E 5 mg, B_1 2.5 mg, B_2 0.9 mg, B_3 20 mg, B_5 3 mg, B_6 2 mg, B_{12} 5 mcg, C 60 mg, biotin 25 mcg, Mn, Ca. Chew. Tab. Bot 100s, 250s. *OTC.*
Use: Mineral, vitamin supplement.

VitalEyes. (Allergan) Vitamins A 10,000 units, C 200 mg, E 100 units,

Zn 40 mg, Cu, Se, Mn. Cap. Bot. 60s. *OTC.*
Use: Mineral, vitamin supplement.

Vital High Nitrogen. (Ross) Amino acids, partially hydrolyzed whey, meat, and soy, hydrolyzed corn starch, sucrose, safflower oil, MCT mono- and diglycerides, soy lecithin, vitamins A, B_1, B_2, B_3, B_5, B_6, B_{12}, C, D, E, K, folic acid, biotin, choline, Ca, P, Mg, Fe, Cu, Zn, Mn, I, Cl. Packet 80 g. *OTC.*
Use: Nutritional supplement.

Vitaline Selenium. (Integrative Therapeutics) Calcium 121 mg, selenium 200 mcg. Cottonseed oil. Gluten free, preservative free, sugar free. Tab. 90s. *OTC.*
Use: Multimineral.

Vitalize SF. (Scot-Tussin) Fe 66 mg, B_1 30 mg, B_6 15 mg, B_{12} 75 mcg, l-lysine 300 mg. Liq. Bot. 120 mL. *OTC.*
Use: Mineral, vitamin supplement.

VitaMedMD Iron 21/7. (Therapeutics MD) Iron 150 mg, vitamins B_{12} 10 mcg, C 200 mg, folic acid 0.8 mg, succinic acid 150 mg, threonic acid 800 mcg. PEG. Tab. **Brown Tab.:** UD 21s. **Purple Tab.:** UD 7s w/folic acid 0.4 mg, succinic acid 150 mg, PEG. *Rx.*
Use: Prenatal vitamin with minerals.

VitaMedMD One Rx. (Therapeutics MD) Folic acid 1 mg (as *Quatrefolic* 600 mcg, folic acid 400 mcg), Fe 30 mg, vitamins D_3 400 units, E 21 units, B_1 1.5 mg, B_2 1.7 mg, B_3 20 mg, B_5 10 mg, B_6 25 mg, B_{12} 8 mcg, C 60 mg, Zn. Biotin 300 mcg, DHA 200 mg. Beeswax, orange oil, rosemary extract, soy, sunflower oil. Cap., softgel. UD 30s. *Rx.*
Use: Prenatal vitamin with minerals.

VitaMedMD Plus Rx. (Therapeutics MD) Folic acid 1mg (as *Quatrefolic* 600 mcg, folic acid 400 mcg), Ca 150 mg, Fe 30 mg, vitamins D_3 600 units, E 30 units, B_1 3 mg, B_2 3.4 mg, B_3 20 mg, B_5 10 mg, B_6 25 mg, B_{12} 12 mcg, C 60 mg, biotin 300 mcg. Cu, I, Zn. **Cap., softgel:** DHA 300 mg, sunflower oil. UD 30s. **Tab.:** Inulin, MCT. UD 30s. *Rx.*
Use: Prenatal vitamin with minerals.

VitaMedMD RediChew Rx. (Therapeutics MD) Folic acid 1 mg (as *Quatrefolic* 600 mcg, folic acid 400 mcg), vitamins D_3 400 units, B_2 1.7 mg, B_6 2 mg, B_{12} 8 mcg. Mannitol. Chew. Tab. UD 30s. *Rx.*
Use: Prenatal vitamin with minerals.

Vitamel with Iron. (Eastwood) Drops 50 mL. Chew. Tab. Bot. 100s. *OTC.*
Use: Mineral, vitamin supplement.

•**vitamin A.** (VYE-ta-min) *USP. Formerly Oleovitamin A.*
Use: Antixerophthalmic vitamin; emollient.
See: Aquasol A.
W/Combinations.
See: Advanced Formula Zenate.
Advera.
Bonamil Infant Formula with Iron.
Boost.
Choice DM.
Fosfree.
Neocate One +.
Nepro.
Ocuvite.
Ocuvite Extra.
Ocuvite PreserVision.
Oncovite.
Ondrox.
Prenatal H.P.
Prenatal Plus.
Prenatal Rx.
Prenatal Z Advanced Formula.
StuartNatal Plus 3.
Theragran AntiOxidant.
Tri-Flor-Vite with Fluoride.

vitamin A. (Various Mfr.) Vitamin A 10,000 IU, 15,000 IU, 25,000 IU. Cap. Bot. 100s, 250s (except 25,000 IU), 500s (10,000 units IU). *Rx-OTC.*
Use: Antixerophthalmic vitamin; emollient.

vitamin A acid.
See: Tretinoin.

vitamin A, alphalin. (Eli Lilly) Vitamin A 50,000 units. Gelseal. Bot. 100s. *Rx.*
Use: Vitamin supplement.

vitamin A, water miscible or soluble. Water-miscible vitamin A.
Use: Vitamin supplement.

vitamin Bc.
See: Folic Acid.

vitamin B combinations.
Use: Nutritional products.
See: Calafol.
Cardiotek Rx.
ComBgen.
DexFol.
Folpace.
W/Vitamin C.
See: Dialyvite Multi-Vitamins for Dialysis Patients.
Dialyvite 3000.
Full Spectrum B.

vitamin B complex. Concentrated extract of dried brewer's yeast and extract of corn processed w/*Clostridium acetobutylicum.*
See: Advanced Formula Zenate.
Advera.
Bonamil Infant Formula with Iron.

Boost.
Fosfree.
Neocate One +.
Nephplex Rx.
Nephron FA.
Nepro.
Ocuvite Extra.
Oncovite.
Prenatal H.P.
Prenatal Plus.
Prenatal Rx.
Prenatal Z Advanced Formula.
StuartNatal Plus 3.

Vitamin B Complex, Betalin Complex, Elixir. (Eli Lilly) Vitamins B_1 2.7 mg, B_2 1.35 mg, B_{12} 3 mcg, B_6 0.555 mg, pantothenic acid 2.7 mg, niacinamide 6.75 mg, liver fraction 500 mg/5 mL, alcohol 17%. Bot. 16 oz. *OTC.*
Use: Vitamin supplement.

Vitamin B Complex, Betalin Complex Pulvules. (Eli Lilly) Vitamins B_1 1 mg, B_2 2 mg, B_6 0.4 mg, pantothenic acid 3.333 mg, niacinamide 10 mg, B_{12} 1 mcg. Cap. Bot. 100s. *OTC.*
Use: Vitamin supplement.

Vitamin B Complex No. 104. (Century) Vitamins B_1 100 mg, B_2 2 mg, B_6 2 mg, d-panthenol 10 mg, niacinamide 125 mg. Vial, benzyl alcohol 1%, gentisic acid ethanolamide 2.5%. Vial 30 mL. *Rx.*
Use: Vitamin supplement.

Vitamin B Complex 100. (McGuff) Vitamin B_1 100 mg, B_2 2 mg, B_3 100 mg, B_5 2 mg, B_6 2 mg/mL. Inj. Vial 10 mL, 30 mL. *Rx.*
Use: Vitamin supplement.

Vitamin B Complex w/Vitamin C. (Century) Vitamins B_1 25 mg, B_2 5 mg, B_6 5 mg, niacinamide 50 mg, panthenol 5 mg, Ca 50 mg, propethylene glycol 300 10%, gentisic acid ethanolamide 2.5%, benzyl alcohol 2%. Vial 30 mL. *Rx.*
Use: Mineral, vitamin supplement.

vitamin B_8.
See: Adenosine Phosphate.

vitamin B_5. Calcium pantothenate.
Use: Vitamin supplement.
See: Calcium Pantothenate.

vitamin B_{15}.
Use: Alleged to increase oxygen supply in blood. Not approved by FDA as a vitamin or drug. Illegal to sell Vitamin B_{15}.

vitamin B_1. Thiamine hydrochloride.
Use: Vitamin supplement.
See: Thiamilate.
Thiamine Hydrochloride.

vitamin B_1 mononitrate. Thiamine mononitrate.
Use: Vitamin supplement.

vitamin B_6. Pyridoxine hydrochloride.
Use: Water-soluble vitamin.
See: Aminoxin.
Pyridoxine Hydrochloride.

vitamin B_6. (Various Mfr.) Vitamin B_6 50 mg, 100 mg, 250 mg, 500 mg. Tab. Bot. 100s, 250s (50 mg, 100 mg only), 1000s (50 mg only). *OTC.*
Use: Water-soluble vitamin.

vitamin B_3. Niacinamide, Nicotinamide.
Use: Vitamin supplement.
See: Niacor.
Niaspan.
Nicotinic Acid (Niacin).
Slo-Niacin.

vitamin B_{12}. Cyanocobalamin. Cobalamine. Vial. Amp.
See: Bedoce.
B-12.
Nascobal.
Sigamine.
Twelve Resin-K.
W/Thiamine, Vitamin B_6.
See: Orexin.

vitamin B_{12}. (Freeda) Vitamin B_{12} 50 mcg (sorbitol, mannitol), 100 mcg, 250 mcg, 500 mcg. Loz. Bot. 100s, 250s (250 mcg, 500 mcg only). *OTC.*
Use: Water-soluble vitamin.

vitamin B-12. (Mason) Vitamin B_{12} **Tab.:** 2,000 mcg. Whey. Preservative free. 60s. **Tab., Sublingual:** 1,000 mcg (dextrose), 5,000 mcg (mannitol). 20s, (5,000 mcg only), 100s (1,000 mcg only). *OTC.*
Use: Water-soluble vitamin.

vitamin B_{12}. (Nature's Blend) Cyanocobalamin 2,500 mcg. Sorbitol. Gluten free and preservative free. Tab., sublingual. *OTC.*
Use: Water-soluble vitamin.

vitamin B_{12}. (Various Mfr.) Cyanocobalamin. **Tab.:** 100 mcg, 500 mcg, 1,000 mcg. 100s. **Inj.: 100 mcg/mL:** Vials 30 mL. **1,000 mcg/mL:** Multidose vials. 10 mL, 30 mL. *Rx.*
Use: Water-soluble vitamin.

vitamin B_{12} a & b.
See: Hydroxocobalamin.

vitamin B_2. Riboflavin.
Use: Vitamin supplement.
See: Riboflavin.

vitamin B_2. (Nature's Blend) Riboflavin 25 mg. Polydextrose, sorbitol. Gluten free and preservative free. Tab. 100s. *OTC.*
Use: Water-soluble vitamin.

vitamin C. Ascorbic acid, sodium ascorbate, calcium ascorbate.
See: Ascocid.

Ascorbic Acid.
Calcium Ascorbate.
C-500.
Cenolate.
C-Gel.
Chewable Vitamin C.
Chew-C.
Complex C.
C-250.
Dull-C.
Hall's Defense.
N'ice.
N'ice with Vitamin C Drops.
SunKist Vitamin C.
Vita-C.
W/Combinations.
See: Advanced Formula Zenate.
Advera.
Allbee-C.
Allbee C-800.
Allbee-T.
Antiox.
Bonamil Infant Formula with Iron.
Boost.
Choice DM.
Chromagen FA.
Chromagen Forte.
C-Max.
Fosfree.
Fruit C 500.
Fruit C 100.
Fruit C 200.
Neocate One +.
Nephplex Rx.
Nephron FA.
Nepro.
Nialexo-C.
Ocuvite.
Ocuvite Extra.
Ocuvite Lutein.
Ocuvite PreserVision.
Oncovite.
Prenatal H.P.
Prenatal Plus.
Prenatal Rx.
Protegra Softgels.
StuartNatal Plus 3.
Theragran Antioxidant.
Thex Forte.
Tri-Flor-Vite with Fluoride.
Vicon-C.
Vicon Forte.
Vicon Plus.
Vi-Zac.
Z-BEC.
W/Vitamin B.
See: Dialyvite Multi-Vitamins for Dialysis Patients.
W/Zinc, Glutathione.
See: Sucrets Defense Kid's Formula.

vitamin C, cevalin. (Eli Lilly) Ascorbic acid 250 mg, 500 mg. Tab. Bot. 100s. *OTC.*
Use: Vitamin supplement.

vitamin D. Cholecalciferol.
Use: Vitamin D supplement.
See: Ergocalciferol.
W/Calcium.
See: Calcium 1000 + D.
W/Combinations.
See: Advanced Formula Zenate.
Advera.
Bonamil Infant Formula with Iron.
Boost.
Caltrate Plus.
Caltrate 600 + D.
Choice DM.
Desert Pure Calcium.
Fosfree.
Neocate One +.
Nepro.
Oesto-Mins.
Oncovite.
Ondrox.
Prenatal Plus.
Prenatal Rx.
StuartNatal Plus 3.
Tri-Flor-Vite with Fluoride.

vitamin D. (Basic Organics) Cholecalciferol (D_3) 2,000 units. Corn oil, soybean oil. Gluten free, preservative free. Cap., softgel. 30s, 60s. *OTC.*
Use: Fat-soluble vitamin.

vitamin D. (Pliva) Vitamin D_2 50,000 units. Soybean oil. Cap. 100s, 1000s. *Rx.*
Use: Vitamin supplement.

vitamin D. (Various Mfr.) Ergocalciferol (D_2) 50,000 units. Cap. Bot. 100s, 1000s. *Rx.*
Use: Vitamin supplement.

vitamin D_1.
See: Dihydrotachysterol.

Vitamin D Supplement Drops. (Hi-Tech) Cholecalciferol (D_3) 400 units per drop. Cherry flavoring, glycerin, polysorbate 80. Soln., Conc. 50 mL w/dropper. *OTC.*
Use: Fat-soluble vitamin.

vitamin D, synthetic.
See: Activated 7-Dehydro-Cholesterol.
Calciferol.

vitamin D_3.
See: Advanced D5000.
Baby Ddrops.
Ddrops.
Decara.
D_3 Dots.
D3-50.
D_3 Healthy Kids.
Delta-D.
Super Strength D-2000 IU.
Thera-D 4000.

Thera-D 2000.
Ultra Strength D2000.
W/Calcium Carbonate.
See: Citrus Calcium with Vitamin D.
D-1000 Extra Strength.
Liquid Calcium with D_3 Maximum Strength.
Super Calcium 600 + D_3 400.

vitamin D_3. (Freeda) Cholecalciferol (D_3) 1000 IU. Sugar free. Tab. Bot. 100s, 500s. *OTC.*
Use: Vitamin supplement.

vitamin D_3. (Integrative Therapeutics) Cholecalciferol (D_3) 2,000 units, 5,000 units. Maltodextrin (2,000 units only), mannitol, sorbitol. Gluten free and preservative free. Chocolate flavor. Chew. Tab. 90s (5,000 units), 120s (2,000 units). *OTC.*
Use: Fat-soluble vitamin.

vitamin D_3. (VitaMed MD) Cholecalciferol (D_3) 1,000 units, 50,000 units. Dye free and gluten free. Cap. 12s (50,000 units), 60s (1,000 units). *OTC.*
Use: Fat-soluble vitamin.

vitamin D-3-cholesterol. Compound of crystalline vitamin D-3 and cholesterol.

vitamin D3 400 IU. (Major) Vitamin D 400 units, calcium 76 mg. Preservative free, sugar free. Tab. 100s. *OTC.*
Use: Fat-soluble vitamin.

vitamin D_2. Activated ergasterol, Ergocalciferol.
See: Calciferol.
Drisdol.
Ergocalciferol Drops.
Viosterol.

•**vitamin E.** (VYE-ta-min) *USP.*
Use: Vitamin E supplement.
See: Aqua-E.
Aquasol E.
Aquavit-E.
Chantel Vitamin E.
E-Oil.
GRX Vitamin E.
Lactinol-E.
Mixed E 400 Softgels.
Mixed E 1000 Softgels.
Natural E 200.
Natural Vitamin E.
Nutr-E-Sol.
One-A-Day Extras Vitamin E.
Soft Sense.
Vitamin E with Mixed Tocopherols.
Vita-Plus E.
Wheat Germ Oil.
W/Combinations.
See: Advanced Formula Zenate.
Advera.
Antiox.
Bonamil Infant Formula with Iron.
Boost.
Choice DM.
Neocate One +.
Nepro.
Ocuvite.
Ocuvite Extra.
Ocuvite Lutein.
Ocuvite PreserVision.
Oncovite.
Ondrox.
Prenatal Plus.
StuartNatal Plus 3.
Theragran AntiOxidant.

vitamin E. (Freeda) Vitamin E 15 IU/ 30 mL. Liq. Bot. 30 mL, 60 mL, 120 mL. *OTC.*
Use: Vitamin supplement.

vitamin E. (Various Mfr.) Vitamin E. **Tab.:** d-alpha tocopherol 100 IU, 200 IU, 400 IU, 500 IU, 800 IU. Bot. 100s, 250s (except 800 IU), 500s (200 IU, 400 IU only). **Cap.:** 100 IU, 200 IU, 400 IU, 1000 IU. Bot. 50s (1000 IU only), 100s, 250s (400 IU only). *OTC.*
Use: Vitamin supplement.

vitamin E, eprolin. (Eli Lilly) Alpha-tocopherol 100 units. Gelseal. Bot. 100s. *OTC.*
Use: Vitamin supplement.

•**vitamin E polyethylene glycol succinate.** (VYE-ta-min E POL-ee-ETH-i-leen GLYE-kol SUX-i-nate) *NF.*
Use: Vitamin supplement.

vitamin E with mixed tocopherols. (Freeda) Vitamin E 100 IU, 200 IU, 400 IU. Tab. Bot. 100s, 250s, 500s (400 IU only). *OTC.*
Use: Vitamin supplement.

vitamin, fat-soluble.
See: Fat-Soluble Vitamins.

vitamin G.
See: Riboflavin.

vitamin K.
See: Mephyton.
Phytonadione.
W/Combinations.
See: Advera.
Bonamil Infant Formula with Iron.
Choice DM.
Neocate One +.

vitamin K. (Nature's Blend) Phytonadione 0.1 mg. Gluten free and preservative free. Tab. 100s. *OTC.*
Use: Fat-soluble vitamin.

vitamin K_1.
See: Phytonadione.

vitamin K_3.
See: Menadione.

vitamin K oxide. Not available, but usually K-1 is desired.

vitamin M.
See: Folic Acid.
vitamin, maintenance formula.
See: Stuart Formula.
vitamin-mineral-supplement liquid. (Morton Grove) Vitamins B_1 0.83 mg, B_2 0.42 mg, B_3 8.3 mg, B_5 1.67 mg, B_6 0.17 mg, B_{12} 0.17 mcg, I, Fe 2.5 mg, Mg, Zn 0.3 mg, Mn, choline, alcohol 18%. Liq. 473 mL. *OTC.*
Use: Mineral, vitamin supplement.
vitamin P. Bioflavonoids.
See: Amino-Opti-C.
Bio-Flavonoid Compounds.
C Factors "1000" Plus.
Ester-C Plus 500 mg Vitamin C.
Ester-C Plus 1000 mg Vitamin C.
Ester-C Plus Multi-Mineral.
Flavons.
Flavons-500.
Hesperidin.
Pan C Ascorbate.
Pan C-500.
Peridin-C.
Quercetin.
Rutin.
Span C.
Super Flavons.
Super Flavons 300.
Tri-Super Flavons 1000.
vitamins.
See: Fat-Soluble Vitamins.
Water-Soluble Vitamins.
vitamins, fat soluble.
See: Calcitriol.
Cholecalciferol.
Dihydrotachysterol.
Doxercalciferol.
Ergocalciferol.
Paricalcitol.
Phytonadione.
Vitamin E.
Vitamin K.
vitamins, stress formula.
See: Probec-T.
Stress Formula with Iron.
Stresstabs 600.
Thera-Combex H-P.
vitamins, water soluble.
See: Aminobenzoate Potassium.
Ascorbic Acid.
Ascorbic Acid Combinations.
Bioflavonoids.
Calcium Ascorbate.
Cyanocobalamin.
Levoleucovorin.
L-methylfolate.
Niacin.
Niacinamide.
Pantothenic Acid.
Pyridoxine Hydrochloride.
Riboflavin.
Sodium Ascorbate.
Thiamin.
vitamins with liver and lipotropic agents.
See: Metheponex.
vitamin T. Sesame seed factor, termite factor.
Use: Claimed to aid proper blood coagulation and promote formation of blood platelets. Not approved by FDA as an active vitamin.
vitamin U. Present in cabbage juice.
Vita Natal. (Scot-Tussin) Folic acid 1 mg. Tab. Bot. 100s. *Rx.*
Use: Vitamin supplement.
Vitaneed. (Biosearch Medical Products) P-beef, Ca and Na caseinates, CHO-maltodextrin. F-partially hydrogenated soy oil, mono- and diglycerides, soy lecithin. Protein 35 g, CHO 125 g, fat 40 g, Na 500 mg, K 1250 mg/L, 1 Cal/mL, 375 mOsm/kg H_2O. Liq. Ready-to-use 250 mL. *OTC.*
Use: Nutritional supplement.
Vitaon. (Vita Elixir) Vitamin B_{12} 25 mcg, thiamine hydrochloride 10 mg, ferric pyrophosphate 250 mg/5 mL. *OTC.*
Use: Vitamin supplement.
Vita Pearl. (vitaMedMD) Folic acid 1.4 mg, iron 30 mg, vitamins D 400 units, E 30 units, B_1 1.7 mg, B_2 2 mg, B_3 20 mg, B_5 10 mg, B_6 25 mg, B_{12} 8 mcg, C 30 mg, I, Zn, biotin 300 mcg, DHA 200 mg. Gluten free, lactose free, sugar free. Beeswax, glycerin, glycerol, sunflower lecithin. Cap., softgel. 30s. *Rx.*
Use: Prenatal vitamin with minerals.
Vita-Plus B12. (Scot-Tussin) Vitamin B_{12} 1000 mcg/mL. Inj. *Rx.*
Use: Vitamin supplement.
Vita-Plus E. (Scot-Tussin) Vitamin E 400 IU as d-alpha tocopheryl acetate. Sugar free. Cap. Bot. 50s. *OTC.*
Use: Vitamin supplement.
Vita-Plus G. (Scot-Tussin) Vitamins A 10,000 units, D 400 units, E_2 2 mg, B_1 5 mg, B_2 2.5 mg, B_3 40 mg, B_6 1 mg, B_{12} 2 mcg, pantothenic acid 4 mg, C 75 mg, Fe, Ca, Zn 0.5 mg, K, Mg, Mn, P. Softgel Cap. Bot. 100s. *OTC.*
Use: Mineral, vitamin supplement.
Vita-Plus H Liquid Sugar Free. (Scot-Tussin) Vitamins B_1 30 mg, l-lysine monohydrochloride 300 mg, B_{12} 75 mcg, B_6 15 mg, iron pyrophosphate soluble 100 mg/5 mL. Bot. 4 oz, 8 oz, pt, gal. *OTC.*
Use: Mineral, vitamin supplement.
Vita-Plus H Softgel. (Scot-Tussin) Fe

13.4 mg, vitamins A 5000 units, D 400 units, E 3 units, B_1 3 mg, B_2 2.5 mg, B_3 20 mg, B_5 5 mg, B_6 1.5 mg, B_{12} 2.5 mcg, C 50 mg, Ca, K, Mg, Mn, P, Zn 1.4 mg. Cap. Bot. 100s. *OTC.*
Use: Mineral, vitamin supplement.

Vita-PMS. (Bajamar Chemical) Vitamins A 2083 units, E 16.7 units, D_3 16.7 units, folic acid 33 mcg, B_1 4.2 mg, B_2 4.2 mg, B_3 4.2 mg, B_5 4.2 mg, B_6 50 mg, B_{12} 10.4 mcg, biotin, C 250 mg, Ca, Mg, I, Fe, Cu, Zn 4.2 mg, Mn, K, Se, Cr, betaine. Tab. Bot. 100s. *OTC.*
Use: Mineral, vitamin supplement.

Vita-PMS Plus. (Bajamar Chemical) Vitamins A 667 units, E 16.7 units, D_3 16.7 units, folic acid 33 mcg, B_1 4.2 mg, B_2 4.2 mg, B_3 4.2 mg, B_5 4.2 mg, B_6 16.7 mg, B_{12} 10.4 mcg, biotin, C 250 mg, Mg, I, Ca, Fe, Cu, Zn 4.2 mg, Mn, K, Se, Cr, betaine. Tab. Bot. 100s. *OTC.*
Use: Mineral, vitamin supplement.

Vita-Ray Creme. (Gordon Laboratories) Vitamins E 3000 units, A 200,000 units/oz w/aloe 10%. Jar 0.5 oz, 2.5 oz. *OTC.*
Use: Emollient.

Vitarex. (Taylor Pharmaceuticals) Vitamins A 10,000 units, D 200 units, B_1 15 mg, B_2 10 mg, B_6 5 mg, B_{12} 5 mcg, C 250 mg, B_3 100 mg, B_5 20 mg, E 15 mg, Fe 15 mg, Ca, Cu, I, K, Mg, Mn, P, Zn 10 mg. Tab. Bot. 100s. *OTC.*
Use: Mineral, vitamin supplement.

Vitazin. (Mesemer) Ascorbic acid 300 mg, niacinamide 100 mg, thiamine mononitrate 20 mg, d-calcium pantothenate 20 mg, riboflavin 10 mg, pyridoxine hydrochloride 5 mg, magnesium sulfate 70 mg, Zn 25 mg. Cap. Bot. 100s. *OTC.*
Use: Mineral, vitamin supplement.

Vita-Zoo. (Towne) Vitamins A 2500 units, D 400 units, E 15 units, C 60 mg, folic acid 0.3 mg, B_1 1.05 mg, B_2 1.2 mg, niacin 13.5 mg, B_6 1.05 mg, B_{12} 4.5 mcg. Tab. Bot. 100s. *OTC.*
Use: Vitamin supplement.

Vita-Zoo Plus Iron. (Towne) Vitamins A 2500 units, D 400 units, E 15 units, C 60 mg, folic acid 0.3 mg, B_1 1.05 mg, B_2 1.2 mg, niacin 13.5 mg, B_6 1.05 mg, B_{12} 4.5 mcg, Fe 15 mg. Tab. Bot. 100s. *OTC.*
Use: Mineral, vitamin supplement.

Vitec. (Pharmaceutical Specialties) Dl-alpha tocopheryl acetate in a vanishing cream base. Cream. 120 g. *OTC.*
Use: Emollient.

Vitelle Irospan. (Fielding) Iron 65 mg (from ferrous sulfate exsiccated), ascorbic acid 150 mg. Sugar. Cap. 60s. *OTC.*
Use: Vitamin and mineral supplement.

Vitelle Lurline PMS. (Fielding) Acetaminophen 500 mg, pamabrom 25 mg, pyridoxine hydrochloride 50 mg. Tab. Bot 50s. *OTC.*
Use: Analgesic combination.

Vitelle Nesentials. (Fielding) Vitamin A 5000 units, D_2 400 units, E 30 units, B_1 3 mg, B_2 3 mg, B_3 25 mg, B_6 2 mg, B_{12} 6 mcg, C 120 mg, Ca, P, Zn. Tab. Bot. 60s. *OTC.*
Use: Vitamin, mineral supplement.

Vitelle Nestabs OTC. (Fielding) Vitamins A 5000 units, C 120 mg, D 400 units, E 30 units, thiamin 3 mg, riboflavin 3 mg, niacinamide 20 mg, B_6 3 mg, folic acid 800 mcg, B_{12} 8 mcg, Ca 200 mg, Fe 29 mg, I, Zn 15 mg. Tab. Bot. 100s. *OTC.*
Use: Vitamin, mineral supplement.

•**vitespen.** (vi-TES-pen) USAN.
Use: Antineoplastic.

Vite With Iron, Children's. (Rugby) Iron 15 mg, vitamins A 2,500 units, D 400 units, E 15 units, B_1 1.05 mg, B_2 1.2 mg, B_3 13.5 mg, B_6 1.05 mg, B_{12} 4.5 mcg, C 60 mg, folic acid 0.3 mg. Cherry flavoring, dextrose, grape flavoring, orange flavoring, sodium benzoate, sugar. Chew. Tab. 100s. *OTC.*
Use: Multivitamin with iron.

Vitrase. (Bausch & Lomb) Hyaluronidase (ovine source) 200 units/mL. Lactose 0.93 mg. Preservative free. Soln. for Inj. Single-use 2 mL vials. *Rx.*
Use: Physical adjunct.

Vitron-C. (Insight Pharmaceuticals) Iron (from ferrous fumarate) 66 mg, ascorbic acid 125 mg. Tab. Bot. 60s. *OTC.*
Use: Mineral and vitamin supplement.

Vituz. (Hawthorn) Chlorpheniramine maleate 4 mg, hydrocodone bitartrate 5 mg. Glycerin, parabens, propylene glycol, saccharin, sucrose. Grape flavor. Soln. 480 mL. *c-III.*
Use: Upper respiratory combination, antitussive combination.

Vivactil. (Barr/Duramed) Protriptyline hydrochloride 5 mg, 10 mg. Lactose. Film-coated. Tab. Bot. 100s, UD 100s (10 mg only). *Rx.*
Use: Antidepressant.

Viva DHA. (Jaymac) Folic acid 1 mg, iron 28 mg, vitamins D 400 units, E 30 units, B_1 3 mg, B_2 3 mg, B_6 20 mg, B_{12} 15 mcg, C 100 mg, Cu, Mg, Zn, omega-3 fatty acids 200 mg (DHA and EPA). Beeswax, glycerol, lecithin, soy. Cap., softgel. 30s. *Rx.*
Use: Prenatal vitamin with minerals.

Viva-Drops. (Vision Pharmaceuticals) Polysorbate 80, sodium chloride, EDTA, retinyl palmitate, mannitol, sodium citrate, pyruvate. Soln. Bot. 10 mL, 15 mL. *OTC.*
Use: Artificial tears.

Vivarin. (Meda Consumer Healthcare) Caffeine 200 mg, dextrose. Tab. Bot. 16s, 24s, 40s, 80s. *OTC.*
Use: CNS stimulant, analeptic.

Vivelle-Dot. (Novartis) Estradiol 0.39 mg (0.025 mg/day), 0.585 mg (0.0375 mg/day), 0.78 mg (0.05 mg/day), 1.17 mg (0.075 mg/day), 1.56 mg (0.1 mg/day). Transdermal system. Calendar pack (8 and 24 [0.39 mg only] systems). *Rx.*
Use: Estrogen, sex hormone.

Vivikon. (AstraZeneca) Vitamins B_1 5 mg, B_2 2 mg, B_6 10 mg, d-panthenol 5 mg, niacinamide 10 mg, procaine hydrochloride 2%/mL. 100 mL. *OTC.*
Use: Vitamin supplement.

Vivitrol. (Alkermes) Naltrexone hydrochloride 380 mg per vial. Carboxymethylcellulose sodium salt, sodium chloride. Susp., ER Inj. Single-use vials. *Rx.*
Use: Antidote, detoxification agent.

Vivonex Flavor Packets. (Procter & Gamble) Nonnutritive flavoring for *Vivonex* diets when consumed orally. Orange-pineapple, lemon-lime, strawberry, and vanilla. Pkg. 60s. *OTC.*
Use: Flavoring.

Vivonex, Standard. (Procter & Gamble) Free amino acid/complete enteral nutrition. Six packets provide kcal 1800, available nitrogen 5.88 g as amino acids 37 g, fat 2.61 g, carbohydrate 407 g, and full day's balanced nutrition. Calorie:nitrogen ratio is 300:1. Unflavored pow. Packet 80 g. Pkg. 6s. *OTC.*
Use: Nutritional supplement.

Vivonex T.E.N. (Procter & Gamble) Free amino acid, high nitrogen/high branched chain amino acid complete enteral nutrition. Ten packets provide kcal 3000, available nitrogen 17 g, amino acids 115 g, fat 8.33 g, carbohydrate 617 g, and full day's balanced nutrition. Calorie:nitrogen ratio is 175:1. Unflavored pow. Packet 80 g. Pkg. 10s. *OTC.*
Use: Nutritional supplement.

Vivotif Berna. (Berna) Typhoid vaccine (oral). *Salmonella typhi* Ty21a (viable) 2 to 6 $\times$ 10^9 colony-forming units and *S. typhi* Ty21a (non-viable) 5 to 50 $\times$ 10^9 colony-forming units, sucrose 26 to 130 mg, ascorbic acid 1 to 5 mg, amino acid mixture 1.4 to 7 mg, lactose 100 to 180 mg, magnesium stearate 3.6 to 4.4 mg. EC Cap. Blister pack 4s. *Rx.*
Use: Immunization.

Vi-Zac. (UCB) Vitamins A 5,000 units, E 50 units, C 500 mg, Zn 18 mg. Lactose. Bot. 60s. *OTC.*
Use: Mineral, vitamin supplement.

Vlemasque. (Dermik) Sulfurated lime topical solution 6% (Vleminck's Soln.), alcohol 7% in drying clay mask. Jar 4 oz. *OTC.*
Use: Dermatologic, acne.

VM. (Last) Vitamins B_1 6 mg, B_2 4 mg, niacinamide 40 mg, Fe 100 mg, Ca 188 mg, P 188 mg, Mn 4 mg, alcohol 12%. Bot. 16 oz. *OTC.*
Use: Mineral, vitamin supplement.

V-Natal. (Virtus Pharmaceuticals) Folate 1 mg, calcium 200 mg, Fe 32 mg, vitamins D 450 units, E 30 units, B_1 3 mg, B_2 3 mg, B_3 20 mg, B_6 50 mg, B_{12} 10 mcg, C 120 mg, choline 55 mg, I, Zn. Film coated. Tab. 90s. *Rx.*
Use: Prenatal vitamin with minerals.

V-Natal DHA. (Virtus Pharmaceuticals)
Tab.: Folic acid 1 mg, calcium 200 mg, Fe 32 mg, vitamins D 450 units, E 30 units, B_1 3 mg, B_2 3 mg, B_3 20 mg, B_6 50 mg, B_{12} 10 mcg, C 120 mg, choline 55 mg, I, Zn. Film coated. UD 30s.
Cap., softgel: DHA 230 mg, EPA 30 mg. Enteric coated. Glycerin. UD 30s. *Rx.*
Use: Prenatal vitamin with minerals.

•**vocimagene amiretrorepvec.** (voe-SIM-a-jeen AM-i-RE-troe-rep-vek) USAN.
Use: Antineoplastic.

•**vofopitant dihydrochloride.** (voe-FOE-pi-tant) USAN.
Use: Antimetic.

•**volasertib.** (VOE-la-SER-tib) USAN.
Use: Antineoplastic.

•**volasertib trihydrochloride.** (VOE-la-SER-tib) USAN.
Use: Antineoplastic.

volatile liquids.
Use: Anesthetic, general.
See: Sevoflurane.
Ultane.

•**volazocine.** (voe-LAY-zoe-SEEN) USAN. Under study.
Use: Analgesic.

Volitane. (Trent) Parethoxycaine 0.2%, hexachlorophene 0.025%, dichlorophene 0.025%. Aerosol spray can 3 oz. *OTC.*
Use: Counterirritant; antiseptic.

•**volociximab.** (voe-loe-SIX-i-mab) USAN.
Use: Antineoplastic.

Vol-Tab Rx. (Trigen Labs) Vitamins A

4,000 units, C 120 mg, D 400 units, E 30 units, B_1 3 mg, B_2 3 mg, B_3 20 mg, B_5 7 mg, B_6 3 mg, B_{12} 8 mcg, biotin 30 mcg, folic acid 1 mg, Ca 200 mg, Fe 29 mg, I, Zn, Mg, Cu. PEG, vegetable oil, polysorbate 80. Tab. 90s. *Rx.*
Use: Prenatal vitamin.

Voltaren. (Endo Pharmaceuticals) Diclofenac sodium 1% (1 g contains diclofenac sodium 10 mg). Isopropyl alcohol, mineral oil. Gel. Tubes. 20 g, 100 g.

Voltaren. (Novartis) Diclofenac sodium. **DR Tab.:** 75 mg. Lactose. Enteric-coated. Bot. 60s, 100s, 1000s, UD 100s. **Ophth. Soln.:** 0.1%. EDTA 1 mg/mL, boric acid, polyoxyl 35 castor oil, sorbic acid 2 mg/mL, tromethamine. 2.5 mL, 5 mL w/dropper. *Rx.*
Use: NSAID; ophthalmic.

Voltaren-XR. (Novartis) Diclofenac sodium 100 mg. Sucrose, cetyl alcohol. ER Tab. Bot. 100s, UD 100s. *Rx.*
Use: Analgesic; NSAID.

Voluven. (Hospira) Hydroxyethyl starch 6 g/100 mL. Sodium chloride 900 mg/100 mL. Inj., Soln. 500 mL. *Rx.*
Use: Plasma expander.

Voluven. (Hospira) Tetrastarch 6 g per 100 mL in sodium chloride 0.9%. Latex free. Inj., Soln. 500 mL single-dose container. *Rx.*
Use: Plasma expander.

vonedrine hydrochloride. Vonedrine (phenylpropylmethylamine) hydrochloride. *OTC.*
Use: Decongestant.

•**vonicog alfa.** (VOE-ni-kog) USAN.
Use: Prophylactic treatment of bleeding episodes and von Willebrand disease.

von Willebrand factor complex/antihemophilic factor.
Use: Antihemophilic agent.
See: Humate-P.

Vopac. (Athlon) Codeine phosphate 30 mg, acetaminophen 650 mg. Tab. 100s, 500s. *c-III.*
Use: Narcotic analgesic.

•**vorapaxar.** (VOR-a-PAX-ar) USAN.
Use: Thrombosis.

•**vorapaxar sulfate.** (VOR-a-PAX-ar) USAN.
Use: Thrombin receptor antagonist.

Voraxaze. (BTG International Inc) Glucarpidase 1,000 units. Lactose. Preservative free. Inj., lyophilized Pow. for Soln. Single-use vial. *Rx.*
Use: Detoxification agent, antidote.

•**voreloxin.** (vor-el-OX-in) USAN.
Use: Antineoplastic.

•**voriconazole.** (vor-i-KON-a-zole) USAN.
Use: Antifungal.
See: Vfend.

voriconazole. (Various Mfr.) Voriconazole. **Tab.:** 50 mg, 200 mg. May contain lactose. 30s. **Pow. for Susp.:** 40 mg/mL (after reconstitution). May contain sodium benzoate, sucrose. Orange flavor. 75 mL. **Inj., lyophilized Pow. for Soln.:** 200 mg. Sulfobutyl ether beta-cyclodextrin sodium 3,200 mg. Single-use vial. *Rx.*
Use: Antifungal, triazole antifungal.

•**vorinostat.** (vore-IN-oh-stat) USAN.
Use: Antineoplastic; histone deacetylase inhibitor.
See: Zolinza.

•**vorozole.** (VORE-oh-zole) USAN.
Use: Antineoplastic.

•**vorsetuzumab.** (VOR-se-TOOZ-ue-mab) USAN.
Use: Antineoplastic.

•**vorsetuzumab mafodotin.** (VOR-se-TOOZ-ue-mab MA-foe-DOE-tin) USAN.
Use: Antineoplastic.

•**vortioxetine.** (VOR-tye-OX-e-teen) USAN.
Use: Antidepressant, anxiolytic.
See: Brintellix.

•**vortioxetine hydrobromide.** (VOR-tye-OX-e-teen) USAN.
Use: Antidepressant, anxiolytic.

•**vosaroxin.** (VOE-sa-ROX-in) USAN.
Use: Antineoplastic.

VōSoL. (ECR Pharmaceuticals) Acetic acid 2%, propylene glycol diacetate 3%, benzethonium chloride 0.02%, sodium acetate 0.015%. Soln.; Otic. 15 mL w/dropper. *Rx.*
Use: Otic preparation.

VōSoL HC. (ECR Pharmaceuticals) Hydrocortisone 1%, acetic acid 2%, benzethonium chloride 0.02%, propylene glycol diacetate 3%. Soln., Otic. 10 mL. *OTC.*
Use: Otic preparation.

VoSpire ER. (Dava) Albuterol (as sulfate) 4 mg, 8 mg. ER Tab. 100s. *Rx.*
Use: Bronchodilator; sympathomimetic.

Votrient. (GlaxoSmithKline) Pazopanib 200 mg (equiv. to pazopanib hydrochloride 216.7 mg). Film coated. Tab. 120s. *Rx.*
Use: Kinase inhibitor, tyrosine kinase inhibitor.

•**votumumab.** (vah-TOOM-uh-mab) USAN.
Use: Monoclonal antibody.

Voxsuprine. (Major) Isoxsuprine hydrochloride 10 mg, 20 mg. Tab. Bot. 100s,

250s, 1000s, UD 100s. *Rx.*
Use: Vasodilator.

VP-CH Plus. (Virtus Pharmaceuticals) Folic acid 1 mg, calcium 104 mg, iron 29 mg, vitamins D 400 units, E 30 units, B_6 25 mg, DHA 265 mg, docusate sodium 50 mg. Beeswax, glycerin, soy lecithin, soybean oil. Cap., softgel. 30s. *Rx.*
Use: Prenatal vitamin with minerals.

VP-CH-PNV. (Virtus Pharmaceuticals) Folic acid 1 mg, Ca 104 mg, Fe 30 mg, vitamins D 400 units, E 30 units, B_6 25 mg, DHA 260 mg, docusate sodium 50 mg. Beeswax, glycerin, soy, soybean oil. Cap., softgel. 30s. *Rx.*
Use: Prenatal vitamin with minerals.

VP-GGR-B6. (Virtus Pharmaceuticals) Folic acid 1.2 mg, Ca 124.1 mg, vitamin B_6 40 mg, ginger root powder extract 100 mg. Tab. 60s. *Rx.*
Use: Prenatal vitamin with minerals.

VP-Heme OB. (Virtus Pharmaceuticals) Folic acid 1 mg, iron 34 mg, vitamins D 400 units, E 10 units, B_1 1.5 mg, B_2 1.6 mg, B_3 17 mg, B_5 10 mg, B_6 50 mg, B_{12} 12 mcg, Cu, I, Se, Zn, biotin 30 mcg. Film coated. Tab. 90s. *Rx.*
Use: Prenatal vitamin with minerals.

VP-Heme OB + DHA Tablets and Softgel Capsules. (Virtus Pharmaceuticals) Folic acid 1 mg, iron 34 mg, vitamins D 400 units, E 10 units, B_1 1.5 mg, B_2 1.6 mg, B_3 17 mg, B_5 10 mg, B_6 50 mg, B_{12} 12 mcg, Cu, I, Se, Zn, biotin 30 mcg. **Tab.:** Film coated. UD 30s. **Cap., softgel:** Omega-3 fatty acids 203 mg (DHA 200 mg, ALA 0.5 mg, and DPA 2.5 mg). Glycerin. Enteric coated. UD 30s. *Rx.*
Use: Prenatal vitamin with minerals.

VP-Heme One. (Virtus Pharmaceuticals) Folic acid 1 mg, iron 28 mg, vitamins D 400 units, E 10 units, B_3 17 mg, B_5 10 mg, B_6 50 mg, B_{12} 12 mcg, C 25 mg, I, Zn, biotin 30 mcg, DHA 200 mg. Glycerin, soybean oil, soy. Cap., softgel. UD 30s. *Rx.*
Use: Prenatal vitamin with minerals.

VP-PNV-DHA. (Virtus Pharmaceuticals) Folic acid 1 mg, calcium 50 mg, Fe 28 mg, vitamins A 2,500 units, D 400 units, E 30 units, B_1 6 mg, B_2 2.2 mg, B_3 20 mg, B_6 16 mg, B_{12} 12 mcg, C 80 mg, Cu, Mg, Zn, DHA 200 mg, EPA 15.8 mg. Beeswax, glycerin, soy lecithin, soybean oil. Cap., softgel. UD 30s. *Rx.*
Use: Prenatal vitamin with minerals.

VPRIV. (Shire Human Genetic Therapies) Velaglucerase alfa 200 units, 400 units. Sucrose 100 mg (200 units), 200 mg (400 units). Preservative free. Single-use vial. *Rx.*
Use: Endocrine and metabolic agent.

VP-Zel Tabs. (Virtus Pharmaceuticals) Vitamins B_3 600 mg, B_6 5 mg, folate 0.5 mcg, Cu, Zn, azelaic acid 5 mg. Film coated. Tab. 60s. *Rx.*
Use: Multivitamin with minerals (except iron).

VSL#3 DS Double Strength. (Sigma-Tau) ≥ 900 billion bacteria blend of *S. thermophilus, B. breve, B. longum, B. infantis, L. acidophilus, L. plantarum, L. paracasei, L. delbrueckii.* Gluten free. Pow.; oral. Sachet (20s). *Rx.*
Use: Probiotic.

VSL#3 Junior. (Sigma-Tau) ≥ 225 billion bacteria blend of *S. thermophilus, B. breve, B. longum, B. infantis, L. acidophilus, L. plantarum, L. paracasei, L. delbrueckii.* Maltose, stevia. Gluten free. Watermelon flavor. Packet. 30s. *OTC.*
Use: Probiotic.

VSL#3 The Living Shield. (Sigma-Tau) **Cap.:** ≥ 112.5 billion bacteria blend of *S. thermophilus, B. breve, B. longum, B. infantis, L. acidophilus, L. plantarum, L. paracasei, L. delbrueckii.* Gluten free. 60s. **Pow.; oral:** ≥ 450 billion bacteria blend of *S. thermophilus, B. breve, B. longum, B. infantis, L. acidophilus, L. plantarum, L. paracasei, L. delbrueckii.* Gluten free. Lemon flavor or unflavored. Sachet (10s, 30s). *OTC.*
Use: Probiotic.

V-Tuss Expectorant. (Vangard Labs, Inc.) Hydrocodone bitartrate 5 mg, pseudoephedrine hydrochloride 60 mg, guaifenesin 200 mg/5 mL, alcohol 12.5%. *c-III.*
Use: Antitussive, decongestant, expectorant.

Vumon. (Bristol-Myers Squibb Oncology/Virology) Teniposide 50 mg (10 mg/mL), benzyl alcohol 30 mg, *Cremophor EL* (polyoxyethylated castor oil), dehydrated alcohol 42.7%. Inj. Amp. 5 mL. *Rx.*
Use: Antineoplastic.

Vusion. (GlaxoSmithKline) Miconazole nitrate 0.25%, zinc oxide 15%, white petrolatum 81.35%. Oint. Tube. 30 g. *Rx.*
Use: Diaper rash combination product.

Vyfemla. (Lupin) Ethinyl estradiol 35 mcg, norethindrone 0.4 mg. Lactose. Tab. 28s w/7 inert tablets (lactose). *Rx.*
Use: Monophasic oral contraceptive.

Vytone. (Artesa Labs) Hydrocortisone acetate 1.9%, iodoquinol 1%. Alcohol, aloe, benzyl alcohol, glycerin, glyceryl,

propylene glycol. Cream. 2 g sachets. *Rx.*
Use: Anti-inflammatory agent, topical corticosteroid.

Vytorin. (Merck/Schering-Plough) Ezetimibe/simvastatin 10 mg/10 mg, 10 mg/20 mg, 10 mg/40 mg, 10 mg/80 mg. Lactose. Tab. 30s, 90s, 500s (10 mg/40 mg, 10 mg/80 mg only), 1,000s (10 mg/10 mg, 10 mg/20 mg only), 2500s (10 mg/80 mg only), 5000s (10 mg/40 mg only), 10,000s (10 mg/10 mg, 10 mg/20 mg only). *Rx.*
Use: Antihyperlipidemic.

Vyvanse. (Shire US) Lisdexamfetamine dimesylate 20 mg, 30 mg, 40 mg, 50 mg, 60 mg, 70 mg. Cap. 100s. *c-II.*
Use: Central nervous system stimulant, amphetamine.

VZIG. (American Red Cross; Mass. Public Health Bio. Lab.) Varicella-Zoster immune globulin. Human globulin fraction of human plasma, primarily IgG 10% to 18% in single-dose vials containing 125 units varicella-zoster virus antibody in 2.5 mg or less. Inj.
Use: Immunization.

W

Wade Gesic Balm. (Wade) Menthol 3%, methyl salicylate 12%, petrolatum base. Tube oz, Jar lb. *OTC.*
Use: Analgesic, topical.

Wade's Drops. Compound benzoin tincture.

Wakespan. (Weeks & Leo) Caffeine 250 mg. TR Cap. Pkg. 15s. *Rx.*
Use: CNS stimulant.

Wal-Finate Allergy. (Walgreen) Chlorpheniramine maleate 4 mg. Tab. Bot. 50s. *OTC.*
Use: Antihistamine.

Wal-Finate Decongestant. (Walgreen) Chlorpheniramine maleate 4 mg, pseudoephedrine sulfate 60 mg. Tab. Bot. 50s. *OTC.*
Use: Antihistamine, decongestant.

Wal-Formula Cough Syrup with D-Methorphan. (Walgreen) Dextromethorphan HBr 15 mg, doxylamine succinate 7.5 mg, sodium citrate 500 mg/10 mL. Syr. Bot. 6 oz, 8 oz. *OTC.*
Use: Antihistamine, antitussive, expectorant.

Wal-Formula M Cough Syrup. (Walgreen) Dextromethorphan HBr 30 mg, pseudoephedrine hydrochloride 60 mg, guaifenesin 200 mg, acetaminophen 500 mg/20 mL. Syr. Bot. 8 oz. *OTC.*
Use: Analgesic, antitussive, decongestant, expectorant.

Wal-Frin Nasal Mist. (Walgreen) Phenylephrine hydrochloride 0.5%, pheniramine maleate 0.2%. Soln. Bot. 0.5 oz. *OTC.*
Use: Antihistamine, decongestant.

Walgreen Artificial Tears. (Walgreen) Hydroxypropyl methylcellulose 0.5%. Soln. Bot. 0.5 oz. *OTC.*
Use: Artificial tears.

Walgreen's Finest Iron. (Walgreen) Iron 30 mg. Tab. Bot. 100s. *OTC.*
Use: Mineral supplement.

Walgreen's Finest Vit B_6. (Walgreen) Pyridoxine hydrochloride 50 mg. Tab. Bot. 100s. *OTC.*
Use: Vitamin supplement.

Walgreen Soda Mints. (Walgreen) Sodium bicarbonate 300 mg. Tab. Bot. 100s, 200s. *OTC.*
Use: Antacid.

Wal-Phed. (Walgreen) Pseudoephedrine hydrochloride. **Syr.:** 30 mg/5 mL. Bot. 4 oz. **Tab.:** 30 mg. Bot. 50s, 100s. *OTC.*
Use: Decongestant.

Wal-Phed Plus. (Walgreen) Pseudoephedrine hydrochloride 60 mg, chlorpheniramine maleate 4 mg. Tab. Bot. 50s. *OTC.*
Use: Antihistamine, decongestant.

Wal-Tussin. (Walgreen) Guaifenesin 100 mg/5 mL. Bot. 4 oz. *OTC.*
Use: Expectorant.

Wampole One-Step hCG. (Wampole) For in vitro detection of hCG in serum and urine. Test. In 3, 24, 96, 500 test kits.
Use: Diagnostic aid, pregnancy.

•**warfarin sodium.** (WORE-fuh-rin) *USP.*
Use: Anticoagulant.
See: Coumadin.
Jantoven.

warfarin sodium. (Various Mfr.) Warfarin sodium 1 mg, 2 mg, 2.5 mg, 3 mg, 4 mg, 5 mg, 6 mg, 7.5 mg, 10 mg. Tab. Bot. 100s, 1000s, 5000s (except 7.5 mg, 10 mg), UD 100s. *Rx.*
Use: Anticoagulant.

Wart Fix. (Last) Castor oil 100%. Bot. 0.3 fl oz. *OTC.*
Use: Dermatologic; wart therapy.

Wart-Off. (Pfizer) Salicylic acid 17% in flexible collodion, alcohol 20.5%, ether 54.2%. Bot. 0.5 oz. *OTC.*
Use: Keratolytic.

wasp venom.
Use: Immunization.
See: Albay.
Pharmalgen.
Venomil.

•**water.** (WA-ter) *USP.*
Use: Pharmaceutic aid.

Water Babies Little Licks by Coppertone. (Schering-Plough) SPF 30, ethylhexyl p-methoxycinnamate, oxybenzone, 2-ethylhexyl salicylate, cherry flavor. Lot. Tube 4.8 g. *OTC.*
Use: Sunscreen.

Water Babies SPF 25 Sunblock. (Schering-Plough) Ethylhexyl p-methoxycinnamate, 2-ethylhexyl salicylate, homosalate, oxybenzone, benzyl alcohol. PABA free, waterproof. Cream. Bot. 90 g. *OTC.*
Use: Sunscreen.

Water Babies UVA/UVB SPF 15 Sunblock. (Schering-Plough) Ethylhexyl p-methoxycinnamate, oxybenzone in lotion base. Lot. Bot. 120 mL. *OTC.*
Use: Sunscreen.

Water Babies UVA/UVB SPF 45 Sunblock. (Schering-Plough) Ethylhexyl p-methoxycinnamate, 2-ethylhexyl salicylate, otocrylene oxybenzone, benzyl alcohol. PABA free, waterproof. Lot. Bot. 120 mL. *OTC.*
Use: Sunscreen.

Water Babies UVA/UVB SPF 30 Sunblock. (Schering-Plough) Ethylhexyl p-methoxycinnamate, 2-ethylhexyl salicylate, homosalate, oxybenzone, benzyl

alcohol. PABA free, waterproof. Lot. Bot. 120 mL, 240 mL. *OTC.*
Use: Sunscreen.

•**water for hemodialysis.** (WA-ter) *USP.*
Use: Hemodialysis.

•**water for injection.** (WA-ter) *USP.*
Use: Pharmaceutic aid (solvent).

watermelon seed extract.
See: Citrin.

W/Phenobarbital, Theobromine.
See: Cithal.

•**water, purified.** (WA-ter) *USP.*
Use: Pharmaceutic aid (solvent).

water-soluble vitamins.
Use: Vitamin supplement.
See: Aminobenzoate Potassium.
Ascorbic Acid.
Ascorbic Acid Combinations.
Bioflavonoids (Vitamin P).
Calcium Ascorbate.
Cyanocobalamin (B_{12}).
Folic Acid and Derivatives.
Leucovorin Calcium.
Levoleucovorin.
Hydroxocobalamin.
Niacin (B_3; Nicotinic Acid).
Niacinamide (Nicotinamide).
Pyridoxine Hydrochloride (B_6).
Riboflavin (B_2).
Sodium Ascorbate.
Thiamin (B_1).
Vitamin B_{12}.
Vitamin C (Ascorbic Acid).

•**wax, carnauba.** (wax kar-NOE-ba) *NF.*
Use: Pharmaceutic aid (tablet coating agent).

•**wax, emulsifying.** *NF.*
Use: Pharmaceutic aid (emulsifying, stiffening agent).

•**wax, microcrystalline.** (wax MYE-kroe-KRIS-ta-lin) *NF.*
Use: Pharmaceutic aid (stiffening, tablet coating agent).

Waxsol. Docusate sodium.

•**wax, white.** *NF.*
Use: Pharmaceutic aid (stiffening agent).

•**wax, yellow.** (wax YEL-oh) *NF.*
Use: Pharmaceutic aid (stiffening agent).

Wayds. (Wayne) Docusate sodium 100 mg. Cap. Bot. 100s. *OTC.*
Use: Laxative.

Wayds-Plus. (Wayne) Docusate w/casanthranol. Cap. Bot. 50s. *OTC.*
Use: Laxative.

Wayne-E. (Wayne) Vitamin E. Cap. **100 units, 200 units:** Bot. 1000s. **400 units:** Bot. 100s. *OTC.*
Use: Vitamin supplement.

Wee Care. (Centurion Labs) Carbonyl iron 15 mg per 1.25 mL. Acesulfame K, glycerin, parabens, potassium sorbate, propylene glycol, sucralose. Wild cherry flavor. Susp. 118 mL. *OTC.*
Use: Trace element.

Wehless. (Roberts) Phendimetrazine tartrate 35 mg. Cap. Bot. 100s. *c-III.*
Use: Anorexiant.

Wehless-105 Timecelles. (Roberts) Phendimetrazine tartrate 105 mg. SA Cap. Bot. 100s. *c-III.*
Use: Anorexiant.

Wehydryl. (Roberts) Diphenhydramine hydrochloride 50 mg/mL. Vial 10 mL. *Rx.*
Use: Antihistamine.

Welchol. (Daiichi Sankyo) Colesevelam hydrochloride. **Tab.:** 625 mg. Film-coated. 180s. **Pow. for Susp.:** 1.875 g, 3.75 g. Aspartame, phenylalanine 24 mg (1.875g), 48 mg (3.75 g). Citrus flavor. Single-dose packet. *Rx.*
Use: Antihyperlipidemic; bile acid sequestrant.

Welders Eye. (Weber) Tetracaine, potassium Cl, boric acid, camphor, glycerin, disodium edetate, benzalkonium Cl as preservatives. Lot. Bot. oz. *OTC.*
Use: Burn therapy.

Wellbutrin. (GlaxoSmithKline) Bupropion hydrochloride 75 mg, 100 mg. Film-coated. Tab. 100s. *Rx.*
Use: Antidepressant.

Wellbutrin SR. (GlaxoSmithKline) Bupropion hydrochloride 100 mg, 150 mg, 200 mg. Film-coated. ER Tab (12 hour). 60s. *Rx.*
Use: Antidepressant.

Wellbutrin XL. (BTA Pharmaceuticals) Bupropion hydrochloride 150 mg, 300 mg. Polyvinyl alcohol. ER Tab (24 hour). 30s, 90s (150 mg only). *Rx.*
Use: Antidepressant.

WellTuss EXP. (Prasco) Dihydrocodeine bitartrate 7.5 mg, guaifenesin 100 mg, pseudoephedrine hydrochloride 15 mg per 5 mL. Sugar, alcohol, and dye free. Menthol, saccharin, sorbitol. Syr. 473 mL. *c-III.*
Use: Antitussive and expectorant combination.

Wera. (Northstar) Ethinyl estradiol 35 mcg, norethindrone 0.5 mg. Lactose, PEG. Tab. 28s w/7 inert tablets (lactose, PEG). *Rx.*
Use: Monophasic oral contraceptive.

Wernet's Adhesive Cream. (Block Drug) Carboxymethylcellulose gum, ethylene oxide polymer, petrolatum in mineral oil

base. Cream. Tube 1.5 oz. *OTC.*
Use: Denture adhesive.

Wernet's Powder. (Block Drug) Karaya gum, ethylene oxide polymer. Bot. 0.63 oz, 1.75 oz, 3.55 oz. *OTC.*
Use: Denture adhesive.

Wes-B/C. (Western Research) Vitamins B_1 15 mg, B_2 10 mg, B_6 5 mg, niacinamide 50 mg, calcium pantothenate 10 mg, C 300 mg. Cap. Bot. 1000s. *OTC.*
Use: Mineral, vitamin supplement.

Wesmatic Forte Tablets. (Wesley) Phenobarbital ⅛ g, ephedrine sulfate 0.25 g, chlorpheniramine maleate 2 mg, guaifenesin 100 mg. Tab. Bot. 100s, 1000s. *Rx.*
Use: Antihistamine, decongestant, expectorant, hypnotic, sedative.

Westcort. (Ranbaxy) Hydrocortisone valerate 0.2% in a hydrophilic base with white petrolatum. **Cream:** Tube. 15 g, 45 g, 60 g, 120 g. **Oint.:** Mineral oil. Tube. 15 g, 45 g, 60 g. *Rx.*
Use: Corticosteroid, topical.

Westhroid. (RLC Labs) Thyroid 16.25 mg (¼ grain) (lactose), 32.5 mg (½ grain), 48.75 mg (¾ grain) (lactose), 65 mg (1 grain), 81.25 mg (1¼ grains) (lactose), 97.5 mg (1½ grains) (lactose), 113.75 mg (1¾ grains) (lactose), 130 mg (2 grains), 146.25 mg (2¼ grains) (lactose), 162.5 mg (2½ grains) (lactose), 194.4 mg (3 grains), 260 mg (4 grains) (lactose), 325 mg (5 grains) (lactose). **Note:** 1 grain = 64.8 mg. Tab. 100s; 30s, 60s, 90s, 990s, 1,000s, 1,008s (16.25 mg, 48.75 mg, 81.25 mg, 97.5 mg, 113.75 mg, 146.25 mg, 162.5 mg, 260 mg, 325 mg). *Rx.*
Use: Thyroid hormone.

Westhroid-P. (RLC Labs) Thyroid desiccated (porcine derived) 16.25 mg (¼ grain), 32.5 mg (½ grain), 48.75 mg (¾ grain), 65 mg (1 grain), 97.5 mg (1½ grains), 130 mg (2 grains). Inulin, lactose. Tab. 30s, 60s, 90s, 100s, 1,000s. *Rx.*
Use: Thyroid hormone.

Wesvite. (Western Research) Vitamins B_1 10 mg, B_2 5 mg, B_6 2 mg, pantothenic acid 10 mg, niacinamide 30 mg, B_{12} 3 mcg, C 100 mg, E 5 units, A 10,000 units, D 400 units, Fe 15 mg, Cu 1 mg, I 0.15 mg, Mn 1 mg, Zn 1.5 mg. Tab. Bot. 1000s. *OTC.*
Use: Mineral, vitamin supplement.

Wetting and Soaking. (Bausch & Lomb) Chlorhexidine gluconate 0.006%, EDTA 0.05%, cationic cellulose derivative polymer. Soln. Bot. 118 mL. *OTC.*
Use: Contact lens care.

Wetting and Soaking. (PBH Wesley Jessen) Buffered, isotonic. Chlorhexidine gluconate 0.005%, EDTA 0.02%, sodium chloride, octylphenoxy (oxyethylene) ethanol, povidone, polyvinyl alcohol, propylene glycol, hydroxyethylcellulose. Soln. Bot. 120 mL. *OTC.*
Use: Contact lens care.

wheat germ oil. (Various Mfr.)
Use: Vitamin supplement

wheat germ oil concentrate. (Thurston) Wheat germ oil concentrate. Perles. 6 min. Bot. 100s. *OTC.*
Use: Cardiovascular agent.

whey protein concentrate (bovine).
See: Bovine Whey Protein Concentrate.

Whirl-Sol. (Sween) Moisturizing bath additive. Bot. 2 oz, 8 oz, 16 oz, 21 oz, gal, 5 gal, 30 gal, 55 gal. *OTC.*
Use: Emollient.

white-faced hornet venom.
Use: Immunization.
See: Albay.
Pharmalgen.
Venomil.

white lotion. Lotio alba.
Use: Astringent.
See: Zinc Sulfide Topical Suspension.

Whitfield's Ointment. (Various Mfr.) Benzoic acid 6%, salicylic acid 3%. Oint. Tube. *OTC.*
Use: Anti-infective, topical.

•**whooping cough vaccine.** *USP.*
See: ActHIB/DTP, Set of DTwP Vial Plus Hib.
Diphtheria and Tetanus Toxoids with Pertussis Vaccine.
Infanrix.
Pertussis Vaccine.
Tripedia.

Whorto's Calamine Lotion. (Whorton Pharmaceuticals, Inc.) Calamine, zinc oxide, glycerin (U.S.P. strength) in carboxymethylcellulose lotion vehicle. Lot. Bot. 4 oz, gal. *OTC.*
Use: Dermatologic; counterirritant.

Wibi. (Valeant Pharmaceuticals) Purified water, SD alcohol 40, glycerin, PEG-4, PEG-6-32 stearate, PEG-6-32, glycol stearate, carbomer 940, PEG-75, methylparaben, propylparaben, triethanolamine, menthol, fragrance. Lot. Bot. 8 oz, 16 oz. *OTC.*
Use: Emollient.

widow spider species antivenin (Latrodectus mactans). (Merck & Co.) Antivenin, *Lactrodectus mactans.*
Use: Immunization.

Wilate. (Octapharma USA) Antihemophilic

factor /von Willebrand factor complex. **450 units/450 units per vial:** Heat treated. Upon reconstitution with the volume of diluent provided (water for injection with 0.1% polysorbate 80), each vial contains VWF:RCo 450 units, factor VIII 450 units, and total protein 7.5 mg or less. Each vial also contains glycine 50 mg, sucrose 50 mg, sodium chloride 117 mg, sodium citrate 14.7 mg, and calcium chloride 0.8 mg. Preservative free. **900 units/900 units per vial:** Heat treated. Upon reconstitution with the volume of diluent provided (water for injection with 0.1% polysorbate 80), each vial contains VWF:RCo 900 units, factor VIII 900 units, and total protein (≤ 15 mg). Each vial also contains glycine 100 mg, sucrose 100 mg, sodium chloride 234 mg, sodium citrate 29.4 mg, and calcium chloride 1.5 mg. Preservative free. Inj., lyophilized Pow. For Soln. Single-dose vial and a vial of diluents, transfer device, and infusion set. *Rx.*
Use: Hematological agent, antihemophilic factor combination.

wild cherry.
Use: Flavored vehicle.

Wilpor-Clear. (Foy Laboratories) Phentermine hydrochloride 30 mg. Cap. Bot. 1000s. *c-iv.*
Use: Anorexiant.

Wilpowr. (Foy Laboratories) Phentermine hydrochloride 30 mg. Cap. Bot. 100s, 500s, 1000s. *c-iv.*
Use: Anorexiant.

WinRho SDF. (Baxter) RH_o(D) immune globulin IV human 1,500 units (300 mcg), 2,500 units (500 mcg), 5,000 units (1,000 mcg), 15,000 units (3,000 mcg). Maltose 10%, polysorbate 80 0.03%. Preservative free. Inj. Soln. Single-dose vial. *Rx.*
Use: Immune globulin.

Wintergreen Sucrets. (GlaxoSmithKline) Dyclonine hydrochloride 0.1%, alcohol 10%, sorbitol. Spray. Bot. 90 mL. *OTC.*
Use: Mouth and throat preparation.

•**witch hazel.** (WICH HAY-zel) *USP.*
Use: Astringent.

witch hazel. (Various Mfr.) Hamamelis water (witch hazel). Bot. 120 mL, 240 mL, 280 mL, 480 mL, 960 mL, gal. *OTC.*
Use: Astringent.

Within. (Bayer Consumer Care) Vitamins A 5000 units, E 30 units, C 60 mg, folic acid 0.4 mg, B_1 1.5 mg, B_2 1.7 mg, niacin 20 mg, B_6 2 mg, B_{12} 6 mcg, pantothenic acid 10 mg, D 400 units, Fe 27 mg, Ca 450 mg, Zn 15 mg. Tab. Bot. 60s, 100s. *OTC.*
Use: Mineral, vitamin supplement.

WNS. (Sanofi-Synthelabo) Sulfamylon hydrochloride. Supp. *Rx.*
Use: Anorectal preparation.

Women's Gentle Laxative. (Goldline Consumer) Bisacodyl 5 mg, lactose, sugar. EC Tab. Pkg. 30s. *OTC.*
Use: Laxative.

Women's Tylenol Multi-Symptom Menstrual Relief. (McNeil Consumer) Acetaminophen 500 mg, pamabrom 25 mg. Tab. Bot. 24s. *OTC.*
Use: Analgesic.

Wonderful Dream. (Kondon) Phenylmercuric nitrate 1:5000, oils of tar, turpentine, olive and linseed, rosin, burgundy pitch, camphor, beeswax, mutton tallow. Salve. 34 g. *OTC.*
Use: Topical.

Wonder Ice. (Pedinol Pharmacal) Menthol in a specially formulated base. Gel. Tube 113 mL. *OTC.*
Use: Liniment.

Wondra. (Procter & Gamble) Petrolatum, lanolin acid, glycerin, stearyl alcohol, cyclomethicone, EDTA, hydrogenated vegetable glycerides phosphate, cetyl alcohol, isopropyl palmitate, stearic acid, PEG-100 stearate, carbomer 934, dimethicone, titanium dioxide, imidazolidinyl urea, parabens. Lot. Bot. 180 mL, 300 mL, 450 mL. *OTC.*
Use: Emollient.

wood charcoal. (Cowley) Wood charcoal. 5 g, 10 g. Tab. Bot. 1000s. *OTC.*

wood creosote.
See: Creosote.

wool fat. Lanolin, Anhydrous.

Wyanoids Relief Factor. (Wyeth) Cocoa butter 79%, shark liver oil 3%, corn oil, EDTA, parabens, tocopherol. Supp. 12s. *OTC.*
Use: Anorectal preparation.

Wydase Lyophilized. (Wyeth) Purified bovine testicular hyaluronidase. Vial 150 units/mL, 1500 units/10 mL with lactose and thimerosal. *Rx.*
Use: Absorption facilitator; hypodermoclysis; urography.

Wydase Stabilized Solution. (Wyeth) Purified bovine testicular hyaluronidase 150 units/mL in sterile saline soln. with sodium Cl, EDTA, thimerosal. Vial 1 mL, 10 mL. *Rx.*
Use: Absorption facilitator; hypodermoclysis; urography.

Wymox. (Wyeth-Ayerst) Amoxicillin trihydrate. **Cap.:** 250 mg Bot. 100s, 500s; 500 mg Bot. 50s, 500s. **Pow. for Oral**

Susp.: 125 mg/5 mL (as trihydrate) when reconstituted; 250 mg/5 mL (as trihydrate) when reconstituted. Bot. 100 mL, 150 mL. Sucrose. *Rx.*
Use: Anti-infective, penicillin.

Wymzya Fe. (Lupin) Ethinyl estradiol 35 mcg, norethindrone 0.4 mg. Lactose, maltodextrin, spearmint flavoring, sucralose. Chew. Tab. 21s (w/7 inert tablets [ferrous fumarate 75 mg, sugar]). *Rx.*
Use: Oral contraceptive.

X

Xalatan. (Pfizer) Latanoprost 0.005%, benzalkonium chloride 0.02%, sodium chloride. Soln. In 2.5 mL fill dropper bottles. *Rx.*
Use: Agent for glaucoma.

•**xaliproden.** (ZAL-ip-roe-den) USAN.
Use: Nootrope.

Xalkori. (Pfizer) Crizotinib 200 mg, 250 mg. Cap. 60s. *Rx.*
Use: Kinase inhibitor, tyrosine kinase inhibitor.

•**xamoterol.** (ZAM-oh-ter-ole) USAN.
Use: Cardiovascular agent.

•**xamoterol fumarate.** (ZAM-oh-ter-ole) USAN.
Use: Cardiovascular agent.

Xanax. (Pfizer) Alprazolam 0.25 mg, 0.5 mg, 1 mg, 2 mg. Lactose. Tab. 100s, 500s, 1000s (except 2 mg), UD 100s (0.25 mg, 0.5 mg only). *c-IV.*
Use: Anxiolytic.

Xanax XR. (Pfizer) Alprazolam 0.5 mg, 1 mg, 2 mg, 3 mg. Lactose. ER Tab. 60s. *c-IV.*
Use: Anxiolytic.

•**xanomeline.** (zah-NO-meh-leen) USAN.
Use: Cholinergic agonist (for Alzheimer disease).

•**xanomeline tartrate.** (zah-NO-meh-leen) USAN.
Use: Cholinergic agonist (for Alzheimer disease).

•**xanoxate sodium.** (ZAN-ox-ate) USAN.
Use: Bronchodilator.

•**xanthan gum.** (ZAN-than) *NF.*
Use: Pharmaceutic aid, suspending agent.

xanthine combinations.
Use: Antiasthmatic combinations.
See: Dyphylline and Guaifenesin.
Theophylline and Guaifenesin.

xanthine derivatives.
See: Aminophylline.
Caffeine.
Dyphylline.
Theobromine.
Theophylline.

•**xanthinol niacinate.** (ZAN-thih-nahl NYE-ah-SIN-ate) USAN.
Use: Vasodilator, peripheral.

xanthiol hydrochloride.
Use: Antinauseant.

xanthotoxin. Methoxsalen.

Xarelto. (Janssen Pharmaceuticals) Rivaroxaban 10 mg, 15 mg, 20 mg. Film coated. Lactose. Tab. 30s, 90s (except 10 mg), UD 100s. *Rx.*
Use: Anticoagulant, selective factor Xa inhibitor.

Xartemis XR. (Mallinckrodt Brand Pharmaceuticals) Acetaminophen 325 mg, oxycodone hydrochloride 7.5 mg. Coated. Edetate disodium, PEG. ER Tab. (contains both immediate-release and extended-release components). 100s. *c-II.*
Use: Opioid analgesic combination.

Xclair. (Align) Isohexadecane, Butyrospermum parkii, ethylhexyl palmitate, glycyrrhetinic acid, cera alba, PEG-30 dipolyhydroxystearate, bisabolol, polyglyceryl-6, polyricinoleate, tocopheryl acetate (antioxidant), castor oil, sodium hyaluronate nylon 12, butylene glycol, magnesium sulfate, piroctone olamine, allantoin, magnesium stearate, disodium EDTA, vitis vinifera, ascorbyl tetraisopalmitate, propyl gallate, telmesteine. Cream. 75 mL. *Rx.*
Use: Dermatological agent, miscellaneous topical combination.

Xeljanz. (Pfizer) Tofacitinib 5 mg (equiv. to tofacitinib citrate 8 mg). Film coated. Lactose, PEG. Tab. 60s, 180s. *Rx.*
Use: Kinase inhibitor, janus kinase inhibitor.

Xeloda. (Genentech) Capecitabine 150 mg, 500 mg. Lactose. Film-coated. Tab. Bot. 60s (150 mg only), 120s (500 mg only). *Rx.*
Use: Antimetabolite, pyrimidine analog.

•**xemilofiban hydrochloride.** (ZEM-i-loe-FYE-ban) USAN.
Use: Treatment of unstable angina; prevention of post-recanalization reocclusion of coronary vessels.

Xenaderm. (Healthpoint) Balsam peru/castor oil/trypsin 87 mg/788 mg/90 units. Safflower oil. Oint. 30 g, 60 g. *Rx.*
Use: Enzyme preparation.

•**xenalipin.** (ZEN-ah-LIH-pin) USAN.
Use: Hypolipidemic.

Xenazine. (Lundbeck) Tetrabenazine 12.5 mg, 25 mg. Lactose. Tab. 112s. *Rx.*
Use: CNS agent.

•**xenbucin.** (ZEN-BYOO-sin) USAN.
Use: Antihyperlipidemic.

Xenical. (Roche) Orlistat 120 mg. Cap. Bot. 90s. *Rx.*
Use: Antiobesity agent; lipase inhibitor.

•**xenon Xe 133.** (ZEE-non) *USP.*
Use: Radiopharmaceutical.

•**xenon Xe 127.** (ZEE-non) *USP.*
Use: Diagnostic aid; medicinal gas; radiopharmaceutical.

Xeomin. (Merz Pharma) IncobotulinumtoxinA 50 units, 100 units. Albumin (human) 1 mg, sucrose 4.7 mg. Preserva-

tive free. Inj., lyophilized Pow. for Soln. Single-use vial. *Rx.*
Use: Botulinum toxin.

Xerac AC. (Person and Covey) Aluminum Cl hexahydrate 6.25% in anhydrous ethanol 96%. Bot 35 mL, 60 mL. *Rx.*
Use: Dermatologic, acne.

Xerese. (Valeant) Acyclovir 5%, hydrocortisone 1%. Cetostearyl alcohol, mineral oil, propylene glycol, white petrolatum. Cream. 2 g, 5 g. *Rx.*
Use: Topical anti-infective, antiviral combination.

Xeroform 3%. (Various Mfr.) Pow. 0.25 lb, 1 lb. Jar 1 lb, 5 lb.
Use: Wound care.

Xero-Lube. (Scherer) Monobasic potassium phosphate, dibasic potassium phosphate, magnesium Cl, potassium Cl, calcium Cl, sodium Cl, sodium fluoride, sorbitol, sodium carboxymethylcellulose, methylparaben. Soln. Bot. 6 oz. *OTC.*
Use: Mouth and throat preparation.

Xgeva. (Amgen) Denosumab 70 mg/mL. Preservative free. Inj., Soln. Single-use vial. *Rx.*
Use: Monoclonal antibody.

Xiaflex. (Auxilium) Collagenase clostridium histolyticum 0.9 mg. Sucrose 18.5 mg. Preservative free. Inj., lyophilized Pow. for Soln. Single-use vial w/diluent (contains 3 mL of calcium chloride dihydrate 0.3 mg/mL in sodium chloride 0.9%). *Rx.*
Use: Enzyme preparation, injectable enzyme combination.

Xibrom. (Ista Pharm) Bromfenac 0.09%. Benzalkonium chloride 0.05 mg/mL, EDTA 0.2 mg/mL, povidone 20 mg/mL, sodium sulfite 0.2 mg/mL, boric acid, sodium borate, sodium hydroxide. Ophth. Soln. Dropper bottles. 5 mL. *Rx.*
Use: Nonsteroidal anti-inflammatory drug, ophthalmic.

Xifaxan. (Salix) Rifaximin 200 mg, 550 mg. EDTA. Film-coated. Tab. 30s, 100s, UD 100s (200 mg); 60s, UD 60s (550 mg). *Rx.*
Use: Anti-infective.

•**xilobam.** (ZIE-low-bam) USAN.
Use: Muscle relaxant.

•**ximelagatran.** (zye-mel-a-GAT-ran) USAN.
Use: Investigational antithrombotic.

Ximino. (Ranbaxy) Minocycline hydrochloride 45 mg, 67.5 mg, 90 mg, 112.5 mg, 135 mg. Lactose. ER Cap. 30s, 500s, UD 10s. *Rx.*
Use: Anti-infective, tetracycline.

•**xipamide.** (ZIP-ah-mide) USAN.
Use: Antihypertensive; diuretic.

Xodol. (Shionogi Pharma) Hydrocodone bitartrate/acetaminophen 7.5 mg/300 mg, 10 mg/300 mg. Tab. 100s, 500s (except 7.5 mg/300 mg). *c-III.*
Use: Narcotic analgesic.

Xofigo. (Bayer) Radium Ra 223 dichloride 1,000 kBq/mL (27 mCi/mL). Sodium. Inj., Soln. Single-use vial. 6 mL. *Rx.*
Use: Radiopharmaceutical.

Xolair. (Genentech) Omalizumab 150 mg (contains 202.5 mg of omalizumab, 145.5 mg of sucrose, 2.8 mg of L-histidine hydrochloride monohydrate, 1.8 mg of L-histidine, and 0.5 mg of polysorbate 20; designed to deliver 150 mg of omalizumab in 1.2 mL after reconstitution). Preservative free. Inj., lyophilized Pow. for Soln. Single-use vials. *Rx.*
Use: Monoclonal antibody.

Xolegel. (GlaxoSmithKline) Ketoconazole 2%. Dehydrated alcohol 34%, glycerin. Gel. Tubes. 2 g, 15 g. *Rx.*
Use: Topical anti-infective, antifungal agent.

Xolegel CorePak. (Barrier Therapeutics) Gel. **Xolegel:** Ketoconazole 2%. Alcohol 34%, glycerin. 45 g. **Xebcort:** Hydrocortisone 1%. Castor oil, menthol, SD alcohol 40-B 20%. 22.7 g. *Rx.*
Use: Antiseborrheic combination.

Xolegel Duo Convenience Pack. (Barrier Therapeutics) **Gel:** Ketoconazole 2%. Alcohol 34%. 15 g. **Shampoo:** Pyrithione zinc 1%. Benzyl alcohol, cetyl alcohol. 120 mL. *Rx.*
Use: Antiseborrheic product.

Xolido. (Enovachem) Lidocaine hydrochloride 2%. Glyceryl, isoparaffin, methylisothiazolinone, sunflower seed oil. Cream. 118 mL. *OTC.*
Use: Amide local anesthetic.

Xolox. (WraSer) Acetaminophen 500 mg, oxycodone hydrochloride 10 mg. Tab. 50s, 100s. *c-II.*
Use: Opioid analgesic combination.

Xopenex. (Sunovion Pharmaceuticals) Levalbuterol. **Soln. for Inhalation:** As levalbuterol hydrochloride. 0.31 mg/3 mL, 0.63 mg/3 mL, 1.25 mg/3 mL. Preservative free, sulfuric acid. UD Vials. 3 mL. **Soln. for Inhalation, concentrate:** 1.25 mg/0.5 mL. Preservative free. UD vials. 0.5 mL. *Rx.*
Use: Bronchodilator, sympathomimetic.

Xopenex HFA. (Sunovion Pharmaceuticals) Levalbuterol (as tartrate) 45 mcg/actuation. Contains no chlorofluorcar-

bons. Aer. Inh. 15 g (200 inhalations). *Rx.*
Use: Bronchodilator, sympathomimetic.

•**xorphanol mesylate.** (ZOR-fa-nol) USAN.
Use: Analgesic.

Xoten-C Pain Relief. (MedChem) Capsaicin 0.001%, menthol 10%, methyl salicylate 20%, cetearyl alcohol, glycerin, trolamine, vitamin E. Lot. 118 mL. *OTC.*
Use: Rub and liniment.

Xoten Pain Relief. (MenChem) Methyl salicylate 6.25%, menthol 12.5%, alcohol, aloe, camphor, eucalyptus, grape seed oil. Lot. 118 mL. *OTC.*
Use: Rub and liniment.

Xpect-AT. (Hawthorn) Carbetapentane citrate 60 mg, guaifenesin 600 mg. ER Tab. 100s. *Rx.*
Use: Upper respiratory combination, antitussive with expectorant.

Xpect-HC. (Hawthorn) Hydrocodone bitartrate 5 mg, guaifenesin 600 mg. ER Tab. 100s. *c-III.*
Use: Antitussive with expectorant.

X-Ray Contrast Media.
See: Iodine Products, Diagnostic.

X•Seb T. (Ivax) Coal tar soln. 10%, salicylic acid 4%. Soln. Bot. 4 oz. *OTC.*
Use: Antiseborrheic.

X•Seb T Plus. (Ivax) Coal tar solution 10%, salicylic acid 0.4%, EDTA. Shampoo. Bot. 118 mL. *OTC.*
Use: Antiseborrheic.

Xtandi. (Astellas Pharma US) Enzalutamide 40 mg. Butylated hydroxytoluene, glycerin, sorbitol. Cap., softgel. 120s. *Rx.*
Use: Hormone, antiandrogen.

Xtracare. (Sween) Bot. 2 oz, 4 oz, 8 oz, 21 oz, gal. *OTC.*
Use: Emollient.

Xtra-Vites. (Barth's) Vitamins A 10,000 units, D 400 units, C 150 mg, B_1 5 mg, B_2 1 mg, niacin 3.33 mg, pantothenic acid 183 mcg, B_6 250 mcg, B_{12} 215 mcg, E 15 units, rutin 20 mg, citrus bioflavonoid complex 15 mg, choline 6.67 mg, inositol 10 mg, folic acid 50 mcg, biotin, aminobenzoic acid. Tab. Bot. 30s, 90s, 180s, 360s. *OTC.*
Use: Vitamin supplement.

X-Trozine. (Shire US) Phendimetrazine tartrate 35 mg. Cap. Tab. Bot. 1000s. *c-III.*
Use: Anorexiant.

X-Trozine S.R. (Shire US) Phendimetrazine tartrate 105 mg. Cap. Bot. 100s, 200s, 1000s. *c-III.*
Use: Anorexiant.

Xulane. (Mylan) Norelgestromin 150 mcg, ethinyl estradiol 35 mcg per 24 hours. Patch; transdermal. 3s. *Rx.*
Use: Contraceptive hormone.

•**xylamidine tosylate.** (zie-LAM-ih-deen TAH-sill-ate) USAN.
Use: Serotonin inhibitor.

•**xylazine hydrochloride.** (ZYE-la-zeen) USAN.
Use: Analgesic.

XyliMelts. (OraHealth) Xylitol 500 mg. Dye free, gluten free, preservative free, soy free, and yeast free. Mint flavor. ER Discs. 40s. *OTC.*
Use: Mouth and throat product.

•**xylitol.** (ZIE-lih-tahl) *NF.*
Use: Pharmaceutic aid, vehicle, sweetened.
See: XyliMelts.

Xylocaine. (APP Pharmaceutical) Lidocaine hydrochloride. **Jelly:** 2%. Parabens. 5 mL, 30 mL. **Top. Soln.:** 4%. Parabens. 50 mL. *Rx-OTC.*
Use: Topical local anesthetic, amide local anesthetic.

Xylocaine. (APP Pharmaceutical) **0.5%:** Multidose vial 50 mL, methylparaben. **1%:** Amp. 20 mL. **2%:** Multidose vial 10 mL, 20 mL, 50 mL, methylparaben. Cartridge 1.8 mL. **0.5% w/epinephrine 1/200,000:** Multidose vial. 50 mL, methylparaben. **1% w/epinephrine 1/100,000:** Multidose vial. 10 mL, 20 mL, 50 mL, methylparaben. **2% w/epinephrine 1/50,000:** Dental cartridge 1.8 mL, sodium metabisulfite. **2% w/epinephrine 1/100,000:** Multidose vial 10 mL, 20 mL, 50 mL, sodium metabisulfite. Cartridge 1.8 mL, sodium bisulfite. **1.5% w/dextrose 7.5%:** Amp. 2 mL. *Rx.*
Use: Anesthetic, local amide.

Xylocaine Hydrochloride 4%. (AstraZeneca) Lidocaine 4%. Soln. Bot. 50 mL. *Rx.*
Use: Anesthetic, local topical.

Xylocaine Hydrochloride IV for Cardiac Arrhythmias. (APP Pharmaceutical) Lidocaine 2% (20 mg/mL). Inj. (for direct IV administration). Amp 5 mL. *Rx.*
Use: Antiarrhythmic agent.

Xylocaine MPF. (APP Pharmaceutical) Lidocaine. **0.5%:** Single-dose vial 50 mL. **1%:** Amp. 2 mL, 5 mL, 30 mL. *PolyAmp DuoFit* 10 mL, 20 mL. Single-dose vial 2 mL, 5 mL, 10 mL, 30 mL. **1.5%:** Amp. 20 mL. *PolyAmp DuoFit* 10 mL, 20 mL. Single-dose vial 5 mL, 10 mL. **2%:** Amp. 2 mL, 10 mL. *PolyAmp DuoFit* 10 mL. Single-dose vial 2 mL,

5 mL, 10 mL. **4%:** Amp. 5 mL. Syr. 5 mL w/laryngotracheal cannula. **1% w/epinephrine 1:200,000:** Amp. 30 mL. Single-dose vial 5 mL, 10 mL, 30 mL, sodium metabisulfite. **1.5% w/epinephrine 1:200,000:** Amp. 5 mL, 30 mL. Single-dose vial 5 mL, 10 mL, 30 mL, sodium metabisulfite. **2% w/epinephrine 1:200,000:** Amp. 20 mL. Single-dose vial 5 mL, 10 mL, 20 mL, sodium metabisulfite. **1.5% w/dextrose 7.5%:** Amp. 2 mL. **5% w/dextrose 7.5%:** Amp. 2 mL. *Rx.*
Use: Anesthetic, local amide.

Xylocaine Ointment. (AstraZeneca) Lidocaine 2.5%, water soluble carbowaxes. Oint. Tube 35 g *OTC.*
Use: Anesthetic, local.

•**xylofilcon A.** (ZILE-oh-FILL-kahn A) USAN.
Use: Contact lens material (hydrophilic).

•**xylometazoline hydrochloride.** (ZYE-loe-me-TAZ-oh-leen) *USP.*
Use: Nasal decongestant, imidazoline.
See: 4-Way Moisturizing Relief.
Otrivin.
Otrivin Pediatric Nasal.

•**xylose.** (ZIE-lohs) *USP.*
Use: Diagnostic aid, intestinal function determination.

Xyntha. (Wyeth) Antihemophilic factor 250 units, 500 units, 1,000 units, 2,000 units, 3,000 units. L-histidine, sucrose. Preservative free and plasma/albumin free. Solvent/detergent treated, nanofiltrated. Inj., lyophilized Pow. for Soln. Kits w/single-use vial and diluent (sodium chloride 0.9% 4 mL). *Rx.*
Use: Antihemophilic agent.

Xyralid. (Auriga) Lidocaine hydrochloride 3%, hydrocortisone acetate 1%. Cetyl alcohol, mineral oil, parabens, stearyl alcohol, white petrolatum. Cream. 85 g. *Rx.*
Use: Anti-inflammatory agent, topical corticosteroid.

Xyralid RC. (Auriga) Hydrocortisone acetate 1%, lidocaine hydrochloride 3%. Cetyl alcohol, glycerin, mineral oil, parabens, stearyl alcohol, urea, white petrolatum. Cream. 7 g w/applicator and cleansing wipes. *Rx.*
Use: Anorectal preparation, steroid-containing product.

Xyrem. (Jazz Pharmaceuticals) Sodium oxybate 500 mg/mL. Sodium 91 mg/mL. Oral Soln. 180 mL with syringe and dosing cups. *c-III.*
Note: Available only through the Xyrem Success Program. Call 1-866-997-3688 for more information.
Use: Psychotherapeutic agent, miscellaneous.

Xyzal. (Sanofi-Aventis) Levocetirizine dihydrochloride. **Oral Soln.:** 2.5 mg/5 mL. Maltitol, parabens, saccharin. 150 mL. **Tab.:** 5 mg. Lactose. Film-coated. 90s, 180s, UD 30s. *Rx.*
Use: Antihistamine, peripherally selective piperazine.

Y

Yager's Liniment. (Yager) Oil of turpentine and camphor w/clove oil fragrance, emulsifier, emollient, ammonium oleate (less than 0.5% free ammonia) penetrant base. *OTC.*
Use: Rubefacient.

Yasmin. (Bayer Healthcare) Ethinyl estradiol 30 mcg, drospirenone 3 mg. Lactose. Film-coated. Tab. Blister pack 28s with 7 inert tabs. *Rx.*
Use: Sex hormone, contraceptive hormone.

yatren.
See: Chiniofon.

YAZ. (Bayer) Drospirenone 3 mg/ethinyl estradiol 0.02 mg. Lactose. Film-coated. Tab. 24s. 4 inert tables. Blister-pack 28s. *Rx.*
Use: Sex hormone, estrogen and progestin combined.

Y-Cof DM Extended-Release. (Larken) Dextromethorphan hydrobromide 30 mg, dexbrompheniramine maleate 6 mg, phenylephrine hydrochloride 20 mg. ER Tab. 100s. *Rx.*
Use: Upper respiratory combination, antitussive combination.

YDP Lice. (Youngs Drug) Synthetic pyrethroid in aerosol. Spray. Can. 5 oz. *OTC.*
Use: Pediculicide, inanimate objects.

yeast adenylic acid. An isomer of adenosine 5-monophosphate, has been found inactive.

yeast, dried.
Use: Protein and vitamin B Complex source.

Yeast-Gard Medicated Disposable Douche. (Lake Consumer) Povidone-iodine 0.3% when reconstituted. Soln. 180 mL twin-pack w/two 5.4 mL medicated douche concentrate packets. *OTC.*
Use: Douche.

Yeast-Gard Medicated Disposable Douche Premix. (Lake Consumer) Octoxynol 9, lactic acid, sodium lactate, sodium benzoate, aloe vera. Soln. 180 mL twin-pack. *OTC.*
Use: Douche.

Yeast-Gard Medicated Douche. (Lake Consumer) Povidone-iodine 10%. Soln. Concentrate. 240 mL. *OTC.*
Use: Douche.

yeast tablets, dried.
Use: Supplementary source of B complex vitamins.
See: Brewer's Yeast.

yeast, torula.
See: Torula Yeast.

Yeast-X. (C.B. Fleet) Pulsatilla 28x. Supp. Pkg. 12s w/applicator. *OTC.*
Use: Vaginal agent.

Yelets. (Freeda) Iron 20 mg, vitamins A 10,000 units, D 400 units, E 10 units, B_1 10 mg, B_2 10 mg, B_3 25 mg, B_5 10 mg, B_6 10 mg, B_{12} 10 mcg, C 100 mg, folic acid 0.1 mg, PABA, lysine, glutamic acid, Ca, I, Mg, Mn, Se, Zn 4 mg. Tab. Bot. 100s, 250s. *OTC.*
Use: Mineral, vitamin supplement.

yellow enzyme.
See: Riboflavin.

•**yellow fever vaccine.** (YEL-oh FEE-ver) *USP.*
Use: Immunization.
See: YF-Vax.

yellow hornet venom.
Use: Desensitizing agent.
See: Albay.
Pharmalgen.
Venomil.

yellow jacket venom.
Use: Desensitizing agent.
See: Albay.
Pharmalgen.
Venomil.

yellow mercuric oxide 1%. (Various Mfr.) Yellow mercuric oxide 1% Oint. Tube 3.5, 3.75, 30 g. *OTC.*
Use: Antiseptic.

yellow mercuric oxide 2%. (Various Mfr.) Yellow mercuric oxide 2%. Oint. Tube 3.5, 3.75, 30 g. *OTC.*
Use: Antiseptic.
See: Stye.

yellow ointment.
Use: Pharmaceutic aid. (ointment base).

yellow wax.
Use: Pharmaceutic aid. (stiffening agent).

Yervoy. (Bristol-Myers Squibb) Ipilimumab 5 mg/mL. Mannitol, polysorbate 80. Preservative free. Inj., Soln.; concentrate. Single-use vial. 10 mL, 40 mL. *Rx.*
Use: Antineoplastic agent, monoclonal antibody.

YF-Vax. (Aventis Pasteur) Yellow fever vaccine not less than 4.74 $\log_{10}$ plaque-forming units (PFU) per 0.5 mL dose when reconstituted. Gelatin, sorbitol. Pow. for Inj., lyophilized. Single-dose vials with 0.6 mL diluent. 5-dose vials with 3 mL of diluent. *Rx.*
Use: Immunization.

Yocon. (Glenwood) Yohimbine hydrochloride 5.4 mg. Tab. Bot. 100s, 1000s. *Rx.*
Use: Anti-impotence agent.

Yodora Deodorant. (Numark) Cream. Jar 2 oz. *OTC.*
Use: Deodorant.

Yodoxin. (Glenwood) Iodoquinol.
Pow.: Bot. 25 g. **Tab.:** 210 mg, 650 mg. Bot. 100s, 1,000s. *Rx.*
Use: Amebicide.

•**yohimbine hydrochloride.** (yoe-HIM-been) *USP.*
Use: Yohimbine has no FDA-sanctioned indications.
See: Aphrodyne.

yohimbine hydrochloride. (Various Mfr.) Indolalkylamine alkaloid. 5.4 mg. Tab. Bot. 100s, 500s, 1000s. *Rx.*
Use: Yohimbine has no FDA-sanctioned indications.

Yohimex. (Kramer) Yohimbine hydrochloride 5.4 mg. Tab. Bot. 100s. *Rx.*
Use: Antiimpotence agent.

ytterbium Yb 169 pentetate injection.
Use: Radiopharmaceutical.

•**yttrium Y 90 clivatuzumab tetraxetan.** (IT-ree-um KLYE-va-TUE-zue-mab) USAN.
Use: Radiopharmaceutical.

•**yttrium Y 90 epratuzumab.** (IT-ree-um e-pra-TOO-zoo-mab) USAN.
Use: Radiopharmaceutical.

•**yttrium Y 90 ibritumomab.** (IT-ree-um ib-ri-TYOO-mo-mab) *USP.*
Use: Radiopharmaceutical.

•**yttrium Y 90 labetuzumab.** (IT-ree-um la-be-TOO-zoo-mab) USAN.
Use: Radiopharmaceutical.

•**yttrium Y 90 tacatuzumab.** (IT-ree-um tak-a-TUE-zoo-mab) USAN.
Use: Radiopharmaceutical.

Z

•**zacopride hydrochloride.** (ZAK-oh-pride) USAN.
Use: Antiemetic; stimulant (peristaltic).

Zaditor. (Novartis Ophthalmics) Ketotifen fumarate 0.025%, glycerol, sodium hydroxide/hydrochloric acid, purified water, benzalkonium chloride 0.01%. Soln. 5 mL. *OTC.*
Use: Antiallergic.

•**zafirlukast.** (zah-FEER-loo-kast) USAN.
Use: Antiasthmatic (leukotriene antagonist).
See: Accolate.

zafirlukast. (Various Mfr.) Zafirlukast 10 mg, 20 mg. May contain lactose, PEG. Tab. 30s, 60s, 100s, 500s, UD 100s. *Rx.*
Use: Leukotriene receptor antagonist.

•**zalcitabine.** (zal-SYE-ta-been) *USP.*
Use: Antiretroviral.

•**zaleplon.** (ZAL-eh-plahn) USAN.
Use: Nonbarbiturate sedative and hypnotic, pyrazolopyrimidine.
See: Sonata.

zaleplon. (Corepharma) Zaleplon 5 mg, 10 mg. Lactose. Cap. 100s. *c-iv.*
Use: Nonbarbiturate sedative and hypnotic, pyrazolopyrimidine.

•**zalospirone hydrochloride.** (zal-OH-spy-rone) USAN.
Use: Anxiolytic.

•**zaltidine hydrochloride.** (ZAHL-tih-deen) USAN.
Use: Antiulcerative.

Zaltrap. (Sanofi-Aventis U.S.) Ziv-aflibercept 25 mg/mL. Sodium chloride 100 mM, sodium citrate 5 mM, sodium phosphate 5 mM, sucrose. Preservative free. Inj., Soln.; concentrate. Single-use vial. 4 mL, 8 mL. *Rx.*
Use: Kinase inhibitor, tyrosine kinase inhibitor.

•**zalutumumab.** (ZAL-ue-TOOM-ue-mab) USAN.
Use: Antineoplastic.

Zamicet. (Hawthorn Pharmaceuticals) Acetaminophen 108.3 mg, hydrocodone bitartrate 3.3 mg per 5 mL. Alcohol 6.7%, edetate disodium, glycerin, methylparaben, saccharin, sorbitol, sucrose. Fruit flavor. Soln., Oral. 473 mL. *c-iii.*
Use: Opioid analgesic combination.

Zanaflex. (Acorda Therapeutics) Tizanidine (as base). **Cap.:** 2 mg (equivalent to tizanidine hydrochloride 2.29 mg), 4 mg (equivalent to tizanidine hydrochloride 4.58 mg), 6 mg (equivalent to tizanidine hydrochloride 6.87 mg). Sugar spheres. 150s. **Tab.:** 4 mg (equivalent to tizanidine hydrochloride 4.58 mg). Lactose. 150s. *Rx.*
Use: Skeletal muscle relaxant.

•**zanamivir.** (zan-AM-ih-veer) USAN.
Use: Antiviral; influenza virus neuraminidase inhibitor.
See: Relenza.

Zanfel. (Zanfel Labs) Polyethylene granules, nonoxynol-9, disodium EDTA, triethanolamine. Cream. Tube. 30 g. *OTC.*
Use: Dermatitis.

Zanfel Wash. (Zanfel Labs) Polyethylene granules, sodium lauroyl sarcosinate, nonoxynol-9, EDTA, triethanolamine. Wash. 30 mL. *OTC.*
Use: Poison ivy treatment.

•**zankiren hydrochloride.** (zan-KIE-ren) USAN.
Use: Antihypertensive.

•**zanolimumab.** (zan-oh-LIM-ue-mab) USAN.
Use: Isoantibody.

Zanosar. (Gensia Sicor) Streptozocin 1 g (100 mg/mL). Pow. for Inj. Vial. *Rx.*
Use: Antineoplastic.

•**zanoterone.** (zan-OH-ter-ohn) USAN.
Use: Antiandrogen.

Zantac. (Covis) Ranitidine hydrochloride 25 mg/mL. Inj., Soln. 2 mL single-dose vial, 6 mL and 40 mL multidose vial (w/phenol 5 mg/mL). *Rx.*
Use: Histamine H_2 antagonist.

Zantac. (GlaxoSmithKline) Ranitidine (as base). **Inj.:** 1 mg/mL, sodium chloride 0.45%. Preservative free. Premixed single-dose plastic containers. 50 mL. 25 mg/mL. Phenol 5 mg/mL. Single-dose vials. 2 mL. Multidose vials. 6 mL. **Syrup:** 15 mg/mL. Alcohol 7.5%, saccharin, sorbitol, parabens. Peppermint flavor. Bot. 480 mL. **Tab.:** 150 mg, 300 mg. Film-coated. 30s (300 mg only), 60s (150 mg only), 180s (150 mg only), 250s (300 mg only), 500s (150 mg only), 1,000s (150 mg only), UD 100s. *Rx.*
Use: Histamine H_2 antagonist.

Zantac EFFERdose. (GlaxoSmithKline) Ranitidine (as base) 25 mg. Aspartame, phenylalanine 2.81 mg, sodium 30.52 mg. Effervescent Tab. 60s. *Rx.*
Use: Histamine H_2 antagonist.

Zantac 150 Maximum Strength. (Boehringer Ingelheim) Ranitidine (as base) 150 mg. Sugar free. Tab. 8s, 24s, 50s, 65s. *OTC.*
Use: Histamine H_2 antagonist.

Zantac 75. (Boehringer Ingelheim) Ranitidine (as base) 75 mg. Sugar free. Tab.

Pkg. 4s, 10s, 20s, 30s, 60s, 80s, 100s. *OTC.*
Use: Histamine H_2 antagonist.

Zantine. (Lexis Laboratories) Dipyridamole 25 mg, 50 mg, 75 mg. Tab. Bot. 1000s. *Rx.*
Use: Coronary vasodilator.

Zarah. (Watson) Drospirenone 3 mg, ethinyl estradiol 30 mcg. Lactose. Tab. Blister card 28s (w/7 inert tablets). *Rx.*
Use: Oral contraceptive.

Zarontin. (Parke-Davis) Ethosuximide. **Cap.:** 250 mg. Bot. 100s. **Syr.:** 250 mg/5 mL. Bot. Pt. *Rx.*
Use: Anticonvulsant.

Zaroxolyn. (UCB Pharma) Metolazone 2.5 mg, 5 mg. Tab. Bot. 100s, 1000s, UD 100s. *Rx.*
Use: Diuretic.

•**zatosetron maleate.** (ZAT-oh-SEH-trahn) USAN.
Use: Antimigraine.

Zavesca. (Actelion) Miglustat 100 mg. Sodium starch glucollate, gelatin. Cap. 90s, blister card 18s. *Rx.*
Use: Gaucher disease.

Z-BEC. (Wyeth) Vitamins E 45 mg, C 600 mg, B_1 15 mg, B_2 10.2 mg, B_3 100 mg, B_6 10 mg, B_{12} 6 mcg, pantothenic acid 25 mg, Zn 22.5 mg. Tab. Bot. 60s, 100s, 500s. *OTC.*
Use: Mineral, vitamin supplement.

Z-Cof DM. (Zyber) Dextromethorphan HBr 15 mg, guaifenesin 200 mg, pseudoephedrine hydrochloride 40 mg per 5 mL. Grape flavor. Alcohol free, sugar free. Syrup. Bot. 473 mL. *Rx.*
Use: Upper respiratory combination, antitussive, expectorant, decongestant.

Z-Cof DMX. (Zyber) Dextromethorphan HBr 15 mg, guaifenesin 200 mg, pseudoephedrine hydrochloride 36 mg per 5 mL. Alcohol free. Menthol, saccharin, sorbitol, glucose, PEG. Grape flavor. Liq. 473 mL. *Rx.*
Use: Upper respiratory combination, antitussive and expectorant combination.

Z-Cof 8 DM. (Zyber) Dextromethorphan hydrobromide 15 mg, guaifenesin 175 mg, pseudoephedrine hydrochloride 30 mg per 5 mL. Acesulfame K, aspartame, methylparaben, phenylalanine 25.26 mg/mL. Alcohol free. Grape flavor. Susp., Oral. 473 mL. *Rx.*
Use: Upper respiratory combination, antitussive and expectorant combination.

Z-Cof I. (Pernix Therapeutics) Dextromethorphan hydrobromide 15 mg, guaifenesin 211 mg, pseudoephedrine hydrochloride 30 mg. Acesulfame K, aspartame, glycerin, methylparaben, phenylalanine 25.26 mg per 5 mL, sodium benzoate. Alcohol free. Grape flavor. Susp. 473 mL. *Rx.*
Use: Upper respiratory combination, antitussive and expectorant combination.

Z-Cof LA. (Zyber) Dextromethorphan HBr 30 mg, guaifenesin 650 mg. SR Tab. 100s. *Rx.*
Use: Upper respiratory combination, antitussive, expectorant.

Z-Cof LAX. (Zyber) Dextromethorphan HBr 30 mg, guaifenesin 835 mg. ER Tab. 100s. *Rx.*
Use: Antitussive with expectorant.

Z-Cof 12 DM. (Pernix Therapeutics) Dextromethorphan hydrobromide 15 mg (as dextromethorphan tannate 30 mg), guaifenesin 175 mg, pseudoephedrine hydrochloride 30 mg (as pseudoephedrine tannate 60 mg) per 5 mL. Alcohol free. Acesulfame K, aspartame, methylparaben. Grape flavor. Susp. 473 mL. *Rx.*
Use: Upper respiratory combination, antitussive and expectorant combination.

Z-Dex. (Trigen Labs) Dextromethorphan hydrobromide 20 mg, guaifenesin 100 mg, phenylephrine hydrochloride 10 mg per 5 mL. Edetate disodium, glycerin, sorbitol. Alcohol free and sugar free. Strawberry flavor. Syr. 473 mL. *Rx.*
Use: Upper respiratory combination, antitussive, expectorant combination.

Z-Dex Pediatric. (Trigen Labs) Dextromethorphan hydrobromide 3 mg, guaifenesin 35 mg, phenylephrine hydrochloride 2.5 mg per 1 mL. Alcohol and sugar free. Parabens, saccharin. Grape flavor. Drops. 30 mL with dropper. *Rx.*
Use: Upper respiratory combination, antitussive and expectorant combination.

Z-Dex 12D. (Trigen Labs) Chlorpheniramine maleate 8 mg, dextromethorphan hydrobromide 30 mg, phenylephrine hydrochloride 20 mg. ER Tab. 100s. *Rx.*
Use: Upper respiratory combination, antitussive combination.

Zeasorb. (Stiefel) Talc, microporous cellulose, acrylamide/sodium acrylate copolymer, chloroxylenol, imidazolidinylurea. Pow. 70.9 g, 312 g. *OTC.*
Use: Dermatologic.

Zeasorb-AF. (GlaxoSmithKline) Miconazole nitrate 2%. Pow. 70 g. *OTC.*
Use: Antifungal, topical.

Zebeta. (Teva Pharmaceuticals) Bisoprolol fumarate 5 mg, 10 mg. Film-coated. Tab. Bot. 30s. *Rx.*
Use: Antiadrenergic/sympatholytic, beta-adrenergic blocker.

Zebutal. (Midlothian Laboratories) Acetaminophen 325 mg, butalbital 50 mg, caffeine 40 mg. Cap. 100s. *Rx.*
Use: Nonnarcotic analgesic with barbiturate.

Ze Caps. (Everett) Vitamin E 200 mg, Zn 9.6 mg as gluconate. Cap. Bot. 60s. *OTC.*
Use: Mineral, vitamin supplement.

Zecuity. (NuPathe) Sumatriptan succinate 6.5 mg per 4 hours (86 mg of total sumatriptan per transdermal patch). Methylparaben. Patch; transdermal. 6s. *Rx.*
Use: Agent for migraine, serotonin 5-HT_1 receptor agonist (triptan).

Zee-Seltzer. (Zee Medical) Aspirin 325 mg, citric acid 1000 mg, sodium bicarbonate 1916 mg, sodium 524 mg. Effervescent Tab. 12s. *OTC.*
Use: Antacid.

Zegerid. (Santarus) **IR Cap.:** Omeprazole/sodium bicarbonate 20 mg/1100 mg, 40 mg/1100 mg. 30s. **Pow. for Oral Susp.:** Omeprazole/sodium bicarbonate 20 mg/1680 mg, 40 mg/1680 mg. Sucrose, sucralose, xanthan gum, xylitol. 30 unit-dose packets. *Rx.*
Use: Proton Pump Inhibitor.

Zegerid OTC. (Schering-Plough) Omeprazole 20 mg/sodium bicarbonate 1,100 mg. Sodium 303 mg. Cap., immediate release. 14s, 42s. *OTC.*
Use: Proton pump inhibitor combination.

•**zein.** (ZEE-in) *NF.*
Use: Pharmaceutic aid (coating agent).

Zelapar. (Valeant Pharmaceuticals) Selegiline hydrochloride 1.25 mg. Aspartame, mannitol, phenylalanine 1.25 mg. Grapefruit flavor. Orally Disintegrating Tab. Blister card. 60s. *Rx.*
Use: Antiparkinson agent.

Zelboraf. (Genentech) Vemurafenib 240 mg. Film coated. Tab. 120s. *Rx.*
Use: Kinase inhibitor, BRAF inhibitor.

Zelnorm. (Novartis) Tegaserod maleate.
Note: Available through investigational limited access program.

Zemaira. (CSL Behring) Alpha-1 proteinase inhibitor (human) 1,000 mg. Preservative free. Inj., lyophilized Pow. for Soln. Single-use vial (w/sodium, mannitol; specific activity is ≥ 0.7 mg of functional alpha-1 proteinase inhibitor per mg of total protein; total alpha-1 proteinase inhibitor functional activity in mg is stated on label of each vial) w/20 mL of diluent (sterile water for inj.) and transfer device. *Rx.*
Use: Respiratory enzyme.

Zemalo. (Alra) Sulfur, zinc oxide, camphor, titanium oxide. Bot. 4 oz, pt, gal. *OTC.*
Use: Dermatologic, counterirritant.

Zema-Pak 10 Day. (Macoven Pharmaceuticals) Dexamethasone 1.5 mg. Lactose, sucrose. Tab. 35s. *Rx.*
Use: Adrenocortical steroid, glucocorticoid.

Zema-Pak 13 Day. (Macoven Pharmaceuticals) Dexamethasone 1.5 mg. Lactose, sucrose. Tab. 51s. *Rx.*
Use: Adrenocortical steroid, glucocorticoid.

Zemplar. (Abbott) Paricalcitol. **Cap.:** 1 mcg, 2 mcg, 4 mcg. Alcohol, medium chain triglycerides. 30s. **Inj.:** 2 mcg/mL, 5 mcg/mL. Single-dose *Fliptop* vials, 1 mL, 2 mL. *Rx.*
Use: Hyperparathyroidism.

Zemuron. (Organon) Rocuronium bromide 10 mg/mL. Inj. Multidose vials. 5 mL, 10 mL. *Rx.*
Use: Muscle relaxant.

Zenatane. (Dr. Reddy's Laboratories) Isotretinoin 10 mg, 20 mg, 40 mg. Edetate disodium, medium chain triglycerides, soybean oil, vegetable oil. Cap., softgel. UD 30s, UD 100s. *Rx.*
Use: First-generation retinoid.

Zenate.
See: Advanced Formula Zenate.

•**zenazocine mesylate.** (zen-AZE-oh-seen) USAN.
Use: Analgesic.

Zenchent. (Actavis) Ethinyl estradiol 35 mcg, norethindrone 0.4 mg. Lactose. Tab. 28s with 7 inert tabs. *Rx.*
Use: Contraceptive hormone, sex hormone.

Zenchent FE. (Actavis) Ethinyl estradiol 35 mcg, norethindrone 0.4 mg. Lactose, maltodextrin, spearmint flavoring, sucralose. Chew. Tab. 21s (w/7 inert tablets [ferrous fumarate 75 mg, sugar, sucralose]). *Rx.*
Use: Monophasic oral contraceptive.

Zencia. (Stratus) Sodium sulfacetamide 9%, sulfur 4%. Aloe, cetyl alcohol, edetate disodium, glyceryl, green tea, parabens, PEG-100, stearyl alcohol. Soap. 473 mL. *Rx.*
Use: Acne product combination.

Zendium. (Oral-B) Sodium fluoride 0.22%. Tube 0.9 oz, 2.3 oz.
Use: Dental caries agent.

Zenieva. (River's Edge) Glycerin, olive oil, squalane, vegetable oil. Fragrance free. Emuls.; Top. Kit w/*Pure* cleanser. 70 g. *Rx.*
Use: Miscellaneous emollient.

•**zeniplatin.** (zen-ih-PLAT-in) USAN.
Use: Antineoplastic.

Zenpep. (Aptalis Pharma US) Lipase/protease/amylase 3,000 units/10,000 units/16,000 units; 5,000 units/17,000 units/27,000 units; 10,000 units/34,000 units/55,000 units; 15,000 units/51,000 units/82,000 units; 20,000 units/68,000 units/109,000 units; 25,000 units/85,000 units/136,000 units. Enteric-coated beads. Castor oil. Cap., delayed release. 12s, 100s, 500s (20,000 units/68,000 units/109,000 units and 25,000 units/85,000 units/136,000 units). *Rx.*
Use: Digestive enzyme.

Zenzedi. (Arbor) Dextroamphetamine sulfate 2.5 mg, 5 mg, 7.5 mg, 10 mg (double scored). Tab. 100s. *c-II.*
Use: Amphetamine.

Zephiran. (Sanofi-Synthelabo) **Aqueous soln.:** Benzalkonium chloride 1:750. Bot. 240 mL, gal. **Disinfectant concentrate:** 17% in 120 mL, gal. **Tincture:** 1:750 in gal. **Tincture spray:** 1:750 in 30 g, 180 g, gal. *OTC.*
Use: Antiseptic; antimicrobial.

Zephiran Towelettes. (Sanofi-Synthelabo) Moist paper towels with soln. of zephiran Cl 1:750. Box 20s, 100s, 1000s. *OTC.*
Use: Antiseptic; antimicrobial.

Zephrex. (Sanofi-Synthelabo) Pseudoephedrine hydrochloride 60 mg, guaifenesin 400 mg. Film-coated. Tab. Bot. 100s. *Rx.*
Use: Decongestant, expectorant.

Zephrex-D. (Westport Pharmaceuticals) Pseudoephedrine hydrochloride 30 mg. Lecithin, PEG, sodium 6 mg, vegetable oil. Tab. UD 24s. *OTC.*
Use: Nasal decongestant, arylalkylamine.

Zephrex LA. (Sanofi-Synthelabo) Pseudoephedrine hydrochloride 120 mg, guaifenesin 600 mg. ER Tab. Bot. 100s. *Rx.*
Use: Decongestant, expectorant.

Zepine. (Foy Laboratories) Reserpine alkaloid 0.25 mg. Tab. Bot. 100s, 500s, 1000s. *Rx.*
Use: Antihypertensive.

•**zeranol.** (ZER-ah-nole) USAN.
Use: Anabolic.

Zestoretic. (AstraZeneca) Lisinopril/hydrochlorothiazide 10 mg/12.5 mg, 20 mg/12.5 mg, 20 mg/25 mg. Mannitol. Tab. Bot. 100s. *Rx.*
Use: Antihypertensive.

Zestril. (AstraZeneca) Lisinopril 2.5 mg, 5 mg, 10 mg, 20 mg, 30 mg, 40 mg. Mannitol. Tab. 100s. *Rx.*
Use: Renin angiotensin system antagonist, angiotensin-converting enzyme inhibitor.

Zetar. (Dermik) Coal tar 1%. Shampoo. Bot. 177 mL. *OTC.*
Use: Antiseborrheic.

Zetia. (Merck/Schering-Plough) Ezetimibe 10 mg. Lactose. Tab. Bot. 30s, 90s, 500s, UD 100s. *Rx.*
Use: Antihyperlipidemic agent.

Zetonna. (Sunovion) Ciclesonide 37 mcg/actuation. Ethanol. Aer.; intranasal. 6.1 g aluminum canister (60 actuations) w/plastic actuator w/dose indicator and cap. *Rx.*
Use: Respiratory inhalant, intranasal steroid.

Zevalin. (Spectrum Pharmaceuticals) Ibritumomab tiuxetan 3.2 mg per 2 mL. Preservative free. Inj., Soln. Single-use vial. 2 mL. Ibritumomab tiuxetan kits w/sodium acetate 50 mM vial, formulation buffer vial (containing albumin [human] 750 mg, sodium chloride 76 mg, sodium phosphate dibasic dodecahydrate 28 mg, pentetic acid 4 mg, potassium phosphate monobasic 2 mg, potassium chloride 2 mg in water for injection 10 mL), empty reaction vial, and 4 identification labels (yttrium-90 chloride sterile solution shipped directly from supplier upon placement of order for ibritumomab kit). *Rx.*
Use: Antineoplastic, monoclonal antibody.

Zflex. (Huckaby Pharmaceuticals) Acetaminophen 500 mg, phenyltoloxamine citrate 55 mg. Tab. 100s. *Rx.*
Use: Nonnarcotic analgesic combination.

Ziac. (Teva) Bisoprolol fumarate/hydrochlorothiazide 2.5 mg/6.25 mg, 5 mg/6.25 mg, 10 mg/6.25 mg. Tab. Bot. 30s, 100s (except 10 mg/6.25 mg). *Rx.*
Use: Antihypertensive.

Ziagen. (ViiV Healthcare) Abacavir sulfate. **Tab.:** 300 mg. Film-coated. Bot. 60s, UD blister packs of 60s. **Oral Soln.:** 20 mg/mL. Parabens, saccharin, sorbitol. Strawberry-banana flavor. Bot. 240 mL. *Rx.*
Use: Antiviral, nucleoside reverse transcriptase inhibitor.

Ziana. (Medicis) Clindamycin phosphate 1.2%, tretinoin 0.025%. EDTA, glycerin,

parabens. Gel. 2 g, 30 g, 60 g. *Rx.*
Use: Topical anti-infective.
•**zibotentan.** (zye-boe-TEN-tan) USAN.
Use: Antineoplastic.
•**ziconotide.** (zi-KOE-noe-tide) USAN.
Use: Analgesic.
See: Prialt.
•**zicronapine.** (zye-KRON-a-peen) USAN.
Use: Antipsychotic.
•**zicronapine succinate.** (zye-KRON-a-peen) USAN.
Use: Antipsychotic.
•**zidometacin.** (ZIE-doe-MEH-tah-sin) USAN.
Use: Anti-inflammatory.
•**zidovudine.** (zie-DOE-view-DEEN) *USP. Formerly Azidothymidine, AZT.*
Use: Antiviral; AIDS; HIV infection.
See: Retrovir.
W/Lamivudine.
See: Combivir.
zidovudine. (Aurobindo Pharma) Zidovudine. **Cap.:** 100 mg. 100s, UD 100s. **Oral Soln.:** 50 mg per 5 mL. Sucrose. Strawberry flavor. 240 mL. *Rx.*
Use: Antiretroviral agent.
zidovudine. (Various Mfr.) Zidovudine 300 mg. Tab. 60s. *Rx.*
Use: Antiretroviral agent.
•**zifrosilone.** (zih-FROE-sih-lone) USAN.
Use: Acetylcholinesterase inhibitor.
Ziks. (Nodum) Methyl salicylate 12%, menthol 1%, capsaicin 0.025%, cetyl alcohol. Cream. Tube. 60 g. *OTC.*
Use: Analgesic.
Zilactin. (Blairex) Benzyl alcohol 10%. Salicylic acid, hydroxypropylcellulose. Gel. 7 g. *OTC.*
Use: Mouth and throat preparation.
Zilactin-B Medicated. (Blairex) Benzocaine 10%. Alcohol 76%. Gel. Tube. 7.5 g. *OTC.*
Use: Anesthetic, local.
Zilactin-L. (Blairex) Benzyl alcohol 10%. SD alcohol 37. Liq. 539 mL. *OTC.*
Use: Topical local anesthetic, amide local anesthetic.
ZilaDent. (Zila) Benzocaine 6%, alcohol 74.9%. Gel. Tube. 7.5 g, single packs. *OTC.*
Use: Anesthetic, local.
•**zilantel.** (ZILL-an-tell) USAN.
Use: Anthelmintic.
•**zileuton.** (ZIE-loo-tone) *USP.*
Use: Leukotriene formation inhibitor.
See: Zyflo.
Zyflo CR.
•**zimeldine hydrochloride.** (zie-MELL-ih-deen) USAN. *Formerly Zimelidine Hydrochloride.*
Use: Antidepressant.
Zims Max Freeze. (Perfecta Products) Menthol 3.7%. Aloe, camphor, isopropyl alcohol, methylparaben, tea tree oil. Gel. 113.4 g. *OTC.*
Use: Emollient.
Zinacef. (Covis) Cefuroxime (as sodium). **Pow. for Inj.:** 750 mg, 1.5 g, 7.5 g. Sodium 2.4 mEq/g. Vials and infusion pack (except 7.5 g). Pharmacy bulk pkg (7.5 g only). **Inj.:** 750 mg, 1.5 g. Sodium 2.4 mEq/g. Premixed, frozen. 50 mL. *Rx.*
Use: Anti-infective, cephalosporin.
zinc. (Various Mfr.) Zinc gluconate 30 mg. Tab. 100s. *OTC.*
Use: Trace element.
•**zinc acetate.** (zink) *USP.* Acetic acid, zinc salt, dihydrate.
Use: Pharmaceutic necessity for zinc-eugenol cement; topical poison ivy product; Wilson disease.
See: Caladryl Clear.
Galzin.
Ivy-Dry.
Ivy-Dry Super.
Nasal•Ease with Zinc.
W/Benzethonium Chloride, Diphenhydramine Hydrochloride.
See: Calagel Maximum Strength.
W/Chloroxylenol, Pramoxine Hydrochloride.
See: Zinotic ES.
W/Diphenhydramine Hydrochloride.
See: Anti-Itch.
Benadryl Extra Strength.
Benadryl Extra Strength Itch Relief Stick.
Benadryl Extra Strength Itch Stopping Cream.
Benadryl Original Strength Itch Stopping Cream.
Benadryl ReadyMist Itch Stopping Spray.
W/Pramoxine Hydrochloride.
See: Calaclear.
Callergy Clear.
Zincate. (Paddock) Zinc sulfate 220 mg (elemental zinc 50 mg). Cap. Bot. 100s, 1000s. *OTC.*
Use: Mineral supplement.
zinc bacitracin. Bacitracin Zinc.
Use: Anti-infective.
•**zinc carbonate.** (zink) *USP.*
Use: Antiseptic, topical; astringent.
•**zinc chloride.** (zink) *USP.*
Use: Astringent; dentin desensitizer.
zinc chloride. (Hospira) Zinc chloride 1 mg/mL (as zinc chloride 2.09 mg/mL). Preservative free. Inj., Soln. Vial.

10 mL. *Rx.*
Use: Intravenous nutritional therapy, trace element.

•**zinc chloride Zn 65.** (zink) USAN.
Use: Radiopharmaceutical.

zinc-eugenol cement.
Use: Dental protectant.

Zincfrin. (Alcon) Phenylephrine hydrochloride 0.12%. Benzalkonium chloride 0.01%, polysorbate 80, zinc sulfate 0.25%. Soln. *OTC.*
Use: Ophthalmic decongestant.

zinc gelatin.
Use: Topical protectant.

Zinc-Glenwood. (Glenwood) Zinc sulfate 220 mg. Cap. Bot. 100s. *OTC.*
Use: Mineral supplement.

•**zinc gluconate.** (zink) *USP.*
Use: Supplement, trace mineral.
See: Cold-Eeze.
Nasal•Ease with Zinc Gluconate.

zinc gluconate. (Various Mfr.) Zinc gluconate. **Loz.:** 10 mg. Cocoa powder, fructose, glycyrrhizic acid, powdered milk, sorbitol. 50s. **Tab.:** 100 mg. May contain polydextrose. Gluten free, preservative free. 100s. *OTC.*
Use: Trace element.

zinc insulin.
See: Insulin Zinc.

Zinc Lozenges with 100 mg Vitamin C. (Windmill) Vitamin C 100 mg, zinc 23 mg. Fructose, sorbitol, dextrose. Preservative free and soy free. Honey-lemon flavor. Loz. 50s. *OTC.*
Use: Multivitamin with minerals.

Zincon. (Medtech) Pyrithione zinc 1%. Propylene glycol. Shampoo. Bot. 118 mL, 240 mL. *OTC.*
Use: Dermatologic agent.

•**zinc oxide.** (zink) *USP.* Flowers of zinc.
Use: Astringent; topical protectant.
See: Calamine.
Delazinc.
W/Combinations.
See: Akne Drying Lotion.
Anusol Ointment.
Balmex.
Bonate.
Columbia Antiseptic Powder.
Desitin.
Dr. Smith's Adult Care.
Dr. Smith's Diaper.
Hemorrhoidal.
Medicated Powder.
Mexsana.
Pazo Hemorrhoid.
Rectal Medicone.
RVPaque.
Saratoga.
Schamberg's.
Soothe & Cool.
Tucks.
Versal.
W/Dimethicone.
See: A & D Zinc Oxide Cream.
W/Menthol.
See: Calmasyn.
Calmoseptine.
W/Talc.
See: Caldesene.

zinc oxide. (Gallipot) Zinc oxide 25%. Petrolatum. Paste, top. 454 g. *OTC.*
Use: Dermatological agent, protectant.

Zinc-Oxyde Plus. (First Aid Research Corporation) Zinc oxide 20%, menthol 0.44%, aloe vera, lt. mineral oil, petrolatum. Fragrance free. Oint. 28 g, 57 g. *OTC.*
Use: Diaper rash product.

zinc phenolsulfonate.
Use: Astringent.

zinc pyrithione.
Use: Bactericide, fungicide, antiseborrheic.
See: Zincon.

•**zinc stearate.** (zink STEER-ate) *USP.* Octadecanoic acid, zinc salt.
Use: Dusting powder; pharmaceutic aid (tablet/capsule lubricant).

zinc sulfanilate. Zinc sulfanilate tetrahydrate. Nizin, Op-Isophrin-Z, Op-Isophrin-Z-M (Broemmel).
Use: Anti-infective.

•**zinc sulfate.** (zink) *USP.* Sulfuric acid, zinc salt (1:1), heptahydrate.
Use: Astringent, ophthalmic.
See: Zinc-Glenwood.
W/Boric Acid, Phenylephrine Hydrochloride.
See: Phenylzin.
W/Calcium Lactate.
See: Zinc-220.
W/Vitamins.
See: Vicon-C.
Vicon Forte.
Vicon Plus.
Vi-Zac.
Z-BEC.

zinc sulfate. (American Regent) Zinc sulfate. **Inj., Soln.:** 1 mg/mL (as zinc sulfate 2.46 mg/mL). Preservative free. Inj., Soln. Single-dose vial. 10 mL. **Inj., Soln., concentrate:** 5 mg/mL (as zinc sulfate 12.32 mg/mL). Preservative free. Vial. 5 mL. *Rx.*
Use: Trace metal.

zinc sulfate. (Various Mfr.) Zinc sulfate 220 mg. Lactose, gelatin. Cap. 100s. *Rx-OTC.*
Use: Nutritional supplement, parenteral.

•**zinc sulfide topical suspension.** (zink) *USP. Formerly White Lotion.* Synonym Lotio alba.
Use: Astringent.

zinc-10-undecenoate.
See: Zinc Undecylenate.

zinc trace metal additive. (I.M.S., Ltd.) Zinc 4 mg/mL. Inj. Vial. 10 mL. *Rx.*
Use: Nutritional supplement, parenteral.

Zinc-220. (Alto) Zinc sulfate 220 mg. Cap. Bot. 100s, 1000s, UD 100s. *OTC.*
Use: Mineral supplement.

•**zinc undecylenate.** (zink uhn-deh-SILL-en-ate) *USP.*
Use: Antifungal.
See: Blis-To-Sol.
W/Undecylenic acid.
See: Cruex Spray Powder
Desenex.

Zincvit. (Kenwood) Vitamin A 5000 units, D_3 50 units, E 50 units, B_1 10 mg, B_2 5 mg, B_6 2 mg, C 300 mcg, B_3 25 mg, Zn 40 mg, Mg 9.7 mg, Mn 1.3 mg, folic acid 1 mg. Cap. Bot. 60s. *Rx.*
Use: Mineral, vitamin supplement.

•**zindotrine.** (ZIN-doe-TREEN) USAN.
Use: Bronchodilator.

Zinecard. (Pfizer) Dexrazoxane (as dexrazoxane hydrochloride) 250 mg, 500 mg. Inj., Lyophilized, Pow. for Soln. Single-use vials with 25-mL vial (250 mg), 50-mL vial (500 mg) sodium lactate injection. *Rx.*
Use: Cytoprotective agent.

•**zinoconazole hydrochloride.** (zih-no-KOE-nah-zole) USAN.
Use: Antifungal.

•**zinostatin.** (ZEE-no-STAT-in) USAN. *Formerly Neocarzinostatin.*
Use: Antineoplastic.

•**zinterol hydrochloride.** (ZIN-ter-ole) USAN.
Use: Bronchodilator.

•**zinviroxime.** (zin-VIE-rox-eem) USAN.
Use: Antiviral.

Zinx Chlor-D. (Auriga) Chlorpheniramine maleate 8 mg, pseudoephedrine hydrochloride 120 mg. ER Cap. 30s, 100s. *Rx.*
Use: Upper respiratory combination, decongestant and antihistamine.

Zinx GCP. (Auriga) Carbetapentane citrate 15 mg, guaifenesin 100 mg, phenylephrine hydrochloride 5 mg per 5 mL. Alcohol free. Maltitol, saccharin, sorbitol. Strawberry flavor. Soln. 118 mL. *Rx.*
Use: Upper respiratory combination, antitussive and expectorant combination.

Zinx PCM. (Auriga) Phenylephrine hydrochloride 10 mg, chlorpheniramine maleate 2 mg, methscopolamine nitrate 1.25 mg per 5 mL. Alcohol, sugar, and dye free. Saccharin, sorbitol. Berry flavor. Oral Susp. 118 mL. *Rx.*
Use: Upper respiratory combination; decongestant, antihistamine, and anticholinergic combination.

Zioptan. (Merck) Tafluprost 0.0015%. Disodium edetate. Preservative free. Soln., Ophth. Single-use container. 0.3 mL. *Rx.*
Use: Agent for glaucoma, prostaglandin agonist.

•**ziprasidone hydrochloride.** (zih-PRAY-sih-dohn) USAN.
Use: Antipsychotic, benzisoxazole derivative.
See: Geodon.

ziprasidone hydrochloride. (Various Mfr.) Ziprasidone (as hydrochloride) 20 mg, 40 mg, 60 mg, 80 mg. May contain lactose. Cap. 30s, 60s, 90s, 100s, 500s, UD 30s, UD 100s. *Rx.*
Use: Antipsychotic agent, benzisoxazole derivative.

•**ziprasidone mesylate.** (zih-PRAY-sih-dohn) USAN.
Use: Antipsychotic.

Zipsor. (Depomed) Diclofenac 25 mg. Isopropyl alcohol, PEG, sorbitol. Cap. 100s. *Rx.*
Use: CNS agent, nonsteroidal anti-inflammatory agent.

zirconium carbonate or oxide.
See: Dermaneed.

Zirgan. (Bausch & Lomb) Ganciclovir 0.15%. Benzalkonium chloride 0.075 mg. Gel; Ophth. Tube. 5 g. *Rx.*
Use: Ophthalmic antiviral agent.

Zithranol. (Elorac) Anthralin 1%. Glyceryl. Shampoo. 85 g. *Rx.*
Use: Antipsoriatic agent.

Zithranol-RR. (Elorac) Anthralin 1.2%. Preservative free. Cream. 15 g, 45 g. *Rx.*
Use: Dermatological agent, anti-psoriatic agent.

Zithromax. (Pfizer) Azithromycin. **Tab.:** 250 mg, 500 mg, 600 mg as dihydrate. Lactose. Film-coated. Bot. 30s, UD 50s (except 600 mg), *Z-Pak* 6s (250 mg only), *TRI-PAK* 3s (500 mg only). **Pow. for Inj.:** 500 mg, sucrose. Lyophilized vials 10 mL, vials 10 mL with 1 *Vial-Mate* adapter. **Pow. for Oral Susp.:** 100 mg/5 mL (as dihydrate) when reconstituted, sucrose. Cherry, banana, and creme de vanilla flavors. 15 mL. 200 mg/5 mL (as dihydrate) when reconstituted, sucrose.

Cherry, banana, and creme de vanilla flavors. 15 mL, 22.5 mL, 30 mL. 1 g/packet as dihydrate, sucrose. Cherry and banana flavors. Single-dose pack, 3s, 10s. *Rx.*
Use: Anti-infective, macrolide.

ziv-aflibercept. (ZIV-a-FLIB-er-sept)
Use: Tyrosine kinase inhibitor.
See: Zaltrap.

Zmax. (Pfizer) Azithromycin 2 g. Microspheres. Sucrose, sodium 148 mg. Cherry and banana flavors. ER Pow. for Oral Susp. Single-dose bottles. 2 g. *Rx.*
Use: Macrolide, anti-infective.

ZNG. (Western Research) Zinc gluconate 35 mg. Tab. *Handicount* 28s (36 bags of 28 tab.). *OTC.*
Use: Mineral supplement.

ZNP Bar. (Stiefel) Pyrithione zinc 2%. Alcohol, castor oil, cetearyl alcohol, glycerin, lactic acid, mineral oil, PEG, titanium dioxide, trisodium EDTA. Soap. 119 g. *OTC.*
Use: Dermatological agent.

ZN-Plus Protein. (Miller Pharmacal Group) Zinc in a zinc-protein complex made with isolated soy protein 15 mg. Tab. Bot. 100s. *OTC.*
Use: Mineral supplement.

Zocor. (Merck) Simvastatin 5 mg, 10 mg, 20 mg, 40 mg, 80 mg. Lactose. Film-coated. Tab. Bot. 1000s, 10,000s (10 mg, 20 mg only), UD 100s, unit-of-use 30s, 90s. *Rx.*
Use: Antihyperlipidemic, HMG-CoA reductase inhibitor.

Zodeac-100. (Econo Med Pharmaceuticals) Fe 60 mg, vitamins A 8000 units, D 400 units, E 30 units, B_1 1.7 mg, B_2 2 mg, B_3 20 mg, B_5 11 mg, B_6 4 mg, B_{12} 8 mcg, C 120 mg, folic acid 1 mg, biotin 300 mcg, Ca, Cu, I, Mg, Zn 15 mg. Tab. Bot. 100s. *Rx.*
Use: Mineral, vitamin supplement.

ZoDen. (Trigen Laboratories) Guaifenesin 20 mg, phenylephrine hydrochloride 1.5 mg. Sorbitol, sucralose. Sugar free, alcohol free. Raspberry flavor. Drops. 30 mL w/dropper. *Rx.*
Use: Upper respiratory combination, decongestant and expectorant combination.

ZoDen DM. (Trigen Laboratories) Chlorpheniramine maleate 1 mg, dextromethorphan hydrobromide 3 mg, phenylephrine hydrochloride 1.5 mg. Parabens, potassium citrate, potassium sorbate, propylene glycol, sorbitol, sucralose. Alcohol free and sugar free. Fruit gum flavor. Liq. Drops. 30 mL w/dropper. *Rx.*
Use: Upper respiratory combination, antitussive combination.

ZoDen PD. (Trigen Laboratories) Diphenhydramine hydrochloride 25 mg, phenylephrine hydrochloride 7.5 mg. Parabens, potassium citrate, potassium sorbate, propylene glycol, sorbitol, sucralose. Alcohol free, gluten free, and sugar free. Fruit candy flavor. Liq. 473 mL. *OTC.*
Use: Upper respiratory combination, decongestant and antihistamine.

ZoDerm. (Doak) Benzoyl peroxide. **Cleanser:** 4.5%, 5.75% (urea 10%, PEG 100, disodium EDTA), 6.5%, 8.5%. Alcohols, EDTA, glycerin, urea. 400 mL (except 5.75%), 473 mL (5.75% only). **Cream:** 4.5%, 6.5%, 8.5%. Alcohols, EDTA, urea. 125 mL. **Gel.:** 4.5%, 6.5%, 8.5%. EDTA, glycerin, urea. 125 mL. *Rx.*
Use: Anti-infective.

Zodryl AC 40. (codaDOSE) Chlorpheniramine maleate 1.11 mg, codeine phosphate 5 mg per 5 mL. Methylparaben, sucralose. Grape flavor. Liq. 118 mL w/oral dispenser. *c-v.*
Use: Upper respiratory combination, antitussive combination.

Zodryl AC 30. (codaDOSE) Chlorpheniramine maleate 1.43 mg, codeine phosphate 5 mg per 5 mL. Methylparaben, sucralose. Grape flavor. Liq. 118 mL w/oral dispenser. *c-v.*
Use: Upper respiratory combination, antitussive combination.

Zodryl AC 35. (codaDOSE) Chlorpheniramine maleate 1.25 mg, codeine phosphate 5 mg per 5 mL. Methylparaben, sucralose. Grape flavor. Liq. 118 mL w/oral dispenser. *c-v.*
Use: Upper respiratory combination, antitussive combination.

Zodryl AC 25. (codaDOSE) Chlorpheniramine maleate 1.665 mg, codeine phosphate 5 mg per 5 mL. Methylparaben, sucralose. Grape flavor. Liq. 118 mL w/oral dispenser. *c-v.*
Use: Upper respiratory combination, antitussive combination.

Zodryl DEC 80. (codaDOSE) Codeine phosphate 5 mg, guaifenesin 100 mg, pseudoephedrine hydrochloride 15 mg. Methylparaben, sucralose. Grape flavor. Susp. 236 mL. *c-v.*
Use: Upper respiratory combination, antitussive and expectorant combination.

Zodryl DEC 50. (codaDOSE) Codeine phosphate 5 mg, guaifenesin 100 mg,

pseudoephedrine hydrochloride 30 mg. Methylparaben, sucralose. Grape flavor. Susp. 236 mL. *c-v*.
Use: Upper respiratory combination, antitussive and expectorant combination.

Zodryl DEC 40. (codaDOSE) Codeine phosphate 5 mg, guaifenesin 100 mg, pseudoephedrine hydrochloride 16.665 mg. Methylparaben, sucralose. Grape flavor. Susp. 118 mL. *c-v*.
Use: Upper respiratory combination, antitussive and expectorant combination.

Zodryl DEC 60. (codaDOSE) Codeine phosphate 5 mg, guaifenesin 100 mg, pseudoephedrine hydrochloride 20 mg. Methylparaben, sucralose. Grape flavor. Susp. 236 mL. *c-v*.
Use: Upper respiratory combination, antitussive and expectorant combination.

Zodryl DEC 30. (codaDOSE) Codeine phosphate 5 mg, guaifenesin 100 mg, pseudoephedrine hydrochloride 21.43 mg. Methylparaben, sucralose. Grape flavor. Susp. 118 mL. *c-v*.
Use: Upper respiratory combination, antitussive and expectorant combination.

Zodryl DEC 35. (codaDOSE) Codeine phosphate 5 mg, guaifenesin 100 mg, pseudoephedrine hydrochloride 18.75 mg. Methylparaben, sucralose. Grape flavor. Susp. 118 mL. *c-v*.
Use: Upper respiratory combination, antitussive and expectorant combination.

Zodryl DEC 25. (codaDOSE) Codeine phosphate 5 mg, guaifenesin 100 mg, pseudoephedrine hydrochloride 25 mg. Methylparaben, sucralose. Grape flavor. Susp. 118 mL. *c-v*.
Use: Upper respiratory combination, antitussive and expectorant combination.

•**zofenoprilat arginine.** (zoe-FEN-oh-PRILL-at AHR-jih-neen) USAN.
Use: Antihypertensive.

•**zofenopril calcium.** (zoe-FEN-oh-PRILL) USAN.
Use: Enzyme inhibitor (angiotensin-converting).

Zofran. (GlaxoSmithKline) Ondansetron hydrochloride. **Tab.:** 4 mg, 8 mg, 24 mg (as hydrochloride dihydrate). Lactose. Bot. 30s, UD 100s, 1 × 3 UD pack (4 mg, 8 mg only); 1 × 1 daily UD pack (24 mg only). **Inj.:** 2 mg/mL (as hydrochloride). Parabens, sodium chloride. Multidose vial. 20 mL. **Oral Soln.:** 4 mg/5 mL (5 mg as hydrochloride dihydrate). Sorbitol, strawberry flavor. Bot. 50 mL. *Rx*.
Use: Antiemetic; antivertigo.

Zofran ODT. (GlaxoSmithKline) Ondansetron hydrochloride (as base) 4 mg, 8 mg. Phenylalanine < 0.03 mg, aspartame, mannitol, parabens. Strawberry flavor. Orally Disintegrating Tab. UD 10s (8 mg only), UD 30s. *Rx*.
Use: Antiemetic; antivertigo.

Zohydro ER. (Zogenix) Hydrocodone bitartrate 10 mg, 15 mg, 20 mg, 30 mg, 40 mg, 50 mg. Sugar. ER Cap. 100s. *c-II*.
Use: Opioid analgesic.

Zoladex. (AstraZeneca) Goserelin acetate 3.6 mg (16-gauge needle), 10.8 mg (14-gauge needle). Implant. Preloaded Syringes. *Rx*.
Use: Hormone, gonadotropin-releasing hormone analog.

•**zolamine hydrochloride.** (zoe-lah-meen) USAN.
Use: Antihistamine; anesthetic, topical.

•**zolazepam hydrochloride.** (zole-AZ-eh-pam) USAN.
Use: Hypnotic; sedative.

•**zoledronate disodium.** (ZOE-leh-droe-nate) USAN.
Use: Bone resorption inhibitor; osteoporosis treatment and prevention.

•**zoledronate trisodium.** (ZOE-leh-droe-nate) USAN.
Use: Bone resorption inhibitor; osteoporosis treatment and prevention.

•**zoledronic acid.** (ZOE-leh-drah-nik) USAN.
Use: Calcium regulator; osteoporosis treatment and prevention; bisphosphonate.
See: Reclast.
Zometa.

zoledronic acid. (Caraco) Zoledronic acid 4 mg (equiv. to zoledronic acid monohydrate 4.264 mg). May contain mannitol, sodium citrate. Inj., lyophilized Pow. for Soln. Single-dose vial w/diluent. *Rx*.
Use: Bisphosphonate.

zoledronic acid. (Various Mfr.) Zoledronic acid. **Inj., Soln., concentrate:** 4 mg per 5 mL (equiv. to zoledronic acid monohydrate 4.264 mg). May contain mannitol, sodium citrate. Single-use vial. 5 mL. **Inj., Soln.:** 4 mg per 100 mL (equiv. to zoledronic acid monohydrate 4.264 mg), 5 mg per 100 mL (equiv. to zoledronic acid monohydrate 5.33 mg). May contain mannitol, sodium citrate.

100 mL ready-to-infuse soln. bag (5 mg per 100 mL), 100 mL single-use bag (4 mg per 100 mL). *Rx.*
Use: Bisphosphonate.

•**zolertine hydrochloride.** (ZOE-ler-teen) USAN.
Use: Antiadrenergic; vasodilator.

•**zolimomab aritox.** (zah-LIM-ah-mab a-rih-TOX) USAN.
Use: Monoclonal antibody (antithrombotic).

Zolinza. (Merck) Vorinostat 100 mg. Cap. 120s. *Rx.*
Use: Antineoplastic, histone deacetylase inhibitor.

•**zolmitriptan.** (zohl-mi-TRIP-tan) USAN.
Tall Man: ZOLMitriptan
Use: Antimigraine agent, serotonin 5-HT_1 receptor agonist.
See: Zomig.
Zomig ZMT.

zolmitriptan. (Various Mfr.) Zolmitriptan. **Tab.:** 2.5 mg, 5 mg. May contain lactose, PEG. UD 6s (2.5 mg), UD 3s (5 mg). **Tab., disintegrating:** 2.5 mg, 5 mg. May contain aspartame, mannitol, phenylalanine. UD 6s (2.5 mg), UD 3s (5 mg). *Rx.*
Use: Agent for migraine, serotonin 5-HT_1 receptor agonist (triptan).

Zoloft. (Pfizer) Sertraline hydrochloride (as base). **Tab.:** 25 mg, 50 mg, 100 mg. Film-coated. Bot. 50s (25 mg only); 100s, 500s, 5000s, UD 100s (50 mg and 100 mg only). **Soln., Oral Conc.:** 20 mg/mL. Menthol, alcohol 12%. Bot. 60 mL. Dropper dispenser contains dry natural rubber. *Rx.*
Use: Antidepressant, selective serotonin reuptake inhibitor.

•**zolpidem tartrate.** (ZOLE-pih-dem) USAN.
Use: Hypnotic; sedative.
See: Ambien.
Ambien CR.
Edluar.
Intermezzo.

zolpidem tartrate. (Various Mfr.) Zolpidem tartrate 5 mg, 10 mg. May contain lactose. Tab. 15s (10 mg only), 30s, 60s (10 mg only), 90s, 100s, 500s, 1,000s, 1,500s, UD 100s. *c-iv.*
Use: Nonbarbiturate sedative/hypnotic, imidazopyridine.

zolpidem tartrate. (Winthrop US) Zolpidem tartrate 6.25 mg, 12.5 mg. May contain lactose, PEG. ER Tab. 100s, 500s, UD 30s (12.5 mg only). *c-iv.*
Use: Nonbarbiturate sedative/hypnotic; imidazopyridine.

Zolpimist. (NovaDel) Zolpidem tartrate 5 mg per actuation. Neotame. Cherry flavor. Spray, Soln.; lingual. 60 metered actuations per container. *c-iv.*
Use: Nonbarbiturate sedative/hypnotic; imidazopyridine.

Zolvit. (ECR Pharmaceuticals) Acetaminophen 100 mg, hydrocodone bitartrate 3.3 mg. Alcohol 7%, glycerin, parabens, propylene glycol, saccharin, sorbitol, sucrose. Tropical fruit punch flavor. Liq. 473 mL. *c-iii.*
Use: Opioid analgesic combination.

•**zomepirac sodium.** (ZOE-mih-PEER-ack) USAN.
Use: Analgesic; anti-inflammatory.

Zometa. (Novartis) Zoledronic acid. **Inj., Soln.:** 4 mg per 100 mL (equiv. to zoledronic acid monohydrate 4.264 mg). Mannitol, sodium citrate. Ready-to-use bottle. 100 mL. **Inj., Soln; Conc.:** 4 mg per 5 mL (as zoledronic acid monohydrate 4.264 mg). Mannitol, sodium citrate. Single-use vial. 5 mL. *Rx.*
Use: Bisphosphonate.

•**zometapine.** (zoe-MET-ah-peen) USAN.
Use: Antidepressant.

Zomig. (Impax Pharmaceuticals) Zolmitriptan. **Nasal Spray:** 2.5 mg, 5 mg. Single-use nasal spray units. **Tab.:** 2.5 mg, 5 mg. Lactose. Film-coated. Blister pack 6s (2.5 mg only), 3s (5 mg only). *Rx.*
Use: Antimigraine agent, serotonin 5-HT_1 receptor agonist.

Zomig ZMT. (AstraZeneca) Zolmitriptan 5 mg. Phenylalanine 5.62 mg, 2.5 mg (5 mg), 2.81 mg (2.5 mg), mannitol, aspartame. Orange flavor. Orally disintegrating Tab. UD 3s (5 mg), UD 6s (2.5 mg). *Rx.*
Use: Antimigraine agent, serotonin 5-HT_1 receptor agonist.

Zonalon. (Medicis Dermatologics) Doxepin hydrochloride 5%. Cetyl alcohol, petrolatum, benzyl alcohol, titanium dioxide. Cream. Tube. 30 g. *Rx.*
Use: Antihistamine, topical.

•**zonampanel.** (zon-AM-pa-nel) USAN.
Use: Ischemic stroke.

Zonatuss. (Vertical Pharmaceutical) Benzonatate 150 mg. Cap. 100s. *Rx.*
Use: Nonnarcotic antitussive.

Zone-A Forte. (Forest) Hydrocortisone 2.5%, pramoxine hydrochloride in a hydrophilic base containing stearic acid 1%, forlan-L, glycerin, triethanolamine, polyoxyl 40 stearate, di-isopropyl adipate, povidone, silicone fluid-200. Paraben free. Lot. Bot. 60 mL. *Rx.*
Use: Corticosteroid; anesthetic, local.

Zone-A Lotion. (Forest) Hydrocortisone acetate 1%, pramoxine hydrochloride 1%. Bot. 2 oz. *Rx.*
Use: Corticosteroid; anesthetic, local.

Zonegran. (Eisai) Zonisamide 25 mg, 50 mg, 100 mg. Cap. Bot. 100s. *Rx.*
Use: Anticonvulsant.

•**zoniclezole hydrochloride.** (zoe-NIH-klih-ZOLE) USAN.
Use: Anticonvulsant.

•**zoniporide mesylate.** (zon-i-POR-ide) USAN.
Use: Cardioprotective agent.

•**zonisamide.** (zoe-NISS-ah-MIDE) USAN.
Use: Anticonvulsant.
See: Zonegran.

zonisamide. (Various Mfr.) Zonisamide 25 mg, 50 mg, 100 mg. May contain lactose (100 mg only). Cap. 30s, 60s, 100s, 250s, 500s, 1000s, UD 100s (100 mg only). *Rx.*
Use: Anticonvulsants.

Zonite Liquid Douche Concentrate. (Menley & James Labs, Inc.) Benzalkonium Cl 0.1%, menthol, thymol, EDTA in buffered soln. Bot. 240 mL, 360 mL. *OTC.*
Use: Vaginal agent.

•**zopolrestat.** (zoe-PAHL-reh-STAT) USAN.
Use: Antidiabetic; aldose reductase inhibitor.

•**zorbamycin.** (zor-ba-MYE-sin) USAN.
Use: Anti-infective.

Zorbtive. (Serono) Somatropin 8.8 mg (≈ 26.4 units). Sucrose, phosphoric acid. Pow. for Inj. Multidose vial with diluent. *Rx.*
Use: Hormone, growth.

ZORprin. (PAR) Aspirin 800 mg. SR Tab. Bot. 100s. *Rx.*
Use: Analgesic.

Zortress. (Novartis) Everolimus 0.25 mg, 0.5 mg, 0.75 mg. Butylated hydroxytoluene, lactose. Tab. UD 60s. *Rx.*
Use: Kinase inhibitor, mTOR inhibitor.

•**zorubicin hydrochloride.** (zoe-ROO-bih-sin) USAN.
Use: Antineoplastic.

Zorvolex. (Iroko Pharmaceuticals) Diclofenac 18 mg, 35 mg. Lactose. Cap. 30s, 90s. *Rx.*
Use: Nonsteroidal anti-inflammatory agent.

Zostavax. (Merck) Oka/Merck varicella-zoster virus (live) 19,400 PFU. Sucrose. Preservative free. Inj., lyophilized. Single-dose vials. 1s, 10s. *Rx.*
Use: Viral vaccine.

zoster vaccine live.
Use: Active immunization agent, viral vaccine.
See: Zostavax.

Zostrix. (Health Care Products) Capsaicin 0.025%. Cream. Tube. 45 g. *Rx.*
Use: Analgesic, topical.

Zostrix Diabetic Foot Pain. (Health Care Products) Capsaicin 0.075%. Benzyl alcohol, cetyl alcohol, glyceryl, PEG-100, white petrolatum. Cream. 56.6 g w/25 applicator pads. *OTC.*
Use: Counterirritant.

Zostrix Diabetic Joint & Arthritis Pain Relief. (Health Care Products) Capsaicin 0.025%. Menthol 2%, alcohols, glyceryl, PEG, petrolatum. Cream. 56.6 g. *OTC.*
Use: Counterirritant.

Zostrix Hot and Cold Therapy. (Health Care Products) **Hot therapy:** Capsaicin 0.025%. Benzyl alcohol, cetyl alcohol, glyceryl, PEG, sorbitol, white petrolatum. Cream. 28.3 g. **Cold therapy:** Menthol 4%. Alcohols, benzyl alcohol, glyceryl, PEG, petrolatum, sorbitol. Cream. 28.3 g. *OTC.*
Use: Counterirritant.

Zostrix-HP. (Health Care Products) *Formerly called Axsain, formerly marketed by Galen.*

Zostrix Maximum Strength. (Health Care Products) Capsaicin 0.075%. Benzyl alcohol, cetyl alcohol, glyceryl, PEG-100, white petrolatum. Cream. 56.6 g w/25 applicator pads. *OTC.*
Use: Counterirritant.

•**zosuquidar trihydrochloride.** (zoe-SOO-kwi-dar) USAN.
Use: Treatment of multidrug resistance.

Zosyn. (Wyeth) Piperacillin sodium/tazobactam sodium. **Inj. Soln.:** 2.25 g/50 mL (2 g/0.25 g) (sodium 5.58 mEq), 3.375 g/50 mL (3 g/0.375 g) (sodium 8.38 mEq), 4.5 g/100 mL (4 g/0.5 g) (sodium 11.17 mEq). *Galaxy* containers. **Pow. for Soln. Inj.:** 2.25 g (2 g/0.25 g) (sodium 5.58 mEq, EDTA 0.5 mg), 3.375 g (3 g/0.375 mg) (sodium 8.38 mEq, EDTA 0.75 mg), 4.5 g (4 g/0.5 g) (sodium 11.17 mEq, EDTA 1 mg), 40.5 g (36 g/4.5 g) (sodium 100.4 mEq). Single-dose vials (except 40.5 g), *ADD-Vantage* vials (except 40.5 g). Bulk vials (40.5 g only). Preservative free. *Rx.*
Use: Extended-spectrum penicillins.

Zotex. (Vertical) Dextromethorphan HBr 20 mg, guaifenesin 100 mg, phenylephrine hydrochloride 10 mg per 5 mL. Parabens, saccharin. Alcohol free,

sugar free. Strawberry flavor. Syrup. 10 mL, 473 mL. *Rx.*
Use: Upper respiratory combination; antitussive, expectorant, decongestant.

Zotex-EX. (Vertical) Dextromethorphan hydrobromide 15 mg, guaifenesin 350 mg, phenylephrine hydrochloride 10 mg. Maltodextrin. Tab. 100s. *Rx.*
Use: Upper respiratory combination, antitussive and expectorant combination.

Zotex-G. (Vertical) Dextromethorphan HBr 15 mg, guaifenesin 133 mg, phenylephrine hydrochloride 10 mg per 5 mL. Sugar and alcohol free. Parabens, saccharin. Grape flavor. Syrup. 10 mL, 473 mL. *Rx.*
Use: Antitussive and expectorant.

Zotex Pediatric. (Vertical) Phenylephrine hydrochloride 2.5 mg/mL, dextromethorphan HBr 3 mg/mL, guaifenesin 35 mg per 1 mL. Sugar and alcohol free. Parabens, saccharin, grape flavor. Drops. 30 mL with dropper. *Rx.*
Use: Upper respiratory combination, antitussive and expectorant combination.

Zoto-HC. (Horizon) Chloroxylenol 1 mg, pramoxine hydrochloride 10 mg, hydrocortisone 10 mg, propylene glycol diacetate 3%. Benzalkonium chloride. Drops. Plastic dropper vials. 10 mL. *Rx.*
Use: Otic preparation.

Zovia 1/50E. (Watson) Ethinyl estradiol 50 mcg, ethynodiol diacetate 1 mg. Lactose. Tab. Pkg. 21s, 28s (with 7 inert tabs.). *Rx.*
Use: Sex hormone, contraceptive hormone.

Zovia 1/35E. (Watson) Ethinyl estradiol 35 mcg, ethynodiol diacetate 1 mg. Lactose. Tab. Pkg. 21s, 28s (with 7 inert tabs.). *Rx.*
Use: Sex hormone, contraceptive hormone.

Zovirax. (Valeant) Acyclovir. **Cap.:** 200 mg. May contain parabens. Bot. 100s, UD 100s. **Tab.:** 400 mg, 800 mg. Bot. 100s, UD 100s (800 mg only). **Cream:** 5% in aqueous cream base, cetostearyl alcohol, mineral oil, white petrolatum. 2 g. **Susp.:** 200 mg/5 mL. Bot. 473 mL. *Rx.*
Use: Antiviral.

Z-Pak.
See: Zithromax.

Z-Pro-C. (Person and Covey) Zinc sulfate 200 mg (elemental zinc 45 mg), ascorbic acid 100 mg. Tab. Bot. 100s. *OTC.*
Use: Mineral, vitamin supplement.

Z-Tuss E. (Magna) Codeine phosphate 9 mg, guaifenesin 200 mg, pseudoephedrine hydrochloride 30 mg. Glycerin, PEG, propylene glycol, saccharin, sorbitol. Sugar free. Cherry flavor. Liq. 473 mL. *c-v.*
Use: Upper respiratory combination, antitussive and expectorant combination.

ZTuss ZT. (Magna) Hydrocodone bitartrate 5 mg, guaifenesin 300 mg. Tab. 100s. *c-III.*
Use: Antitussive with expectorant.

Zubsolv. (Orexo) Buprenorphine hydrochloride/naloxone hydrochloride 1.4 mg/0.36 mg, 5.7 mg/1.4 mg. Mannitol, menthol, sucralose. Menthol flavor. Tab.; sublingual. UD 30s. *c-III.*
Use: Opioid agonist-antagonist analgesic.

•**zucapsaicin.** (zoo-cap-SAY-sin) USAN.
Use: Analgesic, topical.

•**zuclomiphene.** (zoo-KLOE-mih-FEEN) USAN. *Formerly Transclomiphene.*

Zuplenz. (Par) Ondansetron 4 mg, 8 mg. Butylated hydroxytoluene, peppermint flavoring, sucralose. Film; oral. UD 10s. *Rx.*
Use: Antiemetic/antivertigo agent, 5-HT_3 receptor antagonist.

Zurinol. (Major) Allopurinol. Tab. **100 mg:** Bot. 100s, 500s, 1000s, UD 100s. **300 mg:** Bot. 100s, 500s, UD 100s. *Rx.*
Use: Antigout agent.

Z-Xtra. (Magna) Pyrilamine maleate 2.07 mg, benzocaine 2.08 mg, zinc oxide 41.35 mg/mL, apple blossom, silicone, lanolin, and Wysteria oils, isopropanol, camphor, menthol, parabens. Lot. Bot. 118 mL. *OTC.*
Use: Antihistamine, topical.

Zyban. (GlaxoSmithKline) Bupropion hydrochloride 150 mg. Film-coated. ER Tab. 60s. *Rx.*
Use: Smoking deterrent.

Zyclara. (Medicis) Imiquimod 2.5%, 3.75%. Cetyl alcohol, stearyl alcohol, white petrolatum, benzyl alcohol, parabens. Cream. Single-use packet. 28s. *Rx.*
Use: Topical immunomodulator.

Zyderm I. (Inamed) Highly purified bovine dermal collagen 35 mg/mL implant. Sterile syringe 0.1 mL, 0.5 mL, 1 mL, 2 mL.
Use: Collagen implant.

Zyderm II. (Inamed) Highly purified bovine dermal collagen 65 mg/mL implant. Syringe 0.75 mL.
Use: Collagen implant.

Zydone. (DuPont) Hydrocodone bitartrate

5 mg, 7.5 mg, 10 mg, acetaminophen 400 mg. Cap. Bot. 100s, 500s, UD 100s. *c-III.*
Use: Analgesic combination, narcotic.

Zyflo. (Cornerstone Biopharma) Zileuton 600 mg. Film-coated. Tab. 120s. *Rx.*
Use: Leukotriene formation inhibitor.

Zyflo CR. (Cornerstone Biopharma) Zileuton 600 mg. Mannitol. Film-coated. ER Tab. 120s. *Rx.*
Use: Leukotriene formation inhibitor.

Zykadia. (Novartis) Ceritinib 150 mg. Cap. 70s. *Rx.*
Use: Antineoplastic, kinase inhibitor, tyrosine kinase inhibitor.

Zylet. (Bausch & Lomb) Loteprednol 0.5%, tobramycin 0.3%. Benzalkonium chloride 0.01%, edetate disodium, glycerin, povidone, tyloxapol. Ophth. Susp. 2.5 mL, 5 mL, 10 mL. *Rx.*
Use: Ophthalmic steroid antibiotic combination.

Zyloprim. (Faro Pharmaceuticals) Allopurinol 100 mg, 300 mg. Lactose. Tab. Bot. 100s, 500s (300 mg only). *Rx.*
Use: Antigout agent; antimetabolite; purine analog.

Zymacap. (Pharmacia) Vitamins A 5000 units, D 400 units, E 15 mg, C 90 mg, folic acid 400 mcg, B_1 2.25 mg, B_2 2.6 mg, niacin 30 mg, B_6 3 mg, B_{12} 9 mcg, pantothenic acid 15 mg. Cap. Bot. 90s, 240s. *OTC.*
Use: Vitamin supplement.

Zymar. (Allergan) Gatifloxacin 0.3% (3 mg/mL). EDTA, benzalkonium chloride 0.005%. Soln. Dropper Bot. 2.5 mL, 5 mL. *Rx.*
Use: Antibiotic, ophthalmic.

Zymaxid. (Allergan) Gatifloxacin 0.5%. Benzalkonium chloride 0.005%, EDTA. Soln., Ophth. 2.5 mL, 5 mL. *Rx.*
Use: Ophthalmic and otic agent, ophthalmic antibiotic.

Zypram. (Vertical Pharmaceuticals) Hydrocortisone acetate 2.35%, pramoxine hydrochloride 1%. Benzyl alcohol, cetearyl alcohol, glycerin, glyceryl, methylparaben, PEG-12, white petrolatum. Cream. 30 g w/2 wipes and 1 applicator. *Rx.*
Use: Anti-inflammatory agent, topical corticosteroid.

Zyprexa. (Eli Lilly) Olanzapine 2.5 mg, 5 mg, 7.5 mg, 10 mg, 15 mg, 20 mg. Lactose. Tab. 30s, 1,000s (except 2.5 mg and 5 mg), UD 50s (15 mg and 20 mg only), UD 100s (7.5 mg and 15 mg only) *Rx.*
Tall Man: ZyPREXA
Use: Antipsychotic, dibenzapine derivative.

Zyprexa IntraMuscular. (Eli Lilly) Olanzapine 10 mg. Pow. for Inj. Vial. 10 mg. *Rx.*
Tall Man: ZyPREXA
Use: Antipsychotic.

Zyprexa Relprevv. (Eli Lilly) Olanzapine 210 mg, 300 mg, 405 mg. Mannitol. Inj., Pow. for Susp., extended release. Single-use vial w/diluents. *Rx.*
Use: Antipsychotic agent, dibenzapine derivative.

Zyprexa Zydis. (Eli Lilly) Olanzapine 5 mg (phenylalanine 0.34 mg), 10 mg (phenylalanine 0.45 mg), 15 mg (phenylalanine 0.67 mg), 20 mg (phenylalanine 0.9 mg). Aspartame, parabens, mannitol. Tab., orally disintegrating. UD 30s. *Rx.*
Tall Man: ZyPREXA
Use: Antipsychotic, dibenzapine derivative.

Zyrtec Allergy. (McNeil Consumer) Cetirizine hydrochloride 10 mg. **Tab.:** Lactose. 30s. **Tab., orally disintegrating:** Mannitol, sucralose. Citrus flavor. 66s. **Cap., liquid filled:** Glycerin, mannitol, PEG 400, sorbitan, sorbitol. 12s, 25s, 40s, 65s, 70s. *OTC.*
Tall Man: ZyrTEC
Use: Antihistamine, peripherally selective piperazine.

Zyrtec Children's Allergy. (McNeil Consumer) Cetirizine hydrochloride. **Chew. Tab.:** 5 mg, 10 mg. Acesulfame K, maltodextrin, mannitol, sorbitol, lactose. Grape flavor. 5s (5 mg only), 12s (10 mg only). **Syr., Oral:** 1 mg/mL. Parabens, sugar. Grape flavor. Bot. 118 mL. *OTC.*
Tall Man: ZyrTEC
Use: Antihistamine, peripherally selective piperazine.

Zyrtec Children's Hives Relief. (McNeil Consumer) Cetirizine hydrochloride 1 mg/mL. Parabens, sugar. Grape flavor. Syr., Oral. 118 mL. *OTC.*
Tall Man: ZyrTEC
Use: Antihistamine, peripherally selective piperazine.

Zyrtec-D. (McNeil Consumer) Cetirizine hydrochloride 5 mg, pseudoephedrine hydrochloride 120 mg. Lactose. ER Tab. 12s. *OTC.*
Use: Upper respiratory combination, decongestant and antihistamine.

Zyrtec-D 12 Hour. (McNeil Consumer) Pseudoephedrine hydrochloride 120 mg (extended release), cetirizine hydrochloride 5 mg (immediate release). Lactose. ER Tab. Bot. 100s. *Rx.*
Tall Man: ZyrTEC

Use: Upper respiratory combination, decongestant, antihistamine.

Zyrtec Hives Relief. (McNeil Consumer) Cetirizine hydrochloride 10 mg. Lactose. Tab. Blister pack 14s. *OTC.*
Tall Man: ZyrTEC
Use: Antihistamine, peripherally selective piperazine.

Zyrtec Itchy Eye. (McNeil Consumer) Ketotifen 0.025% (as ketotifen fumarate). May contain glycerol, sodium hydroxide and/or hydrochloric acid, benzalkonium chloride 0.01%. Soln., Ophth. 5 mL. *OTC.*
Tall Man: ZyrTEC
Use: Ophthalmic and otic agent, ophthalmic antihistamine.

Zytiga. (Janssen) Abiraterone acetate 250 mg. Lactose. Tab. 120s. *Rx.*
Use: Hormone, antiandrogen.

Zyvox. (Pfizer) Linezolid. **Tab.:** 600 mg. Film coated. PEG, sodium 0.1 mEq. 20s, 100s, UD 30s. **Pow. for Oral Susp.:** 100 mg/5 mL. Sodium 0.4 mEq/5 mL, sucrose, aspartame, mannitol, phenylalanine 20 mg, orange flavor. Bot. 115 mL fill in 240 mL. **Inj.:** 2 mg/mL. Sodium 0.38 mg/mL, sodium citrate. Single-use, ready-to-use bag 100 mL, 200 mL, 300 mL. *Rx.*
Use: Oxalodinone.

ZzzQuil. (Procter & Gamble) Diphenhydramine hydrochloride 8.3 mg per 5 mL. Alcohol, corn syrup, propylene glycol, saccharin, sodium benzoate. Sodium ≈3.83 mg. Liq. 177 mL, 354 mL. *OTC.*
Use: Antihistamine, nonselective ethanolamine.

ZzzQuil Liquicaps. (Procter & Gamble) Diphenhydramine hydrochloride 25 mg. Glycerin, PEG, sorbitol. Cap. 12s, 24s, 48s. *OTC.*
Use: Antihistamine, nonselective ethanolamine.

Reference Information

Standard Medical Abbreviations

Abbreviation	Meaning
≈	approximately equals
Δ	delta
ϵ	epsilon; molar absorption coefficient
Ω	omega; ohm
5-HIAA	5-hydroxyindoleacetic acid
5-HT	5-hydroxytryptamine (serotonin)
6-MP	6-mercaptopurine
17-OHCS	17-hydroxycorticosteroids
α	alpha
A	ampere(s)
Å	angstrom(s)
aa	of each (ana)
āā	of each (ana)
AA	Alcoholics Anonymous; amino acid
AACP	American Association of Clinical Pharmacy; American Association of Colleges of Pharmacy
AARP	American Association of Retired Persons
Ab	antibody
ABGs	arterial blood gases
abs feb	when fever is absent *(absente febre)*
ABVD	Adriamycin (doxorubicin), bleomycin, vinblastine, (and) dacarbazine
ac	before meals or food *(ante cibum)*
ACCP	American College of Clinical Pharmacy
ACD	acid-citrate-dextrose
ACE	angiotensin-converting enzyme
ACEI	angiotensin-converting enzyme inhibitor
ACh	acetylcholine
ACIP	Advisory Committee on Immunization Practices
ACLS	advanced cardiac life support
ACPE	American Council on Pharmaceutical Education
ACS	American Chemical Society
ACT	activated clotting time
ACTH	adrenocorticotropic hormone
a.d.	right ear *(aurio dextra)*

Abbreviation	Meaning
ad to;	to; up to *(ad)*
ADE	adverse drug experience
ADH	antidiuretic hormone
adhib	to be administered *(adhibendus)*
ad lib	as desired, at pleasure *(ad libitum)*
ADLs	activities of daily living
ADME	absorption, distribution, metabolism, and elimination
admov	apply *(admove)*
ADP	adenosine diphosphate
ADR	adverse drug reaction
ADRRS	Adverse Drug Reaction Reporting System
ad sat	to saturation *(ad saturatum, ad saturandum)*
adst feb	when fever is present *(adstante febre)*
ad us.	for external use *(ad usum externum)*
adv	against *(adversum)*
aer	aerosol
Ag	antigen; silver *(argentum)*
agit. Ante us.	shake before using *(agita ante usum)*
agit. Bene	shake well *(agita bene)*
AHA	American Hospital Association
AID	artificial insemination donor
AIDS	acquired immunodeficiency syndrome
AJHP	American Journal of Hospital Pharmacy
ala	alanine
ALL	acute lymphocytic leukemia
ALT	alanine aminotransferase serum (previously SGPT)
alt hor	every other hour *(alternis horis)*
A.M.	before noon; morning *(ante meridiem)*
AMA	American Medical Association
AML	acute myelogenous leukemia
AMP	adenosine monophosphate
ANA	antinuclear antibody(ies)
ANC	acid neutralizing capacity
ANDA	abbreviated new drug application

Abbreviation	Meaning
ANOVA	analysis of variance
ANUG	acute necrotizing ulcerative gingivitis
APA	antipernicious anemia
APAP	acetaminophen
APC	antigen presenting cell(s)
APhA	American Pharmaceutical Association
aPTT	activated partial thromboplastin time
aq.	water *(aqua)*
aq. dest	distilled water *(aqua destillata)*
ARC	AIDS-related complex
ARDS	adult respiratory distress syndrome
ARF	acute renal failure
Arg	arginine
ARV	AIDS-related virus
as	left ear *(aurio sinister)*
ASA	American Society of Anesthesiologists; aspirin
ASHD	arteriosclerotic heart disease
ASHP	American Society of Hospital Pharmacists
Asn	asparagine
Asp	aspartic acid
AST	aspartate aminotransferase, serum (previously SGOT)
atm	standard atmosphere
ATN	acute tubular necrosis
ATP	adenosine triphosphate
ATPase	adenosine triphosphatase
ATPD	ambient temperature and pressure, saturated
at wt	atomic weight
au	both ears *(aures utrae)*
AU	gold *(aurum)*
AUC	area under the plasma concentration-time curve
AV	atrioventricular
A-V	arteriovenous; atrioventricular (block, bundle, conduction, dissociation, extrasystole)
AW	atomic weight
AWP	average wholesale price
ax.	axis
β	beta
BAC	blood-alcohol concentration

Abbreviation	Meaning
BADL	basic activities of daily life
BBB	blood brain barrier
BC	blood culture
BDZ	benzodiazepine
bib	drink *(bibe)*
bid	twice daily; two times a day *(bis in die)*
bm	bowel movement
BMR	basal metabolic rate
bp.	boiling point
BP	blood pressure
BPH	benign prostatic hypertrophy
bpm	beats per minute
BSA	body surface area
BT	bleeding time
BUN	blood urea nitrogen
C	centigrade
C.	*clostridium*
c.	gallon *(cong)*
c̄.	with *(cum)*
°C.	degrees Celsius
Ca	calcium
CA	cancer; carcinoma; cardiac arrest; chronologic age; croup-associated
CAD	coronary artery disease
Cal	Calorie (kilocalorie)
cAMP	cyclic adenosine monophosphate
caps	capsule *(capsula)*
CAS	Chemical Abstracts Service
CAT	computerized axial tomography
cath	catheterize
CBA	cost-benefit analysis
CBC	complete blood count
CC	chief complaint
cc.	cubic centimeter
CCBs	calcium channel blockers
CCU	coronary care unit; critical care unit
CD4	T-helper lymphocytes and macrophages
CDC	Centers for Disease Control and Prevention
CEA	cost effectiveness analysis
CF	cystic fibrosis
CFC	chlorofluorocarbon
CFU	colony-forming units

Abbreviation	Meaning
CHD	coronary heart disease
CHF	congestive heart failure
Ci	curie
CK	creatinine kinase
Cl	chlorine
Cl_{cr}	creatinine clearance
cm	centimeter
Cm	curium
cm^2	square centimeter(s)
cm^3	cubic centimeter
CMA	Certified Medical Assistant
CMC	carpometacarpal
CMI	cell-mediated immunity
CML	chronic myelocytic leukemia
C_{max}	maximum effective plasma concentration
C_{min}	minimum effective plasma concentration
CMT	Certified Medical Transcriptionist
CMV	cytomegalovirus I
CMVIG	cytomegalovirus immune globulin
CN	cranial nerve
CNM	Certified Nurse Midwife
CNS	central nervous system
CO	cardiac output
CO_2	carbon dioxide
CoA	coenzyme A
COG	center of gravity
comp	compound *(compositus)*
COMT	catecholamine-o-methyl transferase
cont rem	let the medicine be continued *(continuetur remedium)*
COPD	chronic obstructive pulmonary disease
CPAP	continuous positive airway pressure
CPK	creatine phosphokinase
CPR	cardiopulmonary resuscitation
CQI	continuous quality improvement
Cr	creatinine; chromium
CrCl	creatinine clearance
CRD	chronic respiratory disease
CRF	chronic renal failure
CRH	corticotropin-releasing hormone

Abbreviation	Meaning
crm	cream
CRNA	Certified Registered Nurse Anesthetist
C&S	culture and sensitivity
CSA	Controlled Substances Act; cyclosporin A
CSF	cerebrospinal fluid; colony-stimulating factors
CSP	cellulose sodium phosphate
ct	clotting time
CT	computerized tomography
CTZ	chemoreceptor trigger zone
cu	cubic
Cu	copper *(cuprum)*
CV	cardiovascular
CVA	cerebrovascular accident
CVP	central venous pressure
CXR	chest x-ray
cyl	cylinder; cylindrical (lens)
cys	cysteine
d.	day *(dies)*
D5W	Dextrose 5% in Water Solution
D10W	Dextrose 10% in Water Solution
D&C	dilation and curettage; designation applied to dyes permitted for use in drugs and cosmetics
D&E	dilation and evacuation
DC	Doctor of Chiropratic
DDS	Doctor of Dental Surgery
DEA	Drug Enforcement Administration
deglut	swallow *(degluttiatur)*
DERM	dermatologic
det	give *(detur)*
DHHS	Department of Health and Human Services
DIC	disseminated intravascular coagulation
dieb alt	every other day *(diebus alternis)*
dil	dilute *(dilue)*
dim	one-half *(dimidius)*
dir prop	with proper direction *(directione propria)*
div in par aeq	divide into equal parts *(divide in partes aequales)*
DIS	drug information source

Abbreviation	Meaning
disp	dispense *(dispensa)*
div	divide
DJD	degenerative joint disease
DKA	diabetic ketoacidosis
dL	deciliter (100 mL)
DMD	Doctor of Dental Medicine
DMSO	dimethyl sulfoxide
DNA	deoxyribonucleic acid
DNR	do not resuscitate
DNS	Director of Nursing Service; Doctor of Nursing Services
DO	Doctor of Osteopathy
DOA	dead on arrival
DP	Doctor of Podiatry
DPH	Doctor of Public Health; Doctor of Public Hygiene
DPI	dry powder inhaler
DPM	Doctor of Physical Medicine; Doctor of Podiatric Medicine
DPS	disintegrations per second
DRG	diagnosis-related groups
DRI	Dietary Reference Intakes
drp	drop(s)
DrPh	Doctor of Public Health; Doctor of Public Hygiene
DRR	Drug Regimen Review
DT	delirium tremens
dtd	give of such a dose *(dentur tales doses)*
DTP	diphtheria, tetanus toxoids & pertussis vaccine
DTRs	deep tendon reflexes
DUB	dysfunctional uterine bleeding
DUE	Drug Usage Evaluations
DUR	Drug Utilization Review
dur dol	while pain lasts *(durante dolore)*
DVA	Department of Veterans Affairs
DVM	Doctor of Veterinary Medicine
DVT	deep venous thrombosis
E.	*Enterococcus*; *Escherichia*
EBV	Epstein-Barr virus
EC	enteric coated
ECG	electrocardiogram
ECT	electroconvulsive therapy
ed.	editor
ED	emergency department; effective dose
ED_{50}	median-effective dose
EDTA	ethylenediamine tetra-acetic acid
EEG	electroencephalogram
EENT	eye, ear, nose, and throat
EF	ejection fraction
eg.	for example *(exempli gratia)*
EIA	enzyme immunoassay
EKG	electrocardiogram
el	elixir
ELISA	enzyme-linked immunosorbent assay
elix	elixir
EMIT	enzyme-multiplied immunoassay test
emp	as directed
ENL	erythema nodosum leprosum
ENT	ear, nose, throat
EPA	Environmental Protection Agency
EPAP	expiratory positive airway pressure
EPO	erythropoietin
EPS	extrapyramidal syndrome (or symptoms)
ER	emergency room; estrogen receptor; extended release; endoplasmic reticulum
ESR	erythrocyte sedimentation rate; electron spin resonance
ESRD	end-stage renal disease
et	and
ET	via endotracheal tube
et al.	for 3 or more coauthors or coworkers *(et alii)*
ex aq	in water
ext rel.	extended release
F	fluorine
f	make; let be made *(fac, fiat, fiant)*
°F	degress Fahrenheit
Fab.	fragment of immunoglobulin G involved in antigen binding
FAO	Food and Agriculture Organizations

Abbreviation	Meaning
FAS	fetal alcohol syndrome
FBS	fasting blood sugar
FDA	Food and Drug Administration
FD&C	designation applied to dyes permitted for use in foods, drugs, and cosmetics; Food, Drug and Cosmetic Act
Fe	iron *(ferrum)*
FEF	forced expiratory flow
FET	forced expiratory time
FEV_1	forced expiratory volume in 1 second
fl oz	fluid ounce(s)
Fru	fructose
FSH	follicle-stimulating hormone
ft.	foot (feet)
ft^2	square foot (feet)
FTC	Federal Trade Commission
FTI	free-thyroxine index
FUO	fever of unknown origin
FVC	forced vital capacity
γ.	gamma
g.	gram *(gramma)*
G-6-P	glucose-6-phosphate
G-6-PD	glucose-6-phosphate dehydrogenase
GABA	gamma-aminobutyric acid
Gal	galactose
gal	gallon
G-CSF	granulocyte colony-stimulating factor
GERD	gastroesophageal reflux disease
GFR	glomerular filtration rate
GGTP	gamma glutamyl transpeptidase
GH	growth hormone
GHRF	growth hormone-releasing factor
GHRH	growth hormone-releasing hormone
GI	gastrointestinal
GLC	gas-liquid chromatography
gln	glutamine
glu	glutamic acid; glutamyl
gly	glycine
Gm	gram *(gramma)*
gr	grain *(granum)*
grad	gradually *(gradatim)*

Abbreviation	Meaning
gran	granule(s)
GRAS	generally regarded as safe
gtt.	a drop *(gutta)*
GU	genitourinary
Gyn	gynecology
H.	*Haemophilus*; *Helicobacter*
h.	hour *(hora)*
H_2	histamine 2
H_2O	water
HA	hyaluronic acid
Hb	hemoglobin
HbF	fetal hemoglobin
HBIG	hepatitis B immune globulin
HCFA	Health Care Financing Administration
HCG	human chorionic gonadotropin
HCl	hydrochloride
HCN	hydrogen cyanide
Hct	hematocrit
hd.	bedtime *(hora decubitus)*
HDL	high-densitiy lipoprotein
HEMA	hematologic
HEME	hematologic
hep.	hepatic
HEPA	high efficiency particulate air
Hg	mercury *(hydragyrum)*
Hgb	hemoglobin
HGH	human pituitary growth hormone
Hib.	*Haemophilus influenzae*
His.	*Haemophilus influenzae* type b
HIV	human immunodeficiency virus
HLA	human leukocyte antigen
HMG-CoA	3-hydroxy-3-methylglutaryl coenzyme A
HMO	health maintenance organization
hor decub	at bedtime *(hora decubitus)*
hor som	at bedtime *(hora somni)*
HPA	hypothalamic-pituitary-adrenocortical (axis)
HPLC	high performance liquid chromatography
HPLC/MS	high performance liquid chromatography/mass spectrometry

Abbreviation	Meaning
HPMC	hydroxypropylmethylcellulose
HPV	human papillomavirus
HR	heart rate
hr	hour
hs	at bedtime *(hora somni)*
HSA	human serum albumin
HSV-1	herpes simplex virus type 1
HSV-2	herpes simplex virus type 2
Hz	hertz
I	iodine
IADL	instrumental activities of daily living
I/O	intake/output
IBW	ideal body weight
IC	intracoronary
ICD	International Classification of Diseases of the World Health Organization
ICF	intracellular fluid
ICP	intracranial pressure
ID	intradermal; infective dose
IDDM	insulin-dependent diabetes mellitus (type 1 diabetes)
IDU	idoxuridine
IFN	interferon
Ig	immunoglobulin
IL	interleukin
Ile	isoleucine
IM	intramuscular
in	inch(es)
in^2	square inch(es)
IND	Investigational New Drug
in d.	daily *(in dies)*
INDA	Investigational New Drug Application
Inh	inhaled
INH	isoniazid
Inhal	inhalation
Inj	injection
INR	International Normalized Ratio
int cib	between meals *(inter cibos)*
IOP	intraocular pressure
IP	intraperitoneal(ly)
IPA	International Pharmaceutical Abstracts
IPPB	intermittent positive pressure breathing
IPV	poliovirus vaccine inactivated
IQ	intelligence quotient
ISA	intrinsic sympathomimetic activity
ISF	interstitial fluid
ISI	Institute for Scientific Information
ISO	International Organization for Standardization
IT	intrathecal(ly)
IU	international unit(s)
IUD	intrauterine device
IV	intravenous
IVF	intravascular fluid
IVP	intravenous piggyback
J	joule(s)
JCAH	Joint Commission on Accreditation of Hospitals
JCAHO	Joint Commission on Accreditation of Healthcare Organizations
K	potassium *(kalium)*; kelvin
kcal	kilocalorie(s)
keV	kiloelectronvolt(s)
kg	kilogram
kJ	kilojoule(s)
Kleb.	*Klebsiella*
KVO	keep vein open
L	liter
L.	*Legionella*; *Listeria*
lb	pound
LBW	low body weight
LD	lethal dose
LD-50	a dose lethal to 50% of the specified animals or microorganisms
LDH	lactate dehydrogenase
LDL	low-density lipoprotein
LE	lupus erythematosus
Leu	leucine
LFT	liver function test
LH	luteinizing hormone
liq	liquid *(liquor)*
LM	Licentiate in Midwifery
LOC	level of consciousness
Lot	lotion
LPN	Licensed Practical Nurse
Lr	lawrencium
LSD	lysergic acid diethylamide

Abbreviation	Meaning
LTCF	long-term care facility
LTM	long-term memory
LUQ	left upper quadrant (of abdomen)
LVEDP	left ventricular end-diastolic pressure
LVET	left ventricular ejection time
LVF	left ventricular function
LVN	Licensed Visiting Nurse; Licensed Vocational Nurse
LVP	large-volume parenterals
Lw	former symbol for lawrencium (see Lr)
Lys	lysine
μm	micrometer
μg	microgram
m	meter
M	mix *(misce)*; molar (strength of a solution)
M.	*Moraxella*; *Mycobacterium*; *Mycoplasma*
m^2	square meter (of body surface area)
m^3	cubic meter(s)
MA	mental age
MAC	maximum allowable cost
MADD	Mothers Against Drunk Driving
man pr	early morning; first thing in the morning *(mane primo)*
MAO	monoamine oxidase
MAOI	monoamine oxidase inhibitor
MAP	mean arterial pressure
max	maximum
MBC	minimum bactericidal concentration
MBD	mimimal brain dysfunction
mcg	microgram
MCH	mean corpuscular hemoglobin
MCHC	mean corpuscular hemoglobin concentration
mCi	millicurie
MCT	medium-chain triglyceride
MCV	mean corpuscular volume
MD	Doctor of Medicine *(Medicinae Doctor)*
MDI	metered-dose inhaler
m dict	as directed *(more dictor)*
MDR	minimum daily requirements
MEC	minimum effective concentration
MEDLARS	Medical Literature Analysis and Retrieval System
MEDLINE	National Library of Medicine medical database
mEq	milliequivalent
Met	methionine
MeV	megaelectronvolt(s)
Mg	magnesium
mg	milligram
MHC	major histocompatibility complex
MI	myocardial infarction
MIA	metabolite bacterial inhibition assay
MIC	minimum inhibitory concentration
MID	minimal inhibitory dose
min	minute; minimum
MIP	maximum inspiratory pressure
mixt	a mixture *(mixtura)*
MJ	mejajoule(s)
mL	milliliter
mm	millimeter
mm^2	square millimeter(s)
mm^3	cubic millimeter(s)
mmHg	millimeters of mercury
mmol	millimole
MMR	measles, mumps and rubella virus vaccine, live
MMWR	Morbidity and Mortality Weekly Report
Mn	manganese
Mo	molybdenum
mo	month
mol	mole(s)
mor dict	in the manner stated *(more dicto)*
mor sol	as usual; as customary *(more solito)*
mOsm	milliosmole
MPH	Master of Public Health
MRI	magnetic resonance imaging
mRNA	messenger RNA
MS	mass spectrometry; mitral stenosis; multiple sclerosis

Abbreviation	Meaning
MW	molecular weight
N	normal (strength of a solution)
N.	*Neisseria*
NA	sodium *(natrium)*
NABP	National Association of Boards of Pharmacy
NABPLEX	National Association of Boards of Pharmacy Licensing Exam
NAD	nicotinamide-adenine dinucleotide phosphate
NADH	reduced form of nicotine adenine dinucleotide
NADP	nicotinamide-adenine dinucleotide phosphate
NADPH	nicotinamide-adenine dinucleotide phosphate (reduced form)
NAPA	*N*-acetyl procainamide
NARD	National Association of Retail Druggists - Now NCPA; National Asssociation of Community Pharmacists
nb.	note well *(nota bene)*
nCi	nanocurie(s)
NCPA	National Association of Community Pharmacists
ND	Doctor of Naturopathic Medicine
NDA	new drug application
NF	National Formulary'
ng.	nanogram
NG	nasogastric
NK	natural killer (cells); killer T cells
NIDDM	non-insulin-dependent diabetes mellitus (type 2 diabetes)
NIH.	National Institutes of Health
NLM	National Library of Medicine
nm	nanometer(s)
NMS	neuroleptic malignant syndrome
NMT	not more than (on prescriptions)
no.	number *(numerus)*
noc.	in the night *(nocturnal)*
noc maneq	at night and in the morning *(nocte maneque)*
non rep	do not repeat; no refills *(non repetatur)*
NPN	nonprotein nitrogen
NPO	nothing by mouth
NS	normal saline (as in solution)
NSAIA	nonsteroidal antiinflammatory agent
NSAID	nonsteroidal antiinflammatory drug
NTD	neural tube defect
O	a pint *(octarius)*
OB/GYN	obstetrics and gynecology
OBRA	Omnibus Budget Reconciliation Act of 1990
OBS	organic brain syndrome
OC	oral contraceptive
Oct	a pint *(octarius)*
od	right eye *(oculus dexter)*
OD	Doctor of Optometry; overdose
Oint	ointment
ol	left eye *(oculus laevus)*
omn hor	at every hour *(omni hora)*
Ophth	ophthalmic
os	left eye *(oculus sinister)*
OSHA	Occupational Safety and Health Administration
OT	occupational therapy
OTC	over-the-counter (nonprescription)
OPV	oral polioviurs vaccine, live
ou	each eye *(oculo uterque)*
o/w	oil-in-water (emulsion)
oz	ounce
P	phosphorus
P	probability
P&T	pharmacy and therapeutics (committee)
Pa	pascal(s)
PA	Physician Assistant; Physician's Assistant
PABA	para-aminobenzoic acid
PAC	premature atrial contraction
$PaCO_2$	arterial plasma partial pressure of carbon dioxide
PAD	premature atrial depolarization
PAF	platelet-activating factor
PaO_2	partial alveolar oxygen
part aeq	equal parts/amounts *(partes aequales)*
part vic	in divided doses *(partitis vicibus)*

Abbreviation	Meaning
PAS	para-aminosalicylic acid
PAW	pulmonary arterial wedge
PAWP	pulmonary arterial wedge pressure
Pb	lead *(plumbum)*
PBP	penicillin-binding protein
pc	after meals *(post cibum; post cibos)*
PCA	patient-controlled analgesia
pCO_2	plasma partial pressure of carbon dioxide
PCP	phencyclidine
PCR	polymerase chain reaction
PDGF	platelet-derived growth factor
PDLL	poorly differentiated lymphocytic lymphoma
PE	pulmonary embolism
PEEP	positive and expiratory pressure
PEG	polyethylene glycol
PERLA	pupils equal, react to light and accommodation
PET	positron emission tomography
pg	picograms(s)
PG	prostaglandin
PGA	prostaglandin A
PGB	prostaglandin B
PGE	prostaglandin E
PGF	prostaglandin F
pH	the negative logarithm of the hydrogen ion concentration
PharmD	Doctor of Pharmacy *(Pharmaciae Doctor)*
PhD	Doctor of Philosophy (Philosophiae Doctor)
Phe	phenylalanine
PhG	German Pharmacopeia *(Pharmacopoeia Germanica)*
PHS	Public Health Service
pKa	the negative logarithm of the dissociation constant
PKU	phenylketonuria
PMA	Pharmaceutical Manufacturers Association
PMH	past medical history
PMI	posterior myocardial infarction
PMN	polymorphonuclear leukocyte

Abbreviation	Meaning
PMR	patient medication record
PMS	premenstrual syndrome
PND	paroxysmal nocturnal dyspnea
po	by mouth; orally *(per os)*
pO_2	oxygen pressure (tension)
POR	problem-oriented medical record
POS	point of service
post cib	after meals *(post cibos)*; pc
PPD	purified protein derivative of tuberculin
PPI	patient package insert
ppm	parts per million
PPO	preferred provider organization
pr	per rectum
Pr.	*Proteus*
prn	as needed; when required *(pro re nata)*
Pro	proline
pro rat. Aet.	According to patient's age *(pro ratione aetatis)*
Ps.	*Pseudomonas*
PSA	prostate-specific antigen
PSP	phenolsulfonphthalein
PSVT	paroxysmal supraventricular tachycardia
pt	pint
PT	prothrombin time; pharmacy and therapeutics; physical therapy
PTH	parathyroid hormone
PTT	partial thromboplastin time
PUD	peptic ulcer disease
pulv	a powder *(pulvis)*
PUVA	oral administration of psoralen and subsequent exposure to ultraviolet light of A wavelenghts (UVA)
PVC	premature ventricular contraction; polyvinyl chloride
PVD	peripheral vascular disease; premature ventricular depolarizations
pwdr	powder
q.	every
Q	volume of blood flow
QA	quality assurance
qad	every other day *(quoque alternis die)*
QC	quality control

Abbreviation	Meaning
qd	every day *(quaque die)*
qh	every hour *(quaque hora)*
q hr	every hour
qid	four times daily *(quarter in die)*
ql	as much as desired *(quantum libet)*
qod	every other day
q 2 hr	every 2 hours
qs	a sufficient quantity *(quantum sufficiat)*; as much as is enough *(quantum satis)*
qs ad	a sufficient quantity to make
qt	quart
qv	as much as you wish *(quam volueris)*
R&D	research and development
RA	rheumatoid arthritis
RAI	radioactive iodine
RAS	renin-angiotension system; reticular-activating system
RAST	radioallergosorbent test
RBC	red blood (cell) count
RDA	Recommended Dietary (Daily) Allowance
RDS	respiratory distress
RDW	red-cell distribution width
RE	reticuloendothelial
rem.	radio equivalent man
REM	rapid eye movement
rep	let it be repeated *(repetatur)*
RES	reticuloendothelial system
RF	releasing factor
Rh	Rhesus (RH blood group)
RIA	radioimmunoassay
RN	Registered Nurse
RNA	ribonucleic acid
ROM	range of motion
RPh	registered pharmacist
rpm	revolutions per minute
rps	revolutions per second
RR	respiratory rate
RT_3U	total serum thyroxine concentration
RUL	right upper lobe (of lung)
RUQ	right upper quadrant (of abdomen)
Rx	prescription only; take; a recipe *(recipe)*
S.	*Salmonella; Serratia*
s	second; without *(sine)*
s̄	without *(sine)*
S&S	signs and symptoms
S-A	sinoatrial
sa	according to art *(secundum artem)*
sat	saturated *(sataratus)*
Sb	antimony *(stibium)*
SBE	self breast examination; subacute bacterial endocarditis
SC	subcutaneous(ly)
S_{cr}	serum creatinine
SD	standard deviation; streptodornase
Se	selenium
sec	second
Ser	serine
sf	sugar free
SGGT	serum gamma-glutamyl transferase
SGOT	(see AST)
SGPT	(see ALT)
Sh.	*Shigella*
SIADH	syndrome of inappropriate secretion of antidiuretic hormone
SIDS	sudden infant death syndrome
Sig	label; let it be printed *(signa)*
SI units	International System of Units
SK	streptokinase
SL	sublingual(ly)
SLE	systemic lupus erythematosus
SMA	sequential multiple analysis
Sn	tin *(stannum)*
SNF	skilled nursing facility
sol	solution *(solutio)*
soln	solution
solv	dissolve
sp	species
SPECT	single photon emission computerized tomography
sp gr	specific gravity

Abbreviation	Meaning
SPF	sun protection factor
sq	square
SR	sedimentation rate; sustained release
ss	one-half *(semis)*
$\bar{s}\bar{s}$	one-half *(semis)*
SSRI	selective serotonin reuptake inhibitors
Staph.	*Staphylococcus*
stat	immediately; at once *(statim)*
STM	short-term memory
STP	standard temperature and pressure
Str.	*Streptococcus*
STD	sexually transmitted disease
supp	suppository *(suppositorium)*
suppl	supplement(s)
susp	suspension
SV	stroke volume
syr	syrup *(syrupus)*
$t_{1/2}$	half-life
T_3	triiodothyronine
T_4	thyroxine
tab	tablet *(tabella)*
tal	such
tal dos	such doses
TB	tuberculosis
TBC	thyroxine-binding globulin
TBP	thyroxine-binding proteins
TBPA	thyroxine-binding prealbumin
TBW	total body weight
TCA	tricyclic antidepressant
TD_{50}	median toxic dose
TEEC	transesophageal echocardiography
TEN	toxic epidermal necrolysis
TENS	transcutaneous electrical nerve stimulation
TG	total triglycerides
THC	tetrahydrocannabinol
Thr	threonine
TIA	transient ischemic attack
tid	three times daily *(ter in die)*
tbsp	tablespoonful
tinct	tincture
TLC	total lung capacity; thin layer chromatography
T_{max}	time to maximum concentration
TMJ	temporomandibular joint
TNF	tumor necrosis factor
TNM	tumor, node, metastasis (tumor staging)
top	topical(ly)
TOPV	trivalent oral polio vaccine
tPA	tissue plasminogen activator
TPN	total parenteral nutrition
TPR	temperature, pulse, respirations
TQM	total quality management
tr	tincture
trit.	triturate *(tritura)*
tRNA	transfer RNA
Trp	tryptophan
TSA	tumor-specific antigens
TSH	thyroid-stimulating hormone
tsp	teaspoonful
TSS	toxic shock syndrome
TSTA	tumor-specific transplantation antigen
TT	thrombin time
TV	tidal volume
Tyr	tyrosine
U	unit
ud.	as directed
UD	unit-dose package
UK	United Kingdom
ung.	ointment *(unguentum)*
URI.	upper respiratory infection
USAN	United States Adopted Name(s)
USP	*United States Pharmacopeia*
USPHS	United States Public Health Service
ut dict	as directed *(ut dictum)*
UTI	urinary tract infection
UVA	ultraviolet A wave
V	volt
VA	Veterans Administration
vag	vaginal(ly)
Val	valine
var	variety
VC	vital capacity

Abbreviation	Meaning
V_c	volume of distribution of the central compartment
V_d	volume of distribution (one compartment)
$V_{d\beta}$	volume of distribution of the β phase
V_{dss}	steady-state apparent volume of distribution
VHDL	very high-density lipoprotein
VLDL	very low-density lipoprotein
VMA	vanillylmandelic acid
vol	volume
VS	vital signs
v/v	volume in volume
v/w	volume in weight
wa	while awake
WBC	white blood (cell) count
WBCT	whole blood clotting time
WDLL	well-differentiated lymphocytic lymphoma
WFI	water for injection
WHO	World Health Organization
wk	week
WNL	within normal limits
w/o	water in oil
wt	weight
w/v	weight in volume
w/w	weight in weight
y/o	years old
yr	year
ZE	Zollinger-Ellison
Zn	zinc

Calculations

To calculate milliequivalent weight:

$$\text{mEq} = \frac{\text{gram molecular weight/valence}}{1000}$$

$$\text{mEq} = \frac{\text{mg}}{\text{eq wt}} \qquad \text{equivalent weight or eq wt} = \frac{\text{gram molecular weight}}{\text{valence}}$$

Commonly Used mEq Weights			
Chloride	35.5 mg = 1 mEq	Magnesium	12 mg = 1 mEq
Sodium	23 mg = 1 mEq	Potassium	39 mg = 1 mEq
Calcium	20 mg = 1 mEq		

To convert temperature:

Fahrenheit to Celsius: (°F – 32) × 5/9 = °C

Celsius to Fahrenheit: (°C × 9/5) + 32 = °F

Celsius to Kelvin: °C + 273 = °K

Temperature Equivalents

°C = 5 ÷ sec × (°F – 32)

°F = 9 ÷ 5 × (°C) + 32

°K = °C + 273

To calculate creatinine clearance (Ccr) from serum creatinine (mL/min):

for males

$$\text{Male: Ccr} = \frac{\text{weight (kg)} \times (140 - \text{age})}{72 \times \text{serum creatinine (mg/dL)}}$$

Female: Ccr = 0.85 × calculation

To calculate ideal body weight (IBW) (kg) in adults:

IBW (kg) (Males) = 50 + (2.3 × Height in inches over 60 inches)

IBW (kg) (Females) = 45.5 kg + (2.3 × Height in inches over 60 inches)

To calculate absolute neutrophil count (ANC):

WBC × (% Segs + % Bands)

To calculate aninon gap:

$Na^+ - (Cl^- \ HCo_3^-)$

Elevated anion gap usually indicates unmeasured anions in the extracellular fluid due to any of the following: methanol, uremia, diabetes, paraldehyde, ischemia, ethylene glycol, salicylates.

To calculate daily fluid requirements (based on patient's weight):

Weight from 0 to 10 kg: 100 kg

Weight from 10 to 20 kg: 50 mL/kg

Weight > 20 kg: 20 mL/kg

To calculate LDL cholesterol:

$LDL_{chol} = (Total_{chol} - HDL_{chol}) - [\text{Triglycerides (must be} < 400)/5]$

To calculate volume status:

BUN: Serum Creatine ratio

* If > 20:1, Patient is volume depleted and requires fluid replacement.

Chem 7 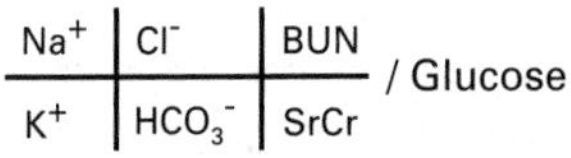

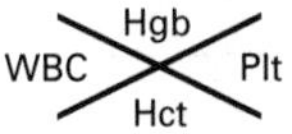

* Glucose: add 1.6 mEq/L Na^+ for every 100 mg/dL glucose is above normal.

To calculate total calcium corrected for albumin:

[Normal albumin – patient's albumin] × 0.8 patient's calcium = corrected calcium

---

Common Systems of Weights and Measures

The listing of common systems of weights and measures is included to aid the practitioner in calculating dosages.

METRIC SYSTEM

Metric Weight			Metric Liquid Measure		
1 femtogram (fg)	= 0.001	pg	1 femtoliter (fL)	= 0.001	pL
1 picogram (pg)	= 0.001	ng	1 picoliter (pL)	= 0.001	nL
1 nanogram (ng)	= 0.001	mcg	1 nanoliter (nL)	= 0.001	μL
1 microgram* (μg [mcg])	= 0.001	mg	1 microliter (μL)	= 0.001	mL
1 milligram (mg)	= 0.001	g	1 milliliter (mL)	= 0.001	L
1 centigram (cg)	= 0.01	g	1 centiliter (cL)	= 0.01	L (= 10 mL)
1 decigram (dg)	= 0.1	g	1 deciliter (dL)	= 0.1	L (= 100 mL)
1 gram (g)	= 1.0	g	1 liter (L)	= 1.0	L (= 1000 mL)
1 dekagram (dag)	= 10.0	g	1 dekaliter (daL)	= 10.0	L
1 hectogram (hg)	= 100.0	g	1 hectoliter (hL)	= 100.0	L
1 kilogram (kg)	= 1000.0	g	1 kiloliter (kL)	= 1000.0	L

* The abbreviation μg or mcg is used for microgram in pharmacy rather than gamma (γ) as in biology.

APOTHECARY SYSTEM*

Apothercary Weight Equivalents			Apothecary Volume Equivalents		
1 grain† (gr)	= 1 gr		1 minim (♏)	= 1 ♏	
1 scruple (℈)	= 20 gr		1 fluidram (fl ʒ)	= 60 ♏	= 8 fl ʒ
1 dram (ʒ)	= 60 gr	= 3 ℈	1 fluid ounce (fl ℥)	= 480 ♏	= 8 fl ℥
1 ounce (℥)	= 480 gr	= 8 ʒ	1 pint (pt or O)	= 7680 ♏	= 16 fl ℥
1 pound (lb)	= 5760 gr	= 12 ℥	1 quart (qt)	= 15630 ♏	= 32 fl ℥
			1 gallon (gal or cong)	= 61440 ♏	= 128 fl ℥

* Used in preparation of pharmaceuticals.

† The grain in each of the above systems has the same value, and thus serves as a basis for the interconversion of the other units.

AVOIRDUPOIS SYSTEM*

Avoirdupois Equivalents		
1 ounce (oz)	= 437.5 grains (gr)	
1 pound (lb)	= 16 ounces (oz)	= 7000 grains (gr)

* Used by manufacturers and wholesalers.

Approximate Practical Equivalents

The listing of approximate practical equivalents is included to aid the practitioner in calculating and converting dosages among the various systems.

Weight Equivalents

1 grain	=	1 gr	=	65 milligrams
1 milligram	=	1 mg	=	0.017 grains
1 gram	=	1 g	=	15.432 grains
1 gram	=	1 g	=	0.035 ounces
1 ounce avoirdupois	=	1 oz	=	28.35 grams
1 ounce apothecary	=	1 ℥	=	31.1 grams
1 pound avoirdupois	=	1 lb	=	454.0 grams
1 pound avoirdupois	=	1 lb	=	0.45 kilograms
1 kilogram	=	1 kg	=	2.20 pounds avoirdupois (lb)

Measure Equivalents

1 milliliter	=	1 mL	=	16.23 minims (♏)
1 cubic centimeter*	=	1 cc	=	1.0 mL
1 fluidram†	=	1 f ʒ	=	3.4 mL
1 teaspoonful†	=	1 tsp	=	5.0 mL
1 tablespoonful	=	1 tbsp	=	15.0 mL
1 fluid ounce	=	1 fl ℥	=	29.57 mL
1 wineglassful	=	2 fl ℥	=	60.0 mL
1 teacupful	=	4 fl ℥	=	120.0 mL
1 tumblerful	=	8 fl ℥	=	240.0 mL
1 pint	=	1 pt or O or Oct	=	473.0 mL
1 quart	=	1 qt	=	946.0 mL
1 liter	=	1 L	=	33.8 fluid ounces (fl ℥)
1 gallon	=	1 gal or C or Cong	=	3785.0 mL

* Cubic centimeter and milliliter are equivalent.

† On prescription a fluidram is assumed to contain a teaspoonful, which is 5 mL.

Weight to Volume Equivalents

1 mg/dL	=	10 μ/mL
1 mg/dL	=	1 mg %
1% solution	=	10 mg per mL
1 ppm	=	1 mg/L

Linear Equivalents

1 millimeter	=	1 mm	=	0.04 inches
1 inch	=	1 in	=	25.4 millimeters
1 inch	=	1 in	=	2.54 centimeters
1 meter	=	1 meter	=	39.37 inches
1 inch	=	1 in	=	0.025 meters

International System of Units

The *Système international d 'unités* (International System of Units) or *SI* is a modernized version of the metric system. The primary goal of the conversion to SI units is to revise the present confused measurement system and to improve test-result communications.

The SI has 7 basic units from which other units are derived:

Base Units of SI		
Physical quantity	Base unit	SI symbol
length	meter	m
mass	kilogram	kg
time	second	s
amount of substance	mole	mol
thermodynamic temperature	kelvin	K
electric current	ampere	A
luminous intensity	candela	cd

Combinations of these base units can express any property, although, for simplicity, special names are given to some of these derived units.

Representative Derived Units		
Derived unit	Name and symbol	Derivation from base units
area	square meter	m^2
volume	cubic meter	m^3.
force	newton (N)	$kg{\bullet}m{\bullet}s^{-2}$
pressure	pascal (Pa)	$kg{\bullet}m^{-1}{\bullet}s^{-2}$ (N/m^2)
work, energy	joule (J)	$kg{\bullet}m^2{\bullet}s^{-2}$ ($N{\bullet}m$)
mass density	kilogram per cubic meter	kg/m^3
frequency	hertz (Hz)	1 $cycles/s^{-1}$
temperature degree	Celsius (°C)	°C = °K – 273.15
concentration		
mass	kilogram/liter	kg/L
substance	mole/liter	mol/L
molality	mole/kilogram	mol/kg
density	kilogram/liter	kg/L

Prefixes to the base unit are used in this system to form decimal multiples and submultiples. The preferred multiples and submultiples listed below change the quantity by increments of 10^3 or 10^{-3}. The exceptions to these recommended factors are within the middle rectangle.

Prefixes and Symbols for Decimal Multiples and Submultiples

Factor	Prefix	Symbol
10^{18}	exa	E
10^{15}	peta	P
10^{12}	tera	T
10^{9}	giga	G
10^{6}	mega	M
10^{3}	kilo	k
10^{2}	hecto	h
10^{1}	deka	da
10^{-1}	deci	d
10^{-2}	centi	c
10^{-3}	milli	m
10^{-6}	micro	μ
10^{-9}	nano	n
10^{-12}	pico	p
10^{-15}	femto	f
10^{-18}	atto	a

To convert drug concentrations to or from SI units:
Conversion factor (CF) = 1000/mol wt
Conversion *to* SI units: μg/mL × CF = μmol/L
Conversion *from* SI units: μmol/L ÷ CF = μg/mL

Normal Laboratory Values

In the following tables, normal reference values for commonly requested laboratory tests are listed in traditional units and in SI units. The tables are a guideline only. Values are method dependent and "normal values" may vary between laboratories.

Blood, Plasma or Serum		
Determination	Reference Value: Conventional units	Reference Value: SI units
Alpha-fetoprotein	Adult: < 15 ng/mL Pregnant (16-18 wk): 38-45 ng/mL	Adult: < 15 mcg/L Pregnant (16-18 wk): 38-45 mcg/L
Ammonia (NH_3) - diffusion	20-120 mcg/dL	12-70 mcmol/L
Ammonia nitrogen	15-45 µg/dL	11-32 µmol/L
Amylase	20-100 units/dL	37-185 U/L
Anion gap (Na^+–[Cl^- + HCO_3^-]) (P)	7-16 mEq/L	7-16 mmol/L
Antinuclear antibodies	negative at 1:10 dilution of serum	negative at 1:10 dilution of serum
Antithrombin III (AT III)	80-120 U/dL	800-1200 U/L
Bicarbonate: Arterial Venous	21-28 mEq/L 22-29 mEq/L	21-28 mmol/L 22-29 mmol/L
Bilirubin: Conjugated (direct) Total	≤ 0.2 mg/dL 0.1-1 mg/dL	≤ 4 mcmol/L 2-18 mcmol/L
Calcitonin: Female Male	≤ 20 pg/mL ≤ 40 pg/mL	≤ 20 ng/L ≤ 40 ng/L
Calcium: Total Ionized	8.6-10.3 mg/dL 4.4-5.1 mg/dL	2.2-2.74 mmol/L 1-1.3 mmol/L
Carbon dioxide content (plasma)	21-32 mmol/L	21-32 mmol/L
Carcinoembryonic antigen	< 3 ng/mL	< 3 mcg/L
Chloride	95-110 mEq/L	95-110 mmol/L
Coagulation screen: Bleeding time Prothrombin time Partial thromboplastin time (activated) Protein C Protein S	 3-9.5 min 10-13 sec 22-37 sec 0.7-1.4 µ/mL 0.7-1.4 µ/mL	 180-570 sec 10-13 sec 22-37 sec 700-1400 U/mL 700-1400 U/mL
Copper, total	70-160 mcg/dL	11-25 mcmol/L
Corticotropin (ACTH [adrenocorticotropic hormone]) - 0800 hr	< 60 pg/mL	< 13.2 pmol/L
Cortisol: 0800 hr 1800 hr 2000 hr	5-30 mcg/dL 2-15 mcg/dL ≤ 50% of 0800 hr	138-810 nmol/L 50-410 nmol/L ≤ 50% of 0800 hr
Creatine kinase: Female Male	20-170 IU/L 30-220 IU/L	0.33-2.83 mckat/L 0.5-3.67 mckat/L
Creatinine kinase isoenzymes, MB fraction	0-12 IU/L	0-0.2 mckat/L
Creatinine	0.5-1.7 mg/dL	44-150 mcmol/L
Fibrinogen (coagulation factor I)	150-360 mg/dL	1.5-3.6 g/L
Follicle-stimulating hormone (FSH): Female Midcycle Male	 2-13 mIU/mL 5-22 mIU/mL 1-8 mIU/mL	 2-13 IU/L 5-22 IU/L 1-8 IU/L
Glucose, fasting	65-115 mg/dL	3.6-6.3 mmol/L
Glucose tolerance test (oral)	mg/dL *Normal* / *Diabetic*	mmol/L *Normal* / *Diabetic*
Fasting	70-105 / > 140	3.9-5.8 / > 7.8
60 min	120-170 / ≥ 200	6.7-9.4 / ≥ 11.1
90 min	100-140 / ≥ 200	5.6-7.8 / ≥ 11.1
120 min	70-120 / ≥ 140	3.9-6.7 / ≥ 7.8

Blood, Plasma or Serum		
	Reference Value	
Determination	Conventional units	SI units
(γ) - Glutamyltransferase (GGT): Male	9-50 units/L	9-50 units/L
Female	8-40 units/L	8-40 units/L
Haptoglobin	44-303 mg/dL	0.44-3.03 g/L
Hematologic tests:		
Fibrinogen	200-400 mg/dL	2-4 g/L
Hematocrit (Hct), female	36%-44.6%	0.36-0.446 fraction of 1
male	40.7%-50.3%	0.4-0.503 fraction of 1
Hemoglobin A_{1C}	4%-6%	0.053-0.075
Hemoglobin (Hb), female	12-16 g/dL	7.49-9.9 mmol/L
male	14-18 g/dL	8.7-11.2 mmol/L
Leukocyte count (WBC)	3800-9800/mcL	3.8-9.8 x 10^9/L
Erythrocyte count (RBC), female	3.5-5 x 10^6/mcL	3.5-5 x 10^{12}/L
male	4.3-5.9 x 10^6/mcL	4.3-5.9 x 10^{12}/L
Mean corpuscular volume (MCV)	80-97.6 mcm^3	80-97.6 fl
Mean corpuscular hemoglobin (MCH)	27-33 pg/cell	1.66-2.09 fmol/cell
Mean corpuscular hemoglobin concentrate (MCHC)	33-36 g/dL	20.3-22 mmol/L
Erythrocyte sedimentation rate (sedrate, ESR)	≤ 30 mm/hr	≤ 30 mm/hr
Erythrocyte enzymes:		
Glucose-6-phosphate dehydrognase (G-6-PD)	250-5000 units/10^6 cells	250-5000 mcunits/cell
Ferritin	10-300 ng/mL	10-300 pmol/L
Folic acid: normal	> 3.1-12.4 ng/mL	7-28.1 nmol/L
Platelet count	150-450 x 10^3/mcL	150-450 x 10^9/L
Reticulocytes	0.5%-1.5% of erythrocytes	0.005-0.015
Vitamin B_{12}	223-1132 pg/mL	165-835 pmol/L
Iron: Female	30-160 mcg/dL	5.4-31.3 mcmol/L
Male	45-160 mcg/dL	8.1-31.3 mcmol/L
Iron binding capacity	220-420 mcg/dL	39.4-75.2 mcmol/L
Isocitrate dehydrogenase	1.2-7 units/L	1.2-7 units/L
Isoenzymes		
Fraction 1	14%-26% of total	0.14-0.26 fraction of total
Fraction 2	29%-39% of total	0.29-0.39 fraction of total
Fraction 3	20%-26% of total	0.20-0.26 fraction of total
Fraction 4	8%-16% of total	0.08-0.16 fraction of total
Fraction 5	6%-16% of total	0.06-0.16 fraction of total
Lactate dehydrogenase	100-250 IU/L	1.67-4.17 mckat/L
Lactic acid (lactate)	6-19 mg/dL	0.7-2.1 mmol/L
Lead	≤ 20 mcg/dL	≤ 2.41 mcmol/L
Lipase	10-150 IU/L	10-150 IU/L
Lipids:		
Total Cholesterol		
Desirable	< 200 mg/dL	< 5.2 mmol/L
Borderline-high	200-239 mg/dL	< 5.2-6.2 mmol/L
High	> 239 mg/dL	> 6.2 mmol/L
LDL		
Desirable	< 130 mg/dL	< 3.36 mmol/L
Borderline-high	130-159 mg/dL	3.36-4.11 mmol/L
High	> 159 mg/dL	> 4.11 mmol/L
HDL		
Low	< 40 mg/dL	
High	≥ 60 mg/dL	
Triglycerides		
Desirable	< 150 mg/dL	
Borderline-high	150-199 mg/dL	
High	200-499 mg/dL	
Very high	> 500 mg/dL	
Magnesium	1.3-2.2 mEq/L	0.65-1.1 mmol/L
Osmolality	280-300 mOsm/kg	280-300 mmol/kg

Blood, Plasma or Serum		
	Reference Value	
Determination	Conventional units	SI units
Oxygen saturation (arterial)	94%-100%	0.94-1 fraction of 1
PCO_2, arterial	35-45 mm Hg	4.7-6 kPa
pH, arterial	7.35-7.45	7.35-7.45
PO_2, arterial: Breathing room air[1] On 100% O_2	80-105 mm Hg > 500 mm Hg	10.6-14 kPa
Phosphatase (acid), total at 37°C	0.13-0.63 IU/L	2.2-10.5 IU/L or 2.2-10.5 mckat/L
Phosphatase alkaline[2]	20-130 IU/L	20-130 IU/L or 0.33-2.17 mckat/L
Phosphorus, inorganic,[3] (phosphate)	2.5-5 mg/dL	0.8-1.6 mmol/L
Potassium	3.5-5 mEq/L	3.5-5 mmol/L
Progesterone Female Follicular phase Luteal phase Male	 0.1-1.5 ng/mL 0.1-1.5 ng/mL 2.5-28 ng/mL < 0.5 ng/mL	 0.32-4.8 nmol/L 0.32-4.8 nmol/L 8-89 nmol/L < 1.6 nmol/L
Prolactin	1.4-24.2 ng/mL	1.4-24.2 mcg/L
Prostate specific antigen	0-4 ng/mL	0-4 ng/mL
Protein: Total Albumin Globulin	6-8 g/dL 3.6-5 g/dL 2.3-3.5 g/dL	60-80 g/L 36-50 g/L 23-35 g/L
Rheumatoid factor	< 60 IU/mL	< 60 kIU/L
Sodium	135-147 mEq/L	135-147 mmol/L
Testosterone: Female Male	6-86 ng/dL 270-1070 ng/dL	0.21-3 nmol/L 9.3-37 nmol/L
Thyroid Hormone Function Tests: Thyroid-stimulating hormone (TSH) Thyroxine-binding globulin capacity Total triiodothyronine (T_3) Total thyroxine by RIA (T_4) T_3 resin uptake	 0.35-6.2 mcU/mL 10-26 mcg/dL 75-220 ng/dL 4-11 mcg/dL 25%-38%	 0.35-6.2 mU/L 100-260 mcg/L 1.2-3.4 nmol/L 51-142 nmol/L 0.25-0.38 fraction of 1
Transaminase, AST (aspartate aminotransferase, SGOT)	11-47 IU/L	0.18-0.78 mckat/L
Transaminase, ALT (alanine aminotransferase, SGPT)	7-53 IU/L	0.12-0.88 mckat/L
Transferrin	220-400 mg/dL	2.20-4.00 g/L
Urea nitrogen (BUN)	8-25 mg/dL	2.9-8.9 mmol/L
Uric acid	3-8 mg/dL	179-476 mcmol/L
Vitamin A (retinol)	15-60 mcg/dL	0.52-2.09 mcmol/L
Zinc	50-150 mcg/dL	7.7-23 mcmol/L

1 Age dependent
2 Infants and adolescents up to 104 U/L
3 Infants in the first year up to 6 mg/dL

Urine		
	Reference value	
Determination	Conventional units	SI units
Calcium[1]	50-250 mcg/day	1.25-6.25 mmol/day
Catecholamines: Epinephrine Norepinephrine	 < 20 mcg/day < 100 mcg/day	 < 109 nmol/day < 590 nmol/day
Catecholamines, 24-hr	< 110 µg	< 650 nmol
Copper[1]	15-60 mcg/day	0.24-0.95 mcmol/day
Creatinine: Child	8-22 mg/kg	71-195 µmol/kg
Adolescent	8-30 mg/kg	71-265 µmol/kg
Female	0.6-1.5 g/day	5.3-13.3 mmol/day
Male	0.8-1.8 g/day	7.1-15.9 mmol/day
pH	4.5-8	4.5-8
Phosphate[1]	0.9-1.3 g/day	29-42 mmol/day
Potassium[1]	25-100 mEq/day	25-100 mmol/day
Protein Total At rest	 1-14 mg/dL 50-80 mg/day	 10-140 mg/L 50-80 mg/day
Protein, quantitative	< 150 mg/day	< 0.15 g/day
Sodium[1]	100-250 mEq/day	100-250 mmol/day
Specific gravity, random	1.002-1.030	1.002-1.030
Uric acid, 24-hr	250-750 mg	1.48-4.43 mmol

[1] Diet Dependent

Drug Levels*			
Drug determination		Reference value: Conventional units	Reference value: SI units
Aminoglycosides	Amikacin		
	(trough)	1-8 mcg/mL	1.7-13.7 mcmol/L
	(peak)	20-30 mcg/mL	34-51 mcmol/L
	Gentamicin		
	(trough)	0.5-2 mcg/mL	1-4.2 mcmol/L
	(peak)	6-10 mcg/mL	12.5-20.9 mcmol/L
	Kanamycin		
	(trough)	5-10 mcg/mL	nd[1]
	(peak)	20-25 mcg/mL	nd
	Netilimicin		
	(trough)	0.5-2 mcg/mL	nd
	(peak)	6-10 mcg/mL	nd
	Streptomycin		
	(trough)	< 5 mcg/mL	nd
	(peak)	20-30 mcg/mL	nd
	Tobramycin		
	(trough)	0.5-2 mcg/mL	1.1-4.3 mcmol/L
	(peak)	6-10 mcg/mL	12.8-21.8 mcmol/L
Antiarrhythmics	Amiodarone	0.5-2.5 mcg/mL	1.5-4 mcmol/L
	Bretylium	0.5-1.5 mcg/mL	nd
	Digitoxin	9-25 mcg/L	11.8-32.8 nmol/L
	Digoxin	0.8-2 ng/mL	0.9-2.5 nmol/L
	Disopyramide	2-8 mcg/mL	6-18 mcmol/L
	Flecainide	0.2-1 mcg/mL	nd
	Lidocaine	1.5-6 mcg/mL	4.5-21.5 mcmol/L
	Mexiletine	0.5-2 mcg/mL	nd
	Procainamide	4-8 mcg/mL	17-34 mcmol/mL
	Propranolol	50-100 ng/mL	190-390 nmol/L
	Quinidine	2-6 mcg/mL	4.6-9.2 mcmol/L
	Tocainide	5-12 mcg/mL	22-52 mcmol/L
	Verapamil	50-200 ng/mL	100-420 nmol/L
Anticonvulsants	Carbamazepine	4-12 mcg/mL	17-51 mcmol/L
	Phenobarbital	10-40 mcg/mL	43-172 mcmol/L
	Phenytoin	10-20 mcg/mL	40-80 mcmol/L
	Primidone	5-15 mg/mL	23-69 mcmol/L
	Valproic Acid	50-100 mcg/L	346-693 mcmol/L
Antidepressants	Amitriptyline	110-250 ng/mL[2]	500-900 nmol/L
	Amoxapine	200-500 ng/mL	637-1594 nmol/L
	Bupropion	50-100 ng/mL	nd
	Clomipramine	80-100 ng/mL	nd
	Desipramine	115-300 ng/mL	281-1125 nmol/L
	Doxepin	30-250 ng/mL	107-537 nmol/L
	Imipramine	100-300 ng/mL	nd
	Maprotiline	200-300 ng/mL	nd
	Nortriptyline	50-150 ng/mL	190-665 nmol/L
	Protriptyline	70-250 ng/mL	266-950 nmol/L
	Trazodone	800-1600 ng/mL	nd

Drug Levels*

Drug determination		Reference value: Conventional units	Reference value: SI units
Antipsychotics	Chlorpromazine	50-300 ng/mL	157-942 nmol/L
	Fluphenazine	5-20 ng/mL	nd
	Haloperidol	5-20 ng/mL	10-30 nmol/L
	Perphenazine	2-6 ng/mL	nd
	Thiothixene	2-57 ng/mL	nd
Miscellaneous	Amantadine	300 ng/mL	nd
	Amrinone	3.7 mcg/mL	nd
	Chloramphenicol	10-20 mcg/mL	31-62 mcmol/L
	Cyclosporine[3]	250-800 ng/mL (whole blood, RIA) 50-300 ng/mL (plasma, RIA)	nd nd
	Ethanol[4]	0 mg/dL	0 mmol/L
	Hydralazine	100 ng/mL	nd
	Lithium	0.6-1.2 mEq/L	0.6-1.2 mmol/L
	Salicylate	100-300 mg/L	724-2172 mcmol/L
	Sulfonamide	5-15 mg/dL	nd
	Theophylline	10-20 mcg/mL	55-110 mcmol/L
	Vancomycin (trough) (peak)	 5-15 ng/mL 20-40 mcg/mL	 nd nd

* The values given are generally accepted as desirable for treatment without toxicity for most patients. However, exceptions are not uncommon.
1 nd = No data available.
2 Parent drug plus N-desmethyl metabolite.
3 24-hour trough values.
4 Toxic: 50-100 mg/dL (10.9–21.7 mmol/L).

The following table is adopted from the Seventh Report of the Joint National Committee on Prevention, Detection, Evaluation, and Treatment of High Blood Pressure, National Institutes of Health.

Classification of Blood Pressure*

Category	Reference value: Systolic (mm Hg)		Reference value: Diastolic (mm Hg)
Normal[1]	< 120	and	< 80
Prehypertension	120-139	or	80-89
High Blood Pressure			
Stage 1 Hypertension	140-159	or	90-99
Stage 2 Hypertension	≥ 160	or	≥ 100

* For adults age 18 and older who are not taking antihypertensive drugs and not acutely ill. When systolic and diastolic blood pressures fall into different categories, the higher category should be selected to classify the individual's blood pressure status. In addition to classifying stages of hypertension on the basis of average blood pressure levels, clinicians should specify presence or absence of target organ disease and additional risk factors.
1 Unusually low readings should be evaluated for clinical significance.

FDA Pregnancy Categories

The rational use of any medication requires a risk vs benefit assessment. Among the myriad of risk factors which complicate this assessment, pregnancy is one of the most perplexing.

The FDA has established five categories to indicate the potential of a systemically absorbed drug for causing birth defects. The key differentiation among the categories rests upon the degree (reliability) of documentation and the risk vs benefit ratio. Pregnancy Category X is particularly notable in that if any data exists that may implicate a drug as a teratogen and the risk vs benefit ratio does not support use of the drug, the drug is contraindicated during pregnancy. These categories are summarized below:

FDA Pregnancy Categories

Pregnancy Category	Definition
A	Controlled studies show no risk. Adequate, well-controlled studies in pregnant women have failed to demonstrate risk to the fetus.
B	No evidence of risk in humans. Either animal findings show risk, but human findings do not; or if no adequate human studies have been done, animal findings are negative.
C	Risk cannot be ruled out. Human studies are lacking, and animal studies are either positive for fetal risk or lacking. However, potential benefits may justify the potential risks.
D	Positive evidence of risk. Investigational or post-marketing data show risk to the fetus. Nevertheless, potential benefits may outweigh the potential risks. If needed in a life-threatening situation or a serious disease, the drug may be acceptable if safer drugs cannot be used or are ineffective.
X	Contraindicated in pregnancy. Studies in animals or humans, or investigational or post-marketing reports have shown fetal risk that clearly outweighs any possible benefit to the patients.

Regardless of the designated pregnancy category or presumed safety, no drug should be administered during pregnancy unless it is clearly needed and potential benefits outweigh potential hazards to the fetus.

Controlled Substances

The Controlled Substances Act of 1970 regulates the manufacturing, distribution, and dispensing of drugs that have abuse potential. The Drug Enforcement Administration (DEA) within the US Department of Justice is the chief federal agency responsible for enforcing the act.

DEA schedules: Drugs under jurisdiction of the Controlled Substances Act are divided into five schedules based on their potential for abuse and physical and psychological dependence. All controlled substances listed in *American Drug Index* are identified by schedule as follows:

Schedule I *(c-i)*: High abuse potential and no accepted medical use (eg, heroin, marijuana, LSD).

Schedule II *(c-ii)*: High abuse potential with severe dependence liability (eg, narcotics, amphetamines, dronabinol, some barbiturates).

Schedule III *(c-iii)*: Less abuse potential than schedule II drugs and moderate dependence liability (eg, nonbarbiturate sedatives, nonamphetamine stimulants, limited amounts of certain narcotics).

Schedule IV *(c-iv)*: Less abuse potential than III drugs and limited dependence liability (eg, some sedatives, antianxiety agents, nonnarcotic analgesics).

Schedule V *(c-v)*: Limited abuse potential. Primarily small amounts of narcotics (codeine) used as antitussives or antidiarrheals. Under federal law, limited quantities of certain *c-v* drugs may be purchased without a prescription directly from a pharmacist if allowed under state statutes. The purchaser must be at least 18 years of age and must furnish suitable identification. All such transactions must be recorded by the dispensing pharmacist.

Registration: Prescribing physicians and dispensing pharmacies must be registered with the DEA, PO Box 28083, Central Station, Washington, DC 20005.

Inventory: Separate records must be kept of purchases and dispensing of controlled substances. An inventory of controlled substances must be made every 2 years.

Prescriptions: Prescriptions for controlled substances must be written in ink and include: Date; name and address of the patient; name, address and DEA number of the physician. Oral prescriptions must be promptly committed to writing. Controlled substance prescriptions may not be dispensed or refilled more than 6 months after the date issued or be refilled more than 5 times. A written prescription signed by the physician is required for schedule II drugs. In case of emergency, oral prescriptions for schedule II substances may be filled; however, the physician must provide a signed prescription within 72 hours. Schedule II prescriptions cannot be refilled. A triplicate order form is necessary for the transfer of controlled substances in schedule II. Forms are available for the individual prescriber at no charge from the DEA.

State Laws: In many cases, state laws are more restrictive than federal laws and therefore impose additional requirements (eg, triplicate prescription forms).

Medical Terminology Glossary

abduction – the act of drawing away from a center.
abstergent – a cleansing application or medicine.
acaricide – an agent lethal to mites.
achlorhydria – the absence of hydrochloric acid from gastric secretions.
acidifier, systemic – a drug used to lower internal body fluid pH in patients with systemic alkalosis.
acidifier, urinary – a drug used to lower the pH of the urine.
acidosis – an accumulation of acid in the body.
acne – an inflammatory disease of the skin accompanied by the eruption of papules or pustules.
active immunity – see Immunity, Active.
acute – a short-term, intense health effect.
acute Hepatitis C – newly acquired symptomatic hepatitis C virus (HCV) infection.
Addison disease – a condition caused by adrenal gland destruction.
adduction – the act of drawing toward a center.
adenitis – a gland or lymph node inflammation.
adjuvant – an agent added to a product formulation that complements or accentuates the active ingredient.
adrenergic – a sympathomimetic drug that activates organs innervated by the sympathetic branch of the autonomic nervous system.
adrenocortical steroid, anti-inflammatory –an adrenal cortex hormone that participates in regulation of organic metabolism and inhibits the inflammatory response to stress; a glucocorticoid.
adrenocortical steroid, salt-regulating –an adrenal cortex hormone that maintains sodium-potassium electrolyte balance by stimulating and regulating sodium retention and potassium excretion by the kidneys.
adrenocorticotropic hormone – an anterior pituitary hormone that stimulates and regulates secretion of the adrenocortical steroids.
adsorbent – an agent that binds chemicals to its surface, thus reducing the bioavailability of toxic substances.
adverse events – undesirable experiences occurring after immunization that may or may not be related to the vaccine.
alkalizer, systemic – a drug that raises internal body fluid pH in patients with systemic acidosis.
allergen – a specific substance that causes an unwanted reaction in the body.
amblyopia – pertaining to a dimness of vision.
amebiasis – an infection with a pathogenic amoeba.
amenorrhea – an abnormal discontinuation of the menses.
amphiarthrosis – a joint in which the surfaces are connected by discs of fibrocartilage.
anabolic – an agent that promotes conversion of a simple substance into more complex compounds; a constructive process for the organism.
analeptic – a potent central nervous system stimulant used to maintain vital functions during severe central nervous system depression.
analgesic – a drug that selectively suppresses pain perception without inducing unconsciousness.
ancyclostomiasis – a disease characterized by the presence of hookworms in the intestine.
androgen – a hormone that stimulates and maintains male secondary sex characteristics.
anemia – a deficiency of red blood cells.
anesthetic, general – a drug that eliminates pain perception by inducing unconsciousness.
anesthetic, local – a drug that eliminates pain perception in a limited area by local action on sensory nerves; a topical anesthetic.
angina pectoris – a sharp chest pain starting in the heart, often spreading down the left arm. A symptom of coronary artery disease.
angiography – visualization of blood vessels upon x-ray following an injection of contrast media.
anhidrotic – a drug that checks perspiration flow from sweat glands; an antidiaphoretic.
anodyne – a drug that acts on the sensory nervous system, either centrally or peripherally, to produce relief from pain.
anorexiant – a drug that reduces appetite.
anorexigenic – an agent that promotes appetite reduction.
antacid – a drug that locally neutralizes excess gastric acid secretions.
antiadrenergic – a drug that prevents response to sympathetic nervous system stimulation and adrenergic drugs; a sympatholytic or sympathoplegic drug.
antiamebic – a drug that kills or inhibits the pathogenic protozoan *Entamoeba histolytica*, the causative agent of amebic dysentery.
antianemic – an agent that treats or prevents anemia.

antiasthmatic – an agent that relieves the symptoms of asthma.
antibacterial – a drug that kills or inhibits pathogenic bacteria, the causative agents of many systemic gastrointestinal and superficial infections.
antibiotic – an agent produced by or derived from living cells of molds, bacteria, or other plants that destroy or inhibit the growth of microbes.
antibody – a protein found in the blood that is produced in response to foreign substances (eg, bacteria or viruses) invading the body. Antibodies protect the body from disease by binding to these organisms and destroying them.
anticholesteremic – a drug that lowers blood cholesterol levels.
anticholinergic – a drug that prevents response to parasympathetic nervous system stimulation and cholinergic drugs; a parasympatholytic or parasympathoplegic drug.
anticoagulant – a drug that inhibits blood clotting.
anticonvulsant – a drug that selectively prevents epileptic seizures.
antidepressant – a psychotherapeutic drug that induces mood elevation, useful in treating depressive neuroses and psychoses.
antidiabetic – a drug used to lower blood sugar or counteract diabetes.
antidote – a drug that prevents or counteracts the effects of poisons or drug overdoses by adsorption in the gastrointestinal tract (general antidotes) or by specific systemic action (specific antidotes).
antieczematic – a topical drug that aids in the control of exudative inflammatory skin lesions.
antiemetic – a drug that prevents or controls vomiting.
antifibrinolytic – a drug that decreases fibrin breakdown.
antifilarial – a drug that kills or inhibits pathogenic filarial worms of the superfamily *Filarioidea*, the causative agents of diseases such as loaiasis.
antiflatulent – an agent that inhibits the excessive formation of gas in the stomach or intestines.
antifungal – a drug that kills or inhibits pathogenic fungi; antimycotic.
antigens – foreign substances (eg, bacteria or viruses) in the body that are capable of causing disease. The presence of antigens in the body triggers an immune response, usually the production of antibodies.
antihelmintic – a drug that kills or expels worm infestations such as pinworms and tapeworms (eg, nematodes, cestodes, trematodes).
antihemophilic – a blood derivative containing the clotting factors absent in the hereditary disease hemophilia.
antihistaminic – a drug that prevents response to histamine, including histamine released by allergic reactions.
antihypercholesterolemic – a drug that lowers blood cholesterol levels, especially elevated levels sometimes associated with cardiovascular disease.
antihypertensive – a drug that lowers blood pressure.
anti-infective, local – a drug that kills a variety of pathogenic microorganisms and is suitable for sterilizing the skin or wounds.
anti-inflammatory – a drug that counteracts or suppresses inflammation.
antileishmanial – a drug that kills or inhibits pathogenic protozoa of the genus *Leishmania*, the causative agents of diseases such as kala azar.
antileprotic – an agent used against leprosy.
antilipemic – an agent that reduces the amount of circulating lipids.
antimalarial – a drug that prevents malaria or inhibits the causative agent (ie, malarial parasites).
antimetabolite – a substance that competes with or replaces a certain metabolite.
antimethemoglobinemic – an agent that reduces the production of methemoglobin.
antimycotic – an agent that inhibits the growth of fungi.
antinauseant – a drug that suppresses nausea.
antineoplastic – a drug that is selectively toxic to rapidly multiplying cells and is useful in destroying malignant tumors.
antioxidant – an agent used to reduce decay or transformation of a material from oxidation.
antiperiodic – a drug that prevents the regular recurrence of a disease or symptom.
antiperistaltic – a drug that inhibits intestinal motility, especially for the treatment of diarrhea.
antipruritic – a drug that prevents or relieves itching.
antipyretic – a drug used to reduce fever; antifebrile; febrifugal.
antirheumatic – a drug that suppresses symptoms of rheumatic disease (eg, reduces the inflammation of rheumatic arthritis).
antirickettsial – a drug that kills or inhibits pathogenic microorganisms of the genus *Rickettsia*, the causative agents of diseases such as typhus (eg, chloramphenicol).
antischistosomal – a drug that kills or inhibits pathogenic flukes of the genus *Schistosoma*, the causative agents of schistosomiasis.

antiseborrheic – a drug that aids in the control of seborrheic dermatitis ("dandruff"); prevents or relieves excessive sebum secretion.
antiseptic – a substance that prevents the growth and development of microorganisms that may lead to infection.
antisialagogue – a drug that diminishes the flow of saliva.
antispasmodic – an agent used to quiet the spasms of voluntary and involuntary muscles; calmative; antihysteric.
antisyphilitic – a remedy used in the treatment of syphilis.
antitoxin – a biological drug containing antibodies against the toxic principles of a pathogenic microorganism, used for passive immunization against the associated disease.
antitrichomonal – a drug that kills or inhibits the pathogenic protozoan *Trichomonas vaginalis*, the causative agent of trichomonal vaginitis.
antitrypanosomal – a drug that kills or inhibits pathogenic protozoa of the genus *Trypanosoma*, the causative agents of diseases such as West African trypanosomiasis.
antitussive – a drug that suppresses coughing; antibechic.
antivenin – a biological drug containing antibodies against the venom of a poisonous animal or insect; an antidote for a venomous bite.
antiviral – literally "against virus;" any medicine capable of destroying or weakening a virus.
anxiety – a feeling of apprehension, uncertainty and fear.
aperient – a mild laxative.
aphasia – the inability to use or understand written and spoken words due to language center injuries in the brain.
aphonia – loss of voice due to disease of the larynx or its innervation.
apnea – the absence of breathing.
areola – a pigmented/depigmented zone surrounding a neoplasm.
arsenical – an agent containing arsenic.
arteriosclerosis – a hardening of the arteries.
arthritis – the inflammation of a joint.
ascariasis – a condition caused by roundworms in the intestine.
ascaricide – an agent that kills roundworms of the genus *Ascaris*.
Aspergillus – a genus of fungi.
astasia – the inability to stand up without help.
asthma – a disease characterized by recurring breathing difficulty due to bronchial muscle constriction.
astringent – an agent that causes tissue contraction, arrests secretion, or controls bleeding.
ataractic – an agent that has a quieting, tranquilizing effect.
ataxia – incoordination, especially of gait.
atheroma – lipid deposits on the inner surface of arteries; a characteristic of atherosclerosis.
atrophy – a wasting away.
avitaminosis – a pathologic state or dysfunction resulting in the body lacking one or more vitamins.
axilla – the armpit.
bacteria – tiny one-celled organisms present throughout the environment that require a microscope to be seen. While not all bacteria are harmful, some cause disease. Examples of bacterial disease include diphtheria, pertussis, tetanus, *Haemophilus influenzae*, and pneumococcus (pneumonia).
bacteriostatic – an agent that inhibits the growth of bacteria.
Basedow disease – a form of hyperthyroidism, also known as Grave disease and Parry disease.
biliary colic – a sharp pain in the upper right side of the abdomen due to a gallstone impaction.
bilirubin – a red bile pigment.
biliuria – the presence of bile in the urine.
blood calcium regulator – a drug that maintains the blood level of ionic calcium, especially by regulating its metabolic disposition elsewhere.
blood volume supporter – an intravenous solution whose solutes are retained in the vascular system to supplement the osmotic activity of plasma proteins.
bradycardia – a slow heart rate.
Bright disease – a disease of the kidneys, including the presence of edema and excessive urine protein formation.
bromidrosis – foul-smelling perspiration.
bronchitis – an inflammation of the bronchi.
bronchodilator – a drug that dilates the bronchus or bronchial tubes (air passages of the lung).
bruit – an abnormal arterial sound audible with a stethoscope.
Buerger disease – a thromboanglitis obliterans inflammation of the walls and surrounding rise of the veins and arteries.
bursitis – an inflammation of the bursa.
callus – a tissue mass that develops at bone fracture sites.
calmative – a sedative.
candidiasis – an infection by the yeastlike genus *Candida*, especially *Candida albicans*.

carbonic anhydrase inhibitor – an enzyme inhibitor, the therapeutic effects of which are diuresis and reduced formation of intraocular fluid.
carcinoma – a malignant growth.
cardiac depressant – a drug that depresses myocardial function so as to suppress rhythmic irregularities characterized by fast heart rate; antiarrhythmic.
cardiac stimulant – a drug that increases the contractile force of the myocardium, especially in weakened conditions such as congestive heart failure; cardiotonic.
cardiopathy – a disease of the heart.
caries – the decay of the teeth.
carminative – an aromatic or pungent drug that mildly irritates the gastrointestinal tract and is useful in the treatment of flatulence and colic. Peppermint Water is a common carminative.
carrier – a person or animal that harbors a specific infectious agent without visible symptoms of the disease. A carrier acts as a potential source of infection.
caruncle – a small, fleshy projection on the skin.
cathartic – an agent having purgative action.
caudal – pertains to the distal end or tail.
caustic – an agent whose effect resembles that of a burn; used to remove abnormal skin growths.
central depressant – a drug that reduces the functional state of the central nervous system and with increasing dosage may induce sedation, hypnosis, and general anesthesia; degree of respiratory suppression is agent dependent.
central stimulant – a drug that increases the functional state of the central nervous system and with increasing dosage may induce restlessness, insomnia, disorientation, and convulsions; degree of respiratory suppression is agent dependent.
cerebrum – the parts of the brain relating to the telecephalon and includes mainly the cerebral cortex and basal ganglia.
cerumen – earwax.
childhood immunizations – a series of immunizations that are given to prevent disease that pose a threat to children. The immunizations in the United States currently include: hepatitis B, diphtheria, tetanus, acellular pertussis, *Haemophilus influenzae* type b, inactivated polio, pneumococcal conjugate, measles, mumps, rubella, varicella, and hepatitis A.
chloasma – a skin discoloration.
cholagogue – a drug that stimulates the emptying of the gallbladder and the flow of bile into the duodenum.
cholecystitis – an inflammation of the gallbladder.
cholecystokinetic – an agent that promotes emptying of the gallbladder.
cholelithiasis – the presence of calculi (stones) in the gallbladder.
choleretic – a drug that increases the production and secretion of bile by the liver.
chorea – a disorder, usually of childhood, characterized by uncontrolled spasmotic muscle movements; sometimes referred to as St. Vitus' dance.
chronic health condition – a health-related state that lasts for a long period of time (eg, multiple sclerosis, asthma).
chronic hepatitis C – liver inflammation in patients with chronic HCV infection; characterized by abnormal levels of liver enzymes.
chymotrypsin – a proteinase in the gastrointestinal tract; its proposed use has been the treatment of edema and inflammation.
cirrhosis – widespread disruption of normal liver structure (scarring of the liver).
claudication – limping.
climacteric – a time period in women just preceding menopause.
clonus – movements noted by rapid muscle contraction then relaxation.
coagulant – an agent that stimulates or accelerates blood clotting.
coccidiostat – a drug used in the treatment of coccidal (protozoal) infections in animals, especially birds; used in veterinary medicine.
colitis – an inflammation of the colon.
colloid – a disperse system of particles larger than those of true solutions but smaller than those of suspensions (1 to 100 millimicrons in size).
collyrium – an eyewash.
colostomy – the surgical formation of a cutaneous opening into the colon.
combination vaccine – two or more vaccines combined and administered at once in order to reduce the number of shots given. For example, the MMR (measles, mumps, rubella) vaccine.
communicable – capable of spreading disease. Also known as infectious.
contagious – capable of being transmitted from one person to another by contact or close proximity.
corticoid – a term applied to hormones of the adrenal cortex or any substance, natural or synthetic, having similar activity.
corticosteroid – a steroid produced by the adrenal cortex.
coryza – acute rhinitis.
counterirritant – an agent (irritant) that causes irritation of the part to which it is applied, and draws blood away from a deep-seated area.

cranial – pertaining to the skull.
crepitation – a crackling sound.
cryptitis – an inflammation of a follicle or glandular tubule, usually in the rectum.
Cryptococcus – a genus of fungi that does not produce spores, but reproduces by budding.
cryptorchidism – the failure of one or both testes to descend.
cutaneous – pertaining to the skin.
cyanosis – a blue or purple skin discoloration due to oxygen deficiency.
cycloplegia – the loss of light accommodation due to loss of control in the eye 's ciliary muscle.
cycloplegic – a drug that paralyzes accommodation of the eye.
cystitis – an inflammation of the bladder.
cystourethography – the examination by x-ray of the bladder and urethra.
cytostasis – a slowing of the movement of blood cells at an inflamed area, sometimes causing capillary blockage.
debridement – the cutting away of dead or excess skin from a wound.
decongestant – a drug that reduces congestion.
decubitus – the patient's position in bed; the act of lying down.
demulcent – an agent generally used internally to sooth and protect mucous membranes.
dermatitis – an inflammation of the skin.
dermatomycosis – a fungal skin infection caused by dermatophytes, yeasts, and other fungi.
detergent – a cleansing or purging agent; an emulsifying agent useful for cleansing wounds and ulcers as well as the skin.
dextrocardia – a condition when the heart is located on the right side of the chest.
diagnostic Aid – a drug used to determine the functional state of a body organ or the presence of a disease.
diaphoretic – a drug used to increase perspiration; hydroticorsudorfice.
diarrhea – an abnormally frequent defecation of semisolid or fluid fecal matter from the bowels.
digestive enzyme – an enzyme used in digestion.
digitalization – the administration of digitalis to obtain a desired tissue level of drug.
diplopia – double vision.
disease – symptomatic sickness, illness, or loss of health.
disinfectant – an agent that destroys pathogenic microorganisms on contact and is suitable for sterilizing inanimate objects.
distal – farthest from a point of reference.
diuretic – a drug that promotes renal excretion of electrolytes and water, thereby increasing urine volume.
dysarthria – a difficulty in speech articulation.
dysmenorrhea – pertaining to painful menstruation.
dysphagia – a difficulty in swallowing.
dyspnea – a difficulty in breathing.
ecbolic – a drug used to stimulate the gravid uterus to the expulsion of the fetus, or to cause uterine contraction; oxytocic.
eclampsia – a toxic disorder occurring late in pregnancy involving hypertension, edema, and renal dysfunction.
ectasia – pertaining to distension or stretching.
ectopic – out of place; not in normal position.
eczema – an inflammatory disease of the skin with infiltrations, watery discharge, scales, and crust.
effervescent – a bubbling; sparkling; giving off gas bubbles.
embolus – a plug (typically a thrombus, bacteria mass, or foreign body) lodged in a vessel; may obstruct circulation.
emetic – a drug that induces vomiting, either locally by gastrointestinal irritation or systemically by stimulation of receptors in the central nervous system.
emollient – a topical drug, especially an oil or fat, used to soften the skin and make it more pliable.
endemic – the continual, low-level presence of disease in a community.
endometrium – the uterine mucous membrane.
enteralgia – an intestinal pain.
enterobiasis – a pinworm infestation.
enuresis – an involuntary urination, as in bedwetting.
epidemic – the occurrence of disease within a specific geographical area or population that is in excess of what is normally expected.
epidemiology – the study of the spread of diseases. Epidemiologists are often sent to investigate outbreaks.
epidermis – the outermost layer of the skin.
episiotomy – a surgical incision of the vulva when deemed necessary during childbirth.
epistaxis – a nosebleed.
erythema – redness.
erythrocyte – a red blood cell.
escharotic – corrosive.
estrogen – a hormone that stimulates and maintains female secondary sex characteristics and functions in the menstrual cycle to promote uterine gland proliferation.

etiology – the cause of a disease.
euphoria – an exaggerated feeling of well-being.
eutonic – a normal muscular tone.
exfoliation – a scaling of the skin.
exophthalmos – a protrusion of the eyeballs.
expectorant – a drug that increases secretion of respiratory tract fluid by lowering its viscosity and promoting its ejection.
extension – the movement of a joint that increases the angle between the bones of the limb at the joint.
exteroceptors – the receptors on the exterior of the body.
fasciculations – the visible twitching movements of muscle bundles.
fibroid – a tumor of fibrous tissue, resembling fibers.
filariasis – the condition of having roundworm parasites reproducing in the body tissues.
fistula – an abnormal opening between one epithelialized surface to another epithelialized body cavity.
flexion – the movement of a joint that decreases the angle between the bones of the limb at the joint.
fulminant – occurring suddenly, with lightning-like rapidity, and with great intensity or severity.
fungistatic – the inhibition of the growth of fungi.
furunculosis – a condition marked by the presence of boils.
gallop rhythm – a heart condition where three separate beats are heard instead of two.
gastralgia – a stomach pain.
gastritis – an inflammation of the stomach lining.
gastrocele – a hernial protrusion of the stomach.
gastrodynia – a pain in the stomach, a stomach ache.
geriatrics – a branch of medicine caring for medical problems of the aged.
germicidal – an agent that kills germs or other pathogenic microorganisms.
gingivitis – an inflammation of the gums.
glaucoma – a disease of the eye evidenced by an increase in intraocular pressure and resulting in hardness of the eye, atrophy of the retina, and eventual blindness.
glossitis – an inflammation of the tongue.
glucocorticoid – a corticoid that increases gluconeogenesis, thereby raising the concentration of liver glycogen and blood sugar.
glycosuria – an abnormal quantity of glucose and carbohydrates in the urine.
gout – a disorder that is characterized by a high uric acid level and sudden onset of recurrent arthritis.
granulation – the formation of small round fleshy granules on a wound as part of the healing process.
Guillain-Barré syndrome – an inflammation of the nerves of unknown cause characterized especially by muscle weakness and paralysis.
hematemesis – the vomiting of blood.
hematinic – an agent that improves blood quality by increasing the hemoglobin concentration and/or the number of red blood cells.
hematopoietic – a drug that stimulates formation of blood cells.
hemiplegia – a condition in which one side of the body is paralyzed.
hemophilia – a sex-linked hereditary blood defect that occurs almost exclusively in males and is characterized by delayed clotting of the blood and consequent difficulty in controlling hemorrhage even after minor injuries.
hemoptysis – the coughing-up of blood.
hemorrhage – an escape of blood through vessel walls; to bleed.
hemostatic – a locally-acting drug that arrests hemorrhage by promoting clot formation or by serving as a mechanical matrix for a clot.
hepatitis – an inflammation of the liver.
hepatitis A – a liver disease caused by the hepatitis A virus (HAV). HAV does not cause a chronic (long-lasting) illness. The virus is transmitted through close intimate contact with an infected person or through ingestion of contaminated food or water.
hepatitis B – a liver disease caused by the hepatitis B virus (HBV). HBV is found in the blood of infected persons and is most commonly transmitted through unprotected sex.
hepatitis B core antibody (anti-HBc) – appears at the onset of symptoms in acute hepatitis B and persists for life. The presence of anti-HBc indicates previous or ongoing infection with HBV.
hepatitis B e antigen (HBeAg) – a secreted product of the nucleocapsid gene of HBV and is found in serum during acute and chronic hepatitis B. Its presence indicated that the virus is replicating and the infected individual is potentially infectious.
hepatitis B immune globulin (HBIG) – a product available for prophylaxis against hepatitis B virus infection. HBIG is prepared from plasma containing high titers of anti-HBs and provides short-term protection (3 to 6 months).

hepatitis B surface antibody (anti-HBs) – the presence of anti-HBs is generally interpreted as indicating recovery and immunity from HBV infection.

hepatitis B surface antigen (HBsAg) – a serologic marker on the surface of HBV. It can be detected in high levels in serum during acute or chronic hepatitis. The body normally produces antibodies to surface antigen as part of the normal immune response to infection.

hepatitis C – a liver disease caused by the hepatitis C virus (HCV), which is found in the blood of persons who have the disease. HCV is spread by contact with the blood of an infected person, most commonly through injection drug use.

hepatitis D – a liver disease caused by hepatitis delta virus (HDV). HDV is a defective virus that needs HBV to exist. HDV is found in the blood of persons infected with the virus and is transmitted in much the same way as HBV is transmitted; however, the case fatality rate with HDV infection is higher than with hepatitis B.

hepatitis E – a disease of the liver caused by the hepatitis E virus (HEV). HEV is transmitted in much the same way as HAV. Hepatitis E, however, does not often originate in the United States. Mortality is high among pregnant women who have hepatitis E.

hepatocellular carcinoma (HCC) – the most common primary malignant liver tumor.

high-risk group – a group in the community with an elevated risk of disease.

histoplasmosis – a lung infection caused by the inhalation of fungus spores, often resulting in pneumonitis.

HIV – human immunodeficiency virus.

Hodgkin disease – a disease marked by chronic lymph node enlargement that may also include spleen and liver enlargement.

hydrocholeresis – the puffing out of a thinner, more watery bile.

hypercholesterolemia – the condition of having an abnormally large amount of cholesterol in the plasma and cells of circulating blood.

hyperemia – an excess of blood in any part of the body.

hyperesthesia – an increase in sensitivity to sensory stimuli.

hyperglycemic – a drug that increases blood glucose levels, especially for the treatment of hypoglycemic states.

hypertension – blood pressure above the normally accepted limits; high blood pressure.

hypertriglyceridemia – an increased level of triglycerides in the blood.

hypnotic – an agent that promotes sleep.

hypodermoclysis – a subcutaneous injection with a solution.

hypoesthesia – a diminished sensation of touch.

hypoglycemic – a drug that lowers blood glucose levels; useful in the control of diabetes mellitus.

hypokalemia – an abnormally small concentration of potassium ions in the blood.

hyposensitize – to reduce the sensitivity to an agent, referring to allergies.

hypotensive – a drug that diminishes tension or pressure to lower blood pressure.

ichthyosis – an inherited skin disease characterized by dryness and scales.

idiopathic – the denoting of a disease of unknown cause.

IDU – injection drug user.

IgM anti-HBc – detected at onset of acute hepatitis B and persists for 3 to 12 months if the disease resolves. In patients who develop chronic hepatitis B, IgM anti-HBc persists at low levels as long as viral replication persists.

ileostomy – the establishment of an opening from the ileum to the outside of the body.

immune globulin (IG) – proteins found in the blood that function as antibodies that fight infection. Previously known as gamma globulin.

immune serum – a biological drug containing antibodies for a pathogenic microorganism, useful for passive immunization against the associated disease.

immune system – the complex system in the body responsible for fighting disease. Its primary function is to identify foreign substances in the body (bacteria, viruses, fungi, or parasites) and develop a defense against them. This defense is known as the immune response. It involves production of protein molecules called antibodies to eliminate foreign organisms that invade the body.

immunity – protection against a disease. There are two types of immunity, passive and active. Immunity is indicated by the presence of antibodies in the blood and can usually be determined with a laboratory test. See Immunity, Active and Passive.

immunity, active – resistance developed in response to an antigen (infecting agent or vaccine) and usually characterized by the presence of antibody produced by the host.

immunity, passive – immunity conferred by an antibody produced in another host.

This type of immunity can be acquired naturally by an infant from its mother or artificially by administration of an antibody-containing preparation (antiserum or immune globulin).

immunization – the process by which a person or animal becomes protected against a disease.

immunizing agent, active – an antigenic preparation (toxoid or vaccine) used to induce formation of specific antibodies against a pathogenic microorganism that provides delayed but permanent protection against the associated disease.

immunizing agent, passive – a biological preparation (antitoxin, antivenin, or immune serum) containing specific antibodies against a pathogenic microorganism that provides immediate but temporary protection against the associated disease.

immunoprophylaxis – preventing the spread of disease by providing physiological immunity.

immunosuppression – when the immune system is unable to protect the body from disease. This condition can be caused by disease (like AIDS) or by certain drugs (like those used in chemotherapy). Individuals whose immune systems are compromised should not receive live, attenuated vaccines.

impetigo – a contagious inflammatory skin infection with isolated pustules, most commonly occurring on the face of young children.

incidence – the number of new disease cases reported in a population over a certain period of time.

incubation period – the time from contact with infectious agents (bacteria or viruses) to onset of disease.

infection – an invasion of an organism by a pathogen such as bacteria or viruses. Some infections lead to disease.

infectious – capable of spreading disease. Also known as communicable.

infectious agents – organisms capable of spreading disease (eg, bacteria or viruses).

insulin – a hormone that promotes use of glucose, protein synthesis, and the formation and storage of neutral lipids; used in the treatment of diabetes mellitus.

inversion – a turning inward.

irrigating solution – a solution for washing wounds or various body cavities.

jaundice – a yellowing of the skin, whites of the eyes, tissues, and certain body fluids, which can result from certain liver diseases, including hepatitis C, or from excessive breakdown of red blood cells due to internal hemorrhage or various other conditions.

keratitis – an inflammation of the cornea.

keratolytic – a topical drug that softens the superficial keratin-containing layer of the skin to promote exfoliation.

lacrimal – pertaining to tears.

laxative – a gentle purgative medicine; mild cathartic.

leishmaniasis – infections transmitted by sand flies.

leukocyte – a white blood cell.

leukocytopenia – a decrease in the number of white blood cells.

leukocytosis – an increased white blood cell count.

leukoderma – an absence of pigment from the skin.

libido – sexual desire.

lipoma – a benign fatty tumor.

lipotropic – a drug, especially one supplementing a dietary factor, that prevents the abnormal accumulation of fat in the liver.

lochia – a vaginal discharge of mucus, blood, and tissue after childbirth.

lues – a plague; specifically syphilis.

macrocyte – a large red blood cell.

malaise – a general feeling of illness.

mastitis – an inflammation of the breast.

melasma – a darkening of the skin.

melena – black feces or black vomit from altered blood in the higher GI tract.

meninges – the membranes covering the brain and spinal cord.

metastasis – the shifting of a disease or its symptoms from one part of the body to another.

microbes – tiny organisms (including viruses and bacteria) that can only be seen with a microscope.

miotics – agents that constrict the pupil of the eye; a myotic.

moniliasis – an infection with any of the species of monilia types of fungi (*Candida*).

morbidity – any departure, subjective or objective, from a state of physiological or psychological well-being.

mortality – the number of deaths in a given time or place.

mucolytic – an agent that can destroy or dissolve mucous membrane secretions.

myalgia – a pain in the muscles.

myasthenia gravis – a chronic progressive muscular weakness caused by myoneural conduction, usually spreading from the face and throat.

myelocyte – an immature white blood cell in the bone marrow.

myelogenous – originating in bone marrow.

myoclonus – involuntary, sudden, rapid, unpredictable jerks.

mydriatic – a drug that dilates the pupil of the eye, usually by anticholinergic or adrenergic mechanisms.
myoneural – pertaining to muscle and nerve.
myopia – nearsightedness.
narcotic – a drug with effects similar to opium and derivatives that produces analgesic effects and has the potential for dependence and tolerance.
neonatal – pertaining to the first four weeks of life.
neoplasm – an abnormal tissue that grows more rapidly than normal and shows a lack of structural organization.
nephritis – an inflammation of the kidney.
nephrosclerosis – a hardening of the kidney tissue.
neuralgia – a pain extending along the course of one or more nerves.
neurasthenia – a condition accompanying or following depression that is characterized by vague fatigue.
neuroglia – the supporting elements of the nervous system.
neuroleptic – a psychotropic drug used to treat psychosis.
neurosis – a psychological or behavioral disorder characterized by anxiety.
NIH – National Institutes of Health.
nocturia – urination at night.
normocytic – erythrocytes that are normal in size, shape, and color.
nosocomial – referring to an infection acquired by a patient while in a hospital.
nuchal – the back of the neck.
nystagmus – a rhythmic oscillation of the eyes.
oleaginous – oily or greasy.
omphalitis – an inflammation of the navel and surrounding area.
onychomycosis – a fungal infection of the nails.
ophthalmic – pertaining to the eye.
oral – pertaining to the mouth.
organism – any living thing. Organisms include humans, animals, plants, bacteria, protozoa, and fungi.
orthopnea – a discomfort in breathing when lying flat.
ossification – a formation of, or conversion to, bone.
osteomyelitis – an inflammation of the marrow of the bone.
osteoporosis – a reduction in bone quantity; skeletal atrophy.
otalgia – pain in the ear; earache.
otitis – inflammation of the ear.
otomycosis – an ear infection caused by fungus.
otorrhea – a discharge from the ear.
outbreak – sudden appearance of a disease in a specific geographic area (eg, neighborhood or community) or population (eg, adolescents).
oxytocic – a drug that selectively stimulates uterine motility and is useful in obstetrics, especially in the control of postpartum hemorrhage.
Paget disease – a skeletal disease in which bone resorption and formation are increased leading to thickening and softening of bones; a disease characterized by lesions around the nipple and areola found in elderly women.
pallor – paleness.
palpitations – an awareness of one's heart action.
pandemic – an epidemic occuring over a very large area.
parasites – any organism that lives in or on another organism without benefiting the host organism; commonly refers to pathogens, most commonly in reference to protozoans and helminths.
parasympatholytic – See Anticholinergic.
parasympathomimetic – See Cholinergic.
parenteral – pertaining to the administration of a drug by means other than through the intestinal tract; subcutaneous, intramuscular, or intravenous drug administration.
parkinsonism – a group of neurological disorders caused by dopamine deficiency marked by hypokinesia, tremor, and muscular rigidity.
paroxysm – a sharp spasm or convulsion.
passive immunity – see Immunity, Passive.
pathogenic – causing an abnormality or disease.
pathogens – bacteria, viruses, parasites, or fungi that can cause disease.
pediatrics – a branch of medicine caring for the medical problems of children from birth through adolescence.
pediculicide – an agent used to kill lice.
pediculosis – an infestation with lice.
pellagra – characterized by GI disturbances, mental disorders, skin redness, and scaling due to niacin deficiency.
pernicious – particularly dangerous or harmful.
phlebitis – an inflammation of a vein.
pleurisy – an inflammation of the membrane surrounding the lungs and the thoracic cavity.
pneumonia – an infection of the lungs.
poikilocytosis – a condition in which pointed or irregularly shaped red blood cells are found in the blood.
polydipsia – excessive thirst.
posology – the science of dosage.

posterior pituitary hormone(s) – a hormone with oxytocic, vasoconstrictor, antidiuretic, and intestinal stimulant properties.

post-exposure prophylaxis (PEP) – prevention or treatment of disease after a possible exposure.

prevalance – the number of disease cases (new and existing) within a population at a given time.

progestin – a hormone that functions in the menstrual cycle and during pregnancy to promote uterine gland secretion and to reduce uterine motility.

pronation – the body's position when lying face downward; rotation of the forearm so the palm on the hand faces backward when the arm is in anatomical position.

prophylactic – a remedy that tends to prevent disease.

protectant – a topical drug that remains on the skin and serves as a physical, protective barrier to the environment.

proteolytic enzyme – an enzyme used to liquify fibrinous or purulent exudates.

psoriasis – an inflammatory skin disease accompanied by itching.

psychotherapy – therapy utilizing communication and interventions with the patient instead of chemical or physical treatments.

ptosis – a drooping or sagging of a muscle or organ, such as the eyelid.

pulmonary – pertaining to the lungs.

purulent – containing or forming pus.

pyelitis – a local inflammation of renal and pelvic cells due to bacterial infection.

pylorospasm – a spasmodic muscle contraction of the pyloric portion of the stomach.

pyoderma – any fever-producing skin infection.

quarantine – to isolate an individual who has or is suspected of having a disease, in order to prevent spreading the disease to others; alternatively, to isolate a person who does not have a disease during a disease outbreak, in order to prevent that person from catching the disease (this is called reverse isolation). Quarantine can be voluntary or ordered by public health officials in times of emergency.

radiopaque medium – a diagnostic drug, opaque to x-rays, whose retention in a body organ or cavity makes x-ray visualization possible.

Raynaud phenomenon – spasms of the digital arteries with blanching and numbness precipitated by cold temperature.

reflex stimulant – a mild irritant suitable for application to the nasopharynx to induce reflex respiratory stimulation.

rheumatoid – resembling rheumatoid arthritis.

rhinitis – an inflammation of the mucous membrane of the nose.

risk – the likelihood that an individual will experience a certain event.

rubefacient – a topical drug that induces mild skin irritation with erythema, sometimes used to relieve the discomfort of deep-seated inflammation.

rubeola/measles – not to be confused with rubella.

saprophytic – receiving nourishment from dead material.

sarcoma – a malignant tumor derived from connective tissue.

scabicide – an insecticide suitable for the erradication of itch mite infestations in humans (scabies).

schistosomacide – an agent that destroys schistosomes; destructive to the trematodic parasites or flukes.

schistosomiasis – an infection with *Schistosoma haematobium.*

scintillation – a visual sensation manifested by an emission of sparks.

sclerosing agent – an irritant suitable for injection into varicose veins to induce their fibrosis and obliteration.

scotomata – an area of varying size and shape within the visual field in which vision is absent or depressed.

seborrhea – a condition arising from an excess secretion of sebum.

sebum – the fatty secretions of sebaceous glands.

sedative – a drug that calms nervous excitement.

seroconversion – development of antibodies in the blood of an individual who previously did not have detectable antibodies.

serology – measurement of antibodies, and other immunological properties, in the blood serum.

side effect – undesirable reaction resulting from immunization or other medication, treatment, etc.

sinusitis – an inflammation of a sinus membrane lining.

skeletal muscle relaxant – a drug that inhibits contraction of voluntary muscles, usually by interfering with their innervation.

smooth muscle relaxant – a drug that inhibits contraction of involuntary (eg, visceral) muscles, usually by action upon their contractile elements.

sociopath – a person designated to have an antisocial personality disorder.

spasmolytic – an agent that relieves spasms and involuntary contractions of a muscle; antispasmodic.

sputum – expectorated mucus.

STD – sexually transmitted disease.

stenosis – the narrowing of the lumen of a blood vessel.
stomachic – a drug that is used to stimulate the appetite and gastric secretion.
stomatitis – an inflammation of the mucous membranes of the mouth.
subcutaneous – underneath the skin.
sudorific – causing perspiration.
superacidity – excessive acidity.
supination – the body 's position when lying face upwards; rotation of the forearm so the palm on the hand faces forward when the arm is in anatomical position.
suppressant – a drug useful in the control, rather than the cure, of a disease; an agent that stops secretion, excretion, or normal discharge.
surfactant – a surface active agent that decreases the surface tension between two miscible liquids; used to prepare emulsions, act as a cleansing agent, etc.
susceptible – unprotected against a certain disease.
synarthrosis (fibrous joint) – a joint in which the bony elements are united by continuous fibrous tissue.
syncope – fainting; loss of consciousness.
synovia – a clear fluid that lubricates the joints; joint oil.
systole – the ventricular contraction phase of a heartbeat.
tachycardia – a rapid contraction rate of the heart.
taeniacide – an agent used to kill tapeworms.
taeniafuge – an agent used to expel tapeworms.
therapeutic – a treatment of disease.
thoracic – pertaining to the chest.
thyroid hormone – a drug containing one or more of the iodinated amino acids that stimulate and regulate the metabolic rate and functional state of body tissues.
thyroid inhibitor – a drug that reduces excessive thyroid hormone production, usually by blocking hormone synthesis.
tics – a repetitive twitching of muscles, often in the face and upper trunk.
tinea – a fungal infection of the skin, hair, or nails.
tonic – continuous muscular contraction.
tonometry – the measurement of tension in some part of the body.
topical – the local external application of a drug to a particular place.
toxoid – a modified toxin, less toxic than the original form, used to induce active immunity to bacterial pathogens.
tranquilizer – a psychotherapeutic drug that promotes tranquility without significant sedation, useful in treating certain neuroses and psychoses.
tremors – involuntary rhythmic tremulous movements.
trichomoniasis – an infection with parasitic flagellate protozoa of the genus *Trichomonas*.
trypanosomiasis – any disease caused by *Trypanosomatidae*.
uricosuric – a drug that promotes renal uric acid excretion; used to treat gout.
urolithiasis – a condition marked by the formation of stones in the urinary tract.
urticaria – a rash or hives.
vaccination – injection of a killed or weakened infectious organism in order to prevent the disease.
vaccine – the preparation of live attenuated or dead pathogenic microorganisms, used to induce active immunity.
vaccine schedule – a chart or plan of vaccinations that are recommended for specific ages and/or circumstances.
vasoconstrictor – an agent used to narrow blood vessels; to constrict blood vessels and reduce tissue congestion in the nose.
vasodilator – a drug that relaxes vascular smooth muscles, especially for the purpose of improving peripheral or coronary blood flow.
vasopressor – an adrenergic drug used systemically to constrict blood vessels and raise blood pressure.
verruca – a wart.
vertigo – dizziness.
vesicant – an agent that, when applied to the skin, causes blistering and the formation of vesicles; an epispastic.
virus – a tiny organism that multiplies within cells and causes disease such as chickenpox, measles, mumps, rubella, pertussis, and hepatitis. Viruses are not affected by antibiotics, the drugs used to kill bacteria.
visceral – pertaining to the internal organs.
vitamin – an organic chemical essential in small amounts for normal body metabolism, used therapeutically to supplement the naturally occurring counterpart in foods.
WHO – World Health Organization.

Oral Dosage Forms That Should Not Be Crushed or Chewed

There are a variety of reasons for crushing tablets or capsule contents prior to administering to patients. Patients may have nasogastric tubes that do not permit the administration of tablets or capsules, an oral solution for a particular medication may not be available from the manufacturer or readily prepared by the pharmacy, patients may have difficulty swallowing capsules or tablets, or mixing of powdered medication with food or drink may make the drug more palatable.

Generally, medications which should not be crushed fall into one of the following categories:

Extended-release products

The formulation of some tablets is specialized as to allow the medication within it to be slowly released into the body. This may be accomplished by centering the drug within the core of the tablet, with a subsequent shedding of multiple layers around the core. Wax melts in the GI tract, releasing drug contained within the wax matrix (eg, OxyCONTIN). Capsules may contain beads that have multiple layers that are slowly dissolved with time.

Common Abbreviations for Extended-Release Products

CD	Controlled dose
CR	Controlled-release
CRT	Controlled-release tablet
LA	Long-acting
SA	Sustained action
SR	Sustained-release
TR	Timed-release
TD	Time delay
XL	Extended-release
XR	Extended-release

Medications that are irritating to the stomach

Tablets that are irritating to the stomach may be enteric-coated which delays release of the drug until the time when it reaches the small intestine. Enteric-coated aspirin is an example of this.

Foul-tasting medication

Some drugs are quite unpleasant to taste so the manufacturer coats the tablet in a sugar coating to increase its palatability. By crushing the tablet, this sugar coating is lost and patients taste the unpleasant tasting medication.

Sublingual medication

Medication intended for use under the tongue should not be crushed. While it appears to be obvious, it is not always easy to determine if a medication is to be used sublingually. Sublingual medications should indicate on the package that they are intended for sublingual use.

Effervescent tablets

These are tablets that, when dropped into a liquid, quickly dissolve to yield a solution. Many effervescent tablets, when crushed, lose their ability to quickly dissolve.

Potentially hazardous substances

Certain drugs, including antineoplastic agents, hormonal agents, some antivirals, some bioengineered agents, and other miscellaneous drugs, are considered potentially hazardous when used in humans based on their characteristics. Examples of these characteristics include carcinogenicity, teratogenicity, reproductive toxicity, organ toxicity at low doses, genotoxicity, or new drugs with structural and toxicity profiles similar to existing hazardous drugs. Exposure to these substances can result in adverse effects and should be avoided. Crushing or breaking a tablet or opening a capsule of a potentially hazardous substance may increase the risk of exposure to the substance through skin contact, inhalation, or accidental ingestion. The extent of exposure, potency, and toxicity of the hazardous substance determines the health risk. Institutions have policies and procedures to follow when handling any potentially hazardous substance. Note: All potentially hazardous substances may not be represented in this table. Refer to institution-specific guidelines for precautions to observe when handling hazardous substances.

Recommendations

1. It is not advisable to crush certain medications.
2. Consult individual monographs prior to crushing a capsule or tablet.
3. If crushing a tablet or capsule is contraindicated, consult with a pharmacist to determine whether an oral solution exists or can be compounded.

Medications that should not be crushed or chewed

Drug product	Dosage form	Reason/Comments*
Accutane	Capsule	Mucous membrane irritant; teratogenic potential
Aciphex	Tablet	Extended-release
Aciphex Sprinkle	Capsule	Slow release. Capsule may be opened and contents sprinkled on soft food (eg, applesauce, fruit- or vegetable-based baby food, yogurt) or emptied into a small amount of liquid (eg, infant formula, apple juice, pediatric electrolyte solution). Granules should not be chewed or crushed.
Actiq	Lozenge	Slow-release. This lollipop delivery system requires the patient to dissolve it slowly.
Actoplus Met XR	Tablet	Variable-release
Actonel	Tablet	Irritant. Chewed, crushed, or sucked tablets may cause oropharyngeal irritation.
Adalat CC	Tablet	Extended-release
Adderall XR	Capsule	Extended-release[a]
Adenovirus (Types 4, 7) Vaccine	Tablet	Teratogenic potential; enteric-coated; do not disrupt tablet to avoid releasing live adenovirus in upper respiratory tract
Advicor	Tablet	Variable-release
Afeditab CR	Tablet	Extended-release
Afinitor	Tablet	Mucous membrane irritant; teratogenic potential; hazardous substance[k]
Aggrenox	Capsule	Extended-release. Capsule may be opened; contents include an aspirin tablet that may be chewed and dipyridamole pellets that may be sprinkled on applesauce.
Alavert Allergy Sinus D-12	Tablet	Extended-release
Allegra-D	Tablet	Extended-release
ALPRAZolam ER	Tablet	Extended-release
Altoprev	Tablet	Extended-release
Ambien CR	Tablet	Extended-release
Amitiza	Capsule	Manufacturer recommended
Amnesteem	Capsule	Mucous membrane irritant; teratogenic potential
Ampyra	Tablet	Extended-release
Amrix	Capsule	Extended-release
Aplenzin	Tablet	Extended-release
Apriso	Capsule	Extended-release[a]; maintain pH at ≤ 6
Aptivus	Capsule	Taste. Oil emulsion within spheres.
Aricept 23 mg	Tablet	Film-coated; chewing or crushing may increase rate of absorption
Arava	Tablet	Teratogenic potential; hazardous substance[k]
Arthrotec	Tablet	Delayed-release; enteric-coated
Asacol	Tablet	Slow-release
Aspirin, Enteric-Coated	Capsule, Tablet	Delayed-release; enteric-coated
Astagraf XL	Capsule	Extended-release

Drug product	Dosage form	Reason/Comments*
Atelvia	Tablet	Extended-release; tablet coating is an important part of the delayed release
Augmentin XR	Tablet	Extended-release[b,h]
AVINza	Capsule	Slow-release[a] (not pudding)
Avodart	Capsule	Capsule should not be handled by pregnant women due to teratogenic potential[j]; hazardous substance[k]
Azulfidine EN	Tablet	Delayed-release
Bayer Aspirin EC	Caplet	Enteric-coated
Bayer Aspirin, Low Dose 81 mg	Tablet	Enteric-coated
Bayer Aspirin, Regular Strength 325 mg	Caplet	Enteric-coated
Biaxin XL	Tablet	Extended-release
Biltricide	Tablet	Taste[h]
Bisac-Evac	Tablet	Enteric-coated[c]
Bisacodyl	Tablet	Enteric-coated[c]
Boniva	Tablet	Irritant. Chewed, crushed, or sucked tablets may cause oropharyngeal irritation.
Bosulif	Tablet	Hazardous substance[k]
Budeprion SR	Tablet	Extended-release
Buproban	Tablet	Extended-release
BuPROPion SR	Tablet	Extended-release
Calan SR	Tablet	Extended-release[h]
Campral	Tablet	Delayed-release; enteric-coated
Caprelsa	Tablet	Teratogenic potential; hazardous substance[k]
Carbatrol	Capsule	Extended-release[a]
Cardene SR	Capsule	Extended-release
Cardizem	Tablet	Not described as slow release but releases drug over 3 hours
Cardizem CD	Capsule	Extended-release
Cardizem LA	Tablet	Extended-release
Cardura XL	Tablet	Extended-release
Cartia XT	Capsule	Extended-release
Casodex	Tablet	Teratogenic potential; hazardous substance[k]
CeeNU	Capsule	Teratogenic potential; hazardous substance[k]
Cefaclor ER	Tablet	Extended-release
Ceftin	Tablet	Taste[b]. Use suspension for children.
Cefuroxime	Tablet	Taste[b]. Use suspension for children.
CellCept	Capsule, Tablet	Teratogenic potential; hazardous substance[i,k]
Charcoal Plus DS	Tablet	Enteric-coated
Chlor-Trimeton 12-Hour	Tablet	Extended-release[b]
Cipro XR	Tablet	Extended-release[b]
Claravis	Capsule	Mucous membrane irritant; teratogenic potential
Claritin-D 12-Hour	Tablet	Extended-release[b]
Claritin-D 24-Hour	Tablet	Extended-release[b]
Colace	Capsule	Taste[e]

Drug product	Dosage form	Reason/Comments*
Colestid	Tablet	Slow-release
Cometriq	Capsule	Teratogenic potential; hazardous substance[k]
Commit	Lozenge	Integrity compromised by chewing or crushing
Concerta	Tablet	Extended-release
ConZip	Capsule	Variable release; tablet disruption may cause overdose
Coreg CR	Capsule	Extended-release[a]; may add contents to chilled applesauce
Cotazym-S	Capsule	Enteric-coated[a]
Covera-HS	Tablet	Extended-release
Creon	Capsule	Extended-release[a]; enteric-coated contents
Crixivan	Capsule	Taste. Capsule may be opened and mixed with fruit puree (eg, banana).
Cyclophosphamide	Capsule, Tablet	Hazardous substance[k]; manufacturer recommendation
Cymbalta	Capsule	Enteric-coated[a]; may add contents to apple juice or applesauce but not chocolate
Cytoxan	Tablet	Drug may be crushed, but manufacturer recommends using injection; hazardous substance[k]
Depakene	Capsule	Slow-release; mucous membrane irritant[b]; hazardous substance[k]
Depakote	Tablet	Delayed-release; hazardous substance[k]
Depakote ER	Tablet	Extended-release; hazardous substance[k]
Depakote Sprinkles	Capsule	Extended-release[a]
Detrol LA	Capsule	Extended-release
Dexedrine	Capsule	Extended-release
Dexilant	Capsule	Delayed-release[a]
Diamox Sequels	Capsule	Extended-release
Dibenzyline	Capsule	Hazardous substance[k]
Diclegis	Tablet	Delayed-release; manufacturer recommendation
Dilacor XR	Capsule	Extended-release
Dilatrate-SR	Capsule	Extended-release
Dilt-CD	Capsule	Extended-release
Dilt-XR	Capsule	Extended-release
Diltia XT	Capsule	Extended-release
Ditropan XL	Tablet	Extended-release
Divalproex ER	Tablet	Extended-release
Donnatal Extentab	Tablet	Extended-release[b]
Doxidan	Tablet	Enteric-coated[c]
Drisdol	Capsule	Liquid-filled[d]
Droxia	Capsule	May be opened; wear gloves to handle; hazardous substance[k]
Duavee	Tablet	Manufacturer recommendation; hazardous substance[k]
Dulcolax	Capsule	Liquid-filled
	Tablet	Enteric-coated[c]

Drug product	Dosage form	Reason/Comments[*]
EC-Naprosyn	Tablet	Delayed-release; enteric-coated
Ecotrin (all products)	Tablet	Enteric-coated
E.E.S.	Tablet	Enteric-coated[b]
Effer-K	Tablet	Effervescent tablet[f]
Effervescent Potassium	Tablet	Effervescent tablet[f]
Effexor XR	Capsule	Extended-release
Embeda	Capsule	Extended-release[a]; do not give via nasogastric tube
E-Mycin	Tablet	Enteric-coated
Enablex	Tablet	Slow-release
Entocort EC	Capsule	Extended-release; enteric-coated[a]
Epanova	Capsule	Manufacturer recommendation
Equetro	Capsule	Extended-release[a]
Ergomar	Tablet	Sublingual form[g]
Erivedge	Capsule	Teratogenic potential[k]
Eryc	Capsule	Enteric-coated
Ery-Tab	Tablet	Delayed-release; enteric-coated
Erythrocin Stearate	Tablet	Enteric-coated
Erythromycin Base	Tablet	Enteric-coated
Erythromycin Delayed-Release	Capsule	Enteric-coated pellets[a]
Etoposide	Capsule	Hazardous substance[k]
Evista	Tablet	Taste; teratogenic potential[j]; hazardous substance[k]
Exalgo	Tablet	Extended-release; breaking, chewing, crushing, or dissolving before ingestion or injecting increases the risk of overdose
Exjade	Tablet	Do not chew or swallow whole; do not give as tablets meant to be given as a liquid
Fareston	Tablet	Teratogenic potential; hazardous substance[k]
Feldene	Capsule	Mucous membrane irritant
Fentanyl	Lozenge	Slow-release; lollipop delivery system requires the patient to slowly dissolve in mouth
Fentora	Tablet	Buccal tablet; swallowing whole or crushing may reduce effectiveness
Feosol	Tablet	Enteric-coated[b]
Fergon	Tablet	Enteric-coated
Ferro-Sequels	Tablet	Slow-release
Fetzima	Capsule	Extended-release
Flagyl ER	Tablet	Extended-release
Fleet Laxative	Tablet	Enteric-coated[c]
Flomax	Capsule	Slow-release
Focalin XR	Capsule	Extended-release[a]
Forfivo XL	Capsule	Extended-release
Fortamet	Tablet	Extended-release
Fosamax	Tablet	Mucous membrane irritant
Fosamax Plus D	Tablet	Mucous membrane irritant
Fulyzaq	Tablet	Delayed-release

Drug product	Dosage form	Reason/Comments*
Gengraf	Capsule	Teratogenic potential; hazardous substance[k]
Geodon	Capsule	Hazardous substance[k]
Gleevec	Tablet	Taste[h]. May be dissolved in water or apple juice; hazardous substance[k]
GlipiZIDE XL	Tablet	Extended-release
Glucophage XR	Tablet	Extended-release
Glucotrol XL	Tablet	Extended-release
Glumetza	Tablet	Extended-release
Gralise	Tablet	Extended-release
Halfprin	Tablet	Enteric-coated
Hetlioz	Capsule	Manufacturer recommendation
Hexalen	Capsule	Teratogenic potential; hazardous substance[k]
Horizant	Tablet	Extended-release
Hycamtin	Capsule	Teratogenic potential; hazardous substance[k]
Hydrea	Capsule	Can be opened and mixed with water; wear gloves to handle; hazardous substance[k]
Iclusig	Tablet	Teratogenic potential; hazardous substance[k]
Imbruvica	Capsule	Teratogenic potential; hazardous substance[k]
Imdur	Tablet	Extended-release[h]
Inderal LA	Capsule	Extended-release
Indomethacin SR	Capsule	Slow-release[a,b]
Inlyta	Tablet	Teratogenic potential; hazardous substance[k]
InnoPran XL	Capsule	Extended-release
Intelence	Tablet	Tablet should be swallowed whole and not crushed; tablet may be dispersed in water
Intermezzo	Tablet	Sublingual form[g]
Intuniv	Tablet	Extended-release
Invega	Tablet	Extended-release
IsoDitrate	Tablet	Extended-release
Isoptin SR	Tablet	Extended-release[h]
Isosorbide Dinitrate Sublingual	Tablet	Sublingual form[g]
ISOtretinoin	Capsule	Mucous membrane irritant
Jalyn	Capsule	Capsule should not be handled by pregnant women due to teratogenic potential[i]; hazardous substance[i,k]
Janumet XR	Tablet	Extended-release
Juxtapid	Capsule	Manufacturer recommendation
Kadian	Capsule	Extended-release[a]. Do not give via nasogastric tubes; may add contents to applesauce without crushing.
Kaletra	Tablet	Film-coated; pregnant women or women who may become pregnant should not handle crushed or broken tablets; active ingredients surrounded by wax matrix to prevent health care exposure

Drug product	Dosage form	Reason/Comments*
Kapidex	Capsule	Delayed-release[a]
Kapvay	Tablet	Extended-release
Kazano	Tablet	Not scored; manufacturer recommended
K-Dur	Tablet	Slow-release
Keppra	Tablet	Taste[b]
Keppra XR	Tablet	Extended-release[b]
Ketek	Tablet	Slow-release
Khedezia	Tablet	Extended-release
Klor-Con	Tablet	Extended-release[b]
Klor-Con M	Tablet	Slow-release[b]; some strengths are scored. To make liquid, place tablet in 120 mL of water; disperse 2 minutes; stir.
K-Lyte/Cl	Tablet	Effervescent tablet[f]
Kombiglyze XR	Tablet	Extended-release; tablet matrix may remain in stool
K-Tab	Tablet	Extended-release[b]
LaMICtal XR	Tablet	Extended-release
Lescol XL	Tablet	Extended-release
Letairis	Tablet	Film-coated; slow release; hazardous substance[k]
Leukeran	Tablet	Teratogenic potential; hazardous substance[k]
Levbid	Tablet	Extended-release[h]
Lialda	Tablet	Delayed-release, enteric-coated
Lithium Carbonate XR	Tablet	Extended-release
Lithobid	Tablet	Extended-release
Lovaza	Capsule	Contents of capsule may erode walls of Styrofoam or plastic materials
Luvox CR	Capsule	Extended-release
Lysodren	Tablet	Hazardous substance[k]
Mag-Tab SR	Tablet	Extended-release
Matulane	Capsule	Teratogenic potential; hazardous substance[k]
Maxiphen DM	Tablet	Slow-release[h]
Mestinon ER	Tablet	Extended-release[b]
Metadate CD	Capsule	Extended-release[a]
Metadate ER	Tablet	Extended-release
Metoprolol ER	Tablet	Extended-release
Micro K Extencaps	Capsule	Extended-release[a,b]
Minocin	Capsule	Slow-release
Mirapex ER	Tablet	Extended-release
Morphine Sulfate Extended-Release	Tablet	Extended-release
Motrin	Tablet	Taste[e]
Moxatag	Tablet	Extended-release
MS Contin	Tablet	Extended-release[b]
Mucinex	Tablet	Slow-release
Mucinex DM	Tablet	Slow-release[b]
Multaq	Tablet	Hazardous substance[k]

Drug product	Dosage form	Reason/Comments*
Myfortic	Tablet	Delayed-release; teratogenic potential; hazardous substance[k]
Myrbetriq	Tablet	Extended-release
Namenda XR	Capsule	Extended-release[a]
Naprelan	Tablet	Extended-release
Neoral	Capsule	Teratogenic potential; hazardous substance[k]
NexIUM	Capsule	Delayed-release[a]
Niaspan	Tablet	Extended-release
Nicotinic Acid	Capsule, Tablet	Slow-release[h]
Nifediac CC	Tablet	Extended-release
Nifedical XL	Tablet	Extended-release
Nifedipine ER	Tablet	Extended-release
Nitrostat	Tablet	Sublingual route[g]
Norpace CR	Capsule	Extended-release; form within a special capsule
Norvir	Tablet	Crushing tablets has resulted in decreased bioavailability of drug[b]
Noxafil	Tablet	Delayed-release
Nucynta ER	Tablet	Extended-release; tablet disruption may cause a potentially fatal overdose
Oleptro	Tablet	Extended-release[h]
Omtryg	Capsule	Manufacturer recommendation
Onglyza	Tablet	Film-coated
Opana ER	Tablet	Extended-release; tablet disruption may cause a potentially fatal overdose
Opsumit	Tablet	Teratogenic potential; hazardous substance[k]
Oracea	Capsule	Delayed-release
Oramorph SR	Tablet	Extended-release[b]
Oravig	Tablet	Buccal tablet
Orphenadrine Citrate ER	Tablet	Extended-release
Otezla	Tablet	Manufacturer recommendation
Oxtellar XR	Tablet	Extended-release
OxyCONTIN	Tablet	Extended-release; surrounded by wax matrix; tablet disruption may cause a potentially fatal overdose
Oxymorphone ER	Tablet	Extended-release
Pancrease MT	Capsule	Enteric-coated[a]
Pancreaze	Capsule	Slow-release[a]; enteric-coated contents
Pancrelipase	Capsule	Slow-release[a]; enteric-coated contents
Paxil CR	Tablet	Extended-release
Pentasa	Capsule	Slow-release[a]
Pertzye	Capsule	Slow-release[a]; enteric-coated contents
Pexeva	Tablet	Film-coated
Plendil	Tablet	Extended-release
Pomalyst	Capsule	Teratogenic potential; hazardous substance[k]; health care workers should avoid contact with capsule contents/body fluids

Drug product	Dosage form	Reason/Comments*
Pradaxa	Capsule	Bioavailability increases by 75% when the pellets are taken without the capsule shell
Prevacid	Capsule	Delayed-release[a]
	Suspension	Slow-release. Contains enteric-coated granules. Not for use in nasogastric tubes; mix with water only.
Prevacid SoluTab	Tablet	Orally disintegrating. Do not swallow; dissolve in water only and dispense via dosing syringe or nasogastric tube.
PriLOSEC	Capsule	Delayed-release
PriLOSEC OTC	Tablet	Delayed-release
Pristiq	Tablet	Extended-release
Procardia XL	Tablet	Extended-release
Procysbi	Capsule	Delayed-release[a]
Propecia	Tablet	Women who are, or may become, pregnant should not handle crushed or broken tablets due to teratogenic potential[j]; hazardous substance[k]
Proscar	Tablet	Women who are, or may become, pregnant should not handle crushed or broken tablets due to teratogenic potential[j]; hazardous substance[k]
Protonix	Tablet	Slow-release
PROzac Weekly	Capsule	Enteric-coated
Purinethol	Tablet	Teratogenic potential[j]; hazardous substance[k]
Pytest	Capsule	Hazardous substance[k]
Qudexy XR	Capsule	Extended-release
QuiNIDine ER	Tablet	Extended-release[h]; enteric-coated
Ranexa	Tablet	Slow-release
Rapamune	Tablet	Hazardous substance[k]; pharmacokinetic NanoCrystal technology may be affected[b]
Rayos	Tablet	Delayed-release; release is dependent upon intact coating
Razadyne ER	Capsule	Extended-release
Renagel	Tablet	Expands in liquid if broken or crushed.
Renvela	Tablet	Enteric-coated[b]; expands in liquid if broken or crushed
Requip XL	Tablet	Extended-release
Rescriptor	Tablet	If unable to swallow, may dissolve 100 mg tablets in water and drink; 200 mg tablets must be swallowed whole
Revlimid	Capsule	Teratogenic potential; hazardous substance[k]; health care workers should avoid contact with capsule contents/body fluids
RisperDAL M-Tab	Tablet	Orally disintegrating. Do not chew or break tablet; after dissolving under tongue, tablet may be swallowed.
Ritalin LA	Capsule	Extended-release[a]
Ritalin SR	Tablet	Extended-release
Rythmol SR	Capsule	Extended-release

Drug product	Dosage form	Reason/Comments*
Ryzolt	Tablet	Extended-release; tablet disruption may cause overdose
SandIMMUNE	Capsule	Teratogenic potential; hazardous substance[k]
Saphris	Tablet	Sublingual form[g]
Sensipar	Tablet	Tablets are not scored and cutting may cause inaccurate dosage
SEROquel XR	Tablet	Extended-release
Sinemet CR	Tablet	Extended-release[h]
Sitavig	Tablet	Buccal tablet; swallowing whole or crushing eliminates or reduces effectiveness
Slo-Niacin	Tablet	Slow-release[h]
Slow-Mag	Tablet	Delayed-release
Solodyn	Tablet	Extended-release
Somnote	Capsule	Liquid-filled
Soriatane	Capsule	Teratogenic potential; hazardous substance[k]
Sprycel	Tablet	Film-coated. Active ingredients are surrounded by a wax matrix to prevent health care exposure. Women who are, or may become pregnant, should not handle crushed or broken tablets; teratogenic potential; hazardous substance[k]
Stavzor	Capsule	Delayed-release; hazardous substance[k]
Stivarga	Tablet	Manufacturer recommendation; teratogenic potential; hazardous substance[k]
Strattera	Capsule	Capsule contents can cause ocular irritation
Sudafed 12-Hour	Capsule	Extended-release[b]
Sudafed 24-Hour	Capsule	Extended-release[b]
Sulfazine EC	Tablet	Delayed-release, enteric-coated
Sular	Tablet	Extended-release
Sustiva	Tablet	Tablets should not be broken (capsules should be used if dosage adjustment needed)
Symax Duotab	Tablet	Controlled-release
Symax SR	Tablet	Extended-release
Syprine	Capsule	Potential risk of contact dermatitis
Tabloid	Tablet	Teratogenic potential; hazardous substance[k]
Tafinlar	Capsule	Teratogenic potential; hazardous substance[k]
Tamoxifen	Tablet	Teratogenic potential; hazardous substance[k]
Targretin	Capsule	Manufacturer recommended; teratogenic potential; hazardous substance[k]
Tasigna	Capsule	Hazardous substance[k]; altering capsule may lead to high blood levels, increasing the risk of toxicity
Taztia XT	Capsule	Extended-release[a]
Tecfidera	Capsule	Manufacturer recommendation; delayed-release; irritant
TEGretol-XR	Tablet	Extended-release[b]

Drug product	Dosage form	Reason/Comments*
Temodar	Capsule	Teratogenic potential; hazardous substance[k]. Note: If capsules are accidentally opened or damaged, rigorous precautions should be taken to avoid inhalation or contact of contents with the skin or mucous membranes.
Tessalon Perles	Capsule	Swallow whole; pharmacologic action may cause choking if chewed or opened and swallowed
Tetracycline	Capsule	Hazardous substance[k]
Thalomid	Capsule	Teratogenic potential; hazardous substance[k]
Theo-24	Capsule	Extended-release[a]; contains beads that dissolve through GI tract
Theochron	Tablet	Extended-release
Theophylline ER	Tablet	Extended-release
Tiazac	Capsule	Extended-release[a]
Topamax	Tablet	Taste
	Capsule	Taste[a]
Toprol XL	Tablet	Extended-release[h]
Toviaz	Tablet	Extended-release
Tracleer	Tablet	Teratogenic potential; hazardous substance[j,k]; women who are, or may be, pregnant should not handle crushed or broken tablets
TRENtal	Tablet	Extended-release
Treximet	Tablet	Unique formulation enhances rapid drug absorption
TriLipix	Capsule	Extended-release
Trokendi XR	Capsule	Extended-release
Tylenol 8-Hour	Caplet	Extended-release
Tylenol Arthritis Pain	Caplet	Controlled-release
Uceris	Tablet	Extended-release; coating on tablet designed to break down at pH of ≥ 7
Ultram ER	Tablet	Extended-release; tablet disruption my cause a potentially fatal overdose
Ultrase	Capsule	Enteric-coated[a]
Ultrase MT	Capsule	Enteric-coated[a]
Ultresa	Capsule	Delayed-release; enteric-coated contents
Uniphyl	Tablet	Slow-release
Urocit-K	Tablet	Wax-coated; prevents upper GI release
Uroxatral	Tablet	Extended-release
Valcyte	Tablet	Irritant potential[b]; teratogenic potential; hazardous substance[k]
Vascepa	Capsule	Manufacturer recommendation
Venlafaxine ER	Tablet	Extended-release
Verapamil SR	Tablet	Extended-release[h]
Verelan	Capsule	Sustained-release[a]
Verelan PM	Capsule	Extended-release[a]
Vesanoid	Capsule	Teratogenic potential; hazardous substance[k]
VESIcare	Tablet	Enteric-coated

Drug product	Dosage form	Reason/Comments*
Videx EC	Capsule	Delayed-release
Vimovo	Tablet	Delayed-release
Viokace	Tablet	Mucous membrane irritant
Viramune XR	Tablet	Extended-release[b]
Voltaren XR	Tablet	Extended-release
VoSpire ER	Tablet	Extended-release
Votrient	Tablet	Crushing significantly increases AUC and T_{max}; hazardous substance[k]; crushed or broken tablets may cause dangerous skin problems
Wellbutrin	Tablet	Film-coated
Wellbutrin SR	Tablet	Extended-release
Wellbutrin XL	Tablet	Extended-release
Xalkori	Capsule	Teratogenic potential; hazardous substance[k]
Xanax XR	Tablet	Extended-release
Xeloda	Tablet	Teratogenic potential; hazardous substance[k]
Xtandi	Capsule	Teratogenic potential; hazardous substance[k]
Zegerid OTC	Capsule	Delayed-release[b]
Zelboraf	Tablet	Teratogenic potential; hazardous substance[k]
Zenpep	Capsule	Delayed-release[a]; enteric-coated contents
Zohydro ER	Capsule	Extended-release; capsule disruption may cause a potentially fatal overdose
Zolinza	Capsule	Irritant; avoid contact with skin or mucous membranes; use gloves to handle; teratogenic potential; hazardous substance[k]
Zomig-ZMT	Tablet	Orally disintegrating form[g]
Zortress	Tablet	Mucous membrane irritant; teratogenic potential; hazardous substance[k]
Zyban	Tablet	Slow-release
Zydelig	Tablet	Manufacturer recommendation
Zyflo CR	Tablet	Extended-release
Zyrtec-D Allergy & Congestion	Tablet	Extended-release
Zytiga	Tablet	Teratogenic potential; hazardous substance[k]; women who are, or may be, pregnant should wear gloves if handling tablets

* Two official USP terms are used to designate special-release medication forms: "extended-release" and "delayed-release." Others such as "sustained-release," "controlled-release," etc, are commonly used on package labeling. The term "slow-release" is being used here to signify all such drugs with a special-release mechanism.

a Capsule may be opened and the contents taken without crushing or chewing; soft food such as applesauce or pudding may facilitate administration; contents may generally be administered via nasogastric tube using an appropriate fluid, provided entire contents are washed down the tube.

b Liquid dosage forms of the product are available; however, dose, frequency of administration, and manufacturers may differ from that of the solid dosage form.

c Antacids and/or milk may prematurely dissolve the coating of the tablet.

d Capsule may be opened and the liquid contents removed for administration.

e The taste of this product would likely be unacceptable to the patient; administration via nasogastric tube should be acceptable.

f Effervescent tablets must be dissolved in the amount of diluent recommended by the manufacturer.

g Tablets are made to disintegrate under (or on) the tongue.

h Tablet is scored and may be broken in half without affecting release characteristics.

i Skin contact may enhance tumor production; avoid direct contact.

j Prescribing information recommends that women who are, or may become, pregnant should not handle medication, especially if crushed or broken; avoid direct contact.

k Potentially hazardous or hazardous substance; refer to institution-specific guidelines for precautions to observe when handling this substance.

References

Mitchell JF. Oral dosage forms that should not be crushed. http://www.ismp.org/tools/DoNotCrush.pdf. Accessed November 11, 2011.

National Institute for Occupational Safety and Health (NIOSH). NIOSH list of antineoplastic and other hazardous drugs in healthcare settings 2012. http://www.cdc.gov/niosh/docs/2012-150/pdfs/2012-150.pdf. Accessed July 11, 2012.

Drug Names That Look Alike and Sound Alike

This list has been prepared to sensitize health care professionals and their support personnel to the need to properly communicate when writing, speaking, reading, and hearing drug names.

No drug name is without problems. Any name can be read, written, or spoken poorly enough so that it can be mistaken for another.

Listed in the accompanying table are drug names in the United States that can look and/or sound alike. Some are dangerously close; whereas others require incomplete prescribing information, poor communication skills, poor listening, poor reading skills, and/or lack of knowledge about the drugs for an error to result.

To reduce errors, practitioners must share the common goal of drug name safety with pharmaceutical manufacturers, the Food and Drug Administration (FDA), the World Health Organization (WHO), the United States Adopted Names (USAN) Council, and the United States Pharmacopeia (USP).

The potential errors can be reduced by:

- Pretesting proposed names for error potential
- Careful selection of brand names and generic names by manufacturers, the FDA, WHO, and USAN Council
- Legible handwriting
- Clear oral communications
- Writing complete drug orders
    - Specifying the dosage form (eg, tablet)
    - Specifying the drug strength (eg, 100 mg)
    - Specifying directions (eg, take one daily with breakfast)
    - Specifying the purpose/indication (eg, take one daily with breakfast to control blood pressure)
- Printing orders for new or rarely prescribed drugs
- Using computer-generated orders
- Using Tall Man letters (eg, diphenhydrAMINE, dimenhyDRINATE)
- Carefully selecting a drug from a computer list
- For those involved in drug dispensing and administration, being aware of the drugs that are available, paying careful attention to the work at hand, and minimizing distractions
- Knowing the patient's condition/problems to ascertain if the drug name that has been read or heard is indicated
- Double-checking completed prescriptions in the pharmacy
- Educating patients about their drug regimens (serves as another final check that the prescription was properly read and dispensed)

Proprietary names are capitalized; other names are in lower case letters.

Accolate . . . . .Accupril
Accolate . . . . .Aclovate
Accupril . . . . .Accolate
Accupril . . . . .Aciphex
acebutolol. . . . . .albuterol
acetylcholine . . . . . . .acetylcysteine
acetylcysteine. . . . . . .acetylcholine
Aciphex . . . . .Accupril
Aciphex . . . . .Aricept
Aclovate . . . . .Accolate
Acnomel. . . . . .Actonel
Actonel. . . . . .Acnomel

Actonel. . . . . .Actos
Actos . . . . .Actonel
Adacel . . . . .Daptacel
Adderall . . . . .Inderal
Adriamycin . . . . .Aredia
Afrin . . . . .aspirin
Aggrastat . . . . .Aggrenox
Aggrastat . . . . .argatroban
Aggrenox . . . . .Aggrastat
Albutein . . . . .albuterol
albuterol . . . . .acebutolol
albuterol . . . . .Albutein
albuterol . . . . .atenolol
Aldactazide . . . . .Aldactone
Aldactone . . . . .Aldactazide
Aldara . . . . .Alora
Alesse . . . . .Aleve
Aleve . . . . .Alesse
Alfenta . . . . .Sufenta
alfentanil. . . . . .Anafranil
alfentanil. . . . . .fentanyl
alfentanil. . . . . .sufentanil
Alkeran. . . . . .Leukeran
Alora . . . . .Aldara
Alora . . . . .Aloxi
Aloxi . . . . .Alora
alprazolam . . . . .alprostadil
alprazolam . . . . .lorazepam
alprostadil. . . . . .alprazolam
Altace. . . . . .alteplase
alteplase. . . . . .Altace
Altocor . . . . .Advicor
Amaryl . . . . .Amerge
Amerge . . . . .Amaryl
amiloride . . . . .amiodarone
amiloride . . . . .amlodipine
amiodarone . . . . .amiloride
amitriptyline . . . . .nortriptyline
amlodipine . . . . .amiloride
amoxapine . . . . .amoxicillin
amoxicillin . . . . .amoxapine
Amrix . . . . .Amvisc
Amvisc . . . . .Amrix
Anafranil. . . . . .alfentanil
Anafranil. . . . . .enalapril
Anafranil. . . . . .nafarelin
Anaprox . . . . .Anaspaz
Anaspaz. . . . . .Anaprox
Antivert. . . . . .Axert
Anusol . . . . .Anusol-HC
Anusol . . . . .Aplisol
Anusol . . . . .Aquasol
Anusol-HC . . . . .Anusol
Aplisol . . . . .Anusol
Aptiom . . . . .Aptivus
Aptivus . . . . .Aptiom
Aquasol . . . . .Anusol
Aralen . . . . .Aranelle
Aranelle . . . . .Aralen
Aranesp . . . . .Aricept
Aredia . . . . .Adriamycin
argatroban . . . . .Aggrastat
Aricept . . . . .Aciphex
Aricept . . . . .Aranesp
Aricept . . . . .Ascriptin
Aricept . . . . .Azilect
Asacol . . . . .Os-Cal
Ascriptin . . . . .Aricept
asparaginase . . . . . . .pegaspargase
aspirin . . . . .Afrin
atenolol . . . . .albuterol
atenolol . . . . .timolol
Atgam . . . . .Ativan
Ativan. . . . . .Atgam
Ativan. . . . . .Avitene
Avalide . . . . .Avandia
Avandamet. . . . . .Avandia
Avandia . . . . .Avalide
Avandia . . . . .Avandamet
Avandia . . . . .Coumadin
Avandia . . . . .Prandin
Aventyl . . . . .Bentyl
Avinza . . . . .Invanz
Avinza . . . . .Evista
Avitene. . . . . .Ativan
Avonex. . . . . .Avelox
Axert . . . . .Antivert
azathioprine . . . . .Azulfidine
azelastine. . . . . .azilsartan
azidothymidine . . . . . .azathioprine
Azilect . . . . .Aricept
azilsartan . . . . .azelastine
azithromycin. . . . . . . .erythromycin
Azulfidine . . . . .azathioprine
bacitracin . . . . .Bactrim
bacitracin . . . . .Bactroban
baclofen . . . . .Bactroban
Bactrim. . . . . .bacitracin

Bactrim	Bactroban
Bactroban	bacitracin
Bactroban	baclofen
Bactroban	Bactrim
Benadryl	benazepril
Benadryl	Bentyl
benazepril	Benadryl
Bentyl	Aventyl
Bentyl	Benadryl
Betadine	betaine
betaine	Betadine
betaxolol	bethanechol
bethanechol	betaxolol
bupivacaine	mepivacaine
bupropion	buspirone
buspirone	bupropion
buspirone	risperidone
butabarbital	butalbital
butalbital	butabarbital
Cafergot	Carafate
Caladryl	calamine
calamine	Caladryl
Calan	Colace
calcitonin	calcitriol
calcitriol	calcitonin
calcium glubionate	calcium gluconate
calcium gluconate	calcium glubionate
Capastat	Cēpastat
Capitrol	captopril
captopril	Capitrol
Carac	Kuric
Carafate	Cafergot
Carbatrol	Cartrol
carboplatin	cisplatin
Cardene	Cardura
Cardene	codeine
Cardizem CD (LA)	Cardizem LA (CD)
Cardura	Cardene
Cardura	Cordarone
Cardura	Coumadin
Cardura	K-Dur
Cardura	Ridaura
carteolol	carvedilol
Cartrol	Carbatrol
carvedilol	carteolol
Casodex	Kapidex
cefotaxime	cefoxitin

cefotaxime	ceftizoxime
cefotaxime	cefuroxime
cefotetan	cefoxitin
cefoxitin	cefotaxime
cefoxitin	cefotetan
ceftazidime	ceftizoxime
ceftizoxime	cefotaxime
ceftizoxime	ceftazidime
cefuroxime	cefotaxime
cefuroxime	deferoxamine
Celebrex	Celexa
Celebrex	Cerebyx
Cēpastat	Capastat
Cerebyx	Celebrex
Cerebyx	Cerezyme
Ceredase	Cerezyme
Cerezyme	Cerebyx
Cerezyme	Ceredase
chlorambucil	Chloromycetin
Chloromycetin	chlorambucil
chlorpromazine	chlorpropamide
chlorpromazine	clomipramine
chlorpromazine	prochlorperazine
chlorpropamide	chlorpromazine
Cidex	Lidex
cimetidine	simethicone
cinoxacin	Ciloxan
cisplatin	carboplatin
Citracal	Citrucel
Citrucel	Citracal
Clarinex	Claritin
Claritin	Clarinex
Clinoril	Clozaril
clomiphene	clomipramine
clomiphene	clonidine
clomipramine	chlorpromazine
clomipramine	clomiphene
clonazepam	clorazepate
clonazepam	lorazepam
clonidine	clomiphene
clonidine	clonazepam
clonidine	quinidine
clotrimazole	co-trimoxazole
Clozaril	Clinoril
Clozaril	Colazal
codeine	Cardene
Colace	Calan
Colazal	Clozaril
Combivent	Combivir

Combivir	Combivent
Compazine	Copaxone
Comvax	Recombivax HB
Copaxone	Compazine
Cordarone	Cardura
Coreg	Corgard
Corgard	Coreg
Cortef	Lortab
co-trimoxazole	clotrimazole
Coumadin	Avandia
Coumadin	Cardura
Covera HS	Provera
Cozaar	Hyzaar
Cozaar	Zocor
cyclobenzaprine	cycloserine
cyclobenzaprine	cyproheptadine
cyclophosphamide	cyclosporine
cycloserine	cyclobenzaprine
cycloserine	cyclosporine
cyclosporine	cyclophosphamide
cyclosporine	cycloserine
cyclosporine	Cyklokapron
Cyklokapron	cyclosporine
cyproheptadine	cyclobenzaprine
dacarbazine	procarbazine
dactinomycin	daptomycin
Dantrium	Daraprim
Daptacel	Adacel
Daraprim	Dantrium
darunavir	Denavir
Darvocet-N	Darvon-N
Darvon	Diovan
Darvon-N	Darvocet-N
daunorubicin	dactinomycin
daunorubicin	doxorubicin
daunorubicin	idarubicin
deferasirox	deferoxamine
deferoxamine	cefuroxime
deferoxamine	deferasirox
Demerol	Detrol
Denavir	darunavir
Depo-Medrol	Solu-Medrol
Dermatop	Dimetapp
desipramine	disopyramide
desipramine	imipramine
Desogen	digoxin
desoximetasone	dexamethasone
Desoxyn	digoxin
dexamethasone	desoximetasone
Dexedrine	Dextran
Dexedrine	Excedrin
Dextran	Dexedrine
DiaBeta	Zebeta
diazepam	diazoxide
diazepam	Ditropan
diazoxide	diazepam
diazoxide	Dyazide
dichloroacetic acid	trichloracetic acid
diclofenac	Diflucan
diclofenac	Duphalac
Diflucan	diclofenac
Diflucan	Diprivan
Diflucan	disulfiram
digoxin	Desogen
digoxin	Desoxyn
digoxin	doxepin
Dilantin	Dilaudid
Dilaudid	Dilantin
dimenhydrinate	diphenhydramine
Dimetapp	Dermatop
Diovan	Darvon
diphenhydramine	dimenhydrinate
Diprivan	Ditropan
Diprosone	dapsone
dipyridamole	disopyramide
disopyramide	desipramine
disopyramide	dipyridamole
disulfiram	Diflucan
dithranol	Ditropan
Ditropan	diazepam
Ditropan	Diprivan
Ditropan	dithranol
dobutamine	dopamine
donepezil	doxepin
dopamine	dobutamine
dopamine	Dopram
Dopram	dopamine
doxapram	doxazosin
doxapram	doxepin
doxapram	doxorubicin
doxazosin	doxapram
doxazosin	doxepin
doxazosin	doxorubicin
doxepin	digoxin
doxepin	donepezil
doxepin	doxapram
doxepin	doxazosin

doxepin . . . . Doxidan
Doxidan . . . . doxepin
Doxil. . . . . Doxy
Doxil. . . . . Paxil
doxorubicin. . . . . dactinomycin
doxorubicin. . . . . daunorubicin
doxorubicin. . . . . doxacurium
doxorubicin. . . . . doxapram
doxorubicin. . . . . doxazosin
doxorubicin. . . . . idarubicin
Doxy. . . . . Doxil
doxycycline . . . . doxylamine
doxylamine. . . . . doxycycline
dronabinol . . . . droperidol
droperidol. . . . . dronabinol
duloxetine. . . . . fluoxetine
Duphalac . . . . diclofenac
Durasal . . . . Durezol
Durezol . . . . Durasal
Dyazide . . . . diazoxide
Dynacin . . . . DynaCirc
DynaCirc . . . . Dynacin
Ecotrin . . . . Edecrin
Edecrin. . . . . Ecotrin
Efavirenz . . . . Etravirine
Eldepryl . . . . enalapril
Eldopaque Forte . . . . Eldoquin Forte
Eldoquin Forte . . . . . . Eldopaque Forte
Elmiron. . . . . Imuran
Enablex . . . . Enbrel
enalapril . . . . Anafranil
enalapril . . . . Eldepryl
Enbrel . . . . Enablex
enflurane . . . . isoflurane
Enjuvia . . . . Januvia
Entex . . . . Tenex
ephedrine. . . . . epinephrine
epinephrine . . . . ephedrine
Epogen . . . . Neupogen
erythromycin. . . . . azithromycin
ethanol . . . . Ethamolin
ethanol . . . . Ethyol
ethosuximide . . . . methsuximide
Ethyol. . . . . ethanol
etidronate. . . . . etomidate
etomidate . . . . etidronate
Etravirine . . . . Efavirenz
Eurax . . . . Evoxac
Eurax . . . . Urex

Evoxac. . . . . Eurax
Excedrin. . . . . Dexedrine
Factrel . . . . Sectral
Fareston. . . . . Fosrenol
Faslodex . . . . Fosamax
Femara . . . . Femhrt
Femhrt . . . . Femara
Femiron . . . . Femring
Femring . . . . Femiron
fentanyl . . . . alfentanil
fentanyl . . . . sufentanil
Feosol . . . . Fer-In-Sol
Fer-In-Sol. . . . . Feosol
Fioricet. . . . . Fiorinal
Fiorinal. . . . . Fioricet
Fiorinal. . . . . Florinef
flavoxate. . . . . fluvoxamine
flecainide . . . . fluconazole
Flexeril . . . . Floxin
Flomax. . . . . Floranex
Flomax. . . . . Fosamax
Floranex. . . . . Flomax
Florinef. . . . . Fiorinal
Floxin . . . . Flexeril
fluconazole. . . . . flecainide
Fludara. . . . . FUDR
Flumadine . . . . flunisolide
Flumadine . . . . flutamide
flunisolide. . . . . Flumadine
flunisolide. . . . . fluocinonide
fluocinolone . . . . fluocinonide
fluocinonide . . . . flunisolide
fluocinonide . . . . fluocinolone
fluoxetine . . . . duloxetine
fluoxetine . . . . fluvastatin
flutamide . . . . Flumadine
fluvastatin. . . . . fluoxetine
fluvoxamine . . . . flavoxate
folic acid. . . . . folinic acid
folinic acid . . . . folic acid
Fortaz. . . . . Forteo
Forteo . . . . Fortaz
Fosamax . . . . Faslodex
Fosamax . . . . Flomax
fosinopril. . . . . lisinopril
Fosrenol . . . . Fareston
Frova . . . . Provera
FUDR. . . . . Fludara
furosemide . . . . Torsemide

glimepiride	glipizide
glipizide	glimepiride
glipizide	glyburide
Glucotrol	glyburide
glyburide	glipizide
glyburide	Glucotrol
GoLYTELY	NuLYTELY
guaifenesin	guanfacine
guanabenz	guanadrel
guanabenz	guanfacine
guanadrel	guanabenz
guanfacine	guaifenesin
guanfacine	guanabenz
guanfacine	guanidine
guanidine	guanfacine
Halcion	Haldol
Haldol	Halcion
Haldol	Stadol
Healon	Hyalgan
heparin	Hespan
Hespan	heparin
Humalog	Humulin
Humulin	Humalog
Hyalgan	Healon
hydralazine	hydroxyzine
hydrochlorothiazide	hydroflumethiazide
hydrocodone	hydrocortisone
hydrocortisone	hydrocodone
hydrocortisone	hydroxychloroquine
hydroflumethiazide	hydrochlorothiazide
hydromorphone	morphine
hydroxychloroquine	hydrocortisone
hydroxyurea	hydroxyzine
hydroxyzine	hydralazine
hydroxyzine	Hydrogesic
hydroxyzine	hydroxyurea
Hytone	Vytone
idarubicin	daunorubicin
idarubicin	doxorubicin
Imdur	Imuran
Imdur	K-Dur
imipramine	desipramine
Imodium	Indocin
Imodium	Ionamin
Imuran	Elmiron
Imuran	Imdur
Imuran	Inderal
indapamide	iopamidol
indapamide	Iopidine
Inderal	Adderall
Inderal	Imuran
Indocin	Imodium
Indocin	Vicodin
Inspra	Spiriva
interferon 2	interleukin 2
interferon alfa-2a	interferon alfa-2b
interferon alfa-2b	interferon alfa-2a
interleukin 2	interferon 2
interleukin 2	interleukin 11
Invanz	Avinza
Invanz	Invega
Invega	Invanz
iodine	Iopidine
Ionamin	Imodium
iopamidol	indapamide
Iopidine	iodipamide
Iopidine	iodine
Iopidine	Lodine
isoflurane	enflurane
Januvia	Enjuvia
Kaletra	Keppra
Kapidex	Casodex
K-Dur	Cardura
Keppra	Kaletra
Klaron	Klor-Con
Klor-Con	Klaron
Kuric	Carac
lactose	lactulose
lactulose	lactose
Lamictal	Lamisil
Lamictal	Lomotil
Lamisil	Lamictal
lamivudine	lamotrigine
lamotrigine	lamivudine
Lasix	Lidex
Lasix	Luxiq
leucovorin	Leukeran
Leukeran	Alkeran
Leukeran	leucovorin
Leukeran	Leukine
Leukine	Leukeran
Leustatin	lovastatin
Levatol	Lipitor
Levbid	Lithobid
Levitra	Lexiva
levothyroxine	liothyronine
Lexiva	Levitra
Lidex	Cidex

Lidex . . . . .Lasix
Lioresal . . . . .lisinopril
liothyronine. . . . . .levothyroxine
Lipitor. . . . . .Levatol
lisinopril . . . . .fosinopril
lisinopril . . . . .Lioresal
Lithobid . . . . .Levbid
Lithobid . . . . .Lithostat
Lithobid . . . . .Lithotabs
Lithostat . . . . .Lithobid
Lithostat . . . . .Lithotabs
Lithotabs . . . . .Lithobid
Lithotabs . . . . .Lithostat
Lomotil . . . . .Lamictal
Lonox. . . . . .Loprox
Loprox . . . . .Lonox
lorazepam . . . . .alprazolam
lorazepam . . . . .clonazepam
Lortab. . . . . .Cortef
Lotensin . . . . .lovastatin
Lotrimin . . . . .Lotrisone
Lotrisone . . . . .Lotrimin
lovastatin . . . . .Leustatin
lovastatin . . . . .Lotensin
Lovenox . . . . .Lotronex
Lunesta . . . . .Neulasta
Lustra. . . . . .Lutera
Lutera. . . . . .Lustra
Luxiq . . . . .Lasix
magnesium sulfate. . .manganese sulfate
manganese sulfate. . .magnesium sulfate
Maxidex . . . . .Maxzide
Maxzide . . . . .Maxidex
Mebaral . . . . .Medrol
Medrol . . . . .Mebaral
medroxy-progesterone . . . . . methylprednisolone
medroxy-progesterone . . . . . methyltestosterone
melphalan . . . . .Mephyton
Mephyton . . . . .melphalan
Mephyton . . . . .mephenytoin
mepivacaine. . . . . . . .bupivacaine
metaproterenol . . . . . .metipranolol
metaproterenol . . . . . .metoprolol
methazolamide . . . . . .metolazone
methenamine . . . . . . .methionine
methionine . . . . .methenamine
methsuximide . . . . . . .ethosuximide
methylprednisolone . .medroxyprogesterone
methyltestosterone. . .medroxyprogesterone
metipranolol . . . . .metaproterenol
metolazone . . . . .methazolamide
metolazone . . . . .metoprolol
metoprolol . . . . .metaproterenol
metoprolol . . . . .metolazone
metoprolol . . . . .misoprostol
metyrapone . . . . .metyrosine
metyrosine . . . . .metyrapone
miconazole. . . . . .Micronor
Micronor. . . . . .miconazole
Midrin. . . . . .Mydfrin
Mifeprex. . . . . .Mirapex
mifepristone . . . . .misoprostol
Minocin . . . . .niacin
MiraLax . . . . .Mirapex
Mirapex . . . . .Mifeprex
Mirapex . . . . .MiraLax
Mircera. . . . . .Mirena
Mirena . . . . .Mircera
misoprostol. . . . . .mifepristone
Monopril. . . . . .Monurol
Monurol . . . . .Monopril
morphine . . . . .hydromorphone
Mucinex . . . . .Mucomyst
Mucomyst. . . . . .Mucinex
Myambutol . . . . .Nembutal
Mycelex . . . . .Myoflex
Mydfrin. . . . . .Midrin
Myleran . . . . .Mylicon
Mylicon. . . . . .Myleran
Myoflex . . . . .Mycelex
nafarelin. . . . . .Anafranil
Naldecon . . . . .Nalfon
Nalfon . . . . .Naldecon
naloxone . . . . .naltrexone
naltrexone . . . . .naloxone
Navane . . . . .Norvasc
Navane . . . . .Nubain
nelfinavir. . . . . .nevirapine
Nembutal . . . . .Myambutol
Neulasta. . . . . .Lunesta
Neulasta. . . . . .Neumega
Neulasta. . . . . .Nuedexta
Neumega . . . . .Neulasta
Neumega . . . . .Neupogen
Neupogen . . . . .Epogen
Neupogen . . . . .Nutramigen

Neurontin	Noroxin
Nevanac	Nexavar
nevirapine	nelfinavir
Nexavar	Nevanac
niacin	Minocin
nicardipine	nifedipine
Nicorette	Nordette
nifedipine	nicardipine
nifedipine	nimodipine
nimodipine	nifedipine
nitroglycerin	nitroprusside
nitroprusside	nitroglycerin
Nitrostat	Hyperstat
Nitrostat	Nystatin
Nordette	Nicorette
Noroxin	Neurontin
Norpace	Norvasc
nortriptyline	amitriptyline
Norvasc	Navane
Norvasc	Norpace
Nubain	Navane
Nuedexta	Neulasta
NuLYTELY	GoLYTELY
Nutramigen	Neupogen
Nystatin	Nitrostat
Occlusal-HP	Ocuflox
OctreoScan	octreotide
OctreoScan	OncoScint
octreotide	OctreoScan
Ocufen	Ocuflox
Ocuflox	Occlusal-HP
Ocuflox	Ocufen
olanzapine	olsalazine
olsalazine	olanzapine
OncoScint	OctreoScan
opium tincture	camphorated tincture of opium (paregoric)
opium tincture, camphorated (paregoric)	opium tincture
Optiray	Optivar
Optivar	Optiray
Orazinc	Orencia
Orencia	Orazinc
Orencia	Orinase
Orinase	Orencia
Ortho-Cept	Ortho-Cyclen
Ortho-Cyclen	Ortho-Cept
Os-Cal	Asacol
oxybutynin	OxyContin
OxyContin	oxybutynin
OxyContin	oxycodone
oxymetazoline	oxymetholone
oxymetholone	oxymetazoline
oxymetholone	oxymorphone
oxymorphone	oxymetholone
Oxytrol	Roxanol
Oxytrol	Uroxatral
paclitaxel	paroxetine
paclitaxel	Paxil
Pamelor	Panlor
Panlor	Pamelor
paregoric	Percogesic
Parlodel	pindolol
paroxetine	paclitaxel
paroxetine	pyridoxine
Paxil	Doxil
Paxil	paclitaxel
Paxil	Plavix
Paxil	Taxol
pazopanib	ponatinib
pegaspargase	asparaginase
penicillamine	penicillin
penicillin	penicillamine
penicillin G potassium	penicillin G procaine
penicillin G procaine	penicillin G potassium
pentosan	pentostatin
pentostatin	pentosan
Percocet	Percodan
Percodan	Percocet
Percodan	Percogesic
Percogesic	Paregoric
Percogesic	Percodan
Perdiem	Pyridium
Peridex	Precedex
phentermine	phentolamine
phentolamine	phentermine
pHisoDerm	pHisoHex
pHisoHex	pHisoDerm
Phos-Flur	PhosLo
PhosLo	Phos-Flur
physostigmine	Prostigmin
physostigmine	pyridostigmine
pindolol	Parlodel
Pitocin	Pitressin
Pitressin	Pitocin
Plaquenil	Plavix
Plavix	Paxil

Plavix	Plaquenil
Polocaine	prilocaine
ponatinib	pazopanib
pralidoxime	Pramoxine
pralidoxime	pyridoxine
Pramoxine	pralidoxime
Prandin	Avandia
Pravachol	Prevacid
Pravachol	propranolol
PreCare	Precose
Precedex	Peridex
Precose	PreCare
prednisolone	prednisone
prednisone	prednisolone
prednisone	primidone
Premarin	Primaxin
Premarin	Remeron
Premphase	Prempro
Prempro	Premphase
Prevacid	Pravachol
Prevacid	Prevpac
Prevpac	Prevacid
prilocaine	Polocaine
prilocaine	Prilosec
Prilosec	prilocaine
Prilosec	Prinivil
Prilosec	Prozac
Primaxin	Premarin
Primaxin	Primacor
primidone	prednisone
Prinivil	Prilosec
Prinivil	Proventil
ProAmatine	protamine
probenecid	Procanbid
Procanbid	probenecid
procarbazine	dacarbazine
prochlorperazine	chlorpromazine
propranolol	Pravachol
propylthiouracil	Purinethol
Proscar	Prozac
Proscar	Psorcon
Prostigmin	physostigmine
protamine	ProAmatine
protamine	Protonix
protamine	Protopam
Protonix	protamine
Protonix	Protopic
Protopam	protamine
Protopic	Protonix
Proventil	Prinivil
Provera	Covera HS
Provera	Frova
Prozac	Prilosec
Prozac	Proscar
Psorcon	Proscar
Purinethol	propylthiouracil
Pyridium	Perdiem
Pyridium	pyridoxine
pyridostigmine	physostigmine
pyridoxine	paroxetine
pyridoxine	pralidoxime
pyridoxine	Pyridium
quinidine	clonidine
quinidine	quinine
quinine	quinidine
Ranexa	Renova
ranitidine	rimantadine
Rapaflo	Rapamune
Rapamune	Rapaflo
Recombivax HB	Comvax
Reglan	Renagel
Regranex	Repronex
Remeron	Premarin
Remeron	Zemuron
Remicade	Renacidin
Renacidin	Remicade
Renagel	Reglan
Renova	Ranexa
Renova	Renvela
Renvela	Renova
Repronex	Regranex
Requip	Risperdal
reserpine	risperidone
Restasis	Retavase
Restoril	Risperdal
Restoril	Zestril
Retavase	Restasis
retinamide	rufinamide
Retrovir	ritonavir
Ribavirin	riboflavin
riboflavin	Ribavirin
rifabutin	rifampin
Rifadin	Rifater
Rifadin	Ritalin
Rifamate	rifampin
rifampin	rifabutin
rifampin	Rifamate
rifampin	rifapentine

rifampin . . . . .rifaximin
Rifater . . . . .Rifadin
rifaximin . . . . .rifampin
rimantadine . . . . .ranitidine
Risperdal . . . . .Requip
Risperdal . . . . .Restoril
risperidone . . . . .reserpine
risperidone . . . . .ropinirole
Ritalin. . . . . .Rifadin
Ritalin LA . . . . .Ritalin SR
Ritalin SR. . . . . .Ritalin LA
ritonavir . . . . .Retrovir
ropinirole . . . . .risperidone
Roxanol . . . . .Oxytrol
Roxanol . . . . .Roxicet
Roxanol . . . . .Uroxatral
Roxicet. . . . . .Roxanol
rufinamide . . . . .retinamide
Rynatan . . . . .Rynatuss
Rynatuss . . . . .Rynatan
Salagen . . . . .selegiline
Sandimmune . . . . . . .Sandostatin
Sandostatin . . . . .Sandimmune
Sarafem . . . . .Serophene
Sectral . . . . .Factrel
Sectral . . . . .Septra
selegiline . . . . .Salagen
Serophene . . . . .Sarafem
sertraline . . . . .Soriatane
simethicone . . . . .cimetidine
Solaraze. . . . . .Soliris
Soliris. . . . . .Solaraze
Solu-Medrol . . . . .Depo-Medrol
somatostatin. . . . . . . .Somatuline
Somatuline. . . . . .somatostatin
somatropin . . . . .sumatriptan
Soriatane . . . . .sertraline
sotalol . . . . .Stadol
Spiriva . . . . .Inspra
Stadol. . . . . .sotalol
Sufenta . . . . .Alfenta
Sufenta . . . . .Survanta
sufentanil . . . . .alfentanil
sulfadiazine . . . . .sulfasalazine
sulfasalazine . . . . . . .sulfadiazine
sumatriptan . . . . .somatropin
Surbex . . . . .Surfak
Surfak . . . . .Surbex
Survanta. . . . . .Sufenta
Synalar. . . . . .Synarel
Synarel. . . . . .Synalar
Tacrine . . . . .Tarceva
Tarceva . . . . .Tacrine
Tarceva . . . . .Tarka
Tarka . . . . .Tarceva
Taxol . . . . .Paxil
Taxol . . . . .Taxotere
Taxotere . . . . .Taxol
Tegretol . . . . .Trental
Tekturna . . . . .Terak
Tenex . . . . .Entex
Tenex . . . . .Xanax
Terak . . . . .Tekturna
terbinafine . . . . .terbutaline
terbutaline . . . . .terbinafine
terbutaline . . . . .tolbutamide
terconazole . . . . .tioconazole
tetracycline. . . . . .tigecycline
thioridazine. . . . . .thiothixene
thiothixene . . . . .thioridazine
tiagabine . . . . .tizanidine
Tiazac . . . . .Ziac
ticarcillin . . . . .tigecycline
tigecycline . . . . .tetracycline
tigecycline . . . . .ticarcillin
timolol . . . . .atenolol
Timoptic . . . . .Viroptic
tioconazole. . . . . .terconazole
tiopronin . . . . .tiotropium
tiotropium . . . . .tiopronin
tizanidine . . . . .tiagabine
TobraDex . . . . .Tobrex
tobramycin . . . . .Trobicin
Tobrex . . . . .TobraDex
tocilizumab. . . . . .tositumomab
tolazamide . . . . .tolbutamide
tolbutamide . . . . .terbutaline
tolbutamide . . . . .tolazamide
Torsemide . . . . .furosemide
tositumomab. . . . . . . .tocilizumab
Tracleer . . . . .Tricor
tramadol. . . . . .Trandate
Trandate. . . . . .tramadol
Trandate. . . . . .Trental
Travatan. . . . . .Xalatan
trazodone . . . . .tramadol
Trental . . . . .Tegretol
Trental . . . . .Trandate

tretinoin	trientine
triamterene	trimipramine
trichloroacetic acid	dichloroacetic acid
Tricor	Tracleer
trientine	tretinoin
trimipramine	triamterene
Trimox	Tylox
Trobicin	tobramycin
Tykerb	Tyzeka
Tylenol	Tylox
Tylox	Trimox
Tylox	Tylenol
Tyzeka	Tykerb
Ultane	Ultram
Ultram	Ultane
Urex	Eurax
Uroxatral	Oxytrol
Uroxatral	Roxanol
Valcyte	Valium
Valcyte	Valtrex
Valium	Valcyte
Valtrex	Valcyte
Vaniqa	Viagra
Vantas	Vantin
Vantin	Vantas
Vasocidin	Vasodilan
Vasodilan	Vasocidin
Verelan	Virilon
Verelan	Vivarin
Verelan	Voltaren
Viagra	Vaniqa
Vicodin	Indocin
Vigamox	Vigomar
Vigomar	Vigamox
vinblastine	vincristine
vinblastine	vinorelbine
vincristine	vinblastine
vinorelbine	vinblastine
Virilon	Verelan
Viroptic	Timoptic
Vivarin	Verelan
Voltaren	Verelan
vorapaxar	Voraxaze
Voraxaze	vorapaxar
Vytone	Hytone
Wellbutrin SR	Wellbutrin XL
Wellbutrin XL	Wellbutrin SR
Xalatan	Travatan
Xanax	Tenex
Xanax	Xenazine
Xanax	Xopenex
Xanax	Zantac
Xeloda	Xenical
Xenazine	Xanax
Xenical	Xeloda
Xopenex	Xanax
Zantac	Xanax
Zantac	Zofran
Zantac	Zyrtec
Zarontin	Zaroxolyn
Zaroxolyn	Zarontin
Zebeta	DiaBeta
Zestril	Restoril
Zestril	Zetia
Zestril	Zostrix
Zetia	Zestril
Ziac	Tiazac
Zocor	Cozaar
Zofran	Zantac
Zofran	Zosyn
Zolinza	Zonalon
Zonalon	Zolinza
ZORprin	Zyloprim
Zostrix	Zestril
Zosyn	Zofran
Zosyn	Zyvox
Zyloprim	ZORprin
Zymar	Zymine
Zymine	Zymar
Zyprexa	Zyrtec
Zyrtec	Zantac
Zyrtec	Zyprexa
Zyvox	Zosyn

This list was compiled by Neil M. Davis, MS, PharmD, FASHP. Suggestions are welcome. If you have any questions, you can reach the author at (561)-865-8726 or by e-mail at neil@medabbrev.com.

Discontinued Drugs

The following is a list of products no longer available in the United States because they were discontinued by the manufacturer or withdrawn from the market.

AA-HC Otic
Abarelix
Abbokinase
Absorbine Footcare Spray Liquid
Absorbine Power Gel
AccuHist DM Pediatric Drops
AccuHist Drops
AccuHist LA
AccuHist PDX
AccuHist Pediatric Drops
Accutane
Accuzyme
Accuzyme SE
Accuzyme Topical Spray
Acetazolamide Tablets
Acetest
Acetohexamide
Aci-Jel Vaginal Gel
Aclaro
Acova
Actisite
Activella
Actonel With Calcium
Acular PF
Adapettes
Adeflor M Tablets
ADEKs
Adenosine Phosphate Injection
Adoxa
Adsorbonac
Advanced-RF NatalCare
ADVIA Centaur HBc IgM
Advicor Tablets
Advil Junior Strength Chewable Tablets
Aeroaid
AeroBid
AeroBid-M
Aerocaine
Afrin Children's
Afrin No-Drip Sinus with Vapornase
Afrin No-Drip 12-Hour Severe Congestion With Menthol
Afrin Saline, Extra Moisturizing Solution
Afrin Sinus with Vapornase
Agenerase
Airet
AK-Dex
Akineton Tablets
AK-Nefrin
AK-Pred
AK-Rinse
AK-Spore H.C. Otic
AK-Tracin Ointment
AK-Trol Ophthalmic Ointment
AK-Trol Ophthalmic Suspension
Akwa Tears
Alacol
Alacol DM Drops
Alacol DM Syrup
Alahist AC
Alamast
Albay
Albutussin
Alcohol 5% and Dextrose 5%
Alcon Saline Solution for Sensitive Eyes
Aldex AN
Aldex DM Tannate
Aldoclor 150
Aldoclor 250
Aldoril D50
Aldoril D30
Aldoril-15
Aldoril-25
Alenaze-D
Alenaze-D NR
Alfenta
Alferon N
Alka-Seltzer Plus Flu
Alkets, Extra Strength Antacid, Chewable Tablets
Allanderm-T
AllanEnzyme
AllanfillEnzyme
AllanHist PDX
AllanVan-DM B.I.D.
AllanVan-S B.I.D.
All Clear
All Clear AR
Allercreme Skin Lotion
Allercreme Ultra Emollient Cream
Allerest Maximum Strength
Allerest PE
Allerfrim
Allergan Enzymatic
Allergen Ear Drops
Allergy Drops
AllerTan
AlleRx
AlleRx-D
AlleRx Dose Pack
Allfen DM
Allfen Jr

Allres Pd
Almora Tablets
Alor 5/500 Tablets
Aloxi Capsules
Alpha-Keri Moisturizing Soap Bar
Alphanate
Alphatrex Cream
Altace Tablets
Altazine
Alu-Cap
Aluminum Acetate Astringent
Alupent Aerosol
Alupent Solution for Inhalation
Alu-Tab
Ambenonium Chloride
Ambifed
Ambifed-G
AMBI 40PSE/400GFN
AMBI 1000/55
AMBI 1000/5
AMBI 60/580
AMBI 60PSE/400GFN
Ambi 10 Cream
AMBI 10PEH/400GFN
Ambi 10 Soap
Amcort Injection
Americaine
Americaine Anesthetic Lubricant
Americaine First Aid Burn
Americaine Hemorrhoidal
Americaine Otic Solutions
Amevive Powder for Injection
Amicar Injection
Amigesic
Aminess
Aminess 5.2%
Aminosyn II 5% in 25% Dextrose
Aminosyn II 7% w/Electrolytes
Aminosyn II 3.5% in 25% Dextrose
Amitone Antacid Chewable Tablets
AmLactin
AmLactin AP Topical Cream
Ammonium Chloride Tablets
AMO Endosol
AMO Endosol Extra
AMO Vitrax
Amoxil Capsules
Amoxil Pediatric Drops
Amphocin
AmVaz
AnaMantle HC
AnaMantle HC 2.5%
Anaplex-DM Cough
Anaplex DMX
Anaplex HD Liquid
Anaspaz
Anbesol Baby
Anbesol Jr.
Anbesol Liquid
Ancef Injection
Ancef Powder for Injection
Andehist DM NR
Andehist-DM Syrup
Andehist Drops
Andehist NR
Andehist Syrup
Android
Andryl 200
Anemagen Capsules
Anemagen OB
Anestafoam
Anexsia Tablets
Anextuss Tablets
Ansaid
Antilirium Injection
Antiminth Oral Suspension
Antispas
Antivenin (Crotalidae) Polyvalent Injection
Anturane Capsules
Anturane Tablets
Anturol
Apatate Tablets
Apexicon
Aphthasol
Apra Children's
Apresazide 50/50
Apresazide 100/50
Apresazide 25/25
Aprodine Syrup
AquaBalm Cream
Aquachloral Supprettes
AquaMEPHYTON Injection
Aquaphyllin Syrup
AquaSite Solution
Aquatensen Tablets
Aralast
Aramine Injection
Arduan Powder for Injection
Aredia
Arfonad
Argesic Cream
Argesic-SA
Aristocort
Aristocort A
Aristocort Forte Injection
Aristocort Intralesional Injection
Artha-G
ArthriCare Double Ice Gel

ArthriCare Odor Free Rub
ArthriCare Triple Medicated Gel
Arthropan
Articaine Hydrochloride
Asacol
Ascriptin A/D
Ascriptin Extra Strength
A-Spas S/L
Aspergum
Aspirin/Pravastatin
Astepro
Atarax Syrup
Atolone
Atridox
Atropine-1
Attenuvax
Atuss DS Tannate
Atuss EX Syrup
Atuss G
Atuss HC
Atuss HD
Atuss HS
Atuss HX
Atuss MS
A-200
Augmentin ES-600
Auralgan
Aurothioglucose Injection
Auroto Otic
Autoplex T
Avar-e Green
Avar Gel
Aveeno Cleansing for Acne-Prone Skin
Aventyl Hydrochloride Pulvules
Aventyl Solution
Azathioprine Sodium Injection
Bactine Pain Relieving Cleansing Wipes
Bactrim IV Infusion
Balacall DM
Balacet 325
Balamine DM
Baltussin HC
Banalg
Banalg Hospital Strength Liniment
Barbidonna Tablets
Barbidonna #2 Tablets
BarnesHind Saline for Sensitive Eyes
Baros Granules
BayRab
BayTet
B-C Bid Tablets
Be-Flex Plus
Belladonna Tincture
Bellamine
Bel-Phen-Ergot SR
Benadryl Allergy
Benadryl Children's Allergy & Cold
Benadryl-D Children's Allergy & Sinus
Benadryl Maximum Strength Cream
Benadryl Maximum Strength Solution (Spray)
Bencort
Bengay SPA Cream
Benoquin
Ben-Tann
Benylin Adult Liquid
Benylin Pediatric Liquid
Benzac AC 2.5
Benzac AC Wash 2.5
Benzac W 5
Benzac W 10
Benzac W 2.5
Benzthiazide
Bepridil Hydrochloride
Betadine First Aid Antibiotics Plus Moisturizer Ointment
Betadine Plus First Aid Antibiotics and Pain Reliever Ointment
Betadine Vaginal Gel
Betagen Ointment
Betagen Solution
BetaTan
BetaVent
Betaxon Ophthalmic Suspension
Betoptic
Bextra Tablets
Bexxar Dosimetric Packaging
Bexxar Therapeutic Packaging
Biavax II Powder for Injection
Bicitra Solution
Bicozene
Bidex-A
Bidex-DMI Tablets
Bidhist
Bidhist-D
Big Shot B-12
Bili-Labstix Reagent Strips
Biocef
Bioclate
Biotel Kidney
Biperiden
Bi-Tann DP
Bitolterol Mesylate
B-Ject-100
Blairex Lens Lubricant
Blinx
Bluboro
Bo-Cal

Bonine Chewable Tablets
Boric Acid
Borofair Otic
Borofax Skin Protectant
Boropak Powder Packets
Bottom Better
BP Allergy Junior
BPM PE DM
BP New Allergy DM
BP Poly-650
BranchAmin 4%
Breezee Mist Antifungal
Brethine Injection
Brethine Tablets
Bretylium Tosylate
Brevibloc Double Strength
Bricanyl
Bromaline
Bromaline DM
Bromatan-DM
Bromatan Plus
Bromday
Bromdex D
Bromfenex
Bromfenex PD
Bromhist-NR
Bromhist PDX Drops
Bromhist Pediatric
Bromo Seltzer
Bromphenex DM
Bromphenex HD Liquid
Bromplex HD
Bronchial
Broncholate Syrup
Brondelate
Bronkids
Brontex Tablets
BrōveX
BrōveX CB
BrōveX CBX
BrōveX CT
BrōveX PB
BrōveX PB C
BrōveX PB CX
BrōveX PB DM
BrōveX PD
BrōveX PSB DM
BrōveX SR
Bucet Capsules
Bucladin-S Softabs
Buclizine
Budeprion SR
Budeprion XL
Bumex
B-Vex D
Byclomine
Calan
Calcifediol
Calciferol Injection
Calcium Caseinate
Cal-Nate Tablets
Caltrate 600
Campath
Capitrol
Capoten
Capozide
Carbaphen 12
Carbastat
Carbetapentane Tannate
Carbinoxamine Compound Drops (Pediatric)
Carbinoxamine Compound Syrup
Carbofed DM Syrup
Carboptic
Carb Pseudo-Tan
Carde
Cardec DM Oral Drops
Cardene Capsules
Cardizem SR Capsules
Carmol 40
Carmol Scalp Treatment
Carmol 10
Carmol 20
Cartrol
Cascara Sagrada Tablets
Casec Powder
Ceclor
Ceclor Pulvules
Cefadyl
Cefamandole Nafate
Cefazolin Sodium
Cefizox
Cefobid
Cefol Filmtab
Cefonicid Sodium
Cefotan
Ceftazidime Injection
Cefzil
Celestone Phosphate Injection
Cenogen-OB Capsules
CenogenUltra
Cenolate
Centergy DM
Centrum Jr. +Extra C
Centrum Jr. + Extra Calcium
Centrum Jr. + Iron
Cēpacol Dual Relief Spray Sore Throat & Cough

Cēpacol Sore Throat Dual Relief Spray
Cēpacol Sore Throat From Post Nasal Drip
Cēpacol Sore Throat Maximum Numbing
Cephadrine Oral
Cephadyn
Cephalexin Hydrochloride Monohydrate
Cephapirin Sodium
Ceptaz
Ceredase
Ceron
Ceron-DM
Certagen Senior Tablets
Certa-Vite
Certa-Vite Golden
Cerumenex Drops (Solution)
Cetamide Ophthalmic Ointment
Ceta-Plus
CharcoAid
CharcoAid 2000
Charcoal and Simethicone
Chardonna-2
Chemstrip bG
Chemstrip 8
Chemstrip 4 the OB
Chemstrip 6
Chemstrip uG
Chigger-Tox+
Children's Advil Chewable Tablets
Children's Benadryl Allergy Fastmelt
Chloral Hydrate Syrup
Chloramphenicol
Chloresium Ointment
Chloresium Solution
Chloresium Tablets
Chlorex-A Tablets
Chlorex-A 12 Suspension
Chloromycetin Powder for Solution
Chloromycetin Sodium Succinate I.V.
Chloroptic S.O.P. Ointment
Chlorpheniramine Maleate/Phenylephrine Hydrochloride ER Capsules
Cholac
Choledyl SA Tablets
Cholinoid
Chorex-5
Choron 10
Chromagen
Chroma-Pak
Ciclopirox Cream
Cidex Solution
Cimetidine Injection
Cimetidine in 0.9% Sodium Chloride
Cinoxacin
Cipro I.V. Injection Concentrate
Cipro XR
Citracal Creamy Bites
Citracal Liquitab
CitraNatal Harmony
Claripel
Clean-N-Soak Solution
Clearplan Easy Kit
Clenia Cream
Clenia Foam
Clinacort Injection
ClindaMax Gel
ClindaMax Lotion
Clindets
Clinistix Reagent Strips
Clinitest
Clofazimine
Codal-DH
Codal-DM
Codeine Phosphate Injection
Codeine Phosphate Solution
Codiclear DH
Codimal DH Syrup
Codimal DM
Codimal PH
Cogentin Tablets
Cognex
Coldmist JR
Coldmist LA
Coldonyl
Colfed-A Capsules
Colfosceril Palmitate
Collastin Oil Free Moisturizer
Collyrium Fresh
ComBgen Tablets
Combiflex
Combiflex ES Tablets
Combipres
Combunox
Comfort Eye Drops
Compazine Injection
Compazine Spansules
Compazine Suppositories
Compazine Syrup
Compazine Tablets
Complete
Complete All-In-One
Complete Weekly Enzymatic Cleaner
Computer Eyes
Comtrex Maximum Strength Nighttime Cold & Cough Tablets
Comtussin HC
Conal
Conceive Ovulation Predictor Cassettes
Confide Reagent Kit for HIV Blood Tests

Cordron-D
Cordron-DM NR
Cordron-D NR
Cordron-HC
Cordron-HC NR
Cormax Cream
Cortamox
Cortatrigen Ear
Cortatrigen Modified Ear Drops
Cortisporin Ophthalmic Suspension
Cortisporin Otic
Cortizone•5 Cream
Corzall
Corzall Plus
Cotrim Pediatric
Cotuss EX
Cotuss HD
Cotuss MS
Coughtuss Liquid
Cough-X Lozenges
CP DEC
CP DEC-DM Drops
C-Phen
C-Phen DM
Crantex
Creamy Tar Shampoo
Crolom
Crysti 1000
C-Tan D
C-Tan D Plus Oral Suspension
C-Tanna 12D
Cuticura Medicated Shampoo
Cuticura Medicated Soap
Cyclocort
Cyklokapron Tablets
Cysto-Conray
Cysto-Conray II
Cystospaz-M Capsules
Cytadren
Cytosar-U Powder for Injection
Cytovene Capsules
Cytoxan
Cytoxan Lyophilized
Cytuss HC
Cytuss-HC NR
Dacriose
Dalalone DP
Dallergy DM
Dallergy JR
Dallergy PE
Danocrine Capsules
Dapiprazole Hydrochloride
Daranide
Darpaz
Darvocet A500
Darvocet-N 50
Darvocet-N 100
Darvon Compound 32
Darvon-N
Darvon Pulvules
Dayalets Filmtabs Tablets
Dazamide Tablets
Debrisan
Decadron Tablets
Decaject-L.A.
De-Chlor HC
De-Chlor MR
De-Chlor NX
Deconamine SR
Deconamine Syrup
Deconex
Deconex IR
Deconomed SR
Deconsal CT
Deconsal II
Defen-LA Tablets
Defy
Degas
Degest 2
Delatest
Delatestryl
Delcort Cream
Deltasone
Demadex Intravenous Solution
Demecarium Bromide
Demulen 1/50
Demulen 1/35
DentiPatch
depMedalone 80
depMedalone 40
Deponit Transdermal Patch
Depopred-80
Depopred-40
Dep-Test
Dermacoat Aerosol
Dermal-Rub Balm
Derma Viva Lotion
Desenex Antifungal, Maximum Strength
Desenex Max
Desenex Powder
Desenex Spray
Despec
Despec Drops
Despec-Tab
Desquam-E 5 Gel
Desquam-X 5
Desquam-X 10 Gel
Desyrel

Desyrel Dividose
Detussin
Dexacine Ophthalmic Ointment
Dexasol
Dexasone L.A. Injection
Dexedrine
Dexone LA
Dexphen w/C
Dextran 70
Dextran 75 Injection
Dex-Tuss
Dex-Tuss DM
Diabinese Tablets
Diamox Tablets
Diasorb
Diastix Reagent Strips
Diatrizoate Meglumine 52% and Diatrizoate Sodium 8%
Diatrizoate Sodium 50%
Diazoxide, Parenteral
Dibent
Dical-D
Dicel
Dicel DM Suspension
Dichlorphenamide
Dicomal DH
Didronel IV Injection
Diethylcarbamazine Citrate
Difil-G forte
Diflucan Injection
Digex
Digibind
Digitek Tablets
Dihistine DH
Dihydrocodeine 3 mg/BPM 4 mg/Phenylephrine Hydrochloride 7.5 mg
DiHydro-CP
DiHydro-PE
Dilacor XR
Dilantin Kapseals
Dilomine
Dilor
Diltia XT
Diltiazem Hydrochloride Tablets
Dimaphen
Dimetane DX
Dimetapp Toddler's Decongestant Plus Cough
Dinate
Diocto C
DiphenMax D
Diphtheria and Tetanus Toxoids, Acellular Pertussis, Haemophilus Influenzae Type B Conjugate Vaccine
Dipivefrin Hydrochloride Ophthalmic Solution
Di-Spaz
Ditropan Syrup
Ditropan Tablets
Diucardin Tablets
Diurigen
Diurigen w/Reserpine 500
Diurigen w/Reserpine 250
Diuril Sodium Intravenous
Diutensen-R
Dobutrex Injection
Dolobid
Dolorac
Dolsed
Domeboro
Donatussin DC
Dopar
Doryx Coated Pellets Delayed-Release Capsules
Dostinex
Dovonex Solution
Doxacurium Chloride
Doxidan
Doxy 200
D-Phen 1000
Dramamine, Children's
Dramamine Liquid
Dristan Fast Acting Formula
Drixomed Tablets
Drotic
Drotrecogin Alfa (Activated)
DroTuss
Dry Eyes Solution
Dryvax
D-Tab
D-Tann
D-Tann AT
D-Tann CD
D-Tann CT
D-Tann DM
D-Test 100
D-Test 200
Duadacin Extra Strength Cold and Flu Tablets
Duet
Duet DHA
Duet DHA ec
Duohist DH
DURAcare II
Duradrin
Duradryl JR Capsules
Durahist
Durahist D

Duraphen II
DuraTan DM
DuraTan Forte
DuraTan PE
Durathate-200 Injection
Duratuss
Duratuss A
Duratuss AC 12 Tannate
Duratuss CS
Duratuss DM
Duratuss GP
Duratuss HD
Duratuss PE Tablets
Durese Tablets
Duricef
Dur-Tann DM
Dyclone
Dyclonine Hydrochloride
Dyline-GG Liquid
Dynabac
DynaCirc
Dynatuss DF
Dynex
Dynex LA
Dynex VR
Dytan
Dytan-CD Suspension
Dytan-CS
Dytan-D
Ear Drops
Ear-Eze
Econopred
Econopred Plus
Ed A-Hist Tablets
ED Chlor-Ped D
ED-TLC
ED Tuss HC
E.E.S. 200
Effervescent Potassium
Effexor
Efudex Occlusion Pack
Elixomin
Elixophyllin GG
Elixophyllin-KI
Elspar
Embeda
Embeline
Embeline E
EMLA Anesthetic Disc
EndaCof
EndaCof-AC
EndaCof-DH
EndaCof DM
EndaCof-PD
EndaCof XP
Endagen-HD
Endal CD
Endal HD
Endal HD Plus
Endal (Nasal Decongestant) Tablets
Endrate Injection
Enduronyl
Enlon Injection
Enlon Plus
Entex HC
Entex LA
Entex Liquid
Entex PSE
EntroEase
EntroEase Dry
Entuss
Enzymatic Cleaner for Extended Wear
Ephedrine Sulfate
Epifrin Solution
Epinal Solution
Epinephrine Hydrochloride Ophthalmic Solution
Epinephrine Hydrochloride Solution
Epinephrine Mist
Epinephryl Borate
Ergamisol Tablets
Ergonovine Maleate
Ergotrate
Eryc
Erygel Gel
Eryzole
Esclim Transdermal System
Esidrix Tablets
Eskalith Tablets
Estar Gel
Estratest
Estratest H.S.
Estrostep 21
Ethaquin
Ethatab
Ethaverine
Ethavex-100
EtheDent Chewable Tablets
Ethezyme
Ethezyme 830
Ethiodol
Ethmozine
ETH-Oxydose
Etrafon (2-10)
Eulexin Capsules
Exact Solution
Excedrin Aspirin Free
ExeClear-C

ExeClear-DM
ExeFen DMX
ExeFen-PD
Exelon Solution
ExeTuss
ExeTuss GP
Ex-Histine
Exna Tablets
Exocaine Plus
Exosurf Neonatal
Extendryl DM
Extendryl G
Extendryl JR
Extendryl SR
Extra Strength Alenic Alka
Extra Strength Dynafed EX
Exubra
Eye Irrigating Wash
Factrel
Fansidar
FemBack Caplets
Femiron Multivitamin and Iron Tablets
Fem-1
Femtrace
Fentanyl Iontophoretic Transdermal System
FeoGen FA
Feostat Tablets, Chewable
Feratab
Fer-Gen-Sol
Feridex I.V.
Ferrex 150 Forte Plus
Ferumoxsil
Fe-Tinic 150
Flagyl IV
Flagyl IV RTU Injection
Flatulex Tablets
Fleet Phospho-Soda
Fleet Prep Kit 1
Fleet Prep Kit 2
Flexaphen
Flex-Care Especially for Sensitive Eyes
Flexeril
Flextra-DS
Flovent Aerosol
Flovent Diskus
Flovent Rotadisk
Floxin Injection
Fludara
Fluorescein Sodium Ophthalmic Solution
Fluori-Methane Spray
Fluor-Op
Fluothane
Flu-Oxinate
Flurate
Flurosyn Ointment
FluTuss HC Liquid
Foamicon
Foille
Foille Plus
Fomivirsen Sodium
Fortovase
Fosamax Oral Solution
Foscavir
Fostril Lotion
4-Way Long Acting Nasal Spray
FreAmine III 8.5% w/Electrolytes
Fumatinic
Fungizone Intravenous
Furacin Soluble Dressing Ointment
Furacin Topical Solution
Furoxane
Gamimune N Injection
Gammar-P I.V.
Gamunex
Ganciclovir Capsules
Ganite
Gani-Tuss-DM NR
Gani-Tuss NR
Gantrisin
Gantrisin Pediatric
Garamycin Injection
Garamycin Ointment
Garamycin Solution
Gas Permeable Daily Cleaner
GastroMARK
Gelclair
Genahist Tablets
Genapap, Children's Elixir
Genapap Extra Strength Tablets
Genapap Infants' Drops
Genaphed Plus
Genasoft
Genaspor Antifungal
Genatuss DM
Genebs
Genebs Extra Strength
GenESA
Geneye Extra
Geneye Ophthalmic Solution
Genoptic
Genoptic S.O.P.
Genotropin Powder for Injection
Genpril
Gentacidin
Gentex HC
Gentex LA
Gentlax Tablets
Gentran 70

Geocillin
Geref
Gerivite Tablets
Gevral Protein
GFN 550/PSE 60/DM 30
GFN 1000/DM 60
GFN 1200/DM 60
Gilphex TR
Gladase
Gladase-C
Glaucon Solution
Glutamic Acid Powder
Glutamic Acid Tablets
Glutethimide
Glutofac-ZX
Glyceryl-T
Gonic
Gonioscopic
GP-500
Granul-Derm
Griseofulvin Microsize
GUAI 800 mg/DM 30 mg
Guaifed
Guaifed-PD
Guaifenesin DM 1000/60
Guaifenex DM
Guaifenex GP
Guaifenex G Tablets (Sustained-release)
Guaifenex LA Tablets (Extended-release)
Guaifenex PSE 85
Guaifenex PSE 120
GuaiMAX-D
Guanabenz Acetate
Guanethidine Monosulfate
Guaphenyl LA
Guiatuss AC
Guiatuss CF Syrup
Guiatuss-DM
Guiatuss PE Liquid
Gynazole-1
Gynodiol
Gynol II Contraceptive
Haldol Decanoate 50
Halenol Children's
Halfan Tablets
HalfLytely
Halofantrine Hydrochloride
Halog Cream
Halotestin Tablets
Halotussin AC Liquid
Halotussin DAC Syrup
Haltran
Hamamelis Water
Healon Yellow Solution
Hemotene
Hepatic-Aid II Instant Drink Powder
Hexabrix
Hexadrol Phosphate
Hibiclens
Hibiclens Sponge Brush
HibTITER
Histacol DM Pediatric Syrup
Histamax D
Hista-Vent DA
Histex
Histex HC
Histex SR
Histinex-D
Histinex HC
Histinex PV
Histolyn-CYL
Histussin D
Histussin HC
Hivid
HMS
Human Albumin Microspheres
Humibid DM Tablets
Humorsol
Humulin 50/50
Humulin L
Humulin U
Hyate:C (Porcine)
Hycodan
Hycotuss Expectorant
Hydase
Hydeltrasol Injection
Hydergine LC
Hydex PD
Hydrap-ES
Hydrate
Hydrocet Capsules
Hydrochlorothiazide/Hydralazine
Hydro Cobex Injection
Hydrocodone Bitartrate and Guaifenesin
Hydrocortone Phosphate Injection
Hydro-Crysti-12 Injection
Hydro-DP
HydroFed
Hydroflumethiazide
Hydro GP
Hydromal
Hydron CP Syrup
Hydron EX
Hydron KGS
Hydron PSC
Hydro-PC II
Hydro-Serp
Hydroserpine

Hydro-Tussin DM Liquid
Hydro-Tussin HC
Hydro-Tussin HD Liquid
Hydro-Tussin HG
Hydro-Tussin XP
Hydroxocobalamin Crystalline
Hydroxyethylcellulose
Hydroxyprogesterone Caproate in Oil
Hygroton
Hy-KXP
Hylaform
Hylorel Tablets
Hylutin Injection
Hypaque-Cysto
Hypaque Meglumine 60%
Hypaque Sodium
Hypaque Sodium 50%
Hyperstat IV Injection
Hyphed
HypoTears PF
Hytakerol Capsules
HyTan Suspension
Hytinic Capsules
Hytone Lotion
Hytuss
Hytuss 2X
Iberet
Iberet-500 Filmtab
Iberet-Folic-500 Filmtab
Icy Hot Stick
Ilotycin
Imovax Rabies I.D.
Impruv Deep Moisturizing
Impruv Natural Repair
Imuran Injection
Inamrinone Lactate
Inapsine
Indamix DM
Inderide
Inderide LA Capsules
Indocin Capsules
Indocin SR
Indocin Suppositories
Indocyanine Green
Inflamase Forte
Inflamase Mild
Influenza A (H1N1) 2009 Monovalent Vaccine
Innohep
Insulin Zinc (Pork)
Intrauterine Progesterone Contraceptive System
Intropin Injection
Inversine
Iobid DM
Iodotope
Ionamin
Ionil-T Plus Shampoo
Ionsys
Iopanoic Acid Iodine
Iophylline
Iosal II
Iothalamate Meglumine
Ioxaglate Meglumine 39.3% and Ioxaglate Sodium 19.6%
Iplex Injection
Iquix
Ircon-FA
Iressa
Ismotic
Isochron
Isoetharine Hydrochloride
Isordil Tembid Tablets
Isuprel Injection
Itchy Eye Drops
Iveegam EN
JE-VAX
J-Max
J-Tan D
J-Tan D HC Liquid
Kantrex
Kaopectate, Maximum Strength
Kapectolin Suspension
Kay Ciel Liquid
Kay Ciel Packets
Keftab
Kemadrin Tablets
Kemstro
Kenaject-40
Kenalog-H
Keralac
Keralac Nailstik
Keri Crème Cream
Keri Light Lotion
Kerol
Kerol AD
Kerol ZX
Keto-Diastix Reagent Strips
Ketostix Reagent Strips
Key-Plex Injection
Key-Pred 50
Key-Pred-SP
Key-Pred 25
K-Lease Capsules
Kleen-Handz
K-Lyte/Cl 25
K-Norm Capsules
Kolephrin GG/DM

Kolyum Liquid
Kovia 6.5
K-Pek
K-Phos M.F.
K + Care
K + Care ET
K + 8
K-Tan
K-Tan 4
Kuric
Kutapressin Injection
Kutrase
Ku-Zyme Capsules
Ku-Zyme HP Capsules
Kwelcof
LactiCare
LactiCare-HC
Lactinol-E Creme
Lactocal-F
Lactrex 12%
Lagesic
Lamprene
Lanoxicaps
Larodopa Tablets
LA-12
LC-65 Solution
Lens Drops
Lens Lubricant
Lens Plus Daily Cleaner
Lens Plus Rewetting Drops
Lente Iletin II Injection
Leustatin
Levall 5.0
Levall 12
Levamisole Hydrochloride
Levlen
Levlite
Levobetaxolol Hydrochloride
Levobupivacaine Hydrochloride
Levocabastine Hydrochloride Ophthalmic Suspension
Levo-Dromoran
Levomethadyl Acetate Hydrochloride
Levsinex Timecaps
Lexxel Extended-Release Tablets
Librium
LidaMantle
LidaMantle HC Relief
Lidocaine Hydrochloride/Hydrocortisone Acetate
Lidosense 4
Lid Wipes-SPF
Lipomul
Liposyn II 20%
Lipram
Lipram 4500 Delayed-Release Capsules
Lipram-PN16 Delayed-Release Capsules
Lipram-PN10 Delayed-Release Capsules
Lipram-PN20 Delayed-Release Capsules
LiQUADD
Liquibid-D
Liquibid-D 1200 Tablets
Liquibid-PD
Liquifilm Tears
Liquifilm Wetting Solution
Liquiprin
Little Noses Gentle Formula, Infants & Children
Liver Derivative Complex
LiveTan DM
Livostin
Lobac Capsules
Lodine Capsules
Lodine XL Tablets
Lodrane
Lodrane D
Lodrane 12 D
Lodrane 24 D
LoHist-LQ
LoHist-PD Pediatric
LoHist 12D
LoKara
Lomefloxacin Hydrochloride
Long Acting Neo-Synephrine II Nose Drops and Nasal Spray
Long Acting Neo-Synephrine II Vapor Spray
Loniten Tablets
Lorabid
Lorcet-HD
Lortab ASA
Lortab 5/500
Lortab 7.5/500
Lortab 10/500
Lortab 2.5/500
Lortuss DM Liquid
Lortuss HC Liquid
Losopan
Losopan Plus
Lotrimin AF Lotion
Lotrimin AF Solution
Lozol
Lubriderm Bath Oil
Lubriderm Cream
Lucidex Tablets
Lufyllin Elixir
Lufyllin-GG Tablets
Lufyllin Injection
Lunelle Injection

Lupron
Lusedra
Lusonal
Luveris
Maalox Antacid/Calcium Supplement Tablets, Chewable
Maalox Antacid Caplets
Maalox Antidiarrheal Tablets
Maalox Antigas Extra Strength Liquid
Maalox Extra Strength Suspension
Maalox Extra Strength Tablets
Maalox Maximum Strength Quick Dissolve Chewable Tablets
Maalox Plus Extra Strength Chewable Tablets
Maalox Plus Tablets
Maalox Quick Dissolve Chewable Tablets
Maalox Suspension
Maalox Tablets
Maalox TC Suspension
Maalox Therapeutic Concentrate Suspension
Macrodex
Magaldrate Plus Suspension
Mag-Cal Tablets
Mag-Caps Capsules
Maginex DS Powder
Maginex Tablets, Enteric-coated
Magnacet
Magnaprin
Magnaprin Arthritis Strength
Magsal
Mallamint Chewable Tablets
Mallazine Eye Drops
Maltsupex Liquid
Maltsupex Tablets
Mandelamine Tablets
Mandol
Maolate
Mapap Infant
Maranox
Marax-DF Syrup
Marax Tab
Marcof Expectorant
Marlin Salt System
Marthritic
Maxaquin Tablets
Maxifed
Maxifed-G
Maxiflu G Tablets
Maximum Strength Allergy Drops
Maximum Strength Anbesol Gel
Maximum Strength Desenex Antifungal
Maxiphen G Tablets
Maxipime
Maxi-Tuss HCG
Maxi-Tuss HCX
Maxivate Lotion
Maxolon
MD-Gastroview Solution
Measles Virus Vaccine, Live Attenuated
Mebaral
Mecasermin Rinfabate
Meda Cap
Medacote
Meda Tab
MED-DM Tablets
Medent-DM
Medent-LDI
Medent PE
Medent PEI
Medicone Ointment
Medicone Suppositories
Medigesic
Mediquell
Medroxyprogesterone Acetate/Estradiol Cypionate
Mefenamic Acid
Mefoxin
Megaton Elixir
Mellaril (all products)
M-End Liquid
M-End Max Liquid
Meni-D
Meperidine Hydrochloride and Promethazine Hydrochloride
Mephentermine
Mephenytoin
Meprozine
Mercurochrome Solution
Mersol Tincture
Meruvax II
Mescolor Tablets
Mesoridazine Besylate
Mestinon Injection
Metahydrin Tablets
Metalone T.B.A.
Metaproterenol Sulfate Solution for Inhalation
Metaraminol Bitartrate
Metatensin
Methalgen
Methenamine Mandelate
Methergine
Methitest Tablets
Methocarbamol Injection
Methoxyflurane
Methyclodine

Methylin ER
Methylin Tablets
Meticorten
Metoclopramide Intensol Concentrated Solution
Metreton Ophthalmic Solution
Micatin Aerosol Spray
Micatin Powder
Miconazole 7
Micro-Guard Powder
Micro-K LS
Micronase Tablets
microNefrin
Migragesic IDA
Mimyx
Mini Two Way Action Tablets
Minizide
Minocin Powder for Injection
Mintezol
MiraSept Disinfecting Solution
MiraSept Rinse and Neutralizer
MiraSept Step 2
Mircera
Mivacron
Moban
Mobigesic Tablets
Moctanin Infusion
Molypen
Momexin
Monarc-M
Monistat-Derm Cream
Monistat-Derm Lotion
Mono-Chlor Liquid
Monochloroacetic Acid
Monocid
Monoctanoin
MouthKote P/R (all products)
MSTA Injection
M.T.E.-5
M.T.E.-5 Concentrated
M.T.E.-4
M.T.E.-4 Concentrated
M.T.E.-7
M.T.E.-6
M.T.E.-6 Concentrated
Mucomyst
Mucosil-10 Solution
Mucosil-20 Solution
Mucus Relief DM
Mudrane
Mudrane GG
Mudrane GG-2
MulTE-PAK-5
MulTE-PAK-4
Multistix SG Reagent Strips
Mumps Skin Test Allergen
Mumpsvax
Murocel Solution
Murocoll-2
Mutamycin
Mycelex-3
Myci-GC
MyDex
MyHist-PD
Mylanta Children's
Mylanta Double Strength Liquid
Mylanta Double Strength Tablets
Mylanta Gas
Mylanta Gas Maximum Strength
Mylanta Gelcaps
Mylanta Lozenges
Mylanta Regular Strength
Mylanta Supreme
Mylanta Tablets
Mylanta Ultra Tabs
Mylocel Tablets
Mylotarg
Myochrysine
Mytelase
Mytrex (all products)
Mytussin AC Cough
Mytussin DAC
Nafazair
NalDex
Nalex-A
Nalex AC
Nalex-A 12
Nalex DH Liquid
Nalex Expectorant
Nalfrx
Nalmefene Hydrochloride
Naphazoline Plus
Naphcon Forte
Naqua Tablets
Narcan
Nariz
Nasacort AQ
Nasarel
Nasatab LA
Nasofed
Nasop Orally Disintegrating Tablets
NataChew
NataFort
Nata Komplete
NatalCare Plus
Natalizumab
NataTab CFe
NataTab Rx

Natru-Vent
Naturetin
Nazarin
Nazarin HC
Nebcin
NegGram
Nembutal Elixir
NeoBenz Micro
NeoDecadron Ophthalmic Solution
Neo-Dexameth
Neo HC
Neoloid Emulsion
Neopap
Neosar Injection
Neosporin AF Aerosol Spray
Neosporin Ophthalmic Ointment
NeoStrata Skin Lightening
Neo-Synephrine
Neo-Synephrine 12-Hour
Neotic
Nephro-Fer
Nephro-Vite + Fe Tablets
Netilmicin Sulfate
Neupro
Neurodep-Caps
Neutra-Phos-K Powder Packets
Neutra-Phos Powder Packets
Neutrexin
Nexiclon XR
Nicomide
Nicosyn Lotion
Nicotrol Transdermal System
Niferex Capsules
Niferex-PN
Nilstat Cream
Nilstat Ointment
Nimotop Capsules
Nitrofurazone Ointment
Nitrofurazone Topical Solution
Nitroglyn Capsules
Nitrong Tablets
NitroQuick
NitroTab
Nizoral Tablets
N-Multistix Reagent Strips
N-Multistix SG
NoHist
NoHist DMX
NoHist-PDX
Nolahist Tablets
Nolvadex
Nomuc-PE
Norel DM
Norel EX
Normodyne Injection
Norplant
Notuss-AC
Notuss-DC
Notuss-Forte
Notuss NX
Notuss NXD
Notuss-PE
Novacet Lotion
Novamine 15%
Novantrone
Novasal Tablets
Novasus
Novocain Solution
NovoLog Mix 70/30 Injection
NPH Iletin II
Nucofed
Nucofed Expectorant
Nucofed Pediatric Expectorant
Nucofed Syrup
Numorphan
Numzident
Numzit Teething Gel
Nupercainal Cream
Nuprin
Nuprin Backache
Nuromax Injection
NutriDox
Nutropin Depot Injection
Nystatin Vaginal Tablets
Ny-Tannic
OCL
Octagam
Octamide PFS
Octicair
OcuClear
OcuCoat PF Solution
OcuCoat Solution
Ocupress Solution
Ocusert Pilo-40
Ocusert Pilo-20
Ocusulf-10
Oforta
Ogen Tablets
Ogen Vaginal
Omnicef
Omontys
OncoScint
Ontak
Onxol
Ony-Clear Solution
Ophthaine
Opti-Clean Solution
Opti-Clean II

Opti-Soft
Optison
Opti-Tears
Opti-Zyme Enzymatic Cleaner Especially for Sensitive Eyes
Orabase Gel
Orasone
Oravig
Oraxyl
Oretic Tablets
Organidin NR
Orinase
Orinase Diagnostic
ORLAAM
Ornex No Drowsiness Maximum Strength
Orthoclone OKT3
Ortho-Est
Ortho-Novum 1/50
Ortho-Novum 10/11
Or-Tyl
Orudis
Orudis KT Tablets
Oruvail
Osmoglyn
Otic-Care
Oti-Med
OtiTricin
Otobiotic Otic
Otocalm Ear
Otocort
Otomycin-HPN
Ovcon-50
Ovrette
OvuGen Kit
OvuKIT Self-Test Kit
OvuQuick Self-Test Kit
Oxacillin Sodium Oral Solution
Oxecta
Oxysept Disinfecting Solution
Oxysept Neutralizer Tablets
Oxysept 2
P_4E_1 Solution
P_1E_1 Solution
P_6E_1 Solution
P_2E_1 Solution
Pacis Powder for Suspension
Packer's Pine Tar
Pain-X
Palcaps 20
Palladone
Palmitate-A 5000
Pamelor Oral Solution
Panacet 5/500 Tablets
Panadol, Children's
Panafil
Panafil SE
Panalgesic Cream
Panasal 5/500 Tablets
Panasol-S
Panatuss DX Liquid
Pan C Ascorbate
Pancof-HC Syrup
Pancof PD Syrup
Pancrease
Pancrecarb MS-8
Pancrecarb MS-4
Pancrecarb MS-16
Pancrelipase Tablets
Pangestyme CN 10 Delayed-Release Capsules
Pangestyme CN 20 Delayed-Release Capsules
Pangestyme EC Delayed-Release Capsules
Pangestyme MT 16 Delayed-Release Capsules
Pangestyme UL 18 Delayed-Release Capsules
Pangestyme UL 12 Delayed-Release Capsules
Pangestyme UL 20 Delayed-Release Capsules
Panlor SS
Pannaz
Pannaz S
Panocaps
Panocaps MT 16
Panocaps MT 20
Panokase Tablets
PanOxyl 5
PanOxyl 10
PAN-2400
Papain-Urea-Chlorophyllin
Papfyll
Pap-Urea Ointment
Paraldehyde
Paral Liquid
Paraplatin
Paredrine
PBM Allergy
P Chlor DM
P Chlor GG
PCM Allergy
PD-Cof Drops
PD-Cof Syrup
PD-Hist • D
Pedameth Liquid
PediaCare Children's Decongestant
PediaCare Children's NightRest Multi-Symptom Cold

Pediaflor Fluoride Drops
Pediahist DM Drops
PediaPhyl D
PediaTan
PediaTan D
Pediatex-CT
Pediatric Bear-E-Bag
Pediatric Triban
Pediazole Granules for Oral Suspension
Pedi-Boro Soak Paks
Pediotic
PE/GG
PE-GUAI
Pemoline
Pentobarbital Sodium Capsules
Pentothal Injection
Pepcid Injection
Perchloracap
Percodan-Demi
Perdiem Overnight Relief
Periactin
Periostat
Permax
Perphenazine Oral Concentrate
Persantine IV
Pfizerpen Injection
Phenabid DM
PhenaVent Capsules
PhenaVent D
PhenaVent LA
PhenaVent PED
Phenerbel-S
Phenergan Suppositories
Phenindamine Tartrate
Phenoptic
Phentermine Resin Complex
Phenylephrine Complex
Phenylephrine Tannate, Chlorpheniramine Tannate and Pyrilamine Tannate
Phenylgesic
Phenyltoloxamine PE CPM
Phenyl-T Oral Suspension
pHisoDerm Cleansing Bar
P-Hist
Phosphocol P 32
Phrenilin
Pilocar
Pilocarpine and Epinephrine Solutions (Ophthalmic Agents for Glaucoma)
Pilopine HS
Pipecuronium Bromide
Piperacillin Sodium Injection
Pitressin Injection
Plaquenil
Plaretase 8000
Platinol-AQ Injection
Plenaxis Powder for Injection
Plendil Extended-Release Tablets
Pneumococcal 7-Valent Conjugate Vaccine
Pneumotussin 2.5 Cough
Pnu-Imune 23 Injection
PNV-DHA Plus
PNV-Iron
Polocaine With Levonordefrin Injection
Polycitra-K Solution
Polycitra-LC Oral Solution
Polycitra Syrup
Polygam S/D
Poly-Hist HC
Poly-Histine
Poly-Hist PD
Polymyxin B Ophthalmic
Polymyxin B Sulfate Sterile Powder for Solution
Poly-Pred Liquifilm
Polysorb Hydrate
Polysporin Ointment
Polysporin Ophthalmic
Polysporin Powder
Poly Tan D
Polythiazide Potassium Perchlorate
Poly-Tussin HD
Poly-Tussin XP
Poly-Vent
Poly-Vent IR
Poly-Vent JR
Poly-Vent Plus
Polyvitamins w/Fluoride 0.5 mg and Iron
Potassium Perchlorate
Pramoxine HC
Pravigard PAC
Prax Cream
Predalone 50 Injection
Predcor-50
Prednicen-M
Prednisol
Prednisol TBA
Prefrin Liquifilm
Pre-Hist-D
Prelone Syrup
PremesisRx
Prenatal-H Capsules
Prenatal MR 90
Prenatal-1 + Iron
Prenatal Plus Improved
Prenatal Plus w/Betacarotene
Prenatal Rx 1
Prenatal S

Prenatal Vitamins Plus
Prenatal Z Advanced Formula
Prenate GT Tablets
Pre-Pen
Pretz-D Solution
Prevacid IV
Prevacid NapraPAC 500
Prevacid NapraPAC 375
Preven
Prevnar
Primacor Injection
Primatene Mist Aerosol Inhalation
Principen
Pro-Banthine
Procainamide Hydrochloride Capsules
Procainamide Hydrochloride Extended-Release Tablets
Procaine Hydrochloride Solution
Procanbid
Prochieve
Pro-Clear
ProctoCream-HC 2.5%
ProctoFoam
Procyclidine
Profasi
Pro-Fast SA Tablets
Profenal
ProFree/GP Weekly Enzymatic Cleaner
Progestasert Intrauterine System
Prolex DH
Prolex DM
Prolex DMX
Prolixin Decanoate
Prometh VC Plain
Promit
ProMod Powder
Pronestyl
Propine Sterile Ophthalmic
Proplex T Injection
Propoxyphene Hydrochloride and Acetaminophen
Propoxyphene Napsylate and Acetaminophen
Proquin XR
Pro-Red
ProSom
Prostigmin
Protirelin
Protropin Powder for Injection
Protuss-D Liquid
Protuss DM Tablets
Protuss Liquid
Proventil Aerosol
Proventil Repetabs Tablets
Proventil Tablets
PSE BPM
PSE Brom DM
PSE CPM
PSE 15/CPM 2
Pseudo Carb Pediatric
Pseudovent Capsules
Pseudovent-PED Capsules
Psoriatec
PsoriGel Gel
P-Tanna 12 Suspension
P-Tann D Suspension
P.T.E.-5
P.T.E.-4
Pulmicort Turbuhaler
Puralube Ophthalmic Ointment
Purge Liquid (castor oil)
P-V-Tussin Syrup
P-V-Tussin Tablets
Pyrelle H.B.
Pyridiate
Q-Tapp
QTest Ovulation Kit
Q-Tussin CF Liquid
Q-Tussin PE
Quadra-Hist D
Quadra-Hist D PED
Quad Tann Pediatric Oral Suspension
Quad-Tuss Tannate Pediatric
Qualaquin
Qual-Tussin DC
Qual-Tussin Pediatric Oral Solution Drops
Quibron
Quibron-T Dividose
Quibron-300
Quibron-T/SR Dividose
Quick CARE Disinfecting Solution
Quick CARE Rinse and Neutralizer
Quinidex Extentabs Tablets
Raniclor
Raptiva
Rauwolfia/Bendroflumethiazide
Rauzide
Rebetron
RE DCP
Redness Reliever
Redur-PCM
Redutemp
Refludan
Reglan Injection
Regular Iletin II Injection
Regular Insulin (Pork)
Regulax SS
Relacon-HC NR

Relafen
Relagesic Liquid
Relasin-HC
Relefact RTH
Relief Ophthalmic Solution
Reluri
Reme Hist DM
Renacidin
RenAmin
Renese-R
Renese Tablets
Reno-Dip
Renografin-60
Reno-60
Reno-30
ReNu Effervescent Enzymatic Cleaner
ReNu Thermal Enzymatic Cleaner
Repan CF
Replens Gel
Repliva 21/7
Rescula Solution
Resectisol
Respa-DM
Respa-1st
Respahist
Respahist-II
Respaire-120 SR
Respaire-60 SR
Respbid Tablets
Resperal
Respi-Tann
Respi-Tann G Suspension
Respi-Tann Pd
Retin-A Solution
RE2+30
RE-U40
Revex
Rēv-Eyes Lyophilized Powder
Rexolate
R-Gel
Rheaban Maximum Strength Tablets
Rhinacon A
Ridenol
RID Mousse
Rinade-B.I.D. Capsules
Rindal HD Plus Syrup
Rindal HPD Syrup
Rinnovi Nail System
Riopan
Ritodrine Hydrochloride
Robafen DM Max
Robitussin Cough & Allergy
Robitussin PE Head and Chest Congestion
Rofecoxib
Roferon-A
Romilar AC
Rondec
Rondec DM Drops
Rondex
Rosac
Rosets
Rosula
Rosula Clarifying Wash
Rosula Cleanser
Rosula NS
R-Tanna
R-Tanna Pediatric
R-Tanna 12
R-Tannic-S A/D Suspension
Rubella and Mumps Virus Vaccine, Live
Rulox #1 Tablets
Rulox #2 Tablets
Rum-K
Ryna-C Liquid
Ryna Liquid
Rynatan
Rynatan Pediatric
Rynatuss
Ryna-12
Ryna-12 S
Ryna-12X
Rynesa 12S
Ryneze
RY-T-12
Ryzolt
Safetussin CD
Sal-Acid
Salflex
Salsitab
Sal-Tropine
Salutensin
Salutensin-Demi
Sanctura XR
Sarna Ultra
Scopace
Seasonale
SecreFlo Intravenous Solution
Sele-Pak
Selepen
Senna Concentrate
Septi-Soft
Septisol
Septocaine Injection
Septra
Septra DS
Septra IV
Seradex-LA
Ser-Ap-Es

Serax
Serentil Tablets
Sermorelin Acetate
Servira
Serzone Tablets
Severe Congestion Tussin
SFC
Sildec
Sildec DM
Silfedrine, Children's
Sil-Tex
Silver Nitrate
Simethicone-Coated Cellulose Suspension
Simuc-GP
Simuc-HD
Simuc Sustained-Release Tablets
Sina-12X
Sinequan Oral Concentrate
Sinuhist
Sinutab Non-Drying
Sinutab Sinus Allergy, Maximum Strength
SINUvent PE
Sitrex
Sitrex PD
Skelaxin Tablets
Slo-Phyllin GG Capsules
Slo-Phyllin GG Syrup
Slo-Phyllin Gyrocaps Capsules
Slow FE
Slow-K Tablets
SLT Lotion
Sno Strips Test
Soac-Lens Solution
Sodium Bicarbonate and Tartaric Acid
Sodium Bicarbonate Injection
Sodium Hyaluronate and Fluorescein Sodium
Sodium Hyaluronate Gel and Lotion
Sodium Phosphate P 32 Injection
Sodium Thiosalicylate
Sofenol 5 Lotion
Solagé
Solganal Injection
Solotuss Suspension
Soltamox
Solurex
Solurex LA
Soluvite-F Drops
Soma Compound
Soma Compound w/Codeine
Somatrem
Sonahist
SonoRx
Soothe Solution
Sorbitrate Chewable Tablets
Sorbitrate Sublingual Tablets
Sorbitrate Tablets
Soriatane CK
Sotalol Hydrochloride Injection
Sparfloxacin
Spectazole
Spectinomycin
Spectrocin Plus Ointment
Spherulin
Stadol
Stadol NS Solution
Staflex
Stamoist E
Statuss Green
Stay-Wet 4
Stay-Wet 3
Sterapred
Sterapred DS
Sterapred-Unipak
SteriNail
Strema
Streptase
Sublimaze
Suboxone Sublingual Tablets
Subutex
Suby's Solution G
Succus Cineraria Maritima Solution
Sudafed Children's Non-Drowsy Cold & Cough
Sudafed PE Nighttime Nasal Decongestant
Sudafed PE Quick-Dissolve Strips
Sudafed Sinus & Cold Non-Drowsy
Sudal 60/500 Tablets
Sudal-12 Tannate Chewable Tablets
SudaTex-DM
SudaTex G
Sudex
Sudodrin
Sulfinpyrazone
Sulfoil Liquid
Sulfoxyl Regular
Sulfoxyl Strong
Sulster Solution
SulZee
Summer's Eve Anti-Itch
Sumycin Syrup
Super Flavons
Super Flavons 300
Supprelin Injections
Suprax Tablets
Supress-PE Pediatric
Susano Elixir
Sustaire Tablets

Su-Tuss DM
Su-Tuss HD
Swim-Ear Liquid
SymPak
Synagis Lyophilized Powder For Injection
Synalar
Synalar-HP Cream
Synophylate-GG
Syntest DS Tablets
Syntest HS Tablets
Synthroid Powder for Injection
Tac-40
Talwin Compound Tablets
Talwin NX
Tanabid SR
TanDur DM
Tannate DMP-DEX
Tannate-12D S
Tannate 12 S
Tannate-V-DM
Tannic-12
Tannihist-12 D
Tavist ND
Tazidime
TearGard
Teargen
Teargen II
Tears Renewed
Teczem
Tedrigen
Tegretol Chewable Tablets
Tempra
Tencon Capsules
Tensilon
Tequin
Terramycin
Teslac
Teslascan
Tesone
Tesone L.A.
Testoderm Transdermal System
Testoject
Testred Cypionate 200
Testrin-P.A.
Tetanus Toxoid, Adsorbed
Tetanus Toxoid, Adsorbed, Purogenated
Tetanus Toxoid Injection
Tetracycline Hydrochloride Fiber
Tetrasine
Tetrasine Extra
T-Gen
Thalitone Tablets
Theobid Duracaps Capsules
Theoclear-80 Syrup
Theoclear L.A. Capsules
Theodrine
Theo-Dur
Theolair Solution
Theolair S.R. Tablets
Theolate
Theomax DF
Theo-Sav Tablets
Theovent Capsules
Theo-X Tablets
Therac Lotion
Theraflu Daytime Severe Cold Packets
Theraflu Nighttime Severe Cold Powder
Theragran-M Caplets
Therapeutic B Complex with Vitamin C
Thiethylperazine Mesylate
Thiopental Sodium
Thorazine
Thrombogen
Thypinone
Thyrel TRH
Tibamine LA
Ticarcillin Disodium
Ticar Powder for Injection
Tilade
Timolide 10-25
Tinactin Solution
Ting
TI-Screen SPF 15 Lotion
TI-Screen SPF 30 Lotion
Titan
TL-Assure
TL-Assure ONE
TL 45%
Tocainide Hydrochloride
Tolazoline Hydrochloride
Tolectin DS Capsules
Tolectin 600
Tolectin 200
Tolinase Tablets
Tonocard Tablets
Toothache Gel
Toradol
Torecan Injection
Tornalate
Torsemide
Tositumomab and Iodine I 131 Tositumomab
Total Solution
Touro Allergy
Touro DM
Touro EX Tablets
Touro LA
Tovalt ODT

Trac Tabs 2X
Tramadol Hydrochloride Tablets
Trandate Injection
Tranxene-SD
Tranxene-SD Half Strength
TraumaCal
Travasol 5.5%
Travasol 3.5% w/Electrolytes
Travatan
Trellium Plus Tablets
Triamcinolone Acetonide Injection
Triamcinolone Diacetate
Triaminic Children's Allergy
Triaminic Children's Nighttime/Daytime Cold & Cough
Triaminic Cold & Allergy
Triaminic Cough & Sore Throat Softchews
Triamonide 40
Triant-HC
Triavil Tablets
Triban
Trichlormethiazide
Tricitrates
Tricodene Cough and Cold
Tricodene Sugar Free Cough & Cold
Tridesilon
Tridil Injection
TriHIBit Injection
Tri-Kort
Tri-Levlen
Trilog
Trilone Injection
Tri-Lo-Sprintec
TriLyte
Trimagen
Trimazide
Trimethaphan Camsylate
Trinalin Repetabs Tablets
Trionate
Triotann Pediatric
Triotann-S Pediatric
Tri-Otic
Tripedia
Triphasil
Triple Tannate Pediatric
Triplex AD
Triplex DM
Tripohist D
Triprolidine Hydrochloride
Triprolidine Tannate
Trital DM
Tri-Vi-Sol With Iron
Tri Vit w/Fluoride
Trizivir
Trobicin Powder for Injection
Trocal
Trovafloxacin Mesylate/Alatrofloxacin Mesylate
Trovan
Trycet
T-Stat Pads
T-Stat Solution
Tubocurarine Chloride Injection
Tucks Clear Gel
Tucks Pads
Tusana-D
Tusdec-DM
Tusdec-HC
Tusnel-HC Liquid
Tussafed HC
Tussafed-HCG
Tussafed-LA
Tussall
Tussall-ER
Tussbid
Tussbid PD
Tuss-DM Tablets
Tussex Cough Syrup
TUSSI-bid
Tussiden DM
Tussi-Organidin-DM NR Liquid
Tussi-Organidin DM-S NR
Tussi-Organidin NR
Tussi-Organidin-S NR Liquid
Tussi-12 D
Tussi-12 DS Suspension
Tussi-12 S
Tussi-12 Tablets
Tussizone-12 RF
Tusso-C
Tusso-HC
Tusso-ZMR
Tusso-ZR
Tuss-Tan
Tuss-Tan Pediatric
Tustan 12S
Twin-K
Tylenol Cough & Sore Throat Daytime
Tylenol Sinus Congestion and Pain Severe
Tylenol With Codeine Elixir
Tylox
Tympagesic
Tysabri Injection
UAD Otic
ULTRAbrom
Ultra Derm Bath Oil
Ultra Derm Lotion
Ultralytic 2

Ultrase
Ultrase MT 18
Ultrase MT 12
Ultrase MT 20
Ultra Tears
Ultravate PAC
Unibase
Uniretic
Unisom With Pain Relief
Uni-Tex 120/10 ER
Unoprostone Isopropyl
Uramaxin Foam
Urea 50% Ointment
Urealac
Urea Nail Gel
Ureaphil
Uridon Modified
Urised
UriSym
Urolene Blue
Vaginex Cream
Valdecoxib
Valrubicin
Valstar Solution
Vanamide
Vanex-HD
Vantin Granules for Suspension
Vaprisol
Varicella-Zoster Immune Globulin (Human)
Vascor Tablets
VasoClear
Vasocon Regular
Vasosulf Solution
VasoTuss HC Tannate Suspension
VaZol-D
Vazotab
Vazotan Tannate
Veetids
Velosulin BR (rDNA) Injection
Venoglobulin-S Powder for Injection
Versed Injection
Versed Syrup
Vesanoid
Viactiv Calcium Flavor Glides
Viadur
Vibramycin Capsules
Vibra-Tabs
Vicam Injection
Vicks Formula 44 Custom Care Dry Cough
Vicks Formula 44e Pediatric Cough & Chest Congestion Relief
Vicks Vitamin C Drops
Vicon-C
Vidarabine
Vigortol
Vinate IC
Viokase 8
Viokase Powder
Viokase 16
Vioxx Suspension
Vioxx Tablets
Vira-A Ointment
ViraTan-DM B.I.D.
Viravan-PDM
Viravan-P Suspension
Viravan-S
Virilon IM Injection
Visine Allergy Relief
Visine Moisturizing
Vision Care Enzymatic Cleaner
Vision Clear
Visonex
Visual-Eyes
Vitazol
Vitelle Nestrex
Vitrasert
Vitussin
Viva CT Prenatal
Vivelle
VoSol-HC Solution
VoSol Solution
V-Tann Suspension
WellTuss HC Liquid
Wet-N-Soak
Wet-N-Soak Plus
Wetting Solution
WHF Lubricating Gel
Wigraine Tablets
Wyamine Sulfate
Wygesic Tablets
Wytensin
Xedec Tablets
Xedec II Tablets
Xigris
XiraHist DM Pediatric
XiraHist Pediatric
XiraTuss
X-Prep Bowel Evacuant Kit-1
X-Prep Liquid
Xylocaine Jelly
Xylocaine Viscous
Yeast-Gard
Your Choice Non-Preserved Saline Solution
Your Choice Sterile Preserved Saline Solution
Yutopar Injection
Zagam
Zazole

Z-Cof HCX
Zeasorb-AF Gel
Zelnorm
Zenapax
Zerit XR Capsules
Zetacet
Zetacet Wash
Zevalin
Zinca-Pak
Zincfrin
Zinc Lozenges
Zingo Intradermal Injection
Zinotic
Zinotic ES
Zinx D-Tuss
Zinx GP
Ziox 405
ZNP Bar Soap
Zodryl AC 80
Zodryl AC 50
Zodryl AC 60
Zodryl DAC 80
Zodryl DAC 50
Zodryl DAC 40
Zodryl DAC 60
Zodryl DAC 30
Zodryl DAC 35
Zodryl DAC 25
Zostrix Neuropathy
Zotex-C
Zotex-D
Zotex GPX
Zotex-PE
Zovirax Powder for Injection, Lyophilized
Z-Tuss AC
ZTuss Expectorant
Zymine
Zymine DXR
Zymine HC
Zymine XR
Zyrphen

Manufacturer and Distributor Listing

3M DENTAL
888-364-3577
800-634-2249
http://www.solutions.3m.com

48878
3M ESPE DENTAL PRODUCTS
651-575-5144
800-634-2248
http://www.solutions.3m.com

07387
3M GLOBAL HEADQUARTERS
888-364-3577
800-228-3957
http://www.3m.com

00089
3M PHARMACEUTICALS
See Graceway Pharmaceuticals, LLC

17518
3M SURGICAL/MEDICAL
800-228-3957
651-733-1110
http://www.solutions.3m.com

42549
4UORTHO
888-316-7846
http://www.4udr.com

63801
7 OAKS PHARMACEUTICAL CORP.
864-850-1700
http://www.7oakspharma.com

40985
21ST CENTURY HEALTHCARE
480-966-8201
800-530-2178
http://www.21stcenturyvitamins.com

93764
A & D MEDICAL
408-263-5333
888-726-9966
http://www.andmedical.com

18754
A AARONS
973-882-1505
http://www.bradpharm.com

12539
AG MARIN PHARMACEUTICALS
305-593-5333
800-241-4603

A.H. ROBINS CONSUMER PRODUCTS
See Wyeth Consumer Health

A.H. ROBINS, INC.
See Wyeth Consumer Health

A.L. LABS
See Alpharma USPD, Inc.

41273
A. NELSON & CO.
800-319-9151
http://www.purabsorb.com

A.P. PHARMA, INC.
650-366-2626
http://www.appharma.com

66591
AAI PHARMA
910-254-7350
800-575-4224
http://www.aaipharma.com

50483
AAPER ALCOHOL & CHEMICAL CO.
502-232-7600
800-456-1017
http://www.pharmcoaaper.com

AASTROM BIOSCIENCES, INC.
734-930-5555

60793
ABANA PHARMACEUTICALS, INC.
See King Pharmaceuticals, Inc.

ABBOTT DIABETES CARE
510-749-5400
888-298-4584
http://www.therasense.com

ABBOTT HOSPITAL PRODUCTS
224-212-2000
800-615-0187
877-946-7747
http://www.hospira.com

ABBOTT LABORATORIES
847-937-6100
800-323-9100
http://www.abbott.com

00074
ABBOTT LABORATORIES PHARMACEUTICAL DIVISION
847-937-6100
800-255-5162
800-633-9110
http://www.abbott.com

29943, 27444
ABBOTT MEDICAL OPTICS
714-247-8200
866-427-8477
http://www.amo-inc.com

ABBOTT NUTRITION
614-624-3191
800-986-8510
http://www.abbottnutrition.com

00074
ABBVIE
800-255-5162
800-633-9110
http://www.abbvie.com

ABGENIX
See Amgen

31060
ABL MEDICAL
801-763-8000
http://www.ablmedical.com

63323
ABRAXIS BIOSCIENCE
310-883-1300
http://www.abraxisbio.com

68817
ABRAXIS ONCOLOGY
908-393-8220
http://www.abraxisbio.com

ACADEMIC PHARMACEUTICALS, INC.
847-735-1170

42907
ACCERA, INC.
303-999-3700
877-649-0004
http://www.accerapharma.com

ACCESS DIABETIC SUPPLY
954-975-0036
800-715-5031
http://www.diabeticsupply.com

67404
ACCESS PHARMACEUTICALS
214-905-5100
http://www.accesspharma.com

16729
ACCORD HEALTHCARE
866-941-7875
919-941-7878
http://www.accord-healthcare.com

ACCUMED
609-883-1818
http://www.accumed.org

ACELLA PHARMACEUTICALS
800-541-4802
678-325-5189
http://www.acellapharma.com

25356
ACETO PHARMA
516-627-6000
http://www.aceto.com

68784
ACINO PRODUCTS
609-695-4300
http://www.acinoproducts.com

00924
ACME UNITED CORP.
203-332-7330
800-835-2263
http://www.acmeunited.com

10144
ACORDA THERAPEUTICS
914-347-4300
800-367-5109
http://www.acorda.com

82607
ACON LABORATORIES
800-838-9502
858-875-8099
http://www.aconlabs.com

45963
ACTAVIS
973-993-4500
800-432-8534
http://www.actavis.us

00228
ACTAVIS ELIZABETH
973-993-4500
800-272-5525
800-432-8534
http://www.actavis.us

46987
ACTAVIS KADIAN
888-496-3082
www.kadian.com

ACTAVIS MID ATLANTIC
973-993-4500
800-432-8534
http://www.actavis.us

67767
ACTAVIS SOUTH ATLANTIC
973-993-4500
800-432-8534
http://www.actavis.us

52152
ACTAVIS TOTOWA
973-993-4500
800-432-8534
http://www.actavis.us

66215
ACTELION PHARMACEUTICALS US, INC.
650-624-6900
866-228-3546
http://www.actelionus.com

52244
ACTIENT PHARMACEUTICALS
847-607-8890
866-931-0717
http://www.actientpharma.com

ACURA PHARMACEUTICALS, INC.
847-705-7709
http://www.acurapharm.com

ACURA PHARMACEUTICALS TECHNOLOGIES
574-842-3305
http://www.acurapharm.com

38739
ADAMIS LABORATORIES, INC.
800-223-6837
561-208-2200

63824
ADAMS RESPIRATORY THERAPEUTICS
See Reckitt Benckiser Pharmaceuticals

ADHEREX TECHNOLOGIES, INC.
919-484-8484
http://www.adherex.com

ADOLOR
484-595-1500
866-423-6567
http://www.adolor.com

ADRIA LABORATORIES
See Pfizer US Pharmaceutical Group

ADVANCE BIOFACTURES CORP.
516-593-7000
http://www.biospecifics.com

17714
ADVANCE
631-981-4600
http://www.advancepharm.com

08541
ADVANCED BIOHEALING
877-422-4463
858-754-3700
http://www.abh.com

ADVANCED BIOTHERAPY, INC.
818-883-6716

55495
ADVANCED MEDICAL ENTERPRISES
787-436-0666
http://www.ameinc.org

ADVANCED MEDICAL OPTICS
See Abbott Medical Optics

10888
ADVANCED NUTRITIONAL TECHNOLOGY
925-828-2128
800-624-6543
http://www.advancednutritionaltech.com

58790
ADVANCED VISION RESEARCH
781-932-8327
800-579-8327
http://www.theratears.com

11042
ADVANCIS PHARMACEUTICAL CORPORATION
See MiddleBrook Pharmaceuticals

ADVANTAGENE
617-916-5445

ADVENTRX PHARMACEUTICALS
858-552-0866
http://www.adventrx.com

76431
AEGERION PHARMACEUTICALS, INC.
617-500-7867
855-305-2347
http://www.aegerion.com

66440
AERO PHARMACEUTICALS, INC.
See Adamis Laboratories, Inc.

AEROVANCE, INC.
510-549-5500

AETERNA ZENTARIS, INC.
418-652-8525

00213
AFFEMANN IMPORTS, INC.
818-348-7767
http://www.affemannimports.com

10572
AFFORDABLE PHARMACEUTICALS
781-848-3062
http://www.affordablepharm.com

AFFYMAX, INC.
650-812-8700
http://www.affymax.com

08554
AGAMATRIX
603-328-6000
http://www.agamatrix.com

60336
AGI DERMATICS
800-590-4244
516-868-9026
http://www.agiderm.com

AGOURON PHARMACEUTICALS
See Pfizer US Pharmaceutical Group

62584, 68084
AHP
800-707-4621
614-492-8177
http://www.healthpak.com

94922
AIDEN INDUSTRIES
877-642-7727
http://www.miaderm.com

38206
AID-PACK USA
See NutraMax Products

89134
AIMSCO/DELTA HI-TECH
801-263-0975
http://www.deltahitechinc.com

59196
AIRPHARMA
913-498-0700
http://www.air-pharma.com

17478, 11098
AKORN, INC.
800-932-5676
847-279-6100
http://www.akorn.com

23360
AKORN STRIDES
847-279-6100
800-932-5676
http://www.akorn.com

41383
AKPHARMA
609-645-6100
800-994-4711
http://www.akpharma.com

24090
AKRIMAX PHARMACEUTICALS
908-372-0506
888-383-1733
http://www.akrimax.com

65162
AKYMA PHARMACEUTICALS
See Amneal Pharmaceuticals

68322
ALAMO PHARMACEUTICALS, LLC
See Avanir Pharmaceuticals

46017
ALAVEN CONSUMER HEALTHCARE, INC. (ACH)
770-916-3920
877-916-3991
http://www.alavench.com

68220
ALAVEN PHARMACEUTICAL, LLC
888-317-0001
800-333-7343
http://www.alavenpharm.com

22400
ALBERTO CULVER
708-450-3000
800-333-6666
http://www.alberto.com

20993
ALCON LABORATORIES, INC.
817-293-0450
800-862-5266
800-451-3937
http://www.alcon.com

00065, 08065
ALCON SURGICAL
817-293-0450
800-862-5266
http://www.alcon.com

00065
ALCON VISION
817-293-0450
800-862-5266
http://www.alcon.com

43234
ALETHEIA
601-667-3584
http://www.altheialabs.com

25682
ALEXION PHARMACEUTICALS
203-272-2596
http://www.alxn.com

50488
ALEXSO
310-253-9761
http://www.alexsoinc.com

ALEXZA PHARMACEUTICALS
650-944-7000
http://www.alexza.com

08514
ALIGN PHARMACEUTICALS
908-834-0960
http://www.alignpharma.com

56121, 66177
ALIGON PHARMACEUTICALS
205-663-0521
http://www.aligoninc.com

68611
ALIMERA SCIENCES
678-990-5740
http://www.alimerasciences.com

53298, 00268, 52709
ALK ABELLO
800-325-7354
512-251-0037
http://www.alk-abello.us

ALK LABORATORIES, INC.
See ALK Abello

65757
ALKERMES
781-609-6000
800-848-4876
http://www.alkermes.com

43351
ALLAIRE PHARMACEUTICALS
732-974-6300
414-434-6617

13279
ALLAN PHARMACEUTICAL, LLC
215-441-9546
877-743-5858
http://www.allanpharmaceutical.com

ALLEGIS PHARMACEUTICALS
601-859-0038
866-468-2419

ALLEN & HANBURYS
See GlaxoSmithKline

ALLENDALE PHARMACEUTICALS, INC.
212-813-2171
888-343-4499
http://www.allendalepharm.com

ALLERCREME
See Carme, Inc.

ALLERDERM LABORATORIES, INC.
800-365-6868
http://www.allerderm.com

00023
ALLERGAN DERMATOLOGICS
714-246-4500
800-347-4500

11980
ALLERGAN, INC.
714-246-4500
800-377-7790
http://www.allergan.com

99965
ALLERGAN OPTICAL
800-433-8871
714-246-4500
http://www.allergan.com

ALLERGY LABORATORIES, INC.
405-235-1451
800-654-3971
http://www.allergylabs.com

49343
ALLERMED
858-292-1060
800-221-2748
http://www.allermed.com

ALLERQUEST
512-251-0037
800-325-7354
http://www.allerquest.com

17355
ALLIANCE LABS
602-276-3434
888-273-9734
http://www.enemeez.com

ALLIANCE PHARMACEUTICAL CORP.
858-410-5200

08462
ALLIANCE TECH MEDICAL
817-326-3183
800-848-8923
http://www.alliancetechmedical.com

68188
ALLIANT PHARMACEUTICALS, INC.
770-817-4500
http://www.alliantpharma.com

ALLIED PHARMACY
817-226-5050

86227
ALLISON MEDICAL
303-795-1618
800-886-1618
http://www.allisonmedical.com

ALLOS THERAPEUTICS
303-426-6262
888-255-6788
http://www.allos.com

54569
ALLSCRIPTS, INC.
847-680-3515
800-654-0889
http://www.allscripts.com

77379, 00311
ALMAY, INC.
919-603-2953
800-992-5629
http://www.almay.com

55349
ALP LIFE SCIENCES
828-357-4300
http://www.alplifesciences.com

ALPHA 1 BIOMEDICALS, INC.
See Arriva Pharmaceuticals, Inc.

49669
ALPHA THERAPEUTIC CORP.
See Grifols USA, Inc.

59743
ALPHAGEN LABORATORIES, INC.
770-475-8973

00228
ALPHARMA PUREPAC PHARMACEUTICALS
See Actavis Elizabeth

63857
ALPHARMA USPD, INC.
See King Pharmaceuticals, Inc.

59390
ALTAIRE
631-722-5988
800-258-2471
http://www.otcdruggist.com

ALTANA, INC.
973-236-9162
800-645-9833
http://www.altana.com

ALTERNA, LLC
973-946-7550
http://www.alternallc.com

91717
ALTERNATIVA NATURAL
631-231-2322
http://www.altnatural.com

00731
ALTO PHARMACEUTICALS, INC.
813-968-0522
800-330-2891
http://www.altopharm.com

ALTUS PHARMA
617-299-2900
888-258-2532

72959
ALVA-AMCO PHARMACAL COMPANIES, INC.
847-663-0700
800-792-2582
http://www.alva-amco.com

47781
ALVOGEN
973-796-3400
http://www.alvogen.com

17314
ALZA CORP.
650-564-5000
800-634-8977
http://www.alza.com

59338
AMAG PHARMACEUTICALS
617-498-3300
http://www.amagpharma.com

52937
AMARIN PHARMA
908-326-2571
http://www.amarincorp.com

66870
AMBI PHARMACEUTICALS, INC.
352-797-5227

10038
AMBIX LABORATORIES
973-890-9002
http://www.ambixlabs.com

AMCON LABORATORIES
314-961-5758
800-255-6161
http://www.amconlabs.com

52054
AMEDRA PHARMACEUTICALS
732-868-1090

61972
AMEND DRUG AND CHEMICAL CORPORATION
See Ruger Chemical Co.

15749
AMERICAN ANTIBIOTICS
727-471-0850
http://www.belcherpharma.com

AMERICAN BIOSCIENCE, INC.
See Abraxis Bioscience

AMERICAN DERMAL CORP.
See Sanofi-Aventis U.S.

62584
AMERICAN HEALTH PACKAGING
614-492-8177
800-707-4621
http://www.americanhealthpackaging.com

00008
AMERICAN HOME PRODUCTS
See Wyeth

73930
AMERICAN INTERNATIONAL INDUSTRIES
323-728-2999
800-621-9585
http://www.aiibeauty.com

AMERICAN LECITHIN COMPANY
203-262-7100
800-364-4416
http://www.americanlecithin.com

AMERICAN MEDICAL INDUSTRIES
605-428-5501

63323
AMERICAN PHARMACEUTICAL PARTNERS, INC.
See APP Pharmaceutical

52769
AMERICAN RED CROSS (NATIONAL HEADQUARTERS)
202-303-5214
800-733-2767
http://www.redcross.org

00517
AMERICAN REGENT, INC.
631-924-4000
800-645-1706
http://www.americanregent.com

41520
AMERICAN SALES COMPANY
716-686-7000
http://www.americansalescompany.net

89137
AMERICAN SCREENING CORP.
866-526-2873
http://www.americanscreeningcorp.com

63921
AMERIDERM LABORATORIES, INC.
973-279-5100
800-455-7211
http://www.ameriderm.com

AMERIFIT BRANDS, INC.
860-894-1285
800-722-3476
http://www.amerifit.com

43975
AMERIGEN PHARMACEUTICALS
732-993-9828
http://www.amerigenpharma.com

62852
AMERILAB TECHNOLOGIES
763-525-1262
http://www.amerilabtech.com

AMERISOURCEBERGEN
610-727-7000
800-829-3132
http://www.amerisourcebergen.com

AMERSHAM HEALTH
44-0-1494-544000

61470
AMERX HEALTH CARE CORP.
727-443-0530
800-448-9599
http://www.amerigel.com

55513
AMGEN
805-447-1000
800-772-6436
http://www.amgen.com

AMICUS THERAPEUTICS, INC.
609-662-2000

52152
AMIDE PHARMACAL
See Actavis Totowa

65162
AMNEAL PHARMACEUTICALS
270-629-2956
866-525-7270
http://www.amneal.com

00548
AMPHASTAR PHARMACEUTICALS, INC.
800-423-4136
http://www.amphastar.com

AMPLIMED CORP.
520-529-1000
http://www.Amplimed.com

00402
AMSCO SCIENTIFIC
See Steris Corp.

68883
AMSINO MEDICAL USA
866-482-1345
http://www.amsinomedusa.com

66780
AMYLIN PHARMACEUTICALS
858-552-2200
800-868-1190
http://www.amylin.com

ANABOLIC LABORATORIES, INC.
949-863-0340
800-445-6849
http://www.anaboliclabs.com

ANAQUEST
See Baxter Healthcare Corporation

10370
ANCHEN PHARMACEUTICALS, INC.
949-837-6178
888-837-6178
http://www.anchen.com

13273
ANDAPHARM
800-408-0143

19100
ANDREW JERGENS CO.
See Kao Brands Company

ANDRULIS PHARMACEUTICAL CORP.
301-419-2400
301-767-1900

ANDRULIS RESEARCH CORP.
301-767-1900

62022
ANDRX LABORATORIES, INC.
See Shionogi Pharma, Inc.

62037
ANDRX PHARMACEUTICALS, INC.
954-382-7600
800-621-7143
http://www.andrx.com

28000
ANESIVA
650-624-9600
http://www.anesiva.com

ANGELINI PHARMACEUTICALS, INC.
201-476-9000

65974
ANGIODYNAMICS
518-798-1215
800-772-6446
http://www.angiodynamics.com

ANI PHARMACEUTICALS
218-634-3500
800-434-1121
http://www.anipharmaceuticals.com

ANIKA THERAPEUTICS, INC.
781-305-9000
http://www.anikatherapeutics.com

65781
ANIMAS DIABETES
610-644-8990
877-767-7373
http://www.animascorp.com

ANORMED, INC.
604-530-1057

70907, 14613, 71483
ANSELL HEALTHCARE, INC.
732-345-5400
http://www.ansell.com

55948
ANTARES PHARMA
763-475-7700
http://www.antarespharma.com

ANTHRA PHARMACEUTICALS, INC.
609-514-1060

ANTIBODIES, INC.
530-758-4400
800-824-8540
http://www.antibodiesinc.com

ANTIGENICS, INC.
212-994-8200
http://www.antigenics.com

ANTISOMA PLC
44-0-20-8799-8200

ANTISOMA RESEARCH, LTD.
44-2-20-8799-8200

ATRIX LABORATORIES, INC.
970-482-5868
http://www.atrixlabs.com

23601
APEX-CAREX HEALTHCARE PRODUCTS
800-328-2935 (Apex)
800-526-8051 (Carex)
http://www.apex-carex.com

APHTON CORP.
305-374-7338

52380, 18407
APLICARE, INC.
203-630-0500
800-760-3236
http://www.aplicare.com

52609
APO PHARMA USA
240-499-7246
http://www.apopharma.com

APOGEE PHARMA
516-622-2208
http://www.apogeepharma.com

60505
APOTEX
954-384-8007
800-706-5575
http://www.apotexcorp.com

APOTHECA
602-252-5244
800-262-5244

25715
APOTHECARY PRODUCTS, INC.
952-890-1940
800-328-2742
http://www.apothecaryproducts.com

APOTHECON, INC.
See Bristol-Myers Squibb Co.

48723, 52925
APOTHECUS PHARMACEUTICAL CORP.
516-624-8200
800-227-2393
http://www.apothecus.com

63323
APP PHARMACEUTICAL
847-969-2700
888-391-6300
http://www.apppharma.com

APPLIED ANALYTICAL INDUSTRIES
910-254-7000
800-575-4224
http://www.aaipharma.com

APPLIED BIOTECH, INC.
858-587-6771
800-257-9525
http://www.abiapogent.com

92896
APPLIED DIABETES RESEARCH
972-241-1884
800-304-7293
http://www.applieddiabetesresearch.org

APPLIED GENETICS, INC.
516-868-9026
http://www.agiderm.com

00847
APPLIED NUTRITION CORPORATION
973-734-0023
800-605-0410
http://www.medicalfood.com

58914
APTALIS PHARMA US, INC.
800-472-2634
800-950-8085
http://www.aptalispharma.com

16110
AQUA PHARMACEUTICALS
610-644-7000
866-665-2782
http://www.aquapharm.com

13310
AR SCIENTIFIC
215-807-1029
877-960-2400
http://www.arscientific.com

ARADIGM CORP.
510-265-9000
http://www.aradigm.com

24338
ARBOR PHARMACEUTICALS
678-334-2420
866-516-4950
http://www.arborpharma.com

51772
ARCHIMEDES PHARMA
908-450-6500
866-435-6775
http://www.archimedespharma.com

90401
ARCHON
800-349-1700
http://www.archonvitamin.com

74312
ARCO PHARMACEUTICALS, INC.
See Natures Bounty

ARCOLA LABORATORIES
See Sanofi-Aventis U.S.

59923
AREVA PHARMACEUTICALS
270-408-4793
http://www.arevapharma.com

ARGINOX PHARMACEUTICALS
888-274-6070

76189
ARIAD PHARMACEUTICALS, INC.
617-494-0400
855-552-7423
http://www.ariad.com

24486
ARISTOS PHARMACEUTICALS
866-280-5755
http://www.aristospharm.com

ARK THERAPEUTICS, LTD.
44-20-7388-7722

08317
ARKRAY USA
952-646-3200
800-818-8877
http://www.arkrayusa.com

ARMOUR PHARMACEUTICAL
See CSL Behring

ARRIVA PHARMACEUTICALS, INC.
510-337-1250
http://www.arrivapharm.com

ARROW INTERNATIONAL CORP. HEADQUARTERS
610-378-0131
800-523-8446
http://www.arrowintl.com

ARTESA LABS
855-899-4237

ARTIELLE IMMUNOTHERAPEUTICS
503-626-1144
http://www.artielle.com

12870
ARZOL
603-352-5242

65557
ASAFI PHARMACEUTICAL
661-294-9509
http://www.asafi.com

89110
ASANTE SOLUTIONS
877-244-8402
http://www.snappump.com

67877
ASCEND LABORATORIES
201-476-1977
http://www.ascendlaboratories.com

17139
ASCEND THERAPEUTICS
703-471-4744
http://www.ascendtherapeutics.com

99207
ASCENT PEDIATRICS, INC.
See Medicis Pharmaceutical Corporation

46698
ASO, LLC
941-379-0300
800-966-8066
http://www.asocorp.com

76388
ASPEN GLOBAL
513-618-3333
866-525-0688
http://www.prasco.com

ASTELLAS PHARMA US, INC.
800-727-7003
800-695-4321
800-888-7704
http://www.astellas.com

00186, 00310
ASTRAZENECA LP
302-886-3000
800-456-3669
http://www.astrazeneca-us.com

38488
ATHENA FEMININE TECHNOLOGIES
866-308-4436
http://www.athenaft.com

59075
ATHENA NEUROSCIENCES, INC.
See Elan Pharmaceuticals

66813
ATHLON PHARMACEUTICALS, INC.
205-986-1111
http://www.athlonpharm.com

59702
ATLEY PHARMACEUTICALS, INC.
804-227-2250
http://www.atley.com

25010
ATON PHARMA
609-671-9010
877-286-6549
http://www.atonrx.com

62107
AUBURN PHARMACEUTICAL
800-222-5609
248-526-3700
http://www.auburnpharm.com

14629
AURIGA PHARMACEUTICALS, INC.
678-282-1600
866-367-8796
http://www.aurigalabs.com

AURIS MEDICAL, INC.
312-283-5633

65862
AUROBINDO PHARMA
732-839-9400
866-850-2876
http://www.aurobindo.com

55150
AUROMEDICS PHARMA
888-238-7880
http://www.auromedics.com

65504
AURORA HEALTHCARE
414-647-3000
http://www.aurorahelathcare.org

42792
AUSTIN PHARMACEUTICALS
AUTOIMMUNE, INC.
626-792-1235
http://www.autoimmuneinc.com

AUTOIMMUNITY RESEARCH FOUNDATION
805-492-3693

66887
AUXILIUM PHARMACEUTICALS, INC.
484-321-5900
877-745-1460
877-663-0412
http://www.auxilium.com

68322
AVANIR PHARMACEUTICALS, LLC
949-389-6700
http://www.avanir.com

AVANT IMMUNOTHERAPEUTICS, INC.
781-433-0771

AVANTOR PERFORMANCE MATERIALS
908-859-2151
800-582-2537
http://www.avantormaterials.com

AVAX TECHNOLOGIES, INC.
913-693-8491
http://www.avax-tech.com

AVENTIS BEHRING
See CSL Behring

AVENTIS PHARMACEUTICALS
See Sanofi-Aventis U.S.

AVICENA GROUP, INC.
415-397-2880
http://www.avicenagroup.com

43684
AVIDAS PHARMACEUTICALS
267-895-1755
http://www.avidaspharma.com

AVIGEN, INC.
510-748-1750
http://www.avigen.com

75854
AVION PHARMACEUTICALS
678-325-5298
888-612-8466

42291
AVKARE
931-292-6222
http://www.avkare.com

76170
AVOCET POLYMER TECHNOLOGIES
815-609-2170
866-352-7227
http://www.avocetcorp.com

58914
AXCAN PHARMA US, INC.
205-991-8085
800-472-2634
http://www.axcan.com

58914
AXCAN SCANDIPHARM
See Axcan Pharma US, Inc.

18860
AZUR PHARMA
215-832-3750
866-833-3560
800-890-3098
http://www.azurpharma.com

63275
B & B PHARMACEUTICALS
303-755-5110
800-499-3100
http://www.bandbpharma.com

00264
B. BRAUN MCGAW
See B. Braun Medical, Inc.

00264
B. BRAUN MEDICAL, INC.
800-854-6851
http://www.bbraunusa.com

00225
B. F. ASCHER AND CO.
913-888-1880
800-324-1880
http://www.bfascher.com

44184
BAJAMAR CHEMICAL CO., INC.
314-721-1896
http://www.vesselvite.com

11414
BAKER CUMMINS DERMATOLOGICALS
See Ivax Pharmaceuticals, Inc.

11414
BAKER NORTON PHARMACEUTICALS
See Ivax Pharmaceuticals, Inc.

50770
BALLARD MEDICAL PRODUCTS
801-572-6800
800-528-5591
http://www.kchealthcare.com

63162
BALLAY PHARMACEUTICALS, INC.
512-847-6458

10888
BANNER PHARMACAPS
336-812-8700
800-447-1140
http://www.banpharm.com

18192
BANYAN TRADING CO.
541-488-9525
800-953-6424
http://www.banyanbotanicals.com

BARBEAU PHARMA, INC.
847-441-4142

08011
BARD
See C.R. Bard

49326
BAROLI
305-772-0665

00555
BARR LABORATORIES, INC.
800-222-0190
http://www.barrlabs.com

BARR PHARMACEUTICALS, INC.
845-362-1100
800-222-0190
http://www.barrlabs.com

BARRE-NATIONAL, INC.
See Alpharma

13478
BARRIER THERAPEUTICS
609-945-1200
http://www.barriertherapeutics.com

10116
BARTOR PHARMACAL CO.
914-967-4219

00078
BASEL PHARMACEUTICALS
See Novartis Pharmaceuticals Corp.

BASF CORPORATION
973-245-6000
800-526-1072
http://www.basf.com

55458
BASIC ORGANICS
614-863-3004
http://www.basicorganics.com

10119
BAUSCH & LOMB PERSONAL PRODUCTS DIVISION
585-338-6000
800-344-8815
http://www.bausch.com

24208
BAUSCH & LOMB PHARMACEUTICALS, INC.
813-975-7770
800-323-0000
http://www.bausch.com

61772
BAUSCH & LOMB SURGICAL
866-393-6642
800-323-0000
http://www.bausch.com

10119, 24208, 61772
BAUSCH & LOMB WORLD HEADQUARTERS
585-338-6000
800-323-0000
http://www.bausch.com

17191
BAXA CORPORATION
303-690-4204
800-567-2292
http://www.baxa.com

10019, 60977
BAXTER HEALTHCARE CORPORATION
847-948-4770
800-933-0303
http://www.baxter.com

60977
BAXTER HEALTHCARE CORPORATION - ANESTHESIA & CRITICAL CARE PHARMACEUTICALS
908-286-7000
800-667-0959
http://www.baxter.com

00944
BAXTER HEALTHCARE CORPORATION - BAXTER BIOSCIENCE
866-424-6724
800-422-9837
800-423-2090
http://www.baxter.com

00338
BAXTER HEALTHCARE CORPORATION - CLINTEC NUTRITION
800-422-2751
http://www.nutriforum.com

00338
BAXTER HEALTHCARE CORPORATION - MEDICATION DELIVERY
847-948-4770
800-933-0303
http://www.baxter.com

64193
BAXTER HYLAND IMMUNO
See Baxter Healthcare Corporation - Baxter Bioscience

60977
BAXTER PHARMACEUTICAL PRODUCTS, INC. (BAXTER PPI)
See Baxter Healthcare Corporation - Anesthesia Critical Care Pharmaceuticals

00941
BAXTER RENAL
847-948-2000
888-736-2543
http://www.baxter.com

42769
BAY PHARMA
410-281-9450

65044
BAYER ALLERGY PRODUCTS
See Hollister-Stier

BAYER CONSUMER CARE DIVISION
973-254-5000
800-331-4536
http://www.bayercare.com

00026
BAYER CORPORATION
412-777-2000
800-468-0894
http://www.bayerus.com

BAYER DIABETES CARE
800-348-8100
http://www.bayerdiabetes.com

00193
BAYER DIAGNOSTICS
877-229-3711
800-248-2637
http://www.bayerdiag.com

50419
BAYER HEALTHCARE PHARMA
973-694-4100
888-842-2937
http://berlex.bayerhealthcare.com

76518, 76385
BAYSHORE PHARMACEUTICALS
1-855-BAY-PHARM
http://www.bayshorepharma.com

BD BIOSCIENCES
877-232-8995
http://www.bdbiosciences.com

BD CONSUMER PRODUCTS DIVISION
410-316-4000
800-638-8663
http://www.bd.com

BD DIAGNOSTIC SYSTEMS & MEDICAL SUPPLIES
800-675-0908
http://www.bd.com

00486
BEACH
813-839-6565
800-322-8210

BECKMAN COULTER
800-742-2345
http://www.beckmancoulter.com

BECKMAN COULTER PRIMARY CARE DIAGNOSTICS
714-993-5321
800-526-3821
http://www.beckmancoulter.com

BECTON DICKINSON
201-847-6800
888-237-2762
http://www.bd.com

76045
BD RX
866-943-8534
http://www.bdrxinc.com

55390
BEDFORD LABORATORIES
440-232-3320
800-562-4797
http://www.bedfordlabs.com

BEIERSDORF JOBST
See BSN Medical

62250
BELCHER PHARMACEUTICALS
727-471-0850
http://www.belcherpharma.com

BELL PHARMACEUTICAL
952-873-2288
800-328-5890

53030
BELMORA
888-470-1526
http://www.belmorallc.com

99731
BENFOTIAMINE, INC.
888-493-8014
http://www.benfotiamine.net

24385
BERGEN BRUNSWIG DRUG CO.
See AmerisourceBergen

50419
BERLEX LABORATORIES, INC.
See Bayer Healthcare Pharma

58337
BERNA
See Crucell Vaccines

BERTEK PHARMACEUTICALS, INC.
See Mylan Pharmaceuticals, Inc.

08515
BESTMED
303-271-0300

53062
BETA DERMACEUTICALS, INC.
210-349-9326
800-434-2382
http://www.beta-derm.com

00283
BEUTLICH PHARMACEUTICALS
847-473-1100
800-238-8542
http://www.beutlich.com

42582
BI-COASTAL PHARMACEUTICAL
732-530-3900
http://www.bicoastalpharm.com

42149
BIGWALL ENTERPRISES
877-365-6274
866-996-9255
http://www.bigwall.us

BIOALLIANCE PHARMA
33-0-1-45-58-76-00
http://www.bioalliancepharma.com

BIOAXONE THERAPEUTICS, INC.
913-693-8491
http://www.bioaxone.com

04142
BIOCODEX, INC.
877-356-7787
650-243-5320
http://www.biocodexusa.com

08216
BIOCORE MEDICAL TECHNOLOGIES
888-565-5243
888-689-5655
http://www.biocore.com

00093
BIOCRAFT LABORATORIES, INC.
See Teva Pharmaceuticals USA

BIOCRYST PHARMACEUTICALS, INC.
205-444-4600
http://www.biocryst.com

BIODEVELOPMENT CORP.
703-006-0290

15594
BIOFILM, INC.
760-727-9030
http://www.astroglide.com

BIOFORM MEDICAL
650-286-4000
866-862-1211
http://www.bioform.com

59627
BIOGEN IDEC
800-456-2255
800-262-2000
http://www.biogenidec.com

BIOGEN PHARMACEUTICALS
818-762-7681

BIOGENEX LABORATORIES
925-275-0550
800-421-4149
http://www.biogenex.com

62436
BIOGLAN PHARMACEUTICALS
See Bradley Pharmaceutical

34061
BIOLIFE, LLC
800-722-7559
http://www.biolife.com

00719
BIOLINE LABS, INC.
888-257-5155
508-880-8990

BIOLITEC PHARMA, LTD.
353-1-463-7415
http://www.biolitecpharma.com

68135
BIOMARIN PHARMACEUTICAL, INC.
415-506-6700
866-274-0606
http://www.bmrn.com

BIOMEDICAL FRONTIERS, INC.
612-378-0228

83059
BIOMERICA, INC.
949-645-2111
800-854-3002
http://www.biomerica.com

BIOMERIEUX
630-628-6055
800-634-7656
http://www.biomerieux-usa.com

BIOMET, INC.
574-267-6639
http://www.biomet.com

BIOMIRA USA, INC.
780-490-2818
877-234-0444
http://www.biomira.com

17700
BIOMOLECULAR SCIENCES, INC.
818-804-5148
800-260-3587
http://www.biomolecularsciences.com

53110
BIONEXUS, LTD.
607-266-9492
800-835-0869
http://www.bionxs.com

62086
BIONICHE PHARMA USA
847-739-3246
888-258-4199
http://www.bioniche.com

08539
BIONIME USA CORPORATION
858-481-8485
866-481-8485
http://www.bionime.com

59741
BIOPHARM LABS
215-949-3711
http://www.bio-pharminc.com

BIOPHARMACEUTICS, INC.
See Feminique Corp.

BIOPHYSICA, INC.
858-452-1523
http://www.biophysica.net

BIO PRODUCTS LABORATORY
44-0-208-258-2200
http://www.bpl.co.uk

BIOPURE CORP.
617-234-6500
http://www.biopure.com

BIOSAFE LABORATORIES
847-234-8111
http://www.ebiosafe.com

BIOSAFE TECHNOLOGIES, INC.
903-463-7321
877-828-4633
http://www.biosafetech.com

BIOSCRIP
952-979-3600
800-444-5951
http://www.bioscrip.com

08611
BIOSENSE MEDICAL DEVICES
877-592-3922

BIOSPECIFICS TECHNOLOGIES CORP.
516-593-7000
http://www.biospecifics.com

BIOSYNEXUS, INC.
301-330-5800
http://www.biosynexus.com

53191
BIO-TECH
479-443-9148
800-345-1199
http://www.bio-tech-pharm.com

BIO-TECHNOLOGY GENERAL CORP.
See Savient Pharmaceuticals, Inc.

59730
BIOTEST PHARMACEUTICALS
561-989-5800
800-458-4244
http://www.biotestpharma.com

55146
BIOTICS RESEARCH
281-344-0909
800-231-5777
http://www.bioticsresearch.com

BIOTRANSPLANT, INC.
617-241-5200

58023
BIOTROL INTERNATIONAL
303-673-0341
800-822-8550
http://www.biotrol.com

64455
BIOVAIL PHARMACEUTICALS, INC.
866-246-8245
908-927-1400
http://www.valeant.com

89130
BIOVENTUS
919-474-6700
800-396-4325
http://www.bioventusglobal.com

66658
BIOVITRUM AB
615-213-0343
http://www.biovitrum.com

BIRA CORP.
724-796-1820

50289
BIRCHWOOD LABORATORIES, INC.
952-937-7900
800-328-6156
http://www.birchlabs.com

12136
BIRD PRODUCTS CORP.
760-778-7200
800-232-7633
http://www.viasyscriticalcare.com

63347
BLAINE LABORATORIES
562-906-4477
800-307-8818
http://www.blainelabs.com

00165
BLAINE PHARMACEUTICALS
859-344-9600
800-633-9353
http://www.blainepharma.com

16728
BLAINES RESEARCH LABS
800-307-8818
562-906-4477
http://www.blaineslabs.com

00154
BLAIR LABORATORIES
See Purdue Frederick Co.

50486
BLAIREX LABS, INC.
812-378-1864
800-252-4739
http://www.blairex.com

51674
BLANSETT PHARMACAL
501-758-8635
800-816-9695
http://www.blansett.com

41388
BLISTEX, INC.
630-571-2870
800-837-1800
http://www.blistex.com

BLOCK DRUG CO., INC.
See GlaxoSmithKline Consumer Healthcare

24658
BLU PHARMACEUTICALS
270-586-6386
877-264-0258
http://www.blurx.us

BLUCO, INC.
734-513-4500
http://www.blucoinc.com

99853
BMS MEDICAL IMAGING
800-299-3431
http://www.radiopharm.com

64681
BMS U.S. MEDICINES GROUP
800-332-2056
212-546-4000
http://www.bms.com

08326, 43820, 00904
BOCA MEDICAL PRODUCTS
800-354-8460
http://www.bocamedical products.com

64376
BOCA PHARMACAL
954-346-8810
800-354-8460
http://www.bocapharmacal.com

50265
BOCAGREENMD
888-543-9160
http://www.bocagreenmd.com

00024
BOCK PHARMACAL CO.
See Sanofi-Aventis U.S.

BODY CHOICE
770-772-2444
http://www.bodychoicenutrition.com

00597
BOEHRINGER INGELHEIM PHARMACEUTICALS, INC.
203-798-9988
800-243-0127
http://www.boehringer-ingelheim.com

BOERICKE & TAFEL
See Natures Way

00220
BOIRON LABORATORIES
800-264-7661
http://www.boironusa.com

00725
BOLAN PHARMACEUTICALS
516-842-8383
800-872-0159

50051
BONNE BELL
216-221-0800
800-321-1006
http://www.bonnebell.com

00074
BOOTS PHARMACEUTICALS, INC.
See Abbott Laboratories Pharmaceutical Division

71401
BOTANICAL LABORATORIES
360-384-5656
800-232-4005
http://www.botlab.com

54288
BPI LABS, LLC
800-426-2457
http://www.bpilabs.com

00270
BRACCO DIAGNOSTICS
609-514-2200
800-631-5245
http://www.bracco.com

BRADLEY PHARMACEUTICALS, INC.
973-882-1505
800-929-9300
http://www.bradpharm.com

52268
BRAINTREE LABORATORIES, INC.
781-843-2202
800-874-6756
http://www.braintreelabs.com

BRAUN
518-828-0450

00264
BRAUN MEDICAL
See B. Braun Medical, Inc.

51991
BRECKENRIDGE
561-443-3314
800-367-3395
http://www.bpirx.com

58659
BRIDGEPORT WHOLESALE PRODUCTS
425-656-0460

10914
BRIGHTON PHARMACEUTICALS
919-459-3950
866-638-7530
http://www.brightonpharma.com

10007
BRIOSCHI
201-796-4226
http://www.brioschi-usa.com

00015
BRISTOL LABS
609-252-4000
800-468-7746

BRISTOL-MYERS ONCOLOGY/VIROLOGY
609-897-2000
800-426-7644
http://www.bms.com

19810
BRISTOL-MYERS PRODUCTS (OTC/CONSUMER AFFAIRS)
See Novartis Pharmaceuticals Corp.

BRISTOL-MYERS SQUIBB COMPANY
212-546-4000
800-321-1335
800-332-2056
http://www.bms.com

15584
BRISTOL-MYERS SQUIBB/GILEAD
650-574-3000
800-445-3235
http://www.gilead.com

16563,11498
BRONSON PHARMACEUTICALS
800-235-3200
http://www.bronsonvitamins.com

42192
BROOKSTONE PHARMACEUTICALS
678-325-5188
800-541-4802
http://www.acellapharma.com

82161
BROWN MEDICAL INDUSTRIES
712-336-4395
800-843-4395
http://www.brownmed.com

63256.
BRYAN CORPORATION
781-935-0004
800-343-7711
http://www.bryancorp.com

63629
BRYANT RANCH PREPACK
818-764-7225
http://www.byrantranch prepack.com

BSN, JOBST
See BSN Medical

19869
BSN MEDICAL
704-554-9933
800-537-1063
http://www.bsnmedical.com

50633
BTG INTERNATIONAL
610-278-1660
http://www.btgplc.com

54396
BTG PHARMACEUTICAL CORPORATION
See Savient Pharmaceuticals, Inc.

BUREL PHARMACEUTICALS
601-855-2016
http://www.burel pharmaceuticals.com

BURROUGHS WELLCOME CO.
See GlaxoSmithKline

C. B. FLEET CO., INC.
See Fleet Laboratories

08011
C. R. BARD
908-277-8000
800-526-4455
http://www.crbard.com

C.R. BARD, INC. UROLOGICAL DIVISION
770-784-6100
800-526-4455
http://www.crbard.com

10486
C S DENT
859-647-0777

59746
CADISTA PHARMACEUTICALS, INC.
800-313-4623
800-308-3985
http://www.cadista.com

55628
CAL PHARMA
562-940-8300
888-551-7778

34362
CALDWELL CONSUMER HEALTH
973-360-1090
888-317-4402
http://www.revivepersonal products.com

08237, 55559
CALGON VESTAL
See ConvaTec

00799
CALMOSEPTINE, INC.
714-840-3405
800-800-3405
http://www.calmoseptine ointment.com

12622
CALWOOD NUTRITIONALS
410-796-5560
800-479-9942
http://www.calwoodnutritionals.com

31722
CAMBER PHARMACEUTICALS
732-377-2029
866-495-1995
http://www.camberpharma.com

CAMBREX BIOSCIENCE
207-594-3400
800-638-8174
http://www.cambrex.com

CAMBRIDGE NEUROSCIENCE
See Baxter Healthcare Corporation

43656
CAMBRIDGE NUTRACEUTICALS
See Baxter Healthcare Corp.

24359
CAMBROOKE FOODS
508-782-2300
866-456-9776
http://www.cambrookefoods.com

38083
CAMPBELL LABS
See Chattem Consumer Products

08396
CAN-AM CARE
678-795-3440
866-202-9067
http://www.canamcare.com

53270
CANGENE BIOPHARMA
410-843-5000
800-441-4225
http://www.cangenebiopharma.com

CANGENE CORP.
204-275-4200
800-226-4363
http://www.cangene.com

42026
CANOPY ROADS PHARMACEUTICALS
770-664-6050
http://www.crpharma.com

CANYON PHARMACEUTICALS
410-771-8606
888-434-7003
http://www.canyonpharma.com

64543
CAPELLON PHARMACEUTICALS, LTD.
817-595-5820
http://www.capellon.com

57664, 32247
CARACO PHARMACEUTICAL LABORATORIES
313-871-8400
800-818-4555
http://www.caraco.com

CARDINAL HEALTH
614-757-5000
800-234-8701
http://www.cardinal.com

08525
CARDIOCOM
952-361-6467
888-243-8881
http://www.cardiocom.com

83076
CARDIOTABS
816-753-4298
800-811-1007
http://www.cardiotabs.com

CAREFUSION
888-876-4287
http://www.carefusion.com

CARESTREAM DENTAL
800-933-8031
http://www.carestreamdental.com

84841
CARGILL
800-221-4455
952-742-7575
http://www.cargill.com

61442,61441
CARLSBAD TECHNOLOGIES
760-431-8284
http://www.carlsbad technologyinc.com

83078
CARMA LABS, INC.
414-421-7707
http://www.carma-labs.com

CARME, INC.
707-226-3900
http://www.senetekplc.net

50000
CARNATION
See Nestle Infant Nutrition

00086
CARNRICK LABORATORIES
See Elan Pharmaceuticals

46287
CAROLINA MEDICAL PRODUCTS COMPANY
252-753-7111
800-227-6637
http://www.carolinamedical.com

53303
CARRINGTON
972-518-1300
800-527-5216
http://www.carringtonlabs.com

11411, 41140.
CARTER PRODUCTS
See Church Dwight

22600
CARTER-WALLACE
See Church Dwight

00037
CARTER-WALLACE, INC.
See Meda Pharmaceuticals

15370
CARWIN ASSOCIATES, INC.
205-525-4566
866-525-4566
http://www.carwinassoc.com

18515
CCA INDUSTRIES, INC.
800-524-2720
http://www.ccaindustries.com

64019
CEBERT PHARMACEUTICALS, INC.
205-981-0201
800-211-0589
http://www.cebert.com

64181
CEDARBURG PHARMACEUTICALS
262-376-1467
http://www.cedarburgpharma.com

CELESTIAL SEASONINGS, INC.
303-530-5300
800-525-0347
http://www.celestialseasonings.com

59572
CELGENE CORP.
908-673-9000
888-423-5436
http://www.celgene.com

65231
CELL PATHWAYS
See OSI Pharmaceuticals

60553
CELL THERAPEUTICS, INC.
206-282-7100
800-215-2355
http://www.celltherapeutics.com

CELLEGY PHARMACEUTICALS, INC.
215-914-0900

CELLTECH PHARMACEUTICAL CO.
See UCB Pharmaceuticals, Inc.

CENTEON
See CSL Behring

00268
CENTER LABORATORIES
See ALK-Abello

CENTERS FOR DISEASE CONTROL AND PREVENTION
404-639-3534
800-311-3435
http://www.cdc.gov

99962
CENTOCOR ORTHO BIOTECH, INC.
888-227-5624
800-457-6399
http://www.centocorortho biotech.com

38083
CENTRAL PHARMACEUTICALS, INC.
See Schwarz Pharma

11528
CENTRIX PHARMACEUTICAL, INC.
205-991-9870
866-991-9870
http://www.cenrx.com

23359
CENTURION LABS, LLC
601-720-0111
http://www.centurionlabs.com

00436
CENTURY
317-849-4210
866-343-2576

63459
CEPHALON
610-883-5710
800-896-5855
http://www.cephalon.com

68330
CEPHAZONE PHARMA
909-392-8900
http://www.cephazone.com

00851
CERA PRODUCTS
843-842-2600
888-237-2598
http://www.ceraproductsinc.com

CERENEX PHARMACEUTICALS
See GlaxoSmithKline

10223
CETYLITE INDUSTRIES, INC.
865-665-6111
800-257-7740
http://www.cetylite.com

40986, 68016
CHAIN DRUG CONSORTIUM
412-828-2061

63868
CHAIN DRUG MARKETING ASSOCIATION, INC.
248-449-9300

CHARLES RIVER LABORATORIES INTERNATIONAL, INC.
978-658-6000
877-CRIVER1 (877-274-8371)
http://www.criver.com

54429
CHASE LABORATORIES
See Banner Pharmacaps

41167
CHATTEM CONSUMER PRODUCTS
423-821-4571
800-366-6833
http://www.chattem.com

CHESAPEAKE BIOLOGICAL LABS, INC.
See Cangene BioPharma

00521
CHESEBROUGH-PONDS USA, INC.
See Unilever Home and Personal Care USA

12462
CHESTER LABS
513-458-3840
800-354-9709
http://www.chester-labs.com

CHEW-RITE CO.
937-746-5509

CHILDRENS HOSPITAL OF COLUMBUS
614-722-2000

CHILTON LABS, INC.
973-575-1992

67066
CHIRHOCLIN
877-272-4888
301-476-8388
http://www.chirhoclin.com

53905
CHIRON THERAPEUTICS
510-655-8730
800-244-7668
http://www.chiron.com

61772
CHIRON VISION
See Bausch & Lomb Surgical

54993
CHRONIMED, INC.
See Bioscrip

96121
CHRONOHEALTH
805-290-4959
866-261-8557

22600
CHURCH DWIGHT
609-683-5900
800-524-1328
http://www.churchdwight.com

00067
CIBA CONSUMER
See Novartis Consumer Health

00078
CIBA-GEIGY PHARMACEUTICALS
See Novartis Pharmaceuticals Corp.

47113
CIBA VISION CORPORATION
770-476-3937
800-845-6585
http://www.cibavision.com

CIMA LABS
952-947-8700
http://www.cimalabs.com

24470
CINTEX
770-744-1202

52544
CIRCA PHARMACEUTICALS, INC.
See Watson Laboratories

CIRRUS HEALTHCARE PRODUCTS, LLC
631-692-7600
800-327-6151
http://www.cirrushealthcare.com

CIS-US, INC.
781-275-7120
800-221-7554
http://www.pharmalucence.com

89128
CITIHEALTH
http://www.NeutekMedical.com

CITRA ANTICOAGULANTS
781-848-2174
800-299-3411
http://www.citraanticoagulants.com

99074
CLARIS LIFESCIENCES LIMITED
732-422-9100
http://www.clarislifesciences.com

45802
CLAY-PARK LABS, INC.
718-901-2800
800-933-5550
http://www.claypark.com

55553
CLINT PHARMACEUTICALS
615-882-0042
800-677-5022
http://www.clintpharmaceuticals.com

CLOSURE MEDICAL CORP.
See Johnson & Johnson

57145
CNS, INC.
952-229-1500
http://www.cns.com

58826
COATS ALOE INTERNATIONAL, INC.
214-340-2563
800-486-2563
http://www.coatsaloe.com

16252
COBALT LABORATORIES, INC.
800-272-5525
239-390-0245
http://www.cobaltlabs.com

43378
CODADOSE
678-866-0172
866-574-8861
http://www.codadose.com

COLGATE-HOYT
See Colgate Oral Pharmaceuticals

00126
COLGATE ORAL PHARMACEUTICALS
213-310-2000
800-226-5428
http://www.colgateprofessional.com

35000
COLGATE-PALMOLIVE CO.
212-310-2000
800-221-4607
http://www.colgateprofessional.com

64682, 27280
COLLAGENEX PHARMACEUTICALS
215-579-7388
888-339-5678
http://www.collagenex.com

COLOPLAST
612-337-7800
800-533-0464
http://www.us.coloplast.com

COLORADO BIOLABS, INC.
970-243-4153
888-442-0067
http://www.coloradobiolabs.com

21406, 55056
COLUMBIA LABORATORIES, INC.
973-994-3999
866-566-5636
http://www.columbialabs.com

11509
COMBE, INC.
914-694-5454
800-873-7400
http://www.combe.com

COMPLIMED MEDICAL RESEARCH GROUP
360-384-5656
888-977-8008
http://www.complimed.com

CONAGRA FUNCTIONAL FOODS, INC.
888-828-4242
http://www.culturelle.com

74108
CONAIR INTERPLAX DIVISION
800-726-6247
http://www.interplak.com

08597, 95863
CONCEIVEX
616-642-6917
888-306-6366
http://www.conceptionkit.com

57648
CONCEPTS IN CONFIDENCE
561-369-1700
800-822-4050
http://www.concepts inconfidence.com

88901
CONCEPTS IN HEALTH
845-727-4900

CON-CISE CONTACT LENS CO.
510-483-9400
800-772-3911
http://www.con-cise.com

20254
CONCORD LABORATORIES
973-227-6757

49281
CONNAUGHT LABS
See Sanofi Pasteur

63032
CONNETICS CORPORATION
See Stiefel Laboratories

00223
CONSOLIDATED MIDLAND CORP.
845-279-6108

97493
CONSUMERS CHOICE SYSTEMS, INC.
425-883-6310
800-479-5232
http://www.womanswellbeing.com

CONTINENTAL CONSUMER PRODUCTS
248-758-1817
800-542-5903

CONTINENTAL QUEST RESEARCH
317-843-2501
800-451-5773
http://www.continentalquest.com

10267
CONTRACT PHARMACAL CORP.
631-231-4610
http://www.cpc.com

CONVATEC
908-904-2200
800-422-8811
http://www.convatec.com

63535
COOKE PHARMA, INC.
See Unither Pharma (United Therapeutics Corp.)

59365
COOPER SURGICAL
203-601-5200
800-480-1985
http://www.coopersurgical.com

59426, 54027
COOPERVISION
949-597-8130
800-538-7850
http://www.coopervision.com

00093
COPLEY PHARMACEUTICAL
See Teva Pharmaceuticals USA

63020
COR THERAPEUTICS, INC.
See Millennium Pharmaceuticals, Inc.

76346
CORCEPT THERAPEUTICS
650-327-3270
http://www.corcept.com

64720
COREPHARMA, LLC
732-868-1090
800-850-2719
http://www.corepharma.com

13548
CORIA LABORATORIES
800-548-5100
http://www.corialabs.com

CORIXA
See GlaxoSmithKline

10122
CORNERSTONE THERAPEUTICS
919-678-6611
888-466-6505
888-661-9260
http://www.crtx.com

COROMEGA CO., INC.
760-599-6088
877-275-3725
http://www.coromega.com

10148
COTHERIX
650-624-6900
877-483-6828
http://www.cotherix.com

COULTER CORP. (BECKMAN COULTER, INC.)
See Beckman Coulter

43199
COUNTY LINE PHARMACEUTICALS
262-439-8109
866-207-5636
http://www.countylinepharma.com

COVIDIEN
508-261-8000
800-722-8772
http://www.covidien.com

08080
COVIDIEN MEDICAL SUPPLIES
508-261-8000
800-962-9888
http://www.covidien.com

24987
COVIS PHARMACEUTICALS
919-535-3049
866-488-4423
http://www.covispharma.com

11025
CREATIVE MEDICAL CORPORATION
787-714-0100

15310
CREEKWOOD PHARMACEUTICAL, INC.
205-995-7390
http://www.crkrx.com

68734
CRITICAL THERAPEUTICS, INC.
781-402-5700
http://www.criticaltherapeutics.com

58337
CRUCELL VACCINES
786-313-8200
800-533-5899
http://www.crucell.com

37379
CSI PHARM
800-654-5635
http://www.csidesigns.com

00053
CSL BEHRING, LLC
610-878-4000
800-683-1288
800-504-5434
http://www.cslbehring.com

33332
CSL BIOTHERAPIES
888-435-8633
http://www.cslbiotherapies-us.com

67919
CUBIST PHARMACEUTICALS, INC.
781-860-8660
866-793-2786
http://www.cubist.com

66220
CUMBERLAND PHARMACEUTICALS, INC.
615-255-0068
866-423-7259
http://www.cumberlandpharma.com

00869
CUMBERLAND SWAN, INC.
See Vijon Laboratories

66860
CURA PHARMACEUTICALS
888-887-7171
732-982-8300
http://www.curapharma.com

08160
CURAMEDICA, LLC
888-613-0729
http://www.curamedica.com

CURASCRIPT
407-804-6700
800-892-9622
http://www.priorityhealthcare.com

55326
CURATEK PHARMACEUTICALS
See 3M Pharmaceuticals

89126
CUSTOM RX TDA
770-401-3853
http://www.topi-click.com

65628
CUTIS PHARMA, INC.
781-935-8141
http://www.cutispharma.com

67159
CV THERAPEUTICS
See Gilead Sciences

CYANOTECH CORP.
808-326-1353
800-395-1353
http://www.cyanotech.com

53409
CYCLIN PHARMACEUTICALS, INC.
800-558-7046
http://www.womenshealth.com

08197
CYGNUS, INC.
650-369-4300
http://www.cygn.com

54799
CYNACON/OCUSOFT
800-233-5469
http://www.ocusoft.com

60258
CYPRESS PHARMACEUTICAL, INC.
601-856-4393
800-856-4393
http://www.cypressrx.com

63004
CYPROS PHARMACEUTICAL CORP.
See Questcor Pharmaceuticals, Inc.

57902
CYTOGEN CORP.
See Eusa Pharma

23731
CYTOSOL LABORATORIES
781-848-9386
800-288-3858

61534
CYTOSOL OPHTHALMICS
828-758-2343
800-234-5166
http://www.cytosol.com

CYTRX CORP.
310-826-5648
http://www.cytrx.com

65759, 10960
D & K HEALTHCARE RESOURCES
314-727-3485
888-727-3485
http://www.dkwd.com
See McKesson

DADE BEHRING
847-267-5300
800-241-0420
http://www.dadebehring.com

63395
DAIICHI PHARMACEUTICAL CORP.
See Daiichi Sankyo, Inc.

63395
DAIICHI SANKYO, INC.
973-944-2600
877-437-7763
http://www.dsi.com

54891
DAKOTA LABORATORIES
877-793-5683

00591, 52544
DANBURY PHARMACAL
951-493-5300
800-338-9066
http://www.watson.com

64875
DANCO LABS, LLC
212-424-1950
877-432-7596
http://www.earlyoptionpill.com

60793
DANIELS PHARMACEUTICALS, INC.
See King Pharmaceuticals, Inc.

89141
DARA BIOSCIENCES, INC.
919-872-5578
http://www.darabiosciences.com

58869
DARTMOUTH PHARMACEUTICALS, INC.
508-295-2200
800-414-3566
http://www.ilovemynails.com

67253
DAVA PHARMACEUTICALS, INC.
201-947-7442
866-947-3282
http://www.davapharm.com

DAVOL
401-463-7000
800-556-6275
http://www.davol.com

58865
DAWN PHARMACEUTICALS, INC.
800-745-3296

52041
DAYTON LABORATORIES
See Propharma

DDN MEDICAL AFFAIRS
414-434-8406
http://www.ddnmedicalaffairs.com

DEGUSSA CORP.
973-541-8000
877-273-2668
http://www.degussa.com

10310
DEL PHARMACEUTICALS
516-844-2020
http://www.dellabs.com

48532
DELMONT LABORATORIES, INC.
610-543-3365
800-562-5541
http://www.delmontlabs.info

00316
DEL-RAY LABORATORY, INC.
423-926-4413
800-877-8869
http://www.crownlaboratories.com

53706
DELTA PHARMACEUTICALS
803-407-7733

00295
DENISON PHARMACEUTICALS
401-723-5500
http://www.hydrolatum.com

DEN-MAT CORPORATION
805-922-8491
800-433-6628

DENTAL HERB CO.
561-241-4262
800-747-4372
http://www.dentalherbcompany.com

13913
DEPOMED, INC.
650-462-5900
866-458-6389
http://www.depomedinc.com

DEPOTECH CORP. (SKYEPHARMA)
858-625-2424
http://www.skyepharma.com

99873
DEPUY MITEK
800-382-4682
508-880-8100
http://www.depuymitek.com

25382
DERMA SCIENCES
609-514-4744
800-825-4325
http://www.dermasciences.com

80208
DERMAIDE RESEARCH
312-649-7220
http://www.dermaide.com

10641
DERMALAB
847-266-0000
http://www.dermalab.com

60974
DERMALOGIX PARTNERS
207-883-4103
800-753-0047
http://www.dermalogix.com

61924
DERMARITE
973-569-9000
800-337-6296
http://www.dermarite.com

00066
DERMIK LABORATORIES, INC. (ARCOLA)
See Valeant Pharmaceuticals International, Inc.

DEROYAL INDUSTRIES, INC.
865-938-7828
888-938-7828
http://www.deroyal.com

08591
DESTAL INDUSTRIES
866-291-2815

16881
DESTON THERAPEUTICS
888-333-1528
http://www.deston.com

08627
DEXCOM, INC.
877-339-2664
http://www.dexcom.com

65430
DEXGEN PHARMACEUTICALS, INC.
732-223-8811
877-339-4361
http://www.dexgen.com

DEXO PHARMA
785-917-9582

49502
DEY L.P.
707-224-3200
800-755-5560

DFB PHARMACEUTICALS
800-441-8227
http://www.dfb.com

55887
DHS, INC.
770-751-1787
800-392-7717

94046
DIABETIC SUPPLY OF SUNCOAST
888-469-3579
http://www.pharmasupply.com

DIAGNOSTICS DEVICES
800-366-5901
http://www.prodigymeter.com

17000
DIAL CORPORATION
480-754-3425
800-258-3425
http://www.dialcorp.com

DIAPHARMA GROUP, INC.
513-860-9324
800-526-5224
http://www.diapharma.com

50419
DIATIDE, INC.
See Berlex

10331
DICKINSON BRANDS, INC.
860-267-2279
888-860-2279
http://www.witchhazel.com

59767
DIGESTIVE CARE, INC.
877-882-5950
http://www.digestivecare.com

55392
DINNO PHARMACEUTICALS
617-645-5552

08587
DINORIO
866-354-3449
http://www.dinorio.com

59009
DISC DISEASE SOLUTIONS
888-495-7440
http://www.discdiseasesolutions.com

DISCOVERY LABORATORIES, INC.
215-488-9300
http://www.discoverylabs.com

DISCUS DENTAL, INC.
800-422-9448
310-845-8600
http://www.discusdental.com

15630
DISETRONIC MEDICAL SYSTEMS
See Roche Insulin Delivery Systems, Inc.

68258
DISPENSING SOLUTIONS, INC.
888-374-7378
770-751-1787
http://www.dispensingsolutionsinc.com

00777
DISTA PRODUCTS CO.
See Eli Lilly and Co.

55812
DIVERSIFIED PHARMACEUTICAL
877-842-4716

DIXON-SHANE
See Amneal Pharmaceuticals

64455
DJ PHARMA, INC.
See Biovail Pharmaceuticals, Inc.

24286
DLC LABORATORIES
562-602-2184
800-858-3889
http://www.dlclabs.com

10337
DOAK DERMATOLOGICS
See Pharmaderm

DONELL DERMEDEX
See Donell, Inc.

DONELL, INC.
212-682-0666
800-324-7455
http://www.donellskin.com

51469
DOVER PHARMACEUTICAL, INC.
781-821-5400
800-777-6847

00514
DOW HICKAM, INC.
See Mylan Pharmaceuticals, Inc.

DOW PHARMACEUTICAL SCIENCES
707-793-2600
877-369-7476
http://www.dowpharm.com

14657
DR. FRESH
866-373-7374
http://www.drfresh.com

55111
DR. REDDY'S LABORATORIES, INC.
866-375-3444
866-733-9352
888-375-3784
http://www.drreddys.com

64061
DREIR PHARMACEUTICALS, INC.
480-607-3584
800-541-4044

58952
DRJ GROUP, INC.
760-635-0174

52316
DSC LABORATORIES
231-777-3012
800-492-5988
http://www.dsclab.com

89411
DSE HEALTHCARE SOLUTIONS, LLC
800-338-8079
732-417-1870
http://www.dsehealth.com

55494
DUCHESNAY USA
484-380-2641
http://www.duchesnayusa.com

25382
DUMEX
See Derma Sciences

50939
DU-MORE
479-631-1088
http://www.dumoreinc.com

00217, 48878
DUNHALL PHARMACEUTICALS, INC.
See Omnii Pharmaceuticals and See Oxypure

DUPONT PHARMACEUTICALS CO.
See Bristol-Myers Squibb Co.

41333
DURACELL
800-551-2355
http://www.duracell.com

51285
DURAMED PHARMACEUTICALS
See Barr Laboratories, Inc.

02340
DUREX CONSUMER PRODUCTS
770-582-2222
888-566-3468
http://www.durex.com

00145
DURHAM PHARMACAL CORP.
See Stiefel Laboratories, Inc.

67308
DUSA PHARMACEUTICALS, INC.
978-657-7500
877-533-DUSA (877-533-3872)
http://www.dusapharma.com

68803
DUTCH OPHTHALMIC
603-778-6929
800-753-8824
http://www.dutchophthalmicusa.com

47783
DUY DRUGS
305-593-5333

47783
DYAX CORPORATION
617-225-2500
800-452-5248
http://www.dyax.com

00168
E. FOUGERA CO.
631-454-7677
800-645-9833
http://www.fougera.com

42367
EAGLE PHARMACEUTICALS
800-910-4917
http://www.eaglepharma.net

EAGLE VISION, INC.
901-380-7000
800-222-7584
http://www.eaglevis.com

EASTMAN KODAK CO.
585-724-4000
800-242-2424
http://www.kodak.com

EATON MEDICAL CORP.
901-274-0000
800-253-5949
http://www.easyeyes.com

51293
ECI PHARMACEUTICALS
954-486-8181
http://www.ecipharma.com

44118
ECKSON LABS
770-744-1202
855-899-4237

76014
ECLAT PHARMACEUTICALS
636-449-1832
http://www.eclatpharma.com

ECOLAB
651-293-2233
800-352-5326
http://www.ecolab.com

ECOLOGICAL FORMULAS, INC.
925-827-2636
800-888-4585
http://www.ecologicalformulas.net

38130
ECONO MED PHARMACEUTICALS
336-226-1091
800-327-6007

55053
ECONOLAB
See Breckenridge Pharmaceutical, Inc.

00095
ECR PHARMACEUTICALS
804-527-1950
800-527-1955
http://www.ecrpharma.com

42799
EDENBRIDGE PHARMACEUTICALS
201-292-1292
http://www.edenbridgepharma.com

49909
EDGEMONT PHARMACEUTICALS
512-550-8555
888-594-4332
http://www.edgemontpharma.com

00485
EDWARDS
662-837-8182
800-543-9560

00433
EDWARDS LIFESCIENCE
800-424-3278
800-882-9837
http://www.edwards.com

55806
EFFCON LABORATORIES
770-579-3558
800-722-2428

62856
EISAI, INC.
888-274-2378
888-793-4724
http://www.eisai.com

24477, 10122
EKR THERAPEUTICS, INC.
888-466-6505
888-661-9260
http://www.crtx.com/about_us/ekr

59075
ELAN PHARMACEUTICALS
800-859-8586
888-638-7605
http://www.elan.com

ELANCO
317-277-3185
800-428-4441
http://www.elanco.com

58298
ELGE
281-232-0463
281-342-8228
http://www.elgeninc.com

00002
ELI LILLY AND COMPANY
317-276-2000
800-545-5979
http://www.lilly.com

00641
ELKINS-SINN, INC.
See West-Ward

42783
ELORAC
847-362-8200

EMD CHEMICALS, INC.
856-423-6300
800-222-0342

EMD SERONO, INC.
781-982-9000
800-283-8088
http://www.emdserono.com

04107, 24155
EMJAY LABORATORIES
See Sheffield Laboratories

91268
EMJOI
212-755-5950
888-310-2493
http://www.emjoi.com

42457
EMMAUS MEDICAL
310-214-0065
877-420-6493
http://www.emmausmedical.com

64068
ENDIT LABORATORIES
910-754-6856
http://www.endit.com

ENDO PHARMACEUTICALS
484-216-4138
800-462-3636
http://www.endo.com

ENDURANCE PRODUCTS COMPANY
503-639-9562
800-964-0876
http://www.endur.com

17433
ENEMEEZ
602-276-3434
888-273-9734
http://www.enemeez.com

76420
ENOVACHEM MANUFACTURING
310-218-4146
http://www.enovachem.com

53703
ENTERA HEALTH
855-436-8372
http://www.enterahealth.com

50081
ENTRA HEALTH SYSTEMS
619-584-6704
877-458-2646
http://www.entrahealthsystems.com

62333
ENVIRODERM PHARMACEUTICALS, INC.
310-768-0700
800-624-9659
http://www.enviroderm.com

57665
ENZON PHARMACEUTICALS, INC.
908-541-8600
866-792-5172
http://www.enzon.com

63948
ENZYMATIC THERAPY
800-558-7372
http://www.enzymatictherapy.com

00185
EON LABS
See Sandoz

42806
EPIC PHARMA
718-949-8607
888-374-2791
http://www.epic-pharma.com

62942
EPIEN MEDICAL
952-746-6770
888-884-4675
http://www.epien.com

18270
EQUIDYNE SYSTEMS
714-447-4474
http://www.injex.com

E.R. SQUIBB & SONS, INC.
See Bristol-Myers Squibb Co.

63135
ESBA LABS
561-746-0365
800-677-9299
http://www.topicaine.com

63475
ESCALON MEDICAL CORP.
800-676-0043
http://www.escalonmed.com

67286
ESP PHARMA
See PDL Biopharma

15456
ESPRIT PHARMA
732-828-9950
http://www.espritpharma.com

54756
ESSENTIAL MEDICAL SUPPLY
800-826-8423

58177
ETHEX CORP.
314-646-3750
800-321-1705
http://www.ethex.com

63713
ETHICON, INC. (JOHNSON & JOHNSON)
908-218-0707
800-255-2500
http://www.ethicon.com

ETI HOLDING
920-469-1313

EURAND AMERICA, INC.
937-898-9669
877-893-0282
http://www.aptalispharma.com

42865
EURAND PHARMACEUTICALS
267-759-9400
888-936-7371
http://www.eurand.com

59652
EURUS PHARMA
855-355-3881
919-645-4990
http://www.euruspharma.com

57902
EUSA PHARMA
215-867-4900
800-833-3533
http://www.eusapharma.com

66521
EVANS VACCINES, LTD.
See Novartis Vaccines and Diagnostics

42700
EVENFLO COMPANY, INC.
937-415-3300
800-233-5921
http://www.evenflo.com

00642
EVERETT
973-324-0200
800-964-9650
http://www.everettlabs.com

EVERIDIS HEALTH SCIENCES
877-776-0101
http://www.everidis.com

17287
EVERTON PHARMACEUTICALS
877-218-3215

42808
EXACT-RX
631-755-1155
http://www.sonarproducts.com

64125
EXCELLIUM PHARMACEUTICAL
973-276-9600

63807
EXCELSIOR MEDICAL CORPORATION
732-776-7525
800-487-4276
http://www.excelsiormedical.com

08287
EXEL INTERNATIONAL
800-940-3935
http://www.exelint.com

76282
EXELAN PHARMACEUTICALS
678-377-0405
855-295-7455
http://www.exelanpharma.com

42388
EXELIXIS, INC.
650-837-7000
855-292-3935
http://www.exelixis.com

60843
EYE CARE & CURE CORPORATION
520-321-1262
800-486-6169
http://www.eyecareandcure.com

68782
EYETECH PHARMACEUTICALS
See OSI Eyetech

10361
E-Z-EM
See Bracco Diagnostics

94542
FACET TECHNOLOGIES
770-590-6400
800-526-2387
http://www.facettechnologies.com

51552
FAGRON
651-681-9517
800-423-6967
http://www.fagron.com

61314
FALCON PHARMACEUTICALS, LTD.
800-343-2133
817-293-0450
http://www.falconpharma.com

58892
FALLENE
800-332-5536
http://www.fallene.com

FARMACON, INC.
203-222-8801

60976
FARO PHARMACEUTICALS, INC.
See Cooper Surgical

61703
FAULDING PHARMACEUTICAL
See Hospira

FDA
301-827-1491
888-463-6332
http://www.fda.gov

50907
FEI PRODUCTS
716-693-6230
877-727-2427
http://www.barrlabs.com

11423
FEMALE HEALTH CO.
312-595-9123
800-884-1601
http://www.femalehealth company.com

08454
FEMCAP
858-481-8837
http://www.femcap.com

00942
FENWAL INTERNATIONAL
847-550-2300
800-333-6925
http://www.fenwalinc.com

48102
FERA PHARMACEUTICALS
414-434-6604
http://www.ferapharma.com

00496
FERNDALE LABORATORIES, INC.
248-548-0900
800-621-6003
http://www.ferndalehealthcare.com

31253, 08439
FERRARIS MEDICAL
http://www.ferrarismedical.com

55566
FERRING PHARMACEUTICALS, INC.
973-796-1600
888-337-7464
http://www.ferringusa.com

08195
FERRIS CORP.
630-887-9797
800-765-9636
http://www.polymem.com

FIBERTONE
See Marlyn Neutraceuticals, Inc.

89122
FIDIA PHARMACEUTICAL USA
862-207-7800
800-242-7494

14428
FIRST AID RESEARCH CORP.
516-783-0274
http://www.firstaidresearch.com

59630
FIRST HORIZON PHARMACEUTICAL
See Sciele Pharma

90891
FIRST QUALITY PRODUCTS
516-829-3030
800-726-6910
http://www.firstquality.com

FISHER SCIENTIFIC INTERNATIONAL
603-926-5911
800-640-0640
http://www.fisherscientific.com

FISKE INDUSTRIES
845-398-3340
http://www.cosmeticsolutions.com

54323
FLANDERS, INC.
843-571-3363
http://www.flanders buttocksointment.com

78573, 86067
FLAVORX
800-884-5771
http://www.flavorx.com

FLEET LABORATORIES
800-999-9711
http://www.cbfleet.com

00256
FLEMING PHARMACEUTICALS
636-343-5306
800-343-0164
http://www.flemingpharma.com

23185
FLENTS PRODUCTS COMPANY
See Apothecary Products, Inc.

FLEX-POWER
510-527-9955
866-353-9769
http://www.flexpower.com

00288
FLUORITAB
231-755-9113

60762
FNC MEDICAL CORPORATION
805-644-7576
800-440-2888
http://www.fncmedical.com

99999
FOCUSED PAIN RELIEF
585-433-2000
877-648-1951
http://www.focusedpainrelief.com

42559
FONTUS PHARMACEUTICALS, INC.
973-265-2777
http://www.fontuspharma.com

98939, 16042
FORA CARE
805-498-8188
http://www.foracare.com

00456
FOREST LABORATORIES, INC.
212-421-7850
800-947-5227
800-678-1605
http://www.forestpharm.com

00456
FOREST LABORATORIES IRELAND, LTD.
See Forest Laboratories, Inc.

00456
FOREST PHARMACEUTICALS, INC.
See Forest Laboratories, Inc.

64814
FORTE PHARMA
See Eon Labs Manufacturing, Inc.

00168
FOUGERA
631-454-7677
800-645-9833
http://www.fougera.com

FOURNIER PHARMA
973-683-0024
http://www.fournierpharma corp.com

58487,10432
FREEDA VITAMINS, INC.
718-433-4337
800-777-3737
http://www.freedavitamins.com

90816, 49230
FRESENIUS
781-699-9000
800-662-1237
http://www.fmcna.com

16167
FROHOCK-STEWART
800-333-6900
http://www.invacare.com

71661
FRUIT OF THE EARTH
972-790-0808
800-527-7731
http://www.fote.com

13551
FSC LABORATORIES
877-387-0021
http://www.fsclabs.com

FUISZ TECHNOLOGIES, LTD.
See Biovail Pharmaceuticals, Inc.

00713
G & W LABS
908-753-2000
800-922-1038
http://www.gwlabs.com

00299
GALDERMA
817-961-5000
866-735-4137
http://www.galdermausa.com

57284
GALEN PHARMA
028-3833-4974
http://www.galen.co.uk

51552
GALLIPOT, INC.
See Fagron

GAMBRO RENAL PRODUCTS
800-232-6800
800-525-2623
http://www.gambro.com

GASTROENTERO-LOGIC, LLC
302-351-4077

57844
GATE PHARMACEUTICALS
215-591-3000
800-292-4283
http://www.tevaselectbrands.com

43386
GAVIS PHARMACEUTICALS
908-603-6080
http://www.gavispharma.com

86040
GC AMERICA
800-323-7063
http://www.gcamerica.com

00407
GE HEALTHCARE
262-544-3011
http://www.gehealthcare.com

00386
GEBAUER
216-581-3030
800-321-9348
http://www.gebauerco.com

48879, 80410, 50804
GEISS DESTIN & DUNN
770-486-0381
866-696-0957
http://www.valuelabels.com

11640
GENAIREX
877-726-4400
http://www.genairex.com

50242
GENENTECH, INC.
650-225-1000
800-821-8590
http://www.gene.com

GENERAL INJECTABLES & VACCINES
276-688-4121
800-521-7468
http://www.giv.com

GENERAL NUTRITION CORP.
412-288-4600
888-462-2548
http://www.gnc.com

10139
GENERAMEDIX, INC.
866-436-3721
877-722-2328
http://www.generamedix.com

GENESIS NUTRITION
732-509-0456
800-451-7933
http://www.genesisnutrition.com

00398
GENESIS PHARMACEUTICALS
973-355-8000
800-459-8663
http://www.glytone-usa.com

68585
GENESIS PRODUCTS
877-266-8292
http://www.genesisproductsinc.com

00302
GENETCO, INC.
800-969-8007
http://www.genetcoinc.com

GENETIC THERAPY, INC.
301-590-2626

00008
GENETICS INSTITUTE
617-876-1170
888-446-3344
http://www.genetics.com

00781
GENEVA DRUGS
See Sandoz Pharmaceuticals-Sandoz Consumer

82915
GENEXEL-SEIN
480-502-6007

15330
GENPHARM, LP
866-436-9155
631-434-2760
http://www.genpharmusa.com

35781
GENSCO LABORATORIES
352-726-6284
http://www.genscolabs.com

00703.
GENSIA SICOR PHARMACEUTICALS, INC.
See Teva Pharmaceuticals USA

66657
GENTA, INC.
908-286-9800
http://www.genta.com

15014
GENTEX PHARMA, LLC
601-201-7231
601-826-0058
http://www.gentexpharma.com

GENVEC, INC.
240-632-5501
240-632-0740
http://www.genvec.com

63861
GENZYME
617-252-7500
888-497-6436
http://www.genzyme.com

58468
GENZYME CORPORATION
617-252-7500
800-326-7002
http://www.genzyme.com

63861
GENZYME TRANSPLANT
617-252-7500
800-376-7002
http://www.genzyme.com

GEODESIC MEDITECH, INC.
858-692-0088
http://www.geodesicmeditech.com

72227
GERBER
231-928-2000
800-284-9488
http://www.gerber.com

54092
GERIATRIC PHARMACEUTICAL CORP.
See Shire US, Inc.

57896
GERI-CARE
718-382-5000
http://www.gericarepharm.com

92771, 54162
GERITREX CORPORATION
914-668-4003
800-736-3437
http://www.geritrex.com

00891
G. HIRSCH & CO.
650-692-8770
800-638-8800
http://www.ghirsch.com

61958
GILEAD SCIENCES
650-574-3000
800-445-3235
http://www.gilead.com

GILLETTE ORAL CARE
617-421-7000
http://www.gillette.com

47400
GILLETTE PERSONAL CARE
617-421-7000
http://www.gillette.com

36819
GINESIS NATURAL PRODUCTS
256-767-8256
800-492-4818
http://www.ginesis.com

63218, 59366
GLADES PHARMACEUTICALS, LLC
888-445-2337
http://www.glades.com

GLAXOSMITHKLINE
888-825-5249
877-311-7515
215-751-4000
http://www.gsk.com

99929
GLAXOSMITHKLINE CONSUMER HEALTHCARE
412-200-4000
800-245-1040
http://www.gsk.com

68462
GLENMARK PHARMACEUTICALS, LTD.
888-721-7115
201-684-8000
http://www.glenmarkpharma.com

41128, 00516
GLENWOOD
201-569-0050
800-542-0772
http://www.glenwood-llc.com

82028
GLOBAL HEALTH, INC.
412-358-9505
http://www.globalhp.com

00115
GLOBAL PHARMACEUTICALS
215-933-0323
800-934-6729
http://www.globalphar.com

26893
GLOBAL PROTECTION COMPANY
617-946-2800
http://www.globalprotection.com

59618
GLOBAL SOURCE
954-747-8977
800-662-7556

33620
GLOVES IN A BOTTLE
818-248-9980
800-600-1881
http://www.glovesinabottle.com

58809
GM PHARMACEUTICALS
888-535-0305
817-303-3800

GML INDUSTRIES, LLC
See Biosafe Technologies, Inc.

60429
GOLDEN STATE MEDICAL SUPPLY
805-477-9866
800-284-8633
http://www.gsms.us

GOLDLINE LABORATORIES, INC.
See Ivax Pharmaceuticals, Inc.

10481
GORDON LABORATORIES
610-734-2011
800-356-7870
http://www.gordonlabs.net

13453
GRACEWAY PHARMACEUTICALS, LLC
See Medicis Pharmaceutical Corporation

12165
GRAHAM FIELD HEALTH PRODUCTS, INC.
800-347-5678
http://www.grahamfield.com

10486
GRANDPA BRANDS COMPANY
859-647-0777
800-684-1468
http://www.grandpabrands.com

00034
GRAY PHARMACEUTICAL CO.
See Purdue Frederick Co.

51301
GREAT SOUTHERN LABORATORIES
281-530-3077
800-747-0783
http://www.greatsouthernlabs.com

GREEN TURTLE BAY VITAMIN CO.
908-277-2240
800-887-8535
http://www.energywave.com

59762
GREENSTONE
212-733-2323
800-438-1985
http://www.greenstonellc.com

22840
GREER LABORATORIES, INC.
828-754-5327
800-378-3906
http://www.greerlabs.com

68516, 61953
GRIFOLS, INC.
888-474-3657
800-421-0008
http://www.grifolsusa.com

GTC BIOTHERAPEUTICS
508-620-9700
800-610-3776
http://www.gtc-bio.com

11399
GTX, INC.
901-523-9700
http://www.gtxinc.com

GUARDIAN DRUG COMPANY
609-860-2600
http://www.guardiandrug.com

00327
GUARDIAN LABORATORIES
See United Guardian Laboratories

GUERBET
812-333-0059
877-729-6679
http://www.guerbet-us.com

62750
GUM-TECH INDUSTRIES, INC.
See Matrixx Initiatives, Inc.

56227
GWM PRODUCTS
855-872-2013
http://www.rtdwounddressing.com

63955
GYNETICS
609-919-1931

08385
H&H WHOLESALE SERVICES, INC.
248-616-3030
800-995-5750
http://www.hhwholesale.com

64285
HAEMACURE CORPORATION
941-364-3700
http://www.haemacure.com

44411
HALL BIOSCIENCE
770-975-7337
http://www.hallbio.com

12164
HALOCARBON PRODUCTS CORPORATION
800-338-5803
http://www.halocarbon.com

18657
HALOZYME THERAPEUTICS
855-495-3639
858-794-8889
http://www.halozyme.com

17478
HAMELN PHARMACEUTICALS GMBH
See Akorn, Inc.

41268
HANNAFORD BROTHERS
800-213-9040
http://www.hannaford.com

HARD TO FIND BRANDS, INC.
724-796-0148
888-796-4832
http://www.hardtofindbrands.com

52512
HARMONY LABORATORIES
704-857-0707
800-245-6284
http://www.harmonylabs.com

67405
HARRIS PHARMACEUTICAL, INC.
239-278-4749
800-983-4708
http://www.harrispharmaceutical.com

HART HEALTH & SAFETY
800-234-4278
http://www.harthealth.com

00904, 61147
HARVARD DRUG CORP.
800-875-0123
http://www.harvardlink.com
http://www.harvarddrugs.com

67754
HARVEST PHARMACEUTICALS, INC.
540-633-7976
800-455-5525
http://www.harvestpharmaceuticals.com

HAUSER PHARMACEUTICAL, INC.
800-441-2309
http://www.hauserpharmaceutical.com

66761
HAW PAR HEALTHCARE
510-887-1899
http://www.hawpar.com

63370
HAWKINS CHEMICAL
612-331-6910
612-617-8544
800-375-0009

63717
HAWTHORN PHARMACEUTICALS, INC.
601-856-4393
800-856-4393
http://www.cypressrx.com

HCD SALES
813-978-3005
800-844-8345
http://www.hcdsales.com

HD SMITH
866-232-1222
800-252-8090
http://www.hdsmith.com

HDC CORPORATION
408-942-7340
800-227-8162
http://www.hdccorp.com

HEALTH ASURE, INC.
831-420-2660
800-635-1233
http://www.healthasure.com

62391
HEALTH CARE LABORATORIES
281-496-9854
800-909-9854
http://www.bioflexor.com

60569, 61787
HEALTH CARE PRODUCTS
866-263-9003
800-899-3116
http://www.diabeticproducts.com

79573
HEALTH ENTERPRISES
508-695-0727
800-633-4243
http://www.healthenterprises.com

HEALTH PRODUCTS CORP.
914-423-2900

HEALTHCARE DIRECT SERVICES
See HCD Sales

HEALTHFIRST CORP.
425-771-5733
800-331-1984
http://www.healthfirst.com

00064
HEALTHPOINT MEDICAL
800-441-8227
http://www.healthpoint.com

93595, 55966
HEALTHSTAR
631-273-2630

50114
HEEL, INC.
505-293-3843
800-621-7644
http://www.heelusa.com

HELENA LABORATORIES
409-842-3714
800-231-5663
http://www.helena.com

HEMACARE CORP.
818-226-1968
http://www.hemacare.com

HEMAGEN DIAGNOSTICS, INC.
443-367-5500
800-495-2180
http://www.hemagen.com

HEMISPHERX BIOPHARMA, INC.
215-988-0080
http://www.hemispherx.net

HENRY SCHEIN, INC.
631-843-5500
800-472-4346
http://www.henryschein.com

00023, 11980
HERBERT LABORATORIES
See Allergan, Inc.

49730
HERCON LABORATORIES CORPORATION
717-764-1191
http://www.herconlabs.com

23155
HERITAGE PHARMACEUTICALS
732-429-1000
866-901-1230
http://www.heritagepharma.com

58060
HEYL CHEM
281-395-7040
866-761-7822
http://www.heyltex.com

10541
HIGH CHEMICAL COMPANY
215-788-3113
800-447-8792
http://www.sarapin.com

HIKMA PHARMACEUTICALS
732-542-1191
http://www.hikma.com

28105
HILL DERMACEUTICALS, INC.
407-323-1187
800-344-5707
http://www.hillderm.com

10542
HILLESTAD PHARMACEUTICALS
800-535-7742
866-358-9773
http://www.hillestadlabs.com

17808
HIMMEL
561-585-0070
800-535-3823
http://www.goliath.ecnext.com

46581
HISAMITSU PHARMACEUTICAL CO., INC.
http://www.salonpas-usa.com

50383
HI-TECH PHARMACAL CO., INC.
631-789-8228
http://www.hitechpharm.com

52959
H.J. HARKINS COMPANY, INC.
805-929-4060

00839
H.L. MOORE DRUG EXCHANGE, INC.
See Moore Medical Corp.

84160, 08522
HMD BIOMEDICAL
321-267-7576
888-446-3246
http://www.hmeproviders.com

HOECHST-MARION ROUSSEL
See Sanofi-Aventis US

95814
HOGIL PHARMACEUTICAL CORP.
914-681-1800
http://www.hogil.com

HOLLES LABORATORIES, INC.
800-356-4015

08380
HOLLISTER
800-323-4060
888-740-8999
http://www.hollister.com

65044
HOLLISTER-STIER LABORATORIES
509-489-5656
800-992-1120
http://www.hollisterstier.com

42828, 08567
HOLLISTER WOUND CARE
800-323-4060
http://www.hollister.com

83170
HOME ACCESS HEALTH CORPORATION
847-781-2500
800-448-8378
http://www.homeaccess.com

21292, 56151
HOME DIAGNOSTICS
954-677-9201
800-342-7226
http://www.niprodiagnostics.com

HONEYWELL HOMMED, LLC
262-783-5440
888-353-5440
http://www.hommed.com

60267
HOPE PHARMACEUTICALS, INC.
800-755-9595
http://www.hopepharm.com

75987
HORIZON PHARMA
224-383-3000
http://www.horizonpharma.com

60904
HORIZON PHARMACEUTICAL CORP.
See Shionigi Pharma, Inc.

19098
HORMEL FOODS
800-523-4635
http://www.hormelfoods.com

61678
HORMEL HEALTHLABS
800-866-7757
http://www.hormelhealthlabs.com

66553
HOSPAK UNIT DOSE PRODUCTS
815-877-6480
815-636-8829

00409
HOSPIRA
224-212-2000
877-946-7747
http://www.hospira.com

00591, 52544
HOUBA (HALSEY DRUG CO.)
See Acura Pharmaceuticals, Inc.

57273, 08489, 08633
HTL-STREFA
770-528-0410
http://www.htl-strefa.com

17238
HUB PHARMACEUTICALS
909-476-8394
800-393-3767
http://www.hubrx.com

65845
HUDSON RCI
951-676-5611
866-246-6990
http://www.hudsonrci.com

44156
HUMANICARE INTERNATIONAL
732-613-9000
800-631-5270
http://www.humanicare.com

03951, 00395
HUMCO HOLDING GROUP, INC.
903-334-6200
800-662-3435
http://www.humco.com

00219
HUMPHREYS PHARMACAL
201-933-7744

31124
HYGENIC CORPORATION
800-321-2135
330-633-8460
http://www.hygeniccorp.com

00944
HYLAND THERAPEUTICS
See Baxter Healthcare Corp.

76325
HYPERION THERAPEUTICS
650-745-7802
888-897-4276
855-823-7878
http://www.hyperiontx.com

75450
HY-VEE
515-267-2800
http://www.hy-vee.com

00186
ICI PHARMACEUTICALS
See AstraZeneca, LP

00187
ICN PHARMACEUTICALS
See Valeant Pharmaceuticals International, Inc.

99733
ICY DIAMOND TOTES
714-393-4886
http://www.icydiamondtotes.com

59627
IDEC PHARMACEUTICALS
See Biogen Idec

24108
IDENIX PHARMACEUTICALS, INC.
617-995-9800
http://www.idenix.com

52565
IGI LABORATORIES
856-697-1441
http://www.igilabs.com

IKARIA
908-238-6600
877-566-9466
http://www.ikaria.com

ILEX CONSUMER GROUP
855-785-6381
http://www.ilexgroup.com

63861
ILEX ONCOLOGY, INC.
See Genzyme Corp.

24430
IMARX THERAPEUTICS
http://www.imarx.com

IMMUCELL CORP.
207-878-2770
800-466-8235
http://www.immucell.com

54129
IMMUNO US, INC. (BAXTER HEALTHCARE CORP.)
See Baxter Healthcare Corp.

IMMUNOGEN
617-995-2500
http://www.immunogen.com

IMMUNOMEDICS, INC.
973-605-8200
http://www.immunomedics.com

28770
IMMUNOTEC RESEARCH, LTD.
450-424-9992
888-917-7779
http://www.immunotec.com

00115
IMPAX LABORATORIES, INC.
510-240-6000
http://www.impaxlabs.com

64896
IMPAX PHARMACEUTICALS
510-240-6000
877-994-6729
http://www.impaxpharma.com

IMS, LTD.
See UCB Pharmaceuticals, Inc.

INAMED CORPORATION
805-683-6761
800-722-2007
http://www.inamed.com

50881
INCYTE CORPORATION
302-498-6700
855-446-2983
http://www.incyte.com

INDEVUS PHARMACEUTICALS, INC.
781-861-8444
800-370-4742
http://www.indevus.com

INFLABLOC PHARMACEUTICALS, INC.
801-464-6100
866-440-7044
http://www.pharmadigm.com

08522
INFOPIA USA
321-267-9911
888-446-3246
http://www.infopiausa.com

61607, 66934
INKINE PHARMACEUTICAL COMPANY, INC.
See Salix Pharmaceuticals, Inc.

INNER HEALTH GROUP
210-661-9257
800-381-4697
http://www.michaelshealth.com

68712
INNOCUTIS
800-449-4468
866-644-6717
http://www.innocutis.com

INNOZEN, INC.
818-593-4880
800-599-8892

INO THERAPEUTICS, INC.
See IKARIA

08489
INPHARMA
877-241-8324

63736
INSIGHT PHARMACEUTICALS
267-852-0505
800-344-7239
http://www.insightpharma.com

16249
INSMED INCORPORATED
804-565-3000
804-565-3079
http://www. insmed.com

58441, 63252
INSOURCE
276-688-0211
800-668-3452
http://www.insourceonline.com

INSPIRE PHARMACEUTICALS, INC.
919-941-9777
http://www.inspirepharm.com

08508
INSULET
781-457-5000
800-591-3455
http://www.myomnipod.com

20482
INSYS THERAPEUTICS
602-910-2617
866-917-2617
http://www.insysrx.com

99732
INTAPORT COMPANY, INC.
732-967-0997
http://www.intaportkb.com

08478, 64895, 08220
INTEGRA LIFESCIENCES CORP.
800-654-2873
800-931-1709
http://www.integra-ls.com

INTEGRATED THERAPEUTICS
See Integrative Therapeutics

88856
INTEGRATIVE HEALTH CONSULTING
See K-Pax Vitamins

INTEGRATIVE THERAPEUTICS
800-917-3696
http://www.integrativeinc.com

10922
INTENDIS, INC.
866-463-3634
http://www.intendis.com

42515
INTERCELL USA, INC.
301-556-4500
http://www.intercell.com

INTERCHEM CORP.
201-261-7333
800-261-7332
http://www.interchem.com

18968
INTERCURE, INC.
201-720-7750
877-988-9388
http://www.intercure.com

54746
INTERFERON SCIENCES
See Hemispherx Biopharma, Inc.

INTERMAX PHARMACEUTICALS, INC.
631-777-3318

64116
INTERMUNE PHARMACEUTICALS
415-466-2200
415-466-2430
http://www.intermune.com

11584
INTERNATIONAL ETHICAL LABS
787-765-3510
800-981-5068
http://www.intetlab.com

INTERNATIONAL LABS, INC.
727-322-7160
http://www.internationallabs.com

00548, 76329
INTERNATIONAL MEDICATION SYSTEMS, LTD.
877-651-2674
800-423-4136
http://www.ims-limited.com

36652
INTERNATIONAL VITAMIN CORP.
732-308-3000
http://www.ivcinc.com

INTERNEURON PHARMACEUTICALS, INC.
See Indevus Pharmaceuticals, Inc.

53746
INTERPHARM LTD.
631-952-0214
http://www.interpharminc.com

00814
INTERSTATE DRUG EXCHANGE
See Henry Schein, Inc.

91536
INVACARE CORPORATION
800-333-6900
http://www.invacare.com

08618
INVACARE SUPPLY GROUP
800-225-4792
http://www.invacaresupplygroup.com

49939
INVADO PHARMACEUTICALS
914-715-6232
866-963-8881
http://www.invadopharmaceuticals.com

INVERESK RESEARCH, INC.
See Charles River Laboratories International, Inc.

38396
INVERNESS MEDICAL INNOVATIONS
781-647-3900
http://www.invernessmedical.com

16874
INVISION PHARMAEUCTICALS
407-499-2225
800-443-4313

99710
INVOLVE PHARMACEUTICALS
248-449-3005

00258
INWOOD LABORATORIES
See Forest Laboratories, Inc.

58768
IOLAB PHARMACEUTICALS
See Ciba Vision Corp.

61646
IOMED
See Iopharm

55532
ION LABS
727-527-1072
877-990-4466
http://www.ionlabs.com

IOP, INC.
714-549-1185
800-535-3545
http://www.iopinc.com

61646
IOPHARM
817-595-5820

54921
IPR PHARMACEUTICALS, INC.
787-750-5353
800-477-6385

15054
IPSEN BIOPHARMACEUTICALS
866-837-2422
http://www.ipsenus.com

55688
IPSEN PHARMACEUTICALS
508-478-8900
http://www.ipsen.com

42211
IROKO PHARMACEUTICALS
267-546-3003
866-916-0576
http://www.iroko.com

IRONWOOD PHARMACEUTICALS, INC.
617-621-7722
http://www.ironwoodpharma.com

08617, 85325
I-SENS
678-417-5990
http://www.i-sens.com

ISIS PHARMACEUTICALS
760-931-9200
http://www.isispharm.com

ISO-TEX DIAGNOSTICS, INC.
281-482-1231
800-613-0600
http://www.isotexdiagnostics.com

67425
ISTA PHARMACEUTICALS, INC.
949-788-6000
800-385-7034
http://www.istavision.com

IVAX CORPORATION
949-455-4700
800-545-8800
http://www.tevausa.com

13613
IVAX DERMATOLOGICALS
305-575-4312

IVAX PHARMACEUTICALS, INC.
305-575-6000
800-327-4114
http://www.ivaxpharmaceuticals.com

12126
IVY CORPORATION
973-575-1990
800-443-8856

59291
IYATA PHARMACEUTICAL
813-740-1810

99940,56091
J & J MEDICAL
732-524-0400
888-222-6036
http://www.jnj.com

16837
J & J MERCK CONSUMER AND SPECIALTY
215-273-7000
800-523-3484
http://www.jnj.com

72904
JACKSON-MITCHELL
209-667-2019
800-891-4628
http://www.meyenberg.com

49938
JACOBUS
609-921-7447

10592
JAMOL LABS
201-262-6363

50458
JANSSEN
800-503-0784
800-526-7736
http://www.janssen.com

57894
JANSSEN BIOTECH
610-651-6000
800-526-7736
http://www.janssenbiotech.com

65847
JANSSEN PHARMACEUTICALS
609-730-2000
800-526-7736
http://www.janssenpharmaceuticalsinc.com

90011
JARROW FORMULAS
310-204-6936
800-726-0886
http://www.jarrow.com

64661
JAYMAC PHARMACEUTICALS, LLC
337-662-5962
800-520-5568
http://www.jaymacpharma.com

68727
JAZZ PHARMACEUTICALS, INC.
650-496-3777
800-520-5568
http://www.jazzpharma.com

18860
JAZZ PHARMACEUTICALS COMMERCIAL CORP
215-832-3767
http://www.jazzpharma.com

51111
J.B. LABORATORIES
616-738-8500
http://www.jblabs.com

68968
JDS PHARMACEUTICALS, LLC
See Noven Pharmaceuticals

50564
JEROME STEVENS
631-567-1113
800-325-9994

42023
JHP PHARMACEUTICALS
877-547-4547
866-923-2547
http://www.jhppharma.com

00304
J.J. BALAN, INC.
See HD Smith

59841
J-MED PHARMACEUTICALS
617-247-0010

60793
JMI-CANTON PHARMACEUTICALS
See King Pharmaceuticals

00204
JOHNSON & JOHNSON
732-524-0400
http://www.jnj.com

58232, 08137
JOHNSON & JOHNSON CONSUMER PRODUCTS COMPANY
800-526-3967
732-524-0400
877-895-3665
http://www.jnj.com

JOHNSON & JOHNSON HEALTHCARE
732-524-0400
http://www.jnj.com

52604
JONES PHARMA INCORPORATED
See King Pharmaceuticals, Inc.

J.R. CARLSON LABORATORIES
847-255-1600
888-234-5656
http://www.carlsonlabs.com

68712
JSJ PHARMACEUTICALS
843-965-8333
800-499-4468
http://www.jsjpharm.com

10106
J.T. BAKER (MALLINCKRODT)
908-859-2151
800-582-2537
http://www.mallbaker.com

59746
JUBILANT PHARMACEUTICALS
800-313-4623
800-308-3985
http://www.cadista.com

KABI PHARMACIA
See Pfizer US Pharmaceutical Group

KABIVITRUM, INC.
See Pfizer US Pharmaceutical Group

66435
KADMON PHARMACEUTICALS
724-778-6100
http://www.kadmon.com

60592
KALCHEM INTERNATIONAL
888-298-9905
http://www.kalchem international.com

KAO BRANDS COMPANY
513-421-1400
800-742-8798
http://www.jergens.com

42043
KARALEX PHARMA
609-759-1777
866-306-0240
http://www.karalexpharma.com

56023
KAREWAY PRODUCT
310-532-0009
http://www.kareway.com

28785
KAZ
800-477-0457
800-541-8001
http://www.kaz.com

76125
KEDRION S.P.A.
855-353-7466
http://www.kedrionusa.com

68387
KELTMAN PHARMACEUTICALS
601-936-7533
800-325-0903
http://www.keltman.com

08219, 08881
KENDALL HEALTHCARE
508-261-8000
800-962-9888
http://www.covidien.com

00482
KENWOOD LABORATORIES
See Bradley Pharmaceutical, Inc.

00369
KEY PHARMACEUTICALS
See Schering-Plough Corp.

32217
KEY2HEALTH
866-584-3101
http://www.key2health.com

62291
KIEL LABORATORIES, INC.
678-450-9187
800-538-3146
http://www.kielpharm.com

36000
KIMBERLY-CLARK
972-281-1200
800-544-1847
http://www.kimberly-clark.com

09038
KIMBERLY-CLARK DIGESTIVE
800-524-3577
http://www.kchealthcare.com

50989
KINESIO HOLDING CORPORATION
505-856-2029
505-797-7818
888-320-8273
http://www.kinesiotaping.com

60793
KING PHARMACEUTICALS, INC.
423-989-8000
800-776-3637
http://www.kingpharm.com

KINGSWOOD LABORATORIES, INC.
317-849-9513
800-968-7772
http://www.moi-stir.com

KINRAY
718-767-1234
800-854-6729
http://www.kinray.com

58223
KIRKMAN LABORATORIES, INC.
503-694-1600
800-245-8282
http://www.kirkmanlabs.com

76218
KLE 2
310-920-8199
310-842-8923
http://www.KLE2.com

28409
KLI CORP.
317-846-7452
800-308-7452
http://www.entertainers-secret.com

46738
KMART CORPORATION
847-286-2500
http://www.searsholdings.com

52187
KMM PHARMACEUTICALS
954-647-2726
http://www.staymacs.com

00074
KNOLL PHARMACEUTICALS
See Abbott Laboratories Pharmaceutical Division

58472
KODAK DENTAL
585-724-5631
800-933-8031
http://www.kodak.com

62515
KONEC, INC.
520-571-9119
http://www.konec-inc.com

00224
KONSYL PHARMACEUTICALS
410-822-5192
800-356-6795
http://www.konsyl.com

60598
KOS PHARMACEUTICALS
See Abbott Laboratories Pharmaceutical Division

66869
KOWA PHARMACEUTICALS AMERICA
334-288-1288
http://www.kowapharma.com

88856
K-PAX VITAMINS
415-381-7565
877-777-5729
http://www.kpaxpharm.com

12546
KRAFT FOODS
877-535-5666
http://www.kraftfoodscompany.com

55505
KRAMER LABORATORIES, INC.
302-223-1287
800-824-4894
http://www.kramerlabs.com

52083
KRAMER-NOVIS
787-767-2072
787-771-9443
http://www.kramernovis.com

62175
KREMERS URBAN
877-332-1714
609-936-5940
http://www.kremersurbanllc.com

33216
KRS GLOBAL BIOTECHNOLOGY
888-242-7996
http://www.gbtbio.com

KV PHARMACEUTICAL COMPANY
314-645-6600
800-234-5874
http://www.kvpharmaceutical.com

68716
KVD PHARMA
908-231-1911
888-477-2220
http://www.gbtbio.com

10702
KVK TECH
215-579-1842
http://www.kvktech.com

LABCORP
405-290-4444
800-634-9330
http://www.labcorp.com

LABOPHARM PHARMACEUTICALS
609-454-0207
877-345-6177
http://www.labopharm.com

LABORATOIRE AGUETTANT
800-422-2751

76336
LABORATOIRE HRA PHARMA
858-335-1300
http://www.pacificlinkconsulting.com

48582
LACLEDE
310-605-4280
877-522-5333
http://www.laclede.com

LACRIMEDICS, INC.
360-376-7095
800-367-8327
http://www.lacrimedics.com

LACTAID, INC.
215-273-7000
800-522-8243
http://www.lactaid.com

10106
LAFAYETTE PHARMACEUTICALS, INC.
See J.T. Baker, Inc.

LAKE CONSUMER PRODUCTS
262-677-5007
800-537-8658
http://www.lakeconsumer.com

LAKE ERIE MEDICAL
734-847-3847
800-284-2130
http://www.lakeeriemedical.com

02110
LANE LABS
201-236-9090
800-526-3005
http://www.lanelabs.com

00527
LANNETT
215-333-9000
800-325-9994
http://www.lannett.com

44677
LANSINOH LABORATORIES
703-299-1100
800-292-4794
http://www.lansinoh.com

LANTHEUS MEDICAL IMAGING
800-362-2668
800-299-3431
http://www.radiopharm.com

68047
LARKEN LABORATORIES, INC.
601-855-7678
888-527-5522
http://www.larkenlabs.com

LA ROCHE-POSAY
888-577-5226
800-560-1803
http://www.laroche-posay.us

16477, 00277
LASER PHARMACEUTICALS
864-286-8229
http://www.laserpharmaceuticals.com

21247
LCM PHAMACEUTICAL
888-411-5465

LECTEC CORPORATION
903-832-0993
http://www.lectec.com

LEDERLE CONSUMER HEALTH
See Wyeth

00008
LEDERLE LABS
See Wyeth

00008
LEDERLE PHARMACEUTICAL DIVISION
See Wyeth

LEDERLE-PRAXIS BIOLOGICALS
See Wyeth

23558
LEE PHARMACEUTICALS
626-442-3141
800-950-5337
http://www.leepharmaceuticals.com

25332
LEGERE PHARMACEUTICALS, INC.
480-991-4033
800-528-3144

12496
LEHN & FINK
See Reckitt Benckiser Pharmaceuticals

05388, 74970, 74980, 41660, 59606, 54499
LEINER HEALTH PRODUCTS
310-835-8400
http://www.leiner.com

10551
LEITNER PHARMACEUTICALS, LLC
866-590-7600
423-989-7238
http://www.leitnerpharma.com

00093
LEMMON CO.
See Teva Pharmaceuticals USA

50222
LEO PHARMA, INC.
973-637-1690
877-494-4536
http://www.leo-pharma.us

62991
LETCO MEDICAL
256-350-1297
800-239-5288
http://www.letcomedical.com

49523
LEX PHARMACEUTICAL
305-888-7375

51862
LIBERTAS PHARMA
678-690-5306
800-987-8566
http://www.libertaspharma.com

08387
LIBERTY MEDICAL SUPPLY
800-705-5797
866-342-2383
http://www.libertymedical.com

00440
LIBERTY PHARMACEUTICAL
866-836-9936
800-615-0721
http://www.libertymedical.com

30610
LIDTKE TECHNOLOGIES
408-858-0502
800-404-8185
http://www.lidtke.com

16055
LIFELINE FOODS
816-279-1651
http://www.lifeline-foods.com

72499
LIFE-LINE NUTRITIONAL PRODUCTS
520-426-3100
800-662-9862
http://www.nationalvitamin.com

53885
LIFESCAN, INC.
800-227-8862
800-524-7226
http://www.lifescan.com

LIFESIGN, LLC
800-526-2125
http://www.lifesignmed.com

LIFESTYLE
732-972-8585
800-622-7376
http://www.purilens.com

64365
LIGAND PHARMACEUTICALS, INC.
858-550-7500
800-964-5836
http://www.ligand.com

66715
LIL DRUG STORE PRODUCTS
800-252-0454
319-393-0454
http://www.lildrugstore.com

LINCOLN DIAGNOSTICS
217-877-2531
800-537-1336
http://www.lincolndiagnostics.com

05632
LINE ONE LABORATORIES
818-886-2288
800-222-9848
http://www.lineonelabsusa.com

54505
LINEAGE THERAPEUTICS
888-894-6528
215-259-3601
http://www.epinephrine autoinject.com

08566
LIONHEARTED INDUSTRIES
480-502-6007

61799
LIPOSOME CO.
See Elan Pharmaceuticals

16110
LIVERITE PRODUCTS
714-259-1800
888-425-5843
http://www.liverite.com

64038
LIVING WELL PHARMACY
310-218-4146
http://www.medchem manufacturing.com

54859
LLORENS PHARMACEUTICAL
305-716-0595
866-595-5598
http://www.llorenspharm.com

00127
LOBANA LABORATORIES (ULMER PHARMACAL)
218-732-2656
800-848-5637
http://www.lobanaproducts.com

34672
LOBOB LABORATORIES
408-432-0580
800-835-6262
http://www.loboblabs.com

55390
LOCH PHARMACEUTICALS
See Bedford Laboratories

09198
LOGAN PHARMACEUTICALS
859-344-9600
888-644-3478

08429
LOGIMEDIX
800-821-0047
http://www.logimedix.com

61480
LOMA LUX LABORATORIES
918-664-9882
800-316-9636
http://www.lomalux.com

12333
LONGS DRUG
800-865-6647
http://www.longs.com

83140, 71249
L'OREAL USA
908-673-3517
800-560-1803
888-577-5226
http://www.laroche-posay.us

71249
LOREAL SUNCARE RESEARCH
212-818-1500
800-322-2036
http://www.lorealusa.com

00273
LORVIC CORP.
See Young Dental Mfg.

67754
LOTUS BIOCHEMICAL CORP.
See Harvest Pharmaceuticals, Inc.

LSI AMERICA CORPORATION
800-720-5936
http://www.ondrox.com

61598
LTC PRODUCTS
513-738-5583
http://www.ltcproducts.net

LUITPOLD PHARMACEUTICALS, INC.
631-924-4000
800-645-1706
http://www.Luitpold.com

55792
LUKARE MEDICAL
855-752-9317

38673
LUMISCOPE
800-672-8293

67386
LUNDBECK, INC.
866-337-6996
866-402-8520
http://www.lundbeckusa.com

10892
LUNSCO, INC.
540-980-4358
800-264-8614

68180
LUPIN PHARMACEUTICALS, INC.
410-576-2000
800-466-1450
http://www.lupinpharmaceuticals.com

LUYTIES PHARMACAL CO.
800-466-3672
http://www.1-800homeopathy.com

00374
LYNE LABS
508-583-8700
800-525-0450
http://www.lyne.com

LYPHO-MED
See Astellas Pharma US, Inc.

67056
MABIS HEALTHCARE
800-526-4753
http://www.mabisdmi.com

33342
MACLEODS PHARMACEUTICALS
414-306-8200
http://www.macleodspharma.com

44183
MACOVEN PHARMACEUTICALS
225-644-2494
877-622-6836
http://www.macovenpharma.com

58407
MAGNA PHARMACEUTICALS, INC.
888-206-5525
502-254-5552
http://www.magnaweb.com

43292
MAGNO-HUMPHRIES LABORATORIES
503-684-5464
800-935-6737
http://www.magno-humphries.com

10705
MAJESTIC DRUG
845-436-0011
800-238-0220
http://www.majesticdrug.com

00904
MAJOR PHARMACEUTICALS
800-616-2471
http://www.major-pharm.com

08278
MALGAM ENTERPRISES, INC.
415-282-2115

MALLINCKRODT
314-654-2000
800-778-7898
http://www.mallinckrodt.com

10106
MALLINCKRODT BAKER, INC.
See Avantor Performance Materials

23635
MALLINCKRODT BRAND PHARMA
314-654-2000
800-554-5343
http://www.mallinckrodt.com

MALLINCKRODT CHEMICAL
314-654-2000
800-325-8888
http://www.mallinckrodt.com

99913
MALLINCKRODT NUCLEAR MEDICINE
314-654-2000
888-744-1414
http://www.mallinckrodt.com

99880
MALLINCKRODT RESPIRATORY
800-635-5267

45043
MANCHESTER PHARMACEUTICALS
970-685-4119
866-758-7068
http://www.manchesterpharma.com

10706
MANNE
843-768-4080
800-517-0228

42998
MARATHON PHARMACEUTICALS, LLC
866-945-7860
http://www.marathonpharma.com

12539
MARIN PHARMACEUTICALS
See A.G. Marin Pharmaceuticals

MARION MERRELL DOW
See Sanofi-Aventis US

25000
MARKSANS PHARMA
516-622-2208
http://www.apogeepharma.com

10135
MARLEX PHARMACEUTICALS
302-328-3355
866-820-7381
http://www.marlexpharm.com

MARLIN INDUSTRIES
805-473-2743
800-423-5926

12939
MARLOP PHARM
908-355-8854

MARLYN NUTRACEUTICALS, INC.
480-991-0200
888-766-4406
http://www.naturally.com

00682
MARNEL PHARMACEUTICALS, INC.
337-232-1396
800-962-7635

00591, 52544
MARSAM PHARMACEUTICALS
See Watson Pharmaceuticals

52555
MARTEC PHARMACEUTICAL, INC.
816-241-4144
800-822-6782
http://www.martec-kc.com

11845
MASON VITAMINS
305-428-6861
888-860-5376
http://www.masonvitamins.com

14362
MASSACHUSETTS PUBLIC HEALTH BIOLOGIC LABORATORIES
617-474-3000
800-457-4626

08496
MASTERS PHARMACEUTICAL
See MHC Medical Products

53905
MATRIX LABORATORIES, INC.
See Chiron Therapeutics

62750
MATRIXX INITIATIVES, INC.
602-385-8888
http://www.matrixxinc.com

41554
MAYBELLINE
800-944-0730

16169
MAYER LABORATORIES
510-229-5300
800-426-6366
http://www.mayerlabs.com

61703
MAYNE PHARMA (USA), INC.
201-225-5500
866-594-8420
http://www.maynepharma.com

MAYO FOUNDATION
507-284-2511
http://www.mayo.edu

00259
MAYRAND, INC.
See Merz Pharmaceuticals

00264
MCGAW, INC.
See B. Braun Medical, Inc.

49072
MCGUFF PHARMACEUTICALS, INC.
714-918-7277
800-603-4795
http://www.mcguff.com

63739, 38703, 49348
MCKESSON CORPORATION
415-983-8300
800-482-3784
http://www.mckesson.com

08692, 08691
MCKESSON/HEALTH MART
415-983-8705
415-983-8300
800-458-4678
http://www.mckesson.com

MCKESSON MEDICAL-SURGICAL
800-700-8737
800-482-3784
http://www.mckgenmed.com

57935
MCNEIL CONSUMER
215-273-7000
800-962-5357
http://www.jnj.com

16837
MCNEIL CONSUMER PHARMACEUTICAL
215-213-7000
877-895-3665
http://www.jnj.com

00045, 00062
MCNEIL PHARMACEUTICAL
See Ortho-McNeil Pharmaceutical

58605
MCR AMERICAN PHARMACEUTICAL
352-754-8587
http://www.mcramerican.com

53014
MD PHARMACEUTICAL
714-751-5881

83903
MDR FITNESS
954-845-9500
800-637-8227
http://www.mdr.com

58607
ME PHARMACEUTICALS, INC.
765-886-5097
866-578-9637
http://www.mepharmusa.com

MEAD JOHNSON LABORATORIES
See Bristol-Myers Squibb Co.

MEAD JOHNSON NUTRITIONALS
812-429-5000
http://www.meadjohnson.com

11883
MEAD-RAYMOND
903-509-0663

00037
MEDA PHARMACEUTICALS
732-564-2200
877-916-3991
http://www.medapharma.us

49741
MEDACTIVE ORAL PHARMACEUTICALS
866-887-4867
http://www.medactive.com

MEDAREX, INC.
609-430-2880
http://www.medarex.com

05313
MEDCARA PHARMACEUTICALS
515-577-6758
855-409-5496
http://www.medcara.com

53276
MED-CHEM PRODUCTS
781-932-5900
http://www.crbard.com

11940
MEDCO LABS
216-292-7546
http://www.medcolabs.com

60793
MEDCO RESEARCH, INC.
See King Pharmaceuticals, Inc.

08212
MEDCON BIOLAB TECHNOLOGIES, INC.
508-839-4203
800-443-6332
http://www.ilexpaste.com

45565
MED-DERM
423-926-4413
800-877-8869
http://www.crownlaboratories.com

67112
MEDECOR PHARMA
877-803-8235
http://www.medecorpharma.com

64253
MEDEFIL, INC.
630-682-4600
http://www.medefil.com

MEDEGEN
901-867-2951
800-233-1987
http://www.medegen.com

20451
MEDELA
877-694-6842
800-435-8316
http://www.medela.com

MEDEVA PHARMACEUTICALS
See UCB Pharmaceuticals, Inc.

MEDI AID CORP.
See Baxa Corp.

MEDICAL ACTION INDUSTRIES
631-231-4600
800-645-7042
http://www.medical-action.com

26974
MEDICAL NUTRITION, INC.
201-569-1188
800-221-0308
http://www.pro-stat.com

08271, 28465
MEDICAL PLASTIC DEVICES
514-694-9835
888-527-2842
http://www.medplas.com

10733
MEDICAL PRODUCTS LABS
800-523-0191
215-677-2700
http://www.medicalproductslaboratories.com

00576
MEDICAL PRODUCTS PANAMERICANA
305-545-6524
305-670-4416

99207
MEDICIS PHARMACEUTICAL CORPORATION
602-808-8800
800-845-1313
800-900-6381
http://www.medicis.com

32671
MEDICORE, INC.
305-558-4000
800-327-8894
http://www.medicore.com

25208
MEDICURE
732-584-5231
866-210-1128
http://www.medicurepharm.com

54365
MEDI-FLEX, INC.
913-451-0880
800-523-0502
http://www.medi-flex.com

43538
MEDIMETRIKS PHARMACEUTICALS
973-882-7512
http://www.medimetriks.com

60574
MEDIMMUNE, INC.
301-398-0000
877-633-4411
http://www.medimmune.com

67150
MEDINICHE
314-542-9539
800-711-4303
http://www.mediniche.com

89117
MEDINVENT
651-236-8545
866-960-9833
http://www.nasoneb.com

00095
MEDI-PLEX PHARM, INC.
See ECR Pharmaceuticals

47682
MEDIQUE PRODUCTS CO.
239-790-1962
800-634-7680
http://www.mediqueproducts.com

38779
MEDISCA, INC.
518-561-0109
800-932-1039
http://www.medisca.com

MEDISENSE, INC.
See Abbott Diabetes Care

12418
MEDIX PHARMACEUTICALS AMERICAS, INC. (MPA)
See Johnson & Johnson Consumer Products Co.

53329,08327
MEDLINE/DERMAL MANAGEMENT
800-633-5463
http://www.medline.com

80196, 08327
MEDLINE INDUSTRIES
800-633-5463
http://www.medline.com

53978
MED-PRO, INC.
308-324-4571
800-447-6060
http://www.med-pro-inc.com

90124, 18122
MEDQUIP
843-815-5301
888-404-5666
http://www.medquip.com

46011
MED-SYSTEMS, INC.
888-547-5492
http://www.sinucleanse.com

MEDTECH
307-733-1680
800-443-4908
http://www.medtechinc.com

MEDTRONIC, INC.
763-514-4000
800-328-2518
http://www.medtronic.com

58281
MEDTRONIC NEUROLOGICAL
800-328-0810
http://www.medtronic.com

66116
MEDVANTX, INC.
858-625-2990
http://www.medvantx.com

13143
MELVILLE BIOLOGICS (PRECISION PHARMA SERVICES)
631-752-7314
http://www.precisionpharma.com

MENICON AMERICA
650-378-1424
800-636-4266
http://www.menicon.com

22200
MENNEN CO.
See Colgate-Palmolive Co.

42279
MENPER DISTRIBUTORS, INC.
305-836-0208
800-560-5223

10742
MENTHOLATUM
716-677-2500
800-688-7660
http://www.mentholatum.com

81317
MENTOR UROLOGY
805-879-6000
800-525-0245
http://www.mentorcorp.com

MERCATOR MEDSYSTEMS, INC.
510-614-4550
http://www.mercatormed.com

00006
MERCK & CO., INC.
800-444-2080
800-994-2111
800-898-8326
908-423-1000
www.merck.com

00006
MERCK SHARP & DOHME
908-423-1000
800-444-2080
http://www.merck.com

00006
MERCK HUMAN HEALTH (A DIVISION OF MERCK & CO.)
215-652-5000
800-672-6372
http://www.merck.com

66582
MERCK/SCHERING-PLOUGH PHARM
866-637-2501
http://www.msppharma.com

62909
MERETEK DIAGNOSTICS, INC.
720-479-6400
888-637-3835
http://www.meretek.com

96095
MERICAL
714-283-9551
http://www.merical.com

00394
MERICON INDUSTRIES, INC.
309-693-2150
800-242-6464
http://www.mericon-industries.com

MERIDIAN MEDICAL TECHNOLOGIES
443-259-7800
800-638-8093
http://www.meridianmeds.com

30727
MERIT PHARMACEUTICALS
323-227-4831
800-696-3748
http://www.meritpharm.com

46783
MERZ AESTHETICS
650-286-4000
http://www.merzaesthetics.com

00259
MERZ PHARMACEUTICALS
336-856-2003
800-637-9872
http://www.merzusa.com

49808
METACON LABS
949-581-4365
866-777-4633
http://www.metaconlabs.com

55571
METAGENICS, INC.
800-692-9400
http://www.metagenics.com

64281
METHAPHARM, INC. (HEAD OFFICE)
954-341-0795
800-287-7686
http://www.methapharm.com

58657
METHOD PHARMACEUTICALS
877-250-3427

08368
METRIKA, INC.
408-524-2255
877-212-4968
http://www.A1cNow.com

86560
MET-RX USA
800-556-3879
http://www.met-rx.com

61738
METTLER ELECTRONICS
714-533-2221
800-854-9305
http://www.mettlerelectronics.com

58063
MGI PHARMA, INC.
952-346-4700
800-562-5580
http://www.mgipharma.com

08496
MHC MEDICAL PRODUCTS
513-354-2694
877-358-4342
http://www.mhcmed.com

MICHIGAN DEPARTMENT OF HEALTH
517-373-3740

MICROGENESYS, INC.
See Protein Sciences Corp.

42632
MICROLIFE
727-451-0484
888-314-2599
http://www.microlife.com

08564
MICROMEDICS
800-624-5662
http://www.micromedics-usa.com

MICRON TECHNOLOGY, INC.
208-368-4000
http://www.micron.com

11042
MIDDLEBROOK PHARMACEUTICALS, INC.
301-944-6600
800-340-3641
http://www.advancispharm.com

15686
MIDLAND PHARMACEUTICAL, LLC
913-233-0054

68308
MIDLOTHIAN LABORATORIES, LLC
334-288-8661
800-344-8661
http://www.midlothianlabs.com

46672
MIKART
404-351-4510
888-4MIKART
http://www.mikart.com

00026
MILES, INC.
See Bayer Corp.

00396
MILEX PRODUCTS, INC.
See Cooper Surgical

18757
MILLENNIUM BIOTECHNOLOGIES
908-604-2500
888-412-9179
http://www.milbiotch.com

63020
MILLENNIUM PHARMACEUTICALS
617-679-7000
800-390-5663
http://www.millennium.com

17204
MILLER
630-871-9557
800-323-2935
http://www.millerpharmacal.com

81361
MILUPA NORTH AMERICA
877-264-5872
http://www.milupana.com

55310
MIMEDX GROUP
678-384-6720
866-477-4219
http://www.mimedx.com

60307
MINRAD, INC.
716-855-1068
800-832-3303
http://www.minrad.com

00485
MISEMER PHARMACEUTICALS, INC.
See Edwards Pharmaceuticals, Inc.

00178
MISSION PHARMACAL
210-696-8400
http://www.missionpharmacal.com

76299
MIST PHARMACEUTICALS
908-282-7208

49771
MOBIUS THERAPEUTICS
314-615-6930
877-393-6486
http://www.mobius therapeutics.com

73107
MOLNLYCKE HEALTHCARE
678-250-7900
800-843-8497
http://www.molnlycke.com

04351
MONAGHAN MEDICAL CORPORATION
518-561-7330
800-833-9653
http://www.monaghanmed.com

61570
MONARCH PHARMACEUTICALS
See King Pharmaceuticals

11868
MONTICELLO DRUG CO.
904-384-3666
800-735-0666
http://www.monticello companies.com

65883
MONTIFF, INC.
310-582-8938

14844
MOOG
801-264-1001
800-970-2337
http://www.moog.com

00839
MOORE MEDICAL CORP.
800-234-1464
http://www.mooremedical.com

MOREPEN, INC.
609-987-1134
http://www.morepen.com

60432
MORTON GROVE PHARMACEUTICALS
800-346-6854
847-967-5600
http://www.mgp-online.com

MORTON INTERNATIONAL
215-592-3000
http://www.rohmhaas.com

MORTON SALT
312-807-2000
http://www.mortonsalt.com

MOTHERSOY INTERNATIONAL, INC.
812-424-5432
888-769-0769
http://www.mothersoy.com

MOUNT SINAI MEDICAL CENTER
212-241-6500
800-637-4624

MOVA PHARMACEUTICAL CORPORATION
905-816-3944
888-728-4366
http://www.patheon.com

89105
MPA-DIABETIC
866-921-0662
http://www.choicedmproducts.com

66977
MPM MEDICAL, INC.
972-893-4090
800-232-5512
http://www.mpmmedicalinc.com

74676
MUELLER
608-643-8530
800-356-9522
http://www.muellersportsmed.com

00150
MURRAY DRUG CORP.
270-753-6654

53489
MUTUAL PHARMACEUTICAL CO., INC. (UNITED RESEARCH LABORATORIES)
215-288-6500
800-523-3684
http://www.urlmutual.com

58204
MVW NUTRITIONALS
855-236-8584
http://www.mvwnutritionals.com

00378
MYLAN
724-514-1800
800-796-9526
http://www.mylan.com

51079
MYLAN INSTITUTIONAL
800-848-0462

49502
MYLAN SPECIALTY LP
908-542-1999
800-848-9213
http://www.mylanspecialty.com

20694
MYOGEN
See Gilead Sciences

59730
NABI
301-770-3099
800-685-5579
http://www.nabi.com

57459
NASTECH PHARMACEUTICAL CO., INC.
425-908-3600
http://www.nastech.com

08164
NATIONAL MEDICAL PRODUCTS, INC.
949-768-1147
http://www.jtip.com

94688
NATIONAL NUTRITION, INC.
717-569-8561
877-271-3570
http://www.medtritionnni.com

54629
NATIONAL VITAMIN
559-781-8871
800-538-5828
http://www.nationalvitamin.com

42937
NATIONWIDE LABORATORIES
732-682-2501

NATREN, INC.
805-371-4737
800-992-3323
http://www.natren.com

47469
NATROL, INC.
818-739-6000
800-262-8765
http://www.natrol.com

94604
NAT-RUL HEALTH PRODUCTS
800-628-7855
http://www.natrulhealth.com

79911
NATURADE
800-421-1830
http://www.naturade.com

NATURALLY VITAMINS CO.
480-991-0200
888-766-4406
http://www.naturallyvitamins.com

93265
NATURE'S BEST
312-245-2834
800-551-2544
http://www.naturesbest enzyme.com

74312
NATURE'S BOUNTY, INC.
631-200-2000
800-433-2990
http://www.naturesbounty.com

94603
NATURE'S HEALTH CONNECTION
606-668-6533
888-600-4642
http://www.australiandream.com

NATURE'S SUNSHINE PRODUCTS, INC.
801-342-4300
800-223-8225
http://www.naturessunshine.com

65203
NATURE'S VISION
269-327-8282
877-740-8180
http://www.naturesvisioninc.com

NATURE'S WAY
801-489-1500
800-926-8883
http://www.naturesway.com

74312
NBTY, INC.
See Nature's Bounty, Inc.

60242
NEIL LABS
609-448-5500
http://www.neillabs.com

05928
NEILMED PHARMACEUTICALS
707-525-3784
877-477-8633
http://www.neilmed.com

72559
NELLSON NEUTRACEUTICAL (FORMERLY NCI MEDICAL FOODS)
626-812-6522
800-869-1515

NEORX CORP.
206-281-7001
http://www.neorx.com

58414
NEOSTRATA
609-520-0715
800-225-9411
http://www.neostrata.com

51759
NEPHROCEUTICALS
937-281-0123
http://www.nephroceuticals.com

00487
NEPHRON PHARMACEUTICALS CORP.
407-246-1389
800-443-4313
http://www.nephronpharm.com

59528
NEPHRO-TECH
785-883-4108
800-879-4755
http://www.nephrotech.com

99825
NESTLE HEALTHCARE NUTRITION
847-317-2800
877-463-7853
http://www.nestleclinical nutrition.com

NESTLE INFANT NUTRITION
800-284-9488
http://www.verybestbaby.com

62860
NEUREX PHARMACEUTICALS
See Elan Pharmaceuticals

NEUROGENESIS
800-345-8912
http://www.neurogenesis.com

14565
NEUROSCI
937-848-9130
http://www.neurosciinc.com

NEUTRACEUTICAL SOLUTIONS, INC.
361-854-0755
800-856-7040
http://www.eliquidsolutions.com

10812
NEUTROGENA CORPORATION
310-642-1150
800-582-4048
http://www.neutrogena.com

NEUTRON TECHNOLOGY CORP.
See Micron Technology, Inc.

50816
NEW AMERICAN THERAPEUTICS
908-282-7450
888-489-5937
http://www.natxcorp.com

NEW HEALTH CORP.
877-263-3555
http://www.newhealthcorp.com

58517
NEW HORIZON RX GROUP
504-465-5545

NEW WORLD TRADING CORP.
407-566-0608

10530
NEXCO PHARMA
713-896-4949
http://www.nexcopharma.com

00722
NEXGEN PHARMA
949-863-0340
949-260-3714
http://www.nexgenpharma.com

58181
NEXTSOURCE BIOTECHNOLOGY
855-672-2468
http://www.nextsource biotechnology.com

61958
NEXSTAR PHARMACEUTICALS, INC.
See Gilead Sciences

24478
NEXTWAVE PHARMACEUTICALS
847-996-6200
http://www.nextwavepharm.com

14789
NEXUS PHARMACEUTICALS
888-806-4606
847-996-3789
http://www.nexuspharma.net

45611
NFI CONSUMER PRODUCTS
800-432-9334
http://www.nfiproducts.com

59016
NICHE PHARMACEUTICALS
817-491-2770
800-677-0355
http://www.niche-inc.com

08384,38384
NIPRO DIAGNOSTICS
800-342-7226
http://www.niprodiagnostics.com

38379,41405
NIPRO MEDICAL CORPORATION
305-599-7174
888-647-7698
http://www.nipro.com

12948
NITROMED, INC.
781-266-4000
http://www.nitromed.com

15662
NNODUM CORPORATION
513-861-2329
888-301-0457
http://www.zikspain.com

51801
NOMAX, INC.
314-961-2500
800-397-0012
http://www.nomax.com

NORAMCO, INC.
706-353-4400
http://www.noramco.com

41805
NORDIC ENTERPRISES
514-419-5160
http://www.newnordic.ca

50445
NORDISK
609-987-5800
http://www.novonordisk-us.com

59730
NORTH AMERICAN BIOLOGICALS, INC.
See Nabi

76906
NORTH AMERICAN HERBAL
800-836-3095
http://www.northamericanherbal.com

62448
NORTH AMERICAN VACCINE, INC.
See Baxter Healthcare Corp.

92942
NORTHERN RESEARCH LABORATORIES, INC.
See Epien Medical

16714
NORTHSTAR RX
480-502-6007
800-206-7821
http://www.northstarrxllc.com

29033
NOSTRUM PHARMACEUTICALS, INC.
732-635-0036
http://www.nostrumpharma.com

08548
NOVA BIOMEDICAL
781-894-0800
800-458-5813
http://www.novabiomedical.com

NOVADEL PHARMA
908-203-4640
http://www.novadel.com

76077
NOVANA MEDICAL
813-855-0700

52308
NOVA ORTHO-MED
800-557-6682
http://www.novamedicalproducts.com

99780
NOVAPLUS
See Novation

00067
NOVARTIS CONSUMER HEALTH
See Novartis Pharmaceuticals Corp.

00212, 41679
NOVARTIS MEDICAL NUTRITION
862-778-8300
888-669-6682
http://www.novartisnutrition.com

58768
NOVARTIS OPHTHALMICS, INC.
866-393-6336
See Novartis Pharmaceuticals Corp.

NOVARTIS PHARMA AG
See Novartis Pharmaceuticals Corp.

00078
NOVARTIS PHARMACEUTICALS CORPORATION
800-526-0175
http://www.pharma.us.novartis.com

NOVATION
888-766-8283
http://www.novationco.com

66500
NOVAVAX
240-268-2000
http://www.novavax.com

68968
NOVEN PHARMACEUTICALS
305-253-5099
888-253-5099
http://www.noven.com

NOVEN THERAPEUTICS, LLC
866-663-2539
800-455-8070
http://www.jdspharma.com

00169, 59060
NOVO NORDISK PHARMACEUTICALS
609-987-5800
800-727-6500
http://www.novonordisk-us.com

49197
NOVOGEN
203-966-2556
http://www.novogen.com

00093
NOVOPHARM USA, INC.
See Teva Pharmaceuticals USA

00159,48932
NOYES
800-522-2469
http://www.pjnoyes.com

68875
NPS PHARMACEUTICALS
855-542-8839
http://www.npsp.com

NU SKIN ENTERPRISES
801-345-1000
800-487-1000
http://www.nuskinenterprises.com

NUGYN, INC.
763-398-0108
877-774-1442
http://www.eros-therapy.com

08910
NULINE PHARMACEUTICALS
914-939-8881
http://www.nulinepharma.com

55499
NUMARK LABS
732-417-1870
800-338-8079
http://www.numarklabs.com

NUPATHE
484-567-0130
http://www.nupathe.com

59547
NURO PHARMA
855-687-6633
http://www.nuropharma.com

07249,00221
NUTRA BALANCE
800-654-3691
317-356-5478
http://www.nutra-balance-products.com

NUTRACEA
877-723-1700
http://www.nutracea.com

NUTRACEUTICAL SOLUTIONS
361-854-0755
800-856-7040
http://www.eliquidsolutions.com

02359
NUTRACEUTICS CORPORATION
877-664-6684
http://www.neutraceutics.com

55970
NUTRAMAX LABORATORIES, INC.
410-776-4000
800-925-5187
http://www.nutramaxlabs.com

NUTRAMAX PRODUCTS
978-282-1800
http://www.nutramax.com

NUTRASAL, LLC
207-856-2222
888-437-5772
http://www.nutrasal.com

NUTRI VENTION
210-661-8589
800-390-7940

26974
NUTRICIA NA
800-221-0308
http://www.pro-stat.com

49735
NUTRICIA NORTH AMERICA
301-795-2300
800-365-7354
http://www.shsna.com

NUTRITION 21
914-701-4500
800-696-0860
http://www.nutrition21.com

59427
NUTRITION WAREHOUSE
800-645-5412

70186
NUTRITIONAL ALLIANCE
954-455-1917
http://www.nutritionalalliance.com

90962
NUTRITIONAL DESIGNS
516-612-4900
888-263-5227
http://www.ndlabs.com

NUVO RESEARCH, INC.
866-949-9277
http://www.nuvoresearch.com

91124
NUVORA, INC.
408-856-2200
877-530-9811
http://www.nuvorainc.com

00407
NYCOMED AMERSHAM
See GE Healthcare

NYCOMED US, INC.
631-454-7677
800-645-9833
http://www.nycomedus.com

76478
OAK PHARMACEUTICALS
800-932-5676
http://www.akorn.com

11169
OAKHURST CO.
516-731-5380
800-831-1135
http://www.oakhurst-medicine.com

OASIS CONSUMER HEALTHCARE
888-963-2747
http://www.oasisdrymouth.com

62032
OBAGI MEDICAL PRODUCTS
562-628-1007
http://www.obagi.com

89114
OCEANA THERAPEUTICS
732-318-3800
866-924-8090
http://www.oceanatherapeutics.com

68682
OCEANSIDE PHARMACEUTICALS
949-461-6199
http://www.oceansidepharmaceuticals.com

55515, 80831.
OCLASSEN PHARMACEUTICALS, INC.
See Watson Pharmaceuticals, Inc.

21406, 55056
O'CONNOR, INC.
See Columbia Laboratories, Inc.

68209
OCTAPHARMA USA, INC.
703-766-4860
866-766-4860
http://www.octapharma.com

53152
OCTOGEN PHARMACAL
770-843-7032
800-729-4613
http://www.octogenpharma.com

54799, 15718
OCUSOFT
800-233-5469
http://www.ocusoft.com

65473
ODYSSEY PHARMACEUTICALS, INC.
877-427-9068
http://www.odysseypharm.com

51660
OHM LABORATORIES, INC.
877-646-5227
http://www.ohmlabs.com

OMNII ORAL PHARMACEUTICALS
561-689-1140
800-445-3386
http://www.4oralcare.com

94030
OMNIS HEALTH
877-450-6734
http://www.omnishealth.com

73796
OMRON MANAGED HEALTHCARE
877-216-1333
847-680-6200
http://www.omronhealthcare.com

16761
ONSET DERMATOLOGICS
401-762-2000
888-713-8154
http://www.onsetdermatologics.com

16781
ONSET THERAPEUTICS
888-713-8154
877-702-0532
http://www.onsettx.com

68305, 93286
ONTOS, INC.
360-740-0888
888-469-7546
http://www.4myskin.com

ONY
716-636-9096
877-274-4669
http://www.onyinc.com

76075
ONYX PHARMACEUTICALS
650-266-0000
877-669-9121
http://www.onyx.com

11916, 64108
OPTICS LABORATORY, INC.
626-350-1926
800-968-6788
http://www.opticslab.com

OPTIKEM INTERNATIONAL
800-525-1752

63369
OPTIMED CONTROLLED RELEASE LAB
See Quality by Design Packaging

50520
OPTIMOX
310-618-9370
800-223-1601
http://www.optimox.com

55933
ORAHEALTH CORPORATION
425-451-9876
877-672-6541
http://www.orahealth.com

00041
ORAL-B LABORATORIES
800-566-7252
http://www.oral-b.com

65976
ORAPHARMA, INC.
215-956-2200
866-273-7846
http://www.orapharma.com

ORASURE TECHNOLOGIES
610-882-1820
800-869-3535
http://www.orasure.com

68820
ORCHID HEALTHCARE
480-502-6007
480-227-7661

54123
OREXO US
855-673-9687
http://www.orexo.com

ORGANOGENESIS, INC.
781-575-0775
http://www.organogenesis.com

00052
ORGANON, INC.
800-222-7579
http://www.organon-usa.com

66203
ORGANON SANOFI
See Organon, Inc.

ORGANON TEKNIKA CORP.
See Biomerieux

15377
ORIGIN BIOMED
902-423-5745
888-234-7256
http://www.originbiomed.com

62161
ORPHAN MEDICAL, INC.
See Jazz Pharmaceuticals

66607
ORPHAN PHARMACEUTICALS USA
See Rare Disease Therapeutics

ORTHO BIOTECH PRODUCTS, LP
See Centocor Ortho Biotech, Inc.

00562
ORTHO-CLINICAL DIAGNOSTICS, INC.
800-828-6316
http://www.orthoclinical.com

99948
ORTHO DERM
800-426-7762
http://www.orthodermatologics.com

00062
ORTHO-MCNEIL PHARMACEUTICAL
800-682-6532
http://www.ortho-mcneil.com

ORTHO NEUTROGENA
800-426-7762
http://www.orthoneutrogena.com

67707
OSCIENT PHARMACEUTICALS
781-398-2300
http://www.oscient.com

65231
OSI PHARMACEUTICALS
631-962-2000
800-572-1932
http://www.osip.com

59857
OSIRIS THERAPEUTICS
443-545-1800
888-674-7471
888-674-9551
http://www.osiris.com

10244
OTIS CLAPP & SONS, INC.
314-344-1100
http://www.otisclapp.com

67817
OTN GENERICS
650-952-8400
800-482-6700
http://www.lynx2otn.com

59148
OTSUKA AMERICA
301-990-0030
800-562-3974
http://www.otsuka.com

67386
OVATION PHARMACEUTICALS, INC.
847-282-1000
888-514-5204
http://www.ovationpharma.com

08470, 08214
OWEN MUMFORD
770-977-2226
800-421-6936
http://www.owenmumford.com

64803
OXFORD PHARMACEUTICAL SERVICES
973-256-0600
http://www.oxfordpharm.com

OXIS INTERNATIONAL
650-212-2568
800-547-3686
http://www.oxisresearch.com

99949
P & G HEALTH
513-983-1100
800-543-7270
http://www.pg.com

99958
P & G PAPER PRODUCTS
513-983-1100
800-543-7270
http://www.pg.com

P & S LABORATORIES, INC.
See Standard Homeopathic Co.

64393
PACIFIC EMERALD CO.
425-485-9208

60758
PACIFIC PHARMA
800-811-4184
714-246-4600

65250
PACIRA PHARMACEUTICALS, INC.
858-625-2424
858-625-2414
http://www.pacira.com

16571
PACK PHARMACEUTICALS, LLC
847-229-0153
800-521-5340
http://www.packpharma.com

00574
PADDOCK LABORATORIES, INC.
866-634-9120
http://www.perrigo.com

38142
PAL MIDWEST, LTD.
815-965-2981
815-332-9405
http://www.rashcream.com

25294
PALCO LABS
831-430-1600
800-346-4488
http://www.palcolabs.com

00516
PALISADES PHARMACEUTICALS, INC.
See Glenwood, Inc.

24518
PALM PHARMACEUTICALS
843-364-3256
http://www.palmpharmaceuticals.com

68134
PALMETTO PHARMACEUTICALS, INC.
864-286-8229

00525
PAMLAB, LLC
985-893-4097
http://www.pamlab.com

PAN AMERICAN LABORATORIES
See Pamlab, LLC

86679
PAPERPAK
See Attends Healthcare Products

49884
PAR PHARMACEUTICAL, INC.
201-802-4000
800-828-9393
http://www.parpharm.com

42702
PARAGON BIOTECK
855-281-1743
888-424-1192
http://paragonbioteck.com

66758
PARENTA PHARMACEUTICALS, INC.
803-461-5500
800-898-9948
http://www.parentarx.com

44229,83490
PARI RESPIRATORY
804-253-7274
http://www.pari.com

PARKE-DAVIS - A PFIZER CO.
See Pfizer US Pharmaceutical Group

64029
PARKEDALE PHARMACEUTICALS
See King Pharmaceuticals, Inc.

00341
PARKER LABORATORIES, INC.
973-276-9500
800-631-8888
http://www.parkerlabs.com

50930
PARNELL
415-256-1800
800-457-4276
http://www.parnellpharm.com

49309
PARTHENON CO., INC.
801-972-5184
800-453-8898
http://www.parthenoninc.com

00418, 11098
PASADENA RESEARCH LABS
See Akorn, Inc.

10866
PASCAL CO., INC.
425-827-4694
800-426-8051
http://www.pascaldental.com

PATHEON
905-821-4001
888-728-4366
http://www.patheon.com

10147
PATRIOT PHARMACEUTICALS, LLC
215-325-7676
800-631-5273
http://www.patriotpharmaceuticals.com

08519
PATTON MEDICAL DEVICES
877-763-7678
http://www.pattonmd.com

PBI
See Upsher-Smith Labs, Inc.

66213
PBM PHARMACEUTICALS
540-832-3282
800-485-9828
http://www.pbmpharmaceuticals.com

PDI - PROFESSIONAL DISPOSABLES INTERNATIONAL, INC.
845-365-1700
http://www.pdipdi.com

PDK LABS, INC.
631-273-2630
http://www.pdklabs.com

55289
PDRX PHARMACEUTICAL
405-942-3040
800-299-7379
http://www.pdrx.com

66346
PEDIAMED PHARMACEUTICALS, INC.
859-282-8582
866-543-6337
http://www.pediamedpharma.com

PEDIATRIC PHARMACEUTICALS
732-603-7708
http://www.pediatricpharm.com

52547
PEDIATRX
866-398-0815
http://www.pediatrx.com

00884
PEDINOL PHARMACAL, INC.
631-293-9500
800-733-4665
http://www.pedinol.com

10974
PEGASUS
850-478-2770
http://www.pegasuslabs.com

25074
PENEDERM, INC.
See Bertek Pharmaceuticals, Inc.

13893
PENN LABORATORIES
877-300-6153
http://www.pennlaboratories.com

60432
PENNEX PHARMACEUTICAL, INC.
See Morton Grove Pharmaceuticals, Inc.

PENTECH PHARMACEUTICALS, INC.
847-255-0303
http://www.pentechinc.com

59316
PERFORMANCE HEALTH PRODUCTS
800-321-2135
877-412-7467
http://www.performancehealth.com

65224
PERNIX THERAPEUTICS, LLC
800-793-2145
http://www.pernixtx.com

00113, 10768
PERRIGO COMPANY
269-673-8451
800-719-9260
http://www.perrigo.com

99278
PERRIGO DIABETES CARE
269-673-8451
800-827-2296
http://www.perrigo.com

00096
PERSON COVEY
818-240-1030
800-423-2341
http://www.personandcovey.com

PERSONAL PRODUCTS CO.
See Johnson & Johnson Healthcare

00927
PFEIFFER CO.
404-614-0255
800-342-6450
http://www.pfeiffer pharmaceuticals.com

12547
PFIZER CONSUMER HEALTH
973-660-5500
800-762-4675
http://www.pfizer.com

PFIZER CONSUMER HEALTHCARE
800-446-9824
973-660-5000
http://www.pfizer.com

PFIZER US PHARMACEUTICAL GROUP
212-733-2323
800-879-3477
http://www.pfizer.com

40042
PHARMAFORCE
614-436-2222
877-788-3232
877-845-6371
http://www.pharmaforceinc.com

PHARMA FRONTIERS
281-775-0609
http://www.pharmafrontier.com

62441
PHARMA MEDICA
905-624-9115
http://www.pharmamedica.com

52959
PHARMA PAC
805-929-1333
800-841-5554
http://www.pharmapac.com

39822
PHARMA-TEK, INC.
See X-Gen Pharmaceuticals, Inc.

45861
PHARMACEUTICA NORTH AMERICA
818-291-0547
877-329-2592
http://www.pnarx.com

00121
PHARMACEUTICAL ASSOCIATES, INC.
864-277-7282
800-845-8210
http://www.pa-inc.net

PHARMACEUTICAL BASICS, INC.
See Upsher-Smith Labs, Inc.

51655
PHARMACEUTICAL CORPORATION OF AMERICA
317-616-4498
800-722-0772

21659
PHARMACEUTICAL LABS, INC.
See Neutraceutical Solutions, Inc.

45334
PHARMACEUTICAL SPECIALTIES, INC.
507-288-8500
800-325-8232
http://www.psico.com

53731
PHARMACEUTIX
800-647-6100
http://www.pharmaceutix health.com

12547
PHARMACIA & UPJOHN CONSUMER HEALTHCARE - A DIVISION OF PFIZER
See Pfizer Consumer Health

PHARMACIA CORP. - A DIVISION OF PFIZER
See Pfizer US Pharmaceutical Group

63704
PHARMACIST PHARMACEUTICAL, LLC
540-375-5415

00462
PHARMADERM
678-287-1500
866-337-6457
http://www.pharmaderm.com

55422, 65937
PHARMAKON LABS
813-886-3216
http://www.pharmakonlabs.com

PHARMALUCENCE
781-275-7120
800-221-7554
http://www.pharmalucence.com

15035
PHARMANEX
801-345-9800
http://www.pharmanex.com

51817
PHARMASCIENCE LAB
514-340-9800
800-363-8805
http://www.pharmascience.com

99734
PHARMASMART INTERNATIONAL
800-781-0323
http://www.pharma-smart.com

48107
PHARMASSURE, INC.
888-462-2548

31604, 78742
PHARMAVITE
818-221-6200
800-423-2405
http://www.pharmavite.com

44178
PHARMAXIS
888-416-1828
http://www.pharmaxis.com.au

PHARMED
800-683-7342
305-592-2324
http://www.pharmed.com

PHARMEDIUM
847-457-2300
800-523-7749
http://www.pharmedium.com

53002
PHARMEDIX
800-486-1811
http://www.pharmedixrx.com

66663
PHARMELLE
See Azur Pharma

00813
PHARMICS, INC.
801-966-4138
800-456-4138
http://www.pharmics.com

67211
PHARMION CORPORATION
See Celgene Corp.

54348
PHARMPAK
415-455-9981
800-541-6315
http://www.pharmpakinc.com

PHOENIX LABORATORIES
516-822-1230

PHOTOCURE ASA
47-22-06-22-10
http://www.photocure.com

PHOTOMEDEX
215-619-3600
http://www.photomedex.com

98152
PHYSICIAN RECOMMENDED NUTRICEUTICALS
800-900-2303
http://www.prnomegahealth.com

54868
PHYSICIANS TOTAL CARE
918-254-2273
800-759-3650
http://www.physicianstotalcare.com

PHYTOPHARMICA, INC.
920-469-1313
800-553-2370
http://www.enzymatictherapy.com

60831
PIERRE FABRE PHARMACEUTICALS
973-898-1042
http://www.pierre-fabre.com

66794, 08367
PIRAMAL CRITICAL CARE
800-414-1901
http://www.piramalusa.com

27843
PIVOTAL THERAPEUTICS
561-288-5231
http://www.pivotaltherapeutics.us

44733
PLAINVIEW HEALTHCARE
800-903-3222
http://www.dairycare.com

PLAYTEX CO.
800-222-0453
http://www.playtex.com

50111
PLIVA, INC.
800-545-8800
http://www.plivainc.com

41100, 11523
PLOUGH, INC.
See Schering-Plough Healthcare Products

37864
PLUS PHARMA
631-543-3334

25197
PMD HEALTHCARE
888-763-4968
http://www.spiropd.com

50991
POLY PHARMACEUTICALS, INC.
601-776-3497
800-882-1041

POLYMEDICA CORPORATION
781-933-2020
800-886-4050
http://www.polymedica.com

POLYMEDICA PHARMACEUTICALS
See Amerifit Brands, Inc.

47144
POLYMER TECHNOLOGY CORP.
978-658-6111
800-323-0000
http://www.polymer.com

08193
POLYMER TECHNOLOGY SYSTEMS
317-870-5610
877-870-5610
http://www.cardiocheck.com

52605
POLYGEN PHARMACEUTICALS
631-392-4045
631-392-4044
http://www.polygenpharma.com

49963
PORTAL PHARMACEUTICALS
787-832-6645

55688
PORTON PRODUCT LIMITED
See Speywood Pharmaceuticals, Inc.

POWDERJECT VACCINES
See Chiron Therapeutics

POYTHRESS
See ECR Pharmaceuticals

68158
PRAECIS PHARMACEUTICALS INCORPORATED
781-795-4100
877-772-3247
http://www.gsk.com

43288
PRAELIA PHARMACEUTICALS
919-435-3130
http://www.praelia.com

62263,63370
PRAGMATIC MATERICALS, INC.
440-349-1313

66993
PRASCO LABORATORIES
513-618-3333
866-525-0688
866-469-1414
http://www.prasco.com

PRATT PHARMACEUTICALS
See Pfizer US Pharmaceutical Group

68094
PRECISION DOSE, INC.
800-397-9228
http://www.precisiondose.com

72058
PRECISION FOODS
800-442-5242
http://www.precisionfoods.com

PREMIER MICRONUTRIENT
615-234-4020
888-606-8883
http://www.premiermicronutrient.com

PRESS CHEMICAL & PHARMACEUTICAL LABORATORIES, INC.
614-863-2802
http://www.epsal.com

75137
PRESTIGE BRANDS INTERNATIONAL
914-524-6810
800-803-4471
http://www.prestigebrands.com

40076
PRESTIUM PHARMA
267-685-0340
http://www.prestiumpharma.com

66378
PRESUTTI LABORATORIES
847-483-6050
http://www.presuttilabs.com

42582
PREVENTION LABORATORIES
800-473-1205
618-252-6922
http://www.preventionlabs.com

00684
PRIMEDICS LABORATORIES
323-770-3005

68040
PRIMUS PHARMACEUTICALS, INC.
480-483-1410
http://www.primusrx.com

39278
PRINCE OF PEACE
800-732-2328
510-887-1799
http://www.popus.com

PRINCETON PHARMACEUTICAL PRODUCTS
See Bristol-Myers Squibb Co.

PRIORITY HEALTHCARE
See Curascript

58417
PRISMIC PHARMACEUTICALS
480-320-1002

PROCTER & GAMBLE COMPANY
513-983-1100
800-543-7270
http://www.pgpharma.com

00149
PROCTER & GAMBLE PHARMACEUTICALS
See Warner Chilcott Pharma

PROCYTE CORPORATION
425-869-1239
http://www.procyte.com

08524
PROGRESSIVE HEALTH SUPPLY
888-887-4772
http://www.progressivehealthsupply.com

66375
PROMEDICA LABS, INC.
973-925-1001

65483
PROMETHEUS LABORATORIES, INC.
858-824-0895
888-423-5227
http://www.prometheuslabs.com

67857
PROMIUS PHARMA, LLC
866-733-3952
http://www.promiuspharma.com

67555
PRONOVA CORPORATION
305-666-4831
866-703-3508
http://www.pronovacorp.com

50313
PROPHARMA
305-592-9216
800-446-0255

65581
PROPST PHARMACEUTICALS
256-704-6394

42747
PROSTRAKAN
908-234-1096
800-726-2876
http://www.prostrakan-usa.com

68905
PROSYNTHESIS LABORATORIES
800-517-5111
http://www.unjury.com

PROTEIN DESIGN LABS, INC.
510-574-1400
http://www.pdl.com

42874
PROTEIN SCIENCES CORPORATION
203-686-0800
800-488-7099
http://www.proteinsciences.com

PROTHERICS, INC.
615-327-1027
888-327-1027
http://www.protherics.com

29978
PROVIDENT PHARMACEUTICALS, LLC
719-278-3988
http://www.providentpharma.com

16241
PRX PHARM
See Par Pharmaceutical, Inc.

89115
PSS WORLD MEDICAL
904-332-3000
800-777-4908
http://www.pssworldmedical.com

PSYCHEMEDICS CORP.
978-206-8220
800-628-8073
http://www.psychemedics.com

65005
PTS LABORATORIES, INC.
562-907-3607
http://www.ptsgeolabs.com

51013
PURACAP PHARMACEUTICAL
908-941-5456
866-770-3027
http://www.puracap.com

00034
PURDUE FREDERICK
203-588-8000
800-877-5666
888-726-7535
http://www.purduepharma.com

59011
PURDUE PHARMA LP
203-588-8000
800-877-5666
888-726-7535
http://www.purduepharma.com

67781
PURDUE PHARMACEUTICAL PRODUCTS
800-877-5666
888-726-7535
http://www.purduepharma.com

PUREPAC PHARMACEUTICAL CO.
See Actavis Elizabeth

PURILENS, INC.
See Lifestyle

PURITANS PRIDE
800-645-9584
http://www.puritan.com

QLT, INC.
604-707-7000
800-663-5486
http://www.qltinc.com

50236
QLT OPHTHALMICS
604-707-7000
http://www.qltinc.com

QLT PHOTOTHERAPEUTICS, INC.
See QLT, Inc.

QOL MEDICAL
866-469-3773
http://www.qolmed.com

Q-PHARMA, INC.
609-883-1818

66774
QUADEX PHARMACEUTICALS, LLC
801-453-9614
http://www.viroxyn.com

QUALICAPS, INC.
336-449-3900
800-227-7853
http://www.qualicaps.com

52917
QUALIS, INC.
515-243-3000

00603
QUALITEST
256-859-4011
800-444-4011
http://www.qualitestrx.com

63369
QUALITY BY DESIGN PACKAGING
812-522-9262
http://www.qbdinc.com

49999
QUALITY CARE PHARM, INC.
See Quality Care Products, LLC

49999
QUALITY CARE PRODUCTS, LLC
419-478-0441
http://qcpmeds.com

63004
QUESTCOR PHARMACEUTICALS, INC.
510-400-0700
800-411-3065
http://www.questcor.com

QUIDEL CORP.
858-552-1100
800-874-1517
http://www.quidel.com

61941
QUIGLEY CORP.
267-880-1100
http://www.quigley.com

94047
QUINCY BIOSCIENCE
608-827-8000
http://www.quincybioscience.com

23710
QUINNOVA PHARMACEUTICALS, INC.
877-660-6263
215-860-6263
http://www.quinnova.com

54391
R & D LABORATORIES, INC.
See Watson Pharmaceuticals

17236
R & S NORTHEAST
215-673-7770
800-262-7770
http://www.rsnortheast.com

12830
R.A. MCNEIL COMPANY
423-493-9170
800-755-3038

53135
RAANI CORPORATION
708-496-8025
http://www.raani.com

RAINBOW LIGHT NUTRITIONAL SYSTEMS
831-420-2660
800-635-1233

10631
RANBAXY LABORATORIES LIMITED
609-720-9200
http://www.ranbaxy.com

63304
RANBAXY PHARMACEUTICALS
609-720-9200
888-726-2299
http://www.ranbaxyusa.com

67216
RANDAL OPTIMAL NUTRIENTS
707-528-1800
800-966-8874
http://www.randalnutritional.com

30103
RANDOB LABORATORIES, LTD.
845-534-2197

49663
RAPTOR PHARMACEUTICAL CORP
877-727-8679
http://www.raptorpharma.com/index.html

66607
RARE DISEASE THERAPEUTICS, INC.
615-399-0700
http://www.raretx.com

68163
RARITAN PHARMACEUTICALS
732-432-8200
http://www.raritanpharm.com

12496
RECKITT BENCKISER PHARMACEUTICALS
973-404-2600
800-333-3899
http://www.reckittbenckiser.com

RECORDATI RARE DISEASES
908-236-0888
866-654-0539
http://www.recordatirarediseases.com

10952
RECSEI LABS
805-964-2912

67857
REDDY PHARMACEUTICAL
See Promius Pharma, LLC

52380, 18407
REDI-PRODUCTS LABS, INC.
See Aplicare Inc.

00091
REED & CARNRICK
See Schwarz

10956
REESE PHARMACEUTICAL CO., INC.
800-321-7178
http://www.reesepharmaceutical.com

REGENERON PHARMACEUTICALS
914-345-7400
http://www.regeneron.com

66779
REGENT LABS, INC.
800-872-1525
http://www.regentlabs.com

42167
RELIAMED
800-409-2848
http://www.reliamedproducts.com

65726
RELIANT PHARMACEUTICALS
See GlaxoSmithKline

REMEL, INC.
800-255-6730
http://www.remel.com

40085
RENAISSANCE PHARMA
267-685-0340
http://www.renaissancepharmainc.com

67066
REPLIGEN
See Chirhoclin

10961
REQUA, INC.
See W.F. Young, Inc.

00433
RESEARCH INDUSTRIES CORP.
See Edwards

RESEARCH TRIANGLE INSTITUTE
919-541-6000
http://www.rti.org

67492
RESICAL, INC.
800-204-6434
http://www.resical.com

60575
RESPA PHARMACEUTICALS, INC.
630-543-3333
http://www.respainc.com

47360
RESPIRATORY DELIVERY SYSTEMS
978-970-1947
http://www.rdsusa.com

08373
RESPIRONICS
724-387-4000
800-345-6443
http://www.respironics.com

00122
REXALL GROUP
See Rexall Sundown, Inc.

30768
REXALL SUNDOWN, INC.
561-241-9400
800-327-0908
http://www.rexallsundown.com

54092
REXAR PHARMACEUTICALS
See Shire US, Inc.

RH PHARMACEUTICALS, INC.
See Cangene Corp.

59258
RHODIA
609-860-4000
http://www.rhodia.com

RHONE-POULENC RORER CONSUMER, INC.
See Sanofi-Aventis US

RHONE-POULENC RORER PHARMACEUTICALS, INC.
See Sanofi-Aventis US

RICHARDSON-VICKS, INC.
See Procter & Gamble Pharmaceuticals

RICHIE PHARMACAL, INC.
502-651-6159
800-627-0250
http://www.richiepharmacal.com

00115
RICHLYN LABORATORIES, INC.
See Global Pharmaceuticals, Inc.

54738
RICHMOND PHARMACEUTICALS
804-270-4498

RICOLA USA, INC.
973-984-6811
http://www.ricolausa.com

54807
R.I.D., INC.
323-268-0635

R.I.J. PHARMACEUTICAL CORP.
845-692-5799
http://www.rijpharm.com

64980
RISING PHARMACEUTICALS, INC.
201-961-9000
http://www.risingpharma.com

76204
RITEDOSE PHARMACEUTICALS
803-806-3300
http://www.ritedose.com

68032
RIVER'S EDGE PHARMACEUTICAL
770-886-3417

54092
ROBERTS PHARMACEUTICAL CORP.
See Shire US, Inc.

50924
ROCHE DIAGNOSTIC SYSTEMS, INC.
See Roche Laboratories

00004
ROCHE LABORATORIES
973-235-5000
800-526-6367
http://www.rocheusa.com

49908
ROCHESTER PHARMACEUTICALS
866-458-1772
http://www.rochesterpharm.com

66358
RODLEN LABORATORIES
847-362-8200

ROERIG
See Pfizer US Pharmaceutical Group

67546
ROMARK LABORATORIES, LC
813-282-8544
http://www.romark.com

10802
ROSEDALE THERAPEUTICS
800-247-4896
http://www.rtherapeutics.com

42037
ROSE LABORATORIES
203-245-1210
800-433-4908

ROSEMONT PHARMACEUTICAL CORP.
See Upsher-Smith Labs, Inc.

64334
ROSE STONE ENTERPRISES
985-892-5939

70074
ROSS PRODUCTS DIVISION, ABBOTT NUTRITIONAL CONSUMER RELATIONS
See Abbott Nutrition

00054
ROXANE LABORATORIES, INC.
800-962-8364
800-562-4797
http://www.roxane.com

00591, 52544
ROYCE LABORATORIES, INC.
See Watson Laboratories

R.P. SCHERER CARDINAL HEALTH
732-537-6200
http://www.cardinal.com

00536
RUGBY LABORATORIES, INC.
678-584-5678
800-645-2158
http://www.watson.com

61972
RUGER CHEMICAL CO.
973-926-0331
800-274-7843
http://www.rugerchemical.com

66794, 08367
RX ELITE
See Piramal Critical Care

17922
RX TIMER CAP, LLC
800-428-7537
http://www.timercap.com

59243
SAGE PHARMACEUTICALS
318-635-1594

53462, 08513
SAGE PRODUCTS
815-455-4700
800-323-2220
http://www.sageproducts.com

25021
SAGENT PHARMACEUTICALS, INC.
847-908-1600
866-625-1618
http://www.sagentpharma.com

64054
SALIENT HCT
847-726-9443

65649
SALIX PHARMACEUTICALS, INC.
919-862-1000
866-435-7981
http://www.salix.com

07411
SALTER LABS
661-854-3166
800-421-0024
http://www.salterlabs.com

66288
SAMSON MEDICAL TECH, LLC
856-751-5051
877-418-3600
http://www.samsonmt.com

00781, 00067
SANDOZ
609-627-8500
800-525-8747
http://www.us.sandoz.com

00067
SANDOZ CONSUMER
See Novartis Pharmaceuticals Corp.

62053
SANGSTAT MEDICAL CORP.
See Genzyme Transplant

65597
SANKYO
See Daiichi Sankyo, Inc.

08313
SANOFI-AVENTIS U.S.
800-207-8049
800-981-2491
http://www.sanofi-aventis.us

49281
SANOFI PASTEUR
570-957-7187
800-822-2463
866-213-4936
http://www.vaccineshoppe.com

SANOFI-SYNTHELABO, INC.
See Sanofi-Aventis U.S.

00024
SANOFI WINTHROP PHARMACEUTICALS
See Sanofi-Aventis U.S.

68012
SANTARUS, INC.
858-314-5700
http://www.santarus.com

65086
SANTEN, INC.
707-254-1750
800-611-2011
http://www.santeninc.com

00281
SAVAGE LABORATORIES
631-454-9071
800-231-0206
http://www.savagelabs.com

54396
SAVIENT PHARMACEUTICALS, INC.
732-418-9300
800-284-2480
http://www.savient.com

46500
S C JOHNSON
262-260-2000
800-494-4855
http://www.scjohnson.com

SCANDINAVIAN FORMULAS, INC.
215-453-2507
800-688-2276
http://www.scandinavianformulas.com

SCHAFFER LABORATORIES
310-325-4200
800-231-6725
http://www.schafferlabs.com

52544
SCHEIN PHARMACEUTICAL, INC.
See Watson Laboratories

00274
SCHERER LABORATORIES, INC.
972-612-6225

00085
SCHERING-PLOUGH CORPORATION
908-298-4000
800-842-4090
http://www.schering-plough.com

41000, 11523
SCHERING-PLOUGH HEALTHCARE PRODUCTS
908-298-4000
800-842-4090
http://www.schering-plough.com

20525
SCHIFF NUTRITION INTERNATIONAL, INC.
801-975-5000
800-435-3948
http://www.schiffnutrition.com

00234, 02340
SCHMID PRODUCTS CO.
See Durex Consumer Products

41000, 11523
SCHOLL, INC.
See Schering-Plough Healthcare Products

33674
SCHWABE NORTH AMERICA, INC.
920-469-1313
800-558-7372
http://www.enzymatictherapy.com

00091
SCHWARZ PHARMA
http://www.schwarzusa.com

SCHWARZKOPF & DEP, INC.
800-326-2855
http://www.henkel.com

SCICLONE PHARMACEUTICALS, INC.
650-358-3456
http://www.sciclone.com

59630
SCIELE PHARMA
See Shionogi US, Inc.

65847
SCIOS, INC.
See Janssen Pharmaceuticals

08589
SCIVOLUTIONS MEDICAL
704-853-0100
http://www.scivolutionsmedical.com

00372
SCOT-TUSSIN PHARMACAL, INC.
401-942-8555
800-638-7268
http://www.scot-tussin.com

66424
SDA LABORATORIES, INC.
203-861-0005

08471
SEA-BAND
401-841-5900
http://www.sea-band.com

SEARLE
See Pfizer US Pharmaceutical Group

51144
SEATTLE GENETICS
425-527-4000
http://www.seagen.com

15127
SELECT BRAND
501-296-3373
http://www.usadrug.com

63402
SEPRACOR PHARMACEUTICALS
508-481-6700
800-245-5961
http://www.sepracor.com

SEPTODONT, INC.
302-328-1102
800-872-8305
http://www.septodontinc.com

17314
SEQUUS PHARMACEUTICALS, INC.
See Alza Corp.

50694
SERES LABORATORIES
707-526-4526
http://www.sereslabs.com

44087
SERONO LABORATORIES, INC.
See EMD Serono

11026
SEYER PHARMATEC, INC.
787-286-3223
888-782-3585
http://www.spharmatec.com

SHAKLEE CORP.
925-924-2000
800-928-0327
http://www.shaklee.com

49813
SHEAR KERSHMAN LABS
636-519-8900
http://www.shearkershman.com

SHEFFIELD PHARMACEUTICALS
860-442-4451
800-222-1087
http://www.sheffield-pharmaceuticals.com

17474, 08219
SHERWOOD DAVIS & GECK
See Kendall Health Care Products

SHIELD MANUFACTURING, INC.
716-694-7100
800-828-7669
http://www.shieldsports.com

45809, 59630
SHIONOGI, INC.
800-461-3696
http://www.shionogi.com

45809
SHIONOGI USA, INC.
See Shionogi Pharma, Inc.

54092
SHIRE US, INC.
484-595-8800
800-536-7878
http://www.shire.com

49735
SHS NORTH AMERICA
See Nutricia North America

00703
SICOR PHARMACEUTICALS, INC.
888-838-2872
800-545-8800
http://www.tevausa.com

50111
SIDMAK LABORATORIES, INC.
See Pliva, Inc.

42794
SIGMAPHARM LABORATORIES
215-352-6655
http://www.sigmapharm.com

45749, 54482
SIGMA-TAU PHARMACEUTICALS, INC.
301-948-1041
800-447-0169
http://www.sigmatau.com

45129
SIGVARIS
770-631-1778
800-322-7744
http://www.sigvarisusa.com

54838
SILARX PHARMACEUTICALS, INC.
845-352-4020
888-974-5279
http://www.silarx.com

SILVERGATE PHARMACEUTICALS
855-379-0382

53799, 94841
SIMILASAN
303-539-4060
800-240-9780
http://www.similasanusa.com

98302
SIMPLE DIAGNOSTICS
877-342-2385
http://www.simplediagnostics.com

88888
SIMPLY BARCODES
877-872-2060
404-885-6066

65880
SIRIUS LABORATORIES, INC.
978-657-7500
877-533-3872
http://www.siriuslabs.com

24839
SJ PHARMACEUTICALS
877-604-7575
http://www.sjpharma.com

67402
SKINMEDICA, INC.
760-448-3600
866-867-0110
http://www.skinmedica.com

SKYEPHARMA INC.
See Pacira Pharmaceuticals, Inc.

SLATE PHARMACEUTICALS
919-682-8800
http://www.slatepharma.com

08436
SLIM FAST FOODS CO.
561-833-9920
800-726-9866
http://www.slim-fast.com

SMITH & NEPHEW, INC. ENDOSCOPY
978-749-1000
http://www.smith-nephew.com

08363
SMITH & NEPHEW, INC. ORTHO
901-396-2121
800-821-5700
http://www.smith-nephew.com

40565, 50484
SMITH & NEPHEW WOUND MANAGEMENT
721-392-1261
800-876-1261
http://www.snwmd.com

58291
SNUVA, INC.
708-725-3783
800-250-4258
http://www.snuva.com

66658
SOBI
610-228-2042
866-276-2078
http://www.sobi.com

57771
SOLACE NUTRITION
888-876-5223
http://www.solacenutrition.com

43547
SOLCO HEALTHCARE
787-656-0909
http://www.legacypharm.com

SOLGAR CO., INC.
201-944-2311
800-645-2246
http://www.solgar.com

10454
SOLSTICE NEUROSCIENCES
267-620-8000
866-220-5042
http://www.solsticeneuro.com

94922
SOLUBLE SYSTEMS
757-877-8899
http://www.solublesystems.com

00032
SOLVAY PHARMACEUTICALS
See Abbott Laboratories

42847
SOMAXON PHARMACEUTICALS
858-876-6500
http://www.somaxon.com

63669, 61577
SOMBRA COSMETICS
505-888-0288
800-225-3963
http://www.sombrausa.com

39506
SOMERSET PHARMACEUTICALS
813-288-0040
800-892-8889
http://www.somersetpharm.com

58676
SOURCECF
267-759-9400
888-419-8357
http://www.sourcecf.com

45713, 61118
SOUTHWEST TECHNOLOGIES
816-221-2442
800-247-9951
http://www.elastogel.com

58016
SOUTHWOOD PHARMACEUTICALS
800-442-4443
http://www.southwoodhealthcare.com

SOVEREIGN PHARMACEUTICALS
817-284-0429
http://www.sovpharm.com

66530
SPEAR DERMATOLOGY PRODUCTS
973-895-6447
http://www.speardermatology.com

38415
SPECIALTY MEDICAL SUPPLIES
954-752-5603
http://www.specialtymedicalmanufacturingsupplies.com

49452
SPECTRUM CHEMICAL MANUFACTURING CORP.
310-516-8000
800-813-1514
http://www.spectrumchemical.com

68152
SPECTRUM PHARMACEUTICALS
702-835-6300
http://www.sppirx.com

38472
SPENCO MEDICAL CORPORATION
254-772-6000
800-877-3626
http://www.spenco.com

SPEYWOOD PHARMACEUTICALS, INC.
See Ipsen, Inc.

12258
S.S.S. COMPANY
404-521-0857
800-237-3843
http://www.ssspharmaceuticals.com

ST. JUDE MEDICAL, INC.
651-483-2000
800-328-9634

67253
STADA PHARMACEUTICALS, INC.
See Dava Pharmaceuticals

99929
STANBACK CO. (GLAXOSMITHKLINE)
See GlaxoSmithKline Consumer Healthcare, LP

STANDARD DRUG CO. & FAMILY PHARMACY
217-629-9884
800-632-9884

STANDARD HOMEOPATHIC CO. (HYLAND'S)
310-768-0700
800-624-9659
http://www.hylands.com

00076
STAR PHARMACEUTICALS, INC.
See Esprit Pharma

STASON PHARMACEUTICALS, INC.
949-380-4327
http://www.stasonpharma.com

16590
STAT RX USA
770-227-0065

51383
STEADMED MEDICAL
817-885-8273
855-888-8273
http://www.steadmed.com

51318.
STELLAR PHARMACAL CORP.
See Esprit Pharma

STEPHAN COMPANY
954-971-0600
800-327-4963
http://www.thestephanco.com

STERICYCLE
847-367-9493
866-783-7422
http://www.stericycle.com

52544
STERIS CORP.
440-354-2600
800-548-4873
http://www.steris.com

STERLING HEALTH
972-991-9293
http://www.sterlinghealthcenter.com

00024
STERLING WINTHROP
See Sanofi-Aventis US

54879
STI PHARMA
215-710-3270
866-426-2431
http://www.stipharmallc.com

STIEFEL CONSUMER HEALTHCARE
305-443-3800
http://www.stiefel.com

00145
STIEFEL LABORATORIES, INC.
888-784-3335
http://www.stiefel-us.com

14168
STONEBRIDGE PHARMACEUTICALS
888-445-2337
http://www.stiefel.com

58980
STRATUS PHARMACEUTICALS
305-254-6793
800-442-7882
http://www.stratuspharmaceuticals.com

00310
STUART PHARMACEUTICALS
See AstraZeneca, LP

17350
SUCAMPO PHARMACEUTICALS, INC.
301-961-3400
http://www.sucampo.com

SUGEN, INC. (INFORMAGEN, INC.)
See Pfizer US Pharmaceutical Group

SUMMA RX LABORATORIES
940-325-0771
800-527-7319
http://www.summalabs.com

11086, 94731
SUMMERS LABS
610-454-1471
800-533-7546
http://www.sumlab.com

SUMMIT INDUSTRIES, INC.
773-588-2444
800-729-9729
http://www.summitindustries.net

00078
SUMMIT PHARMACEUTICALS
See Novartis Pharmaceuticals Corp.

14508
SUN PHARMACEUTICAL INDUSTRIES
313-871-8400
800-818-4555
http://www.caraco.com

22252, 22319
SUNBEAM
800-435-1250
http://www.sunbeamhealth.com

63402
SUNOVION PHARMACEUTICALS
508-481-6700
800-739-0565
http://www.sunovion.com

33413
SUNRISE MEDICAL
631-435-1515
800-782-0282
http://www.sunriselab.com

41167
SUNSOURCE
423-821-4571

62701
SUPERGEN
925-560-0100
800-353-1075
http://www.supergen.com

17772
SUPERNUS PHARMACEUTICALS
301-838-2500
http://www.supernus.com

48503
SURGICAL APPLIANCE INDUSTRIES
800-888-0458
800-888-0867
http://www.surgicalappliance.com

60232
SWISS-AMERICAN PRODUCTS
972-385-2900
800-633-8872
http://www.elta.net

18867
SWISS BIOCEUTICAL
775-841-7020

SYNCOM PHARMACEUTICALS, INC.
973-787-2405
800-400-0056
http://www.syncom.com

55513
SYNERGEN, INC.
See Amgen, Inc.

00004
SYNTEX LABORATORIES
See Roche Laboratories

66576
SYNTHO PHARMACEUTICALS, INC.
631-755-9898
http://www.synthopharmaceutical.com

63672
SYNTHON PHARMACEUTICALS, INC.
919-493-6006
919-536-1323
http://www.synthon-usa.com

SYVA CO.
See Dade Behring

51224
TAGI PHARMA
815-624-7685
http://www.tagipharma.com

64764
TAKEDA PHARMACEUTICALS
224-554-6500
877-825-3327
http://www.tpna.com

76181
TALEC PHARMA
636-449-1830

13533
TALECRIS BIOTHERAPEUTICS, INC.
919-316-6300
800-243-4153
http://www.talecris.com

20536
TALON THERAPEUTICS
650-588-6404
702-835-6300
http://www.talontx.com

89152
TANDEM DIABETES CARE
858-366-6900
877-801-6901
http://www.tandemdiabetes.com

75486
TANNING RESEARCH LABS, INC.
386-677-9559
800-874-4844
http://www.htropic.com

TANOX, INC.
713-578-4000
http://www.tanox.com

00300
TAP PHARMACEUTICAL PRODUCTS, INC.
847-582-2000
800-621-1020
http://www.tap.com

16730
TARGET
612-696-5941
http://investors.target.com

TARGETED GENETICS CORP.
206-623-7612
800-828-6022
http://www.targen.com

TARGETED MEDICAL PHARMA
310-474-9809
http://www.ptlcentral.com

TARMAC PRODUCTS, INC.
305-557-6423
http://www.tarmacproducts.com

51672
TARO PHARMACEUTICALS USA, INC.
914-345-9001
800-544-1449
http://www.tarousa.com

11098
TAYLOR PHARMACAL
See Akorn, Inc.

67336
TEAMM PHARMACEUTICALS, INC.
919-481-9020
866-481-9020
http://www.teammpharma.com

51879, 83626
TEC LABORATORIES, INC.
541-926-4577
800-482-4464
http://www.teclabsinc.com

08605,93573
TECHNOLOGICAL INVESTMENTS, LLC
512-255-2271
http://www.medi-fridge.com

59519
TELCARE
240-396-6003
http://www.telcare.com

TELLURIDE PHARM. CORP.
908-369-1800
http://www.tellpharm.com

TEL-TEST, INC.
281-482-2762
800-631-0600
http://www.tel-test.com

68436
TERAL
787-383-2781

15054
TERCICA
650-624-4900
http://www.tercica.com

53225
TERRAIN PHARMACEUTICALS
925-866-4163
http://www.TerrainRx.com

08418, 08970
TERUMO MEDICAL CORPORATION
732-302-4900
800-888-3786
http://www.terumomedical.com

TESTPAK, INC.
973-887-4440
http://www.testpak.com

TEVA MARION PARTNERS
816-508-5000
800-221-4026
http://www.tevausa.com

68546
TEVA NEUROSCIENCE
888-838-2872
http://www.tevaneuro.com

00093
TEVA PHARMACEUTICALS USA
215-591-3000
888-838-2872
800-545-8800
http://www.tevausa.com

59310
TEVA RESPIRATORY
888-482-9522

99976
TEVA/WOMENS HEALTH
201-930-3300
800-227-7522
800-222-0190
http://www.tevawomenshealth.com

00217
T E WILLIAMS
719-687-8770
800-755-7659

29273
TG UNITED PHARMACEUTICALS
352-799-9813
http://www.tgunited.com

51672
THAMES PHARMACAL, INC.
See Taro Pharmaceuticals USA, Inc.

08348
THAYER MEDICAL
800-250-3330
http://www.thayermedical.com

78112, 75137
THE DENOREX CO.
866-840-0011
http://www.denorex.com

57464
THE F. C. STURTEVANT COMPANY
914-337-5131
888-871-5661
http://www.columbiapowder.com

11694
THE KEY COMPANY
314-965-7629
314-965-6699
800-325-9592
http://www.thekeycompanyusa.com

65293
THE MEDICINES COMPANY
973-290-6000
800-388-1183
http://www.themedicinescompany.com

54633
THE PODIATREE COMPANY
855-763-8733
http://www.thepodiatreecompany.com

99735
THE THERAPLEX COMPANY, LLC
888-437-2753
http://www.theraplex.com

53097
THEPHARMANETWORK
201-476-1977
http://www.ascendlaboratories.com

64067
THERAKOS, INC.
610-280-1000
http://www.therakos.com

50803
THERAPEARL, LLC
877-732-7509
http://www.therapearl.com

THERAPEUTIC ANTIBODIES, INC.
See Protherics, Inc.

THERASENSE
See Abbott Diabetes Care

THERAVANCE
855-633-8479
http://www.theravance.com

64011
THER-RX CORPORATION
314-646-3700
877-567-7676
http://www.ther-rx.com

11926
THOMPSON MEDICAL CO., INC.
See Chattem Consumer Products

66435
THREE RIVERS PHARMACEUTICALS
See Kadmon Pharmaceuticals

24856
THROMBOGENICS, INC.
732-590-2900
866-945-9808
http://www.thrombogenics.com

23589
TIBER LABORATORIES
770-886-3417
678-208-0388
http://www.tiberlabs.com

66403
TIGER BALM
510-887-1899
http://www.tigerbalm.com

49483
TIME-CAP LABS
631-753-9090
http://www.timecaplabs.com

14654, 54023
TISHCON CORP.
516-333-3050
800-848-8442
http://www.tishcon.com

46963
TISSUE SEAL
877-754-6458
http://www.tissueseal.com

TOMS OF MAINE, INC.
207-985-2944
800-367-8667
http://www.tomsofmaine.com

36800
TOPCO
847-676-3030
888-423-0139
http://www.topco.com

58211
TOPIX PHARMACEUTICALS
631-226-7979
800-445-2595

38423
TOPOTARGET
866-914-2922
http://www.topotarget.com

13668
TORRENT PHARMACEUTICALS
269-544-2299
http://www.torrentpharma.com

50201
TOWER LABORATORIES
860-767-2127
http://www.towerlabs.com

62511
TRANSDERMAL TECHNOLOGIES, INC.
561-848-2345
800-282-5511
http://www.transdermal technologies.com

TRASK NUTRITION
877-760-9258
800-579-3131
http://www.fibromalic.com

TRI TECH LABORATORIES
434-845-7073
http://www.tritechlabs.com

14290
TRIAX PHARMACEUTICALS, LLC
908-372-0500
866-453-0577
http://www.triaxpharma.com

13811
TRIGEN LABORATORIES
732-721-0070
888-987-4436
http://www.trigenlab.com

68752
TRIMARC LABORATORIES
405-942-3289
http://www.trimarclabs.com

TRIMED LAB, INC.
732-249-6363

54295
TRINITY PHARMACEUTICALS
412-342-5502
http://www.trinitypharmallc.com

61355
TRINITY TECHNOLOGIES
781-235-2223
http://www.trinitytechnologies.com

27808
TRIS PHARMA
732-940-2800
http://www.trispharma.com

79511
TRITON CONSUMER PRODUCTS, INC.
847-228-7650
800-942-2009
http://www.mg217.com

55859
TROPHIKOS
877-421-7160
http://www.trophikos.com

10025
TROPICAL PHARMACAL
787-737-8445

50247
TRUTEK CORP.
908-685-1111
http://www.trutekcorp.com

00463
TRUXTON
856-933-2333
http://www.truxtonpharma.com

TWEEZERMAN
516-676-7772
800-645-3340
http://www.tweezerman.com

27434
TWINLAB CORP.
631-467-3140
800-645-5626
http://www.twinlab.com

64915
TYLER, INC.
See Integrative Therapeutics

53335
TYSON NUTRACEUTICALS
310-325-5600
http://www.tyson nutraceuticals.com

00456
UAD LABORATORIES, INC.
See Forest Pharmaceuticals, Inc.

UCB PHARMACEUTICALS, INC.
770-970-7500
866-822-0068
http://www.ucb-usa.com

62592
UCYCLYD PHARMA, INC.
888-829-2593
http://www.medicis.com

51079, 08459
UDL LABORATORIES, INC.
800-848-0462
http://www.udllabs.com

00127
ULMER PHARMACAL CO.
800-848-5637
http://www.lobanaproducts.com

55093
ULTIMARK PRODUCTS
877-489-6073
http://www.ultimarkproducts.com

08222, 08474, 57515
ULTIMED
651-291-7909
877-854-3434
http://www.diabetes-care.com

ULURU, INC.
214-905-5145
http://www.uluruinc.com

23535,29300
UNICHEM, INC.
866-562-4616
866-931-0704
http://www.unichemusa.com

60814
UNICITY
800-864-2489
801-226-2600
http://www.makelifebetter.com

59640
UNICO HOLDINGS, INC.
800-367-4477
561-582-3030
http://www.unico-holdings.com

UNIFIRST CORPORATION
800-225-3364
http://www.unifirst.com

62305
UNIGEN PHARMACEUTICAL
410-751-2108
360-486-8200
http://www.unigenpharma.com

UNILEVER HOME AND PERSONAL CARE USA
203-661-2000
800-243-5320
http://www.unilever.com

41785
UNIMED PHARMACEUTICALS
See Solvay Pharmaceuticals

08479
UNIPATH DIAGNOSTICS CO.
See Inverness Medical Innovations

59707
UNIQUEONE PHARMACEUTICAL & MEDICAL SUPPLIES
See One Pharma & Medical Supply Co.

00327
UNITED GUARDIAN LABORATORIES
631-273-0900
800-645-5566
http://www.u-g.com

00677
UNITED RESEARCH LABORATORIES (URL)
See Mutual Pharmaceutical Co., Inc.

63261
UNITED STATES SURGICAL CORP.
203-845-1000
800-722-8772
http://www.ussurg.com

66302
UNITED THERAPEUTICS CORP.
301-608-9292
877-864-8437
http://www.unither.com

63535
UNITHER PHARMA (UNITED THERAPEUTICS CORP.)
301-608-9292
888-808-6838
http://www.unitedtherapeutics.com

59730
UNIVAX BIOLOGICS
See Nabi

UPJOHN CO.
See Pfizer US Pharmaceutical Group

00245
UPSHER-SMITH PHARMACEUTICALS
763-315-2000
800-654-2299
http://www.upsher-smith.com

65580
UPSTATE PHARMA, LLC
770-970-7500
800-477-7877
http://www.ucbpharma.com

92293
UROCARE PRODUCTS, INC.
909-621-6013
800-423-4441
http://www.urocare.com

UROCOR, INC.
See LabCorp

UROLOGIX
763-475-1400
800-475-1403
http://www.urologix.com

US BIOSCIENCE
216-765-5000
800-321-9322
http://www.usbio.com

US DENTEK CORP.
800-433-6835
http://www.usdentek.com

08463
US DIAGNOSTICS
866-216-5303

68728
US FOODS & PHARMACEUTICALS
866-678-4436
608-278-1293
http://www.usfp.com

13774
US MEDICAL INSTRUMENTS
619-661-5500
http://www.usmedical instruments.com

US NEUTRACEUTICALS, LLC
352-357-2004
877-876-8872
http://www.usnutra.com

52747
US PHARMACEUTICAL CORPORATION
770-987-4745
http://www.uspco.com

00187
VALEANT PHARMACEUTICALS INTERNATIONAL, INC.
877-361-2719
800-548-5100
949-461-6000
800-321-4576
http://www.valeant.com

55592
VALERA PHARMACEUTICALS
See Indevus Pharmaceuticals

08560
VALERITAS
908-927-9920
866-881-1209
http://www.valeritas.com

30698
VALIDUS PHARMACEUTICALS
866-825-4387
http://www.validuspharma.com

54627
VALMED, INC.
508-845-3438

VALUE IN PHARMACEUTICALS
800-724-3784
http://www.vippharm.com

00615
VANGARD
800-825-4123

67537
VARSITY LABORATORIES
205-986-1111

65199
VATRING PHARMACEUTICALS
276-322-1888

75959
VAYA PHARMA
864-200-2710
866-225-0695
http://www.vayapharma.com

VENTANA MEDICAL SYSTEMS, INC.
520-887-2155
800-227-2155
http://www.ventanamed.com

11391
VENTLAB CORPORATION
336-753-5000
800-593-4654
http://www.ventlab.com

67887
VERACITY PHARMACEUTICALS, INC.
954-426-1919
800-354-8460
http://www.veracitypharma.com

16887
VERNALIS PHARMACEUTICALS
See Ipsen Pharmaceuticals

61748
VERSAPHARM
770-499-8100
800-548-0700
http://www.versapharm.com

VERTEX PHARMACEUTICALS, INC.
617-576-3111
http://www.vpharm.com

67000
VERUM PHARMACEUTICALS
See Victory Pharmaceuticals

13436
VERUS PHARMACEUTICALS, INC.
866-634-8774
http://www.veruspharm.com

78112, 75137
VETCO, INC.
516-755-1155
800-754-8853
http://www.littleremedies.com

00702
VHA, INC.
972-830-0626
800-842-5146
http://www.vha.com

57141
VIACTIV LIFESTYLE
877-842-2842
http://www.viactiv.com

VIASYS HEALTHCARE
610-862-0800
866-484-2797
http://www.viasyscriticalcare.com

00149
VICKS HEALTH CARE PRODUCTS
See Procter & Gamble Pharmaceuticals

00149
VICKS PHARMACY PRODUCTS
See Procter & Gamble Pharmaceuticals

67000
VICTORY PHARMA, INC.
858-350-4217
866-427-6819
http://www.victorypharma.com

42238
VIDARA THERAPEUTICS
http://www.vidararx.com

67204
VINDEX PHARMACEUTICALS, INC.
901-759-4970
http://www.vindexpharm.com

00254
VINTAGE PHARMACEUTICALS, INC.
704-596-9440

53459
VIP INTERNATIONAL
718-390-0490

00187
VIRATEK
See Valeant Pharmaceuticals International, Inc.

VIREXX
See Paladin Labs

66593
VIROPHARMA, INC.
610-458-7300
888-651-0201
http://www.viropharma.com

76439
VIRTUS PHARMACEUTICALS
813-283-1344
http://www.virtusrx.com

68013
VISION PHARMA
732-974-6300
http://www.visionpharma.com

54891
VISION PHARMACEUTICALS, INC.
605-996-3356
800-325-6789
http://www.visionpharm.com

61971
VISTA PHARMACEUTICALS
973-736-1952
973-736-4457
http://www.vistapharmaceuticals.com

98669
VISTAKON PHARMACEUTICALS, LLC
904-443-1000
800-843-2020
http://www.vistakonpharmaceuticals.com

66689, 67043
VISTAPHARM, INC.
205-981-1387
877-437-8567
http://www.vistapharm.com

49727
VITA-RX CORP.
706-568-1881

08321
VITAL CARE GROUP
305-620-4007
800-392-4547
http://www.vitalcare.com

08166
VITAL SIGNS, INC.
973-790-1330
800-932-0760
http://www.vital-signs.com

54022
VITALINE
800-917-3696

VITALITY, INC.
See Vital Care Group

82966
VITAMIN HEALTH
888-890-3937
http://www.vitaminhealthbrands.com

VITAMIN RESEARCH PRODUCT, INC.
775-884-8210
800-877-2447
http://www.vrp.com

62541
VIVUS, INC.
650-934-5200
888-345-6873
http://www.vivus.com

WAKEFIELD PHARMACEUTICALS, INC.
See Ivax Pharmaceuticals, Inc.

81131, 49035
WAL-MART
800-925-6278
888-922-0400
http://www.walmartstores.com

40805
WAL-MED, INC.
253-845-6633
877-542-3688
http://www.wallace-medical.com

00017
WAMPOLE LABORATORIES
See Inverness Medical Innovations

00047
WARNER CHILCOTT LABORATORIES
973-442-3200
800-521-8813
http://www.warnerchilcott.com

12546
WARNER LAMBERT AMERICAN CHICLE
973-540-2000
800-524-2624

59930
WARRICK PHARMACEUTICAL CORP.
See Schering-Plough Corp.

00591, 52544
WATSON LABORATORIES
800-272-5525
http://www.watsonpharm.com

00591, 52544
WATSON PHARMACEUTICALS, INC.
800-272-5525
http://www.watsonpharm.com

71603
W.E. BASSETT
203-929-8483
http://www.trim.com

77890
WEGMANS
609-223-2486
http://www.irvingconsumerproducts.com

55946
WELEDA
800-241-1030
http://www.usa.weleda.com

89129
WELLDOC
443-692-3100
http://www.welldoc.com

65197
WELLSPRING PHARMACEUTICAL
941-552-7880
877-273-1396
http://www.wellspringpharm.com

00917
WESLEY PHARMACAL, INC.
215-953-1680

00006
WEST POINT PHARMA
See Merck & Co.

53240
WESTPORT PHARMACEUTICALS
877-801-8409

64727
WESTERN RESEARCH LABORATORIES
See RLC Labs

00143, 00641
WEST-WARD
732-542-1191
800-631-2174
http://www.west-ward.com

00072
WESTWOOD SQUIBB PHARMACEUTICALS
See Bristol-Myers Squibb Co.

11444
W.F. YOUNG
800-628-9653
http://www.absorbine.com

44567
WG CRITICAL CARE
888-493-0861
http://www.wgcriticalcare.com

WHITBY PHARMACEUTICALS, INC.
See UCB Pharmaceuticals, Inc.

72695
WHITE LABS, INC.
858-693-3441
888-593-2785
http://www.whitelabs.com

00317
WHORTON PHARMACEUTICALS, INC.
205-786-2584

35046
WINDMILL CONSUMER PRODUCTS
973-575-6591
800-822-4320
http://www.windmillvitamins.com

51101
WILLIAM LABORATORIES, INC.
860-749-1350
800-767-7643
http://www.williamlabs.com

52536
WILSHIRE PHARMACEUTICALS
678-334-2420
877-495-6856
http://www.wilshirerx.com

00427
WINSTON LABORATORIES
847-362-8200
http://www.winstonlabs.com

52047
WINTEC
636-257-5400

00955
WINTHROP, US
800-372-6634
800-362-7466
http://www.winthropus.com

12120
WISCONSIN PHARMACAL
262-677-4121
800-558-6614
http://www.pharmacalway.com

WM. WRIGLEY JR. CO.
312-644-2121
800-974-4539
http://www.wrigley.com

64679
WOCKHARDT USA
973-257-4960
800-346-6854
http://www.wockhardtusa.com

WOLLFOAM COMPANY
516-731-5380

64248
WOMEN FIRST HEALTHCARE
See Mutual Pharmaceutical Co., Inc.

64836
WOMENS CAPITAL CORP.
See Barr Laboratories, Inc.

08111, 61168
WOODSIDE BIOMEDICAL
See Abbott Hospital Products

60193
WOODWARD LABORATORIES, INC.
948-598-2400
800-780-6999
http://www.woodwardlabs.com

66992
WRASER PHARMACEUTICALS
601-605-0664
888-252-3901
http://www.wraser.com

00008
WYETH
800-666-7248
800-999-9384
http://www.wyeth.com

WYETH CONSUMER HEALTH
See Pfizer Consumer Health

11511
WYNNPHARM
732-544-4080
800-214-9600
http://www.wynnpharm.com

XACTDOSE, INC.
See Alpharma

66479
XANODYNE PHARMACEUTICALS, INC.
859-371-6383
877-926-6396
http://www.xanodyne.com

00187
XCEL PHARMACEUTICALS
See Valeant Pharmaceuticals International, Inc.

XENOPORT
877-936-6778

39822
X-GEN PHARMACEUTICALS, INC.
607-562-2700
866-390-4411
http://www.x-gen.us

76234
XOMA
510-204-7200
800-544-9662
http://www.xoma.com

42195
XSPIRE PHARMA
601-990-9497
http://www.xspirerx.com

00116
XTTRIUM LABORATORIES
773-268-5800
800-587-3721
http://www.xttrium.com

XUBEX
407-478-2663
866-699-8239
http://www.xubex.com

55212
YASOO HEALTH
919-439-2960
http://www.yasoo.com

YOUNG AGAIN PRODUCTS
910-371-6775
877-950-4400
http://www.youngagainproducts.com

00273, 60077
YOUNG DENTAL MFG.
314-344-0010
800-325-1881
http://www.youngdental.com

89901
ZANFEL LABORATORIES, INC.
800-401-4002
http://www.zanfel.com

ZARS PHARMA
801-350-0202
http://www.zars.com

90389
ZEE MEDICAL, INC.
800-841-8417
http://www.zeemedical.com

ZENITH LABORATORIES
See Ivax Pharmaceuticals, Inc.

18011
ZERXIS PHARMA, LLC
985-893-4097
http://www.pamlab.com

51284
ZILA, INC.
602-266-6700
866-945-2776
http://www.zila.com

85836
ZIMMER
516-313-2693

00053
ZLB BEHRING
See CSL Behring

44206
ZLB BIOPLASMA
See CSL Behring

64909
ZOETICA PHARMACEUTICAL GROUP
See Dava Pharmaceuticals, Inc.

43376
ZOGENIX
858-259-1165
866-964-3649
http://www.zogenix.com

ZONAGEN, INC.
281-719-3400
http://www.zonagen.com

65224
ZYBER PHARMACEUTICALS, INC.
See Pernix Therapeutics, LLC

68382
ZYDUS PHARMACEUTICALS USA, INC.
877-993-8779
http://www.zydususa.com

23594
ZYLERA PHARMACEUTICALS
919-443-2575
http://www.zylera.com

ZYMETX, INC.
405-809-1314
888-817-1314
http://www.zymetx.com

28400
ZYMOGENETICS, INC.
206-442-6600
888-784-7662
http://www.zymogenetics.com